Biological Psychiatry

Volume II

Biological Psychiatry
Volume II

Edited by

Prof. Dr. Hugo D'haenen

Head of the Psychiatric Department,
Academic Hospital, and Professor of Psychiatry,
Free University of Brussels, Belgium

Prof. Dr. J.A. den Boer

Professor of Biological Psychiatry,
Department of Psychiatry,
University Hospital Groningen,
The Netherlands

Prof. P. Willner

University of Wales,
Swansea, UK

JOHN WILEY & SONS, LTD

Copyright © 2002 John Wiley & Sons Ltd, The Atrium, Southern Gate, Chichester,
West Sussex PO19 8SQ, England

Telephone (+44) 1243 779777

Email (for orders and customer service enquiries): cs-books@wiley.co.uk
Visit our Home Page on www.wileyeurope.com or www.wiley.com

Other Wiley Editorial Offices

John Wiley & Sons Inc., 111 River Street, Hoboken, NJ 07030, USA

Jossey-Bass, 989 Market Street, San Francisco, CA 94103-1741, USA

Wiley-VCH Verlag GmbH, Boschstr. 12, D-69469 Weinheim, Germany

John Wiley & Sons Australia Ltd, 33 Park Road, Milton, Queensland 4064, Australia

John Wiley & Sons (Asia) Pte Ltd, 2 Clementi Loop #02-01, Jin Xing Distripark, Singapore 129809

John Wiley & Sons Canada Ltd, 22 Worcester Road, Etobicoke, Ontario, Canada M9W 1L1

British Library Cataloguing in Publication Data

A catalogue record for this book is available from the British Library

ISBN 0-471-49198-5

Typeset in 9/10pt Times from the authors' disks by Laserwords Private Limited, Chennai, India
Index produced by Indexing Specialists (UK) Ltd, Hove, East Sussex
Printed and bound in Great Britain by TJ International, Padstow, Cornwall
This book is printed on acid-free paper responsibly manufactured from sustainable forestry in which at least two trees are planted for each one used for paper production.

Contents

VOLUME II

XVIII

Mood Disorders

XVIII-1

Animal Models of Depression: A Diathesis/Stress Approach

Paul Willner and Paul J. Mitchell

INTRODUCTION

Animal models of depression are used both as screening tests to discover and develop novel antidepressant drug therapies, and as simulations for investigating various aspects of the neurobiology of depressive illness, including the neuropharmacological mechanisms mediating the effects of antidepressant treatments. These different functions of animal models have different and, to some extent, conflicting requirements.

A simulation of depression aims to mimic aspects of the clinical situation, and should embody a degree of complexity, to permit investigation of the validity of the model. In addition, if a model is to be used to investigate antidepressant actions, a slow onset comparable to the clinical time course is highly desirable, and the model should therefore exhibit differences (either in direction of response, or in response magnitude) between single (acute) and repeated (chronic or continuous) treatment regimes. By contrast, the only essential requirement for antidepressant screening tests is that they make accurate predictions of antidepressant activity. For practical reasons, they should also be cheap, robust, reliable and easy to use (Danysz *et al.*, 1991; Willner, 1991a), and for all of these subsidiary reasons, a screening test should in principle be as simple as possible. However, the view that such screening tests should also respond acutely has changed during the past decade, in line with the drive from the clinic to identify rapid-onset antidepressant treatments. By necessity this approach involves the assessment of drug action associated with chronic/continuous drug treatment regimes and an acute response is thus of little value. Appropriate screening tests to be used relatively early during drug development should therefore have the ability to identify the time course of drug action associated with repeated treatment schedules.

The present chapter is concerned primarily to evaluate the suitability of the available animal models as research tools, and we therefore focus initially on issues relating to the validity of the available models as simulations of depression.

VALIDITY

In line with current thinking, our assessment of the validity of animal models of depression addresses the three dimensions of predictive, face and construct validity (Willner, 1984, 1991a). The concept of predictive validity implies that manipulations known to influence the pathological state should have similar effects in the model. Face validity refers to a phenomenological similarity between the model and the disorder being modelled. Construct validity implies that the model has a sound theoretical rationale. Some reviewers have advocated the primacy of one of these approaches (predictive validity: Geyer and Markou, 1995; face validity: Weiss and Kilts, 1998; construct validity, Sarter and Bruno, Chapter III). In principle, we share Sarter and Bruno's position, that construct validity is the most important of the three dimensions. In practice, however, the construct validity of animal models of depression is difficult to determine, and therefore we favour a balanced approach in which a view of the validity of a model is formed only after considering all three sources of evidence. We therefore begin by reviewing briefly the three sets of validation criteria, as they apply to animal models of depression.

Predictive Validity

In practice, the predictive validity of animal models of depression is determined solely by their response to antidepressant drugs. A valid test should be sensitive and specific: it should respond to effective antidepressant treatments ('true positive' effects), including electroconvulsive shock (ECS), and should fail to respond to ineffective agents ('true negative' effects). A model with high predictive validity should therefore maximize identification of both 'true positives' and 'true negatives', but should minimize identification of 'false positives' and 'false negatives'. Furthermore, positive responses should occur at behaviourally selective doses (i.e. those which do not generally disrupt behaviour, or induce motor impairment) that are within or close to the clinical range, and should be demonstrable with a range of structurally diverse compounds. It should be recognized that no animal model has a 100% prediction rate although some complex experimental paradigms have approached this level of predictive ability. Part of the problem lies not so much with the preclinical model but with the fact that there are several grey areas in the clinical literature where it is not known whether certain drugs (e.g. anticholinergics) possess antidepressant activity or not. It is generally agreed that the most effective treatment for depressive illness is electroconvulsive therapy (ECT). A suitable starting point to test the validity of an animal model should therefore be to demonstrate a positive response to repeated ECS. Failure to respond appropriately to ECS would severely question the predictive validity of the model.

About 30% of depressed patients fail to respond to antidepressant drug treatment, while the response rate for ECT is slightly higher. The occurrence of refractory patients probably reflects the heterogeneity of depressive illness. Nevertheless, a model that did not respond to the benchmark tricyclic antidepressants (TCAs), selective serotonin reuptake inhibitors (SSRIs), or the recently developed serotonin–noradrenaline reuptake inhibitors (SNRIs)

Biological Psychiatry: Edited by H. D'haenen, J.A. den Boer and P. Willner. ISBN 0-471-49198-5

would not be taken seriously. This situation is unlikely to change in the absence of well-established therapies for tricyclic-resistant depression.

Beyond the clinically established antidepressant treatments (TCAs, monoamine oxidase inhibitors (MAOIs), SSRIs, SNRIs and some atypical antidepressants, such as mianserin) are a wide range of newer compounds for which antidepressant activity has been claimed, ranging from pharmacologically-selective compounds that are probably effective (e.g. α_2-adrenoceptor antagonists; ligands for serotonin (5-hydroxytryptamine; 5-HT) receptor subtypes including $5HT_{1A}$ receptor ligands that possess agonist activity (and partial agonists), ligands for $5\text{-}HT_{2A}$ and $5\text{-}HT_{2C}$ receptor subtypes, and *N*-methyl-D-aspartate (NMDA) receptor ligands), through preparations of mixed pharmacological activity (e.g. SSRI with selective $5\text{-}HT_{1A}$ receptor antagonist activity) to compounds of uncertain status (e.g. phosphodiesterase inhibitors, calcium antagonists, anticonvulsants). Even in the case of the SSRIs, whose antidepressant efficacy is beyond doubt, it is still uncertain whether their spectrum of activity is identical to that of the TCAs. Therefore, while a well-rounded description of an animal model of depression should include an account of its pharmacological profile broader than that provided by its response to traditional antidepressants, the contribution of these newer compounds to validation is limited.

To some extent, similar uncertainties exist in relation to drugs which are ineffective as antidepressants. The 'false positives' most commonly encountered in animal models of depression are psychomotor stimulants, anticholinergics and opiates. However, prior to the development of antidepressants, drugs from all three of these classes were regularly prescribed for the relief of depression (see Willner, 1985). Indeed, certain opiates (e.g. buprenorphine) have antidepressant activity (Emrich *et al.*, 1983), but anticholinergics and stimulants have never been properly assessed, as their use was discontinued prior to the introduction of blind clinical trials. Again, the uncertain status of these compounds to some extent undermines their value as definitive standards of negative control.

Finally, the response to antidepressant drugs is insufficient to define an animal model of depression. Some antidepressants are active in some animal models of anxiety and panic, following chronic treatment (Bodnoff *et al.*, 1988; Fontana *et al.*, 1989), and indeed, are increasingly seen as the drugs of choice in many forms of anxiety (see Den Boer, Chapter XIX-13). It is therefore crucial for establishing the predictive validity of an animal model of depression to demonstrate that the model does not respond to benzodiazepines.

Face Validity

To assess face validity, the extent of similarity between the model and the disorder is examined, on as wide as possible a range of symptoms and signs. However, not all symptoms of a psychiatric condition carry equal weight and for an animal model to be valid, a resemblance to the clinically defined core symptoms of the disorder carries more weight than a resemblance to any subsidiary symptoms (Abramson and Seligman, 1978). The most recent edition of the *Diagnostic and Statistical Manual* (DSM-IV) provides a framework within which to assess these similarities. However, not all of the clinical symptoms of depression can be modelled in animals; symptoms conveyed by subjective verbal report (e.g. excessive guilt, feelings of worthlessness, suicide ideation) are in principle excluded (Willner, 1984, 1990).

A DSM-IV diagnosis of major depression requires the presence of at least one of two core symptoms: loss of interest or pleasure (anhedonia) and depressed mood. Of these two core symptoms, anhedonia can be modelled in animals, but depressed mood cannot. In assessing the face validity of animal models of depression, anhedonia therefore assumes a central position. The problem here, however, is that anhedonia is also a core symptom of schizophrenia. Drug-induced reversal of anhedonia in animal models, while highly encouraging, should thus be considered in relation to DSM-IV criteria for both depressive illness and schizophrenia.

The subsidiary symptoms of depression in DSM-IV that are amenable to modelling in animals include psychomotor changes, fatigue or loss of energy (which might be modelled as decreased persistence), and disturbances of sleep or food intake. Interestingly, psychomotor activity, sleep and appetite may be increased or decreased, and diametrically opposite changes in locomotion have both been cited in support for the validity of a model. This lack of precision, together with the fact that the clinical phenomena of psychomotor retardation and agitation (which are considerably more complex than gross changes in locomotor activity) may even coexist (Nelson and Charney, 1981), suggests that simulations in which a change in locomotor activity is the major, or only, behavioural feature should not be taken too seriously. Unfortunately, it is precisely these behaviours that feature most prominently in many animal models of depression (Willner, 1991b).

Because the pharmacotherapy of depression typically requires chronic drug treatment, the validity of an animal model is called into question by an acute response to conventional (e.g. TCA) antidepressant treatment. There is some evidence of very early antidepressant responses in clinical studies designed explicitly to detect them (e.g. Frazer *et al.*, 1985; see also Willner, 1989a) but even so, repeated treatment is required for a full response. Acute treatment refers to a single bolus dose of drug and any acute treatment effects are usually observed within minutes or hours following the bolus dose. Multiple acute doses may be administered, over a short period, simply to increase levels of drug in the biophase without evoking secondary adaptive changes in neurotransmitter mechanisms. In contrast, chronic treatment refers to repeated bolus doses administered for extended periods (days, weeks, months). Chronic treatment effects may be associated with drug-induced adaptive changes in neurotransmitter-receptor-mediated systems, rather than increased drug levels in the plasma. Thus, in comparison to chronic treatment effects, an acute response in an animal model may be opposite, orthogonal (due to side effects, e.g. sedation) or absent. Irrespective of how it responds to acute antidepressant treatment, to be valid, an animal model of depression must respond to chronic treatment. Furthermore, since tolerance does not occur to the clinical effects of antidepressants, the response in the model must be maintained until the cessation of antidepressant treatment. This test has not been universally applied to animal models of depression, but in general, those models to which the test has been applied have passed it, though tolerance to antidepressant effects has been reported in some behavioural paradigms (e.g. Cuomo *et al.*, 1983; Niesink and van Ree, 1982).

Construct Validity

An evaluation of the theoretical rationale of an animal model requires a means of bringing the theoretical accounts of both the disorder itself and the disordered behaviour exhibited by the model into alignment. However, any evaluation of animal models of depression is intrinsically limited by the rudimentary state of theories of the pathology of depression. Indeed, there is little in the extensive literature describing neurochemical abnormalities or biochemical markers reportedly associated with depression that can be usefully employed to provide a theoretical standard against which to validate animal models. Even the most basic questions of whether the level of activity in monoaminergic systems is elevated or decreased in depression were and remain controversial (Willner, 1985).

Similar problems arise in relation to modelling the aetiology of depression. It is now clear that a variety of different factors are implicated in the aetiology of depression: 'psychological' factors include undesirable life events, chronic mild stress, adverse childhood experiences, and personality traits such as introversion and impulsiveness; 'biological' factors include genetic influences, and a variety of physical illnesses and medications (see Akiskal, 1985, 1986; Willner, 1985 for reviews). However, for most of these factors, there is little theoretical understanding of the processes by which they influence the physiological processes underlying mood. In certain cases, the immediate precipitant of a depression may be clearly identified: for example, seasonal affective disorder (SAD) and post-partum depression. More usually, the pathogenesis of depression is better understood as the result of an accumulation of a number of different risk factors (Akiskal, 1985; Aneshensel and Stone, 1982; Brown and Harris, 1978). This point has been largely overlooked in the construction of animal models of depression, which in general have assumed a single causal factor. This may be counterproductive, since few of the identified aetiological factors appear sufficiently potent to precipitate depression in an otherwise risk-free individual.

Although attempts to assess the theoretical rationale of animal models are limited by this lack of theoretical structure at the clinical level, a number of generalizations are possible. The major group of animal models of depression are based on responses to stressors of various kinds, and are usually justified by reference to the role of stressful life events in the aetiology of depression (Brown and Harris, 1978, 1988; Lloyd, 1980). However, if very severe acute stress is used (e.g. Weiss *et al.*, 1982), the relevance of these procedures to depression, rather than, for example, to posttraumatic stress disorder (PTSD) is questionable. Furthermore, the adverse consequences of life events endure for a prolonged period of six to twelve months, in part by exacerbating ongoing life difficulties (Brown, 1989; Brown and Harris, 1988). Thus, life events should not be viewed as acute stressors (indeed, in the case of bereavement, a diagnosis of depression is explicitly excluded during the period of acute loss); from this perspective, it may be more appropriate to use chronic stress regimes, rather than acute stressors, to model the aetiological role of life events. Other factors have been identified that confer a long-lasting vulnerability to depression, in particular, an inadequate level of social support, which to a large extent arises from inadequate socialization (Aneshensel and Stone, 1982; Brown, 1989; Brown and Harris, 1978, 1988; see Willner, 1989b). From these starting points, a number of animal models of depression have been developed that are based on the adverse effects of social isolation. However, with the exception of some of the primate studies (see below), these models have largely ignored both the complexity of childhood social deprivation phenomena and the mediation of their effects through later social relationships.

Although assessment of the theoretical rationale of animal models of depression is limited by the paucity of theory, construct validity can also be evaluated at the level of constructs: that is, whether the behavioural phenomena are correctly described. This approach is best exemplified by the extensive experimental analysis of whether 'learned helplessness' is an appropriate term to describe the impairments of escape learning that follow exposure to inescapable electric shock (Seligman, 1975). The term 'learned helplessness' implies that the animals perform poorly because they have learned that their responses are ineffective in controlling their environment (Seligman, 1975). However, inescapable shock has a variety of other, simpler effects that could also explain many of the behavioural impairments, such as decreased locomotor activity (Anisman *et al.*, 1979; Glazer and Weiss, 1976) and analgesia (Lewis *et al.*, 1980). In addition, while inescapable shock results in 'cognitive' impairment (Jackson *et al.*, 1978) such behavioural effects arise from impairment at the level of attentional processing rather than 'helplessness' (Minor *et al.*, 1984). Thus, there are many reasons to question whether the learned helplessness procedure does in fact produce 'helplessness'.

Anhedonia is another construct that has been subjected to this kind of experimental attention. In this case, the question is whether the animals are failing to perform rewarded behaviour because they are insensitive to rewards or for some other reason. This question has been most extensively investigated in relation to the effects of chronic sequential exposure to a variety of mild stressors (chronic mild stress; CMS). CMS has been shown to cause an antidepressant-reversible decrease in the consumption of dilute sucrose solutions, which is hypothesized to reflect a decrease in the reward value of the sucrose (Willner, 1997; Willner *et al.*, 1987). Initial studies showed that, in contrast to the effect on dilute solutions of sucrose or saccharin, CMS did not decrease the intake of plain water, food pellets or concentrated sucrose solutions; thus the effects are not simply nonspecific changes in consummatory behaviour (Muscat and Willner, 1992). Some studies have suggested that decreases in sucrose intake reflect loss of body weight (e.g. Matthews *et al.*, 1995), but there is ample evidence (reviewed in Willner, 1997) to reject this suggestion, including the fact that the effects are seen in the absence of body weight changes. Furthermore, the effects of CMS are not confined to consummatory behaviours. CMS also attenuated or abolished place preferences established using a variety of natural or drug rewards. However, drug-induced place aversions were unaffected by CMS. Thus, the effect of CMS on place conditioning cannot be explained by nonspecific motivational impairments or a failure of associative learning (reviewed in Willner, 1997). Finally, CMS has also been shown to cause an increase in the threshold for brain-stimulation reward (Moreau *et al.*, 1992). Together, these results support the position that CMS causes a generalized decrease in sensitivity to rewards, and that under appropriate experimental conditions, decreases in sucrose intake provide a simple means of detecting this anhedonia.

These examples of successful experimental analyses of construct validity contrast sharply with a third example, the 'behavioural despair' test (Porsolt *et al.*, 1979). This term was introduced to describe the immobility seen in rats or mice forced to swim in a confined space, based on the assumption that when the animals adopted an immobile posture, they had 'despaired of' escaping. Unfortunately, this interpretation is not susceptible to experimental analysis. Consequently, although the test continues to be very widely used, the name 'behavioural despair' has been largely abandoned, and replaced instead by the theoretically neutral term 'the forced swim test'.

Heterogeneity of Depression

It has frequently been remarked (e.g. Fibiger, 1991) that the approach adopted in successive editions of the DSM, which identifies psychiatric disorders by the presence of a sufficient number of symptoms from a longer list, results in very different clinical presentations receiving the same diagnosis. However, discussion of the heterogeneity of depression is several decades older than the DSM system. It has been recognized since the 1920s that there are at least two forms of depression, but only one of them has enjoyed general agreement as to its nature (Willner, 1985). This is the syndrome that has been known, variously, as autonomous depression, endogenous depression, endogenomorphic depression and, more recently, melancholia. Because a consensus exists as to its existence and symptom profile, melancholia has emerged as the major subtype of depression, and its definition in DSM-IV is somewhat more restrictive than that of the parent syndrome, major depressive disorder.

Little attention has been paid to the question of subtypes of depression in the development of animal models, which have tended to focus either on an undifferentiated depressive state or on melancholia. Melancholia is defined, in DSM-IV (major depressive episode with melancholic features), by the presence of anhedonia, which is also the only core symptom of major depression that is amenable to modelling in animals. Anhedonia may be readily modelled as decreased sensitivity to rewards, although, as noted above, this construct is considerably more complex than a simple decrease in the performance of a rewarded behaviour. In relation to the other symptoms that can be modelled, the diagnosis of melancholia specifies the direction of changes in appetite and sleep (decreased), although, as in the diagnosis of major depressive disorder, psychomotor changes could be in either direction (retardation or agitation). In many empirical studies, psychomotor retardation has emerged as the symptom most characteristic of melancholia, while psychomotor agitation tends to be more closely associated with psychotic features such as delusions of guilt (Nelson and Charney, 1981). Nevertheless, there is considerable overlap between these two groups of symptoms, and agitated melancholias are not uncommon. Unlike non-melancholic depressions, melancholia is characterized by a decrease in the latency to enter the first period of rapid eye movement (REM) sleep (Kupfer and Thase, 1983) and an increased activity of the hypothalamic–pituitary–adrenal (HPA) system, usually detected by the dexamethasone suppression test (DST) (Carroll, 1982). In a valid simulation of melancholia, these biological markers would be expected to coexist alongside decreased sensitivity to rewards. However, the specificity of both of these markers for melancholia is less than originally claimed.

Unlike melancholia, no consensus exists that non-melancholic depression is a homogeneous entity, and this issue has been extensively debated. Within the 'non-melancholic' spectrum, two syndromes have been described that are of interest in the present context. One of these is not recognized in DSM-IV, but has features which suggest that it might represent a coherent biological entity. This is a form of depression in which central 5HT activity is decreased, as indicated by low concentrations of the 5HT metabolite 5-hydroxyindole acetic acid (5-HIAA) in cerebrospinal fluid. These depressions are characterized by high levels of anxiety and agitation, and Van Praag (1994) has suggested that these symptoms are primary, with depressed mood as a secondary response to a failure to cope with the consequences. It has been suggested that some animal models of depression, which are characterized by high levels of locomotor activity and/or aggression, may represent models of this subtype. There is as yet little further evidence on which to judge the validity of these claims.

A second 'non-melancholic' subtype of depression is delusional depression (previously known as psychotic depression). Delusional depression (DSM-IV major depressive episode with psychotic features) is difficult to translate into behavioural terms, being differentiated from non-delusional depression only by a greater association with psychomotor agitation (Nelson and Charney, 1981). Delusional depressions are pharmacologically distinct in that they respond to ECT or combinations of TCAs with neuroleptics, but not to TCAs alone (Nelson, 1987). The development of an animal model that responds to ECS but not to TCAs has not yet been achieved.

Bipolar disorder is another well-defined diagnostic category for which there are no animal models. There are a number of animal models of mania (see Lyon, 1991), but the alternation of depressive-like and manic-like behaviours in an animal model has not yet been systematically addressed. Indeed, the episodic nature of unipolar depression (e.g. brief recurrent depression) also remains to be explored in animal models.

THE DIATHESIS/STRESS CONCEPT

It is widely assumed that individuals within the population vary in their risk of contracting psychiatric disorders, and that such disorders are typically precipitated by external or internal (e.g. hormonal) events. The term diathesis refers to a predisposition to contract the disorder, while the term stress refers simply to the precipitant (note that the term 'stress' is used here in a different sense from the usual). A predisposition to become depressed (a depressive diathesis) may arise in a variety of ways, which may involve different levels of explanation. For example, a number of genetic diatheses have been identified, particularly in relation to bipolar disorder (see Souery *et al.*, Chapter XVIII-10). Some early life experiences are also known to increase the risk for depression, particularly parental deprivation (Robertson and Bowlby, 1952). The mechanisms by which these experiences increase the risk of depression (and other psychiatric disorders) are largely unknown, but probably involve psychological and psychosocial constructs. For example, parental deprivation may decrease the ability to form close relationships, and so dilute the quality of social support available in later life. Early life experiences also determine characteristic styles of processing information in relation to the self. For example, the negative thinking that characterizes the depressed person is thought to reflect the activation of a negative 'cognitive schema', learned through adverse childhood experiences such as rejection, criticism, or living with a depressed parent (Beck, 1967).

It follows from the diathesis/stress concept that a person who has a weak depressive diathesis would only succumb to an intense stress, whereas a person with a strong depressive diathesis may succumb to minor or trivial stresses. As these minor events might be relatively common, a depressive diathesis might result in a chronic presentation that looks very similar to an acute major depressive episode. Indeed, there is a depressive (gloomy, pessimistic, introverted) personality type, and where the symptoms are intense and disabling, this is classified as a depressive personality disorder. (This syndrome, present in DSM-III-R, was removed from DSM-IV as a clinical diagnosis, but is retained for research purposes.) A depressive personality disorder can shade into dysthymia, a more intense and more variable presentation. The diagnostic criteria for dysthymia include a number of somatic symptoms that are absent in the criteria for depressive personality disorder, but DSM-IV comments: 'It remains controversial whether the distinction between depressive personality disorder and dysthymic disorder is useful. The research criteria given for this proposed disorder differ from the diagnostic criteria for dysthymic disorder by their emphasis on cognitive, interpersonal, and intrapsychic personality traits.' This emphasis means that the symptoms of depressive personality disorder fall outside the scope of animal models. Dysthymia, however, can be modelled in animals. Dysthymia may be present from early childhood, or may have a more definable later onset. In either case, the distinction between dysthymia and a major depressive episode rests largely on the fact that dysthymia is less intense, and of chronic duration. In other respects, major depression and dysthymia are very similar in their presentation (for example, DSM-IV specifies that there are even common abnormalities in sleep electroencephalogram (EEG) recordings). Indeed, the only significant differences are in some of the subjective symptoms that are not amenable to animal modelling, such as excessive guilt and suicidal ideation, which are less prominent in dysthymia.

Thus, depressive diatheses may present as 'silent' until activated by stress (e.g. a genetic risk factor that does not directly elicit depressive symptoms, or a tendency towards depressive thinking that is well controlled), as a sub-syndromal depressive condition, or as a chronic condition that is difficult to distinguish from a major depressive episode. Consequently, animal models of a depressive diathesis could appear either as essentially 'normal' animals that are more sensitive to a precipitant used to induce 'depressive' behaviour, or could present 'depressive' features in the absence of any specific experimental manipulation.

In surveying changes over time in the landscape of animal models of depression, the major recent development has been a growth in the number of models that are better thought of as models of a predisposition to depression rather than as a depressive response to a precipitating event. We have therefore adopted this distinction as the organizing principle of this chapter. In the remainder of the chapter, we discuss first those models of depression that are based on exposure to adversity, and later, models that create or uncover a depressive diathesis. For the sake of completeness, we also mention briefly some of the pharmacological screening tests that were among the earliest animal models of depression to be developed.

MODELS OF DEPRESSION AS A RESPONSE TO ADVERSITY (i.e. STRESS)

A variety of adverse events have been used to produce animal models of depression, based on the observation that in general, the behavioural effects of stress are reversible by antidepressant drugs. However, the extent to which these effects meet the criteria for predictive validity, and the quality of the resulting models in terms of face and construct validity, varies greatly. For ease of presentation, we have grouped the models reviewed according to the nature of the stressor: acute experimenter-applied stressors; chronic experimenter-applied stressors; and models based on social stress and social isolation.

Acute Stress Models

Learned Helplessness Models

As noted earlier, the learned helplessness paradigm is based on the observation that animals exposed to uncontrollable stress (usually electric shocks) are subsequently impaired in learning to escape shock, an effect that is not seen in animals exposed to comparable, or indeed, identical, patterns of controllable shock. The protective effect of control appears to result from lower levels of fear (Jackson and Minor, 1988), which raises important questions about the relationship between depression and anxiety. Seligman (1975) proposed that exposure to uncontrollable stress provides the basis, in animals as in people, for learning that stress is uncontrollable (helplessness), and that this learning has a number of debilitating consequences, including depression. However, this interpretation has been the subject of considerable controversy, in both the human (Abramson *et al.*, 1978, 1989) and the animal literature (Minor *et al.*, 1984, 1988; Weiss *et al.*, 1982) and is probably incorrect (see above, and Willner, 1986, 1990). Nevertheless, the learning difficulties that follow exposure to uncontrollable shock are reversed with reasonable selectively by multiple acute, subchronic (3–5 days), treatment with TCAs or atypical antidepressants (Sherman *et al.*, 1982). SSRIs also appear to be effective, but only within a limited dose range (Martin *et al.*, 1989), as well as a number of other potential antidepressants such as 5-HT_{1A} receptor agonists (Giral *et al.*, 1988), β-adrenoceptor agonists (Martin *et al.*, 1986a), although some of these effects have been disputed (Christensen and Geoffroy, 1991), and extracts of St John's wort (*Hypericum perforatum*) (Gambarana *et al.*, 1999a; Kumar *et al.*, 2001). Interestingly, chronic, but not acute, treatment with lithium prevents the development of learned helplessness in rodents (Teixeira *et al.*, 1995). There are a few false positives, including the 5-HT_2 receptor antagonist, methysergide (Brown *et al.*, 1982), *p*-chlorophenylalanine (*p*CPA) (Edwards *et al.*, 1986) and piracetam (Cavoy *et al.*, 1988), while neuroleptics, stimulants, sedatives and anxiolytics are generally ineffective (Porsolt *et al.*, 1991; Sherman *et al.*, 1982).

The learned helplessness paradigm shows many symptomatic parallels to major depression—much so that it has been suggested that rodents subjected to uncontrollable shock could meet DSM diagnostic criteria (Weiss *et al.*, 1982)! However, the learned helplessness paradigm is implemented in a variety of different ways in different laboratories, and the version of the paradigm giving rise to the broadest range of symptoms (Weiss *et al.*, 1982) uses extremely high shock levels (4–6 ma) which are of doubtful relevance to depression. Furthermore, the effects of this regime largely dissipate within 2–3 days, and the effects of antidepressant pretreatment have not been studied using this procedure. The effects of antidepressants have typically been studied using shocks of a considerably lower intensity (1.0–1.5 ma) which cause a far less pervasive pattern of behavioural impairment.

Paradoxically, the effects of milder shock intensities are of longer duration, making it possible to interpose multiple acute (subchronic) drug treatment (typically for 3–5 days) between the initial uncontrollable shock session and the learning test. Furthermore, the duration of learned helplessness may be prolonged indefinitely by repeatedly exposing the subjects to the environment in which inescapable shock had occurred (Maier, 2001), which strengthens the face validity of this model of depression. However, a further problem is that different components of the learned helplessness syndrome may be related to different aspects of the induction procedure. For example, a long-term (7 weeks) suppression of home-cage locomotor activity has been reported following a single shock session (Desan *et al.*, 1988), but this effect is unrelated to shock controllability, and so clearly distinct from other learned helplessness phenomena (Woodmansee *et al.*, 1991). It is clear that the learned helplessness paradigm should more correctly be considered as a mixture of paradigms, and care should be taken in generalizing conclusions between them.

Among the consequences of low-intensity uncontrollable (but not controllable) shock is a poor performance of rewarded behaviour, which, as noted above, may be of particular relevance to melancholia. One manifestation of this effect is a long-lasting decrease in responding for brain-stimulation reward (intracranial self-stimulation; ICSS), in mice, which is specific to certain electrode placements, and therefore suggests a subsensitivity within part of the brain mechanism of reward, rather than, for example, a motor impairment (Zacharko *et al.*, 1983, 1987). Normal sensitivity to ICSS was restored by chronic, but not acute, treatment with TCAs (Zacharko and Anisman, 1991; Zacharko *et al.*, 1983). Interestingly, a long-lasting anhedonia is seen only if the animals are tested in the immediate aftermath of stress; otherwise the effect dissipates rapidly (Zacharko *et al.*, 1983). A related observation is that mild stressors, which are without effect in normal animals, may reinstate behavioural deficits resulting from an initial exposure to severe stress (Anisman and Zacharko, 1982). These studies suggest that it may be possible to develop conditioning models to explain how the risk of depression is elevated for several months in the aftermath of a stressful life event.

Another important observation is that uncontrollable electric shock has variable behavioural effects (most of which are antidepressant-reversible) in different inbred mouse strains. To take an extreme example, in the C57BL/67 strain, uncontrollable shock severely impaired subsequent learning to escape shock, but had no effect on responding for brain-stimulation reward, while the DBA/2J strain showed exactly the opposite pattern of deficits (Shanks and Anisman, 1988; Zacharko *et al.*, 1987). These studies may provide a starting point from which to investigate the physiological mechanisms underlying individual differences in responses to stress.

Vollmayr and Henn (2001) have recently described a procedure in which mild shocks induce learned helplessness in only some of the subjects, which may mimic the variable human predisposition for depressive illness. This procedure has been used as the basis for a selective breeding programme, which has produced a 'congenital learned helplessness' (cLH) and a 'congenital non-learned helplessness' strain. An impressive recent neuroimaging study of cLH rats reported that metabolism was decreased in dorsal frontal, medial orbital and anterior cingulated cortex, but increased in the subgenual region of the cingulated cortex (Shumake *et al.*, 2000); exactly these changes have been described in depressed patients (Drevets and Raichle, 1998; Mayberg *et al.*, 1999). However, there are also anomalies: in particular, cLH rats show a decreased adrenocortical response to stress (King *et al.*, 2001). There is also uncertainty as to just what is being selected in the cLH breeding programme. cLH animals have been shown to exhibit stress-induced analgesia (King *et al.*, 2001), raising the possibility that an increase in pain threshold might provide a very simple explanation of their escape learning impairments. And given the separation of shock-induced escape deficits and anhedonia in inbred mouse strains (Shanks and Anisman, 1988; Zacharko *et al.*, 1987), there is no reason to assume that the cLH strain, which was bred by selecting on the basis of shock-induced escape deficits, would also exhibit shock-induced anhedonia.

There is a relatively extensive literature dealing with the neurochemical bases of stress-induced motor inactivation (see Maier, 1984; Willner, 1985). Briefly, the debilitating effect of uncontrollable stress on later performance may be reversed by agonists at μ-opioid, dopamine (DA), α_1- and β-adrenergic receptors or by anticholinergic drugs; conversely, helplessness may be simulated pharmacologically by drugs that reduce DA and/or noradrenalin (NA) function, or by drugs that increase cholinergic function (Anisman and Zacharko, 1982; Besson *et al.*, 1996, 1998, 1999). Any influence of DA neurotransmission on learned helplessness appears to be mediated by the D1 dopamine receptor (Gambarana *et al.*, 1995a, b). Furthermore, reduced catecholamine neurotransmission, either by inhibition of catecholamine synthesis with α-methyl-ρ-tyrosine (De Montis *et al.*, 1993) or by treatment with α_1- and β-adrenoceptor antagonists (as well as the opiate receptor antagonist naloxone) has been shown to block the therapeutic effect of TCAs (Martin *et al.*, 1986b). Similarly, blockade of NMDA-receptor-mediated neurotransmission also blocks TCA-induced reversal of learned helplessness (Meloni *et al.*, 1993). Gamma-aminobutyric acid (GABA) neurotransmission also seems to be involved in learned helplessness behaviour. Thus a long-term increase in $GABA_B$ neurotransmission is associated with exacerbation of learned helplessness, while the action of antidepressant drugs in this model is associated with a long-term reduction in $GABA_B$ neurotransmission (Nakagawa *et al.*, 1996a, b). In contrast, studies of the role of 5-HT in learned helplessness are inconsistent (see Willner, 1990). Some 5HT receptor agonists may reverse learned helplessness, while 5-HT lesions did not prevent the action of TCAs in this model (Soubrie *et al.*, 1986). The induction of behavioural depression/learned helplessness may be regulated, at least in part, by serotonergic input into the hippocampal CA3 subfield. Papolos *et al.* (1996) have shown that intracerebroventricular administration of an antisense oligonucleotide to the $5\text{-}HT_{2A}$ receptor reduced receptor density in the CA3 area and induced learned helplessness behaviour.

Forced Swim Test

In the forced swim test, rats or mice are forced to swim in a confined space. While mice are subjected to a single swim test following a single drug administration, rats are generally subjected to two tests, usually spaced 24 h apart, to generate increased immobility scores. The onset of immobility exhibited by rats in the second test is delayed by pretreatment with a wide variety of antidepressants, usually administered in a multiple acute (subacute) treatment schedule consisting of three injections over the time period between the two swim sessions. The fact that the forced swim test responds to acute drug treatment has been a frequent source of criticism. Small antidepressant effects may be present after a single high dose. Larger effects are observed after multiple acute treatments at lower doses, but these changes may simply reflect an elevation of brain drug concentrations.

Effective treatments include TCAs, MAOIs, most atypical antidepressants, the selective NA reuptake inhibitor, reboxetine (Connor *et al.*, 1999), $5\text{-}HT_{1A}$, $5\text{-}HT_{1B}$ and $5\text{-}HT_{2C}$ receptor agonists (Cryan and Lucki, 2000; O'Neill and Conway, 2001), extracts of St John's wort (*Hypericum perforatum*) (Butterweek *et al.*, 1997), ECS and REM sleep deprivation (Borsini and Meli, 1988; Porsolt, 1981; Porsolt *et al.*, 1991). The test is not usually sensitive to SSRIs (Borsini, 1995; Borsini and Meli, 1988; Connor *et al.*, 2000), although activity of these compounds has sometimes been reported, and this appears to reflect a subtle technical change, an increase in the water depth (e.g. Cryan and Lucki, 2000; van der Heyden *et al.*, 1991). There have also been a variety of other negative reports; nevertheless, some 90% of clinically active antidepressants are active in the forced swim test, with the proportion rising in studies using chronic drug treatment (Borsini and Meli, 1988; Porsolt *et al.*, 1991). It has been suggested that both serotonergic and noradrenergic systems may be involved in mediating antidepressant-induced reductions in immobility; serotonergic-mediated effects result from increased swimming time while noradrenergic-mediated effects reflect increased climbing behaviour (Detke *et al.*, 1995).

Reduced immobility scores have also been observed following treatment with neurosteroids (Reddy *et al.*, 1998), neuropeptide Y (Stogner and Holmes, 2000) and NMDA receptor antagonists (Panconi *et al.*, 1993; van der Bos *et al.*, 1992). The effect of NMDA receptor antagonists is to reduce calmodulin-mediated activation of nitric oxide (NO) synthase. Likewise, NO synthase inhibitors have been reported to be as effective in reducing immobility as imipramine (Harkin *et al.*, 1999a). In rat studies, selective antagonists for subtypes of the cholecystokinin (CCK) receptor have both been shown to reduce immobility score. However, these positive effects are dependent on time of drug administration. Thus, the CCK_A antagonist devazepide is only effective when given before the conditioning pre-test (Hernando *et al.*, 1996) while the CCK_B antagonist L-365,260 is effective when given immediately prior to the re-test (Hernando *et al.*, 1994). These observations suggest a role for CCK in behavioural adaptations to acute stress.

On the negative side, while the test successfully discriminates antidepressants from neuroleptics and anxiolytics (Porsolt *et al.*, 1977), false positives have been reported for stimulants, convulsants, anticholinergics, antihistamines, pentobarbital, opiates, a variety of brain peptides (see above) and a number of other drugs (Borsini and Meli, 1988; Porsolt *et al.*, 1991). Some false positive responses have been reported to disappear if chronic drug treatment is used, or the duration of the test is prolonged (Kawashima *et al.*, 1986; Kitada *et al.*, 1981), but the generality of these effects has not been established.

While the predictive validity of the forced swim test may be better than has sometimes been assumed, its face and construct validity are minimal. The only symptomatic resemblance to depression is an inability or reluctance to maintain effort. Interestingly, positive responses to antidepressant drug treatment (i.e. reduced immobility) are only observed if subjects are forced to swim in water at least 10 °C below core body temperature (P.J. Mitchell, personal observations) and consequently develop severe hypothermia. If mice are forced to swim in water maintained at body temperature then immobility still occurs, but the response to antidepressant treatment is abolished. These observations clearly implicate the importance of severe cold stress and the consequent induction of hypothermia in this model, which further weakens the parallel with depression.

The theoretical rationale of this test derives entirely from its supposed relationship to learned helplessness. However, the relationship between the two models is unclear. Prior inescapable, but not escapable, shock has been found to increase immobility in the forced swim test, (Nomura *et al.*, 1982; Weiss *et al.*, 1981), but in view of the consistent finding of decreased motor activity following inescapable shock (see Anisman and Zacharko, 1982), it would be surprising were this not the case. The reciprocal finding has not been demonstrated: forced swimming did not impair subsequent escape performance in a shock avoidance task in which performance deficits are typically seen following inescapable shock (O'Neill and Valentino, 1982).

Nevertheless, the two tests do seem to share similar physiological substrates. Immobility in the swim test is also reversed by stimulating 5-HT_{1A}, 5-HT_{1B} and 5-HT_{2C} receptors (Cryan and Lucki, 2000; O'Neill and Conway, 2001; van der Heyden *et al.*, 1991), DA or α_1-adrenergic receptors or by anticholinergics, and potentiated by treatments that decrease the activation of DA (e.g. amisulpride: Papp and Wieronska, 2000) or NA systems or increase cholinergic transmission. Similarly, the therapeutic actions of antidepressants in this model are blocked by DA receptor antagonists and by treatments that reduce NA function, including neurotoxic destruction of the ascending NA pathways and α_1-adrenoceptor antagonists. As in the learned helplessness test, impairment of 5HT transmission neither increases immobility nor blocks its reversal by antidepressants (see Borsini and Meli, 1988; Willner, 1990).

Tail-Suspension Test

A number of variants of the forced swim test have been proposed. One of these, the tail-suspension test, has been claimed to be ethically superior to the forced swim test, as stress levels appear to be reduced (Porsolt *et al.*, 1986; Steru *et al.*, 1985). In this model, mice suspended by the tail show a temporal pattern of struggling followed by immobility, similar to that seen in the forced swimming test. Antidepressants, at strikingly low doses, have been shown to increase the duration of mobility and also, in an automated version of the test, to increase the power of the movements (though the latter effect is rather less convincing). Effective agents include TCAs, MAOIs and atypical antidepressants; the latter include mianserin, the selective NA reuptake inhibitor, reboxetine (Wong *et al.*, 2000), extracts of St John's wort (*Hypericum perforatum*) (Butterweek *et al.*, 1997), the NMDA receptor antagonist MK-801 (Panconi *et al.*, 1993) and, significantly, some (but by no means all) 5-HT uptake inhibitors (David *et al.*, 2001; Perrault *et al.*, 1992; but see also Fujishiro *et al.*, 2001; Teste *et al.*, 1993), which are usually ineffective in the forced swim test (see above). Immobility was also reduced by stimulant drugs, but was potentiated by neuroleptics or anxiolytics (Porsolt *et al.*, 1986; Steru *et al.*, 1985).

While it is tempting to see the tail-suspension test as a more sensitive version of the forced swim test, there are subtle differences between them, which are not at present understood but involve significant mediation by a noradrenergic-receptor-mediated mechanism(s) (Ferrari *et al.*, 1991). In particular, 5HT_{1A} receptor agonists are active in the forced swim test, but are ineffective in the tail-suspension test (Porsolt *et al.*, 1991), whereas the mixed 5-$HT_{1A/1B}$ receptor agonist RU 24969 was active in the latter. Like the forced swim test, the face and construct validity of the tail-suspension test are minimal.

Restraint Stress

Rats subjected to 2 h restraint stress exhibit hypolocomotion when examined in an open field 24 h later. Chronic treatment with desmethylimipramine (desipramine, DMI) or sertraline prior to restraint stress reverses the hypolocomotion (Kennett *et al.*, 1987). There is little basis on which to evaluate the validity of this model, which is included here simply to illustrate the generality of the reversibility of stress effects by antidepressants. Note, however, that, unlike the models described earlier, which respond to acute antidepressant treatment, this model requires chronic treatment.

Chronic Stress Models

Chronic Severe Stress

Repeated presentation of the same stressor usually leads to adaptation. However, adaptation can be prevented by presenting a variety of stressors in an unpredictable sequence. Katz and colleagues showed that three weeks of exposure to electric shocks, immersion in cold water, immobilization, reversal of the light/dark cycle and a variety of other stressors caused a decrease in the activating effect of acute stress in an open field test. However, the activating effect of acute stress was maintained in animals receiving daily antidepressant treatment during the chronic stress period; the effects of administering antidepressants after exposure to stress have not been studied in this model. A variety of antidepressant drugs, as well as ECS, were found to prevent the effect of chronic stress, but the MAOI tranylcypromine was ineffective. Various non-antidepressants failed to prevent the effect of stress. In addition to causing changes in open field activity, chronic stress also increased plasma corticosteroid levels. This effect showed the same spectrum of pharmacological sensitivity, with the exception that an anticholinergic was also effective (Katz *et al.*, 1981; see Willner, 1990 for review). Similar effects have also been reported in mice; corticosteroid levels and the response to an acute stress were normalized by TCAs, but not by the SSRI fluoxetine (Soblosky and Thurmond, 1986).

A further effect observed in rats after chronic stress was a failure to increase fluid consumption when saccharine was added to the drinking water, suggesting that chronic stress might cause anhedonia; this deficit was partially restored by imipramine (Katz, 1982). The chronic stress model has been used very little since the original series of publications, in part because the levels of severity employed raise serious ethical problems. However, a variant of the model has been devised which employs very mild stressors, and this model is described next.

Chronic Mild Stress (CMS)

The CMS model was developed in an attempt to achieve the same endpoints as the chronic stress model, but in a more ethically acceptable manner. The procedure involves relatively continuous exposure of rats or mice to a variety of mild stressors, such as periods of food and water deprivation, small temperature reductions, changes of cage mates, and other similarly innocuous manipulations. Over a period of weeks of chronic exposure to the mild stress regime, rats gradually reduced their consumption of a preferred dilute sucrose solution, and in untreated animals this deficit persisted for several weeks following the cessation of stress (Willner *et al.*, 1987, 1991). As discussed earlier (see the section on Construct Validity, above), a variety of studies have been performed to confirm that these effects reflect a generalized insensitivity to reward; in particular, chronic mild stress also impairs responsiveness to reward as assessed by different methods, including suppression of place preference conditioning (Papp *et al.*, 1991, 1992, 1993) and increased threshold for ICSS (Moreau *et al.*, 1992). Studies of the effects of the individual elements of the chronic mild stress regime revealed that one element, social housing (in animals usually housed individually), was particularly potent, but no individual element (including social housing) was either necessary to induce anhedonia or sufficient to maintain anhedonia for a prolonged period (Muscat and Willner, 1992).

Antidepressant treatment has no effect on sucrose consumption or ICSS threshold in non-stressed animals, but following the reduction of sucrose intake by stress, normal behaviour was gradually restored by chronic treatment (2–5 weeks) with a wide variety of antidepressants, including TCAs, SSRIs, a specific NA reuptake inhibitor (maprotiline), MAO-A inhibitors, atypical antidepressants such as mianserin, buspirone, and amisulpride, and ECS. Also effective were some agents of uncertain antidepressant status, such as antihistaminic and anticholinergic drugs. Ineffective drugs include the anxiolytic chlordiazepoxide, various neuroleptics, amphetamine and morphine (reviewed by Willner, 1997; Willner and Papp, 1997). Fluoxetine, maprotiline and mianserin (but not chlordiazepoxide) were also found to restore the rewarding properties of food, as assessed in the place conditioning paradigm (Cheeta *et al.*, 1994; Muscat *et al.*, 1992). In contrast to the extensive array of drugs correctly classified in CMS experiments, very few false positives or false negatives have been reported.

The reversal of an established behavioural deficit during the continued presence of the stressor is an important feature of this model: if, as seems likely, chronic stress does play a role in the aetiology of melancholia (e.g. Aneshensel and Stone, 1982; Monroe *et al.*, 1985; Rodgers, 1991), its continued presence during antidepressant therapy would usually be the norm. Also important is the extended time course of antidepressant action, which makes it feasible to detect rapid onset of action. Many novel agents have been identified as potential antidepressants using the CMS procedure, and these include some that appear to act more rapidly than TCAs or SSRIs, including the D2/D3 receptor antagonist amisulpride (Papp and Wieronska, 2000), the glycine antagonist 1-aminocyclopropanecarboxylic acid (ACPC) (Papp and Moryl, 1996), the $5HT_{1A}$ receptor agonist BIMT-17 (D'Aquila *et al.*, 1997), and the SNRI venlafaxine (M. Papp, personal communication). Potentiation of antidepressant action by lithium and pindolol has also been reported (Sluzewska and Szczawinska, 1996a, b). In at least three instances (the D2/D3 receptor agonist pramipexole, the corticosterone synthesis inhibitor ketoconazole, and the catechol-*O*-methyl transferase (COMT) inhibitor tolcapone), the antidepressant effect of these compounds was demonstrated in the clinic only after these actions had been predicted in the CMS model (see Willner, 1997).

In addition to decreasing responsiveness to rewards, CMS also causes the appearance of many other symptoms of major depressive disorder. Behavioural changes in animals exposed to CMS include decreases in sexual, aggressive and investigative behaviours, and decreases in locomotor activity. These are seen during the dark phase of the light–dark cycle, which is the rat's active period; EEG measures of active waking are also decreased during the dark phase. In contrast, CMS did not cause the appearance of an 'anxious' profile in two animal models of anxiety, the elevated plus-maze and the social interaction test, suggesting that the behavioural changes are specific for depression. Animals exposed to CMS show an advanced phase shift of diurnal rhythms, diurnal variation, with symptoms worst at the start of the dark (active) phase, and a variety of sleep disorders characteristic of depression, including decreased REM sleep latency, an increased number of REM sleep episodes, and more fragmented sleep patterns. They also gain weight more slowly, leading to a relative loss of body weight, and show signs of increased activity in the HPA axis, including adrenal hypertrophy and corticosterone hypersecretion. Abnormalities have also been detected in the immune system, including an increase in serum, decreases in thymus weight, natural killer cell activity and reactivity to T-cell mitogens, and an increase in acute phase proteins that was reversed by chronic antidepressant treatment. Taken together with the generalized decrease in responsiveness to rewards, these parallels to the symptoms of depression, and in particular, to melancholia, are both extensive and comprehensive (reviewed by Willner, 1997). Indeed, it is arguable that the only symptoms of depression that have not been demonstrated in animals exposed to CMS are those uniquely human symptoms that are only accessible to verbal enquiry. Even without these symptoms, a rat exposed to CMS could, in principle, legitimately attract a DSM-IV diagnosis of either major depressive disorder or major depressive disorder with melancholic features.

Studies of the neural basis of the CMS-induced anhedonia have focused primarily on the mesolimbic DA system. The behavioural changes in animals subjected to CMS are accompanied by a decrease in D2/D3-receptor binding and D2-mRNA expression in the nucleus accumbens, and a pronounced functional subsensitivity to the rewarding and locomotor stimulant effects of the D2/D3 receptor agonist quinpirole, administered systemically or within the nucleus accumbens. All of these effects are also reversed by chronic antidepressant treatment (Dziedzicka-Wasylewska *et al.*, 1997; Willner and Papp, 1997). In other studies, animals successfully treated with antidepressants were treated acutely with D2/D3 receptor antagonists, at low doses that were without effect in non-stressed animals or in untreated stressed animals. This treatment reversed the effects of a wide variety of antidepressants on rewarded behaviour (Willner and Papp, 1997). These data argue strongly that an increase in D2/D3 receptor responsiveness may be responsible for the therapeutic action of antidepressants in this model (Willner and Papp, 1997). A similar reversal of SSRI action by the D2 antagonist sulpiride has been observed in a clinical study, as predicted from the CSM data (see Willner, 1997).

A recent CMS study suggests a neural mechanism that could mediate the negative information processing bias characteristic of depression (Beck, 1967). In this study, DA release in nucleus accumbens and prefrontal cortex was monitored by microdialysis following exposure to a palatable reward and a stressor (tail pinch). CMS markedly inhibited DA release in response to rewards, but potentiated responses to the stressor; and both of these effects of CMS were reversed by chronic treatment with the TCA, DMI (Di Chiara *et al.*, 1999).

While the CMS model has a great many positive features, and is probably the most valid animal model of depression currently available (see below), a major drawback is that the model has proven extremely difficult to implement reliably, and while many laboratories have succeeded in doing so, many others have not. The reasons for this lack of reliability have been extensively debated (see Willner, 1997), but as yet are unresolved.

Stress Induction and Mild Stress Maintenance

Tagliamonte and colleagues have described a model that represents a cross between learned helplessness and CMS. In this procedure, an altered state is first induced by acute exposure to a session of moderately intense inescapable tail shock, and then maintained, apparently indefinitely, by exposure to milder stressors (brief restraint, a small number of shocks, or exposure to the inescapable shock apparatus), presented at two-day intervals. This treatment resulted in an impairment of shock escape learning, as in learned helplessness, and a failure to learn a simple maze task reinforced by a highly palatable food (vanilla sugar), as in CMS. Both of these deficits were prevented by chronic pretreatment with TCAs or fluoxetine (De Montis *et al.*, 1995; Ghiglieri *et al.*, 1997). The stress procedure also decreased basal levels of extracellular DA in the nucleus accumbens shell, and this change also was prevented by chronic TCA treatment (Gambarana *et al.*, 1999b).

We noted earlier (see the section on Construct Validity, above) that the effect of severe life events to precipitate depression was best characterized as an acute severe stress followed by a chronic increase in mild stress. Stress induction followed by mild stress maintenance exactly parallels these processes, and is the only animal model of depression to do so. This procedure could potentially provide a more reliable and robust alternative to the CMS procedure, but few data are as yet available. In particular, while antidepressants have been shown to prevent the development of behavioural abnormalities, they have not as yet been shown to reverse an established deficit. Also, the portability of the procedure to other laboratories has not yet been demonstrated.

Withdrawal from Chronic Psychomotor Stimulants (Amphetamine and Cocaine)

A number of studies have reported that responding for ICSS was reduced in the days following withdrawal from chronic amphetamine treatment. In these studies, amphetamine was administered to rats for between 4 and 10 days, typically using several administrations each day, at increasing doses (Barrett and White, 1980; Kokkinidis and Zacharko, 1980; Leith and Barrett, 1976; Simpson and Annau, 1977). The threshold for ICSS was elevated following amphetamine withdrawal, confirming that the rate reduction reflects a subsensitivity to brain-stimulation reward rather than a depression of motor activity (Cassens *et al.*, 1981; Leith and Barrett, 1980). After 14 days of amphetamine treatment, the decreased sensitivity to ICSS did not recover during 18 days of further testing (Leith and Barrett, 1980) reflecting subsensitivity of reward systems rather than simple depression of motor activity. In a single pharmacological study, this effect was alleviated by two days of imipramine or amitriptyline treatment, and with continued treatment, normal responding was restored (Kokkinidis *et al.*, 1980).

In a variant of this procedure, animals self-administer cocaine, rather than being administered amphetamine (Koob, 1989). In these experiments, the threshold for brain-stimulation reward, administered through electrodes in the posterior lateral hypothalamus, was obtained using a discrete trial procedure (Kornetsky and Esposito, 1981), which is sensitive to changes in reward value, but not to changes in motor performance (Markou *et al.*, 1989). Following 24 h of cocaine self-administration, ICSS thresholds were elevated for several hours (Koob, 1989), indicating that cocaine withdrawal induced a state of anhedonia. Acute administration of the DA receptor agonist bromocriptine restored ICSS thresholds to normal (Markou and Koob, 1989). Only one conventional antidepressant has been tested in this procedure: repeated administration of the TCA DMI was reported to shorten the duration of post-cocaine anhedonia (Markou *et al.*, 1992).

It has frequently been assumed that stimulant drug treatment is a form of stress, since in many respects stimulant treatment and stress appear to be interchangeable (Antelman *et al.*, 1980; Post, 1975). Indeed, withdrawal from chronic cocaine treatment in rats is associated with intense anxiety-related behaviour and extrahypothalamic-limbic corticotropin-releasing hormone (CRH) hypersecretion (Sarnyai *et al.*, 1995). The similarities between stress and stimulant withdrawal are thought to arise from the fact that, like stimulant drugs, stressors activate the mesolimbic and mesocortical DA projections (Blanc *et al.*, 1980). Independent of a relationship to stress, there is an obvious parallel between the effects of stimulant withdrawal and the depressions that frequently follow the cessation of chronic stimulant use (Watson *et al.*, 1972), although in the animal model, the time course is rather more compressed.

As the stimulant withdrawal models are based exclusively upon changes in ICSS behaviour, their construct validity depends largely on the assumption that brain-stimulation reward activates natural reward pathways (Hoebel, 1976). Although early studies suggested that ICSS had unusual properties compared to natural rewards (for example, rapid extinction), it was later recognized that these properties derive from differences in the experimental procedures typically employed (such as the delay of reinforcement); when such extraneous factors are equated, ICSS appears very comparable to a high-incentive natural reward presented under conditions of low drive (see Gibson *et al.*, 1965). These parallels, together with the observation that responding for ICSS performance is influenced by many of the factors that control responding for natural rewards, have justified the assumption that the ICSS electrode stimulates directly the neural substrates that are activated indirectly by natural rewards (Hoebel, 1976). A degree of caution is required, since although people implanted with ICSS electrodes report a variety of pleasurable sensations, they also report other reasons for stimulating, such as curiosity (Atrens, 1984; Valenstein, 1973). Nevertheless, the commonality of anatomical substrate between ICSS and other types of reward supports the use of this procedure as an animal model of hedonic behaviour (see also Koob, 1989; Wise, 1989). However, the relationship of drug-induced depressions to major depressive disorder is uncertain, and the validity of this model is therefore questionable.

Social Dominance Models

Parallels have often been noted between depressive and submissive behaviours (Gardner, 1982; Price, 1972), and a number of laboratories have attempted to model depression by using animals of low social rank. Subordinates, and those who have lost status as a result of defeat in social conflict situations, are at greater risk for psychopathology. Biological similarities between defeated animals and human depression have frequently been noted (see Gilbert and Allan, 1998; Henry, 1982; Toates, 1995), and there is considerable evidence that depressed individuals see themselves as inferior and behave submissively (reviewed by Gilbert and Allan, 1998). Indeed, social skills training, of which assertiveness training represents a major component, is used clinically as a psychotherapy for depression, which has been found to be as effective as TCA treatment (e.g. Hersen *et al.*, 1984). Like the chronic mild stress procedure, animal models based on social dominance employ realistic inducing conditions, which are of particular ecological relevance.

Social Defeat

Social defeat is a potent stressor, and repeated defeat is a form of chronic stress, which is associated with a decrease in aggressive behaviour (Albonetti and Farabollini, 1994). A single social defeat has been reported to produce a gradual, but long-lasting, increase in immobility in the forced swim test, which was prevented by chronic treatment with clomipramine (Koolhaas *et al.*, 1990). A similar model has been developed in submissive C57BL/6J mice: a single defeat by a dominant male mouse of the same strain was reported to cause a gradual increase over weeks in passive behaviour in response to a mild stressor, which could be antagonized by clomipramine; defeated animals also had higher immobility times in the forced swim test (Korte *et al.*, 1991). In a chronic version of a similar procedure, mice were housed in social contact, but were physically separated except for one daily 3-minute encounter. Again, increased immobility in the forced swim test was observed in repeatedly defeated animals, and this effect was prevented by chronic treatment with imipramine (Kudryatseva *et al.*, 1991), though in this study, imipramine did not normalize social behaviour in the defeated animals (Kudryatseva *et al.*, 1991).

In a modified rat model, defeat of dominant pair-housed rats by rats of a different, more aggressive strain resulted in the loss of dominant status relative to their previously submissive partners, which was restored by chronic imipramine treatment (Willner *et al.*, 1995). This loss of status was accompanied by the abolition of morphine-induce place conditioning, most likely reflecting a decrease in hedonic tone (Coventry *et al.*, 1997). This suggests that it may be appropriate to view submission models, potentially, as models of melancholia. However, more evidence is needed for any firm conclusion.

In a modified murine social defeat paradigm, subordinate mice subjected to repeated social defeat showed reduced growth compared to dominant subjects, together with citalopram-sensitive anxiogenic-like behaviour (Keeney and Hogg, 1999; Keeney *et al.*, 2001). The defeated mice exhibited a maintained increase in both core temperature and circulating corticosterone levels indicative of chronic stress, although social defeat had no effect on either ethanol consumption or immobility time measured in the forced swim test. Similarly, a single social defeat of Lewis rats resulted in hypophagia and weight loss, together with increased measures of anxiety, and these effects were reduced following acute fluoxetine treatment (Berton *et al.*, 1999).

Overall, these various studies suggest that social defeat may in principle provide a valid and ecologically sound model of depression. However, a variety of procedures have been used, and at present, the data are not entirely consistent.

Social Hierarchy

Rats housed in closed groups develop a social hierarchy and the relative social position of each group member may be identified by assessing each individual's level of success during agonistic encounters with other group members. If rats are housed in triads then a social hierarchy consisting of a dominant, subdominant and subordinate develops. Chronic administration (2-week) of either clomipramine or mianserin to the subdominant animal results in an increase in that subject's rank position at the expense of the level of dominance enjoyed by the dominant group member (Mitchell and Redfern, 1992a). The increase in the social position of the antidepressant-treated subdominant rat is likely to be related to increased assertiveness expressed during social encounters. An attractive feature of this model is that daily assessment of social structure allows the time course of antidepressant-induced elevation of social position to be determined.

However, not all features of subordinate animals are necessarily of relevance to depression, and the relationship between social dominance and social competition is potentially problematic. In group-housed rats competing for limited access to a high-incentive reward, the performance of subordinate animals was improved by acute or chronic anxiolytic treatment (Gentsch *et al.*, 1990; Joly and Sanger, 1991), suggesting that the social competition test is relevant to anxiety rather than depression. Consistent with this view is the observation that chronic treatment with *m*-chlorophenylpiperazine (*m*CPP), a major metabolite of the antidepressant trazodone, which also possesses antidepressant activity, failed to increase the performance subdominant rats in a social competition test (Moledina *et al.*, 2000) at a dose previously shown to increase the aggressive behaviour of resident rats in a resident–intruder test (see below) (Mitchell and Redfern, 2000). However, the benzodiazepine anxiolytic diazepam, which improves performance in a social competition test, did not increase aggressive behaviour in dyadic encounters, after either acute or chronic administration (Mitchell and Redfern, 1992b). Further studies will be necessary to confirm this ineffectiveness of anxiolytics in social dominance tests.

The Resident–Intruder Test

Antidepressant treatment has consistently been shown to have profound effects on rat, but not necessarily mouse, social and agonistic behaviour. While acute treatment with pharmacologically disparate antidepressant drugs (including TCAs, MAOIs, SSRIs, SNRIs, 5-HT_{1A} receptor agonists and partial agonists, and 5-HT_{2C} receptor agonists) commonly reduces the aggressive behaviour of resident rats when confronted with an unknown conspecific intruder, chronic antidepressant treatment (including repeated ECS) increases such aggressive behaviour (Cobain *et al.*, 1994a, b; Mitchell and Fletcher, 1993, 1994; Mitchell and Forster, 1992; Mitchell and Hogg, 2001a, b; Mitchell and Redfern, 1992b, 1997a, b, 2000; Willner *et al.*, 1981). These observations are consistent with the view that aggression is the only type of rodent social behaviour consistently increased following chronic treatment with antidepressants (File and Tucker, 1986).

The fact that chronic antidepressant treatment increases aggressive behaviour appears at first sight to be incompatible with the use of SSRIs in the clinical treatment of impulsive aggression (Coccaro and Kavoussi, 1997; Evenden, 1999a; Fava and Rosenbaum, 1993). However, this is a clinical, rather than an experimental, paradox, since clinically, antidepressants both increase aggression in submissive depressed individuals (manifest as a reversal of intropunitive aggression and/or impaired sociability: see Dixon *et al.*, 1989; Kaplan *et al.*, 1961; Priest *et al.*, 1980) and decrease pathological aggression (e.g. Hollander, 1999; Vartiainen *et al.*, 1995). A resolution of this paradox may be that antidepressant treatment increases assertiveness, since this would increase low levels of social dominance while at the same time decreasing high levels of physical aggression. Hence, the ability of chronic antidepressant treatment to increase aggression in rats may reflect the increased assertiveness and associated externalization of emotions expressed during recovery from depressive illness. Such increased assertive/aggressive behaviour is consistent with the effects of such treatment in the social hierarchy model (see above). However, face validity of the resident–intruder model is reduced by the fact that the test involves 'normal' unmanipulated animals; non-depressed people do not respond to antidepressant treatment. Interestingly, and in contrast to the rat studies, the aggressive behaviour of male mice in resident–intruder studies is particularly sensitive to anxiolytic, rather than antidepressant, drug activity (e.g. Lumley *et al.*, 2000).

By programming daily dyadic encounters, the resident–intruder paradigm can be used to compare the rate of onset of antidepressant-induced elevation in aggression between antidepressant treatments and to assess the utility of potential adjuvant treatment to accelerate antidepressant-related changes in rodent behaviour. Indeed, the first published studies to demonstrate the ability of a selective 5-HT_{1A} receptor antagonist (WAY-100635) to accelerate time-dependent antidepressant-induced behavioural changes used the resident–intruder test (Mitchell and Redfern, 1997b).

Social Separation

The presumed aetiological role in depression of loss events, and particularly loss of a loved one, has led to the development of a number of animal models of depression based on separation phenomena.

Although the evolutionary proximity of primates has led some authors to consider primate separation models to be of particular importance (e.g. Everitt and Keverne, 1979), they have produced remarkably little of value. Precisely because of their evolutionary proximity, the use of primates sacrifices many of the advantages of animal models, such as the easing of ethical constraints, and the possibility of testing adequately sized groups of subjects.

Neonatal Isolation

The most familiar of these models involve non-human primates, either infants isolated from their parents, or juveniles isolated from their peer group. The separation response consists of an initial stage of 'protest', characterized by agitation, sleeplessness and distress calls, followed by 'despair', characterized by a decrease in activity, appetite, play and social interaction, and the assumption of a hunched posture and 'sad' facial expression (see Henn and McKinney, 1987; Suomi, 1976). These symptoms are strikingly similar to those of 'anaclitic depression' in institutionalized children (Robertson and Bowlby, 1952). However, while parental loss in childhood, and loss events such as bereavement in adults, are implicated in the aetiology of depression, they also increase the risk of a variety of other psychiatric and non-psychiatric disorders (Brown *et al.*, 1973; Schmale, 1973). The nature of the separation response is sensitive to the environment in which the experiments are carried out (e.g. Reite *et al.*, 1981; Suomi, 1976), and the incidence of 'depressive' behaviours may in some experiments be as low as 15% (Lewis *et al.*, 1976).

The few pharmacological studies using these models have not been impressive. Very few published studies have attempted to use antidepressant treatments to modify primate separation behaviour, and because of the expense of using primates, the size of experimental groups in most studies has usually been too small to provide reliable data. Chronic treatment with DMI (Hrdina *et al.*, 1979), imipramine (Suomi *et al.*, 1978), oxaprotiline (McKinney and Kraemer, 1989) and ECS (Lewis and McKinney, 1976) have been reported to reverse some, but not all, of the effects of separation in monkeys. Trifluoperazine, amphetamine and diazepam did not affect responses to social isolation in chimpanzees (Menzel *et al.*, 1963, Turner *et al.*, 1969), but some therapeutic effects of chlorpromazine were seen in rhesus monkeys (McKinney *et al.*, 1973). 'Depressive'—like behaviours in singly-housed rhesus monkeys are associated with decreased concentrations of NA in the cerebrospinal fluid, with relatively little effect on DA or 5HT (Kraemer *et al.*, 1989). Following a return to social housing, NA levels normalize, but the animals remain hypersensitive to pharmacological challenges of the NA system (Kraemer *et al.*, 1984a, b).

In fact, separation phenomena of 'protest' followed by 'despair' are present to some extent in many other species, including cats, dogs, rodents and precocial birds (Katz, 1981; McKinney and Bunney, 1969), and several of these phenomena have also been used as the basis for the development of animal models of depression. One of these, the reactivation of distress calling in one-week-old chicks, appears to perform relatively well as an antidepressant screening test (Lehr, 1989). The vocalizations of guinea-pig pups separated from their mothers also respond to antidepressants, and this test was used successfully to detect antidepressant-like activity of the Substance P neurokinin 1 (NK1) receptor antagonists (Rupniak *et al.*, 2000).

Adult Isolation

Chronic (4–6 weeks) isolation of adult rats has been found to cause a disruption of cooperative social behaviour (Berger and Schuster, 1982) reminiscent of the poor social performance of depressed people (Lewinsohn, 1974). In a single study of the effects of antidepressant treatment, the impairment of social cooperation in isolated rats was reversed by chronic treatment with either imipramine or fluoxetine, and the effect of imipramine in this model was abolished by the 5-HT antagonist metergoline (Willner *et al.*, 1989).

MODELS OF PREDISPOSITION TO DEPRESSION (i.e. DIATHESIS)

Depressive diatheses have been modelled genetically, genomically, developmentally and by brain lesioning. These areas are reviewed in turn.

Genetic Models

Selective Breeding for Muscarinic Hypersensitivity (FSL)

The Flinders Sensitive Line (FSL) rat is the result of selective breeding for sensitivity to the hypothermic effect of cholinergic agonists and is based on the hypothesis that central cholinergic systems are important in depression since increased cholinergic sensitivity has been reported in depressed patients. Although bred for cholinergic hypersensitivity, FSL animals also show a number of other pharmacological abnormalities, including serotonergic hypersensitivity and dopaminergic hyposensitivity (Overstreet and Janowsky, 1991). Relative to the control Flinders Resistant Line, FSL animals have a number of characteristics reminiscent of depression, including cholinergic supersensitivity, increased REM sleep and reduced locomotor activity, which is further pronounced following electric footshock (Overstreet, 1993). FSL animals also show greater immobility in the forced swim test (Overstreet and Janowsky, 1991). This behaviour was normalized by chronic treatment with a high dose of imipramine, and partly reversed by DMI or sertraline, but was not restored by chronic amphetamine or scopolamine (Overstreet, 1991; Overstreet *et al.*, 1995; Schiller *et al.*, 1992). FSL rats also exhibit a greater vulnerability to the suppressive effect of chronic mild stress on responsiveness to sweet reward (Pucilowski *et al.*, 1991, 1993) but behave normally in the elevated plus-maze, a putative animal model of anxiety (Overstreet, 1991).

While these observations are consistent with a depressive diathesis and greater behavioural responsiveness to stress, other data are not. FSL rats have markedly elevated levels of 5-HT, NA and DA in specific brain areas, which are normalized during chronic treatment with DMI (Zangen *et al.*, 1997, 1999), and hypothalamic levels of CRH and circulating levels of adrenocorticotrophic hormone (ACTH) are lower in FSL rats (Owens *et al.*, 1991), indicating reduced HPA axis activity, in contrast to the increased HPA axis activity observed in depression. Similarly, acute and chronic treatments with nicotine, a non-antidepressant, both exhibit an antidepressant-like effect on the behaviour of FSL rats in the forced swim test (Tizabi *et al.*, 1999), which was blocked by prior treatment with the nicotinic receptor antagonist mecamylamine (Tizabi *et al.*, 2000). It should be noted that the major pharmacological evidence supporting the FSL strain as a model of depression derives from studies using the forced swim test, which is itself of questionable validity.

The Roman Low-Avoidance (RLA) Strain

The Roman low-avoidance (RLA) rat strain has been selectively bred for poor avoidance in the shuttle box paradigm, while the Roman high-avoidance (RHA) counterparts have been selectively bred for their good performance in that task. Compared to RHA rats, the behaviour of RLA rats expressed in the open-field, elevated plus-maze and hole-board tests are consistent with high levels of emotionality (Escorihuela *et al.*, 1999) and reflect differences in response to or the ability to cope with stress. In contrast, RLA and RHA rats react similarly to social defeat (Meerlo *et al.*, 1997). This latter finding suggests that the RLA strain is likely to prove of limited relevance to depression.

The Fawn-Hooded Strain

The Fawn-Hooded (FH) rat strain exhibits hypercortisolaemia and blunted response to dexamethasone-induced suppression of cortisol secretion (Owens and Nemeroff, 1991) consistent with the hyperactivity of the HPA axis which is observed in depressive illness. The elevated levels of plasma cortisol are reduced by chronic treatment with the TCAs imipramine and clomipramine, and with the MAO-A inhibitor clorgyline (Aulakh *et al.*, 1993). FH rats also exhibit reduced growth rate consistent with an abnormality of the hypothalamic-somatotrophic (HSM) axis (Gomez *et al.*, 1999). FH rats exhibit increased immobility in the forced swim test in some studies (but not all; see Hall *et al.*, 1998a; Lahmame *et al.*, 1996) and increased ethanol intake and preference (Overstreet *et al.*, 1992). Furthermore, ethanol consumption in FH rats is increased by social isolation (Hall *et al.*, 1998b). Recent studies also indicate higher levels of anxiety in FH rats (Hall *et al.*, 2000; Kantor *et al.*, 2001) together with impaired social behaviour (Kantor *et al.*, 2000). These observations indicate that the FH rat may be a suitable model of comorbid depressive illness, alcoholism and anxiety, but clearly, much more work would be needed to substantiate this conclusion.

Like FSL rats, FH rats exhibit cholinergic supersensitivity (Overstreet *et al.*, 1992). In contrast, FH rats exhibit functional hyposensitivity to a variety of 5-HT and NA receptor agonists (Aulakh *et al.*, 1994, 1996) reflecting altered serotonergic and noradrenergic function in the FH strain.

Genomic Models

HPA Transgenic

In depressive illness, the secretion of CRH from the paraventricular nucleus of the hypothalamus is under the control of a glucocorticoid-receptor-mediated inhibitory feedback system. Conditions of extreme, prolonged stress cause reduced sensitivity of the glucocorticoid receptor, thereby reducing the effectiveness of the feedback loop, resulting in hypercortisolaemia. A transgenic mouse strain expressing glucocorticoid-receptor antisense has been described which exhibits dysfunction of the HPA axis in a manner similar to that seen in depressive illness (Montkowski *et al.*, 1995; Pepin *et al.*, 1992a). Chronic treatment with antidepressants reduces plasma cortisol and ACTH levels (Montkowski *et al.*, 1995; Pepin *et al.*, 1992b), by increasing glucocorticoid-receptor mRNA expression (Barden, 1996), with a subsequent elevation of glucocorticoid-receptor activity resulting in increased sensitivity of the HPA axis to glucocorticoid negative feedback (Barden, 1999). However, while behavioural and neuroendocrine responses to stress are modified in transgenic mice (Farisse *et al.*, 1999; Linthorst *et al.*, 2000), the direction of these changes is inconsistent with a model of depressive illness: relative to wild-type controls, transgenic mice exhibit reduced immobility in the forced swim test and less anxiety-related behaviour on the elevated plus-maze but increased aggressive behaviour (Beaulieu *et al.*, 1993; Montkowski *et al.*, 1995). All of these changes are in the opposite direction to those expected.

5-HT Transporter Knockout

The serotonin reuptake transporter (5-HTT) is pivotal in the inactivation and control of serotonergic neurotransmission, and blockade of the serotonin transporter is the principal target of the TCA, SSRI and SNRI drugs. Investigations of subjects which lack the serotonergic transporter, while not a model of depression, may provide an insight into the adaptive mechanisms associated with a permanent lack of serotonin reuptake. Recent studies suggest that 5-HTT knockout mice show regional differences from wild-type mice in terms of 5-HT_{1A} receptor protein and mRNA expression (reduced in dorsal raphe, hypothalamus, amygdala and septum, but increased in hippocampus: Fabre *et al.*, 2000; Lanfumey *et al.*, 2000; Li *et al.*, 2000), which are associated with reduced functional sensitivity to the hypothermic effects of the 5-HT_{1A} receptor agonist 8-hydroxy-2-(di-*n*-propylamino)tetraline (8-OH-DPAT) (Li *et al.*, 1999). Similarly, 5-HT_{2A} receptor density is also reduced in 5-HTT knockout mice (Rioux *et al.*, 1999). Interestingly, the desensitization of 5-HT_{1A} autoreceptors in 5-HTT knockout mice is further enhanced by exposure to stressful conditions (Lanfumey *et al.*, 2000).

CRH Receptor Subtype Knockouts

CRH is a critical coordinator of the HPA axis and subtypes of CRH receptors, CRH-R1 and CRH-R2, are found throughout the central nervous system and peripheral tissue. CRH has higher affinity for the CRH-R1 receptor, while urocortin (a CRH-related peptide) exhibits 40-fold selectivity for the CRH-R2 receptor. CRH-R1 knockout mice exhibit anxiolytic-like behaviour, which may be due to impaired spatial recognition memory (Contarino *et al.*, 1999), together with characteristic responses to stress (Timpl *et al.*, 1998) indicative of disrupted HPA axis (Smith *et al.*, 1998). In contrast, CRH-R2 knockout mice exhibit increased anxiety-like behaviour and are hypersensitive to stress (Bale *et al.*, 2000).

Tachykinin Receptor Knockout

The NK1 receptor is expressed in brain areas associated with the control and management of depressive illness, anxiety, stress and sensitivity to the rewarding properties of food and drugs of abuse. Indeed, antagonists at the NK1 receptor have been suggested as potential antidepressant drugs with a novel mode of action (Froger *et al.*, 2001; Rupniak *et al.*, 2000, 2001). The NK1 receptor knockout mouse is not an animal model of depression. Rather, these mice show behavioural changes similar to those elicited by antidepressants in normal mice, including a decrease in neonatal vocalization following maternal separation, decreased aggressive behaviour in the resident–intruder test, and decreased immobility in the forced swim and tail-suspension tests (Rupniak *et al.*, 2001). NK1 receptor knockout mice also exhibit a loss of the rewarding properties of morphine, together with reduced physical response to opiate withdrawal, but their response to cocaine is unchanged (Murtra *et al.*, 2000), suggesting that this may reflect a specific interaction with opioid systems, rather than a general effect on brain reward mechanisms.

Developmental Models

Neonatal Antidepressant Treatment

Neonatal treatment of rat pups with the TCA clomipramine has been reported to cause a spectrum of symptoms reminiscent of depression, including decreases in sexual and aggressive behaviour, a shortening of REM sleep latency, and subsensitivity to ICSS. Treated animals were also hyperactive in some tests (Vogel *et al.*, 1990, 1996). Animals were typically tested when mature, at ages that varied between tests. Most of the behavioural and sleep abnormalities were present on first testing at approximately 3 months; however, the ICSS abnormalities were absent at 4–5 months, but present at 6–8 months. ICSS was not tested in older animals, but some other abnormalities appeared to normalize at around 11 months (Vogel *et al.*, 1990). These effects are probably not specific to clomipramine, since neonatal treatment with DMI, zimeldine or the SSRI Lu 10-134-C has also been reported to increase immobility in the forced swim test in adult rats (Hansen *et al.*, 1997; Hilakivi and Hilakivi, 1987; Velazquez-Moctezuma and Diaz Ruiz, 1992), while neonatal treatment with the SSRI citalopram similarly reduces adult aggressive behaviour (Manhaes de Castro *et al.*, 2001). Zimeldine, like clomipramine, but not DMI, also disrupts adult rat sleep patterns by shortening the duration of REM sleep bouts (Frank and Heller, 1997). In contrast, neonatal treatment with scopolamine, a cholinergic receptor antagonist, suppressed REM sleep, as observed with neonatal clomipramine treatment, but unlike clomipramine, facilitated adult male sexual behaviour. These results suggest that the neonatal clomipramine-induced reduction in male sexual behaviour is not due to early REM sleep deprivation (Velazquez-Moctezuma *et al.*, 1993).

As yet, information concerning the pharmacological responsiveness of this model is minimal: some effects of imipramine and REM sleep deprivation have been reported, but the numbers of subjects tested were too low to allow reliable conclusions to be drawn (Vogel *et al.*, 1990). While this model appears to have good face validity, in terms of the range of symptoms displayed and the insidious onset of anhedonia, the mechanisms by which neonatal antidepressant treatment has adverse effects in mature animals are unknown. In particular, it is unclear what, if any, is the relationship between neonatal antidepressant treatment and the aetiology of depression in humans. The extent to which the symptoms can be reversed by antidepressants is uncertain. Nevertheless, these studies raise the disconcerting possibility that a breast-fed infant could develop a susceptibility to melancholia by ingesting TCAs prescribed to the nursing mother for the relief of post-partum depression.

Prenatal/Neonatal Stress

Prenatally stressed (PS) rats (where the dam is subjected to repeated footshock during the early stages of pregnancy) exhibit elevated activity of the HPA axis and defensive behaviour before weaning, and the heightened defensive behaviour, as well as exaggerated behavioural, physiological and neuroendocrine responses to stressful stimuli, persists into adulthood (Takahashi *et al.*, 1992; Ward *et al.*, 2000; White and Birkle, 2001). Current behavioural data suggest similarities between the behavioural profiles of PS rats and the anxiogenic changes in behaviour induced by yohimbine and idazoxan (White and Birkle, 2001); these data indicate high levels of anxiety in PS rats. However, female, but not male, PS mice exhibit an antidepressant-reversible increase in immobility time in the forced swim test, indicating that PS might induce a gender-dependent increase in the risk of depression-like behaviour (Alonso *et al.*, 1999; 2000).

Neonatal stress in non-human primates has been shown to induce hypersecretion of CRH (Coplan *et al.*, 1996) and abnormal social behaviour in adulthood, indicative of enhanced response to stressors (Clarke and Schneider, 1993). Similarly, neonatal stress in rat pups, achieved by maternal separation, also increases CRH levels in adulthood (Ladd *et al.*, 1996).

Waiting Behaviour

Two procedures have been described in which antidepressants increase the ability of rats to withhold responses. They are not based on developmental—or indeed, any other—manipulations, but they do involve constitutional predispositions, and are reported at this point for convenience.

In one paradigm (differential reinforcement of low rate-72 s; DRL-72) premature responding delays the delivery of reward, and the ability of drugs to improve performance in this model has been claimed to be an efficient antidepressant screening test (Seiden *et al.*, 1985), although this has been disputed (Pollard and Howard, 1986). In the second paradigm, a larger reward may be earned by waiting; again, the improvement of performance in this model appears to be a specific property of a wide range of antidepressants (Bizot *et al.*, 1988a). Drugs which possess 5-HT_{1A} receptor agonist activity are antidepressant-like in both of these waiting paradigms (Archer, 1991; Bizot *et al.*, 1988b; Kostowski *et al.*, 1992; Richards *et al.*, 1994), and in the DRL-72 test, antidepressant effects were blocked by a 5-HT receptor antagonist (Marek *et al.*, 1989). The relevance of these behaviours to depression is unclear. In a different schedule designed to examine accurate estimation of time intervals, acute treatment with antidepressant drugs (imipramine, clomipramine and zimeldine) failed to modify timing accuracy (Bayley *et al.*, 1998) suggesting that improvement in performance on DRL schedules, including SSRIs (Sokolowski and Seiden, 1999), is most likely due to reduced rate of lever-pressing rather than improved timing.

Clinical evidence strongly suggests that similar disorders of 5-HT function cut across diagnostic boundaries, and are expressed as 'pathologically impulsive behaviour' rather than as any particular disorder (Soubrie, 1986; Willner, 1989b). Indeed, mice lacking the 5-HT_{1B} receptor (5-HT_{1B} knockout mice) exhibit more impulsive aggressive behaviour, drink more ethanol and acquire cocaine self-administration faster than wild-type mice (Brunner and Hen, 1997; Scearce-Levie *et al.*, 1999), which reflects (in part at least) reduced 5-HT function (Evenden, 1999b), and may provide an animal model of addiction and motor impulsivity. In vervet monkeys (*Cercopithecus aethiops sabaeus*) there appears to be a clear inverse relationship between serotonin turnover and social impulsivity (Fairbanks *et al.*, 2001). The inability to withhold responses in the two rodent 'waiting' models may constitute instances of impulsive behaviour, and as such, the effect of antidepressants in these paradigms may not relate specifically to depression.

The constitutional predisposition referred to earlier is that antidepressant effects in the DRL vary considerably between rats of different strains, or rats of the same strain obtained from different suppliers (Balcells-Olivero *et al.*, 1998).

Lesion Model

Olfactory Bulbectomy

The other major animal model of depression is based on the destruction of the olfactory bulb in rats, which disrupts the limbic-hypothalamic axis. Bulbectomized (OB) animals display a variety of behavioural changes, including irritability, hyperactivity, and an impairment of passive avoidance learning (Cairncross *et al.*, 1979). Recent observations suggest that OB rats exhibit increased reactivity together with a reduced rate of habituation to novel stimuli (Mar *et al.*, 2000) together with changes in the immune system and NA, DA, 5-HT, GABA, cholinergic and glutaminergic neurotransmitter systems (Kelly *et al.*, 1997). They also show an elevation of circulating corticosteroid levels (as do stressed animals), which appears to be an increased corticosteroid response to stress rather than an increase in basal levels (Broekkamp *et al.*, 1986). These changes are reversed by antidepressants, including compounds with 5-HT_{1A} receptor agonist activity (Borsini *et al.*, 1997; McGrath and Norman, 1999), SNRIs (McGrath and Norman, 1998) and selective NA reuptake inhibitors (Harkin *et al.*, 1999b) in addition to the TCAs. The most specific antidepressant effect is the reversal of the passive avoidance learning deficit (Cairncross *et al.*, 1979; Van Riezen and Leonard, 1990), although attenuation of hyperactivity in the open field is nowadays the most commonly used behavioural predictor of antidepressant activity (Kelly *et al.*, 1997). However, while all TCA and atypical antidepressants appear to be effective in this test, MAOIs are not (Jesberger and Richardson, 1986). While repeated administration of TCAs is necessary to normalize behaviour in this model, a limited number of studies suggest that some SSRIs act after acute treatment (Joly and Sanger, 1986; Lloyd *et al.*, 1982). Recent studies suggest that the OB rat model of depression is insensitive to the potential rapid-onset antidepressant action induced by concomitant treatment with 5-HT_{1A} receptor antagonists (Cryan *et al.*, 1998, 1999). The implication that the model involves primarily serotonergic mechanisms is supported by the observation that the effects of subchronic treatment with imipramine and mianserin were reversed by acute administration of the 5-HT_2 receptor antagonist metergoline (Broekkamp *et al.*, 1980).

Although pharmacologically specific for antidepressants, the face validity of the olfactory bulbectomy model appears slight. Unlike the stress models, the bulbectomized rat resembles an agitated hyposerotonergic, rather than a retarded, depression (Lumia *et al.*, 1992), but beyond hyperactivity, it is difficult to discern any further points of behavioural resemblance. Indeed, increased irritability and aggression together with exaggerated reactivity to auditory and tactile stimulation may reflect additional septal damage. Nevertheless, bulbectomized rats do resemble depressed humans on a surprisingly wide range of peripheral neurochemical and immunological markers, such as abnormalities of platelet 5HT transport and neutrophil phagocytosis (Leonard, 1991).

PHARMACOLOGICAL SCREENING TESTS

Finally, we mention briefly some older tests, now little used, based on interactions between antidepressants and a range of other pharmacological agents. Generally speaking, the predictive validity of these tests is poor, and their face and construct validity as simulations of depression is minimal or zero.

Reserpine and Tetrabenazine Reversal

The rationale behind the reserpine model of depression is from clinical observations of patients treated with reserpine for hypertension who subsequently developed signs of depressive illness. Later observations indicated that the symptoms induced by reserpine in laboratory animals (including ptosis, hypothermia and sedation) were due to depletion of central monoamines. It is generally accepted that an ability to reverse the reserpine syndrome is due to reduced inactivation of central monoamines, either by inhibiting monoamine reuptake or by inhibiting the enzyme monoamine oxidase. Indeed, the classical TCAs in use today were developed on the basis of their positive effects in this model. False negatives include iprindole, mianserin, rolipram and SSRIs, while false positives include stimulants, anticholinergics and analgesics. This model possesses little or no face or construct validity to depression. Even so, it is still used in drug development although its use is largely limited to confirmation of pharmacological activity, in relation to monoamine reuptake inhibition (Rogoz *et al.*, 1999a, b; Wong *et al.*, 2000) and MAOI activity (e.g. Caille *et al.*, 1996; Iwata *et al.*, 1997; Kato *et al.*, 1998).

Tetrabenazine is chemically related to reserpine and likewise depletes central, although not peripheral, stores of NA and 5-HT. It therefore similarly induces sedation and hypothermia. Consequently the validity profile of this model is no better than that of reserpine. It is still used in drug development but, again, simply to confirm pharmacological activity (e.g. Darias *et al.*, 1999; Ferris *et al.*, 1995).

5-HTP Potentiation

5-Hydroxytryptophan (5-HTP) is the immediate precursor of 5-HT, and the consequences of 5-HTP loading in animals are behaviours associated with 5-HT excess (hypothermia, sedation, head-twitch response), which may be potentiated by drugs which attenuate 5-HT inactivation. As with other pharmacological screening tests this model has no validity as a model of depression, and is largely employed in mechanistic studies to confirm pharmacological activity (Ferris *et al.*, 1995; Porsolt, *et al.*, 2000).

Yohimbine Potentiation

Yohimbine preferentially inhibits presynaptic α_2-adrenoceptors, so increasing the release of NA and causing behavioural excitation and increased heart rate and blood pressure. A combination of increased NA release together with reduced NA inactivation following antidepressant treatment results in a lethal cocktail and it is this phenomena that is employed in this test. Almost all antidepressants potentiate the lethal effects of yohimbine, but how such effects are related to depressive illness is unclear, and the test has no validity as a model. As with other pharmacological screening models, the use of yohimbine potentiation is primarily limited to mechanistic studies (e.g. Eguchi *et al.*, 1997).

Apomorphine and Clonidine Antagonism

On acute treatment, some antidepressants, including TCAs, NA reuptake inhibitors, the SNRI venlafaxine (Redrobe *et al.*, 1998) and β-adrenoceptor agonist drugs, antagonize the hypothermia induced by a single high dose of apomorphine (Puech *et al.*, 1981). On chronic treatment, TCAs, MAOIs and some atypical drugs antagonize the hypolocomotion and/or hypothermia induced by a single dose of clonidine (e.g. Kostowski and Malatynska, 1983; Kostowski and Obersztyn, 1988; von Voigtlander *et al.*, 1978). False positives in both cases include the psychostimulants amphetamine, *p*-chloro-methyl-amphetamine (PCA) and L-dihydroxyphenylalanine (L-DOPA), while MAOIs, SSRIs and atypical drugs are generally inactive (Maj *et al.*, 1986; Pawlowski and Mazela, 1986).

Potentiation of Apomorphine- and Clonidine-Induced Aggression

Acute treatment of rats with apomorphine or of mice with clonidine increases aggressive behaviour. Prior chronic, but not acute, treatment with antidepressants usually potentiates apomorphine- or clonidine-induced aggression (Maj, 1984; Maj *et al.*, 1979, 1980, 1981, 1982). False negatives in these tests include the SSRIs (e.g. Matto *et al.*, 1998a), while false positives include examples of 5-HT antagonists and neuroleptics (Maj, 1984; Maj *et al.*, 1982). The aggressive behaviour induced by daily administration of apomorphine was attenuated by acute treatment with trazodone at non-sedative doses, which had little or no effects on forced swim behaviour or on levels of anxiety, while chronic treatment with trazodone slowed the development of apomorphine-induced aggression (Rudissaar *et al.*, 2001). Other studies (e.g. Matto *et al.*, 1998b) suggest that 5-HT reuptake inhibition has no major effect on apomorphine-induced aggressive behaviour. Available data for clonidine-induced aggression are rather equivocal (e.g. Rogoz *et al.*, 1999a, b) although this behaviour was potentiated by venlafaxine (Maj and Rogoz, 1999). The predictive validity of these tests is limited, and their face and construct validity, non-existent.

EVALUATION

Table XVIII-1.1 presents a summary of the models surveyed, showing our evaluation of each model against the accepted validation criteria. (The pharmacological screening tests are excluded, as they have little or no validity on any of the criteria.) The first three columns score each model on a scale of 0 to 3, using the following scoring system:

0	no positive evidence, or no excess of positive evidence over negative
+	small amount of positive evidence or small excess of positive evidence over negative
++	moderate amount of positive evidence or large excess of positive evidence over negative
+++	large amount of positive evidence, with little or no negative evidence

(A score of 3 does not, however, imply, that there is no room for improvement.) The fourth column presents an overall validity estimate arrived at by summing across columns 1–3.

It should be borne in mind that these judgements to some extent reflect the authors' subjective impressions, and they should not be taken too seriously.

With this caveat, we draw the following conclusions:

1. Easily ahead of the pack, the CMS model scores a maximum 9, against a highest score of 5 for any of the other models. We reiterate, however, that this strength is to some extent offset by the limited reliability of the procedure.

Table XVIII-1.1 Evaluation of animal models of depression

Animal model	Validity PV	FV	CV	Sum	Evaluation Depression	Melancholia	Sensitivity to chronic drug treatment
Stress models							
Acute stress models							
Learned helplessness	++	++	+	5	++	++	+
Forced swim	++	0	0	2	+	0	0
Tail suspension	++	0	0	2	+	0	0
Restraint stress	+	+	0	2	+	0	+
Chronic stress models							
Chronic severe stress	+	++	+	4	++	+	++
Chronic mild stress	+++	+++	+++	9	+++	+++	+++
Induction and maintenance	+	++	++	5	++	++	0
Psychostimulant withdrawal	+	+	+	3	+	+	+
Social dominance models							
Social defeat	+	+	+	3	+	+	+
Social hierarchy	+	++	++	5	++	0	+++
Resident–intruder	+++	+	+	5	++	0	+++
Social isolation models							
Neonatal isolation	+	++	+	4	++	0	+
Adult isolation	+	+	+	3	+	0	+
Diathesis models							
Genetic models							
Muscarinic hypersensitivity (FSL)	+	++	0	3	+	+	0
Roman Low-Avoidance	0	0	0	0	0	0	0
Fawn-Hooded	+	+	0	2	+	0	+
Genomic models							
HPA transgenic	+	0	+	2	+	0	+
5-HT transporter knockout	0	0	0	0	0	0	0
CRH receptor subtypes knockouts	0	0	0	0	0	0	0
Tachykinin receptor knockout	0	0	0	0	0	0	0
Developmental models							
Neonatal antidepressant treatment	0	++	+	3	+	0	0
Prenatal/neonatal stress	0	+	0	1	0	0	0
Waiting behaviour	++	0	0	2	+	0	0
Lesion model							
Olfactory bulbectomy	++	+	+	4	++	0	++

PV, predictive validity; FV, face validity; CV, construct validity; sum = PV + FV + CV.
See text for an explanation of the scoring system.

2. High overall scores (4–5) are achieved by models from all of the groups classified as 'stress' models, but by only one of the 'diathesis' models, olfactory bulbectomy.
3. This means that the genetic, genomic and developmental models all require further development. In the case of genomic models in particular, it would not be surprising to see this achieved rapidly.
4. Good predictive validity can be achieved in the absence of face and construct validity. Thus, scores of 2/3 for predictive validity are awarded to the forced swim, tail-suspension and waiting behaviour models, which score 0 elsewhere. (Note, however, that the high score for the forced swim test refers to the modification of this procedure introduced by Lucki and colleagues [e.g. Cryan and Lucki, 2000; Detke *et al.*, 1995], which responds to SSRIs. We would only award 1/3 to the traditional version of this test.)

The next two columns present estimates of the overall validity of each model, on a scale of 0–3, in relation to major depressive disorder, and to melancholia. We must emphasize that a score of +++ means only that a model performs better than those scored ++, which in turn perform better than those scored +; there is no implication that a model receiving a score of 3 cannot be improved. We also note that in some cases (e.g. social defeat) the low score reflects a paucity of positive evidence, rather than the presence of negative evidence. In making the overall estimates, we have weighted face and construct validity a little more highly than predictive validity. In estimating validity with respect to melancholia we have weighted the available information in relation to the specific feature of melancholia. Again, the CMS model stands out as the only model receiving a +++ rating in both categories. Seven further models perform relatively well as simulations of depression (score ++): learned helplessness, chronic severe stress (note, however, that ethical considerations would usually rule this model out of use), the induction and maintenance model, social hierarchy, resident–intruder test, neonatal isolation, and olfactory bulbectomy. Two of these models, learned helplessness and induction and maintenance, also perform well as models of melancholia. It should also be noted that the simple metric used to compute the overall ratings does not take account of discrepancies between the different components of the assessment. In particular, the ++ rating for the resident–intruder model derives largely from the excellent predictive validity of this model, face and construct validity being very limited.

The final column evaluates each model against the criterion that is central to current efforts in drug development, sensitivity to chronic drug treatment, by which we mean that the model responds to chronic, but not acute, treatment with conventional antidepressants. The importance of this feature is that only when a model displays a gradual onset of action is it possible to detect a more rapid onset. The estimates in the table are conservative, in the sense that some of the models (e.g. induction and maintenance) have the capability, potentially, to demonstrate a gradual onset of action, since they have an extended time course, but this has not yet been investigated. The three models for which the clearest evidence for gradual onset of action has been obtained are CMS, social hierarchy and the resident–intruder test.

SIMULATIONS OF DEPRESSIVE ILLNESS VERSUS DRUG SCREENING TESTS

While the focus of this chapter has been on the development of simulations of depression, to be used as research tools, many of the same behavioural models are also used for drug development purposes. The universal use of cheap, quick drug screening tests by the pharmaceutical industry since the beginning of the 1970s resulted in a large array of antidepressant drugs being discovered, all of which have pharmacological and therapeutic profiles qualitatively similar to that of the archetypal TCA, imipramine, or MAOI, isoniazid. Unfortunately, the success of such acute treatment screening tests (e.g. the pharmacological procedures reviewed, or the forced swim test) not only restricted the development of animal models with improved face and construct validity, but has also largely been responsible for delaying the development of animal models in which antidepressants are active only following their chronic administration. The majority of models used routinely as antidepressant screening tests, and which respond acutely to drug treatment, are of no value in the drive to identify rapid-onset antidepressant drugs and are of limited or minimal validity as simulations of depression (cf. Willner, 1984). Generally, the use of drug screening models has simply resulted in the identification of further 'me-too' compounds (compounds of novel chemical structure whose acute pharmacological profile is similar to that of compounds already available to the clinician), provides no information on speed of onset of desirable drug activity, has been of very limited use in furthering our knowledge of the mechanisms associated with the psychopathology of depressive illness or adaptive changes associated with the recovery process from depression, and has largely failed to identify novel mechanisms and targets for future drug discovery.

In order to ascertain whether views within the pharmaceutical industry are changing, one of us (P.W.) conducted a small survey, which was carried out in the summer of 1999. A total of 28 questionnaires were sent out to companies with a known interest in CNS pharmacology, asking about the use of 12 named behavioural tests in antidepressant development, and the respondent's level of confidence in the outcome of each test. Assurances were given about anonymity, confidentiality and the absence of any commercial interest on the part of the investigator. Fourteen replies (50%) were received, of which twelve provided usable data. Six tests were reported to be in routine use by six or more (i.e. >50%) of the respondents: forced swim test in rats and mice, tail-suspension test, CMS; DRL-72s, and social separation. The first five of these tests are evaluated here (Table XVIII-1.1) as providing reasonably good predictive information, while varying considerably in their validity as simulations of depression. (The sixth test, social separation, performs less well, but it was realized subsequently that different companies were using very different tests under this general heading, none of which alone met the 50% criterion.)

Confidence in a positive outcome that a novel agent detected by the model would be an effective antidepressant in clinical trials was rated on a scale of 0 (not at all confident) to 6 (totally confident). All of the models achieved a mean rating of 3, with the exception of CMS, which was rated 5. It would appear that drug industry scientists are well aware of the literature summarized in Table XVIII-1.1.

It has traditionally been a major consideration in the design of antidepressant screening tests that they respond to acute or subacute drug administration. As a direct consequence, they are incapable, by virtue of their design, of responding to the major current challenge of discovering new antidepressants that have a shorter onset of action. By contrast, it is implicit in their protracted time course that chronic realistic animal models do have the capacity to detect a rapidly acting novel antidepressant. In fact, most pharmaceutical companies have now abandoned the high-volume, random screening approach in favour of the development of a small number of compounds specifically designed to meet predetermined pharmacological criteria. In such a programme, the place of behavioural screening methods shifts from the discovery phase to the development phase, and the logistical disadvantages of using complex, chronic models are small, relative to the costs of testing an ineffective drug in the clinic.

WHERE NEXT?

We conclude with some comments on likely future developments in this area. The greatest immediate contribution of animal models of depression is likely to be in relation to the elucidation of the mechanisms of action of antidepressant drugs. Thirty years of clinical experience has given rise to two widely accepted axioms: that only rarely do antidepressants cause discernible clinical improvement within the first two weeks of treatment, and that they are devoid of mood-elevating effects in normal human subjects. The clinical requirement for chronic treatment regimes has led to a considerable literature describing the effects of chronic antidepressant administration in normal animals, and numerous changes in pre- and/or postsynaptic receptor function have been reported, in a variety of systems. These descriptive studies are an essential first step towards establishing mechanisms of antidepressant action. However, the inability to determine which of the many effects of antidepressants are responsible for their therapeutic actions constitutes a fundamental limitation of this approach, which has not been widely recognized. The development of chronic animal models, in which an abnormal state is induced and maintained for a prolonged period during which 'therapy' can be administered, provides a powerful methodology for investigating these problems.

Although they have as yet made little impact, it is to be expected that genomic models will play a significant role in these developments. However, it will be important not to lose sight of the fact that genetic and genomic models are mostly of relevance to depressive diatheses. Studies in which valid and realistic models of depressive diatheses are combined with valid and realistic stress models are awaited with interest.

REFERENCES

Abramson, L.Y. and Seligman, M.E.P., 1978. Modeling psychopathology in the laboratory: history and rationale. In: Maser, J.D. and Seligman, M.E.P. (eds), *Psychopathology: Experimental Models*, pp. 1–26. W.H. Freeman, San Francisco, CA.

Abramson, L.Y., Seligman, M.E.P. and Teasdale, J.D., 1978. Learned helplessness in humans: critique and reformulation. *J. Abnorm. Psychol.*, **87**, 49–74.

Abramson, L.Y., Metalsky, G. and Alloy, L.B., 1989. Hopelessness depression: a theory-based subtype of depression. *Psychol. Rev.*, **96**, 358–72.

Akiskal, H.S., 1985. Interaction of biologic and psychologic factors in the origin of depressive disorders. *Acta Psychiatr. Scand.*, **71**, 131–9.

Akiskal, H.S., 1986. A developmental perspective on recurrent mood disorders: a review of studies in man. *Psychopharmacol. Bull.*, **22**, 579–86.

Albonetti, M.E. and Farabollini, F., 1994. Social stress by repeated defeat: effects on social behaviour and emotionality. *Behav. Brain Res.*, **62**, 187–93.

Alonso, S.J., Castellano, M.A., Quintero, M. and Navarro, E., 1999. Action of antidepressant drugs on maternal stress-induced hypoactivity in female rats. *Meth. Find. Exp. Clin. Pharmacol.*, **21**, 291–5.

Alonso, S.J., Damas, C. and Navarro, E., 2000. Behavioral despair in mice after prenatal stress. *J. Physiol. Biochem.*, **56**, 77–82.

Aneshensel, C.S. and Stone, J.D., 1982. Stress and depression: a test of the buffering model of social support. *Arch. Gen. Psychiatr.*, **39**, 1392–6.

Anisman, H.A. and Zacharko, R.M., 1982. Depression: the predisposing influence of stress. *Behav. Brain Sci.*, **5**, 89–137.

Anisman, H., Irwin, J. and Sklar, L.S., 1979. Deficits of escape performance following catecholamine depletion: implications for behavioural deficits induced by uncontrollable stress. *Psychopharmacology*, **64**, 163–70.

Antelman, S.M., Eichler, A.J., Black, C.A. and Kocan, D., 1980. Interchangeability of stress and amphetamine sensitization. *Science*, **207**, 329–31.

Archer, T., 1991. Animal models and drug screens for depression: pragmatism and the validity requirement. In: Olivier, B., Mos, J. and Slangen, J. (eds), *Animal Models in Psychopharmacology*, pp. 243–50. Birkhauser, Basel.

Atrens, D.M., 1984. Self-stimulation and psychotropic drugs: a methodological and conceptual critique. In: Bond, N.S. (ed.), *Animal Models in Psychopathology*, pp. 227–56. Academic Press, Sydney.

Aulakh, C.S., Hill, J.L. and Murphy, D.L., 1993. Attenuation of hypercortisolemia in fawn-hooded rats by antidepressant drugs. *Eur. J. Pharmacol.*, **240**, 85–8.

Aulakh, C.S., Tolliver, T., Wozniak, K.M., Hill, J.L. and Murphy, D.L., 1994. Functional and biochemical evidence for altered serotonergic function in the fawn-hooded rat strain. *Pharmacol. Biochem. Behav.*, **49**, 615–20.

Aulakh, C.S., Mazzola-Pomietto, P. and Murphy, D.L., 1996. Long-term antidepressant treatment restores clonidine's effect on growth hormone secretion in a genetic animal model of depression. *Pharmacol. Biochem. Behav.*, **55**, 265–8.

Balcells-Olivero, M., Cousins, M.S. and Seiden, L.S., 1998. Holtzman and Harlan Sprague–Dawley rats: differences in DRL 72-sec performance and 8-hydroxy-di-propylamino tetralin-induced hypothermia. *J. Pharmacol. Exp. Ther.*, **286**, 742–52.

Bale, T.L., Contarino, A., Smith, G.W., Chan, R., Gold, L.H., Sawchenko, P.E., Koob, G.F., Vale, W.W. and Lee, K.F., 2000. Mice deficient for corticotropin-releasing hormone receptor-2 display anxiety-like behaviour and are hypersensitive to stress. *Nat. Genet.*, **24**, 410–4.

Barden, N., 1996. Modulation of glucocorticoid receptor gene expression by antidepressant drugs. *Pharmacopsychiatry*, **29**, 12–22.

Barden, N., 1999. Regulation of corticosteroid receptor gene expression in depression and antidepressant action. *J. Psychiat. Neurosci.*, **24**, 25–39.

Barrett, R.J. and White, D.K., 1980. Reward system depression following chronic amphetamine: antagonism by haloperidol. *Pharmacol. Biochem. Behav.*, **13**, 555–9.

Bayley, P.J., Bentley, G.D. and Dawson, G.R., 1998. The effects of selected antidepressant drugs on timing behaviour in rats. *PsychoPharmacology (Berl)*, **136**, 114–22.

Beaulieu, S., Rousse, I., Gratton, A., Barden, N. and Rochford, J., 1993. Behavioural characterization of a transgenic mouse model of impaired type II glucocorticoid receptor function. *Soc. Neurosci. Abstr.*, **19**, 489.8.

Beck, A.T., 1967. *Depression: Clinical, Experimental and Theoretical Aspects*. Harper & Row, New York.

Berger, B.D. and Schuster, R., 1982. An animal model of social interaction: implications for the analysis of drug action. In: Spiegelstein, M.Y. and Levy, A. (eds), *Behavioral Models and the Analysis of Drug Action*, pp. 415–28. Elsevier, Amsterdam.

Berton, O., Durand, M., Aguerre, S., Mormede, P. and Chaouloff, F., 1999. Behavioral, neuroendocrine and serotonergic consequences of single social defeat and repeated fluoxetine pretreatment in the Lewis rat strain. *Neuroscience*, **92**, 327–41.

Besson, A., Privat, A.M., Eschalier, A. and Fialip, J., 1996. Effects of morphine, naloxone and their interaction in the learned-helplessness paradigm in rats. *Psychopharmacology (Berl)*, **123**, 71–8.

Besson, A., Privat, A.M., Eschalier, A. and Fialip, J., 1998. Reversal of learned helplessness by morphine in rats: involvement of a dopamine mediation. *Pharmacol. Biochem. Behav.*, **60**, 519–25.

Besson, A., Privat, A.M., Eschalier, A. and Fialip, J., 1999. Dopaminergic and opioidergic mediations of tricyclic antidepressants in the learned helplessness paradigm. *Pharmacol. Biochem. Behav.*, **64**, 541–8.

Bizot, J.C., Thiebot, M.H., Le Bihan, C., Soubrie, P. and Simon, P., 1988a. Effects of imipramine-like drugs and serotonin uptake blockers on delay of reward in rats: possible implication in the behavioral mechanism of action of antidepressants. *J. Pharmacol. Exp. Ther.*, **286**, 1144–51.

Bizot, J.C., Thiebot, M.H. and Puech, A.J., 1988b. Effects of 5-HT-related drugs on waiting capacities in rats. *Psychopharmacology*, **96**, S5.

Blanc, G., Herve, D., Simon, H., Lisoprawski, A., Glowinski, J. and Tassin, J.P., 1980. Response to stress of mesocortical frontal dopaminergic neurons in rats after long-term isolation. *Nature*, **284**, 265–76.

Bodnoff, S.R., Suranyi-Codotte, B., Aitken, D.H., Quirion, R. and Meaney, M.Y., 1988. The effects of chronic antidepressant treatment in an animal model of anxiety. *Psychopharmacology*, **95**, 298–302.

Borsini, F., 1995. Role of the serotonergic system in the forced swimming test. *Neurosci. Biobehav. Rev.*, **19**, 377–95.

Borsini, F. and Meli, A., 1988. Is the forced swimming test a suitable model for revealing antidepressant activity? *Psychopharmacology*, **94**, 147–60.

Borsini, F., Cesana, R., Kelly, J., Leonard, B.E., McNamara, M., Richards, J. and Seiden, L., 1997. BIMT 17: a putative antidepressant with a fast onset of action? *Psychopharmacology (Berl)*, **134**, 378–86.

Broekkamp, C.L., Garrigou, D. and Lloyd, K.G., 1980. Serotonin-mimetic and antidepressant drugs on passive avoidance learning by olfactory bulbectomized rats. *Pharmacol. Biochem. Behav.*, **13**, 643–6.

Broekkamp, C.L., O'Connor, W.T., Tonnaer, J.A.D.M., Rijk, H.W. and Van Delft, A.M.L., 1986. Corticosterone, choline acetyltransferase and noradrenaline levels in olfactory bulbectomized rats in relation to changes in passive avoidance acquisition and open field activity. *Physiol. Behav.*, **37**, 429–34.

Brown, G.W., 1989. A psychosocial view of depression. In: Bennett, D.H. and Freeman, H. (eds), *Community Psychiatry*, pp. 71–114. Churchill-Livingstone, London.

Brown, G.W. and Harris, T., 1978. *Social Origins of Depression*. Tavistock, London.

Brown, G.W. and Harris, T. (eds), 1988. *Life Events and Illness*. Guilford Press, New York.

Brown, G.W., Sklair, F., Harris, T.O. and Birley, J.L.T., 1973. Life events and psychiatric disorders. I. Some methodological issues. *Psychol. Med.*, **3**, 74–87.

Brown, L., Rosellini, R.A., Samuels, O.B. and Riley, E.P., 1982. Evidence for a serotonergic mechanism of the learned helplessness phenomenon. *Pharmacol. Biochem. Behav.*, **17**, 877–83.

Brunner, D. and Hen, R., 1997. Insights into the neurobiology of impulsive behavior from serotonin receptor knockout mice. *Ann. N. Y. Acad. Sci.*, **836**, 81–105.

Butterweck, V., Wall, A., Lieflander-Wulf, U., Winterhoff, H. and Nahrstedt, A., 1997. Effects of the total extract and fractions of *Hypericum perforatum* in animal assays for antidepressant activity. *Pharmacopsychiatry*, **30**(suppl 2), 117–24.

Caille, D., Bergis, O.E., Frankhauser, C., Gardes, A., Adam, R., Charieras, T., Grosset, A., Rovei, V. and Jarreau, F.X., 1996. Befloxatone, a new reversible and selective monoamine oxidase-A inhibitor. II Pharmacological profile. *J. Pharmacol. Exp. Ther.*, **277**, 265–77.

Cairncross, K.D., Cox, B., Forster, C. and Wren, A.F., 1979. Olfactory projection systems, drugs and behaviour: a review. *Psychoneuroendocrinology*, **4**, 253–72.

Carroll, B.J., 1982. The dexamethasone suppression test for melancholia. *Br. J. Psychiat.*, **140**, 292–304.

Cassens, G.P., Actor, C., Kling, M. and Schildkraut, J.J., 1981. Amphetamine withdrawal effects threshold of intracranial self-stimulation. *Psychopharmacology*, **73**, 318–22.

Cavoy, A., Ennaceur, A. and Delacour, J., 1988. Effects of piracetam on learned helplessness in rats. *Physiol. Behav.*, **42**, 545–9.

Cheeta, S., Broekkamp, C. and Willner, P., 1994. Stereospecific reversal of stress-induced anhedonia by mianserin and its (+)-enantiomer. *Psychopharmacology*, **116**, 523–8.

Christensen, A.V. and Geoffroy, M., 1991. The effect of different serotonergic drugs in the learned helplessness model of depression. In: Olivier, B., Mos, J. and Slangen, J. (eds), *Animal Models in Psychopharmacology*, pp. 205–9. Birkhauser, Basel.

Clarke, A.S. and Schneider, M.L., 1993. Prenatal stress has long-term effects on behavioral responses to stress in juvenile rhesus monkeys. *Dev. Psychobiol.*, **26**, 293–304.

Cobain, M.R., Forster, E.A., Mitchell, P.J. and Fletcher, A., 1994a. Effect of acute treatment with selective 5-HT_{1A} ligands on the agonistic behaviour of rats. *J. Psychopharmacol.*, Abstract Book BAP/ISBP meeting, Abstract 24.

Cobain, M.R., Forster, E.A., Mitchell, P.J. and Fletcher, A., 1994b. The antidepressant effect of 5-HT_{1A} ligands is mediated by agonist activity at 5-HT_{1A} receptors. *J. Psychopharmacol.*, Abstract Book BAP/ISBP meeting, Abstract 25.

Coccaro, E.F. and Kavoussi, R.J., 1997. Fluoxetine and impulsive aggressive behaviour in personality-disordered subjects. *Arch. Gen. Psychiat.*, **54**, 1081–8.

Connor, T.J., Kelliher, P., Harkin, A., Kelly, J.P. and Leonard, B.E., 1999. Reboxetine attenuates forced swim test-induced behavioural and neurochemical alterations in the rat. *Eur. J. Pharmacol.*, **379**, 125–33.

Connor, T.J., Kelliher, P., Shen, Y., Harkin, A., Kelly, J.P. and Leonard, B.E., 2000. Effect of subchronic antidepressant treatments on behavioral, neurochemical, and endocrine changes in the forced-swim test. *Pharmacol. Biochem. Behav.*, **65**, 591–7.

Contarino, A., Dellu, F., Koob, G.F., Smith, G.W., Lee, K.F., Vale, W. and Gold, L.H., 1999. Reduced anxiety-like and cognitive performance in mice lacking the corticotropin-releasing factor receptor 1. *Brain Res.*, **835**, 1–9.

Coplan, J.D., Andrews, M.W., Rosenblum, L.A., Owens, M.J., Friedman, S., Gorman, J.M. and Nemeroff, C.B., 1996. Persistent elevations of cerebrospinal fluid concentrations of corticotropin-releasing factor in adult nonhuman primates exposed to early-life stressors — implications for the pathophysiology of mood and anxiety disorders. *Proc. Natl. Acad. Sci. USA*, **93**, 1619–23.

Coventry, T.L., D'Aquila, P.S., Brain, P. and Willner, P., 1997. Social influences on morphine conditioned place preference. *Behav. Pharmacol.*, **8**, 575–84.

Cryan, J.F. and Lucki, I., 2000. Antidepressant-like behavioral effects mediated by 5-hydroxytryptamine(2C) receptors. *J. Pharmacol. Exp. Ther.*, **295**, 1120–6.

Cryan, J.F., McGrath, C., Leonard, B.E. and Norman, T.R., 1998. Combining pindolol and paroxetine in an animal model of chronic antidepressant action — can early onset of action be detected? *Eur. J. Pharmacol.*, **352**, 23–8.

Cryan, J.F., McGrath, C., Leonard, B.E. and Norman, T.R., 1999. Onset of the effects of the 5-HT_{1A} antagonist, WAY-100635, alone, and in combination with paroxetine, on olfactory bulbectomy and 8-OH-DPAT-induced changes in the rat. *Pharmacol. Biochem. Behav.*, **63**, 333–8.

Cuomo, V., Cagiano, R., Brunello, N., Fumagalli, R. and Racagni, G., 1983. Behavioural changes after acute and chronic administration of typical and atypical antidepressants in rat: Interactions with reserpine. *Neurosci. Lett.*, **40**, 315–9.

Danysz, W., Archer, T. and Fowler, C.J., 1991. Screening for new antidepressant compounds. In: Willner, P. (ed.), *Behavioural Models in Psychopharmacology: Theoretical, Industrial and Clinical Perspectives*, pp. 126–56. Cambridge University Press, Cambridge.

D'Aquila, P., Monleon, S., Borsini, F., Brain, P. and Willner, P., 1997. Anti-anhedonic actions of the novel serotonergic agent flibanserin, a potential rapidly-acting antidepressant. *Eur. J. Pharmacol.*, **340**, 121–32.

Darias, V., Abdala, S., Martin-Herrera, D. and Vega, S., 1999. Study of the antidepressant activity of 4-phenyl-2-thioxo-benzo[4,5]thieno[2,3-d]pyrimidine derivatives. *Arzneimittelforschung*, **49**, 986–91.

David, D.J., Nic Dhonnchadha, B.A., Jolliet, P., Hascoet, M. and Bourin, M., 2001. Are there gender differences in the temperature profile of mice after acute antidepressant administration and exposure to two animal models of depression? *Behav. Brain Res.*, **119**, 203–11.

De Montis, M.G., Gambarana, C. and Meloni, D., 1993. Alpha-methyl-para-tyrosine antagonizes the effect of chronic imipramine on learned helplessness in rats. *Eur. J. Pharmacol.*, **249**, 179–83.

De Montis, M.G., Gambarana, C., Ghiglieri, O. and Tagliamonte, A., 1995. Reversal of stable behavioural modifications through NMDA receptor inhibition in rats. *Behav. Pharmacol.*, **6**, 562–7.

Desan, P.H., Silbert, L.H. and Maier, S.F., 1988. Long-term effects of inescapable stress on daily running activity and antagonism by desipramine. *Pharmacol. Biochem. Behav.*, **30**, 21–9.

Detke, M.J., Rickels, M. and Lucki, I., 1995. Active behaviors in the rat forced swimming test differentially produced by serotonergic and noradrenergic antidepressants. *Psychopharmacology*, **121**, 66–72.

Di Chiara, G., Loddo, P. and Tanda, G., 1999. Reciprocal changes in prefrontal and limbic dopamine responsiveness to aversive and rewarding stimuli after chronic mild stress: implications for the psychobiology of depression. *Biol. Psychiat.*, **46**, 1624–33.

Dixon, A.K., Fisch, H.U., Huber, C. and Walser, A., 1989. Ethological studies in animals and man: their use in psychiatry. *Pharmacopsychiatry*, **22**(suppl 1), 44–50.

Drevets, W.C. and Raichle, M.E., 1998. Reciprocal suppression of regional cerebral blood flow during emotional versus higher cognitive processes: implications for interactions between emotion and cognition. *Cognition and Emotion*, **12**, 353–85.

Dziedzicka-Wasylewska, M., Willner, P. and Papp, M., 1997. Changes in dopamine receptor mRNA expression following chronic mild stress and chronic antidepressant treatment. *Behav. Pharmacol.*, **8**, 607–18.

Edwards, E., Johnson, J., Anderson, D., Turano, P. and Henn, F.A., 1986. Neurochemical and behavioral consequences of mild uncontrollable shock: effects of PCPA. *Pharmacol. Biochem. Behav.*, **25**, 415–21.

Eguchi, J., Inomata, Y., Yuasa, T., Egawa, M. and Saito, K., 1997. Pharmacological profile of the novel antidepressant 4-(2-fluorophenyl)-6-methyl-2-(1-piperazinyl)thieno-[2,3-d]pyrimidine monohydrate hydrochloride. *Arzneimittelforschung*, **47**, 1337–47.

Emrich, H.M., Vogt, P. and Herz, A., 1983. Possible antidepressant effects of opioids: action of buprenorphine. *Ann. N. Y. Acad. Sci.*, **398**, 108–12.

Escorihuela, R.M., Fernandez-Teruel, A., Gil, L., Aguilar, R., Tobena, A. and Driscoll, P., 1999. Inbred Roman high- and low-avoidance rats: differences in anxiety, novelty-seeking, and shuttlebox behaviors. *Physiol. Behav.*, **67**, 19–26.

Evenden, J., 1999a. Impulsivity: a discussion of clinical and experimental findings. *J. Psychopharmacol*, **13**, 180–92.

Evenden, J., 1999b. Varieties of impulsivity. *Psychopharmacology (Berl)*, **146**, 348–61.

Everitt, B.J. and Keverne, E.B., 1979. Models of depression based on behavioural observations of experimental animals. In: Paykel, E.S. and Coppen, A. (eds), *Psychopharmacology of Affective Disorders*, pp. 41–59. Oxford University Press, Oxford.

Fabre, V., Beaufour, C., Evrard, A., Rioux, A., Hanoun, N., Lesch, K.P., Murphy, D.L., Lanfumey, L., Hamon, M. and Martres, M.P., 2000. Altered expression and functions of serotonin 5-HT_{1A} and 5-HT_{1B} receptors in knock-out mice lacking the 5-HT transporter. *Eur. J. Neurosci.*, **12**, 2299–310.

Fairbanks, L.A., Melega, W.P., Jorgensen, M.J., Kaplan, J.R. and McGuire, M.T., 2001. Social impulsivity inversely associated with CSF 5-HIAA and fluoxetine exposure in vervet monkeys. *Neuropsychopharmacology*, **24**, 370–8.

Farisse, J., Boulenguez, P., Semont, A., Hery, F., Barden, N., Faudon, M. and Hery, M., 1999. Regional serotonin metabolism under basal and restraint stress conditions in the brain of transgenic mice with impaired glucocorticoid receptor function. *Neuroendocrinology*, **70**, 413–21.

Fava, M. and Rosenbaum, J.F., 1993. Psychopharmacology of pathologic aggression. *Harvard Rev Psychiat*, **1**, 244–6.

Ferrari, F., Cassinadri, M., Tartoni, P.L. and Tampieri, A., 1991. Effects of B-HT 920 in the tail-suspension test. *Pharmacol. Res.*, **24**, 75–81.

Ferris, R.M., Brieaddy, L., Mehta, N., Hollingsworth, E., Rigdon, G., Wang, C., Soroko, F., Wastila, W. and Cooper, B., 1995. Pharmacological properties of 403U76, a new chemical class of 5-hydroxytryptamine- and noradrenaline-reuptake inhibitor. *J. Pharm. Pharmacol.*, **47**, 775–81.

Fibiger, H.C., 1991. The dopamine hypotheses of schizophrenia and depression: contradictions and speculations. In: Willner, P. and Scheel-Kruger, J. (eds), *The Mesolimbic Dopamine System: From Motivation to Action*, pp. 615–37. John Wiley & Sons, Chichester.

File, S.E. and Tucker, J.C., 1986. Behavioral consequences of antidepressant treatment in rodents. *Neurosci. Bio. Behav. Rev.*, **10**, 123–34.

Fontana, D.J., Carbary, T.J. and Commisaris, R.L., 1989. Effects of acute and chronic anti-panic drug administration on conflict behavior in the rat. *Psychopharmacology*, **98**, 157–62.

Frank, M.G. and Heller, H.C., 1997. Neonatal treatments with the serotonin uptake inhibitors clomipramine and zimelidine, but not the noradrenaline uptake inhibitor desipramine, disrupt sleep patterns in adult rats. *Brain Res.*, **768**, 287–93.

Frazer, A., Lucki, I. and Sills, M., 1985. Alterations in monoamine-containing neuronal function due to administration of antidepressants repeatedly to rats. *Acta Pharmacol. Toxicol.*, **56**(suppl 1), 21–34.

Froger, N., Gardier, A.M., Moratalla, R., Alberti, I., Lena, I., Boni, C., De Felipe, C., Hunt, S.P., Jacquot, C., Hamon, M. and Lanfumey, L., 2001. 5-Hydroxytryptamine (5-HT)1A autoreceptor adaptive changes in P (neurokinin 1) receptor knock-out mice mimic antidepressant desensitization. *J. Neurosci.*, **21**, 8188–97.

Fujishiro, J., Imanishi, T., Baba, J. and Kosaka, K., 2001. Comparison of noradrenergic and serotonergic antidepressants in reducing immobility time in the tail suspension test. *Jpn J. Pharmacol.*, **85**, 327–30.

Gambarana, C., Ghiglieri, O., Tagliamonte, A., D'Alessandro, N. and de Montis, M.G., 1995a. Crucial role of D1 dopamine receptors in mediating the antidepressant effect of imipramine. *Pharmacol. Biochem. Behav.*, **50**, 147–51.

Gambarana, C., Ghiglieri, O. and de Montis, M.G., 1995b. Desensitization of the D1 dopamine receptors in rats reproduces a model of escape deficit reverted by imipramine, fluoxetine and clomipramine. *Prog. Neuropsychopharmacol. Biol. Psychiat.*, **19**, 741–55.

Gambarana, C., Ghiglieri, O., Tolu, P., De Montis, M.G., Giachetti, D., Bombardelli, E. and Tagliamonte, A., 1999a. Efficacy of an *Hypericum perforatum* (St. John's wort) extract in preventing and reverting a condition of escape deficit in rats. *Neuropsychopharmacology*, **21**, 247–57.

Gambarana, C., Masi, F., Tagliamonte, A., Scheggi, S., Ghiglieri, O. and De Montis, M.G., 1999b. A chronic stress that impairs reactivity in rats also decreases dopaminergic transmission in the nucleus accumbens: a microdialysis study. *J. Neurochem.*, **72**, 2039–46.

Gardner, R., 1982. Mechanisms in manic-depressive disorder: an evolutionary model. *Arch. Gen. Psychiat.*, **39**, 1436–41.

Gentsch, C., Lichsteiner, M. and Feer, H., 1990. Competition for sucrose-pellets in triads of male Wistar rats: effects of acute and subchronic chlordiazepoxide. *Psychopharmacology*, **100**, 530–4.

Geyer, M.A. and Markou, A., 1995. Animal models of psychiatric disorders. In: Bloom, F.E. and Kupfer, D. (eds), *Psychopharmacology: The Fourth Generation of Progress*, pp. 787–98. Raven, New York.

Ghiglieri, O., Gambarana, C., Scheggi, S., Tagliamonte, A., Willner, P. and De Montis, G., 1997. Palatable food induces an appetitive behaviour in satiated rats which can be inhibited by chronic stress. *Behav. Pharmacol.*, **8**, 619–28.

Gibson, W.E., Reid, L.D., Sakai, M. and Porter, P.B., 1965. Intracranial reinforcement compared with sugar-water reinforcement. *Science*, **148**, 1357–8.

Gilbert, P. and Allan, S., 1998. The role of defeat and entrapment (arrested flight) in depression: an exploration of an evolutionary view. *Psychol. Med.*, **28**, 585–98.

Giral, P., Martin, P., Soubrie, P. and Simon, P., 1988. Reversal of helpless behaviour in rats by putative $5HT_{1A}$ agonists. *Biol. Psychiat.*, **23**, 237–42.

Glazer, H.I. and Weiss, J.M., 1976. Long-term interference effect: an alternative to 'learned helplessness'. *J. Exp. Psychol. Anim. Behav. Proc.*, **2**, 201–13.

Gomez, F., Grauges, P., Lopez-Calderon, A. and Armario, A., 1999. Abnormalities of hypothalamic-pituitary-adrenal and hypothalamic-somatotrophic axes in Fawn-Hooded rats. *Eur. J. Endocrinol.*, **141**, 290–6.

Hall, F.S., Huang, S., Fong, G.F. and Pert, A., 1998a. The effects of social isolation on the forced swim test in Fawn Hooded and Wistar rats. *J. Neurosci. Meth.*, **79**, 47–51.

Hall, F.S., Huang, S., Fong, G.W., Pert, A. and Linnoila, M., 1998b. Effects of isolation-rearing on voluntary consumption of ethanol, sucrose and saccharin solutions in Fawn Hooded and Wistar rats. *Psychopharmacology (Berl)*, **139**, 210–6.

Hall, F.S., Huang, S., Fong, G.W., Sundstrom, J.M. and Pert, A., 2000. Differential basis of strain and rearing effects on open-field behaviour in Fawn Hooded and Wistar rats. *Physiol. Behav.*, **71**, 525–32.

Hansen, H.H., Sanchez, C. and Meier, E., 1997. Neonatal administration of the selective serotonin reuptake inhibitor Lu 10-134-C increases forced swimming-induced immobility in adult rats: a putative animal model of depression? *J. Pharmacol. Exp. Ther.*, **283**, 1333–41.

Harkin, A.J., Bruce, K.H., Craft, B. and Paul, I.A., 1999a. Nitric oxide synthase inhibitors have antidepressant-like properties in mice. 1 Acute treatments are active in the forced swim test. *Eur. J. Pharmacol.*, **372**, 207–13.

Harkin, A., Kelly, J.P., McNamara, M., Connor, T.J., Dredge, K., Redmond, A. and Leonard, B.E., 1999b. Activity and onset of action of reboxetine and effect of combination with sertraline in an animal model of depression. *Eur. J. Pharmacol.*, **364**, 123–32.

Henn, F.A. and McKinney, W.T., 1987. Animal models in psychiatry. In: Meltzer, H.Y. (ed.), *Psychopharmacology: The Third Generation of Progress*, pp. 697–704. Raven, New York.

Henry, J.P., 1982. The relation of social to biological processes in disease. *Soc. Sci. Med.*, **16**, 369–80.

Hernando, F., Fuentes, J.A., Roques, B.P. and Ruiz-Gayo, M., 1994. The CCKB receptor antagonist, L-365,260, elicits antidepressant-type effects in the forced-swim test in mice. *Eur. J. Pharmacol.*, **261**, 257–63.

Hernando, F., Fuentes, J.A. and Ruiz-Gayo, M., 1996. Impairment of stress adaptive behaviours in rats by the CCKA receptor antagonist, devazepide. *Br. J. Pharmacol.*, **118**, 400–6.

Hersen, M., Bellack, A.S., Himmelhoch, J.M. and Thase, M.E., 1984. Effect of social skill training, amitriptyline and psychotherapy in unipolar depressed women. *Behav. Ther.*, **15**, 21–40.

Hilakivi, L.A. and Hilakivi, I., 1987. Increased adult behavioural 'despair' in rats neonatally exposed to desipramine or zimelidine: an animal model of depression. *Pharmacol. Biochem. Behav.*, **28**, 267–9.

Hoebel, B.G., 1976. Brain-stimulation reward and aversion in relation to behaviour. In: Wauquier, A. and Rolls, E. (eds), *Brain-Stimulation Reward*, pp. 331–72. North Holland, New York.

Hollander, E., 1999. Managing aggressive behavior in patients with obsessive-compulsive disorder and borderline personality disorder. *J. Clin. Psychiat.*, **60**, S38–S44.

Hrdina, P.D., Von Kulmiz, P. and Stretch, R., 1979. Pharmacological modification of experimental depression in infant macaques. *Psychopharmacology*, **64**, 89–93.

Iwata, N., Puchler, K. and Plenker, A., 1997. Pharmacology of the new reversible inhibitor of monoamine oxidase A, RS-8359. *Int. Clin. Psychopharmacol.*, **12**(suppl 5), S3–10.

Jackson, R.L. and Minor, T.R., 1988. Effects of signaling inescapable shock on subsequent escape learning: implications for theories of coping and 'learned helplessness'. *J. Exp. Psychol.: Anim. Behav. Proc.*, **14**, 390–400.

Jackson, R.L., Maier, S.F. and Rapoport, P.M., 1978. Exposure to inescapable shock produces both activity and associative deficits in rats. *Learn. Motiv.*, **9**, 69–98.

Jesberger, J.A. and Richardson, J.S., 1986. Effects of antidepressant drugs on the behavior of olfactory bulbectomized and sham-operated rats. *Behav. Neurosci.*, **100**, 256–74.

Joly, D. and Sanger, D.J., 1986. The effects of fluoxetine and zimelidine on the behavior of olfactory bulbectomized rats. *Pharmacol. Biochem. Behav.*, **24**, 199–204.

Joly, D. and Sanger, D.J., 1991. Social competition in rats: a test sensitive to acutely administered anxiolytics. *Behav. Pharmacol.*, **2**, 205–13.

Kantor, S., Anheuer, Z.E. and Bagdy, G., 2000. High social anxiety and low aggression in Fawn-Hooded rats. *Physiol. Behav.*, **71**, 551–7.

Kantor, S., Graf, M., Anheuer, Z.E. and Bagdy, G., 2001. Rapid desensitisation of $5\text{-}HT_{1A}$ receptors in Fawn-Hooded rats after chronic fluoxetine treatment. *Eur. Neuropsychopharmacol.*, **11**, 15–24.

Kaplan, S.M., Kravetz, R.S. and Ross, W.D., 1961. The effects of imipramine on the depressive components of medical disorders. *Proc. 3rd World Congress Psychiatry*, **2**, 1362–7.

Kato, M., Katayama, T., Iwata, H., Yamamura, M., Matsuoka, Y. and Narita, H., 1998. *In vivo* characterization of T-794, a novel reversible inhibitor of monoamine oxidase-A, as an antidepressant with a wide safety margin. *J. Pharmacol. Exp. Ther.*, **284**, 983–90.

Katz, R.J., 1981. Animal models and human depressive disorders. *Neurosci. Biobehav. Rev.*, **5**, 231–46.

Katz, R.J., 1982. Animal model of depression: pharmacological sensitivity of a hedonic deficit. *Pharmacol. Biochem. Behav.*, **16**, 965–8.

Katz, R.J., Roth, K.A. and Carroll, B.J., 1981. Acute and chronic stress effects on open field activity in the rat: implications for a model of depression. *Neurosci. Biobehav. Rev.*, **5**, 247–51.

Kawashima, K., Araki, H. and Aihara, H., 1986. Effect of chronic administration of antidepressants on duration of immobility in rats forced to swim. *Jpn J. Pharmacol.*, **40**, 199–204.

Keeney, A.J. and Hogg, S., 1999. Behavioural consequences of repeated social defeat in the mouse: preliminary evaluation of a potential animal model of depression. *Behav. Pharmacol.*, **10**, 753–64.

Keeney, A.J., Hogg, S. and Marsden, C.A., 2001. Alterations in core body temperature, locomotor activity, and corticosterone following acute and repeated social defeat of male NMRI mice. *Physiol. Behav.*, **74**, 177–84.

Kelly, J.P., Wrynn, A.S. and Leonard, B.E., 1997. The olfactory bulbectomized rat as a model of depression: an update. *Pharmacol. Ther.*, **74**, 299–316.

Kennett, G.A., Dourish, C.T. and Curzon, G., 1987. Antidepressant-like action of 5-HT_{1A} agonists and conventional antidepressants in an animal model of depression. *Eur. J. Pharmacol.*, **134**, 265–74.

King, J.A., Abend, S. and Edwards, E., 2001 Genetic predisposition and the development of posttraumatic stress disorder in an animal model. *Biol. Psychiatr.*, **50**, 231–7.

Kitada, Y., Miyauchi, T., Satoh, A. and Satoh, S., 1981. Effects of antidepressants in the rat forced swimming test. *Eur. J. Pharmacol.*, **72**, 145–52.

Kokkinidis, L. and Zacharko, R.M., 1980. Response sensitization and depression following long-term amphetamine treatment in a self-stimulation paradigm. *Psychopharmacology*, **68**, 73–6.

Kokkinidis, L., Zacharko, R.M. and Predy, P.A., 1980. Post-amphetamine depression of self-stimulation responding from the substantia nigra: reversal by tricyclic antidepressants. *Pharmacol. Biochem. Behav.*, **13**, 379–83.

Koob, G.F., 1989. Anhedonia as an animal model of depression. In: Koob, G.F., Ehlers, C.L. and Kupfer, D.J. (eds), *Animal Models of Depression*, pp. 162–83. Birkhauser, Basel.

Koolhaas, J.M., Hermann, P.M., Kemperman, C., Bohus, B., van der Hoofdakker, R.H. and Beersma, D.G.M., 1990. Single social defeat in male rats induces a gradual but long lasting behavioral change: a model of depression? *Neurosci. Res. Commun.*, **7**, 35–41.

Kornetsky, C. and Esposito, R.U., 1981. Reward and detection thresholds for brain stimulation: dissociative effects of cocaine. *Brain Res.*, **209**, 496–500.

Korte, S.M., Smit, J., Bouws, G.A.H., Koolhaas, J.M. and Bohus, B., 1991. Neuroendocrine evidence for hypersensitivity in serotonergic neuronal system after psychosocial stress of defeat. In: Olivier, B., Mos, J. and Slangen, J. (eds), *Animal Models in Psychopharmacology*, pp. 199–203. Birkhauser, Basel.

Kostowski, W. and Malatynska, E., 1983. Antagonism of behavioural depression produced by clonidine in the Mongolian gerbil: a potential screening test for antidepressant drugs. *Psychopharmacology (Berl)*, **79**, 203–8.

Kostowski, W. and Obersztyn, M., 1988. Chronic administration of desipramine and imipramine but not zimelidine attenuates clonidine-induced depression of avoidance behavior in rats. *Pol. J. Pharmacol. Pharm.*, **40**, 341–9.

Kostowski, W., Dyr, W., Krzascik, P., Jarbe, T. and Archer, T., 1992. 5-Hydroxytryptamine1A receptor agonists in animal models of depression and anxiety. *Pharmacol. Toxicol.*, **71**, 24–30.

Kraemer, G.W., Ebert, M.H., Lake, C.R. and McKinney, W.T., 1984a. Hypersensitivity to d-amphetamine several years after early social deprivation in rhesus monkeys. *Psychopharmacology*, **82**, 266–71.

Kraemer, G.W., Ebert, M.H., Lake, C.R., McKinney, W.T., 1984b. Cerebrospinal fluid measures of neurotransmitter changes associated in the pharmacological alteration of the despair response to social separation in rhesus monkeys. *Psychiat. Res.*, **11**, 303–15.

Kraemer, G.W., Ebert, M.H., Schmidt, D.E. and McKinney, W.T., 1989. A longitudinal study of the effect of different rearing conditions on cerebrospinal fluid norepinephrine and biogenic amine metabolism in rhesus monkeys. *Neuropsychopharmacology*, **2**, 175–89.

Kudryatseva, N.N., Bakshtanovskaya, I.V. and Koryakina, L.A., 1991. Social model of depression in mice of C57BL/6J strain. *Pharmacol. Biochem. Behav.*, **38**, 315–20.

Kumar, V., Singh, P.N. and Bhattacharya, S.K., 2001. Anti-stress activity of Indian *Hypericum perforatum L. Indian. J. Exp. Biol.*, **39**, 344–9.

Kupfer, D.J. and Thase, M.E., 1983. The use of the sleep laboratory in the diagnosis of affective disorders. *Psychiat. Clin. North Am.*, **6**, 3–25.

Ladd, C.O., Owens, M.J. and Nemeroff, C.B., 1996. Persistent changes in corticotropin-releasing factor neuronal systems induced by maternal deprivation. *Endocrinology*, **137**, 1212–18.

Lahmame, A., Gomez, F. and Armario, A., 1996. Fawn-hooded rats show enhanced active behaviour in the forced swimming test, with no evidence for pituitary-adrenal axis hyperactivity. *Psychopharmacology (Berl)*, **125**, 74–8.

Lanfumey, L., Mannoury La Cour, C., Froger, N. and Hamon, M., 2000. 5-HT-HPA interactions in two models of transgenic mice relevant to major depression. *Neurochem. Res.*, **25**, 1199–1206.

Lehr, E., 1989. Distress-call reactivation in isolated chicks: a behavioural indicator with high selectivity for antidepressants. *Psychopharmacology*, **97**, 145–6.

Leith, N.J. and Barrett, R.J., 1976. Amphetamine and the reward system: evidence for tolerance and post-drug depression. *Psychopharmacology*, **46**, 19–25.

Leith, N.J. and Barrett, R.J., 1980. Effects of chronic amphetamine or reserpine on self-stimulation: animal model of depression? *Psychopharmacology*, **72**, 9–15.

Leonard, B., 1991. The olfactory bulbectomized rat as a model of depression. *Eur. Neuropsychopharmacol.*, **1**, 297–8.

Lewinsohn, P.M., 1974. A behavioural approach to depression. In: Friedman, R.J. and Katz, M.M. (eds), *The Psychology of Depression: Contemporary Theory and Research*, pp. 157–85. Winston/Wiley, New York.

Lewis, J.K. and McKinney, W.T., 1976. Effects of electroconvulsive shock on the behaviour of normal and abnormal rhesus monkeys. *Behav. Psychiat.*, **37**, 687–93.

Lewis, J.K., McKinney, W.T., Young, L.D. and Kraemer, G.W., 1976. Mother–infant separation in rhesus monkeys as a model of human depression: a reconsideration. *Arch. Gen. Psychiat.*, **33**, 699–705.

Lewis, J.W., Cannon, J.T. and Liebeskind, J.C., 1980. Opioid and non-opioid mechanisms of stress-induced analgesia. *Science*, **208**, 623–5.

Li, Q., Wichems, C., Heils, A., Van De Kar, L.D., Lesch, K.P. and Murphy, D.L., 1999. Reduction of 5-hydroxytryptamine $(5\text{-HT})_{1A}$-mediated temperature and neuroendocrine responses and 5-HT_{1A} binding sites in 5-HT transporter knockout mice. *J. Pharmacol. Exp. Ther.*, **291**, 999–1007.

Li, Q., Wichems, C., Heils, A., Lesch, K.P. and Murphy, D.L., 2000. Reduction in the density and expression, but not G-protein coupling, of serotonin receptors (5-HT_{1A}) in 5-HT transporter knock-out mice: gender and brain region differences. *J. Neurosci.*, **20**, 7888–95.

Linthorst, A.C., Flachskamm, C., Barden, N., Holsboer, F. and Reul, J.M., 2000. Glucocorticoid receptor impairment alters CNS responses to a psychological stressor: an *in vivo* microdialysis study in transgenic mice. *Eur. J. Neurosci.*, **12**, 283–91.

Lloyd, C., 1980. Life events and depressive disorder reviewed. *Arch. Gen. Psychiat.*, **37**, 529–48.

Lloyd, K.G., Garrigou, D. and Broekkamp, C.L.E., 1982. The action of monoaminergic, cholinergic and gabaergic compounds in the olfactory bulbectomized rat model of depression. In: Langer, S.Z., Takahashi, R., Segawa, T. and Briley, M. (eds), *New Vistas in Depression*, pp. 179–86. Pergamon Press, New York.

Lumia, A.R., Teicher, M.H., Salchli, F., Ayers, E. and Possidente, B., 1992. Olfactory bulbectomy as a model for agitated hyposerotonergic depression. *Brain Res.*, **587**, 181–5.

Lumley, L.A., Charles, R.F., Charles, R.C., Hebert, M.A., Morton, D.M. and Meyerhoff, J.L., 2000. Effects of social defeat and of diazepam on behavior in a resident–intruder test in male DBA/2 mice. *Pharmacol. Biochem. Behav.*, **67**, 433–47.

Lyon, M., 1991. Animal models of mania and schizophrenia. In: Willner, P. (ed.), *Behavioural Models in Psychopharmacology: Theoretical, Industrial and Clinical Perspectives*, pp. 253–310 Cambridge University Press, Cambridge.

Maier, S.F., 1984. Learned helplessness and animal models of depression. *Prog. Neuropsychopharmacol. Biol. Psychiat.*, **8**, 435–46.

Maier, S.F., 2001. Exposure to the stressor environment prevents the temporal dissipation of behavioral depression/learned helplessness. *Biol. Psychiat.*, **49**, 763–73.

Maj, J., 1984. Central effects following repeated treatment with antidepressant drugs. *Pol. J. Pharmacol. Pharm.*, **36**, 87–99.

Maj, J. and Rogoz, Z., 1999. Pharmacological effects of venlafaxine, a new antidepressant, given repeatedly, on the alpha 1-adrenergic, dopamine and serotonin systems. *J. Neural. Transm.*, **106**, 197–211.

Maj, J., Mogilnicka, E. and Kordecka, A., 1979. Chronic treatment with antidepressant drugs: potentiation of apomorphine-induced aggressive behaviour in rats. *Neurosci. Lett.*, **13**, 337–41.

Maj, J., Mogilnicka, E. and Kordecka-Magiera, A., 1980. Effects of chronic administration of antidepressant drugs on aggressive behavior induced by clonidine in mice. *Pharmacol. Biochem. Behav.*, **13**, 153–4.

Maj, J., Mogilnicka, E., Klimek, V. and Kordecka-Magiera, A., 1981. Chronic treatment with antidepressants: potentiation of clonidine-induced aggression in mice via noradrenergic mechanism. *J. Neural. Transm.*, **52**, 189–97.

Maj, J., Rogoz, Z., Skuza, G. and Sowinska, H., 1982. Effects of chronic treatment with antidepressants on aggressiveness induced by clonidine in mice. *J. Neural. Transm.*, **55**, 19–25.

Maj, J., Michaluk, J., Rawlow, A., Rogoz, Z. and Skuza, G., 1986. Central action of the antidepressant drug pirlindole. *Arzneimittelforschung*, **36**, 1198–1201.

Manhaes de Castro, R., Barreto Medeiros, J.M., Mendes da Silva, C., Ferreira, L.M., Guedes, R.C., Cabral Filho, J.E. and Costa, J.A., 2001. Reduction of intraspecific aggression in adult rats by neonatal treatment with a selective serotonin reuptake inhibitor. *Braz. J. Med. Biol. Res.*, **34**, 121–4.

Mar, A., Spreekmeester, E. and Rochford, J., 2000. Antidepressants preferentially enhance habituation to novelty in the olfactory bulbectomized rat. *Psychopharmacology (Berl)*, **150**, 52–60.

Marek, G.J., Li, A. and Seiden, L.S., 1989. Selective 5-hydroxytryptamine-2 antagonists have antidepressant-like effects on differential-reinforcement-of-low rate 72-s schedule. *J. Pharmacol. Exp. Ther.*, **250**, 60–71.

Markou, A. and Koob, G.F., 1989. Bromocriptine reverses post-cocaine anhedonia in a rat model of cocaine withdrawal. *American College of Neuropsychopharmacology, Abstracts*, 157.

Markou, A., Hanley, S.J., Chehade, A.K. and Koob, G.F., 1989. Effects of performance and reward manipulations on current-intensity thresholds and other measures derived from a discrete-trial self-stimulation procedure in rats. *Soc. Neurosci. Abstr.*, **15**, 35.

Markou, A., Hauger, R.L. and Koob, G.F., 1992. Desmethylimipramine attenuates cocaine withdrawal in rats. *Psychopharmacology (Berl)*, **109**, 305–14.

Martin, P., Soubrie, P. and Simon, P., 1986a. Shuttle-box deficits induced by inescapable shocks in rats: reversal by the beta-adrenoreceptor stimulants clenbuterol and salbutamol. *Pharmacol. Biochem. Behav.*, **24**, 177–81.

Martin, P., Soubrie, P. and Simon, P., 1986b. Noradrenergic and opioid mediation of tricyclic-induced reversal of escape deficits caused by inescapable shock pretreatment in rats. *Psychopharmacology*, **90**, 90–4.

Martin, P., Laporte, A.M., Soubrie, P., El Mestikawy, S. and Hamon, S., 1989. Reversal of helpless behaviour by serotonin reuptake inhibitors. In: Bevan, P., Cools, A.R. and Archer, T. (eds), *Behavioural Pharmacology of 5HT*, pp. 231–4. Lawrence Erlbaum, New York.

Matthews, K., Forbes, N. and Reid, I.C., 1995. Sucrose consumption as a hedonic measure following chronic unpredictable mild stress. *Physiol. Behav.*, **57**, 241–8.

Matto, V., Skrebuhhova, T. and Allikmets, L., 1998a. The effect of antidepressants on rat aggressive behavior in the electric footshock and apomorphine-induced aggressiveness paradigms. *Meth. Find. Exp. Clin. Pharmacol.*, **20**, 329–37.

Matto, V., Allikmets, L. and Skrebuhhova, T., 1998b. Apomorphine-induced aggressiveness and [^{3}H]citalopram binding after antidepressant treatment in rats. *Pharmacol. Biochem. Behav.*, **59**, 747–52.

Mayberg, H.S., Liotti, M., Brannan, S.K., McGinnis, S., Mahurian, R.K., Jerabek, P.A., Silva, J.A., Tekell, J.L., Martin, C.C., Lancaster, J.L. and Fox, P.T., 1999. Reciprocal limbic-cortical function and negative mood: converging PET findings in depression and normal sadness. *Am. J. Psychiat.*, **156**, 675–82.

McGrath, C. and Norman, T.R., 1998. The effect of venlafaxine treatment on the behavioural and neurochemical changes in the olfactory bulbectomised rat. *Psychopharmacology (Berl)*, **136**, 394–401.

McGrath, C. and Norman, T.R., 1999. (+)-S-20499 — a potential antidepressant? A behavioural and neurochemical investigation in the olfactory bulbectomised rat. *Eur. Neuropsychopharmacol.*, **9**, 21–7.

McKinney, W.T. and Bunney, W.E., 1969. Animal model of depression: review of evidence and implications for research. *Arch. Gen. Psychiat.*, **21**, 240–8.

McKinney, W.T. and Kraemer, G.W., 1989. Effects of oxaprotiline on the response to peer separation in rhesus monkeys. *Biol. Psychiat.*, **25**, 818–21.

McKinney, W.T., Young, L.D. and Suomi, S.J., 1973. Chlorpromazine treatment of disturbed monkeys. *Arch. Gen. Psychiat.*, **29**, 490–4.

Meerlo, P., Overkamp, G.J. and Koolhaas, J.M., 1997. Behavioural and physiological consequences of a single social defeat in Roman high- and low-avoidance rats. *Psychoneuroendocrinology*, **22**, 155–68.

Meloni, D., Gambarana, C., De Montis, M.G., Dal Pra, P., Taddei, I. and Tagliamonte, A., 1993. Dizoclipine antagonizes the effect of chronic imipramine on learned helplessness in rats. *Pharmacol. Biochem. Behav.*, **46**, 423–6.

Menzel, E.W., Davenport, R.K. and Rogers, C.M., 1963. Effects of environmental restriction upon the chimpanzee's responsiveness to objects. *J. Comp. Physiol. Psychol.*, **56**, 78–85.

Minor, T.R., Jackson, R.L. and Maier, S.F., 1984. Effects of task-irrelevant cues and reinforcement delay on choice-escape learning following inescapable shock: evidence for a deficit in selective attention. *J. Exp. Psychol.: Anim. Behav. Proc.*, **10**, 543–56.

Minor, T.R., Pelleymounter, M.A. and Maier, S.F., 1988. Uncontrollable shock, forebrain norepinephrine, and stimulus selection during choice-escape learning. *Psychobiology*, **16**, 135–45.

Mitchell, P.J. and Fletcher, A., 1993. Venlafaxine exhibits pre-clinical antidepressant activity in the resident–intruder social interaction-paradigm. *Neuropharmacology*, **32**, 1001–9.

Mitchell, P.J. and Fletcher, A., 1994. Repeated electroconvulsive shock increases aggressive behaviour in resident rats. *Soc. Neurosci. Abstr.*, **20**, 385 (abstract 164.12).

Mitchell, P.J. and Forster, E.A., 1992. Gepirone exhibits antidepressant-like activity on the social/agonistic behaviour of resident rats. *J. Psychopharmacol.*, Abstract Book BAP/EBPS meeting, **A84** (abstract 335).

Mitchell, P.J., Hogg, S., 2001a. Escitalopram: behavioural model predicts antidepressant activity. *World J. Biol. Psychiat.*, **2**(suppl 1), abstract P024-21.

Mitchell, P.J. and Hogg, S., 2001b. Escitalopram: rapid antidepressant activity in rats. *World J. Biol. Psychiat.*, **2**(suppl 1), abstract P024-19.

Mitchell, P.J. and Redfern, P.H., 1992a. Chronic treatment with clomipramine and mianserin increases the hierarchical position of subdominant rats housed in triads. *Behav. Pharmacol.*, **3**, 239–47.

Mitchell, P.J. and Redfern, P.H., 1992b. Acute and chronic antidepressant drug treatments induce opposite effects in the social behaviour of rats. *J. Psychopharmacol.*, **6**, 241–57.

Mitchell, P.J. and Redfern, P.H., 1997a. Effects of citalopram and paroxetine on rodent social and agonistic behaviour. *J. Psychopharmacol.*, **11**(suppl), A41 (abstract 161).

Mitchell, P.J. and Redfern, P.H., 1997b. Potentiation of the time-dependent, antidepressant-induced changes in the agonistic behaviour of resident rats by the 5-HT_{1A} receptor antagonist, WAY-100635. *Behav. Pharmacol.*, **8**, 585–606.

Mitchell, P.J. and Redfern, P.H., 2000. Effects of *m*-chlorophenylpiperazine and mesulergine on rodent agonistic behaviour. *J. Psychopharmacol.*, **14**(suppl), A32 (abstract PD2).

Moledina, A., Mitchell, P.J. and Redfern, P.H., 2000. Effects of *m*-chlorophenylpiperazine on social competition in male Wistar rats. *J. Psychopharmacol.*, **14**(suppl), A39 (abstract PD28).

Monroe, S.M., Thase, M.E., Hersen, M., Himmelhochh, J.M. and Bellack, A.S., 1985. Life events and the endogenous-nonendogenous distinction in the treatment and posttreatment course of depression. *Comp. Psychiat.*, **26**, 175–86.

Montkowski, A., Barden, N., Wotjak, C., Stec, I., Ganster, J., Meaney, M., Engelman, M., Reul, J.M.H.M., Landgraf, R. and Holsboer, F., 1995. Long-term antidepressant treatment reduces behavioural deficits in transgenic mice with impaired glucocorticoid receptor function. *J. Neuroendocrinol.*, **7**, 841–5.

Moreau, J.-L., Jenck, F., Martin, J.R., Mortas, P. and Haefely, W.E., 1992. Antidepressant treatment prevents chronic unpredictable mild stress-induced anhedonia as assessed by ventral tegmental self-stimulation behavior in rats. *Eur. Neuropsychopharmacol.*, **2**, 43–9.

Murtra, P., Sheasby, A.M., Hunt, S.P.and De Felipe, C., 2000. Rewarding effects of opiates are absent in mice lacking the receptor for substance P. *Nature*, **405**, 180–3.

Muscat, R. and Willner, P., 1992. Suppression of sucrose drinking by chronic mild unpredictable stress: a methodological analysis. *Neurosci. Biobehav. Rev.*, **16**, 519–24.

Muscat, R., Papp, M. and Willner, P., 1992. Reversal of stress-induced anhedonia by the atypical antidepressants, fluoxetine and maprotiline. *Psychopharmacology (Berl)*, **109**, 433–8.

Nakagawa, Y., Ishima, T., Ishibashi, Y., Tsuji, M. and Takashima, T., 1996a. Involvement of GABAB receptor systems in experimental depression: baclofen but not bicuculline exacerbates helplessness in rats. *Brain Res.*, **741**, 240–5.

Nakagawa, Y., Ishima, T., Ishibashi, Y., Tsuji, M. and Takashima, T., 1996b. Involvement of GABAB receptor systems in action of antidepressants. II: Baclofen attenuates the effect of desipramine whereas muscimol has no effect in learned helplessness paradigm in rats. *Brain Res.*, **728**, 225–30.

Nelson, J.C., 1987. The use of antipsychotic drugs in the treatment of depression. In: Zohar, J. and Belmaker, R.H. (eds), *Treating Resistant Depression*, pp. 131–46. PMA, New York.

Nelson, J.C. and Charney, D.S., 1981. The symptoms of major depression. *Am. J. Psychiat.*, **138**, 1–13.

Niesink, R.J.M. and van Ree, J.M., 1982. Antidepressant drugs normalize the increased social behaviour of pairs of male rats induced by short term isolation. *Neuropharmacology*, **21**, 1343–8.

Nomura, A., Shimizu, J., Kamateni, H., Kinjo, M., Watanabe, M. and Nakazawa, T., 1982. Swimming mice: in search of an animal model for human depression. In: Langer, S.Z., Takahashi, R., Segawa, T. and Briley, M. (eds), *New Vistas in Depression*, pp. 203–10. Pergamon, New York.

O'Neill, K.A. and Valentino, D., 1982. Escapability and generalization: effect on behavioural despair. *Eur. J. Pharmacol.*, **78**, 379–80.

O'Neill, M.F. and Conway, M.W., 2001. Role of 5-HT_{1A} and 5-HT_{1B} receptors in the mediation of behavior in the forced swim test in mice. *Neuropsychopharmacology*, **24**, 391–8.

Overstreet, D.H., 1991. A behavioral, psychopharmacological and neurochemical update on the Flinders Sensitive Line rat, a potential genetic animal model of depression. *Behav. Genet.*, **21**, 67–74.

Overstreet, D.H., 1993. The Flinders sensitive line rats: a genetic animal model of depression. *Neurosci. Biobehav. Rev.*, **17**, 51–68.

Overstreet, D.H. and Janowsky, D.S., 1991. A cholinergic supersensitivity model of depression. In: Boulton, A., Baker, G. and Martin-Iverson, M. (eds), *Neuromethods*, vol. 20: *Animal Models in Psychiatry*, pp. 81–114. Birkhauser, Basel.

Overstreet, D.H., Rezvani, A. and Janowsky, D.S., 1992. Genetic animal models of depression and ethanol preference provide support for cholinergic and serotonergic involvement in depression and alcoholism. *Biol. Psychiat.*, **31**, 919–36.

Overstreet, D.H., Pucilowski, O., Rezvani, A.H. and Janowsky, D.S., 1995. Administration of antidepressants, diazepam and psychomotor stimulants further confirms the utility of Flinders Sensitive Line rats as an animal model of depression. *Psychopharmacology (Berl)*, **121**, 27–37.

Owens, M.J. and Nemeroff, C.B., 1991. Physiology and pharmacology of corticotropin-releasing factor. *Pharmacol. Rev.*, **43**, 425–73.

Owens, M.J., Overstreet, D.H., Knight, D.L., Rezvani, A.H., Ritchie, J.C., Bissette, G., Janowsky, D.S. and Nemeroff, C.B., 1991. Alterations in the hypothalamic–pituitary–adrenal axis in a proposed animal model of depression with genetic muscarinic supersensitivity. *Neuropsychopharmacology*, **4**, 87–93.

Panconi, E., Roux, J., Altenbaumer, M., Hampe, S. and Porsolt, R.D., 1993. MK-801 and enantiomers: potential antidepressants or false positives in classical screening models? *Pharmacol. Biochem. Behav.*, **46**, 15–20.

Papolos, D.F., Yu, Y.M., Rosenbaum, E. and Lachman, H.M., 1996. Modulation of learned helplessness by 5-hydroxytryptamine2A receptor antisense oligodeoxynucleotides. *Psychiat. Res.*, **63**, 197–203.

Papp, M. and Moryl, E., 1996. Antidepressant-like effects of l-aminocyclopropanecarboxylic acid and d-cycloserine in an animal model of depression. *Eur. J. Pharmacol.*, **316**, 145–51.

Papp, M. and Wieronska, J., 2000. Antidepressant-like activity of amisulpride in two animal models of depression. *J. Psychopharmacol.*, **14**, 46–52.

Papp, M., Willner, P. and Muscat, R., 1991. An animal model of anhedonia: attenuation of sucrose consumption and place preference conditioning by chronic unpredictable mild stress. *Psychopharmacology*, **104**, 255–9.

Papp, M., Lappas, S., Muscat, R. and Willner, P., 1992. Attenuation of place preference conditioning but not place aversion conditioning by chronic mild stress. *J. Psychopharmacol.*, **6**, 352–6.

Papp, M., Muscat, R. and Willner, P., 1993. Subsensitivity of rewarding and locomotor stimulant effects of a dopamine agonist following chronic mild stress. *Psychopharmacology*, **110**, 152–8.

Pawlowski, L. and Mazela, H., 1986. Effects of antidepressant drugs, selective noradrenaline or 5-hydroxytryptamine uptake inhibitors, on apomorphine-induced hypothermia in mice. *Psychopharmacology (Berl)*, **88**, 240–6.

Pepin, M.C., Pothier, F. and Barden, N., 1992a. Impaired type II glucocorticoid-receptor function in mice bearing antisense RNA transgene. *Nature*, **355**, 725–8.

Pepin, M.C., Pothier, F. and Barden, N., 1992b. Antidepressant drug action in a transgenic mouse model of endocrine changes seen in depression. *Mol. Pharmacol.*, **42**, 991–5.

Perrault, G., Morel, E., Zivkovic, B. and Sanger, D.J., 1992. Activity of litoxetine and other serotonin uptake inhibitors in the tail suspension test in mice. *Pharmacol. Biochem. Behav.*, **42**, 45–7.

Pollard, G.T. and Howard, J.L., 1986. Similar effects of antidepressant and non-antidepressant drugs on behavior under an interresponse-time >72-s schedule. *Psychopharmacology*, **89**, 253–8.

Porsolt, R.D., 1981. Behavioural despair. In: Enna, S.J., Malick, J.B. and Richelson, E. (eds), *Antidepressants: Neurochemical, Behavioural and Clinical Perspectives*, pp. 121–39. Raven Press, New York.

Porsolt, R.D., LePichon, M. and Jalfre, M., 1977. Depression: a new animal model sensitive to antidepressant treatment. *Nature*, **266**, 730–2.

Porsolt, R.D., Bertin, A., Blavet, M., Deniel, M. and Jalfre, M., 1979. Immobility induced by forced swimming in rats: effects of agents which modify central catecholamine and serotonin activity. *Eur. J. Pharmacol.*, **57**, 201–10.

Porsolt, R.D., Chermat, R., Simon, P. and Steru, L., 1986. The tail suspension test: computerized device for evaluating psychotropic activity profiles. *Psychopharmacology*, **89**, S28.

Porsolt, R.D., Lenegre, A. and McArthur, R.A., 1991. Pharmacological models of depression. In: Olivier, B., Mos, J. and Slangen, J.L. (eds), *Animal Models in Psychopharmacology*, pp. 137–59. Birkhauser, Basel.

Porsolt, R.D., Roux, S. and Drieu, K., 2000. Evaluation of a ginko biloba extract (Egb 761) in functional tests for monoamine oxidase inhibition. *Arzneimittelforschung*, **50**, 232–5.

Post, M.D., 1975. Cocaine psychoses: a continuum model. *Am. J. Psychiat.*, **132**, 225–31.

Price, J.S., 1972. Genetic and phylogenetic aspects of mood variation. *Int. J. Mental Hlth.*, **1**, 124–44.

Priest, R.G., Beaumont, G. and Raptopoulos, P., 1980. Suicide, attempted suicide and antidepressant drugs. *J. Int. Med. Res.*, **8**(suppl 3), 8–13.

Pucilowski, O., Danysz, W., Overstreet, D.H., Rezvani, A.H., Eichelman, B. and Janowsky, D.S., 1991. Decreased hyperthermic effect of MK-801 in selectively bred hypercholinergic rats. *Brain Res. Bull.*, **26**, 621–5.

Pucilowski, O., Overstreet, D.H., Rezvani, A.H. and Janowsky, D.S., 1993. Chronic mild stress-induced anhedonia: greater effect in a genetic rat model of depression. *Physiol. Behav.*, **54**, 1215–20.

Puech, A.J., Chermat, R., Poncelet, M., Doare, L. and Simon, P., 1981. Antagonism of hypothermia and behavioral response to apomorphine: a simple, rapid and discriminating test for screening antidepressants and neuroleptics. *Psychopharmacology (Berl)*, **75**, 84–91.

Reddy, D.S., Kaur, G. and Kulkarni, S.K., 1998. Sigma (sigma1) receptor mediated anti-depressant-like effects of neurosteroids in the Porsolt forced swim test. *Neuroreport*, **9**, 3069–73.

Redrobe, J.P., Bourin, M., Colombel, M.C. and Baker, G.B., 1998. Dose-dependent noradrenergic and serotonergic properties of venlafaxine in animal models indicative of antidepressant activity. *Psychopharmacology*, **138**, 1–8.

Reite, M., Short, R., Seiler, C. and Pauley, J.D., 1981. Attachment, loss and depression. *J. Child. Psychol. Psychiat.*, **22**, 141–69.

Richards, J.B., Sabol, K.E., Hand, T.H., Jolly, D.C., Marek, G.J. and Seiden, L.S., 1994. Buspirone, gepirone, ipsapirone, and zalospirone have distinct effects on the differential-reinforcement-of-low-rate 72-s schedule when compared with 5-HTP and diazepam. *Psychopharmacology (Berl)*, **114**, 39–46.

Rioux, A., Fabre, V., Lesch, K.P., Moessner, R., Murphy, D.L., Lanfumey, L., Hamon, M. and Martres, M.P., 1999. Adaptive changes of serotonin 5-HT_{2A} receptors in mice lacking the serotonin transporter. *Neurosci. Lett.*, **262**, 113–16.

Robertson, J. and Bowlby, J., 1952. Responses of young children to separation from their mothers. *Cour du Centre Internationale de L'Enfance*, **2**, 131–42.

Rodgers, B., 1991. Models of stress, vulnerability and affective disorder. *J. Affect. Disord.*, **21**, 1–13.

Rogoz, Z., Wrobel, A., Krasicka-Domka, M. and Maj, J., 1999a. Pharmacological profile of reboxetine, a representative of new class of antidepressant drugs, selective noradrenaline reuptake inhibitor (NARI), given acutely. *Pol. J. Pharmacol.*, **51**, 399–404.

Rogoz, Z., Skuza, G. and Maj, J., 1999b. Pharmacological profile of milnacipran, a new antidepressant, given acutely. *Pol. J. Pharmacol.*, **51**, 317–22.

Rudissaar, R., Pruus, K., Vaarmann, A., Pannel, P., Skrebuhhova-Malmros, T., Allikmets, L. and Matto, V., 2001. Acute trazodone and quipazine treatment attenuates apomorphine-induced aggressive behaviour in male rats without major impact on emotional behaviour or monoamine content post mortem. *Pharmacol. Res.*, **43**, 349–58.

Rupniak, N.M., Carlson, E.C., Harrison, T., Oates, B., Seward, E., Owens, S., de Felipe, C., Hunt, S. and Wheeldon, A., 2000. Pharmacological blockade or genetic deletion of substance P (NK_1) receptors attenuates neonatal vocalization in guinea-pigs and mice. *Neuropharmacology*, **39**, 1413–21.

Rupniak, N.M.J., Carllson, E.J., Webb, J.K., Harrison, T., Porsolt, R.D., Roux, S., de Felipe, C., Hunt, S.P., Oates, B. and Wheeldon, A., 2001. Comparison of the phenotype of NK1R-/- mice with pharmacological blockade of the substance P (NK_1) receptor in assays for antidepressant and anxiolytic drugs. *Behav. Pharmacol.*, **12**, 497–508.

Sarnyai, Z., Biro, E., Gardi, J., Vecsernyes, M., Julesz, J. and Telegdy, G., 1995. Brain corticotropin-releasing factor mediates 'anxiety-like' behavior induced by cocaine withdrawal in rats. *Brain Res.*, **675**, 89–97.

Scearce-Levie, K., Chen, J.P., Gardner, E. and Hen, R., 1999. 5-HT receptor knockout mice: pharmacological tools or models of psychiatric disorders. *Ann. N. Y. Acad. Sci.*, **868**, 701–15.

Schiller, G.D., Pucilowski, O., Wienicke, C. and Overstreet, D.H., 1992. Immobility-reducing effects of antidepressants in a genetic animal model of depression. *Brain Res. Bull.*, **28**, 821–3.

Schmale, A.H., 1973. Adaptive role of depression in health and disease. In: Scott, J.P. and Senay, E. (eds), *Separation and Depression*, pp. 187–214. American Association for the Advancement of Science, Washington, DC.

Seiden, L.S., Dahms, J.L. and Shaughnessy, R.A., 1985. Behavioral screen for antidepressants: the effects of drugs and electroconvulsive shock on performance under a differential-reinforcement-of-low-rate schedule. *Psychopharmacology*, **86**, 55–60.

Seligman, M.E.P., 1975. *Helplessness: On Depression, Development and Death*. W.H. Freeman, San Francisco, CA.

Shanks, N. and Anisman, H., 1988. Stressor-provoked behavioral changes in six strains of mice. *Behav. Neurosci.*, **102**, 894–905.

Sherman, A.D., Sacquitne, J.L. and Petty, F., 1982. Specificity of the learned helplessness model of depression. *Pharmacol. Biochem. Behav.*, **16**, 449–54.

Shumake, J., Poremba, A., Edwards, E. and Gonzalez-Lima, F., 2000 Congenital helpless rats as a genetic model for cortex metabolism in depression. *Neuroreport*, **11**, 3793–8.

Simpson, D.M. and Annau, Z., 1977. Behavioural withdrawal following several psychoactive drugs. *Pharmacol. Biochem. Behav*, **7**, 59–64.

Sluzewska, A. and Szczawinska, K., 1996a. Lithium potentiation of antidepressants in chronic mild stress model of depression in rats. *Behav. Pharmacol.*, **7**(suppl 1), 105.

Sluzewska, A. and Szczawinska, K., 1996b. The effects of pindolol addition to fluvoxamine and buspirone in chronic mild stress model of depression. *Behav. Pharmacol.*, **7**(suppl 1), **105**.

Smith, G.W., Aubry, J.M., Dellu, F., Contarino, A., Bilezikjian, L.M., Gold, L.H., Chen, R., Marchuk, Y., Hauser, C., Bentley, C.A., Sawchenko, P.E., Koob, G.F., Vale, W. and Lee, K.F., 1998. Corticotropin releasing factor receptor-1-deficient mice display decreased anxiety, impaired stress response, and aberrant neuroendocrine development. *Neuron*, **20**, 1093–102.

Soblosky, J.S. and Thurmond, J.B., 1986. Biochemical and behavioral correlates of chronic stress: effects of tricyclic antidepressants. *Pharmacol. Biochem. Behav.*, **24**, 1361–8.

Sokolowski, J.D. and Seiden, L.S., 1999. The behavioral effects of sertraline, fluoxetine, and paroxetine differ on the differential-reinforcement-of-low-rate 72-second operant schedule in the rat. *Psychopharmacology (Berl)*, **147**, 153–61.

Soubrie, P., 1986. Reconciling the role of central serotonin neurons in human and animal behaviour. *Behav. Brain. Sci.*, **9**, 319–64.

Soubrie, P., Martin, P., El Mestikawy, S., Thiebot, M.H., Simon, P. and Hamon, M., 1986. The lesion of serotonergic neurons does not prevent antidepressant-induced reversal of escape failures produced by inescapable shocks in rats. *Pharmacol. Biochem. Behav.*, **25**, 1–6.

Steru, L., Chermat, R., Thierry, B. and Simon, P., 1985. The tail suspension test: a new method for screening antidepressants in mice. *Psychopharmacology*, **85**, 367–70.

Stogner, K.A. and Holmes, P.V., 2000. Neuropeptide-Y exerts antidepressant-like effects in the forced swim test in rats. *Eur. J. Pharmacol.*, **387**, R9–R10.

Suomi, S.J., 1976. Factors affecting responses to social separation in rhesus monkeys. In: Serban, G. and Kling, A. (eds), *Animal Models in Human Psychobiology*, pp. 9–26. Plenum Press, New York.

Suomi, S.J., Seaman, S.F., Lewis, J.K., DeLizio, R.B. and McKinney, W.T., 1978. Effects of imipramine treatment on separation-induced social disorders in rhesus monkeys. *Arch. Gen. Psychiat.*, **35**, 321–5.

Takahashi, L.K., Turner, J.G. and Kalin, N.H., 1992. Prenatal stress alters brain catecholaminergic activity and potentiates stress-induced behavior in adult rats. *Brain Res.*, **574**, 131–7.

Teixeira, N.A., Pereira, D.G. and Hermini, A.H., 1995. Chronic but not acute Li^+ treatment prevents behavioral depression in rats. *Braz. J. Med. Biol. Res.*, **28**, 1003–7.

Teste, J.F., Pelsy-Johann, I., Decelle, T. and Boulu, R.G., 1993. Anti-immobility activity of different antidepressant drugs using the tail suspension test in normal or reserpinized mice. *Fundam. Clin. Pharmacol.*, **7**, 219–26.

Timpl, P., Spanagel, R., Sillaber, I., Kresse, A., Reul, J.M., Stalla, G.K., Blanquet, V., Steckler, T., Holsboer, F. and Wurst, W., 1998. Impaired stress response and reduced anxiety in mice lacking a functional corticotropin-releasing hormone receptor. *Nat. Genet.*, **19**, 162–6.

Tizabi, Y., Overstreet, D.H., Rezvani1, A.H., Louis, V.A., Clark, E. Jr, Jonowsky, D.S. and Kling, M.A., 1999. Antidepressant effects of nicotine in an animal model of depression. *Psychopharmacology (Berl)*, **142**, 193–9.

Tizabi, Y., Rezvani1, A.H., Russell, L.T., Tyler, K.Y. and Overstreet, D.H., 2000. Depressive characteristics of FSL rats: involvement of central nicotinic receptors. *Pharmacol. Biochem. Behav.*, **66**, 73–7.

Toates, F., 1995. *Stress: Conceptual and Biological Aspects*. John Wiley & Sons, Chichester.

Turner, C., Davenport, R. and Rogers, C., 1969. The effect of early deprivation on the social behaviour of adolescent chimpanzees. *Am. J. Psychiat.*, **125**, 1531–6.

Valenstein, E.S., 1973. *Brain Control: A Critical Examination of Brain Stimulation and Psychosurgery*. John Wiley & Sons, New York.

van den Bos, R., Charria Ortiz, G.A. and Cools, A.R., 1992. Injections of the NMDA-antagonist D-2-amino-7-phosphonoheptanoic acid (AP-7) into the nucleus accumbens of rats enhance switching between cue-directed behaviours in a swimming test procedure. *Behav. Brain. Res.*, **48**, 165–70.

van der Heyden, J.A.M., Olivier, B. and Zethof, T.J.J., 1991. The behavioural despair model as a predictor of antidepressant activity: effects of serotonergic drugs. In: Olivier, B., Mos, J. and Slangen, J. (eds), *Animal Models in Psychopharmacology*, pp. 211–15. Birkhauser, Basel.

Van Praag, H.M., 1994. 5-HT-related anxiety- and/or aggression-driven depression. *Int. Clin. Psychopharmacol.*, **9**(suppl 1), 5–6.

Van Riezen, H. and Leonard, B.E., 1990. Effects of psychotropic drugs on the behaviour and neurochemistry of olfactory bulbectomized rats. In: File, S.E. (ed.), *Psychopharmacology of Anxiolytics and Antidepressants*, pp. 231–50. Pergamon Press, New York.

Vartiainen, H., Tiihonen, J., Putkonen, A., Koponen, H., Virkkunen, M., Hakola, P. and Lehto, H., 1995. Citalopram, a selective serotonin reuptake inhibitor, in the treatment of aggression in schizophrenia. *Acta Psychiat. Scand.*, **91**, 348–51.

Velazquez-Moctezuma, J. and Diaz Ruiz, O., 1992. Neonatal treatment with clomipramine increased immobility in the forced swim test: an attribute of animal models of depression. *Pharmacol. Biochem. Behav.*, **42**, 737–9.

Velazquez-Moctezuma, J., Aguilar-Garcia, A. and Diaz Ruiz, O., 1993. Behavioral effects of neonatal treatment with clomipramine, scopolamine, and idazoxan in male rats. *Pharmacol. Biochem. Behav.*, **46**, 215–17.

Vogel, G., Neill, D., Hagler, M. and Kors, D., 1990. A new animal model of endogenous depression: a summary of present findings. *Neurosci. Biobehav. Rev.*, **14**, 85–91.

Vogel, G., Hagler, M., Hennessey, A. and Richard, C., 1996. Dose-dependent decrements in adult male rat sexual behavior after neonatal clorimipramine treatment. *Pharmacol. Biochem. Behav.*, **54**, 605–9.

Vollmayr, B. and Henn, F.A., 2001. Learned helplessness in the rat: improvements in validity and reliability. *Brain Res. Brain Res. Protoc.*, **8**, 1–7.

von Voigtlander, P.F., von Triezenberg, H.G. and Losey, E.G., 1978. Interactions between clonidine and antidepressant drugs: a method for identifying antidepressant-like agents. *Neuropharmacology*, **17**, 375–81.

Ward, H.E., Johnson, E.A., Salm, A.K. and Birkle, D.L., 2000. Effects of prenatal stress on defensive withdrawal behavior and corticotropin releasing factor systems in rat brain. *Physiol. Behav.*, **70**, 359–66.

Watson, R., Hartman, E. and Schildkraut, J.J., 1972. Amphetamine withdrawal: affective state, sleep patterns and MHPG excretion. *Am. J. Psychiat.*, **129**, 263–9.
Weiss, J.M. and Kilts, C.D., 1998. Animal models of depression and schizophrenia. In: Schatzberg, A.F. and Nemeroff, C.B. (eds), *Textbook of Psychopharmacology*, pp. 89–131. American Psychiatric Press, Washington DC.
Weiss, J.M., Goodman, P.A., Losito, B.G., Corrigan, S., Charry, J.M. and Bailey, W.H., 1981. Behavioural depression produced by an uncontrollable stressor: relationship to noreprinephrine, dopamine, and serotonin levels in various regions of rat brain. *Brain. Res. Rev.*, **3**, 167–205.
Weiss, J.M., Bailey, W.H., Goodman, P.A., Hoffman, L.J., Ambrose, M.J., Salman, S. and Charry, J.M., 1982. A model for neurochemical study of depression. In: Spiegelstein, M.Y. and Levy, A. (eds), *Behavioural Models and the Analysis of Drug Action*, pp. 195–223. Elsevier, Amsterdam.
White, D.A. and Birkle, D.L., 2001. The differential effects of prenatal stress in rats on the acoustic startle reflex under baseline conditions and in response to anxiogenic drugs. *Psychopharmacology (Berl)*, **154**, 169–76.
Willner, P., 1984. The validity of animal models of depression. *Psychopharmacology*, **83**, 1–16.
Willner, P., 1985. *Depression: A Psychobiological Synthesis*. John Wiley & Sons, New York.
Willner, P., 1986. Validating criteria for animal models of human mental disorders: learned helplessness as a paradigm case. *Prog. Neuropsychopharmacol. Biol. Psychiat.*, **10**, 677–90.
Willner, P., 1989a. Sensitization to the actions of antidepressant drugs. In: Emmett-Oglesby, M.W. and Goudie, A.J. (eds), *Psychoactive Drugs: Tolerance and Sensitization*, pp. 407–59. Humana Press, Clifton, NJ.
Willner, P., 1989b. Towards a theory of serotonergic dysfunction in depression. In: Archer, T., Bevan, P. and Cools, A. (eds), *Behavioural Pharmacology of 5-HT*, pp. 157–78. Lawrence Erlbaum, New York.
Willner, P., 1990. Animal models of depression: an overview. *Pharmacol. Ther.*, **45**, 425–55.
Willner, P., 1991a. Behavioural models in psychopharmacology. In: Willner, P. (ed.), *Behavioural Models in Psychopharmacology: Theoretical, Industrial and Clinical Perspective*, pp. 3–18. Cambridge University Press, Cambridge.
Willner, P., 1991b. Animal models as simulations of depression. *Trends Pharmacol. Sci.*, **12**, 131–6.
Willner, P., 1997. Validity, reliability and utility of the chronic mild stress (CMS) model of depression: a ten-year review and evaluation. (Plus 17 peer commentaries and author's response). *Psychopharmacology*, **134**, 319–77
Willner, P. and Papp, M., 1997. Animal models to detect antidepressants: are new strategies necessary to detect new agents? In: Skolnick, P. (ed.), *Antidepressants: New Pharmacological Strategies*, pp. 213–34. Humana Press, Totowa, NJ.
Willner, P., Theodorou, A. and Montgomery, A.M.J., 1981. Subchronic treatment with the tricyclic antidepressant DMI increases isolation-induced fighting in rats. *Pharmacol. Biochem. Behav.*, **14**, 475–9.
Willner, P., Towell, A., Sampson, D., Sophokleous, S. and Muscat, R., 1987. Reduction of sucrose preference by chronic mild unpredictable stress, and its restoration by a tricyclic antidepressant. *Psychopharmacology*, **93**, 358–64.
Willner, P., Sampson, D., Phillips, G., Fichera, R., Foxlow, P. and Muscat, R., 1989. Effects of isolated housing and chronic antidepressant treatment on cooperative social behaviour in rats. *Behav. Pharmacol.*, **1**, 85–90.
Willner, P., Sampson, D., Papp, M., Phillips, G. and Muscat, R., 1991. Animal models of anhedonia. In: Soubrie, P. (ed.), *Animal Models of Psychiatric Disorders*, vol. 3, *Anxiety, Depression and Mania*, pp. 71–99. Karger, Basel.
Willner, P., D'Aquila, P.S., Coventry, T. and Brain, P., 1995. Loss of social status: preliminary evaluation of a novel animal model of depression. *J. Psychopharmacol.*, **9**, 207–13.
Wise, R.A., 1989. The brain and reward. In: Liebmann, J.M. and Cooper, S.J. (eds), *The Neuropharmacological Basis of Reward*, pp. 377–424. Oxford University Press, Oxford.
Wong, E.H., Sonders, M.S., Amara, S.G., Tinholt, P.M., Piercey, M.F., Hoffmann, W.P., Hyslop, D.K., Franklin, S., Porsolt, R.D., Bonsignori, A., Carfagna, N. and McArthur, R.A., 2000. Reboxetine: a pharmacologically potent, selective, and specific norepinephrine reuptake inhibitor. *Biol. Psychiat.*, **47**, 818–29.
Woodmansee, W.W., Silbert, L.H. and Maier, S.F., 1991. Stress-induced changes in daily activity in the rat are modulated by different factors than are stress-induced escape-learning deficits. *Soc. Neurosci. Abstr.*, **17**, 146.
Zacharko, R.M. and Anisman, H., 1991. Stressor-provoked alterations of intracranial self-stimulation in the mesocortiolimbic dopamine system: an animal model of depression. In: Willner, P. and Scheel-Kruger, J. (eds), *The Mesolimbic Dopamine System, From Motivation to Action*, pp. 411–42. John Wiley & Sons, Chichester.
Zacharko, R.M., Bowers, W.J., Kokkinidis, L. and Anisman, H., 1983. Region-specific reductions of intracranial self-stimulation after uncontrollable stress: possible effects on reward processes. *Behav. Brain. Res.*, **9**, 129–41.
Zacharko, R.M., Lalonde, G.T., Kasian, M. and Anisman, H., 1987. Strain-specific effects of inescapable shock on intracranial self-stimulation from the nucleus accumbens. *Brain Res.*, **426**, 164–8.
Zangen, A., Overstreet, D.H. and Yadid, G., 1997. High serotonin and 5-hydroxyindoleacetic acid levels in limbic brain regions in a rat model of depression: normalization by chronic antidepressant treatment. *J. Neurochem.*, **69**, 2477–83.
Zangen, A., Overstreet, D.H. and Yadid, G., 1999. Increased catecholamine levels in specific brain regions of a rat model of depression: normalization by chronic antidepressant treatment. *Brain Res.*, **824**, 243–50.

XVIII-2

Monoaminergic Transmitter Systems

Alexander Neumeister and Dennis S. Charney

INTRODUCTION

There is considerable evidence available in the literature supporting the idea that brain monoamine systems play a key role in the pathogenesis of affective disorders, in particular depression. These hypotheses have primarily taken the form of proposing abnormal regulation in serotonin (5-HT) (Coppen, 1967) and the catecholamines norepinephrine (NE) (Bunney and Davis, 1965; Schatzberg and Schildkraut, 1995) and dopamine (DA) (Kapur and Mann, 1992)in depression. Early studies have focused largely on levels of monoamines and their receptors and have stimulated several theories about the pathophysiology of depression, including the monoamine deficiency and receptor sensitivity hypotheses. However, we have to acknowledge today that these hypotheses have not provided us with an ultimate explanation about the role of monoamines in depression. Nor can the pathophysiology of depression be explained simply by dysregulation of 5-HT and/or NE or DA transmission. Recent advances in molecular and cellular neurobiology have offered new insights into mechanisms possibly involved in the pathophysiology of depression, and also into the mechanisms of action of antidepressant treatment modalities (for reviews see Duman *et al.*, 1997; Manji *et al.*, 2001; Sulser, 1989). These studies have shown that chronic antidepressant treatment regulates intracellular signal transduction pathways and the expression of specific target genes.

The purpose of this chapter is to provide a concise review of clinical studies on the role of 5-HT and NE transmission in depression. However, several caveats need to be considered. First, depression is not a homogeneous disorder, and classifying a given patient with depression is a clinical decision and remains a subjective interpretation of a syndrome, even though the decision should be based on established diagnostic criteria such as DSM-IV criteria (American Psychiatric Association, 1994). However, identifying homogeneous groups of patients with depression has proven to be a virtually impossible task. This might explain some of the variability of biological findings in depression and the lack of consistent replication of many intriguing findings. Second, almost all patients being studied in clinical studies have been exposed to different pharmacological and non-pharmacological treatments before entering studies. This may confound the results of clinical and preclinical studies. Finally, there is no methodological homogeneity in processing experimental samples and assays. It is remarkable that despite these methodological problems a number of neurochemical findings have been replicated in the past in patients with depression and have provided researchers with insight into the underlying biology of this devastating illness.

SEROTONIN

Serotoninergic neurons are located in the brainstem where they can project to virtually every part of the central nervous system, often modulating neuronal responses to other neurotransmitters. As a result of this widespread projection pattern, 5-HT is known to be involved in the regulation of a wide variety of functions, including mood, anxiety, aggression, sleep, arousal, appetite and sexual function. However, it has to be acknowledged that the precise details of the mechanisms involved are not fully understood. Interest into the potential role of 5-HT in the pathophysiology of psychiatric disorders was spurred by the observation that hallucinogens such as lysergic acid diethylamide and psilocybin inhibit the peripheral actions of 5-HT. This led to the hypothesis that brain serotonergic function might be altered in patients with psychiatric disorders (Gaddum and Hameed, 1954; Wooley and Shaw, 1954). Further evidence for the importance of serotonergic mechanisms in depression was inferred by the observation that imipramine improved mood and boosted psychomotor activity (Kuhn, 1958). This initial observation of the antidepressant properties of imipramine led to more intensive testing in clinical trials of this compound and later the other tricyclic antidepressants and monoamine oxidase inhibitors for the treatment of depression. The results from these clinical trials, indicating that the action of antidepressant drugs involves enhancement of brain serotonergic activity, and further evidence for dysfunction at multiple levels in the serotonergic system of depressed patients culminated in the 'serotonin hypothesis' of depression (Maes and Meltzer, 1995). Whether this serotonergic dysfunction is the primary cause of depression or is a necessary risk factor remains unclear and is the subject of intensive research.

Seasonality of Serotonergic Function

One factor that has to be considered when evaluating the potential role of 5-HT in depression is the seasonal variation in central and peripheral 5-HT function in humans. There is considerable evidence in the literature suggesting a seasonal variation in several phenomena, such as mood, feeding behaviour and suicide, and that these phenomena may be related to changes in central and peripheral 5-HT function (Maes *et al.*, 1995). In healthy subjects and non-psychiatric patients several studies have described seasonal variations in central and peripheral 5-HT function. Studies of humans distinguish whether measures are static (e.g. biochemical levels in body fluids or blood elements) or dynamic (e.g. neuroendocrine responses to pharmacologic challenges).

Several lines of evidence based on static measures support the hypothesis of seasonal fluctuations of 5-HT function in humans: (1) hypothalamic 5-HT concentrations in human post-mortem brain specimens are decreased in winter after values peak in autumn (Carlsson *et al.*, 1980), (2) levels of plasma tryptophan, the precursor of 5-HT, show a bimodal seasonal pattern (Maes *et al.*, 1995), (3) platelet 5-HT uptake and ^{3}[H]-imipramine binding show a seasonal pattern, albeit with some differences in seasonal peaks and troughs (Arora and Meltzer, 1988; DeMet *et al.*, 1989; Tang

Biological Psychiatry: Edited by H. D'haenen, J.A. den Boer and P. Willner. ISBN 0-471-49198-5

and Morris, 1985; Whitaker *et al.*, 1984), (4) levels of 5-HT and its metabolites in cerebrospinal fluid show seasonal fluctuations, varying with latitude and population studied (Asberg *et al.*, 1981; Brewerton *et al.*, 1988), (5) serum melatonin concentrations demonstrate summer and winter peaks in healthy males (Arendt *et al.*, 1977), and (6) recently Neumeister *et al.* (2000) reported *in vivo* a significant reduced availability of hypothalamic 5-HT transporter sites in winter compared with summer in healthy female subjects (Figure XVIII-2.1).

There are few reports in the literature about seasonal variations in 5-HT function using dynamic measures. Joseph-Vanderpool *et al.* (1993) report a seasonal variation in behavioural responses to the administration of *meta*-chlorophenylpiperazine (mCPP) in patients with SAD, with higher 'activation/euphoria' scores in SAD patients during winter compared with summer or after successful light therapy. More recently, Cappiello *et al.* (1996) demonstrated a seasonal variation in neuroendocrine (prolactin) responses to intravenous tryptophan administration in unipolar, non-melancholic depressed patients. Interestingly, seasonality was more pronounced in female than in male patients. No such seasonal variability was found in bipolar, melancholic or psychotic patients or in healthy controls.

Altogether, substantial evidence is published in the literature arguing for a seasonal variation of central and peripheral 5-HT function in patients suffering from depression and also in healthy controls. Thus, we can hypothesize that seasonality of central and peripheral 5-HT function is physiological. It is not clear whether seasonal 5-HT fluctuations may represent a predisposing factor for depression with and without a seasonal pattern. It has to be said that the variability in the specific seasonal peaks and nadirs reported by different research groups reflects the use of different study designs, methodologies, sample sizes and measures of 5-HT function. Consequently, further studies are needed to clarify the role of seasonal variations in central and peripheral 5-HT function in the regulation of human behaviour and in the pathogenesis of mood disorders.

Tryptophan-Depletion Studies

The situation regarding how to evaluate the potential role of 5-HT in depression has been hampered by the fact that, until recently, it has not been possible to measure brain 5-HT directly, which means that researchers had to rely on indirect evidence for the involvement of this transmitter in the pathogenesis of depression and its role in antidepressant treatment modalities. Over the past few years, neurotransmitter depletion paradigms have provided another means of examining the potential role of 5-HT systems in the pathophysiology of depression and their role in pharmacological and non-pharmacological treatment modalities for depression.

The aim of tryptophan depletion is to lower brain 5-HT by depleting its precursor tryptophan. Most of the tryptophan in plasma is protein-bound, with only about 5% being left free and available to be transported into the brain across the blood–brain barrier by an active protein shuttle for which five other large amino acids (valine, leucine, isoleucine, phenylalanine and tyrosine) also compete. Once in the brain, the initial step in the biosynthesis of 5-HT is the conversion of L-tryptophan to 5-hydroxytryptophan, a reaction catalysed by the rate-limiting enzyme tryptophan hydroxylase (Fernstrom, 1983). The Michaelis constant for tryptophan hydroxylase is higher than tryptophan concentration in the brain, suggesting that under physiological conditions the activity of this enzyme is limited by the availability of the substrate (Friedman *et al.*, 1972). Animal studies have shown that the synthesis and content of 5-HT in rat brain vary in parallel with brain tryptophan concentrations (Fernstrom and Wurtman, 1971). Moreover, it has been shown that increase in brain tryptophan concentration raises 5-HT release *in vitro* (Auerbach and Lipton, 1985; Schaechter and Wurtman, 1989) and *in vivo* (Carboni *et al.*, 1989; Sharp *et al.*, 1992), although some studies disagree with these findings (Elks *et al.*, 1979; Marsden *et al.*, 1979). In summary, the concentration of brain 5-HT depends upon the availability of its precursor tryptophan.

Preclinical data show that the acute administration of a tryptophan-free amino acid mixture of essential amino acids produces a rapid and substantial decrease in plasma tryptophan levels, associated with a decrease in brain tryptophan, brain 5-HT and 5-HIAA levels in rats (Gessa *et al.*, 1974). Studies in humans show profound decreases of plasma tryptophan levels (Bell *et al.*, 2001; Moore *et al.*, 2000; Neumeister *et al.*, 1997b) and cerebrospinal fluid levels of 5-HIAA (Carpenter *et al.*, 1998; Moreno *et al.*, 2000b; Williams *et al.*, 1999) after oral administration of an amino acid mixture without tryptophan (Table XVIII-2.1).

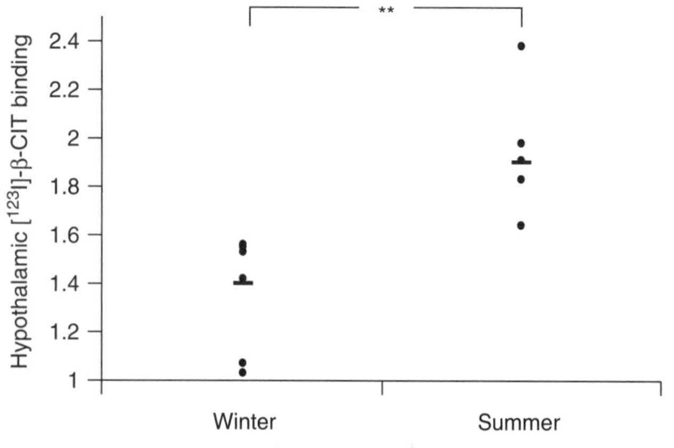

Figure XVIII-2.1 Hypothalamic serotonin transporter availability is significantly reduced in winter compared with summer in healthy female controls, as studied *in vivo* using [^{123}I]-β-CIT single photon emission computed tomography (SPECT) (Neumeister *et al.*, 2000)

Table XVIII-2.1 Amino acids used for tryptophan depletion versus sham depletion

Makes one beverage	
L-Alanine	5.5 g
Glycine	3.2 g
L-Histidine	3.2 g
L-Isoleucine	8.0 g
L-Leucine	13.5 g
L-Lysine	11.0 g
L-Phenylalanine	5.7 g
L-Proline	12.2 g
L-Serine	6.9 g
L-Threonine	6.9 g
L-Tyrosine	6.9 g
L-Valine	8.9 g
L-Methionine	12.0 g
L-Arginine	19.6 g
L-Cysteine	10.8 g
During sham depletion the beverage contains additional amino acid:	
L-Tryptophan	2.3 g

Three mechanisms appear to be responsible for the transient decrease in brain 5-HT activity during tryptophan depletion: (1) the amino acid mixture (Table XVIII-2.1) that is given to the subjects during tryptophan depletion stimulates protein synthesis in the liver, which uses up plasma tryptophan, (2) the amino acid mixture contains large amounts of the other neutral amino acids, which compete with tryptophan for the transport across the blood–brain barrier and thus restrict uptake of tryptophan into the brain and (3) a recent study showed an increase of plasma neopterin levels induced by tryptophan depletion (Stastny *et al.*, submitted). It has been shown that increased neopterin levels may facilitate catabolism of free plasma tryptophan, possibly via an interferon γ-induced activation of the tryptophan-cleaving cellular enzyme indoleamine 2,3-dioxygenase (Mellor and Munn, 1999). These mechanisms lead to the rapid and substantial, albeit transient, reduced synaptic availability of 5-HT in the brain.

The value of a depletion paradigm depends on whether the method is reliable, reversible and specific. All three issues have been addressed in several studies and have shown that the tryptophan-depletion method fulfils all three requirements for a meaningful research tool (Delgado *et al.*, 1990; Ellenbogen *et al.*, 1996; Moja *et al.*, 1989; Smith *et al.*, 1987). In particular, studies in monkeys (Young *et al.*, 1989) and humans (Moreno *et al.*, 2000b; Neumeister *et al.*, 1998c) showed that tryptophan depletion did not change the metabolism of other neurotransmitters, whereas levels of tryptophan and 5-HIAA in plasma and cerebrospinal fluid, respectively, were lowered. Thus, if the effects of tryptophan depletion can be attributed to changes in a transmitter system in the brain, it is probably 5-HT systems that are affected.

Tryptophan-Depletion Studies in Healthy Subjects

Studies of tryptophan depletion in healthy subjects have shown conflicting results. Healthy male subjects with their baseline ratings of depression in the upper normal range exhibit a transient worsening of their mood during tryptophan depletion, although never amounting to clinical depression (Smith *et al.*, 1987; Young *et al.*, 1985). In contrast, healthy male subjects who were euthymic at baseline and who were rigorously screened for any psychiatric or somatic illness remained unaffected by tryptophan depletion (Abbott *et al.*, 1992). Healthy male controls with a multigenerational family history for major affective disorders reported a greater reduction in mood induced by tryptophan depletion than healthy controls without a positive family history (Benkelfat *et al.*, 1994). Tryptophan-depletion studies in female subjects with no personal history of depression showed an increased risk to develop depressive symptoms during tryptophan depletion. In some tryptophan-depletion studies in healthy female controls family histories of affective disorders were assessed and were positive (Klaassen *et al.*, 1999), negative (Ellenbogen *et al.*, 1996; Klaassen *et al.*, 1999), or unknown (Weltzin *et al.*, 1995). These studies showed consistently an increased risk for an exacerbation of depressive symptoms during tryptophan depletion with more pronounced effects when the family history for affective disorders is positive. This is supported by a recent study in unaffected relatives of patients with bipolar affective disorders, who experience a transient lowering of their mood after tryptophan depletion (Quintin *et al.*, 2001). However, another study reported no mood-lowering effects of tryptophan depletion in healthy females with a negative family history of depression (Delgado *et al.*, 1989), and several studies report no mood-lowering effects of tryptophan depletion in healthy female subjects (Salomon *et al.*, 1997; Voderholzer *et al.*, 1998).

Other studies have focused on the memory and cognitive effects of tryptophan depletion, and have shown that tryptophan depletion impairs long-term memory formation and interferes with the process of memory consolidation (Riedel *et al.*, 1999; Schmitt *et al.*, 2000). It is noteworthy that tryptophan depletion did not affect other measures of frontal functioning. Sleep disturbances represent another key symptom of depression, so studies have been conducted to determine whether tryptophan depletion is capable of inducing sleep abnormalities, including changes in sleep continuity or architecture. Studies reported reduced REM latency after tryptophan depletion (Bhatti *et al.*, 1998; Moja *et al.*, 1979), but not unequivocally (Voderholzer *et al.*, 1998). The combination of tryptophan depletion plus administration of the 5-HT1A receptor agonist ipsapirone produced a significant suppression of REM sleep whereas tryptophan depletion alone did not significantly alter any REM sleep measure (Moore *et al.*, 2001). This differs markedly from the consistent tryptophan-depletion-induced REM-disinhibiting effect seen in medicated depressed patients. Another area of interest is whether reduced 5-HT activity during tryptophan depletion results in increased aggression since reduced brain serotonergic activity is believed to be associated with aggressive behaviour. It was shown that tryptophan depletion induces a rise in ratings of aggression in subjects with high-trait aggression but has little effect in those with low-trait aggression (Bjork *et al.*, 2000). Another study found an association between decreased serotonergic transmission and increased aggression in women who have been studied during the late luteal phase of their menstrual cycle (Bond *et al.*, 2001). Significantly, acute ethanol consumption may be associated with a decrease in tryptophan availability, and may induce aggressive behaviour in susceptible individuals (Badawy *et al.*, 1995).

Behavioural responses to tryptophan depletion in healthy subjects show a high variability. There are subgroups of subjects who appear to be at a greater risk to develop depressive symptoms during tryptophan depletion. Possible explanations include a positive family history of depression, gender and possibly high, albeit not reaching the levels of clinical depression, baseline ratings of depression. Studies that have included men and women have reported a gender difference, with a tendency for tryptophan depletion to produce more prominent mood-lowering effects in women, despite similar effects of tryptophan depletion on plasma tryptophan levels. This suggests that women may be more susceptible to the effects of tryptophan depletion than men. This is of particular interest considering the results of a positron emission tomography study of humans showing gender differences in 5-HT metabolism, with tryptophan depletion producing greater biochemical effects in women than in men (Nishizawa *et al.*, 1997). However, it has to be acknowledged that uptake of alpha-methyl L-tryptophan is not clearly established as a reliable indicator of 5-HT synthesis.

An intriguing finding is the association between the allelic distribution of the serotonin transporter gene promoter polymorphism (5-HTTLPR) and the behavioural responses to tryptophan depletion in a group of healthy women with and without family history of depression (Neumeister *et al.*, in press). The study showed subjects with the short allele of the 5-HTTLPR at increased risk to develop depressive symptoms during tryptophan depletion relative to subjects who are homozygous for the long allele. Future epidemiological studies will have to confirm the relevance of this finding, and will answer the clinically and scientifically relevant question as to whether the short allele of the 5-HTTLPR polymorphisms is associated with an increased risk for developing depression, as the authors had hypothesized. Brain imaging studies may be helpful in studying the underlying neural processes.

Tryptophan-Depletion Studies in Depression

To test the hypothesis that decreased 5-HT function is associated with depression, several studies were performed including untreated, symptomatic depressed patients prior to initiation of an antidepressant treatment (Delgado *et al.*, 1994; Neumeister *et al.*,

1997c; Price *et al.*, 1997, 1998). It was hypothesized that tryptophan depletion would lead to an exacerbation of the depressive syndrome. However, the results of these studies were somewhat unexpected. Consistently, it was shown that tryptophan depletion did not exacerbate depressive symptoms in these subjects. Remarkably, in two studies (Delgado *et al.*, 1994; Price *et al.*, 1998) some patients showed an improvement of their condition on the day after tryptophan depletion. The failure to aggravate depression by depleting brain 5-HT can be explained by the hypothesis that brain 5-HT function is already maximally dysfunctional in depressed patients and thus further lowering of 5-HT activity has no further effects on depressive symptoms. Alternatively, it can be hypothesized that disturbed 5-HT function does not explain the biological basis of depression, and that there is no direct relationship between severity of depressive symptoms and brain 5-HT function. A possible explanation for the improvement in symptoms the day after tryptophan depletion is an upregulation of postsynaptic 5-HT receptors because of the decreased release of 5-HT at the synapse during tryptophan depletion. Typically, 5-HT levels are restored the day after tryptophan depletion and the net effect is an enhancement of brain 5-HT function, resulting in an improvement of the patient's condition.

A recent study (Berman *et al.*, in press) evaluated whether combined tryptophan depletion and catecholamine depletion compared with tryptophan depletion and sham depletion would aggravate the depressive syndrome in unmedicated, symptomatic depressed patients. The authors report a progressive decrease in Hamilton depression scores in both groups with no difference between the combined monoamine-depletion group and the tryptophan-depletion group. This finding that simultaneous disruptions of 5-HT function and catecholamine function do not exacerbate depressive symptoms in untreated symptomatic depressed subjects supports the hypothesis that monoamines have an indirect role in regulating mood in actively depressed patients.

Intensive research using tryptophan depletion has been done during the past few years to study the role of 5-HT in the mechanism of action of antidepressant drugs, and non-pharmacological treatments for depression, such as light therapy and sleep deprivation. The hypothesis of these studies was that antidepressant treatments lead to an enhancement of brain 5-HT function and that tryptophan depletion will disrupt the antidepressant effects. This has now been tested in multiple studies, and researchers have found that tryptophan depletion reverses the antidepressant effects of antidepressant medications, in particular of agents with a predominantly serotonergic mode of action (Aberg-Wistedt *et al.*, 1998; Bremner *et al.*, 1997; Delgado *et al.*, 1990, 1999; Spillmann *et al.*, 2001). It should be noted, however, that tryptophan depletion causes clinically relevant symptoms only in about 50–60% of the patients, and one study reported no mood effects of tryptophan depletion at all (Moore *et al.*, 1998). However, the majority of studies clearly demonstrated that the depressive symptoms evoked by tryptophan depletion were often similar to those the patients had experienced during their depressive episode. As noted above, the behavioural responses to tryptophan depletion were substantially more prominent in subjects who had been successfully treated with selective 5-HT reuptake inhibitors (SSRIs) relative to the responses in those subjects who had responded to a treatment with noradrenergic antidepressants (Delgado *et al.*, 1999; Miller *et al.*, 1996a). This finding, and the finding that catecholamine depletion predominantly induces a depressive relapse in subjects treated with noradrenergic antidepressants, suggests that enhanced serotonergic or noradrenergic transmission is necessary to maintain the antidepressant responses to SSRIs or noradrenergic agents, respectively (Figure XVIII-2.2). Other variables that may affect the reoccurrence of depressive symptoms during tryptophan depletion are the length of the remitted state of the patient, with a greater likelihood of depressive symptom exacerbation when the duration of remission is short, the number of previous depressive episodes, and the pattern of response to the antidepressant treatment. Patients who responded to treatment with placebo seem to be less vulnerable to the effects of tryptophan depletion than 'true' drug responders. This suggests that antidepressants induce biological changes in the neuron that make the subjects less vulnerable to acute changes in brain 5-HT function.

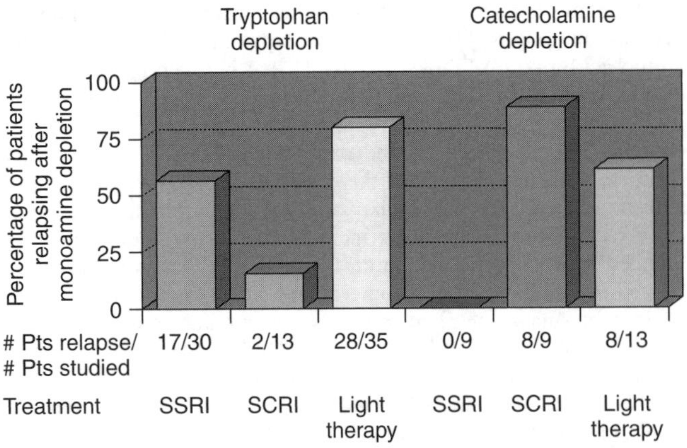

Figure XVIII-2.2 Tryptophan depletion induces a depressive relapse predominantly in patients remitted on selective serotonin reuptake inhibitors (SSRIs), but not in patients remitted on selective catecholamine reuptake inhibitors (SCRIs). In contrast, catecholamine depletion induces an exacerbation of depressive symptoms in patients remitted on SCRIs but not in patients remitted on SSRIs. Patients remitted on light therapy show a depressive relapse in both, tryptophan depletion and catecholamine depletion

Non-pharmacological, albeit biologically based, treatments for depression include light therapy and sleep deprivation. Light therapy is the treatment of first choice for patients suffering from seasonal depressions during autumn and winter, and has been shown to be effective in non-seasonal depression when given in conjunction with other antidepressant treatment modalities (Neumeister *et al.*, 1999b). Tryptophan depletion (Neumeister *et al.*, 1997a, 1998c) and catecholamine depletion (Neumeister *et al.*, 1998c) reversed the antidepressant effects of light therapy, suggesting that both transmitter systems are involved in the mechanism of action of light therapy. Several lines of evidence suggest that sleep deprivation exerts its antidepressant effects by enhancing serotonergic transmission. To test this hypothesis, patients who responded to a single night of total sleep deprivation underwent tryptophan depletion or sham depletion (Neumeister *et al.*, 1998b). It was expected that tryptophan depletion would reverse the antidepressant effects of sleep deprivation. Unexpectedly, tryptophan depletion did not reverse the antidepressant effects of sleep deprivation, but rather prevented the otherwise naturally occurring depressive relapse after the recovery night. The authors concluded that it seems to be unlikely that serotonin alone mediates the antidepressant effects of sleep deprivation; however, serotonergic mechanisms may play an important role.

The effects of tryptophan depletion in formerly depressed, fully remitted patients, off medication is of particular interest to understand the role of 5-HT in the pathogenesis of the disorder. It might be expected that these subjects are specifically vulnerable to the depressiogenic effects of tryptophan depletion. The majority of the studies (Moreno *et al.*, 1999; Neumeister *et al.*, 1998a; Smith *et al.*, 1997) reported a depressive relapse induced by tryptophan depletion whereas subjects remained well during sham depletion. However, two studies found no exacerbation of depression during tryptophan depletion (Lam *et al.*, 2000; Leyton *et al.*, 1997). These discrepancies may be explained by the differing length of remission among the different studies, and by differing study populations. Furthermore, a recent study in remitted depressed patients shows, similar to the effects of antidepressant treatment, that tryptophan depletion is associated with a decrease in 5-HT$_2$ receptor binding (Yatham *et al.*, 2001). This might have explained the failure of tryptophan depletion to exacerbate depressive symptoms in this study. The depressive relapse induced by tryptophan depletion in remitted patients off therapy suggests that at least a subgroup of patients with depression remain vulnerable to changes in 5-HT function. Interestingly, two studies showed that the majority of subjects who relapsed during tryptophan depletion experienced further depressive episodes in the near future (Moreno *et al.*, 2000a; Neumeister *et al.*, 1999a). Thus, tryptophan depletion may be capable of predicting the future course of depression.

Altogether, tryptophan-depletion studies have been shown to provide a way of examining the role of 5-HT in the pathophysiology of depression and the mechanism of action of antidepressants. The behavioural responses to tryptophan depletion provide insight into the underlying biology of depression, and suggest that serotonergic mechanisms may play a key role in the disorder. Many questions remain unanswered but tryptophan depletion may be a research tool to study gene–environment interactions in the future, and therefore may lead to further understanding of the processes involved in the pathophysiology of depression.

Serotonin 1A Receptor Function in Depression

Most 5-HT receptors belong to the family of G protein-coupled receptors (GPCRs), a large group of proteins that transduce signals through coupling to guanine nucleotide-binding regulatory proteins. Serotonin receptors are classified into seven groups according to their ligand-binding affinity profiles, molecular structures and intracellular transduction mechanisms. The human 5-HT$_1$ receptor subfamily includes 5-HT$_{1A}$, 5-HT$_{1B}$, 5-HT$_{1D}$, 5-HT$_{1E}$ and 5-HT$_{1F}$ receptors. Multiple lines of evidence suggest that 5-HT$_{1A}$ receptor functions are abnormal in depression. The data supporting this hypothesis have been obtained by assessing neuroendocrine and temperature responses to 5-HT$_{1A}$ receptor agonists in depressed subjects versus healthy controls (Lesch, 1992), measuring 5-HT$_{1A}$ receptor density in brain tissue acquired post-mortem (Bowen *et al.*, 1989; Lopez *et al.*, 1998) and examining 5-HT$_{1A}$ receptor functions in rats following administration of antidepressant drugs (Artigas *et al.*, 1996; Chaput *et al.*, 1991; Haddjeri *et al.*, 1998).

Human 5-HT$_{1A}$ receptors are expressed presynaptically on 5HT cell bodies in the raphe (somatodendritic autoreceptors) and postsynaptically in other brain regions (Azmitia and Whitaker-Azmitia, 1991). In humans and monkeys, the density of 5-HT$_{1A}$ receptors is very high in the raphe and parts of the hippocampal formation, high in hypothalamus, insula, temporal, cingulate and ventral prefrontal cortices, moderately high in occipital and parietal cortices, and very low in the cerebellum, striatum, thalamus and white matter. In the cortex, hippocampus and amygdala postsynaptic 5-HT$_{1A}$ receptors are located on pyramidal cells and interneurons, and stimulation of these receptors generally inhibits glutamate-mediated depolarization of parent neuron (Azmitia and Whitaker-Azmitia, 1991; Sprouse and Aghajanian, 1988).

5-HT$_{1A}$ autoreceptors constitute an important control point for serotonergic activity in the brain. Stimulation of presynaptic 5-HT$_{1A}$ autoreceptors similarly inhibits the 5-HT neuron firing in the raphe, reducing 5HT release, and can reduce 5HT synthesis via inhibition of tryptophan hydroxylase (Briley and Moret, 1993; Chaput and de Montigny, 1988; Chaput *et al.*, 1986; Sprouse and Aghajanian, 1988). Postsynaptic 5-HT$_{1A}$ receptors are also abundantly expressed by astrocytes and some other glia (Azmitia *et al.*, 1996). These 5-HT$_{1A}$ receptors are expressed by the majority of astrocytes in frontal and limbic cortex, but essentially none of the astroglia in striatum, thalamus or cerebellum (Whitaker-Azmitia *et al.*, 1993). Stimulation of astrocyte-based 5-HT$_{1A}$ sites causes astrocytes to acquire a more mature morphology and to release the trophic factor S-100B, which promotes growth and arborization of serotonergic axons (Whitaker-Azmitia and Azmitia, 1989; Whitaker-Azmitia *et al.*, 1990). S-100B is primarily released by astroglia in the developing brain, when it plays a role in the development of the serotonergic system. S-100B also plays a role in maintaining the cytoskeleton in adult animals by promoting tubulin polymerization and inhibiting PKC-mediated breakdown of microtubules (Azmitia, 1999). In addition, stimulation of neuron-based 5-HT$_{1A}$ receptors inhibits PKA-mediated disassociation of the proteins comprising the tubulin polymers of the cytoskeleton. Administration of 5-HT$_{1A}$ receptor antagonists, antibodies to S-100B or agents that deplete 5-HT all produce similar losses of dendrites, spines and/or synapses in adult and developing animals, effects which are blocked by administration of 5-HT$_{1A}$ receptor agonists or SSRIs. The role of postsynaptic 5-HT$_{1A}$ receptor function in maintenance of the cytoskeleton has led to the hypothesis that a reduction of 5-HT$_{1A}$ receptor function may comprise a risk factor for the neuropathological abnormalities identified in limbic and paralimbic cortical areas in mood disorders (reduced cortex volume, reduced synaptic proteins, increased neuronal density, reduced glial counts) (Drevets, 2000; McEwen, 1999).

5-HT$_{1A}$ Receptor Imaging in Depression

Positron emission tomography (PET) studies obtained *in vivo* show evidence of reduced pre- and postsynaptic 5-HT$_{1A}$ receptor binding in depression. Drevets and colleagues (Drevets *et al.*, 1999) demonstrated that the mean 5-HT$_{1A}$ receptor binding potential (BP) was reduced in the mesiotemporal cortex and raphe in unmedicated depressives relative to controls using PET and [*carbonyl*-^{11}C]WAY-100635. A similar reduction was evident in the parietal cortex, striate cortex and left orbital cortex/ventrolateral prefrontal cortex. These data were consistent with those of Sargent *et al.* (2000), who found decreased 5-HT$_{1A}$ receptor BP in unmedicated depressives relative to healthy controls in the raphe, mesiotemporal cortex, insula, anterior cingulate, temporal polar cortex, ventrolateral prefrontal cortex and orbital cortex. A subgroup of the subjects were scanned both pre- and post-paroxetine treatment, and 5-HT$_{1A}$ receptor BP did not significantly change in any area.

These data were compatible with 5-HT$_{1A}$ receptor agonist challenge results showing that unmedicated depressed subjects have blunted hypothermic and adrenocorticotropin (ACTH) and cortisol release in response to ipsapirone or buspirone, relative to healthy controls (Lesch, 1992). The degree of blunting correlated with depression severity (Rausch *et al.*, 1990). Since 5-HT$_{1A}$-receptor-stimulation-induced hypothermia and ACTH/cortisol release are thought to distinguish pre- and postsynaptic 5-HT$_{1A}$ receptor stimulation, respectively, in humans and rats, these findings were compatible with the PET data implicating both pre- and postsynaptic 5-HT$_{1A}$ receptors in depression. Abnormally decreased 5-HT$_{1A}$ receptor BP in depression may reflect either downregulation of receptor density or a reduction in the number of brain cells expressing 5-HT$_{1A}$ receptors. The likelihood that abnormal 5-HT$_{1A}$ receptor binding in primary mood disorders is accounted for by differences in nonspecific binding is reduced by the high selectivity of [*carbonyl*-^{11}C]WAY-100635 for 5-HT$_{1A}$ receptors. Furthermore, reduced [^{11}C]WAY-100635 binding in depression is not expected to reflect a compensatory response to abnormal 5-HT release, or an effect of endogenous 5-HT concentrations on radiotracer binding. The 5-HT$_{1A}$ receptor density and mRNA expression appear insensitive to reducing 5-HT transmission by lesioning the raphe or administering PCPA, or to pharmacologically induced increases in 5-HT concentrations. Moreover, in baboons administration of agents which increase 5-HT release, including fenfluramine, citalopram, and amphetamine, does not alter [^{11}C]WAY-100635 binding (Parsey *et al.*, 1998). The insensitivity to endogenous 5-HT is partly related to the ~50-fold greater 5-HT_{1A} receptor affinity of WAY-100635 relative to endogenous 5-HT (based upon K_D).

Altogether, reductions in 5-HT_{1A} receptor binding in depression may reflect alterations in the cellular elements that express these receptors, or in the factors that downregulate genetic expression of these receptors. Preclinical and clinical data suggest that 5-HT_{1A} receptors play a key role in the regulation of brain 5-HT activity and thus may be a target for novel antidepressant and antianxiety drugs with a more directed mechanism of action and possibly with a more favourable side effect profile.

NORADRENALIN

There is much data available supporting the hypothesis of a noradrenergic deficiency in depression (Delgado, 2000; Heninger *et al.*, 1996). The original catecholamine deficiency hypothesis of depression proposed that depression is a result of decreased catecholaminergic activity, whereas mania is associated with a relative excess (Schildkraut, 1965). In early reports urinary levels of MHPG were found to be significantly lower in patients with unipolar depression relative to healthy controls. However, these findings have not been consistently replicated. The original concept that depression is associated with decreased levels of catecholamines (for overview see Schatzberg and Schildkraut, 1995) as assessed with measurements of norepinephrine and its metabolites in peripheral samples has been invaluable in developing concepts of the biological mechanisms underlying depressive disorders and has served as a rich source from which researchers have generated testable experimental hypotheses. A recent study showing pronounced and sustained central hypernoradrenergic function in depression with melancholic features (Wong *et al.*, 2000) supports these early observations. New techniques such as brain imaging or depletion paradigms have provided new insight into the role of catecholaminergic mechanisms in the pathophysiology of mood disorders. Such studies have confirmed initial hypotheses that have suggested a pivotal role for noradrenergic systems in the pathophysiology of depression.

Catecholamine Depletion Studies

Of various methods employed for modifying the functions of sympathetic nervous systems, a unique and successful one has been the inhibition of catecholamine biosynthesis by α-methyl-para-tyrosine (AMPT) (Engelman *et al.*, 1968a; Sjoerdsma *et al.*, 1965). AMPT decreases norepinephrine and dopamine levels via inhibition of tyrosine hydroxylase, a rate-limiting enzyme in the synthesis of both transmitters (Widerlov and Lewander, 1978). AMPT is adequately absorbed from the gastrointestinal tract and the degree of inhibition achieved in man approximates the values, which could be predicted from the plasma levels of the drug (Engelman *et al.*, 1968b). In clinical investigations, AMPT (in dosages ranging from 1 g per day to 4 g per day) leads to profound decreases in urinary excretion of catecholamine metabolites and cerebrospinal fluid levels of the dopamine metabolite homovanillic acid (HVA) with no change in the 5-HT metabolite 5-hydroxyindoleacetic acid (5-HIAA) (Brodie *et al.*, 1971; Engelman *et al.*, 1968a; Sjoerdsma *et al.*, 1965). A maximal reduction of catecholamine metabolites during AMPT treatment occurs after 2–3 days of treatment (Bunney *et al.*, 1971; Engelman *et al.*, 1968b). It has been shown that about 20% of the urinary MHPG is derived from the central nervous system pool (Potter *et al.*, 1984).

Catecholamine Depletion Studies in Healthy Subjects

In order to evaluate the role of catecholamines in regulation of mood, anxiety and alertness, and its potential role in the pathogenesis of psychiatric disorders, it is also important to study the effects of catecholamine depletion in healthy volunteers. Treatment with AMPT has been shown to induce pronounced increases in sleepiness and mild increases in negative mood and anxiety, when administered to healthy male controls (McCann *et al.*, 1995). Significantly, replacement of catecholamine stores with L-DOPA reversed the effects of catecholamine depletion, and was associated with a more rapid recovery from AMPT's effects than when subjects were treated with AMPT alone. Another study of the same group comparing the psychological effects of AMPT alone versus AMPT plus 40.5 hours of total sleep deprivation (McCann *et al.*, 1993) suggests that catecholamines may be involved in mood changes during sleep deprivation. Combined treatment with AMPT and sleep deprivation led to significant increases in negative mood, whereas no treatment alone produced consistent mood changes. With the use of a different methodology to deplete catecholamines, by administering an amino acid mixture deficient of phenylalanine and tyrosine, Leyton and colleagues (Leyton *et al.*, 2000b) induced lowered mood and energy and increased irritability scores in a group of healthy women. Interestingly, the behavioural changes induced by catecholamine depletion were similar to those found during tryptophan depletion in the same group of subjects. In both conditions, the behavioural effects were more pronounced following exposure to aversive psychological events. Another study suggests that acutely decreased catecholamine transmission may disrupt mechanisms mediating alcohol self-administration (Leyton *et al.*, 2000a). Altogether, these studies support the role of catecholamines in a variety of human behaviours and also suggest that disturbed catecholamine transmission may predispose humans to various psychiatric disorders, including depression and different anxiety disorders.

Catecholamine Depletion Studies in Depression

The role of norepinephrine and dopamine in the pathogenesis of depression and in the mechanisms of action of antidepressant drugs have been subjects of intensive research during the past decades. A comprehensive overview of catecholaminergic function in depression is beyond the scope of this chapter. The purpose of the present chapter is to show the biochemical and behavioural effects of catecholamine depletion in depressed patients in different states of their illness, and their implications in our understanding of the pathogenesis of depression and its treatment. In the initial studies performed by Bunney and colleagues at the National Institute of Health (Bunney *et al.*, 1971) the authors demonstrated the antimanic effects of AMPT in a small group of manic patients, whereas three of four unipolar psychotic depressed patients showed an increase of depression on AMPT. However, small sample sizes and the lack of a control group or a placebo condition limit the interpretation of these initial findings. More recent studies addressing these methodological shortcomings showed that drug-free, untreated, symptomatic depressed patients had significant increased visual analogue ratings of 'tired' and decreased ratings of 'energetic'. However, there was no alteration in mood reported by the authors (Miller *et al.*, 1996b). This finding suggests that a simple norepinephrine or dopamine deficiency hypothesis is insufficient to explain the neurobiological basis of depression. Rather, the role of noradrenergic systems needs to be considered in relationship to many other neurobiological factors that may be involved in the pathogenesis of depression. An alternative explanation could be that during a depressive state the catecholamine systems are already maximally dysfunctional and thus further manipulations do not worsen the condition of the patient.

Studies of the effects of AMPT on patients remitted on antidepressants or remitted depressed patients off medications provided further insight into the pathogenesis of depression and mechanisms of action of different antidepressants. Depressed patients in remission and on noradrenergic antidepressants (desipramine and mazindol) experienced a depressive relapse during catecholamine depletion, whereas those patients whose remissions were maintained with the selective 5-HT reuptake inhibitors (SSRIs) fluoxetine and sertraline remained well during catecholamine depletion (Miller *et al.*, 1996a). The administration of AMPT induced core symptoms of depression, such as depressed mood, loss of interest, anhedonia, cognitive disturbances, and sense of worthlessness and failure. Another study reported the reoccurrence of depressive symptoms induced by catecholamine depletion in a group of patients with seasonal affective disorder/winter type remitted on light therapy (Neumeister *et al.*, 1998c), supporting recent findings of reduced dopaminergic function in untreated patients with winter depression (Neumeister *et al.*, 2001). These findings disagree with a small study of three depressed patients with a favourable treatment response to imipramine (Shopsin *et al.*, 1975). However, beside the sample size of that study being small and there being no control situation, it has to be considered that imipramine is a potent 5-HT reuptake inhibitor as well as a norepinephrine reuptake inhibitor. The findings that catecholamine depletion disrupts the antidepressant effects of catecholaminergic, but not serotonergic, antidepressants, whereas tryptophan depletion reverses the antidepressant effects of serotonergic antidepressants, but not catecholaminergic antidepressants (Delgado *et al.*, 1999), argue against a single monoamine-related mechanism of action of antidepressants. However, such studies suggest that enhanced catecholamine function is important to maintain response to noradrenergic antidepressants, and enhanced serotonergic function is important to maintain response to serotonergic antidepressants.

State-related changes in catecholamine function have been described in depressed subjects, whereas enduring abnormalities have been less reliably identified. Recent catecholamine depletion studies in fully remitted, medication-free, formerly depressed subjects showed a depressive relapse in these subjects during catecholamine depletion, but not during sham depletion (Berman *et al.*, 1999; Lam *et al.*, 2001). The authors argue that the reoccurrence of depressive symptoms during catecholamine depletion may represent a reliable marker for a history of depression, and may well be a trait marker for the disorder. Further studies are needed to clarify the importance of these findings.

α_2-Adrenergic Receptors

Neurotransmission in the noradrenergic system is mediated by a number of different neurotransmitter receptors whose function has been implicated in either the pathophysiology of depression or in the mechanism of action of antidepressants (Duman and Nestler, 1995). The α_2-adrenergic receptors (α_2-AR) have been the focus of considerable research on their role in the pathophysiology of depression. The α_2-ARs are a heterogeneous group of receptors that bind to the naturally occurring ligands epinephrine and norepinephrine (O'Dowd *et al.*, 1989; Venter *et al.*, 1989). α_2-ARs mediate their functions through the G_i class of G proteins (Lefkowitz and Caron, 1988; Limbird, 1988). The α_2-ARs are located on nerve terminals and on the cell bodies and/or dendrites, and participate in local and neuronal feedback inhibition (Cedarbaum and Aghajanian, 1977; Hein *et al.*, 1999; Langer, 1997; Miller, 1998; Stjarne, 1989). Activation of these receptors by endogenous ligands or α_2-agonists, e.g. clonidine, decreases noradrenalin release and the firing rate of the neurons (Engberg and Eriksson, 1991; Hein *et al.*, 1999; MacDonald *et al.*, 1991) and results in bradycardia, hypotension, hypothermia, locomotor inhibition, anxiolysis, analgesia and sedation (Aantaa and Scheinin, 1993; Altman *et al.*, 1999; Hein *et al.*, 1999; Lakhlani *et al.*, 1997; Puke and Wiesenfeld-Hallin, 1993; Rohrer and Kobilka, 1998; Ruffolo *et al.*, 1993; Sallinen *et al.*, 1999). Clonidine is a partial agonist at brain α_2-ARs, but also has high affinity for non-adrenergic imidazoline-binding sites. It has been shown that the distribution of non-adrenergic [^{3}H]-clonidine binding sites is correlated but distinct from that of α_2-ARs, and that the affinity of these sites is distinct from α_2-AR sites (Piletz *et al.*, 2000). Blockade of α_2-ARs by α_2-antagonists, e.g. yohimbine, increases the firing rate and responsiveness of neurons to stimulation (Simson and Weiss, 1987; Tjurmina *et al.*, 1999) and promotes release of noradrenalin (Freedman and Aghajanian, 1984; Grossman *et al.*, 1991; Scheinin *et al.*, 1988; Starke *et al.*, 1975). It has to be acknowledged that interpretation of data from yohimbine challenge studies is complicated by mixed drug effects due to the blockade of both pre- and postsynaptic α_2-ARs in the hypothalamus and presynaptic D_2 dopaminergic autoreceptors in the pituitary (Meltzer *et al.*, 1983). In addition, yohimbine exhibits affinity to 5-HT$_{1A}$ receptors, although yohimbine is tenfold selective for human α_{2A}-ARs versus human 5-HT$_{1A}$ receptors (Newman-Tancredi *et al.*, 1998). In addition to these α_2-auto-AR, α_2-heteroreceptors have been identified, which are located elsewhere than on noradrenergic neurons. These heteroreceptors are involved in the regulation of release of a variety of neurotransmitters, including serotonin (Gobert *et al.*, 1997, 1998; Mongeau *et al.*, 1993; Raiteri *et al.*, 1990), dopamine (Gobert *et al.*, 1997, 1998; Trendelenburg *et al.*, 1994), and histamine (Gulat-Marnay *et al.*, 1989). Activation of α_2-ARs by α_2-agonists reduces the turnover of norepinephrine, serotonin and dopamine in the brain.

It has been demonstrated that α_2-ARs mediate a variety of physiological functions and pharmacological effects in the central nervous system, mainly by inhibiting neuronal firing and release of noradrenalin and other neurotransmitters. A wide range of functions in peripheral tissues is also mediated by α_2-ARs, including regulation of noradrenalin release from sympathetic nerves, smooth muscle contraction, platelet aggregation, insulin secretion, glomerular filtration and energy metabolism (Ruffolo *et al.*, 1993).

The α_2-ARs have been the focus of considerable research on their role in the pathogenesis of depression (Charney *et al.*, 1981; Cohen *et al.*, 1980; McKenna *et al.*, 1992; Piletz *et al.*, 1986; Smith *et al.*, 1983). An increase in the density of platelet α_2-ARs has been reported in drug-free depressives. Also, the platelet aggregation response has been reported as being enhanced in depression. The findings of increased α_2-AR density in depression, both in the central nervous system and in the periphery, have not been consistently replicated. Blunted growth hormone responses have been reported in depressive patients in different states — untreated, treated with antidepressants, and when being remitted. This argues that alterations in α_2-AR function may be a trait characteristic in at least a subgroup of depressed patients.

SUMMARY

The data obtained from studies evaluating the role of monoamines in the pathophysiology of mood disorders, in particular depression, and in antidepressant treatments provide evidence that monoamines do not have a direct effect on regulating mood, but rather have a modulator role on other neurobiological systems. However, there is substantial evidence that adequate monoaminergic activity in the brain is necessary to achieve and maintain an antidepressant response to antidepressant treatments. Future research should try to further increase our knowledge about the interactions between serotonergic and noradrenergic transmitter systems and other neurobiological systems. This may become of clinical relevance since preclinical studies have revealed potential molecular and anatomic sites that could contribute to the development of future generations of antidepressant agents.

REFERENCES

Aantaa, R. and Scheinin, M., 1993. Alpha 2-adrenergic agents in anaesthesia. *Acta Anaesthesiol. Scand.*, **37**, 433–48.

Abbott, F.V., Etienne, P., Franklin, K.B., Morgan, M.J., Sewitch, M.J. and Young, S.N., 1992. Acute tryptophan depletion blocks morphine analgesia in the cold-pressor test in humans. *Psychopharmacology*, **108**, 60–6.

Aberg-Wistedt, A., Hasselmark, L., Stain-Malmgren, R., Aperia, B., Kjellman, B.F. and Mathé, A.A., 1998. Serotonergic 'vulnerability' in affective disorder: a study of the tryptophan depletion test and relationships between peripheral and central serotonin indexes in citalopram-responders. *Acta Psychiat. Scand.*, **97**, 374–80.

Altman, J.D., Trendelenburg, A.U., MacMillan, L., Bernstein, D., Limbird, L., Starke, K., Kobilka, B.K. and Hein, L., 1999. Abnormal regulation of the sympathetic nervous system in alpha2A-adrenergic receptor knockout mice. *Molec. Pharmacol.*, **56**, 154–61.

American Psychiatric Association, 1994. *Diagnostic and Statistical Manual of Mental Disorders*, 4th edn, American Psychiatric Association, Washington, DC.

Arendt, J., Wirz-Justice, A. and Bradtke, J., 1977. Circadian, diurnal and circannual rhythms of serum melatonin and platelet serotonin in man. *Chronobiologia*, **4**, 96–7.

Arora, R.C. and Meltzer, H.Y., 1988. Seasonal variation of imipramine binding in the blood platelets of normal controls and depressed patients. *Biol. Psychiat.*, **23**, 217–26.

Artigas, F., Romero, L., de Montigny, C. and Blier, P., 1996. Acceleration of the effect of selected antidepressant drugs in major depression by 5-HT1A antagonists. *Trends Neurosci.*, **19**, 378–83.

Asberg, M., Bertilsson, L., Rydin, E., Schalling, D., Thoren, P. and Traskman-Bendz, L., 1981. Monoamine metabolites in cerebrospinal fluid in relation to depressive illness, suicidal behavior and personality. In: Angrist, B., Burrows, G.D. and Lader, M. (eds), *Recent Advances in Neuropsychopharmacology* pp. 257–71. Pergamon Press, Oxford.

Auerbach, S. and Lipton, P., 1985. Regulation of serotonin release from the *in vitro* rat hippocampus: effects of alterations in levels of depolarization and in rates of serotonin metabolism. *J. Neurochem.*, **44**, 1116–30.

Azmitia, E.C., 1999. Serotonin neurons, neuroplasticity, and homeostasis of neural tissue. *Neuropsychopharmacology*, **21**, 33S–45S.

Azmitia, E.C. and Whitaker-Azmitia, P.M., 1991. Awakening the sleeping giant: anatomy and plasticity of the brain serotonergic system. *J. Clin. Psychiat.*, **52**(suppl), 4–16.

Azmitia, E.C., Gannon, P.J., Kheck, N.M. and Whitaker-Azmitia, P.M., 1996. Cellular localization of the 5-HT1A receptor in primate brain neurons and glial cells. *Neuropsychopharmacology*, **14**, 35–46.

Badawy, A.A., Morgan, C.J., Lovett, J.W., Bradley, D.M. and Thomas, R., 1995. Decrease in circulating tryptophan availability to the brain after acute ethanol consumption by normal volunteers: implications for alcohol-induced aggressive behaviour and depression. *Pharmacopsychiatry*, **28**(suppl 2), 93–7.

Bell, C., Abrams, J. and Nutt, D., 2001. Tryptophan depletion and its implications for psychiatry. *Br. J. Psychiat.*, **178**, 399–405.

Benkelfat, C., Ellenbogen, M.A., Dean, P., Palmour, R.M. and Young, S.N., 1994. Mood-lowering effect of tryptophan depletion. Enhanced susceptibility in young men at genetic risk for major affective disorders. *Arch. Gen. Psychiat.*, **51**, 687–97.

Berman, R.M., Narasimhan, M., Miller, H.L., Anand, A., Cappiello, A., Oren, D.A., Heninger, G.R. and Charney, D.S., 1999. Transient depressive relapse induced by catecholamine depletion: potential phenotypic vulnerability marker? *Arch. Gen. Psychiat.*, **56**, 395–403.

Berman, R.M., Sanacora, G., Anand, A., *et al.* (in press) Monoamine depletion in unmedicated depressed subjects. *Biol. Psychiat.*

Bhatti, T., Gillin, J.C., Seifritz, E., Moore, P., Clark, C., Golshan, S., Stahl, S., Rapaport, M. and Kelsoe, J., 1998. Effects of a tryptophan-free amino acid drink challenge on normal human sleep electroencephalogram and mood. *Biol. Psychiat.*, **43**, 52–9.

Bjork, J.M., Dougherty, D.M., Moeller, F.G. and Swann, A.C., 2000. Differential behavioral effects of plasma tryptophan depletion and loading in aggressive and nonaggressive men. *Neuropsychopharmacology*, **22**, 357–69.

Bond, A.J., Wingrove, J. and Critchlow, D.G., 2001. Tryptophan depletion increases aggression in women during the premenstrual phase. *Psychopharmacology (Berl)*, **156**, 477–80.

Bowen, D.M., Najlerahim, A., Procter, A.W., Francis, P.T. and Murphy, E., 1989. Circumscribed changes of the cerebral cortex in neuropsychiatric disorders of later life. *Proc. Natl Acad. Sci. USA*, **86**, 9504–8.

Bremner, J.D., Innis, R.B., Salomon, R.M., Staib, L.H., Ng, C.K., Miller, H.L., Bronen, R.A., Krystal, J.H., Duncan, J., Rich, D., Price, L.H., Malison, R., Dey, H., Soufer, R. and Charney, D.S., 1997. Positron emission tomography measurement of cerebral metabolic correlates of tryptophan depletion-induced depressive relapse. *Arch. Gen. Psychiat.*, **54**, 364–74.

Brewerton, T.D., Berrettini, W.H., Nurnberger, J.I., Jr and Linnoila, M., 1988. Analysis of seasonal fluctuations of CSF monoamine metabolites and neuropeptides in normal controls: findings with 5HIAA and HVA. *Psychiat. Res.*, **23**, 257–65.

Briley, M. and Moret, C., 1993. Neurobiological mechanisms involved in antidepressant therapies. *Clin. Neuropharmacol.*, **16**, 387–400.

Brodie, H.K., Murphy, D.L., Goodwin, F.K. and Bunney, W.E., Jr, 1971. Catecholamines and mania: the effect of alpha-methyl-para-tyrosine on manic behavior and catecholamine metabolism. *Clin. Pharmacol. Ther.*, **12**, 218–24.

Bunney, W.E., Jr and Davis, J.M., 1965. Norepinephrine in depressive reactions a review. *Arch. Gen. Psychiat.*, **13**, 483–94.

Bunney, W.E., Jr, Brodie, H.K., Murphy, D.L. and Goodwin, F.K., 1971. Studies of alpha-methyl-para-tyrosine, L-dopa, and L-tryptophan in depression and mania. *Am. J. Psychiat.*, **127**, 872–81.

Cappiello, A., Malison, R.T., McDougle, C.J., Vegso, S.J., Charney, D.S., Heninger, G.R. and Price, L.H., 1996. Seasonal variation in neuroendocrine and mood responses to i.v. L-tryptophan in depressed patients and healthy subjects. *Neuropsychopharmacology*, **15**, 475–83.

Carboni, E., Cadoni, C., Tanda, G.L. and Di Chiara, G., 1989. Calcium-dependent, tetrodotoxin-sensitive stimulation of cortical serotonin release after a tryptophan load. *J. Neurochem.*, **53**, 976–8.

Carlsson, A., Svennerholm, L. and Winblad, B., 1980. Seasonal and circadian monoamine variations in human brains examined post mortem. *Acta Psychiat. Scand.*, **280**(suppl), 75–85.

Carpenter, L.L., Anderson, G.M., Pelton, G.H., Gudin, J.A., Kirwin, P.D., Price, L.H., Heninger, G.R. and McDougle, C.J., 1998. Tryptophan depletion during continuous CSF sampling in healthy human subjects. *Neuropsychopharmacology*, **19**, 26–35.

Cedarbaum, J.M. and Aghajanian, G.K., 1977. Catecholamine receptors on locus coeruleus neurons: pharmacological characterization. *Eur. J. Pharmacol.*, **44**, 375–85.

Chaput, Y. and de Montigny, C., 1988. Effects of the 5-hydroxytryptamine receptor antagonist, BMY 7378, on 5-hydroxytryptamine neurotransmission: electrophysiological studies in the rat central nervous system. *J. Pharmacol. Exp. Ther.*, **246**, 359–70.

Chaput, Y., de Montigny, C. and Blier, P., 1986. Effects of a selective 5-HT reuptake blocker, citalopram, on the sensitivity of 5-HT autoreceptors: electrophysiological studies in the rat brain. *Naunyn-Schmiedebergs Arch. Pharmacol.*, **333**, 342–8.

Chaput, Y., de Montigny, C. and Blier, P., 1991. Presynaptic and postsynaptic modifications of the serotonin system by long-term administration of antidepressant treatments. An *in vivo* electrophysiologic study in the rat. *Neuropsychopharmacology*, **5**, 219–29.

Charney, D.S., Heninger, G.R., Sternberg, D.E., Redmond, D.E., Leckman, J.F., Maas, J.W. and Roth, R.H., 1981. Presynaptic adrenergic receptor sensitivity in depression. The effect of long-term desipramine treatment. *Arch. Gen. Psychiat.*, **38**, 1334–40.

Cohen, R.M., Campbell, I.C., Cohen, M.R., Torda, T., Dickar, D., Siever, L.J. and Murphy, D.L., 1980. Presynaptic noradrenergic regulation during depression and antidepressant drug treatment. *Psychiat. Res.*, **3**, 93–105.

Coppen, A., 1967. The biochemistry of affective disorders. *Br. J. Psychiat.*, **113**, 1237–64.

Delgado, P.L., 2000. Depression: the case for a monoamine deficiency. *J. Clin. Psychiat.*, **61**, 7–11.

Delgado, P.L., Charney, D.S., Price, L.H., Landis, H. and Heninger, G.R., 1989. Neuroendocrine and behavioral effects of dietary tryptophan restriction in healthy subjects. *Life Sci.*, **45**, 2323–32.

Delgado, P.L., Charney, D.S., Price, L.H., Aghajanian, G.K., Landis, H. and Heninger, G.R., 1990. Serotonin function and the mechanism of antidepressant action. Reversal of antidepressant-induced remission by rapid depletion of plasma tryptophan. *Arch. Gen. Psychiat.*, **47**, 411–8.

Delgado, P.L., Price, L.H., Miller, H.L., Salomon, R.M., Aghajanian, G.K., Heninger, G.R. and Charney, D.S., 1994. Serotonin and the neurobiology of depression: effects of tryptophan depletion in drug-free depressed patients. *Arch. Gen. Psychiat.*, **51**, 865–74.

Delgado, P.L., Miller, H.L., Salomon, R.M., Licinio, J., Krystal, J.H., Moreno, F.A., Heininger, G.R. and Charney, D.S., 1999. Tryptophan-depletion challenge in depressed patients treated with desipramine or fluoxetine: implications for the role of serotonin in the mechanism of antidepressant action. *Biol. Psychiat.*, **46**, 212–20.

DeMet, E.M., Chicz-DeMet, A. and Fleischmann, J., 1989. Seasonal rhythm of platelet 3H-imipramine binding in normal controls. *Biol. Psychiat.*, **26**, 489–95.

Drevets, W.C., 2000. Neuroimaging studies of mood disorders. *Biol. Psychiat.*, **48**, 813–29.

Drevets, W.C., Frank, E., Price, J.C., Kupfer, D.J., Holt, D., Greer, P.J., Huang, Y., Gautier, C. and Mathis, C., 1999. PET imaging of serotonin 1A receptor binding in depression. *Biol. Psychiat.*, **46**, 1375–87.

Duman, R.S. and Nestler, E.J., 1995. Signal transduction pathways for catecholamine receptors. In: Bloom, F.E. and Kupfer, D.J. (eds), *Psychopharmacology, The Fourth Generation of Progress*, pp. 303–20. Raven Press, New York.

Duman, R.S., Heninger, G.R. and Nestler, E.J., 1997. A molecular and cellular theory of depression. *Arch. Gen. Psychiat.*, **54**, 597–606.

Elks, M.L., Youngblood, W.W. and Kizer, J.S., 1979. Serotonin synthesis and release in brain slices: independence of tryptophan. *Brain Res.*, **172**, 471–86.

Ellenbogen, M.A., Young, S.N., Dean, P., Palmour, R.M. and Benkelfat, C., 1996. Mood response to acute tryptophan depletion in healthy volunteers: sex differences and temporal stability. *Neuropsychopharmacology*, **15**, 465–74.

Engberg, G. and Eriksson, E., 1991. Effects of alpha 2-adrenoceptor agonists on locus coeruleus firing rate and brain noradrenaline turnover in *N*-ethoxycarbonyl-2-ethoxy-1,2-dihydroquinoline (EEDQ)-treated rats. *Naunyn Schmiedebergs Arch. Pharmacol.*, **343**, 472–7.

Engelman, K., Horwitz, D., Jequier, E. and Sjoerdsma, A., 1968a. Biochemical and pharmacologic effects of alpha-methyltyrosine in man. *J. Clin. Invest.*, **47**, 577–94.

Engelman, K., Jequier, E., Udenfriend, S. and Sjoerdsma, A., 1968b. Metabolism of alpha-methyltyrosine in man: relationship to its potency as an inhibitor of catecholamine biosynthesis. *J. Clin. Invest.*, **47**, 568–76.

Fernstrom, J.D., 1983. Role of precursor availability in control of monoamine biosynthesis in brain. *Physiol. Rev.*, **63**, 484–546.

Fernstrom, J.D. and Wurtman, R.J., 1971. Brain serotonin content: physiological dependence on plasma tryptophan levels. *Science*, **173**, 149–52.

Freedman, J.E. and Aghajanian, G.K., 1984. Idazoxan (RX 781094) selectively antagonizes alpha 2-adrenoceptors on rat central neurons. *Eur. J. Pharmacol.*, **105**, 265–72.

Friedman, P.A., Kappelman, A.H. and Kaufman, S., 1972. Partial purification and characterization of tryptophan hydroxylase from rabbit hindbrain. *J. Biol. Chem.*, **247**, 4165–73.

Gaddum, J.H. and Hameed, K.A., 1954. Drugs which antagonize 5-hydroxytryptamine. *Br. J. Pharmacol.*, **9**, 240–8.

Gessa, G.L., Biggio, G., Fadda, F., Corsini, G.U. and Tagliamonte, A., 1974. Effect of the oral administration of tryptophan-free amino acid mixtures on serum tryptophan, brain tryptophan and serotonin metabolism. *J. Neurochem.*, **22**, 869–70.

Gobert, A., Rivet, J.M., Cistarelli, L., Melon, C. and Millan, M.J., 1997. Alpha2-adrenergic receptor blockade markedly potentiates duloxetine- and fluoxetine-induced increases in noradrenaline, dopamine, and serotonin levels in the frontal cortex of freely moving rats. *J. Neurochem.*, **69**, 2616–9.

Gobert, A., Rivet, J.M., Audinot, V., Newman-Tancredi, A., Cistarelli, L. and Millan, M.J., 1998. Simultaneous quantification of serotonin, dopamine and noradrenaline levels in single frontal cortex dialysates of freely-moving rats reveals a complex pattern of reciprocal auto- and heteroreceptor-mediated control of release. *Neuroscience*, **84**, 413–29.

Grossman, E., Rea, R.F., Hoffman, A. and Goldstein, D.S., 1991. Yohimbine increases sympathetic nerve activity and norepinephrine spillover in normal volunteers. *Am. J. Physiol.*, **260**, R142–7.

Gulat-Marnay, C., Lafitte, A., Arrang, J.M. and Schwartz, J.C., 1989. Modulation of histamine release and synthesis in the brain mediated by alpha 2-adrenoceptors. *J. Neurochem.*, **53**, 513–8.

Haddjeri, N., Blier, P. and de Montigny, C., 1998. Long-term antidepressant treatments result in a tonic activation of forebrain 5-HT1A receptors. *J. Neurosci.*, **18**, 10150–6.

Hein, L., Altman, J.D. and Kobilka, B.K., 1999. Two functionally distinct alpha2-adrenergic receptors regulate sympathetic neurotransmission. *Nature*, **402**, 181–4.

Heninger, G.R., Delgado, P.L. and Charney, D.S., 1996. The revised monoamine theory of depression: a modulatory role for monoamines, based on new findings from monoamine depletion experiments in humans. *Pharmacopsychiatry*, **29**, 2–11.

Joseph-Vanderpool, J.R., Jacobsen, F.M., Murphy, D.L., Hill, J.L. and Rosenthal, N.E., 1993. Seasonal variation in behavioral responses to m-CPP in patients with seasonal affective disorder and controls. *Biol. Psychiat.*, **33**, 496–504.

Kapur, S. and Mann, J.J., 1992. Role of the dopaminergic system in depression. *Biol. Psychiat.*, **32**, 1–17.

Klaassen, T., Riedel, W.J., van Someren, A., Deutz, N.E., Honig, A. and van Praag, H.M., 1999. Mood effects of 24-hour tryptophan depletion in healthy first-degree relatives of patients with affective disorders. *Biol. Psychiat.*, **46**, 489–97.

Kuhn, R., 1958. The treatment of depressive states with G22355 (imipramine hydrochloride). *Am. J. Psychiat.*, **115**, 459–64.

Lakhlani, P.P., MacMillan, L.B., Guo, T.Z., McCool, B.A., Lovinger, D.M., Maze, M. and Limbird, L.E., 1997. Substitution of a mutant alpha2a-adrenergic receptor via 'hit and run' gene targeting reveals the role of this subtype in sedative, analgesic, and anesthetic-sparing responses *in vivo*. *Proc. Natl Acad. Sci. USA*, **94**, 9950–5.

Lam, R.W., Bowering, T.A., Tam, E.M., Grewal, A., Yatham, L.N., Shiah, I.S. and Zis, A.P., 2000. Effects of rapid tryptophan depletion in patients with seasonal affective disorder in natural summer remission. *Psychol. Med.*, **30**, 79–87.

Lam, R.W., Tam, E.M., Grewal, A. and Yatham, L.N., 2001. Effects of alpha-methyl-para-tyrosine-induced catecholamine depletion in patients with seasonal affective disorder in summer remission. *Neuropsychopharmacology*, **25**, S97–S101.

Langer, S.Z., 1997. 25 years since the discovery of presynaptic receptors: present knowledge and future perspectives. *Trends Pharmacol. Sci.*, **18**, 95–9.

Lefkowitz, R.J. and Caron, M.G., 1988. Adrenergic receptors. Models for the study of receptors coupled to guanine nucleotide regulatory proteins. *J. Biol. Chem.*, **263**, 4993–6.

Lesch, K., 1992. The ipsapirone/5-HT_{1A} receptor challenge in anxiety disorders and depression. In: Stahl, S., Hesselink, J.K., Gastpar, M. and Traber, J. (eds), *Serotonin 1A Receptors in Depression and Anxiety*, pp. 135–162. Raven Press, New York.

Leyton, M., Young, S.N., Blier, P., Ellenbogen, M.A., Palmour, R.M., Ghadirian, A.M. and Benkelfar, C., 1997. The effect of tryptophan depletion on mood in medication-free, former patients with major affective disorder. *Neuropsychopharmacology*, **16**, 294–7.

Leyton, M., Young, S.N., Blier, P., Baker, G.B., Pihl, R.O. and Benkelfat, C., 2000a. Acute tyrosine depletion and alcohol ingestion in healthy women. *Alcohol Clin. Exp. Res.*, **24**, 459–64.

Leyton, M., Young, S.N., Pihl, R.O., Etezadi, S., Lauze, C., Blier, P., Baker, G.B. and Benkelfar, C., 2000b. Effects on mood of acute phenylalanine/tyrosine depletion in healthy women. *Neuropsychopharmacology*, **22**, 52–63.

Limbird, L.E., 1988. Receptors linked to inhibition of adenylate cyclase: additional signaling mechanisms. *Faseb J.*, **2**, 2686–95.

Lopez, J.F., Chalmers, D.T., Little, K.Y. and Watson, S.J., 1998. Regulation of serotonin 1A, glucocorticoid, and mineralocorticoid receptor in rat and human hippocampus: implications for neurobiology of depression. *Biol. Psychiat.*, **43**, 547–573.

MacDonald, E., Scheinin, M., Scheinin, H. and Virtanen, R., 1991. Comparison of the behavioral and neurochemical effects of the two optical enantiomers of medetomidine, a selective alpha-2-adrenoceptor agonist. *J. Pharmacol. Exp. Ther.*, **259**, 848–54.

Maes, M. and Meltzer, H.Y., 1995. The serotonin hypothesis of major depression. In: Bloom, F.E. and Kupfer, D.J. (eds), *Psychopharmacology: The Fourth Generation of Progress*, pp. 933–44. Raven Press, New York.

Maes, M., Scharpé, S., Verkerk, R., D'Hondt, P., Peeters, D., Cosyns, P., Thompson, P., De Meyer, F., Wauters, A. and Neels, H., 1995. Seasonal variation in plasma L-tryptophan availability in healthy volunteers. relationships to violent suicide occurrence. *Arch. Gen. Psychiat.*, **52**, 937–46.

Manji, H.K., Drevets, W.C. and Charney, D.S., 2001. The cellular neurobiology of depression. *Nat. Med.*, **7**, 541–7.

Marsden, C.A., Conti, J., Strope, E., Curzon, G. and Adams, R.N., 1979. Monitoring 5-hydroxytryptamine release in the brain of the freely moving unanaesthetized rat using *in vivo* voltammetry. *Brain Res.* **171**, 85–99.

McCann, U.D., Penetar, D.M., Shaham, Y., Thorne, D.R., Sing, H.C., Thomas, M.L., Gillin, J.C. and Belenky, G., 1993. Effects of catecholamine depletion on alertness and mood in rested and sleep deprived normal volunteers. *Neuropsychopharmacology*, **8**, 345–56.

McCann, U.D., Thorne, D., Hall, M., Popp, K., Avery, W., Sing, H., Thomas, M. and Belenky, G., 1995. The effects of L-dihydroxyphenylalanine on alertness and mood in alpha-methyl-para-tyrosine-treated healthy humans. Further evidence for the role of catecholamines in arousal and anxiety. *Neuropsychopharmacology*, **13**, 41–52.

McEwen, B.S., 1999. Stress and hippocampal plasticity. *A. Rev. Neurosci.*, **22**, 105–22.

McKenna, K.F., Baker, G.B., Coutts, R.T. and Greenshaw, A.J., 1992. Chronic administration of the antidepressant-antipanic drug phenelzine and its *N*-acetylated analogue: effects on monoamine oxidase, biogenic amines, and alpha 2-adrenoreceptor function. *J. Pharmacol. Sci.*, **81**, 832–5.

Mellor, A.L. and Munn, D.H., 1999. Tryptophan catabolism and T-cell tolerance: immunosuppression by starvation? *Immunol. Today*, **20**, 469–73.

Meltzer, H.Y., Simonovic, M. and Gudelsky, G.A., 1983. Effect of yohimbine on rat prolactin secretion. *J. Pharmacol. Exp. Ther.*, **224**, 21–7.

Miller, H.L., Delgado, P.L., Salomon, R.M., Berman, R., Krystal, J.H., Heninger, G.R. and Charney, D.S., 1996a. Clinical and biochemical effects of catecholamine depletion on antidepressant-induced remission of depression. *Arch. Gen. Psychiat.*, **53**, 117–28.

Miller, H.L., Delgado, P.L., Salomon, R.M., Heninger, G.R. and Charney, D.S., 1996b. Effects of alpha-methyl-para-tyrosine (AMPT) in drug-free depressed patients. *Neuropsychopharmacology*, **14**, 151–7.

Miller, R.J., 1998. Presynaptic receptors. *A. Rev. Pharmacol. Toxicol.*, **38**, 201–27.

Moja, E.A., Mendelson, W.B., Stoff, D.M., Gillin, J.C. and Wyatt, R.J., 1979. Reduction of REM sleep by a tryptophan-free amino acid diet. *Life Sci.*, **24**, 1467–70.

Moja, E.A., Cipolla, P., Castoldi, D. and Tofanetti, O., 1989. Dose-response decrease in plasma tryptophan and in brain tryptophan and serotonin after tryptophan-free amino acid mixtures in rats. *Life Sci.*, **44**, 971–6.

Mongeau, R., Blier, P. and de Montigny, C., 1993. *In vivo* electrophysiological evidence for tonic activation by endogenous noradrenaline of alpha 2-adrenoceptors on 5-hydroxytryptamine terminals in the rat hippocampus. *Naunyn Schmiedebergs Arch. Pharmacol.*, **347**, 266–72.

Moore, P., Gillin, C., Bhatti, T., Demodena, A., Seifritz, E., Clark, C., Stahl, S., Rapaport, M. and Kelsoe, J., 1998. Rapid tryptophan depletion, sleep electroencephalogram, and mood in men with remitted depression on serotonin reuptake inhibitors. *Arch. Gen. Psychiat.*, **55**, 534–9.

Moore, P., Landolt, H.P., Seifritz, E., Clark, C., Bhatti, T., Kelsoe, J., Rapaport, M. and Gillin, J.C., 2000. Clinical and physiological consequences of rapid tryptophan depletion. *Neuropsychopharmacology*, **23**, 601–22.

Moore, P., Seifritz, E., Schlosser, A., Greenfield, D., Stahl, S., Rapaport, M. and Kelsoe, J., 2001. Rapid tryptophan depletion plus a serotonin 1A agonist. Competing effects on sleep in healthy men. *Neuropsychopharmacology*, **25**(suppl 1), S40–4.

Moreno, F.A., Gelenberg, A.J., Heninger, G.R., Potter, R.L., McKnight, K.M., Allen, J., Phillps, A.P. and Delgado, P.L., 1999. Tryptophan depletion and depressive vulnerability. *Biol. Psychiat.*, **46**, 498–505.

Moreno, F.A., Heninger, G.R., McGahuey, C.A. and Delgado, P.L., 2000a. Tryptophan depletion and risk of depression relapse: a prospective study of tryptophan depletion as a potential predictor of depressive episodes. *Biol. Psychiat.*, **48**, 327–9.

Moreno, F.A., McGavin, C., Malan, T.P., Gelenberg, A.J., Heninger, G.R., Mathé, A.A. and Delgado, P.L., 2000b. Tryptophan depletion selectively reduces CSF 5-HT metabolites in healthy young men: results from single lumbar puncture sampling technique. *Int. J. Neuropsychopharmacol.*, **3**, 277–83.

Neumeister, A., Praschak-Rieder, N., Besselmann, B., Rao, M.L., Gluck, J. and Kasper, S., 1997a. Effects of tryptophan depletion on drug-free patients with seasonal affective disorder during a stable response to bright light therapy. *Arch. Gen. Psychiat.*, **54**, 133–8.

Neumeister, A., Praschak-Rieder, N., Hesselmann, B., Tauscher, J. and Kasper, S., 1997b. [The tryptophan depletion test. Basic principles and clinical relevance]. *Nervenarzt*, **68**, 556–62.

Neumeister, A., Praschak-Rieder, N., Hesselmann, B., Vitouch, O., Rauh, M., Barocka, A. and Kasper, S., 1997c. Rapid tryptophan depletion in drug-free depressed patients with seasonal affective disorder. *Am. J. Psychiat.*, **154**, 1153–5.

Neumeister, A., Praschak-Rieder, N., Hesselmann, B., Vitouch, O., Rauh, M., Barocka, A. and Kasper, S., 1998a. Effects of tryptophan depletion in fully remitted patients with seasonal affective disorder during summer. *Psychol. Med.*, **28**, 257–64.

Neumeister, A., Praschak-Rieder, N., Hesselmann, B., Vitouch, O., Rauh, M., Barocka, A., Tauscher, J. and Kasper, S., 1998b. Effects of tryptophan depletion in drug-free depressed patients who responded to total sleep deprivation. *Arch. Gen. Psychiat.*, **55**, 167–72.

Neumeister, A., Turner, E.H., Matthews, J.R., Postolache, T.T., Barnett, R.L., Rauh, M., Vetticad, R.G., Kasper, S. and Rosenthal, N.E., 1998c. Effects of tryptophan depletion vs catecholamine depletion in patients with seasonal affective disorder in remission with light therapy. *Arch. Gen. Psychiat.*, **55**, 524–30.

Neumeister, A., Habeler, A., Praschak-Rieder, N., Willeit, M. and Kasper, S., 1999a. Tryptophan depletion: a predictor of future depressive episodes in seasonal affective disorder? *Int. Clin. Psychopharmacol.*, **14**, 313–5.

Neumeister, A., Stastny, J., Praschak-Rieder, N., Willeit, M. and Kasper, S., 1999b. Light treatment in depression (SAD, s-SAD and non-SAD). In: Holick, M.F. and Jung, E.G. (eds), *Biologic Effects of Light*, pp. 409–16. Kluwer Academic, Basel.

Neumeister, A., Pirker, W., Willeit, M., Praschak-Rieder, N., Asenbaum, S., Brücke, T. and Kasper, S., 2000. Seasonal variation of availability of serotonin transporter binding sites in healthy female subjects as measured by [123I]-2 beta-carbomethoxy-3 beta-(4-iodophenyl)tropane and single photon emission computed tomography. *Biol. Psychiat.*, **47**, 158–60.

Neumeister, A., Willeit, M., Praschak-Rieder, N., Asenbaum, S., Stastny, J., Hilger, E., Pirker, W., Konstantinidis, A. and Kasper, S., 2001. Dopamine transporter availability in symptomatic depressed patients with seasonal affective disorder and healthy controls. *Psychol. Med.*, **31**, 1467–73.

Neumeister, A., Konstantinidis, A., Stastny, J., *et al.* (in press) An association between serotonin transporter gene promotor polymorphism (5-HTTLPR) and behavioral responses to tryptophan depletion in healthy women with and without family history of depression. *Arch. Gen. Psychiat.*

Newman-Tancredi, A., Nicolas, J.P., Audinot, V., Gauaudan, S., Verriéle, L., Touzard, M., Chaput, C., Richard, N. and Millan, M.J., 1998. Actions of alpha2 adrenoceptor ligands at alpha2A and 5-HT1A receptors: the antagonist, atipamezole, and the agonist, dexmedetomidine, are highly selective for alpha2A adrenoceptors. *Naunyn Schmiedebergs Arch. Pharmacol.*, **358**, 197–206.

Nishizawa, S., Benkelfat, C., Young, S.N., Leyton, M., Mzengeza, S., de Montigny, C., Blier, P. and Diksic, M., 1997. Differences between males and females in rates of serotonin synthesis in human brain. *Proc. Natl Acad. Sci. USA*, **94**, 5308–13.

O'Dowd, B.F., Lefkowitz, R.J. and Caron, M.G., 1989. Structure of the adrenergic and related receptors. *A. Rev. Neurosci.*, **12**, 67–83.

Parsey, R.V., Hwang, D., Simpson, N., Kegeles, L., Anjivel, S., Zea-Ponce, Y., Lombardo, I., Popilskis, S., Van Heertum, R., Mann, J.J. and Laruelle, M., 1998. Kinetic derivation of serotonin 5HT-1A receptor binding potential with [C-11]carbonyl-WAY 100635 and competition studies with endogenous serotonin. *J. Nucl. Med.*, **39**(5 suppl), 167P.

Piletz, J.E., Schubert, D.S. and Halaris, A., 1986. Evaluation of studies on platelet alpha 2 adrenoreceptors in depressive illness. *Life Sci.*, **39**, 1589–616.

Piletz, J.E., Ordway, G.A., Zhu, H., Duncan, B.J. and Halaris, A., 2000. Autoradiographic comparison of [3H]-clonidine binding to non-adrenergic sites and alpha(2)-adrenergic receptors in human brain. *Neuropsychopharmacology*, **23**, 697–708.

Potter, W.Z., Karoum, F. and Linnoila, M., 1984. Common mechanism of action of biochemically 'specific' antidepressants. *Prog. Neuropsychopharmacol. Biol. Psychiat.*, **8**, 153–61.

Price, L.H., Malison, R.T., McDougle, C.J., McCance-Katz, E.F., Owen, K.R. and Heninger, G.R., 1997. Neurobiology of tryptophan depletion in depression: effects of m-chlorophenylpiperazine (mCPP). *Neuropsychopharmacology*, **17**, 342–50.

Price, L.H., Malison, R.T., McDougle, C.J., Pelton, G.H. and Heninger, G.R., 1998. The neurobiology of tryptophan depletion in depression: effects of intravenous tryptophan infusion. *Biol. Psychiat.*, **43**, 339–47.

Puke, M.J. and Wiesenfeld-Hallin, Z., 1993. The differential effects of morphine and the alpha 2-adrenoceptor agonists clonidine and dexmedetomidine on the prevention and treatment of experimental neuropathic pain. *Anesth. Analg.*, **77**, 104–9.

Quintin, P., Benkelfat, C., Launay, J.M., Arnulf, I., Pointereau-Bellenger, A., Barbault, S., Alvarez, J.C., Varoquaux, O., Perez-Diaz, F., Jouvent, R. and Leboyer, M., 2001. Clinical and neurochemical effect of acute tryptophan depletion in unaffected relatives of patients with bipolar affective disorder. *Biol. Psychiat.*, **50**, 184–90.

Raiteri, M., Maura, G., Folghera, S., Cavazzani, P., Andrioli, G.C., Schlicker, E., Schalnus, R. and Göthert, M., 1990. Modulation of 5-hydroxytryptamine release by presynaptic inhibitory alpha 2-adrenoceptors in the human cerebral cortex. *Naunyn Schmiedebergs Arch. Pharmacol.*, **342**, 508–12.

Rausch, J.L., Stahl, S.M. and Hauger, R.L., 1990. Cortisol and growth hormone responses to the 5-HT1A agonist gepirone in depressed patients. *Biol. Psychiat.*, **28**, 73–8.

Riedel, W.J., Klaassen, T., Deutz, N.E., van Someren, A. and van Praag, H.M., 1999. Tryptophan depletion in normal volunteers produces selective impairment in memory consolidation. *Psychopharmacology (Berl)*, **141**, 362–9.

Rohrer, D.K. and Kobilka, B.K., 1998. G protein-coupled receptors: functional and mechanistic insights through altered gene expression. *Physiol. Rev.*, **78**, 35–52.

Ruffolo, R.R., Jr, Nichols, A.J., Stadel, J.M. and Hieble, J.P., 1993. Pharmacologic and therapeutic applications of alpha 2-adrenoceptor subtypes. *A. Rev. Pharmacol. Toxicol.*, **33**, 243–79.

Sallinen, J., Haapalinna, A., MacDonald, E., Viitarnaa, T., Lahdesmaki, J., Rybnikova, E., Pelto-Huikko, M., Kobilka, B.K. and Scheinin, M., 1999. Genetic alteration of the alpha2-adrenoceptor subtype c in mice affects the development of behavioral despair and stress-induced increases in plasma corticosterone levels. *Molec. Psychiat.*, **4**, 443–52.

Salomon, R.M., Miller, H.L., Krystal, J.H., Heninger, G.R. and Charney, D.S., 1997. Lack of behavioral effects of monoamine depletion in healthy subjects. *Biol. Psychiat.*, **41**, 58–64.

Sargent, P.A., Kjaer, K.H., Bench, C.J., Rabiner, E.A., Messa, C., Meyer, J., Gunn, R.N., Grasby, P.N. and Cowen, P.J., 2000. Brain serotonin1A receptor binding measured by positron emission tomography with [11C]WAY-100635: effects of depression and antidepressant treatment. *Arch. Gen. Psychiat.*, **57**, 174–80.

Schaechter, J.D. and Wurtman, R.J., 1989. Tryptophan availability modulates serotonin release from rat hypothalamic slices. *J. Neurochem.*, **53**, 1925–33.

Schatzberg, A.F. and Schildkraut, J.J., 1995. Recent studies on norepinephrine systems in mood disorders. In: Bloom, F.E. and Kupfer, D.J. (eds), *Psychopharmacology: The Fourth Generation of Progress*, pp. 911–20. Raven Press, New York.

Scheinin, H., MacDonald, E. and Scheinin, M., 1988. Behavioural and neurochemical effects of antipamezole, a novel alpha 2-adrenoceptor antagonist. *Eur. J. Pharmacol.*, **151**, 35–42.

Schildkraut, J.J., 1965. The catecholamine hypothesis of affective disorders: a review of supporting evidence. *Am. J. Psychiat.*, **122**, 509–22.

Schmitt, J.A., Jorissen, B.L., Sobczak, S., van Boxtel, M.P.J., Hogervorst, E., Deutz, N.E.P. and Riedel, W., 2000. Tryptophan depletion impairs memory consolidation but improves focussed attention in healthy young volunteers. *J. Psychopharmacol.*, **14**, 21–9.

Sharp, T., Bramwell, S.R. and Grahame-Smith, D.G., 1992. Effect of acute administration of L-tryptophan on the release of 5-HT in rat hippocampus in relation to serotoninergic neuronal activity: an *in vivo* microdialysis study. *Life Sci.*, **50**, 1215–23.

Shopsin, B., Gershon, S., Goldstein, M., Friedman, E. and Wilk, S., 1975. Use of synthesis inhibitors in defining a role for biogenic amines during imipramine treatment in depressed patients. *Psychopharmacol. Commun.*, **1**, 239–49.

Simson, P.E. and Weiss, J.M., 1987. Alpha-2 receptor blockade increases responsiveness of locus coeruleus neurons to excitatory stimulation. *J. Neurosci.*, **7**, 1732–40.

Sjoerdsma, A., Engelman, K., Spector, S. and Udenfriend, S., 1965. Inhibition of catecholamine synthesis in man with alpha-methyl-tyrosine, an inhibitor of tyrosine hydroxylase. *Lancet*, **2**, 1092–4.

Smith, C.B., Hollingsworth, P.J., Garcia-Sevilla, J.A. and Zis, A.P., 1983. Platelet alpha 2 adrenoreceptors are decreased in number after antidepressant therapy. *Prog. Neuropsychopharmacol. Biol. Psychiat.*, **7**, 241–7.

Smith, K.A., Fairburn, C.G. and Cowen, P.J., 1997. Relapse of depression after rapid depletion of tryptophan. *Lancet*, **349**, 915–9.

Smith, S.E., Pihl, R.O., Young, S.N. and Ervin, F.R., 1987. A test of possible cognitive and environmental influences on the mood lowering effect of tryptophan depletion in normal males. *Psychopharmacology*, **91**, 451–7.

Spillmann, M.K., Van der Does, A.J., Rankin, M.A., Vuola, R.D., Alpert, J.E., Nierenberg, A.A., Rosenbaum, J.F., Hayden, D. and Schoenfeld, D., 2001. Tryptophan depletion in SSRI-recovered depressed outpatients. *Psychopharmacology (Berl)*, **155**, 123–7.

Sprouse, J.S. and Aghajanian, G.K., 1988. Responses of hippocampal pyramidal cells to putative serotonin 5-HT1A and 5-HT1B agonists: a comparative study with dorsal raphe neurons. *Neuropharmacology*, **27**, 707–15.

Starke, K., Borowski, E. and Endo, T., 1975. Preferential blockade of presynaptic alpha-adrenoceptors by yohimbine. *Eur. J. Pharmacol.*, **34**, 385–8.

Stastny, J., Konstantindis, A., Schwarz, M.J., *et al.* (submitted) Effects of tryptophan depletion and catecholamine depletion on immune parameters in patients with seasonal affective disorder in remission with light therapy. *Biol. Psychiat.*

Stjarne, L., 1989. Basic mechanisms and local modulation of nerve impulse-induced secretion of neurotransmitters from individual sympathetic nerve varicosities. *Rev. Physiol. Biochem. Pharmacol.*, **112**, 1–137.

Sulser, F., 1989. New perspectives on the molecular pharmacology of affective disorders. *Eur. Arch. Psychiat. Neurol. Sci.*, **238**, 231–9.

Tang, S.W. and Morris, J.M., 1985. Variation in human platelet 3H-imipramine binding. *Psychiat. Res.*, **16**, 141–6.

Tjurmina, O.A., Goldstein, D.S., Palkovits, M. and Kopin, I.J., 1999. Alpha2-adrenoceptor-mediated restraint of norepinephrine synthesis, release, and turnover during immobilization in rats. *Brain Res.*, **826**, 243–52.

Trendelenburg, A.U., Starke, K. and Limberger, N., 1994. Presynaptic alpha 2A-adrenoceptors inhibit the release of endogenous dopamine in rabbit caudate nucleus slices. *Naunyn Schmiedebergs Arch. Pharmacol.*, **350**, 473–81.

Venter, J.C., Fraser, C.M., Kerlavage, A.R. and Buck, M.A., 1989. Molecular biology of adrenergic and muscarinic cholinergic receptors. A perspective. *Biochem. Pharmacol.*, **38**, 1197–208.

Voderholzer, U., Hornyak, M., Thiel, B., Huwig-Poppe, C., Kiemen, A., König, A., Backhaus, J., Riemann, D., Berger, M. and Hohagen, F., 1998. Impact of experimentally induced serotonin deficiency by tryptophan depletion on sleep EEG in healthy subjects. *Neuropsychopharmacology*, **18**, 112–24.

Weltzin, T.E., Fernstrom, M.H., Fernstrom, J.D., Neuberger, S.K. and Kaye, W.H., 1995. Acute tryptophan depletion and increased food intake and irritability in bulimia nervosa. *Am. J. Psychiat.*, **152**, 1668–71.

Whitaker, P.M., Warsh, J.J., Stancer, H.C., Persad, E. and Vint, C.K., 1984. Seasonal variation in platelet 3H-imipramine binding: comparable values in control and depressed populations. *Psychiat. Res.*, **11**, 127–31.

Whitaker-Azmitia, P.M. and Azmitia, E.C., 1989. Stimulation of astroglial serotonin receptors produces culture media which regulates growth of serotonergic neurons. *Brain Res.*, **497**, 80–5.

Whitaker-Azmitia, P.M., Murphy, R. and Azmitia, E.C., 1990. Stimulation of astroglial 5-HT1A receptors releases the serotonergic growth factor, protein S-100, and alters astroglial morphology. *Brain Res.*, **528**, 155–8.

Whitaker-Azmitia, P.M., Clarke, C. and Azmitia, E.C., 1993. Localization of 5-HT1A receptors to astroglial cells in adult rats: implications for neuronal-glial interactions and psychoactive drug mechanism of action. *Synapse*, **14**, 201–5.

Widerlov, E. and Lewander, T., 1978. Inhibition of the *in vivo* biosynthesis and changes of catecholamine levels in rat brain after alpha-methyl-*p*-tyrosine; time- and dose-response relationships. *Naunyn Schmiedebergs Arch. Pharmacol.*, **304**, 111–23.

Williams, W.A., Shoaf, S.E., Hommer, D., Rawlings, R. and Linnoila, M., 1999. Effects of acute tryptophan depletion on plasma and cerebrospinal fluid tryptophan and 5-hydroxyindoleacetic acid in normal volunteers. *J. Neurochem.*, **72**, 1641–7.

Wong, M.L., Kling, M.A., Munson, P.J., Listwak, S., Licinio, J., Prolo, P., Karp, B., McCutcheon, I.E., Geracioti, T.D., Jr, DeBellis, M.D., Rice, K.C., Goldstein, D.S., Veldhuis, J.D., Chrousos, G.P., Oldfield, E.H., McCann, S.M. and Gold, P.W., 2000. Pronounced and sustained central hypernoradrenergic function in major depression with melancholic features: relation to hypercortisolism and corticotropin-releasing hormone. *Proc. Natl Acad. Sci. USA*, **97**, 325–30.

Wooley, D.W. and Shaw, E., 1954. A biochemical and pharmacological suggestion about certain mental disorders. *Proc. Natl Acad. Sci. USA*, **40**, 228–31.

Yatham, L.N., Liddle, P.F., Shiah, I.S., Lam, R.W., Adam, M.J., Zis, A.P. and Ruth, T.J., 2001. Effects of rapid tryptophan depletion on brain 5-HT(2) receptors: a PET study. *Br. J. Psychiat.*, **178**, 448–53.

Young, S.N., Smith, S.E., Pihl, R.O. and Ervin, F.R., 1985. Tryptophan depletion causes a rapid lowering of mood in normal males. *Psychopharmacology*, **87**, 173–7.

Young, S.N., Ervin, F.R., Pihl, R.O. and Finn, P., 1989. Biochemical aspects of tryptophan depletion in primates. *Psychopharmacology*, **98**, 508–11.

XVIII-3

Evidence for GABAergic and Glutamatergic Involvement in the Pathophysiology and Treatment of Depressive Disorders

Gerard Sanacora

The majority of neurons in the brain use either γ-aminobutyric acid (GABA) or glutamate as their primary neurotransmitter. In effect these two neurotransmitters serve to regulate the excitability of almost all neurons in the brain. Therefore, it is not surprising that they are implicated in a broad range of both physiological and pathophysiological events related to brain function. Although the past three decades of research has emphasized the role of the biogenic amines and hypothalamic–pituitary–adrenal (HPA) axis in the neurobiology of mood disorders, emerging evidence now suggests that the amino acid neurotransmitter systems also contribute to the pathophysiology and pharmacological treatment of depression.

Newly developed neurochemical imaging techniques and advances in molecular pharmacology are now providing novel methods to study the amino acid neurotransmitter systems. Through the use of these modalities and novel pharmaceutical agents we are now beginning to uncover the extent to which these ubiquitous systems are related to depression and other mood disorders. In the following pages we will examine the evidence supporting the involvement of the GABAergic and glutamatergic systems in the neurobiology of mood disorders.

EVIDENCE SUPPORTING GABAERGIC CONTRIBUTIONS TO THE NEUROBIOLOGY OF DEPRESSION

Dysregulation of GABAergic neurotransmission is increasingly implicated in the neurobiology of mood disorders (Lloyd *et al.*, 1989; Petty, 1995; Sanacora *et al.*, 2000; Shiah and Yatham, 1998). Supporting evidence comes in the form of (1) animal studies showing stress-related changes in GABAergic function, and the ability of GABA modulating agents to alter animal models of depression, (2) demonstration of GABAergic abnormalities in depressed patients, and (3) GABAergic effects of antidepressant and mood stabilizing medications.

GABA and Animal Models of Stress and Depression

Multiple lines of evidence suggest stress is a major precipitating factor in the development of depressive episodes. Existing animal studies suggest that stress-related effects on the GABAergic neurotransmitter system may contribute to this relationship. Several studies have found decreased cortical $GABA_A$ receptor function following exposure to short-term stress in various rodent models (Biggio *et al.*, 1984; Concas *et al.*, 1988; Sanna *et al.*, 1992; Serra *et al.*, 1991). Additionally, stressful early life events can result in long-lasting changes in $GABA_A$ receptor function that appear related to altered expression of adult behaviours (Caldji *et al.*, 2000). Lower GABA concentrations, synthesis rates, and neurotransmitter uptake have also been reported in acute stress paradigms (Acosta *et al.*, 1993; Borsini *et al.*, 1988). Chronic stress produced similar changes in GABAergic function, including decreases in brain GABA concentrations, glutamic acid decarboxylase (GAD) activity, GABA uptake, and regional $GABA_A$ receptor binding (Acosta and Rubio, 1994; Insel, 1989; Weizman *et al.*, 1989). Interestingly, the time course of these events corresponds to changes in neuroactive steroid concentrations, which may serve as endogenous mediators of homeostatic function by maintaining GABAergic regulation during prolonged stress (Barbaccia *et al.*, 1996, 1997).

The role of GABA in the regulation of the HPA axis is now drawing increasing attention (Barbaccia *et al.*, 1996, 1997; Boudaba *et al.*, 1996; Calogero *et al.*, 1988; Owens *et al.*, 1991). Local circuits from within the hypothalamus provide a rich supply of GABAergic innervation directly on to the corticotropin-releasing hormone (CRH) containing parvocellular region of the paraventricular nucleus (PVN) (Herman and Cullinan, 1997). These stress-activated PVN-projecting GABAergic pathways appear to play a prominent role in modulating the HPA axis response to stress (Bowers *et al.*, 1998). Disruption of this system could be related to the abnormal HPA stress responses commonly observed in mood-disordered individuals.

The ability of GABA modulating agents to alter the expression of stress responses and animal models of depression further suggest a role for the inhibitory neurotransmitter system in the neurobiology of mood disorders. Initial studies by Sherman and Petty demonstrating the ability of intrahippocampal GABA injections both to prevent and reverse the induction of learned helplessness provided the initial link to the GABAergic system (Sherman and Petty, 1980). Other studies demonstrating decreased Ca^{++}-dependent GABA release from the hippocampus of helpless animals, and inhibition of imipramine's 'antidepressant-like' effects on learned helplessness behaviour by intrahippocampal administration of the GABA antagonist bicuculline (Petty and Sherman, 1981), provided additional evidence that GABA-mediated mechanisms are associated with the development of depression-like behaviours in this model.

Transient GABA reductions were reported in several brain regions following the initial session of the forced swimming test (FST) (Borsini *et al.*, 1988), another frequently used animal model of depression and a test of antidepressant activity. Similar to the actions of other antidepressant agents, GABA agonists reduce

Biological Psychiatry: Edited by H. D'haenen, J.A. den Boer and P. Willner. ISBN 0-471-49198-5

the immobility time during the forced swimming test (Borsini *et al.*, 1986; Poncelet *et al.*, 1987). Inhibiting GABA breakdown by administering the GABA-transaminase (GABA-T) inhibitor amino-oxyacetic acid prior to the first forced swim session elevated GABA levels, and decreased immobility time (Borsini *et al.*, 1988), suggesting that the immobility time associated with the FST is mediated in part through the GABAergic system.

Like the learned helplessness and FST models, the olfactory bulbectomized rat, another commonly used behavioural model of depression, also appears sensitive to modulation by GABA mimetics. The passive avoidance deficit (Lloyd *et al.*, 1983, 1987), muricidal behaviour (Delini-Stula and Vassout, 1978) and open field behaviour (Leonard, 1984), measures frequently used as tests of antidepressant-like activity, are all reversed following the administration of GABA agonists. In other studies $GABA_B$ binding was demonstrated to be significantly decreased in the frontal cortex of these animals (Lloyd *et al.*, 1987). GABA mimetics also produce antidepressant-like activity in other tests of antidepressant activity such as the paradoxical sleep and 5-HTP head twitch (for review see Lloyd *et al.*, 1989).

Evidence of GABAergic Abnormalities in Mood Disorder Patients

There are several forms of evidence suggesting possible widespread abnormalities of GABAergic function to mood disorders. However, the most convincing evidence linking the GABAergic system to the neurobiology of mood disorders are the studies showing decreased GABA in the plasma, cerebrospinal fluid (CSF) and cerebral cortex of depressed individuals.

CSF

Gold and colleagues first reported decreased CSF GABA levels in mood disorder patients (Gold *et al.*, 1980). They found significantly lower CSF GABA concentrations in mood disorder patients compared to a group of subjects undergoing a neurological evaluation and a group of psychotic subjects. A second CSF study (Post *et al.*, 1980) reported a non-significant trend toward lower GABA levels in 16 depressed patients, compared to 8 manic patients and 41 healthy comparison subjects. A third study (Gerner and Hare, 1981) highlighted the complexities of CSF GABA studies. It compared CSF GABA levels from groups of depressed, schizophrenic, manic and anorexia nervosa patients to the levels of healthy comparison subjects using two samples of CSF. Consistent with the initial study by Gold *et al.*, only the depressed subjects exhibited lower CSF GABA than the healthy comparison subjects when the sample was obtained from the first 12 cm^3 collected. However, when the second aliquot of CSF (15–26 cm^3, the same as in the Post *et al.*, study) was used, the trend was no longer statistically significant (Gerner *et al.*, 1984). Gerner later replicated the findings of decreased GABA concentrations in a larger study measuring CSF levels in 41 depressed patients and 38 controls. Consistent with the previous studies, lower CSF GABA levels were not observed in patients diagnosed with schizophrenia or mania. A Japanese study also reported significantly lower CSF GABA levels in depressed patients compared to a mixed group of healthy comparison subjects and hospitalized patients without neuropsychiatric illness (Kasa *et al.*, 1982). A later study by Roy and collaborators (Roy *et al.*, 1991b) also found lower CSF GABA levels in patients with a current depressive episode. However, when they controlled for age and gender there was no significant difference. Only the subgroup of patients with unipolar

Table XVIII-3.1 Review of CSF GABA studies in depression

	Comparison subjects				Depressed patients		
Reference	CSF Sample (cc)	Sample size	Gender	CSF GABA level ($pmol\ ml^{-1}$) mean ± SEM	Sample size	Gender	CSF GABA level ($pmol\ ml^{-1}$) mean ± SEM
Gold *et al.* (1980)	0–10	20 (neurologic patients)	M = 4 F = 16	218 ± 26	MDE = 17 UP = 10 BP = 5 ETOH = 1 OBS = 1	M = 1 F = 16	122 ± 10*
Post *et al.* (1980)	16–28	41 (healthy)	M = 26 F = 15	232 ± 13	MDE = 16 (sub-type not specified)	M = 6 F = 10	214 ± 13
Gerner and Hare (1981)	1–12 15–26	29 (healthy)	M = 14 F = 15	183 ± 12 200 ± 11	MDE = 24 UP = 19 BP = 5	M = 11 F = 13	134 ± 5* 172 ± 10
Zimmer *et al.* (1981)	1–6	6 (surgical patients)	Not specified	360 ± 29	DS = 6 (sub-type not specified)	M = 3 F = 3	280 ± 45
Kasa *et al.* (1982)	5–10	24 (mixed group of healthy subjects and hospital patients without neurologic and psychiatric disorders)	Not specified	138 ± 12	MDE = 13 (sub-type not specified)	M = 11 F = 2	96 ± 39*
Gerner *et al.* (1984)	0–12	38 (healthy)	M = 18 F = 20	190 ± 5	MDE = 41 Up = 30 BP = 10	M = 18 F = 23	140 ± 6*
Roy *et al.* (1991b)	1–10	20 (healthy)	M = 8 F = 12	145 ± 10	MDE = 25 UP = 18 BP = 7	M = 4 F = 21	119 ± 33

Note: *Sig. $P < 0.05$. M = male, F = female, MDE = major depressive episode, DS=depressive syndrome, UP = unipolar depression, BP = bipolar depression, OBS = organic brain syndrome, ETOH = alcohol related.

melancholic depression had significantly lower GABA levels than all other groups. Finally, a study by Zimmer and colleagues reported a non-significant decrease in CSF GABA levels with depressive mood states in a small group of poorly defined subjects (Zimmer *et al.*, 1980).

In summary, all of the CSF studies to date have found at least a trend toward decreased GABA concentrations in depressed subjects (see Table XVIII-3.1). A meta-analysis of this data (Petty *et al.*, 1993c) revealed a highly significant difference between depressed and comparison subjects. Interestingly, the finding appears to be relatively specific to depression. No significant differences were observed in schizophrenic, anorectic or manic subjects (Gerner and Hare, 1981; Gerner *et al.*, 1984; Gold *et al.*, 1980; Post *et al.*, 1980). In further support of this specificity, Roy and colleagues (Roy *et al.*, 1991a) reported CSF GABA levels to be selectively decreased in depressed alcoholic patients compared to non-depressed alcoholics. Unfortunately, lack of diagnostic specificity in these early studies and the grouping of unipolar and bipolar patients into a common class does not allow for tests of further specificity. The fact that none of the studies examined remitted patients also leaves the state versus trait dependence issue unresolved.

Plasma Levels

There are several reports of decreased plasma GABA levels in individuals with affective disorders, with the majority of studies from a single laboratory (Berrettini *et al.*, 1982a, 1986; Petty and Schlesser, 1981; Petty and Sherman, 1984; Petty *et al.*, 1990, 1992, 1993b). In general, these findings suggest a trait-dependent reduction in plasma GABA levels in patients with mood disorders. This is best noted by a markedly increased percentage of individuals having plasma GABA concentrations below 100 pmol ml^{-1}. Unlike the CSF studies, there is no clear evidence of specificity between active episodes and remitted states, or between depressed and manic states. However, the group of patients with the lowest GABA levels had more severe melancholic-like symptoms. Similar to the CSF studies, the lower GABA concentrations were somewhat specific to mood disorders. No change in plasma GABA was observed in patients with schizophrenia, generalized anxiety disorder, eating disorders or panic disorder (Petty and Sherman, 1984; Goddard *et al.*, 1996; Roy-Byrne *et al.*, 1992; Petty, 1994 for review see). However, lower plasma GABA levels were seen in alcoholism (Petty *et al.*, 1993a), Parkinson's disease (Manyam, 1982) and premenstrual dysphoric disorder (Halbreich *et al.*, 1996).

Post-Mortem and Biopsy Studies

Post-mortem studies consisting mostly of depressed suicide victims have not provided consistent evidence of GABAergic abnormalities. No significant differences were found in $GABA_B$ binding in a post-mortem sample of 16 suicide victims compared to 20 controls (Arranz *et al.*, 1992). This is consistent with earlier post-mortem studies that showed no change in $GABA_B$ binding sites in depressed suicide victims (Cross *et al.*, 1988). $GABA_A$-benzodiazepine binding was increased by 18% in the frontal cortex of 21 depressed suicide victims compared to 21 age- and sex-matched controls (Cheetham *et al.*, 1988).

Biopsy and post-mortem data on GABA concentrations also remains inconclusive, an outcome that may be due in part to the dramatic post-mortem increase in the activity of GABA's primary synthetic enzyme GAD. A negative correlation was found between GABA concentrations and severity of depression in a study measuring GABA levels from cortex removed during psychosurgery (Honig *et al.*, 1988). However, Korpi *et al.* (1988) found no significant differences in brain GABA levels of suicide victims. Similar inconsistencies are seen regarding GAD activity levels. An early study reported significantly lower rates of GABA synthesis in several brain regions from elderly depressed patients compared to control subjects (Perry *et al.*, 1977). Consistent with this, a single study found lower plasma GAD activity in depressed patients (Kaiya *et al.*, 1982). However, Cheetham *et al.* (1988) found no significant differences in GAD activity in depressed suicide victims, and a more recent study reported a significant increase in the expression of the GAD_{67} isoform of the enzyme in the prefrontal cortex of depressed patients (Toth *et al.*, 1999). No differences were found in the one study investigating the activity of GABA-T activity in depressed and non-depressed suicide victims (Sherif *et al.*, 1991), although lower platelet GABA-T activity was found in euthymic medication-free bipolar patients (Berrettini *et al.*, 1982b). Recent studies by Rajkowska and colleagues suggest that mood disorders are associated with reduced numbers of neurons in layer II in regions of the frontal cortex (Rajkowska *et al.*, 1999), and preliminary findings further demonstrate an associated reduction of calbindin-immunoreactive neurons in layer II depressed subjects (Personal Communication Dr. Rajkowska).

In vivo Brain Studies of GABA

Advances in magnetic resonance spectroscopy (MRS) have made it possible to measure GABA concentrations *in vivo*. Using this methodology, decreased GABA concentrations were demonstrated in the occipital cortex of depressed subjects (Figure XVIII-3.1) (Sanacora *et al.*, 1999a). In two other preliminary studies the occipital GABA concentrations were found to be normalized following treatment with either electroconvulsive therapy (Sanacora *et al.*, 1999b) or selective serotonin reuptake inhibitor (SSRI) medications (Sanacora *et al.*, 2002). Since these initial MRS studies were limited to the occipital cortex it is difficult to determine the pathophysiological significance of the findings. However, in light of the previous reports that consistently demonstrated decreased GABA concentrations in the plasma and CSF of depressed patients, the studies suggest that widespread alterations of GABAergic function are associated with major depression. In a single preliminary report using SPECT imaging of radiolabelled Iomazenil to examine benzodiazepine binding, no significant difference was observed between depressed subjects and a historical group of healthy control subjects despite the presence of lower occipital cortex GABA concentrations (Kugaya *et al.*, 2001).

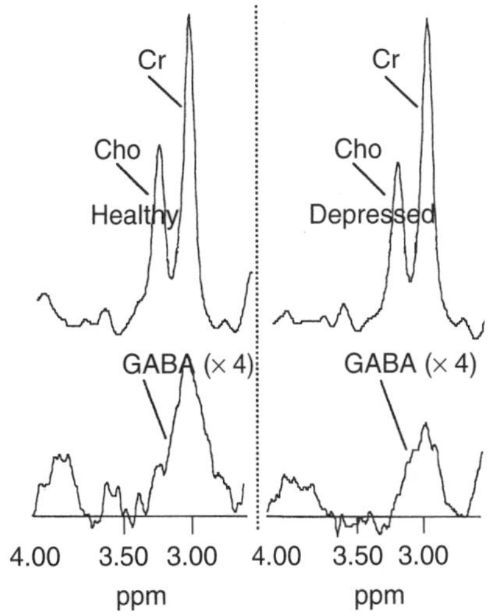

Figure XVIII-3.1 *In vivo* 1H-MRS spectra from representative healthy and depressed subjects. The relative differences in occipital cortex GABA between these two subjects is illustrated by the size of the GABA peaks on the spectra

Pharmacological Challenges

The use of pharmacological challenge studies to investigate GABAergic involvement in depression has yielded inconsistent findings. Administration of the $GABA_B$ agonist baclofen is known to increase growth hormone secretion from the anterior pituitary (Koulu *et al.*, 1979; Müller, 1987). Two studies have shown this effect to be blunted in depressed individuals, suggesting altered $GABA_B$ function in depression (Marchesi *et al.*, 1991; O'Flynn and Dinan, 1993). However, two other studies found no significant difference between healthy comparison and depressed subjects in response to a baclofen challenge (Davis *et al.*, 1997; Monteleone *et al.*, 1990).

Findings Related to Endogenous Modulators of GABA Function

Neuroactive steroids are metabolites of progesterone and deoxycorticosterone that interact with the $GABA_A$/benzodiazepine receptor complex. Decreased plasma levels of several neuroactive steroids possessing potentiating effects on the $GABA_A$ receptor were observed along with a concomitant increase in two neurosteroids that may act as functional GABA antagonists in depressed individuals (Romeo *et al.*, 1998). Treatment with antidepressant medication appears to reverse this disequilibrium. This effect of antidepressant medications on neuroactive steroid concentrations is consistent with an earlier rodent study demonstrating increased neuroactive steroids concentrations in response to fluoxetine treatment (Uzunov *et al.*, 1996), and may contribute to the mechanism of antidepressant action by altering GABAergic transmission. Furthermore, the involvement of neuroactive progesterone metabolites in the pathophysiology of depression also suggests one possible explanation for the elevated rates of depression in the post-partum period (O'Hara *et al.*, 1984), and elevated rates of depressive symptoms in the late luteal phase of the menstrual cycle (Rubinow *et al.*, 1984).

Genetic Studies

Attempts to examine the relationship between the GABAergic system and mood disorders using genetic analysis studies are yet to yield convincing evidence (Table XVIII-3.2). Puertollano and colleagues reported an association between manic-depressive illness and tetranucleotide repeat polymorphisms at the GABRB1 gene in a study of a subpopulation of Spanish females (Puertollano *et al.*, 1997). Oruc *et al.* (1996) failed to detect a significant association with GABRA1 and GABAR3 and bipolar disorder. A third study by Serretti and colleagues (Serretti *et al.*, 1998) also failed to find an association between depressive symptomatology and the GABRA1 gene in a group of unipolar and bipolar depressed patients. Petty and colleagues recently provided preliminary evidence suggesting that regulation of plasma GABA levels may be under the control of a single gene, inherited in a recessive manner (Petty *et al.*, 1999). This is consistent with an older study that showed a statistically significant correlation between plasma GABA concentrations of depressed subjects and first-degree relatives (Petty, 1994).

GABA's Role in the Treatment of Mood Disorders

The delayed clinical response to tricyclic antidepressants (TCA), SSRI and monoamine oxidase inhibitors (MAOI) suggests that other neurotransmitter systems in addition to the monoamines may be involved in the mechanism of antidepressant action. Several studies have sought to examine the possible involvement of the GABAergic system in this regard.

Receptors

Chronic administration of all three classes of antidepressants (TCA, SSRI, MAOI) and ECT have been reported to enhance $GABA_B$ receptor binding in animal studies (for review see Lloyd *et al.*, 1987). However, contrasting findings have also been reported (Cross and Horton, 1988; McManus and Greenshaw, 1991; Monteleone *et al.*, 1990; Szekely *et al.*, 1987). The upregulation of $GABA_B$ receptors appears dependent on chronic administration of antidepressant medications, as no changes were seen after acute administration. Interestingly, other neuroleptic, anxiolytic and psychostimulant medications failed to show similar effects (Lloyd *et al.*, 1987), but mood stabilizing agents such as sodium valproate, carbamazepine and lithium did enhance $GABA_B$ binding (Motohashi *et al.*, 1989).

Using the olfactory bulbectomized rat model Joly and colleagues (Joly *et al.*, 1987) reported that only desipramine 'responders' displayed a significant increase in $GABA_B$ receptor binding, thus suggesting a functional relationship between the increase in $GABA_B$ receptors and behaviour. Interpretation of the above findings is complicated by a recent study by Beck and colleagues suggesting that the potency of $GABA_B$ transmission is decreased following chronic fluoxetine treatment in selected subfields of the rat hippocampus as measured by baclofen-stimulated hyperpolarization (Beck *et al.*, 1997).

There are two reports of long-term antidepressant administration resulting in downregulation of $GABA_A$ receptors (Suranyi-Cadotte *et al.*, 1984; Suzdak and Gianutsos, 1985). However, these finding were not replicated in a later study (Kimber *et al.*, 1987), and increased numbers of benzodiazepine receptors were found in selected areas of rat brain following chronic administration of sertraline (Giardino *et al.*, 1993). Chronic administration of

Table XVIII-3.2 Summary of findings in depressed subjects

	Levels relative to controls	Comments	References
Plasma GABA	↓	Consistent findings of low plasma GABA with one exception.	Petty (1994), Petty and Schlesser (1981), Petty *et al.* (1992), Rode *et al.* (1991)
CSF GABA	↓	4 of 7 studies found significantly lower GABA concentrations, others reported trend toward lower GABA in depression.	Gerner and Hare (1981), Gerner *et al.* (1984), Gold *et al.* (1980), Kasa *et al.* (1982), Post *et al.* (1980), Roy *et al.* (1991b), Zimmer *et al.* (1981)
Brain GABA	↓	Inconsistent findings with limited post-mortem studies, *In vivo* MRS study highly significant	Honig *et al.* (1989), Korpi *et al.* (1988), Sanacora *et al.* (199b)
GABAergic neurons	↓	Single study results	Rajkowska *et al.* (1999) (Personal Communication Dr. Rajkowska)

imipramine, phenelzine and buspirone resulted in altered $GABA_A$ receptor subunit patterns in rat brains (Tanay *et al.*, 1996), but no consistent pattern of change was observed.

GABA Levels

Several older studies found elevated GABA levels and enhanced GABA release in rat brains following high-dose acute administration of TCAs and MAOIs, and daily electroconvulsive shock (Bowdler *et al.*, 1983; Korf and Venema, 1983; Patel *et al.*, 1975; Perry and Hansen, 1973; Popov and Matthies, 1969). However, other studies found GABA levels to be generally unaltered by antidepressant administration (Olsen *et al.*, 1978; Pilc and Lloyd, 1984). More recent studies consistently find the MAOI phenelzine to increase GABA levels in the rat brain (Baker *et al.*, 1991; McKenna *et al.*, 1994; McManus *et al.*, 1992). The increased GABA levels do not appear the direct result of changes in synthetic or catabolic enzyme gene expression since phenelzine produced no effect on the steady-state levels of mRNAs that encode for GABA-T, GAD_{65} or GAD_{67} (Lai *et al.*, 1998). However, the elevated brain GABA levels do appear in part related to the anxiolytic properties of the drug in animal models (Paslawski *et al.*, 1996). The true relevance of the elevated GABA levels to phenelzine's antidepressant actions remains unknown. Seemingly in contrast to the above findings, Giardino and colleagues (Giardino *et al.*, 1996) found chronic sertraline treatment to decrease GAD expression in several rat brain regions. As mentioned above, recent MRS findings suggest that GABA concentrations in the occipital cortex are elevated following treatment with antidepressant agents.

Effectiveness of Mood Stabilizers and Antidepressants with GABAergic Activity

GABA Analogues

Several studies suggest that compounds that enhance GABAergic transmission possess antidepressant properties. As noted above, GABA agonists have antidepressant-like activity in several animal models used to assess antidepressant action (Lloyd *et al.*, 1989). These findings prompted clinical investigation of GABA-enhancing drugs as antidepressants. Due to the pharmacological limitations of many of these compounds, their use in clinical trials is limited. However, progabide and fengabine (SL 79229) are two GABA-mimetic compounds that reached clinical trials as antidepressant agents. Both of these compounds appeared to be effective antidepressants in multiple controlled clinical trials, in some reports having equal efficacy to TCAs (for compilation of studies see Bartholini *et al.*, 1986). However, development of these compounds was halted due to unfavourable side-effect profiles, and no recent work has been reported as a follow-up to these initial studies.

Benzodiazepines and Anticonvulsants

The benzodiazepine class of $GABA_A$ agonists appear to be ineffective as antidepressant agents in general (Schatzberg and Cole, 1978; Tiller *et al.*, 1989). However, the efficacy of the triazolobenzodiazepine alprazolam remains contested (Petty *et al.*, 1995). Interestingly, valproic acid, a compound that appears to increase GABAergic transmission through multiple mechanisms (Löscher, 1993), has proven mood stabilizing properties (Bowden *et al.*, 1994), and possible efficacy in unipolar major depression (Davis *et al.*, 1996). Other anticonvulsants (gabapentin and topiramate) with GABAergic activity have recently attracted attention as possible mood stabilizing, and antidepressant drugs (Brown *et al.*, 1999; Post *et al.*, 1997). However, the clinical effectiveness of these treatments awaits further study.

In conclusion, the evidence supporting the hypothesis that the GABAergic system contributes to the mechanism of action of antidepressant medications remains preliminary and contestable.

GLUTAMATE

Given that glutamate is the principal excitatory neurotransmitter in the mammalian brain it is likely to contribute to a wide array of both normal and abnormal brain functions. Its involvement has been previously implicated in the pathophysiology of several neurodegenerative disorders as well as schizophrenia, obsessive compulsive disorder and alcohol dependence (Carlsson, 2001; Danbolt, 2001; Tsai and Coyle, 1998). Supporting evidence for glutamate's role in the pathophysiology of mood disorders comes from (1) animal studies showing stress-related changes in glutamatergic function, and its possible relationship to excitotoxicity, (2) demonstration of glutamatergic abnormalities in depressed patients, (3) glutamatergic effects of antidepressant and mood stabilizing medications and (4) the effectiveness of glutamate modulating agents in the treatment of depression.

Stress-Related Effects

Glutamatergic neurotransmission appears intimately involved in a stress-responsive cascade of events that result in neurotoxicity (Sapolsky, 2000). Stress has been shown to increase synaptic glutamate concentrations in the hippocampus and prefrontal cortex (Moghaddam, 1993; Moghaddam *et al.*, 1994), and to alter glutamate receptor function in the hippocampus and hypothalamus (Bartanusz *et al.*, 1995; Nowak *et al.*, 1995b). If this model is correct, stress-responsive neurotoxicity may help explain several recent findings demonstrating altered hippocampal and cortical morphology (Bremner *et al.*, 2000; Sheline *et al.*, 1996) and histology (Ongür *et al.*, 1998; Rajkowska *et al.*, 1999), associated with major depression. In support of this hypothesis, studies using glutamate transporter GLT-1 knockout mice with excessive synaptic glutamate have demonstrated pathological destruction of hippocampal neurons (Tanaka *et al.*, 1997).

Other data suggests that glutamatergic activity is closely tied to the stress-responsiveness of the paralimbic–HPA axis, and that glutamate is capable of stimulating CRF release into the portal circulation (Cratty and Birkle, 1999; Feldman and Weidenfeld, 1997; Ziegler and Herman, 2000). Consistent with glutamate's proposed role in the regulation of the stress response, *N*-methyl-D-aspartate (NMDA) receptor antagonists reduce immobility time on the FST (Maj *et al.*, 1992) and prevent many of the behavioural deficits associated with chronic stress (Ossowska *et al.*, 1997).

Evidence of Glutamatergic Abnormalities in Mood Disorder Patients

Plasma

Studies regarding plasma levels of glutamate in mood disorders remain inconclusive. An early study by Kim and colleagues (Kim *et al.*, 1982) reported elevated glutamate levels in a group of depressed patients, but could not separate the effect from the use of antidepressant medications. Altamura and colleagues (Altamura *et al.*, 1993) also initially reported elevated plasma glutamate levels in a group of mood disorder patients but in a later study found no significant differences in plasma glutamate concentrations comparing unmedicated patients with major depression to healthy controls (Altamura *et al.*, 1995). However, employing a linear discriminant analysis, the group did find a highly significant separation between major depressed subjects and normal volunteers, using glycine, glutamate and taurine as discriminatory variables. In more recent studies, Mauri and colleagues (Mauri *et al.*, 1998) found elevated plasma and platelet levels of glutamate in depressed patients compared to controls, but Maes *et al.* (1998) found no difference in serum glutamate levels from depressed patients compared to age- and sex-matched controls. Interestingly, however, they did find significantly reduced serum glutamate levels following a 5-week period of treatment with antidepressants.

CSF

Very few CSF studies have addressed the glutamatergic system in relation to depression. Levine and colleagues used MRS technology to demonstrate significantly higher CSF glutamine concentrations in the CSF of 18 hospitalized patients with acute unmedicated severe depression compared to 22 control subjects (Levine *et al.*, 2000). In a second study, Hiraoka and colleagues (Hiraoka *et al.*, 1989) reported that mean CSF glutamine levels in functional psychosis (schizophrenia, manic-depressive illness and other psychoses) did not differ from those of neurotic patients, patients with cerebrovascular disorders or patients with metabolic neuropathy.

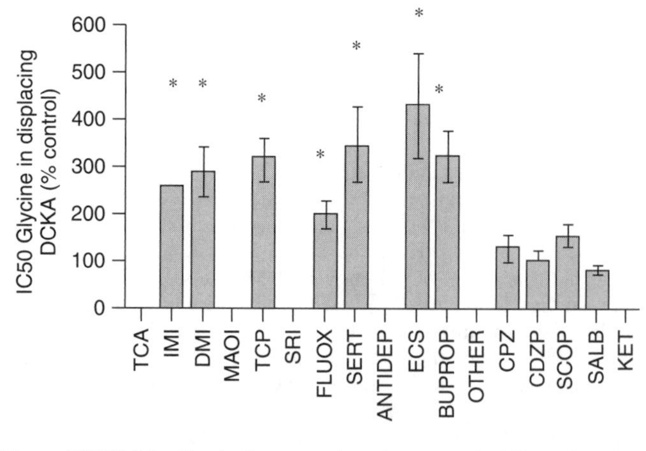

Figure XVIII-3.2 Graph demonstrating the general ability of various antidepressant treatments to reduce the potency of glycine in displacing DCKA binding on NMDA receptors. Adapted from Paul *et al.* (1994)

Brain

A single study examining neurosurgical samples from chronically depressed subjects did not find a significant difference in frontal cortex glutamate concentrations (Francis *et al.*, 1989). Another study also failed to find any significant difference in the binding of a non-competitive antagonist to the NMDA receptor among depressed suicide victims and an age-matched comparison group (Holemans *et al.*, 1993). However, Nowak and colleagues reported that the proportion of high-affinity, glycine displaceable [3H]CGP-39653 binding to glutamate receptors was reduced in age- and post-mortem interval-matched suicide victims (Nowak *et al.*, 1995a).

In vivo measures of excitatory amino acids in the brain can be made with the use of 1H-MRS. Using standard clinical field strength magnets, the visibility of these metabolites are limited by several factors that make it extremely difficult to assign unequivocal resonance peaks. This has led to the use of a combined measure termed Glx that contains glutamate, glutamine and GABA, of which the greatest proportion reflects the glutamate concentration. In one of the more unique studies, Cousins and Harper used this methodology to demonstrate temporary decreases in Glx levels coinciding with a patient's transient experience of suicidal depression following Taxol and Neupogen chemotherapy (Cousins and Harper, 1996). More recently, Auer and colleagues (Auer *et al.*, 2000) reported decreased Glx measures in the anterior cingulate cortex of severely depressed subjects. A preliminary study by Michael and colleagues also showed a similar decrease in baseline anterior cingulate Glx levels that later increased following treatment with ECT (Michael *et al.*, 2001). Interestingly, no decrease was seen in a group of bipolar depressed subjects participating in this study. Consistent with the idea that Glx measures may differ between unipolar and bipolar depressed patients, elevated levels of Glx were found in both the frontal lobe and basal ganglia of depressed bipolar children compared to a control group (Castillo *et al.*, 2000).

Glutamatergic Effects of Antidepressant and Mood Stabilizing Agents

A growing body of research suggests that the NMDA class of glutamate receptors may be involved in the mechanism of action of antidepressants (Skolnick, 1999). Downregulation of the glycine-B site of NMDA receptors appears to be a common feature of current antidepressant treatments. As shown in Figure XVIII-3.2, tricyclics, serotonin reuptake inhibitors, electroconvulsive stimuli and bupropion selectively reduced the potency of glycine to inhibit [3H]-5,7-dichlorkynurenic acid (5,7-DCKA) binding to the glycine-B site of the NMDA receptor, a change consistent with downregulation of NMDA receptor function (Paul *et al.*, 1994). In this study, the NMDA antagonist ketamine did not modify sensitivity to glycine, although it directly reduced NMDA receptor function through blockade of the calcium channel within the NMDA receptor complex. The tricyclic antidepressant desipramine, which has direct NMDA receptor antagonism at therapeutic doses (Reynolds and Miller, 1988; White *et al.*, 1990), reduces the potency of glycine to displace 5,7-DCKA binding similarly to other antidepressants and it additionally reduces the density of 5,7-DCKA binding sites (Paul *et al.*, 1994). Interestingly, pretreatment of mice with desipramine was shown to significantly reduce NMDA-induced biting and scratching behaviour (Mjellem *et al.*, 1993).

Several mood stabilizing compounds also appear to attenuate glutamatergic function. Repeated administration of lithium, the prototype mood stabilizer, may promote the uptake of glutamate from the synapse (Dixon and Hokin, 1998), attenuate the function of glutamate receptors (Nonaka *et al.*, 1998) and reduce the function of intracellular signalling cascades that are activated by the binding of glutamate to its receptors (Manji and Lenox, 1999). Anticonvulsant and voltage-sensitive calcium channel antagonist mood stabilizers appear to reduce glutamate release (Cunningham and Jones, 2000), and to inhibit intracellular signalling downstream from glutamate receptors (Manji *et al.*, 1999).

NMDA Antagonist as Antidepressant Agents

Animal Studies

A growing body of preclinical research suggests that NMDA glutamate receptor antagonists exhibit antidepressant-like effects in animal models. Non-competitive NMDA antagonists (amantadine and memantine), competitive NMDA receptor antagonists (CGP 37849) and glycine-B partial agonists (ACPC) have antidepressant-like effects in several tests, including the Porsolt swim test (Moryl *et al.*, 1993; Przegalinski *et al.*, 1997), the tail suspension test (Trullas and Skolnick, 1990) and the chronic mild stress paradigm (Ossowska *et al.*, 1997; Papp and Moryl, 1994).

The mechanisms through which NMDA receptor antagonism exerts this effect are not yet clear. However, several possible pathways exist. For example, NMDA antagonists are known to downregulate β-adrenergic receptors, in a manner similar to other antidepressants (Wedzony *et al.*, 1995). NMDA receptor antagonists also enhance serotonergic function (Lejeune *et al.*, 1994; Pallotta *et al.*, 1998) by several mechanisms, including increasing the number of 5-HT1A receptors (Wedzony *et al.*, 1997). Alternatively, the mechanism may be the result of a more direct effect on cortical excitability in critical regions of brain activity.

Treatment of Humans with Glutamate Modulating Agents

In humans, the antidepressant activity of NMDA receptor antagonists has received little rigorous evaluation. Initial studies by Crane suggested that D-cycloserine (DCS), an antibiotic developed to treat tuberculosis with indirect NMDA receptor antagonist-like effects mediated through the glycine-B site, possessed antidepressant activity (Crane, 1959, 1961). He reported beneficial effects with respect to depressed mood, insomnia and reduced appetite in depressed tuberculosis patients treated with DCS in doses of 500 mg per day. Interestingly, the rapid onset of antidepressant activity was a striking feature of DCS effects in these patients.

Case reports and preliminary studies suggest that amantadine, a low-affinity non-competitive antagonist of the NMDA receptor, has clinical efficacy in treating depressive symptoms provide additional evidence of the antidepressant activity of NMDA receptor antagonists (Dietrich *et al.*, 2000, Ferszt *et al.*, 1999, Huber *et al.*, 1999). Memantine, a related non-competitive NMDA receptor antagonist, also shows signs of behavioural improvement across a number of dimensions in patients with neuropsychiatric disorders, including mood and motor activity (Ambrozi and Danielczyk, 1988; Görtelmeyer and Erbler, 1992).

Most recently, a placebo-controlled pilot study suggested that the administration of single doses of ketamine 0.5 mg kg^{-1}, intravenously, had antidepressant effects in depressed patients (Berman *et al.*, 2000). Ketamine infusion produced mild psychosis and euphoria that dissipated within 120 minutes, while the antidepressant effects of ketamine infusion emerged over the first 180 minutes and persisted over 72 hours (Figure XVIII-3.3).

Although the clinical evidence supporting the antidepressant efficacy of NMDA antagonists remains limited, if effective, NMDA antagonists may show unique onset rapidity of clinical efficacy.

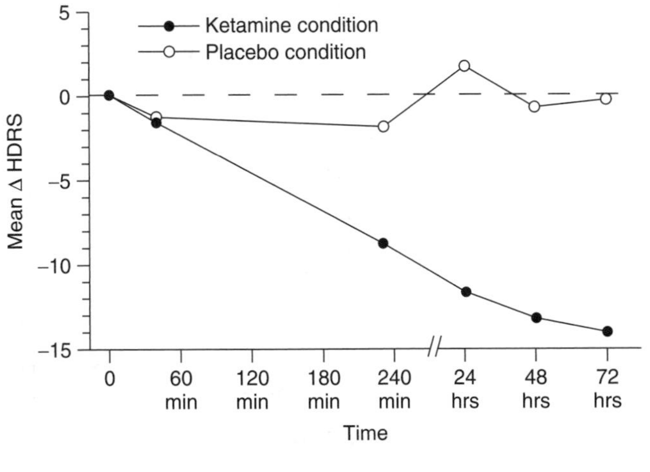

Figure XVIII-3.3 Graph illustrating the decrease in depressive symptom severity as measured by the Hamilton depression rating scale (HDRS) in seven subjects following either administration of placebo (open circle) or ketamine (closed circle) over a 72-hour period. Adapted from Berman *et al.* (2000)

CONCLUSION

Increasing evidence from several lines of research suggests that the major amino acid neurotransmitter systems contribute to the pathophysiology of mood disorders and the mechanisms of antidepressant and mood stabilizing actions. Relatively recent advances in magnetic resonance spectroscopy, along with an increased understanding of amino acid physiology and pharmacology, have now made it possible to begin our investigation into the role these systems may play in the pathophysiology and treatment of mood disorders.

The convergence of this evidence with other studies showing glial deficits and neuronal atrophy associated with stress and depression suggests that a common link may exist. Mismatches between inhibitory and excitatory drive are likely to promote atrophy and neurotoxicity, and may also be related to the reports of altered energy metabolism and cortical excitability that are commonly associated with mood disorders.

REFERENCES

Acosta, G.B. and Rubio, M.C., 1994. GABAA receptors mediate the changes produced by stress on GABA function and locomotor activity. *Neurosci. Lett.*, **176**(1), 29–31.

Acosta, G.B., Otero, Losada, M.E. and Rubio, M.C., 1993. Area-dependent changes in GABAergic function after acute and chronic cold stress. *Neurosci. Lett.*, **154**(1–2), 175–8.

Altamura, C.A., Mauri, M.C., Ferrara, A., Moro, A.R., D'Andrea, G. and Zamberlan, F., 1993. Plasma and platelet excitatory amino acids in psychiatric disorders. *Am. J. Psychiat.*, **150**(11), 1731–3.

Altamura, C., Maes, M., Dai, J. and Meltzer, H.Y., 1995. Plasma concentrations of excitatory amino acids, serine, glycine, taurine and histidine in major depression. *Eur. Neuropsychopharmacol.*, **5**(suppl), 71–5.

Ambrozi, L. and Danielczyk, W., 1988. Treatment of impaired cerebral function in psychogeriatric patients with memantine—results of a phase II double-blind study. *Pharmacopsychiatry*, **21**(3), 144–6.

Arranz, B., Cowburn, R., Eriksson, A., Vestling, M. and Marcusson, J., 1992. Gamma-aminobutyric acid-B (GABAB) binding sites in postmortem suicide brains. *Neuropsychobiology*, **26**(1–2), 33–6.

Auer, D.P., Pütz, B., Kraft, E., Lipinski, B., Schill, J. and Holsboer, F., 2000. Reduced glutamate in the anterior cingulate cortex in depression: an *in vivo* proton magnetic resonance spectroscopy study. *Biol. Psychiat.*, **47**(4), 305–13.

Baker, G.B., Wong, J.T., Yeung, J.M. and Coutts, R.T., 1991. Effects of the antidepressant phenelzine on brain levels of gamma-aminobutyric acid (GABA). *J. Affect. Disord.*, **21**(3), 207–11.

Barbaccia, M.L., Roscetti, G., Trabucchi, M., Mostallino, M.C., Concas, A., Purdy, R.H. and Biggio, G., 1996. Time-dependent changes in rat brain neuroactive steroid concentrations and GABAA receptor function after acute stress. *Neuroendocrinology*, **63**(2), 166–72.

Barbaccia., M.L., Roscetti., G., Trabucchi., M., Purdy, R.H., Mostallino, M.C., Concas, A. and Biggio, G., 1997. The effects of inhibitors of GABAergic transmission and stress on brain and plasma allopregnanolone concentrations. *Br. J. Pharmacol.*, **120**(8), 1582–8.

Bartanusz, V., Aubry, J.M., Pagliusi, S., Jezova, D., Baffi, J. and Kiss, J.Z., 1995. Stress-induced changes in messenger RNA levels of *N*-methyl-D-aspartate and AMPA receptor subunits in selected regions of the rat hippocampus and hypothalamus. *Neuroscience*, **66**(2), 247–52.

Bartholini, G., Lloyd, K.G. and Morselli, P.L. (eds), 1986. *GABA and Mood Disorders: Experimental and Clinical Research*. Raven Press, New York.

Beck, S.G., Birnstiel, S., Choi, K.C. and Pouliot, W.A., 1997. Fluoxetine selectively alters 5-hydroxytryptamine1A and gamma-aminobutyric acidB receptor-mediated hyperpolarization in area CA1, but not area CA3, hippocampal pyramidal cells. *J. Pharmacol. Exp. Ther.*, **281**(1), 115–22.

Berman, R.M., Cappiello, A., Anand, A., Oren, D.A., Heninger, G.R., Charney, D.S. and Krystal, J.H., 2000. Antidepressant effects of ketamine in depressed patients. *Biol. Psychiat.*, **47**(4), 351–4.

Berrettini, W.H., Nurnberger, J.I., Jr, Hare, T., Gershon, E.S. and Post, R.M., 1982a. Plasma and CSF GABA in affective illness. *Br. J. Psychiat.*, **141**, 483–7.

Berrettini, W.H., Umberkoman-Wiita, B., Nurnberger, J.I. Jr, Vogel, W.H., Gershon, E.S. and Post, R.M., 1982b. Platelet GABA-transaminase in affective illness. *Psychiat. Res.*, **7**(2), 255–60.

Berrettini, W.H., Nurnberger, J.I., Jr, Hare, T.A., Simmons-Alling, S. and Gershon, E.S., 1986. CSF GABA in euthymic manic-depressive patients and controls. *Biol. Psychiat.*, **21**(8–9), 844–6.

Biggio, G., Concas, A., Serra, M., Salis, M., Corda, M.G., Nurchi, V., Crisponi, C. and Gessa, G.L., 1984. Stress and beta-carbolines decrease the density of low affinity GABA binding sites; an effect reversed by diazepam. *Brain Res.*, **305**(1), 13–8.

Borsini, F., Evangelista, S. and Meli, A., 1986. Effect of GABAergic drugs in the behavioral 'despair' test in rats. *Eur. J. Pharmacol.*, **121**(2), 265–8.

Borsini, F., Mancinelli, A., D'Aranno, V., Evangelista, S. and Meli, A., 1988. On the role of endogenous GABA in the forced swimming test in rats. *Pharmacol. Biochem. Behav.*, **29**(2), 275–9.

Boudaba, C., Szabó, K. and Tasker, J.G., 1996. Physiological mapping of local inhibitory inputs to the hypothalamic paraventricular nucleus. *J. Neurosci.*, **16**(22), 7151–60.

Bowden, C.L., Brugger, A.M., Swann, A.C., Calabrese, J.R., Janicak, P.G., Petty, F., Dilsaver, S.C., Davis, J.M., Rush, A.J. and Small, J.G., 1994. Efficacy of divalproex vs lithium and placebo in the treatment of mania. The Depakote Mania Study Group. *JAMA*, **271**(12), 918–24.

Bowdler, J.M., Green, A.R., Minchin, M.C. and Nutt, D.J., 1983. Regional GABA concentration and [3H]-diazepam binding in rat brain following repeated electroconvulsive shock. *J. Neural Transm.*, **56**(1), 3–12.

Bowers, G., Cullinan, W.E. and Herman, J.P., 1998. Region-specific regulation of glutamic acid decarboxylase (GAD) mRNA expression in central stress circuits. *J. Neurosci.*, **18**(15), 5938–47.

Bremner, J.D., Narayan, M., Anderson, E.R., Staib, L.H., Miller, H.L. and Charney, D.S., 2000. Hippocampal volume reduction in major depression. *Am. J. Psychiat.*, **157**(1), 115–8.

Brown, E.S., Suppes, T., McElroy, S., Kmetz, G., Frye, M., Denicoff, K., Keck, P., Nolen, W., Kupka, R., Altshuler, L., Rochussen, J., Haytef, J., Leverich, G. and Post, R., 1999. A pilot trial of adjunctive topiramate in the treatment of bipolar disorder. In: *54th Annual Convention and Scientific Program*, 13–15 May, p. 78. Society of Biological Psychiatry, Washington, DC.

Caldji, C., Francis, D., Sharma, S., Plotsky, P.M. and Meaney, M.J., 2000. The effects of early rearing environment on the development of GABAA and central benzodiazepine receptor levels and novelty-induced fearfulness in the rat. *Neuropsychopharmacology*, **22**(3), 219–29.

Calogero, A.E., Gallucci, W.T., Chrousos, G.P. and Gold, P.W., 1988. Interaction between GABAergic neurotransmission and rat hypothalamic corticotropin-releasing hormone secretion *in vitro*. *Brain Res.*, **463**(1), 28–36.

Carlsson, M.L., 2001. On the role of prefrontal cortex glutamate for the antithetical phenomenology of obsessive compulsive disorder and attention deficit hyperactivity disorder. *Prog. Neuropsychopharmacol. Biol. Psychiat.*, **25**(1), 5–26.

Castillo, M., Kwock, L., Courvoisie, H. and Hooper, S.R., 2000. Proton MR spectroscopy in children with bipolar affective disorder: preliminary observations. *Am. J. Neuroradiol.*, **21**(5), 832–8.

Cheetham, S.C., Crompton, M.R., Katona, C.L., Parker, S.J. and Horton, R.W., 1988. Brain GABAA/benzodiazepine binding sites and glutamic acid decarboxylase activity in depressed suicide victims. *Brain Res.*, **460**(1), 114–23.

Concas, A., Serra, M., Atsoggiu, T. and Biggio, G., 1988. Foot-shock stress and anxiogenic beta-carbolines increase t-[35S]butylbicyclophosphorothionate binding in the rat cerebral cortex, an effect opposite to anxiolytics and gamma-aminobutyric acid mimetics. *J. Neurochem.*, **51**(6), 1868–76.

Cousins, J.P. and Harper, G., 1996. Neurobiochemical changes from Taxol/Neupogen chemotherapy for metastatic breast carcinoma corresponds with suicidal depression. *Cancer Lett.*, **110**(1–2), 163–7.

Crane, G.E., 1959. Cycloserine as an antidepressant agent. *Am. J. Psychiat.*, **115**, 1025–6.

Crane, G.E., 1961. The psychotropic effects of cycloserine: a new use for an antibiotic. *Comprehensive Psychiat.*, **2**, 51–9.

Cratty, M.S. and Birkle, D.L., 1999. *N*-methyl-D-aspartate (NMDA)-mediated corticotropin-releasing factor (CRF) release in cultured rat amygdala neurons. *Peptides*, **20**(1), 93–100.

Cross, J.A. and Horton, R.W., 1988. Effects of chronic oral administration of the antidepressants, desmethylimipramine and zimelidine on rat cortical GABAB binding sites: a comparison with 5-HT2 binding site changes. *Br. J. Pharmacol.*, **93**(2), 331–6.

Cross, J.A., Cheetham, S.C., Crompton, M.R., Katona, C.L. and Horton, R.W., 1988. Brain GABAB binding sites in depressed suicide victims. *Psychiat. Res.*, **26**(2), 119–29.

Cunningham, M.O. and Jones, R.S., 2000. The anticonvulsant, lamotrigine decreases spontaneous glutamate release but increases spontaneous GABA release in the rat entorhinal cortex *in vitro*. *Neuropharmacology*, **39**(11), 2139–46.

Danbolt, N.C., 2001. Glutamate uptake. *Prog. Neurobiol.*, **65**(1), 1–105.

Davis, L.L., Kabel, D., Patel, D., Choate, A.D., Foslien-Nash, C., Gurguis, G.N., Kramer, G.L. and Petty, F., 1996. Valproate as an antidepressant in major depressive disorder. *Psychopharmacol. Bull.*, **32**(4), 647–52.

Davis, L.L., Trivedi, M., Choate, A., Kramer, G.L. and Petty, F., 1997. Growth hormone response to the GABAB agonist baclofen in major depressive disorder. *Psychoneuroendocrinology*, **22**(3), 129–40.

Delini–Stula, A. and Vassout, A., 1978. Influence of baclofen and GABA-mimetic agents on spontaneous and olfactory-bulb-ablation-induced muricidal behaviour in the rat. *Arzneimittelforschung*, **28**(9), 1508–9.

Dietrich, D.E., Kleinschmidt, A., Hauser, U., Schneider, U., Spannhuth, C.W., Kipp, K., Huber, T.J., Wieringa, B.M., Emrich, H.M. and Johannes, S., 2000. Word recognition memory before and after successful treatment of depression. *Pharmacopsychiatry*, **33**(6), 221–8.

Dixon, J.F. and Hokin, L.E., 1998. Lithium acutely inhibits and chronically up-regulates and stabilizes glutamate uptake by presynaptic nerve endings in mouse cerebral cortex. *Proc. Natl Acad. Sci. USA*, **95**(14), 8363–8.

Feldman, S. and Weidenfeld, J., 1997. Hypothalamic mechanisms mediating glutamate effects on the hypothalamo-pituitary-adrenocortical axis. *J. Neural Transm.*, **104**(6–7), 633–42.

Ferszt, R., Kühl, K.P., Bode, L., Severus, E.W., Winzer, B., Berghöfer, A., Beelitz, G., Brodhun, B., Müller-Oerlinghausen, B. and Ludwig, H., 1999. Amantadine revisited: an open trial of amantadinesulfate treatment in chronically depressed patients with Borna disease virus infection. *Pharmacopsychiatry*, **32**(4), 142–7.

Francis, P.T., Poynton, A., Lowe, S.L., Najlerahim, A., Bridges, P.K., Bartlett, J.R., Procter, A.W., Bruton, C.J. and Bowen, D.M., 1989. Brain amino acid concentrations and Ca^{2+}-dependent release in intractable depression assessed antemortem. *Brain Res.*, **494**(2), 315–24.

Gerner, R.H. and Hare, T.A., 1981. CSF GABA in normal subjects and patients with depression, schizophrenia, mania, and anorexia nervosa. *Am. J. Psychiat.*, **138**(8), 1098–101.

Gerner, R.H., Fairbanks, L., Anderson, G.M., Young, J.G., Scheinin, M., Linnoila, M., Hare, T.A., Shaywitz, B.A. and Cohen, D.J., 1984. CSF neurochemistry in depressed, manic, and schizophrenic patients compared with that of normal controls. *Am. J. Psychiat.*, **141**(12), 1533–40.

Giardino, L., Zanni, M., Velardo, A., Amato, G. and Calzà, L., 1993. Effect of sertraline treatment on benzodiazepine receptors in the rat brain. *J. Neural Transm. Gen. Sect.*, **94**(1), 31–41.

Giardino, L., Zanni, M., Bettelli, C., Savina, M.A. and Calzà, L., 1996. Regulation of glutamic acid decarboxylase mRNA expression in rat brain after sertraline treatment. *Eur. J. Pharmacol.*, **312**(2), 183–7.

Goddard, A.W., Narayan, M., Woods, S.W., Germine, M., Kramer, G.L., Davis, L.L. and Petty, F., 1996. Plasma levels of gamma-aminobutyric acid and panic disorder. *Psychiat. Res.*, **63**(2–3), 223–5.

Gold, B.I., Bowers, M.B., Jr, Roth, R.H. and Sweeney, D.W., 1980. GABA levels in CSF of patients with psychiatric disorders. *Am. J. Psychiat.*, **137**(3), 362–4.

Görtelmeyer, R. and Erbler, H., 1992. Memantine in the treatment of mild to moderate dementia syndrome. A double-blind placebo-controlled study. *Arzneimittelforschung*, **42**(7), 904–13.

Halbreich, U., Petty, F., Yonkers, K., Kramer, G.L., Rush, A.J. and Bibi, K.W., 1996. Low plasma gamma-aminobutyric acid levels during the late luteal phase of women with premenstrual dysphoric disorder. *Am. J. Psychiat.*, **153**(5), 718–20.

Herman, J.P. and Cullinan, W.E., 1997. Neurocircuitry of stress: central control of the hypothalamo-pituitary-adrenocortical axis. *Trends Neurosci.*, **20**(2), 78–84.

Hiraoka, A., Miura, I., Tominaga, I. and Hattori, M., 1989. Capillary-isotachophoretic determination of glutamine in cerebrospinal fluid of various neurological disorders. *Clin. Biochem.*, **22**(4), 293–6.

Holemans, S., De Paermentier, F., Horton, R.W., Crompton, M.R., Katona, C.L. and Maloteaux, J.M., 1993. NMDA glutamatergic receptors, labelled with [3H]MK-801, in brain samples from drug-free depressed suicides. *Brain Res.*, **616**(1–2), 138–43.

Honig, A., Bartlett, J.R., Bouras, N. and Bridges, P.K., 1988. Amino acid levels in depression: a preliminary investigation. *J. Psychiat. Res.*, **22**(3), 159–64.

Huber, T.J., Dietrich, D.E. and Emrich, H.M., 1999. Possible use of amantadine in depression. *Pharmacopsychiatry*, **32**(2), 47–55.

Insel, T.R., 1989. Decreased *in vivo* binding to brain benzodiazepine receptors during social isolation. *Psychopharmacology (Berl)*, **97**(2), 142–4.

Kaiya, H., Namba, M., Yoshida, H. and Nakamura, S., 1982. Plasma glutamate decarboxylase activity in neuropsychiatry. *Psychiat. Res.*, **6**(3), 335–43.

Kasa, K., Otsuki, S., Yamamoto, M., Sato, M., Kuroda, H. and Ogawa, N., 1982. Cerebrospinal fluid gamma-aminobutyric acid and homovanillic acid in depressive disorders. *Biol. Psychiat.*, **17**(8), 877–83.

Kim, J.S., Schmid–Burgk, W., Claus, D. and Kornhuber, H.H., 1982. Increased serum glutamate in depressed patients. *Arch. Psychiatr. Nervenkr.*, **232**(4), 299–304.

Kimber, J.R., Cross, J.A. and Horton, R.W., 1987. Benzodiazepine and GABAA receptors in rat brain following chronic antidepressant drug administration. *Biochem. Pharmacol.*, **36**(23), 4173–5.

Korf, J. and Venema, K., 1983. Desmethylimipramine enhances the release of endogenous GABA and other neurotransmitter amino acids from the rat thalamus. *J. Neurochem.*, **40**(4), 946–50.

Korpi, E.R., Kleinman, J.E. and Wyatt, R.J., 1988. GABA concentrations in forebrain areas of suicide victims. *Biol. Psychiat.*, **23**(2), 109–14.

Koulu, M., Lammintausta, R. and Dahlström, S., 1979. Stimulatory effect of acute baclofen administration on human growth hormone secretion. *J. Clin. Endocrinol. Metab.*, **48**(6), 1038–40.

Kugaya, A., Sanacora, G., Verhoeff, N., Fujita, M., Seneca, N., Khan, S., Anand, A., Degen, K., Mason, G., Zoghbi, S., Baldwin, R., Seibyl, J. and Innis, R., 2001. *In vivo* cortical benzodiazepine receptor binding and GABA levels in patients with unipolar major depression. *J. Nucl. Med.*, **42**(suppl), S61.

Lai, C.T., Tanay, V.A., Charrois, G.J., Baker, G.B. and Bateson, A.N., 1998. Effects of phenelzine and imipramine on the steady-state levels of mRNAs that encode glutamic acid decarboxylase (GAD67 and GAD65), the GABA transporter GAT-1 and GABA transaminase in rat cortex. *Naunyn-Schmiedebergs Arch. Pharmacol.*, **357**(1), 32–8.

Lejeune, F., Gobert, A., Rivet, J.M. and Millan, M.J., 1994. Blockade of transmission at NMDA receptors facilitates the electrical and synthetic activity of ascending serotoninergic neurones. *Brain Res.*, **656**(2), 427–31.

Leonard, B.E., 1984. The olfactory bulbectomized rat as a model of depression. *Pol. J. Pharmacol. Pharm.*, **36**(5), 561–9.

Levine, J., Panchalingam, K., Rapoport, A., Gershon, S., McClure, R.J. and Pettegrew, J.W., 2000. Increased cerebrospinal fluid glutamine levels in depressed patients. *Biol. Psychiat.*, **47**(7), 586–93.

Lloyd, K.G., DeMontis, G., Broekkamp, C.L., Thuret, F. and Worms, P., 1983. Neurochemical and neuropharmacological indications for the involvement of GABA and glycine receptors in neuropsychiatric disorders. *Adv. Biochem. Psychopharmacol.*, **37**, 137–48.

Lloyd, K.G., Morselli, P.L. and Bartholini, G., 1987. GABA and affective disorders. *Med. Biol.*, **65**(2–3), 159–65.

Lloyd, K.G., Zivkovic, B., Scatton, B., Morselli, P.L. and Bartholini, G., 1989. The gabaergic hypothesis of depression. *Prog. Neuropsychopharmacol. Biol. Psychiat.*, **13**(3–4), 341–51.

Löscher, W., 1993. Effects of the antiepileptic drug valproate on metabolism and function of inhibitory and excitatory amino acids in the brain. *Neurochem. Res.*, **18**(4), 485–502.

Maes, M., Verkerk, R., Vandoolaeghe, E., Lin, A. and Scharpe, S., 1998. Serum levels of excitatory amino acids, serine, glycine, histidine, threonine, taurine, alanine and arginine in treatment-resistant depression: modulation by treatment with antidepressants and prediction of clinical responsivity. *Acta Psychiat. Scand.*, **97**(4), 302–8.

Maj, J., Rogóz, Z., Skuza, G. and Sowinska, H., 1992. Effects of MK-801 and antidepressant drugs in the forced swimming test in rats. *Eur. Neuropsychopharmacol.*, **2**(1), 37–41.

Manji, H.K. and Lenox, R.H., 1999. Ziskind–Somerfeld Research Award. Protein kinase C signaling in the brain: molecular transduction of mood stabilization in the treatment of manic-depressive illness. *Biol. Psychiat.*, **46**(10), 1328–51.

Manji, H.K., Bebchuk, J.M., Moore, G.J., Glitz, D., Hasanat, K.A. and Chen, G., 1999. Modulation of CNS signal transduction pathways and gene expression by mood-stabilizing agents: therapeutic implications. *J. Clin. Psychiat.*, **60**(suppl 2), 27–39; discussion 40–1, 113–6.

Manyam, B.V., 1982. Low CSF gamma-aminobutyric acid levels in Parkinson's disease. Effect of levodopa and carbidopa. *Arch. Neurol.*, **39**(7), 391–2.

Marchesi, C., Chiodera, P., De, Ferri, A., De Risio, C., Dassó, L., Menozzi, P., Volpi, R. and Coiro, V., 1991. Reduction of GH response to the GABA-B agonist baclofen in patients with major depression. *Psychoneuroendocrinology*, **16**(6), 475–9.

Mauri, M.C., Ferrara, A., Boscati, L., Bravin, S., Zamberlan, F., Alecci, M. and Invernizzi, G., 1998. Plasma and platelet amino acid concentrations in patients affected by major depression and under fluvoxamine treatment. *Neuropsychobiology*, **37**(3), 124–9.

McKenna, K.F., McManus, D.J., Baker, G.B. and Coutts, R.T., 1994. Chronic administration of the antidepressant phenelzine and its *N*-acetyl analogue: effects on GABAergic function. *J. Neural Transm.*, **41**(Suppl), 115–22.

McManus, D.J. and Greenshaw, A.J., 1991. Differential effects of antidepressants on GABAB and beta-adrenergic receptors in rat cerebral cortex. *Biochem. Pharmacol.*, **42**(8), 1525–8.

McManus, D.J., Baker, G.B., Martin, I.L., Greenshaw, A.J. and McKenna, K.F., 1992. Effects of the antidepressant/antipanic drug phenelzine on GABA concentrations and GABA-transaminase activity in rat brain. *Biochem. Pharmacol.*, **43**(11), 2486–9.

Michael, N., Erfurth, A., Pecuch, P., Ohrmann, P., Wolgast, M., Arolt, V., Heindel, W. and Pfleiderer, B., 2001. Clinical response to electroconvulsive therapy (ECT) restores reduced glutamate/glutamine levels in the left anterior cingulum of severely depressed patients. In: *World Congress of Biological Psychiatry*, Vol. 2, p. 191S. Berlin.

Mjellem, N., Lund, A. and Hole, K., 1993. Reduction of NMDA-induced behaviour after acute and chronic administration of desipramine in mice. *Neuropharmacology*, **32**(6), 591–5.

Moghaddam, B., 1993. Stress preferentially increases extraneuronal levels of excitatory amino acids in the prefrontal cortex: comparison to hippocampus and basal ganglia. *J. Neurochem.*, **60**(5), 1650–7.

Moghaddam, B., Bolinao, M.L., Stein–Behrens, B. and Sapolsky, R., 1994. Glucocorticoids mediate the stress-induced extracellular accumulation of glutamate. *Brain Res.*, **655**(1–2), 251–4.

Monteleone, P., Maj, M., Iovino, M. and Steardo, L., 1990. GABA, depression and the mechanism of action of antidepressant drugs: a neuroendocrine approach. *J. Affect. Disord.*, **20**(1), 1–5.

Moryl, E., Danysz, W. and Quack, G., 1993. Potential antidepressive properties of amantadine, memantine and bifemelane. *Pharmacol. Toxicol.*, **72**(6), 394–7.

Motohashi, N., Ikawa, K. and Kariya, T., 1989. GABAB receptors are upregulated by chronic treatment with lithium or carbamazepine. GABA hypothesis of affective disorders? *Eur. J. Pharmacol.*, **166**(1), 95–9.

Müller, E.E., 1987. Neural control of somatotropic function. *Physiol. Rev.*, **67**(3), 962–1053.

Nonaka, S., Hough, C.J. and Chuang, D.M., 1998. Chronic lithium treatment robustly protects neurons in the central nervous system against excitotoxicity by inhibiting *N*-methyl-D-aspartate receptor-mediated calcium influx. *Proc. Natl Acad. Sci. USA*, **95**(5), 2642–71.

Nowak, G., Ordway, G.A. and Paul, I.A., 1995a. Alterations in the *N*-methyl-D-aspartate (NMDA) receptor complex in the frontal cortex of suicide victims. *Brain Res.*, **675**(1–2), 157–64.

Nowak, G., Redmond, A., McNamara, M. and Paul, I.A., 1995b. Swim stress increases the potency of glycine at the *N*-methyl-D-aspartate receptor complex. *J. Neurochem.*, **64**(2), 925–7.

O'Flynn, K. and Dinan, T.G., 1993. Baclofen-induced growth hormone release in major depression: relationship to dexamethasone suppression test result. *Am. J. Psychiat.*, **150**(11), 1728–30.

O'Hara, M.W., Neunaber, D.J. and Zekoski, E.M., 1984. Prospective study of postpartum depression: prevalence, course, and predictive factors. *J. Abnorm. Psychol.*, **93**(2), 158–71.

Olsen, R.W., Ticku, M.K., Van Ness, P.C. and Greenlee, D., 1978. Effects of drugs on gamma-aminobutyric acid receptors, uptake, release and synthesis *in vitro*. *Brain Res.*, **139**(2), 277–94.

Ongür, D., Drevets, W.C. and Price, J.L., 1998. Glial reduction in the subgenual prefrontal cortex in mood disorders. *Proc. Natl Acad. Sci. USA*, **95**(22), 13290–5.

Oruc, L., Furac, I., Croux, C., Jakovljevic, M., Kracun, I., Folnegovic, V. and Van Broeckhoven, C., 1996. Association study between bipolar disorder and candidate genes involved in dopamine-serotonin metabolism and GABAergic neurotransmission: a preliminary report [letter]. *Psychiatr. Genet.*, **6**(4), 213–7.

Ossowska, G., Klenk–Majewska, B. and Szymczyk, G., 1997. The effect of NMDA antagonists on footshock-induced fighting behavior in chronically stressed rats. *J. Physiol. Pharmacol.*, **48**(1), 127–35.

Owens, M.J., Vargas, M.A., Knight, D.L. and Nemeroff, C.B., 1991. The effects of alprazolam on corticotropin-releasing factor neurons in the rat brain: acute time course, chronic treatment and abrupt withdrawal. *J. Pharmacol. Exp. Ther.*, **258**(1), 349–56.

Pallotta, M., Segieth, J. and Whitton, P.S., 1998. *N*-methyl-D-aspartate receptors regulate 5-HT release in the raphe nuclei and frontal cortex of freely moving rats: differential role of 5-HT1A autoreceptors. *Brain Res.*, **783**(2), 173–8.

Papp, M. and Moryl, E., 1994. Antidepressant activity of non-competitive and competitive NMDA receptor antagonists in a chronic mild stress model of depression. *Eur. J. Pharmacol.*, **263**(1–2), 1–7.

Paslawski, T., Treit, D., Baker, G.B., George, M. and Coutts, R.T., 1996. The antidepressant drug phenelzine produces antianxiety effects in the plus-maze and increases in rat brain GABA. *Psychopharmacology (Berl)*, **127**(1), 19–24.

Patel, G.J., Schatz, R.P., Constantinides, S.M. and Lal, H., 1975. Effect of desipramine and pargyline on brain gamma-aminobutyric acid. *Biochem. Pharmacol.*, **24**(1), 57–60.

Paul, I.A., Nowak, G., Layer, R.T., Popik, P. and Skolnick, P., 1994. Adaptation of the *N*-methyl-D-aspartate receptor complex following chronic antidepressant treatments. *J. Pharmacol. Exp. Ther.*, **269**(1), 95–102.

Perry, E.K., Gibson, P.H., Blessed, G., Perry, R.H. and Tomlinson, B.E., 1977. Neurotransmitter enzyme abnormalities in senile dementia. Choline acetyltransferase and glutamic acid decarboxylase activities in necropsy brain tissue. *J. Neurol. Sci.*, **34**(2), 247–65.

Perry, T.L. and Hansen, S., 1973. Sustained drug-induced elevation of brain GABA in the rat. *J. Neurochem.*, **21**(5), 1167–75.

Petty, F., 1994. Plasma concentrations of gamma-aminobutyric acid (GABA) and mood disorders: a blood test for manic depressive disease? *Clin. Chem.*, **40**(2), 296–302.

Petty, F., 1995. GABA and mood disorders: a brief review and hypothesis. *J. Affect. Disord.*, **34**(4), 275–81.

Petty, F. and Schlesser, M.A., 1981. Plasma GABA in affective illness. A preliminary investigation. *J. Affect. Disord.*, **3**(4), 339–43.

Petty, F. and Sherman, A.D., 1981. GABAergic modulation of learned helplessness. *Pharmacol. Biochem. Behav.*, **15**(4), 567–70.

Petty, F. and Sherman, A.D., 1984. Plasma GABA levels in psychiatric illness. *J. Affect. Disord.*, **6**(2), 131–8.

Petty, F., Kramer, G.L., Dunnam, D. and Rush, A.J., 1990. Plasma GABA in mood disorders. *Psychopharmacol. Bull.*, **26**(2), 157–61.

Petty, F., Kramer, G.L., Gullion, C.M. and Rush, A.J., 1992. Low plasma gamma-aminobutyric acid levels in male patients with depression. *Biol. Psychiat.*, **32**(4), 354–63.

Petty, F., Fulton, M., Moeller, F., Kramer, G., Wilson, L., Fraser, K. and Isbell, P., 1993a. Plasma gamma-aminobutyric acid (GABA) is low in alcoholics. *Psychopharmacol. Bull.*, **29**(2), 277–81.

Petty, F., Kramer, G.L., Fulton, M., Moeller, F.G. and Rush, A.J., 1993b. Low plasma GABA is a trait-like marker for bipolar illness. *Neuropsychopharmacology*, **9**(2), 125–32.

Petty, F., Kramer, G.L. and Hendrickse, W., 1993c. In: Mann, J.J. and Kupler, D.J. (eds), *Biology of Depressive Disorders*, Part A, *A Systems Perspective*, pp. 79–108. Plenum Press, New York.

Petty, F., Trivedi, M.H., Fulton, M. and Rush, A.J., 1995. Benzodiazepines as antidepressants: does GABA play a role in depression? *Biol. Psychiat.*, **38**(9), 578–91.

Petty, F., Fulton, M., Kramer, G.L., Kram, M., Davis, L.L. and Rush, A.J., 1999. Evidence for the segregation of a major gene for human plasma GABA levels *Molec. Psychiat.*, **4**(6), 587–9.

Pilc, A. and Lloyd, K.G., 1984. Chronic antidepressants and GABA 'B' receptors: a GABA hypothesis of antidepressant drug action. *Life Sci.*, **35**(21), 2149–54.

Poncelet, M., Martin, P., Danti, S., Simon, P. and Soubrié, P., 1987. Noradrenergic rather than GABAergic processes as the common mediation of the antidepressant profile of GABA agonists and imipramine-like drugs in animals. *Pharmacol. Biochem. Behav.*, **28**(3), 321–6.

Popov, N. and Matthies, H., 1969. Some effects of monoamine oxidase inhibitors on the metabolism of gamma-aminobutyric acid in rat brain. *J. Neurochem.*, **16**(3), 899–907.

Post, R.M., Ballenger, J.C., Hare, T.A., Goodwin, F.K., Lake, C.R., Jimerson, D.C. and Bunney, W.E.J., 1980. Cerebrospinal fluid GABA in normals and patients with affective disorders. *Brain Res. Bull.*, **5**(suppl 2), 755–9.

Post, R.M., Leverich, G.S., Denicoff, K.D., Frye, M.A., Kimbrell, T.A. and Dunn, R., 1997. Alternative approaches to refractory depression in bipolar illness. *Depress. Anxiety*, **5**(4), 175–89.

Przegalinski, E., Tatarczynska, E., Deren–Wesoek, A. and Chojnacka-Wojcik, E., 1997. Antidepressant-like effects of a partial agonist at strychnine-insensitive glycine receptors and a competitive NMDA receptor antagonist. *Neuropharmacology*, **36**(1), 31–7.

Puertollano, R., Visedo, G., Zapata, C. and Fernández-Piqueras, J., 1997. A study of genetic association between manic-depressive illness and a highly polymorphic marker from the GABRbeta-1 gene. *Am. J. Med. Genet.*, **74**(3), 342–4.

Rajkowska, G., Miguel–Hidalgo, J.J., Wei, J., Dilley, G., Pittman, S.D., Meltzer, H.Y., Overholser, J.C., Roth, B.L. and Stockmeier, C.A., 1999. Morphometric evidence for neuronal and glial prefrontal cell pathology in major depression. *Biol. Psychiat.*, **45**(9), 1085–98.

Reynolds, I.J. and Miller, R.J., 1988. Tricyclic antidepressants block *N*-methyl-D-aspartate receptors: similarities to the action of zinc. *Br. J. Pharmacol.*, **95**(1), 95–102.

Rode, A., Bidzinski, A. and Puzynski, S., 1991. Poziom GABA w osoczu chorych na depresje endogenna i w czasie leczenia tymoleptykami. [GABA levels in the plasma of patients with endogenous depression and during the treatment with thymoleptics]. *Psychiatr. Pol.*, **25**(3–4), 4–7.

Romeo, E., Ströhle, A., Spalletta, G., di Michele, F., Hermann, B., Holsboer, F., Pasini, A. and Rupprecht, R., 1998. Effects of antidepressant treatment on neuroactive steroids in major depression. *Am. J. Psychiat.*, **155**(7), 910–3.

Roy, A., DeJong, J., Lamparski, D., George, T. and Linnoila, M., 1991a. Depression among alcoholics. Relationship to clinical and cerebrospinal fluid variables. *Arch. Gen. Psychiat.*, **48**(5), 428–32.

Roy, A., Dejong, J. and Ferraro, T., 1991b. CSF GABA in depressed patients and normal controls. *Psychol. Med.*, **21**(3), 613–8.

Roy–Byrne, P.P., Cowley, D.S., Hommer, D., Greenblatt, D.J., Kramer, G.L. and Petty, F., 1992. Effect of acute and chronic benzodiazepines on plasma GABA in anxious patients and controls. *Psychopharmacology (Berl)*, **109**(1–2), 153–6.

Rubinow, D.R., Roy–Byrne, P., Hoban, M.C., Gold, P.W. and Post, R.M., 1984. Prospective assessment of menstrually related mood disorders. *Am. J. Psychiat.*, **141**(5), 684–6.

Sanacora, G., Mason, G.F., Rothman, D.L., Behar, K.L., Hyder, F., Petroff, O.A., Berman, R.M., Charney, D.S. and Krystal, J.H., 1999a. Reduced cortical gamma-aminobutyric acid levels in depressed patients determined by proton magnetic resonance spectroscopy. *Arch. Gen. Psychiat.*, **56**(11), 1043–7.

Sanacora, G., Mason, G.F., Rothman, D.L., Berman, R., Charney, D.S., Ciarcia, J.J. and Krystal, J.H., 1999b. ECT effects on cortical GABA levels as determined by 1H-MRS. In: *International Society for Magnetic Resonance in Medicine*, Philadelphia, PA.

Sanacora, G., Mason, G.F. and Krystal, J.H., 2000. Impairment of GABAergic transmission in depression: new insights from neuroimaging studies. *Crit. Rev. Neurobiol.*, **14**(1), 23–45.

Sanacora, G., Mason, G.F., Rothman, D.L and Krystal, J.H., 2002. Increased occipital cortex GABA concentrations following in depressed patients after therapy with selective serotonin reuptake inhibitors. *American Journal of Psychiatry*, **159**(4), 663–665.

Sanna, E., Cuccheddu, T., Serra, M., Concas, A. and Biggio, G., 1992. Carbon dioxide inhalation reduces the function of GABAA receptors in the rat brain. *Eur. J. Pharmacol.*, **216**(3), 457–8.

Sapolsky, R.M., 2000. The possibility of neurotoxicity in the hippocampus in major depression: a primer on neuron death. *Biol. Psychiat.*, **48**(8), 755–65.

Schatz, R.A. and Lal, H., 1971. Elevation of brain GABA by pargyline: a possible mechanism for protection against oxygen toxicity. *J. Neurochem.*, **18**(12), 2553–5.

Schatzberg, A.F. and Cole, J.O., 1978. Benzodiazepines in depressive disorders. *Arch. Gen. Psychiat.*, **35**(11), 1359–651.

Serra, M., Sanna, E., Concas, A., Foddi, C. and Biggio, G., 1991. Footshock stress enhances the increase of [35S]TBPS binding in the rat cerebral cortex and the convulsions induced by isoniazid. *Neurochem. Res.*, **16**(1), 17–22.

Serretti, A., Macciardi, F., Cusin, C., Lattuada, E., Lilli, R., Di Bella, D., Catalano, M. and Smeraldi, E., 1998. GABAA alpha-1 subunit gene not associated with depressive symptomatology in mood disorders. *Psychiatr. Genet.*, **8**(4), 251–4.

Sheline, Y.I., Wang, P.W., Gado, M.H., Csernansky, J.G. and Vannier, M.W., 1996. Hippocampal atrophy in recurrent major depression. *Proc. Natl Acad. Sci. USA*, **93**(9), 3908–13.

Sherif, F., Marcusson, J. and Oreland, L., 1991. Brain gamma-aminobutyrate transaminase and monoamine oxidase activities in suicide victims. *Eur. Arch. Psychiat. Clin. Neurosci.*, **241**(3), 139–44.

Sherman, A.D. and Petty, F., 1980. Neurochemical basis of the action of antidepressants on learned helplessness. *Behav. Neural. Biol.*, **30**(2), 119–34.

Shiah, I. and Yatham, L.N., 1998. GABA function in mood disorders: an update and critical review. *Life Sci.*, **63**(15), 1289–303.

Skolnick, P., 1999. Antidepressants for the new millennium. *Eur. J. Pharmacol.*, **375**(1–3), 31–40.

Suranyi-Cadotte, B.E., Dam, T.V. and Quirion, R., 1984. Antidepressant–anxiolytic interaction: decreased density of benzodiazepine receptors in rat brain following chronic administration of antidepressants. *Eur. J. Pharmacol.*, **106**(3), 673–5.

Suzdak, P.D. and Gianutsos, G., 1985. Parallel changes in the sensitivity of gamma-aminobutyric acid and noradrenergic receptors following chronic administration of antidepressant and GABAergic drugs. A possible role in affective disorders. *Neuropharmacology*, **24**(3), 217–22.

Szekely, A.M., Barbaccia, M.L. and Costa, E., 1987. Effect of a protracted antidepressant treatment on signal transduction and [3H](-)-baclofen binding at GABAB receptors. *J. Pharmacol. Exp. Ther.*, **243**(1), 155–9.

Tanaka, K., Watase, K., Manabe, T., Yamada, K., Watanabe, M., Takahashi, K., Iwama, H., Nishikawa, T., Ichihara, N., Kikuchi, T., Okuyama, S., Kawashima, N., Hori, S., Takimoto, M. and Wada, K., 1997. Epilepsy and exacerbation of brain injury in mice lacking the glutamate transporter GLT-1. *Science*, **276**(5319), 1699–1702.

Tanay, V.A., Glencorse, T.A., Greenshaw, A.J., Baker, G.B. and Bateson, A.N., 1996. Chronic administration of antipanic drugs alters rat brainstem GABAA receptor subunit mRNA levels. *Neuropharmacology*, **35**(9–10), 1475–82.

Tiller, J.W., Schweitzer, I., Maguire, K.P. and Davis, B., 1989. Is diazepam an antidepressant? *Br. J. Psychiat.*, **155**, 483–9.

Toth, Z., Bunney, W.E., Potkin, S.G. and Jones, E.G., 1999. Gene expression for glutamic acid decarboxylase is increased in prefrontal cortex of depressed patients. In: *Society for Neuroscience 29th Annual Meeting*, Miami Beach, FL, p. 2097.

Trullas, R. and Skolnick, P., 1990. Functional antagonists at the NMDA receptor complex exhibit antidepressant actions. *Eur. J. Pharmacol.*, **185**(1), 1–10.

Tsai, G. and Coyle, J.T., 1998. The role of glutamatergic neurotransmission in the pathophysiology of alcoholism. *A. Rev. Med.*, **49**, 173–84.

Uzunov, D.P., Cooper, T.B., Costa, E. and Guidotti, A., 1996. Fluoxetine-elicited changes in brain neurosteroid content measured by negative ion mass fragmentography. *Proc. Natl Acad. Sci. USA*, **93**(22), 12599–604.

Wedzony, K., Klimek, V. and Nowak, G., 1995. Rapid down-regulation of beta-adrenergic receptors evoked by combined forced swimming test and CGP 37849 — a competitive antagonist of NMDA receptors. *Pol. J. Pharmacol.*, **47**(6), 537–40.

Wedzony, K., Mackowiak, M., Czyrak, A., Fija, K. and Michalska, B., 1997. Single doses of MK-801, a non-competitive antagonist of NMDA receptors, increase the number of 5-HT1A serotonin receptors in the rat brain. *Brain Res.*, **756**(1–2), 84–91.

Weizman, R., Weizman, A., Kook, K.A., Vocci, F., Deutsch, S.I. and Paul, S.M., 1989. Repeated swim stress alters brain benzodiazepine receptors measured *in vivo*. *J. Pharmacol. Exp. Ther.*, **249**(3), 701–7.

White, G., Lovinger, D.M., Peoples, R.W. and Weight, F.F., 1990. Inhibition of *N*-methyl-D-aspartate activated ion current by desmethylimipramine. *Brain Res.*, **537**(1–2), 337–9.

Ziegler, D.R. and Herman, J.P., 2000. Local integration of glutamate signaling in the hypothalamic paraventricular region: regulation of glucocorticoid stress responses. *Endocrinology*, **141**(12), 4801–4.

Zimmer, R., Teelken, A.W., Meier, K.D., Ackenheil, M. and Zander, K.J., 1980. Preliminary studies on CSF gamma-aminobutyric acid levels in psychiatric patients before and during treatment with different psychotropic drugs. *Prog. Neuropsychopharmacol.*, **4**(6), 613–20.

XVIII-4

Peptidergic Transmitter Systems

Jeffrey H. Meyer

Peptides refer to short proteins consisting of chains of less than 100 amino acids. There are as many as 250 peptide neurotransmitters in the brain (see Table XVIII-4.1 for a partial list). Some, such as corticotrophin-releasing factor, have been extensively investigated with respect to mood disorders, but most have not.

Peptides may function as neurotransmitters, neuromodulators and neurohormones. Neurotransmitters are synthesized in presynaptic neurons, and are released after depolarization by presynaptic neurons in sufficient amounts to have effects upon postsynaptic neurons. Neurotransmitters have immediate effects upon postsynaptic neurons and are removed by the synaptic cleft. Neuromodulators have longer term effects upon neurons. For example, a neuromodulator may stimulate a receptor coupled to an effector that influences a second messenger, leading to a cascade that changes ongoing cellular functioning. Neurohormones are similar to neuromodulators except that neurohormones are released into blood, cross the blood–brain barrier, and then bind to receptors.

In this chapter, abnormalities of peptidergic transmitter systems in mood disorders are reviewed. Abnormal peptidergic functioning may involve neurotransmitter, neuromodulator and neurohormone effects. There will be some discussion regarding the role of specific peptidergic transmitter systems in clinical treatment.

OPIOIDS

It is well known that opioid agonist administration can influence mood, and cause analgesia in humans. Given that these behavioural states are dysregulated during depressive episodes, there has been some interest in measuring abnormalities of opioid receptors during mood disorders.

Table XVIII-4.1 A partial list of peptides in the central nervous system

Adrenocorticotrophic hormone
Androgens
Bradykinin
Calcitonin
Cholecystokinin
Corticotrophin-releasing hormone
Cortisol
Oestrogens
Glucagon
Growth hormone
Insulin
Nerve growth factor
Neuropeptide Y
Opioids
Oxytocin
Somatostatin
Substance P
Vasoactive intestinal peptide
Vasopressin

The major classes of opioid receptors are delta (δ), kappa (κ), and mu (μ). Two reports have found an increase in μ opioid receptor density in multiple brain regions of suicide victims (Gabilondo *et al.*, 1995; Gross-Isseroff *et al.*, 1990). The earlier study sampled depressed patients. In the later study, the diagnosis was not always known; however, among those in which the diagnosis was known, most had depression. These reports are consistent with preliminary, *in vivo*, imaging investigations. There is one published abstract reporting an increase in μ opioid receptor binding potential in an [^{11}C] carfentanil positron emission tomography study of depression (Zubieta *et al.*, 1995). The binding potential is proportional to receptor density and affinity (Meyer and Ichise, 2001; Mintun *et al.*, 1984).

Increased μ opioid receptor density should enhance the effects of endogenous opioids and it may seem counterintuitive that increased μ opioid receptor density is observed in depressive episodes. It is possible that these findings may be secondary to lower endogenous opioids or other abnormalities that affect the regulation of this receptor (Law and Loh, 1999).

CHOLECYSTOKININ (CCK)

Cholecystokinin is a family of short-chain peptides which bind to CCK receptors. CCK receptors are categorized into CCK_A and CCK_B receptors. CCK is of interest in mood disorders because anxiety symptoms often occur comorbidly with depressive episodes, and peptides that have CCK_B receptor agonist properties provoke panic attacks (Bradwejn and Koszycki, 1994; Rehfeld, 2000). A second reason for the interest in CCK in mood disorders is that CCK can modulate the release of dopamine in the nucleus accumbens and influence reward behaviours in animal models (Vaccarino, 1994).

Studies sampling CCK in cerebrospinal fluid tend to find no differences between depressed and healthy subjects (Gerner and Yamada, 1982; Gjerris and Rafaelsen, 1984; Gjerris *et al.*, 1984; Rafaelsen and Gjerris, 1985). One study associated state anxiety level with several CCK peptides in a large sample of depressed patients (Lofberg *et al.*, 1998). It has been reported that CCK receptors are increased in frontal cortex of young suicide victims (Harro *et al.*, 1992). The most common diagnosis of a suicide victim is a major depressive episode and major depressive disorder (Barraclough *et al.*, 1974; Robins *et al.*, 1959) so it may be that this abnormality occurs during depressive episodes. Post-mortem investigations of CCK have found no changes in entorhinal cortex concentrations in depressed subjects (Perry *et al.*, 1981) and no changes in several cortex and limbic regions in suicide victims (Kleinman *et al.*, 1985).

Biological Psychiatry: Edited by H. D'haenen, J.A. den Boer and P. Willner. ISBN 0-471-49198-5

These findings suggest that most CCK peptides are not globally altered during depressive episodes. They do not clarify whether CCK peptides may be altered in small, specific subregions such as the shell of the nucleus accumbens. Thus it is theoretically possible that CCK peptides may have a role within specific neurochemical brain circuits and contribute to pathological behaviour such as impaired reward.

Even if it is eventually found that CCK peptides do not contribute to the pathophysiology of depression, CCK antagonists might be considered as possible treatments to enhance reward or reduce anxiety. The main barrier to the clinical development of such compounds is that they often do not penetrate the blood–brain barrier (Wilson *et al.*, 2001).

CORTICOTROPHIN-RELEASING FACTOR

Corticotrophin-releasing factor (CRF) binds to CRF_1 and CRF_2 receptors. Hypersecretion of CRF is known to occur during depressive episodes. Evidence for this includes increased cerebrospinal fluid CRF in depressed patients (Banki *et al.*, 1987; France *et al.*, 1988; Nemeroff *et al.*, 1984) as well as several findings in suicide victims. In suicide victims, cerebrospinal fluid CRF was increased, and CRF receptor density was decreased in multiple brain regions (Arato *et al.*, 1989; Hucks *et al.*, 1997; Nemeroff *et al.*, 1988). These findings suggest that CRF is higher throughout the central nervous system during depressive episodes (Nemeroff *et al.*, 1988).

Increased CRF appears to affect other hormones during depressive episodes. The adrenocorticotrophic hormone (ACTH) response to CRF is blunted (Hartline *et al.*, 1996; Pariante *et al.*, 1995) and the decreased ACTH responsiveness to CRF can be considered a consequence of chronically excessive CRF stimulation. Since CRF stimulates ACTH and ACTH stimulates cortisol secretion, the increased cortisol secretion observed during depressive episodes is most likely attributable to increased CRF during depressive episodes.

In addition to effects upon ACTH and cortisol secretion, CRF may influence anxiety systems and have specific behavioural effects during depressive episodes. CRF has been implicated in stress response behaviours in animal models. Stressors increase the synthesis of CRF and CRF administration increases stress-related behaviours (Gray and Bingaman, 1996; Lightman *et al.*, 1993). Some of these effects may be consequent to CRF release in the hypothalamic–pituitary axis because exploratory behaviours are reduced after CRF administration to the hypothalamus (Menzaghi *et al.*, 1993).

CRF release in the amygdala may also contribute to these stress behaviours. Stress paradigms appear to activate CRF releasing neurons in the amygdala and CRF administered to the amygdala increases stress behaviours (Gray and Bingaman, 1996; Honkaniemi, 1992). CRF-containing neurons in the amygdala project to other limbic regions that contribute to the stress response (septum, hypothalamus, vagal nucleus) (Gray and Bingaman, 1996).

Glucocorticoids suppress CRF by providing negative feedback to the secretion of CRF, and this feedback is impaired during depression (Carroll, 1976; Carroll *et al.*, 1976). It has been postulated that one mechanism of antidepressants is to enhance this inhibitory feedback upon CRF secretion by increasing glucocorticoid receptor expression (Barden *et al.*, 1995; McQuade and Young, 2000). A number of antidepressants, including desipramine, imipramine, moclobemide and lithium, increase mRNA of type II glucocorticoid receptors (Barden *et al.*, 1995; McQuade and Young, 2000; Pepin *et al.*, 1989).

Another interesting direction of clinical treatment is the use of CRF antagonists to treat mood disorders. An open trial of a CRF_1 antagonist in patients with depressive episodes reported promising results with good tolerability and a reasonable response rate (Zobel *et al.*, 2000).

CORTISOL

Cortisol is a peptide that binds to both glucocorticoid and mineralocorticoid receptors. Increased cortisol levels in the serum and cerebrospinal fluid may be the most replicated finding in depressive episodes (Holsboer, 2000). It has also been demonstrated that cortisol secretion is resistant to inhibition by dexamethasone during depressive episodes (Carroll, 1976; Carroll *et al.*, 1976). Adrenal gland size is also reported to be enlarged during depressive episodes (Nemeroff *et al.*, 1992; Rubin *et al.*, 1995, 1996).

In animal models, it has been demonstrated that increased stress may result in a number of changes in cells within the hippocampus: decreased number of granule cells, decreased neurogenesis of granule cells, increased death of neurons, and atrophy of neuronal dendrites (Duman *et al.*, 2000; Fuchs and Flugge, 1998; Sapolsky, 2000). It is thought that cortisol is in part responsible for mediating these effects because stress raises cortisol levels and some of these hippocampal changes occur after high doses of glucocorticoids (Fuchs and Flugge, 1998; Sapolsky, 2000).

There are several observations of changes in depression that have been attributed to increased stress and/or increased glucocorticoids because they resemble such effects observed in the hippocampus in animal models (Duman *et al.*, 1997; Fuchs and Flugge, 1998; Sapolsky, 2000). Post-mortem investigation of both unipolar and bipolar illnesses reports decreased neuronal size, and neuronal and glial densities in some cortex layers within Brodmann's area 9 of the prefrontal cortex (Rajkowska *et al.*, 1999, 2001). Hippocampal volume as measured using structural magnetic resonance imaging (MRI) is reported to be lower in major depressive disorder (Bremner *et al.*, 2000; Sheline *et al.*, 1996, 1999).

Increased stress during depressive episodes may be causing increased cortisol. The increased cortisol during depressive episodes could then be contributing to the post-mortem and MRI changes reflecting cell loss (Bremner *et al.*, 2000; Rajkowska *et al.*, 1999, 2001; Sheline *et al.*, 1996, 1999). Increased cortisol is not specific to mood disorders and can be found in other psychiatric illnesses, most notably bulimia. Even so, the effects of high cortisol may be an important part of the pathophysiology of this illness.

VASOPRESSIN AND OXYTOCIN

Arginine vasopressin (AVP) is a neuropeptide and hormone which binds to V_1, V_2 and V_3 receptor subtypes. V_3 (also known as V_{1B}) receptors can be found in the anterior pituitary and are of particular interest in mood disorders (Thibonnier *et al.*, 1998, 2001). V_1 receptors are mostly in vasculature and V_2 receptors are mostly renal (Thibonnier *et al.*, 1998, 2001). The reason why AVP has been investigated in mood disorders is that it participates in stress responses and modulates the hypothalamic–pituitary cortisol axis. In rodent models, vasopressin secretion is increased after immobilization and novelty stress, and especially after repeated immobilization stress (Bartanusz *et al.*, 1993; Chen and Herbert, 1995; Gibbs, 1986; Ivanyi *et al.*, 1991). These findings are consistent with a report that stressful events can increase vasopressin secretion in humans (Meyerhoff, 1990).

Vasopressin can enhance the function of the hypothalamic–pituitary axis to secrete cortisol. Vasopressin facilitates CRF-stimulated ACTH production. The mechanism for enhancing the effect of CRF may involve increased production of CRF itself and/or increased synthesis of CRF_1 receptors (Aguilera *et al.*, 2001; Bartanusz *et al.*, 1993; Gibbs, 1986).

Since increased CRF secretion occurs during depressive episodes, investigators have been interested in assessing whether increased AVP secretion may contribute to increased CRF secretion observed during depressive episodes. Serum and cerebrospinal fluid levels during depressive episodes are not consistently different from those of healthy subjects (Inder *et al.*, 1997; Legros and Ansseau, 1992; Legros *et al.*, 1993; Pitts *et al.*, 1995; van Londen *et al.*, 1997); however, one study did correlate CRF levels with AVP levels during depressive episodes (Pitts *et al.*, 1995). Within specific brain structures such as the paraventricular nucleus of the hypothalamus and the suprachiasmatic nucleus, increased numbers of AVP secreting neurons are reported (Purba *et al.*, 1996; Zhou *et al.*, 2001). While the role of the latter finding is still unclear, the increased numbers of AVP secreting neurons in the hypothalamus may be important: increased arginine vasopressin release could facilitate activation of the hypothalamic–pituitary axis for cortisol production.

Oxytocin (OT) may have a similar role to AVP in major depressive disorder. The role of this peptide during stress and its influence upon ACTH secretion appear to be similar to AVP (Callahan *et al.*, 1992; Gibbs, 1986; Ivanyi *et al.*, 1991). OT secretion is increased during stressful conditions and OT can facilitate CRF stimulation of ACTH (Callahan *et al.*, 1992; Gibbs, 1986; Ivanyi *et al.*, 1991).

Since increased CRF secretion occurs during depressive episodes, investigators have been interested in assessing whether increased OT secretion also occurs during depressive episodes. Cerebrospinal fluid and serum measures of OT are not consistently abnormal during depressive episodes (Legros and Ansseau, 1992; Legros *et al.*, 1993; Pitts *et al.*, 1995; van Londen *et al.*, 1997). There is one report of increased OT cell numbers in the paraventricular nucleus of the hypothalamus during depressive episodes (Zhou *et al.*, 2001). It is possible that OT will have a role as a facilitator of CRF stimulation during depressive episodes.

NEUROPEPTIDE Y

Neuropeptide Y is a 36-amino acid neurotransmitter with five receptor subtypes. There are some reports that neuropeptide Y is reduced in the cerebrospinal fluid and plasma of patients with depressive episodes (Hashimoto *et al.*, 1996; Nilsson *et al.*, 1996; Westrin *et al.*, 1999; Widerlov *et al.*, 1988). Neuropeptide Y is also reported to be lower in the prefrontal cortex of suicide victims (Widdowson *et al.*, 1992). Neuropeptide Y mRNA was reported to be lower in the prefrontal cortex of subjects with bipolar disorder (Widdowson *et al.*, 1992) and a post hoc analysis showed increased Y_2 mRNA expression in layer IV of the prefrontal cortex in suicide victims (Caberlotto and Hurd, 2001).

An interesting argument has been made that neuropeptide Y may be inadequately inhibiting CRF secretion during depressive episodes (Antonijevic *et al.*, 2000). The role of neuropeptide Y in mood disorders is still an area of ongoing investigation.

SUBSTANCE P

Substance P is classified with the tachykinin family and binds to neurokinin (NK_1) receptors. There is only limited evidence to suggest that there are abnormalities of the function of this peptide in mood disorders: one study found an elevation of substance P and/or substance P related peptides in cerebrospinal fluid of patients with major depressive disorder, and a second found no difference in substance P levels in major depressive disorder or bipolar disorder (Berrettini *et al.*, 1985; Rimon *et al.*, 1984). One study found no difference in substance P concentrations in a number of different brain regions in suicide victims as compared to healthy subjects (Kleinman *et al.*, 1985). One study found no overall difference in NK_1 density in the anterior cingulate gyrus in patients with a history of unipolar or bipolar disorder (Burnet and Harrison, 2000). In this study a secondary analysis found a decrease in the ratio of NK_1 density between superficial and deep layers in patients with a history of unipolar disorder. Further studies are needed to replicate this post hoc finding, to determine if there are substance P or NK_1 receptor abnormalities in other brain regions, and to address whether any such changes are related to the specific state of illness, i.e. depressive episode.

Although substance P might not play a role in mood disorders, NK_1 antagonists may have useful antidepressant properties. In behavioural models in animals, NK_1 antagonists reduce stress-induced vocalizations, enhance memory performance and reduce anxiety behaviours (Hasenohrl *et al.*, 2000; Kramer *et al.*, 1998). In addition, NK_1 antagonists promote cell growth and survival, and enhance recovery from lesions (Barker, 1996). All of these properties would seem favourable for the treatment of depressive episodes.

One clinical trial of an NK_1 antagonist found a similar rate of antidepressant response as compared to paroxetine and a significantly better response rate than placebo (Kramer *et al.*, 1998). Replication of this finding will be important as the placebo response rate was very high in this study.

NEUROTROPHINS

Brain-derived neurotrophic factor (BDNF) is a peptide within the family of neurotrophins and it binds to the tyrosine kinase receptor trkB. Neurotrophins and BDNF are released in the brain after damaging process such as seizures, hypoglycaemia and ischaemia (Lindvall *et al.*, 1994). Under such conditions, BDNF and neurotrophins demonstrate neuroprotective effects, and contribute to the formation of new synapses (Lindsay *et al.*, 1994; Lindvall *et al.*, 1994).

Neurotrophins are involved in processes of neuronal plasticity that occur in response to changes in perceptual stimuli (Thoenen, 1995). It is possible that processes which interfere with neurotrophin function will interfere with neuronal plasticity. This may be very relevant to stress during depressive episodes as it has been demonstrated that elevated stress may decrease hippocampal BDNF levels in animals (Duman *et al.*, 1997).

Neurotrophins may mediate some therapeutic effects of antidepressants. Long-term antidepressant (serotonin and norepinephrine reuptake inhibitors, monoamine oxidase inhibitors) administration to animals increases the expression of BDNF and trkB (Duman *et al.*, 1997). This finding may be relevant to clinical treatment of depression: a recent post-mortem study found elevated BDNF levels in the cerebellum in antidepressant-treated patients with major depressive disorder (Bayer *et al.*, 2000).

CONCLUSIONS

The relationship between peptides and mood disorders is a new frontier that bears further investigation. Studies of peptides in mood illnesses in humans have mostly sampled unipolar depression, and the relevance of these investigations to bipolar disorder is not known. The relationship between most peptides and mood disorders has not been studied.

Some peptides, such as CRF, may play a role in behavioural symptoms of depression, whereas peptides such as cortisol and NGF may contribute to pathological changes observed. Intervening with treatments to reverse abnormalities of these neuropeptides should result in new therapeutic opportunities for mood disorders.

Other peptides (such as substance P) may have no role in the pathophysiology of the illness, yet their antagonists could influence either symptoms or pathology and have important therapeutic properties. Most current antidepressant medications share considerable commonality because they bind to monoamine receptors or influence monoamines. For treatment-refractory patients, new classes of antidepressants could be extremely important.

REFERENCES

Aguilera, G., Rabadan-Diehl, C. and Nikodemova, M., 2001. Regulation of pituitary corticotropin releasing hormone receptors. *Peptides*, **22**, 769–74.

Antonijevic, I.A., Murck, H., Bohlhalter, S., Frieboes, R.M., Holsboer, F. and Steiger, A., 2000. Neuropeptide Y promotes sleep and inhibits ACTH and cortisol release in young men. *Neuropharmacology*, **39**, 1474–81.

Arato, M., Banki, C.M., Bissette, G. and Nemeroff, C.B., 1989. Elevated CSF CRF in suicide victims. *Biol. Psychiat.*, **25**, 355–9.

Banki, C.M., Bissette, G., Arato, M., O'Connor, L. and Nemeroff, C.B., 1987. CSF corticotropin-releasing factor-like immunoreactivity in depression and schizophrenia. *Am. J. Psychiat.*, **144**, 873–7.

Barden, N., Reul, J.M. and Holsboer, F., 1995. Do antidepressants stabilize mood through actions on the hypothalamic–pituitary–adrenocortical system? *Trends Neurosci.*, **18**, 6–11.

Barker, R., 1996. Tachykinins, neurotrophism and neurodegenerative diseases: a critical review on the possible role of tachykinins in the aetiology of CNS diseases. *Rev. Neurosci.*, **7**, 187–214.

Barraclough, B., Bunch, J., Nelson, B. and Sainsbury, P., 1974. A hundred cases of suicide: clinical aspects. *Br. J. Psychiat.*, **125**, 355–73.

Bartanusz, V., Jezova, D., Bertini, L.T., Tilders, F.J., Aubry, J.M. and Kiss, J.Z., 1993. Stress-induced increase in vasopressin and corticotropin-releasing factor expression in hypophysiotrophic paraventricular neurons. *Endocrinology*, **132**, 895–902.

Bayer, T.A., Schramm, M., Feldmann, N., Knable, M.B. and Falkai, P., 2000. Antidepressant drug exposure is associated with mRNA levels of tyrosine receptor kinase B in major depressive disorder. *Prog. Neuropsychopharmacol. Biol. Psychiat.*, **24**, 881–8.

Berrettini, W.H., Rubinow, D.R., Nurnberger, J.I., Jr, Simmons-Alling, S., Post, R.M. and Gershon, E.S., 1985. CSF substance P immunoreactivity in affective disorders. *Biol. Psychiat.*, **20**, 965–70.

Bradwejn, J. and Koszycki, D., 1994. The cholecystokinin hypothesis of anxiety and panic disorder. *Ann. N. Y. Acad. Sci.*, **713**, 273–82.

Bremner, J.D., Narayan, M., Anderson, E.R., Staib, L.H., Miller, H.L. and Charney, D.S., 2000. Hippocampal volume reduction in major depression. *Am. J. Psychiat.*, **157**, 115–8.

Burnet, P.W.J. and Harrison, P.J., 2000. Substance P (NK1) receptors in the cingulate cortex in unipolar and bipolar mood disorder and schizophrenia. *Biol. Psychiat.*, **47**, 80–3.

Caberlotto, L. and Hurd, Y.L., 2001. Neuropeptide Y Y(1) and Y(2) receptor mRNA expression in the prefrontal cortex of psychiatric subjects. Relationship of Y(2) subtype to suicidal behavior. *Neuropsychopharmacology*, **25**, 91–7.

Callahan, M.F., Thore, C.R., Sundberg, D.K., Gruber, K.A., O'Steen, K. and Morris, M., 1992. Excitotoxin paraventricular nucleus lesions: stress and endocrine reactivity and oxytocin mRNA levels. *Brain Res.*, **597**, 8–15.

Carroll, B.J., 1976. Limbic system–adrenal cortex regulation in depression and schizophrenia. *Psychosom. Med.*, **38**, 106–21.

Carroll, B.J., Curtis, G.C. and Mendels, J., 1976. Neuroendocrine regulation in depression. II. Discrimination of depressed from nondepressed patients. *Arch. Gen. Psychiat.*, **33**, 1051–8.

Chen, X. and Herbert, J., 1995. Alterations in sensitivity to intracerebral vasopressin and the effects of a V1a receptor antagonist on cellular, autonomic and endocrine responses to repeated stress. *Neuroscience*, **64**, 687–97.

Duman, R., Heninger, G. and Nestler, E., 1997. A molecular and cellular theory of depression. *Arch. Gen. Psychiat.*, **54**(7), 597–606.

Duman, R.S., Malberg, J., Nakagawa, S. and D'Sa, C., 2000. Neuronal plasticity and survival in mood disorders. *Biol. Psychiat.*, **48**, 732–9.

France, R.D., Urban, B., Krishnan, K.R., Bissett, G., Banki, C.M., Nemeroff, C. and Speilman, F.J., 1988. CSF corticotropin-releasing factor-like immunoactivity in chronic pain patients with and without major depression. *Biol. Psychiat.*, **23**, 86–8.

Fuchs, E. and Flugge, G., 1998. Stress, glucocorticoids and structural plasticity of the hippocampus. *Neurosci. Biobehav. Rev.*, **23**, 295–300.

Gabilondo, A.M., Meana, J.J. and Garcia-Sevilla, J.A., 1995. Increased density of mu-opioid receptors in the postmortem brain of suicide victims. *Brain Res.*, **682**, 245–50.

Gerner, R.H. and Yamada, T., 1982. Altered neuropeptide concentrations in cerebrospinal fluid of psychiatric patients. *Brain Res.*, **238**, 298–302.

Gibbs, D.M., 1986. Vasopressin and oxytocin: hypothalamic modulators of the stress response: a review. *Psychoneuroendocrinology*, **11**, 131–9.

Gjerris, A. and Rafaelsen, O.J., 1984. Catecholamines and vasoactive intestinal polypeptide in cerebrospinal fluid in depression. *Adv. Biochem. Psychopharmacol.*, **39**, 159–60.

Gjerris, A., Rafaelsen, O.J., Vendsborg, P., Fahrenkrug, J. and Rehfeld, J.F., 1984. Vasoactive intestinal polypeptide decreased in cerebrospinal fluid (CSF) in atypical depression. Vasoactive intestinal polypeptide, cholecystokinin and gastrin in CSF in psychiatric disorders. *J. Affect. Disord.*, **7**, 325–37.

Gray, T.S. and Bingaman, E.W., 1996. The amygdala: corticotropin-releasing factor, steroids, and stress. *Crit. Rev. Neurobiol.*, **10**, 155–68.

Gross-Isseroff, R., Dillon, K.A., Israeli, M. and Biegon, A., 1990. Regionally selective increases in mu opioid receptor density in the brains of suicide victims. *Brain Res.*, **530**, 312–6.

Harro, J., Marcusson, J. and Oreland, L., 1992. Alterations in cholecystokinin receptors in suicide victims. *Eur. Neuropsychopharmacol.*, **2**, 57–63.

Hartline, K., Owens, M. and Nemeroff, C., 1996. Postmortem and cerebrospinal fluid studies of corticotrophin-releasing factor in humans. *Ann. N. Y. Acad. Sci.*, **780**, 96–105.

Hasenohrl, R., De Souza-Silva, M., Nikolaus, S., Tomaz, C., Brandao, M., Schwarting, R. and Huston, J., 2000. Substance P and its role in neural mechanisms governing learning, anxiety and functional recovery. *Neuropeptides*, **34**, 272–80.

Hashimoto, H., Onishi, H., Koide, S., Kai, T. and Yamagami, S., 1996. Plasma neuropeptide Y in patients with major depressive disorder. *Neurosci. Lett.*, **216**, 57–60.

Holsboer, F., 2000. The corticosteroid receptor hypothesis of depression. *Neuropsychopharmacology*, **23**, 477–501.

Honkaniemi, J., 1992. Colocalization of peptide- and tyrosine hydroxylase-like immunoreactivities with Fos-immunoreactive neurons in rat central amygdaloid nucleus after immobilization stress. *Brain Res.*, **598**, 107–13.

Hucks, D., Lowther, S., Crompton, M.R., Katona, C.L. and Horton, R.W., 1997. Corticotropin-releasing factor binding sites in cortex of depressed suicides. *Psychopharmacology (Berl)*, **134**, 174–8.

Inder, W.J., Donald, R.A., Prickett, T.C., Frampton, C.M., Sullivan, P.F., Mulder, R.T. and Joyce, P.R., 1997. Arginine vasopressin is associated with hypercortisolemia and suicide attempts in depression. *Biol. Psychiat.*, **42**, 744–7.

Ivanyi, T., Wiegant, V.M. and de Wied, D., 1991. Differential effects of emotional and physical stress on the central and peripheral secretion of neurohypophysial hormones in male rats. *Life Sci.*, **48**, 1309–16.

Kleinman, J.E., Hong, J., Iadarola, M., Govoni, S. and Gillin, C.J., 1985. Neuropeptides in human brain — postmortem studies. *Prog. Neuropsychopharmacol. Biol. Psychiat.*, **9**, 91–5.

Kramer, M., Cutler, N., Feighner, J., Shrivastava, R., Carman, J., Sramek, J., Reines, S., Liu, G., Snavely, D., Wyatt-Knowles, E., Hale, J., Mills, S., MacCoss, M., Swain, C., Harrison, T., Hill, R., Hefti, F., Scolnick, E., Cascieri, M., Chicchi, G., Sadowski, S., Williams, A., Hewson, L., Smith, D., Carlson, E., Hargreaves, R. and Rupniak, N., 1998. Distinct mechanism for antidepressant activity by blockade of central substance P receptors. *Science*, **281**, 1640–5.

Law, P.Y. and Loh, H.H., 1999. Regulation of opioid receptor activities. *J. Pharmacol. Exp. Ther.*, **289**, 607–24.

Legros, J.J. and Ansseau, M., 1992. Neurohypophyseal peptides and psychopathology. *Prog. Brain Res.*, **93**, 455–60.

Legros, J.J., Ansseau, M. and Timsit-Berthier, M., 1993. Neurohypophyseal peptides and psychiatric diseases. *Regul. Pept.*, **45**, 133–8.

Lightman, S.L., Harbuz, M.S., Knight, R.A. and Chowdrey, H.S., 1993. CRF mRNA in normal and stress conditions. *Ann. N. Y. Acad. Sci.*, **697**, 28–38.

Lindsay, R.M., Wiegand, S.J., Altar, C.A. and DiStefano, P.S., 1994. Neurotrophic factors: from molecule to man. *Trends Neurosci.*, **17**, 182–90.

Lindvall, O., Kokaia, Z., Bengzon, J., Elmer, E. and Kokaia, M., 1994. Neurotrophins and brain insults. *Trends Neurosci.*, **17**, 490–6.

Lofberg, C., Agren, H., Harro, J. and Oreland, L., 1998. Cholecystokinin in CSF from depressed patients: possible relations to severity of depression and suicidal behaviour. *Eur. Neuropsychopharmacol.*, **8**, 153–7.

McQuade, R. and Young, A.H., 2000. Future therapeutic targets in mood disorders: the glucocorticoid receptor. *Br. J. Psychiat.*, **177**, 390–5.

Menzaghi, F., Heinrichs, S.C., Pich, E.M., Weiss, F. and Koob, G.F., 1993. The role of limbic and hypothalamic corticotropin-releasing factor in behavioral responses to stress. *Ann. N. Y. Acad. Sci.*, **697**, 142–54.

Meyer, J. and Ichise, M., 2001. Modelling of receptor ligand data in PET and SPECT imaging: a review of major approaches. *J. Neuroimaging*, **11**, 30–9.

Meyerhoff, J., 1990. Neuroendocrine responses to emotional stress: possible interactions between circulating factors and anterior pituitary hormone release. In: Porter, J. and Jezova, D. (eds), *Circulating Regulatory Factors and Neuroendocrine Function*, pp. 91–111. New York, Plenum Press.

Mintun, M.A., Raichle, M.E., Kilbourn, M.R., Wooten, G.F. and Welch, M.J., 1984. A quantitative model for the *in vivo* assessment of drug binding sites with positron emission tomography. *Ann. Neurol.*, **15**, 217–27.

Nemeroff, C.B., Owens, M.J., Bissette, G., Andorn, A.C. and Stanley, M., 1988. Reduced corticotropin releasing factor binding sites in the frontal cortex of suicide victims. *Arch. Gen. Psychiat.*, **45**, 577–9.

Nemeroff, C.B., Widerlov, E., Bissette, G., Walleus, H., Karlsson, I., Eklund, K., Kilts, C.D., Loosen, P.T. and Vale, W., 1984. Elevated concentrations of CSF corticotropin-releasing factor-like immunoreactivity in depressed patients. *Science*, **226**, 1342–4.

Nemeroff, C.B., Krishnan, K.R., Reed, D., Leder, R., Beam, C. and Dunnick, N.R., 1992. Adrenal gland enlargement in major depression. A computed tomographic study. *Arch. Gen. Psychiat.*, **49**, 384–7.

Nilsson, C., Karlsson, G., Blennow, K., Heilig, M. and Ekman, R., 1996. Differences in the neuropeptide Y-like immunoreactivity of the plasma and platelets of human volunteers and depressed patients. *Peptides*, **17**, 359–62.

Pariante, C., Nemeroff, C. and Miller, A., 1995. Glucocorticoid receptors in depression. *Isr. J. Med. Sci.*, **31**, 705–12.

Pepin, M.C., Beaulieu, S. and Barden, N., 1989. Antidepressants regulate glucocorticoid receptor messenger RNA concentrations in primary neuronal cultures. *Brain Res. Molec. Brain Res.*, **6**, 77–83.

Perry, R.H., Dockray, G.J., Dimaline, R., Perry, E.K., Blessed, G. and Tomlinson, B.E., 1981. Neuropeptides in Alzheimer's disease, depression and schizophrenia. A post-mortem analysis of vasoactive intestinal peptide and cholecystokinin in cerebral cortex. *J. Neurol. Sci.*, **51**, 465–72.

Pitts, A.F., Samuelson, S.D., Meller, W.H., Bissette, G., Nemeroff, C.B. and Kathol, R.G., 1995. Cerebrospinal fluid corticotropin-releasing hormone, vasopressin, and oxytocin concentrations in treated patients with major depression and controls. *Biol. Psychiat.*, **38**, 330–5.

Purba, J.S., Hoogendijk, W.J., Hofman, M.A. and Swaab, D.F., 1996. Increased number of vasopressin- and oxytocin-expressing neurons in the paraventricular nucleus of the hypothalamus in depression. *Arch. Gen. Psychiat.*, **53**, 137–43.

Rafaelsen, O.J. and Gjerris, A., 1985. Neuropeptides in the cerebrospinal fluid (CSF) in psychiatric disorders. *Prog. Neuropsychopharmacol. Biol. Psychiat.*, **9**, 533–8.

Rajkowska, G., Miguel-Hidalgo, J.J., Wei, J., Dilley, G., Pittman, S.D., Meltzer, H.Y., Overholser, J.C., Roth, B.L. and Stockmeier, C.A., 1999. Morphometric evidence for neuronal and glial prefrontal cell pathology in major depression. *Biol. Psychiat.*, **45**, 1085–98.

Rajkowska, G., Halaris, A. and Selemon, L.D., 2001. Reductions in neuronal and glial density characterize the dorsolateral prefrontal cortex in bipolar disorder. *Biol. Psychiat.*, **49**, 741–52.

Rehfeld, J.F., 2000. Cholecystokinin and panic disorder — three unsettled questions. *Regul. Pept.*, **93**, 79–83.

Rimon, R., Le Greves, P., Nyberg, F., Heikkila, L., Salmela, L. and Terenius, L., 1984. Elevation of substance P-like peptides in the CSF of psychiatric patients. *Biol. Psychiat.*, **19**, 509–16.

Robins, E., Murphy, G., Wilkinson, R., Gassner, S. and Kayes, J., 1959. Some clinical considerations in the prevention of suicide based on a study of 134 successful suicides. *Am. J. Publ. Hlth.*, **49**(7), 888–99.

Rubin, R.T., Phillips, J.J., McCracken, J.T. and Sadow, T.F., 1996. Adrenal gland volume in major depression: relationship to basal and stimulated pituitary-adrenal cortical axis function. *Biol. Psychiat.*, **40**, 89–97.

Rubin, R.T., Phillips, J.J., Sadow, T.F. and McCracken, J.T., 1995. Adrenal gland volume in major depression. Increase during the depressive episode and decrease with successful treatment. *Arch. Gen. Psychiat.*, **52**, 213–8.

Sapolsky, R.M., 2000. Glucocorticoids and hippocampal atrophy in neuropsychiatric disorders. *Arch. Gen. Psychiat.*, **57**, 925–35.

Sheline, Y.I., Wang, P.W., Gado, M.H., Csernansky, J.G. and Vannier, M.W., 1996. Hippocampal atrophy in recurrent major depression. *Proc. Natl. Acad. Sci. USA*, **93**, 3908–13.

Sheline, Y.I., Sanghavi, M., Mintun, M.A. and Gado, M.H., 1999. Depression duration but not age predicts hippocampal volume loss in medically healthy women with recurrent major depression. *J. Neurosci.*, **19**, 5034–43.

Thibonnier, M., Conarty, D.M., Preston, J.A., Wilkins, P.L., Berti-Mattera, L.N. and Mattera, R., 1998. Molecular pharmacology of human vasopressin receptors. *Adv. Exp. Med. Biol.*, **449**, 251–76.

Thibonnier, M., Coles, P., Thibonnier, A. and Shoham, M., 2001. The basic and clinical pharmacology of nonpeptide vasopressin receptor antagonists. *A. Rev. Pharmacol. Toxicol.*, **41**, 175–202.

Thoenen, H., 1995. Neurotrophins and neuronal plasticity. *Science*, **270**, 593–8.

Vaccarino, F.J., 1994. Nucleus accumbens dopamine–CCK interactions in psychostimulant reward and related behaviors. *Neurosci. Biobehav. Rev.*, **18**, 207–14.

van Londen, L., Goekoop, J.G., van Kempen, G.M., Frankhuijzen-Sierevogel, A.C., Wiegant, V.M., van der Velde, E.A. and De Wied, D., 1997. Plasma levels of arginine vasopressin elevated in patients with major depression. *Neuropsychopharmacology*, **17**, 284–92.

Westrin, A., Ekman, R. and Traskman-Bendz, L., 1999. Alterations of corticotropin releasing hormone (CRH) and neuropeptide Y (NPY) plasma levels in mood disorder patients with a recent suicide attempt. *Eur. Neuropsychopharmacol.*, **9**, 205–11.

Widdowson, P.S., Ordway, G.A. and Halaris, A.E., 1992. Reduced neuropeptide Y concentrations in suicide brain. *J. Neurochem.*, **59**, 73–80.

Widerlov, E., Lindstrom, L.H., Wahlestedt, C. and Ekman, R., 1988. Neuropeptide Y and peptide YY as possible cerebrospinal fluid markers for major depression and schizophrenia, respectively. *J. Psychiat. Res.*, **22**, 69–79.

Wilson, A.A., Jin, L., Garcia, A., DaSilva, J.N. and Houle, S., 2001. Carbon-11 labelled cholecystokininB antagonists: radiosynthesis and evaluation in rats. *Life Sci.*, **68**, 1223–30.

Zhou, J.N., Riemersma, R.F., Unmehopa, U.A., Hoogendijk, W.J., van Heerikhuize, J.J., Hofman, M.A. and Swaab, D.F., 2001. Alterations in arginine vasopressin neurons in the suprachiasmatic nucleus in depression. *Arch. Gen. Psychiat.*, **58**, 655–62.

Zobel, A.W., Nickel, T., Kunzel, H.E., Ackl, N., Sonntag, A., Ising, M. and Holsboer, F., 2000. Effects of the high-affinity corticotropin-releasing hormone receptor 1 antagonist R121919 in major depression: the first 20 patients treated. *J. Psychiat. Res.*, **34**, 171–81.

Zubieta, J., Treisman, G., Fishman, M., Dannals, R., Ravert, H. and Frost, J., 1995. Increased mu opioid receptor binding in unmedicated major depression: a PET study with [11C] carfentanil (abstract). *J. Nucl. Med.*, **36**, 21.

XVIII-5

Neuroendocrinology of Mood Disorders

Dorothy K.Y. Sit and Anthony J. Rothschild

INTRODUCTION

The major mood disorders are associated with specific, highly reproducible neuroendocrine alterations, and conversely, certain endocrine disorders (e.g. hypothyroidism and Cushing's disease) are associated with higher than expected rates of mood disturbances. Neuroendocrine abnormalities have been thought to provide a 'window on the brain', revealing clues regarding the pathophysiology of central nervous system dysfunction. This neuroendocrine strategy is based on extensive research which indicates that the secretion of peripheral endocrine hormones is largely controlled by the respective pituitary trophic hormone. The pituitary hormones are in turn regulated by hypothalamic release and release-inhibiting hormones. Mood disorders are associated with multiple alterations, specifically of the hypothalamic–pituitary–adrenal (HPA), hypothalamic–pituitary–thyroid (HPT) and growth hormone axes. In this chapter, we review the research on the alterations of these axes and also discuss the roles of melatonin, dehydroepiandrosterone, parathyroid hormone and gonadal hormones in the pathophysiology of mood disorders.

HYPOTHALAMIC–PITUITARY–ADRENAL AXIS

Introduction

Hypercortisolism has been prevailingly linked to the hormonal stress response found in patients experiencing affective disorders, especially in depression. Stressful life events may trigger a psychiatric condition in susceptible individuals, perhaps indicating a response of the HPA axis. Current research, however, is now aimed at understanding the mechanism by which the HPA axis may be causally linked to the pathophysiology of mood disorders. A growing body of preclinical and clinical research continues to provide information on the close ties between abnormalities in the HPA axis and various regions of the brain, with their subsequent influence to alter function of crucial neurotransmitters (and their receptors), relevant to the development of affective disorders.

HPA Axis Function

Corticosteroids and Mood Effects

Cortisol and the HPA axis play a crucial role in the stress response system, acting as an important interface between the central nervous system and the peripheral endocrine response system (Holsboer, 2001). Each hormone in the HPA axis cascade, as well as the other neuropeptides, possesses important effects not only on behaviour and emotions, but have significant roles in modulating the immune, endocrine and autonomic nervous systems. Cortisol enhances the availability of glucose, the main nutrient for all cells, including those found in the brain. Hypercortisolism, as a reflection of a hyperactive HPA axis state, now is postulated to be causally linked to the pathophysiology of depression.

Patients with depression and documented hypercortisolism often present with vegetative changes, such as sleep disturbance and energy reduction, decreased attention and cognition, psychosis, suicidality, anxiety, psychomotor disturbances or decreased libido (Wolkowitz, 1994). More recent literature hypothesizes that current antidepressants stimulate corticosteroid receptor expression, causing enhanced negative feedback on the HPA axis restoring appropriate corticotropin-releasing hormone (CRH) and cortisol levels. By reducing the levels of circulating cortisol, mood and vegetative symptoms may improve.

Historically, medically ill patients who were prescribed steroids such as prednisone, dexamethasone, cortisone and other synthetic corticosteroids for various medical conditions reportedly developed behavioural and emotional changes, such as mood lability, depression, hypomania, memory and attention changes, or psychosis. Those treated with exogenous corticosteroids seem to present with hypomania, while those with an underlying condition that produces increased endogenous steroids present with depression (Plihal *et al.*, 1996). Patients with Cushing's syndrome (non-adrenocorticotropic hormone [ACTH] related) and disease (increased ACTH) develop depression at similar incidence rates, even though the disease origins are different, implying that cortisol contributes to the development of psychiatric symptoms (Murphy, 1991).

Of note, patients with Addison's disease, an immune-related disorder leading to adrenocortical insufficiency, may also develop depression which responds to cortisol and other hormone replacement therapy (Leigh and Kramer, 1984). DeBattista *et al.* (2000) reported on 22 patients with non-psychotic depression who were randomly assigned to a one-day treatment with either ovine CRH, hydrocortisone or saline. Depression rating scales given immediately prior to treatment and the day following treatment demonstrated a rapid and robust reduction in depressive symptoms. Arana *et al.* (1995) and Dinan *et al.* (1997) described brief open-label trials using high-dose dexamethasone for the treatment of depression, reporting significant symptom improvement. On the otherhand, Wolkowitz *et al.* (1996) found the contrary, albeit in a very small sample size of five patients. Wolkowitz and Reus, (1999) postulated that both anti-glucocorticoid treatment and brief high-dose steroid treatment may have similar effects on the HPA axis, such as lowering of cortisol levels through upregulation of brain corticosteroid receptors; altering levels of the other adrenal steroid hormones; and increase in ACTH levels (after dexamethasone's initial inhibitory effect on ACTH production is worn off).

The HPA Axis, Serotonin, and Hippocampal Pathophysiology

It appears that corticosteroids influence brain function through the modulation of gene expression, and direct cell membrane effects

Biological Psychiatry: Edited by H. D'haenen, J.A. den Boer and P. Willner. ISBN 0-471-49198-5

(McEwen *et al.*, 1979). The mechanisms by which hypercortisolism leads to affective disorders, such as depression, may be explained by effects of increased CRH, enhanced secretion of ACTH from the pituitary, increased adrenal steroid output, and impaired response to negative feedback at the levels of the hypothalamus, pituitary, adrenals and hippocampus. The hippocampus is implicated in its role of regulating the HPA axis. This stems from findings of increased expression of mineralocorticoid (type I) and glucocorticoid (type II) receptors in the hippocampus (Jacobson and Sapolsky, 1991), along with evidence of increased HPA stress reactions after hippocampal damage, and hippocampal glucocorticoid receptor blocking (Feldman and Conforti, 1980; Sapolsky *et al.*, 1984). In fact, type I receptors are predominantly found in the hippocampus, while type II receptors are distributed in many regions of the brain, including the hippocampus (Joels and Dekloet, 1992; McEwen *et al.*, 1992).

The hippocampus is densely distributed with serotonin 1A receptors, and there is early evidence that interactions between corticosteroids and the 5-HT 1A receptor (Lopez *et al.*, 1998; Meijer *et al.*, 1998) may contribute to the pathophysiology of affective disorders. In fact, 5-HT 1A receptor density reduction and downregulation appear to be mediated by the mineralocorticoid receptors (Meijer *et al.*, 1997), while adrenalectomy appeared to reverse the decrease in hippocampal 5-HT 1A receptor levels (Lopez, 1998).

With the advent of more suitable positron emission tomography (PET) imaging tracers, decreased pre- and postsynaptic binding of 5-HT 1A receptors in depressed patients have been detected. Serotonin 2A receptors demonstrated equivocal results, perhaps due to the heterogeneity of depressive disorders and varying severity of presentations. Much data also indicate a decreased density in serotonin transporters in the brains of depressed patients (Ellis and Salmond, 1994). Post-mortem studies of suicide victims examining postsynaptic 5-HT 1A receptor density in the hippocampus and frontal cortex reported inconsistent results (Lowther *et al.*, 1997; Stockmeier *et al.*, 1997). The reports of increased 5-HT 1A receptor sites among individuals who have completed suicide may suggest that these receptors are more regulated by steroid levels in the hippocampus and, less so, in other parts of the brain. Also, tracers used in PET studies of patients (antagonistic action binding to receptors in high- and low-affinity states) differ from those used in post-mortem studies (agonist action with high-affinity binding).

MRI studies of depressed patients showed decreased hippocampal size, correlating with lifetime duration of illness and treatment resistance (Shah *et al.*, 1999; Sheline *et al.*, 1999). McEwen (2000) summarized the possible causes for hippocampal atrophy, and noted evidence of its reversibility after treatment. Reduction in the volume of Ammon's horn or dentate gyrus may occur secondary to reduced dendrite branching, impaired neurogenesis, decreased neuronal survival rate or permanent neuron loss. Atrophy of other areas of the brain, such as the prefrontal cortex (Drevets *et al.*, 1997) and amygdala (Sheline *et al.*, 1998), has been linked to depressive disorders. Glial cell loss appears to contribute to atrophy of the prefrontal cortex, amygdala and possibly hippocampus, which has also been associated with depression.

For further details, Fujita *et al.* (2000) completed an excellent review of the literature on the role of the hippocampus in depression pathophysiology.

The D-fenfluramine challenge test is used in studies as an indirect indicator of central serotonergic functioning, by measuring the prolactin (PRL) response to D-fenfluramine (serotonin releasing agent) exposure. O'Keane *et al.* (1992) reported that a fenfluramine-induced prolactin response was augmented after antidepressant treatment with medications including tricyclic agents and serotonin reuptake inhibitors, as have other groups (Charney *et al.*, 1984; Kasper *et al.*, 1990; Maes *et al.*, 1991; Price *et al.*, 1989). Shapira *et al.* (1993) found that an increased prolactin response to D-fenfluramine occurred after lithium treatment for depression, which persisted even after medication cessation.

On the other hand, in a double-blinded randomized control trial comparing patients before and after treatment with two SSRIs, fluoxetine and fluvoxamine, Kavoussi *et al.* (1999) observed a lack of enhancement of the PRL response after an 8-week period of treatment. This group postulated that study patients may have been less severely depressed, and free of Axis I and II comorbidities. Indeed, certain patients had normal PRL responses to D-fenfluramine even prior to the intervention. They explained that SSRI treatment may have prevented D-fenfluramine uptake into presynaptic neurons, thus lessening the release of 5-HT from these neurons, and thereby reducing the PRL response. Lastly, the question was raised that the action of certain SSRIs, such as fluvoxamine, may preferentially downregulate 5-HT 2 receptors (Spigset and Mjorndal, 1997). Recent literature has suggested that the PRL response to D-fenfluramine may be mediated by the 5-HT2 Rec (Coccaro *et al.*, 1996).

Mannel *et al.* (1997) found the fenfluramine test not to be a useful tool for the prediction of therapeutical outcome, upon measuring PRL and cortisol responses in euthymic patients (combination of unipolar, bipolar and schizoaffective diagnoses), treated on long-term lithium or carbamazepine prophylaxis. However, they observed a trend that blunted cortisol release in response to the FEN challenge seemed to occur in those responding to lithium or carbamazepine treatment, which may reflect better mood stabilization.

Dopamine and the HPA Axis

As described in the previous section, psychotic depression appears to be associated with hypercortisolaemia and activation of the dopamine system (Schatzberg and Rothschild, 1988; Schatzberg *et al.*, 1985) while suppression of glucocorticoid (GC) release reduces dopamine activity (Piazza *et al.*, 1996). In plasma homovanillic acid (HVA) (metabolite of dopamine) studies, there is evidence of increased central dopamine activity (Aberg-Widtedt *et al.*, 1985; Devanand *et al.*, 1985; Sweeney *et al.*, 1978), while others have found the absence of effect (Wolkowitz *et al.*, 1987). Plasma HVA is derived from peripheral noradrenergic neurons and limits interpretation of these results. Measures of CSF HVA levels may be more suggestive of presynaptic dopamine activity (Pitchot *et al.*, 1992), but psychomotor activity may interfere with CSF HVA measurements (van Praag *et al.*, 1975).

Other groups have administered dopamine agonists (APOmorphine), to observe prolactin and growth hormone responses, as an indirect indicator of dopamine receptor activity in depressed patients (Duval *et al.*, 2000) and depressed, suicidal patients (Pitchot *et al.*, 2001). Results are interpreted with difficulty due to their indirect indication of central neurotransmitter activity at the hypothalamic level.

Of interest, Cyr *et al.* (2001) reported their findings in transgenic mice bearing blocked GC receptor expression, compared to control mice. They were able to show increased amphetamine-induced locomotor activity, with increased concentrations of striatal dopamine and its metabolites, dihydroxyphenylacetic acid and HVA. Transgenic mice exhibited increased D1 and D2 receptor binding. Upon exposure to amitriptyline, increased dopamine-specific transporter binding occurred (restoring dopamine uptake into synaptosomes), and upon exposure to fluoxetine, reduced striatal D1 and D2 receptor levels were observed. These results seem to indicate that increased GC levels in these transgenic mice was associated with hyperactive dopamine activity, and corrected following antidepressant exposure.

Measures of HPA Axis Function

Dexamethasone-Suppression Test (DST)

The cortisol response to challenge with the exogenous corticosteroid dexamethasone is measured to determine the intact function of the HPA axis response, by suppressing cortisol release. Patients with psychiatric disorders, particularly major depression, often fail to suppress their cortisol production, or will escape from suppression abnormally early. According to the DST protocol published by Carroll *et al.* (1981), dexamethasone 1.0 mg was administered at 11 p.m., and blood samples for serum cortisol were taken the following day, at 8 a.m., 4 p.m. and 11 p.m. The greatest sensitivity was obtained when all three samples were collected (Rush *et al.*, 1996). For convenience, outpatients are usually tested in the afternoon, thus losing sensitivity of the test results. Carroll *et al.* (1981) defined the criterion for a normal response to the DST as a cortisol level of $5.0\,\mu g\,dl^{-1}$, using the modified Murphy competitive protein finding technique (Murphy, 1968). Rubin *et al.* (1987) suggested a cortisol level cut-off of $3.5\,\mu g\,dl^{-1}$, with the more specific radioimmunoassay (RIA) technique. Rush *et al.* (1996) reported that a limit of $4.0\,\mu g\,dl^{-1}$, would achieve a 96% specificity of the DST. Rothschild *et al.* (1982) described how cortisol levels with a threshold of $15\,\mu g\,dl^{-1}$ would attain a high specificity and high predictive value for psychotic depression, and may be more clinically useful in confirming this particular diagnosis.

Interestingly, depressed patients found to be DST cortisol suppressors have higher plasma dexamethasone concentrations than DST non-suppressors (Carson *et al.*, 1988), with dexamethasone plasma levels rising with treatment (Holsboer *et al.*, 1986b). This may indicate a hypercortisolaemic induction of liver enzymes, to augment dexamethasone metabolism (Holsboer *et al.*, 1986a).

Other Measures of HPA Activity

Salivary cortisol has proven to be an accurate and valid measure of free cortisol (Kirschbaum and Hellhammer, 1994), and is closely correlated with serum and plasma cortisol levels before and after the DST. Normal values may range from 1 to $25\,nmol\,l^{-1}$. Difficulties in interpreting salivary cortisol results arise from the use of different cut-off values in different laboratories, and measurements made at different times of the day.

The 24-hour urinary-free cortisol (UFC) sample appears to closely reflect circulating unbound plasma cortisol production, and is a helpful indicator of adrenal cortical activity (Carroll *et al.*, 1976). Total creatinine is also determined, as a measure of renal function. Normal UFC excretion is 40–50 μg in 24 hours, versus $>90\,\mu g$ in 24 hours in the (non-psychotically) depressed.

Finally, age may be an important contributing factor to increased cortisol levels, determined in the DST (Halbreich *et al.*, 1984), although others have not found this to be a significant factor (Schweitzer *et al.*, 1991). In certain studies, the population of older adults who have documented cognitive decline exhibit higher levels of 24-hour UFC, with women more than men demonstrating memory impairments (as tested by verbal free recall and spatial recognition performance, implying encoding deficits) associated with increased UFC (Seeman *et al.*, 1997).

The DST and Mood Disorders

Schatzberg *et al.* (1983) reported that using a plasma cortisol level cut-off of $15\,\mu g\,dl^{-1}$, the frequency of DST non-suppression in the group with psychotic depression (PD) was greater than in those with non-PD (71.4% versus 58.1%). Rothschild *et al.* (1982) examined patients with schizophrenia and psychotic symptoms, to compare DST responses of PD patients. None of the schizophrenic patients had DST non-suppression, while half of the PD patients showed elevated post-dexamethasone cortisol levels, $>14\,\mu g\,dl^{-1}$. A meta-analysis of 14 studies, carried out by Nelson and Davis (1997), found the DST non-suppression rate at 64% in PD patients, versus 41% in non-PD patients. In addition, there was no difference in the rate of DST non-suppression among the endogenously depressed versus those with non-endogenous depression (39% versus 36%). Patients with psychotic depression exhibit the most replicable findings of DST non-suppression, in addition to elevated post-dexamethasone cortisol levels and high levels of 24-hour UFC. Schatzberg *et al.* (1985) and Schatzberg and Rothschild (1988) hypothesized that in certain depressed patients, the hypercortisolaemic state enhanced dopamine activity, leading to psychotic symptoms.

Cassidy *et al.* (1998) reported on the cortisol responses to DST in bipolar manic patients, and although the sample size was small, mixed manic patients seemed to exhibit greater degrees of non-suppression than pure manic patients do. With disease remission, cortisol suppression became restored. Cassidy's (1998) study also summarized the literature published on the effects of mania on DST non-suppression, reporting the frequency to be from 0% to 70%. Drawing conclusions here may be difficult, due to numerous methodologic differences, such as the dexamethasone dose chosen and time of blood draw.

As for dysthymic disorder, the rate of DST non-suppression falls between that observed in patients with major depression and healthy controls. Howland and Thase (1991) reported on a meta-analysis of ten studies comparing DST results in patients with dysthymic disorder, major depression and other psychiatric diagnoses. They found that 14% of dysthymic individuals, 59% of major depressive patients and 6% of healthy controls demonstrated DST non-suppression, with no significant difference reported between the rate in dysthymics and that in controls. Interestingly, Ravindran *et al.* (1994) found the rate of non-suppression in the DST in dysthymic patients was 7%, and the non-suppressors proved to be more successful responders to antidepressant therapy (with fluoxetine).

DST and Outcome of Mood Disorders

Deshauer *et al.* (1999) observed the pattern of DST cortisol response, in a four-year follow-up study, of 19 completely remitted, unipolar depressed and bipolar disorder patients on lithium prophylaxis. Those with initial DST non-suppression demonstrated persisting HPA dysregulation (more females than males), despite symptom remission. Ribeiro *et al.* (1993) reported on a meta-analysis of long-term outcomes of depressed patients, describing those with DST non-suppression at post-treatment evaluations to have poorer outcomes.

Rothschild *et al.* (1993) found significant positive correlation between higher cortisol activity at one-year post-treatment, and impaired social and occupational functioning as measured by the Social Adjustment Scale — Self Report (SAS-SR) (Weissman *et al.*, 1978). Likely, impaired functioning was linked to cognitive deficits associated with the hypercortisolaemia. Belanoff *et al.* (2001) provide an excellent review on the effects of cortisol on cognition. Chronic hypercortisolaemia has been linked to neurotoxic effects, especially in the hippocampus, which possesses numerous glucocorticoid receptors (McEwen *et al.*, 1991). Preclinical evidence from rat and primate studies suggested evidence of hippocampal neuron loss (Sapolsky *et al.*, 1990). Cushing's syndrome patients, who have an endogenous overproduction of cortisol, demonstrated depressive symptoms, impaired cognition and decreased hippocampal volume (Starkman *et al.*, 1992). Of interest, after treatment of patients with Cushing's disease (microsurgical resection of pituitary adenomas), the hippocampal volume was increased by up to 10% (Starkman *et al.*, 1999). Further discussion on the HPA axis and hippocampal function will follow below.

DEX/CRH Test

Heuser *et al.* (1994) summarized their experience with the dexamethasone (DEX) suppression/CRH challenge test, to assess HPA axis abnormalities, by first pretreating patients with DEX 1.5 mg orally at 23 : 00 h the previous night. This is followed the next day with administering human CRH (hCRH) 100 μg intravenously, with blood samples drawn for serum cortisol and ACTH every 15 minutes from 14 : 00 to 18 : 00 h. This group reported that from a sample of 140 psychiatric patients with various diagnoses, including major depression, mania, panic disorder and schizophrenia, cortisol and ACTH release were significantly greater than healthy controls. The sensitivity of this test was 80% for major depression, exceeding that of the standard DST, which reportedly has sensitivity of 44% from a meta-analysis of available data (Arana and Forbes, 1991), depending on age, depression severity and DEX dose. Normal controls demonstrated suppression of ACTH and cortisol release.

With this test, DEX suppresses the HPA axis at the pituitary level, but does not suppress the release of CRH or vasopressin from the hypothalamus. Depressed patients may have altered glucocorticoid feedback regulation, such that pre-administered DEX was paradoxically unable to suppress ACTH and cortisol release after the hCRH bolus. In animals exposed to chronic stress conditions, vasopressinergic regulation of the pituitary–adrenal system takes over (de Goeij *et al.*, 1992). Likewise, psychiatric illness may lead to an increased hypothalamic CRH and vasopressin production, resulting in augmented ACTH and corticosteroid release, and a transient CS receptor desensitization.

Thus in a DEX-pretreated depressed patient, ACTH release in response to administered CRH would be greater than in a control patient, because of synergistic action between the CRH given and the increased available vasopressin (von Bardeleben *et al.*, 1985). Limitations include the cumbersome nature of the test, which requires intravenous administration of both DEX and human CRH, and frequent blood monitoring thereafter; and although the test is fairly sensitive for depression, the specificity remains low.

Rybakowski and Twardowska (1999) used this test to compare 16 bipolar and 24 unipolar depressed patients, with 20 healthy controls, finding that HPA dysregulation was more pronounced in patients with bipolar depression, as shown by significantly higher cortisol levels during the acute episode and in remission. Holsboer *et al.* (1995) reported that healthy probands at high risk for psychiatric disorders developed an increase in plasma cortisol response to the DEX/hCRH challenge test, at levels between depressed patients and the controls without family history.

The results of the DEX/CRH test, administered to inpatients with depression at the time of treatment initiation and at time of discharge, seemed to suggest that those individuals with increased cortisol response at discharge time exhibited a higher risk of relapse in the next six months, versus those with low cortisol responses (more appropriate response) (Zobel *et al.*, 1999), although this report did not report the average length of hospitalization for observed patients.

Of interest, Holsboer *et al.* (1995) and Krieg *et al.* (2001) (in the Munich vulnerability study) described their findings of cortisol response to the DEX/CRH challenge in apparently healthy relatives of patients being treated for acute major depression. In the Krieg study, those relatives with increased cortisol response exhibited higher scores on psychometric scales measuring 'rigidity' and 'autonomic lability', and 32% of first-degree healthy relatives had depression-like features in other neuroendocrine and polysomnographic (EEG) measures. Their prospective study continues to monitor these relatives, in order to determine whether these measures are able to predict risk for developing affective disorders in the relatives of patients already being treated.

CRH

Corticotrophin-releasing hormone is a neuropeptide with numerous sites of action in the endocrine, autonomic and immune systems, modulating various behaviours, e.g. anxiety-related behaviour, food intake, reproduction, arousal and motor function. CRH is released from the paraventricular nucleus (PVN) of the hypothalamus into portal vessels, and triggers release of ACTH from the anterior pituitary. From preclinical evidence, it is postulated that CRH behaves as a neurotransmitter, which acts at different sites in the brain to exert neuroendocrine and behavioural effects. CRH activates the HPA axis to cause increased corticosteroid release. Increased cortisol levels feed back into a circuit via three possible routes: negative feedback at the level of the PVN neurons and anterior pituitary (Swanson and Simmons, 1989), positive feedback at the level of the central nucleus of the amygdala (CeA) and the dorsal PVN (Swanson and Simmons, 1989), and negative feedback through the ventral hippocampus to the bed nucleus of the stria terminalis (BNST) (Herman *et al.*, 1992).

CRH projections from the central nucleus of the amygdala, PVN and BNST terminate in the locus ceruleus (Van Bockstaele *et al.*, 1998), and may be responsible for enhanced arousal to stressors with an emotional component, as well as affect attention. CRH interacts with serotonin at the level of the raphe nuclei (Price *et al.*, 1998), to influence behaviours and emotions (via serotonin innervations in the forebrain). CRH may also affect dopamine neurons in the substantia nigra, thereby modulating dopaminergic activity in the striatum.

For more detail, Steckler and Holsboer (1999) provide an excellent overview of preclinical data pertaining to CRH receptor subtypes and their link to emotion and other affective conditions. The activation of CRH receptors allows CRH to exert its influence on behaviour. Importantly, two receptors have been found thus far, CRH1 and CRH2. In preclinical studies, CRH2-alpha is expressed more in subcortical regions of the brain (lateral septum, ventromedial hypothalamus, dorsal raphe nucleus), and may be more responsible for behaviours such as feeding, reproduction and defence. CRH2-beta is expressed in non-neuronal tissue, such as the choroid plexus, arterioles, cardiac and skeletal muscle (Steckler and Holsboer, 1999). CRH1 receptors are found in the pituitary, cerebellum and frontal cortex, and seem to modulate the cognitive processes, e.g. attention, executive function, emotional experience, and perhaps learning and memory.

Urocortin is a neuropeptide that is 45% homologous to CRH, which binds more potently to the CRH2-alpha receptor, than CRH (Donaldson *et al.*, 1996). Binding of the different CRH receptor subtypes likely activates different functions. However, urocortin does not appear to mediate ACTH release from the anterior pituitary at baseline, after induced stress and adrenalectomy, according to preclinical studies (Turnbull *et al.*, 1999).

Ongoing basic and clinical research studies are being undertaken to further understand the effects of glucocorticoids on CRH gene expression, and the implications of CRH on fear and anxiety. Much continues to be reported on the neurobiology of stress and anxiety, including HPA dysregulation secondary to stress, and the resulting predisposition to or development of abnormal autonomic, CNS, neuroendocrine and immune system responses. Important reports and reviews include Schulkin *et al.* (1998), McEwen (2000), Thrivikraman *et al.* (2000) and Liu *et al.* (1997).

CRH, ACTH and Cortisol Responses in Mood Disorders

Symptoms of stress activation and melancholic depression have common features such as anxiety and fear, constricted affect, stereotyped thinking, including guilt preoccupations, pessimism for the future, and sense of worthlessness. There may be evidence of physiological hyperarousal, autonomic and neuroendocrine activation, along with inhibited appetite, libido, and growth and reproduction (Gold *et al.*, 1988). Early studies by Gold *et al.* (1984), Holsboer *et al.* (1984) and Nemeroff *et al.* (1984, 1988) implicated CRH in the hypercortisolaemia found in depression: Gold and colleagues, in their study of HPA responses to ovine CRH, to glucocorticoid antagonists such as mifepristone, arginine vasopressin and to continuous infusions of CRH; Nemeroff and colleagues, in reporting elevated cerebrospinal fluid (CSF) CRH levels in depressed patients, and later describing reduced CRH receptors in the cerebral cortex of post-mortem suicide victims; and Holsboer and colleagues, in replicating findings of pituitary inhibition by hypercortisolaemia.

Norepinephrine (NE) is a neurotransmitter with numerous functions, inhibiting feeding, grooming and sleep behaviours. It activates the amygdala to enhance the coding of emotionally connected memories. NE inhibits medial prefrontal cortex functions, such as shifting mood states, developing novel versus well-rehearsed behaviours, and inhibiting the HPA axis and brainstem autonomic activity (Arnsten *et al.*, 1999; Gold and Chrousos, 1999). NE appears to stimulate the HPA axis, under chronic stress situations. Sympathetic inputs to the adrenal system are activated, thus sustaining hypercortisolaemia (Gold and Chrousos, 1999). CRH may also play a role in the learning and storage of fear responses in the amygdala. Rodent and primate research have shown that central administration of CRH activates the HPA axis, leading to sympathetic nervous system activation (Britton *et al.*, 1982; Brown *et al.*, 1982; Sirinathsinghji *et al.*, 1983; Sutton *et al.*, 1982).

Wong *et al.* (2000) postulated that melancholic depression activated a stress response via the NE-locus ceruleus and CRH systems. A study of 10 melancholic, depressed, medication-free patients and 14 healthy controls found that depressed patients exhibited elevated CSF NE (even during sleep), indicating central noradrenergic activation in depression.

The observation of elevated plasma cortisol may have resulted from possible direct NE activation of hypothalamic CRH neurons (Calogero *et al.*, 1988), NE activation of the amygdala and, subsequently, the HPA axis (Goldstein *et al.*, 1996), NE inhibition of the medial prefrontal cortex, which inhibits the HPA axis (Arnsten *et al.*, 1999), and sympathetic modulation of adrenal secretion during stress (Arnsten *et al.*, 1999). In fact, increased cortisol has been documented to directly activate brainstem noradrenergic neurons via CRH (Wong *et al.*, 2000). On the other hand, this study reported that CSF CRH levels and plasma ACTH levels were within 'normal' range. This actually represents inappropriately elevated levels of CSF CRH and plasma ACTH, in the setting of hypercortisolaemia (Kling *et al.*, 1991), thus indicating a possible dysfunction in the glucocorticoid negative feedback on hypothalamic CRH neurons, or an override of the negative feedback by CSF NE excitation.

Earlier, Gold *et al.* (1995) linked similar depressive states, those of atypical depression, seasonal affective disorder and depression accompanying Cushing's disease. Such patients usually describe symptoms of lethargy, fatigue, hypersomnia, hyperphagia and increased mood reactivity. It was postulated that with chronic hypercortisolism, these patients developed a central, hypothalamic CRH deficiency, with low ACTH levels, and a blunted response to exogenous CRH.

Vieta *et al.* (1999) compared the ACTH and free cortisol response to hCRH in 42 lithium-treated bipolar manic and hypomanic patients in remission with 21 healthy controls, and reported high baseline and peak ACTH levels in the patients. At six months follow-up, using stepwise logistic regression, the measured ACTH area under the curve, after CRH stimulation, documented a significant prediction of manic relapse with a sensitivity of 56% and specificity of 92%. After a 12-month follow-up, again enhanced ACTH response was found and the ACTH AUC predicted mania with sensitivity 75% and specificity 91%. Gold *et al.* (1984) did not find significant difference between remitted bipolar and healthy control patients (and between manic euthymic bipolar patients); however, samples sizes were small.

Heim *et al.* (2001) reported on HPA axis responses to provocation challenge tests (CRH stimulation and ACTH stimulation tests) in survivors of childhood abuse, finding that women with a history of abuse but without major depression exhibited greater ACTH responses to ovine CRH. Depressed women with and without histories of abuse both exhibited blunted ACTH responses, likely indicating CRH receptor downregulation, secondary to intrinsic chronic CRH hypersecretion from the hypothalamus. In addition, the women with abuse histories and major depression exhibited more comorbid post-traumatic stress disorder (PTSD) and recent chronic mild stress than the same cohort, without major depression. Heim *et al.* (2000) also reported on autonomic responses and ACTH and cortisol levels, after psychological laboratory stress exposure, to similar cohorts of women with a history of childhood abuse. Here, women with abuse histories, regardless of coexisting depressed mood, exhibited increased ACTH but normal cortisol responses, compared with healthy controls and depressed women without childhood abuse.

CRH Antagonists in Treatment of Depression and Anxiety Disorders

Holsboer (1999) argued that a number of clinical conditions, including anxiety, depression and alcohol withdrawal, are accompanied by an exaggerated stress response, and that certain psychiatric conditions, such as psychotic depression, seem to exhibit enhanced dopamine neurotransmission secondary to elevated cortisol. The longer-term administration of the antidepressant trimipramine appeared efficacious in treating psychotic depression, via suppression of the HPA system (Holsboer-Trachsler *et al.*, 1994). Preclinical studies to decrease CRH1 receptor function by blockade, or suppression of synthesis through receptor gene deletion, have resulted in decreased anxiety in stressed animal models. Therefore, it would seem appropriate and promising to explore the development of modalities to block the central hyperdrive mechanism of the HPA axis, inferred to be responsible for the production of anxiety and depressive symptoms (such as suppressing CRH gene activation and release, and inducing CRH receptor blockade).

In rodents, CRH1 seems to modulate anxiety, possibly through its regulation of the HPA axis, as demonstrated by the anxiolytic effects of CRH1 antagonists (Arborelius *et al.*, 2000). This study reported that in rats, chronic administration of the CRH1 antagonist CP-154,156 decreased CRH production in the paraventricular nucleus of the hypothalamus, rather than alter the synthesis of CRH1 receptors, and did not cause adrenal insufficiency.

Zobel *et al.* (2000) described the effects of administering the CRH1 receptor antagonist R121919, to 20 patients for the treatment of major depression, over a period of 30 days. Patients were randomized to two groups; one group received the lower dose of 40 mg per day, and the second group was started on 40 mg per day and titrated up to 80 mg per day. At the end of the study, depression and anxiety scores improved significantly. At the same time, CRH1 receptor blockade did not seem to impair the release of ACTH and cortisol, as shown by results of CRH challenge tests given both before and after the study.

CRH1 antagonists appear to shorten the time of onset of antidepressants, exerting antidepressant effects, and may also be beneficial in treating insomnia, which frequently accompanies anxiety and mood disorders. There are concerns, however, that in the setting of a hyperactive HPA axis (as found in depression), the CRH receptors may be downregulated or desensitized, thus resulting in the blunted ACTH response to CRH (Holsboer, 1999). Upon exposing the depressed patient to CRH1 antagonists, which would block the already desensitized CRH receptors, cognitive impairment may be induced or worsened, because of the interaction of CRH with the cholinergic systems, at the cortical level.

There are many other possible applications for CRH1 receptor antagonists, not only for treatment of depression, but also for the treatment of substance abuse (especially drug-seeking behaviour), anxiety disorders (including PTSD) and eating disorders. Further preclinical and clinical studies to clarify the function of these receptors and their subtypes, as well as the effect of various neuropeptides on receptor activity, are needed.

Anti-Glucocorticoid Agents

Cushing's patients, managed with either surgical intervention, or anti-glucocorticoid agents such as ketoconazole, metyrapone and aminoglutethimide, remit from depression up to a rate of 70% (Nieman *et al.*, 1985; Sonino *et al.*, 1993). Wolkowitz *et al.* (1999a) reported on their double-blind trial using ketoconazole versus placebo for the treatment of depression over a four-week period, and reported significant improvements in depressive symptoms, in those patients with an underlying hypercortisolaemic state. Ghadirian *et al.* (1995) reported the use of the three anti-glucocorticoid agents mentioned above in the treatment of depression, in an open-label, two-month trial. They described 60% of the patient sample with a greater than 50% reduction in depression symptomatology, and 50% with sustained remission at eight months follow-up. Most recently, the anti-progesterone and anti-glucocorticoid agent mifepristone, also known as RU-486, has been found to rapidly reverse symptoms in patients with primary psychotic depression (see Belanoff *et al.*, 2001 for review) and psychotic depression secondary to Cushing's syndrome (Van der Lely *et al.*, 1991).

The HPA Axis and PTSD

Quite recent literature has been published on the HPA responses in adult survivors of child abuse, thus adding important information to already present literature documenting HPA axis changes in male combat veterans and Holocaust survivors, with PTSD. As in depression, patients with PTSD hypersecrete CRH, as proven by elevated levels of CRH found in the cerebrospinal fluid (Baker *et al.*, 1999). On the other hand, there is evidence suggesting that PTSD patients possess an HPA axis with an exaggerated negative feedback mechanism.

For example, male combat veterans have decreased 24-hour UFC excretion (Mason *et al.*, 1986; Yehuda *et al.*, 1990) and lower plasma cortisol levels measured in the morning and throughout the day (Boscarino, 1996; Yehuda *et al.*, 1994). Likewise, Holocaust survivors demonstrated lower 24-hour UFC (Yehuda *et al.*, 1995).

Other studies report combat veterans with higher baseline plasma cortisol levels than controls, but no differences in baseline plasma ACTH levels, in the ACTH response to stress as well as in the cortisol response to stress (Liberzon *et al.*, 1999). Surprisingly, prepubertal children with PTSD demonstrate elevated 24-hour UFC, as compared to healthy controls and children with only a primary anxiety disorder. Combat veterans also exhibited greater plasma cortisol suppression to lower doses of dexamethasone (Yehuda *et al.*, 1995).

Heim *et al.* (2000) measured the HPA axis response (afternoon plasma ACTH and cortisol levels) and autonomic response (heart rate) to a standardized psychosocial laboratory stressor, consisting of an anticipation and preparation phase, followed by 10 minutes of public speaking and mental arithmetic task performance before an audience. Women with a history of childhood abuse exhibited increased pituitary–adrenal and autonomic responses, particularly those with concurrent major depression. This increased reactivity may occur from CRH hypersecretion, as a persisting consequence of past abuse, and may predispose such individuals to developing certain affective disorders. If this is the case, it may also suggest a choice of therapy, such as the use of CRH antagonists for treatment of depression in this patient population.

Heim *et al.* (2001) elaborated on the above study, by comparing a cohort of adult survivors of childhood abuse (with and without major depression) to healthy controls, by measuring plasma ACTH and cortisol responses to the ovine CRH challenge, and plasma cortisol responses to the ACTH challenge. They discovered that abused women without depression exhibited greater than usual ACTH responses to the exogenous CRH, contrasting with both non-abused and abused women with depression, who demonstrated blunted ACTH responses to CRH. In the ACTH stimulation test, abused women without depression had lower baseline and stimulated plasma concentrations, as compared to healthy controls, and to non-abused and abused women with depression. Newport and Nemeroff (2000) provide an excellent review of the neurobiology of PTSD.

Combining current clinical and preclinical data from rat (Plotsky *et al.*, 1993), and primate studies (Coplan *et al.*, 1996), early life stress may cause alterations at the adrenal level leading to an underlying hypocortisolaemic state, as found in patients with PTSD. Second, childhood trauma may also result in the development of a hyperreactive HPA axis towards stress in adulthood, with an underlying sensitization of the anterior pituitary to CRH. This may lead to increased CRH release in times of stress, perhaps contributing to pituitary downregulation and observed hypocortisolism. At the same time, abused women with depression may have developed an override of this pituitary downregulation, explaining their blunted ACTH response to the CRH challenge. Further preclinical and clinical studies are necessary to confirm and clarify the meaning of the above findings.

DEHYDROEPIANDROSTERONE AND DHEA(S)

Dehydroepiandrosterone (DHEA) and its sulphated metabolite, DHEA(S), are adrenocortical steroids, which serve as the precursor to testosterone and oestrogen. Circulating plasma and CSF levels peak in the mid-20s, and decline with age, reaching a nadir at age 65–70 years (Azuma *et al.*, 1993), when age-related illnesses increase substantially. DHEA(S) appears to decrease in settings of medical illness as well as with chronic stress (Spratt *et al.*, 1993), in contrast to cortisol, which tends to increase or remain unchanged. In fact the plasma ratio of DHEA(S) to cortisol falls with chronic stress and increasing age (Fava *et al.*, 1989; Goodyer *et al.*, 1998; McKenna *et al.*, 1997; Reus *et al.*, 1993; Wolkowitz *et al.*, 1992).

Hypotheses for mechanism of action of DHEA, from preclinical studies, include: transformation of this compound to testosterone or oestrogen (which both have mood enhancing effects), the effect of DHEA on increasing the bioavailability of gonadal steroids (Barrett-Connor *et al.*, 1999; Morrison, 1997; Morrison *et al.*, 1998; Yaffe *et al.*, 1998a), antagonistic effects on cortisol production (Browne *et al.*, 1992; Osran *et al.*, 1993), GABA antagonistic effects (Friess *et al.*, 1995; Majewska, 1992; Spivak, 1994; Steffensen, 1995; Yoo *et al.*, 1996), GABA inverse agonist effect of DHEA(S) (Friess *et al.*, 1995; Majewska, 1992), which may then cause a secondary increase in other GABA agonist neurosteroids, potentiation of NMDA neurotransmission (Bergeron *et al.*, 1996) and of NMDA-induced hippocampal release of norepinephrine (Majewska, 1995; Monnet *et al.*, 1995) and lastly, increased serotonin and dopamine brain levels (Abadie *et al.*, 1993; Murray and Gillies, 1997; Porter and Svec, 1995). DHEA(S) has been reported to increase hippocampal cholinergic function (Rhodes *et al.*, 1996, 1997), and enhance neuronal excitation (Carette and Poulain, 1984; Diamond *et al.*, 1995; Meyer and Gruol, 1994; Spivak, 1994).

In human studies, depression has been linked to lowered levels of DHEA(S) (Legrain *et al.*, 1995; Yaffe *et al.*, 1998a), with lower morning DHEA : cortisol ratios being reported in depressed patients (Osran *et al.*, 1993). Goodyer *et al.* (1996) found DHEA hyposecretion in morning measurements, with cortisol hypersecretion in evenings to be significantly correlated with the diagnosis and severity of depressive episodes in children and adolescents. Among post-partum women, Buckwalter *et al.* (1999), found higher DHEA levels were associated with less depression, interpersonal sensitivity and better short-term memory function; it was hypothesized that DHEA might play a role in regulating mood and cognition in pregnancy, although this remains to be tested.

More recently, Michael *et al.* (2000) reported on decreased levels of salivary DHEA in adults with major depression, with lower morning DHEA correlating with improved Hamilton Depression Scale (HAM-D) scores. This is suggestive that DHEA(S) changes reflect actual mood changes, rather than a simple medication-related effect. In this study, they recruited individuals with current major depression (mostly on antidepressants), remitted depression and still taking antidepressants, and a normal control group. Interestingly, the remitted patients demonstrated DHEA levels between the group with depression and the control group. In the data analysis, when depressed patients on treatment were separated from those patients not taking medications, there was no significant effect on DHEA levels; however, numbers were not large. Further studies on the possible interrelated effects of DHEA and cortisol are implicated, especially in light of preclinical literature reporting the actions of DHEA to antagonize damaging effects of steroids on hippocampal neurons (Kimonides *et al.*, 1999), the antidepressant effects of DHEA (Wolkowitz *et al.*, 1999b) and the ability to predict the course of adolescent depression from cortisol/DHEA measurements (Goodyer *et al.*, 1998).

Low plasma DHEA(S) has been reported with anxiety (Diamond *et al.*, 1989), perceived stress (Labbate *et al.*, 1995), cynicism and hostility (Fava *et al.*, 1987; Littman *et al.*, 1993). In contrast, higher DHEA(S) has been associated with more 'expansive personality ratings' (Hermida *et al.*, 1985) and healthier psychological profiles (Fava *et al.*, 1992). Other literature describe contrary findings, with depressed patients exhibiting increased urinary or serum DHEA(S) levels (Heuser *et al.*, 1998; Tollefson *et al.*, 1990) or unchanged levels (Fava *et al.*, 1989; Reus *et al.*, 1993; Shulman *et al.*, 1992).

Increased DHEA to cortisol ratios have also been found in panic disorder patients (Fava *et al.*, 1989). Herbert *et al.* (1996) reported that adolescents with depression and comorbid panic or phobic disorder did not exhibit low DHEA levels in morning samples.

Studies have explored the link between higher DHEA(S) levels and improved cognition and general functioning, especially among the elderly (Berkman *et al.*, 1993; Berr *et al.*, 1996; Cawood and Bancroft, 1996; Flood and Roberts, 1988; Kalmijn *et al.*, 1998; Ravaglia *et al.*, 1996, 1997; Reus *et al.*, 1993). Other studies report no effect or contrary findings, with the absence of association between DHEA(S) and cognition in women (Yaffe *et al.*, 1998b) or inverse association between DHEA(S) and declining cognition in female versus male nursing home patients (Morrison *et al.*, 1998, 2000) and female versus male Alzheimer's disease patients (Miller *et al.*, 1998).

Open-label studies showed that treatment with DHEA resulted in mood improvement, and increased interest, energy and activity levels, in healthy subjects (Morales *et al.*, 1994) and depressed patients (Wolkowitz *et al.*, 1997). Wolkowitz *et al.* (1999b) performed a double-blinded trial with 22 depressed patients, who were either already on antidepressants (with persisting depressive symptoms) or were medication-free. Patients were randomized to DHEA 90 mg per day or placebo for six weeks. Greater than 50% decreases in Hamilton Depression Rating Scale, with documented statistical significance, were reported in 5 of 11 patients treated with DHEA, compared to none of the 11 patients treated with placebo. This is a preliminary study, and larger scale trials may provide more useful information. For dysthymic patients, Bloch *et al.* (1999) treated non-medicated patients in a 12-week double-blinded placebo-controlled study, with DHEA (90 mg daily for three weeks, then increased to 450 mg daily for another three weeks), or placebo for six weeks and was able to show a robust antidepressant response with DHEA.

GROWTH HORMONE, PROLACTIN, AND OTHER ANTERIOR PITUITARY ABNORMALITIES

Alterations in the production of other anterior pituitary hormones, including growth hormone and prolactin, are associated with mood alterations. This would include conditions of over- and underproduction of such hormones.

Growth Hormone

The pulsatile release of growth hormone (GH) is regulated by the stimulatory effect of GH releasing hormone (GHRH), and the inhibitory effect of somatostatin (which itself is regulated by insulin-like growth factor-I) (Scanlon *et al.*, 1996). The secretion of GH can be increased in response to falls in blood glucose level, exercise, sleep, stress and alpha-adrenergic agonists; its release may be inhibited by beta-adrenergic agonists.

Overproduction of GH frequently occurs secondary to pituitary adenoma, rarely, hyperplasia, and results in acromegaly in adults and gigantism in children. Physical manifestations include skeletal overgrowth, especially of the hands, feet, skull and lower jaw, symptoms of headache, decreased libido, kyphosis and joint pains, and the development of hypertension, hypogonadism and diabetes mellitus (Lishman, 1998). Patients may present with psychiatric disorders, such as depression (Fava *et al.*, 1993; Ferrier, 1987). However, Abed *et al.* (1987) failed to confirm an increased rate of depression when compared with the general population.

GH deficiency causes growth failure and short stature in children, with psychiatric sequelae, including distorted body image and low self-esteem. In adults, decreased sense of well-being (Holmes and Shalet, 1995), anhedonia, fatigue and social isolation may improve from hormone replacement with recombinant GH (Degerblad *et al.*, 1990).

Neuroendocrine researchers use GH as an indirect indicator of neurotransmitter function (Porter *et al.*, 1998). Studies of children, adolescents and adults with major depression found altered responses of GH to clonidine (alpha-2 agonist)(Dolan and Calloway, 1986) and L-tryptophan (serotonin precursor) (Price *et al.*, 1991), possibly suggesting reductions in alpha-2 adrenergic and serotonin receptor functions.

Birmaher *et al.* (2000) reported a decreased GH response to GHRH in acutely depressed and recovered children and adolescents, as compared to healthy controls. Dahl *et al.* (2000) also reported low GH response to GHRH in acutely depressed children, as well as those in remission. Coplan *et al.* (2000) reported on ten-year follow-up data of now young adults, with and without major depression; those adults with lifetime depression exhibited lower levels of GH in the 100 minutes before sleep onset, in adolescence; those with a history of suicide attempts during adolescence had greater 24-hour GH release. Chronically elevated levels of corticosteroids may inhibit neurotransmitter actions, in addition to directly affecting pituitary secretion of GH, as reported by Watson *et al.* (2000).

Prolactin

Prolactin, which is secreted by the anterior pituitary gland, is under tonic inhibition from dopamine released by the hypothalamus (Lishman, 1998). Serotonin, acetylcholine, thyrotrophin-releasing hormone (TRH), oestrogen, endogenous opiates, stressors and nipple stimulation all promote prolactin release (Rafuls *et al.*, 1987). Symptoms of hyperprolactinaemia commonly arise from prolactin-secreting adenomas, and may result in amenorrhea, galactorrhea, infertility and impotence (more in men). In addition, psychiatric manifestations, such as depression, anxiety and irritability, may occur. Mood changes appear to respond better to treatment with dopamine agonists (such as bromocriptine) to reduce prolactin levels, rather than antidepressants, which seem to be less effective (Fava, 1993). Diagnosis is made from serum screening for prolactin elevation, and confirmed with imaging studies. Transsphenoidal resection or radiotherapy to remove or shrink the adenoma are other possible treatment options.

Prolactin responses to dopamine agonists are used to indirectly measure serotonin activity, as was discussed earlier in the chapter.

HYPOPITUITARISM

This is a state which can be caused by pituitary tumours (craniopharyngioma in children), post-partum ischaemic necrosis of the anterior pituitary gland (Sheehan's syndrome) or, very rarely, secondary to a basal skull fracture (Lishman, 1998). Symptoms often exist for an extended period of time prior to diagnosis, and can include weakness, fatigue, cold sensitivity, decreased libido, amenorrhea, impotence and weight loss. Facial expressions are diminished, and the development of depression, irritability, apathy, somnolence, memory impairment and metabolic changes can occur before the onset of delirium. This presents secondary to concurrent infection, and manifests with hypoglycaemia, hypotension and hypocortisolaemia. Differential diagnosis should include hypothyroidism, Addison's disease (hyperpigmentation would be prominent), delirium, dementia and anorexia nervosa (AN) (apathy and somnolence are usually not found in cases of AN). With hormone replacement therapy, including cortisol or prednisolone, thyroxine and gonadal hormones, symptoms typically resolve.

PARATHYROID HORMONE (PTH)

The parathyroid glands are situated on the thyroid but function discretely from the thyroid axis. The synthesis and release of PTH is modulated by serum calcium levels, in which elevated calcium inhibits PTH release, while low serum calcium causes increased PTH synthesis and release. Increased serum phosphate causes an increase in PTH release (by decreasing serum calcium levels, such as in cases of renal failure). The commonest cause of hyperparathyroidism is the benign adenoma of a parathyroid gland; it is rarely associated with multiple endocrine neoplasia (MEN type I — associated with pancreatic and pituitary tumours, or MEN type II — associated with thyroid cancer and pheochromocytoma) (Lishman, 1998). Mood symptoms are a frequent presentation, with reports of up to two-thirds of patients experiencing psychiatric changes (Petersen, 1968). These can include amotivation, depression, lethargy, memory impairment, irritability and explosive outbursts (Petersen, 1968). Patients may complain of anorexia, nausea, headache, thirst and polyuria. Physical symptoms of renal calculi, bony deformities and fracture, myopathy of proximal muscles, hypotonia and corneal calcifications may develop (Lishman, 1998). Laboratory abnormalities associated with hyperparathyroidism include elevated serum calcium levels and low serum phosphate, (serum albumin values will need to be considered). Radioimmunoassay of parathyroid hormone levels will confirm diagnosis. Alkaline phosphatase is raised secondary to bony involvement; renal calculi, and calcifications in the caudate and frontal lobes may be identified on imaging. Occasionally, EEG will exhibit widespread slow activity, along with paroxysms of frontal delta waves (Lishman, 1998). Surgical resection of the adenoma improves most symptoms, but depression and other psychiatric manifestations may require treatment with psychotropic medications for complete symptom resolution.

Hypoparathyroidism can occur following neck surgery, and after thyroidectomy (occurring in up to 50% of these patients). Symptoms frequently arise from chronic tetany; signs and symptoms may include perioral, hand and feet numbness and tingling, muscle cramps, limb stiffness, carpopedal spasms, and even laryngeal stridor. Presenile cataracts, seizures, macrocytic anaemia, and prolonged QT interval are other possible manifestations (Brown, 1984). Psychiatric changes occur in up to 50% of these cases, as reported by Denko and Kaelbling (1962), and may present with delirium, difficulty concentrating, emotional lability and cognitive impairment. Other symptoms include depression, anxiety, irritability and social isolation. Psychosis, obsessions and derealization rarely occur (Denko and Kaelbling, 1962; Rafuls *et al.*, 1987). Calcium and vitamin D replacement successfully treat the above symptoms.

MELATONIN AND AFFECTIVE DISORDERS

Melatonin is an indolamine derivative of serotonin, produced in the pineal body, and secreted into the bloodstream and cerebrospinal fluid. Melatonin receptors are found in the hypothalamus, cerebellum and pineal body itself. Secretions usually peak at night and reach a nadir during the daytime. Melatonin appears to lower body temperature at night and increase sedation (Shafii and Shafii, 1990).

Nurnberger *et al.* (2000) attempted to replicate observations made in the past (Lewy *et al.*, 1980; Wetterberg *et al.*, 1981; Wetterbuerg *et al.*, 1979), that bipolar patients exhibit supersensitivity to the suppression of melatonin production by light, as this may be a marker for genetic vulnerability for affective disorders (Nurnberger *et al.*, 1988). Results from Nurnberger's more recent study observed no difference in light-induced melatonin suppression among bipolar, unipolar and healthy patients. Cortisol levels were similar in all three groups of patients. Lithium and propranolol did not produce any effect, despite past research documenting beta-adrenergic influence on melatonin production (Connolly and Lynch, 1983). Among bipolar I patients, they were able to document significantly lower melatonin levels on nights with light exposure, as well as a later peak time for melatonin on dark nights. On the other hand, both Lam *et al.* (1990) and Whalley *et al.* (1991) were not able to confirm that bipolar patients exhibited increased light sensitivity. Indeed, medication effects may account for these differences, and further study would be merited.

HYPOTHALAMIC–PITUITARY–THYROID AXIS AND MOOD DISORDERS

Thyroid dysfunction has been reported to affect up to 6% of the general population, with psychiatric patients exhibiting higher rates of abnormal thyroid metabolism, and women demonstrating a higher incidence than men (Whybrow, 1995). Joffe and Levitt (1993) have edited an excellent text on this topic, with more detailed overview on such related issues.

Historically, links between thyroid diseases and psychiatric disorders include Caleb Parry's (1825) report that 'nervous affectations' seemed to often occur with thyroid disorders. Gull (1873) reported observations of myxoedema resulting in psychosis. Later, the Clinical Society of London (1888) reported that 36% of myxoedematous patients developed 'delusions and hallucinations', and Asher (1949) coined the description 'myxoedema madness'. Robert Graves (1940) reported the case of a woman with 'symptoms ... suppose to be hysterical', who developed 'tachycardia, weakness, exophthalmos, and thyromegaly'.

Hypothyroidism

Hypothyroidism can be classified according to the level of dysfunction in the HPT axis, primary hypothyroidism referring to abnormal function of the thyroid gland (accountable for 95% of cases), secondary hypothyroidism as pituitary dysfunction, and tertiary hypothyroidism as hypothalamic dysfunction (Gharib and Abboud, 1987). Idiopathic, autoimmune, iatrogenic (psychotropic culprits, such as lithium and carbamazepine) and iodine deficiency causes explain most cases of hypothyroidism. Hashimoto's thyroiditis, an immune-related condition, is associated with elevated TSH and decreased thyroid hormone release, producing thyroid gland enlargement.

Primary hypothyroidism is subdivided into three grades. Grade I is characterized by increased levels of thyroid-stimulating hormone (TSH), decreased free thyroxine index (FTI) and an increased TSH response to thyrotrophin-releasing hormone (TRH), along with clinical findings such as weight gain, dry skin, hoarse voice, cold intolerance, fatigue, constipation, menstrual disturbances, psychomotor retardation and cognitive disturbances. Grade II hypothyroid patients have increased TSH, normal FTI, increased TSH response to TRH, but few clinical findings. Patients with Grade III hypothyroidism present with normal TSH, normal FTI, but an increased TSH response to TRH stimulation, with a clinically euthyroid presentation (Evered, 1973; Wenzel *et al.*, 1974). Traditionally, Grades II and III hypothyroidism are considered 'subclinical' forms, but ongoing reports of clinical psychiatric sequelae from these states, e.g. major depression, may imply the contrary (Haggerty and Prange, 1995; Joffe and Levitt, 1993).

The thyroid axis interacts closely with the sympathetic nervous system, with thyroid hormones potentiating central and peripheral sympathetic–adrenergic activity (Emlen *et al.*, 1972). Hypothyroidism is associated with a decrease in the number and activity of beta-adrenergic receptors, in particular. Thyroid hormones affect second-messenger systems, such as the phosphoinositol and adenyl cyclase pathways, which may influence alpha and beta adrenoreceptor activity. There appears to be a reduction in messenger RNA coding for the beta-adrenergic receptors responding to epinephrine and norepinephrine, as shown in rat studies (Gross *et al.*, 1980; Mason *et al.*, 1987; Sandrini *et al.*, 1991).

Lithium acts to inhibit the conversion of thyroxine (T4) to triiodothyronine (T3), and inhibit iodine uptake, thyroid hormone production and thyroid secretion by the thyroid gland (Burrow *et al.*, 1971; Carlson *et al.*, 1973). Patients treated with lithium may develop decreased total T4, decreased free T3, increased TSH, exaggerated TSH response to TRH challenge, anti-thyroid antibodies, and clinical evidence of hypothyroidism and/or goitre. Lithium appears to suppress thyroid function, albeit on a temporary basis. It is usually a reversible condition upon cessation of this medication (Joffe and Levitt, 1993). It would likely be prudent to screen the above laboratory tests prior to initiation of lithium, and intermittently throughout the course of treatment.

Carbamazepine has reportedly been shown to decrease thyroid function in patients treated for seizure disorders and affective illness (Ericsson *et al.*, 1985; Larkin *et al.*, 1989; Tanaka *et al.*, 1987). This occurs more often in responders than non-responders of the medication, is unrelated to the mean dose or blood level of the anti-epileptic (Roy-Byrne *et al.*, 1984), and may be a result of a reduced TSH response to TRH (Joffe *et al.*, 1984). On the other hand, valproic acid has not been demonstrated to affect thyroid function (Ericsson *et al.*, 1985; Larkin *et al.*, 1989).

Lastly, electroconvulsive therapy may cause a rise in serum TSH, during treatment, and may be correlated with seizure length (Aperia *et al.*, 1985a, b; Papakostas *et al.*, 1991). Phototherapy has not been shown to affect thyroid function tests (Bauer *et al.*, 1993; Joffe, 1991).

Hyperthyroidism

Hyperthyroidism is commonly caused by Graves' disease, an autoimmune process associated with increased circulating thyroid hormones, and with higher incidence in females than males (6 : 1 ratio). Toxic multinodular goitre, a non-malignant condition in which thyroid nodules produce excessive thyroid hormones, and overtreatment of hypothyroidism are other possible causes for hyperthyroidism. This results in physical, cognitive and affective symptoms, including increased motor activity (tremulousness, tremor, restlessness), tachycardia, weight loss, anorexia, heat intolerance, menstrual irregularities, exophthalmos, mood lability, distractibility and decreased concentration, impaired short-term memory, and, in extreme conditions, frank delusions and hallucinations (Kamlana and Holms, 1986; MacCrimmon *et al.*, 1979). A small minority of patients, especially the elderly, presents with contrasting symptoms of apathy, lethargy, depression and social isolation (Peake, 1981). Complaints of depressed mood and anxiety may occur (Wilson *et al.*, 1962).

Hyperthyroidism is diagnosed by decreased TSH (<0.2), elevated total T4 and elevated free T3. The TRH challenge test can be used to prove a hyperthyroid state, by administering 500 μg TRH intravenously, and measuring TSH levels at baseline, and every 15 minutes, for the first hour. Usually, women and men show peak values of $>6\,\mathrm{uU\,ml^{-1}}$, following the challenge test; men older than 40 years tend to exhibit a rise of $>2\,\mathrm{uU\,ml^{-1}}$. In the absence of pituitary disease, suppressed TSH response indicates thyrotoxicosis; if TSH response to the TRH challenge is within normal limits, a hyperthyroid condition is unlikely.

Joffe and Singer (1987) reported no change in thyroid function in depressed patients treated with phenelzine; however, monoamine oxidase inhibitors cause increased circulating catecholamines, and it may be suggested to avoid this class of medication in patients with a history of hyperthyroidism. Thyroid hormones activate the sympathetic nervous system, including the autonomic nervous system and central adrenergic inputs. These effects have long been recognized in the cardiovascular system (Harrison, 1964). Of note, hyperthyroidism may increase myocardial sensitivity to catecholamines, leading to cardiac toxicity in those patients with increased serum thyroid levels and elevated catecholamines (Larsen and Ingbar, 1992).

There have also been noted associations between hyperthyroidism and tricyclic antidepressant toxicity (Prange *et al.*, 1969). Hoeflich *et al.* (1992) were not able to observe adverse effects on thyroid function in depressed patients (both responders and non-responders) treated with either maprotiline or fluvoxamine for four weeks. Shelton *et al.* (1993) compared the thyroid function of depressed patients treated with desipramine or fluoxetine, reporting 26% of study patients exhibited baseline abnormalities in thyroid levels, and a small but statistically significant increase in total T4 in those treated with desipramine, and a decline in T3 in those who responded to fluoxetine but not desipramine. McCowen *et al.* (1997) found that sertraline may adversely affect thyroid function.

Mood Disorders and Thyroid Function

Depression

Although patients with unipolar major depression commonly present in euthyroid states, at ranges in both upper and lower limits of normal, various other abnormalities have also been reported. These may include elevated T4 levels, decreased serum T3, blunted TSH response to TRH challenge, and evidence of subclinical hypothyroidism (Joffe and Levitt, 1992; Sullivan *et al.*, 1997). According to Kirkegaard and Faber (1998), this normalized in responders to treatment with fluvoxamine after only one month, suggesting interactions between the hypothalamic–pituitary–thyroid (HPT) axis and serotonin neurotransmission. Linnoila *et al.* (1979) and Kirkegaard and Faber (1981) reported increased serum levels of reverse T3 (the hormonally inactive form of T3) in acutely depressed individuals, with return to normal values upon recovery from depression, thus implying a state-dependent change.

Up to 15–20% of depressed patients exhibit subclinical hypothyroidism (Haggerty and Prange, 1995), with women patients more at risk for impaired thyroid function (Gold *et al.*, 1981). Prange and Loosen (1984) reported 25–33% of major depressive patients show blunted TSH response to TRH challenge. This could suggest a feedback mechanism involved in a chronically activated HPT axis (Banki, 1988), a response to a transient thyroxaemic condition (Loosen and Prange, 1982) or a response to hypercortisolaemia associated with depression (Re *et al.*, 1976).

Frye *et al.* (1999b) were not able to predict TRH hypersecretion and subsequent pituitary downregulation (with blunted TSH release) in patients with depression.

Of interest, there exist numerous reports of increased prevalence of anti-thyroid antibodies among depressed patients, 8–20% (Gold *et al.*, 1982; Haggerty *et al.*, 1991; Joffe, 1987; Nemeroff *et al.*, 1985) versus 5% in the general population (Tunbridge and Caldwell, 1991). The clinical significance remains unclear, since this is often accompanied by normal serum thyroid concentrations.

More recently, Joffe's group (Joffe, 1999; Joffe and Marriot, 2000) examined the relationship between basal thyroid hormone levels and the long-term course of depression and stage of treatment-resistant depression (Thase and Rush, 1995), reporting that time to recurrence of major depression was inversely related to T3 but not to T4 levels, supporting past findings that peripheral thyroid levels do not necessarily correlate with antidepressant treatment resistance (Vandoolaeghe *et al.*, 1997).

Also, the blunting of the TSH response to TRH challenge has been reported in acute and abstinent alcohol-dependent patients (Loosen, 1988; Loosen *et al.*, 1992), as well as in panic disorder patients (Fishman *et al.*, 1985; Stein and Uhde, 1988).

Bipolar Disorders

Whybrow and Prange (1981) hypothesized that mobilization of thyroid hormones in the CNS would augment recovery from depression, and, conversely, excessive mobilization would increase the risk of mania in certain individuals. In addition, thyroid hormones may have a central neuromodulatory role, through its actions on central beta-adrenergic receptors (Whybrow and Prange, 1981). However, measurements of peripherally measured hormone levels may not be an accurate reflection of central activity. Manic patients can develop a relative hyperthyroxinaemia with a slightly increased total or free T3/T4 (Bauer and Whybrow, 1988). Lee *et al.* (2000) reported on their study of 46 bipolar manic patients, followed for their thyroid indices, at baseline and one and six months after lithium treatment. Despite the absence of a placebo control group, they found that a reduction in free T4 levels and free T3 levels correlated with a drop in psychotic symptoms, as measured by the Brief Psychiatric Rating Scale (Overall and Gorham, 1962) scores, after one month of lithium treatment. In fact, a progressive reduction in TSH levels was documented throughout the six months of treatment. These observational results seem to support but not necessarily confirm Whybrow and Prange's theory.

Around 10–15% of patients with bipolar disorder are classified with the rapid-cycling subtype (experiencing four or more affective episodes yearly) (American Psychiatric Association, 1994), with women representing up to 80–95% of the patients categorized to this subtype. Various studies report both association and lack of association between hypothyroidism and rapid-cycling bipolar disorder (Cho *et al.*, 1979; Cowdry *et al.*, 1983; Joffe, 1988; Wehr, 1988). Bauer and Whybrow (1990) reported evidence of overt, mild and subclinical hypothyroidism in this sub-group. Gender (female sex) and length of treatment with lithium may be predisposing factors to developing thyroid abnormalities; Bartalena *et al.* (1990) found decreased total and free serum thyroid hormone levels in female bipolar patients, whether or not they were rapid-cyclers, and there was no difference between these two groups, in anti-thyroid antibody titres, presence of goitres and thyroid hormone indices.

Chang *et al.* (1998) reported an increase in mean TSH, and decreased T4 levels, in mixed manic patients, as compared to patients with pure mania, but no significant differences in T3 concentration or in previous exposure to lithium, agreeing with past reports that mixed mania may be more commonly associated with thyroid dysfunction. Frye *et al.* (1999a) found that lithium-treated bipolar patients, with lower free T4 concentrations, exhibited more affective episodes and greater severity of depression, but again causal links remain unclear.

Thyroid Treatment Modalities for Psychiatric Conditions

Major Depression

TRH is a neuropeptide produced by the hypothalamus, which regulates the thyroid axis by controlling the secretion of TSH and thus regulating thyroid hormone synthesis and release. Kastin *et al.* (1972) and Prange *et al.* (1972) reported antidepressant effects from TRH administered intravenously to patients with unipolar depression. However, numerous studies attempting to replicate these results demonstrated minimal or no benefit (Kiely *et al.*, 1976; Mountjoy *et al.*, 1974; Vogel *et al.*, 1977).

T3, a metabolite of T4 with a shorter half-life, appears to be the more biologically active form of thyroid hormone. It has been used as monotherapy treatment of depression, but there is little data supporting its efficacy (Feldmesser-Reiss, 1958; Flach *et al.*, 1958). Stern *et al.* (1991, 1993) performed double-blinded trials on ECT patients with unipolar, bipolar and schizoaffective depressions, who were pretreated with T3, and found improvements in mood and cognition. On the other hand, it is possible that cognitive improvements resulted from a reduction in the number of ECT treatments necessary for remission of the acute episode in those receiving T3 (Joffe and Sokolov, 1994; Sackeim, 1994).

T3 has been most studied as an adjuvant to antidepressant therapy. At doses of 25–50 μg per day, T3 was reported to accelerate the response to antidepressants (Prange *et al.*, 1969; Wheatley, 1972), and convert non-responders to responders (see Aronson *et al.*, 1996 for meta-analysis). Joffe *et al.* (1993) reported that T3 augmentation appeared equally efficacious as lithium, with both medications proving to be more useful than placebo. In fact, two-thirds of tricyclic antidepressant (TCA)-resistant patients responded successfully to T3 augmentation. Of interest, Joffe and Singer (1990) reported on a double-blind trial comparing T3 with T4 augmentation (in the absence of a placebo), and found that T3-treated patients responded at a higher rate than T4-treated individuals (53% versus 19%). Targum *et al.* (1984) reported on the use of T4 augmentation for TCA-resistant depressed patients, but also diagnosed a number of the study patients to have baseline subclinical hypothyroidism.

Case reports on the association of T3 augmentation with the development of angina exacerbation and paroxysmal atrial fibrillation in elderly patients (Cole *et al.*, 1993; Gitlin, 1986) warrant that caution be used when prescribing thyroid hormones.

Bipolar Disorders

A higher prevalence of hypothyroidism has been found in both the rapid- and non-rapid-cycling patients (Bartalena *et al.*, 1990; Joffe *et al.*, 1988; Wehr *et al.*, 1988), as discussed above. In a small sample sized study, Baumgartner *et al.* (1994) treated refractory bipolar patients (non-rapid-cycling) with T4, given 250–500 μg daily, and found significant response to T4, as measured by frequency of relapse and length of hospitalization. However, a significant portion of the study patients was described to also have subclinical hypothyroidism.

The use of T4 at doses up to 500 μg per day has been studied in the treatment of rapid-cycling bipolar disorder, with variable responses, from complete remission to minimal improvement (Bauer and Whybrow, 1990; Leibow, 1983; Stancer and Persad, 1982). Such therapy has been reportedly well tolerated, but there remain concerns about iatrogenically induced hyperthyroid states, and the accompanying risk, albeit theoretical, e.g. osteoporosis. Whybrow (1994) followed up patients from the 1990 study with serial bone densitometries, and discovered a net increase in bone density. However, these patients were also treated with lithium, and it is plausible that lithium may be protective against osteoporosis (Whybrow, 1994). Replication studies using larger numbers of patients, preferably with blinded and randomized controlled trials, are necessary.

GONADAL HORMONES AND MOOD DISORDERS

This topic is covered in greater detail in Chapter XVIII-12. However, this is an area that is being avidly studied in both preclinical and clinical settings. Important data continues to be published on the neurobiological mechanisms of action of these hormones — oestrogen (McEwen *et al.*, 1979), luteinizing hormone (Meller *et al.*, 2001), follicular-stimulating hormone and androgenic steroids (Weber *et al.*, 2000).

Progesterone along with its 5alpha-reduced metabolites, pregnanolone and allopregnanolone, has demonstrated anxiolytic, hypnotic and anaesthetic actions through GABA-A receptor modulation, thereby increasing chloride ion neuronal membrane permeability and reducing neuron excitability (Finn and Gee, 1994; Freeman *et al.*, 1993; Majewska, 1992; Majewska *et al.*, 1986; Wang *et al.*, 1996). Pregnenolone sulphate and dehydroepiandrosterone sulphate (DHEAS) (both 3beta-hydroxy-5-ene steroids) act on GABA-A receptors via *N*-methyl-D-aspartate (NMDA) receptor-mediated intracellular calcium influx across neuronal membranes (Bicikova *et al.*, 2000). Evidence is being gathered to support the roles of gonadal hormones in modulating dopaminergic (Woolley and McEwen, 1994), serotonergic (Biegon, 1990; Biegon *et al.*, 1983), noradrenergic (Biegon *et al.*, 1983) and other neurotransmitter systems.

Bloch *et al.* (2000) investigated the possible role of gonadal steroid level changes in post-partum depression (PPD). Hormonal changes in pregnancy and parturition were artificially simulated in healthy, euthymic, non-pregnant women, with and without history of PPD. Findings suggested a differential sensitivity to the mood-destabilizing effects of gonadal steroids in women with a history of PPD. A year earlier, Buckwalter *et al.* (1999) published their findings on 19 women who were followed during and after pregnancy. Steroid hormone levels were compared to patients' cognitive functioning and mood symptoms. During pregnancy, higher progesterone levels seemed to be associated with greater mood disturbances (particularly with obsessive-compulsive type symptoms), and higher DHEAS with better mood. Two months after delivery, higher testosterone levels was more associated with greater mood disturbances. While cognitive changes (particularly, verbal memory) were documented during pregnancy, they occurred independent of mood changes. Young *et al.* (2000) found that in comparing a sample of 25 depressed with 25 non-depressed women (all premenopausal, aged 20–49), the depressed women exhibited lower oestradiol levels, and a shorter half-life of the luteinizing hormone. Study limitations included a small sample size, and the fact that patients were enrolled at random phases of the menstrual cycle. Attempts were made to control for cycle variability by matching each depressed patient with a control patient, who was similar in age and in menstrual cycle day. This is one example of the intrinsic difficulty facing researchers investigating gonadal hormones and their links to various psychiatric and cognitive conditions.

Further literature has been published on the use of gonadal steroids in treating mood and anxiety disorders, focusing on their efficacy in treating post-partum affective disorders (Gregoire *et al.*, 1996; Sichel *et al.*, 1995), premenstrual syndrome and premenstrual dysphoric disorders (Magos *et al.*, 1986; Watson *et al.*, 1989), and perimenopausal and menopausal depressions (Best *et al.*, 1992; Ditkoff *et al.*, 1991; Limouzin-Lamothe *et al.*, 1994; Oppenheim, 1983; Schneider *et al.*, 1977; Wiesbader and Karzrok, 1938). Lastly, a body of data is accumulating on the effects of the gonadal steroids on mood and aggressive disorders in men (Pope *et al.*, 2000).

Soares *et al.* (2001) reported on their 12-week, double-blind, randomized, placebo-controlled trial of 17beta-oestradiol transdermal patch (100 μg) for the treatment of perimenopausal women with major depression, dysthymic disorder or minor depression for 50 women. Remission from depression was reported in 68% of treated women, versus 20% in the placebo-treated group. Results may be considered difficult to interpret, due to small sample size, broad diagnostic entry criteria (both minor and major depressive disorders) and vague exclusion criteria. The study did attempt to address safety concerns of the transdermal oestrogen patch, referring to published studies of the use of this patch in women with severe PMS (Smith *et al.*, 1995) and post-partum depression (Ahokas *et al.*, 1999). On the other hand, they did not refer to safety data on the use of the patch for perimenopausal women. A last possible concern would be the use of unopposed oestrogen therapy in patients with intact uteri. Albeit the study was limited to only 12 weeks, the risk of endometrial cancer increases by a factor of eight to ten in women who use unopposed oestrogen for at least ten years (Grady *et al.*, 1995).

Among the postmenopausal population in the United States, approximately 38% use hormone replacement therapy (Keating *et al.*, 1999). Manson and Martin (2001) provided an excellent review on this topic, addressing the conundrum of such widespread use of HRT, despite the lack of conclusive data regarding benefits and risks of such treatment, since much collected data were from observational studies. The safety issues of prescribing hormone replacement are closely following along, with recent literature seeking to answer concerns of increased risk for venous thrombosis in women on low-dose oral contraceptives (Vanderbroucke *et al.*, 2001), risk of endometrial cancer recurrence in HRT patients (Suriano *et al.*, 2001), safety of HRT in breast cancer survivors (O'Meara *et al.*, 2001) and possible risk for developing ovarian cancer in women already on HRT (Rodriguez *et al.*, 2001). All of these issues must be carefully considered in the face of potentially increased use of gonadal steroids in the treatment of psychiatric disorders. However, literature on the use of oestrogen and progesterone for treatment of perimenopausal and postmenopausal symptoms is now reporting that a lower dose of combination therapy is equally efficacious (Archer *et al.*, 2001; Utian *et al.*, 2001).

The cognitive benefits of oestrogen and oestrogenic-receptor modulators are also being actively studied. LeBlanc *et al.* (2001) performed a systematic review and meta-analysis on 29 studies and reported difficulty in combining studies on cognition, due to the heterogeneous nature of the study designs. They did perform a meta-analysis on the observational studies, finding that HRT may decrease the risk of dementia (summary odds ratio of 0.66), but reiterated concerns of methodological limitations in most studies. Mulnard *et al.* (2000), of the multi-centred Alzheimer's Disease

Cooperative Study, reported on their randomized, double-blinded, placebo-controlled trial conducted between 1995 and 1999, on 120 women with mild to moderate AD. It was found that oestrogen replacement given for a one-year period did not slow disease progression, nor did it improve global, cognitive or functional outcomes of patients in the study, and acknowledged the need for much more research. Yaffe *et al.* (2001) reported that use of the selective oestrogen-receptor modulator raloxifene (for treatment of postmenopausal women with osteoporosis), over a three-year period, did not improve cognitive scoring.

Gender Differences and Age-Related Changes in the HPA Axis

Seeman *et al.* (2001) tested the hypothesis that women exhibit greater age-related HPA axis reactivity to challenge (using a standardized 30 minute cognitive challenge). A group of 26 younger subjects (9 men and 17 women), in their 20s were compared to 14 older subjects (7 men and 7 women) in their 60s. Baseline salivary cortisol levels were measured and repeated during and following a battery of cognitive tests. These tests were administered in a fast-paced, time-limited fashion, and designed to increase both HPA and sympathetic nervous system activity. Results from previously published data showed that older age was associated with higher baseline cortisol (Deuschle *et al.*, 1997; van Cauter *et al.*, 1996); women exhibited shorter nocturnal nadirs, higher morning cortisol levels, and higher mean 24-hour readings (van Cauter *et al.*, 1996). Postmenopausal women showed greater HPA reactivity to CRH challenge (Heuser *et al.*, 1994) and less feedback inhibition (blunted ACTH decline) in response to cortisol infusion, at the level of the pituitary. In the younger age group, some studies reported that men tended to exhibit greater cortisol response (Kirshbaum *et al.*, 1992), while others found no significant gender difference (Gallucci *et al.*, 1993; Stoney *et al.*, 1987; Streeten *et al.*, 1984).

The question of the possible role gonadal hormones may play in shifting the HPA axis of older women to greater reactivity was raised, since higher oestrogen levels have been linked to decreased blood pressure (von Eiff, 1971) and decreased HPA reactivity (Bonen *et al.*, 1991; Marinari *et al.*, 1976). This may be counteracted in settings of higher progesterone levels (Kirshbaum *et al.*, 1999). On the other hand, hormone replacement therapy has been linked to blunted cortisol responses to cognitive and physical stress tests in postmenopausal women (Lindheim *et al.*, 1992, 1994). In addition to the lack of feedback inhibition to cortisol in older women, a greater increase in the ACTH response to CRH or vasopressin challenge has also been observed (Born *et al.*, 1995). Preclinical studies have suggested oestrogenic regulation of the hippocampus and hypothalamus, due to the presence of oestrogen receptors in these regions (Teyler and DiScenna, 1986), oestrogenic regulation of synaptogenesis in the CA1 region of the hippocampus (McEwen *et al.*, 1994) and induction of other electrical activity and membrane changes in the hippocampus and hypothalamus by oestrogen (Foy *et al.*, 1982; Minami *et al.*, 1990; Wong and Moss, 1991).

SUMMARY

Numerous factors may contribute to the pathophysiology of mood disorders, including the pathophysiology of the brain's adaptation to stress, (allostatic load) (McEwen and Stellar, 1993; Sterling and Eyer, 1988), the possible role of chronic stress on hippocampal damage and dysfunction (which may result in psychiatric symptoms) (McEwen, 2000), as well as the effects of genetic predisposition and developmental stresses (Liu *et al.*, 1997). It remains challenging and at times, controversial, to draw firm conclusions from observations of the endocrine abnormalities associated with mood disorders. The stress effect arising from these psychiatric conditions can precipitate significant and widespread metabolic/endocrine changes ('state' markers). Researchers are now attempting to differentiate this from causal factors ('trait' markers) for such endocrine changes, to determine which are associated with the pathophysiological mechanisms of mood disorders.

REFERENCES

Abadie, J.M., Wright, B., Correa, G., Browne, E.S., Porter, J.R. and Svec, F., 1993. Effect of dehydroepiandrosterone on neurotransmitter levels and appetite regulation of the obese Zucker rat. The Obesity Research Program. *Diabetes*, **42**:662–9.

Abed, R.T., Clark, J., Elbadawy, M.H. and Cliffe, M.J., 1987. Psychiatric morbidity in acromegaly. [Erratum appears in *Acta Psychiat. Scand.*, 1987, **76**(6):735]. *Acta Psychiat. Scand.*, **75**(6):635–9.

Aberg-Widtedt, A., Widedt, B. and Bertilsson, L., 1985. Higher CSF levels of HVA and 5-H1AA in delusional compared to nondelusional depression [letter]. *Arch. Gen. Psychiat.*, **42**:925–6.

Ahokas, A., Kaukoranta, J. and Aito, M., 1999. Effect of oestradiol on postpartum depression. *Psychopharmacology*, **146**(1):108–10.

American Psychiatric Association, 1994. *Diagnostic and Statistical Manual of Mental Disorders*, 4th edn. (DSM-IV) American Psychiatric Association, Washington, DC.

Aperia, B., Bergman, H., Engelbrektson, K., Thoren, M. and Wetterberg, L., 1985a. Effects of electroconvulsive therapy on neuropsychological function and circulating levels of ACTH, cortisol, prolactin, and TSH in patients with major depressive illness. *Acta Psychiat. Scand.*, **72**(6):536–41.

Aperia, B., Thoren, M. and Wetterberg, L., 1985b. Prolactin and thyrotropin in serum during electroconvulsive therapy in patients with major depressive illness. *Acta Psychiat. Scand.*, **72**(3):302–8.

Arana, G.W. and Forbes, R.A., 1991. Dexamethasone for the treatment of depression: a preliminary report. *J. Clin. Psychiat.*, **52**:304–6.

Arana, G.W., Santos, A.B., Laraia, M.T., McLeod-Bryant, S., Beale, M.D., Rames, L.J., Roberts, J.M., Dias, J.K. and Molloy, M., 1995. Dexamethasone for the treatment of depression: a randomized, placebo-controlled, double-blind trial. *Am. J. Psychiat.*, **152**:265–7.

Arborelius, L., Skelton, K.H., Thrivikraman, K.V., Plotsky, P.M., Schulz, D.W. and Owens, M.J., 2000. Chronic administration of the selective corticotropin-releasing factor 1 receptor antagonist CP-154,526: behavioral, endocrine and neurochemical effects in the rat. *J. Pharmacol. Exp. Ther.*, **294**:588–97.

Archer, D.F., Dorin, M., Lewis, V., Schneider, D.L. and Pickar, J.H., 2001. Effects of lower doses of conjugated equine estrogens and medroxyprogesterone acetate on endometrial bleeding. *Fertil. Steril.*, **75**(6):1080–7.

Arnsten, A.F., Mathew, R., Ubriani, R., Taylor, J.R. and Li, B.M., 1999. Alpha-1 noradrenergic receptor stimulation impairs prefrontal cortical cognitive function. *Biol. Psychiat.*, **45**(1):26–31.

Aronson, R., Offman, H.J., Joffe, R.T. and Naylor, C.D., 1996. Triiodothyronine augmentation in the treatment of refractory depression: a meta-analysis. *Arch. Gen. Psychiat.*, **53**:842–8.

Asher, R., 1949. Myxoedematous madness. *Br. Med. J.*, **22**:555–62.

Azuma, T., Matsubara, T., Shima, Y., Haeno, S., Fujimoto, T., Tone, K., Shibata, N. and Sakoda, S., 1993. Neurosteroids in cerebrospinal fluid in neurologic disorders. *J. Neurol. Sci.*, **120**:87–92.

Baker, D.G., West, S.A., Nicholson, W.E., Ekhator, N.N., Kasckow, J.W., Hill, K.K., Bruce, A.B., Orth, D.N. and Geracioti, T.D., Jr, 1999. Serial CSF corticotropin-releasing hormone levels and adrenocortical activity in combat veterans with posttraumatic stress disorder. *Am. J. Psychiat.*, **156**(4):585–8.

Banki, C.M., Bissette, G., Arato, M. and Nemeroff, C.B., 1988. Elevation of immunoreactive CSF TRH in depressed patients. *Am. J. Psychiat.*, **145**:1526–31.

Barrett-Connor, E., Von Muhlen, D.G. and Kritz-Silverstein, D., 1999. Bioavailable testosterone and depressed mood in older men: the Rancho Bernardo Study. *J. Clin. Endocrinol. Metabol.*, **84**:573–7.

Bartalena, L., Pellegrini, L., Meschi, M., Antonangeli, L., Bogazzi, F., Dell'Osso, L., Pinchera, A. and Placidi, G.F., 1990. Evaluation of thyroid function in patients with rapid cycling and non-rapid-cycling bipolar disorder. *Psychiat. Res.*, **34**:13–17.

Bauer, M.S. and Whybrow, P.C., 1988. Thyroid hormones and the central nervous system in affective illness: Interactions that may have clinical significance. *Integ. Psychiat.*, **6**:75–100.

Bauer, M.S. and Whybrow, P.C., 1990. Rapid cycling bipolar affective disorder. II. Treatment of refractory rapid cycling with high-dose levothyroxine: a preliminary study. *Arch. Gen. Psychiat.*, **47**:435–40.

Bauer, M.S., Kurtz, J., Winokur, A., Phillips, J., Rubin, L.B. and Marcus, J.G., 1993. Thyroid function before and after four-week light treatment in winter depressives and controls. *Psychoneuroendocrinology*, **18**:437–43.

Baumgartner, A., Bauer, M.S. and Hellweg, R., 1994. Treatment of intractable non-rapid cycling bipolar affective disorder with high-dose thyroxine: an open clinical trial. *Neuropsychopharmacology*, **10**:183–9.

Belanoff, J.K., Gross, K., Yager, A. and Schatzberg, A.F., 2001. Corticosteroids and cognition. *J. Psychiat. Res.*, **35**:127–45.

Bergeron, R., de Montigny, C. and Debonnel, G., 1996. Potentiation of neuronal NMDA response induced by dehydroepiandrosterone and its suppression by progesterone: effects mediated via sigma receptors. *J. Neurosci.*, **16**:1193–1202.

Berkman, L.F., Seeman, T.E., Albert, M., Blazer, D., Kahn, R., Mohs, R., Finch, C., Schneider, E., Cotman, C. and McClearn, G., 1993. High, usual and impaired functioning in community-dwelling older men and women: findings from the MacArthur Foundation Research Network on Successful Aging. *J. Clin. Epidemiol.*, **46**:1129–40.

Berr, C., Lafont, S., Debuire, B., Dartigues, J.F. and Baulieu, E.E., 1996. Relationships of dehydroepiandrosterone sulfate in the elderly with functional, psychological, and mental status, and short-term mortality: a French community-based study. *Proc. Natl Acad. Sci. USA*, **93**:13410–15.

Best, N.R., Rees, M.P., Barlow, D.H. and Cowen, P.J., 1992. Effect of estradiol implant on noradrenergic function and mood in menopausal subjects. *Psychoneuroendocrinology*, **17**:87–93.

Bicikova, M., Tallova, J., Hill, M., Krausova, Z. and Hampl, R., 2000. Serum concentrations of some neuroactive steroids in women suffering from mixed anxiety-depressive disorder. *Neurochem. Res.*, **25**:1623–7.

Biegon, A., 1990. Effects of steroid hormones on the serotonergic system. *Ann. N. Y. Acad. Sci.*, **600**:427–32.

Biegon, A., Reches, A., Snyder, L. and McEwen, B.S., 1983. Serotonergic and noradrenergic receptors in the rat brain: modulation by chronic exposure to ovarian hormones. *Life Sci.*, **32**(17):2015–21.

Birmaher, B., Dahl, R.E., Williamson, D.E., Perel, J.M., Brent, D.A., Axelson, D.A., Kaufman, J., Dorn, L.D., Stull, S., Rao, U. and Ryan, N.D., 2000. Growth hormone secretion in children and adolescents at high risk for major depressive disorder. *Arch. Gen. Psychiat.*, **57**:867–72.

Bloch, M., Schmidt, P.J., Danaceau, M.A., Adams, L.F. and Rubinow, D.R., 1999. Dehydroepiandrosterone treatment of midlife dysthymia. *Biol. Psychiat.*, **45**(12):1533–41.

Bloch, M., Schmidt, P.J., Danaceau, M., Murphy, J., Nieman, L. and Rubinow, D.R., 2000. Effects of gonadal steroids in women with a history of postpartum depression. *Am. J. Psychiat.*, **157**:924–30.

Bonen, A., Haynes, F.W. and Graham, T.E., 1991. Substrate and hormonal responses to exercise in women using oral contraceptives. *J. Appl. Physiol.*, **70**(5):1917–27.

Born, J., Ditschuneit, I., Schreiber, M., Dodt, C. and Fehm, H.L., 1995. Effects of age and gender on pituitary–adrenocortical responsiveness in humans. *Eur. J. Endocrinol.*, **132**(6):705–11.

Boscarino, J.A., 1996. Post-traumatic stress disorder, exposure to combat, and lower plasma cortisol among Vietnam veterans — findings and clinical implications. *J. Consult. Clin. Psychol.*, **64**:191–201.

Britton, D.R., Koob, G.F., Rivier, J. and Vale, W., 1982. Intraventricular corticotropin-releasing factor enhances behavioral effects of novelty. *Life Sci.*, **31**(4):363–7.

Brown, G.M., 1984. Psychiatric and neurologic aspects of endocrine disease. In: Brown, G.M., Koslow, S.H. and Reichlin, S. (eds), *Neuroendocrinology and Psychiatric Disorders*, pp. 185–93. Raven Press, New York.

Brown, M.R., Fisher, L.A., Spiess, J., Rivier, C., Rivier, J. and Vale, W., 1982. Corticotropin-releasing factor: actions on the sympathetic nervous system and metabolism. *Endocrinology*, **111**(3):928–31.

Browne, E.S., Wright, B.E., Porter, J.R. and Svec, F., 1992. Dehydroepiandrosterone: antiglucocorticoid action in mice. *Am. J. Med. Sci.*, **303**:366–71.

Buckwalter, J.G., Stanczyk, F.Z., McCleary, C.A., Bluestein, B.W., Buckwalter, D.K., Rankin, K.P., Chang, L. and Goodwin, T.M., 1999. Pregnancy, the postpartum, and steroid hormones: effects on cognition and mood. *Psychoneuroendocrinology*, **24**:69–84.

Burrow, G.N., Burke, W.R., Himmelhoch, J.M., Spencer, R.P. and Hershman, J.M., 1971. Effect of lithium on thyroid function. *J. Clin. Endocrinol. Metab.*, **32**:647–52.

Calogero, A.E., Gallucci, W.T., Chrousos, G.P. and Gold, P.W., 1988. Catecholamine effects upon rat hypothalamic corticotropin-releasing hormone secretion *in vitro*. *J. Clin. Invest.*, **82**:839–46.

Carette, B. and Poulain, P., 1984. Excitatory effect of dehydroepiandrosterone, its sulphate ester and pregnenolone sulphate, applied by iontophoresis and pressure, on single neurons in the septo-preoptic area of the guinea pig. *Neurosci. Lett.*, **45**:205–10.

Carlson, H.E., Tample, R. and Robbins, J., 1973. Effect of lithium on thyroxine disappearance in man. *J. Clin. Endocrinol. Metab.*, **36**:1249–54.

Carroll, B.J., Curtis, G.C., Davies, B.M., Mendels, J. and Sugerman, A.A., 1976. Urinary free cortisol excretion in depression. *Psychol. Med.*, **6**(1):43–50.

Carroll, B.J., Feinberg, M., Greden, J.F., Tarika, J., Albala, A.A., Haskett, R.F., James, N.M., Kronfol, Z., Lohr, N., Steiner, M., de Vigne, J.P. and Young, E., 1981. A specific laboratory test for the diagnosis of melancholia: standardization, validation and clinical utility. *Arch. Gen. Psychiat.*, **38**:15–22.

Carson, S.W., Halbreich, U., Yeh, C.M., Asnis, G. and Goldstein, S., 1988. Cortisol suppression per nanogram per milliliter of plasma dexamethasone in depressive and normal subjects. *Biol. Psychiat.*, **24**:569–77.

Cassidy, F., Ritchie, J.C. and Carroll, B.J., 1998. Plasma dexamethasone concentration and cortisol response during manic episodes. *Biol. Psychiat.*, **43**:747–54.

Cawood, E.H. and Bancroft, J., 1996. Steroid hormones, the menopause, sexuality and well-being of women. *Psychol. Med.*, **26**:925–36.

Chang, K.D., Keck, P.E., Stanton, S.P., McElroy, S.L., Strakowski, S.M. and Geracioti, T.D., 1998. Differences in thyroid function between bipolar manic and mixed states. *Biol. Psychiat.*, **43**:730–3.

Charney, D.S., Heninger, G.R. and Sternberg, D.E., 1984. Serotonin function and mechanism of action of antidepressant treatment: effects of amitriptyline and desipramine. *Arch. Gen. Psychiat.*, **41**:359–65.

Cho, J.T., Bone, S., Dunner, D.L., Colt, E. and Fieve, R., 1979. The effect of lithium treatment on thyroid function in patients with primary affective disorder. *Am. J. Psychiat.*, **136**:115–16.

Clinical Society of London, 1888. Report on myxoedema. *Trans. Clin. Soc. London*, **2**(suppl):18.

Coccaro, E.F., Kavoussi, R.J., Oakes, M., Cooper, T.B. and Hauger, R.L., 1996. 5-HT2A/2C blockade by amesergide fully attenuates prolactin response to d-fenfluramine challenge in physically healthy human subjects. *Psychopharmacology (Berl)*, **126**:24–30.

Cole, P.A., Bostwick, J.M. and Fajtova, V.T., 1993. Thyrotoxicosis in a depressed patient on l-triiodothyronine [letter]. *Psychosomatics*, **34**(6):539–40.

Connolly, M.S. and Lynch, C.B., 1983. Classical genetic analysis of circadian body temperature rhythms in mice. *Behav. Genet.*, **13**:491–500.

Coplan, J.D., Andrews, M.W., Rosenblum, L.A., Owens, M.J., Friedman, S., Gorman, J.M. and Nemeroff, C.B., 1996. Persistent elevations of cerebrospinal fluid concentrations of corticotropin-releasing factor in adult nonhuman primates exposed to early-life stressors: implications for the pathophysiology of mood and anxiety disorders. *Proc. Natl Acad. Sci. USA.*, **93**:1619–23.

Coplan, J.D., Wolk, S.I., Goetz, R.R., Ryan, N.D., Dahl, R.E., Mann, J. and Weissman, M.M., 2000. Nocturnal growth hormone secretion studies in adolescents with or without major depression re-examined: integration of adult clinical follow-up data. *Biol. Psychiat.*, **47**:594–604.

Cowdry, R.W., Wehr, T.A., Zis, A.P. and Goodwin, F., 1983. Thyroid abnormalities associated with rapid-cycling bipolar illness. *Arch. Gen. Psychiat.*, **40**:414–20.

Cyr, M., Morissette, M., Barden, N., Beaulieu, S., Rochford, J. and Di Paolo, T., 2001. Dopaminergic activity in transgenic mice underexpressing glucocorticoid receptors: effect of antidepressants. *Neuroscience*, **102**:151–8.

Dahl, R.E., Birmaher, B., Williamson, D.E., Dorn, L., Perel, J., Kaufman, J., Brent, D.A., Axelson, D.A. and Ryan, N.D., 2000. Low growth hormone response to growth hormone-releasing hormone in child depression. *Biol. Psychiat.*, **48**:981–8.

DeBattista, C., Posener, J.A., Kalehzan, B.M. and Schatzberg, A.F., 2000. Acute antidepressant effects of intravenous hydrocortisone and CRH in depressed patients: a double-blind, placebo-controlled study. *Am. J. Psychiat.*, **157**:1334–7.

Degerblad, M., Almkvist, O., Grundiz, R., Hall, K., Kaijser, L., Knutsson, E., Ringertz, H. and Thoren, M., 1990. Physical and psychological capabilities during substitution therapy with recombinant growth hormone in adults with growth hormone deficiency. *Acta Endocrinol.*, **123**:185–93.

De Goeij, D.C., Jezova, D. and Tilders, F.J., 1992. Repeated stress enhances vasopressin synthesis in corticotropin releasing factor neurons in the paraventricular nucleus. *Brain Res.*, **577**(1):165–8.

Denko, J.D. and Kaelbling, R., 1962. The psychiatric aspects of hypoparathyroidism. *Acta Psychiat. Scand.*, **38**:7–10.

Deshauer, D., Grof, E., Alda, M. and Grof, P., 1999. Patterns of DST positivity in remitted affective disorders. *Biol. Psychiat.*, **45**:1023–9.

Deuschle, M., Gotthardt, U., Schweiger, U., Weber, B., Korner, A., Schmider, J., Standhardt, H., Lammers, C.H. and Heuser, I., 1997. With aging in humans the activity of the hypothalamus–pituitary–adrenal system increases and its diurnal amplitude flattens. *Life Sci.*, **61**(22):2239–46.

Devanand, D.P., Bowers, M.B., Hoffman, F.J. and Nelson, J.C., 1985. Elevated plasma homovanillic acid in depressed females with melancholia and psychosis. *Psychiat. Res.*, **15**:1–4.

Diamond, D.M., Branch, B.J., Fleshner, M. and Rose, G.M., 1995. Effects of dehydroepiandrosterone sulfate and stress on hippocampal electrophysiological plasticity. *Ann. N. Y. Acad. Sci.*, **774**:304–7.

Diamond, P., Brisson, G.R., Candas, B. and Peronnet, F., 1989. Trait anxiety, submaximal physical exercise and blood androgens. *Eur. J. Appl. Physiol. Occupat. Physiol.*, **58**:699–704.

Dinan, T.G., Lavelle, E., Cooney, J., Burnett, F., Scott, L., Dash, A., Thakore, J. and Berti, C., 1997. Dexamethasone augmentation in treatment-resistant depression. *Acta Psychiat. Scand.*, **95**:58–61.

Ditkoff, E.C., Crary, W.G., Cristo, M. and Lobo, R., 1991. Estrogen improves psychological function in asymptomatic postmenopausal women. *Obstet. Gynecol.*, **78**:991–5.

Dolan, R.J. and Calloway, S.P., 1986. The human growth hormone response to clonidine: relationship to clinical and neuroendocrine profile in depression. *Am. J. Psychiat.*, **143**:772–4.

Donaldson, C.J., Sutton, S.W., Perrin, M.H., Corrigan, A.Z., Lewis, K.A., Rivier, J.E., Vaughan, J.M. and Vale, W.W., 1996. Cloning and characterization of human urocortin [Erratum appears in *Endocrinology*, 1996, **137**(9):3896]. *Endocrinology*, **137**(5):2167–70.

Drevets, W.C., Price, J.L., Simpson, J.R., Todd, R.D., Reich, T., Vannier, M. and Raichle, M.E., 1997. Subgenual prefrontal cortex abnormalities in mood disorders. *Nature*, **386**:824–7.

Duval, F., Mokrani, M.C., Crocq, M.A., Bailey, P.E., Diep, T.S., Correa, H. and Macher, J.P., 2000. Dopaminergic function and the cortisol response to dexamethasone in psychotic depression. *Prog. Neuro-Psychopharmacol. Biol. Psychiat.*, **24**(2):207–25.

Ellis, P.M. and Salmond, C., 1994. Is platelet imipramine binding reduced in depression? A meta-analysis. *Biol. Psychiat.*, **36**(5):292–9.

Emlen, W., Segal, D. and Mandell, A., 1972. Thyroid state: effects on pre- and post-synaptic central noradrenergic mechanisms. *Science*, **175**:79–82.

Ericsson, U.B., Bjerre, I., Forsgren, M. and Ivarsson, S.A., 1985. Thyroglobulin and thyroid hormones in patients on long-term treatment with phenytoin, carbamazepine, and valproic acid. *Epilepsia*, **26**:594–6.

Evered, D.C., Ormstron, B.J., Smith, P.A., Hall, R. and Bird, T., 1973. Grades of hypothyroidism. *Br. Med. J.*, **1**:657–62.

Fava, M., Littman, A. and Halperin, P., 1987. Neuroendocrine correlates of the Type A behavior pattern: a review and new hypothesis. *Int. J. Psychiat. Med.*, **17**:289–307.

Fava, M., Rosenbaum, J.F., MacLaughlin, R.A., Tesar, G.E., Pollack, M.H., Cohen, L.S. and Hirsch, M., 1989. Dehydroepiandrosterone-sulfate/cortisol ratio in panic disorder. *Psychiat. Res.*, **28**(3):345–50.

Fava, M., Littman, A., Lamon-Fava, S., Milani, R., Shera, D., MacLaughlin, R., Cassem, E., Leaf, A., Marchio, B., Bolognesi, E. and Guaraldi, G.P., 1992. Psychological, behavioral, and biochemical risk factors for coronary artery disease among American and Italian male corporate managers. *Am. J. Cardiol.*, **70**:1412–16.

Fava, G.A., Sonino, N. and Morphy, M.A., 1993. Psychosomatic view of endocrine disorders. *Psychother. Psychosom.*, **59**:20–33.

Feldman, S. and Conforti, N., 1980. Participation of the dorsal hippocampus in the glucocorticoid feedback effect on adrenocortical activity. *Neuroendocrinology*, **30**:52–5.

Feldmesser-Reiss, E.E., 1958. The application of triiodothyronine in the treatment of mental disorders. *J. Nerv. Ment. Dis.*, **127**:540.

Ferrier, I.N., 1987. Endocrinology and psychosis. *Br. Med. Bull.*, **43**:672–88.

Finn, D.A. and Gee, K.W., 1994. The estrus cycle, sensitivity to convulsants and the anticonvulsant effect of a neuroactive steroid. *J. Pharmacol. and Exp. Ther.*, **27**(1):164–70.

Fishman, S.M., Sheehan, D.V. and Carr, D.B., 1985. Thyroid indices in panic disorder. *J. Clin. Psychiat.*, **46**:432–3.

Flach, F.F., Celian, C.I. and Rawson, R.W., 1958. Treatment of psychiatric disorders with triiodothyronine. *Am. J. Psychiat.*, **114**:841.

Flood, J.F. and Roberts, E., 1988. Dehydroepiandrosterone sulfate improves memory in aging mice. *Brain Res.*, **448**:178–81.

Foy, M.R., Teyler, T.J. and Vardaris, R.M., 1982. Delta 9-THC and 17-beta-estradiol in hippocampus. *Brain Res. Bull.*, **8**(4):341–5.

Freeman, F.W., Purdy, R.H., Coutifaris, C., Rickels, K. and Paul, S.M., 1993. Anxiolytic metabolites of progesterone: correlation with mood and performance on measures following oral progesterone administration to healthy female volunteers. *Neuroendocrinology*, **58**:478–84.

Friess, E., Trachsel, L., Guldner, J., Schier, T., Steiger, A. and Holsboer, F., 1995. DHEA administration increases rapid eye movement sleep and EEG power in the sigma frequency range. *Am. J. Physiol.*, **268**:E107–13.

Frye, M.A., Denicoff, K.D., Bryan, A.L., Smith-Jackson, E.E., Ali, S.O., Luckenbaugh, D., Leverich, G.S. and Post, R.M., 1999a. Association between lower serum free T4 and greater mood instability and depression in lithium-maintained bipolar patients. *Am. J. Psychiat.*, **156**:1909–14.

Frye, M.A., Dunn, R.T., Gary, K.A., Kimbrell, T.A., Callahan, A.M., Luckenbaugh, D.A., Cora-Locatellit, G., Vanderham, E.V., Winokur, A. and Post, R.M., 1999b. Lack of correlation between cerebrospinal fluid thyrotropin-releasing hormone (TRH) and TRH-stimulated thyroid-stimulating hormone in patients with depression. *Biol. Psychiat.*, **45**:1049–52.

Fujita, M., Charney, D.S. and Innis, R.B., 2000. Imaging serotonergic neurotransmission in depression: hippocampal pathophysiology may mirror global brain alterations. *Biol. Psychiat.*, **48**:810–12.

Gallucci, W.T., Baum, A., Laue, L., Rabin, D.S., Chrousos, G.P., Gold, P.W. and Kling, M.A., 1993. Sex differences in sensitivity of the hypothalamic–pituitary–adrenal axis. *Health Psychol.*, **12**(5):420–5.

Ghadirian, A.M., Englesmann, F., Dhar, V., Filipini, D., Keller, R., Chouinard, G. and Murphy, B.E.P., 1995. The psychotropic effects of inhibitors of steroid biosynthesis in depressed patients refractory to treatment. *Biol. Psychiat.*, **37**:369–75.

Gharib, H. and Abboud, C.F., 1987. Primary idiopathic hypothalamic hypothyroidism. *Am. J. Med.*, **83**:171–4.

Gitlin, M.J., 1986. L-triiodothyronine-precipitated angina and clinical response. *Biol. Psychiat.*, **21**(5–6):543–5.

Gold, M.S., Pottash, A.L.C. and Extein, I., 1981. Hypothyroidism and depression. *JAMA*, **245**:1919–22.

Gold, M.S., Pottash, A.L.C. and Extein, I., 1982. Symptomless autoimmune thyroiditis in depression. *Psychiat. Res.*, **6**:261–9.

Gold, P.W. and Chrousos, G.P., 1999. The endocrinology of melancholic and atypical depression: relation to neurocircuitry and somatic consequences. *Proc. Assoc. Amer. Physicians*, **111**(1):22–34.

Gold, P.W., Chrousos, G., Kellner, C., Post, R., Roy, A., Augerinos, P., Schulte, H., Oldfield, E. and Loriaux, D., 1984. Psychiatric implication of basic and clinical studies of corticotrophic releasing factor. *Am. J. Psychiat.*, **141**:619–24.

Gold, P.W., Goodwin, F.K. and Chrousos, G.P., 1988. Clinical and biochemical manifestations of depression (first of two parts). *N. Engl J. Med.*, **319**:348–53.

Gold, P.W., Licinio, J., Wong, M.-L. and Chrousos, G.P., 1995. Corticotropin releasing hormone in the pathophysiology of melancholic and atypical depression and in the mechanism of action of antidepressant drugs. *Ann. N. Y. Acad. Sci.*, **771**:716–29.

Goldstein, L.E., Rasmusson, A.M., Bunney, B.S. and Roth, R.H., 1996. Role of the amygdala in the coordination of behavioral, neuroendocrine, and prefrontal cortical monoamine responses to psychological stress in the rat. *J. Neurosci.*, **16**(15):4787–98.

Goodyer, I.M., Herbert, J., Altham, P.M.E., Secher, S. and Shiers, H.M., 1996. Adrenal secretion during major depression in 8 to 16 year olds. I. Altered diurnal rhythms in salivary cortisol and dehydroepiandrosterone (DHEA): at presentation. *Psychol. Med.*, **26**:245–56.

Goodyer, I.M., Herbert, J. and Altham, P.M., 1998. Adrenal steroid secretion and major depression in 8 to 16 year olds. III. Influence of cortisol/DHEA ratio at presentation on subsequent rates of disappointing life events and persistent major depression. *Psychol. Med.*, **28**:265–73.

Grady, D., Gebretsadik, T., Kerlikowske, K., Ernster, V. and Petitti, D., 1995. Hormone replacement therapy and endometrial cancer risk: a meta-analysis. *Obstet. Gynecol.*, **85**(2):304–13.

Graves, R., 1940. Clinical lectures. *Med. Classics*, **5**:35.

Gregoire, A.J., Kumar, R., Everitt, B., Henderson, A.F. and Studd, J.W., 1996. Transdermal oestrogen for treatment of severe postnatal depression. *Lancet*, **347**(9006):930–3.

Gross, G., Brodde, O. and Schumann, H., 1980. Decreased number of adrenoceptors in the cerebral cortex of hypothyroid rats. *Eur. J. Pharmacol.*, **61**:191–7.

Gull, W., 1873. On a cretinoid state supervening in adult life. *Trans. Clin. Soc. London*, **7**:180–5.

Haggerty, J.J., Jr and Prange, A.J., 1995. Borderline hypothyroidism and depression. *A. Rev. Med.*, **46**:37–46.

Halbreich, U., Asnis, G.M., Zumoff, B., Nathan, R.S. and Shindledecker, R., 1984. Effect of age and sex on cortisol secretion in depressives and normals. *Psychiat. Res.*, **13**:221–9.

Hamilton, M., 1960. A rating scale for depression. *J. Neurol. Neurosurg. Psychiat.*, **23**:56–62.

Harrison, T.S., 1964. Adrenal medullary and thyroid relationships. *Physiol. Rev.*, **44**:161.

Heim, C., Newport, D.J., Heit, S., Graham, Y.P., Wilcox, M., Bonsall, R., Miller, A. and Nemeroff, C.B., 2000. Pituitary–adrenal and autonomic responses to stress in women after sexual and physical abuse in childhood. *JAMA*, **284**:592–7.

Heim, C., Newport, D.J., Bonsall, R., Miller, A.H. and Nemeroff, C.B., 2001. Altered pituitary–adrenal axis responses to provocative challenge tests in adult survivors of childhood abuse. *Am. J. Psychiat.*, **158**:575–81.

Herbert, J., Goodyer, I.M., Altham, P.M.E., Pearson, J., Secher, S.M. and Shiers, H.M., 1996. Adrenal secretion and major depression in 8 to 16 year olds. II. Influence of co-morbidity at presentation. *Psychol. Med.*, **26**:257–63.

Herman, J.P., Cullinan, W.E., Young, E.A., Akil, H. and Watson, S.J., 1992. Selective forebrain fiber tract lesions implicate ventral hippocampal structures in tonic regulation of paraventricular nucleus corticotropin-releasing hormone (CRH) and arginine vasopressin (AVP) mRNA expression. *Brain Res.*, **592**(1–2):228–38.

Hermida, R.C., Halberg, F. and del Pozo, F., 1985. Chronobiologic pattern discrimination of plasma hormones, notably DHEA-S and TSH, classifies an expansive personality. *Chronobiologia*, **12**(2):105–36.

Heuser, I., Yassouridis, A. and Holsboer, F., 1994. The combined dexamethasone/CRH test: a refined laboratory test for psychiatric disorders. *J. Psychiat. Res.*, **28**:341–56.

Heuser, I., Deuschle, M., Luppa, P., Schweiger, U., Standhardt, H. and Weber, B., 1998. Increased diurnal plasma concentrations of dehydroepiandrosterone in depressed patients. *J. Clin. Endocrinol. Metabol.*, **83**:3130–3.

Hoeflich, G., Kasper, S., Danos, P. and Schmidt, R., 1992. Thyroid hormones, body temperature, and antidepressant therapy. *Biol. Psychiat.*, **31**:859–62.

Holmes, S.J. and Shalet, S.M., 1995. Factors influencing the desire for long-term growth hormone replacement in adults. *Clin. Endocrinol.*, **43**:151–7.

Holsboer, F., 1999. The rationale for corticotropin-releasing hormone receptor (CRH-R) antagonists to treat depression and anxiety. *J. Psychiat. Res.*, **33**:181–214.

Holsboer, F., 2001. Stress, hypercortisolism and corticosteroid receptors in depression: implications for therapy. *J. Affect. Disord.*, **62**:77–91.

Holsboer, F., Muller, O.A., Doerr, H.G., Sippel, W.G., Stalla, G.K., Gerken, A., Steiger, A., Boll, E. and Benkert, O., 1984. ACTH and multisteroid responses to corticotropin-releasing factor in depressive illness: relationship to multisteroid responses after ACTH stimulation and dexamethasone suppression. *Psychoneuroendocrinology*, **9**:147–60.

Holsboer, F., Wiedemann, K. and Boll, E., 1986a. Shortened dexamethasone half-life in depressed dexamethasone non-suppressors. *Arch. Gen. Psychiat.*, **43**:813–15.

Holsboer, F., Wiedemann, K., Gerken, A. and Boll, E., 1986b. The plasma dexamethasone variable in depression: test–retest studies and early biophase kinetics. *Psychiat. Res.*, **17**:97–103.

Holsboer, F., Lauer, C.J., Schreiber, W. and Krieg, J.-C., 1995. Altered hypothalamic–pituitary–adrenocortical regulation in healthy subjects at high familial risk for affective disorders. *Neuroendocrinology*, **62**:340–7.

Holsboer-Trachsler, E., Hemmeter, U., Hatzinger, M., Seifritz, E., Gerhard, U. and Hobi, V., 1994. Sleep deprivation and bright light as potential augmenters of antidepressant drug treatment — neurobiological and psychometric assessment of course. *J. Psychiat. Res.*, **28**:381–99.

Howland, R.H. and Thase, M.E., 1991. Biological studies of dysthymia. *Biol. Psychiat.*, **30**(3):283–304.

Jacobson, L. and Sapolsky, R.M., 1991. The role of the hippocampus in feedback regulation of the hypothalamic–pituitary–adrenal axis. *Endocrinol. Rev.*, **12**:118–34.

Joffe, R.T., 1987. Antithyroid antibodies in major depression. *Acta Psychiat. Scand.*, **76**:598–9.

Joffe, R.T., 1988. Triiodothyronine potentiation of the antidepressant effect of phenylzine. *J. Clin. Psychiat.*, **49**(10):409–10.

Joffe, R.T., 1991. Thyroid function and phototherapy in seasonal affective disorder [letter]. *Am. J. Psychiat.*, **148**:393.

Joffe, R.T., 1999. Peripheral thyroid hormone levels in treatment resistant depression. *Biol. Psychiat.*, **45**:1053–5.

Joels, M. and DeKloet, E.R., 1992. Control of neuronal excitability by corticosteroid hormones. *Trends Neurosci.*, **15**:25–30.

Joffe, R.T. and Levitt, A.J., 1992. Major depression and subclinical (grade 2) hypothyroidism. *Psychoneuroendocrinology*, **17**:215–21.

Joffe, R.T. and Levitt, A.J., 1993. The thyroid and depression. In: Joffe, R.T. and Levitt, A.J. (eds), *The Thyroid Axis and Psychiatric Illness*, pp. 195–253. American Psychiatric Press, Washington, DC.

Joffe, R.T. and Marriot, M., 2000. Thyroid hormone levels and recurrence of major depression. *Am. J. Psychiat.*, **157**:1689–91.

Joffe, R.T. and Singer, W., 1987. Effect of phenelzine on thyroid function in depressed patients. *Biol. Psychiat.*, **22**:1033–5.

Joffe, R.T. and Singer, W., 1990. A comparison of triiodothyronine and thyroxine in the potentiation of tricyclic antidepressants. *Psychiat. Res.*, **32**(3):241–51.

Joffe, R.T. and Sokolov, S., 1994. The thyroid and electroconvulsive treatment. *Psychopharmacol. Bull.*, **30**:485–7.

Joffe, R.T., Gold, P.W., Uhde, T.W. and Post, R.M., 1984. The effects of carbamazepine on the thyrotropin response to thyrotropin-releasing hormone. *Psychiat. Res.*, **12**:161–6.

Joffe, R.T., Kutcher, S.P. and MacDonald, C., 1988. Thyroid function and bipolar affective disorder. *Psychiat. Res.*, **25**:117–21.

Joffe, R.T., Levitt, A.J., Bagby, R.M., MacDonald, C. and Singer, W., 1993. Predictors of response to lithium and triiodothyronine augmentation of antidepressants in tricyclic non-responders. *Br. J. Psychiat.*, **163**:574–8.

Kalmijn, S., Launer, L.J., Stolk, R.P., de Jong, F.H., Pols, H.A., Hofman, A., Breteler, M.M. and Lamberts, S.W., 1998. A prospective study on cortisol, dehydroepiandrosterone sulfate, and cognitive function in the elderly. *J. Clin. Endocrinol. Metab.*, **83**:3487–92.

Kamlana, S.H. and Holms, L., 1986. Paranoid reaction and underlying thyrotoxicosis. *Br. J. Psychiat.*, **149**:376–7.

Kasper, S., Vieira, A., Schmidt, R. and Richter, P., 1990. Multiple hormones responses to stimulation with dl-fenfluramine in patients with major depression before and after antidepressive treatment. *Pharmacopsychiat.*, **23**:76–84.

Kastin, A.J., Ehrensing, R.H., Schalch, D.S. and Anderson, M.S., 1972. Improvement in mental depression with decreased thyrotropin response after administration of thyrotropin releasing hormone. *Lancet*, **2**:740–2.

Kavoussi, R.J., Hauger, R.L. and Coccaro, E.F., 1999. Prolactin response to d-fenfluramine in major depression before and after treatment with serotonin reuptake inhibitors. *Biol. Psychiat.*, **45**:295–9.

Keating, F.S., Manassiev, N. and Stevenson, J.C., 1999. Maximising the use of HRT: focus on hysterectomised women. *Curr. Med. Res. Opin.*, **15**(4):290–7.

Kiely, W.F., Adrian, A.D., Lee, J.H. and Nicoloff, J.T., 1976. Therapeutic failure of oral thyrotropin-releasing hormone in depression. *Psychosom. Med.*, **38**:233–41.

Kimonides, V.G., Spillantini, M.G., Sofroniew, M.V., Fawcett, J.W. and Herbert, J., 1999. Dehydroepiandrosterone antagonizes the neurotoxic effects of corticosterone and translocation of stress-activated protein kinase 3 in hippocampal primary cultures. *Neuroscience*, **89**:429–36.

Kirkegaard, C. and Faber, J., 1981. Altered serum levels of thyroxine, triiodothyronines and diiodothyronines in endogenous depression. *Acta Endocrinol.*, **96**:199–207.

Kirkegaard, C. and Faber, J., 1998. The role of thyroid hormones in depression. *Eur. J. Endocrinol.*, **138**:1–9.

Kirschbaum, C. and Hellhammer, D.H., 1994. Salivary cortisol in psychoneuroendocrine research: recent developments and applications. *Psychoneuroendocrinology*, **19**:313–33.

Kirschbaum, C., Wust, S. and Hellhammer, D., 1992. Consistent sex differences in cortisol responses to psychological stress. *Psychosomat. Med.*, **54**(6):648–57.

Kirschbaum, C., Kudielka, B.M., Gaab, J., Schommer, N.C. and Hellhammer, D.H., 1999. Impact of gender, menstrual cycle phase, and oral contraceptives on the activity of the hypothalamus–pituitary–adrenal axis. *Psychosomat. Med.*, **61**(2):154–62.

Kling, M.A., Roy, A., Doran, A.R., Calabrese, J.R., Rubinow, D.R., Whitfield, H.J., Jr, May, C., Post, R.M., Chrousos, G.P. and Gold, P.W., 1991. Cerebrospinal fluid immunoreactive corticotropin-releasing hormone and adrenocorticotropin secretion in Cushing's disease and major depression: potential clinical implications. *J. Clin. Endocrinol. Metab.*, **72**:260–71.

Krieg, J.-C., Lauer, C.J., Schreiber, W., Modell, S. and Holsboer, F., 2001. Neuroendocrine, polysomnographic and psychometric observations in healthy subjects at high familial risk for affective disorders: the current state of the 'Munich Vulnerability Study'. *J. Affect. Disord.*, **62**:33–7.

Labbate, L.A., Fava, M., Oleshansky, M., Zoltec, J., Littman, A. and Harig, P., 1995. Physical fitness and perceived stress: relationships with coronary artery disease risk factors. *Psychosomatics*, **36**:555–60.

Lam, R.W., Berkowitz, A.L., Berga, S.L., Clark, C.M., Kripke, D.F. and Gillin, J.C., 1990. Melatonin suppression in bipolar and unipolar mood disorders. *Psychiat. Res.*, **33**:129–34.

Larkin, J.G., Macphee, G.J., Beastall, G.H. and Brodie, M.J., 1989. Thyroid hormone concentrations in epileptic patients. *Eur. J. Clin. Pharmacol.*, **36**:213–16.

Larsen, P. and Ingbar, S.H., 1992. The thyroid gland. In: Wilson, J.D. and Foster, D.W. (eds), *Williams' Textbook of Endocrinology*, pp. 357–413. W.B. Saunders, Philadelphia, PA.

LeBlanc, E.S., Janowsky, J., Chan, B.K.S. and Nelson, H.D., 2001. Hormone replacement therapy and cognition: systemic review and meta-analysis. *JAMA*, **285**:1489–99.

Lee, S., Chow, C.C., Wing, Y.K., Shek, A.C.C., Mak, T.W.L., Ahuja, A., Lee, D.T.S. and Leung, T.Y.S., 2000. Thyroid function and psychiatric morbidity in patients with manic disorder receiving lithium therapy. *J. Clin. Psychopharmacol.*, **20**:204–9.

Legrain, S., Berr, C., Frenoy, N., Gourlet, V., Debuire, B. and Baulieu, E.E., 1995. Dehydroepiandrosterone sulfate in a long-term care aged population. *Gerontology*, **41**:343–51.

Leibow, D., 1983. L-thyroxine for rapid-cycling bipolar illness [letter]. *Am. J. Psychiat.*, **140**(9):1255.

Leigh, H. and Kramer, S.I., 1984. The psychiatric manifestations of endocrine disease. *Adv. Intern. Med.*, **29**:413–45.

Lewy, A.J., Wehr, T.A., Goodwin, F.K., Newsome, D.A. and Markey, S.P., 1980. Light suppresses melatonin secretion in humans. *Science*, **210**:1267–9.

Liberzon, I., Abelson, J.L., Flagel, S.B., Raz, J. and Young, E.A., 1999. Neuroendocrine and psychophysiologic responses in PTSD: a symptom provocation study. *Neuropsychopharmacology*, **21**(1):40–50.

Limouzin-Lamothe, M., Mairon, N., LeGal, J. and LeGal, M., 1994. Quality of life after the menopause: influence of hormonal replacement therapy. *Am. J. Obstet. Gynecol.*, **170**:618–24.

Lindheim, S.R., Legro, R.S., Bernstein, L., Stanczyk, F.Z., Vijod, M.A., Presser, S.C. and Lobo, R.A., 1992. Behavioral stress responses in premenopausal and postmenopausal women and the effects of estrogen. *Am. J. Obstet. Gynecol*, **167**(6):1831–6.

Lindheim, S.R., Legro, R.S., Morris, R.S., Wong, I.L., Tran, D.Q., Vijod, M.A., Stanczyk, F.Z. and Lobo, R.A., 1994. The effect of progestins on behavioral stress responses in postmenopausal women. *J. Soc. Gynecol. Invest.*, **1**(1):79–83.

Linnoila, M., Lamberg, B.A., Rosberg, G., Karonen, S.L. and Welin, M.G., 1979. Thyroid hormones and TSH, prolactin, and LH responses to repeated TRH and LRH injections in depressed patients. *Acta Psychiat. Scand.*, **59**:536–44.

Lishman, W.A., 1998. Endocrine diseases and metabolic disorders. In: *Organic Psychiat.: The Psychological Consequences of Cerebral Disorder*. Blackwell Science, Oxford.

Littman, A.B., Fava, M., Halpern, P., Lamon-Fava, S., Drews, F.R., Oleshansky, M.A., Bielenda, C.C. and MacLaughlin, R.A., 1993. Physiologic benefits of a stress reduction program for healthy middle-aged army officers. *J. Psychosom. Res.*, **37**:345–54.

Liu, D., Diorio, J., Tannenbaum, B., Caldji, C., Francis, D., Freedman, A., Sharma, S., Pearson, D., Plotsky, P.M. and Meaney, M.J., 1997. Maternal care, hippocampal glucocorticoid receptors, and hypothalamic–pituitary–adrenal responses to stress. *Science*, **277**:1659–62.

Loosen, P.T., 1988. Thyroid function in affective disorders and alcoholism [review]. In: Brown, W.A. (ed.), *Endocrinology of Neuropsychiatric Disorders*, pp. 55–82. W. B. Saunders, Philadelphia, PA.

Loosen, P.T. and Prange, A.J., 1982. The serum thyrotropin (TSH) response to thyrotropin-releasing hormone (TRH) in psychiatric patients: a review. *Am. J. Psychiat.*, **139**:405–16.

Loosen, P.T., Sells, S., Geracioti, T.D. *et al.*, 1992. Thyroid hormones and alcoholism. In: Watson, R.R. (ed.), *Drug and Alcohol Abuse Review,* Vol. 3: *Alcohol Abuse Treatment*, pp. 283–306. Human Press, Totowa, NJ.

Lopez, J.F., Chalmers, D.T., Little, K.Y. and Watson, S.J., 1998. Regulation of serotonin-1A, glucocorticoid and mineralocorticoid receptor in rat and human hippocampus: implications for the neurobiology of depression. *Biol. Psychiat.*, **43**:547–73.

Lowther, S., De Paermentier, F., Cheetham, S.C., Crompton, M.R., Katona, C.L. and Horton, R.W., 1997. 5-HT1A receptor binding sites in post-mortem brain samples from depressed suicides and controls. *J. Affect. Disord.*, **42**:199–207.

MacCrimmon, D.J., Wallace, J.E., Goldberg, W.M. and Streiner, D.L., 1979. Emotional disturbance in cognitive deficits in hyperthyroidism. *Psychosom. Med.*, **41**:31–40.

Maes, M., D'Hondt, P., Suy, E., Minner, B., Vandervorst, C. and Raus, J., 1991. HPA axis hormones and prolactin responses to dextro-fenfluramine in depressed patients and healthy controls. *Prog. Neuropsychopharmacol. Biol. Psychiat.*, **15**:781–90.

Magos, A.L., Brincat, M. and Studd, J.W.W., 1986. Treatment of the premenstrual syndrome by subcutaneous oestradiol implants and cyclical oral norethisterone: placebo controlled study. *Br. Med. J.*, **292**:1629–33.

Majewska, M.D., 1992. Neurosteroid: endogenous bimodal modulators of the GABA-A receptor. Mechanism of action and physiological significance. *Prog. Neurobiol.*, **38**:379–95.

Majewska, M.D., 1995. Neuronal actions of dehydroepiandrosterone: possible roles in brain development, aging, memory, and affect. *Ann. N. Y. Acad. Sci.*, **7774**:111–20.

Majewska, M.D., Harrison, N.L., Schwartz, R.D., Barker, J.L. and Paul, S.M., 1986. Metabolites of steroid hormones are barbiturate-like modulators of the aminobutyric acid receptors. *Science*, **232**:1004–7.

Mannel, M., Muller-Oerlinghausen, B., Czernik, A. and Sauer, H., 1997. 5-HT brain function in affective disorder: d,l-fenfluramine-induced hormone release and clinical outcome in long-term lithium/carbamazepine prophylaxis. *J. Affect. Disord.*, **46**:101–13.

Manson, J.E. and Martin, K.A., 2001. Postmenopausal hormone-replacement therapy. *N. Engl J. Med.*, **345**:34–40.

Marinari, K.T., Leshner, A.I. and Doyle, M.P., 1976. Menstrual cycle status and adrenocortical reactivity to psychological stress. *Psychoneuroendocrinology*, **1**(3):213–18.

Mason, G.A., Walker, C.H., Prange, A.J.J. and Bondy, S.C., 1987. GABA uptake is inhibited by thyroid hormones: implications for depression. *Psychoneuroendocrinology*, **12**:53–9.

Mason, J.W., Giller, E.L., Kosten, T.R., Ostroff, R. and Podd, L., 1986. Urinary-free cortisol in post-traumatic stress disorder. *J. Nerv. Ment. Dis.*, **174**:145–9.

McCowen, K.C., Garber, J.R. and Spark, R., 1997. Elevated serum thyrotropin in thyroxine-treated patients with hypothyroidism given sertraline [Letter]. *N. Engl J. Med.*, **337**(14):1010–1.

McEwen, B.S., 2000. Effects of adverse experiences for brain structure and function. *Biol. Psychiat.*, **48**:721–31.

McEwen, B.S. and Stellar, E., 1993. Stress and the individual: mechanisms leading to disease. *Arch. Intern. Med.*, **153**:2093–101.

McEwen, B.S., Davis, P.G., Parsons, B. and Pfaff, W.G., 1979. The brain as a target a for steroid hormone action. *A. Rev. Neurosci.*, **2**:65–112.

McEwen, B.S., Coirini, H., Danielsson, A., Frankfurt, M., Gould, E., Mendelson, S., Schumacher, M., Segarra, A. and Woolley, C., 1991. Steroid and thyroid hormones modulate a changing brain. *J. Steroid Biochem. Molec. Biol.*, **40**(1–3):1–14.

McEwen, B.S., Angulo, J., Cameron, H., Chao, H., Daniels, D., Gannon, M., Gould, E., Mendelson, S., Sakai, R., Spencer, R. and Woolley, C., 1992. Paradoxical effects of adrenal steroids on the brain: protection versus degeneration. *Biol. Psychiat.*, **31**:177–99.

McEwen, B.S., Cameron, H., Chao, H.M., Gould, E., Luine, V., Magarinos, A.M., Pavlides, C., Spencer, R.L., Watanabe, Y. and Woolley, C., 1994. Resolving a mystery: progress in understanding the function of adrenal steroid receptors in hippocampus. *Prog. Brain Res.*, **100**:149–55.

McKenna, T.J., Fearon, U., Clarke, D. and Cunningham, S.K., 1997. A critical review of the origin and control of adrenal androgens. *Baillieres Clin. Obstet. Gynaecol.*, **11**:229–48.

Meijer, O.C., Van Oosten, R.V. and DeKloet, E.R., 1997. Elevated basal trough levels of corticosterone suppress hippocampal 5-hydroxytryptamine(1A) receptor expression in adrenally intact rats: implication for the pathogenesis of depression. *Neuroscience*, **80**:419–26.

Meijer, O.C., de Lange, E.C., Breimer, D.D., de Boer, A.G., Workel, J.O. and de Kloet, E.R., 1998. Penetration of dexamethasone into brain glucocorticoid targets is enhanced in mdr1 A P-glycoprotein knockout mice. *Endocrinology*, **139**:1789–93.

Meller, W.H., Grambsch, P.L., Bingham, C. and Tagatz, G.E., 2001. Hypothalamic pituitary gonadal axis dysregulation in depressed women. *Psychoneuroendocrinology*, **26**:253–9.

Meyer, J.H. and Gruol, D.L., 1994. Dehydroepiandrosterone sulfate alters synaptic potentials in area CA1 of the hippocampal slice. *Brain Res.*, **633**, 253–61.

Michael, A., Jenaway, A., Paykel, E.S. and Herbert, J., 2000. Altered salivary dehydroepiandrosterone levels in major depression in adults. *Biol. Psychiat.*, **48**:989–95.

Miller, T.P., Taylor, J., Rogerson, S., Mauricio, M., Kennedy, Q., Schatzberg, A., Tinklenberg, J. and Yesavage, J., 1998. Cognitive and noncognitive symptoms in dementia patients: relationship to cortisol and dehydroepiandrosterone. *Int. Psychogeriat.*, **10**:85–96.

Minami, T., Oomura, Y., Nabekura, J. and Fukuda, A., 1990. 17 beta-estradiol depolarization of hypothalamic neurons is mediated by cyclic AMP. *Brain Res.*, **519**(1–2):301–7.

Monnet, F.P., Mahe, V., Robel, P. and Baulieu, E.E., 1995. Neurosteroids, via sigma receptors, modulate the [3H]norepinephrine release evoked by *N*-methyl-d-aspartate in the rat hippocampus. *Proc. Natl Acad. Sci. USA*, **92**:3774–8.

Morales, A.J., Nolan, J.J., Nelson, J.C. and Yen, S.S.C., 1994. Effects of replacement dose dehydroepiandrosterone in men and women of advancing age. *J. Clin. Endocrinol. Metab.*, **78**:1360–7.

Morrison, M.F., 1997. Androgens in the elderly: will androgen replacement therapy improve mood, cognition, and quality of life in aging men and women? *Psychopharmacol. Bull.*, **33**:293–6.

Morrison, M.F., Katz, I.R., Parmelee, P., Boyce, A.A. and TenHave, T., 1998. Dehydroepiandrosterone sulfate (DHEAS) and psychiatric and laboratory measures of frailty in a residential care population. *Am. J. Geriat. Psychiat.*, **6**:277–84.

Morrison, M.F., Redei, E., TenHave, T., Parmelee, P., Boyce, A.A., Sinha, P.S. and Katz, I.R., 2000. Dehydroepiandrosterone sulfate and psychiatric measures in a frail, elderly residential care population. *Biol. Psychiat.*, **47**:144–50.

Mountjoy, C.Q., Price, J.S. and Weller, M., 1974. A double-blind crossover sequential trial of oral thyrotropin-releasing hormone in depression. *Lancet*, **2**:958–60.

Mulnard, R.A., Cotman, C.W., Kawas, C., van Dyck, C.H., Sano, M., Doody, R., Koss, E., Pfeiffer, E., Jin, S., Gamst, A., Grundman, M., Thomas, R. and Thal, L.J., 2000. Estrogen replacement therapy for treatment of mild to moderate Alzheimer disease: a randomized controlled trial. Alzheimer's Disease Cooperative Study [Erratum appears in *JAMA*, 2000, **284**(20):2597]. *JAMA*, **283**(8):1007–15.

Murphy, B.E.P., 1968. Clinical evaluation of urinary cortisol determination by competitive protein-binding radioassay. *J. Clin. Endocrinol. Metab.*, **28**:343–8.

Murphy, B.E.P., 1991. Steroids and depression. *J. Steroid Biochem. Molec. Biol.*, **38**(5):537–59.

Murray, H.E. and Gillies, G.E., 1997. Differential effects of neuroactive steroids on somatostatin and dopamine secretion from primary hypothalamic cell cultures. *J. Neuroendocrinol.*, **9**(4):287–95.

Nelson, J.C. and Davis, J.M., 1997. Dexamethasone suppression test studies in psychotic depression: a meta-analysis. *Am. J. Psychiat.*, **154**:1497–1503.

Nemeroff, C.B., Widerlov, E., Bissette, G., Wallevs, H., Karlsson, I., EKlund, K., Kilts, C.D., Loosen, P.T. and Vale, W., 1984. Elevated concentrations of CSF corticotropin releasing factor-like immunoreactivity in depressed patients. *Science*, **227**:1342–4.

Nemeroff, C.B., Simon, J.S., Haggerty, J.J. and Evans, D.L., 1985. Antithyroid antibodies in depressed patients. *Am. J. Psychiat.*, **142**:840–3.

Nemeroff, C.B., Owens, M.J., Bissette, G., Andorn, A.C. and Stanley, M., 1988. Reduced corticotropin releasing factor binding sites in the frontal cortex of suicide victims. *Arch. Gen. Psychiat.*, **45**(6):577–9.

Newport, D.J. and Nemeroff, C.B., 2000. Neurobiology of posttraumatic stress disorder. *Curr. Opin. Neurobiol.*, **10**:211–18.

Nieman, L.K., Chrousos, G.P., Kellner, C., Spitz, I.M., Nisula, B.C., Cutler, G.B., Merriam, G.R., Bardin, C.W. and Loriaux, D.L., 1985. Successful treatment of Cushing's syndrome with the glucocorticoid antagonist RU 486. *J. Clin. Endocrinol. Metab.*, **61**:536–40.

Nurnberger, J.I., Jr, Berrettini, W., Tamarkin, L., Hamovit, J., Norton, J. and Gershon, E., 1988. Supersensitivity to melatonin suppression by light in young people at high risk for affective disorder: a preliminary report. *Neuropsychopharmacology*, **1**:217–23.

Nurnberger, J.I., Jr, Adkins, S., Lahiri, D.K., Mayeda, A., Hu, K., Lewy, A., Miller, A., Bowman, E.S., Miller, M.J., Rau, N.L., Smiley, C. and Davis-Singh, D., 2000. Melatonin suppression by light in euthymic bipolar and unipolar patients. *Arch. Gen. Psychiat.*, **57**:572–9.

O'Keane, V., McLoughlin, D. and Dinan, T.G., 1992. D-fenfluramine induced prolactin and cortisol release in major depression: response to treatment. *J. Affect. Disord.*, **26**:143–50.

O'Meara, E.S., Rossing, M.A., Daling, J.R., Elmore, J.G., Barlow, W.E. and Weiss, N.S., 2001. Hormone replacement therapy after a diagnosis of breast cancer in relation to recurrence and mortality. *J. Natl Cancer Ins.*, **93**(10):754–62.

Oppenheim, G., 1983. Estrogen in the treatment of depression: neuropharmacological mechanisms. *Biol. Psychiat.*, **18**(6):721–5.

Osran, H., Reist, C., Chen, C.C., Lifrak, E.T., Chicz-DeMet, A. and Parker, L.N., 1993. Adrenal androgens and cortisol in major depression. *Am. J. Psychiat.*, **150**:806–9.

Overall, J. and Gorham, D., 1962. The brief psychiatric rating scale. *Psychol. Rep.*, **10**:799–812.

Papakostas, Y., Markianos, M., Papadimitriou, G., Lykouras̆, L. and Stefanis, C., 1991. Thyrotropin and prolactin responses to ECT in schizophrenia and depression. *Psychiat. Res.*, **37**:5–10.

Parry, C.H., 1825. *Collections from the Unpublished Writings of the Late C.H. Parry*, Vol. II. Underwoods, London.

Peake, R.L., 1981. Recurrent apathetic hyperthyroidism. *Arch. Intern. Med.*, **141**:258–62.

Petersen, P., 1968. Psychiatric disorders in primary hyperparathyroidism. *J. Clin. Endocrinol. Metab.*, **28**(10):1491–5.

Piazza, P.V., Rouge-Pont, F., Deroche, V., Maccari, S., Simon, H. and Le Moal, M., 1996. Glucocorticoids have state-dependent stimulant effects on the mesencephalic dopaminergic transmission. *Proc. Natl Acad. Sci. USA*, **93**:8716–20.

Pitchot, W., Hansenne, M., Gonzales Moreno, A. and Ansseau, M., 1992. Suicidal behavior and growth hormone response to apomorphine test. *Biol. Psychiat.*, **31**:1213–19.

Pitchot, W., Reggers, J., Pinto, E., Hansenne, M., Fuchs, S., Pirard, S. and Ansseau, M., 2001. Reduced dopaminergic activity in depressed suicides. *Psychoneuroendocrinology*, **26**:331–5.

Plihal, W., Krug, R., Pietrowsky, R., Fehm, H.L. and Born, J., 1996. Corticosteroid receptor mediated effects on mood in humans. *Psychoneuroendocrinology*, **21**:515–23.

Plotsky, P.M., Thrivikraman, K.V. and Meaney, M.J., 1993. Central and feedback regulation of hypothalamic corticotropin-releasing factor secretion. *Ciba Found. Symp.*, **172**:59–75.

Pope, H.G., Kouri, E.M. and Hudson, J.I., 2000. Effects of testosterone on mood and aggression in men. *Arch. Gen. Psychiat.*, **57**:133–40.

Porter, J.R. and Svec, F., 1995. DHEA diminishes fat food intake in lean and obese Zucker rats. *Ann. N. Y. Acad. Sci.*, **774**:329–31.

Porter, R., McAllister-Williams, R., Lunn, B. and Young, A., 1998. 5-Hydroxytryptamine receptor function in man is reduced by acute administration of hydrocortisone. *Psychopharmacology*, **139**:243–50.

Prange, A.J. and Loosen, P.T., 1984. Aspects of thyroid axis function in depression. In: Shah, V.S. and Donald, A.G. (eds), *Psychoneuroendocrine Dysfunction*, p. 41. Plenum Press, New York.

Prange, A.J., Jr, Wilson, I.C., Raybon, S.M. and Lipton, M.A., 1969. Enhancement of the imipramine antidepressant activity by thyroid hormone. *Am. J. Psychiat.*, **126**(4):457–69.

Prange, A.J., Lara, P.P. Wilson, I.C., Alltop, L.B. and Breese, G.R., 1972. Effects of thyrotropin-releasing hormone in the treatment of depression. *Lancet*, **2**:999–1001.

Price, L.H., Charney, D.S., Delgado, P.L., Anderson, G.M. and Heninger, G.R., 1989. Effects of desipramine and fluvoxamine treatment on the prolactin response to tryptophan. Serotonergic function and the mechanism of antidepressant action. *Arch. Gen. Psychiat.*, **46**:625–31.

Price, L.H., Charney, D.S., Delgado, P.L. and Heninger, G.R., 1991. Serotonin function and depression: neuroendocrine and mood responses to intravenous l-tryptophan in depressed patients and healthy comparison subjects. *Am. J. Psychiat.*, **148**:1518–25.

Price, L.H., Malison, R.T., McDougle, C.J., Pelton, G.H. and Heninger, G.R., 1998. The neurobiology of tryptophan depletion in depression: effects of intravenous tryptophan infusion. *Biol. Psychiat.*, **43**(5):339–47.

Rafuls, W.A., Extein, I., Gold, M.S. *et al.*, 1987. Neuropsychiatric aspects of endocrine disorders. In: Hales, R.E. and Yudofsky, S.C. (eds), *The American Psychiatric Press Textbook of Neuropsychiat*, pp. 307–25. American Psychiatric Press, Washington, DC.

Ravaglia, G., Forti, P., Maioli, F., Boschi, F., Bernardi, M., Pratelli, L., Pizzoferrato, A. and Gasbarrini, G., 1996. The relationship of dehydroepiandrosterone sulfate (DHEAS) to endocrine-metabolic parameters and functional status in the oldest-old. Results from an Italian study on healthy free-living over ninety-year-olds. *J. Clin. Endocrin. Metabol.*, **81**:1173–8.

Ravaglia, G., Forti, P., Maioli, F., Boschi, F., Cicognani, A., Bernardi, M., Pratelli, L., Pizzoferrato, A., Porcu, S. and Gasbarrini, G., 1997. Determinants of functional status in healthy Italian nonagenarians and centenarians: a comprehensive functional assessment by the instruments of geriatric practice. *J. Am. Geriat. Soc.*, **45**:1196–1202.

Ravindran, A.V., Bialik, R.J. and Lapierre, Y.D., 1994. Primary early onset dysthymia, biochemical correlates of the therapeutic response to fluoxetine: I. Platelet monoamine oxidase and the dexamethasone suppression test. *J. Affect. Dis.*, **31**:111–17.

Re, R.N., Kourides, I.A., Ridgway, E.D., Weintraub, B.D. and Maloff, F., 1976. The effect of glucocorticoid administration on human pituitary secretion of thyrotropin and prolactin. *J. Clin. Endocrinol. Metab.*, **43**:338–46.

Reus, V.I., Wolkowitz, O.M., Roberts, E., Chan, T., Turetsky, N., Manfredi, F. and Weingartner, H., 1993. Dehydroepiandrosterone (DHEA) and memory in depressed patients. *Neuropsychopharmacology*, **9**:66S.

Rhodes, M.E., Li, P.K., Flood, J.F. and Johnson, D.A., 1996. Enhancement of hippocampal acetylcholine release by the neurosteroid dehydroepiandrosterone sulfate: an *in vivo* microdialysis study. *Brain Res.*, **733**:284–6.

Rhodes, M.E., Li, P.K., Burke, A.M. and Johnson, D.A., 1997. Enhanced plasma DHEAS, brain acetylcholine and memory mediated by steroid sulfatase inhibition. *Brain Res.*, **733**:28–32.

Ribeiro, S.C.M., Tandon, R., Grunhaus, L. and Greden, J.F., 1993. The dexamethasone suppression test as a predictor of outcome in depression: a meta-analysis. *Am. J. Psychiat.*, **150**:1618–29.

Rodriguez, C., Patel, A.V., Calle, E.E., Jacob, E.J. and Thun, M.J., 2001. Estrogen replacement therapy and ovarian cancer mortality in a large prospective study of US women. *JAMA*, **285**:1460–5.

Rothschild, A.J., Schatzberg, A.F., Rosenbaum, A.H., Stahl, J.B. and Cole, J.O., 1982. The dexamethasone suppression test as a discriminator among sub-types of psychotic patients. *Br. J. Psychiat.*, **141**:471–4.

Rothschild, A.J., Samson, J.A., Bond, T.C., Luciana, M.M., Schildkraut, J.J. and Schatzberg, A.F., 1993. Hypothalamic–pituitary–adrenal axis activity and one-year outcome in depression. *Biol. Psychiat.*, **34**:392–400.

Roy-Byrne, P.P., Joffe, R.T., Uhde, T.W. and Post, R.M., 1984. Carbamazepine and thyroid function in affectively ill patients. Clinical and theoretical implications. *Arch. Gen. Psychiat.*, **41**:1150–3.

Rubin, R.T., Poland, R.E., Lesser, I.M., Winston, R.A. and Blodgett, A.N.A., 1987. Neuroendocrine aspects of primary endogenous depression. I: Cortisol secretory dynamics in patients and matched controls. *Arch. Gen. Psychiat.*, **44**:328–36.

Rush, A.J., Giles, D.E., Schlesser, M.A., Orsulak, P.J., Parker, C.R., Jr, Weissenburger, J.E., Crowley, G.T., Khatami, M. and Vasavada, N., 1996. The dexamethasone suppression test in patients with mood disorders. *J. Clin. Psychiat.*, **57**:470–84.

Rybakowski, J.K. and Twardowska, K., 1999. The dexamethasone/CRH test in depression in bipolar and unipolar affective illness. *J. Psychiat. Res.*, **33**:363–70.

Sachar, E.J., Hellman, L., Fukuskima, D.K. and Gallagher, T.F., 1970. Cortisol production in depressive illness. *Arch. Gen. Psychiat.*, **23**:289–98.

Sackeim, H.A., 1994. Central issues regarding the mechanism of action of electroconvulsive therapy: directions for future research. *Psychopharmacol. Bull.*, **30**:281–303.

Sandrini, M., Marrama, D., Vergoni, A. and Bertolini, A., 1991. Effects of thyroid status on the characteristics of alpha1, alpha2, beta, imipramine, and GABA receptors in the rat brain. *Life Sci.*, **48**:659–66.

Sapolsky, R.M., 2000. The possibility of neurotoxicity in the hippocampus in major depression: a primer on neuron death. *Biol. Psychiat.*, **48**:755–65.

Sapolsky, R.M., Krey, L.C. and McEwen, B.S., 1984. Glucocorticoid-sensitive hippocampal neurons are involved in terminating the adrenocortical stress response. *Proc. Natl Acad. Sci.*, **81**:6174–7.

Sapolsky, R.M., Uno, H., Rebert, C.S. and Finch, C.E., 1990. Hippocampal damage associated with prolonged glucocorticoid exposure in primates. *J. Neurosci.*, **10**(9):2897–902.

Scanlon, M.F., Issa, B.G. and Dieguez, C., 1996. Regulation of growth hormone secretion. *Horm. Res.*, **46**:149–54.

Schatzberg, A.F. and Rothschild, A.J., 1988. The roles of glucocorticoid and dopaminergic systems in delusional (psychotic) depression. *Ann. N. Y. Acad. Sci.*, **537**:462–71.

Schatzberg, A.F., Rothschild, A.J., Stahl, J.B., Bond, T.C., Rosenbaum, A.H., Lofgren, S.B., MacLaughlin, R.A., Sullivan, M.A. and Cole, J.O., 1983. The dexamethasone suppression test: identification of sub-types of depression. *Am. J. Psychiat.*, **140**:88–91.

Schatzberg, A.F., Rothschild, A.J., Langlais, P.J., Bird, E.D. and Cole, J.O., 1985. A corticosteroid/dopamine hypothesis for psychotic depression and related states. *J. Psychiat. Res.*, **19**:57–64.

Schneider, M.A., Brotherton, P.L. and Hailes, J., 1977. The effects of exogenous oestrogens on depression in menopausal women. *Med. J. Aus.*, **2**:162–3.

Schulkin, J., Gold, P.W. and McEwen, B.S., 1998. Induction of corticotropin-releasing hormone gene expression by glucocorticoids: implication for understanding the states of fear and anxiety and allostatic load. *Psychoneuroendocrinology*, **23**:219–43.

Schweitzer, I., Tucknell, V.M., Maguire, K.P., Tiller, J.W., Harrison, L.C. and Davies, B.M., 1991. Plasma cortisol and 11-deoxycortisol activity in depressed patients and normal volunteers. *Psychoneuroendocrinology*, **16**:375–82.

Seeman, T.E., McEwen, B.S., Singer, B.H., Albert, M.S. and Rowe, J.W., 1997. Increase in urinary cortisol excretion and memory declines: MacArthur studies of successful aging. *J. Clin. Endocrinol. Metab.*, **82**:2458–65.

Seeman, T.E., McEwen, B.S., Rowe, J.W. and Singer, B.H., 2001. Allostatic load as a marker of cumulative biological risk: MacArthur studies of successful aging. *Proc. Natl Acad. Sci. USA*, 4770–5.

Shafii, M. and Shafii, S.L. (eds), 1990. *Biological Rhythms, Mood Disorder, Light Therapy and the Pineal Gland*. American Psychiatric Press, Washington, DC.

Shah, P.J., O'Carroll, R.E., Rogers, A., Moffoot, A.P. and Ebmeier, K.P., 1999. Abnormal response to negative feedback in depression. *Psychol. Med.*, **29**(1):63–72.

Shapira, B., Cohen, J., Newman, M.E. and Lerer, B., 1993. Prolactin response in fenfluramine and placebo challenge following maintenance pharmacotherapy withdrawal in remitted depressed patients. *Biol. Psychiat.*, **33**:531–5.

Sheline, Y.I., Gado, M.H. and Price, J.L., 1998. Amygdala core nuclei volumes are decreased in recurrent major depression. *Neuro-Report*, **9**:2023–8.

Sheline, Y.I., Sanghavi, M., Mintun, M.A. and Gado, M.H., 1999. Depression duration but not age predicts hippocampal volume loss in medically healthy women with recurrent major depression. *J. Neurosci.*, **19**:5034–3.

Shelton, R.C., Winn, S., Ekhatore, N. and Loosen, P.T., 1993. The effects of antidepressants on the thyroid axis in depression. *Biol. Psychiat.*, **33**:120–6.

Shulman, L.H., DeRogatis, L., Spielvogel, R., Miller, J.L. and Rose, L.I., 1992. Serum androgens and depression in women with facial hirsutism. *J. Am. Acad. Dermatol.*, **27**:178–81.

Sichel, D.A., Cohen, L.S., Robertson, L.M., Ruttenberg, A. and Rosenbaum, J.F., 1995. Prophylactic estrogen in recurrent postpartum affective disorder. *Biol. Psychiat.*, **38**(12):814–8.

Sirinathsinghji, D.J.S., Rees, L.H., Rivier, J. and Vale, W., 1983. Corticotropin-releasing factor is a potent inhibitor of sexual receptivity in the female rat. *Nature*, **305**:232–5.

Smith, R.N., Studd, J.W., Zamblera, D. and Holland, E.F., 1995. A randomised comparison over 8 months of 100 micrograms and 200 micrograms twice weekly doses of transdermal oestradiol in the treatment of severe premenstrual syndrome. *Br. J. Obstet. Gynaecol.*, **102**:475–84.

Soares, C.D.N., Almeida, O.P., Joffe, H. and Coehn, L.S., 2001. Efficacy of estradiol for the treatment of depressive disorders in perimenopausal women. *Arch. Gen. Psychiat.*, **58**:529–34.

Sonino, N., Fava, G.A., Belluardo, P., Girelli, M.E. and Boscaro, M., 1993. Course of depression in Cushing's syndrome: response to treatment and comparison with Grave's disease. *Horm. Res.*, **39**:202–6.

Spigset, O. and Mjorndal, T., 1997. Effect of fluvoxamine on platelet 5-HT2A receptors as studied by [3H] lysergic acid diethyl-amide binding in healthy volunteers. *Psychopharmacology (Berl)*, **133**:39–42.

Spivak, C.E., 1994. Desensitization and noncompetitive blockade of GABA-A receptors in ventral midbrain neurons by a neurosteroid dehydroepiandrosterone sulfate. *Synapse*, **16**:113–22.

Spratt, D.I., Longcope, C., Cox, P.M., Bigos, S.T. and Welbur-Welling, C., 1993. Differential changes in serum concentrations of androgens and estrogens (in relation with cortisol) in post-menopausal women with acute illness. *J. Clin. Endocrinol. Metab.*, **76**:1542–7.

Stancer, H.C. and Persad, E., 1982. Treatment of intractable rapid-cycling manic-depressive disorder with levothyroxine. *Arch. Gen. Psychiat.*, **49**:311–12.

Starkman, M.N., Gebarski, S.S., Berent, S. and Schteingart, D., 1992. Hippocampal formation volume, memory dysfunction and cortisol levels in patients with Cushing's syndrome. *Biol. Psychiat.*, **32**:756–65.

Starkman, M.N., Giordani, B., Gebarski, S.S., Berent, S., Schork, M.A. and Schteingart, D.E., 1999. Decrease in cortisol reverses human hippocampal atrophy following treatment of Cushing's disease. *Biol. Psychiat.*, **46**:1595–1602.

Steckler, T. and Holsboer, F., 1999. Corticotropin-releasing hormone receptor subtypes and emotion. *Biol. Psychiat.*, **46**(11):1480–508.

Steffensen, S.C., 1995. Dehydroepiandrosterone sulfate suppresses hippocampal recurrent inhibition and synchronizes neuronal activity to theta rhythm. *Hippocampus*, **5**:320–8.

Stein, M.B. and Uhde, T.W., 1988. Thyroid indices in panic disorder. *Am. J. Psychiat.*, **145**:745–7.

Sterling, P. and Eyer, J., 1988. Allostasis: a new paradigm to explain arousal pathology. In: Fisher, S. and Resaon, J. (eds), *Handbook of Life Stress, Cognition, and Health*, pp. 629–49. John Wiley & Sons, New York.

Stern, R.A., Nevels, C.T., Shelhorse, M.E., Porohaska, N.L., Mason, G.A. and Prange, A.J.J., 1991. Antidepressant and memory effects of combined thyroid hormone treatment in electroconvulsive therapy: preliminary findings. *Biol. Psychiat.*, **30**:623–7.

Stern, R.A., Steketee, M.C., Durr, A.L., Prange, A.J.J. and Golden, R.N., 1993. Combined use of thyroid hormone and ECT. *Convul. Ther.*, **9**:285–92.

Stockmeier, C.A., Dilley, G.E., Shapiro, L.A., Overholser, J.C., Thompson, P.A.A. and Meltzer, H.Y., 1997. Serotonin receptors in suicide victims with major depression. *Neuropsychopharmacology*, **16**:162–73.

Stockmeier, C.A., Shapiro, L.A., Dilley, G.E., Kolli, T.N., Friedman, L. and Rajkowska, G., 1998. Increase in serotonin-1A autoreceptors in the midbrain of suicide victims with major depression — postmortem evidence for decreased serotonin activity. *J. Neurosci.*, **18**:7394–401.

Stoney, C.M., Davis, M.C. and Matthews, K.A., 1987. Sex differences in physiological responses to stress and in coronary heart disease: a causal link? *Psychophysiology*, **24**(2):127–31.

Streeten, D.H., Anderson, G.H. Jr, Dalakos, T.G., Seeley, D., Mallov, J.S., Eusebio, R., Sunderlin, F.S., Badawy, S.Z. and King, R.B., 1984. Normal and abnormal function of the hypothalamic–pituitary–adrenocortical system in man. *Endoc. Rev.*, **5**(3):371–94.

Sullivan, P.F., Wilson, D.A., Mulder, R.T. and Joyce, P.R., 1997. The hypothalamic–pituitary–thyroid axis in major depression. *Acta Psychiat. Scand.*, **95**:370–8.

Suriano, K.A., McHale, M., McLaren, C.E., Li, K.T., Re, A. and DiSaia, P.J., 2001. Estrogen replacement therapy in endometrial cancer patients: a matched control study. *Obstet Gynecol*, **97**:555–560.

Sutton, R.E., Koob, G.F., Lemoal, M., Rivier, J. and Vale, W., 1982. Corticotropin-releasing factor produces behavioral activation in rats. *Nature*, **297**:331–3.

Swanson, L.W. and Simmons, D.M., 1989. Differential steroid hormone and neural influences on peptide mRNA levels in CRH cells of the paraventricular nucleus: a hybridization histochemical study in the rat. *J. Comp. Neurol.*, **285**(4):413–35.

Sweeney, D., Nelson, C., Bowers, M., Mass, J. and Heninger, G., 1978. Delusional versus nondelusional depression: neurochemical differences [letter]. *Lancet*, **2**:100–1.

Tanaka, K., Kodama, S., Yokoyama, S., Komatsu, M., Konishi, H., Momota, K. and Matsuo, T., 1987. Thyroid function in children with long-term anticonvulsant treatment. *Pediat. Neurosci.*, **13**:90–4.

Targum, S.D., Greenberg, R.D., Harmon, R.L., Kessler, K., Salerian, A.J. and Fram, D.H., 1994. Thyroid hormone and the TRH stimulation test in refractory depression. *J. Clin. Psychiat.*, **45**:345–6.

Teyler, T.J. and DiScenna, P., 1986. The hippocampal memory indexing theory. *Behav. Neurosci.*, **100**(2):147–54.

Thase, M.E. and Rush, H.A., 1995. Treatment-resistant depression. In: Bloom, F.E. and Kupfer, D.J. (eds), *Psychopharmacology, the Fourth Generation of Progress*, pp. 1081–98. Raven Press, New York.

Thrivikraman, K.V., Nemeroff, C.B. and Plotsky, P.M., 2000. Sensitivity to glucocorticoid-mediated fast-feedback regulation of the hypothalamic–pituitary–adrenal axis is dependent upon stressor specific neurocircuitry. *Brain Res.*, **870**:87–101.

Tunbridge, W.M.G. and Caldwell, G., 1991. The epidemiology of thyroid diseases. In: Braverman, L.E. and Utiger, R.D. (eds), *The Thyroid Gland*, p. 287. J.B. Lippincott, Philadelphia, PA.

Turnbull, A.V. and Rivier, C.L., 1999. Regulation of the hypothalamic–pituitary–adrenal axis by cytokines: actions and mechanisms of action. *Physiol. Rev.*, **79**(1):1–71.

Turnbull, A.V., Vaughan, J., Rivier, J.E., Vale, W.W. and Rivier, C., 1999. Urocortin is not a significant regulator of intermittent electrofootshock-induced adrenocorticotropin secretion in the intact male rat. *Endocrinology*, **140**(1):71–8.

Utian, W.H., Shoupe, D., Bachmann, G., Pinkerton, J.V. and Pickar, J.H., 2001. Relief of vasomotor symptoms and vaginal atrophy with lower doses of conjugated equine estrogens and medroxyprogesterone acetate. *Fertil. Steril.*, **75**(6):1065–79.

Van Bockstaele, E.J., 1998. Morphological substrates underlying opioid, epinephrine and gamma-aminobutyric acid inhibitory actions in the rat locus coeruleus. *Brain Res. Bull.*, **47**(1):1–15.

Van Cauter, E., Leproult, R. and Kupfer, D.J., 1996. Effects of gender and age on the levels and circadian rhythmicity of plasma cortisol. *J. Clin. Endocrinol. Metab.*, **81**(7):2468–73.

Vanderbroucke, J.P., Rosing, J., Bloemenkamp, K.W.M., Middeldorp, S., Helmerhorst, F.M., Bouma, B.N. and Rosendaal, F.R., 2001. Oral contraceptives and the risk of venous thrombosis. *N. Engl J. Med.*, **344**:1527–33.

Van Der Lely, A.J., Foeken, K., van der Mast, R.C. and Lamberts, S.W., 1991. Rapid reversal of acute psychosis in the Cushing syndrome with the cortisol-receptor antagonist mifepristone (RU 486). *Ann. Intern. Med.*, **114**:143–4.

Vandoolaeghe, E., Maes, M., Vandevyvere, J. and Neels, H., 1997. Hypothalamic–pituitary–thyroid axis function in treatment-resistant depression. *J. Affect. Disord.*, **43**:143–50.

Van Praag, H.M., Korf, J., Lakke, J.P.W.F. and Schut, T., 1975. Dopamine metabolism in depression, psychoses, and Parkinson's disease: the problem of specificity of biological variables in behavior disorders. *Psychol. Med.*, **5**:138–46.

Vieta, E., Martinez-de-Osaba, M.J., Colom, F., Martinez-Aran, A., Benbarre, A. and Gasto, C., 1999. Enhanced corticotropin response to corticotropin-releasing hormone as a predictor of mania in euthymic bipolar patients. *Psychol. Med.*, **29**:971–8.

Vogel, H.P., Benkert, B.F., Illig, R., Muller-Oerlinghausen, B. and Poppenberg, A., 1977. Psychoendocrinological and therapeutic effects of TRH in depression. *Acta Psychiat. Scand.*, **56**:223–32.

von Bardeleben, U., Holsboer, F., Stalla, G.K. and Muller, A.O., 1985. Combined administration of human corticotropin-releasing factor and vasopressin induces cortisol escape from dexamethasone suppression in healthy subjects. *Life Sci.*, **37**:1613–18.

von Eiff, A.W., Plotz, E.J., Beck, K.J. and Czernik, A., 1971. The effect of estrogens and progestins on blood pressure regulation of normotensive women. *Am. J. Obstet. Gynecol.*, **109**(6):887–92.

Wang, M., Seippel, L., Purdy, R. and Backstrom, T., 1996. Relationship between symptom severity and steroid variation in women with premenstrual syndrome: study on serum pregnanolone, pregnanolone sulfate, 5-alpha-pregnane-3,20-dione and 3-alpha-hydroxy-5alpha-pregnan-20-one. *J. Clin. Endocrinol. Metab.*, **81**:1076–82.

Watson, N.R., Studd, J.W.W., Savvas, M., Garnett, T. and Baber, R.J., 1989. Treatment of severe premenstrual syndrome with oestradiol patches and cyclical oral norethisterone. *Lancet*, **2**:730–2.

Watson, S., Porter, R.J. and Young, A.H., 2000. Effect of hydrocortisone on the pituitary response to growth hormone releasing hormone. *Psychopharmacology*, **152**:40–6.

Weber, B., Lewicka, S., Dueschle, M., Colla, M. and Heuser, I., 2000. Testosterone, androstenedione and dihydrotestosterone concentrations are elevated in female patients with major depression. *Psychoneuroendocrinology*, **25**:765–71.

Wehr, T.A., Sack, D.A., Rosenthal, N.E. and Cowdry, R.W., 1988. Rapid-cycling affective disorder: contributing factors and treatment responses in fifteen patients. *Am. J. Psychiat.*, **145**:179–84.

Weissman, M.M., Prusoff, B.A., Thompson, W.D., Harding, P.S. and Myers, J.K., 1978. Social adjustment by self-report in a community sample and in psychiatric outpatients. *J. Nerv. Ment. Dis.*, **166**:317–26.

Wenzel, K.W., Meinhold, H., Raffenberg, M., Adkofer, F. and Schleusener, H., 1974. Classification of hypothyroidism in evaluating patients after radioactive therapy by serum cholesterol, T3 uptake, total T4, FT4-index, total T3, basal TSH, and TRH test. *Eur. J. Clin. Invest.*, **4**:141–8.

Wetterberg, L., Aperia, B., Beck-Friis, J., Kjellman, F., Ljunggren, J.-G., Petterson, U., Sjolin, A., Tham, A. and Unden, F., 1981. Pineal–hypothalamic–pituitary function in patients with depressive illness. In: Fuxe, K., Gustafsson, J.A. and Wetterberg, L. (eds), *Steroid Hormone Regulation of the Brain*, pp. 397–403. Pergamon Press, Oxford.

Wetterbuerg, L., Beck-Friis, J., Aperia, B. and Petterson, U., 1979. Melatonin/cortisol ratio in depression [letter]. *Lancet*, **2**:1361.

Whalley, L.J., Perini, T., Whering, A. and Bennie, J., 1991. Melatonin response to bright light in recovered, drug-free bipolar patients. *Psychiat. Res.*, **38**:13–19.

Wheatley, D., 1972. Potentiation of amitriptyline by thyroid hormone. *Arch. Gen. Psychiat.*, **26**:229–33.

Whybrow, P.C., 1994. The therapeutic use of triiodothyronine and high dose thyroxine in psychiatric disorder (review). *Acta Medica Aust.*, **21**:47–52.

Whybrow, P.C., 1995. Sex differences in thyroid axis function: relevance to affective disorder and its treatment. *Depression*, **3**:33–42.

Whybrow, P.C. and Prange, A.J.J., 1981. A hypothesis of thyroid–catecholamine receptor interaction. *Arch. Gen. Psychiat.*, **38**:106–13.

Wiesbader, H. and Karzrok, R., 1938. Menopause: consideration of symptoms, etiology and treatment by means of estrogens. *Endocrinology*, **23**:32–8.

Wilson, W., Johnson, J. and Smith, R., 1962. Affective changes in thyrotoxicosis and experimental hypermetabolism. *Recent Adv. Biol. Psychiat.*, **4**:234–42.

Wolkowitz, O.M., 1994. Prospective controlled studies of the behavioral and biological effects of exogenous corticosteroids. *Psychoneuroendocrinology*, **19**:233–55.

Wolkowitz, O.M. and Reus, V.I., 1999. Treatment of depression with antiglucorticoid drugs. *Psychosom. Med.*, **61**:698–711.

Wolkowitz, O.M., Doran, A.R., Breier, A., Roy, A., Jimerson, D.C., Sutton, M.E., Golden, R.N., Paul, S.M. and Pickar, D., 1987. The effects of dexamethasone on plasma homovanillic acid and 3-methoxy-4-hydroxyphenylglycol: evidence for abnormal corticosteroid–catecholamine interactions in major depression. *Arch. Gen. Psychiat.*, **44**:782–9.

Wolkowitz, O.M., Reus, V.I., Manfredi, F., Ingbar, J. and Brizendine, L., 1992. Antiglucorticoid strategies in hypercortisolemic states. *Psychopharmacol. Bull.*, **28**:247–51.

Wolkowitz, O.M., Reus, V.I., Manfredi, F., Chan, T., Ormiston, S. and Johnson, R., 1996. Dexamethasone for depression. *Am. J. Psychiat.*, **153**:1111–12.

Wolkowitz, O.M., Reus, V.I., Roberts, E., Manfredi, F., Chan, T., Raum, W.J., Ormiston, S., Johnson, R., Canick, J., Brizendine, L. and Weingartner, H., 1997. Dehydroepiandrosterone (DHEA) treatment of depression. *Biol. Psychiat.*, **41**:311–18.

Wolkowitz, O.M., Reus, V.I., Chan, T., Manfredi, F., Raum, W., Johnson, R. and Canick, J., 1999a. Antiglucocorticoid treatment of depression: double-blind ketoconazole. *Biol. Psychiat.*, **45**:1070–4.

Wolkowitz, O.M., Reus, V.I., Keebler, A., Nelson, N., Friedland, M., Brizendine, L. and Roberts, E., 1999b. Double-blind treatment of major depression with dehydroepiandrosterone. *Am. J. Psychiat.*, **156**:646–9.

Wong, M. and Moss, R.L., 1991. Electrophysiological evidence for a rapid membrane action of the gonadal steroid, 17 beta-estradiol, on CA1 pyramidal neurons of the rat hippocampus. *Brain Res.*, **543**(1):148–52.

Wong, M.-L., Kling, M.A., Munson, P.J., Listwak, S., Licinio, J., Prolo, P., Karp, B., McCutcheon, I.E., Geracioti, T.D., DeBellis, M.D., Rice, K.C., Goldstein, D.S., Veldhuis, J.D., Chrousos, G.P., Oldfield, E.H., McCann, S.M. and Gold, P.W., 2000. Pronounced and sustained central hypernoradrenergic function in major depression with melancholic features: relation to hypercortisolism and corticotropin-releasing hormone. *Proc. Natl Acad. Sci. USA*, **97**:325–30.

Woolley, C.S., Gould, E. and McEwen, B.S., 1990. Exposure to excess glucocorticoids alters dendritic morphology of adult hippocampal pyramidal neurons. *Brain Res.*, **531**:225–31.

Woolley, C.S. and McEwen, B.S., 1994. Estradiol regulates hippocampal dendritic spine density via an *N*-methyl-D-aspartate receptor-dependent mechanism. *J. Neurosci.*, **14**(12):7680–7.

Yaffe, K., Ettinger, B., Pressman, A., Seeley, D., Whooley, M., Schaefer, C. and Cummings, S., 1998a. Neuropsychiatric function and dehydroepiandrosterone sulfate in elderly women: a prospective study. *Biol. Psychiat.*, **43**:694–700.

Yaffe, K., Sawaya, G., Lieberburg, I. and Grady, D., 1998b. Estrogen therapy in post-menopausal women: effects on cognitive function and dementia. *JAMA*, **279**:688–95.

Yaffe, K., Krueger, K., Sarkar, S., Grady, D., Barrett-Connor, E., Cox, D.A. and Nickelsen, T., 2001. Cognitive function in postmenopausal women treated with raloxifene. *N. Engl J. Med.*, **344**:1207–13.

Yehuda, R., Southwick, S.M., Nussbaum, G., Wahby, V., Giller, E.L. and Mason, J., 1990. Low urinary cortisol excretion in patients with post-traumatic stress disorder. *J. Nerv. Ment. Dis.*, **178**:366–9.

Yehuda, R., Teicher, M.H., Levengood, R.A., Trestman, R.L. and Siever, L.J., 1994. Circadian regulation of basal cortisol levels in post-traumatic stress disorder. *Ann. N. Y. Acad. Sci.*, **746**:378–80.

Yehuda, R., Kahana, B., Binder-Brynes, K., Southwick, S.M., Mason, J.W. and Giller, E.L., 1995. Low urinary cortisol excretion in Holocaust survivors with post-traumatic stress disorder. *Am. J. Psychiat.*, **152**:982–6.

Yoo, A., Harris, J. and Dubrovsky, B., 1996. Dose–response study of dehydroepiandrosterone sulfate on dentate gyrus long-term potentiation. *Exp. Neurol.*, **137**:151–6.

Young, E.A., Midgley, A.R., Carlson, N.E. and Brown, M.B., 2000. Alteration in the hypothalamic–pituitary–ovarian axis in depressed women. *Arch. Gen. Psychiat.*, **57**:1157–62.

Zobel, A.W., Yassouridis, A., Frieboes, R.-M. and Holsboer, F., 1999. Prediction of medium-term outcome by cortisol response to the combined dexamethasone-CRH test in patients with remitted depression. *Am. J. Psychiat.*, **156**:949–51.

Zobel, A.W., Nickel, T., Kunzel, H.E., Ackl, N., Sonntag, A., Ising, M. and Holsboer, F., 2000. Effects of the high-affinity corticotropin-releasing hormone receptor 1 antagonist R121919 in major depression: the first 20 patients treated. *J. Psychiat. Res.*, **34**:171–81.

XVIII-6

Psychophysiology of Mood Disorders

Silvana Galderisi

INTRODUCTION

Mood disorders are markedly heterogeneous with respect to signs, symptoms, course, response to therapeutic interventions and outcome. Attempts at reducing heterogeneity by subgrouping subjects on the basis of clinical aspects is a valuable strategy; however, the scarce impact on everyday practice of most clinical subtypes underscores its limitation. External validation of clinical subtypes (demonstrating that they are characterized by different psychophysiological patterns) has been an important goal of psychophysiological research in mood disorders. Several other conceptual strategies can be identified throughout the reviewed literature: the search for trait or state markers, the attempt at clarifying pathogenetic mechanisms of the observed dysfunctions, and the identification of early predictors of course, outcome or response to different therapeutic interventions.

On the whole, however, the field has suffered from the lack of unifying hypotheses and systematic research, which is reflected in the fact that relevant reviews, including the present one, are organized according to the different techniques applied in the investigations. Moreover, evaluation and comparison of different findings is often hampered by poor characterization of studied populations with respect to relevant or confounding variables such as symptoms, clinical subtypes, medication (or other therapeutic intervention) history, or substance abuse or dependence.

This chapter is organized in two main sections, peripheral and central measures, each including several subsections dealing with specific measures or techniques.

As previous excellent reviews of the topic are available (Goodwin and Jamison, 1990; Henriques and Davidson, 1989; Zahn, 1986), an attempt has been made to cover the relevant literature with particular attention to more recent findings. Furthermore, since some readers might be unfamiliar with specific technical issues, when deemed appropriate a brief definition and description of the psychophysiological measures or techniques discussed in the section is provided.

PERIPHERAL PSYCHOPHYSIOLOGICAL INDICES IN RESEARCH ON MOOD DISORDERS

Disturbances of several physiological functions, such as sleep, appetite, sexual drive, sweat secretion and chronobiological rhythms, are commonly found in mood disorders and indicate a dysregulation of the autonomous system in affected subjects. Despite the large number of studies focusing on autonomic measures, much remains to be done to characterize this dysregulation. Investigations based on the concomitant evaluation of several autonomic parameters are promising; their integration with central measures, as well as with neuroendocrine and neurochemical measures, may contribute greatly to progress in this field of research.

Electrodermal Activity

Electrodermal activity (EDA) has been largely investigated as a measure of tonic and phasic arousal. Different variables can be evaluated, including the skin conductance level (SCL; the tonic level, generally measured after a resting period, before the first stimulus presentation), the spontaneous skin conductance responses (SSCRs; nonspecific fluctuations of activity independent of external stimuli), the skin conductance orienting responses (SCORs; related to external stimuli) and habituation (reduction in response to repeated stimulation). For each of these indices the eventual asymmetry pattern can be assessed.

Low baseline EDA has been frequently found in depressed patients when compared with healthy subjects. Such a reduction has been observed for both SCL and SCORs (Dawson *et al.*, 1977, 1985; Iacono *et al.*, 1983; 1984; Schnur *et al.*, 1995; Storrie *et al.*, 1981; Ward *et al.*, 1983; Zahn, 1986). Negative or discrepant findings have also been reported: Toone *et al.* (1981) found no difference between unmedicated subjects with depression and healthy comparison subjects; Albus *et al.* (1982) found higher SCL in drug-free depressed patients as compared with controls; Levinson (1991) reported higher SCL and a trend toward more SSCRs in a group of depressed patients (including schizoaffective depressed subjects), and interpreted the finding as the result of a hyperarousal condition. Faster habituation of the SCOR has been demonstrated in depressive patients (Frith *et al.*, 1982; Thorell, 1987). However, findings have been inconsistent (Miquel *et al.*, 1999; Storrie *et al.*, 1981). Methodological issues might partly account for the observed discrepancies, while the confounding role of clinical heterogeneity in tested populations is not strongly supported by available findings. In fact, the reduction of EDA activity and reactivity in subjects with mood disorders appears rather independent of subjects' clinical characteristics. Low SCL has been found in both medicated and unmedicated depressed subjects (Iacono *et al.*, 1983; Storrie *et al.*, 1981; Thorell *et al.*, 1987; Ward and Doerr, 1986), in unipolar and bipolar patients (Williams *et al.*, 1985) and in acutely ill depressed and manic patients, as well as after clinical recovery associated with antidepressant treatment or electroconvulsive therapy (Dawson *et al.*, 1977; Storrie *et al.*, 1981), in both suppressors and non-suppressors to the dexamethasone suppression test (DST) (Williams *et al.*, 1985), and in subclinically depressed versus non-depressed college students (Gehricke and Shapiro, 2001). However, EDA reduction seems to be even more pronounced in endogenous patients and in patients with symptoms of inhibition (Dawson *et al.*, 1977; Lader and Wing, 1969; Thorell *et al.*, 1987; Williams *et al.*, 1985).

EDA stability across different clinical subtypes of affective disorders has prompted research on its potential diagnostic utility. Reduced SCL as a diagnostic index of depression was investigated by several authors (Dawson *et al.*, 1985; Iacono *et al.*, 1983; Ward

Biological Psychiatry: Edited by H. D'haenen, J.A. den Boer and P. Willner. ISBN 0-471-49198-5

et al., 1983), who reported a sensitivity ranging from 65% to 96%, a specificity from 46% to 89% and an efficiency from 64% to 88%. Dawson *et al.* (1985) also investigated SCOR as a diagnostic marker and reported a sensitivity of 85%, a specificity of 75% and an efficiency of 80%. In an attempt to improve discrimination among different diagnoses, some authors have used multi-component recording to measure the orienting response (OR). In particular, the finger pulse amplitude response (FPAR) has often been used in association with the SCOR, as it represents the OR of an autonomic system component which is physiologically and biochemically independent of the EDA system (Bernstein *et al.*, 1981; Fowles, 1986). The use of multi-component recording to measure OR might also foster understanding of the pathophysiological mechanisms of abnormal OR in psychiatric disorders. Empirical findings suggest that when OR is jointly indexed by both SCOR and FPAR, subjects with depression can be differentiated much better from subjects with schizophrenia (Bernstein *et al.*, 1988): in fact, while the latter exhibit reduced responding across all OR components, suggesting a central OR deficit related to attentional dysfunction, the former showed a high rate of non-responding only in the electrodermal component, interpreted by Bernstein *et al.* (1988) as related to a peripheral deficit involving the EDA system. More recently the authors confirmed previous findings (Bernstein *et al.*, 1995) and proposed that a reduction in cholinergically mediated activity, rather than a central deficit of OR, may be implicated in autonomic findings in depression. The hypothesis is based on the fact that, besides FPAR, other aspects of the OR component have been found unimpaired in depressives (e.g. pupillary dilatation response or P300), while other cholinergically mediated systems appear dysfunctional (e.g. salivation reduction, reduced blood flow response in the forearm during mental tasks, reduced variability of the respiratory sinus arrhythmia in the resting ECG). The hypothesis remains difficult to reconcile with evidence for a functional excess of central cholinergic activity in depression. It should be mentioned, however, that measuring SCOR and FPAR in concert, Levinson (1991) failed to differentiate subjects with schizophrenia from those with depression, while Schnur *et al.* (1999) could not differentiate patients with schizophrenia from those with mania.

The possibility that different pathophysiological mechanisms underlie EDA reduction in subjects with schizophrenia and those with mood disorders is also suggested by the findings of Katsanis and co-workers, showing that in subjects with mood disorders, in contrast with what is observed in those with schizophrenia, there is no relationship between season of birth and EDA reduction (Katsanis *et al.*, 1992). Similarly, Bernstein *et al.* (1988) pointed out that in schizophrenics the frequency of electrodermal responding varies with the task relevance of the stimulus, while in depression no relationship is observed, suggesting that SCOR deficit is centrally determined in schizophrenia but not in depression, where a peripheric cholinergic defect might be implicated.

Bilateral recordings of EDA in subjects with mood disorders have shown higher activity from the left than from the right hand (Gruzelier and Venables, 1974; Myslobosky and Horesh, 1978; Schneider, 1983). The asymmetry pattern has been interpreted as the result of either a hypoactivation or a hyperactivation of the right hemisphere in depressive disorders. Conflicting interpretations originate from the difficulty of disentangling the relative activating or inhibitory contribution of each hemisphere to EDA from either hand. Lenhart and Katkin (1986) recorded, in adjunct to bilateral EDA, conjugate lateral eye movements in a group of college students with subsyndromal depression. They confirmed the previously reported pattern of EDA asymmetry (L > R) and found a bias toward left-tending conjugate lateral eye movements. Findings were interpreted as reflecting right-hemisphere hyperexcitability in affective illness.

The EDA asymmetry pattern L > R was also found in high-risk subjects, the offspring of parents with bipolar affective disorders (Zahn *et al.*, 1989). However, in the latter study it was limited to the recording task period and concomitant with high self-ratings of depressed mood, which led the authors to conclude that, rather than being a stable property of the nervous system, it should be considered as a state marker of depression. Several studies failed to find any asymmetry in bilateral EDA recordings of patients with affective disorders (Iacono and Tuason, 1983; Storrie *et al.*, 1981; Toone *et al.*, 1981).

Cardiovascular Measures

Heart rate (HR), heart rate orienting responses (HRORs) and heart rate variability (HRV) have been the most frequently used indices. Systolic, diastolic and mean blood pressure, as well as forearm blood flow, have also been investigated in some studies.

The main findings in subjects with depression included an elevated resting heart rate and/or HRORs (Carney *et al.*, 1988; Dawson *et al.*, 1977, 1985; Lahmeyer and Bellur, 1987; Lehofer *et al.*, 1997) and a reduced HR variability (Carney *et al.*, 1995a; Dallack and Roose, 1990). Discrepant findings have also been reported (Jacobsen *et al.*, 1984; Lader and Wing, 1969; Yeragani *et al.*, 1991). Medication status, concomitant anxiety and failure to adequately match subjects for age and sex might account for the discrepancies.

Research on HRV has received particular attention, due to its medical implications: reduced HRV as a result of diminished cardiac vagal tone was shown to be a strong predictor of sudden death in subjects with myocardial infarction; subjects with depressive disorders have an increased incidence of mortality for cardiovascular diseases, and reduced HRV might represent a predisposing factor (for review see Dalack and Roose, 1990).

As a measure of HRV the respiratory sinus arrhythmia (RSA; the variation in heart rate associated with respiratory cycles) has been employed in some studies. It is used to assess cardiac parasympathetic tone. Spectral analysis of beat-to-beat variations in HR and blood pressure (BP) has also been applied to describe sympathetic and parasympathetic contributions to cardiovascular regulation (Malliani *et al.*, 1991; Tulen, 1993). Three spectral peaks are identified: a low-frequency peak (around 0.04 Hz), which for HR is associated with both sympathetic and parasympathetic activity, while for BP reflects variations in peripheral vasomotor activity; a mid-frequency peak (around 0.1 Hz), associated with the baroreflex response (and reflecting mainly sympathetic activity, although for HR the parasympathetic contribution cannot be excluded); and a high-frequency peak (around 0.20–0.35 Hz), which for HR reflects the RSA and therefore the parasympathetic tone, while for BP mainly results from mechanical effects of respiration.

Tulen *et al.* (1996) investigated autonomic regulation in 16 drug-free female depressed patients, divided into high and low on trait anxiety (HTA, LTA), during supine rest, orthostatic challenge, and post-orthostatic challenge supine rest. Spectral analysis of fluctuations in HR and BP was employed. They found that patients did not differ from controls during supine rest; during the orthostatic challenge they did not show the normal increase of BP mid-frequency band fluctuations, suggesting a reduced sympathetic activation, and exhibited a reduction of HR variations, pointing to a strong vagal inhibition. The latter effect was more marked in HTA patients; during the post-orthostatic supine rest patients showed a significant increase in HR variability, in the absence of clear changes in BP variability, suggesting a predominant cardiac vagal increase. The authors conclude that an impairment of orthostatic reflex in depressed patients is suggested, with a prevalence of parasympathetic over sympathetic dysfunction, especially in HTA patients.

Lehofer *et al.* (1997) studied both RSA and HR in 23 unmedicated and 23 medicated DSM-III depressed subjects, melancholic subtype, and 46 healthy comparison subjects. HR was higher in both medicated and unmedicated depressed subjects, while RSA was lower only in medicated patients versus comparison subjects. They concluded that there is no difference in vagal tone between unmedicated depressives and healthy controls, and therefore higher HR in unmedicated patients might be due to either an increased sympathetic tone or an increased 'autonomous' heart rate (which, together with the vagal and sympathetic activity, contributes to the heart frequency). It is independent of autonomic nervous system control, is about 100 beats per minute and is found in transplanted heart patients (Bernardi *et al.*, 1989). Moser *et al.* (1998) came to a similar conclusion measuring heart rate, RSA, pulsewave velocity (a measure of the sympathetic tone in the cardiovascular system) and BP in 26 patients suffering from major depression, melancholic type, who had been unmedicated for at least three months, and 26 comparison healthy subjects. Patients exhibited a higher HR, and no difference in cardiac vagal tone or sympathetic cardiovascular tone. Taken together, the results indicate that autonomous heart rate is higher in subjects with depression; whether this is due to a less well-trained heart resulting from reduced physical exercise or is a physiological state or trait marker of depression is left open by the authors.

Austen and Wilson (2001) measured RSA in unmedicated subjects with subsyndromal seasonal affective disorder (SAD) and healthy comparison subjects in both winter and non-winter periods. They found a significant group–season interaction due to significant higher RSA scores in winter only in subjects with SAD. For HR, SCL and diastolic blood pressure, instead, only an effect of the season was found: in both SAD and control subjects HR decreased while SCL and blood pressure increased during winter. According to the authors, increased RSA, due to an increased vagal tone, may parallel the sleep symptom observed in SAD (increased sleep), thus suggesting a similarity with the hibernation process and different underlying mechanisms with respect to non-seasonal depression. As also proposed by the authors, further research across a year-long period is needed to confirm and extend these observations across groups, and eventually confirm that SAD is a different disorder from non-seasonal depression.

Dysregulation of the autonomic nervous system has been considered a leading candidate mechanism for the association between depression and increased medical morbidity and mortality in patients with coronary heart disease (CHD) (Carney *et al.*, 1999). In a group of 50 depressed and 39 medically comparable CHD non-depressed subjects, Carney *et al.* (1999) found an elevated resting HR and an exaggerated HR response to orthostatic challenge in the former group. However, the mechanism underlying the observed autonomic dysfunction remains unclear: in fact, the two groups did not differ in resting or standing plasma levels of norepinephrine, excluding an increased sympathetic activity; at the same time, studies of HRV in depressed CHD patients have found no support for lower vagal tone in these subjects (Carney *et al.*, 1995b).

Eye Movements

Although included in the section on peripheral measures, the study of eye movements is not relevant to autonomic dysregulation. Eye movement investigations, in fact, provide important clues to central nervous system functioning. Increasingly sophisticated studies enable attempts to relate the results of electrophysiological recordings to the topology of brain function, as well as to brain imaging findings.

The majority of eye movement studies carried out in subjects with affective disorders have focused on the smooth pursuit eye movement system; a minority have investigated saccadic eye movements.

Smooth pursuit eye movements (SPEMs) occur when a moving object (target) is fixated and followed by the eyes. More often visual targets oscillating in a uniform sinusoidal or pendular manner have been used. Saccades are the brief rapid movements of the eyes aimed at bringing the eye focus from one point to another of the visual field.

SPEMs have been largely investigated in subjects with schizophrenia, in which their dysfunction is regarded as a promising biological marker of the disorder (Holzman, 1987; Holzman *et al.*, 1973, 1974; Iacono and Clementz, 1992). Several studies have also found SPEM abnormalities in subjects with affective disorders, calling into question the diagnostic specificity of SPEM dysfunction.

Studies contrasting subjects with affective disorders to healthy comparison groups have reported abnormal SPEMs in patients (Holzman, 1985; Iacono *et al.*, 1982; Klein *et al.*, 1976; Levin *et al.*, 1981; Salzman *et al.*, 1978; Shagass *et al.*, 1974). Several studies have reported no striking difference between subjects with mood disorders (both bipolar and unipolar) and those with schizophrenia on eye-tracking performance (Amador *et al.*, 1991; Friedman *et al.*, 1992; Iacono *et al.*, 1992; Küfferle *et al.*, 1990; Levin *et al.*, 1981; Lipton *et al.*, 1980; Sweeney *et al.*, 1999; Yee *et al.*, 1987), while others did find significant differences (Cegalis and Sweeney, 1981; Iacono and Koenig, 1983; Iacono *et al.*, 1982; Muir *et al.*, 1992). Heterogeneity in recording techniques, experimental paradigms, evaluated measures, patients' diagnosis or medication status may account for discrepancies.

Some studies used global performance measures (qualitative ratings of eye tracking or quantitative global evaluation, which assess the similarity between the target trace and the eye movement trace), while others used quantitative measures of SPEM-specific characteristics, such as gain (eye velocity/target velocity), anticipatory saccade (AS) rate (frequency of large saccades that take the eyes ahead of target), square wave jerk (SWJ) rate (frequency of pairs of small saccades, in opposite directions, separated by approximately 200 ms) or corrective catch-up saccade (CUS) rate (frequency of saccades occurring when a low pursuit gain causes the eyes to fall behind the target in order to quickly take the eyes to the target). ASs and SWJs are intrusive saccades, while CUSs are corrective saccades.

The increasing use of more sophisticated methods is relevant to the diagnostic issue: global measures might be less sensitive than specific quantitative measures. Patients in different diagnostic categories might have globally abnormal eye tracking; however, the specific pattern of abnormalities might help discriminating among them.

Friedman *et al.* (1995), in a study including 26 unmedicated schizophrenics, 14 unmedicated subjects with affective disorders (mostly unipolar), never treated with lithium, and 45 healthy subjects, used two global measures — qualitative rating and root mean square (RMS), which is a measure of the extent to which the eye position and target position differ over time — and six quantitative measures — CUS rate, CUS amplitude, gain, SWJ rate, AS number, and total time scored. They found that (1) RMS error and qualitative measures did not differentiate subjects with schizophrenia or affective disorders from healthy comparison groups, and (2) patients with affective disorders were not impaired on eye-tracking measures, whereas patients with schizophrenia were impaired in terms of gain, CUS rate and total time scored. They concluded that unmedicated subjects with affective disorders never exposed to lithium treatment perform an easy SPEM task as well as comparison subjects, that SPEM abnormalities are specific to schizophrenia and that specific quantitative ratings are more sensitive than global ones.

Friedman *et al.* (1992) reported that subjects with schizophrenia and those with affective disorders did not differ on SWJ and AS rate; the same group (Abel *et al.*, 1991) had previously found that CUS rate at the target velocity of 20°/s differentiated the two diagnostic groups, being significantly higher in subjects with schizophrenia. Each diagnostic group showed a different abnormality pattern when compared with healthy subjects. Similar findings were reported by Flechtner *et al.* (1997), who studied 43 subjects with schizophrenia, 34 with major depression and 42 healthy comparison subjects, and found that the two patient groups did not differ on gain, intrusive saccades and AS, while CUS rate was significantly higher in subjects with schizophrenia than in those with depression.

Sweeney *et al.* (1999) have recently stressed the importance of studying eye tracking by using experimental paradigms providing assessment of the pursuit across different target velocities and evaluating other important SPEM components, such as pursuit initiation or performance in conditions of low stimulus position predictability. In a carefully designed study, they tested 32 subjects with schizophrenia (20 drug-naïve, 12 drug-free for 28 days), 35 with affective disorders (26 unipolar, 9 bipolar, all drug-free for 28 days) and 24 comparison healthy subjects. All patients were tested during acute episodes of illness. No abnormality showed a diagnostic specificity.

As mentioned above, several variables may affect eye movements. Substances with a depressant effect on the central nervous system (such as barbiturates, chloral hydrate, alcohol and benzodiazepines) may either superimpose nystagmus or increase saccadic events during pursuit or fixation, whereas neuroleptics, tricyclics and monoamine oxidase inhibitors do not seem to influence SPEMs (Holzman *et al.*, 1975, 1991; Levy *et al.*, 1984). In studies involving subjects with affective disorders, lithium treatment in particular has been regarded as an important confounding variable (Iacono *et al.*, 1982; Levy *et al.*, 1985). According to Corbett *et al.* (1989) the oculomotor effects of lithium include nystagmus, saccade pursuit, saccadic dysmetria and oculogyric crises. Holzman *et al.* (1991), in a study in which subjects with affective disorders were tested prior to starting lithium and then at weekly intervals after beginning treatment, reported that, in the context of clinical improvement, lithium administration degraded SPEMs and the nature of the degradation was idiosyncratic, involving different changes in different subjects and including gain decrements, increase in total number of saccades (but not AS) and fixation instability. Gooding *et al.* (1993), however, in a carefully designed study, found no lithium effect on SPEMs.

Eye-tracking abnormalities were also investigated in the offspring of probands with either unipolar or bipolar depression. In the unaffected offspring of subjects with bipolar disorder no impairment of eye tracking was found (Holzman *et al.*, 1984; Iacono *et al.*, 1992; Levy *et al.*, 1983), suggesting that the dysfunction represents a trait marker in schizophrenia and a state-related measure in mood disorders. Such a conclusion is not completely supported by a study carried out in the offspring of schizophrenic, unipolar depressed and bipolar probands from the New York High-Risk Project (Rosenberg *et al.*, 1997). In that study, in fact, a significant global performance deficit was demonstrated in the offspring of depressed probands and of schizophrenic probands, but not in those of bipolar patients. However, only the offspring of probands with schizophrenia had a higher mean frequency of anticipatory saccades. The authors suggested that the familial specificity of global eye-tracking deficit to schizophrenia might be limited with respect to unipolar major depression.

Visual fixation — that is, the ability to maintain gaze on a stationary target — has also been investigated in subjects with affective disorders. Amador *et al.* (1991, 1995) found fixation abnormalities in subjects with schizophrenia and their first-degree relatives, but not in those with depression. Gooding *et al.* (2000) did not find any fixation abnormality in either subjects with schizophrenia or those with bipolar I disorder. The latter study used a different recording technique (infrared scleral reflection instead of electro-oculogram recording) and added quantitative to qualitative evaluation.

Several studies showed no latency or accuracy abnormality of saccadic eye movements in subjects with bipolar affective disorders versus healthy comparison groups (Crawford *et al.*, 1995; Sereno and Holzman, 1995; Tien *et al.*, 1996). Some other studies, while confirming saccade accuracy, reported increased saccadic latency in bipolar versus healthy subjects (Park and Holzman, 1992; Yee *et al.*, 1987). An increased error rate on antisaccade tasks has also been reported in bipolar versus healthy comparison subjects (Sereno and Holzman, 1995; Tien *et al.*, 1996). Relatively few studies have investigated saccadic eye movements in depressed subjects. Fukushima *et al.* (1990) reported that medicated depressed patients had a normal saccade latency and were able to suppress reflexive saccades during an antisaccade task. Done and Frith (1989) found a normal saccade latency during a visually guided saccade task in a small group of drug-free depressed subjects, but a prolonged latency during a voluntary saccade task. Sweeney *et al.* (1998) administered a battery of oculomotor tasks (selected to assess the functional integrity of frontostriatal circuitry and of the cerebellar vermis) to 29 unmedicated inpatients with unipolar major depression and 19 comparison subjects. In the patient group, in comparison with healthy subjects, they found no abnormality of saccade latency, an impaired ability to suppress saccades to peripheral targets in the antisaccade task, more saccadic intrusions during fixation and a mild saccadic dysmetria during sensorially guided eye movements. Since lesions of the cerebellar vermis disrupt saccade accuracy but not necessarily latency or velocity, the impaired accuracy observed in depressed patients is compatible with a dysfunction of the cerebellar vermis. The remaining abnormalities are interpreted as the result of prefrontal dysfunction. The authors conclude that a functional disturbance of the dorsolateral prefrontal cortex may be common to both bipolar and unipolar patients, whereas the cerebellar vermis dysfunction seems characteristic of unipolar patients. It is worthy of notice that abnormalities of the cerebellar vermis have been reported by both structural and functional brain imaging studies in depressed patients (Dolan *et al.*, 1992; Shah *et al.*, 1992).

Bipolar patients receiving neuroleptic treatment were less accurate than neuroleptic-free patients on saccades directed towards remembered or predicted targets, which presumably require an internal representation of the stimulus (Crawford *et al.*, 1995).

CENTRAL PSYCHOPHYSIOLOGICAL INDICES IN RESEARCH ON MOOD DISORDERS

Central indices have been extensively used in the psychophysiological research on mood disorders. The huge literature on the EEG, ERPs and sleep parameters in affective disorders cannot be exhaustively reviewed for obvious space limitations. In the following section, the main results will be summarized and discussed in the light of their contribution to the generation of hypotheses on the pathophysiology of these disorders.

Quantitative Electroencephalogram (QEEG)

QEEG in Depressive Disorders

QEEG research in depressive disorders did not report consistent findings. Most replicated results include an increase of alpha (Brenner *et al.*, 1986; John *et al.*, 1988; Schaffer *et al.*, 1983; von Knorring, 1983) and/or beta (Flor-Henry *et al.*, 1979; John *et al.*, 1988; Knott and Lapierre, 1987a) activity in depressed patients, when compared with healthy subjects. Increased slow-wave activity, generally observed in subjects with dementia, has been found in elderly depressed patients by some authors, though to a lesser degree than in dementia (Brenner *et al.*, 1986; Have *et al.*, 1991; Nystrom *et al.*, 1986). Studies investigating early- and late-onset depressed patients failed to find differences between the two groups, but reported a relationship between increased delta wave activity and poor performance on several neurocognitive tests in patients with late-onset depression (Dahabra *et al.*, 1998; Visser *et al.*, 1985).

Lateralized findings have also been inconsistent. An increase of beta activity, predominantly over the left side, was reported in depressed when compared to healthy subjects, suggesting left hemisphere overactivation (Flor-Henry and Koles, 1984; Kemali *et al.*, 1981; Matousek *et al.*, 1981). Some authors reported an increase of alpha activity and a polymodal distribution of the mean alpha amplitude over the right hemisphere in depressed compared to healthy subjects, suggesting a reduced activation and a disorganization of this hemisphere (von Knorring, 1983; von Knorring *et al.*, 1983).

An asymmetric increase of the alpha activity over the left frontal regions was reported by some studies in currently or previously depressed patients (Baehr *et al.*, 1998; Gotlib *et al.*, 1998; Henriques and Davidson, 1990, 1991) and in subclinically depressed students (Davidson *et al.*, 1987; Schaffer *et al.*, 1983). Children of depressed mothers, who might be at risk for affective disorders, were shown to have greater alpha activity over the left than over the right frontal regions (Tomarken *et al.*, 1994). The increase of alpha was interpreted as a sign of decreased left frontal activation with a deficit in approach-related behaviours (Davidson, 1992). The opposite asymmetry pattern was observed for the parietal regions, with an increase of alpha power over the right-hemisphere leads, in currently or previously depressed subjects (Davidson *et al.*, 1987; Henriques and Davidson, 1990). The increase of alpha over the right parietal regions might be associated with cognitive deficits, suggesting right posterior dysfunction in depression (Davidson *et al.*, 1987; Tucker *et al.*, 1981). For the parietal asymmetry pattern, however, conflicting results were reported by some studies in either depressed students or subjects with major depression. Some of them failed to find any abnormality in parietal regions (Henriques and Davidson, 1991; Schaffer *et al.*, 1983), while others found a bilateral increase of alpha (Pollock and Schneider, 1989, 1990) or a right posterior alpha reduction (Pozzi *et al.*, 1995; Suzuki *et al.*, 1996). According to Bruder *et al.* (1997) the presence of anxiety in the clinical picture might influence the laterality pattern observed over the posterior regions. In fact, non-anxious depressed patients showed more alpha activity (less activation) over the right than over the left posterior leads, whereas anxious depressed patients showed the opposite pattern. Two studies reported a failure to suppress alpha activity over the right posterior regions in depressed subjects during the performance of a spatial task (Henriques and Davidson, 1997; Reid *et al.*, 1995), suggesting that a cognitive challenge might be necessary to disclose the right-hemisphere deficit in posterior regions. Suicidal ideation might also influence the posterior asymmetry pattern. In fact, preliminary findings suggest that adolescent depressed and non-depressed suicide attempters have more alpha activity over the left than the right frontal regions, but differ in the direction of the asymmetry over the posterior regions: a greater alpha activity over the left than the right posterior leads was related to suicidal intent, but not to depression severity (Graae *et al.*, 1996).

So far the topographic analysis of the brain electrical activity from multilead recordings by means of the identification of the brain electrical microstates (BEMs) has not received great attention in relation to mood disorders. BEMs are stable segments of scalp electric fields in the sub-second range, and reflect the coordinated activation of neuronal circuits involved in mentation (Koenig and Lehmann, 1996; Lehmann *et al.*, 1987). The main quantitative parameters of the BEMs include the duration, the spatial variance (i.e. spatial changes per time unit), the topographic characteristics of the field, as assessed by the locations of the positive and negative centroids (the centre of gravity of the positive and negative areas, respectively), and the field strength. With respect to healthy comparison subjects, depressive patients showed a reduced duration of the brain electrical microstate more represented in subjects' mentation and a larger spatial variance. However, the topographic characteristics of the identified microstates were similar in the two groups (Strik *et al.*, 1995). The findings were interpreted as the electrophysiological correlates of impaired attention and automatic processing in depressive patients.

QEEG in Bipolar Disorder

Only a few QEEG studies have been carried out in acute, drug-free subjects during a manic episode, probably because of the difficulty of obtaining cooperation from these patients. Flor-Henry and Koles (1984) found a decrease of alpha power in manic patients with respect to healthy subjects, suggesting an overarousal in the former group. Shagass *et al.* (1984) found that patients with mania have higher EEG frequencies and greater variability than those with depression, and interpreted the results as a sign of overarousal in mania. In bipolar subjects left hemisphere abnormalities have been reported, akin to those in schizophrenia (Davidson, 1987; Flor-Henry, 1987).

A study on the adult offspring of subjects with bipolar disorder, comparing the ill siblings (subjects who met the DSM-III criteria for bipolar disorder) with those who were well, showed a reduction of alpha activity in the ill group (Knott and Lapierre, 1987b). However, in the ill-sibling group, all subjects were asymptomatic at the moment of assessment, some were on maintenance treatment or had been treated with antidepressants and observed a very short wash-out period (72 hours) before assessment, leaving open the possibility that study findings were influenced by drug treatment.

QEEG and Treatment Responsiveness

A few investigations were aimed at assessing the usefulness of QEEG in the prediction of response to antidepressant drugs. Knott *et al.* (1985) with an open-label paradigm found a lower relative theta power in the baseline recording of depressed subjects with a favourable clinical response to imipramine, with respect to non-responders to the same drug. Cook *et al.* (1999) used a new measure, combining relative and absolute power, the cordance, in the theta band to investigate QEEG correlates of response to fluoxetine in unipolar depression, with a double-blind, placebo-controlled paradigm. Significantly more depressed subjects with high cordance in theta band were responders to fluoxetine in comparison to those with low cordance. Since previous studies showed that cordance correlates with brain metabolism (Leuchter *et al.*, 1999), the results were interpreted as suggesting that only depressed subjects with low baseline dysregulation respond to treatment.

Galderisi *et al.* (1996) used a test-dose procedure to study the QEEG changes associated with clinical response to moclobemide in unipolar depressed patients. A single dose of 200 mg moclobemide induced a transient increase of theta activity (observed up to the third hour after drug administration), a slight augmentation of alpha and a sustained increase of beta activity (observed up to the sixth hour after drug administration). Drug-induced increase of beta was found to correlate with the decrease of depression psychopathological ratings observed after 42 days of treatment.

In a group of drug-free, acute patients with mania, Small *et al.* (1999) reported more baseline fast theta activity (6–8 Hz) in non-responders to pharmacotherapy than in responders. After treatment, non-responders had more delta and theta over frontal and temporal regions, as well as more beta1 activity over left temporal leads.

Event-Related Potentials (ERPs)

ERPs in Depressive Affective Disorders

For nearly all ERP components discrepant findings were reported in depressed subjects (Bruder *et al.*, 1995, 1998; el Massioui and Lesevre, 1988; Kayser *et al.*, 2000; Ogura *et al.*, 1993; Pierson *et al.*, 1996; Zahn, 1986).

The contingent negative variation (CNV) is a slow negative potential occurring within the interval between a warning stimulus and an imperative signal which prompts the subject's response. The CNV has generators in the prefrontal cortex and shows a brainstem cholinergic modulation (Halgren, 1990). It is thought to be related to the orientation, expectation and preparation for the motor act (Wascher *et al.*, 1997).

The CNV was found to be reduced in depressed when compared with healthy subjects (Ashton *et al.*, 1988; Sartory, 1985; Shagass, 1983). However, other studies failed to find the CNV reduction (Elton, 1984; Knott and Lapierre, 1987a). A study subdividing depressed patients into two groups, one with retardation/blunted affect and the other with anxiety/impulsiveness, found a reduced CNV only in the former group versus healthy subjects (Pierson *et al.*, 1996). An augmented CNV amplitude was demonstrated in a subgroup of depressed patients with increased reactivity to apomorphine, underscoring the clinical-biological heterogeneity of depressive disorders (Timsit-Berthier, 1986). A reduction of the P1-N1 component amplitude was reported in depressed compared to healthy subjects (el Massioui and Lesevre, 1988; Pierson *et al.*, 1996), suggesting a disturbance in early sensory processing. The finding was not replicated by other studies (Bruder *et al.*, 1995; 1998).

For N2, an ERP component thought to index both automatic orienting and initial effortful stimulus evaluation (Bruder *et al.*, 1998), a reduced amplitude was observed in depressed versus healthy subjects, when using emotional faces; differences were maximal over right parietal regions, indicating a posterior right-hemisphere deficit (Deldin *et al.*, 2000).

Several studies examined the P3 component of the ERPs in depression. This component includes (1) the P3a subcomponent, with a centro-frontal amplitude maximum, which represents an orienting response, and (2) the P3b subcomponent, with a centro-parietal maximum, which is related to the categorization and completion of the task. The P3 amplitude was found to be reduced in depressed versus healthy subjects (Bruder *et al.*, 1998; Pfefferbaum *et al.*, 1984; Roth *et al.*, 1981; Thier *et al.*, 1986). However, according to some studies (Gangadhar *et al.*, 1993; Picton, 1992), the reduction was not seen during episode remission. Other studies reported a normal P3 amplitude in depressives (Bange and Bathien, 1998; Giedke *et al.*, 1980; Sara *et al.*, 1994). Depressed subjects with retardation/blunted affect presented a reduced P3a amplitude, while those with agitation/impulsiveness did not (Partiot *et al.*, 1993). Since P3a is related to the orienting, the authors interpreted the results as evidence of disturbed automatic processing in depression with retardation and blunted affect. In a subsequent study, in which a more complex task was used, a group of retarded/blunted depressives showed a reduction of both P3a and P3b amplitude with respect to anxious/impulsive patients and healthy subjects (Pierson *et al.*, 1996). Actually, in the anxious/impulsive group the P3b amplitude was even larger than in healthy subjects, suggesting that the combination of the two subgroups may cancel out differences between patients and comparison groups. Kayser *et al.* (2000) investigated the P3 during passive viewing of faces with negative and neutral emotional valence in depressed and healthy subjects. The P3b showed an amplitude reduction in depressed compared to healthy subjects. Furthermore, the P3b showed an amplitude enhancement over right posterior leads for negative as compared to neutral faces, only in healthy subjects. Depressed patients presented a similar effect for the P3a component. The authors hypothesized that an early stimulus categorization (indexed by the P3a) was followed by inhibition of further affective processing (indexed by the P3b) in depressed subjects. The study findings gave further support to the presence of a reduced activation of right posterior areas in depressed subjects.

Discrepant findings were reported for P3 latency increase (which might index cognitive deterioration) in depressed subjects (Blackwood *et al.*, 1987; Dahabra *et al.*, 1998; Pfefferbaum *et al.*, 1984; Roth *et al.*, 1991). Bruder (1995) criticized the use of very easy tasks in studies reporting negative results and demonstrated a longer P3 latency in depressed subjects, with respect to a comparison group, only for a right-hemisphere task (Bruder, 1995). In a previous study, comparing subgroups of depressed subjects, Bruder *et al.* (1991) reported an increase of P3 latency in subjects with typical as compared with those with atypical depression only during the performance of a right-hemisphere task. Thus, discrepancies concerning P3 latency might be related to the use of tasks of different complexity and to the heterogeneity of depressive disorders.

ERPs in Bipolar Disorder

A reduced sensory gating, as measured by the suppression of the amplitude of the auditory P50 in response to the second of paired stimuli, was observed in manic patients, akin to findings in schizophrenia. However, in mania the abnormality is limited to acute symptomatic phases, while in schizophrenia it is a trait characteristic (Franks *et al.*, 1983; Freedman *et al.*, 1987). A study found that although the abnormality was present in bipolar subjects with manic or depressive episodes as well as in schizophrenics, only in subjects with mania it was associated with increased plasma levels of the norepinephrine metabolite 3-methoxy-4-hydroxyphenylglycol (Baker *et al.*, 1990). Knott and Lapierre (1987b) reported an increased amplitude of the auditory P1 in the ill group compared with the well group in the adult offspring of bipolar subjects, suggesting an increased arousal in the ill group. The P200 component, thought to reflect the evaluation of stimuli physical characteristics and with generators in modality-specific cortical areas, was found to be reduced in bipolar I and schizophrenic patients with a negative family history compared to those with a positive family history for psychotic disorders (Tabarés-Seisdedos *et al.*, 2001). The two groups also differed in the presence of a larger right Sylvian fissure in patients with a negative family history. All patients were treated at the moment of testing.

Asymmetry indices might be useful in discriminating bipolar depressed from both unipolar depressed and healthy subjects (Bruder *et al.*, 1992). As a matter of fact, bipolar depressed subjects had a lower N1 amplitude for stimuli presented to the left than for those presented to the right visual hemifield. The same asymmetry was not found in either unipolar depressed or healthy subjects. In the same study, bipolar subjects were tested in a dot enumeration task and showed a reduced left visual field accuracy which was responsible for the absence of the visual field asymmetry found in both unipolar depressed and comparison subjects. The findings were interpreted as signs of reduced right-hemisphere arousal due to a dysfunction of the arousal/attentional system in the same hemisphere.

A few studies examined the P3 component in patients with mania. Salisbury *et al.* (1999) investigated P3 in treated patients with schizophrenia and bipolar disorder with psychotic features, and in healthy comparison subjects. They found a P3 amplitude reduction in both patient groups, with respect to healthy subjects. Maximum reduction of P3 amplitude was found over the left temporal lead in patients with schizophrenia and over the midline frontal lead in those with bipolar disorder. A study comparing bipolar and healthy subjects reported an amplitude reduction over the frontal regions and a more posterior location of the P3 topography in the patient group, suggesting a reduced inhibitory frontal control in mania (Strik *et al.*, 1998). In line with a frontal deficit are recent findings of a functional imaging study showing a reduction of frontal activity in mania (Blumberg *et al.*, 2000).

ERPs and Treatment Responsiveness

The intensity dependence of the N1/P2 component of the auditory ERPs has been used to predict clinical response to treatment with lithium or antidepressants in subjects with mood disorders. The slope of the amplitude/stimulus intensity function (ASF) is an index of the amplitude changes due to increasing stimulus intensity: the steeper the slope, the greater the amplitude changes of the studied ERP components due to increasing stimulus intensity. The concept of intensity dependence has substituted that of augmenting/reducing introduced by Buchsbaum and Silverman (1968). Several authors reported that subjects showing a steeper pre-treatment ASF exhibited a favourable response to lithium treatment (Baron *et al.*, 1975; Buchsbaum *et al.*, 1971, 1979; Hegerl *et al.*, 1986, 1987; Nurnberger *et al.*, 1979). Hegerl and Juckel (1993) argued that the intensity dependence of the N1/P2 auditory ERP component is modulated by the serotonergic system: a strong intensity dependence of this component indicates a low central serotonergic activity. Among the findings supporting this hypothesis, the relationship between ASF slope and response to fluvoxamine is relevant to the present review. The effects of a fluvoxamine test dose on the ASF slope was related to clinical response to the same drug: patients with a flattening of the ASF slope induced by the fluvoxamine test dose were responders to the subsequent fluvoxamine therapy (Hegerl and Juckel, 1993). Subsequent research by Hegerl's group confirmed the role of serotonin in the modulation of ASF (Hegerl and Juckel, 1993; Juckel *et al.*, 1997, 1999). They showed that a strong pre-treatment ASF of the N1/P2 predicts a favourable clinical response to specific serotonin reuptake inhibitors (SSRI) in depressed patients (Gallinat *et al.*, 2000; Hegerl *et al.*, 2001).

A study showed an increase in the amplitude of the visual P3b and a significant decrease in its latency in depressed patients, after 6 weeks of treatment with moclobemide with respect to baseline (Galderisi *et al.*, 1996). The latency modification of the component was independent of changes in psychopathological scores.

Ancy *et al.* (1996) showed a larger baseline P300 amplitude in responders than in non-responders to ECT.

Sleep Studies

Sleep disturbances are common in affective disorders, with a prevalence of insomnia in the majority of subjects and hypersomnia in some subtypes of affective disorders (Armitage and Hoffmann, 1997; Reynolds and Kupfer, 1987; Riemann *et al.*, 2001). Insomnia represents a risk factor for depression (Ford and Kamerow, 1989; Livingston *et al.*, 1993; Schramm *et al.*, 1995) and increases the risk of suicide (Wingard and Berkman, 1983). Sleep deprivation may alleviate depressive symptoms (Wirz-Justice and Van der Hoofdakker, 1999; Wu and Bunney, 1990) and trigger mania in bipolar subjects (Wehr, 1991). In line with the latter observation, insomnia was shown to be a risk factor for mania (Barbini *et al.*, 1996). These data underscore the importance of sleep to mood disturbances.

Normal sleep includes alternating episodes of rapid eye movement (REM) sleep and non-REM (NREM) sleep. The latter includes four stages of progressively deeper sleep (stages 1–4). The deepest stages (3 and 4) represent the so-called slow-wave sleep (SWS). A sleep cycle of about 90 minutes includes both NREM and REM episodes. Within the cycle, SWS predominates during the first part of the night, while REM sleep predominates during the last part of the night.

An endogenous circadian clock, involved in biological circadian rhythms (such as body temperature and melatonin secretion) and thought to be located in the suprachiasmatic nucleus of the hypothalamus, regulates REM sleep and sleep spindles (12–15 Hz EEG oscillations with prevalent occurrence in stage 2 of the non-REM sleep). The circadian clock is entrained by time cues so that the sleep–wake cycle is synchronized to the day–night cycle and biological rhythms are synchronized with one another. A forced desynchronization in healthy subjects between the circadian internal clock and day–night cycle influences mood (Boivin *et al.*, 1997). There is also strong evidence that the balance between cholinergic and aminergic neurotransmitter systems regulates REM propensity. In particular, serotonergic tone regulates the level of activity of the cholinergic pontine neurons that stimulate REM sleep (Rye, 1997). Sleep spindles are associated with low levels of hyperpolarization of thalamocortical GABAergic neurons, while SWS is associated with high levels of hyperpolarization of the same neurons and a complete inhibition of the thalamic relay (McCormick and Bal, 1997; Steriade *et al.*, 1993). Homeostatic mechanisms (e.g. enhancement of the propensity to sleep by prolonged wakefulness) determine the amount of SWS and contribute to the regulation of sleep spindles and the progression from spindles to SWS (Borbely, 1998; Dijk and Czeisler, 1995).

Power spectral analysis of the sleep EEG demonstrated that SWS sleep is characterized by high amplitude delta, which is inversely related to beta activity (Merica and Fortune, 1997; Portas *et al.*, 1997). The increase of low-frequency (in the theta-alpha range) power during extended wakefulness might be associated with the homeostatic process of sleepiness promotion (Cajochen *et al.*, 1999). An association between beta frequency and cortisol secretion was demonstrated (Chapotot *et al.*, 1998), suggesting a relationship between arousal and HPA axis function. Beta activity during non-REM sleep was found to be inversely correlated with subjective sleep quality (Nofzinger *et al.*, 2000).

It has been recently hypothesized that non-REM sleep involves the deactivation of the ventromedial prefrontal cortex, mediating a dissociation of higher order cortex from sensory cortex, which might be essential in restorative sleep (Nofzinger *et al.*, 2000).

Sleep Disturbances in Unipolar Depression

Sleep alterations in depression include reduced sleep time and sleep fragmentation, reduced REM latency (<65 min), increased percentage of time spent in REM sleep in the first part of the night and increased REM density (i.e. density of rapid eye movements during REM sleep), and reduced SWS, particularly during the first sleep cycle (Benca *et al.*, 1992; Lauer *et al.*, 1991; Reynolds and Kupfer, 1987; see also Brunello *et al.*, 2000; Riemann *et al.*, 2001, for reviews).

Most of these sleep abnormalities, probably with the only exception of increased REM density, are not specific to depressive patients (Benca *et al.*, 1992; Lauer *et al.*, 1991; Reynolds and Kupfer, 1987), and are more prominent in older than in young depressed subjects (Riemann *et al.*, 2001). The relationships of sleep abnormalities with severity of depression, endogenous or psychotic features, and the course of the illness remain controversial (Buysse *et al.*, 1994; Frank *et al.*, 1992; Kerkhofs *et al.*, 1988; Hubain *et al.*, 1995, 1996; Kupfer *et al.*, 1984, 1990; Riemann and Berger, 1989; Rush *et al.*, 1986; Thase *et al.*, 1986, 1995). Patients with seasonal affective disorders, which often present daytime sleepiness and fatigue, do not show the same sleep abnormalities reported in those with non-seasonal major depression (Anderson *et al.*, 1994; Brunner *et al.*, 1996; Palchikov *et al.*, 1997; Partonen *et al.*, 1993). However, they might have a disturbance in homeostatic processes as expressed by a lower increase of theta-alpha power during extended wakefulness, with respect to healthy controls (Cajochen *et al.*, 2000).

It is not clear whether some of the described sleep abnormalities might be present during phases of remission (Riemann and Berger, 1989; Rush *et al.*, 1986; Steiger *et al.*, 1989). Discrepancies in the findings might be related to the medication status of the subjects (REM sleep is likely to rebound at initial withdrawal from antidepressants) or to the definition of remission adopted by the different investigations. A reduced REM latency in remitted depressed subjects was found to be related to the risk of relapses (Buysse *et al.*, 1997; Giles *et al.*, 1987).

Cholinergic stimulation by arecoline administration was found to induce shorter latency REM episodes in remitted depressed subjects than in healthy comparison groups (Nurnberger *et al.*, 1989; Sitaram *et al.*, 1980). Relatives of depressed subjects without a personal lifetime history of affective disorders showed the same response to the cholinergic challenge (Krieg *et al.*, 2001; Schreiber *et al.*, 1992; Sitaram *et al.*, 1982); however, a study found that affectively ill relatives had shorter latency REM episodes than well relatives (Sitaram *et al.*, 1987), suggesting that the cholinergic hypersensitivity is both a trait and a state marker.

Increased REM density and reduced SWS were also reported in non-depressed subjects with a family history of affective disorders, suggesting that these abnormalities represent a vulnerability marker (Giles *et al.*, 1989; Krieg *et al.*, 2001; Lauer *et al.*, 1995).

Studies using power spectral analysis have reported that high pre-treatment delta activity, irrespective of sleep stage, is associated with clinical responsiveness (Kupfer *et al.*, 1994). The decrease of slow-wave activity in the first with respect to the second non-REM episode was found to be related to poor clinical response to both pharmacotherapy and psychotherapy (Ehlers *et al.*, 1996; Thase *et al.*, 1998).

Buysse *et al.* (1997) found that the upper frequency part of the delta activity (2–3 Hz) is related to the acute depressed state, while the lower part (0.5–1 Hz) is related to the risk of recurrence.

A study has reported an increase of beta activity in non-REM sleep in depressed as compared with healthy subjects, which was related to increased relative glucose metabolism in ventromedial prefrontal cortex (Nofzinger *et al.*, 2000).

Period analysis of the EEG has also been used to study sleep dysregulation in depression, particularly disturbances of ultradian rhythms (90 minutes, which is approximately the period of a sleep cycle). The main findings include a lower interhemispheric coherence in the beta and theta frequency range and reduced intrahemispheric coherence between delta and beta bands (Armitage *et al.*, 1992, 1993, 1995). The same abnormalities were found in remitted, previously depressed, drug-free patients (Armitage *et al.*, 1993), as well as in healthy relatives of affective patients (Armitage *et al.*, 2000). The authors interpret the data as evidence of dysregulated ultradian rest–activity cycle as a vulnerability marker of depression (Armitage *et al.*, 2000).

Sleep Disturbances in Subjects with Bipolar Affective Disorders

Several studies comparing age-matched unipolar and bipolar depressed subjects did not find any difference in sleep abnormalities (Duncan *et al.*, 1979; Feinberg and Carrol, 1984; Kerkhofs *et al.*, 1988; Lauer *et al.*, 1992).

Sleep architecture in bipolar depressed subjects with hypersomnia was found to be normal (Thase *et al.*, 1989).

Manic patients have severe sleep disorders but are difficult to investigate and only a few studies were carried out. Some of them reported a normal sleep architecture, while others found reduced REM latency and increased REM density with respect to healthy comparison groups (Gann *et al.*, 1993; Goodwin and Jamison, 1990; Hudson *et al.*, 1988, 1992). Unlike depressed patients, manic patients do not show reduced SWS (Hudson *et al.*, 1988, 1992).

CONCLUSIONS

In conclusion, a great amount of work has been carried out, but few questions have been clearly addressed and answered. Several limitations in many of the reviewed studies have hampered the possibility of fully exploiting the potential of such valuable work; the most important among them are the lack of strong hypotheses, the poor characterization of populations under investigation and the application of experimental paradigms using tasks which are far too simple to disclose cognitive-emotional dysfunctions specific to these disorders.

Some efforts must be acknowledged, such as the identification of psychophysiological markers of vulnerability to mood disorders and predictors of illness course, response to treatment and outcome. Vulnerability markers have been identified by research on eye tracking, quantitative EEG asymmetry and sleep architecture, while ERP studies have found predictors of response to SSRI drugs and sleep studies have characterized predictors of both course and treatment responsiveness. The clinical relevance of these research findings urges further investigation to confirm and extend the available evidence.

Much work has also been devoted to the search for a diagnostic marker, but no conclusion can be drawn. EDA reduction, REM dysregulation and the reduction of SWS are examples of proposed diagnostic markers for affective disorders. However, their efficiency was not systematically assessed and, when evaluated, has not always appeared satisfactory; according to some data it might be improved by the combination of multiple indices. Attempts at using psychophysiological indices to validate clinical subtypes (e.g. unipolar/bipolar, typical/atypical, endogenous/non-endogenous) have not been systematic, preventing clear conclusions. The use of psychophysiological indices to identify more homogeneous phenotypes might be a promising alternative strategy, which has not been adequately explored so far.

A few studies (e.g. those investigating ERP asymmetry during emotional activation) have designed experimental paradigms using tasks aimed at disclosing specific cognitive-emotional dysfunctions of affective disorders, yielding consistent findings. A larger application of these experimental paradigms is highly advisable.

Findings provided by EEG asymmetry studies in depression deserve special attention for their internal consistency and coherence with both neuropsychological and brain imaging findings (Bench *et al.*, 1992; 1993; Delvenne *et al.*, 1990; Fox, 1994; Passero *et al.*, 1995; Schlegel *et al.*, 1989). Future EEG and ERP studies in mood disorders might take advantage from the application of advanced electrophysiological topographic and tomographic techniques, such as the brain electrical microstates and low resolution electromagnetic tomography (LORETA) (Pascual-Marqui *et al.*, 1994).

An important limitation of psychophysiological research in mood disorders has been the poor control of confounding variables, such as medication status, age, gender, handedness, state or trait anxiety. This limitation has plagued early investigations in this field, and, surprisingly, can still be found in more recent work, despite clear demonstrations of the strong influence that such confounders exert on psychophysiological indices.

A task of future research should be the disambiguation of important empirical findings, such as those concerning EDA asymmetry, interpreted as either a hypoactivation or a hyperactivation of the right hemisphere.

Further progress of the whole research field might be fostered by studies carried out in a more comprehensive perspective—that is, combining, for example, clinical, psychophysiological, neuroendocrinological and brain imaging techniques.

REFERENCES

Abel, L.A., Friedman, L., Jesberger, J., Malki, A. and Meltzer, H.Y., 1991. Quantitative assessment of smooth pursuit gain and catch-up saccades in schizophrenia and affective disorders. *Biological Psychiatry*, **29**, 1063–72.

Albus, M., Engel, R.R., Muller, F., Zander, K.-J. and Ackenheil, M., 1982. Experimental stress situations and the state of autonomic arousal in schizophrenic and depressive patients. *International Pharmacopsychiatry*, **17**, 129–35.

Amador, X.F., Sackeim, H.A., Mukherjee, S., Halperin, R., Neeley, P., Maclin, E. and Schnur, D., 1991. Specificity of smooth pursuit eye movement and visual fixation abnormalities in schizophrenia — comparison to mania and normal controls. *Schizophrenia Research*, **5**, 135–44.

Amador, X.F., Malaspina, D., Sackeim, H.A., Coleman, E.A., Kaufmann, C.A., Hasan, A. and Gorman, J.M., 1995. Visual fixation and smooth pursuit eye movement abnormalities in patients with schizophrenia and their relatives. *Journal of Neuropsychiatry and Clinical Neurosciences*, **7**, 197–206.

Ancy, J., Gangadhar, B.N. and Janakiramaiah, N.N., 1996. 'Normal' P300 amplitude predicts rapid response to ECT in melancholia. *Journal of Affective Disorders*, **41**, 211–21.

Anderson, J.I., Rosen, L.N., Mendelson, W.B., Jacobsen, F.M., Skwerer, R.G., Joseph-Vanderpool, J.R., Duncan, C.C., Wehr, T.A. and Rosenthal, N.E., 1994. Sleep in fall/winter seasonal affective disorder: effects of light and changing season. *Journal of Psychosomatic Research*, **38**, 323–37.

Armitage, R. and Hoffmann, R., 1997. Sleep electrophysiology of major depressive disorders. *Current Review of Mood and Anxiety Disorders*, **1**, 139–51.

Armitage, R., Roffwarg, H.P., Rush, A.J., Calhoun, J.S., Purdy, D.G. and Giles, D.E., 1992. Digital period analysis of sleep EEG in depression. *Biological Psychiatry*, **31**, 52–68.

Armitage, R., Roffwarg, H.P. and Rush, A.J., 1993. Digital period analysis of EEG in depression: periodicity, coherence, and interhemispheric relationships during sleep. *Progress in Neuropsychopharmacology and Biological Psychiatry*, **17**, 363–72.

Armitage, R., Hudson, A., Trivedi, M. and Rush, A.J., 1995. Sex differences in the distribution of EEG frequencies during sleep: unipolar depressed outpatients. *Journal of Affective Disorders*, **34**, 121–9.

Armitage, R., Emslie, G.J., Hoffmann, R.F., Weinberg, W.A., Kowatch, R.A., Rintelmann, J. and Rush, J., 2000. Ultradian rhythms and temporal coherence in sleep EEG in depressed children and adolescents. *Biological Psychiatry*, **47**, 338–50.

Ashton, H., Golding, J.F., Marsh, V.R., Thompson, J.W., Hassanyeh, F. and Tyrer, S.P., 1988. Cortical evoked potentials and clinical rating scales as measures of depressive illness. *Psychological Medicine*, **18**, 305–7.

Austen, M.L. and Wilson, G.V., 2001. Increased vagal tone during winter in subsyndromal seasonal affective disorder. *Biological Psychiatry*, **50**, 28–34.

Baehr, E., Rosenfeld, J.P., Baehr, R. and Earnest, C., 1998. Comparison of two EEG asymmetry indices in depressed patients vs. normal controls. *International Journal of Psychophysiology*, **31**, 89–92.

Baker, N.J., Staunton, M., Adler, L.E., Gerhardt, G.A., Drebing, C., Waldo, M., Nagamoto, H. and Freedman, R., 1990. Sensory gating deficits in psychiatric in-patients: relation to catecholamine metabolites in different diagnostic groups. *Biological Psychiatry*, **27**, 519–28.

Bange, F. and Bathien, N., 1998. Visual cognitive dysfunction in depression: an event-related potential study. *Electroencephalography and Clinical Neurophysiology*, **108**, 472–81.

Barbini, B., Bertelli, S., Colombo, C. and Smeraldi, E., 1996. Sleep loss, a possible factor in augmenting manic episode. *Psychiatry Research*, **65**, 121–5.

Baron, M., Gershon, E.S., Rudy, V., Jones, W.Z. and Buchsbaum, M.S., 1975. Lithium carbonate response in depression. *Archives of General Psychiatry*, **32**, 1107–11.

Benca, R.M., Obermeyer, W.H., Thisted, R.A. and Gillin, J.C., 1992. Sleep and psychiatric disorders. A meta-analysis. *Archives of General Psychiatry*, **49**, 651–68.

Bench, C.J., Friston, K.J., Brown, R.G., Scott, L.C., Frackowiak, R.S.J. and Dolan, R.J., 1992. The anatomy of melancholia — focal abnormalities of cerebral blood flow in major depression. *Psychological Medicine*, **22**, 607–15.

Bench, C.J., Friston, K.J., Brown, R.G., Frackowiak, R.S. and Dolan, R.J., 1993. Regional cerebral blood flow in depression measured by positron emission tomography the relationship with clinical dimensions. *Psychological Medicine*, **23**, 579–90.

Bernardi, L., Keller, F., Sanders, M., Reddy, P.S., Griffith, B., Meno, F. and Pinsky, M.R., 1989. Respiratory sinus arrhythmia in the denervated human heart. *Journal of Applied Physiology*, **67**, 1447–55.

Bernstein, A.S., Taylor, K.W., Starkey, P., Juni, S., Lubowsksy, J. and Paley, H., 1981. Bilateral skin conductance, finger pulse volume, and EEG orienting response to tones of differing intensities in chronic schizophrenics and controls. *Journal of Nervous and Mental Disease*, **169**, 513–28.

Bernstein, A.S., Reidel, J.A., Graae, F., Seidman, D., Steele, H., Connolly, J. and Lubowsky, J., 1988. Schizophrenia is associated with altered orienting activity, depression with electrodermal (cholinergic?) deficit and normal orienting response. *Journal of Abnormal Psychology*, **97**, 3–12.

Bernstein, A.S., Schnur, D.B., Bernstein, P., Yeager, A., Wrable, J. and Smith, S., 1995. Differing patterns of electrodermal and finger pulse responsivity in schizophrenia and depression. *Psychological Medicine*, **25**, 51–62.

Blackwood, D., Whalley, L., Christie, J., Blackburn, I., St Clair, D. and McInnes, A., 1987. Changes in auditory P3 event-related potential in schizophrenia and depression. *British Journal of Psychiatry*, **150**, 154–60.

Blumberg, H.P., Stern, E., Martinez, D., Ricketts, S., de Asis, J., White, T., Epstein, J., McBride, P.A., Eidelberg, D., Kocsis, J.H. and Silbersweig, D.A., 2000. Increased anterior cingulate and caudate activity in bipolar mania. *Biological Psychiatry*, **48**, 1045–52.

Boivin, D.B., Czeisler, C., Dijk, D.J., Duffy, J.F., Folkard, S., Minors, D.S., Totterdell, P. and Waterhouse, J.M., 1997. Complex interaction of the sleep–wake cycle and circadian phase modulates mood in healthy subjects. *Archives of General Psychiatric*, **54**, 145–52.

Borbely, A.A., 1998. Processes underlying sleep regulation. *Hormone Research*, **49**, 114–17.

Brenner, R.P., Ulrich, R.F., Spiker, D.G., Sclabassi, R.J., Reynolds, C.F., Marin, R.S. and Boller, F., 1986. Computerized EEG spectral analysis in elderly normal, demented and depressed subjects. *Electroencephalography and Clinical Neurophysiology*, **64**, 438–92.

Bruder, G.E., 1995. Cerebral laterality and psychopathology: perceptual and event-related potential asymmetries in affective and schizophrenic disorders. In: Davidson, R.J. and Hugdahl, K. (eds), *Brain Asymmetry*, pp. 661–91. MIT Press, Cambridge, MA.

Bruder, G.E., Toewy, J.P., Stewart, J.W., Friedman, D., Tenke, C. and Quitkin, F.M., 1991. Event-related potentials in depression: influence of task, stimulus hemifield and clinical features on P3 latency. *Biological Psychiatry*, **30**, 233–46.

Bruder, G.E., Stewart, J.W., Towey, J.P., Friedman, D., Tenke, C.R., Voglmaier, M.M., Leite, P., Cohen, P. and Quitkin, M., 1992. Abnormal cerebral laterality in bipolar depression: convergence of behavioral and brain event-related potential findings. *Biological Psychiatry*, **32**, 33–47.

Bruder, G.E., Tenke, C.E., Stewart, J.W., Towey, J.P., Leite, P., Voglmaier, M. and Quitkin, F.M., 1995. Brain event-related potentials to complex tones in depressed patients: relations to perceptual asymmetry and clinical features. *Psychophysiology*, **32**, 373–81.

Bruder, G.E., Fong, R., Tenke, C.E., Leite, P., Towey, J.P., Stewart, J.E., McGrath, P.J. and Quitkin, F.M., 1997. Regional brain asymmetries in major depression with or without an anxiety disorder: a quantitative electroencephalographic study. *Biological Psychiatry*, **41**, 939–48.

Bruder, G.E., Tenke, C.E., Towey, J.P., Leite, P., Fong, R., Stewart, J.E., McGrath, P.J. and Quitkin, F.M., 1998. Brain ERPs of depressed patients to complex tones in an oddball task: relation of reduced P3 asymmetry to physical anhedonia. *Psychophysiology*, **35**, 54–63.

Brunello, N., Armitage, R., Feinberg, I., Holsboer-Trachsler, E., Léger, D., Linkowski, P., Mendelson, W.B., Racagni, G., Saletu, B., Sharpley, A.L., Turek, F., Van Cauter, E. and Mendlewicz, J., 2000. Depression and sleep disorders: clinical relevance, economic burden and pharmacological treatment. *Neuropsychobiology*, **42**, 107–19.

Brunner, D.P., Kräuchi, K., Dijk, D.J., Leonhardt, G., Haugh, H.J. and Wirz-Justice, A., 1996. Sleep EEG in seasonal affective disorder and control women: effects of midday light treatment and sleep deprivation. *Biological Psychiatry*, **40**, 485–96.

Buchsbaum, M.S. and Silverman, J., 1968. Stimulus intensity control and the cortical evoked response. *Psychosomatic Medicine*, **30**, 12–22.

Buchsbaum, M.S., Goodwin, F., Murphy, D. and Borge, G., 1971. AER in affective disorders. *American Journal of Psychiatry*, **128**, 19–25.

Buchsbaum, M.S., Carpenter, W.T., Fedio, P., Goodwin, F.K., Murphy, D.L. and Post, R.M., 1979. Hemispheric differences in evoked potential enhancement by selective attention to hemiretinally presented stimuli in schizophrenic, affective and post-temporal lobectomy patients. In: Gruzelier, J. and Flor-Henry, P. (eds), *Hemispheric Asymmetries of Function in Psychopathology*, pp. 317–28. Elsevier, Amsterdam.

Buysse, D.J., Kupfer, D.J., Frank, E., Monk, T. and Ritenour, A., 1994. Do electroencephalographic sleep studies predict recurrence in depressed patients successfully treated with psychotherapy? *Depression*, **2**, 105–8.

Buysse, D.J., Frank, E., Lowe, K.K., Cherry, C.R. and Kupfer, D.J., 1997. Electroencephalographic sleep correlates of episode and vulnerability to recurrence in depression. *Biological Psychiatry*, **41**, 406–18.

Cajochen, C., Foy, R. and Dijk, D.J., 1999. Frontal predominance of a relative increase in sleep delta and theta EEG activity after sleep loss in humans. *Sleep Research Online*, **2**, 65–9.

Cajochen, C., Brunner, D.P., Kräuchi, K., Graw, P. and Wirz-Justice, A., 2000. EEG and subjective sleepiness during extended wakefulness in seasonal affective disorder: circadian and homeostatic influences. *Biological Psychiatry*, **47**, 610–17.

Carney, R.M., Rich, M.W., TeVelde, A., Saini, J., Clark, K. and Freeland, E., 1988. The relationship between heart rate, heart rate variability and depression in patients with coronary artery disease. *Journal of Psychosomatic Research*, **32**, 159–64.

Carney, R.M., Saunders, R.D., Freedland, K.E., Stein, P., Rich, M.W. and Jaffe, A.S. (1995a) Depression is associated with reduced heart rate variability in patients with coronary heart disease. *American Journal of Cardiology*, **76**, 562–4.

Carney, R.M., Freedland, K.E., Rich, M.W. and Jaffe, A.S. (1995b) Depression as a risk factor for cardiac events in established coronary hearth disease: a review of possible mechanisms. *Annals of Behavioral Medicine*, **17**, 142–9.

Carney, R.M., Freedland, K.E., Veith, R.C., Cryer, P.E., Skala, J.A., Lynch, T. and Jaffe, A.S., 1999. Major depression, heart rate, and plasma norepinephrine in patients with coronary heart disease. *Biological Psychiatry*, **45**, 458–63.

Cegalis, J.A. and Sweeney, J.A., 1981. The effect of attention on smooth pursuit eye movements of schizophrenics. *Journal of Psychiatry Research*, **16**, 145–61.

Chapotot, F., Gronfier, C., Jouny, C., Muzet, A. and Brandenberger, G., 1998. Cortisol secretion is related to electroencephalographic alertness in human subjects during daytime wakefulness. *Journal of Clinical Endocrinology and Metabolism*, **83**, 4263–8.

Cook, I.A., Leuchter, A.F., Witte, E., Abrams, M., Uijtdehaage, S.H.J., Stubbeman, W., Rosenberg-Thompson, S. and Anderson-Hanley, C., 1999. Neuropsychologic predictors of treatment response to fluoxetine in major depression. *Psychiatry Research*, **85**, 263–73.

Corbett, J.J., Jacobson, D.M., Thompson, H.S., Hart, M.N. and Albert, D.W., 1989. Downbeating nystagmus and other ocular motor defects caused by lithium toxicity. *Neurology*, **39**, 481–7.

Crawford, T.J., Haeger, B., Kennard, C., Reveley, M.A. and Henderson, L., 1995. Saccadic abnormalities in psychotic patients. II. The role of neuroleptic treatment. *Psychological Medicine*, **25**, 473–83.

Dahabra, S., Ashton, C.H., Bahrainian, M., Britton, P.G., Ferrier, I.N., McAllister, V.A., Marsh, V.R. and Moore, P.B., 1998. Structural and functional abnormalities in elderly patients clinically recovered from early- and late-onset depression. *Biological Psychiatry*, **44**, 34–46.

Dalack, G.W. and Roose, S.P., 1990. Perspectives on the relationship between cardiovascular disease and affective disorder. *Journal of Clinical Psychiatry*, **51**, 4–9.

Davidson, R.J., 1987. Cerebral asymmetry and the nature of emotion: implications for the study of individual differences and psychopathology. In: Takahashi, R., Flor-Henry, P., Gruzelier, J. and Niwa, S. (eds), *Cerebral Dynamics, Laterality and Psychopathology*, pp. 71–83. Elsevier, Amsterdam.

Davidson, R.J., 1992. Anterior cerebral asymmetry and the nature of emotion. *Brain and Cognition*, **20**, 125–51.

Davidson, R.J., Chapman, J.P. and Chapman, L.J., 1987. Task-dependent EEG asymmetry discriminates between depressed and non-depressed subjects. *Psychophysiology*, **24**, 585.

Dawson, M.E., Schell, A.M. and Catania, J.J., 1977. Autonomic correlates of depression and clinical improvement following electroconvulsive shock therapy. *Psychophysiology*, **14**, 569–78.

Dawson, M.E., Schell, A.M., Braaten, J.R. and Catania, J.J., 1985. Diagnostic utility of autonomic measures for major depressive disorders. *Psychiatry Research*, **15**, 261–70.

Deldin, P.J., Keller, J., Gergen, J.A. and Miller, G.A., 2000. Right-posterior face processing anomaly in depression. *Journal of Abnormal Psychology*, **109**, 116–21.

Delvenne, V., Delecluse, F., Hubain, P.P., Schoutens, A., De Maertelaer, V. and Mendlewicz, J., 1990. Regional cerebral blood flow in patients with affective disorders. *British Journal of Psychiatry*, **157**, 359–65.

Dijk, D.J. and Czeisler, C.A., 1995. Contribution of the circadian pacemaker and the sleep homeostat to sleep propensity, sleep structure, electroencephalographic slow waves, and sleep spindle activity in humans. *Journal of Neuroscience*, **15**, 3526–38.

Dolan, R.J., Bench, C.J., Brown, R.G., Scott, L.C., Friston, K.J. and Frackowiak, R.S.J., 1992. Regional cerebral blood flow abnormalities in depressed patients with cognitive impairment. *Journal of Neurology, Neurosurgery and Psychiatry*, **55**, 768–73.

Done, D.J. and Frith, C.D., 1989. Automatic and strategic volitional saccadic eye movements in psychotic patients. *Archives of Psychiatric and Neurological Sciences*, **239**, 27–32.

Duncan, W.C., Pettigrew, K.D. and Gillin, J.C., 1979. REM architecture changes in bipolar and unipolar depression. *American Journal of Psychiatry*, **136**, 1424–7.

Ehlers, C.L., Haustad, J.W. and Kupfer, D.J., 1996. Estimation of the time course of slow wave sleep over the night in depressed patients: effects of clomipramine and clinical response. *Biological Psychiatry*, **39**, 171–81.

el Massioui, F. and Lesevre, N., 1988. Attention impairment and psychomotor retardation in depressed patients: an event-related potential study. *Electroencephalography and Clinical Neurophysiology*, **70**, 46–55.

Elton, M., 1984. A longitudinal investigation of event-related potentials in depression. *Biological Psychiatry*, **19**, 1635–49.

Feinberg, J. and Carrol, B.J., 1984. Biological 'markers' for endogenous depression. *Archives of General Psychiatry*, **41**, 1080–5.

Flechtner, K.-M., Steinacher, B., Sauer, R. and Mackert, A., 1997. Smooth pursuit eye movements in schizophrenia and affective disorder. *Psychological Medicine*, **27**, 1411–9.

Flor-Henry, P., 1987. Cerebral dynamics, laterality and psychopathology: a commentary. In: Takahashi, R., Flor-Henry, P., Gruzelier, J. and Niwa, S. (eds), *Cerebral Dynamics, Laterality and Psychopathology*, pp. 3–21. Elsevier, Amsterdam.

Flor-Henry, P. and Koles, Z.J., 1984. Statistical quantitative EEG studies of depression, mania, schizophrenia and normals. *Biological Psychology*, **19**, 257–79.

Flor-Henry, P., Koles, Z.J., Howarth, B.G. and Burton, L., 1979. Neurophysiological studies of schizophrenia, mania and depression. In: Gruzelier, J. and Flor-Henry, P. (eds), *Hemisphere Asymmetries of Function in Psychology*, pp. 189–222. Elsevier, Amsterdam.

Ford, D.E. and Kamerow, D.B., 1989. Epidemiologic study of sleep disturbances and psychiatric disorders. An opportunity for prevention? *Journal of the American Medical Association*, **262**, 1479–84.

Fowles, D.C., 1986. The eccrine system and electrodermal activity. In: Coles, M.G.H., Donchin, E. and Porges, S.W. (eds), *Psychophysiology, Systems, Processes, and Applications*, pp. 508–610. Guilford Press, New York.

Fox, N.A., 1994. Dynamic cerebral processes underlying emotion regulation. In: Fox, N.A. (ed.), *The Development of Emotion Regulation. Biological and Behavioral Consideration*, Monographs of the Society for Research in Child Development, pp. 152–66. University of Chicago Press, Chicago, IL.

Frank, E., Kupfer, D.J., Hamer, T., Grochocinski, V.J. and McEachran, A.B., 1992. Maintenance treatment and psychobiologic correlates of endogenous subtypes. *Journal of Affective Disorders*, **25**, 181–90.

Franks, R., Adler, L., Waldo, M., Alpert, J. and Freedman, R., 1983. Neurophysiological studies of sensory gating in mania: comparison with schizophrenia. *Biological Psychiatry*, **18**, 989–1005.

Freedman, R., Adler, L.E., Gerhardt, G.A., Waldo, M., Baker, N., Rose, G.M., Drebing, C., Nagamoto, H., Bickford-Wimer, P. and Franks, R., 1987. Neurobiological studies of sensory gating in schizophrenia. *Schizophrenia Bulletin*, **13**, 669–78.

Friedman, L., Abel, L.A., Jesberger, J.A., Malki, A. and Meltzer, H.Y., 1992. Saccadic intrusions into smooth pursuit in patients with schizophrenia or affective disorder and normal controls. *Biological Psychiatry*, **31**, 1110–8.

Friedman, L., Jesberger, J.A., Siever, L.J., Thompson, P., Mohs, R. and Meltzer, H.Y., 1995. Smooth pursuit performance in patients with affective disorders or schizophrenia and normal controls: analysis with specific oculomotor measures, RMS error and qualitative ratings. *Psychological Medicine*, **25**, 387–403.

Frith, C., Stevens, M., Johnstone, E. and Crow, T., 1982. Skin conductance habituation during acute episodes of schizophrenia: quantitative differences from anxious and depressed patients. *Psychological Medicine*, **12**, 575–83.

Fukushima, J., Morita, N., Fukushima, A.K., Chiba, T., Tanaka, S. and Yamashita, I., 1990. Voluntary control of saccadic eye movements in patients with schizophrenic and affective disorders. *Journal of Psychiatry Research*, **24**, 9–24.

Galderisi, S., Mucci, A., Bucci, P., Mignone, M.L. and Maj, M., 1996. Influence of moclobemide on cognitive functions of nine depressed patients: pilot trial with neurophysiological and neuropsychological indices. *Neuropsychobiology*, **33**, 48–54.

Gallinat, J., Bottlender, R., Juckel, G., Munke-Puchner, A., Stotz, G., Kuss, H.J., Mavrogiorgou, P. and Hegerl, U., 2000. The loudness dependency of the auditory evoked N1/P2-component as a predictor of the acute SSRI response in depression. *Psychopharmacology*, **148**, 404–11.

Gangadhar, B.N., Ancy, J., Janakiramaiah, N. and Umapathy, C., 1993. P300 amplitude in non-bipolar, melancholic depression. *Journal of Affective Disorders*, **28**, 57–60.

Gann, H., Riemann, D., Hohagen, F., Strauss, L.G., Dressing, H., Müller, W.E. and Berger, M., 1993. 48-hour rapid cycling: results of psychometric, polysomnographic, PET imaging and neuroendocrine longitudinal investigations in a single case. *Journal of Affective Disorders*, **28**, 133–40.

Gehricke, J.-G. and Shapiro, D., 2001. Facial and autonomic activity in depression: social context differences during imagery. *International Journal of Psychophysiology*, **41**, 53–64.

Giedke, H., Bolz, J. and Heimann, H., 1980. Evoked potentials, expectancy wave, and skin resistance in depressed patients and healthy controls. *Pharmacopsychiatry*, **13**, 91–101.

Giles, D.E., Jarrett, R.B., Roffwarg, H.P. and Rush, A.J., 1987. Reduced rapid eye movement latency: a predictor of recurrence in depression. *Neuropsychopharmacology*, **1**, 33–9.

Giles, D.E., Jarrett, R.B., Biggs, M.M., Rush, A.J. and Roffwarg, H.P., 1989. Longitudinal assessment of EEG sleep in depression and clinical remission. *Sleep Research*, **18**, 175.

Gooding, D.C., Iacono, W.G., Katsanis, J., Meiser, M. and Grove, W.M., 1993. The association between lithium carbonate and smooth pursuit eye tracking among first-episode patients with psychotic affective disorders. *Psychophysiology*, **30**, 3–9.

Gooding, D.C., Grabowski, J.A. and Hendershot, C.S., 2000. Fixation stability in schizophrenia, bipolar, and control subjects. *Psychiatry Research*, **97**, 119–28.

Goodwin, F. and Jamison, K., 1990. *Manic-Depressive Illness*. Oxford University Press, New York.

Gotlib, I.H., Ranganath, C. and Rosenfeld, J.P., 1998. Frontal EEG alpha asymmetry, depression, and cognitive functioning. *Cognition and Emotion*, **12**, 449–78.

Graae, F., Tenke, C., Bruder, G., Rotheram, M.J., Piacentini, J., Castro-Blanco, D., Leite, P. and Towey, J., 1996. Abnormality of EEG alpha asymmetry in female adolescent suicide attempters. *Biological Psychiatry*, **40**, 706–13.

Gruzelier, J. and Venables, P., 1974. Bimodality and lateral asymmetry of skin conductance orienting activity in schizophrenics: replication and evidence of lateral asymmetry in patients with depression and disorders of personality. *Biological Psychiatry*, **8**, 55–73.

Halgren, E., 1990. Evoked potentials. In: Boulton, A.A., Baker, G. and Vanderwolf, C. (eds), *Neuromethods,* vol. 15, *Neurophysiological Techniques: Applications to Neural Systems*, pp. 147–275. Humana, Clifton, NJ.

Have, G., Kolbeinsson, H. and Petursson, H. (1991)Dementia and depression in old age: psychophysiological aspects. *Acta Psychiatrica Scandinavica*, **83**, 329–33.

Hegerl, U. and Juckel, G., 1993. Intensity dependence of auditory evoked potentials as an indicator of central serotonergic neurotransmission: a new hypothesis. *Biological Psychiatry*, **33**, 173–87.

Hegerl, U., Gallinat, J. and Juckel, G., 2001. Event-related potentials. Do they reflect central serotonergic neurotransmission and do they predict clinical response to serotonin agonists? *Journal of Affective Disorders*, **62**, 93–100.

Hegerl, U., Ulrich, G. and Müller-Oerlinghausen, B., 1986. Augmenting-reducing response to auditory evoked potentials and its relationship to the prophylaptic effect of lithium salt. *Pharmacopsychiatry*, **19**, 274–5.

Hegerl, U., Ulrich, G. and Müller-Oerlinghausen, B., 1987. Auditory evoked potentials and response to lithium prophylaxis. *Pharmacopsychiatry*, **20**, 213–6.

Henriques, J.B. and Davidson, R.J., 1989. Affective disorders. In: Turpin, G. (ed.), *Handbook of Clinical Psychophysiology* pp. 357–92. John Wiley & Sons, Chichester.

Henriques, J.B. and Davidson, R.J., 1990. Regional brain electrical asymmetries discriminate between previously depressed and healthy control subjects. *Journal of Abnormal Psychology*, **99**, 22–31.

Henriques, J.B. and Davidson, R.J., 1991. Left frontal hypoactivation in depression. *Journal of Abnormal Psychology*, **100**, 535–45.

Henriques, J.B. and Davidson, R.J., 1997. Brain electrical asymmetries during cognitive task performance in depressed and non-depressed subjects. *Biological Psychiatry*, **42**, 1039–50.

Holzman, P.S., 1985. Eye movement dysfunctions and psychosis. *International Review of Neurobiology*, **27** 179–205.

Holzman, P.S., 1987. Recent studies of psychophysiology in schizophrenia. *Schizophrenia Bulletin*, **13**, 49–75.

Holzman, P.S., Proctor, L.R. and Hughes, D.W., 1973. Eye-tracking patterns in schizophrenia. *Science*, **181**, 179–81.

Holzman, P.S., Proctor, L.R., Levy, D.L., Yasillo, N.J., Meltzer, H.Y. and Hurt, S.W., 1974. Eye-tracking dysfunctions in schizophrenic patients and their relatives. *Archives of General Psychiatry*, **31**, 143–51.

Holzman, P.S., Levy, D.L., Uhlenhuth, L.R., Proctor, L.R. and Freedman, D.X., 1975. Smooth-pursuit eye movements and diazepam, CPZ, and secobarbital. *Psychopharmacologia*, **44**, 111–15.

Holzman, P.S., Solomon, C.M., Levin, S. and Waternaux, C.S., 1984. Pursuit eye movement dysfunctions in schizophrenia: family evidence for specificity. *Archives of General Psychiatry*, **41**, 136–9.

Holzman, P.S., O'Brian, C. and Waternaux, C., 1991. Effects of lithium treatment on eye movements. *Biological Psychiatry*, **29**, 1001–15.

Hubain, P.P., Sourey, D., Jonck, L., Staner, L., Van Veeren, C., Kerkhofs, M., Mendlewicz, J. and Linkowski, P., 1995. Relationship between the Newcastle scale and sleep polysomnographic variables in major depression: a controlled study. *European Neuropsychopharmacology*, **5**, 129–34.

Hubain, P., Van Veeren, C., Staner, L., Mendlewicz, J. and Linkowski, P., 1996. Neuroendocrine and sleep variables in major depressed in-patients: role of severity. *Psychiatry Research*, **63**, 83–92.

Hudson, J.I., Lipinski, J.F., Frankenburg, F.R., Grochocinski, V.J. and Kupfer, D.J., 1988. Electroencephalographic sleep in mania. *Archives of General Psychiatry*, **45**, 267–73.

Hudson, J.I., Lipinski, J.F., Keck, P.E., Aizley, H.G., Likas, S.E., Rothschild, A., Waternaux, C.M. and Kupfer, D.J., 1992. Polysomnographic characteristics of young manic patients. *Archives of General Psychiatry*, **49**, 378–83.

Iacono, W.G. and Clementz, B.A., 1992. A strategy for elucidating genetic influences on complex psychopathological syndromes (with special references to ocular motor function and schizophrenia) In: Chapman, L.J., Chapman, J.P. and Fowels, D.C. (eds), *Progress in Experimental Personality and Psychopathology Research: Frontiers of Psychopathology*, vol. 16, pp. 11–65. Springer, New York.

Iacono, W.G. and Koenig, W.G.R., 1983. Features that distinguish the smooth-pursuit eye-tracking performance of schizophrenic, affective-disorder, and normal individuals. *Journal of Abnormal Psychology*, **92**, 29–41.

Iacono, W.G. and Tuason, V.B., 1983. Bilateral electrodermal asymmetry in euthymic patients with unipolar and bipolar affective disorders. *Biological Psychiatry*, **18**, 303–15.

Iacono, W.G., Peloquin, L.J., Lumry, A.E., Valentine, R.H. and Tuason, V.B., 1982. Eye tracking in patients with unipolar and bipolar affective disorders in remission. *Journal of Abnormal Psychology*, **91**, 35–44.

Iacono, W.G., Lykken, D.T., Peloquin, L.J., Lumry, A.E., Valentine, R.H. and Tuason, V.B., 1983. Electrodermal activity in euthymic unipolar and bipolar affective disorders. *Archives of General Psychiatry*, **40**, 557–65.

Iacono, W.G., Lykken, D.T., Haroian, K.P., Peloquin, L.J., Valentine, R.H. and Tuason, V.B., 1984. Electrodermal activity in euthymic patients with affective disorders: one-year retest stability and the effects of stimulus intensity and significance. *Journal of Abnormal Psychology*, **93**, 304–11.

Iacono, W.G., Moreau, M., Beiser, M., Fleming, A.E. and Lin, T.Y., 1992. Smooth-pursuit eye tracking in first-episode psychotic patients and their relatives. *Journal of Abnormal Psychology*, **101**, 104–16.

Jacobsen, J., Hauksson, P. and Vestergaard, P., 1984. Heart rate variation in patients treated with antidepressants. An index of anticholinergic effects? *Psychopharmacology*, **84**, 544–8.

John, E.R., Prichep, L.S., Fridman, J. and Easton, P., 1988. Neurometrics: computer-assisted differential diagnosis of brain dysfunctions. *Science*, **239**, 162–9.

Juckel, G., Molnar, M., Hegerl, U., Csepe, V. and Karmos, G., 1997. Auditory-evoked potentials as indicator of brain serotonergic activity — first evidence in behaving cats. *Biological Psychiatry*, **41**, 1181–95.

Juckel, G., Hegerl, U., Molnar, M., Csepe, V. and Karmos, G., 1999. Auditory evoked potentials reflect serotonergic neuronal activity — a study in behaving cats administered drugs acting on 5-HT1A autoreceptors in the dorsal raphe nucleus. *Neuropsychopharmacology*, **21**, 710–6.

Katsanis, J., Ficken, J., Iacono, W.G. and Beiser, M., 1992. Season of birth and electrodermal activity in functional psychoses. *Biological Psychiatry*, **31**, 841–55.

Kayser, J., Bruder, G.E., Tenke, C.E., Stewart, J.W. and Quitkin, F.M., 2000. Event-related potentials (ERPs) to hemifield presentations of emotional stimuli: differences between depressed patients and healthy adults in P3 amplitude and asymmetry. *International Journal of Psychophysiology*, **36**, 211–36.

Kemali, D., Vacca, L., Marciano, F., Nolfe, G. and Iorio, G., 1981. CEEG findings in schizophrenics, depressives, obsessives, heroin addicts and normals. *Advances in Biological Psychiatry*, **6**, 17–28.

Kerkhofs, M., Kempenaers, C., Linkowski, P., de Maertelaer, V. and Mendlewicz, J., 1988. Multivariate study of sleep EEG in depression. *Acta Psychiatrica Scandinavica*, **77**, 463–8.

Klein, R.H., Salzman, L.F., Jones, F. and Ritzler, B., 1976. Eye tracking in psychiatric patients and their offspring. *Psychophysiology*, **13**, 186.

Knott, V. and Lapierre, Y. (1987a) Electrophysiological and behavioural correlates of psychomotor responsivity in depression. *Biological Psychiatry*, **22**, 313–24.

Knott, V.J. and Lapierre, Y.D. (1987b) Computerized EEG correlates of depression and antidepressant treatment. *Progress in Neuropsychopharmacology and Biological Psychiatry*, **11**, 213–21.

Knott, V., Waters, B., Lapierre, Y. and Gray, R., 1985. Neurophysiological correlates of sibling pairs discordant for bipolar affective disorder. *American Journal of Psychiatry*, **142**, 248–50.

Koenig, T. and Lehmann, D., 1996. Microstates in language-related brain potential maps show noun-verb differences. *Brain and Language*, **53**, 169–82.

Krieg, J.-C., Laurere, C.J., Schreiber, W., Modell, S. and Holsboer, F., 2001. Neuroendocrine, polysomnographic and psychometric observations in healthy subjects at high familial risk for affective disorders: the current state of the 'Munich vulnerability study'. *Journal of Affective Disorders*, **62**, 33–7.

Küfferle, B., Friedmann, A., Topitz, A., Földes, P., Kutzer, M. and Steinberger, K., 1990. Smooth pursuit eye movements in schizophrenia: influences of neuroleptic treatment and the question of specificity. *Psychopathology*, **23**, 106–14.

Kupfer, D.J., Ulrich, R.F., Coble, P.A., Jarrett, D.B., Grochocinski, V.J., Doman, J., Matthews, G. and Bórbely, A.A., 1984. Application of automated REM and slow wave sleep analysis: I. Normal and depressed subjects. *Psychiatry Research*, **13**, 325–34.

Kupfer, D.J., Frank, E., McEachran, A.B. and Grochocinski, V.J., 1990. Delta sleep ratio: a biological correlate of early recurrence in unipolar affective disorder. *Archives of General Psychiatry*, **477**, 1100–5.

Kupfer, D.J., Ehlers, C.L., Frank, E., Grochocinski, V.J., McEachran, A.B. and Buhari, A., 1994. Persistent effects of antidepressants: EEG sleep studies in depressed patients during maintenance treatment. *Biological Psychiatry*, **35**, 781–93.

Lader, M.H. and Wing, L., 1969. Physiological measures in agitated and retarded depressed patients. *Psychiatry Research*, **7**, 89–95.

Lahmeyer, H.W. and Bellur, S.N., 1987. Cardiac regulation and depression. *Psychiatry Research*, **21**, 1–6.

Lauer, C.J., Rieman, D., Wiegand, M. and Berger, M., 1991. From early to late adulthood: changes in EEG sleep of depressed patients and healthy volunteers. *Biological Psychiatry*, **29**, 979–93.

Lauer, C.J., Wiegand, M. and Krieg, J.C., 1992. All-night electroencephalographic sleep and cranial computed tomography in depression. *European Archives of Psychiatry and Clinical Neuroscience*, **242**, 59–68.

Lauer, C.J., Schreiber, W., Holsboer, F. and Krieg, J.C., 1995. In quest of identifying vulnerability markers for psychiatric disorders by all-night polysomnography. *Archives of General Psychiatry*, **52**, 145–53.

Lehmann, D., 1987. Principles of spatial analysis. In: Gevins, A.S. and Redmond, A. (eds), *Methods of Analysis of Brain Electrical and Magnetic Signals. Handbook of Electroencephalography and Clinical Neurophysiology*, vol. 1, pp. 309–54. Elsevier, Amsterdam.

Lehofer, M., Moser, M., Hoehn-Saric, R., McLeod, D., Liebmann, P., Drnovsek, B., Egner, S., Hildebrandt, G. and Zapotoczky, H.-G., 1997. Major depression and cardiac autonomic control. *Biological Psychiatry*, **42**, 914–19.

Lenhart, R.E. and Katkin, E.S., 1986. Psychophysiological evidence for cerebral laterality effects in a high-risk sample of students with subsyndromal bipolar depressive disorder. *American Journal of Psychiatry*, **143**, 602–7.

Leuchter, A.F., Uijtdehaage, S.H.J., Cook, I.A., O'Hara, R. and Mandelkers, M., 1999. Relationship between brain electrical activity and cerebral energy utilization in normal subjects. *Psychiatry Research: Neuroimaging Section*, **90**, 125–40.

Levin, S., Lipton, R.B. and Holzman, P.S., 1981. Pursuit eye movement in psychopathology: effects of target characteristics. *Biological Psychiatry*, **16**, 255–67.

Levinson, D.F., 1991. Skin conductance orienting response in unmedicated RDC schizophrenic, schizoaffective, depressed, and control subjects. *Biological Psychiatry*, **30**, 663–83.

Levy, D.L., Lipton, R.B., Yasillo, N.J., Peterson, J., Pandey, G.N. and Davis, J.M., 1984. Psychotropic drug effects on smooth pursuit eye movements: a summary of recent findings. In: Gale, A.G. and Johnson, F. (eds), *Theoretical and Applied Aspects of Eye Movement Research*, pp. 497–505. North-Holland, Amsterdam.

Levy, D.L., Dorus, E., Shaughnessy, R., Yasillo, N.J., Pandey, G.N., Janical, P.G., Gibbons, R.D., Gaviria, M. and Davis, J.M., 1985. Pharmacologic evidence for specificity of pursuit dysfunction to schizophrenia: lithium carbonate associated abnormal pursuit. *Archives of General Psychiatry*, **42**, 335–41.

Levy, J., Heller, W., Banich, M.T. and Burton, L.A., 1983. Are variations among right-handed individuals in perceptual asymmetries caused by characteristic arousal differences between hemispheres? *Journal of Experimental Psychology*, **9**, 329–59.

Lipton, R.B., Levin, S. and Holzman, P.S., 1980. Horizontal and vertical pursuit eye movements, the oculocephalic reflex, and the functional psychoses. *Psychiatry Research*, **3**, 193–203.

Livingston, G., Blizard, B. and Mann, A., 1993. Does sleep disturbance predict depression in elderly people? A study in inner London. *British Journal of General Practice*, **43**, 445–8.

Malliani, A., Pagani, M., Lombardi, F. and Cerutti, S., 1991. Cardiovascular neural regulation explored in the frequency domain. *Circulation*, **84**, 482–92.

Matousek, M., Capone, C. and Okawa, M., 1981.Measurement of the interhemispheral differences as a diagnostic tool in psychiatry. *Advances in Biological Psychiatry*, **6**, 76–80.

McCormick, D.A. and Bal, T., 1997. Sleep and arousal: thalamocortical mechanisms. *Annual Review in Neuroscience*, **20**, 185–215.

Merica, H. and Fortune, R.D., 1997. A neuronal transition probability model for the evolution of power in the sigma and delta frequency bands of sleep EEG. *Physiological Behaviour*, **62**, 585–9.

Miquel, M., Fuentes, I., Garcia-Merita, M. and Rojo, L., 1999. Habituation and sensitization processes in depressive disorders. *Psychopathology*, **32**, 35–42.

Moser, M., Lehofer, M., Hoehn-Saric, R., McLeod, D.R., Hildebrandt, G., Steinbrenner, B., Voica, M., Liebmann, P. and Zapotoczky, G., 1998. Increased heart rate in depressed subjects in spite of unchanged autonomic balance? *Journal of Affective Disorders*, **48**, 115–24.

Muir, W.J., St Clair, D.M., Blackwood, D.H.R., Roxburgh, H.M. and Marshall, I., 1992. Eye-tracking dysfunction in the affective psychoses and schizophrenia. *Psychological Medicine*, **22**, 573–80.

Myslobosky, M.S. and Horesh, N., 1978. Bilateral electrodermal activity in depressive patients. *Biological Psychology*, **6**, 111–20.

Nofzinger, E.A., Price, J.C., Meltzer, C.C., Buysse, D.J., Villemagne, V.L., Miewald, J.M., Sembrat, R.C., Steppe, D.A. and Kupfer, D.J., 2000. Towards a neurobiology of dysfunctional arousal in depression: the

relationship between beta EEG power and regional cerebral glucose metabolism during NREM sleep. *Psychiatry Research: Neuroimaging Section*, **98**, 71–91.
Nurnberger, J., Gershon, E., Murphy, D., Buchsbaum, M.S., Hamovit, J., Lamour, M., Rappaport, J. and Gershon, E., 1979. Biological and clinical predictors of lithium response in depression. In: Cooper, R., Gershon, E., Kline, G. and Schou, R. (eds), *Lithium—Controversies and Unresolved Issues*, pp. 241–56. Excerpta Medica, Amsterdam.
Nurnberger, J., Berrettini, W., Mendelson, W., Sack, D. and Gershon, E.S., 1989. Measuring cholinergic sensitivity: I. Arecoline effects in bipolar patients. *Biological Psychiatry*, **25**, 610–7.
Nystrom, C., Matousek, M. and Hallstrom, T., 1986. Relationships between EEG and clinical characteristics in major depressive disorder. *Acta Psychiatrica Scandinavica*, **73**, 390–4.
Ogura, C., Nageishi, Y., Omura, F., Fukao, K., Ohta, H., Kishimoto, A. and Matsubayashi, M., 1993. N200 component of event-related potentials in depression. *Biological Psychiatry*, **33**, 720–6.
Palchikov, V.E., Zolotarev, D.Y., Danilenko, K.V. and Putilov, A.A., 1997. Effects of the seasons and of bright light administered at different times of day on sleep EEG and mood in patients with seasonal affective disorder. *Biological Rhythms Research*, **28**, 166–84.
Park, S. and Holzman, P.S., 1992. Schizophrenics show spatial working memory deficits. *Archives of General Psychiatry*, **49**, 975–82.
Partiot, A., Pierson, A., Le Houezec, J., Dodin, V., Renault, B. and Jouvent, R., 1993. Loss of automatic processes and blunted-affect in depression: a P3 study. *European Psychiatry*, **8**, 309–18.
Partonen, T., Appelberg, B. and Partinen, M., 1993. Effects of light treatment on sleep structure in seasonal affective disorder. *European Archives of Psychiatry and Clinical Neuroscience*, **242**, 310–13.
Pascual-Marqui, R.D., Michel, C.M. and Lehmann, D., 1994. Low resolution electromagnetic tomography: a new method for localizing electrical activity in the brain. *International Journal of Psychophysiology*, **7**, 49–65.
Passero, S., Nardini, M. and Battistini, N., 1995. Regional cerebral blood flow changes following chronic administration of antidepressant drugs. *Progress in Neuro-Psychopharmacology and Biological Psychiatry*, **19**, 627–36.
Pfefferbaum, A., Wenegrat, B., Ford, J.M., Roth, W.T. and Kopell, B.S., 1984. Clinical applications of the P3 component of event-related potentials. *Electroencephalography and Clinical Neurophysiology*, **59**, 104–24.
Picton, T.W., 1992. The P300 wave of the human event-related potential. *Journal of Clinical Neurophysiology*, **9**, 456–79.
Pierson, A., Ragot, R., Van Hooff, J., Partiot, A., Renault, B. and Jouvent, R., 1996. Heterogeneity of information-processing alterations according to dimensions of depression: an event-related potentials study. *Biological Psychiatry*, **40**, 98–115.
Pollock, V.E. and Schneider, L.S., 1989. Topographic electroencephalographic alpha in recovered depressed elderly. *Journal of Abnormal Psychology*, **98**, 268–73.
Pollock, V.E. and Schneider, L.S., 1990. Quantitative, waking EEG research on depression. *Biological Psychiatry*, **27**, 757–80.
Portas, C.M., Thakkar, M., Rainnie, D.G., Greene, R.W. and McCarley, R.W., 1997. Role of adenosine in behavioral state modulation: a microdialysis study in the freely moving cat. *Neuroscience*, **79**, 225–35.
Pozzi, D., Golimstock, A., Petracchi, M., Garcia, H. and Starkstein, S., 1995. Quantified electroencephalographic changes in depressed patients with and without dementia. *Biological Psychiatry*, **38**, 677–83.
Rechlin, T., 1994. Decreased parameters of heart rate variation in amitriptyline treated patients: lower parameters in melancholic depression than in neurotic depression—a biological marker? *Biological Psychiatry*, **36**, 705–7.
Reid, S.A., Allen, J.J.B. and Duke, L.M., 1995. Differences in task-specific EEG activity of depressed and non-depressed subjects. *Psychophysiology*, **32**, S61.
Reynolds, C.F.,III and Kupfer, D.J., 1987. Sleep research in affective illness: state of the art circa 1987. *Sleep*, **10**, 199–215.
Riemann, D. and Berger, M., 1989. EEG sleep in depression and in remission and the REM sleep response to the cholinergic agonist RS 86. *Neuropsychopharmacology*, **2**, 145–52.
Riemann, D., Berger, M. and Voderholzer, U., 2001. Sleep and depression—results from psychobiological studies: an overview. *Biological Psychology*, **57**, 67–103.
Rosenberg, D.R., Sweeney, J.A., Squires-Wheeler, E., Keshavan, M.S., Cornblatt, B.A. and Erlenmeyer-Kimling, L., 1997. Eye-tracking dysfunction in offspring from the New York High-Risk Project: diagnostic specificity and the role of attention. *Psychiatry Research*, **66**, 121–30.
Roth, W.T., Pfefferbaum, A., Kelly, A.T., Berger, R.A. and Kopell, B.S., 1981. Auditory ERPs in schizophrenia and depression. *Psychiatry Research*, **4**, 199–212.
Roth, W.T., Goodale, J. and Pfefferbaum, A., 1991. Auditory event-related potentials and electrodermal activity in medicated and unmedicated schizophrenics. *Biological Psychiatry*, **29**, 585–99.
Rush, A.J., Erman, M.K., Giles, D.E., Schlesser, M.A., Carpenter, G., Vasavada, K. and Roffwarg, H.P., 1986. Polysomnographic findings in recently drug-free and clinically remitted depressed patients. *Archives of General Psychiatry*, **43**, 878–84.
Rye, D.B., 1997. Contributions of the pedunculopontine region to normal and altered REM sleep. *Sleep*, **20**, 757–88.
Salisbury, D.F., Shenton, M.E. and McCarley, R.W., 1999. P300 topography differs in schizophrenia and manic psychosis. *Biological Psychiatry*, **45**, 98–106.
Salzman, L.F., Klein, R.H. and Strauss, J.S., 1978. Pendulum eye-tracking in remitted psychiatric patients. *Psychiatry Research*, **14**, 121–6.
Sara, G., Gordon, E., Kraiuhin, C., Coyle, S., Howson, A. and Meares, R., 1994. The P300 ERP component: an index of cognitive dysfunction in depression? *Journal of Affective Disorders*, **31**, 29–38.
Sartory, G., 1985. The contingent negative variation (CNV) in psychiatric states. In: Papakostopoulos, D., Butler, S. and Martin, I. (eds), *Clinical and Experimental Neuropsychophysiology*, pp. 286–311. Croom Helm, London.
Schaffer, C.E., Davidson, R.J. and Saron, C., 1983. Frontal and parietal electroencephalogram asymmetry in depressed and non-depressed subjects. *Biological Psychiatry*, **18**, 753–62.
Schlegel, S., Adenhoff, J.B., Eissner, D., Lindner, P. and Nickel, O., 1989. Regional cerebral blood flow in depression: associations with psychopathology. *Journal of Affective Disorders*, **17**, 211–18.
Schneider, S.J., 1983. Multiple measures of hemispheric dysfunction in schizophrenia and depression. *Psychological Medicine*, **13**, 287–97.
Schnur, D.B., Bernstein, A.S., Yeager, A., Smith, S. and Bernstein, P., 1995. The relationship of the skin conductance and finger pulse amplitude components of the orienting response to season of birth in schizophrenia and depression. *Biological Psychiatry*, **37**, 34–41.
Schnur, D.B., Smith, S., Smith, A., Marte, V., Horwitz, E., Sackeim, H.A., Mukherjee, S. and Bernstein, A.S., 1999. The orienting response in schizophrenia and mania. *Psychiatry Research*, **88**, 41–54.
Schramm, E., Hoaghen, F., Käppler, C., Grasshoff, U. and Berger, M., 1995. Mental comorbidity of chronic insomnia in general practice attenders using DSM-III-R. *Acta Psychiatrica Scandinavica*, **91**, 10–17.
Schreiber, W., Lauer, C.J., Krumrey, K., Holsboer, F. and Krieg, J.-C., 1992. Cholinergic REM sleep induction test in subjects at high risk for psychiatric disorders. *Biological Psychiatry*, **32**, 79–90.
Sereno, A.B. and Holzman, P.S., 1995. Antisaccades and smooth pursuit eye movements in schizophrenia. *Biological Psychiatry*, **37**, 394–401.
Shagass, C., 1983. Contingent negative variation and other slow potentials in adult psychiatry. In: Hughes, J.R. and Wilson, W. (eds), *EEG and Evoked Potentials in Psychiatry and Behavioral Neurology*, pp. 149–68. Butterworths, Boston, MA.
Shagass, C., Amadeo, M. and Overton, D.A., 1974. Eye-tracking performance in psychiatric patients. *Biological Psychiatry*, **9**, 245–60.
Shagass, C., Roemer, R.A., Straumanis, J.J. and Josiassen, R.C., 1984. Psychiatric diagnostic discriminations with combinations of quantitative EEG variables. *British Journal of Psychiatry*, **144**, 581–92.
Shah, S.A., Doraiswamy, P.M., Husain, M.M., Escalona, P.R., Na, C., Figiel, G.S., Patterson, L.J., Ellinwood, E.H. Jr, McDonald, W.M. and Boyko, O.B., 1992. Posterior fossa abnormalities in major depression: a controlled magnetic resonance imaging study. *Acta Psychiatrica Scandinavica*, **85**, 474–9.
Sitaram, N., Nurnberger, J.I. and Gershon, E.S., 1980. Faster cholinergic REM sleep induction in euthymic patients with primary affective illness. *Science*, **20**, 200–2.
Sitaram, N., Nurnberger, J.I., Gershon, E.S. and Gillin, J., 1982. Cholinergic regulation of mood and REM sleep: potential model and marker of vulnerability to affective disorder. *American Journal of Psychiatry*, **139**, 571–6.
Sitaram, N., Dube, S., Keshavan, M., Davies, A. and Reynal, P., 1987. The association of supersensitive cholinergic REM-induction and affective illness within pedigrees. *Psychiatry Research*, **21**, 487–97.

Small, J.G., Milstein, V., Malloy, F.W., Medlock, C.E. and Klapper, M.H., 1999. Clinical and quantitative EEG studies of mania. *Journal of Affective Disorders*, **53**, 217–24.

Steiger, A., von Bardeleben, U., Herth, T. and Holsboer, F., 1989. Sleep EEG and nocturnal secretion of cortisol and human growth hormone in male patients with endogenous depression before treatment and after recovery. *Journal of Affective Disorders*, **16**, 189–95.

Steriade, M., McCormick, D.A. and Sejnowski, T.J., 1993. Thalamocortical oscillations in the sleeping and aroused brain. *Science*, **262**, 679–85.

Storrie, M.C., Doerr, H.O. and Johnson, M.H., 1981. Skin conductance characteristics of depressed subjects before and after therapeutic intervention. *Journal of Nervous and Mental Disease*, **69**, 176–9.

Strik, W.K., Dierks, T., Becker, T. and Lehmann, D., 1995. Larger topographical variance and decreased duration of brain electric microstates in depression. *Journal of Neural Transmission: General Section*, **99**, 213–22.

Strik, W.K., Ruchsow, M., Abele, S., Fallgatter, A.J. and Mueller, T.J., 1998. Distinct neurophysiological mechanisms for manic and cycloid psychoses: evidence from a P300 study on manic patients. *Acta Psychiatrica Scandinavica*, **98**, 459–66.

Suzuki, H., Mori, T., Kimura, M. and Endo, S., 1996. Quantitative EEG characteristics of the state depressive phase and the state of remission in major depression. *Seishin Shinkeigaku Zasshi*, **98**, 363–7.

Sweeney, J.A., Strojwas, M.H., Mann, J.J. and Thase, M.E., 1998. Prefrontal and cerebellar abnormalities in major depression: evidence from oculomotor studies. *Biological Psychiatry*, **43**, 584–94.

Sweeney, J.A., Luna, B., Haas, G.L., Keshavan, M.S., Mann, J.J. and Thase, M.E., 1999. Pursuit tracking impairments in schizophrenia and mood disorders: step-ramp studies with unmedicated patients. *Biological Psychiatry*, **46**, 671–80.

Tabarés-Seisdedos, R., Balanzá-Martínez, V., Pallardó, Y., Salazar-Fraile, J., Selva, G., Vilela, C., Vallet, M., Leal, C. and Gómez-Beneyto, M., 2001. Similar effect of family history of psychosis on Sylvian fissure size and auditory P200 amplitude in schizophrenic and bipolar subjects. *Psychiatry Research: Neuroimaging Section*, **108**, 29–38.

Thase, M.E., Kupfer, D.J. and Ulrich, R.F., 1986. Electroencephalographic sleep in psychotic depression. *Archives of General Psychiatry*, **43**, 886–93.

Thase, M.E., Himmelhoch, J.M., Mallinger, A.G., Jarrett, D.B. and Kupfer, D.J., 1989. Sleep EEG and DST findings in anergic bipolar depression. *American Journal of Psychiatry*, **146**, 329–33.

Thase, M.E., Kupfer, D.J., Buysse, D.J., Frank, E., Simons, A.D., McEachran, A.B., Rashid, K.F. and Grochocinski, V.J., 1995. Electroencephalographic sleep profiles in single-episode and recurrent unipolar forms of major depression: I. Comparison during acute depressive states. *Biological Psychiatry*, **38**, 506–15.

Thase, M.E., Fasiczka, A.L., Berman, S.R., Simons, A.D. and Reynolds, C.F., 1998. Electroencephalographic sleep profiles before and after cognitive behavior therapy of depression. *Archives of General Psychiatry*, **55**, 138–44.

Thier, P., Axmann, D. and Giedke, H., 1986. Slow brain potentials and psychomotor retardation in depression. *Electroencephalography and Clinical Neurophysiology*, **63**, 570–81.

Thorell, L.H., 1987. Electrodermal activity in suicidal and nonsuicidal depressive patients and in matched healthy subjects. *Acta Psychiatrica Scandinavica*, **76**, 420–30.

Thorell, L.H., Kjellman, B.F. and d'Elia, G., 1987. Electrodermal activity in antidepressant medicated and unmedicated depressive patients and in matched healthy subjects. *Acta Psychiatrica Scandinavica*, **76**, 684–92.

Tien, A.Y., Ross, D.E., Pearlson, G. and Strauss, M.E., 1996. Eye movements and psychopathology in schizophrenia and bipolar disorder. *Journal of Nervous and Mental Disease*, **184**, 331–8.

Timsit-Berthier, M., 1986. Contingent negative variation (CNV) in psychiatry. In: McCallum, W.C., Zappoli, R. and Denoth, F. (eds), *Cerebral Psychophysiology: Studies in Event-related Potentials*, pp. 429–38. Elsevier, Amsterdam.

Tomarken, A.J., Simien, S. and Garber, J., 1994. Resting frontal brain asymmetry discriminates adolescent children of depressed mothers from low-risk controls. *Psychophysiology*, **31**, S97.

Toone, B.K., Cooke, E. and Lader, M.H., 1981. Electrodermal activity in the affective disorders and schizophrenia. *Psychological Medicine*, **11**, 497–508.

Tucker, D.M., Stenslie, C.E., Roth, R.S. and Shearer, S.L., 1981. Right frontal lobe activation and right hemisphere performance. *Archives of General Psychiatry*, **38**, 169–74.

Tulen, J.H.M., 1993. Catecholamines, mood and cardiovascular control, PhD Thesis, Erasmus University, Rotterdam.

Tulen, J.H.M., Bruijn, J.A., de Man, K.J., van der Velden, E., Pepplinkhuizen, L. and Man in 't Veld, A.J., 1996. Anxiety and autonomic regulation in major depressive disorder: an exploratory study. *Journal of Affective Disorders*, **40**, 61–71.

Visser, S.L., Van Tilburg, W., Hooijer, C., Jonker, C. and De Rijke, W., 1985. Visual evoked potentials (VEPs) in senile dementia (Alzheimer type) and in non-organic behavioral disorders in the elderly: comparison with EEG parameters. *Electroencephalography and Clinical Neurophysiology*, **60**, 115–21.

von Knorring, L., 1983. Interhemispheric EEG differences in affective disorders. In: Flor-Henry, P. and Gruzelier, J. (eds), *Laterality and Psychopathology*, pp. 315–26. Elsevier, New York.

von Knorring, L., Perris, C., Goldstein, L., Kemali, D., Monakhov, K. and Vacca, L., 1983. Intercorrelation between different computer-based measures of the EEG alpha amplitude and its variability over time and their validity in differentiating healthy volunteers from depressed patients. In: Mendlewicz, J. and Van Praag, M. (eds), *Advances in Biological Psychiatry*, pp. 172–81. Karger, New York.

Ward, N.G. and Doerr, H.O., 1986. Skin conductance. A potentially sensitive and specific marker for depression. *Journal of Nervous and Mental Disease*, **174**, 553–9.

Ward, N.G., Doerr, H.O. and Storrie, M.C., 1983. Skin conductance — a potentially sensitive test for depression. *Psychiatry Research*, **10**, 292–302.

Wascher, E., Verleger, R., Vieregge, P., Jaskowski, P., Koch, S. and Kömpf, D., 1997. Responses to cued signals in Parkinson's disease. Distinguishing between disorders of cognition and of activation. *Brain*, **120**, 1355–75.

Wehr, T.A., 1991. Sleep loss as a possible mediator of disease causes of mania. *British Journal of Psychiatry*, **159**, 576–8.

Williams, K.M., Iacono, W.G. and Remick, R.A., 1985. Electrodermal activity among subtypes of depression. *Biological Psychiatry*, **20**, 158–62.

Wingard, D.L. and Berkman, L.F., 1983. Mortality risk associated with sleeping patterns among adults. *Sleep*, **6**, 102–7.

Wirz-Justice, A. and Van der Hoofdakker, R.H., 1999. Sleep deprivation in depression: what do we know, where do we go? *Biological Psychiatry*, **46**, 445–53.

Wu, J.C. and Bunney, W.R., Jr, 1990. The biological basis of an antidepressant response to sleep deprivation and relapse: review and hypothesis. *American Journal of Psychiatry*, **147**, 14–21.

Yee, R.D., Balogh, R.W., Marder, S.R., Levy, D.L., Sakala, S.M. and Honrubia, V., 1987. Eye movements in schizophrenia. *Investigative Ophthalmology and Visual Science*, **28**, 366–74.

Yeragani, V.K., Pohl, R., Balon, R., Ramesh, C., Glitz, D. and Jung, I., 1991. Heart rate variability in patients with major depression. *Psychiatry Research*, **37**, 35–46.

Zahn, T.P., 1986. Psychophysiological approaches to psychopathology. In: Coles, M.G.H., Donchin, E. and Porges, S.W. (eds), *Psychophysiology: Systems, Processes, and Applications*, pp. 545–58. Guilford Press, New York.

Zahn, T.P., Nurnberger, J.I. and Berrettini, W.H., 1989. Electrodermal activity in young adults at genetic risk for affective disorder. *Archives of General Psychiatry*, **46**, 1120–4.

XVIII-7

The Neuropsychology of Mood Disorders: Affect, Cognition and Neural Circuitry

Aprajita Mohanty and Wendy Heller

Research in the past decade has greatly enhanced our understanding of the neural processes that implement cognitive, emotional and physiological functions in mood disorders. Abnormalities or disturbances in these functions have been shown to be associated with corresponding abnormalities in regional brain functions (Heller and Nitschke, 1998). This has led to increased research efforts focused on linking theories of cognitive neuropsychology to the anatomy and physiology of related brain function in mood disorders.

Despite extensive evidence indicating impairment of cognitive functioning in depression, this area is largely ignored, especially in diagnostic evaluation (Austin *et al.*, 1992). The current *Diagnostic and Statistical Manual of Mental Disorders* (DSM-IV; American Psychiatric Association, 1994) identifies cognitive factors (e.g. indecisiveness, difficulties in thought and concentration) as fundamental components of depressive episodes and dysthymia. Neuropsychological studies have identified a variety of other cognitive characteristics associated with depressed moods. For example, depression is associated with deficits in executive functioning (Channon and Green, 1999; Freidman, 1964; Goodwin, 1997; Raskin *et al.*, 1982; Silberman *et al.*, 1983), memory (Burt *et al.*, 1995), attention (Mialet *et al.*, 1996), and visuospatial processing (Asthana *et al.*, 1998). Depression-related cognitive deficits range in severity from mild subclinical impairments to pervasive global deficits, often referred to as pseudodementia (Abrams and Taylor, 1987; Golinkoff and Sweeny, 1989; Watts *et al.*, 1990). The term pseudodementia was coined to describe patients with affective disorders who display an unusually large number of cognitive deficits that are typically associated with organic brain disease (Kiloh, 1961). The conjunction of depression and cognitive impairments of various types poses a clinical diagnostic problem because it increases the likelihood of a variety of misdiagnoses, including degenerative dementia, stroke or learning disability (Marsden and Harrison, 1972).

Abnormal patterns of brain activity and function associated with depression have been demonstrated in research using a variety of techniques, such as neuropsychological testing (Miller *et al.*, 1995; Rubinow and Post, 1992; Silberman and Weingartner, 1986), lesion techniques (Lipsey *et al.*, 1983; Robinson and Price, 1982; Robinson *et al.*, 1984), electrophysiological techniques (Deldin *et al.*, 2000; Heller *et al.*, 1995; Henriques and Davidson, 1990), and haemodynamic techniques (Baxter *et al.*, 1989; Bench *et al.*, 1992, 1993; George *et al.*, 1994a). Parallel findings to those obtained in depressed populations have been described in normal individuals following induction of depressed mood (Davidson *et al.*, 1979, 1985) as well as individuals scoring high on measures of depressed affect (Tomarken *et al.*, 1992). Despite substantial evidence indicating that the same brain regions implicated as abnormal in depression are also fundamental for various aspects of cognitive processing, the implications of these neuropsychological findings for cognitive processing in depression have rarely been studied (Rubinow and Post, 1992).

In this chapter, we review the evidence and describe the nature of the cognitive characteristics that have been identified in depression. In addition, we provide a brief discussion of the neural mechanisms likely to be associated with these cognitive characteristics. Before discussing the nature of cognition in depression we review a number of important factors that are likely to impact cognitive function in depression. These factors can introduce important methodological confounds in studies examining the relationship between depression and cognitive impairment, thus weakening the conclusions drawn from the results of clinical neuropsychological studies (Murphy and Sahakian, 2001).

GENERAL COGNITIVE DEFICITS AND CHARACTERISTICS OF DEPRESSION

Cognitive deficits in depression are influenced by the clinical characteristics of the disorder, such as the presence of specific symptoms, depression subtype and symptom severity. For example, cognitive deficits in depression have been found to vary with the presence of psychotic symptoms.

Cognition and Psychosis

Studies show that depressed patients with psychotic features such as delusions and hallucinations have more structural brain abnormalities than normal controls (Lesser *et al.*, 1991), show neuropsychological performance comparable to that of patients with schizophrenia (Jeste *et al.*, 1996; Nelson *et al.*, 1998) and are more impaired than patients with non-psychotic depression and normal controls (Basso and Bornstein, 1999; Jeste *et al.*, 1996; Lesser *et al.*, 1991; Nelson *et al.*, 1998) on a broad range of neuropsychological measures such as attention, response inhibition, verbal declarative memory and visuospatial abilities. It is important to keep in mind that drug effects can be a possible confounding factor in these studies as the selected clinical groups differed in the types and dosages of psychotropic medications with which they were being treated. Studies have shown that some psychotropic medications can impair or, conversely, improve neuropsychological test performance (Spohn and Strauss, 1989). Furthermore, individuals with psychotic depression may have more severe depressive symptoms, more frequent recurrence of depressive episodes and longer episodes, poorer response to pharmacotherapy, more hyperactive hypothalamus–pituitary–adrenal (HPA) activity (Coryell *et al.*,

Biological Psychiatry: Edited by H. D'haenen, J.A. den Boer and P. Willner. ISBN 0-471-49198-5

1996) and more structural brain abnormalities such as cortical atrophy (Gewirtz *et al.*, 1994). To the degree that these factors have a detrimental influence on cognitive function, individuals with psychotic features will present with more deficits.

Cognition and Subtypes of Depression

Cognitive deficits have also been found to vary with subtypes of depression. For example, Austin *et al.* (1999) reported that although depressed individuals were impaired on most mnemonic tasks, on simple reaction time and on Trails B of the Trail Making Test, melancholic patients defined by narrower criterion were additionally impaired on the Wisconsin Card Sorting Task (WCST) and on digit symbol substitution. In contrast, the cognitive performance of the more narrowly defined non-melancholic patients was largely unimpaired. Silberman *et al.* (1985) reported that patients exhibiting an abnormal dexamethasone suppression test (DST) response, usually seen in endogenous depression, showed more cognitive impairment than those with less evidence of physiological dysfunction. Using the Newcastle scale to define subjects with endogenous and non-endogenous depression, Cornell *et al.* (1984) reported impairment of complex reaction time only in subjects with endogenous depression.

Cognition and Severity of Depression

The relationship between depression subtype and cognitive deficits is confounded by depression severity, which can also affect cognitive functioning. For example, while Austin *et al.* (1992, 1999) reported frontal deficits only in individuals narrowly diagnosed with endogenous or melancholic depression, the differences disappeared after controlling for depression severity (Austin *et al.*, 1999). Individuals with melancholia showed poorer performance on cognitive tasks in the morning, when mood is reported to be more depressed, compared to evening — whereas controls displayed the opposite pattern (Moffoot *et al.*, 1994). The impact of severity has also been studied by correlating scores on clinical scales such as the Hamilton Depression Scale (Hamilton, 1960) with cognitive performance scores (for review, see Austin *et al.*, 2001). Using this method, studies have shown that severely depressed patients, especially those with significant psychomotor impairment, are more cognitively impaired (Austin *et al.*, 1992; Tarbuck and Paykel, 1995). Thus, depression severity appears to contribute to the neuropsychological deficits seen in individuals with depression. However, this does not imply that cognitive deficits occur only in acute stages; some research has shown that cognitive deficits might persist even after symptom remission (Trichard *et al.*, 1995).

Cognition and Treatment of Depression

Individuals with depression generally receive a combination of medications — including mood stabilizers, antidepressants, neuroleptics and benzodiazepines — which could have an impairing effect on neuropsychological performance. It is possible that differences observed between patients and controls, or patients in different stages of bipolar illness, are confounded by different medication regimens (Murphy and Sahakian, 2001). There is some evidence to suggest that different antidepressants may exert different effects on cognitive functioning. For example, amitriptyline, mianserin and trazodone have been reported to have adverse effects on a range of cognitive processes, including memory. The detrimental impact of these drugs was found to be more marked immediately following administration, and the effects wore off with time (Thompson, 1991). Studies have also shown that compared to depressed patients not treated with ECT, patients treated with ECT showed explicit memory deficits (Squire *et al.*, 1984). In general, however, prolonged antidepressant treatments appear to be associated with improved cognitive function as depressive symptoms remit (Frith *et al.*, 1983).

Cognition and Motivation

Some studies have argued that cognitive deficits in depression reflect motivational impairments (Hockey, 1986). In support of this notion, depressed patients show deficits in effortful as compared to automatic cognitive tasks, including problem solving, explicit memory, general learning and reading (for review, see Hartlage *et al.*, 1993; see also Klein and Seligman, 1976; Klein *et al.*, 1976; Price *et al.*, 1978). For example, depression has been found to be associated with impaired performance on verbal recall but unimpaired performance on verbal recognition (Roy-Byrne *et al.*, 1986) and with impaired explicit memory performance but intact implicit memory performance (Danion *et al.*, 1995; Ilsley *et al.*, 1995).

Several hypotheses have been proposed to explain the impairment of controlled operations in depression. These include lack of availability of cognitive resources due to decreased arousal (Gjerde, 1983), inadequate allocation of available resources due to an emphasis on irrelevant thoughts (Ellis and Ashbrook, 1988) or self-focused worries (Ingram, 1990), lack of initiative in the use of strategies required for information processing (Hertel and Hardin, 1990), or activation of automatic processes in depression (such as depressive ideation and depressive biases) which interfere with controlled processes (Mialet *et al.*, 1996).

Some researchers have suggested that abnormal responsivity to negative feedback, a commonly reported phenomenon in depression, may contribute to poor performance on some cognitive tasks. They (e.g. Elliott *et al.*, 1996) have argued that deficits in executive functions in depression are mediated by a highly specific form of motivational deficit involving the response of patients to perceived failure. Using conditional probability analyses, their study demonstrated that failure on one item of a test dramatically increased the chance of failure on the subsequent item in patients with depression. On both the Tower of London test and matching to sample tests, both of which provide feedback on performance, depressed patients showed a significant tendency to respond incorrectly after negative feedback. According to Elliott *et al.* (1996) the over-sensitivity to negative feedback is a highly specific form of motivational impairment that interacts with and exacerbates the neuropsychological deficits seen in depression. This impairment in the ability to alter behaviour in response to feedback could also account for the higher rates of perseverative errors seen in the performance of depressed individuals on executive functioning tasks (Channon, 1996).

Although motivational factors are likely to play a role in most aspects of performance, current perspectives do not support the notion that deficits in motivation alone can account for the patterns of cognitive deficit in depression (Heller and Nitschke, 1998; Hertel and Rude, 1991; Richards and Ruff, 1989). Heller and Nitschke (1998) argued that most of the data can be accounted for by impairments in functions of the prefrontal cortex (to be reviewed in more detail in subsequent sections of this chapter).

Cognition and Anxiety

A great deal of research has suggested that depression and anxiety are accompanied by distinct physiological, cognitive and emotional characteristics that appear to reflect the activity and function of different brain regions (Heller and Nitschke, 1997, 1998; Heller *et al.*, 1995; see also Chapter XIX-8). An important implication of these findings would be that a number of neuropsychological and neurophysiological studies may have been compromised by a failure to account for the substantial comorbidity of depression and anxiety (Keller *et al.*, 2000). In light of these findings, it is important to consider the comorbidity of anxiety and depression in studies of cognition as disparate patterns of activation in anxiety and depression may differentially affect cognitive functioning.

From this review it is evident that differences observed between patients and controls, or between patients in different stages of depression, may be confounded by different factors such as clinical features of depression, medication regimens and comorbidity of depression with anxiety. Although these methodological problems bring unavoidable complications into investigations of disordered mood and cognition, it is important to adopt measures that control for potential confounds (Murphy and Sahakian, 2001). These measures include careful choice of controls, matching patients and controls on age and premorbid intelligence, and matching patients on measures of phase of illness, severity of depression, treatment regimen, comorbid conditions, etc.

NEUROPSYCHOLOGICAL FUNCTIONING IN DEPRESSION

Executive Functioning

Executive functions are known to rely on anterior regions of the brain (Banich, 1997; Heller and Nitschke, 1997) and include judgement, planning, abstract thinking, metacognition (i.e. 'thinking about thinking'), cognitive flexibility (i.e. flexibility in strategy use), verbal fluency, initiative, and the ability to generate alternate strategies and to direct behaviour in a goal-directed manner. Examples might include the ability to shift response set and modify strategies in task performance (Cicerone *et al.*, 1983), the evaluation of a situation and the use of cues and extra information in the environment to guide behaviour (Alivisatos and Milner, 1989), and the ability to monitor behaviour or performance accurately (Luria, 1966).

Miyake *et al.* (2000) argued that executive functions involve three important target functions — shifting, updating and inhibition — which are clearly distinguishable but are also moderately correlated constructs. Shifting involves shifting back and forth between multiple tasks, operations or mental sets (Monsell, 1996), updating requires monitoring and coding incoming information for relevance to the task at hand and revising the items held in working memory by replacing old, irrelevant information with new, relevant information (Morris and Jones, 1990), and inhibition involves the ability to deliberately inhibit dominant, automatic or prepotent responses when necessary (Miyake *et al.*, 2000). Furthermore, these executive functions were seen to contribute differentially to performance on specific tasks. More specifically, WCST performance was related most to shifting, Tower of Hanoi to inhibition, random number generation to inhibition and updating, and operation span to updating.

Individuals with depression display deficient performance on a number of set-shifting tasks such as the WCST and 'Go–No Go' tasks (Jones *et al.*, 1988). Deficits on the WCST were correlated with the severity of depression and were less severe than those demonstrated by patients with schizophrenia (Merriam *et al.*, 1999). However, another study showed that both schizophrenic and depressed individuals showed very little difference in their deficient performance on frontal lobe tasks like WCST, the Trail Making Test, and a verbal fluency test (Franke *et al.*, 1993). Channon (1996) reported that dysphoric subjects were poorer than controls in sorting to correct categories and had higher rates of both perseverative and non-perseverative errors on the WCST. The dysphoric subjects also had greater difficulties in shifting sets correctly. Unipolar depressed patients have been seen to show deficits on other attentional set-shifting tasks such as intradimensional/extradimensional (ID/ED) set shift (Purcell *et al.*, 1997). Thus, the majority of evidence points towards deficits on set-shifting tasks in depression.

A number of studies have also shown that depression is associated with impairment in working memory (Elliott *et al.*, 1996). Working memory is conceptualized as a limited capacity mental workspace involving holding task-relevant information online as well as simultaneous manipulation and updating of its contents by executive processes. Thus, working memory is presumed to be supported by an attentional control system, or 'central executive', probably localized to dorsolateral prefrontal cortex (Nitschke *et al.*, 2000; Pelosi *et al.*, 2000). Measuring event-related potentials (ERPs) as a neurophysiological correlate of working memory impairment, Pelosi *et al.* (2000) reported that individuals with depression showed deficits on a working memory task that were accompanied by ERP abnormalities consistent with dysfunction of a central executive system.

Individuals with depression also show impaired performance on tasks that test inhibitory aspects of executive functioning such as the Tower of London planning test (Elliott *et al.*, 1996, 1997). Similar results have been reported for the Stroop colour-word test (Degl'Innocenti *et al.*, 1998; Trichard *et al.*, 1995). In summary, findings from a wide variety of neuropsychological tasks indicate that depression is associated with deficits on important executive functions including set shifting, inhibition and updating.

Researchers have also investigated whether executive functioning deficits are a persistent feature of depression. A residual deficit in executive function appears to be seen in some patients with a history of depression. Paradiso *et al.* (1997) reported neurocognitive impairment in individuals after recovery from unipolar depression which was most noticeable on set-shifting tasks and was not related to medication status. Beats *et al.* (1996) also showed that deficits such as slowed simple and choice reaction times, perseveration on the set-shifting task and impaired verbal fluency did not fully remit upon recovery. Similarly, Trichard *et al.* (1995) in a study of executive functioning in middle-aged individuals with severe depression reported improved performance on the verbal fluency task but not the Stroop task upon recovery. Currently, it appears that residual deficits in mnemonic and executive functions persist in some patients with a history of depression. However, the relationship of these deficits to epidemiological variables such as age, treatment, duration and chronicity of illness, and number of episodes remains to be more clearly determined (Austin *et al.*, 2001).

Neural Correlates of Executive Function

The cognitive findings described above showing deficits in multiple domains of executive function are consistent with evidence from a variety of neuropsychological techniques indicating abnormal function of anterior brain regions in depression. Studies have identified abnormal patterns of asymmetric brain activity as well as abnormal levels of brain activity in a number of regions in prefrontal cortex, including dorsolateral, medial, orbitofrontal and anterior cingulate regions.

Abnormal patterns of asymmetric activity in anterior brain regions are demonstrated by lesion studies showing that left hemisphere strokes are significantly associated with the development of symptoms of depression (Lipsey *et al.*, 1983; Robinson *et al.*, 1983). Furthermore, significant correlations have been reported between the severity of depression and proximity of the lesion to the anterior pole of the left hemisphere (Lipsey *et al.*, 1983; Robinson and Price, 1982; Robinson *et al.*, 1984, 1985). The finding of asymmetric activity in anterior brain regions in depression has been substantiated by psychophysiological studies. In studies of EEG alpha, depression has been associated with less left than right anterior activity (Henriques and Davidson, 1990, 1991;

Schaffer *et al.*, 1983). Similarly, evidence from a variety of resting and cognitive activation paradigms has shown that depression is associated with altered regional cerebral blood flow (rCBF) and metabolism in prefrontal cortex, anterior cingulate gyrus and basal ganglia (for review, see Videbech, 2000). Consistent with EEG findings, positron emission tomography (PET) studies have reported a decrease in regional rCBF in the left dorsolateral prefrontal cortex in depression (Baxter *et al.*, 1989; Bench *et al.*, 1992, 1993; George *et al.*, 1993, 1994a; Martinot *et al.*, 1990).

In addition, specific changes in the medial prefrontal cortex have been associated with cognitive impairment in depression. The medial prefrontal region is characterized by reciprocal connections with other higher order association areas, mainly dorsolateral and caudal orbitomedial prefrontal cortex as well as anterior cingulate cortex (Kendell and Gourlay, 1970). In a study comparing patterns of rCBF in depressed patients with cognitive impairment to those of equally depressed patients without cognitive impairment, Dolan *et al.* (1992) reported decreased rCBF in the medial prefrontal brain region in the depressed cognitively impaired group. Similarly, significant decreases in rCBF in medial frontal gyrus were reported in patients with depression-related cognitive impairment (Bench *et al.*, 1992) and there was a significant correlation between a measure of global cognitive function and rCBF decreases in medial prefrontal cortex in patients meeting criteria for primary depression (Bench *et al.*, 1993).

Dolan *et al.* (1994) conducted a principal component analysis on two subtests discriminating most between depressed patients, non-patients and patients with cognitive impairment, which resulted in a two-factor solution (memory and attention) accounting for 50% of the variance in test scores. Increasing neuropsychological impairment on both factors was associated with decreased rCBF in the medial prefrontal and the frontal polar cortex. These findings were interpreted by Dolan and colleagues to indicate that the medial prefrontal cortex could mediate psychological components such as executive functions that are common to both attention and memory. In addition, each factor showed unique patterns of correlations with posterior brain regions. The memory factor was associated with rCBF in the retrosplenial precuneus and posterior cingulate cortices, regions implicated in auditory and verbal long-term memory (Grasby *et al.*, 1993). The attention factor was associated with rCBF in the posterior brain region extending from inferior post-central gyrus to the inferior parietal lobule.

Contrary to findings of decreased activity in particular brain regions, some studies have shown increased rCBF in areas of left prefrontal cortex, including ventrolateral prefrontal cortex, frontal polar cortex, medial orbital cortex, and the pregenual portion of the anterior cingulate gyrus as well as the left amygdala in individuals with familial pure depressive disease (FPDD), defined as primary major depression in an individual with a first-degree relative with primary depression. In light of these conflicting findings, Drevets and Raichle (1995) propose that the findings of decreased frontal flow and metabolism can be attributed to confounds introduced by medication effects and decreased frontal lobe size, as reported in post-mortem and MRI studies (Bowen *et al.*, 1989; Coffey *et al.*, 1993). They suggest using methods that correct PET measurements for volumetric differences. While these cautions are appropriate, a resolution of these inconsistencies awaits further research.

Drevets and Raichle (1998) also argue that different brain regions are involved in emotional versus cognitive conditions, and that there is a reciprocal relationship between them (Drevets and Raichle, 1998). Across a number of PET studies, they observed that regions implicated in emotional processing, such as the orbitofrontal cortex (OFC), ventral prefrontal cortex and amygdala show increased activity during emotional states but decreased activity during performance of cognitive tasks. Conversely, a complementary set of regions including dorsal anterior cingulate and dorsolateral prefrontal cortex show increased activity during attentionally demanding cognitive tasks, but decreased activity during experimentally induced and pathological emotional states such as depression. Drevets and Raichle (1998) hypothesize that suppression of neural activity in certain cognitive processing regions during intense emotional states could be a possible mechanism by which severe depression may interfere with cognitive performance.

An alternative to this cognition–emotion reciprocity position is the idea that tasks typically classified as 'cognitive' and 'emotional' may rely, at least in part, on common, overlapping neural systems due to their common, overlapping behavioural functions (Compton *et al.*, submitted; Heller and Nitschke, 1997; Miller, 1996; Nitschke *et al.*, 2000). We have argued that, because of the overlap in 'cognitive' and 'emotional' functions implemented by many brain regions, patterns of brain activity associated with changes in emotional state provide an important means for exploring the cognitive characteristics of emotional disorders (Heller and Nitschke, 1997; Miller, 1996; Nitschke *et al.*, 2000).

Earlier, we reviewed evidence examining the impact of abnormal response to feedback on cognitive functioning in depression. Some researchers have argued that cognitive deficits in depression are related to dysregulation of the neurobiological reinforcement and reward systems (Beats *et al.*, 1996; Elliott *et al.*, 1996, 1997). Using PET, Elliott *et al.* (1998) showed that behavioural response to feedback in depression is associated with attenuated activation in medial caudate and orbitofrontal cortex, regions that are implicated in reward mechanisms (Schultz *et al.*, 1992).

In summary, studies show that executive functioning deficits in depression are associated with abnormal patterns of brain activation in prefrontal brain regions. In future research, it will be important to examine more precisely how emotion modulates cognition and vice versa in depression. Further investigation into reciprocal brain mechanisms as well as integrated brain mechanisms for emotion and cognition could have important implications for cognitive deficits in depression. Another potentially important line of research appears to be that of the role of brain systems that regulate reinforcement and reward in depression.

Memory

Evidence from a large number of studies indicates that individuals with depression perform comparatively poorly on memory tasks. A meta-analytic study (Burt *et al.*, 1995) synthesizing 147 recall and recognition studies in clinically depressed and non-depressed samples revealed a significant, stable association between depression and memory impairment. Furthermore, the study showed that memory impairment in depression is linked to particular aspects of memory as well as particular subtypes of depression. Specifically, depression is associated with deficits on explicit, but not implicit, memory tasks. It is also associated with a tendency to remember negative material better than positive material.

Depression has been associated with impaired performance on tests of short-term memory, verbal and visual recognition memory, spatial working memory, and immediate or delayed recall (Cutting, 1979; Massman *et al.*, 1992; Richards and Ruff, 1989). Two main theoretical frameworks have been proposed to explain memory deficits in depression. According to one model, they can be attributed to impairment in effortful processing related to reduced attentional resources (Ellis and Ashbrook, 1988). Support for this model comes from studies that show that depressed individuals are more likely to show deficits on effortful or controlled tasks than on recognition tasks or tests of implicit memory (Denny and Hunt, 1992; Hertel and Hardin, 1990; Ilsley *et al.*, 1995; Hertel and Milan, 1994; Roy-Byrne *et al.*, 1986).

In contrast, Hertel (1994) proposed that attentional resources are intact in depression, but what is missing is the initiative to control them. This model is strongly supported by studies that show that use of attentional control strategies such as focusing attention on the task and monitoring relevance of the past (Hertel, 1994) can result in improvement of memory deficits in depression. Similarly, a study conducted by Weingartner *et al.* (1981) reported that depressed individuals failed to use encoding operations that are useful in reorganizing input to facilitate later recall. This is consistent with findings that depressed patients perform more poorly than normal controls on memory tasks involving intentional coding strategies than on tasks in which memory is encoded incidentally (Hartlage *et al.*, 1993).

A phenomenon that is commonly demonstrated in memory studies in depression is that of mood congruency, that is, enhanced encoding and/or retrieval of negatively valenced material while the individual is in the corresponding mood state. The biasing effect of mood on recall of autobiographical memories has been demonstrated in studies of clinically depressed individuals (Clark and Teasdale, 1982, Gilligan and Bower, 1984; Williams and Scott, 1988). For example, Lloyd and Lishman (1975) reported that the speed of retrieval of unpleasant memories in depressed individuals correlated positively with severity of depression. Similarly, Williams (1992) showed that depressed individuals demonstrate a biased pattern of recall with fewer memories of positive experiences.

However, biased recall of negative memories could be attributed to depressed patients actually having more depressing experiences or, conversely, being more likely to interpret neutral experiences in a negative way. Some studies have tried to resolve this ambiguity by using mood induction techniques and randomly assigning normal individuals to 'happy' and 'sad' conditions with the aim of controlling the number of depressing experiences across groups. Results from these studies show that when mood is 'sad', people tend to recall more negative personal memories and fewer positive personal memories, whereas the trend is reversed when mood is more positive (Teasdale and Fogarty, 1979; Teasdale *et al.*, 1980). A similar experiment was conducted on individuals with clinical depression characterized by diurnal mood swings. Results showed that when patients were more depressed, negative memories were more probable and positive memories were less probable, whereas the pattern was reversed for patients in a more positive mood (Clark and Teasdale, 1982).

Similar to findings on autobiographical memory, the biased recall of mood congruent information in depression has also been demonstrated for explicit memory tasks, which are tasks that require conscious recollection of facts or episodes. Studies with normal individuals with varying levels of depression (Gotlib and McCann, 1984) as well as clinically depressed individuals (Bradley and Mathews, 1983; Dunbar and Lishman, 1984) provide evidence for increased recall of negative material and/or decreased recall of positive materials. Depressed mood has been shown to be associated with higher recall for negative content than positive content in incidental free-recall paradigms (Gotlib *et al.*, 2000). The memory bias for negative material appears to be specific to depression-relevant stimuli (Gotlib *et al.*, 2000). For example, Watkins *et al.* (1992) found that depressed individuals exhibited a bias for depression-relevant but not threat-related words. Although there is substantial evidence indicative of memory bias related to explicit memory in depression, there is little evidence supporting this bias on implicit memory tasks (Gotlib *et al.*, 2000; for review see Roediger and McDermott, 1992).

Some researchers hypothesize that the enhanced recall of negative memories and material in depressed mood may provide a cognitive mechanism for the maintenance of depression (Teasdale, 1983), and cognitive theories of depression (Beck, 1967) assert that negatively biased information processing may constitute a vulnerability factor for the onset and/or maintenance of depression. Gotlib and Krasnoperova (1998) reviewed research focusing on information-processing paradigms to examine depression-associated biases in attention to, and memory for, negative information. They concluded that there is strong evidence that depression is associated with concurrent information-processing biases and that some aspects of cognitive functioning, particularly those involving memory processes, may represent a vulnerability factor for depression. Thus, the research on memory biases in depression has potential clinical implications as these maladaptive biases may represent an enduring cognitive characteristic that can be measured and utilized as an indicator of vulnerability for depression (Dalgleish and Watts, 1990).

Neural Correlates of Memory

The cognitive findings described in the previous section are consistent with the neuropsychological data suggesting deficits in a variety of executive functions associated with prefrontal cortex, as reviewed above. Impairment in the strategic use of information, inappropriate deployment of attentional resources, and inadequate maintenance and updating of online material could account for many of the observed memory deficits (for review, see Heller and Nitschke, 1997). A recent study by Herrmann *et al.* (2001) also emphasized the importance of prefrontally mediated executive control strategies in efficient episodic memory retrieval. Additional support comes from an electrophysiological study conducted by Etienne *et al.* (1999), which reported that participants higher in depression did not initiate frontal lobe functions in anticipation of the task that would later improve their memory performance. However, when asked to attend to stimuli, high-depressed individuals showed an association between better memory performance and increased frontal activity. Thus, deficits could be attributed to a lack of initiative in the use of frontally-mediated strategies that are required for memory processing.

The extensive literature on cognitive biases in depression is also highly relevant to the relationship between anterior brain asymmetry and emotional valence (Heller and Nitschke, 1997). There is considerable evidence from a variety of research paradigms that anterior brain asymmetries are associated with valence (for review, see Heller, 1990) with relatively more right than left anterior activity associated with unpleasant affect and sad mood states. This model of asymmetric brain activity would lead us to predict an increased bias towards negatively valenced material and a bias in the opposite direction for positively valenced material, a pattern that is commonly seen in depression.

Besides the anterior brain regions, posterior brain regions have also been implicated in memory deficits in depression. Beats *et al.* (1996) argue that the profile of memory deficits seen in depression can best be characterized by temporal lobe dysfunction in addition to frontostriatal dysfunction. Austin *et al.* (1992) reported that depression-related clinical variables were significantly associated with tests of temporal lobe function such as pattern recognition, spatial span and delayed match to sample task (DMST). A study by Sweeney *et al.* (2000) showed that deficits in bipolar and non-bipolar depressed patients were restricted to episodic memory, suggestive of a more selective dysfunction in mesial temporal lobe function during episodes of depression. It is also possible that these memory deficits are a function of poor visuospatial spatial functioning rather than memory *per se*. Visuospatial functions, implemented in the posterior brain regions, are commonly impaired in depression and could lead to poor encoding resulting in impairment in memory retrieval.

Researchers have also hypothesized that hippocampal dysfunction may contribute to the verbal declarative memory deficits observed in depression. Depressed individuals have smaller left hippocampal volume (Bremner *et al.*, 2000; Mervaala *et al.*, 2000) and exhibit reduced grey matter density in the left temporal cortex, including the hippocampus (Shah *et al.*, 1998). Additionally, neuropsychological impairment in depressed individuals has been shown to be associated with smaller left hippocampal volume (Shah *et al.*, 1998; von Gunten *et al.*, 2000). Individuals with a history of major depressive episodes but who are currently in remission show significantly smaller left and right hippocampal volumes with no difference in total cerebral volumes (Sheline *et al.*, 1996). It has been hypothesized that hippocampal volume loss in depression is due to neuronal cell death in the hippocampus resulting from adverse effects of stress hormones (Bemelmans *et al.*, 1996). Brown *et al.* (1999) reviewed studies to examine the hypothesis that hypercortisolaemia leads to hippocampal dysfunction and found cognitive impairment consistent with hippocampal dysfunction in depression, bipolar disorder, Cushing's disease, and in those individuals receiving exogenous corticosteroids. It will also be important in future research to take into account the comorbidity of anxiety with depression, because hippocampal involvement has been reported in post-traumatic stress disorder (see Chapter XIX-8).

Attention

Impaired attention has been considered one of the cardinal features of clinical depression. Decreased concentration is an important criterion for the diagnosis of depression in DSM-IV (American Psychiatric Association, 1994). In a thorough review of the attention literature in depression, Mialet *et al.* (1996) reported that impairment was consistently observed on tasks such as simple and choice reaction time tasks (Cornell *et al.*, 1984), the Digit Symbol Subtest (Austin *et al.*, 1992), the Continuous Performance Task (Cornblatt *et al.*, 1989) and sustained attention tasks (Mialet *et al.*, 1996).

Despite the claim that attentional biases are more common in anxious individuals and memory biases more common in depressed individuals (Dalgleish and Watts, 1990; Mathews and MacLeod, 1994), a number of studies have reported an attentional bias for negatively valenced stimuli in depression. Studies have shown that both depressed non-patients and clinically depressed patients took longer to name the colours of tachistoscopically presented depression-relevant words than neutral words (Gotlib and Cane, 1987; Gotlib and McCann, 1984). Furthermore, this bias was not evident after symptomatic recovery. Depressed individuals were also slower on a reaction time task when the distractor words were negative than when they were positive or neutral (Ingram *et al.*, 1994; McCabe and Gotlib, 1993). Similarly, studies have shown that on an emotional dot probe task depressed individuals were faster to detect a dot that replaced negative stimuli (e.g. words and emotion faces) than a dot that replaced positive stimuli (Krasnoperova *et al.*, 1998; Mathews *et al.*, 1996). However, a number of studies failed to find the association between depression and attentional bias to negative stimuli (Clark *et al.*, 1983; Mogg *et al.*, 1993, 2000). Due to substantial comorbidity between depression and anxiety, the possibility that attentional biases observed are not due to depression but to accompanying anxiety cannot be ruled out.

ERP studies have also demonstrated deficits in attentional processing in depression. For example, N2b, an ERP measure of selective attention, was enhanced in non-patients with dysthymia and anhedonia (Fernandes *et al.*, 1999; Giese-Davis *et al.*, 1993) and in patients with major depression (Keller *et al.*, 1999). Due to substantial comorbidity of anxiety and depression, Mohanty *et al.* (2000) used self-report scales that have been shown to distinguish between anxiety, depression and negative affect (Nitschke *et al.*, 2001) to determine which among these is related to the attentional deficit measured by N2b enhancement. The results indicate that it is negative affect, not something specific to depression or anxiety, that carries the N2b enhancement.

Two main hypotheses have been proposed to explain attention disturbances in depression; the resource allocation hypothesis, discussed in detail in earlier sections, and the distractor inhibition hypothesis (Ellis, 1991; Ellis and Ashbrook, 1988; Hertel and Rude, 1991). According to the distractor inhibition hypothesis, depressed individuals show an impaired ability to suppress external and internal distractors, resulting in inappropriate allocation of resources. The increased interference seen on attentional tasks requiring distractor inhibition such as the colour-word Stroop task (Raskin *et al.*, 1982; Trichard *et al.*, 1995) led Lemelin *et al.* (1997) to hypothesize that there is a difficulty in inhibiting distractors in depression. Support was provided for this hypothesis by a study using a negative priming paradigm which demonstrated that depressed patients had reduced ability to inhibit features of a distractor (MacQueen *et al.*, 2000).

Neural Correlates of Attention

An area that has been strongly implicated in both attentional and emotional processing is the anterior cingulate cortex. Bush *et al.* (2000) conducted a meta-analysis of activations and deactivations in the anterior cingulate during cognitive and emotional studies. They reported that the dorsal portion of the anterior cingulate was activated by Stroop and Stroop-like divided attention tasks as well as by complex response selection tasks. This area was deactivated (reduced blood flow or MR signal) by emotional tasks. The rostral ventral portion of the anterior cingulate was activated by tasks that relate to emotional content or symptom provocation (e.g. anxiety and induced sadness in depressed subjects) whereas this region was deactivated by cognitively challenging tasks. The reciprocal suppression of the so-called cognitive subdivision during intense emotional states such as severe depression (Bench *et al.*, 1992; Mayberg, 1997) or film-induced negative emotion could have important implications for attentional deficits in depression. Studies have shown that the cingulate gyrus is important in directed attention and in choosing the appropriate response in the presence of distractions or competing responses (Bench *et al.*, 1993; George *et al.*, 1994b). In a study designed to investigate the neural regions that could be involved in an attentional task in depression and normal controls, George *et al.* (1997) used a Stroop interference task and a modified Stroop interference task consisting of sad words. Results showed that control subjects activated the left anterior cingulate gyrus during a response interference task, whereas depressed individuals failed to show a corresponding increase in activity in this area. Instead, depressed individuals showed increased activation in the dorsolateral prefrontal cortex and visual cortex.

Mayberg (1997) postulated that the dorsal anterior cingulate (in conjunction with the dorsolateral prefrontal cortex) modulates the cognitive and psychomotor aspects of depression while the ventral anterior cingulate appears to modulate the vegetative, autonomic and affective aspects of depression, via the modulation of subgenual prefrontal cortex. Mayberg *et al.* (1999) reported increases in limbic–paralimbic blood flow (subgenual cingulate, anterior insula) and decreases in neocortical regions (right dorsolateral prefrontal, inferior parietal) during depression. After recovery, the reverse pattern, with limbic metabolic decreases and neocortical increases, was seen. A significant correlation between subgenus cingulate and right dorsolateral prefrontal activity was also demonstrated in both conditions. According to Mayberg and colleagues, the reciprocal regional relationship between ventral limbic and dorsal cortical compartments suggests that the negative influence of depressed mood on attention can be attributed to abnormal functional connections between these regions rather than concurrent changes in both sites independently.

Visuospatial Functioning

Depressed individuals have been shown to display deficits on tasks associated with cognitive functions implemented by right posterior regions of the brain (Heller and Nitschke, 1997). Individuals with depression show impaired performance on right hemisphere tasks such as judgement of line orientation, three-dimensional constructional praxis, spatial association learning, and subtests of the WAIS-R performance scale (Flor-Henry, 1976; Asthana *et al.*, 1998; Silberman and Weingarter, 1986). Furthermore, severity of depression has been found to correlate with performance on tests of visuospatial function such as spatial span, pattern recognition and delayed matching to sample (Elliott *et al.*, 1996).

NEUROPSYCHOLOGICAL FUNCTIONING IN MANIA

In contrast to the extensive literature describing the cognitive characteristics of depression, only a few studies have focused on the nature of cognitive impairment accompanying mania. According to Murphy *et al.* (2001) possible explanations for the scarcity of research in this area include practical problems in using standardized neuropsychological assessment procedures in mania, as well as the nature of a manic episode, which may prevent individuals from serving as reliable participants. In general, findings from a variety of studies show that mania is associated with impaired performance on neuropsychological tasks of attention (Bulbena and Berrios, 1993; Taylor and Abrams, 1986), memory, including pattern and spatial recognition memory as well as delayed visual recognition (Bulbena and Berrios, 1993; Bunney and Hartman, 1965; Henry *et al.*, 1971; Johnson and Magaro, 1987; Murphy *et al.*, 1999; Taylor and Abrams, 1986), and visuospatial functioning (Bulbena and Berrios, 1993; Taylor and Abrams, 1986). Some researchers attribute memory deficits in mania to altered patterns of verbal associations (Henry *et al.*, 1971), loosening of associations, and overinclusiveness, which results in an impaired ability to filter environmental stimuli (Andreason and Powers, 1974).

Another major area of functioning that is affected in mania is executive functioning. Individuals with mania exhibit disruptions in social behaviour and decision making similar to those observed in individuals with frontal cortical lesions (Bechara *et al.*, 1994). Mania is associated with deficits on executive functioning tasks such as attentional set-shifting tasks (Clark *et al.*, 2000; Morice, 1990), planning ability (Murphy *et al.*, 1999) and decision making (Clark *et al.*, 2000; Murphy *et al.*, 2001). Ferrier *et al.* (1999) also reported residual impairment in executive function in individuals with euthymic bipolar disorder after controlling for age, premorbid intelligence and depression symptoms.

Depression and mania are associated with distinct physiological, emotional and cognitive characteristics that seem to reflect the activity and function of different brain regions. Gainotti (1972) reported dramatic differences between patients with right brain damage, who exhibited cheerful and euphoric emotions (the 'indifference reaction'), and patients with left brain damage, who exhibited distressed and tearful emotions (the 'catastrophic reaction'). Similarly, another lesion study showed that mania was associated with damage to areas of the right hemisphere that are connected with the limbic system whereas depression was associated with damage to anterior cortical and subcortical regions of the left hemisphere (Robinson *et al.*, 1988). These findings suggest that brain mechanisms implemented in the right hemisphere are associated with negative affect while those associated with positive affect are implemented in the left hemisphere (Shackman, 2000). This is based on the assumption that focal brain lesions act as deactivating forces in the region in which they are located (Heller, 1990). Conversely, in normal individuals, one would expect that negative affect would be associated with increased activity in the right hemisphere while positive affect would be associated with increased activity in the left hemisphere.

Studies examining physiological activity during different emotions have shown that individuals who show greater left anterior activity report increased positive affect, engage in more approach behaviours, and respond more intensely to positive than negative stimuli, whereas individuals who show increased right hemisphere activity report more negative affect, engage in more avoidance behaviours, and respond more to negative than positive stimuli (for review, see Davidson, 1995). Consistent with these findings, the prefrontal cortex has been found to be differentially involved in negative and positive emotions, with increased left anterior activation during positive affect and increased right-sided activation during negative affect (Davidson, 1992, 1998; Davidson *et al.*, 1990).

Some studies comparing the performance of individuals on a range of neuropsychological tests report no differences between mania and depression (Bulbena and Berrios, 1993; Goldberg *et al.*, 1993). These findings have led to the hypothesis that similar neuropsychological processes are involved in mania and depression despite different clinical presentations (Murphy and Sahakian, 2001). However, differences in cognitive functioning between mania and depression emerged on a shifting task using affective stimuli (Murphy *et al.*, 1999). Individuals with mania were impaired in their ability to inhibit behavioural responses and focus attention, while depressed individuals were impaired in their ability to shift the focus of their attention. Furthermore, individuals with mania tended to show a bias towards positive stimuli while depressed individuals displayed a bias towards negative stimuli. These findings are in line with the prediction that different patterns of lateralized prefrontal activity would cause differences in cognitive performance, at least for affective stimuli, between mania and depression (Murphy *et al.*, 1999). Differences in performance were also seen on a recognition memory task, with a more conservative response bias associated with depression and a more liberal response bias associated with mania (Corwin *et al.*, 1990). Thus, cognitive performance in depression and mania seems to be influenced by the affective nature of the task as well as affective responses to task stimuli.

CONCLUSION

We have reviewed extensive evidence from a variety of sources suggesting that depression is associated with biases or deficits in cognitive functioning. Areas of cognitive functioning that are impaired in depression include executive functioning, attention, working memory, memory, particularly explicit memory, and visuospatial functioning. Further research aimed at the identification of moderator variables such as depression severity, psychosis, patient status and medication status is required to clarify the extent and nature of the relationship between depression and the aforementioned cognitive deficits.

Evidence from a variety of techniques such as neuropsychological testing, as well as lesion, electrophysiological and haemodynamic measurement, has implicated the role of different brain regions in cognitive functioning in depression. In general, cognitive deficits are associated with abnormal patterns of activity in anterior brain regions, particularly dorsolateral prefrontal, medial prefrontal, orbitofrontal and anterior cingulate cortex. Additionally, memory, attentional and visuospatial deficits appear to be related to abnormal activity in posterior brain regions, including the temporal lobe, and limbic structures such as the hippocampus.

Despite extensive evidence indicating of cognitive functioning deficits in depression, researchers examining the neuropsychology of depression have focused largely on the relationship of regional brain activity to emotion and not cognition (Heller and Nitschke, 1997). For a better understanding of cognitive neuropsychological disturbances in depression it is important to develop a comprehensive theoretical formulation elucidating the relationship between various brain regions and cognition. Examples of theoretical formulations relating regional brain activity and cognition in emotional disorders include Heller (1990, 1993), Davidson (1998), Drevets and Raichle (1998) and Mayberg (1997). For better characterization of cognitive deficits in depression it is also important to examine how emotion modulates cognition and vice versa. More specifically, studies designed to investigate reciprocal brain mechanisms as well as integrated brain mechanisms for emotion and cognition have important implications for cognitive deficits in depression. Insights into these issues could also benefit research on the cognitive correlates of mania. For example, earlier studies using affectively neutral stimuli have yielded findings suggesting similarities in cognitive dysfunction for mania and depression. However, recent studies utilizing experimental designs that require both cognitive and emotional processing have indicated biases in information processing and abnormal responses to feedback that appear to be consistent with distinct patterns of regional brain activity in mania and depression.

The association between neuropsychological impairment and depression has a number of clinical and research implications. According to Austin *et al.* (2001), both affective disturbance and cognitive impairment need to be considered as equally important manifestations of depressive disorder. They propose that cognitive testing can be used as a helpful adjunct in clinical evaluation of patients both at initial episode and following recovery. Cognitive testing in depression has potential as an evaluative tool because performance on cognitive tests has been shown to be sensitive to a variety of depression-related clinical variables such as severity (Moffoot *et al.*, 1994), presence of psychosis (Basso and Bornstein, 1999) and depression subtype (Silberman *et al.*, 1985). Despite evidence supporting sensitivity of cognitive measures to depression, it is still debatable whether cognitive deficits such as memory impairment are specific to depression or a reflection of a more general form of psychopathology (Burt *et al.*, 1995). Thus, an important diagnostic issue for clinicians is to determine whether findings of impaired memory in depression are specific to depression and distinctive enough to be used for purposes such as differentiating between depression and dementia (Burt *et al.*, 1995).

An area of research that has immense clinical utility involves the role of cognitive biases and deficits in the onset, course and maintenance of depression. For example, cognitive precursors such as information-processing biases may taint perceptions of previously depressed individuals and predispose them to the mood disturbance (Mathews and MacLeod, 1994). According to another cognitive perspective, known as the diathesis-stress model of cognitive vulnerability (Beck *et al.*, 1979), depression-relevant experiences trigger latent negative thoughts, leading to an increased risk of depression. Mineka and Gilboa (1998) argue that cognitive biases may play a threefold role, in which they mediate the course of emotional disorders, predict vulnerability to relapse, and contribute to the onset of depression.

In conclusion, an understanding of the neuropsychological concomitants of depression has the potential not only to enhance basic scientific knowledge of the disorder but also has important implications for intervention. Since researchers have proposed that cognitive characteristics such as executive functioning deficits, memory biases and attentional deficits play an important role in increasing risk for, as well as the maintenance of, depression (Mineka and Gilboa, 1998), treatment strategies aimed at improving neurocognitive functioning in these domains may prove to be beneficial in depression. Support for such strategies comes from treatment of schizophrenia and organic brain syndromes where neurocognitive rehabilitation programmes focusing on cognitive flexibility, working memory and planning ability have been shown to be effective (Delahunty and Morice, 1996; Garety *et al.*, 2000; Moore *et al.*, 2001; Morice and Delahunty, 1993). Similarly, research on patterns of abnormal brain activity in depression may contribute to an understanding of the mechanisms underlying pharmacological and psychological treatment in depression. For example, Mayberg *et al.* (1999) has suggested that the neural pathology associated with depression can be addressed via a top-down (psychotherapeutic) or bottom-up (pharmacological) intervention strategy, based on a model of reciprocal relationships between limbic and prefrontal cortical regions. Bench *et al.* (1995) reported that recovery from depression was associated with increases in rCBF in the same areas in which focal decreases in rCBF were described in the depressed state. Another example comes from the field of transcranial magnetic stimulation (TMS), a method that allows noninvasive stimulation of regions of the cerebral cortex. Using this method, researchers have demonstrated that left dorsolateral prefrontal cortex TMS resulted in significant decreases on measures of depression (Pascual-Leone *et al.*, 1996). Future research might capitalize on these findings by using cognitive and emotional activation paradigms to activate regions of the brain such as the left dorsolateral prefrontal cortex, and examining the effect of these manipulations on both depressed mood and cognitive deficits in depression.

REFERENCES

Abrams, R. and Taylor, M.A., 1987. Cognitive dysfunction in melancholia. *Psychological Medicine*, **17**, 359–62.

Alivisatos, B. and Milner, B., 1989. Effects of frontal or temporal lobectomy on the use of advance information in a choice reaction time task. *Neuropsychologia*, **27**, 495–503.

American Psychiatric Association, 1994. *Diagnostic and Statistical Manual of Mental Disorders*, 4th edn. APA, Washington, DC.

Andreasen, N.J.C. and Powers, P.S., 1974. Overinclusive thinking in mania and schizophrenia. *British Journal of Psychiatry*, **125**, 452–6.

Asthana, H.S., Mandal, M.K., Khurana, H. and Haque-Nizamie, S., 1998. Visuospatial and affect recognition deficit in depression. *Journal of Affective Disorders*, **48**, 57–62.

Austin, M.P., Ross, M., Murray, C., O'Carroll, R.E., Ebmeier, K.P. and Goodwin, G.M., 1992. Cognitive function in major depression. *Journal of Affective Disorders*, **25**, 21–9

Austin, M.P., Mitchell, P., Wilhelm, K., Parker, G., Hickie, I., Brodaty, H., Chan, J., Eyers, K., Milic, M. and Hadzi-Pavlovic, D., 1999. Cognitive function in depression: a distinct pattern of frontal impairment in melancholia? *Psychological Medicine*, **29**, 73–85.

Austin, M.P., Mitchell, P. and Goodwin, G.M., 2001. Cognitive deficits in depression: possible implications for functional neuropathology. *British Journal of Psychiatry*, **178**, 200–6.

Banich, M.T., 1997. *Neuropsychology: The Neural Bases of Mental Function*. Houghton Mifflin, Boston, MA.

Basso, M.R. and Bornstein, R.A., 1999. Neuropsychological deficits in psychotic versus nonpsychotic unipolar depression. *Neuropsychology*, **13**, 69–75.

Baxter, L.R., Schwartz, J.M., Phelps, M.E., Mazziotta, J.C., Guze, B.H., Selin, C.E., Gerner, R.H. and Sumida, R.M., 1989. Reduction of prefrontal cortex glucose metabolism common to three types of depression. *Archives of General Psychiatry*, **46**, 243–50.

Beats, B.C., Sahakian, B.J. and Levy, R., 1996. Cognitive performance in tests sensitive to frontal lobe dysfunction in the elderly depressed. *Psychological Medicine*, **26**, 591–603.

Bechara, A., Damasio, A.R., Damasio, H. and Anderson, S.W., 1994. Insensitivity to future consequences following damage to human prefrontal cortex. *Cognition*, **50**, 7–15.

Beck, A.T., 1967. *Depression: Causes and Treatments*. University of Pennsylvania Press, Philadelphia, PA.

Beck, A.T., Rush, A.J., Shaw, B.F. and Emery, G., 1979. *Cognitive Therapy of Depression*. Basic Books, New York.

Bemelmans, K.J., Goekoop, J.G. and van Kempen, G.M.J., 1996. Recall performance in acutely depressed patients and plasma cortisol. *Biological Psychiatry*, **39**, 750–2.
Bench, C.J., Friston, K.J., Brown, R.G., Scott, L.C., Frackowiak, R.S. and Dolan, R.J., 1992. The anatomy of melancholia — focal abnormalities of cerebral blood flow in major depression. *Psychological Medicine*, **22**, 605–17.
Bench, C.J., Frith, C.D., Grasby, P.M., Friston, K.J., Paulesu, P., Frackowiak, R.S.J. and Dolan, R.J., 1993. Investigations of the functional anatomy of attention using the Stroop test. *Neuropsychologia*, **31**, 907–2.
Bench, C.J., Frankowiak, R.S.J. and Dolan, R.J., 1995. Changes in regional cerebral blood flow on recovery from depression. *Psychological Medicine*, **25**, 247–61.
Bowen, D.M., Najlerahim, A., Procter, A.W., Francis, P.T. and Murphy, E., 1989. Circumscribed changes of the cerebral cortex in neuropsychiatric disorders of later life. *Proceedings of National Academy of Sciences*, **86**, 9504–8.
Bradley, B.P. and Mathews, A., 1983. Negative self-schemata in clinical depression. *British Journal of Clinical Psychology*, **22**, 171–83.
Bremner, J.D., Narayan, M., Anderson, E.R., Staib, L.H., Miller, H.L. and Charey, D.S., 2000. Hippocampal volume reduction in major depression. *American Journal of Psychiatry*, **157**, 115–7.
Brown, E.S., Rush, A.J. and McEwen, B.S., 1999. Hippocampal remodeling and damage by corticosteroids: implications for mood disorders. *Neuropsychopharmacology*, **21**, 474–84.
Bulbena, A. and Berrios, G.E., 1993. Cognitive function in the affective disorders: a prospective study. *Psychopathology*, **26**, 6–12.
Bunney, W.E.J. and Hartmann, E.L., 1965. A study of a patient with 48-hour manic depressive cycles, I. An analysis of behavioral factors. *Archives of General Psychiatry*, **12**, 611–18.
Burt, D.B., Zembar, M.J. and Niederehe, G., 1995. Depression and memory impairment: a meta-analysis of the association, its pattern, and specificity. *Psychological Bulletin*, **117**, 285–305.
Bush, G., Luu, P. and Posner, M.I., 2000. Cognitive and emotional influences in anterior cingulate cortex. *Trends in Cognitive Science*, **4**, 215–22.
Channon, S., 1996. Executive dysfunction in depression: the Wisconsin card sorting test. *Journal of Affective Disorders*, **39**, 107–14.
Channon, S. and Green, P.S.S., 1999. Executive function in depression: the role of performance strategies in aiding depressed and non-depressed patients. *Journal of Neurology, Neurosurgery and Psychiatry*, **66**, 162–71.
Cicerone, K.D., Lazar, R.M. and Shapiro, W.R., 1983. Effects of frontal lobe lesions on hypothesis sampling during concept formation. *Neuropsychologia*, **21**, 513–24.
Clark, D.M. and Teasdale, J.D., 1982. Diurnal variation in clinical depression and accessibility of memories of positive and negative experiences. *Journal of Abnormal Psychology*, **91**, 87–95.
Clark, D.M., Teasdale, J.D., Broadbent, D.E. and Marti, M., 1983. Effect of mood on lexical decisions. *Bulletin of the Psychonomic Society*, **21**, 175–8.
Clark, L., Iverson, S.D. and Goodwin, G.M., 2000. A neuropsychological investigation of prefrontal cortex function in acute mania. *Journal of Psychopharmacology*, **14**, A22.
Coffey, C.E., Wilkinson, W.E., Weiner, R.D., Parashos, I.A., Djang, W.T., Webb, M.C., Figiel, G.S. and Spritzer, C.E., 1993. Quantitative cerebral anatomy in depression: a controlled magnetic resonance imaging study. *Archives of General Psychiatry*, **50**, 7–16.
Compton, R.J., Banich, M.T., Mohanty, A., Milham, M.P., Miller, G.A., Scalf, P.E. and Heller, W. (submitted) Paying attention to emotion: An fMRI investigation of cognitive and emotional stroop tasks.
Cornblatt, B.A., Lenzenweger, M.F. and Erlennmeyer-Kimmling, K.L., 1989. The continuous performance test, identical pair version: II. Contrasting attentional profile in schizophrenic and depressed patients. *Psychiatry Research*, **29**, 65–86.
Cornell, D.G., Suarez, R. and Berent, S., 1984. Psychomotor retardation in melancholic and nonmelancholic depression: cognitive and motor components. *Journal of Abnormal Psychology*, **93**, 150–7
Corwin, J., Peselow, E., Feenan, K., Rotrosen, J. and Fieve, R., 1990. Disorders of decision in affective disease: an effect of β-adrenergic dysfunction? *Biological Psychiatry*, **27**, 813–33.
Coryell, W., Leon, A., Winokur, G., Endicott, J., Keller, M., Akiskal, H. and Solomon, D., 1996. Importance of psychotic features to long-term course in major depressive disorder. *American Journal of Psychiatry*, **153**, 483–9.
Cutting, J., 1979. Memory in functional psychosis. *Journal of Neurology, Neurosurgery, and Psychiatry*, **42**, 1031–7.
Dalgleish, T. and Watts, F.N., 1990. Biases of attention and memory in disorders of anxiety and depression. *Clinical Psychology Review*, **10**, 589–604.
Danion, J.M., Kauffmann-Muller, F., Grange, D., Zimmerman, M.A. and Greth, P., 1995. Affective valence of words, explicit and implicit memory in clinical depression. *Journal of Affective Disorders*, **34**, 227–34.
Davidson, R.J., 1992. Emotion and affective style: hemispheric substrates. *Psychological Science*, **3**, 39–43.
Davidson, R.J., 1995. Cerebral asymmetry, emotion and affective style. In: Davidson, R.J. and Hughdahl, K. (eds), *Brain Asymmetry*, pp. 361–87. MIT Press, Cambridge, MA.
Davidson, R.J., 1998. Affective style and affective disorders: perspectives from affective neuroscience. *Cognition Emotion*, **12**, 307–20.
Davidson, R.J., Schwartz, G.E., Saron, C., Benett, J. and Goleman, D.J., 1979. Frontal versus parietal EEG asymmetry during positive and negative affect. *Psychophysiology*, **16**, 202–3.
Davidson, R.J., Schaffer, C.E. and Saron, C., 1985. Effects of lateralized presentations on self reports of emotion and EEG asymmetry in depressed and non-depressed subjects. *Psychophysiology*, **22**, 353–64.
Davidson, R.J., Ekman, P., Saron, C.D., Senulis, J.A. and Friesen, W.V., 1990. Approach-withdrawal and cerebral asymmetry: emotional expression and brain physiology: I. *Journal of Personality and Social Psychology*, **58**, 330–41.
Degl'Innocenti, A., Agren, H. and Backman, L., 1998. Executive deficits in major depression. *Acta Psychiatrica Scandinavica*, **97**, 182–8
Delahunty, A. and Morice, R., 1996. Rehabilitation of frontal/executive impairments in schizophrenia. *Australian and New Zealand Journal of Psychiatry*, **30**, 760–7.
Deldin, P.J., Keller, J., Gergen, J.A. and Miller, G.A., 2000. Right-posterior face processing anomaly in depression. *Journal of Abnormal Psychology*, **109**, 116–21.
Denny, E.B. and Hunt, R.R., 1992. Affective valence and memory in depression: dissociation of recall and fragment completion. *Journal of Abnormal Psychology*, **101**, 575–80.
Dolan, R.J., Bench, C.J., Brown, R.G., Scott, L.C., Friston, K.J. and Frackowiak, R.S.J., 1992. Regional cerebral blood flow abnormalities in depressed patients with cognitive impairment. *Journal of Neurology, Neurosurgery and Psychiatry*, **55**, 768–73
Dolan, R.J., Bench, C.J., Brown, R.G., Scott, L.C. and Frackowiak, R.S.J., 1994. Neuropsychological dysfunction in depression: the relationship to regional cerebral blood flow. *Psychological Medicine*, **24**, 849–57.
Drevets, W.C., 1999. Prefrontal cortical-amygdalar metabolism in major depression. *Annals of New York Academy of Sciences*, **877**, 614–37.
Drevets, W.C. and Raichle, M.E., 1995. Positron emission tomographic imaging studies of human emotional disorders. In: Gazzaniga, M.S. (ed), *The Cognitive Neurosciences*, pp. 1153–64. MIT Press, Cambridge, MA.
Drevets, M.C. and Raichle, M.E., 1998. Reciprocal suppression of regional cerebral blood flow during emotional versus higher cognitive processes: implications for interactions between emotion and cognition. *Cognition and Emotion*, **12**, 353–85.
Dunbar, G.C. and Lishman, W.A., 1984. Depression, recognition-memory and hedonic tone: a signal detection analysis. *British Journal of Psychiatry*, **144**, 376–82.
Ellis, H.C., 1991. Focused attention and depressive deficits in memory. *Journal of Experimental Psychology: General*, **120**, 310–12.
Ellis, H.C. and Ashbrook, P.W., 1988. Resource allocation model of the effects of depressed mood states on memory. In: Fiedler, K. and Forgas, J. (eds), *Affect, Cognition and Social Behavior*, pp. 25–43. Toronto, Hogrefe.
Ellis, H.C. and Ashbrook, P.W., 1989. The 'state' of mood and memory research: a selective review. *Journal of Social Behavior and Personality*, **4**, 1–21.
Elliott, R., Sahakian, B.J., McKay, A.P., Herrod, J.J., Robbins, T.W. and Paykel, E.S., 1996. Neuropsychological impairments in unipolar depression: the influence of perceived failure on subsequent performance. *Psychological Medicine*, **26**, 975–90.
Elliott, R., Baker, S.C., Rogers, R.D., O'Leary, D.A., Paykel, E.S., Frith, C.D., Dolan, R.J. and Sahakian, B.J., 1997. Prefrontal dysfunction in depressed patients performing a complex planning task: a study using positron emission tomography. *Psychological Medicine*, **27**, 931–42.

Elliott, R., Sahakian, B.J., Michael, A., Paykel, E.S. and Dolan, R.J., 1998. Abnormal neural response to feedback on planning and guessing tasks in patients with unipolar depression. *Psychological Medicine*, **28**, 559–71.

Etienne, M.A., Heller, W., Nitschke, J.B. and Miller, G.A., 1999. Frontal brain activity is related to memory performance in depression. Poster session presented at annual meeting of Society for Research in Psychopathology, Montreal, Quebec, Canada.

Fernandes, L.O.L., Keller, J., Giese-Davis, J.E., Hicks, B.D., Klein, D.N. and Miller, G.A., 1999. Converging evidence for a cognitive anomaly in early psychopathology. *Psychophysiology*, **36**, 511–21.

Ferrier, I.N., Stanton, B.R., Kelly, T.P. and Scott, J., 1999. Neuropsychological function in euthymic patients with bipolar disorder. *British Journal of Psychiatry*, **175**, 246–51.

Flor-Henry, P., 1976. Lateralized temporal limbic dysfunction and psychopathology. *Annals of New York Academy of Sciences*, **280**, 777–95.

Franke, P., Maier, W., Hardt, J., Frieboes, R., Lichtermann, D. and Hain, C., 1993. Assessment of frontal lobe functioning in schizophrenia and unipolar major depression. *Psychopathology*, **26**, 76–84.

Friedman, A.S., 1964. Minimal effects of severe depression on cognitive functioning. *Journal of Abnormal and Social Psychology*, **69**, 237–43.

Frith, C.D., Stevens, M., Johnstone, E.C., Deakin, J.F., Lawler, P. and Crow, T.J., 1983. Effects of ECT and depression on various aspects of memory. *British Journal of Psychiatry*, **142**, 610–17.

Ganiotti, G., 1972. Emotional behavior and hemisphere side of the lesion, *Cortex*, **8**, 41–55.

Garety, P.A., Fowler, D. and Kuipers, E., 2000. Cognitive-behavioral therapy for medication-resistant symptoms. *Schizophrenia Bulletin*, **26**, 73–86.

George, M.S., Ketter, T.A. and Post, R.M., 1993. SPECT and PET imaging in mood disorders. *Journal of Clinical Psychiatry*, **54**, 6–13.

George, M.S., Ketter, T.A. and Post, R.M., 1994a. Prefrontal cortex dysfunction in clinical depression. *Depression*, **2**, 59–72.

George, M.S., Ketter, T.A., Parekh, P.I. *et al.*, 1994b. Regional brain activity when selecting a response despite interference: an $H_2\,^{15}O$ PET study of the Stroop and an emotional Stroop. *Human Brain Mapping*, **1**, 194–209.

George, M.S., Ketter, T.A., Parekh, P.I., Rosinsky, N., Ring, H.A., Pazzaglia, P.J., Marangell, L.B., Callahan, A.M. and Post, R.M., 1997. Blunted left cingulate activation in mood disorder subjects response interference task (the Stroop). *Journal of Neuropsychiatry and Clinical Neurosciences*, **9**, 55–63.

Gewirtz, G., Squires-Wheeler, E., Sharif, Z. and Honer, W.G., 1994. Results of computerised tomography during first admission for psychosis. *British Journal of Psychiatry*, **164**, 789–95.

Giese-Davis, J., Miller, G.A. and Knight, R., 1993. Memory template comparison processes in anhedonia and dysthymia. *Psychophysiology*, **30**, 646–56.

Gilligan, S.C. and Bower, G.H., 1984. Cognitive consequences of emotional arousal. In: Izard, C., Kagan, J. and Zajonc, R. (eds), *Emotions, Cognitions, and Behavior*, pp. 547–88. Cambridge University Press, New York.

Gjerde, P.F., 1983. Attentional capacity dysfunction and arousal in schizophrenia. *Psychological Bulletin*, **93**, 57–72.

Goldberg, T.E., Gold, J.M., Greenberg, R., Griffin, S., Schulz, S.C., Pickar, D., Kleinman, J.E. and Weinberger, D.R., 1993. Contrasts between patients with affective disorders and patients with schizophrenia on a neuropsychological test battery. *American Journal of Psychiatry*, **150**, 1355–62.

Golinkoff, M. and Sweeney, J.A., 1989. Cognitive impairments in depression. *Journal of Affective Disorders*, **17**, 105–12.

Goodwin, G.M., 1997. Neuropsychological and neuroimaging evidence for the involvement of the frontal lobes in depression. *Journal of Psychopharmacology*, **11**, 115–22.

Gotlib, I.H. and Cane, D.B., 1987. Construct accessibility and clinical depression: a longitudinal investigation. *Journal of Abnormal Psychology*, **96**, 199–204.

Gotlib, I.H. and Krasnoperova, E., 1998. Biased information processing as a vulnerability factor for depression. *Behavior Therapy*, **29**, 603–17.

Gotlib, I.H. and McCann, C.D., 1984. Construct accessibility and depression: an examination of cognitive and affective factors. *Journal of Personality and Social Psychology*, **47**, 427–39.

Gotlib, I.H., Gilboa, E. and Sommerfeld, B.K., 2000. Cognitive functioning depression: nature and origins. In: Davidson, R.J. (ed.), *Wisconsin Symposium on Emotion,* Vol. 1, *Anxiety, Depression, and Emotion*, pp. 133–63. Oxford University Press, New York.

Grasby, P.M., Frith, C.D., Friston, K.J., Bench, C., Frackowiak, R.S.J. and Dolan, R.J., 1993. Functional mapping of brain areas implicated in auditory memory function. *Brain*, **116**, 1–20.

Hamilton, M., 1960. A rating scale for depression. *Journal of Neurology, Neurosurgery, and Psychiatry*, **23**, 56–62.

Hartlage, S., Alloy, L.B., Vazquez, C. and Dykman, B., 1993. Automatic and effortful processing in depression. *Psychological Bulletin*, **113**, 247–78.

Heller, W., 1990. The neuropsychology of emotion: developmental patterns and implications for psychopathology. In: Stein, N.L., Leventhal, B. and Trabasso, T. (eds), *Psychological and Biological Approaches to Emotion*, pp. 167–211. Lawrence Eribaum, Hillsdale, NJ.

Heller, W., 1993. Neuropsychological mechanisms of individual differences in emotion, personality, and arousal. *Neuropsychology*, **7**, 1–14.

Heller, W. and Nitschke, J.B., 1997. Regional brain activity in emotion: a framework for understanding cognition in depression. *Cognition and Emotion*, **11**, 638–61.

Heller, W. and Nitschke, J.B., 1998. The puzzle of regional brain activity in depression and anxiety: the importance of subtypes and comorbidity. *Cognition and Emotion*, **12**, 421–47.

Heller, W., Etienne, M.A. and Miller, G.A., 1995. Patterns of perceptual asymmetry in depression and anxiety: implications for neuropsychological models of emotion and psychopathology. *Journal of Abnormal Psychology*, **104**, 327–33.

Heller, W., Nitschke, J.B., Etienne, M.A. and Miller, G.A., 1997. Patterns of regional brain activity differentiate types of anxiety. *Journal of Abnormal Psychology*, **106**, 376–85.

Henriques, J.B. and Davidson, R.J., 1990. Regional brain electrical asymmetries discriminate between previously depressed and healthy control subjects. *Journal of Abnormal Psychology*, **99**, 22–31.

Henriques, J.B. and Davidson, R.J., 1991. Left frontal hypoactivation in depression. *Journal of Abnormal Psychology*, **100**, 535–45.

Henry, G., Weingartner, H.G. and Murphy, D., 1971. Idiosyncratic patterns of learning and word association during mania. *American Journal of Psychiatry*, **128**, 564–73.

Herrmann, M., Rotte, M., Grubich, C., Ebert, A.D., Schiltz, K., Muente, T.F. and Heinze, H.J., 2001. Control of semantic interference in episodic memory retrieval is associated with an anterior cingulate-prefrontal activation pattern. *Human Brain Mapping*, **13**, 94–103.

Hertel, P.T., 1994. Depression and memory: are impairments remediable through attentional control? *Current Direction in Psychological Science*, **3**, 190–4.

Hertel, P.T. and Hardin, T.S., 1990. Remembering with and without awareness in a depressed mood: evidence of deficits in initiative. *Journal of Experimental Psychology: General*, **119**, 45–59.

Hertel, P.T. and Milan, S., 1994. Depressive deficits in recognition: dissociation of recollection and familiarity. *Journal of Abnormal Psychology*, **103**, 736–42.

Hertel, P.T. and Rude, S.S., 1991. Depressive deficits in memory: focusing attention improves subsequent recall. *Journal of Experimental Psychology: General*, **120**, 301–9.

Hockey, R., 1986. Stress and cognitive components of skilled performance. In: Hamilton, V. and Warburton, D. (eds), *Human Stress and Cognition*, pp. 141–78. John Wiley & Sons, Chichester.

Ilsley, J.E., Moffoot, A.P.R. and O'Carroll, R.E., 1995. An analysis of memory dysfunction in major depression. *Journal of Affective Disorders*, **35**, 1–9.

Ingram, R.E., 1990. Depressive cognition: models, mechanisms, and methods. In: Ingram, R.E. (ed.), *Contemporary Psychological Approaches to Depression: Theory, Research, and Treatment*, pp. 169–95. Plenum Press, New York.

Ingram, R.E., Bernet, C.Z. and McLaughlin, S.C., 1994. Attentional allocation processes in individuals at risk for depression. *Cognitive Therapy and Research*, **18**, 317–32.

Jeste, D.V., Heaton, S.C., Paulsen, J.S., Ercoli, L., Harris, M.J. and Heaton, R.K., 1996. Clinical and neuropsychological comparison of psychotic depression with nonpsychotic depression and schizophrenia. *American Journal of Psychiatry*, **153**, 490–6.

Johnson, M.H. and Magaro, P.A., 1987. Effects of mood severity on memory processes in depression and mania. *Psychological Bulletin*, **101**, 28–40.

Jones, B.P., Henderson, M. and Welch, C.A., 1988. Executive functions in unipolar depression before and after electroconvulsive therapy. *International Journal of Neuroscience*, **38**, 287–97.

Keller, J., Isaacks, B.G., Wesemann, D., Gergen, J.A. and Miller, G.A., 1999. Diagnostic and cognitive specificity of memory deficits in psychopathology. Paper presented at the annual meeting of the Cognitive Neuroscience Society, Washington, DC.

Keller, J., Nitschke, J.B., Bhargava, T., Deldin, P.J., Gergen, J.A., Miller, G.A. and Heller, W., 2000. Neuropsychological differentiation of depression and anxiety. *Journal of Abnormal Psychology*, **109**, 3–10.

Kendell, R.E. and Gourlay, J., 1970. The clinical distinction between the affective psychoses and schizophrenia. *British Journal of Psychiatry*, **117**, 261–6.

Kiloh, L.G., 1961. Pseudo-dementia. *Acta Psychiatrica Scandinavica*, **37**, 336–50.

Klein, D.C. and Seligman, M.E., 1976. Reversal of performance deficits and perceptual deficits in learned helplessness and depression. *Journal of Abnormal Psychology*, **85**, 11–26.

Klein, D.C., Fencil-Morse, E. and Seligman, M.E., 1976. Learned helplessness, depression, and the attribution of failure. *Journal of Personality and Social Psychology*, **33**, 508–16.

Krasnoperova, E., Neubauer, D.L. and Gotlib, I.H., 1998. Attentional biases for negative interpersonal stimuli in clinical depression and anxiety. Unpublished manuscript, Stanford University.

Lemelin, S., Baruch, P., Vincent, A., Everett, J. and Vincent, P., 1997. Distractibility and processing resource deficit in major depression: evidence for two deficient attentional processing models. *Journal of Nervous and Mental Diseases*, **185**, 542–8.

Lesser, I.M., Miller, B.L., Boone, K.B., Hill-Gutierrez, E.H., Mehringer, C.M., Wong, K. and Mena, I., 1991. Brain injury and cognitive function in late-onset psychotic depression. *Journal of Neuropsychiatry and Clinical Neurosciences*, **3**, 33–40.

Lipsey, J.R., Robinson, R.G., Pearlson, G.D., Rao, K. and Price, T.R., 1983. Mood change following bilateral hemisphere brain injury. *British Journal of Psychiatry*, **143**, 266–73.

Lloyd, G.G. and Lishman, W.A., 1975. Effect of depression on the speed of recall of pleasant and unpleasant experiences. *Psychological Medicine*, **5**, 173–80.

Luria, A.R., 1966. *Higher Cortical Functions in Man*. Basic Books, New York.

MacQueen, G.M., Tipper, S.P., Young, L.T., Joffe, R.T. and Levitt, A.J., 2000. Impaired distractor inhibition on a selective attention task in unmedicated, depressed subjects. *Psychological Medicine*, **30**, 557–64.

Marsden, C.D. and Harrison, M.J.G., 1972. Outcome of investigation of patients with presenile dementia. *British Medical Journal*, **2**, 249–52.

Martinot, J., Hardy, P., Feline, A., Huret, J., Mazoyer, B., Attar-Levy, D., Pappata, S. and Syrota, A., 1990. Left prefrontal glucose hypometabolism in the depressed state: a confirmation. *American Journal of Psychiatry*, **147**, 1313–17.

Massman, P.J., Delis, D.C., Butters, N., Dupont, R.M. and Gillin, J.C., 1992. The subcortical dysfunction hypothesis of memory deficits in depression: neuropsychological validation in a subgroup of patients. *Journal of Clinical and Experimental Neuropsychology*, **14**, 687–706.

Mathews, A. and MacLeod, C., 1994. Cognitive approaches to emotion and emotional disorders. *Annual Review of Psychology*, **45**, 25–50.

Mathews, A., Ridgeway, V. and Williamson, D.A., 1996. Evidence for attention to threatening stimuli in depression. *Behavior Research and Therapy*, **34**, 695–705.

Mayberg, H.S., 1997. Limbic-cortical dysregulation: a proposed model of depression. *Journal of Neuropsychiatry and Clinical Neurosciences*, **9**, 471–81.

Mayberg, H.S., Liotti, M., Brannan, S.K., McGinnis, S., Mahurin, R.K., Jerabek, P.A., Silva, J.A., Tekell, J.L., Martin, C.C., Lancaster, J.L. and Fox, P.T., 1999. Reciprocal limbic-cortical function and negative mood: converging PET findings in depression and normal sadness. *American Journal of Psychiatry*, **156**, 675–82.

McCabe, S.B. and Gotlib, I.H., 1993. Attentional processing in clinically depressed subjects: a longitudinal investigation. *Cognitive Therapy and Research*, **17**, 359–77.

Merrian, E.P., Thase, M.E., Haas, G.L., Keshavan, M.S. and Sweeney, J.A., 1999. Prefrontal cortical dysfunction in depression determined by Wisconsin Card Sorting test performance. *American Journal of Psychiatry*, **156**, 780–2.

Mervaala, E., Fohr, J., Kononen, M., Valkonen-Korhonen, M., Vainio, P., Partanen, K., Partanen, J., Tiihonen, J., Viinamaki, H., Karjalainen, A.K. and Lehtonen, J., 2000. Quantitative MRI of the hippocampus and the amygdala in severe depression. *Psychological Medicine*, **30**, 117–25.

Mialet, J.-P., Pope, H.G. and Yurgelun-Todd, D., 1996. Impaired attention in depressive states: a non-specific deficit? *Psychological Medicine*, **26**, 1009–20.

Miller, E.N., Fujioka, T.A., Chapman, I.J. and Chapman, J.P., 1995. Hemispheric asymmetries of function in patients with major affective disorders. *Journal of Psychiatric Research*, **29**, 173–83.

Miller, G.A., 1996. How we think about cognition, emotion, and biology in psychopathology. *Psychophysiology*, **33**, 615–28.

Mineka, S. and Gilboa, E., 1998. Cognitive biases in anxiety and depression. In: Flack, W.F. Jr and Laird, J.D. (eds), *Emotions in Psychopathology: Theory and Research*, pp. 216–28. Oxford University Press, New York.

Miyake, A., Friedman, N., Emerson, M., Witzki, A.H. and Howerter, A., 2000. The unity and diversity of executive functions and their contributions to complex 'frontal lobe' tasks: a latent variable analysis. *Cognitive Psychology*, **41**, 49–100.

Moffoot, A.P.R., O'Carroll, R.E., Bennie, J., Carroll, S., Dicj, H., Ebmeier, K.P. and Goodwin, G.M., 1994. Diurnal variation of mood and neuropsychological function in major depression with melancholia. *Journal of Affective Disorders*, **32**, 257–69.

Mogg, K., Bradley, B.P., Williams, R. and Matthews, A., 1993. Subliminal processing of emotional information in anxiety and depression. *Journal of Abnormal Psychology*, **102**, 304–11.

Mogg, K., Millar, N. and Bradley, B.P., 2000. Biases in eye movements to threatening facial expressions in generalized anxiety disorder and depressive disorder. *Journal of Abnormal Psychology*, **109**, 695–704.

Mohanty, A., Herrington, J.D., Fisher, J.E., Koven, N.S., Keller, J., Gergen, J.A., Heller, W. and Miller, G.A., 2000. Distinguishing cognitive deficits: negative affect in depression. Poster session presented at the annual meeting of the Society for Research in Psychopathology, Boulder, CO

Monsell, S., 1996. Control of mental processes. In: Bruce, V. (ed.), *Unsolved Mysteries of the Mind: Tutorial Essays in Cognition*, pp. 93–148. Erlbaum Taylor and Francis, Hove.

Moore, S., Sandman, C.A., McGrady, K. and Kesslak, J.P., 2001. Memory training improves cognitive ability in patients with dementia. *Neuropsychological Rehabilitation*, **11**, 245–61.

Morice, R., 1990. Cognitive inflexibility and pre-frontal dysfunction in schizophrenia and mania. *British Journal of Psychiatry*, **157**, 50–4.

Morice, R. and Delahunty, A., 1993. Integrated psychological therapy for schizophrenia. *British Journal of Psychiatry*, **163**, 414.

Morris, N. and Jones, D.M., 1990. Memory updating in working memory: the role of the central executive. *British Journal of Psychology*, **81**, 111–21.

Murphy, F.C. and Sahakian, B.J., 2001. Neuropsychology of bipolar disorder. *British Journal of Psychiatry*, **178**, 120–7.

Murphy, F.C., Sahakian, B.J., Rubinsztein, J.S., Michael, A., Rogers, R.D., Robbins, T.W. and Paykel, E.S., 1999. Emotional bias and inhibitory control processes in mania and depression. *Psychological Medicine*, **29**, 1307–21.

Murphy, F.C., Rubinsztein, J.S., Michael, A., Rogers, R.D., Robbins, T.W., Paykel, E.S. and Sahakian, B.J.I., 2001. Decision-making cognition in mania and depression. *Psychological Medicine*, **31**, 679–93.

Nelson, E., Sax, K.W. and Strakowski, S.M., 1998. Attentional performance in patients with psychotic and nonpsychotic major depression and schizophrenia. *American Journal of Psychiatry*, **155**, 137–9.

Nitschke, J.B., Heller, W. and Miller, G.A., 2000. Anxiety, stress, and cortical brain function. In: Borod, J.C. (ed.), *The Neuropsychology of Emotion*, pp. 298–319. Oxford University Press, New York.

Nitschke, J.B., Heller, W., Imig, J.C., McDonald, R.P. and Miller, G.A., 2001. Distinguishing dimensions of anxiety and depression. *Cognitive Therapy and Research*, **25**, 1–22.

Paradiso, S., Lamberty, G.J., Garvey, M.J. and Robinson, R.G., 1997. Cognitive impairment in the euthymic phase of chronic unipolar depression. *Journal of Nervous and Mental Disease*, **185**, 748–54.

Pascual-Leone, A., Rubio, B., Pallardo, F. and Catala, M.D., 1996. Rapid-rate transcranial magnetic stimulation of left dorsolateral prefrontal cortex in drug-resistant depression. *Lancet*, **348**, 233–7.

Pelosi, L., Slade, T., Blumhardt, L.D. and Sharma, V.K., 2000. Working memory dysfunction in major depression: an event-related potential study. *Clinical Neurophysiology*, **111**, 1531–43.

Price, K.P., Tryon, W.W. and Raps, C.S., 1978. Learned helplessness and depression in a clinical population: a test of two behavioral hypotheses. *Journal of Abnormal Psychology*, **87**, 113–21.

Purcell, R., Maruff, P., Kyrios, M. and Pantelis, C., 1997. Neuropsychological function in young patients with unipolar major depression. *Psychological Medicine*, **27**, 1277–85.

Raskin, A., Friedman, A.S. and DeMascio, A., 1982. Cognitive and performance deficits in depression. *Psychopharmacology Bulletin*, **18**, 196–202.

Richards, P.M. and Ruff, R.M., 1989. Motivational effects on neuropsychological functioning: Comparison of depressed versus nondepressed individuals. *Journal of Consulting and Clinical Psychology*, **57**, 396–402.

Robinson, R.G. and Price, T.R., 1982. Post-stroke depressive disorders: a follow-up study of 103 patients. *Stroke*, **13**, 635–41.

Robinson, R.G., Starr, L.B., Kubos, K.L. and Price, T.R., 1983. A two-year longitudinal study of post stroke mood disorders: findings during the initial evaluation. *Stroke*, **14**, 736–41.

Robinson, R.G., Kubos, K.L., Starr, L.B., Rao, K. and Price, T.R., 1984. Mood disorders in stroke patients. *Brain*, **107**, 81–93.

Robinson, R.G., Lipsey, J.R., Bolla-Wilson, K., Bolduc, P.L., Pearlson, G.D., Rao, K. and Price, T.R., 1985. Mood disorders in left-handed stroke patients. *American Journal of Psychiatry*, **142**, 1424–9.

Robinson, R.G., Boston, J.D., Starkstein, S.E. and Price, T.R., 1988. Comparison of mania and depression after brain injury: causal factors. *American Journal of Psychiatry*, **145**, 172–8.

Roediger, H.L. and McDermott, K.B., 1992. Depression and implicit memory: a commentary. *Journal of Abnormal Psychology*, **101**, 587–91.

Roy-Byrne, P.P., Weingartner, H., Bierer, L.M., Thompson, K. and Post, R.M., 1986. Effortful and automatic cognitive processes in depression. *Archives of General Psychiatry*, **43**, 265–7.

Rubinow, D.R. and Post, R.M., 1992. Impaired recognition of affect in facial expression in depressed patients. *Biological Psychiatry*, **31**, 947–53.

Schaffer, C.E., Davidson, R.J. and Saron, C., 1983. Frontal and parietal electroencephalogram asymmetry in depressed and nondepressed subjects. *Biological Psychiatry*, **18**, 753–62.

Schultz, W., Apicella, P., Scarnati, E. and Ljungberg, T., 1992. Neuronal activity in monkey ventral striatum related to the expectation of reward. *Journal of Neuroscience*, **12**, 4595–610.

Shackman, A.J., 2000. Anterior cerebral asymmetry, affect, and psychopathology: commentary on the withdrawal-approach model. In: R.J. Davidson (ed.), *Anxiety, Depression, and Emotion*, pp. 109–32. Oxford University Press, Oxford.

Shah, P.J., Ebmeier, K.P., Glabus, M.F. and Goodwin, G.M., 1998. Cortical grey matter reductions associated with treatment-resistant chronic unipolar depression: controlled magnetic resonance imaging study. *British Journal Psychiatry*, **172**, 527–32.

Sheline, Y.I., Wang, P.W., Gado, M.H., Csernansky, J.G. and Vannier, M.W., 1996. Hippocampal atrophy in recurrent major depression. *Proceeding of the National Academy of Sciences*, **93**, 3908–13.

Silberman, E.K. and Weingartner, H., 1986. Hemispheric lateralization of functions related to emotion. *Brain and Cognition*, **5**, 322–53.

Silberman, E.K., Weingartner, H. and Post, R.M., 1983. Thinking disorder in depression: logic and strategy in an abstract reasoning task. *Archives of General Psychiatry*, **40**, 775–80.

Silberman, E.K., Weingartner, H., Targum, S.D. and Byrnes, S., 1985. Cognitive functioning in biological subtypes of depression. *Biological Psychiatry*, **20**, 654–61.

Spohn, H.E. and Strauss, M.E., 1989. Relation of neuroleptic and anticholinergic medication to cognitive functions in schizophrenia. *Journal of Abnormal Psychology*, **98**, 367–80.

Squire, L.R., Cohen, N.J. and Zouzounis, J.A., 1984. Preserved memory in retrograde amnesia: sparing of a recently acquired skill. *Neuropsychologia*, **22**, 145–52.

Sweeney, J.A., Kmiec, J.A. and Kupfer, D.A., 2000. Neuropsychological impairments in bipolar and unipolar mood disorders on the CANTAB neurocognitive battery. *Biological Psychiatry*, **48**, 674–85.

Tarbuck, A.F. and Paykel, E.S., 1995. Effects of major depression on the cognitive function of younger and older subjects. *Psychological Medicine*, **25**, 285–95.

Taylor, M.A. and Abrams, R., 1986. Cognitive dysfunction in mania. *Comprehensive Psychiatry*, **27**, 186–91.

Teasdale, J.D., 1983. Negative thinking in depression: cause, effect, or reciprocal relationship. *Advances in Behaviour Research and Therapy*, **5**, 3–25.

Teasdale, J.D. and Fogarty, S.J., 1979. Differential effects of induced mood on retrieval of pleasant and unpleasant events from episodic memory. *Journal of Abnormal Psychology*, **88**, 248–57.

Teasdale, J.D., Taylor, R. and Fogarty, S.J., 1980b. Effects of induced elation–depression on the accessibility of memories of happy and unhappy experiences. *Behaviour Research and Therapy*, **18**, 339–46.

Thompson, P.J., 1991. Antidepressants and memory: a review. *Human Psychopharmacology*, **6**, 79–90.

Trichard, C., Martinot, J.L., Alagille, M., Masure, M.C., Hardy, P., Ginestet, D. and Feline, A., 1995. Time course of prefrontal lobe dysfunction in severely depressed in-patients: a longitudinal neuropsychological study. *Psychological Medicine*, **25**, 79–85.

Tomarken, A.J., Davidson, R.J., Wheeler, R.E. and Doss, R.C., 1992. Individual differences in anterior brain asymmetry and fundamental dimensions of emotion. *Journal of Personality and Social Psychology*, **62**, 676–87.

Videbech, P., 2000. PET measurements of brain glucose metabolism and blood flow in major depressive disorder: a critical review. *Acta Psychiatrica Scandinavica*, **101**, 11–20.

Watkins, P.C., Mathews, A., Williamson, D.A. and Fuller, R.D., 1992. Mood-congruent memory in depression: emotional priming or elaboration? *Journal of Abnormal Psychology*, **101**, 581–6.

Watts, F.N., Dalgleish, T., Bourke, P. and Healy, D., 1990. Memory deficit in clinical depression: processing resources and the structure of materials. *Psychological Medicine*, **20**, 345–9.

Weingartner, H., Cohen, R.M., Murphy, D.L., Martello, J. and Gerdt, C., 1981. Cognitive processes in depression. *Archives of General Psychiatry*, **38**, 42–7.

Williams, J.M.G., 1992. Autobiographical memory and emotional disorders. In: Christianson, S.A. (ed.), *The Handbook of Emotion and Memory: Research and Theory*, pp. 451–77. Lawrence Erlbaum, Hillsdale, NJ.

Williams, J.M.G. and Scott, J., 1988. Autobiographical memory in depression. *Psychological Medicine*, **18**, 689–95.

von Gunten, A., Fox, N.C., Cipolotti, L. and Ron, M.A., 2000. A volumetric study of hippocampus and amygdala in depressed patients with subjective memory problems. *Journal of Neuropsychiatry and Clinical Neurosciences*, **12**, 493–8.

XVIII-8

Functional Neuroscience of Mood Disorders

Michel Le Moal and Willy Mayo

INTRODUCTION

The evolution of criteria, symptoms and models for diagnosing mood disorders, as reflected in classical twentieth-century textbooks, has been a long process, if we consider Kraepelin's (1921) phenomenological characterizations to constitute a historical landmark. This is especially true for classification and the progressive importance of biological theories. A depressive state is considered to result from either endogenous determinants or a reaction to environmental or life events and a failure to adapt. The evolution from the first edition of the *Diagnostic and Statistical Manual of Mental Disorders* (DSM-I) (American Psychiatric Association, 1952) to the fourth edition (DSM-IV) (American Psychiatric Association, 1994) illustrates, through the push for more reliable and valid diagnoses and for a change to a categorical system (notably for research), profound changes due largely to the new pharmacological thought and its aminergic theories and derivatives. However, it remains clear that the parallel neurobiological investigation on mood has not played a pivotal role, and that pathophysiological mechanisms have still not been identified, at least in a specific manner, in relation to the categories proposed by the last DSM (Boland and Keller, 1999). Moreover, the relation between the genetic aspects of susceptibility to mood disorders (mainly bipolar) and possible defects at the neuronal levels have not yet been demonstrated. These problems are now at the forefront of psychiatric research. Thanks to advances in statistical analysis combined with powerful new biotechnology methods, hypotheses can now be explored more rapidly. Replicated linkage has, at present, proposed susceptibility loci on chromosomes X, 18 and 21, but a single locus genetic model is in no way responsible for unipolar, bipolar and recurrent disorders (for review, see Sanders *et al.*, 1999), leading to multifactorial vulnerabilities, including environmental factors as well as many genes. Finally, promising data from brain-imaging techniques have opened a new era to help identify circuitries involved in the physiopathology and proposed new neuroanatomies of mood disorders (Manji *et al.*, 2001). However, these investigations raise methodological problems.

NEUROSCIENCE OF MOOD DISORDERS: THEORETICAL AND METHODOLOGICAL CONSIDERATIONS

Difficulties for an Experimental Psychopathology of Mood Disorders

Basic and experimental neurosciences and clinical neuropsychiatry have joined forces over the past decade to promote the biological foundations of mental illness. The task is so difficult that it can be considered, together with the mind–consciousness problem, as the last frontier in biomedical research and the definitive inclusion of psychiatry in medical sciences. In spite of significant advances that have transformed the clinical perspectives in neurology and related disorders (obsessive–compulsive disorders and Tourette's syndrome are good examples), the growing tendency to 'neurologize' classic psychiatric syndromes, such as the various forms of schizophrenia, has not yet led to universal consensus regarding the aetiology and pathophysiology of such major mental illnesses.

From a neurobiological standpoint, and in the perspective of the neuroanatomical bases of the syndromes, three main general questions remain to be solved. First, when considering a given syndrome or disorder, or a specific mental disease, the symptoms that define the disease still have to be related to a given (or a set of related) 'normal' integrated functions. In other words, a continuum from physiology to pathology and vice versa is expected and, if so, then these functional dimensions should correlate with anatomical loci. The neurobiological interpretations of the symptoms have to be placed within the framework of the structure–function paradigm (Pearlson, 1999), in which modern neurosciences and neuropsychology have made enormous progress, even regarding mental functions and higher cognitive processes. The neuropsychological paradigm first applied to the neurology of cortical functions is now open to psychiatric symptoms. For instance, the disinhibition syndrome characteristic of acute mania will be referred to a similar syndrome sometimes seen after frontal brain injury, and mania will be attributed to a dysfunction of this region.

Second, by the same token, using working hypotheses inspired by experimental medicine, and considering that the concept of experimental psychopathology results directly from the structure–function paradigm, the neurobiologist could create appropriate animal models of the given illness by manipulating either the function or the underlying structure. In this context, the interpretation of experimental conditions is limited by the fact that most of the major human mental disorders do not exist *per se* in animals. Moreover, two other problems render experimental psychopathology difficult: on the one hand, manipulation of the model to obtain all the basic symptoms or dimensions that could characterize the illness or syndrome is theoretically impossible because they are known mainly by subjective report, and on the other hand, these basic symptoms may also be found in other heterogeneous disorders, because of the difficulty of defining mental illness, as reflected by ever changing concepts in psychiatry, or due to the clinical reality of considerable comorbidities. For instance, many depressed patients display anxiety symptoms, while anxiety and depression are also considered separately in DSM-IV.

Third, the pharmacological paradigm is not totally satisfying. It is based on a well-known working hypothesis: (1) the active drug acts on neuronal systems that are defective and part of the pathophysiology of the disease; (2) it is of major interest to discover the site of action of therapeutic drugs, and these sites or structures have generally been characterized as being the specific

Biological Psychiatry: Edited by H. D'haenen, J.A. den Boer and P. Willner. ISBN 0-471-49198-5

neurotransmitter systems; and (3) the more a given drug acts on many transmitter systems, the better is its therapeutic efficacy. However, the transmitter systems cannot be considered as the anatomical locus of the mental functions whose defects are reflected in the symptoms; in other words, it is difficult to imagine that the serotoninergic neurons are the anatomical substrates of symptoms characteristic of mood disorders. Of course, it is possible that the primary defect has taken place at this level, but that the symptoms result from the dysfunction of the region modulated by these neurons whose cell bodies are located in the reticular formation and related structures (Le Moal, 1995; Le Moal and Simon, 1991).

From the Physiology of Emotion to the Pathophysiology of Mood

Mood disorders have — as a trivial definition — a disturbance of mood as the predominant feature (DSM-IV). The term 'mood' refers to something based on an empirical consensus but nevertheless represents a construct with multiple facets that needs to be clarified according to its roots (old English *mod*, meaning mind, soul, courage, or German *mut*, meaning mental disposition, spirit, courage, or an Indo-European prefix, *me-*, adding the sense of strong activity, energy), leading to the general definition of a particular state of mind or feeling, humour, temper or spirit. According to common sense, mood is a mixture of feeling, humour and state of mind, i.e. a state of emotional tone and cognition. The construct emotion is not considered in the DSM-IV or in classical psychiatric dictionaries as concerns its generally understood meaning (strong feelings aroused to the point of awareness, complex reactions with both physical and mental manifestations, whatever the specific labels used, e.g. fear, anger, love, hate). Conversely, the neurobiologist deals with emotion and the construct affect but not mood. After two decades in which studies on emotion were not a central theme in neurosciences — a topic blunted largely by a hard-line, reductionistic, new-wave computational cognition that neglected feelings and emotions as important aspects of everyday life — a huge amount of knowledge has now been accumulated (LeDoux, 2000), and publications have acknowledged the neurobiology of emotion, or affective neuroscience, as a major discipline (Damasio, 1994; Damasio, 2000; Lane and Nadel, 2000; LeDoux, 1996; Pankseep, 1998; Rolls, 2001). Classically, specialists attempt to identify genetically dictated emotional operating systems considered to exist in both animal and human brains, and to evaluate how emotional feelings are generated. The vast difference in cognitive abilities among species contrasts with the homology in mammals concerning ancient subcortical evolutionarily derived systems. The problem is to appraise whether these data have something to do with mood, and whether they represent the neurophysiological foundations of mood disorders. As stated by Pankseep (1998; p. 5), 'Clinical psychology and psychiatry attempt to deal at a practical level with the underlying disturbances in brain mechanisms, but neither possesses an adequate neuroconceptual foundation for the sources of emotionality upon which systematic understanding can be constructed.' It is a challenge for this decade to relate modern cognitive neuropsychology to a new 'neuropsychology of emotion' (Lane and Nadel, 2000) and a neuropsychology of mood disorders.

NEUROSCIENCE AND NEUROENDOCRINOLOGY OF EMOTIONS

Anatomical Networks

Early in the twentieth century, neurophysiologists and clinicists suggested that emotions originated from (or were processed) at a subcortical level (Dupré-Devaux, 1901; Nothnagel, 1889) and that this subcortical 'emotional' level would be under the control of the cortex (Cannon, 1929). During the same period, Bard (1928) demonstrated in animals the critical role of a subcortical structure, namely the hypothalamus. These data were confirmed in humans through the observations of Foerster and Gagel (1933), indicating that lesions located in the hypothalamus could induce profound emotional disturbances. However, the first description of a network devoted to the processing of emotions was due to Papez (1937). For Papez, the 'stream of feeling' flows through interconnected medial structures. External inputs through primary sensory cortices reach the hippocampus, and via the mammillary bodies this information arrives at the hypothalamus. For Papez, the hypothalamus still represents the core structure of the emotional circuitry; its role is to associate an emotional value with the sensory afferents and to induce the associated motor response. From mammillary bodies, information can also reach the cingulate gyrus, and through the retrosplenial cortex it induces a feedback on the hippocampal formation. Interestingly, a direct route has also been described from the thalamic nuclei to the hypothalamus, possibly explaining the relatively quick and direct processing of some emotional information (Figure XVIII-8.1).

A few years later, Yakovlev (1948) suggested that emotional and motivational expressions are controlled by a 'middle layer' of the brain composed of partially myelinated long neurons located in the limbic thalamus, basal ganglia and hippocampal and olfactory structures. Yakovlev also dissociated a mediodorsal pathway from a basolateral pathway. The mediodorsal pathway centred on the hippocampus is similar to the circuit of Papez and seems to be involved mainly in memory functions (Livingston and Escobar, 1971). The basolateral pathway, more involved in mood regulation, involves the amygdala and its connections with the hypothalamus, dorsomedial thalamus and orbitofrontal cortex. The functional anatomy of emotional processes proposed by Papez and Yakovlev was reanalysed by McLean (1949) as the concept of the limbic system (referring to the *grand lobe limbique* initially identified by Broca in 1878). This limbic system concept is still in debate (Kötter and Meyer, 1992; LeDoux, 1991), but the recurrent problem in the search for neural substrates of emotions again lies in the definition of the word and the construct of emotion itself (Lewis and Haviland, 1992). Currently, only the circuits involved in the detection and response to danger seem to be well defined. The core structure is the amygdala: the lateral part receives cortical sensory or hippocampal inputs, and the central part controls fear responses by way of projections to the brainstem areas. The crucial role of the amygdala was evidenced by numerous studies in animals (Gloor, 1960; Kaada, 1951) and, more recently, by the experiments of LeDoux (for review, see LeDoux, 2000). These experiments also emphasize the previously suggested dual networks of Papez, i.e. a direct thalamolimbic pathway and a classical thalamocorticolimbic pathway (Figure XVIII-8.1b).

The Monoaminergic Hypothesis

Among the neurotransmitter circuits of the brain studied for their possible roles in mood disorders, monoaminergic systems have been implicated repeatedly since the 1960s. In 1965, the hypothesis of a deficit in monoamines — mainly noradrenaline — was proposed for the first time (Bunney and Davis, 1965; Schildkraut, 1965). This hypothesis was supported by evidence of low urinary levels of 3-methoxy-4-hydroxyphenylglycol (MHPG), the principal metabolite of noradrenaline, in depressed patients (mainly in bipolar depression) compared with control subjects (Maas *et al.*, 1972), and by the fact that antidepressant drugs (tricyclics and monoamine oxidase inhibitors) are known to increase noradrenergic transmission. As well as the depressive phase of bipolar disorders,

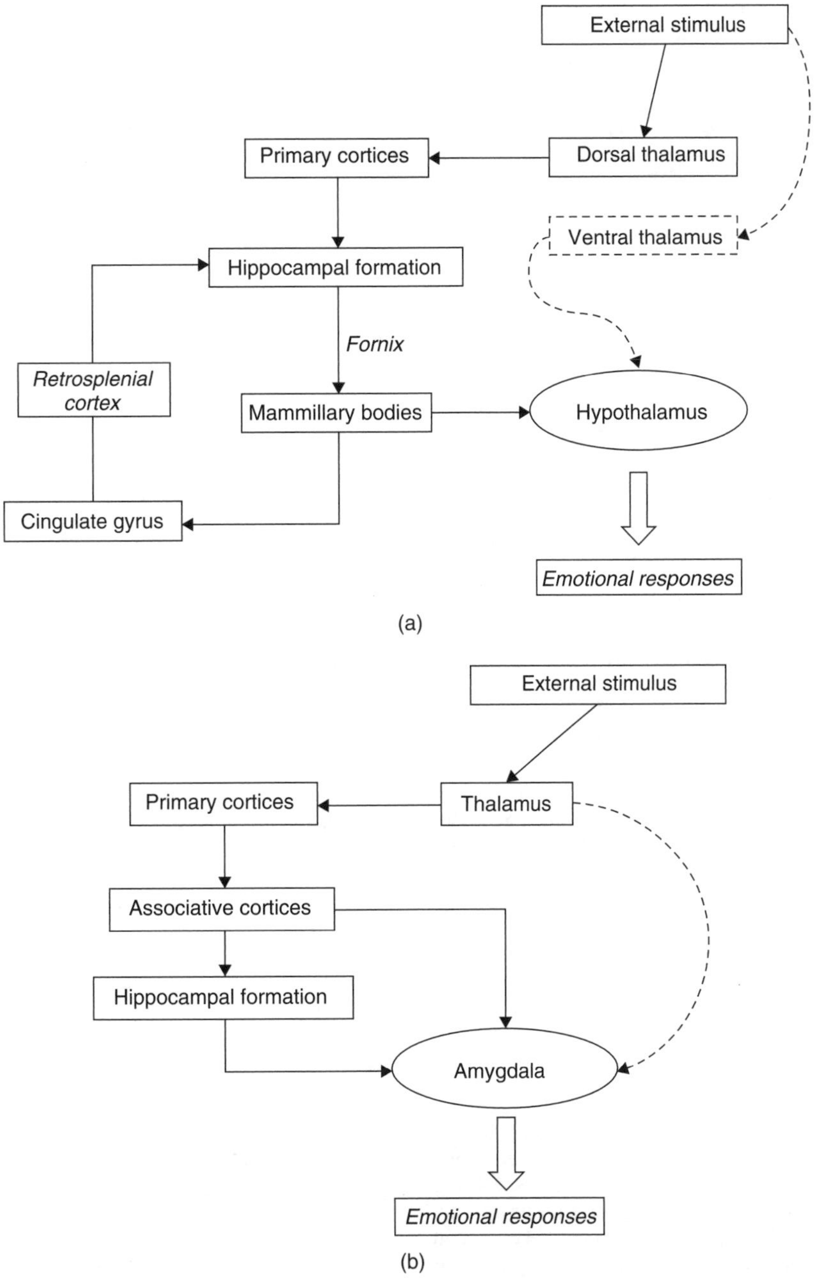

Figure XVIII-8.1 Models of anatomical networks integrating cortical and subcortical structures that could associate emotional values with sensorial afferents. (a) the model of Papez; (b) the model of LeDoux

the noradrenaline hypothesis was proposed to explain the manic phase of the illness in terms of increased noradrenaline activity (Schildkraut, 1965), and was supported more recently by Maj *et al.* (1984) and Swann *et al.* (1987). Further evidence came from the use of α-methylparatyrosine (AMPT), a competitive inhibitor of the rate-limiting enzyme for the synthesis of noradrenaline that reinstalls depressive symptoms in patients previously treated with noradrenaline uptake inhibitors (Miller *et al.*, 1996). Interestingly, AMPT has a far less significant effect in normal subjects, and is ineffective in patients treated with selective serotonin reuptake inhibitors (SSRIs) (Delgado *et al.*, 1993), indicating that noradrenaline alterations alone are not sufficient to induce depression. α2-Adrenergic and β-adrenergic receptors seem to be implicated in the pathophysiology of depression. Indeed, an increase of α2 receptors has been described both peripherally (platelets) and centrally (Garcia-Sevilla *et al.*, 1987; Meana *et al.*, 1992), indicating increased sensitivity of these receptors, inducing a decrease of the activity of noradrenergic neurons. β-Adrenergic receptors have also been implicated in depression, but there are many discrepancies in the reports available.

A serotonin (5-hydroxytryptamine, 5-HT) hypothesis for depression was also proposed to explain the pathophysiology of the disease as well as the mechanisms of antidepressants. This hypothesis is supported by various observations. Concerning precursor availability, there are data indicating that plasma concentrations of L-tryptophan are lower in some depressive subjects compared with

Table XVIII-8.1 Relationships between the HPA axis, neurotransmitter systems and some trophic factors on the hippocampal formation integrity in depression, antidepressant treatments and stress. The data refer to a cellular hypothesis of depression in which neural plasticity plays a crucial role. Neuronal atrophy or death in the hippocampal formation and prefrontal cortex contribute to the pathophysiology of mood disorders. The stress factor and life events may contribute to differential individual vulnerabilities to subsequent stressors and to depressive trends. It is possible that antidepressant treatments could oppose these adverse cellular effects, resulting in loss of neuronal plasticity by increasing either neurogenesis or cell survival. The molecular mechanisms underlying these effects include the role of cAMP signal transduction cascade and neurotrophic factors (after Duman and Charney, 1999)

				Hippocampal plasticity	
	Hormones (glucocorticoids, CRF)	Neurotransmitters (5-HT, noradrenaline)	Trophic factors (BDNF)	Neurogenesis (DG)	Cell number (CA3) or volume
Depression	↗	↘	?	?	↘
Antidepressant treatment (SSRl, lithium, ECS)	↘	↗	↗	↗	↗
Stress	↗	↘?	↘	↘	↘

DG, dentate gyrus; ECS, electroconvulsive shock.

normal subjects (Meltzer and Lowy, 1987). These lower levels of the precursor could lead to decreased serotonin synthesis in the central nervous system (CNS), and experimental reductions of plasma L-tryptophan can induce some symptoms of depression (Delgado *et al.*, 1989) or reverse the action of SSRIs (but not noradrenergic antidepressants) (Delgado *et al.*, 1999). Concerning the evaluation of metabolites, there are no clear data linking the cerebrospinal fluid (CSF) concentrations of 5-hydroxyindoleacetic acid (5-HIAA) and the depressive symptoms, except for impulsive suicidal behaviour (Asberg *et al.*, 1976; Roy *et al.*, 1989). A decrease in the binding of the serotonin transporter (SERT) in platelets of depressed subjects compared with normal subjects was reported frequently (Ellis and Salmond, 1994), and this decrease was also observed in the occipital cortex of depressed subjects (Perry *et al.*, 1983). A decrease in SERT binding has been described in suicide victims in the frontal cortex (Stanley *et al.*, 1982) and in the ventrolateral prefrontal cortex (Arango *et al.*, 1995). Concerning the possible alteration of serotonin receptors in depression, the complexity of these receptors must be taken into account (there are at least seven receptor families with multiple members in each family) (Saxena, 1995). Nevertheless, most research has focused on 5-HT$_{2A}$ and more recently on 5-HT$_{1A}$ receptors. 5-HT$_{1A}$ receptors are found mainly in the CNS, whereas 5-HT$_{2A}$ receptors are found in various central and peripheral tissues. Many studies report an increase in the binding of 5-HT$_{2A}$ receptors in platelets of depressed subjects compared with normal subjects, and treatment of depressed patients with antidepressants downregulates 5-HT$_{2A}$ receptors in platelets (Biegon *et al.*, 1990; Cowen *et al.*, 1987). The 5-HT$_{1A}$ receptor, which controls the rate of firing of 5-HT neurons, exhibits a reduced binding in the frontal cortex of depressed medicated subjects compared with controls, suggesting a downregulation effect of antidepressants (Yates *et al.*, 1990). Altogether, these studies evidence the implication of noradrenaline and 5-HT systems in the pathophysiology of depression and an alteration of their functioning with compounds having antidepressant properties.

The pathogenesis of mood disorders cannot be explained only in terms of altered noradrenaline and/or 5-HT neurotransmission. Indeed, an involvement of dopamine was suggested several years ago (Serra *et al.*, 1979). Subsequent animal and clinical studies have suggested that drugs that increase dopamine levels (amphetamine, cocaine) induce mood elation, while drugs that decrease dopamine levels (reserpine) and dopamine receptor blockers (neuroleptics) can depress mood and induce dysphoria, respectively (for review, see Willner, 1995). Chronic antidepressant treatments increase the sensitivity to dopamine receptor stimulations, possibly trough an increase of D2/D3 receptor function and a decrease in D1 receptor number and activity (D'Aquila *et al.*, 2000). Interestingly, these changes occur mainly in the mesolimbic dopaminergic system. This system is crucial for reward-related behaviour and incentive motivation (Le Moal, 1995), which are altered in depression. In this circuit, the modulation of the dopaminergic transmission in the nucleus accumbens may represent 'a common final pathway responsible for at least part of the spectrum of behavioural actions of antidepressant drugs' (Willner, 1995); interestingly, recent imaging studies report significant modifications of the volume of this nucleus in mood disorders (see Anatomical considerations following postmortem studies below).

It remains to be determined whether the aminergic changes are a primary cause, a consequence, or only a part of a complex chain of pathophysiological events. Answering this question would help us to understand the real place of antidepressants as therapeutic agents. These agents will be taken into account when neuroplastic changes due to therapeutics are considered (see Table XVIII-8.1).

The Hypothalamic-pituitary-adrenal Axis, Stress, and the Neurotrophic Hypothesis

Patients suffering from depression exhibit some symptoms that indicate a deregulation of the main neuroendocrinological system implicated in the stress response, the hypothalamic-pituitary-adrenal (HPA) axis, notably hypercortisolaemia and the absence of suppression in the dexamethasone suppression test. Corticotropin-releasing factor (CRF) is a peptide involved in the regulation of the HPA axis, and its physiology is affected in depression. In depressed patients, there is an increase of CRF concentrations in the CSF (Nemeroff *et al.*, 1984), and these concentrations can be normalized by various antidepressant treatments (De Bellis *et al.*, 1993; Nemeroff *et al.*, 1991). Thus, an alteration of HPA axis regulation in depression could magnify some deleterious effects of stress (Figure XVIII-8.2).

It is well known that stress can induce neuronal atrophy in some limbic structures, particularly the hippocampus (Sapolsky *et al.*, 1990), and a reduced hippocampal volume has been described in depressed patients (Sheline *et al.*, 1996). Furthermore, it is now established that stress and the associated glucocorticoid release decreases neurogenesis in the hippocampus (Gould *et al.*, 1997; Tanapat *et al.*, 2001). Conversely, antidepressant treatments increase hippocampal neurogenesis (cell proliferation

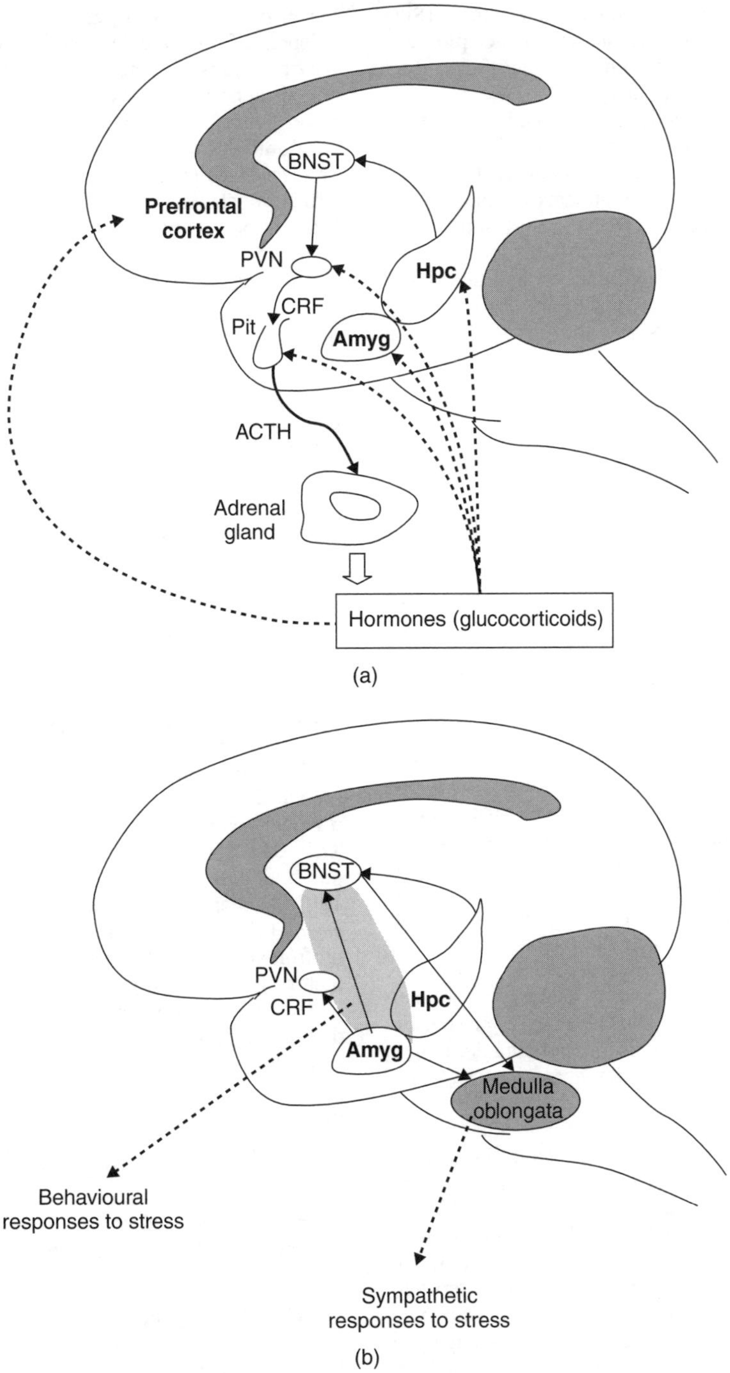

Figure XIII-8.2 The brain stress systems. (a) HPA axis stress system: Stressful stimuli increase CRF, which in turn stimulates adrenocorticotropic hormone (ACTH) release from the pituitary, which results in enhanced release of glucocorticoids from the adrenal gland. High levels of glucocorticoids, through negative feedback, decrease CRF synthesis at the level of the paraventricular nucleus (PVN) but activate CRF activity at the level of the central nucleus of the amygdala. (b) Extrahypothalamic stress system: Stressful stimuli also activate CRF systems in the basal forebrain, notably the bed nucleus of the stria terminalis and the central nucleus of the amygdala, to help mediate behavioural responses to stressors and to mediate sympathetic activation associated with stressors Amyg, amygdala; BNST, bed nucleus of the stria terminalis; Hpc, hippocampus; Pit, pituitary gland Redrawn from Koob and Le Moal (2001)

and cell survival) (Malberg *et al.*, 2000). The mechanisms underlying such actions of antidepressants are still unknown. Antidepressants may normalize the HPA axis activity, which may lead to an upregulation of brain-derived neurotrophic factor (BDNF), reported to be increased in the hippocampus of subjects treated with antidepressants (Nibuya *et al.*, 1995), possibly by an activation of the cyclic adenosine monophosphate (cAMP)–cyclic adenosine monophosphate response element binding protein (CREB) cascade. BDNF is known to enhance the growth and survival of 5-HT cells (Mamounas *et al.*, 1995), and to increase synaptic strength in the hippocampus (Kang and Schuman, 1995), and it is downregulated in the latter by stress (Smith *et al.*, 1995). In some animal models of depression, BDNF seems to have antidepressant-like effects (Siuciak *et al.*, 1996). Imaging methods have shown smaller pituitary volumes in bipolar but not unipolar disorders, suggesting a dysfunction in the HPA axis (Sassi *et al.*, 2001).

According to the neurotrophic hypothesis, depression may result from damage of hippocampal neurons, possibly stress-induced and amplified by the hypercorticosterolaemia of depressed patients (Table XVIII-8.1). Some antidepressant treatments could enhance the expression of neurotrophic factors (BDNF), thus stimulating hippocampal neurons. Nevertheless, this hypothesis only seems to be related to depression associated with stress, and additional studies are required to understand better the link between the neuroprotective role of antidepressants and the compensation of hippocampal atrophy.

MORPHOLOGICAL STUDIES IN A NEUROPSYCHOLOGICAL CONTEXT

Anatomical Considerations Following Post-Mortem Studies

Post-mortem studies may provide evidence for the hypothesis that structural-morphological changes are responsible for the chronic functional disorders (for review, see Baumann and Bogerts, 2001). In contrast to schizophrenia and other major psychoses, little has been done to investigate the neurohistological correlates of mood disorders. Studies resulting from subjects who committed suicide frequently suffer from the lack of robust amnestic and retrospective diagnosis that establishes firmly the existence of a chronic monopolar or bipolar disorder. Future studies should use well-characterized brain specimens, well-constructed experimental designs, and well-controlled confounds (for review, see Lewis, 2002). However, investigations suggest structural disturbances in the parahippocampal cortical regions with malformations in the entorhinal lamination (Bernstein *et al.*, 1998), reduction in size (Altshuler *et al.*, 1990), and alterations in the temporal lobe. The prefrontal regions have also been investigated, and a decrease in laminar thickness was found without a change in laminar density (Goodwin, 1997; Rajkowska, 1997), while layer-specific reduction of interneurons was noticed in the anterior cingular cortex (Vincent *et al.*, 1997). No firm data or significant investigations can be reported concerning the cytoarchitecture of monoaminergic neurons, although some studies favour a role for indolaminergic neurons with a reduced neuron number in the ventral subnuclei of the dorsal raphe nucleus in major depression without a clear generalization for bipolar disorder (Baumann and Bogerts, 2001).

Volume measures have been undertaken for large regions, such as the telencephalic basal ganglia and limbic regions (Baumann *et al.*, 1999b; Baumann *et al.*, 1999c), but possible post-mortem artefacts (autolysis, medication, age, gender) have to be excluded. Results suggest that predominantly limbic-affiliated basal ganglia are involved in the pathology of mood disorders, irrespective of the diagnosis of polarity: there are reduced volumes in the right putamen, right and left pallidum (external part), and, in the most affected patients, the left nucleus accumbens. Moreover, the data suggest a trend towards reduction of the left amygdala in current major depression but not in bipolar disorder. These studies do not evidence changes in the volume of the hippocampus, stria terminalis, temporal horn or thalamus. In major depression, the right hypothalamus was smaller.

In parallel, brainstem structures have been explored, in particular for a possible pathomorphology of the aminergic nuclei. In the locus coeruleus, the main source of forebrain noradrenergic innervation, the total number of neurons was higher bilaterally in bipolar disorder (Baumann *et al.*, 1999c), in particular in the rostral two-thirds and in the dorsal part. This finding is considered to be consistent with others (for review, see Baumann and Bogerts, 2001). Fewer tyrosine hydroxylase-immunoreactive neurons were found in a depressed non-suicide group compared with depressed suicide and control groups (Baumann *et al.*, 1999a). The cytoarchitecture of the dorsal raphe has also been investigated, and the ventral part shows fewer neurons, especially of the ovoid and round types, in patients with unipolar or bipolar mood disorders; a compensatory adaptive process is noticed in the form of increased nucleolar size. Such structural changes may contribute to an impaired serotoninergic innervation of brain regions supposed to be involved in the pathophysiology of mood disorders (Arango *et al.*, 1990; Baumann and Bogerts, 2001).

Structural Imaging

Structural imaging for evaluating morphology changes includes computed tomography (CT) and magnetic resonance imaging (MRI). These studies are just beginning to guide proposals for functional and structural models. Most of the studies reveal significant prevalence of hyperdensities in deep and periventricular white matter, which have also been found in the thalamus, basal ganglia, putamen and globus pallidus, especially in elderly subjects during their first experience of unipolar depression (Chimowitz *et al.*, 1992; Drevets *et al.*, 1999; Krishnan *et al.*, 1988; Soares and Mann, 1997), in the course of late-life unipolar depression (Lidaka *et al.*, 1996). One group of subjects, who experienced their first major depressive episode later in life and exhibited cerebrovascular defects as an aetiological factor, had left frontal lobe and striatum hyperdensities (Greenwald *et al.*, 1996; Greenwald *et al.*, 1998). These anatomical characteristics do not seem to be found in bipolar disorder. In parallel, neuromorphometric explorations report regional volumetric reductions in the temporal and frontal cortices. There are some data on volumetric reduction of the hippocampus and amygdala in unipolar depression (Botteron and Figiel, 1997; Duman and Charney, 1999; Pearlson *et al.*, 1997; Sheline *et al.*, 1996), and the same type of information was found for the prefrontal cortex (Drevets *et al.*, 1997a). Observations are contradictory for the basal ganglia.

The safer conclusion deduced from structural neuroimaging is that some structural changes can be observed in unipolar depression, essentially in late-onset cases, while in other pathological situations, and in young or adult subjects or bipolar episodes, brain morphology seems to be relatively preserved (Soares and Mann, 1997). The regions targetted were those shown to participate in emotional processing (thalamus, basal ganglia, frontal lobe, hippocampus, amygdala), with the exception of the hypothalamus, brainstem nuclei and regions related to neuroendocrine-autonomic systems less tractable to neuroimaging approaches.

Functional Imaging

Functional imaging is open to new concepts closer to behavioural physiology, revealing physiological correlates of depressive states but also of asymptomatic situations. As discussed previously, the theoretical assumption is that mood disorders correspond in terms of symptoms to the disruption of emotional processes normally depressed or regulated in normal subjects, and reflect the passage from homeostatic regulation to allostasis and pathology (Koob and Le Moal, 2001). Again, such a hypothesis includes the fact that hyperemotional situations experienced by normal subjects (fear, anxiety, sadness) are correlated with metabolic and blood flow–haemodynamic changes that might be related functionally to pathophysiological changes thought to take place in mood disorders (Banki *et al.*, 1992). It is becoming possible to quantify neuroreceptor binding and neurochemical abnormalities, and such an approach aims to provide neuroimaging bases for research concerning vulnerability. In practice, as regards mood disorders, the literature is composed essentially of glucose metabolism and blood-flow studies. The elevation or decrease of the latter may reflect an increase or inhibition of neurotransmitter functioning, regardless of the cause, and comparison with normal-state or healthy subjects aims to provide evidence on correlative changes due to depressive symptomatology (affective, cognitive, behavioural).

Reviews of more than 30 studies confirm that deficits are present when these parameters are examined regionally (Soares and Mann, 1997). A decrease in the cerebral frontal cortex was observed and confirmed with a variety of methodologies, as well as abnormalities in the basal ganglia and thalamic and cerebellar areas, in both unipolar and bipolar patients. This seems to correlate with the severity of the illness, especially for the frontal cortex. Data concerning the temporal lobe and other limbic regions, such as the hippocampus and amygdala, are more conflicting, at least for bipolar patients.

Integration of Different Approaches

Integration of data from functional and structural imaging is not easy. With respect to the main structural characteristics, the following points can be observed: (1) increased incidence of white-matter lesions in bipolar subjects and hyperdensities in unipolar major depressions; (2) smaller basal ganglia in unipolar patients and smaller cerebellum in unipolar and bipolar patients; and (3) conflicting findings for smaller frontal lobe in unipolar patients. The complex symptomatology and the various syndromes that characterize mood disorders suggest the existence of an extensive network and subtle imbalances and dynamics between regions as well as between neurotransmitters due to various causes, such as genetic-developmental, environmental and vascular ageing, and these aetiologies penetrate the circuits in different loci (Figure XVIII-8.3). Moreover, a dysfunction at one level of the circuit results in dysfunction in other areas. These modular systems could also be involved in other pathologies or comorbidities, such as Tourette's syndrome or obsessive–compulsive disorders.

The prefrontal cortex, the most consistently identified functional neuroimaging finding, represents a set of regions and plays a role in cognitive processes, working memory, planning, control and inhibition, attentional set shifting, motivation and mood regulation (George, 1994; Weinberger, 1993). Its dysfunction, lesion or atrophy seems consistent with a role in the pathophysiology of mood disorders. It is proposed that depressed mood and psychomotor retardation are related to changes in the dorsolateral part but also in the anterior cingulate due to its extensive connections with the limbic regions: suicide is related to the ventral prefrontal and anxiety to the posterior cingulate. Such phrenological approaches are still working hypotheses.

However, contradictions do exist, especially when neuropsychological data are confronted with possible underlying neurostructural abnormalities. Rubinsztein *et al.* (2001), departing from the observations that decision-making and task-related activation are associated with activation in the ventral prefrontal cortex and the anterior cingulated gyrus, investigated these regions in manic, unipolar depressive, and control subjects. They showed that during appropriate tasks, activation was increased in the left dorsal anterior cingulate, but decreased in the right frontal polar region, in the manic patients compared with the control patients. Moreover, less activation was noticed in the inferior frontal gyrus. Depressed patients did not show significant task-related differences in activation compared with control subjects. These patterns point to abnormal responses in specific frontal regions in manic patients and are consistent with neuropsychological observations in patients with lesions in the ventromedial prefrontal cortex. However, in a parallel study, another group did not reach the same conclusions (Clark *et al.*, 2001). In this context, the authors wanted to describe the neuropsychological profile of severe acute mania using a range of tasks selected primarily for the detection of localized neural disruption within the prefrontal cortex. They showed that manic patients did not resemble patients with ventromedial prefrontal cortex damage, and concluded that this region is not implicated as a locus of pathology in mania.

Coupled with the cortical regions, functional abnormalities are noticed in the basal ganglia in unipolar and even bipolar depression.

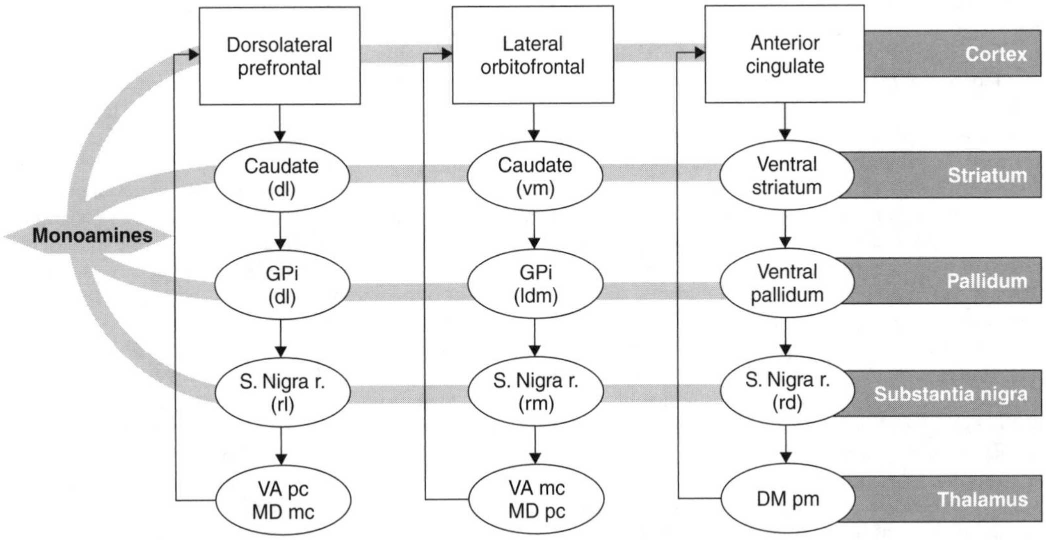

Figure XVIII-8.3 Modular organization of thalamocorticostriatal circuits. Note that each circuit engages specific regions at five levels of integration of the forebrain, and that the monoamines regulate the functioning of each circuit and allow each element to function in relation to the others. Interestingly, monoamines modulate numerous structures included in classical emotional anatomical networks. dl, dorsolateral; DM, dorsomedial; GPi, internal segment of globus pallidus; ldm, lateral dorsomedial; MD mc, medialis dorsalis pars magnocellularis; MD pc, medialis dorsalis pars parvocellularis; pm, posteromedial; rd, rostrodorsal; rl, rostrolateral; rm, rostromedial; S. Nigra r, substantia nigra pars reticulata; VA mc, ventralis anterior pars magnocellularis; VA pc, ventral anterior pars compacta; vl, ventrolateral; vm, ventromedial Redrawn from Alexander *et al.* (1986) and Le Moal (1995)

Atrophies have been noted in the caudate and putamen. Specific neurological diseases of these areas are associated with prefrontal mood changes. Moreover, the caudate and putamen have major connections with the medial temporal structures, hippocampus and amygdala, which in turn have relations with the frontal cortex. The metabolic rate in the amygdala region predicts severity of depression in depressed patients (Abercrombie *et al.*, 1996); in this circuit, potential white-matter abnormalities may contribute to the pathogenesis. An increasingly well-documented role of the amygdala-hippocampal complex has been described in dementia subsequent to recurrent stress, HPA feedback inhibition and neuronal destructions (McEwen and Sapolsky, 1995) (see Figure XVIII-8.2). This process may occur in depression characterized by HPA axis overactivity, and indeed hippocampal atrophy seems to exist in depression, although this is disputed in the literature (Pearlson *et al.*, 1997; Sheline *et al.*, 1996). The cerebellum and brainstem structures are connected with the limbic regions, and structural abnormalities have been described. In total, many studies are in agreement regarding a frontotemporal-basal ganglia circuitry in primary depression. In general, data also imply connected circuitries in major unipolar depression: a limbic (amygdala)-thalamo-(mediodorsal)-corticofrontal circuit and a limbic-striatal-pallidal-thalamic circuit (Cummings, 1993; George *et al.*, 1993a; Grodd *et al.*, 1995; Guze and Gitlin, 1994; Gyulai *et al.*, 1997; Schneider *et al.*, 1995). Cellular physiologists propose the existence of excitatory projections and subsequent increase of synaptic transmission from the limbic and frontal regions. These converging data, mainly from functional imaging techniques, remain to be interpreted in the course of major depression. Indeed, these imaging abnormalities may reflect neuromodulator dysfunction, and/or real concomitants of one or some of the symptoms of a general emotional state and/or a general pathophysiological trait and a vulnerability to depression, and/or a neuroplasticity and circuit reorganization (see Table XVIII-8.1).

Again, the main problem that confronts these neuroanatomical findings is the correspondence between what is known from behavioural physiology and neuropsychology on the one hand and symptoms on the other hand, i.e. neural and biological substrates or correlates of the various emotions and mood disorders expressed by the symptom that characterizes the different forms of depression.

Regarding the prefrontal cortex, interesting data are provided by imaging changes (increase or decrease in the imaging aspect) according to the mental state, cognitive operations, positive or negative emotions and, even more interestingly, when cognition and emotion interact in the same region. These functional correlations facilitate interpretations of the pathological changes from the symptom point of view. In view of these neuropsychological dysfunctions, reduced blood flow in the dorsomedial frontal cortex may be related to the classic impaired attentional and memory processing observed in major depression, while slowing of cognitive processes is confined to reduced dorsolateral functioning (Dolan *et al.*, 1994), regions where increased blood flow was observed in normal subjects who increased their mental activity. Moreover, the orbital subregion is assumed to play a role in modulating psychological perseveration and emotional states, and increased blood flow is observed in ventrolateral, pregenual anterior cingulate and orbital subregions during emotional processing and obsessive–compulsive states and during experimentally induced anxiety. These regions also constitute part of the circuitries described for obsessive–compulsive disorders, due to their connections with the amygdala, accumbens and hypothalamus, and decreased blood flow appears in the course of active pharmacological treatments. It has been shown that these orbital cortical regions are activated during depression in order to modulate — or inhibit — emotional responses, or to break perseverative problems and negative thoughts (Drevets and Botteron, 1997). Finally, some authors described increased functional imaging correlates with severity of symptoms (Abercrombie *et al.*, 1996; Drevets *et al.*, 1997b; Drevets and Raichle, 1992). Regional glucose metabolism in the right amygdala was shown to predict the severity of predispositional negative affect in depressed patients (Abercrombie *et al.*, 1996).

HYPOTHESIS AND CONCLUSION

Research into the pathophysiological bases of mood disorders is progressing at each level of organization under investigation (Manji *et al.*, 2001): (1) the genetic-molecular level (transcription factors, mRNA stabilization, nuclear import/export) and the subsequent gene expression-transcriptome processes; (2) the cellular level with signal transduction and modulation processes (cytoskeletal events, G-proteins, protein kinase C (PKC) and other substrates); (3) the system levels, neuronal circuits, and circadian and neurovegetative regulations (neuroplasticity processes); and (4) the cognitive-affective interactions. However, from molecular genetics (Craddock and Jones, 2001) to structural and functional defects, very little is known that might suggest a possible lead or causality between these levels.

A functional neuroanatomy of mood disorders (Soares and Mann, 1997) has emerged recently, and data obtained from morphological and imaging techniques are confronted and interpreted on the grounds of affective neuroscience. A frontolimbic-basal ganglia circuitry has been proposed, but such a structural approach needs to be refined. The regions involved account for two of the main groups of symptoms on the cognitive side (Austin *et al.*, 2001) and on the affective side, both interacting in everyday life (Buck, 1999; Cacioppo and Gardner, 1999; van Weelden, 1997). In summary, the prefrontal cortex is believed to play a role in volition, control and inhibition, working memory, and perhaps motivation and mood regulation. Dysfunction of the dorsolateral part orients the pathology to psychomotor slowing and depressed mood. Anxiety seems to be related to the posterior cingulate and also the amygdala. It is clear that the hierarchical position of these cortical regions results in dysfunction in the other areas. Defects in another group of regions seem to be present in unipolar and — in some studies — bipolar mood disorders, and are translated into psychomotor and cognitive symptoms. Both the putamen and caudate have many relations with the amygdala and hippocampus, suggesting possible trouble in affective, cognitive and inhibition abilities, the appearance of anxiety thus rendering comorbidities plausible. The amygdala-hippocampal complex may be subjected to structural abnormalities, in which overactivity of the HPA axis might have a role (McEwen and Sapolsky, 1995). Many studies have noted lateralization of functional or structural abnormalities; these data are very important (the classic interhemispheric differentiation of mood disorders after stroke) and need more clarification. Needless to say, autonomic, motivational and hormonal symptoms might be caused by sympathetic hormonal peripheral systems.

Neuropathological and imaging techniques have provided data that strengthen working hypotheses for future investigations. Again, as in pathologies such as anxiety, obsessive–compulsive disorders (Baxter *et al.*, 1992), Tourette's syndrome (George *et al.*, 1993b; Lombroso and Leckman, 1999), and drug dependence (Koob and Le Moal, 1997; Koob and Le Moal, 2001), a network including the prefrontal cortex, basal ganglia and limbic regions, including the anterior cingulate cortex (Bush *et al.*, 2000), is undoubtedly implicated (Figure XVIII-8.4).

Neuroimaging (structural and functional) abnormalities observed *in vivo* suggest neurohistological alterations linking macro- and micropathology: the basal ganglia are smaller, and structural changes are observed in noradrenergic and serotonergic nuclei (Baumann and Bogerts, 2001). However, clear distinctions between

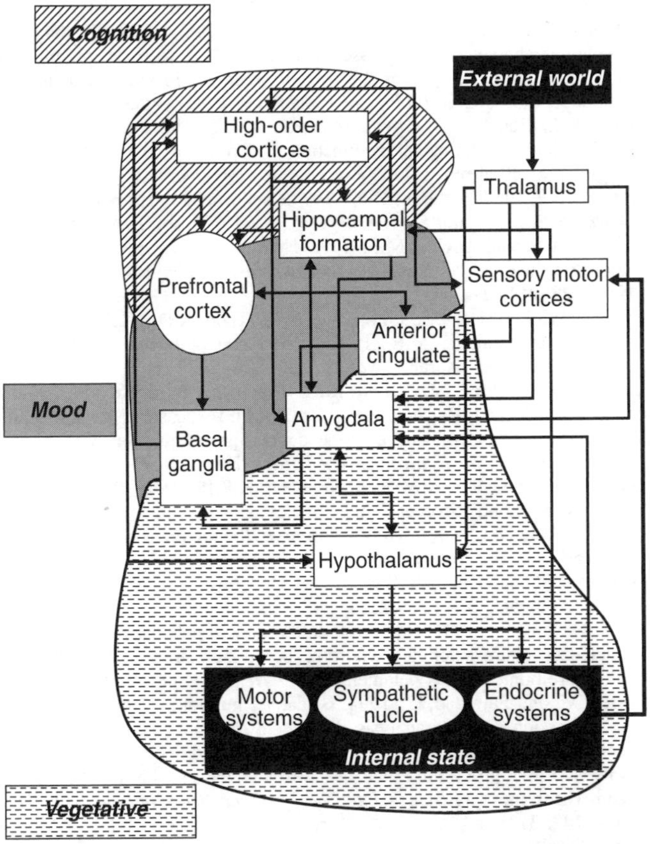

Figure XVIII-8.4 Neuroanatomical model of the central processing of emotions. Parts of these circuits are related mainly (but not exclusively) to cognitive, mood or vegetative processing and are modulated by monoamines (cf. Figure XVIII-8.3). The different circuits presented here are involved in the dialogue between the external and the internal world. External input, such as sensory information, via a classical thalamic relay, could be processed by the cortex or directly by the amygdala. The amygdala can also be influenced by the internal state (mainly by way of hormonal signalling) and, in turn, through the hypothalamus, which modulates this internal state. The evaluation of the nature of information is mainly via the prefrontal cortex, while comparison between this information and previous personal experiences involves the hippocampal formation. The prefrontal cortex and hippocampus are interconnected closely with the amygdala, and these three structures emerge as a possible mood-processing network integrating cognitive and vegetative inputs in order to make sense of the dialogue between the external and internal worlds

unipolar and bipolar syndromes, between the variety of syndromes and collateral symptoms, between acute and chronic defects, between early and late onset, and between the various aetiologies are needed for future investigations. Hemispheric lateralization dysfunction in the limbic system has been observed and merits confirmation. Besides the variety of technical manifestations and the problem of comorbidity (Nathan and Langenbucher, 1999), refinements of the techniques and methodologies will allow a more precise dissection of the circuitries, substructures or functional modules involved, such as the frontal cortex (Schoenbaum and Setlow, 2001), amygdala (Davis, 1998) or basal ganglia (Le Moal, 1995) in both acute and chronic depression.

There is still a gap between the enormous advances that have been made in past decades in affective neurosciences and a neuroscientifically based physiopathology of mood disorders, in particular in terms of structure–function relationships. It is possible that different circuitries are recruited for different emotional expression of feelings in normal subjects. For instance, experiments in humans support the hypothesis of a left hemisphere specialization for positive emotional expression and a right hemisphere specialization for expression of a negative emotion (Lee *et al.*, 1993). Moreover, there may be relationships between emotional and pre-existing personality traits, especially the harm avoidance dimension, which covaries with mood and anxiety (Svrakic *et al.*, 1992). During the past few years, progress has been made concerning (1) the neurofunctional and neuroadaptive changes, considered longitudinally, in the course of the illness, before and during mood disorders, and also in the recovery phases, in parallel with symptom evaluation; and (2) the neurofunctional changes due to pharmacotherapeutic agents or to behavioural-cognitive therapies, from disorder to recovery. Although differences in overall efficacy among groups receiving lithium, imipramine or paroxetin were not statistically significant, these drugs may affect the brain in different ways, the same being true for the mechanisms of mood stabilizers, which also have underappreciated neuroprotective effects (Manji *et al.*, 2001).

Further knowledge concerning the neurobiology and neuroanatomy of mood disorders will benefit from intense collaborative efforts in imaging techniques, neuropharmacology, physiological approaches and behavioural neurosciences.

REFERENCES

Abercrombie, H.C., Larson, C.L., Ward, R.T., Shaefer, S.M., Holden, J.E., Perlman, S.B., Turski, P.A., Krahn, D.D. and Davidson, R.J., 1996. Metabolic rate in the amygdala predicts negative affect and depression severity in depressed patients: an FDG-PET study. *Neuroimage*, **3**, S217.

Altshuler, L.L., Casanova, M.F., Goldberg, T.E. and Kleinman, J.E., 1990. The hippocampus and parahippocampus in schizophrenia, suicide, and control brains. *Archives of General Psychiatry*, **47**, 1029–1034.

American Psychiatric, 1952. *Diagnostic and Statistical Manual of Mental Disorders*, 1st edn. American Psychiatric, Washington, DC.

American Psychiatric, 1994. *Diagnostic and Statistical Manual of Mental Disorders*, 4th edn. American Psychiatric Association, Washington, DC.

Arango, V., Ernsberger, P., Marzuk, P.M., Chen, J.S., Tierney, H., Stanley, M., Reis, D.J. and Mann, J.J., 1990. Autoradiographic demonstration of increased serotonin 5-HT2 and beta-adrenergic receptor binding sites in the brain of suicide victims. *Archives of General Psychiatry*, **47**, 1038–1047.

Arango, V., Underwood, M.D., Gubbi, A.V. and Mann, J.J., 1995. Localized alterations in pre- and postsynaptic serotonin binding sites in the ventrolateral prefrontal cortex of suicide victims. *Brain Research*, **688**, 121–133.

Asberg, M., Traskman, L. and Thoren, P., 1976. 5-HIAA in the cerebrospinal fluid. A biochemical suicide predictor? *Archives of General Psychiatry*, **33**, 1193–1197.

Austin, M.P., Mitchell, P. and Goodwin, G.M., 2001. Cognitive deficits in depression: possible implications for functional neuropathology. *British Journal of Psychiatry*, **178**, 200–206.

Banki, C.M., Karmacsi, L., Bissette, G. and Nemeroff, C.B., 1992. Cerebrospinal fluid neuropeptides in dementia. *Biological Psychiatry*, **32**, 452–456.

Bard, P., 1928. A diencephalic mechanism for the expression of rage with special reference to the sympathetic nervous system. *American Journal of Physiology*, **84**, 490.

Baumann, B. and Bogerts, B., 2001. Neuroanatomical studies on bipolar disorder. *British Journal of Psychiatry Supplement*, **41**, S142–S147.

Baumann, B., Danos, P. and Diekmann, S., 1999a. Impact of suicide and diagnosis on tyrosine hydroxylase expressing neurons in the locus caeruleus of patients with mood disorders. *European Archives of Psychiatry and Clinical Neuroscience*, **249**, 212–219.

Baumann, B., Danos, P., Krell, D., Diekmann, S., Leschinger, A., Stauch, R., Wurthmann, C., Bernstein, H.G. and Bogerts, B., 1999b. Reduced volume of limbic system-affiliated basal ganglia in mood disorders: preliminary data from a postmortem study. *Journal of Neuropsychiatry and Clinical Neurosciences*, **11**, 71–78.

Baumann, B., Danos, P., Krell, D., Diekmann, S., Wurthmann, C., Bielau, H., Bernstein, H.G. and Bogerts, B., 1999c. Unipolar-bipolar dichotomy of mood disorders is supported by noradrenergic brainstem system morphology. *Journal of Affective Disorders*, **54**, 217–224.

Baxter, L.R.J., Schwartz, J.M., Bergman, K.S., Szuba, M.P., Guze, B.H., Mazziotta, J.C., Alazraki, A., Selin, C.E., Ferng, H.K., *et al.*, 1992. Caudate glucose metabolic rate changes with both drug and behavior therapy for obsessive-compulsive disorder. *Archives of General Psychiatry*, **49**, 681–689.

Bernstein, H.G., Krell, D., Baumann, B., Danos, P., Falkai, P., Diekmann, S., Henning, H. and Bogerts, B., 1998. Morphometric studies of the entorhinal cortex in neuropsychiatric patients and controls: clusters of heterotopically displaced lamina II neurons are not indicative of schizophrenia. *Schizophrenia Research*, **33**, 125–132.

Biegon, A., Essar, N., Israeli, M., Elizur, A., Bruch, S. and Bar-Nathan, A.A., 1990. Serotonin 5-HT2 receptor binding on blood platelets as a state dependent marker in major affective disorder. *Psychopharmacologia*, **102**, 73–75.

Boland, R.J. and Keller, M.B., 1999. Diagnostic classification of mood disorders: historical context and implications for neurobiology. In: Charney, D.S., Nestler, E.J. and Bunney, B.S. (eds), *Neurobiology of Mental Illness*, pp. 291–298. Oxford University Press, New York.

Botteron, K.N. and Figiel, G.S., 1997. The neuromorphometry of affective disorders. In: Krishnan, K.R.R. and Doraiswamy, P.M. (eds), *Brain Imaging in Clinical Psychiatry*, pp. 145–184. Marcel Dekker, New York.

Broca, P., 1878. Le grand lobe limbique et la scissure limbique dans la série des mammiféres. *Revue Anthropologique*, **21**, 384–498.

Buck, R., 1999. The biological affects: a typology. *Psychological Review*, **106**, 301–336.

Bunney, W.E. and Davis, M., 1965. Norepinephrine in depressive reactions. *Archives of General Psychiatry*, **13**, 137–152.

Bush, G., Luu, P. and Posner, M.I., 2000. Cognitive and emotional influences in anterior cingulate cortex. *Trends in Cognitive Sciences*, **4**, 215–222.

Cacioppo, J.T. and Gardner, W.L., 1999. Emotion. *Annual Review of Psychology*, **50**, 191–214.

Cannon, W.B., 1929. *Bodily Changes in Pain, Hunger, Fear and Rage*. Appleton, New York.

Chimowitz, M.I., Estes, M.L., Furlan, A.J. and Awad, I.A., 1992. Further observations on the pathology of subcortical lesions identified on magnetic resonance imaging. *Archives of Neurology*, **49**, 747–752.

Clark, L., Iversen, S.D. and Goodwin, G.M., 2001. A neuropsychological investigation of prefrontal cortex involvement in acute mania. *American Journal of Psychiatry*, **158**, 1605–1611.

Cowen, P.J., Charig, E.M., Fraser, S. and Elliott, J.M., 1987. Platelet 5-HT receptor binding during depressive illness and tricyclic antidepressant treatment. *Journal of Affective Disorders*, **13**, 45–50.

Craddock, N. and Jones, I., 2001. Molecular genetics of bipolar disorder. *British Journal of Psychiatry*, **178**, S128–S133.

Cummings, J.L., 1993. The neuroanatomy of depression. *Journal of Clinical Psychiatry*, **54**(Suppl), 14–20.

D'Aquila, P.S., Collu, M., Gessa, G.L. and Serra, G., 2000. The role of dopamine in the mechanism of action of antidepressant drugs. *European Journal of Pharmacology*, **405**, 365–373.

Damasio, A.R., 1994. *Descartes' Error: Emotion, Reason, and the Human Brain*. Grosset & Putnam, New York.

Damasio, A.R., 2000. *The Feelings of What Happens*. William Heinemann, London.

Davis, M., 1998. Are different parts of the extended amygdala involved in fear versus anxiety? *Biological Psychiatry*, **44**, 1239–1247.

De Bellis, M.D., Gold, P.W., Geracioti, T.D.J., Listwak, S.J. and Kling, M.A., 1993. Association of fluoxetine treatment with reductions in CSF concentrations of corticotropin-releasing hormone and arginine vasopressin in patients with major depression. *American Journal of Psychiatry*, **150**, 656–657.

Delgado, P.L., Charney, D.S., Price, L.H., Landis, H. and Heninger, G.R., 1989. Neuroendocrine and behavioural effects of dietary tryptophan restriction in healthy subjects. *Life Sciences*, **45**, 2323–2332.

Delgado, P.L., Miller, H.L., Salomon, R.M., Licinio, J., Heninger, G.R., Gelenberg, A.J. and Charney, D.S., 1993. Monoamines and the mechanism of antidepressant action: effects of catecholamine depletion on mood of patients treated with antidepressants. *Psychopharmacology Bulletin*, **29**, 389–396.

Delgado, P.L., Miller, H.L., Salomon, R.M., Licinio, J., Krystal, J.H., Moreno, F.A., Heninger, G.R. and Charney, D.S., 1999. Tryptophan-depletion challenge in depressed patients treated with desipramine or fluoxetine: implications for the role of serotonin in the mechanism of antidepressant action. *Biological Psychiatry*, **46**, 212–220.

Dolan, R.J., Bench, C.J., Brown, R.G., Scott, L.C. and Frackowiak, R.S., 1994. Neuropsychological dysfunction in depression: the relationship to regional cerebral blood flow. *Psychological Medicine*, **24**, 849–857.

Drevets, W.C. and Botteron, K.N., 1997. Neuroimaging in psychiatry. In: Guze, S.B. (ed.), *Adult Psychiatry*, pp. 53–81. Mosby Press, St Louis.

Drevets, W.C. and Raichle, M.E., 1992. Neuroanatomical circuits in depression: implications for treatment mechanisms. *Psychopharmacology Bulletin*, **28**, 261–274.

Drevets, W.C., Price, J.L., Simpson, J.R.J., Todd, R.D., Reich, T., Vannier, M. and Raichle, M.E., 1997a. Subgenual prefrontal cortex abnormalities in mood disorders. *Nature*, **386**, 824–827.

Drevets, W.C., Price, J.L., Todd, R.D., Reich, T., Bardgett, M.E., Csernansky, J.G. and Raichle, M.E., 1997b. PET measures of amygdala metabolism in bipolar and unipolar depression: correlation with plasma cortisol. *Society for Neuroscience Abstract*, **23**(2), 1407.

Drevets, W.C., Gadde, K.M. and Krishnan, K.R.R., 1999. Neuroimaging studies of mood disorders. In: Charney, D.S., Nestler, E.J. and Bunney, B.S. (eds), *Neurobiology of Mental Illness*, pp. 394–418. Oxford University Press, New York.

Duman, R.S. and Charney, D.S., 1999. Cell atrophy and loss in major depression. *Biological Psychiatry*, **45**, 1083–1084.

Dupré-Devaux, A., 1901. Rire et pleurer spasmodiques par ramollissement nucléocapsulaire antérieur: syndrome pseudobulbaire par désintégration lacunaire bilatérale des putamens. *Revue Neurologique*, **9**, 919.

Ellis, P.M. and Salmond, C., 1994. Is platelet imipramine binding reduced in depression? A meta-analysis. *Biological Psychiatry*, **36**, 292–299.

Foerster, O. and Gagel, O., 1933. Ein Fall von Ependymocyste des III. Ventrikels: Ein Beitrag zur Frage der Beziehungen psychischer Storungen zum Hirnstamm. *Zeitschrift Fur Die Gesampte Neurologie und Psychiatrie*, **149**, 312.

Garcia-Sevilla, J.A., Udina, C., Fuster, M.J., Alvarez, E. and Casas, M., 1987. Enhanced binding of [3H] (-) adrenaline to platelets of depressed patients with melancholia: effect of long-term clomipramine treatment. *Acta Psychiatrica Scandinavica*, **75**, 150–157.

George, M.S., 1994. The emerging neuroanatomy of depression. *Psychiatry Annual*, **24**, 635–636.

George, M.S., Ketter, T.A. and Post, R.M., 1993a. SPECT and PET imaging in mood disorders. *Journal of Clinical Psychiatry*, **54**(Suppl), 6–13.

George, M.S., Trimble, M.R., Ring, H.A., Sallee, F.R. and Robertson, M.M., 1993b. Obsessions in obsessive-compulsive disorder with and without Gilles de la Tourette's syndrome. *American Journal of Psychiatry*, **150**, 93–97.

Gloor, P., 1960. Amygdala. In: Field, J. and Magoun, H.W. (eds), *Handbook of Physiology: Neurophysiology*. American Physiological Society, Washington, DC.

Goodwin, G.M., 1997. Neuropsychological and neuroimaging evidence for the involvement of the frontal lobes in depression. *Journal of Psychopharmacology*, **11**, 115–122.

Gould, E., McEwen, B.S., Tanapat, P., Galea, L.A. and Fuchs, E., 1997. Neurogenesis in the dentate gyrus of the adult tree shrew is regulated by psychosocial stress and NMDA receptor activation. *Journal of Neuroscience*, **17**, 2492–2498.

Greenwald, B.S., Kramer-Ginsberg, E., Krishnan, R.R., Ashtari, M., Aupperle, P.M. and Patel, M., 1996. MRI signal hyperintensities in geriatric depression. *American Journal of Psychiatry*, **153**, 1212–1215.

Greenwald, B.S., Kramer-Ginsberg, E., Krishnan, K.R., Ashtari, M., Auerbach, C. and Patel, M., 1998. Neuroanatomic localization of magnetic resonance imaging signal hyperintensities in geriatric depression. *Stroke: a Journal of Cerebral Circulation*, **29**, 613–617.

Grodd, W., Schneider, F., Klose, U. and Nagele, T., 1995. Functional magnetic resonance tomography of psychological functions exemplified by experimentally induced emotions. *Der Radiologe*, **35**, 283–289.

Guze, B.H. and Gitlin, M., 1994. The neuropathologic basis of major affective disorders: neuroanatomic insights. *Journal of Neuropsychiatry and Clinical Neurosciences*, **6**, 114–121.

Gyulai, L., Alavi, A., Broich, K., Reilley, J., Ball, W.B. and Whybrow, P.C., 1997. I-123 iofetamine single-photon computed emission tomography in rapid cycling bipolar disorder: a clinical study. *Biological Psychiatry*, **41**, 152–161.

Kaada, B.R., 1951. Somato-motor, autonomic and electrocorticographic responses to electrical stimulation of 'rhinencephalic' and other forebrain structures in primates, cat and dog. *Acta Physiologica Scandinavica*, **24**, 1–285.

Kang, H. and Schuman, E.M., 1995. Long-lasting neurotrophin-induced enhancement of synaptic transmission in the adult hippocampus. *Science*, **267**, 1658–1662.

Koob, G.F. and Le Moal, M., 1997. Drug abuse: hedonic homeostatic dysregulation. *Science*, **278**, 52–58.

Koob, G.F. and Le Moal, M., 2001. Drug addiction, dysregulation of reward, and allostasis. *Neuropsychopharmacology*, **24**, 97–129.

Kötter, R. and Meyer, N., 1992. The limbic system: a review of its empirical foundation. *Behavioural Brain Research*, **52**, 105–127.

Kraepelin, E., 1921. *Manic-Depressive Insanity and Paranoia*. E & S Livingstone, Edinburgh.

Krishnan, K.R., Goli, V., Ellinwood, E.H., France, R.D., Blazer, D.G. and Nemeroff, C.B., 1988. Leukoencephalopathy in patients diagnosed as major depressive. *Biological Psychiatry*, **23**, 519–522.

Lane, R.D. and Nadel, I., 2000. *Cognitive Neuroscience of Emotion*. Oxford University Press, New York.

LeDoux, J.E., 1991. Emotion and the limbic system concept. *Concepts in Neuroscience* 169–199.

LeDoux, J.E., 1996. *The Emotional Brain: the Mysterious Underpinnings of Emotional Life*. Simon & Schuster, New York.

LeDoux, J.E., 2000. Emotion circuits in the brain. *Annual Review of Neuroscience*, **23**, 155–184.

Lee, G.P., Loring, D.W. and Meador, K.J., 1993. Influence of premorbid personality and location of lesion on emotional expression. *International Journal of Neuroscience*, **72**, 157–165.

Le Moal, M., 1995. Mesocorticolimbic dopaminergic neurons. Functional and regulatory roles. In: Bloom, F.E. and Kupfer, D.J. (eds), *Psychopharmacology: the Fourth Generation of Progress*, pp. 283–294. Raven Press, New York.

Le Moal, M. and Simon, H., 1991. Mesocorticolimbic dopaminergic network: functional and regulatory roles. *Physiological Reviews*, **71**, 155–234.

Lewis, D.A., 2002. The human brain revisited: opportunities and challenges in postmortem studies of psychiatric disorders. *Neuropsychopharmacology*, **26**, 143–154.

Lewis, M. and Haviland, J., 1992. *Handbook of Emotions*. Guilford, New York.

Lidaka, T., Nakajima, T., Kawamoto, K., Fukuda, H., Suzuki, Y., Maehara, T. and Shiraishi, H., 1996. Signal hyperintensities on brain magnetic resonance imaging in elderly depressed patients. *European Neurology*, **36**, 293–299.

Livingston, K.E. and Escobar, A., 1971. Anatomical bias of the limbic system concept. *Archives of Neurology*, **24**, 17–21.

Lombroso, P.J. and Leckman, J.F., 1999. The neurobiology of Tourette's syndrome and ticrelated disorders in children. In: Charney, D.S., Nestler, E.J. and Bunney, B.S. (eds), *Neurobiology of Mental Illness*, pp. 779–787. Oxford University Press, New York.

Maas, J.W., Fawcett, J.A. and Dekirmenjian, H., 1972. Catecholamine metabolism, depressive illness, and drug response. *Archives of General Psychiatry*, **26**, 252–262.

MacLean, P.D., 1949. Psychosomatic disease and the visceral brain: recent developments bearing on the Papez theory of emotion. *Psychosomatic Medicine*, **11**, 338–353.

Maj, M., Ariano, M.G., Arena, F. and Kemali, D., 1984. Plasma cortisol, catecholamine and cyclic AMP levels, response to dexamethasone suppression test and platelet MAO activity in manic-depressive patients. A longitudinal study. *Neuropsychobiology*, **11**, 168–173.

Malberg, J.E., Eisch, A.J., Nestler, E.J. and Duman, R.S., 2000. Chronic antidepressant treatment increases neurogenesis in adult rat hippocampus. *Journal of Neuroscience (Online)*, **20**, 9104–9110.

Mamounas, L.A., Blue, M.E., Siuciak, J.A. and Altar, C.A., 1995. Brain-derived neurotrophic factor promotes the survival and sprouting of serotonergic axons in rat brain. *Journal of Neuroscience*, **15**, 7929–7939.

Manji, H.K., Moore, G.J. and Chen, G., 2001. Bipolar disorder: leads from the molecular and cellular mechanisms of action of mood stabilisers. *British Journal of Psychiatry*, **178**, S107–S119.

McEwen, B.S. and Sapolsky, R.M., 1995. Stress and cognitive function. *Current Opinion in Neurobiology*, **5**, 205–216.

Meana, J.J., Barturen, F. and Garcia-Sevilla, J.A., 1992. Alpha 2-adrenoceptors in the brain of suicide victims: increased receptor density associated with major depression. *Biological Psychiatry*, **31**, 471–490.

Meltzer, H.Y. and Lowy, M.T., 1987. The serotonin hypothesis of depression. In: Meltzer, H.Y. (ed.), *Psychopharmacology: the Third Generation of Progress*, pp. 513–526. Raven Press, New York.

Miller, H.L., Delgado, P.L., Salomon, R.M., Berman, R., Krystal, J.H., Heninger, G.R. and Charney, D.S., 1996. Clinical and biochemical effects of catecholamine depletion on antidepressant-induced remission of depression. *Archives of General Psychiatry*, **53**, 117–128.

Nathan, P.E. and Langenbucher, J.W., 1999. Psychopathology: description and classification. *Annual Review of Psychology*, **50**, 79–107.

Nemeroff, C.B., Widerlov, E., Bissette, G., Walleus, H., Karlsson, I., Eklund, K., Kilts, C.D., Loosen, P.T. and Vale, W., 1984. Elevated concentrations of CSF corticotropin-releasing factor-like immunoreactivity in depressed patients. *Science*, **226**, 1342–1344.

Nemeroff, C.B., Bissette, G., Akil, H. and Fink, M., 1991. Neuropeptide concentrations in the cerebrospinal fluid of depressed patients treated with electroconvulsive therapy. Corticotrophin-releasing factor, beta-endorphin and somatostatin. *British Journal of Psychiatry*, **158**, 59–63.

Nibuya, M., Morinobu, S. and Duman, R.S., 1995. Regulation of BDNF and trkB mRNA in rat brain by chronic electroconvulsive seizure and antidepressant drug treatments. *Journal of Neuroscience*, **15**, 7539–7547.

Nothnagel, H., 1889. *Topische Diagnostik der Nervenkrankheiten, Eine Klinische Studie*. Hirschwald, Berlin.

Pankseep, J., 1998. *Affective Neuroscience*. Oxford University Press, New York.

Papez, J.W., 1937. A proposed mechanism of emotion. *Archives of Neurology and Psychiatry*, **38**, 725–733.

Pearlson, G.D., 1999. Structural and functional brain changes in bipolar disorder: a selective review. *Schizophrenia Research*, **39**, 133–140.

Pearlson, G.D., Barta, P.E., Powers, R.E., Menon, R.R., Richards, S.S., Aylward, E.H., Federman, E.B., Chase, G.A., Petty, R.G. and Tien, A.Y., 1997. Medial and superior temporal gyral volumes and cerebral asymmetry in schizophrenia versus bipolar disorder. *Biological Psychiatry*, **41**, 1–14.

Perry, E.K., Marshall, E.F., Blessed, G., Tomlinson, B.E. and Perry, R.H., 1983. Decreased imipramine binding in the brains of patients with depressive illness. *British Journal of Psychiatry*, **142**, 188–192.

Rajkowska, G., 1997. Morphometric methods for studying the prefrontal cortex in suicide victims and psychiatric patients. *Annals of the New York Academy of Sciences*, **836**, 253–268.

Rolls, E.T., 2001. *The Brain and Emotion*. Oxford University Press, New York.

Roy, A., De Jong, J. and Linnoila, M., 1989. Cerebrospinal fluid monoamine metabolites and suicidal behavior in depressed patients. A 5-year follow-up study. *Archives of General Psychiatry*, **46**, 609–612.

Rubinsztein, J.S., Fletcher, P.C., Rogers, R.D., Ho, L.W., Aigbirhio, F.I., Paykel, E.S., Robbins, T.W. and Sahakian, B.J., 2001. Decision-making in mania: a PET study. *Brain: a Journal of Neurology*, **124**, 2550–2563.

Sanders, A.R., Detera-Wadleigh, S.D. and Gershon, E.S., 1999. Molecular genetics of mood disorders. In: Charney, D.S., Nestler, E.J. and Bunney, B.S. (eds), *Neurobiology of Mental Illness*, pp. 299–316. Oxford University Press, New York.

Sapolsky, R.M., Uno, H., Rebert, C.S. and Finch, C.E., 1990. Hippocampal damage associated with prolonged glucocorticoid exposure in primates. *Journal of Neuroscience*, **10**, 2897–2902.

Sassi, R.B., Nicoletti, M., Brambilla, P., Harenski, K., Mallinger, A.G., Frank, E., Kupfer, D.J., Keshavan, M.S. and Soares, J.C., 2001. Decreased pituitary volume in patients with bipolar disorder. *Biological Psychiatry*, **50**, 271–280.

Saxena, P.R., 1995. Serotonin receptors: subtypes, functional responses and therapeutic relevance. *Pharmacology and Therapeutics*, **66**, 339–368.

Schildkraut, J.J., 1965. The catecholamine hypothesis of affective disorders: a review of supporting evidence. *American Journal of Psychiatry*, **122**, 509–522.

Schneider, F., Gur, R.E., Mozley, L.H., Smith, R.J., Mozley, P.D., Censits, D.M., Alavi, A. and Gur, R.C., 1995. Mood effects on limbic blood flow correlate with emotional self-rating: a PET study with oxygen-15 labeled water. *Psychiatry Research*, **61**, 265–283.

Schoenbaum, G. and Setlow, B., 2001. Integrating orbitofrontal cortex into prefrontal theory: common processing themes across species and subdivisions. *Learning and Memory*, **8**, 134–147.

Serra, G., Argiolas, A., Klimek, V., Fadda, F. and Gessa, G.I., 1979. Chronic treatment with antidepressants prevents the inhibitory effect of small doses of apomorphine on dopamine synthesis and motor activity. *Life Sciences*, **25**, 415–423.

Sheline, Y.I., Wang, P.W., Gado, M.H., Csernansky, J.G. and Vannier, M.W., 1996. Hippocampal atrophy in recurrent major depression. *Proceedings of the National Academy of Sciences of the United States of America*, **93**, 3908–3913.

Siuciak, J.A., Lewis, D.R., Wiegand, S.J. and Lindsay, R.M., 1996. Antidepressant-like effect of brain-derived neurotrophic factor (BDNF). *Pharmacology, Biochemistry and Behavior*, **56**, 131–137.

Smith, M.A., Makino, S., Kvetnansky, R. and Post, R.M., 1995. Stress and glucocorticoids affect the expression of brain-derived neurotrophic factor and neurotrophin-3 mRNAs in the hippocampus. *Journal of Neuroscience*, **15**, 1768–1777.

Soares, J.C. and Mann, J.J., 1997. The anatomy of mood disorders–review of structural neuroimaging studies. *Biological Psychiatry*, **41**, 86–106.

Stanley, M., Virgilio, J. and Gershon, S., 1982. Tritiated imipramine binding sites are decreased in the frontal cortex of suicides. *Science*, **216**, 1337–1339.

Svrakic, D.M., Przybeck, T.R. and Cloninger, C.R., 1992. Mood states and personality traits. *Journal of Affective Disorders*, **24**, 217–226.

Swann, A.C., Koslow, S.H., Katz, M.M., Maas, J.W., Javaid, J., Secunda, S.K. and Robins, E., 1987. Lithium carbonate treatment of mania. Cerebrospinal fluid and urinary monoamine metabolites and treatment outcome. *Archives of General Psychiatry*, **44**, 345–354.

Tanapat, P., Hastings, N.B., Rydel, T.A., Galea, L.A. and Gould, E., 2001. Exposure to fox odor inhibits cell proliferation in the hippocampus of adult rats via an adrenal hormone-dependent mechanism. *Journal of Comparative Neurology*, **437**, 496–504.

Van Weelden, P.W., 1997. Memory for emotions. *New Ideas in Psychology*, **15**, 55–70.

Vincent, S.L., Todtenkopf, M.S. and Benes, F.M., 1997. A comparison of the density of pyramidal and nonpyramidal neurons in the anterior cingulate cortex of schizophrenics and manic-depressives. *Society for Neuroscience Abstract*, **23**, 2199.

Weinberger, D.R., 1993. A connectionist approach to the prefrontal cortex. *Journal of Neuropsychiatry and Clinical Neurosciences*, **5**, 241–253.

Willner, P., 1995. Dopamine in mood disorders. In: Bloom, F.E. and Kupfer, D.J. (eds), *Psychopharmacology: the Fourth Generation of Progress*, pp. 921–931. Raven Press, New York.

Yakovlev, P.I., 1948. Motility, behavior and the brain: stereodynamic organization and neural coordinates of behavior. *Journal of Nervous and Mental Disease*, **107**, 313–335.

Yates, M., Leake, A., Candy, J.M., Fairbairn, A.F., McKeith, I.G. and Ferrier, I.N., 1990. 5HT2 receptor changes in major depression. *Biological Psychiatry*, **27**, 489–496.

XVIII-9

Brain Imaging in Mood Disorders

Klaus P. Ebmeier and Dina Kronhaus

INTRODUCTION

Depression, as the reversible psychiatric condition par excellence, is clearly an ideal object for functional neuroimaging studies. In theory, patients return to their initial (healthy) brain state so that any image changes observed during an affective episode should mark the brain structures and circuits involved in the expression of symptoms and signs. Authors have imaged patients when ill and after recovery and used a number of strategies to exploit short-term fluctuations of symptoms. Such fluctuations occur naturally, as in the typical diurnal variations of mood (Moffoot *et al.*, 1994b), or they can be provoked by interventions, such as mood induction (Baker *et al.*, 1997), sleep deprivation (Ebert *et al.*, 1994a) or tryptophan depletion (Smith *et al.*, 1999b). If, on the other hand, anatomical changes did exist in depression, they would be predicted in cases of treatment resistance (Shah *et al.*, 1998), in secondary or late-onset depression (Ebmeier *et al.*, 1998), or possibly a priori in certain patients with a genetic predisposition for the illness (Drevets *et al.*, 1998).

Anatomical systems involved are likely to be medial limbic, with the anterior cingulate cortex and orbitofrontal cortex playing a prominent role (Ebert and Ebmeier, 1996). There is also the well-rehearsed hypothesis of hypercortisolaemia, which occurs frequently in depression and, at least in animal models, leads to hippocampal damage. Hippocampal damage, in turn, would release the pituitary secretion of adrenocorticotropic hormone (ACTH) from hippocampal suppression and result in a positive feedback loop (Sapolsky *et al.*, 1986). This mechanism may not be specific to depression (Welberg *et al.*, 2001), as some authors have also used it to explain cognitive impairment or dementia (Hibberd *et al.*, 2000) and the sequelae of severe psychological trauma (Bremner *et al.*, 1995).

Neuropsychological tasks have been employed in imaging studies to activate brain systems thought to be implicated in depression, in particular using 'frontal' (e.g. word-generation) or 'temporal' (memory) tasks. In such experiments, limited task performance may be responsible for group differences. Attempts to control for such performance differences include pacing tasks at a speed that all patients can manage, and post-hoc correlation of brain activity with task performance, e.g. by using analysis of covariance. A further complication of functional imaging protocols is that it is now very difficult to recruit untreated patients in a psychiatric setting. Primary-care physicians have usually already treated their patients with a standard antidepressant (e.g. a selective serotonin reuptake inhibitor, SSRI) by the time of referral. The cost and effort required to recruit patients at the primary-care level is usually seen as prohibitive. For this reason, many studies contain samples of medicated patients and have to be interpreted with caution. It also cannot be excluded that changes in brain activity or even brain anatomy may be caused by medication (DelBello *et al.*, 1999).

Medication is, of course, a particular problem for receptor ligand studies. Based on effective pharmacological treatment, there are a variety of hypotheses, particularly involving the serotonergic and noradrenergic transmitter systems, which are theoretically amenable to *in vivo* testing with neuroimaging (Delgado *et al.*, 1990). Not only the availability of untreated patients but also the availability of receptor ligands has limited such research. The latter may be partially responsible for the dearth of noradrenaline ligand studies. Not all ligands are suitable; their use may be limited by their specificity for the receptor concerned, their affinity (i.e. the likelihood to be displaced by endogenous ligand) and their nondisplaceable (non-specific) binding fraction. In spite of these limitations, first results are now emerging that test some of the extant pharmacological hypotheses in depression.

Rather than giving a balanced review of all studies carried out in the field, we will focus on certain themes and future prospects that appear to be emerging. Our selection will no doubt be idiosyncratic, but we hope that we have captured the important paradigms and paths of current research. In order to limit the size of the chapter, we will focus on key publications of the last 5 years (at the time of writing), as earlier literature has been summarized well in a number of other reviews (Davidson *et al.*, 1999; Drevets, 1998; Kennedy *et al.*, 1997; Norris *et al.*, 1997; Stoll *et al.*, 2000; Videbech, 1997; Videbech, 2000). Rather than systematically dividing the imaging literature by image modality or diagnosis, we will attempt to present a logical narrative, proceeding from simple (e.g. neurochemical) hypotheses, such as the dopamine theory of psychomotor retardation in depression, to more complex models. Hypotheses that are, in a sense, post-hoc, i.e. exploit the natural history of depressive symptoms and their treatment, will be followed by experimental approaches, which imply complex neuronal systems and attempt to activate selectively such systems that are thought to be implicated in the expression of depressive symptoms. Mania is a rare condition that is very difficult to study with neuroimaging techniques, and reports are rare (Al-Moussawi *et al.*, 1996). This illness will, therefore, not be discussed, except when included in studies of bipolar depressed patients.

PHARMACOLOGY

Dopamine and Motor Function

Although dopamine is not thought to be involved primarily in the treatment and the experience of symptoms of depression, it may play an important role in the brain reward systems and in movement control. It has been implicated in retarded depression, both by the reduction of the dopamine metabolite homovanillic acid in cerebrospinal fluid (Jimerson, 1987) and by increased D2 receptor binding, particularly in psychomotor retarded patients (Ebmeier and

Biological Psychiatry: Edited by H. D'haenen, J.A. den Boer and P. Willner. ISBN 0-471-49198-5

Ebert, 1997). Increased postsynaptic receptor binding is interpreted mainly as evidence of reduced dopaminergic activity with resulting receptor supersensitivity or, alternatively, reduced displacement of the radioligand by endogenous dopamine (Shah *et al.*, 1997). Sleep deprivation, which may have an amphetamine-like effect, is associated with displacement of such ligands from their binding sites in the neostriatum (Ebert and Berger, 1998). Whether reduced availability of dopamine is ubiquitous in depression is, however, doubtful. At least one single photon emission computed tomography (SPECT) study (Klimke *et al.*, 1999) ($n = 15$) found a reduction in ligand binding to D2 receptors that normalized on clinical recovery and predicted response to SSRIs. Paillere-Martinot *et al.* (2001) reported a reduction in left caudate 18F-dihydroxyphenylalanine (DOPA) positron emission tomography (PET) only in blunted and retarded, but not in impulsive and anxious, depression. Examining presynaptic loci, 15 drug-naive patients with major depression showed significant increases in SPECT striatal dopamine transporter (DAT) binding capacity (Laasonen-Balk *et al.*, 1999). This may be interpreted similarly to the findings in D2 receptors, as a correlate of reduced availability of dopamine (see above). This effect, however, was not reported in 31 drug-naive children. Serotonin transporter (SERT) binding (see below) but not DAT binding in the hypothalamus and midbrain was increased (Dahlstrom *et al.*, 2000). Interestingly, during acute cocaine abstinence ($n = 28$), associated with depressive symptoms and a 20% increase in striatal DAT binding capacity measured by SPECT, there was a negative correlation of tracer binding with Hamilton depression scores (Malison *et al.*, 1998a), suggesting an adaptive response. Basal ganglia involvement in depression is demonstrated not only by abnormal dopamine ligand studies but also by imaging studies examining brain activation and blood flow. Hickie *et al.* (1999) reported a correlation between (delayed) reaction time and (reduced) left neostriatal activation from simple to choice reaction time tasks in psychomotor retarded patients. Finally, basal ganglia pathology may predispose to late-onset or secondary depression, as suggested by magnetic resonance imaging (MRI) lesion studies (Lauterbach *et al.*, 1997) and MRI studies of iron deposition (Steffens *et al.*, 1998).

Noradrenaline

Although noradrenaline has been implicated in depression for many years (Zis and Goodwin, 1982), there have been relatively few neuroimaging studies. After driving the noradrenergic system with clonidine, an $\alpha 2$ agonist, a study in six depressed and six healthy women found an increase in right prefrontal perfusion only in the depressed group, suggesting either presynaptic subsensitivity or a local supersensitivity of postsynaptic alpha2 receptors (Fu *et al.*, 2001). This may not be a specific finding, as Moffoot reported similar results for patients with Korsakoff psychosis (Moffoot *et al.*, 1994a).

Serotonin

Serotonergic Activation, Treatment Effects and Response

In accordance with the theoretical and practical importance of SSRIs in the treatment of depression, a number of studies have examined the effects of SSRIs on brain function, both explicitly and by comparing patients when they are ill and recovered. Mayberg *et al.* (1997) examined 18 hospitalized patients with unipolar depression and reported that rostral (anterior) cingulate (Brodman's area 24a,b) metabolism predicted response (hypermetabolism) and lack of response (hypometabolism) to fluoxetine. In a repeat measures study (Brody *et al.*, 1999), 16 depressed outpatients were imaged with 18F-fluorodeoxyglucose (FDG)–PET before and after treatment with paroxetine. SSRI responders showed a reduction in ventral prefrontal perfusion, but (left) ventral anterior cingulate reduction before treatment predicted a better response. These findings could be in contradiction to the data of Mayberg *et al.* (1997). However, patients in that study were more clinically unwell, different SSRIs were used, and the target areas do not seem to be congruent.

In reversal of SSRI treatment, depletion of serotonin by a low-tryptophan amino acid drink can lead to a temporary lowering of mood in recovered depressed patients. Smith *et al.* (1999b) found that 'increasing levels of depression after tryptophan depletion were associated with diminished neural activity in ventral anterior cingulate, orbitofrontal cortex and caudate nucleus regions' during paced verbal fluency performance. In addition, depressive relapse attenuated cognitive task-related activation in the anterior cingulate. This study illustrates potential complications in design arising when behavioural conditions are mixed with pharmacological interventions in neuroimaging: although not obvious in this study, the pharmacological interventions may affect task performance as well as mood. The separation of drug and clinical effects, and the statistical definition of the interaction between the two, are, up to a point, arbitrary. The same group also confirmed the specific hypothesis that mood deterioration induced by low-tryptophan drink would increase activity in the projection from the habenula to the raphe, structures that are part of the feedback loop controlling the release of 5-hydroxytryptamine (5-HT) throughout the brain (Morris *et al.*, 1999). A reliable differential effect of the indirect serotonin agonist fenfluramine on brain perfusion in healthy volunteers and depressed patients has not been established. A study of 13 depressed and 18 healthy women showed identical effects in both diagnostic groups after intravenous infusion (Meyer *et al.*, 1998).

Serotonin Transporter

After an initial rush of interest in the association of certain SERT alleles with depression, a number of imaging studies have used SERT ligands with patients (Battersby *et al.*, 2001). Such studies are understandably difficult to conduct, as medicated patients cannot be used. Unipolar depressed patients exhibited a characteristic reduction of 18% in SERT in the brainstem, where the highest concentrations of receptors can be found, compared with healthy volunteers (Malison *et al.*, 1998b). Patients with seasonal affective disorder showed reduced SERT binding capacity in the thalamus and hypothalamus but not in the midbrain or pons (Willeit *et al.*, 2000). This effect, however, was reversed in the hypothalamus and midbrain, where increased SERT binding correlated with concurrent depression in a group of drug-naive children ($n = 41$). Increased binding could be attributed to a reduction of serotonin within the synaptic cleft (thus allowing increased tracer binding), with developmental differences accounting for contradictory results for transporter binding in adults and children (Dahlstrom *et al.*, 2000).

5-HT2 Receptor

Post-mortem studies have suggested that a history of depression and, in particular, suicidal behaviour is associated with an increase in 5-HT2 receptors (Mann *et al.*, 1999). In contrast, a study of six drug-free, depressed patients examined with 18F-altanserin PET reported reduced binding in the right posterolateral orbitofrontal cortex and anterior insula with trends on the left side (Biver *et al.*, 1997). This apparent contradiction may be explained by receptor downregulation due to medication: eight of ten depressed patients who improved with desipramine showed a decrease in 18F-setoperone binding to the 5-HT2 receptor in many cortical areas

(Yatham *et al.*, 1999). Further, an 18F-setoperone study before and after 6 weeks of paroxetine medication in 19 depressed patients suggested a reduced binding capacity after treatment, which was found mainly in patients younger than 30 years of age. A study of 14, better controlled, drug- and self-harm-free (>6 months) depressed patients showed no abnormalities in prefrontal 18F-setoperone binding (Meyer *et al.*, 1999). Similarly, 11 elderly depressed patients did not show an *in vivo* reduction of 18F-altanserin binding capacity (Meltzer *et al.*, 1999).

5-HT1a Receptor

Rueter *et al.* (1998) have argued that antidepressant effects are due to a desensitization of 5-HT1a somatodendritic autoreceptors in the rat. This is responsible for the return to normal firing rate levels in the dorsal raphe nucleus. A single study has confirmed the hypothesized reduction in 5-HT1a binding capacity in depressed patients (Lesch *et al.*, 1990) using the PET ligand 11C-WAY-100635. Twelve primarily depressed patients with a family history of the illness showed reductions in binding capacity in the brainstem raphe, medial temporal cortex and possibly other cortical areas. This effect was greatest in bipolar patients and patients with a family history of bipolar illness (Drevets *et al.*, 1999).

'NATURAL EXPERIMENTS': CLINICAL PROFILES, TREATMENT RESPONSE AND TREATMENT RESISTANCE

What can neuroimaging studies tell us about depression that clinical description could not? Comparison of pretreatment and post-treatment neural activity is the most obvious way to associate *in vivo* neurobiological markers with depressive symptoms, cognitive ability or deficits. There is also mounting evidence for a correspondence between pretreatment metabolism in specific areas and treatment outcome. Characteristic changes in perfusion may help to classify patients with similar neuropathology. Changes in functional circuitry may emerge as predictors of treatment response and residual dysfunction whenever remission is not synonymous with recovery. Because substantial placebo or spontaneous remission effects contribute to the drug treatment of depression, it is unclear whether changes in cortical dynamics upon recovery are associated with the nature or the extent of drug-induced changes (Andrews, 2001).

Neuroanatomical and functional deficits may already be identifiable as vulnerability factors in patients' families. They may, at the other extreme, be the correlate of lingering abnormalities, such as perturbed cortical dynamics and impaired cognitive performance that are present beyond remission (Abas *et al.*, 1990). Persistent abnormalities can be a consequence of several factors. First, chronic administration of antidepressant, anticonvulsant or antipsychotic medication may contribute to the enduring brain changes (DelBello *et al.*, 1999). Second, impaired function during (or between) clinical episodes may compromise a system that is already fragile or affected in some way, and thus cause enduring damage (Sapolsky *et al.*, 1986). Finally, since affective disorders are often characterized by recurrent episodes over time, the normal process of ageing may be a confounder or may interact with the illness process (Kapur *et al.*, 1994). The interpretation of treatment progress in depression is also not straightforward. Change in behaviour, cognition or motor activity may not necessarily imply an associated modification in functional circuitry with return to normal activity (Goodwin *et al.*, 1993). Psychopharmacological agents target one or more neurotransmitter systems. Nonetheless, if the activity of one of the widely projecting neurotransmitter systems (dopamine, noradrenaline, 5-HT) increases, then global cortical dynamics will also be affected. Functional connectivity changes in mood disorders will be associated with abnormalities at rest (baseline) or, more likely, an abnormal pattern of recruitment during cognitive or motor activity. Where structural abnormalities have been reported in unipolar and bipolar depression, it is not unreasonable to assume that baseline and task-associated functional connectivity changes may occur. Brain imaging provides an assessment tool for the course of both illness-induced changes and active mechanism of recovery or compensation. In accordance with Alexander's (Alexander *et al.*, 1986) and Swerdlow and Koob's (1987) theories of functional cortico-subcortical loops, cortical areas (such as the frontal, temporal and parietal cortices), subcortical areas (such as the basal ganglia and thalamus), and most of all areas related to the limbic system (such as the anterior cingulate, hippocampus and amygdala) will be affected.

In order to better understand blood-flow abnormalities in affective disorders and consequent remission effected by different forms of treatment, findings can be separated into a number of distinct categories: pretreatment perfusion, post-treatment perfusion, activity in responders and non-responders, and the comparison of either or both with control subjects. Some studies do not include healthy volunteers; therefore, it is impossible to tell whether remission is associated with normalization of perfusion. The use of diverse methodologies in clinical studies makes the comparison between their findings difficult. The neuroanatomical maps or delineation of specific brain regions (Brodman's areas) used to localize activation may not be identical throughout the literature. Despite anatomical proximity, these areas may have very different connectivity patterns. For example, the medial or orbital frontal networks receive input from very different areas of the cortex (Barbas *et al.*, 1999; Bhashghaei and Barbas, 2001). Methodological constraints on studies in a clinical setting include great variations in the size of samples, which are often small and occasionally non-uniform in terms of age, medication and clinical history. Medication can influence outcomes in both neuropsychological and imaging studies, although the duration of medication effects is not known (Elliott *et al.*, 1998). An agreed standard for response to medication lies around 6 weeks, but it may take longer to establish remission. Therefore, brain imaging carried out at a later stage (Pizzagalli *et al.*, 2001) may be recording the long-term behavioural gain of therapeutic intervention, rather than incidental drug effects.

An alternative to measuring regional metabolic changes is to examine functional connectivity. Mallet *et al.* (1998) found decreased interhemispheric connectivity along with reduced connectivity within the right hemisphere (in a cortical–subcortical as well as anterior–posterior orientation) in schizophrenia, obsessive–compulsive disorder and unipolar depression. In depressed subjects, these deficits were mostly resolved on remission. A distinct 'melancholic pattern' was noted, with decreased correlation between the orbitofrontal cortex and the dorsolateral prefrontal cortex compared with controls and non-melancholic depressed subjects (Mallet *et al.*, 1998).

TREATMENT METHODS

Sleep Deprivation

Up to 60% of patients can improve after a night of total sleep deprivation (TSD) (Ebert and Berger, 1998). In contrast to the delayed cumulative effects of antidepressant medication, TSD has an immediate effect that does not appear to extend beyond the next full night's sleep (Ebert and Berger, 1998). The experimental advantage of TSD is that patients do not have to be medicated to show a short-term clinical improvement. The effects of TSD have been explained by increased dopamine release in the basal ganglia, which results in increased displacement of the D2/D4 receptor radio ligand 123I-iodobenzamide (IBZM) by endogenous dopamine, i.e. reduced ligand binding (Ebert *et al.*, 1994b). However, an allele of the D4 dopamine receptor, which has been suggested previously to increase susceptibility to this treatment, was not linked to treatment response in 124 bipolar patients (Serretti *et al.*, 1999). A growing body of evidence is documenting hyperperfusion in the medial prefrontal cortex as a state or trait related change (Ebert and Berger, 1998; Ebert *et al.*, 1996). Allied with limbic hyperperfusion, a number of studies describe dorsolateral prefrontal cortex hypoperfusion in depression and during mood induction in normal volunteers (Mayberg *et al.*, 1999). The early sleep-deprivation literature reported increased perfusion in the orbitofrontal cortex that was found in the right anterior cingulate and bilateral orbitofrontal cortex and basal cingulate. Increased right hippocampal pretreatment flow was associated with greater treatment response (Ebert *et al.*, 1994a). Similar findings, indicating the association between successful drug treatment and pretreatment limbic hyperperfusion, have since been reported by a number of groups. Comparing glucose metabolism in hospitalized unipolar patients, Mayberg *et al.* (1997) reported hyperperfusion in the rostral anterior cingulate (Brodman's area 24a/b) to be indicative of a favourable treatment outcome. Although subsequent non-responders were reported to be marginally more impaired than responders on neuropsychological performance, no other correlation between perfusion and clinical ratings was found. Hypoperfusion in responders was greater than in non-responders in the dorsolateral prefrontal cortex (Brodman's area 45/46), anterior insula and inferior parietal cortex (Brodman's area 40). Pretreatment premotor cortex activation, on the other hand, was greater in responders.

The prognostic capacity of anterior cingulate activity with reference to the extent of treatment response can also be measured with electroencephalography (EEG) (Smith *et al.*, 1999a). Higher θ (6.5–8 Hz) activity in the rostral cingulate was associated with a greater response after 4–6 months of treatment with nortriptyline. A greater degree of response was associated with increased pretreatment θ activity in the medial frontal cortex (Brodman's area 24, 32), consistent with previous functional imaging reports (Mayberg *et al.*, 1997).

Pretreatment metabolism in the medial prefrontal cortex (Brodman's area 32), ventral anterior cingulate (Brodman's area 24) and posterior subcallosal gyrus (Brodman's area 25) was found to be higher in responders to TSD than in non-responders and healthy volunteers (Wu *et al.*, 1999). Normalization upon recovery was noted with decreased flow in the medial prefrontal cortex (Brodman's area 32) and the frontal pole (Brodman's area 10). All depressed subjects had a lower striatal (putamen) metabolic rate than controls, which persisted after treatment and, by contrast, decreased in normal volunteers. Frontal and occipital cortex metabolism was also higher in both groups before treatment. The activity in the right lateral prefrontal cortex (Brodman's area 46) and higher superior temporal cortex and right insula increased in responders. Perfusion was decreased in the lateral prefrontal cortex of controls. Moreover, in comparison with control subjects, the neuropsychological performance of all depressed patients deteriorated markedly after a night of TSD. Normal subjects performing a verbal learning task following 35 hours of sleep deprivation exhibited a pattern of increased activation in the prefrontal and parietal cortices, whereas activity in their temporal lobe was decreased (Drummond *et al.*, 2000). Decline in subjects' performance of a free recall task was correlated positively with activation of their parietal lobe. Bilateral prefrontal cortex activation, which was related closely to personal perception of fatigue, was interpreted as a competitive mechanism associated with the homeostatic urge for sleep. Compensation for decreased temporal lobe activity appears to be achieved by increased perfusion in the bilateral parietal lobes in verbal tasks, which are not associated with this area in the control condition. Just as TSD created characteristic changes in blood flow during the verbal learning challenge, elevated pretreatment regional cerebral blood flow (rCBF) in the right orbitofrontal cortex and basal cingulate of patients was normalized in responders to partial sleep deprivation (in the latter part of the night). Post-treatment left inferior temporal flow was correlated with treatment response (Volk *et al.*, 1997).

In summary, these studies appear to suggest that elevated metabolism and blood flow in the prefrontal or medial prefrontal cortex areas is an adaptive marker aiding response to different forms of therapeutic intervention, especially sleep deprivation. Depressed patients may share an abnormal functional network (decreased flow in subcortical structures) (Wu *et al.*, 1999) or persistent abnormalities throughout the temporal cortex (where structural changes have also been reported) (Shah *et al.*, 1998; Sheline *et al.*, 1998; Sheline *et al.*, 1999) that may accommodate behavioural changes by compensating for hypoperfusion elsewhere. In certain patients, this mechanism may later cease to be effective.

Sleep disturbance during rapid eye movement (REM) and non-rapid eye movement (NREM) sleep are well documented in patients suffering from affective disorders (Kupfer and Reynolds, 1992). Ho *et al.* (1996) studied the δ stage of slow-wave (high-amplitude) sleep of NREM sleep with FDG–PET in depression and found that metabolism was elevated in the occipital and parietal cortices to a greater degree than elsewhere. Limbic structures, such as the posterior cingulate, amygdala and hippocampus, were more active in depressed patients; however, metabolism in midline structures and the neostriatum (including the medial prefrontal cortex, medial thalamus, anterior cingulate, bilateral caudate, putamen and the head of the caudate) was reduced compared with controls. In conjunction with an EEG investigation, Nofzinger *et al.* (2000) studied the link between β EEG frequency (characterized by higher frequency and lower amplitude) and glucose metabolism in different areas of the cortex, defined on the basis of findings from control data. β-Wave frequency had been coupled previously with secretion of cortisol (Chapotot *et al.*, 1998) and, in this study, was present for longer in depressed subjects and was associated negatively with subjective sleep quality. No hypofrontality was found in this study; however, orbitofrontal cortex (including Brodman's areas 11, 25, 32) metabolism was higher in depressed patients than in controls, which may be indicative of dysfunctional arousal. Finally, the contrast between waking and REM sleep revealed that, unlike controls, depressed subjects failed to recruit anterior paralimbic areas (right parahippocampal gyrus, right insula and anterior cingulate). Instead, temporal-limbic areas (amygdala, subiculum, inferior temporal cortex, sensorimotor cortex) were activated (Nofzinger *et al.*, 1999).

Light Therapy

In patients suffering from seasonal affective disorder, light therapy produced dissimilar blood-flow changes in responders and non-responders. Responders expressed a globally increased activity, measured with hexamethyl-propyleneamine-oxim (HMPAO)–SPECT, relative to the cerebellum mainly in the frontal and cingulate cortices along with the thalamus (Vasile *et al.*, 1997).

Pharmacotherapy

Ogura *et al.* (1998) found in an HMPAO–SPECT study of patients with major depression that the severity of depression was correlated negatively with perfusion in the left superior frontal, right lateral temporal and right parietal cortex. After treatment with tricyclic antidepressants (clomipramine and amoxapine), remitted patients' perfusion did not differ significantly from that of controls.

Brody *et al.* (1999) reported that a better response to the serotonin reuptake inhibitor paroxetine was associated with lower pretreatment glucose uptake in the left ventral anterior cingulate. In responders, values returned to normal in the ventrolateral prefrontal cortex and orbitofrontal cortex, but not in the dorsolateral prefrontal cortex or inferior frontal gyrus. Hamilton depression score changes were correlated with changes in glucose metabolism in some areas (ventrolateral prefrontal cortex and inferior frontal gyrus). Remission was associated with increased baseline perfusion in the left premotor and supplementary motor areas, along with decreased left ventral anterior cingulate metabolism (Brody *et al.*, 1999). These findings do not fit the Mayberg *et al.* (1997) study, but patients in Brody's study were more depressed and the researchers identified an area that lies ventral to Mayberg's 'rostral cingulate'.

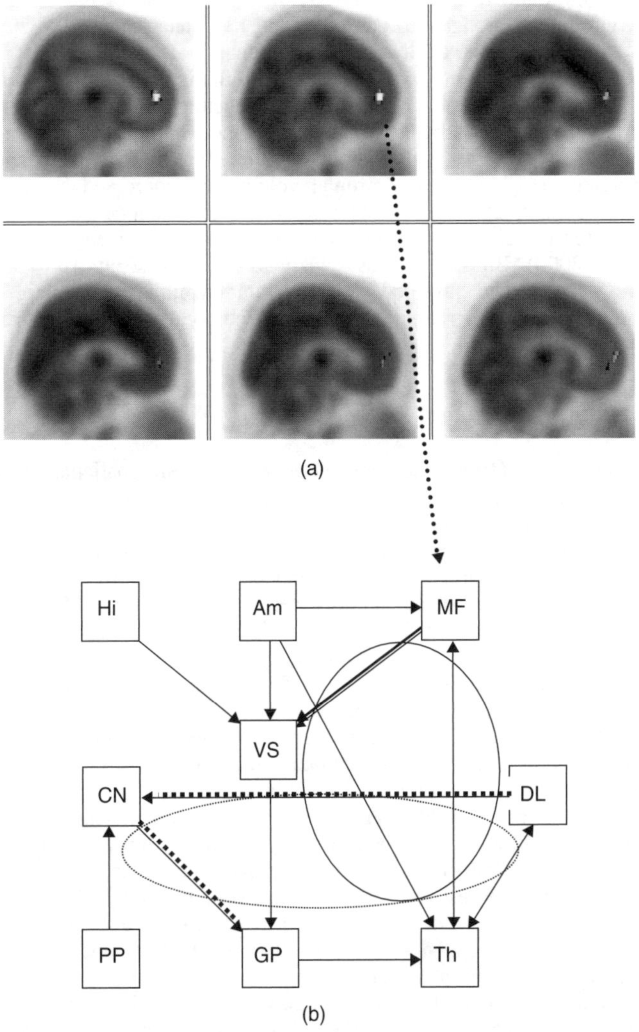

Figure XVIII-9.1 Effect of one session of TMS (5–20 Hz at 80% motor threshold over the left dorsolateral prefrontal cortex) on rCBF during a word-generation task. (a) Statistical parametric map of areas with $P < 0.01$ for effect size (z) and contiguous area (k), using Statistical Parametric Mapping, version 1996. (b) Neuroanatomical projections. Am, amygdala; CN, caudate nucleus; DL, dorsolateral prefrontal cortex; GP, globus pallidus; Hi, hippocampus; MF, medial orbitofrontal cortex; PP, posterior parietal cortex; Th, thalamus; VS, ventral striatum; Dotted ellipse, dorsolateral prefrontal loop; continuous ellipse, limbic loop; dotted arrow DL to CN, increase in regression coefficient *c* with significance levels in left dorsolateral loop ($c = 2.45$, $P < 0.05$); dotted arrow CN to GP, increase in regression coefficient *c* with significance levels in left dorsolateral loop ($c = 2.15$, $P = 0.05$); continuous arrow MF to VS, bilateral limbic loop (left: $c = 2.51$, $P < 0.05$; right: $c = 2.89$, $P < 0.05$) (See Colour Plate XVIII-9.1)

Physical Therapies

Electroconvulsive treatment (ECT) is by itself anticonvulsant, which suggests a reduction in cortical activity after a course of treatments (Ketter *et al.*, 1999; Post *et al.*, 2000). Using glucose uptake as a measure of cortical activity 5 days after a course of bilateral ECT in ten patients, Nobler *et al.* (2001) were able to support this hypothesis. Yatham *et al.* (2000) had previously failed to detect a significant change in five patients 1 week after a course of ECT. This is likely to be an effect of insufficient power.

Transcranial magnetic stimulation (TMS) has been used extensively to investigate cortical function in healthy volunteers and psychiatric patients (George *et al.*, 1998). A number of the simple hypotheses underlying the use of TMS in the treatment of psychiatric illness are based on the assumption that low-frequency TMS suppresses cortical activity (quenching) while high-frequency stimulation increases cortical excitability. Speer *et al.* (2000) were able to support this notion using 1- and 20-Hz stimulation over the left dorsolateral prefrontal cortex in a cross-over study of ten depressed patients. They found rCBF increases under the stimulation site and in associated paralimbic structures after 20-Hz stimulation and decreases in more restricted frontal, temporal and subcortical structures after 1-Hz stimulation. Similarly, Zheng (2000) found increases in cerebral perfusion in areas remote from the stimulation site after stimulation over the left dorsolateral prefrontal cortex.

In a parallel design study comparing 5, 10 and 20 Hz applied over the left dorsolateral prefrontal cortex in depressed patients, we found localized increases in the anterior cingulate after the first day's treatment, in combination with increased functional connectivity in the ipsilateral dorsolateral prefrontal loop and bilateral in the cingulate (limbic) loop (Figure XVIII-9.1).

In summary, recent studies have suggested an association between anatomical and functional changes in different prefrontal areas and their associated structures on one hand and disordered cognition and affect on the other. Such changes have been documented extensively in cingulate activity following successful treatment (e.g. Ebert *et al.*, 1996; Mayberg *et al.*, 1999; Volk *et al.*, 1997). Cingulate pretreatment perfusion differentiates between responders and non-responders (Mayberg *et al.*, 1997; Wu *et al.*, 1999). Furthermore, abnormalities in glial density (Drevets, 1999) and even changes in neuronal size (Rajkowska *et al.*, 1999) were found in the prefrontal cortex of unipolar patients (as discussed below). Finally, the cingulate is activated differentially in cognitive tasks (e.g. Stroop) involving attention or motivation (Whalen *et al.*, 1998), possibly denoting subregions that can be involved in specific tasks, promising a more differentiated understanding of the cognitive and emotional aspects of depression.

EFFECTS OF AGE, CHRONICITY AND TREATMENT RESISTANCE: IRREVERSIBLE AND REVERSIBLE CHANGES

Depression has been perceived as a transitory state where, on remission, brain function and altered or compromised cognition return to normal. This is no longer considered to be accurate in every case. Neuropsychological studies have discovered persistent abnormalities in cognitive performance, pertaining to the duration and severity of the illness (Abas *et al.*, 1990; Shah *et al.*, 1998). A number of imaging studies have also found potentially enduring deficits (e.g. Abas *et al.*, 1990; Shah *et al.*, 1998; Sheline *et al.*, 1999). Shah *et al.* (1998), in addition to a mere group difference, described a correlation between abnormal verbal memory and left medial temporal lobe grey matter deficits in the impaired group. Just as for certain unipolar depressed patients, structural abnormalities in bipolar depression include white-matter lesions, decreased cerebellar size, and sulcal as well as ventricular enlargement (see

Stoll *et al.*, 2000 for review). Structural MRI in 24 hospitalized bipolar patients (Strakowski *et al.*, 1999) revealed an increase in amygdala size with a similar trend in the globus pallidus, thalamus and striatum. These changes did not appear to correlate with other clinical measures, such as illness duration, medication, substance abuse, or the presence of previous episodes, although antipsychotic use would be a likely candidate.

Pathological studies have shown an excess of atheromatous disease in elderly depressed patients (Thomas *et al.*, 2001). In fact, some authors used the term 'MRI-defined vascular depression' (Krishnan *et al.*, 1997) to describe a group of elderly depressed patients with mainly later age of onset, nonpsychotic subtype, functional disability, anhedonia and a relative absence of family history (Krishnan *et al.*, 1997). Although these patients did not have a significantly worse prognosis than nonvascular depressives, a subgroup with late onset of the illness did (Krishnan *et al.*, 1998). In a large epidemiological study of cardiovascular health, small vascular lesions of the basal ganglia but not severity of white-matter lesions were associated with increased reporting of depressive symptoms as measured by the Centre for Epidemiological Studies Depression Scale (Steffens *et al.*, 1999). In a subsample, however, the MRI vascular changes in basal ganglia and non-basal ganglia structures appeared to exert their effects on depressive symptoms via the functional consequences of vascular disease, such as physical disability and cognitive impairment (Sato *et al.*, 1999). On the other hand, a case–control study of 96 elderly patients with late- and early-onset depression found the former to be associated with more white-matter hyperintensities, enlarged ventricles and hypertension (Lavretsky *et al.*, 1998).

MRI white-matter hyperintensities thus appear to be a hallmark of late-onset depression. Hyperintensities are also associated with treatment resistance (Lavretsky *et al.*, 1999; Simpson *et al.*, 1998) and future residual dysfunction, as well as cognitive decline (Hickie *et al.*, 1997; Jenkins *et al.*, 1998; Kramer-Ginsberg *et al.*, 1999) White-matter lesions seem to go with medical comorbidity, relatively independently of whole-brain and frontal atrophy, which are also more common in late-life depression (Kumar *et al.*, 2000). In particular, frontal lobe atrophy is correlated with severity of depression (Kumar *et al.*, 1998). A recent Newcastle study found that frontal white-matter changes were also more common in depressed patients with dementia. Finally, white-matter changes and frontal atrophy may be more common in depressed elderly patients with delusions (Kim *et al.*, 1999; O'Brien *et al.*, 1997a).

A combined MRI and SPECT study conducted in Edinburgh suggested greater temporal perfusion abnormalities in late- than early-onset depression and an association between cognitive deterioration and deep white-matter changes (Ebmeier *et al.*, 1997b; Ebmeier *et al.*, 1998). Similar (left medial) temporal lobe changes were reported in late-onset depression (Greenwald *et al.*, 1997), suggesting a possible link between late-onset depression and Alzheimer's disease. A large study comparing 61 depressed patients with 77 demented patients suggests, however, that temporal lobe volumetry can distinguish clearly been these two groups (O'Brien *et al.*, 1997b). Similar results were obtained using hippocampal width alone (Ebmeier *et al.*, 1997b).

Research in younger but also elderly depressed patients suggests that there may be a subgroup with long-lasting or treatment-resistant illness who show (medial) temporal lobe structural and functional changes (Shah and Ebmeier, 1998; Sheline *et al.*, 1999; Vakili *et al.*, 2000). Although there is little corroborating clinical evidence, some authors have argued that hypercortisolaemia associated with clinical depression may be responsible for the hippocampal damage observed in elderly patients. Contrary to this assumption, there is some limited evidence that temporal lobe changes are more common in late onset, i.e. shorter-lasting, depression (Ebmeier *et al.*, 1998; Lavretsky *et al.*, 1998).

Age Effects

As in younger patients, in elderly patients variation of depressive symptoms is associated with changes of brain activity in (medial) prefrontal structures. This can be shown in sleep-deprivation studies (Smith *et al.*, 1999a), in follow-up studies of depressed patients (Halloran *et al.*, 1999), in cross-sectional studies of clinical correlates in elderly depression (Awata *et al.*, 1998; Ebmeier *et al.*, 1997b) and even Alzheimer's disease (Hirono *et al.*, 1998).

Depression in children and adolescents has been attracting researchers' attention in recent years. Although the prevalence of affective disorders in childhood is now accepted to be on a par with the adult form of the illness, the contribution of the child's environment, along with cognitive and neuroanatomical developmental factors, is unclear. Data on functional brain activity in early-onset depression are consistent with findings in adults reporting left anterolateral hypoperfusion. Nonetheless, it is not certain whether the association between haemodynamic response and neural activity are analogous across the lifespan (Davidson and Slagter, 2000). Decreased frontal volume and increased choline-to-creatinine ratios in the anterior medial frontal lobe have been reported in depressed children and adolescents (reviewed in Steingard, 2000). Bipolar, just as schizophrenic, adolescents ($n = 35$) were reported to have reduced intracranial volume with enlarged ventricles and increased frontal and temporal sulci (Friedman *et al.*, 1999).

Treatment Resistance

Shah *et al.* (1998) demonstrated in 20 young patients with treatment-resistant unipolar depression, all of whom had been ill for more than 2 years, that temporal lobe structures, including the hippocampus, were reduced in grey matter density. The reduction in left medial temporal lobe grey matter density was correlated with poor performance in an auditory verbal memory task. Mervaala *et al.* (2000) examined 34 drug-resistant patients with major depression and were able to replicate findings of reduction in volume of left hippocampus. In addition, the choline/creatinine ratio in mesial temporal lobe was raised, suggesting membrane breakdown. Sheline *et al.* (1999) imaged 24 women with recurrent major depression and found that bilateral hippocampi were reduced in volume in proportion to illness duration and after controlling for age effects. Interestingly, patients also performed poorly in a verbal memory task, which may be a correlate of hippocampal reductions. Vakili *et al.* (2000) measured hippocampal volumes in 38 patients with primary depression. Although as a group patients had normal-sized hippocampi, treatment response to 20 mg fluoxetine for 8 weeks was associated with a relatively larger right hippocampus in women. Somewhat at variance with these results, a study focusing on temporal lobe epilepsy patients reported amygdala enlargement to be associated with dysthymia and depressive symptoms (Tebartz van Elst *et al.*, 1999; Tebartz van Elst *et al.*, 2000). The discrepancy may be explained by different pathology underlying mood changes in epilepsy, by divergent changes in amygdala and hippocampus, or by a different timepoint in the natural history of depression. Ketter *et al.* (2001) examined 43 treatment-resistant bipolar patients and found a contrast between cortical and subcortical glucose metabolism (18FDG–PET). Normalized effects indicating increased metabolism were reported in subcortical areas (ventral striatum and right amygdala) as well as in the posterior cortex, thalamus and cerebellum. Depressed bipolar patients also showed an absolute prefrontal, temporal and anterior paralimbic hypometabolism. Elevated metabolism in posterior cortical areas (including posterior thalamus and cerebellum) persisted beyond remission (i.e. in euthymic patients), indicating a trait marker unique to bipolar patients. Cognitive task activation (in this case, an auditory task) may be recruiting qualitatively different circuits in patients and controls, a concern shared by all studies employing neuropsychological activation paradigms (Ketter *et al.*, 2001).

Cellular Changes

Both neuronal and glial volume changes have been reported. The latter can be a consequence of a number of factors. As a result of the chronic use of antipsychotic medication, increased volume of glial cells was noted in the prefrontal cortex of rhesus monkeys (Selemon *et al.*, 1999). Reports of laminar as well as regionally specific patterns of glial but also neuronal reduction, where neurons decreased both in size (dorsolateral prefrontal cortex) and density (orbitofrontal cortex), was observed in the prefrontal cortex of unipolar patients (Rajkowska *et al.*, 1999). By contrast, post-mortem studies in both unipolar and bipolar patients with a family history of depression have not revealed any differences in the neuronal population, while glial density was decreased; glial volume of schizophrenic patients was unchanged (Drevets *et al.*, 1997; Ongur *et al.*, 1998). Finally, age-associated glial changes in primate grey matter reached statistical significance only in the cingulate (Sloane *et al.*, 2000). It is apparent that some association between changes in glial density and pathological or restorative processes has been established in patients suffering from affective disorders. Nonetheless, it is still unclear whether these changes are adaptive, compensatory or incidental. Further, the functional effect of such changes is still undetermined.

The association between neuronal activity and the metabolic processes measured by various functional brain-imaging modalities (haemodynamic response in functional magnetic resonance imaging (fMRI), glucose utilization in FDG–PET, and so forth), is not without question. Furthermore, it is apparent that astrocytes as well as neurons may contribute to the signal changes observed in FDG–PET (Magistretti and Pellerin, 1996; Magistretti and Pellerin, 1999). In the presence of glial reduction in anterolimbic structures reported by a number of groups (Drevets *et al.*, 1998; Rajkowska *et al.*, 1999), it is unknown whether, and to what extent, glucose utilization and its associated PET signal are altered as a result.

Lithium and valproate have been suggested to have neurotrophic and neuroprotective effects. An increase of 3% in the cortical grey matter volume of bipolar patients after 4 weeks of lithium administration is attributed to neurotrophic factors rather than to cell swelling (Moore *et al.*, 2000). Mood stabilizers could be involved in the regulation of gene expression by increasing levels of mRNA for PEBP2β (polyomavirus enhancer-binding protein 2 beta subunit), which controls coding for the neuroprotective protein BCL2 (B cell lymphoma protein 2) in the frontal cortex. Increased neuronal survival and increased regeneration are all effected by BCL2 upregulation, protecting against excitotoxic damage (Chen *et al.*, 1999; Chen and Chuang, 1999). It is unclear whether recent post-mortem findings of increased neuronal numbers throughout the hypothalamus and the dorsal raphe could be related to chronic use of medication (Rajkowska *et al.*, 1999).

Small structures such as the brainstem raphe nuclei are imaged with difficulty. It is, therefore, fortuitous that ultrasound sonography can be applied using a preauricular acoustic bone window to image the mesencephalic brainstem with structures such as the red nucleus and the rostral pontine brainstem. Becker *et al.* (1995) examined 40 unipolar, 40 bipolar depressive and 40 schizophrenic inpatients, as well as 40 healthy volunteers. Reduced midline echogenicity relative to the red nucleus, which can be interpreted as structural disruption of the raphe nuclei, was found only in the unipolar depressed patients.

EXPERIMENTAL APPROACHES TO DEPRESSION: COMPLEX MODELS

Cognitive performance in depression and its relationship with the disturbance of emotion or mood have been examined in a number of contexts. Along with an investigation of cognitive impairment in subjects suffering from affective disorders, there is a large body of literature reporting different procedures of precipitating depressed or dysphoric mood in healthy subjects (mood induction). A number of conceptual questions are inherent in this literature. Above all, it is unclear to what extent sad mood is analogous with clinical depression. The transient time course of the neuropsychological impairment brought about by mood induction is usually far shorter than the experience of clinical depression. Similarly, induced mood may be of a different quality from morbid depression, although biological symptoms, such as depressive retardation, can be observed after experimental mood induction (Ebert *et al.*, 1996). The absence of biological markers often associated with depression (such as hypercortisolaemia), along with structural and functional differences, hinder direct comparison. In this sense, even if the neural systems recruited in healthy controls during mood induction are analogous to the neuroanatomical circuit activated in depressed patients at rest, the dynamics of the circuit may be different in the two conditions due to selective dysfunction in specific components or the connectivity between these. It is even possible that some of the differences between patients and controls can be explained by simple mechanisms, e.g. that depressed patients are slower to recruit the appropriate neuronal systems or their components.

Since neuropsychological studies are described in detail in Chapter XVIII-7 and XIX-8 of this book, we will focus on neuronal systems implicated by clinical and mood-induction paradigms. We will try to integrate structural and functional findings reported earlier in the chapter in an attempt to assemble some of the complex interactions between specific structures and the systems they comprise in the manifestation of affective illness.

Neuropsychological studies suggest that cognitive deficits may be the consequence of competition between cognitive and affective functional resources. If this holds true, such that neural pathways identified in the induction paradigm are analogous to those affected in the specific mood disorder they are trying to emulate, then transient sadness or elation in normal volunteers can provide a useful insight into the neural correlate of cognitive performance in mood disorders. However, covariation between the degree of depression, impaired task performance and (in-)activity of relevant functional circuits does not necessarily imply a causal relationship between the three. Thus, apparently similar short-term deficits of neuronal activity observed both in clinical depression and after mood induction could be grounded in dissimilar processes. In the long term, these may be of no consequence for healthy volunteers, but they could result in the significant deficits noted in patients with recurrent and severe depression (Shah *et al.*, 1998).

The following section includes studies emphasizing perfusion changes associated with emotional states. Most studies report impaired cognitive performance as a consequence of transient mood change, although their methods may differ greatly. Anatomical structures that are classically grouped under the definition of 'limbic lobe' are involved in circuits responsible for both cognitive function and the generation of affect. These include the cingulate cortex, hippocampus, amygdala and thalamus, as well as other prefrontal and subcortical structures. Both mood-induction and clinical studies report altered dynamics in the limbic and prefrontal circuits, comprising activation or deactivation under specific conditions, compensatory effects, and the interplay between different regions (e.g. cortical and subcortical, limbic and dorsolateral prefrontal cortex, etc). The role of the cingulate has been emphasized by authors such as MacLean (1985). He saw the phylogenetic emergence of the cingulate cortex as fundamental to the development of maternal care in mammals. There is therefore a convergence of paradigms (Stevens and Price, 2000) between psychodynamic speculation about attachment and loss (Bowlby, 1969) and the understanding of limbic brain function in depression (Ebert *et al.*, 1996).

Such theories are now amenable to empirical testing. Lorberbaum *et al.* (1999) employed fMRI in four recently confined mothers listening to recordings of infants' cries and white noise as a control condition. Increased brain activity could be demonstrated in the anterior cingulate and right medial prefrontal cortex. These regional activations are probably not very specific, as similar areas are activated during pain and are thought to be related to affective and attentional concomitants of pain sensation (Peyron *et al.*, 2000; Schnitzler and Ploner, 2000). However, with careful experimental procedures, hypotheses about the specific role of the medial prefrontal cortex in emotion are testable, in principle.

Supporting the imaging studies in humans, there is also an animal model of congenitally helpless rats with reductions in brain activity in the dorsal frontal, medial orbital and anterior cingulate cortex, combined with increases in the subgenual cingulate (Shumake *et al.*, 2000).

Mood Induction and Neuropsychological Paradigms

Neuropsychological studies use cognitive tasks in order to recruit associated functional circuits through their component structures. Specific functional vulnerability can be described by either impaired performance of a particular task or impaired activation of characteristic circuits or their constituents. Neuropsychological tasks have been designed to probe activity in brain regions associated with them. Frontal areas are activated by tasks such as the Wisconsin card sorting test (WCST) or the Tower of London (TOL) task, both of which involve the application and manipulation of rules, adaptive skills and flexibility necessary for set shifting. Tasks that involve memory are expected to be particularly sensitive to structural and/or functional discontinuity in (mesial) temporal structures, such as the hippocampus. Finally, the involvement of subcortical structures in the experience of clinical and experimental mood is expressed by both perseverative responses (the inability to change strategies) and psychomotor slowing, experienced predominantly by melancholic patients (Austin *et al.*, 1999; Austin *et al.*, 2001). It appears that similar limbic-subcortical circuits are involved in different experimental mood-induction procedures; however, different substructures may be affected, possibly due to inconsistent methodology of experimental paradigms and the different affects involved.

Studies: Mood Induction

Baker *et al.* (1997) induced sad and elated mood in controls and examined brain activity following performance of a verbal fluency task. They reported anatomical dissociation between mood and cognitive function. Both mood states curtailed the activity normally associated with the verbal fluency task throughout the left prefrontal, premotor and cingulate cortex, as well as the thalamus. Reduced activation in the rostral medial orbitofrontal cortex and anterior cingulate was associated uniquely with sad mood.

Mayberg *et al.* (1999) proposed a simplified model of brain responses. They hypothesized a general increase in limbic-paralimbic perfusion coupled with a decrease in neocortical perfusion to accompany induction of sadness in healthy volunteers, while reciprocal changes were predicted during the resolution of dysphoric symptoms in depressed patients. These authors also observed an inverse correlation between right dorsolateral prefrontal and subgenual cingulate perfusion, supporting this notion. These finding can be interpreted as corollary evidence for the inverse relationship between depressed mood and attention.

Beauregard *et al.* (1998) studied patients' and controls' ($n = 7$) responses to mood induction. Transient sadness (triggered by film clips with emotional content) produced activation in the medial and inferior prefrontal, middle temporal cortex, cerebellum and caudate. Significantly greater activation in the left medial prefrontal cortex (Brodman's area 8) and right cingulate gyrus (Brodman's area 32) was observed in depressed patients, suggesting that these two structures may have a role in pathological sadness.

Elliott *et al.* (1997) postulated a catastrophic reaction to failure as a specific neuropsychological mechanism underlying poor performance in depression. They examined performance feedback responses in six patients and controls. Depressed patients did not share the expected activation in the medial caudate and ventromedial orbitofrontal cortex found in controls. Patients' brains were, therefore, insensitive to changes in both task and feedback conditions, consistent with the a priori hypothesis.

Schneider *et al.* (1996) found activation in a network related to performance feedback during the attempt at solving unsolvable anagrams; perfusion increased in healthy subjects ($n = 12$) in the mammillary bodies and the amygdala, and decreased in hippocampus. Solvable tasks were associated with increased perfusion in the latter. Increased frontal and temporal perfusion was associated with both conditions.

The Stroop interference task has been typically associated with activation of the cingulate gyrus (Pardo *et al.*, 1990). A different activation pattern was observed in depressed patients ($n = 11$), who failed to activate the left cingulate in comparison with control subjects. Reduced perfusion in patients' right cingulate was balanced by stronger activation of the left dorsolateral prefrontal cortex and the visual cortex (George *et al.*, 1997). A variant of the Stroop interference task (the emotional counting Stroop paradigm) showed a unique activation of the rostral anterior cingulate using fMRI in normal volunteers (Whalen *et al.*, 1998). Comparing perfusion between trials containing affective (such as murder) and neutral words, associated negative content with increased perfusion in the anterior cingulate without a change in reaction time. Performance of this form of the Stroop task compared with fixation *per se* was associated with overall decreased perfusion. These findings may suggest an association between pathological anxiety and an inability to reduce cingulate activation during task compared with fixation.

Correlation between higher global perfusion and increased cognitive demands was associated with task switching. The superior parietal cortex was reported to have a specific role in task switching, although this effect may be task specific (Kimberg *et al.*, 2000). Illness severity in this subtype correlates with increased perfusion in frontolimbic structures parahippocampal gyrus and cingulate (Ebmeier *et al.*, 1997a).

Induction of depressed and elated mood can, at times, be associated with overlapping or diverging neural circuitry. Dissociable recruitment of subcortical and cortical structures in healthy subjects ($n = 16$) during experience of both positive and negative affect was associated with specific changes in subcortical structures (especially the amygdala) but not frontotemporal structures (Schneider *et al.*, 1995). Both happy and sad mood correlated with increased blood oxygen level-dependent (BOLD) fMRI response in the left amygdala of healthy subjects ($n = 12$) (Schneider *et al.*, 1997). De Raedt *et al.* (1997) used a modified Velten procedure to induce mood both 'within and out of the realm of attention'. The latter involved a combination of dichotic listening and subliminal stimulation. Right lateral reduction in thalamic perfusion was found during both conditions compared with responses to neutral stimuli. Increased hippocampal perfusion was limited to subliminal stimulation conditions.

Divergent circuits were found in the evaluation of negative versus positive affective content. While the former was associated with increased perfusion in the right frontal gyrus and thalamus, the latter produced activation of the bilateral insula and the right inferior frontal gyrus. Neither showed associated changes in amygdala perfusion (Teasdale *et al.*, 1999). In a different study, subcortical limbic structures (amygdala, associative cortex, primary visual cortex, cerebellum) were activated through evaluation of unpleasant stimuli, while pleasant stimuli activated cortical structures (medial prefrontal cortex, dorsolateral prefrontal cortex, and the right orbitofrontal cortex, Paradiso *et al.*, 1999). Spatiotemporal differences in activation of the neuroanatomical correlate of positive and negative affect, expressed through characteristic activation of either orbitofrontal cortex or prefrontal cortex, were shown in healthy volunteers ($n = 10$). Recruitment of the medial prefrontal network in the context of negative affective content was established faster than the activation of the lateral prefrontal circuit, which was associated with positive affect (Northoff *et al.*, 2000). Finally, retrieval of episodic memories with affective content was associated with activation of anterior temporal lobe and left amygdala (Dolan *et al.*, 2000), a pattern mirrored by McGaugh and Cahill (1997) and Hamann and Adolphs (1999) in encoding of similar memories.

Hypofrontality along with specific prefrontal deficits have been reported extensively in the literature. Both depressed ($n = 6$) and control subjects performing the TOL task exhibited a pattern of deactivating the medial prefrontal cortex, superior temporal gyrus and posterior cingulate. For control subjects, increased difficulty was associated with a linear augmentation in the recruitment of the appropriate functional circuitry. By contrast, depressed patients presented with decreased activity in the rostral prefrontal cortex, caudate nucleus and anterior cingulate, without the expected compensation by the dorsolateral prefrontal cortex (Elliott *et al.*, 1997). Parietal cortex activation did not reach threshold in this experiment. Neural dissociation between cognitive and affective activation denoted specific activity-related changes in the medial frontal cortex. A reduction from baseline activity in the medial prefrontal cortex was linked to cognitive activation. Practice was associated with decreased perfusion in the medial prefrontal cortex, while performance anxiety was linked to increased perfusion in the same region. In a different experiment, elevated perfusion in the medial prefrontal cortex was reported during the anticipation of painful stimuli, and was correlated negatively with anxiety rating (i.e. increased anxiety produced a smaller reduction from baseline). Corresponding changes in flow were noted in the hypothalamus and midbrain. Thus, a decrease from baseline activity in the prefrontal cortex is thought to be a consequence of recruiting the network related to attention (Simpson *et al.*, 2001a; Simpson *et al.*, 2001b).

Systems

We conclude the chapter by discussing the neuronal circuits or systems putatively linked with affective illness. To the best of our current knowledge, there is no clear or direct correspondence between neurobiological factors and their effect on emotional experience or expression. Structural changes in areas such as the hippocampus, prefrontal cortex, cingulate or amygdala are perfect candidates for theories of dysfunctional loci. However, as we have indicated throughout this chapter, neurobiological abnormalities are not entirely predictive of functional deficits. Furthermore, dysfunction in affective disorders may involve long-term mechanisms of compensation and deterioration over time, which may not be explicit in present theories of unipolar and bipolar depression.

The limbic system is, of course, a natural candidate for many neuroimaging investigations. The evolutionary angle described earlier in this chapter (Bowlby, 1969; MacLean, 1985) places structures associated closely with environmental feedback, particularly in a social context, at the locus of a system associated with integrating internal and external states. For example, specific behaviours or neuropsychological tasks yield an associated activation in structures such as the cingulate gyrus (maternal separation cry, Stroop), amygdala (fear), hippocampus (autobiographical memories) and dorsolateral prefrontal cortex (TOL task), to name but a few. It is important to note that in brain regions not classically associated with the limbic system (and thus not salient in many investigations), such as the parietal cortex, reports of functional abnormalities are increasing (Davidson *et al.*, 1999; Drummond *et al.*, 2000; Ho *et al.*, 1996; Mayberg, 1997) Since regions of functional interest are often defined a priori in neuroimaging studies, a bias towards the well-documented structural and functional changes in limbic regions may be perpetuated.

Behavioural response to long-term stress in a social context seems to be adaptive, in the sense that initial alarm and resistance will ultimately lead to exhaustion and acceptance (Selye, 1936). Similarly, rank theories in mood disorders postulate acknowledgement of subordinate status and a 'yielding' motor response in the presence of higher rank (Stevens and Price, 2000). The limbic system is therefore assumed to unite behaviour and neuroanatomy, where conflict between external and internal input can be resolved, a role associated particularly with the cingulate. The impact on both psychomotor and prefrontal-cognitive associated capacity is inherent in these theories.

Expanding Papez's early theories of limbic circuit connectivity and function, current neuroimaging tools are instrumental in facilitating both understanding and advancement of functional circuitry in depression and mania. Careful attention to experimental design (such as activation under different experimental conditions), as well as the development of new chemical tracers and more powerful imaging technology, will contribute towards a better appreciation of the various phases associated with affective disorders. We are nearing a qualitative coupling between systems with either function or dysfunction. This is achieved by direct and indirect comparison between patients and healthy control subjects performing tasks under similar conditions. Nonetheless, quantitative knowledge regarding activity in distinct systems is, for now, sketchy.

Common to both prefrontal and limbic structures is the overlap between sensory and affective processes (LeDoux, 1996), where a visceral system provides feedback through endocrine and other neurobiological mechanisms. It is possible that inhibition by the prefrontal cortex may be involved in feedback control (not only the classically inhibitory orbitofrontal cortex but also the lateral prefrontal cortex, both denoting different strategies of associative learning) (Roberts and Wallis, 2000). Consequently, activity, or lack thereof, in frontal regions may lead to limbic hyperperfusion via nonlinear excitatory or inhibitory operational modes.

Hypofrontality has been reported extensively in different contexts. Thus, the interaction between cognitive and affective circuits with the frontal cortex has been described by neuroanatomical (Barbas *et al.*, 1999; Price *et al.*, 1996), neuropsychological and neuroimaging studies (Mayberg *et al.*, 1997; Rogers *et al.*, 1998). These circuits appear to have functional as well as structural regional specificity, whereby connectivity to other (remote) regions throughout the cortex and the subcortex are clearly defined.

The limbic system has been separated into affective and cognitive components, supported by neuroanatomical studies in humans and primates (e.g. Devinsky *et al.*, 1995; Mayberg *et al.*, 1999; Mega *et al.*, 1997; Price, 1999a). The integration of viscerosensory and affective information, yielding endocrine and motor changes (Price, 1999b) contributes to an extended network, which cannot be explicable by lesion studies alone (Frith and Dolan, 1998).

A number of compensatory mechanisms can be deduced from the extensive neuroimaging literature in the field. The amygdala and orbitofrontal cortex appear to activate in synergy, where the orbitofrontal cortex is activated more strongly in response to amygdala dysfunction (Drevets, 1999). In healthy subjects, compensatory strategies require greater activity in the prefrontal and parietal cortices to balance for decreased temporal lobe perfusion and associated performance deficits after a night of TSD (Drummond *et al.*, 2000). By contrast, Elliott *et al.* (1997) showed that depressed patients lacked an adaptive capacity, which was expressed by their inability to recruit prefrontal as well as subcortical structures during performance of the TOL task. Further, correspondence between hyperperfusion in the cognitive and affective divisions of the cingulate reported by Mayberg *et al.* (1999) could arguably have a compensatory role in depression and recovery.

Therefore, a hyperactive limbic (or 'ventral'; see Mayberg *et al.*, 1999) system was noted by a number of groups, where increased perfusion can imply higher probability for response to treatment (Mayberg *et al.*, 1997; Wu *et al.*, 1999) or, alternatively, increased likelihood of more severe illness (Austin *et al.*, 1992). In the long term, connections to temporal (amygdala, hippocampus), parietal, prefrontal and subcortical structures will help us understand the extent to which an extended network can compensate for limbic hyperperfusion.

Blood flow and glucose metabolism in subcortical structures, the dorsolateral prefrontal cortex and the cingulate have been linked extensively with affective disorders through neurological and movement disorders, lesion studies, functional activation and imaging at rest (Cummings, 1993; Mega and Cummings, 1994, Soares and Mann, 1997). Furthermore, basal ganglia and frontal lesions carry a higher probability for cognitive impairment (Rogers *et al.*, 1998; Videbech, 1997). It is apparent that subcortical involvement can be associated with increased pathophysiology (e.g. psychomotor retardation), recurrent episodes and cognitive decline (Hickie *et al.*, 1997; Hickie *et al.*, 1999; Simpson *et al.*, 1998). The anterior cingulate may play a cardinal role in this context, due to its widespread connections and functional association with the prefrontal cortex (Ebert *et al.*, 1996; Koski and Paus, 2000). This is, at present, not clearly specified, ranging from theories of a 'somatic marker' (Damasio, 1994), motivation, attention and error detection (Carter *et al.*, 1999) due to its specificity in the integration of cognition and affect. It is confounded by the structural changes in specific subgroups of unipolar and bipolar patients (Drevets *et al.*, 1997). Finally, since hippocampal volume reduction is associated with the severity of depressive illness (Sheline *et al.*, 1999) and, by association (Drummond *et al.*, 2000), transient hypoactivity in the temporal cortex, its function may be balanced by prefrontal and parietal regions.

It would be interesting to probe such functional correspondences between two or more structures in a clinical context.

To conclude, a unified theory of affective disorders is developing through the application of different imaging methods and consideration of both animal and human neuroanatomical data. Future studies will no doubt consider a larger, distributed functional network, coupled with better understanding of the long-term effects of clinical deterioration, medication and the ageing process. What emerges, is a functional interplay of brain modules that are associated with specific mood states, attention, non-specific emotional factors, and certain aspects of the neuropsychological tasks used. We now have the tools to test relevant hypotheses in the living brain. The groundwork will have to be done with fMRI and possibly TMS in healthy volunteers, although in the last analysis, studies in sufficiently large, homogeneous and representative groups of patients will be necessary. The understanding that has come from studies so far is that dimensions of mood are indeed interlinked closely with cognitive categories, and that experimental studies may necessitate our rethinking of clinical and psychological constructs.

REFERENCES

Abas, M.A., Sahakian, B.J. and Levy, R., 1990. Neuropsychological deficits and CT scan changes in elderly depressives. *Psychological Medicine*, **20**, 507–520.

Alexander, G.E., DeLong, M.R. and Strick, P.L., 1986. Parallel organisation of functionally segregated circuits linking basal ganglia and cortex. *Annual Review of Neuroscience*, **9**, 357–381.

Al-Moussawi, A.H., Evans, N., Ebmeier, K.P., Roeda, D., Chaloner, F. and Ashcroft, G.W., 1996. Limbic system dysfunction in schizophrenia and mania — a study using 18F-fluorodeoxyglucose and positron emission tomography. *British Journal of Psychiatry*, **169**, 509–516.

Andrews, G., 2001. Placebo response in depression: bane of research, boon to therapy. *British Journal of Psychiatry*, **178**, 192–194.

Austin, M.-P., Dougall, N.J., Ross, M., Murray, C.L., O'Carroll, R.E., Moffoot, A., Ebmeier, K.P. and Goodwin, G.M., 1992. Single photon emission tomography with 99mTc-exametazime in major depression and the pattern of brain activity underlying the endogenous/neurotic continuum. *Journal of Affective Disorders*, **26**, 31–43.

Austin, M.-P., Mitchell, P., Wilhelm, K., Parker, G., Hickie, I., Brodaty, H., Chan, J., Eyers, K., Milic, M. and Hadzi-Pavlovic, D., 1999. Cognitive function in depression: a distinct pattern of frontal impairment in melancholia? *Psychological Medicine*, **29**, 73–85.

Austin, M.-P., Mitchell, P. and Goodwin, G.M., 2001. Cognitive deficits in depression. *British Journal of Psychiatry*, **178**, 200–206.

Awata, S., Ito, H., Konno, M., Ono, S., Kawashima, R., Fukuda, H. and Sato, M., 1998. Regional cerebral blood flow abnormalities in late-life depression: relation to refractoriness and chronification. *Psychiatry and Clinical Neurosciences*, **52**, 97–105.

Baker, S.C., Frith, C.D. and Dolan, R.J., 1997. The interaction between mood and cognitive function studied with PET. *Psychological Medicine*, **27**, 565–578.

Barbas, H., Ghashghaei, H., Dombrowski, S.M. and Rempel-Clower, N.L., 1999. Medial prefrontal cortices are unified by common connections with superior temporal cortices and distinguished by input from memory-related areas in the rhesus monkey. *Journal of Comparative Neurology*, **410**, 343–367.

Battersby, S., Ogilvie, A.D., Blackwood, D.H.R., Shen, S., Muqit, M.M., Muir, W.J., Teague, P., Goodwin, G.M. and Harmar, A.J., 2001. Presence of multiple functional polyadenylation signals and a single nucleotide polymorphism in the 3′ untranslated region of the human serotonin transporter gene. *Journal of Neurochemistry*, **72**, 1384–1388.

Beauregard, M., Leroux, J.M., Bergman, S., Arzoumanian, Y., Beaudoin, G., Bourgouin, P. and Stip, E., 1998. The functional neuroanatomy of major depression: an fMRI study using an emotional activation paradigm. *Neuroreport*, **9**, 3253–3258.

Becker, G., Becker, T., Struck, M., Lindner, A., Burzer, K., Retz, W., Bogdahn, U. and Beckmann, H., 1995. Reduced echogenicity in brainstem raphe specific to unipolar depression: a transcranial color-coded real-time sonography study. *Biological Psychiatry*, **38**, 180–184.

Bhashghaei, H.T. and Barbas, H., 2001. Neural interaction between the basal forebrain and functionally distinct prefrontal cortices in the rhesus monkey. *Neuroscience*, **103**, 593–614.

Biver, F., Wikler, D., Lotstra, F., Damhaut, P., Goldman, S. and Mendlewicz, J., 1997. Serotonin 5-HT2 receptor imaging in major depression: focal changes in orbito-insular cortex. *British Journal of Psychiatry*, **171**, 444–448.

Bowlby, J., 1969. *Attachment and Loss*. Tavistock Institute of Human Relations, London.

Bremner, J.D., Randall, P., Scott, T.M., Bronen, R.A., Seibyl, J.P., Southwick, S.M., Delaney, R.C., McCarthy, G., Charney, D.S. and Innis, R.B., 1995. MRI-based measurement of hippocampal volume in patients with combat related post-traumatic stress disorder. *American Journal of Psychiatry*, **152**, 973–981.

Brody, A.L., Saxena, S., Silverman, D.H., Alborzian, S., Fairbanks, L.A., Phelps, M.E., Huang, S.C., Wu, H.M., Maidment, K. and Baxter, L.R.J., 1999. Brain metabolic changes in major depressive disorder from pre- to post-treatment with paroxetine. *Psychiatry Research*, **91**, 127–139.

Carter, C.S., Botvinick, M.M. and Cohen, J.D., 1999. The contribution of the anterior cingulate cortex to executive processes in cognition. *Reviews in the Neurosciences*, **10**, 49–57.

Chapotot, F., Gronfier, C., Jouny, C., Muzet, A. and Brandenberger, G., 1998. Cortisol secretion is related to electroencephalographic alertness in human subjects during daytime wakefulness. *Journal of Clinical Endocrinology and Metabolism*, **83**, 4263–4268.

Chen, G., Zeng, W.Z., Yuan, P.X., Huang, L.D., Jiang, Y.M., Zhao, Z.H. and Manji, H.K., 1999. The mood-stabilizing agents lithium and valproate robustly increase the levels of the neuroprotective protein bcl-2 in the CNS. *Journal of Neurochemistry*, **72**, 879–882.

Chen, R.W. and Chuang, D.M., 1999. Long term lithium treatment suppresses p53 and Bax expression but increases Bcl-2 expression — a prominent role in neuroprotection against excitotoxicity. *Journal of Biological Chemistry*, **274**, 6039–6042.

Cummings, J.L., 1993. Frontal-subcortical circuits and human-behavior. *Archives of Neurology*, **50**, 873–880.

Dahlstrom, M., Ahonen, A., Ebeling, H., Torniainen, P., Heikkila, J. and Moilanen, I., 2000. Elevated hypothalamic/midbrain serotonin (monoamine) transporter availability in depressive drug-naive children and adolescents. *Molecular Psychiatry*, **5**, 514–522.

Damasio, A.R., 1994. *Descartes Error: Emotion Reason and the Human Brain*, GP Putbans Sons, New York.

Davidson, R.J. and Slagter, H.A., 2000. Probing emotion in the developing brain: functional neuroimaging in the assessment of the neural substrates of emotion in normal and disordered children and adolescents. *Mental Retardation and Developmental Disabilities Research Reviews*, **6**, 166–170.

Davidson, R.J., Abercrombie, H., Nitschke, J.B. and Putnam, K., 1999. Regional brain function, emotion and disorders of emotion. *Current Opinion in Neurobiology*, **9**, 228–234.

DelBello, M.P., Strakowski, S.M., Zimmerman, M.E., Hawkins, J.M. and Sax, K.W., 1999. MRI analysis of the cerebellum in bipolar disorder: a pilot study. *Neuropsychopharmacology*, **21**, 63–68.

Delgado, P.L., Charney, D.S., Price, L.H., Aghajanian, G.K., Landis, H. and Heninger, G.R., 1990. Serotonin function and the mechanism of antidepressant action. *Archives of General Psychiatry*, **47**, 411–417.

De Raedt, R., D'haenen, H., Everaert, H., Cluydts, R. and Bossuyt, A., 1997. Cerebral blood flow related to induction of a depressed mood within and out of the realm of attention in normal volunteers. *Psychiatry Research*, **74**, 159–171.

Devinsky, O., Morrell, M.J. and Vogt, B.A., 1995. Contributions of anterior cingulate cortex to behavior. *Brain*, **118**, 279–306.

Dolan, R.S., Lane, R., Chua, P. and Fletcher, P., 2000. Dissociable temporal lobe activations during emotional episodic memory retrieval. *Neuroimage*, **11**, 203–209.

Drevets, W.C., 1998. Functional neuroimaging studies of depression: the anatomy of melancholia. *Annual Review of Medicine*, **49**, 341–361.

Drevets, W.C., 1999. Prefrontal cortical-amygdalar metabolism in major depression. *Annals of the New York Academy of Sciences*, **877**, 614–637.

Drevets, W.C., Price, J.L., Simpson, J.R., Todd, R.D., Reich, T., Vannier, M. and Raichle, M.E., 1997. Subgenual prefrontal cortex abnormalities in mood disorders. *Nature*, **386**, 824–827.

Drevets, W.C., Ongur, D. and Price, J.L., 1998. Neuroimaging abnormalities in the subgenual prefrontal cortex: implications for the pathophysiology of familial mood disorders. *Molecular Psychiatry*, **3**, 220–226.

Drevets, W.C., Frank, E., Price, J.C., Kupfer, D.J., Holt, D., Greer, P.J., Huang, Y., Gautier, C. and Mathis, C., 1999. PET imaging of serotonin 1A receptor binding in depression. *Biological Psychiatry*, **46**, 1375–1387.

Drummond, S.P.A., Brown, G.G., Gillin, J.C., Stricker, J.L., Wong, E.C. and Buxton, R.B., 2000. Altered brain response to verbal learning following sleep deprivation. *Nature*, **403**, 655–657.

Ebert, D. and Berger, M., 1998. Neurobiological similarities in antidepressant sleep deprivation and psychostimulant use: a psychostimulant theory of antidepressant sleep deprivation. *Psychopharmacology*, **140**, 1–10.

Ebert, D. and Ebmeier, K.P., 1996. The role of the cingulate gyrus in depression: from functional anatomy to neurochemistry. *Biological Psychiatry*, **39**, 1044–1050.

Ebert, D., Feistel, H., Barocka, A. and Kaschka, W., 1994a. Increased limbic blood-flow and total sleep-deprivation in major depression with melancholia. *Psychiatry Research-Neuroimaging*, **55**, 101–109.

Ebert, D., Feistel, H., Kaschka, W., Barocka, A. and Pirner, A., 1994b. Single-photon emission computerized-tomography assessment of cerebral dopamine D2 receptor blockade in depression before and after sleep-deprivation–preliminary results. *Biological Psychiatry*, **35**, 880–885.

Ebert, D., Feistel, H., Loew, T. and Pirner, A., 1996. Dopamine and depression-D2 receptor SPECT before and after antidepressant therapy. *Psychopharmacology*, **126**, 91–94.

Ebmeier, K.P. and Ebert, D., 1997. Imaging functional change and dopaminergic activity in depression. In: Beninger, R.J., Palomo, T. and Archer, T. (eds), *Dopamine Disease States*, Vol. 3, pp. 511–522. Cerebro y Mente Press, Madrid.

Ebmeier, K.P., Cavanagh, J.T.O., Moffoot, A.P.R., Glabus, M.F., O'Carroll, R.E. and Goodwin, G.M., 1997a. Cerebral perfusion correlates of depressed mood. *British Journal of Psychiatry*, **170**, 77–81.

Ebmeier, K.P., Prentice, N., Ryman, A., Halloran, E., Rimmington, J.E., Best, J.K. and Goodwin, G.M., 1997b. Temporal lobe abnormalities in dementia and depression: a study using high resolution single photon emission tomography and magnetic resonance imaging. *Journal of Neurology, Neurosurgery, and Psychiatry*, **63**, 597–604.

Ebmeier, K.P., Glabus, M.F., Prentice, N., Ryman, A. and Goodwin, G.M., 1998. A voxel-based analysis of cerebral perfusion in dementia and depression of old age. *Neuroimage*, **7**, 199–208.

Elliott, R., Baker, S.C., Rogers, R.D., O'Leary, D.A., Paykel, E.S., Frith, C.D., Dolan, R.J. and Sahakian, B.J., 1997. Prefrontal dysfunction in depressed patients performing a complex planning task: a study using positron emission tomography. *Psychological Medicine*, **27**, 931–942.

Elliott, R., Sahakian, B.J., Michael, A., Paykel, E.S. and Dolan, R.J., 1998. Abnormal neural response to feedback on planning and guessing tasks in patients with unipolar depression. *Psychological Medicine*, **28**, 559–571.

Friedman, L., Findling, R.L., Kenny, J.T., Swales, T.P., Stuve, T.A., Jesberger, J.A., Lewin, J.S. and Schulz, S.C., 1999. An MRI study of adolescent patients with either schizophrenia or bipolar disorder as compared to healthy control subjects. *Biological Psychiatry*, **46**, 78–88.

Frith, C. and Dolan, R.J., 1998. Images of psychopathology. *Current Opinion in Neurobiology*, **8**, 259–262.

Fu, C.H., Reed, L.J., Meyer, J.H., Kennedy, S., Houle, S., Eisfeld, B.S. and Brown, G.M., 2001. Noradrenergic dysfunction in the prefrontal cortex in depression. *Biological Psychiatry*, **49**, 317–325.

George, M.S., Ketter, T.A., Parekh, P.I., Rosinsky, N., Ring, H.A., Pazzaglia, P.J., Marangell, L.B., Callahan, A.M. and Post, R.M., 1997. Blunted left cingulate activation in mood disorder subjects during a response interference task (the stroop). *Journal of Neuropsychiatry and Clinical Neurosciences*, **9**, 55–63.

George, M.S., Nahas, Z., Speer, A.M., Kimbrell, T.A., Wassermann, E.M., Lawandales, C.C., Molloy, M., Bohning, D., Risch, S.C. and Post, R.M., 1998. Transcranial magnetic stimulation (TMS)–a new method for investigating the neuroanatomy of depression. In: Ebert, D. and Ebmeier, K.P. (eds), *Biological Psychiatry: New Models for Depression*, Vol. 19, Karger, Basel.

Goodwin, G.M., Austin, M.-P., Dougall, N.J., Ross, M., Murray, C.L., O'Carroll, R.E., Moffoot, A., Prentice, N. and Ebmeier, K.P., 1993. State changes in brain activity shown by the uptake of 99mTc-exametazime with single photon emission tomography in major depression before and after treatment. *Journal of Affective Disorders*, **29**, 243–253.

Greenwald, B.S., Kramer-Ginsberg, E., Bogerts, B., Ashtari, M., Aupperle, P., Wu, H., Allen, L., Zeman, D. and Patel, M., 1997. Qualitative magnetic resonance imaging findings in geriatric depression. Possible link between later-onset depression and Alzheimer's disease? *Psychological Medicine*, **27**, 421–431.

Halloran, E., Prentice, N., Murray, C.L., O'Carroll, R.E., Glabus, M.F., Goodwin, G.M. and Ebmeier, K.P., 1999. Follow-up study of depression in the elderly. Clinical and SPECT data. *British Journal of Psychiatry*, **175**, 252–258.

Hamann, S.B. and Adolphs, R., 1999. Normal recognition of emotional similarity between facial expressions following bilateral amygdala damage. *Neuropsychologia*, **37**, 1135–1141.

Hibberd, C., Yau, J.L. and Seckl, J.R., 2000. Glucocorticoids and the ageing hippocampus. *Journal of Anatomy*, **197**, 553–562.

Hickie, I., Scott, E., Wilhelm, K. and Brodaty, H., 1997. Subcortical hyperintensities on magnetic resonance imaging in patients with severe depression — a longitudinal evaluation. *Biological Psychiatry*, **42**, 367–374.

Hickie, I., Ward, P., Scott, E., Haindl, W., Walker, B., Dixon, J. and Turner, K., 1999. Neo-striatal rCBF correlates of psychomotor slowing in patients with major depression. *Psychiatry Research*, **92**, 75–81.

Hirono, N., Mori, E., Ishii, K., Ikejiri, Y., Imamura, T., Shimomura, T., Hashimoto, M., Yamashita, H. and Sasaki, M., 1998. Frontal lobe hypometabolism and depression in Alzheimer's disease. *Neurology*, **50**, 380–383.

Ho, A.P., Gillin, J.C., Buchsbaum, M.S., Wu, J.C., Abel, L. and Bunney, W.E., 1996. Brain glucose metabolism during non-rapid eye movement sleep in major depression — a positron emission tomography study. *Archives of General Psychiatry*, **53**, 645–652.

Jenkins, M., Malloy, P., Salloway, S., Cohen, R., Rogg, J., Tung, G., Kohn, R., Westlake, R., Johnson, E.G. and Richardson, E., 1998. Memory processes in depressed geriatric patients with and without subcortical hyperintensities on MRI. *Journal of Neuroimaging*, **8**, 20–26.

Jimerson, D.C., 1987. Role of dopamine mechanisms in the affective disorders. In: Meltzer, H.Y. (ed.), *Psychopharmacology: the Third Generation of Progress*, pp. 505–511. Raven Press, New York.

Kapur, S., Meyer, J., Houle, S. and Brown, G., 1994. Functional anatomy of the dopaminergic system: PET study in humans. *Neuropsychopharmacology*, **19**(3S), Part 2, 17S.

Kennedy, S.H., Javanmard, M. and Vaccarino, F.J., 1997. A review of functional neuroimaging in mood disorders: positron emission tomography and depression. *Canadian Journal of Psychiatry*, **42**, 467–475.

Ketter, T.A., Kimbrell, T.A., George, M.S., Dunn, R.T., Speer, A.M., Benson, B.E., Willis, M.W., Danielson, A., Frye, M.A., Herscovitch, P. and Post, R.M., 2001. Effects of mood and subtype on cerebral glucose metabolism in treatment-resistant bipolar disorder. *Biological Psychiatry*, **49**, 97–109.

Ketter, T.A., Kimbrell, T.A., George, M.S., Willis, M.W., Benson, B.E., Danielson, A., Frye, M.A., Herscovitch, P. and Post, R.M., 1999. Baseline cerebral hypermetabolism associated with carbamazepine response, and hypometabolism with nimodipine response in mood disorders. *Biological Psychiatry*, **46**, 1364–1374.

Kim, D.K., Kim, B.L., Sohn, S.E., Lim, S.W., Na, D.G., Paik, C.H., Krishnan, K.R. and Carroll, B.J., 1999. Candidate neuroanatomic substrates of psychosis in old-aged depression. *Progress in Neuropsychopharmacology and Biological Psychiatry*, **23**, 793–807.

Kimberg, D.Y., Aguirre, G.K. and D'Esposito, M., 2000. Modulation task-related neural activity in task-switching: an fMRI study. *Cognitive Brain Research*, **10**, 189–196.

Klimke, A., Larisch, R., Janz, A., Vosberg, H., Muller-Gartner, H.W. and Gaebel, W., 1999. Dopamine D-2 receptor binding before and after treatment of major depression measured by [I-123]IBZM SPECT. *Psychiatry Research—Neuroimaging*, **90**, 91–101.

Koski, L. and Paus, T., 2000. Functional connectivity of the anterior cingulate cortex within the human frontal lobe: a brain-mapping meta-analysis. *Experimental Brain Research*, **133**, 55–65.

Kramer-Ginsberg, E., Greenwald, B.S., Krishnan, K.R., Christiansen, B., Hu, J., Ashtari, M., Patel, M. and Pollack, S., 1999. Neuropsychological functioning and MRI signal hyperintensities in geriatric depression. *American Journal of Psychiatry*, **156**, 438–444.

Krishnan, K.R., Hays, J.C. and Blazer, D.G., 1997. MRI-defined vascular depression. *American Journal of Psychiatry*, **154**, 497–501.

Krishnan, K.R., Hays, J.C., George, L.K. and Blazer, D.G., 1998. Six-month outcomes for MRI-related vascular depression. *Depression and Anxiety*, **8**, 142–146.

Kumar, A., Jin, Z., Bilker, W., Udupa, J. and Gottlieb, G., 1998. Late-onset minor and major depression: early evidence for common neuroanatomical substrates detected by using MRI. *Proceedings of the National Academy of Sciences of the United States of America*, **95**, 7654–7658.

Kumar, A., Bilker, W., Jin, Z. and Udupa, J., 2000. Atrophy and high intensity lesions: complementary neurobiological mechanisms in late-life major depression. *Neuropsychopharmacology*, **22**, 264–274.

Kupfer, D.J. and Reynolds, C.F., 1992. Sleep and affective disorders. In: Paykel, E.S. (ed.), *Handbook of Affective Disorders*, 2nd edn, pp. 311–323. Churchill Livingstone, Edinburgh.

Laasonen-Balk, T., Kuikka, J., Viinamaki, H., Husso-Saastamoinen, M., Lehtonen, J. and Tiihonen, J., 1999. Striatal dopamine transporter density in major depression. *Psychopharmacology*, **144**, 282–285.

Lauterbach, E.C., Jackson, J.G., Wilson, A.N., Dever, G.E. and Kirsh, A.D., 1997. Major depression after left posterior globus pallidus lesions. *Neuropsychiatry, Neuropsychology, and Behavioral Neurology*, **10**, 9–16.

Lavretsky, H., Lesser, I.M., Wohl, M. and Miller, B.L., 1998. Relationship of age, age at onset, and sex to depression in older adults. *American Journal of Geriatric Psychiatry*, **6**, 248–256.

Lavretsky, H., Lesser, I.M., Wohl, M., Miller, B.L. and Mehringer, C.M., 1999. Clinical and neuroradiologic features associated with chronicity in late-life depression. *American Journal of Geriatric Psychiatry*, **7**, 309–316.

LeDoux, J., 1996. *The Emotional Brain*. Simon & Schuster, New York.

Lesch, K.P., Mayer, S., Disselkamp-Tietze, J., Hoh, A., Schoelnhammer, G. and Schulte, H.M., 1990. Subsensitivity of the 5-hydroxytryptamine1A (5HT1A) receptor mediated hypothermic response to ipsapirone in unipolar depression. *Life Sciences*, **46**, 1271–1277.

Lorberbaum, J.P., Newman, J.D., Dubno, J.R., Horwitz, A.R., Nahas, Z., Teneback, C.C., Bloomer, C.W., Bohning, D.E., Vincent, D., Johnson, M.R., Emmanuel, N., Brawman-Mintzer, O., Book, S.W., Lydiard, R.B., Ballenger, J.C. and George, M.S., 1999. Feasibility of using fMRI to study mothers responding to infant cries. *Depression and Anxiety*, **10**, 99–104.

MacLean, P.D., 1985. Brain evolution relating to family, play, and the separation call. *Archives of General Psychiatry*, **42**, 405–417.

Magistretti, P.J. and Pellerin, L., 1996. The contribution of astrocytes to the 18F-2-deoxyglucose signal in PET activation studies. *Molecular Psychiatry*, **1**, 445–452.

Magistretti, P.J. and Pellerin, L., 1999. Cellular mechanisms of brain energy metabolism and their relevance to functional brain imaging. *Philosophical Transactions of the Royal Society of London. Series B: Biological Sciences*, **354**, 1155–1163.

Malison, R.T., Best, S.E., van Dyck, C.H., McCance, E.F., Wallace, E.A., Laruelle, M., Baldwin, R.M., Seibyl, J.P., Price, L.H., Kosten, T.R. and Innis, R.B., 1998a. Elevated striatal dopamine transporters during acute cocaine abstinence as measured by [123I] beta-CIT SPECT. *American Journal of Psychiatry*, **155**, 832–834.

Malison, R.T., Price, L.H., Berman, R., van Dyck, C.H., Pelton, G.H., Carpenter, L., Sanacora, G., Owens, M.J., Nemeroff, C.B., Rajeevan, N., Baldwin, R.M., Seibyl, J.P., Innis, R.B. and Charney, D.S., 1998b. Reduced brain serotonin transporter availability in major depression as measured by [123I]-2 beta-carbomethoxy-3 beta-(4-iodophenyl)tropane and single photon emission computed tomography. *Biological Psychiatry*, **44**, 1090–1098.

Mallet, L., Mazoyer, B. and Martinot, J.L., 1998. Functional connectivity in depressive, obsessive-compulsive, and schizophrenic disorders: an explorative correlational analysis of regional cerebral metabolism. *Psychiatry Research—Neuroimaging*, **82**, 83–93.

Mann, J.J., Oquendo, M., Underwood, M.D. and Arango, V., 1999. The neurobiology of suicide risk: a review for the clinician. *Journal of Clinical Psychiatry*, **60**(Suppl 2), 7–11.

Mayberg, H.S., 1997. Limbic-cortical dysregulation: a proposed model of depression. *Journal of Neuropsychiatry*, **9**, 471–481.

Mayberg, H.S., Brannan, S.K., Mahurin, R.K., Jerabek, P.A., Brickman, J.S., Tekell, J.L., Silva, J.A., McGinnis, S., Glass, T.G., Martin, C.C. and Fox, P.T., 1997. Cingulate function in depression: a potential predictor of treatment response. *Neuroreport*, **8**, 1057–1061.

Mayberg, H.S., Liotti, M., Brannan, S.K., McGinnis, S., Mahurin, R.K., Jerabek, P.A., Silva, J.A., Tekell, J.L., Martin, C.C., Lancaster, J.L. and Fox, P.T., 1999. Reciprocal limbic-cortical function and negative mood: converging PET findings in depression and normal sadness. *American Journal of Psychiatry*, **156**, 675–682.

McGaugh, J.L. and Cahill, L., 1997. Interaction of neuromodulatory systems in modulating memory storage. *Behavioral Brain Research*, **83**, 31–38.

Mega, M.S. and Cummings, J.L., 1994. Frontal-subcortical circuits and neuropsychiatric disorders. *Journal of Neuropsychiatry and Clinical Neurosciences*, **6**, 358–370.

Mega, M.S., Cummings, J.L., Salloway, S. and Malloy, P., 1997. The limbic system: an anatomic, phylogenetic, and clinical perspective. *Journal of Neuropsychiatry and Clinical Neurosciences*, **9**, 315–330.

Meltzer, C.C., Price, J.C., Mathis, C.A., Greer, P.J., Cantwell, M.N., Houck, P.R., Mulsant, B.H., Ben-Eliezer, D., Lopresti, B., DeKosky, S.T. and Reynolds, C.F., 1999. PET imaging of serotonin type 2A receptors in late-life neuropsychiatric disorders. *American Journal of Psychiatry*, **156**, 1871–1878.

Mervaala, E., Fohr, J., Kononen, M., Valkonen-Korhonen, M., Vainio, P., Partanen, K., Partanen, J., Tiihonen, J., Viinamaki, H., Karjalainen, A.K. and Lehtonen, J., 2000. Quantitative MRI of the hippocampus and amygdala in severe depression. *Psychological Medicine*, **30**, 117–125.

Meyer, J.H., Kennedy, S. and Brown, G.M., 1998. No effect of depression on [(15)O]H2O PET response to intravenous D-fenfluramine. *American Journal of Psychiatry*, **155**, 1241–1246.

Meyer, J.H., Kapur, S., Houle, S., DaSilva, J., Owczarek, B., Brown, G.M., Wilson, A.A. and Kennedy, S.H., 1999. Prefrontal cortex 5-HT2 receptors in depression: an [18F]setoperone PET imaging study. *American Journal of Psychiatry*, **156**, 1029–1034.

Moffoot, A., O'Carroll, R.E., Murray, C., Dougall, N., Ebmeier, K.P. and Goodwin, G.M., 1994a. Clonidine infusion increases uptake of 99mTc-exametazime in anterior cingulate cortex in Korsakoff's psychosis. *Psychological Medicine*, **24**, 53–61.

Moffoot, A.P.R., O'Carroll, R.E., Bennie, J., Carroll, S., Dick, H., Ebmeier, K.P. and Goodwin, G.M., 1994b. Diurnal variation of mood and cognitive function in major depression with melancholia. *Journal of Affective Disorders*, **32**, 257–269.

Moore, G.J., Bebchuk, J.M., Hasanat, K., Chen, G., Seraji-Bozorgzad, N., Wilds, I.B., Faulk, M.W., Koch, S., Glitz, D.A., Jolkovsky, L. and Manji, H.K., 2000. Lithium increases *N*-acetyl-aspartate in the human brain: *in vivo* evidence in support of bcl-2's neurotrophic effects? *Biological Psychiatry*, **48**, 1–8.

Morris, J.S., Smith, K.A., Cowen, P.J., Friston, K.J. and Dolan, R.J., 1999. Covariation of activity in habenula and dorsal raphe nuclei following tryptophan depletion. *Neuroimage*, **10**, 163–172.

Nobler, M.S., Oquendo, M.A., Kegeles, L.S., Malone, K.M., Campbell, C., Sackeim, H.A. and Mann, J.J., 2001. Decreased regional brain metabolism after ECT. *American Journal of Psychiatry*, **158**, 305–308.

Nofzinger, E.A., Nichols, T.E., Meltzer, C.C., Price, J., Steppe, D.A., Miewald, J.M., Kupfer, D.J. and Moore, R.Y., 1999. Changes in forebrain function from waking to REM sleep in depression: preliminary analyses of [18F]FDG PET studies. *Psychiatry Research*, **91**, 59–78.

Nofzinger, E.A., Price, J.C., Meltzer, C.C., Buysse, D.J., Villemagne, V.L., Miewald, J.M., Sembrat, R.C., Steppe, D.A. and Kupfer, D.J., 2000. Towards a neurobiology of dysfunctional arousal in depression: the relationship between beta EEG power and regional cerebral glucose metabolism during NREM sleep. *Psychiatry Research*, **98**, 71–91.

Norris, S.D., Krishnan, K.R.R. and Ahearn, E., 1997. Structural changes in the brain of patients with bipolar affective disorder by MRI: a review of the literature. *Progress in Neuropsychopharmacology and Biological Psychiatry*, **21**, 1323–1337.

Northoff, G., Richter, A., Gessner, M., Schlagenhauf, F., Fell, J., Baumgart, F., Kaulisch, T., Kotter, R., Stephan, K.E., Leschinger, A., Hagner, T., Bargel, B., Witzel, T., Hinrichs, H., Bogerts, B., Scheich, H. and Heinze, H.J., 2000. Functional dissociation between medial and lateral prefrontal cortical spatiotemporal activation in negative and positive emotions: a combined fMRI/MEG study. *Cerebral Cortex*, **10**, 93–107.

O'Brien, J.T., Ames, D., Schweitzer, I., Desmond, P., Coleman, P. and Tress, B., 1997a. Clinical, magnetic resonance imaging and endocrinological differences between delusional and non-delusional depression in the elderly. *International Journal of Geriatric Psychiatry*, **12**, 211–218.

O'Brien, J.T., Desmond, P., Ames, D., Schweitzer, I., Chiu, E. and Tress, B., 1997b. Temporal lobe magnetic resonance imaging can differentiate Alzheimer's disease from normal ageing, depression, vascular dementia and other causes of cognitive impairment. *Psychological Medicine*, **27**, 1267–1275.

Ogura, A., Morinobu, S., Kawakatsu, S., Totsuka, S. and Komatani, A., 1998. Changes in regional brain activity in major depression after successful treatment with antidepressant drugs. *Acta Psychiatrica Scandinavica*, **98**, 54–59.

Ongur, D., Drevets, W.C. and Price, J.L., 1998. Glial reduction in the subgenual prefrontal cortex in mood disorders. *Proceedings of the National Academy of Sciences of the United States of America*, **95**, 13290–13295.

Paillere-Martinot, M.-L., Bragulat, V., Artiges, E., Dolle, F., Hinnen, F., Jouvent, R. and Martinot, J.-L., 2001. Decreased presynaptic dopamine function in the left caudate of depressed patients with affective flattening and psychomotor retardation. *American Journal of Psychiatry*, **158**, 314–316.

Papez, J.W., 1937. A proposed mechanism of emotion. *Archives of Neurology and Psychiatry*, **38**, 725–743.

Paradiso, S., Johnson, D.L., Andreasen, N.C., O'Leary, D.S., Watkins, G.L., Ponto, L.L.B. and Hichwa, R.D., 1999. Cerebral blood flow changes associated with attribution of emotional valence to pleasant, unpleasant, and neutral visual stimuli in a PET study of normal subjects. *American Journal of Psychiatry*, **156**, 1618–1629.

Pardo, J.V., Pardo, P.J., Janer, K.W. and Raichle, M.E., 1990. The anterior cingulate cortex mediates processing selection in the Stroop attentional conflict paradigm. *Proceedings of the National Academy of Sciences of the United States of America*, **87**, 256–259.

Peyron, R., Laurent, B. and Garcia-Larrea, L., 2000. Functional imaging of brain responses to pain. A review and meta-analysis. *Neurophysiology Clinics*, **30**, 263–288.

Pizzagalli, D., Pascual-Marqui, R.D., Nitschke, J.B., Oakes, T.R., Larson, C.L., Abercrombie, H.C., Schaefer, S.M., Koger, J.V., Benca, R.M. and Davidson, R.J., 2001. Anterior cingulate activity as a predictor of degree of treatment response in major depression: evidence from brain electrical tomography analysis. *American Journal of Psychiatry*, **158**, 405–415.

Post, R.M., Speer, A.M., Weiss, S.R.B. and Li, H., 2000. Seizure models: anticonvulsant effects of ECT and rTMS. *Progress in Neuropsychopharmacology and Biological Psychiatry*, **24**, 1251–1273.

Price, J.L., 1999a. Networks within the orbital and medial prefrontal cortex. *Neurocase*, **5**, 231–241.

Price, J.L., 1999b. Prefrontal cortical networks related to visceral function and mood. *Annals of the New York Academy of Science*, **877**, 383–396.

Price, J.L., Carmichael, S.T. and Drevets, W.C., 1996. Networks related to the orbital and medial prefrontal cortex: a substrate for emotional behavior? *Progress in Brain Research*, **107**, 523–536.

Rajkowska, G., Miguel-Hidalgo, J.J., Wei, J.R., Dilley, G., Pittman, S.D., Meltzer, H.Y., Overholser, J.C., Roth, B.L. and Stockmeier, C.A., 1999. Morphometric evidence for neuronal and glial prefrontal cell pathology in major depression. *Biological Psychiatry*, **45**, 1085–1098.

Roberts, A.C. and Wallis, J.D., 2000. Inhibitory control and affective processing in the prefrontal cortex: neuropsychological studies in the common marmoset. *Cerebral Cortex*, **10**, 252–262.

Rogers, M.A., Bradshaw, J.L., Pantelis, C. and Phillips, J.G., 1998. Frontostriatal deficits in unipolar major depression. *Brain Research Bulletin*, **47**, 297–310.

Rueter, L.E., de Montigny, C. and Blier, P., 1998. Electrophysiological characterization of the effect of long-term duloxetine administration on the rat serotonergic and noradrenergic systems. *Journal of Pharmacology and Experimental Therapeutics*, **285**, 404–412.

Sapolsky, R.M., Krey, L.C. and McEwen, B., 1986. The neuroendocrinology of stress and ageing: the glucocorticoid cascade hypothesis. *Endocrine Reviews*, **7**, 284–301.

Sato, R., Bryan, R.N. and Fried, L.P., 1999. Neuroanatomic and functional correlates of depressed mood: the Cardiovascular Health Study. *American Journal of Epidemiology*, **150**, 919–929.

Schneider, F., Gur, R.E., Mozley, L.H., Smith, R.J., Mozley, P.D., Censits, D.M., Alavi, A. and Gur, R.C., 1995. Mood effects on limbic blood flow correlate with emotional self-rating: a PET study with oxygen-15 labeled water. *Psychiatry Research—Neuroimaging*, **61**, 265–283.

Schneider, F., Grodd, W. and Machulla, H.J., 1996. Behavioral neuroimaging with positron emission tomography and magnetic resonance imaging. *Nervenarzt*, **67**, 721–729.

Schneider, F., Grodd, W., Weiss, U., Klose, U., Mayer, K.R., Nagele, T. and Gur, R.C., 1997. Functional MRI reveals left amygdala activation during emotion. *Psychiatry Research—Neuroimaging*, **76**, 75–82.

Schnitzler, A. and Ploner, M., 2000. Neurophysiology and functional neuroanatomy of pain perception. *Journal of Clinical Neurophysiology*, **17**, 592–603.

Selemon, L.D., Lidow, M.S. and Goldman-Rakic, P.S., 1999. Increased volume and glial density in primate prefrontal cortex associated with chronic antipsychotic drug exposure. *Biological Psychiatry*, **46**, 161–172.

Selye, H., 1936. A syndrome produced by diverse nocuous agents. *Nature*, **138**, 32.

Serretti, A., Benedetti, F., Colombo, C., Lilli, R., Lorenzi, C. and Smeraldi, E., 1999. Dopamine receptor D4 is not associated with antidepressant activity of sleep deprivation. *Psychiatry Research*, **89**, 107–114.

Shah, P. and Ebmeier, K.P., 1998. Structural and functional brain markers of age of onset and chronicity in major depressive disorder. In: Ebert, D. and Ebmeier, K.P. (eds), *New Models for Depression*, Vol. 19, pp. 136–152. Karger, Basel.

Shah, P.J., Ogilvie, A., Goodwin, G.M. and Ebmeier, K.P., 1997. Clinical and psychometric correlates of dopamine D2 binding in depression. *Psychological Medicine*, **27**, 1247–1256.

Shah, P.J., Ebmeier, K.P., Glabus, M.F. and Goodwin, G.M., 1998. Cortical grey matter reductions associated with treatment resistant chronic unipolar depression: a controlled MRI study. *British Journal of Psychiatry*, **172**, 527–532.

Sheline, Y.I., Gado, M.H. and Price, J.L., 1998. Amygdala core nuclei volumes are decreased in recurrent major depression. *Neuroreport*, **9**, 2023–2028.

Sheline, Y.I., Sanghavi, M., Mintun, M.A. and Gado, M.H., 1999. Depression duration but not age predicts hippocampal volume loss in medically healthy women with recurrent major depression. *Journal of Neuroscience*, **19**, 5034–5043.

Shumake, J., Poremba, A., Edwards, E. and Gonzalez-Lima, F., 2000. Congenital helpless rats as a genetic model for cortex metabolism in depression. *Neuroreport*, **11**, 3793–3798.

Simpson, S., Baldwin, R.C., Jackson, A. and Burns, A.S., 1998. Is subcortical disease associated with a poor response to antidepressants? Neurological, neuropsychological and neuroradiological findings in late-life depression. *Psychological Medicine*, **28**, 1015–1026.

Simpson, J.R., Drevets, W.C., Snyder, A.Z., Gusnard, D.A. and Raichle, M.E., 2001a. Emotion-induced changes in human medial prefrontal cortex: II. During anticipatory anxiety. *Proceedings of the National Academy of Sciences of the United States of America*, **98**, 688–693.

Simpson, J.R., Snyder, A.Z., Gusnard, D.A. and Raichle, M.E., 2001b. Emotion-induced changes in human medial prefrontal cortex: I. During cognitive task performance. *Proceedings of the National Academy of Sciences of the United States of America*, **98**, 683–687.

Sloane, J.A., Hollander, W., Rosene, D.L., Moss, M.B., Kemper, T. and Abraham, C.R., 2000. Astrocytic hypertrophy and altered GFAP degradation with age in subcortical white matter of the rhesus monkey. *Brain Research*, **862**, 1–10.

Smith, G.S., Reynolds, C.F., Pollock, B., Derbyshire, S., Nofzinger, E., Dew, M.A., Houck, P.R., Milko, D., Meltzer, C.C. and Kupfer, D.J., 1999a. Cerebral glucose metabolic response to combined total sleep deprivation and antidepressant treatment in geriatric depression. *American Journal of Psychiatry*, **156**, 683–689.

Smith, K.A., Morris, J.S., Friston, K.J., Cowen, P.J. and Dolan, R.J., 1999b. Brain mechanisms associated with depressive relapse and associated cognitive impairment following acute tryptophan depletion. *British Journal of Psychiatry*, **174**, 525–529.

Soares, J.C. and Mann, J.J., 1997. The anatomy of mood disorders — review of structural neuroimaging studies. *Biological Psychiatry*, **41**, 86–106.

Speer, A.M., Kimbrell, T.A., Wassermann, E.M., D'Repella, J., Willis, M.W., Herscovitch, P. and Post, R.M., 2000. Opposite effects of high and low frequency rTMS on regional brain activity in depressed patients. *Biological Psychiatry*, **48**, 1133–1141.

Steffens, D.C., Tupler, L.A., Ranga, K. and Krishnan, R., 1998. Magnetic resonance imaging signal hypointensity and iron content of putamen nuclei in elderly depressed patients. *Psychiatry Research*, **83**, 95–103.

Steffens, D.C., Helms, M.J., Krishnan, K.R. and Burke, G.L., 1999. Cerebrovascular disease and depression symptoms in the cardiovascular health study. *Stroke*, **30**, 2159–2166.

Steingard, R.J., 2000. The neuroscience of depression in adolescence. *Journal of Affective Disorders*, **61**, 15–21.

Stevens, A. and Price, J., 2000. Disorders of attachment and rank. In: *Evolutionary Psychiatry*, 2nd edn, Routledge, London.

Stoll, A.L., Renshaw, P.F., Yurgelun-Todd, D.A. and Cohen, B.M., 2000. Neuroimaging in bipolar disorder: what have we learned? *Biological Psychiatry*, **48**, 505–517.

Strakowski, S.M., DelBello, M.P., Sax, K.W., Zimmerman, M.E., Shear, P.K., Hawkins, J.M. and Larson, E.R., 1999. Brain magnetic resonance imaging of structural abnormalities in bipolar disorder. *Archives of General Psychiatry*, **56**, 254–260.

Swerdlow, N.R. and Koob, G.F., 1987. Dopamine, schizophrenia, mania, and depression: toward a unified hypotheses of cortico-striato-pallido-thalamic function. *Behavioural and Brain Sciences*, **10**, 197–245.

Teasdale, J.D., Howard, R.J., Cox, S.G., Ha, Y., Brammer, M.J., Williams, S.C.R. and Checkley, S.A., 1999. Functional MRI study of the cognitive generation of affect. *American Journal of Psychiatry*, **156**, 209–215.

Tebartz van Elst, L., Woermann, F.G., Lemieux, L. and Trimble, M.R., 1999. Amygdala enlargement in dysthymia — a volumetric study of patients with temporal lobe epilepsy. *Biological Psychiatry*, **46**, 1614–1623.

Tebartz van Elst, L., Woermann, F., Lemieux, L. and Trimble, M.R., 2000. Increased amygdala volumes in female and depressed humans. A quantitative magnetic resonance imaging study. *Neuroscience Letters*, **281**, 103–106.

Thomas, A.J., Ferrier, I.N., Kalaria, R.N., Perry, R.H., Brown, A. and O'Brien, J.T.O., 2001. A neuropathological study of vascular factors in late-life depression. *Journal of Neurology, Neurosurgery and Psychiatry*, **70**, 83–87.

Vakili, K., Pillay, S.S., Lafer, B., Fava, M., Renshaw, P.F., Bonello-Cintron, C.M. and Yurgelun-Todd, D.A., 2000. Hippocampal volume in primary unipolar major depression: a magnetic resonance imaging study. *Biological Psychiatry*, **47**, 1087–1090.

Vasile, R.G., Sachs, G., Anderson, J.L., Lafer, B., Matthews, E. and Hill, T., 1997. Changes in regional cerebral blood flow following light treatment for seasonal affective disorder: responders versus non-responders. *Biological Psychiatry*, **42**, 1000–1005.

Videbech, P., 1997. MRI findings in patients with affective disorder: a meta-analysis. *Acta Psychiatrica Scandinavica*, **96**, 157–168.

Videbech, P., 2000. PET measurements of brain glucose metabolism and blood flow in major depressive disorder: a critical review. *Acta Psychiatrica Scandinavica*, **101**, 11–20.

Volk, S.A., Kaendler, S.H., Hertel, A., Maul, F.D., Manoocheri, R., Weber, R., Georgi, K., Pflug, B. and Hor, G., 1997. Can response to partial sleep deprivation in depressed patients be predicted by regional changes of cerebral blood flow? *Psychiatry Research—Neuroimaging*, **75**, 67–74.

Welberg, L.A., Seckl, J.R. and Holmes, M.C., 2001. Prenatal glucocorticoid programming of brain corticosteroid receptors and corticotrophin-releasing hormone: possible implications for behaviour. *Neuroscience*, **104**, 71–79.

Whalen, P.J., Bush, G., McNally, R.J., Wilhelm, S., McInerney, S.C., Jenike, M.A. and Rauch, S.L., 1998. The emotional counting Stroop paradigm: a functional magnetic resonance imaging probe of the anterior cingulate affective division. *Biological Psychiatry*, **44**, 1219–1228.

Willeit, M., Praschak-Rieder, N., Neumeister, A., Pirker, W., Asenbaum, S., Vitouch, O., Tauscher, J., Hilger, E., Stastny, J., Brucke, T. and Kasper, S., 2000. [123I]-beta-CIT SPECT imaging shows reduced brain serotonin transporter availability in drug-free depressed patients with seasonal affective disorder. *Biological Psychiatry*, **47**, 482–489.

Wu, J., Buchsbaum, M.S., Gillin, J.C., Tang, C., Cadwell, S., Wiegand, M., Najafi, A., Klein, E., Hazen, K. and Bunney, W.E., 1999. Prediction of antidepressant effects of sleep deprivation by metabolic rates in the ventral anterior cingulate and medial prefrontal cortex. *American Journal of Psychiatry*, **156**, 1149–1158.

Yatham, L.N., Liddle, P.F., Dennie, J., Shiah, I.S., Adam, M.J., Lane, C.J., Lam, R.W. and Ruth, T.J., 1999. Decrease in brain serotonin 2 receptor binding in patients with major depression following desipramine treatment: a positron emission tomography study with fluorine-18-labeled setoperone. *Archives of General Psychiatry*, **56**, 705–711.

Yatham, L.N., Clark, C.C. and Zis, A.P., 2000. A preliminary study of the effects of electroconvulsive therapy on regional brain glucose metabolism in patients with major depression. *Journal of ECT*, **16**, 171–176.

Zheng, X.M., 2000. Regional cerebral blood flow changes in drug-resistant depressed patients following treatment with transcranial magnetic stimulation: a statistical parametric mapping analysis. *Psychiatry Research—Neuroimaging*, **100**, 75–80.

Zis, A.P. and Goodwin, F.K., 1982. The amine hypothesis. In: Paykel, E.S. (ed.), *Handbook of Affective Disorders*, pp. 175–190. Guildford Press, New York.

XVIII-10

Molecular Genetics in Mood Disorders

D. Souery, S. Linotte and J. Mendlewicz

INTRODUCTION

Despite intensive search for biological underpinnings, the aetiology of major mood disorders remains unknown. More work on the neurobiology of these disorders is clearly indicated. Twin and family studies have consistently demonstrated a genetic component to the disorders. Decades of research into the genetic aetiology of mood disorders provide evidence in favour of a complex mode of inheritance unlikely to be determined by single gene dysfunction, and apparently non-Mendelian patterns of inheritance. Part of the complexity of the genetic variance lies in the heterogeneity of the disorders — the depressive patient, for example, can be characterized by a variety of different symptoms and identifying features that may represent different subtypes. Different genetic mechanisms may be involved: epistasis, locus heterogeneity, allelic heterogeneity, dynamic mutations, imprinting and mitochondrial gene mutation (these issues are reviewed in Chapter XII). In terms of phenotype, there are also a variety of non-genetic factors that lessen our ability to detect genes in mental disorders: phenocopies, clinical heterogeneity, assessment bias, population stratification and lack of appropriate control groups.

Of the genetic mechanisms listed above, it is possible that more than one may be involved in the transmission of psychiatric disorders. In complex disorders the correspondence between gene and phenotype is not necessarily direct: a given genotype may give rise to a variety of phenotypes according to other genes present and environmental factors, or different genotypes may give rise to the same phenotype. Despite these complex characteristics, family- and population-based studies have provided substantial evidence that genetic factors contribute to the expression of the disorders. Recent molecular genetic approaches indicate that several chromosomal regions may be involved in the aetiology of mood disorders.

The initial molecular genetic studies of Bipolar disorder (BPAD), considered as the core phenotype of mood disorders, involved the parametric linkage studies of large families. Linkage examines the cosegregation of a genetic marker and disease in affected individuals within families; that is, the non-random sharing of marker alleles between affected members of each family (Smeraldi and Macciardi, 1995). Two genetic loci are linked if they are located closely together on a chromosome. In linkage analysis, the frequency of meiotic recombinations as an expression of the distance between marker locus and the gene under investigation is used for gene mapping (see Chapter XII). Given the difficulties inherent in detecting genes of small to modest effect using the linkage approach, the candidate gene association method offers an alternative strategy of studying genetic factors involved in complex diseases in which the mode of transmission is not known. Association between diseases and marker may be found if the gene itself, or a locus in linkage disequilibrium with the marker, is involved in the pathophysiology of the disease (Hodge, 1994). Thus, an association may imply a direct effect of the gene tested, or the effect of another gene close to the marker examined. The candidate gene approach is a useful method to investigate association between markers and disease. A candidate gene refers to a region of the chromosome which is potentially implicated in the aetiology of the disorder concerned. The possibility of false-positive results must be taken into account, as a very large number of candidate genes now exist. The probability that each of these genes is involved in the aetiology of the disorder is relatively low.

The candidate gene approach can be extended to phenotypes not directly linked to the diagnoses of mood disorders. The therapeutic effect of psychotropic drugs may be considered to investigate genetic polymorphisms (psychopharmacogenetics). In recent years, research in psychopharmacogenetics has focused on evaluating functional polymorphisms both in genes coding for drug-metabolizing enzymes and in genes coding for other enzymes or receptors involved in the mechanism of action of psychoactive drugs. In this context, the use of new technologies is rapidly evolving. Gene expression patterns in response to drug treatments can be investigated by new techniques such as DNA microarrays. Microarrays are powerful tools for investigating the mechanism of drug action by measuring changes in mRNA levels in brain tissues before and after exposure to treatment (Debouck and Goodfellow, 1999).

This chapter reviews the current methodologies and study tools used to search for molecular genetic factors in mood disorders and the chromosomal regions of interest already investigated for bipolar (BPAD) and unipolar (UPAD) mood disorders.

CANDIDATE CHROMOSOMAL REGIONS AND CANDIDATE GENES

Chromosome X

A systematic review of the literature on linkage studies in BPAD (Turecki *et al.*, 1996) indicated that the proportion of positive DNA findings is higher for X markers compared to other chromosomal regions. Mendlewicz *et al.* (1987) first reported possible genetic linkage between BPAD and coagulation Factor IX (F9) located at Xq27 in 11 pedigrees. The same genetic marker was also tested in a French pedigree where linkage was confirmed (Lucotte *et al.*, 1992). Linkage with DNA markers on the X chromosome has been excluded, however, in other pedigrees (Berrettini *et al.*, 1990; Bredbacka *et al.*, 1993; Gejman *et al.*, 1990). A study published in 1987 by Baron *et al.* (1987) demonstrated positive linkage for glucose 6 phosphate dehydrogenase (G6PD), but later results from the same author did not support this finding (Baron *et al.*, 1993), although G6PD was slightly positive for linkage in one family. In a more recent study (De Bruyn *et al.*, 1994), several DNA markers in the Xq27–28 region were tested in nine bipolar families.

Biological Psychiatry: Edited by H. D'haenen, J.A. den Boer and P. Willner. ISBN 0-471-49198-5

Results suggestive of linkage were found in four bipolar I (BPI) families with the markers F9, F8 and DXS52. Pekkarinen *et al.* (1995) evaluated 27 polymorphic markers on the X chromosome (Xq25–28 region) in one large Finnish family, and found the highest lod scores when using a narrower phenotype definition (BPI and BPII only). Linkage was found between a marker located on Xq26 (AFM205wd2) and BPAD. This marker is located about 7 cM centromeric to the F9 locus. The initial genome screen for BPAD in the NIMH genetics initiative of 97 pedigrees also revealed positive though small lod scores on the X chromosome (Xp22 and Xq26–28) (Stine *et al.*, 1997). All these results are extremely suggestive of X linkage and in particular, the Xq26–28 region should be considered a strong candidate for genetic studies in BPAD.

The associations between BPAD and polymorphic DNA markers in the pseudoautosomal region of the X chromosome have also been investigated. Yoneda *et al.* (1992) reported an association between the A4 allele of the marker DXYS20 in this chromosomal region in Japanese BPAD patients. This has not been replicated in European populations, however (Nöthen *et al.*, 1993; Parsian and Todd, 1994).

The MAOA and MAOB genes which code for the enzymes that degrade biogenic amines, including neurotransmitters implicated in the pathophysiology of mood disorders, such as norepinephrine, dopamine and serotonin, are both located on the X chromosome and tightly linked to each other (Xp11.12–Xp11.4). Lim *et al.* (1994a, 1995) reported a weak but significant association for three different polymorphisms of MAOA, yet not for MAOB, in a sample of 57 BPAD patients compared to population controls not assessed for psychiatric status. A weak association was found for MAOA and bipolar disorder by Kawada *et al.* (1995), but different alleles were more frequent in the patient population compared to the previous report. A series of negative reports followed, leaving the question open as to the usefulness of the MAO genes in psychiatric genetics research (Craddock *et al.*, 1995a; Muramatsu *et al.*, 1997; Nöthen *et al.*, 1995).

Chromosome 18

Berrettini *et al.* (1994) first reported linkage of BPAD to chromosome 18 DNA markers in a systematic genome survey of 22 families including 156 subjects with bipolar disorder. Although the overall lod score for the pedigree series was negative, results of two-point linkage analysis in individual families indicated possible linkage with some marker loci in the 18p11 region. Non-parametric analysis (affected pedigree member and affected sib-pair analysis) of this sample confirmed the observation of linkage (Gershon *et al.*, 1996). These results suggested the existence of a susceptibility gene in the pericentromic region that can not be fully evaluated by classic linkage analysis. These results may be of interest because genes coding for the alpha unit of a GTP binding protein involved in neurotransmission, a corticotrophin receptor gene, and RED-1 containing triplet repeats have been mapped to this region. Stine *et al.* (1996) studied 28 nuclear families for markers on chromosome 18 and also found evidence for linkage and allele sharing between sib-pairs at 18p11.22–p11.21. This study replicated the findings of Berrettini and colleagues, yet also demonstrated evidence for linkage and parent-of-origin effect in a region located on the long arm of chromosome 18, a sex-averaged distance 30 cM away. An excess of paternally but not maternally transmitted alleles from the D18S41 was observed.

In a study of five rigorously defined, high-density German families, no robust evidence for linkage for the pericentromeric region could be found, although one family showed slightly elevated lod scores under a recessive mode of inheritance for D18S40 (Maier *et al.*, 1995). Linkage to the pericentromeric region of chromosome 18 was excluded in three large Old Order Amish families (Pauls *et al.*, 1995), and in two large Belgian pedigrees (De Bruyn *et al.*, 1996). In the Belgian pedigrees, while negative lod scores were found for a marker located in the pericentromeric region, linkage and segregation analysis in one family suggested that the 18q region of the chromosome (18q21.33–q23) might contain a susceptibility locus for BPAD (De Bruyn *et al.*, 1996). Freimer *et al.* (1996), using both linkage and association strategies, reported evidence of linkage with markers in this region (18q22) in a Costa Rican pedigree with a common founder. A subsequent study further supported the interest of the 18q23 region, showing linkage among six pedigrees (Coon *et al.*, 1996). An additional study of 173 affected subjects using the multilocus affected pedigree member method demonstrated a susceptibility gene in the pericentromeric region, and multilocus analysis by the affected sib-pair method also showed evidence for linkage (Berrettini *et al.*, 1997). Yet despite slight allele sharing with two markers on chromosome 18 (D18S40 on 18p and D18S70 on 18q) in the NIMH genetics initiative BPAD pedigrees, linkage to chromosome 18 was not confirmed in this large genome scan (Detera-Wadleigh *et al.*, 1997). Furthermore, Knowles *et al.* (1998) found no evidence for significant linkage between bipolar disorder and chromosome 18 pericentromeric markers in another large sample (1013 genotyped individuals) using ten highly polymorphic markers.

Chromosome 5

Preliminary linkage data including three DNA markers on this chromosome (D5S39, D5S43 and D5S62) suggested linkage with BPAD (Coon *et al.*, 1993). Two of these markers, D5S62 and D5S43, are located on the distal region of the long arm of chromosome 5 (5q35-qter). This region contains candidate genes for mood disorders such as the alpha-1 protein subunit of the GABA A receptor (GABRA1) and the 5-HT1A receptor (5-HTR1A). These two markers, however, had exclusion lod scores in a previous study of 14 families (Detera-Wadleigh *et al.*, 1992). Similarly, strongly negative lod scores were found in a linkage study covering the 5-HTR1A locus in five pedigrees (Curtis *et al.*, 1993). The dopamine transporter gene (DAT1) is located in a different region of chromosome 5 (5p15.3). This marker has been investigated in association studies with BPAD yet no association has been found (Gomez-Casero *et al.*, 1996; Manki *et al.*, 1996; Souery *et al.*, 1996a). Kelsoe *et al.* (1996) reported possible linkage, however, between a locus near the dopamine transporter (DAT) and BPAD, under a dominant transmission model giving a modest lod score of 2.38. Replication of this finding was shown in another linkage analysis subsequently (Waldman *et al.*, 1997).

Chromosome 11

Chromosome 11 has been thoroughly investigated in mood disorders because of the presence of candidate genes involved in catecholamine neurotransmission such as tyrosine hydroxylase (TH, 11p15), tyrosinase (11q14-21), dopamine receptor D2 (DRD2, 11q22-23), dopamine receptor D4 (DRD4, 11p15.5) and tryptophan hydroxylase (TPH, 11p15). Overall, results of linkage studies indicate that the TH gene does not contribute a major gene effect to BPAD (Souery *et al.*, 1996b). A possible role for the TH gene was also examined in BPAD association studies, all on moderate to small sample sizes. Meta-analysis of the results (Furlong *et al.*, 1999) does not support the TH gene having a major role in the aetiology of BPAD, while data suggest that this candidate gene should be examined in larger samples of UPAD for which this marker may confer susceptibility to the disease.

Linkage to the dopamine 2 receptor (DRD2) has been excluded in a number of studies (Byerley *et al.*, 1990; Ewald *et al.*, 1994;

Holmes *et al.*, 1991; Kelsoe *et al.*, 1993; Nanko *et al.*, 1994). Most association studies have similarly showed no association between the gene for this receptor and BP (Craddock *et al.*, 1995b; Manki *et al.*, 1996; Souery *et al.*, 1996a).

Linkage to the DRD4 receptor gene has not been definitively excluded (Nanko *et al.*, 1994; Sidenberg *et al.*, 1994), and a few association studies have found positive results. For unipolar patients alone, an excess of short exon III repeats (2–4 repeats) has been found to be significantly more frequent than in controls (Manki *et al.*, 1996). The 7 repeat allele was associated with bipolar disorder, and an excess of allele 3 among controls in another study, yet negative results were then found in a larger sample by the same group (Lim *et al.*, 1994b). Serretti *et al.* (1998) recently reported an excess of allele 7 among mood disorder patients with delusional features, suggesting its importance in psychoses, not necessarily mood disorders.

Serotonin Markers and Mood Disorders

Dysfunction of the serotonergic system has long been suspected in major depression and related disorders. Depression can be treated successfully with selective drugs which target serotonin receptors. The serotonin transporter may also be involved in susceptibility to mood disorders and in the response to treatment with these drugs. Allelic association has been suggested between the serotonin transporter gene (located on chromosome 17q11.1–12) and UPAD (Ogilvie *et al.*, 1996). The presence of one allele of this gene was significantly associated with a risk of UPAD. This study also included a group of BPAD patients although no associations were found with this marker in this patient group compared to normal controls. This preliminary finding may add to our understanding of the possibility of polygenic inheritance in mood disorders. These findings were replicated in two different samples, again showing an association between this marker and UPAD (major depression with melancholia) (Gutierrez *et al.*, 1998a) and no association with a group of BPAD patients (Gutierrez *et al.*, 1998b). A higher frequency of the 12-repeat allele of the variable number tandem repeat (VNTR) polymorphism has been associated with mood disorders in a number of studies (Battersby *et al.*, 1996; Collier *et al.*, 1996; Rees *et al.*, 1997), with results being the most significant for bipolar subjects. The 9 repeat allele has been shown to be significantly associated with unipolar depression, on the other hand (Battersby *et al.*, 1996; Ogilvie *et al.*, 1996).

A linkage study with the functional variant of the serotonin transporter gene in families with BPAD could not exclude linkage (Ewald *et al.*, 1998b). More interestingly, a polymorphism within the promoter region of the serotonin transporter gene has been associated with treatment response to fluvoxamine, a typical serotonin reuptake inhibitor (SSRI) in major depression with psychotic features (Smeraldi *et al.*, 1998). This promising preliminary finding requires to be confirmed. The tryptophan hydroxylase (TPH) gene, which codes for the rate-limiting enzyme of serotonin metabolism, is also an important candidate gene for mood disorders and suicidal behaviour. Bellivier *et al.*, (1998b) reported a significant association between genotypes at this marker and BPAD; no association was found with suicidal behaviour. In a previous study in depressed patients suicidal behaviour has been associated with one variant of this gene (Mann *et al.*, 1997).

Chromosome 4

Possible candidate genes on chromosome 4 include the dopamine receptor D5 (DRD5) and the alpha adrenergic 2C receptor (ADRA2C) genes. Using both linkage and sib-pair methods to evaluate six families, positive results have been found for the loci for DRD5 and ADRA2C (Byerley *et al.*, 1994), although this was not fully replicated in a later study with a larger sample size (Blackwood *et al.*, 1996). Linkage was found between a locus on chromosome 4p (D4S394, 4p16) and BPAD in the latter study, yielding a robust two-point lod score of 4.1 under a model that allowed for heterogeneity. Although the region of 4p16 contains the genes for both DRD5 and ADRA2C, specific markers for these genes were not significant for linkage in this study. Although linkage was not found in the NIMH initiative for any region on chromosome 4, modest elevation of allele frequencies was found for markers on both arms of the chromosome, D4S2397 and D4S391 on 4p and DS1647 4q (Detera-Waldeigh *et al.*, 1997).

Other possible candidate genes mapped to chromosome 4 include those coding for protein subunits of the heteromeric GABA A receptor: the alpha 2 protein subunit (GABRA2) and the beta 1 subunit (GABRB1), located at 4p13–12. This region was excluded for linkage in a large family in the Blackwood *et al.* (1996) study, but perhaps could be examined more fully.

Chromosome 21

Straub *et al.* (1994) detected linkage with the locus for liver-type phosphofructokinase enzyme (PFLK) on chromosome 21 (21q22.3) in one large, multigenerational bipolar family. Initial results from 47 families assessed in this genome survey did not support linkage with this marker, however. Follow-up linkage analysis of an extended sample of 57 families on the 373 most informative individuals, using markers less than 2 cM apart, found evidence of linkage (lod score 3.35) at marker D21S1260, which is 5 cM proximal to PFKL (Aita *et al.*, 1998). Linkage between bipolar disorder and the PFLK region has also been confirmed in other studies (Ewald *et al.*, 1996, Smyth *et al.*, 1997), although negative results have also been reported (Byerley *et al.*, 1995; Vallada *et al.*, 1996). Further confirmation of linkage to this region with a large sample size, and a later report of excess allele sharing of a cluster of markers within a 9 cM interval on 21q (D21S1254, D21S65, D21S1440 and D21S1254), were found in the NIMH Genetics Initiative bipolar pedigrees (Detera-Waldeigh *et al.*, 1996, 1997). Linkage to a larger region proximal to the gene for PFKL, 21q21–22, has also been reported by a number of groups (Kwok *et al.*, 1999, LaBuda *et al.*, 1996). Taken together, these results indicate that the region of interest on 21q remains large, although no discrete locus or obvious candidate gene has been identified as of yet.

Chromosome 12

Darier's disease (keratosis follicularis), a rare autosomal dominant skin disorder associated with increased prevalence of epilepsy and mental retardation, whose gene has been mapped to chromosome 12q23–24.1 was found to cosegregate with bipolar disorder in one pedigree (Craddock *et al.*, 1994). The Darier's disease region has been investigated in several family studies in BPAD, suggesting a possible linkage (Barden *et al.*, 1996; Craddock *et al.*, 1994; Dawson *et al.*, 1995; Ewald *et al.*, 1998a). Two of these studies have been able to report significant lod scores greater than 3 (Barden *et al.*, 1996; Ewald *et al.*, 1998). To further test the hypothesis that genes containing expanded trinucleotide repeats may contribute to the genetic aetiology of BPAD, loci within this region containing CAG/CTG repeat expansions have also been investigated, but no association was found with BPAD (Franks *et al.*, 1999).

ANTICIPATION AND EXPANDED TRINUCLEOTIDE REPEAT SEQUENCES

Anticipation implies that a disease occurs at a progressively earlier age of onset and with increased severity in successive generations.

This may explain deviations from Mendelian inheritance observed in some inherited diseases. This phenomenon has been observed in several neurological diseases, including myotonic dystrophy, fragile X syndrome, Huntington's disease and spinobulbar muscle atrophy (Paulson and Fischbeck, 1996; Trottier *et al.*, 1995). Anticipation has been found to correlate with a new class of mutations, expanded trinucleotide repeat sequences. An expanded repeat sequence is unstable and may increase in size across generations, leading to an increased disease severity of the disorder. CAG repeats are detected by the repeat expansion detection (RED) method. Such unstable mutations could also be an alternative explanation in addition to environmental factors for discordance between monozygotic twins for mood disorders, where the repeat amplification might be different during mitosis in each of the two twins. A shortcoming of anticipation studies involves ascertainment bias. Earlier age of onset and/or increased severity in successive generations may be related to increased sensitivity to diagnosis in offspring of affected parents. It may appear that parents have a later age of onset compared to children, but perhaps parents with an earlier age of onset were not able to reproduce at all. Social and environmental factors in the younger generation may favour earlier detection, and expression of the disease is not necessarily related to observed repeats. Cohort effects can be controlled for in statistical analyses, however, such as examining age at onset in an entire generation compared to the difference observed between probands and parents.

Most unstable nucleotide repeat diseases showing anticipation also demonstrate imprinting, or parent-of-origin effect. Mood disorders have not yet unequivocally shown such an effect, although this does not necessarily exclude the possibility that anticipation occurs.

Evidence for anticipation has been observed in BPAD (Grigoroiu-Serbanescu *et al.*, 1997; McInnis *et al.*, 1993; Nylander *et al.*, 1994; Ohara *et al.*, 1998) and in UPAD (Engström *et al.*, 1995). Correlation between anticipation observed at the phenotypic level with the number of dynamic mutations may be the only way to confirm the implication of this phenomenon in mood disorders. One study highlighted an association between the number of CAG trinucleotide repeats and severity of BPAD illness in Swedish and Belgian patients (Lindblad *et al.*, 1995). This study, replicated subsequently in a different sample (O'Donovan *et al.*, 1995; Oruc *et al.*, 1997), showed for the first time in a major psychiatric disorder that the length of CAG repeats were significantly higher in BPAD compared to normal controls. These molecular genetic findings may indicate a genetic basis for anticipation in BPAD. However, no correlation has been found between CAG/CTG repeats and phenotypic measures of severity in a sample of 133 unrelated BPAD patients (Craddock *et al.*, 1997) and in several independent studies (Guy *et al.*, 1999; Li *et al.*, 1998; Vincent *et al.*, 1996; Zander *et al.*, 1998). This hypothesis has recently been tested in a sample of two-generation pairs with BPAD. Globally, no significant differences were found in the mean number of CAG repeats between parent and offspring generations. A significant increase in CAG repeats between parents and offspring was observed, however, when the phenotype increased in severity, i.e. changed from major depression, single episode or unipolar recurrent depression to BPAD (Mendlewicz *et al.*, 1997). A significant increase in CAG repeat length between generations was also found in female offspring with maternal inheritance, but not in male offspring. This is the first evidence of genetic anticipation in BPAD families and should be followed by the identification of loci within the genome containing triplet repeats. CTG18.1 on chromosome 18q21.1 and ERDA1 on chromosome 17q21.3 are two repeat loci recently identified (Lindblad *et al.*, 1998) which can be investigated in such study. In this study, several hundreds of candidate loci containing repeats were screened in a set of BPAD patients but expanded alleles at ERDA1 and CTG18.1 loci were found to be associated with BPAD phenotype. The authors observed that in a Swedish sample, including both unrelated and familial cases, 89% of expanded RED products correlate with expansions at these two loci and that expansion at the CTG18.1 locus was associated to the phenotype. Using the same method in a Belgian sample, Verheyen *et al.* (1999) demonstrated that 86% of the RED expansions could be accounted for by ERDA1 and CTG18.1 repeats. Expanded alleles at ERDA1 were found to be more frequent in bipolar patients. Eight CAG/CTG triplet repeats located in the 18q21.33–q23 region, identified as a candidate region in bipolar families, have been investigated in bipolar disorder by Goossens *et al.* (2000), but no expansion has been found in the bipolar family and the case-control sample investigated.

CONCLUSIONS

The physical mapping of the human genome provides an immense factory providing thousands of genes which will accelerate the identification of genes responsible for mood disorders and will contribute to significant advances in the awareness of diagnosis (diagnostic process and early recognition), pathophysiology, epidemiology and treatment issues. During the past two decades, the search for genes for mood disorders has mainly contributed to better understand and confirm the genetic complexities inherent in these disorders. The large amount of results available and the difficulty of digesting them corroborate this observation. The major contribution of these findings should be integrated in the context of the worldwide efforts to identify the thousands of genes of the human genome. The majority of these genes will be identified within the next few years. Several consistent hypotheses are currently being tested and will, hopefully, speed up the process of narrowing the important regions when the complete genome map becomes available. The most promising chromosomal regions have been localized on chromosomes 4, 5, 11, 12, 18, 21 and X. A number of candidate genes have also been investigated, some of which are directly linked to neurobiological hypotheses of the aetiology of mood disorders. In parallel, specific hypotheses have been implicated, such as anticipation and dynamic mutations. Further research should concentrate on these hypotheses and confirm positive findings through interdisciplinary and multicentre projects.

REFERENCES

Aita, V.M., Liu, J., Terwilllinger, J.D. *et al.*, 1998. A follow-up linkage analysis of chromosome 21 continues to provide evidence for a putative bipolar affective disorder locus. *Am. J. Med. Genet. (Neuropsychiat. Genet.)*, **81**(6), 476.

Barden, N., Plante, M., Rochette, D., Gagne, B. *et al.*, 1996. Genome wide microsatellite marker linkage study of bipolar affective disorders in a very large pedigree derived from a homogeneous population in Quebec points to susceptibility locus on chromosome 12. *Psychiat. Genet.*, **6**, 145–6.

Baron, M., Risch, N., Hamberge, R. *et al.*, 1987. Genetic linkage between X-chromosome markers and bipolar affective illness. *Nature*, **326**, 289–92.

Baron, M., Freimer, N.F., Risch, N. *et al.*, 1993. Diminished support for linkage between manic depressive illness and X-chromosome markers in three Israeli pedigrees. *Nature Genet.*, **3**, 49–55.

Battersby, S., Ogilvie, A.D., Smyth, C.A. *et al.*, 1996. Structure of a variable number tandem repeat of the serotonin transporter gene and association with affective disorder. *Psychiat. Genet.*, **6**, 177–81.

Bellivier, F., Henry, C., Szuke, A., Schurhoff, F. *et al.*, 1998a. Serotonin transporter gene polymorphisms in patients with unipolar or bipolar depression. *Neurosci. Lett.*, **255**(3), 143–6.

Bellivier, F., Leboyer, M., Courtet, P., Buresi, C. *et al.*, 1998b. Association between the tryptophan hydroxylase gene and manic-depressive illness. *Arch. Gen. Psychiat.*, **55**, 33–7

Berrettini, W.H., Goldin, L.R., Gelernter, J. *et al.*, 1990. X chromosome markers and manic-depressive illness: rejection of linkage to Xq28 in nine bipolar pedigrees. *Arch. Gen. Psychiat.*, **47**, 366–73.

Berrettini, W.H., Ferraro, T.N., Goldin, L.R. *et al.*, 1994. Chromosome 18 DNA markers and manic-depressive illness: evidence for a susceptibility gene. *Proc. Natl Acad. Sci. USA*, **91**, 5918–22.

Berrettini, W.H., Ferraro, T.N., Goldin, L.R., Detera-Wadleigh, S.D., Choi, H., Muniec, D., Guroff, J.J., Kazuba, D.M., Nurnberger, J.I., Jr, Hsieh, W.T., Hoehe, M.R. and Gershon, E.S., 1997. A linkage study of bipolar illness. *Arch. Den. Psychiat.*, **54**(1), 27–35.

Blackwood, D., He, L., Morris, S. *et al.*, 1996. A locus for bipolar affective disorder on chromosome 4p. *Nature Genet.*, **12**, 427–30.

Bredbacka, P.E., Pekkarinen, P., Peltonen, L. *et al.*, 1993. Bipolar disorder in an extended pedigree with a segregation pattern compatible with X-linked transmission: exclusion of the previously reported linkage to F9. *Psychiat. Genet.*, **3**, 79–87.

Byerley, W., Leppert, M., O'Connell, P. *et al.*, 1990. D_2 dopamine receptor gene not linked to manic-depression in three families. *Psychiat. Genet.*, **1**, 55–62.

Byerley, W., Hoff, M., Holik, J. *et al.*, 1994. A linkage study with D_5 dopamine and α_{2C}-adrenergic receptor genes in six multiplex bipolar pedigrees. *Psychiat. Genet.*, **4**, 121–4.

Byerley, W., Holik, J., Hoff, M. *et al.*, 1995. Search for a gene predisposing to manic-depression on chromosome 21. *Am. J. Med. Genet.*, **60**(3), 231–3.

Collier, D.A., Stober, G., Li, T. *et al.*, 1996. A novel functional polymorphism within the promoter of the serotonin transporter gene: possible role in susceptibility to affective disorders. *Molec. Psychiat.*, **1**, 453–60.

Coon, H., Jensen, S., Hoff, M. *et al.*, 1993. A genome-wide search for genes predisposing to manic-depression, assuming autosomal dominant inheritance. *Am. J. Hum. Genet.*, **52**, 1234–49.

Coon, H., Hoff, M., Holik, J., Hadley, D. *et al.*, 1996. Analysis of chromosome 18 DNA markers in multiplex pedigrees with manic depression. *Biol. Psychiat.*, **39**, 689–96.

Craddock, N., McGuffin, P. and Owen, M., 1994. Darier's disease cosegregating with affective disorder. *Brit. J. Psychiat.*, **165**(2), 272.

Craddock, N., Daniels, J., Roberts, E., Rees, M. *et al.*, 1995a. No evidence for allelic association between bipolar disorder and monoamine oxidase A gene polymorphisms. *Am. J. Med. Genet.*, **60**, 322–4.

Craddock, N., Roberts, Q., Williams, N., McGuffin, P. *et al.*, 1995b. Association study of bipolar disorder using a functional polymorphism (Ser311 → Cys) in the dopamine D2 receptor gene. *Psychiat. Genet.*, **5**(2), 63–5.

Craddock, N., McKeon, P., Moorhead, S., Guy, C. *et al.*, 1997. Expanded CAG/CTG repeats in bipolar disorder: no correlation with phenotypic measures of illness severity. *Biol. Psychiat.*, **42**(10), 876–81.

Curtis, D., Brynjolfsson, J., Petursson, H. *et al.*, 1993. Segregation and linkage analysis in five manic depression pedigrees excludes the 5HT1a receptor gene (HTR1A). *Ann. Hum. Genet.*, **57**, 27–39.

Dawson, E., Parfitt, E., Roberts, Q. *et al.*, 1995. Linkage studies of bipolar disorder in the region of Darier's disease gene on chromosome 12q23-24.1 *Am. J. Med. Genet. (Neuropsychiat. Genet.)*, **60**(2), 94–102.

Debouck, C. and Goodfellow, P.N., 1999. DNA microarrays in drug discovery and development. *Nature Genet.*, **21**(1 suppl), 48–50.

De Bruyn, A., Raeymaekers, P., Mendelbaum, K. *et al.*, 1994. Linkage analysis of bipolar illness with X-chromosome DNA markers: a susceptibility gene in Xq27-28 cannot be excluded. *Am. J. Med. Genet.*, **54**, 411–19.

De Bruyn, A., Souery, D., Mendelbaum, K. *et al.*, 1996. Linkage analysis of 2 families with bipolar illness and chromosome 18 markers. *Biol. Psychiat.*, **39**, 679–88.

Detera-Wadleigh, S.D., Berrettini, W.H., Goldin, L.R. *et al.*, 1992. A systematic search for a bipolar predisposing locus on chromosome 5. *Neuropsychopharmacology*, **6**, 219–29.

Detera-Waldeigh, S.D., Badner, J.A., Goldin, L.R. *et al.*, 1996. Affected sib-pair analyses reveal support of prior evidence for a susceptibility locus for bipolar disorder, on 21q. *Am. J. Hum. Genet.*, **58**, 1279–85.

Detera-Wadleigh, S.D., Badner, J.A., Yoshikawa, T. *et al.*, 1997. Initial genome screen for bipolar disorder in the NIMH genetics initiative pedigrees: chromosomes 4, 7, 9, 18, 19, 20 and 21q. *Am. J. Med. Genet. (Neuropsychiat. Genet.)*, **74**, 254–62.

Engström, C., Thornlund, A.S., Johansson, E.L. *et al.*, 1995. Anticipation in unipolar affective disorder. *J. Affect. Disord.*, **35**(1–2), 31–40

Ewald, H., Mors, O., Friedrich, U. *et al.*, 1994. Exclusion of linkage between manic depressive illness and tyrosine hydroxylase and dopamine D_2 receptor genes. *Psychiat. Genet.*, **4**, 13–22.

Ewald, H., Eiberg, H., Mors, O. *et al.*, 1996. Linkage study between manic-depressive illness and chromosome 21. *Am. J. Med. Genet.*, **67**(2), 218–24.

Ewald, H., Degn, B., Mors, O., Kruse, T.A., 1998a. Significant linkage between bipolar affective disorder and chromosome 12q24. *Psychiat. Genet.*, **8**, 131–40.

Ewald, H., Flint, T., Degn, B., Mors, O., Kruse, T.A., 1998b. A functional variant of the serotonin transporter gene in families with bipolar affective disorder. *J. Affect. Disord.*, **48**, 135–44.

Franks, E., Guy, C., Jacobsen, N., Bowen, T., Owen, M.J. *et al.*, 1999. Eleven trinucleotide repeat loci that map to chromosome 12 excluded from involvement in the pathogenesis of bipolar disorder. *Am. J. Med. Genet.*, **5**, 67–70.

Freimer, N., Reus, V., Escamilla, M. *et al.*, 1996. Genetic mapping using haplotype, association and linkage methods suggests a locus for severe bipolar disorder (BPI) at 18q22–q23. *Nature Genet.*, **12**, 436–44.

Furlong, R.A., Rubinsztein, J.S., Ho, L., Walsh, C., Coleman, T.A. *et al.*, 1999. Analysis and metaanalysis of two polymorphisms within the tyrosine hydroxylase gene in bipolar and unipolar affective disorders. *Am. J. Med. Genet.*, **5**, 88–94.

Gejman, P.V., Detera-Wadleigh, S., Martinez, M.M. *et al.*, 1990. Manic depressive illness not linked to factor IX in a independent series of pedigrees. *Genomics*, **8**, 648–55.

Gershon, E.S., Badner, J.A., Detera-Waldeigh, S.D. *et al.*, 1996. Maternal inheritance and chromosome 18 allele sharing in unilineal bipolar illness pedigrees. *Am. J. Med. Genet. (Neuropsychiat. Genet.)*, **67**, 202–7.

Gomez-Casero, E., Perez de Castro, I., Saiz-Ruiz, J. *et al.*, 1996. No association between particular DRD3 and DAT gene polymorphisms and manic-depressive illness in a Spanish sample. *Psychiat. Genet.*, **6**(4), 209–12.

Goossens, D., Villafuerte, S., Tissir, F., Van Gestel, S. *et al.*, 2000. No evidence for the involvement of CAG/CTG repeats from within 18q21.33–q23 in bipolar disorder. *J. Eur. J. Hum. Genet.*, **8**(5), 385–8.

Greenberg, D.A., 1993. Linkage analysis of 'necessary' disease loci versus 'susceptibility' loci. *Am. J. Hum. Genet.*, **52**(1), 135–43.

Grigoroiu-Serbanescu, M., Wickramaratne, P.J., Hodge, S.E., Milea, S. and Mihailescu, R., 1997. Genetic anticipation and imprinting in bipolar I illness. *Br. J. Psychiat.*, **170**, 162–6.

Gutierrez, B., Pintor, L., Gasto, C., Rosa, A. *et al.*, 1998a. Variability in the serotonin transporter gene and increased risk for major depression with melancholia. *Hum. Genet.*, **103**, 319–22.

Gutierrez, B., Arranz, M.J., Collier, D.A., Valles, V. *et al.*, 1998b. Serotonin transporter gene and risk for bipolar affective disorder: an association study in Spanish population. *Biol. Psychiat.*, **43**, 843–7.

Guy, C.A., Bowen, T., Jones, I., McCandless, F., Owen, M.J., Craddock, N. and O'Donovan, M.C., 1999. CTG18.1 and ERDA-1 CAG/CTG repeat size in bipolar disorder. *Neurobiol. Dis.*, **6**, 302–7.

Hodge, S.E., 1994. What association analysis can and cannot tell us about the genetics of complex disease. *Am. J. Med. Genet.*, **54**, 318–23.

Holmes, D., Brynjolfsson, J., Brett, P. *et al.*, 1991. No evidence for a susceptibility locus predisposing to manic depression in the region of the dopamine (D_2) receptor gene. *Br. J. Psychiat.*, **158**, 635–41.

Kawada, Y., Hattori, M., Dai, X.Y., Nanko, S. *et al.*, 1995. Possible association between monoamine oxidase A gene and bipolar affective disorder. *Am. J. Hum. Genet.*, **56**, 335–6.

Kelsoe, J.R., Kristbjanarson, H., Bergesch, P. *et al.*, 1993. A genetic linkage study of bipolar disorder and 13 markers on chromosome 11 including the D2 dopamine receptor. *Neuropsychopharmacology*, **9**(4), 293–301.

Kelsoe, J.R., Sadovnick, A.D., Kristbjarnarson, H. *et al.*, 1996. Possible locus of bipolar disorder near the dopamine transporter on chromosome 5 *Am. J. Med. Genet.*, **67**(6), 533–40.

Knowles, J.A., Rao, P.A., Cox-Matise, T. *et al.*, 1998. No evidence for significant linkage between bipolar affective disorder and chromosome 18 pericentromeric markers in a large series of multiplex pedigrees. *Am. J. Hum. Genet.*, **62**, 916–24.

Kwok, J.B., Adams, L.J., Salmon, J.A. *et al.*, 1999. Nonparametric simulation-based statistical analyses for bipolar affective disorder locus on chromosome 21q22.3. *Am. J. Med. Genet.*, **88**(1), 99–102.

LaBuda, M.C., Maldonado, M., Marshall, D., Otten, K., Gerhard, D.S., 1996. A follow-up report of a genome search for affective disorder predisposition loci in the Old Order Amish. *Am. J. Hum. Genet.*, **59**, 1343–62.

Li, T., Vallada, H.P., Liu, X., Xie, T. *et al.*, 1998. Analysis of CAG/CTG repeat size in Chinese subjects with schizophrenia and bipolar disorder using the repeat expansion detection method. *Biol. Psychiat.*, **44**, 1160–5.

Lim, L.C.C., Powell, J.F. and Murray, R., 1994a. Monoamine oxidase A gene and bipolar affective disorder. *Am. J. Hum. Genet.*, **54**, 1122–4.

Lim, L.C.C., Nöthen, M.M., Körner, J. *et al.*, 1994b. No evidence of association between Dopamine D_4 receptor variants and bipolar affective disorder. *Am. J. Med. Genet.*, **54**, 259–63.

Lim, L.C.C., Powell, J., Sham, P., Castle, D. *et al.*, 1995. Evidence for a genetic association between alleles of monoamine oxidase A gene and bipolar disorder. *Am. J. Med. Genet.*, **60**, 325–31.

Lindblad, K., Nylander, P.O., De Bruyn, A. *et al.*, 1995. Detection of expanded CAG repeats in bipolar affective disorder using the repeat expansion detection (RED) method. *Neurobiol. Dis.*, **2**, 55–62.

Lindblad, K., Nylander, P.O., Zander, C. *et al.*, 1998. Two commonly expanded CAG/CTG repeat loci: involvement in affective disorders? *Molec. Psychiat.*, **3**(5), 405–10.

Lucotte, G., Landoulsi, A., Berriche, S. *et al.*, 1992. Manic depressive illness is linked to factor IX in a French pedigree. *Ann. Génét.*, **35**, 93–5.

Maier, W., Hallmayer, J., Zill, P. *et al.*, 1995. Linkage analysis between pericentromeric markers on chromosome 18 and bipolar disorder: a replication test. *Psychiat. Res.*, **59**, 7–15.

Manki, H., Shigenobu, K., Muramatsu, T. *et al.*, 1996. Dopamine D2, D3 and D4 receptor and transporter gene polymorphims and mood disorders. *J. Affect. Dis.*, **40**, 7–13.

Mann, J.J., Malone, K.M., Nielsen, D.A., Goldman, D., Edos, J. and Gelernter, J., 1997. Possible association of a polymorphism of the tryptophan hydroxylase gene with suicidal behavior in depressed patients. *Am. J. Psychiat.*, **154**(10), 1451–3.

McInnis, M.G., McMahon, F.J., Chase, G.A. *et al.*, 1993. Anticipation in bipolar affective disorder. *Am. J. Hum. Genet.*, **53**, 385–90.

Mendlewicz, J., Lipp, O., Souery, D. *et al.*, 1997. Expanded trinucleotide CAG repeats in families with bipolar affective disorder. *Biol. Psychiat.*, **42**(12), 1115–22.

Mendlewicz, J., Simon, P., Sevy, S. *et al.*, 1987. Polymorphic DNA marker on chromosome and manic-depression. *Lancet*, **1**, 1230–2.

Muramatsu, T., Matsushita, S., Kanba, S. *et al.*, 1997. Monoamine oxidase genes polymorphisms and mood disorder. *Am. J. Med. Genet.*, **74**, 494–6.

Nanko, S., Fukuda, R., Hattori, M. *et al.*, 1994. Linkage studies between affective disorder and dopamine D2, D3, and D4 receptor gene loci in four Japanese pedigrees. *Psychiat. Res.*, **52**(2), 149–57.

Nöthen, M.M., Eggermann, K., Albus, M. *et al.*, 1995. Association analysis of the monoamine oxidase A gene in bipolar affective disorder by using family-based internal controls. *Am. J. Hum. Genet.*, **57**, 975–7.

Nöthen, M.M., Cichon, S., Erdmann, J. *et al.*, 1993. Pseudoautosomal marker DXYS20 and manic depression. *Am. J. Hum. Genet.*, **52**, 841–2.

Nylander, P.O., Engström, C., Chotai, J. *et al.*, 1994. Anticipation in Swedish families with bipolar affective disorder. *J. Med. Genet.*, **9**, 686–9.

O'Donovan, M.C., Guy, C., Craddock, N. *et al.*, 1995. Expanded CAG repeats in schizophrenia and bipolar disorder. *Nature Genet.*, **10**, 380–1.

Ogilvie, A.D., Battersby, S., Bubb, V.J. *et al.*, 1996. Polymorphism in serotonin transporter gene associated with susceptibility to major depression. *Lancet*, **347**, 731–3.

Ohara, K., Suzuki, Y., Ushimi, Y., Yoshida, K. and Ohara, K., 1998. Anticipation and imprinting in Japanese familial mood disorders. *Psychiat. Res.*, **79**(3), 191–8.

Oruc, L., Lindblad, K., Verheyen, G. *et al.*, 1997. CAG expansions in bipolar and unipolar disorders. *Am. J. Hum. Genet.*, **60**, 730–2.

Parsian, A. and Todd, R.D., 1994. Bipolar disorder and the pseudoautosomal region: an association study. *Am. J. Med. Genet.*, **54**, 5–7.

Pauls, D.L., Ott, J., Paul, S.M. *et al.*, 1995. Linkage analyses of chromosome 18 markers do not identify a major susceptibility locus for bipolar affective disorder in the Old Order Amish. *Am. J. Med. Gen.*, **57**, 636–43.

Paulson, H.L. and Fischbeck, K.H., 1996. Trinucleotide repeats in neurogenetic disorders. *A. Rev. Neurosci.*, **19**, 79–107.

Plomin, R., Owen, M.J. and McGuffin, P., 1994. The genetic basis of complex human behaviors. *Science*, **264**(5166), 1733–9.

Pekkarinen, P., Terwilliger, J., Bredbacka, P.-E. *et al.*, 1995. Evidence of a predisposing locus to bipolar disorder on Xq24-q27.1 in an extended Finnish pedigree. *Genome Res.*, **5**, 105–15.

Propping, P., Nöthen, M.M., Fimmers, R. *et al.*, 1993. Linkage versus association studies in complex diseases. *Pychiatr. Genet.*, **3**, 136.

Rees, M., Norton, N., Jones, I. *et al.*, 1997. Association study of bipolar disorder at the human serotonin transporter gene (hSERT; 5HTT). *Molec. Psychiat.*, **2**, 398–402.

Serretti, A., Macciardi, F., Cusin, C. *et al.*, 1998. Dopamine receptor D4 gene is associated with delusional symptomatology in mood disorders. *Psychiat. Res.*, **80**(2), 129–36.

Sidenberg, D.G., King, N., Kennedy, J.L., 1994. Analysis of new D_4 dopamine receptor (DRD4) coding region variants and TH microsatellite in the old Amish family (00A110). *Psychiatr. Genet.*, **4**, 95–9.

Smeraldi, E. and Macciardi, F., 1995. Association and linkage studies in mental illness. In: Papadimitriou, G.N. and Mendlewicz, J. (eds), *Genetics of Mental Disorders* Part I: *Theoretical Aspects*. Baillière's Clinical Psychiatry, International Practice and Research, Vol. 1, no. 1, pp. 97–110. Baillière Tindall, London.

Smeraldi, E., Zanardi, R., Benedetti, F., Di Bella, D. *et al.*, 1998. Polymorphism within the promoter of the serotonin transporter gene and antidepressant efficacy of fluvoxamine. *Molec. Psychiat.*, **3**, 508–11.

Smyth, C., Kalsi, G., Curtis, D. *et al.*, 1997. Two-locus admixture linkage analysis of bipolar and unipolar affective disorder supports the presence of susceptibility loci on chromosomes 11p15 and 21q22. *Genomics*, **39**, 271–98.

Souery, D., Lipp, O., Mahieu, B. *et al.*, 1996a. Association study of bipolar disorder with candidate genes involved in catecholamine neurotransmission: DRD2, DRD3, DAT1 and TH genes. *Am. J. Med. Genet. (Neuropsychiatr. Genet.)*, **67**(6), 551–5.

Souery, D., Papadimitriou, G.N. and Mendlewicz, J., 1996b. New genetic approaches in affective disorders. In: Papadimitriou, G.N. and Mendlewicz, J. (eds), *Genetics of Mental Disorders* Part II: *Clinical Issues*. Baillière's Clinical Psychiatry, International Practice and Research, Vol. 2, no. 1. Baillière Tindall, London.

Stine, C., Xu, J., Koskela, R. *et al.*, 1996. Evidence for linkage of bipolar disorder to chromosome 18 with parent-of-origin effect. *Am. J. Hum. Genet.*, **57**, 1384–94.

Stine, O.C., McMahon, F.J., Chen, L. *et al.*, 1997. Initial genome screen for bipolar disorder in the NIMH genetics initiative pedigrees: chromosomes 2, 11, 13, 14 and X. *Am. J. Med. Genet.*, **74**, 263–9.

Straub, R.E., Lehner, Th., Luo, Y. *et al.*, 1994. A possible vulnerability locus for bipolar affective disorder on chromosome 21q22.3. *Nature Genet.*, **8**, 291–6.

Terwilliger, J.D. and Ott, J., 1992. A haplotype-based haplotype relative risk statistic. *Hum. Hered.*, **42**, 337–46.

Trottier, Y., Lutz, Y., Stevanin, G. *et al.*, 1995. Polyglutamine expansion as a pathological epitope in Huntington's disease and four dominant cerebellar ataxias. *Nature*, **378**(6555), 403–6.

Turecki, G., Rouleau, G.A., Mari, J.J. *et al.*, 1996. A systematic evaluation of linkage studies in bipolar disorder. *Acta Psychiat. Scand.*, **93**, 317–26.

Vallada, H., Craddock, N., Vasques, L. *et al.*, 1996. Linkage studies in bipolar affective disorder with markers on chromosome 21. *J. Affect. Disord.*, **41**(3), 217–21.

Verheyen, G.R., Del-Favero, J., Mendlewicz, J., Lindblad, K., Van Zand, K., Aalbregtse, M., Schalling, M. and Van Broeckhoven, C., 1999. Molecular interpretation of expanded RED products in bipolar disorder by CAG/CTG repeats located at chromosomes 17q and 18q. *Neurobiol. Dis.*, **6**, 424–32.

Vincent, J.B., Klempan, T., Parikh, S.S. *et al.*, 1996. Frequency analysis of large CAG/CTG trinucleotide repeats in schizophrenia and bipolar affective disorder. *Molec. Psychiat.*, **1**, 141–8.

Waldman, I.D., Robinson, B.F., Feigon, S.A. *et al.*, 1997. Linkage disequilibrium between the dopamine transporter gene (DAT1) and bipolar disorder: extending the transmission disequilibrium test to examine genetic heterogeneity. *Genet. Epidemiol.*, **14**, 699–704.

Yoneda, H., Sakai, T., Ishida, T. *et al.*, 1992. An association between manic-depressive illness and a pseudoautosomal DNA marker. *Am. J. Hum. Genet.*, **51**, 1172–3.

Zander, C., Schurhoff, F., Laurent, C., Chavand, O. *et al.*, 1998. CAG repeat sequences in bipolar affective disorder: no evidence for association in a French population. *Am. J. Med. Genet.*, **81**, 338–41.

XVIII-11

Neonatal Developmental Neuroplasticity: A Critical Contribution from Environment

Robert M. Post

INTRODUCTION

Hubel and Wiesel won the Nobel Prize for medicine with their elegant dissection of the impact of visual deprivation on the biochemistry, physiology and microstructure of the ocular dominance columns in the visual cortex (Hubel and Wiesel, 1979). They elucidated a gradient of progressively more profound and irreversible effects in the normal development of visual pathways and processing as a function of depriving environmental input by reducing visual input in one eye to virtually zero by suturing it shut. Not only was there dysfunction and atrophy of the ocular dominance columns related to the deprived eye, but a compensatory increase in those columns synaptically related to the eye that continued to have normal visual stimulation (Wiesel and Hubel, 1965; Hubel and Wiesel, 1979, 1998).

Similar, and perhaps even more complex, interactions appear to be occurring in diencephalic, paralimbic and cortical circuits involved in mediating the normal processes of maternal infant nurturing and bonding. The lack of normal developmental trajectories in this domain have been repeatedly linked to vulnerability to depression in adults later in life (Emde *et al.*, 1965; Powell *et al.*, 1967; Brown *et al.*, 1973a, b; Breier *et al.*, 1988). Thus, the neuropsychobiology of such early environmental insults is of particular interest to the topic of this chapter, and re-emphasizes a role for environmental contingencies as well as genetic inheritance in vulnerability to affective illness.

Depression Recurrence

The work of Kendler and associates provides a particularly cogent set of examples of both gene and environmental effects. As illustrated in Figure XVIII-11.1, a variety of early environmental losses or adversities are risk factors for subsequent depressions (Kendler *et al.*, 1993). In addition, concurrent stresses and losses interact with these earlier vulnerabilities in the precipitation of affective episodes. Moreover, minor or neurotic depressions are precursors to more major depressions, and major depressions are a key risk factor for subsequent major depressive recurrences, all within the background of genetic vulnerability to the recurrent affective disorders. Whether such dual contributions would meet the more formal criteria enunciated earlier by Boomstra and Martin for gene–environment interactions remains to be delineated, and in this chapter we will use the term interactions loosely only to imply that effects of both inherited and environmental domains can be discernible.

Suicidality in Bipolar Illness

A similar interactive schema is evident in the risk factors for suicidality in patients with bipolar disorder (Leverich *et al.*, 2002a, b). A family history of severe suicides attempted or completed, as well as a family history of substance abuse, interacts with a variety of environmental experiential variables as precursors of suicide attempts (Figure XVIII-11.2). An increased incidence of suicide attempts is affected by genetics, course of illness variables, psychiatric Axis I and Axis II comorbidities, medical comorbidities, and a history of early extreme stressors and environmental adversities (physical or sexual abuse in childhood or adolescence), as well as more proximal stressors such as loss of significant others and lack of adequate access to mental and medical health care.

Thus, paradigms in unipolar depression and in suicidality in patients with bipolar illness both indicate powerful interactions of genetic and environmental variables. On the experiential side, both paradigms suggest components of episode sensitization and stress sensitization.

Episode Sensitization

Perhaps the best clinical evidence for the occurrence of episode sensitization is the study of Kessing *et al.* (1998) of more than 20 000 patients hospitalized for depression or mania. These investigators found that for both unipolar and bipolar patients, the best predictor of incidence and time to relapse was the number of prior episodes, supporting the hypothesis that episodes beget episodes. However, one has to caution that it is possible that those patients who are most vulnerable to recurrence were preselected and one may have a poor prognosis subgroup in those who have the most prior episodes and subsequent recurrences. Kessing and associates present statistical reasons to suggest that this is not the case (Kessing, 1998; Kessing *et al.*, 1998), but such a proposition could only be resolved with a randomized prospective study of adequate versus inadequate long-term prophylaxis to see whether the intervening occurrence of episodes did change the future course; this study is not really possible given the ethical constraints against inadequate prophylaxis.

The studies of Brown and colleagues (Harris *et al.*, 1986, 1987; Bifulco *et al.*, 1987) are among the most elegant in demonstrating the interaction of proximal and distal stressors in the occurrence of depression. Brown and colleagues found that a variety of risk factors in single mothers appeared to be associated with the occurrence of depression upon the occurrence of a proximal stressor. One of these factors, again related to loss of a significant other (in this case loss of one's mother in childhood), could act as a predictor of subsequent depression. This occurred with a variety of other modulating variables including lack of a confidant, having more than four children at home to care for, and lack of employment. The study of Breier *et al.* (1988) is particularly revealing in terms of the potential lasting effects of early

Biological Psychiatry: Edited by H. D'haenen, J.A. den Boer and P. Willner. ISBN 0-471-49198-5

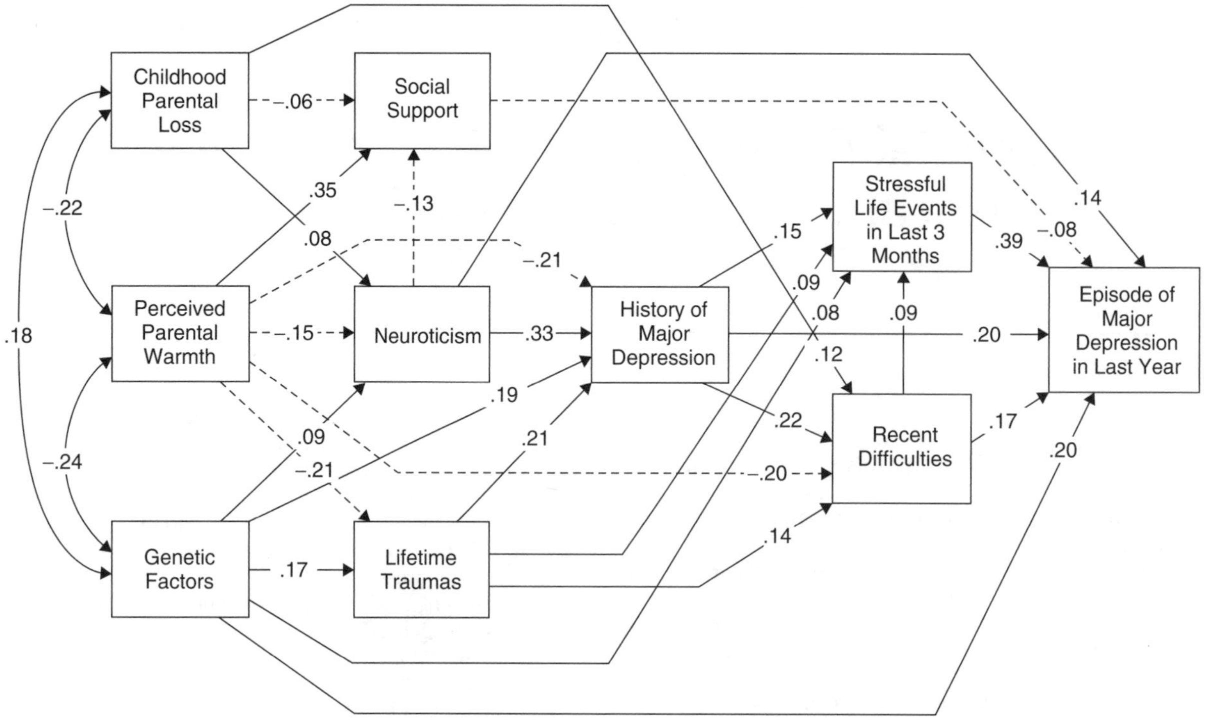

Figure XVIII-11.1 Kendler's path estimates of the best-fitting model of prediction of major depression in 1360 female twins. Early and recent life events (left, top two boxes) interacting with genetic vulnerability (left, bottom box) predispose to early mild symptoms and episodes (neuroticism box) and more major depression (middle box and last box on right). Episode occurrence further increases vulnerability to recurrence (middle box to last box on right). The values along the double-headed arrows between the independent variables (at the left side of the figure) are correlation coefficients. The values along the single-headed arrows are path or standardized regression coefficients indicating the weight of the relationships. The black single-headed arrows represent positive path coefficients. Negative path coefficients are depicted by striped paths (see Kendler *et al.*, 1993, for details). Reprinted with permission from the *American Journal of Psychiatry*, © 1993

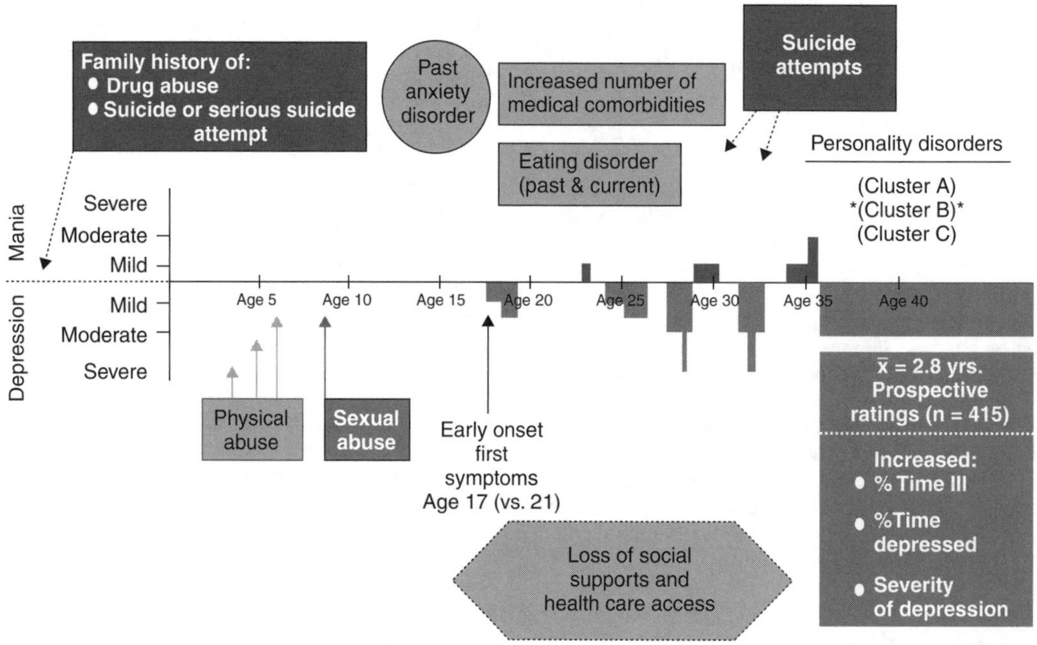

Figure XVIII-11.2 Schema of factors associated with suicide attempts in 632 patients with bipolar illness in the Stanley Foundation Bipolar Network (from Leverich *et al.*, 2002a, b)

parental loss. These investigators found that loss of a parent in childhood increased the incidence of adult depression only if the surviving parent failed to adequately substitute for the loss of the other. These data are particularly important, indicating that a variety of factors can be involved within any given risk factor as to whether or not it becomes a crucial determinant of increasing the risk of episode recurrence or of a suicidal act. The studies of Brown and colleagues in unipolar depression (Harris *et al.*, 1986, 1987; Bifulco *et al.*, 1987) and of Leverich and colleagues for suicidality in bipolar depressed patients (Leverich *et al.*, 2002a, b) re-emphasize this point, that lack of a confidant may be a particularly important mediating factor. Given a variety of stressors, the lack of availability of others to share perspectives, give their insights, and provide psychological and physical support, appears to be critically important.

Stress Sensitization

A variety of empirical investigations in affective illness suggest stress sensitization. The first (noted above) suggests that several types of early-life stressors are pertinent to later affective illness onset. In addition, numerous studies document that proximal stressors or psychosocial precipitants are more obvious in initial episodes of affective disorder than in later ones in which the episodes often occur more autonomously (reviewed in Post, 1992). Although the literature is not completely in agreement in this regard (Hammen and Gitlin, 1997), the majority of studies do suggest that early compared with later episodes are more likely to be associated with stressors. These observations thus validate Kraepelin (1921) and others' original view that:

> we must regard all alleged injuries as possibly sparks for the discharge of individual attacks, but that the real cause of the malady must be sought in *permanent internal changes*, what at least very often, perhaps always, are innate.
>
> in spite of the removal of the discharging cause, the attack follows its independent development. But, finally, the appearance of wholly similar attacks on wholly dissimilar occasions or quite without external occasion shows that even there where there has been external influence, it must not be regarded as a necessary presupposition for the appearance of the attack.
>
> Unfortunately the powerlessness of our efforts to cure must only too often convince us that the attacks of manic-depressive insanity may be to an astonishing degree *independent of external influences*. (Kraepelin, 1921, pp. 180–1)

Stress sensitization may not be unique to unipolar and bipolar disorders; evidence is emerging that it plays a role in the occurrence of the full-blown post-traumatic stress disorder (PTSD) syndrome. Several investigators have indicated that in patient populations who did develop PTSD after a given stressor compared with those who did not, there is a greater history of prior early stressors (Bremner *et al.*, 1993; Yehuda *et al.*, 1995; Breslau *et al.*, 1999). Together, these data in affective illness and in PTSD suggest that early stressors provide an area of vulnerability upon which the more proximal stressors act and interact. Should this prove to be true, the neurobiological and neuropsychological mechanisms that could underlie these types of stress sensitization phenomena deserve exploration.

EARLY MATERNAL SEPARATION

Maternal separation and parental neglect have long been recognized as potential risk factors for depression. Spitz and others studied anaclitic depression (Emde *et al.*, 1965; Harmon *et al.*, 1982), and Harlow and associates described some of the catastrophic and lasting consequences of social and environmental deprivation (Harlow *et al.*, 1965; Suomi *et al.*, 1970; Young *et al.*, 1973). Kuhn and Schanberg were among the first to demonstrate the physiological potency of even transient aberrations in the normal maternal–infant relationship (Kuhn *et al.*, 1978). They observed that the failure to show normal trajectories of growth and development in neonatal rat pups separated from their mothers could be ameliorated by the appropriate amount of touch and licking substitution (Pauk *et al.*, 1986). Separated animals did not show a failure to secrete adequate levels of growth hormone, but that growth hormone could not activate the critical enzyme for neural development, ornithine decarboxylase (Kuhn *et al.*, 1978). If neonatal rat pups were stroked lightly with a toothbrush on the ventral surface of their abdomens, they showed normal growth and normal amounts of ornithine decarboxylase activity induced by growth hormone (Pauk *et al.*, 1986). The ethological background of this interaction was determined to involve the fact that the neonate rodent has a neurogenic bladder and urinates only when the mother licks the ventral surface of the abdomen. This urine is then further licked by the mother to enhance the neonatal maternal bond at the level of smell and taste, as well as sound and touch.

Based on these preclinical observations, Kuhn and Shanberg moved to the neonatal nursery and demonstrated that properly handled premature infants grew better than those who were less handled in their incubators (Field *et al.*, 1986). At the same time, Levine and colleagues (Stanton *et al.*, 1988; Levine *et al.*, 1991) were demonstrating the consequences of single brief periods (24 hours) of maternal deprivation in neonatal rat pups, which were long-lasting alterations in behaviour and endocrinology. Some of the fundamental neurobiological mechanisms in those alterations have begun to be revealed; these animals remain hypercortisolaemic and anxious in open field tests and show a variety of changes in acute signal transduction chemicals and neurotrophic factors (Suchecki *et al.*, 1993; Rots *et al.*, 1996; Smith *et al.*, 1997; Zhang *et al.*, 1998, 2002).

For example, in rat pups separated for one day on day 11 of their life and then sacrificed on day 12, there was an increased induction of mRNA for nerve growth factor (NGF) and c-jun (Zhang *et al.*, 1998) and a decrease in hippocampal brain-derived neurotropic factor (BDNF), calcium-calmodulin kinase II (CaMKII), and nitric oxide synthase (NOS) (Zhang *et al.*, 2002; Xing *et al.*, 1998) (Figure XVIII-11.3a). In common with these changes is an approximate doubling in the rate of apoptosis observed throughout the brain, which correlates with the degree of increase in growth hormone in white matter areas of brain (Zhang *et al.*, 2002), raising the question of why increases in growth hormone might be associated with increases in cell death measured by the apoptag technique. It appears that the high-affinity receptor for NGF, the Trk-A receptor, is not adequately developed at this neonatal age and the low affinity p75 growth factor receptor predominates. When activated, the p75 receptor mediates an increase in apoptosis (Barrett, 2000). Zhang and associates (Zhang *et al.*, 2002) have observed that apoptosis occurs in both neuronal and glial cells.

Although these acute observations remain to be followed longitudinally, and the long-term consequences on brain microstructure and behaviour remain to be elucidated, they do provide another plausible mechanism (in addition to genetic deficits and other prenatal alterations) for the reported deficits in neurons or glia in selected areas of the brain in patients with schizophrenic, unipolar and bipolar affective disorders (Selemon *et al.*, 1995, 1998; Drevets *et al.*, 1998; Ongur *et al.*, 1998; Rajkowska *et al.*, 1999; Knable, 1999). In addition, they provide another plausible mechanism for the near uniform reports that patients with schizophrenia

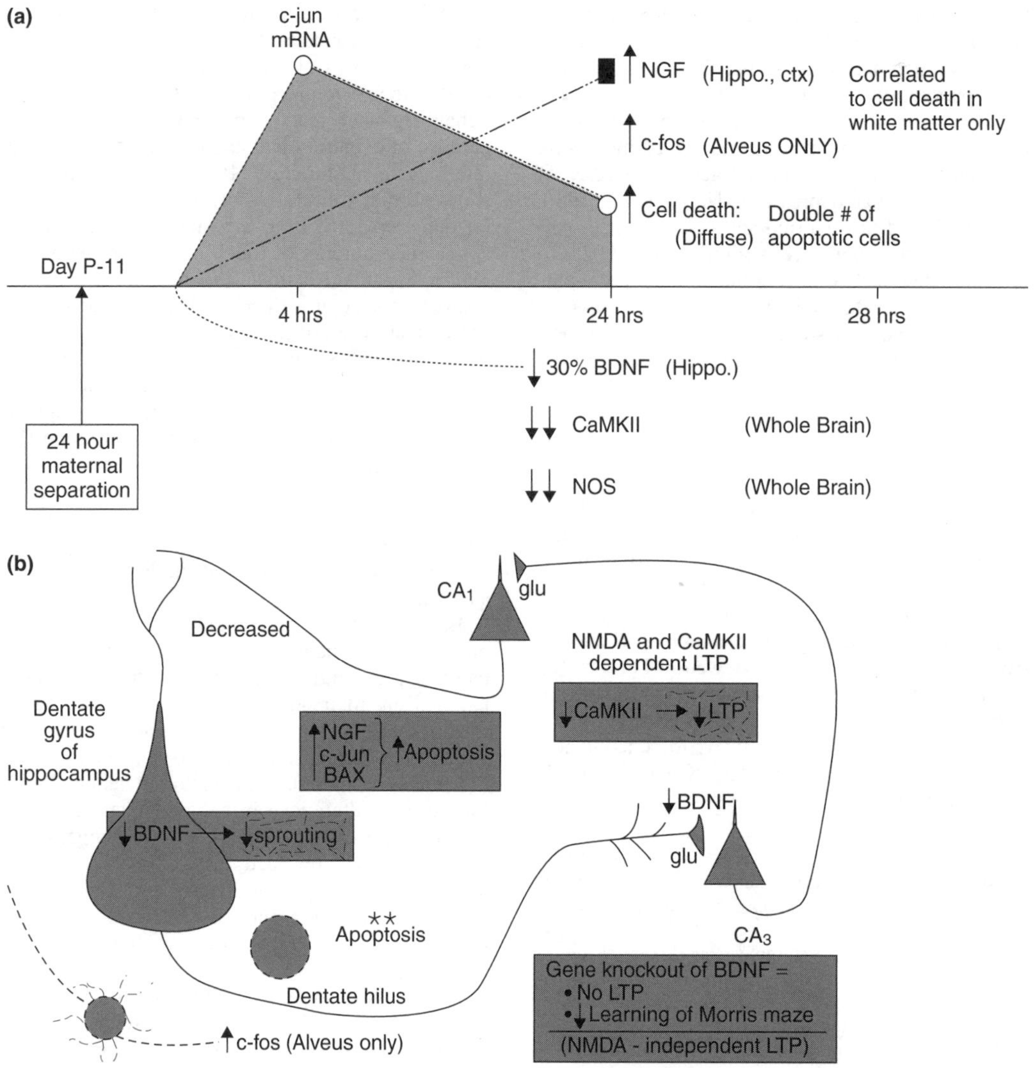

Figure XVIII-11.3 (a) Effects of maternal separation in neonatal rat pups on neurotrophins, transcription factors and gene expression (compiled using data from Zhang *et al.*, 1998, 2002). NGF, nerve growth factor; Hippo., hippocampus; ctx, cortex; BDNF, brain-derived neurotrophic factor; CaMKII, calcium-calmodulin kinase II; NOS, nitric oxide synthase. (b) Potential hippocampal effects of neonatal maternal separation. BDNF, brain-derived neurotrophic factor; NGF, nerve growth factor; NMDA, *N*-methyl-D-aspartate; glu, glutamate; CaMKII, calcium-calmodulin kinase II; LTP, long-term potentiation

often have significantly smaller brain sizes than comparative control populations (Lawrie and Abukmeil, 1998). Although it is not clear what factors mediate such processes, the potential impact of environmental deprivation should now be added to those of genetic determinants so beautifully demonstrated in the twin studies of Weinberger and colleagues (Suddath *et al.*, 1990; Berman *et al.*, 1992; Weinberger *et al.*, 1992; Torrey *et al.*, 1995), who found that in identical twins discordant for schizophrenia, the ill twin almost always had increased ventricle size. Ventricular size was highly correlated within twin pairs, showing the effect of genetics, but additional environmental vulnerabilities appeared to be at work in increasing the risk for becoming ill in those who had another factor associated with the larger ventricular size (Suddath *et al.*, 1990).

The maternal-separation-induced decrements in hippocampal BDNF are equally interesting in relation to a number of reports of smaller hippocampal size in patients with either affective disorders (Sheline *et al.*, 1996; Bremner *et al.*, 2000) or PTSD (Bremner *et al.*, 1995, 1997; Gurvits *et al.*, 1996; Stein *et al.*, 1997), although there are notable exceptions in this regard (Hauser *et al.*, 2000; Vakili *et al.*, 2000). Could a sufficiently consistent or recurrent stress-induced decrement in BDNF early in life be associated with the relatively small hippocampal size (Figure XVIII-11.3b)? Moreover, even if the size of the hippocampus were normal, recent evidence suggests that BDNF is important to the development of normal learning and memory, as reflected in a variety of behavioural tests, and for the normal development of long-term potentiation (LTP) in the hippocampus (Korte *et al.*, 1996, 1998), the best studied model of learning and memory (Malenka and Nicoll, 1999). Similarly, animals deficient in CaMKII have impaired LTP (Silva *et al.*, 1992).

One can only wonder whether the acute decrements in these two substances (CaMKII and BDNF) after maternal separation stress could occur at a critical developmental juncture and result in sustained deficits (Figure XVIII-11.3b). Recent data of Xing and colleagues show that CaMKII amRNA is significantly decreased in the prefrontal cortex of patients with bipolar illness compared with normal controls (Xing *et al.*, 2002). Could such a defect in this and related signal transduction systems necessary for adequate learning and memory be a factor in the many different types of evidence of frontal dysfunction in patients with bipolar illness? The fact that CaMKII is decreased in the prefrontal cortices of patients with bipolar illness, and that it can be acutely decreased in rat pups undergoing a single day of maternal deprivation stress, at least opens the possibility of both genetic and environmental influences on such a critical intracellular transduction system.

Increases and decreases in intracellular calcium are crucial to reading the input on a single neuron and translating it into synaptic and neuronal output. On the synaptic level, increases or decreases in intracellular calcium can be associated with LTP or long-term depression (LTD), respectively (Malenka *et al.*, 1989; Bolshakov and Siegelbaum, 1994), and at a cellular level can be associated with neurotrophic, apoptotic and excitotoxic effects. Thus, neural excitability as well as neural life and death are intimately related to reading intracellular calcium signals. Could a 30% deficit of CaMKII in prefrontal cortex (Xing *et al.*, 2002), one of the most critical kinases involved in calcium homeostasis based on either genetic and/or environmental determinants, account for some of the dysregulations in cognition and affect in patients with bipolar illness?

REPEATED MATERNAL DEPRIVATION: BRIEF SEPARATIONS VERSUS LONGER SEPARATIONS

The work of Plotsky and Meaney reveals a number of striking principles about the quality, quantity, timing and duration of stressors as crucial variables in determining the eventual neurobiological and behavioural outcomes. Repeated maternal deprivation stress lasting 15 minutes produces animals that are relatively hypocorticosteronaemic and are protected against age-related memory defects as adults in association with lesser degrees of hippocampal atrophy. In contrast, animals subjected to repeated maternal deprivation stress of 3 hours' duration remain anxious in the open field and are hypercorticosteronaemic throughout their lives (Plotsky and Meaney, 1993). In addition, they are more prone to alcohol- and cocaine-self-administration than their litter mate non-separated controls. Strikingly, all of these alterations are reversible with treatment with serotonin-selective reuptake inhibitors (SSRIs), although if the SSRI is discontinued, the full syndrome returns (Huot *et al.*, 2001; Meaney *et al.*, 2002).

Many of these behavioural and biochemical changes mirror those induced in the model of Barden and associates (Pepin *et al.*, 1992; Beaulieu *et al.*, 1994) in which transgenic mice were developed to have a deficient number of type II glucocorticoid receptors (Figure XVIII-11.4). These animals are hypercortisolaemic and anxious in a variety of open field tests and also normalize much of their behaviour and biochemistry with antidepressant treatment. These convergent data of a transgenic model and an environmentally-induced model emphasize not only the potential for each to affect a relatively similar behavioural syndrome, but also suggest the strong potential for genetic and environmental interactions.

Thus, one could conceptualize that an animal with a genetically low level of glucocorticoid receptors that are subthreshold for inducing hypercortisolaemia and anxious behaviours might, under the proper provocation stress, exceed that threshold and manifest new behavioural and biochemical pathologies. It is interesting that this anxious, hypercortisolaemic syndrome is driven by glucocorticoid receptor deficiencies in one instance, and by glucocorticoid excess with subsequent compensatory receptor downregulation in the other, again suggesting the possibility of multiple pathophysiological routes to similar behavioural and biochemical pathologies. An example of such common phenotypic manifestations arising from very different transmitter and receptor alterations is clearly evident in the case of diabetes mellitus, wherein one can develop the illness because of either a deficiency in the hormone insulin, or because of a variety of defects in the insulin receptor activation

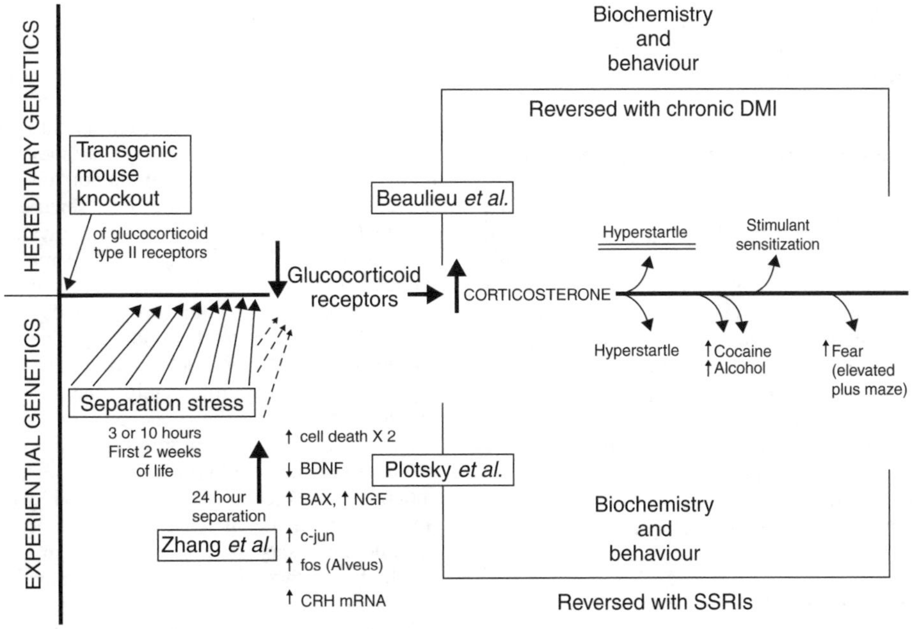

Figure XVIII-11.4 Convergent genetic and environmental models of depression. Either heredity or experiential genetics may lead to compounding behavioural and biochemical end-points similar to those seen in depression and reversible by antidepressants. DMI, desipramine; BDNF, brain-derived neurotrophic factor; NGF, nerve growth factor; CRH, corticotropin-releasing hormone; SSRIs, serotonin-selective reuptake inhibitors

and its associated downstream effects (insulin resistance) despite normal to high levels of circulating insulin.

In addition to this type of mechanistic heterogeneity, the work of Plotsky and Meaney has further elucidated mechanisms of individual differences in response to maternal deprivation stress. They noted that the potential mechanism of protection against age-related memory decline in the 15-minute separated animals was that their mothers engaged in increased licking behaviour upon return of the rat pup to the litter (Liu *et al.*, 1997). Conversely, in the 3-hour deprivation experience, the mother apparently fails to recognize the previously separated neonate as her own and continues to run about the cage in a somewhat frantic and agitated manner, sometimes virtually trampling her offspring. If the mother is given a substitute litter during the time that the 3-hour deprived rat pup is removed, her behaviour remains normal upon its return, and the 3-hour separated animal does not show the typical neurobehavioural effects of repeated 3-hour separations (Anisman *et al.*, 1998). These data, again, point to crucial interactions of parent and child in the evolution of pathological behavioural and biochemical syndromes. If the brief separation is accompanied by increased licking behaviour, animals show long-term benefit. Furthermore, if the 3-hour separated animal is spared some of the traumatic effects that occur as a sequel, it is spared the long-term adverse consequences. These effects are also dependent on the time-course of neural development because animals that are separated as adolescents instead of neonates tend to show the opposite long-term behavioural and biochemical outcomes.

Given the potential potent and long-lasting effects of degree of maternal licking behaviour upon reunion, Meaney and colleagues sought to ascertain whether normal variations in maternal licking behaviour were associated with individual variability in corticosterone levels and anxiety behaviours. Indeed, they found that low-licking mothers tended to have highly anxious, highly corticosteronaemic offspring. Conversely, mothers with naturally high levels of the licking behaviour tended to have low anxious, low corticosteronaemic offspring (Liu *et al.*, 1997).

These familial traits could thus have a hereditary genetic or experientially mediated impact on gene expression. In a series of studies, these investigators elegantly demonstrated that the latter was the case. In cross-fostering studies, offspring of low-licking mothers were reared by high-licking mothers and, in fact, manifested the biobehavioural signature typical of high-licking offspring, i.e. low levels of corticosterone and low levels of anxiety. Conversely, when offspring from a naturally high-licking mother were cross-fostered by a low-licking one, high levels of corticosterone and high levels of anxiety behaviour were evident (Francis *et al.*, 1999)

Most strikingly, the signature of the second generation followed not the familial pattern, but that induced by the cross-fostering. That is, animals destined to be hypercorticosteronaemic and anxious who were cross-fostered by a high-licking mother had the opposite behavioural signature themselves as adults, and when they later had their offspring, they continued to manifest low corticosterone and anxiety. Thus, a multi-generational change in the biobehavioural signature was induced, based only on a single change in maternal rearing behaviour in one generation (Francis *et al.*, 1999). These data must give one pause about the interpretation of hypothetically hereditary genetic traits which, without the appropriate controls, may on closer examination (such as this one) turn out to depend on familial- and experience-based alterations in gene expression.

Biochemistry of Longer Separations

The neurobiological mechanisms mediating high corticosterone and high anxiety behaviours in the 3-hour separated animals are beginning to be revealed, including distinct changes in the expression of corticotropin-releasing hormone (CRH) in the amygdala and hypothalamus, and a variety of other changes in neuroendocrine and peptide set-points that are permanently altered by repeated maternal deprivation (Plotsky and Meaney, 1993). Other neurobiological changes include a decrease in tone of the inhibitory GABA/benzodiazepine system and increased corticotropin-releasing factor (CRF) and noradrenaline (NA) (Ladd *et al.*, 2000). What is clear from these studies is that some of these stress-related changes in neurobiology can be manifest over the entire life span of the organism. This appears to result from altered levels of gene transcription in critical developmental pathways which, with the proper timing, duration, quality and severity, may change neurobiological set-points in responsivity in an enduring fashion.

Thus, these data provide a plausible set of mechanisms for explaining how early environmental adversity could impart long-lasting effects on biochemistry as well as neuropsychological approaches to self, others, and the environment in parentally neglected and/or traumatized individuals. They also provide a multitude of potential compensatory mechanisms that could alter or even completely reverse this neurobehavioural signature. In the case of the briefly separated rat pup, increased evoked maternal behaviour results in long-lasting stress immunization and less decline in hippocampal function in old age (Plotsky and Meaney, 1993). It is also possible that individual differences in endogenous compensatory mechanisms could similarly play a role as to whether or not a stressor was sufficient to induce the neurochemical change.

Pathological versus Adaptive Changes in Gene Expression

The kindling model clearly elucidates the induction of endogenous compensatory mechanisms at the level of gene expression (Figure XVIII-11.5). Amygdala-kindled seizures evoke a series of alterations that appear related to the primary pathological process of kindling progression and maintenance of the pathological kindled 'memory trace'. At the same time, each seizure evokes a transient increase in a variety of endogenous anticonvulsant factors (Post and Weiss, 1992), including an increase in benzodiazepine and $GABA_A$ receptors as well as increases in neuropeptides that are potentially anticonvulsant by themselves such as thyrotropin-releasing hormone (TRH), cholecystokinin (CCK), neuropeptide Y (NPY) as well as the proconvulsant CRF.

The importance of these adaptations is indicated by the 'time-off from last seizure' effect (Weiss *et al.*, 1995; Post and Weiss, 1996). If an anticonvulsant (such as carbamazepine or diazepam) is given the day after an amygdala-kindled seizure, the drugs are highly effective in their acute anticonvulsant properties. However, if sufficient time from the last seizure is allowed to elapse (without intervening seizures being given) then the same doses of drug are no longer effective, apparently because the seizure-induced endogenous anticonvulsant mechanisms have dissipated over this period. An interval of four days or greater is necessary for carbamazepine to lose its effectiveness, and ten days for diazepam. Levels of TRH and TRH mRNA increase in the hippocampus for approximately four days after amygdala-kindled or electroconvulsive seizures, and benzodiazepine and $GABA_A$ receptor increases slightly longer.

That these data could reflect physiologically relevant endogenous anticonvulsant mechanisms is suggested by two sets of observations (in addition to the increases lasting about the appropriate length of time necessary to observe the 'time-off' effect). Wan *et al.* (1998) found that intra-hippocampal injections of TRH are indeed anticonvulsant against amygdala-kindled seizures. Moreover, in animals that have become tolerant to the anticonvulsant effects of carbamazepine or diazepam, even a full-blown seizure is insufficient to induce the increases in TRH mRNA, suggesting that loss of this and other related compensatory anticonvulsant adaptations could be

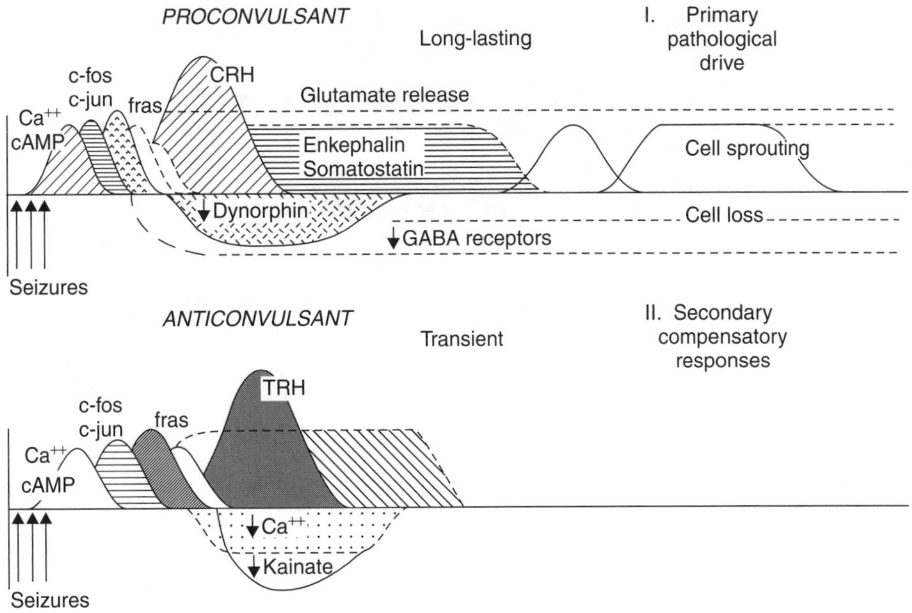

Figure XVIII-11.5 Schematic illustration of potential genomic, neurotransmitter and peptidergic alterations that follow repeated kindled seizures. Putative mechanisms related to the primary pathological drive (i.e. kindled seizure evolution) are illustrated on top and those thought to be related to the secondary compensatory responses (i.e. anticonvulsant effects) are shown on the bottom. The horizontal line represents time. Sequential transient increases in second messengers and immediate early genes (IEGs) are followed by longer lasting alterations in peptides, neurotransmitters and receptors or their mRNAs, as illustrated above the line, whereas decreases are shown below the line. Given the potential unfolding of these competing mechanisms in the evolution of seizure disorders, the question arises regarding whether parallel opposing processes also occur in the course of affective illness or other psychiatric disorders. Endogenous adaptive changes (bottom) may be exploited in the design of the new treatment strategies

linked to a loss of efficacy in instances of tolerance development as well (Figure XVIII-11.6) (Weiss *et al.*, 1995).

The idea that TRH represents an entire class of endogenous compensatory anticonvulsant mechanisms led us to follow up on the earlier observations of Prange and associates (1972) of the acute antidepressant effects of parenteral TRH. Given the evidence for TRH hypersecretion in some depressed patients based on increased levels in the spinal fluid or a blunting of the TSH response to TRH (Loosen and Prange, 1982; Banki *et al.*, 1988), we wondered whether this heightened TRH activity in depression could also represent a depression-induced endogenous antidepressant adaptation.

We thus administered 500 μg of TRH intrathecally in the context of a routine lumbar puncture (LP) in patients with refractory affective disorders and saw substantial antidepressant and antianxiety effects compared with a sham control injection (Marangell *et al.*, 1997). These data are consistent with the notion that increases in TRH observed in some depressed patients are endogenous antidepressant adaptations that, if sufficient, might normally lead to the spontaneous termination of a depressive episode. Although this proposition remains to be definitively tested and demonstrated, the data are not inconsistent with such a viewpoint.

The suggestion that changes in stress or depressive-episode-induced alterations in gene expression may either be part of a primary pathological process or a compensatory adaptation could help account for the inherent intermittency or cyclicity of the recurrent affective disorders (Figure XVIII-11.7) (Post and Weiss, 1996). One could postulate that during periods of relative wellness, the compensatory adaptions (as augmented [or not] by exogenous medications) would be sufficient to counter the underlying pathological processes.

Pathological alteration in gene expression might be driven by either those mediated by the hereditary genetic background or by experientially induced alterations. Similarly, the degree or set-point of the endogenous antidepressant mechanisms could also be determined by either genetic or environmental processes or their interaction (Figure XVIII-11.8). Thus, a predominance of depressive biological processes rather than those pushing to euthymia could be based on relatively low levels of a given compensatory neurochemical element, predisposing to, but not sufficient to result in, depressions. These could be further lowered and eroded by single or repeated episodes of extreme environmental adversity, such that they fail to exceed the threshold for adequate endogenous mechanisms maintaining euthymia.

Such a balance of pathological versus adaptive factors could also take place at the level of reaction to more proximal stressors that could influence the onset of a given affective episode. If appropriate medical and social supports are available, a stressor may not have the same pathological potency. This is most readily elucidated in the learned helplessness model, wherein the animal that receives the stressful tail shock and is able to terminate it by pressing a lever does not show helpless behaviour or the associated biochemical alterations. In contrast, the yoked control animal that receives exactly the same timing, magnitude and duration of the tail shock stress, but does not have the mechanism available for turning it off (ability to act/cope), develops the helpless neurobehavioural syndrome (Seligman and Maier, 1967; Seligman *et al.*, 1980). Thus, resistance to stress-induced behavioural changes could be built in at the level of either decreased pathological neurochemical response or increased compensatory adaptations, each mediated on either a genetic or environmental basis (or their interaction) (Figures XVIII-11.4 and XVIII-11.8). Both of these pathological or adaptive mechanisms could be enhanced or minimized with the appropriate targetted medication, or other somatic or psychotherapeutic treatment interventions.

Such a 'push–pull' model is reminiscent of the emerging perspective on the development of a variety of malignancies. In

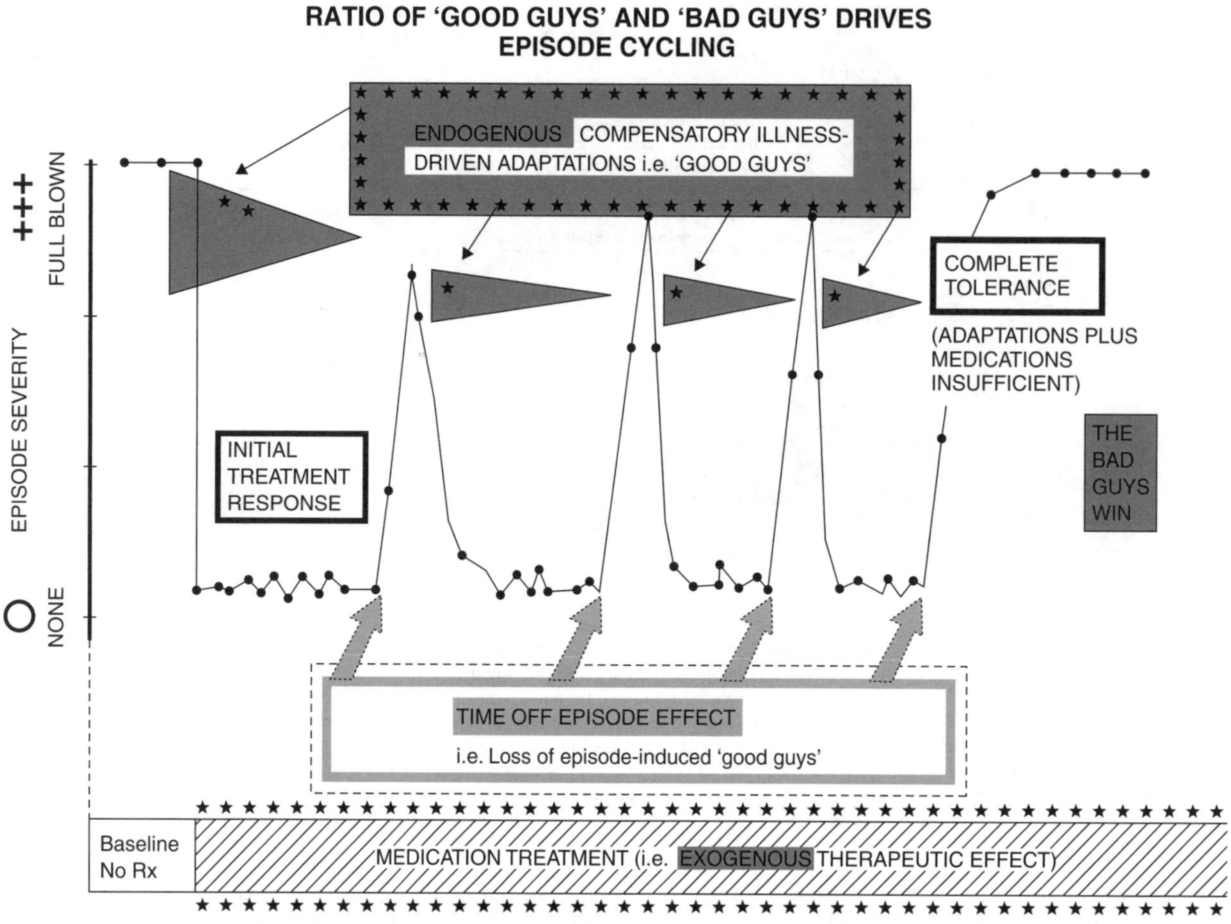

Figure XVIII-11.6 Hypothetical schema of the role of endogenous regulatory factors in the generation and progression of illness cyclicity. After an illness episode, adaptive compensatory mechanisms are induced (i.e. 'good guys'; shaded triangle with two stars), which together with drug treatment suppress the illness (initial treatment response; box). The 'good guys' dissipate with time (i.e. the 'time-off seizure' effect), and episodes of illness re-emerge. Although this re-elicits illness-related compensatory mechanisms, the concurrent drug treatment prevents some of the illness-induced adaptive responses from occurring (smaller triangles with one star). As tolerance proceeds (associated with the loss of adaptive mechanisms) faster illness re-emergence occurs. Thus, the drug is becoming less effective in the face of less robust compensatory mechanisms. The primary pathology is progressively re-emerging, driven by both additional stimulations and episodes (i.e. the kindled memory trace, or the 'bad guys') along with a loss of illness-induced adaptations. Because this cyclic process is presumably driven by the ratio of the 'bad versus good guys' at the level of changes in gene expression, we postulate that such fluctuations in the 'battle of the oncogenes' arising out of illness and treatment-related variables could account for individual patterns in illness cyclicity

the case of colon cancer, a sequence of five to more than a dozen changes in gene expression are required for the full-blown metastatic lesion (Gryfe *et al.*, 1997). These involve both increases in cellular activating, replicating and survival factors, as well as losses of neuroprotective and apoptotic (cell death) factors on the basis of multiple somatic mutations (Figure XVIII-11.9). With enough of this combination of enhanced mechanisms for cell replication and loss of compensatory tumour suppressor and cell death factors, the tumour can progress from a benign hyperplastic lesion to that of an adenoma, full-blown carcinoma, and finally, one with full metastatic malignancy. In the case of a malignancy, these positive and negative effects on gene expression enhancing cell replication and survival occur via the mechanism of somatic mutations, either genetically predisposed from the onset or arising spontaneously.

In a parallel fashion, at the level of experientially induced changes in gene expression interacting with hereditary genetic vulnerabilities, we could envision a similar cumulative progression to full-blown affective illness associated with increased likelihood of suicide attempts, treatment resistance and, ultimately, treatment refractoriness. As with the accumulating somatic mutations in the evolution of a cancer, in affective illness these might involve both increases in virulence of pathological mechanisms and, at the same time, a sequence of losing adaptive and protective mechanisms. This loss of protective factors could arise at the level of endogenous compensatory mechanisms (such as those represented by TRH), or those exogenously provided (such as those represented by some types of medications as well as social and psychotherapeutic support). Just as the animal that learns it is able to terminate the tail shock by pressing a lever does not develop the learned helplessness syndrome, if one approaches severe stressors and losses as adversities to which one can adapt (by virtue of positive distal factors derived from an optimal upbringing or by virtue of proximal factors such as new therapeutic insights), significant degrees of affective dysregulation may not occur (Figure XVIII-11.2 and Figure XVIII-11.8).

Such modulatory influences could, hypothetically, occur with appropriate psychotherapeutic intervention in a dynamic and supportive fashion, or with specific cognitive-behavioural interventions tuned to just these sets of issues and proactive problem solving toward them. However, if one has lost a parent early in life, one

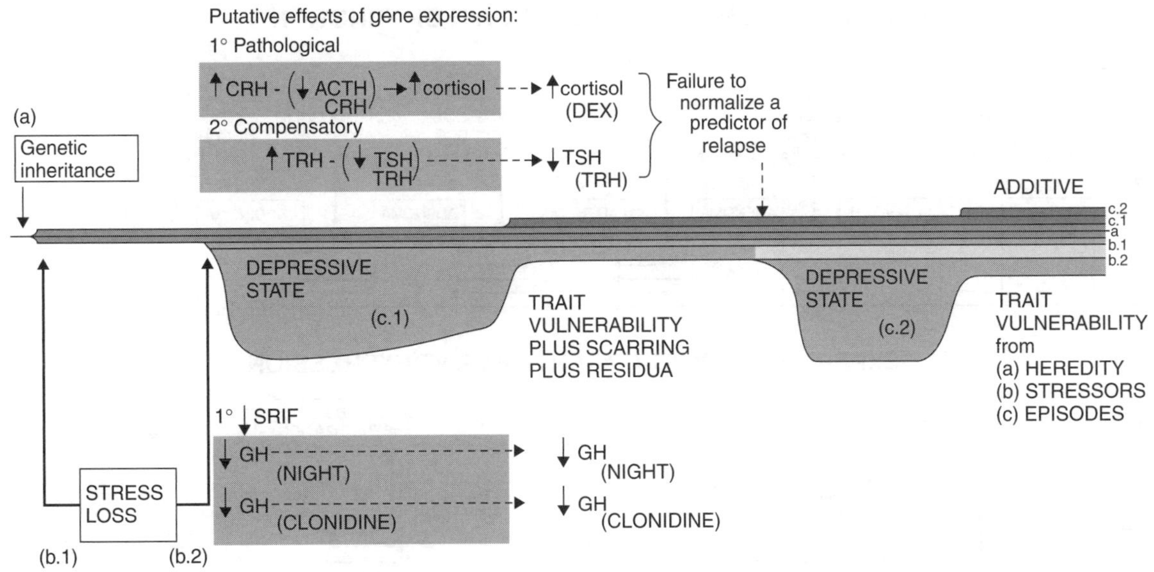

Figure XVIII-11.7 Accumulating experiential genetic vulnerability in recurrent affective illness. Schematic of how initial stressors may leave behind trait vulnerabilities (at the level of alterations in gene expression). With appropriate reactivation by stress of relevant neurobiological systems, the threshold for neuropeptide and hormonal changes associated with a depressive episode may be exceeded. These episode-related alterations may be normalized with the termination of episode but in some instances may persist and add further trait vulnerabilities toward recurrence (c) in addition to the genetic (a) and stressor (b) changes. CRH, corticotropin-releasing hormone; ACTH, adrenocorticotropin-releasing hormone; TRH, thyrotropin-releasing hormone; TSH, thyroid stimulating hormone; DEX, dexamethasone; GH, growth hormone; SRIF, somatostatin

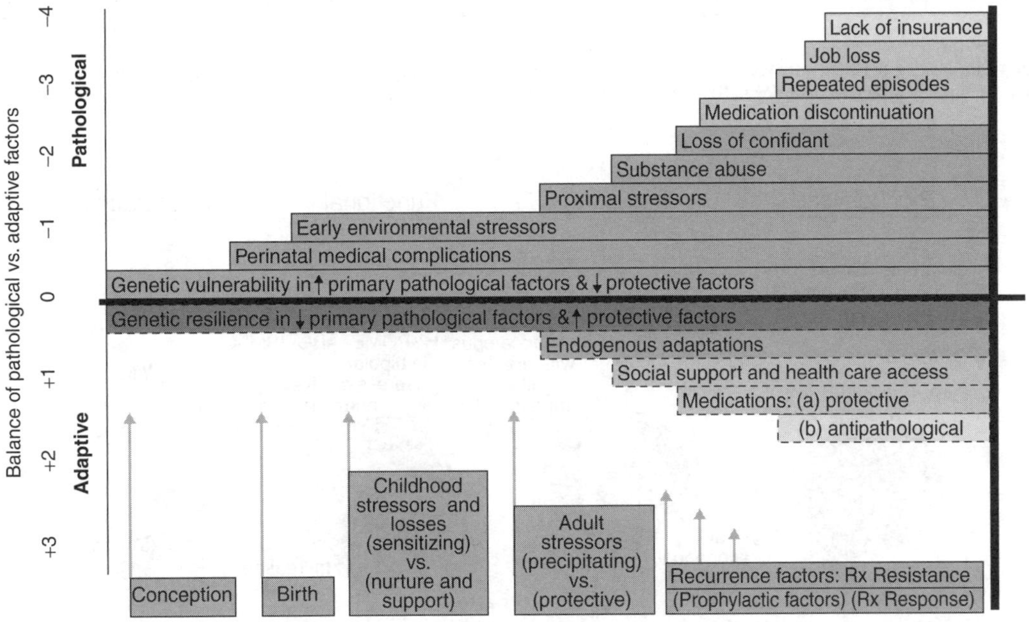

Figure XVIII-11.8 Ratio of pathological versus adaptive factors in determining illness episodes and well intervals

might have the dual liability of the loss itself and the associated failure to have the adaptive developmental benefits of that positive parental experience (in the absence of another stepping in to fill the role). If, in addition, one also loses more proximal social supports through lack of a confidant or inadequate access to health care resources, even malleable problems may appear unsolvable, particularly in the context of an inherent or experientially based set of depressive cognitions.

BRAIN MICROSTRUCTURE CHANGES: ENVIRONMENTAL AND PHARMACOLOGICAL INFLUENCES

A variety of micro- and macrostructural alterations have been described in unipolar and bipolar disorder (Figure XVIII-11.10), including altered cellular arrangements in frontal cortex and decreased glia in the subgenual part of the anterior cingulate gyrus

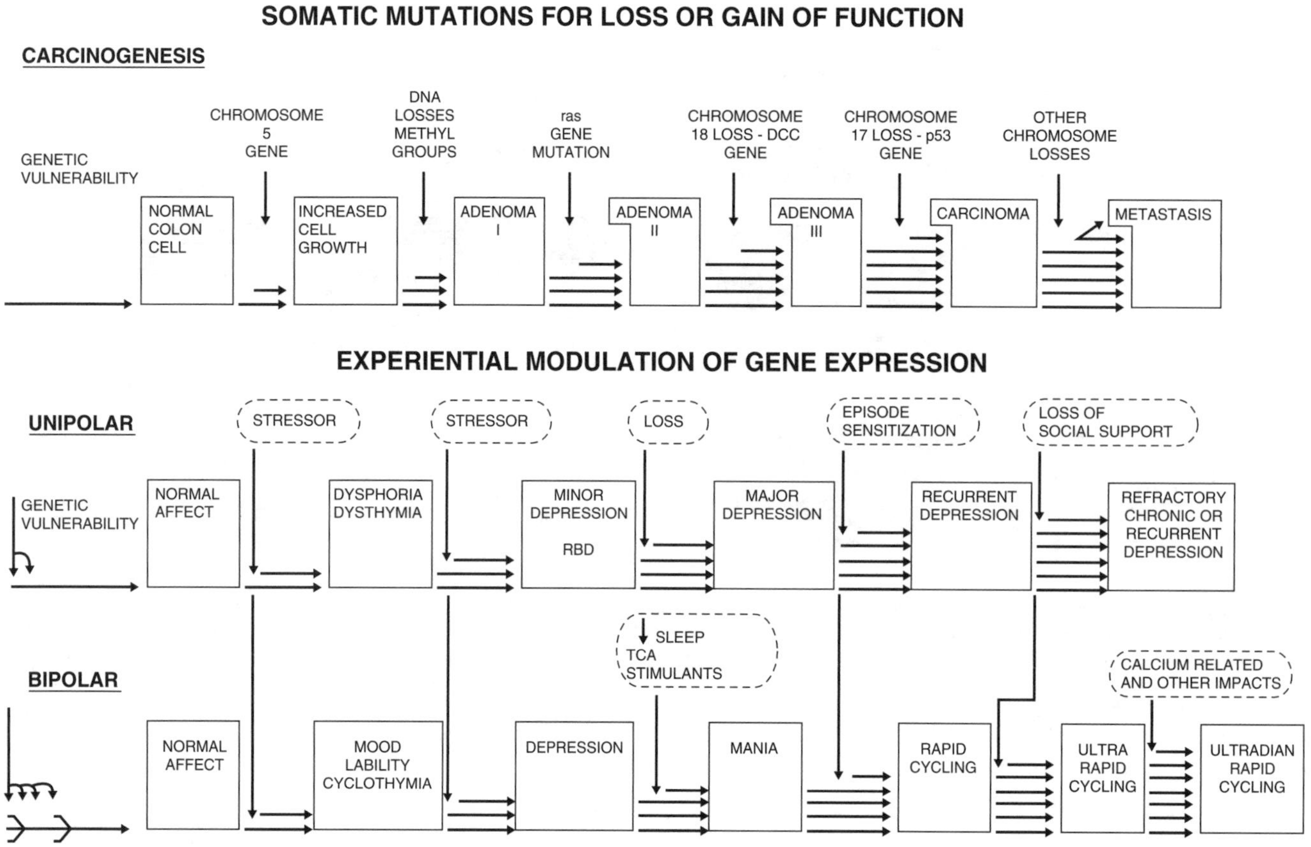

Figure XVIII-11.9 Similarities between somatic mutations in gene expression underlying carcinogenesis and experiential modulation of gene expression observed in unipolar or bipolar affective disorder. RBD, recurrent brief depression; TCA, tricyclic antidepressant

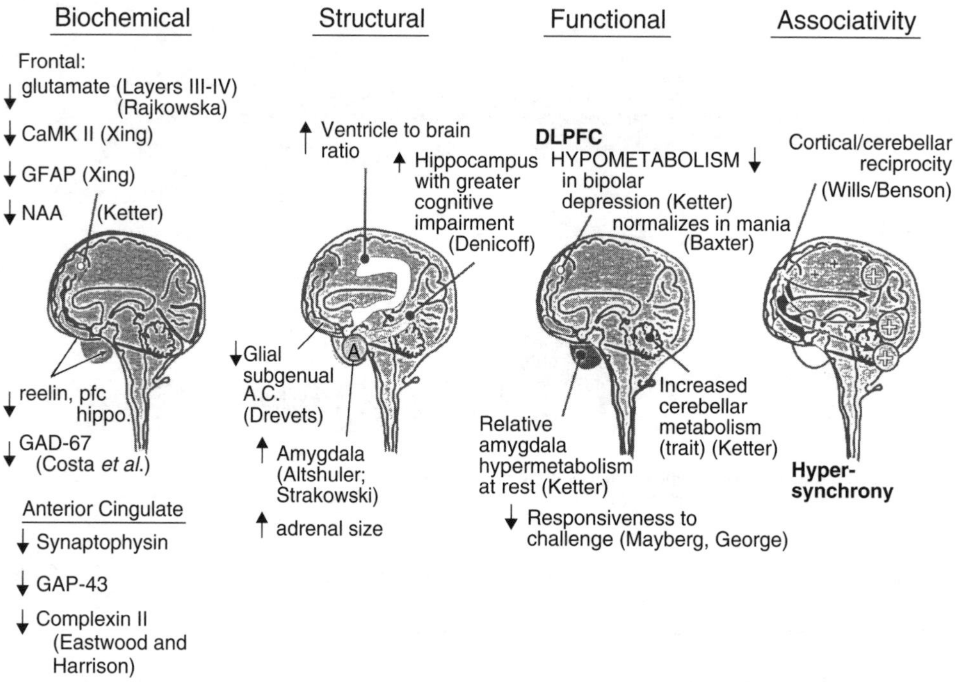

Figure XVIII-11.10 Biochemical, structural, and functional abnormalities in bipolar illness. CaMKII, calcium-calmodulin kinase II; GFAP, glial fibrillary acidic protein; NAA, *N*-acetylaspartate; pfc, prefrontal cortex; hippo., hippocampus; GAD-67, glutamic acid decarboxylase-67; GAP-43, growth associated protein-43; A.C., anterior cortex

(Drevets *et al.*, 1998; Rajkowska, 2000). Alterations in hippocampal size have been reported, as have increases in the size of the amygdala in two studies (Altshuler *et al.*, 1998; Strakowski *et al.*, 1999), but not in all cases (Pearlson *et al.*, 1997). We allude to these structural changes not because they have been definitively demonstrated, but only because they are likely to be contributing factors to the cascade of psychological and neurobiological processes that could be part of the mechanisms involved in illness vulnerability and progression. They may also be markers of high genetic vulnerability (the findings of Drevets *et al.* (1998) were limited to those patients with positive familial histories for affective disorder) or environmental impacts (not unlike the observations of Hubel and Weisel noted previously).

It may be particularly important to conceptualize even these structural alterations as potentially plastic and remediable rather than permanent and immutable. We know that environmental contingencies can be arranged to enhance cell survival, neurogenesis and the increased ratio of progenitor cells converting to neurons as opposed to glia. The latter finding is demonstrated in the studies of Kempermann *et al.* (1998) in which rearing in an enriched environment led to the increase of neural to glial ratio. Similarly, environmental adversity has been shown to decrease the rate of neurogenesis (Gould and Tanapat, 1999), which is estimated to occur in the adult rodent hippocampus at the rate of some 9000 cells per day (Cameron and McKay, 2001). Just as this neurogenesis appears bidirectionally malleable by environmental experiential mechanisms, it also appears to be alterable by pharmacology.

It is perhaps not a coincidence that the antidepressants as a class appear to induce stress counter-regulatory mechanisms at the level of gene expression for neurotrophic factors such as BDNF and neurotrophin-3 (NT3). The studies of Smith and associates at the NIMH (Smith *et al.*, 1995a, b) and those of Duman and colleagues (Nibuya *et al.*, 1995; Duman *et al.*, 1997; Duman, 1998) have revealed that antidepressants exert opposite effects to those of stress on these neurotrophic factors. Moreover, if an animal is stressed while on chronic antidepressant treatment, some of the stress-induced alterations are partially ameliorated or blocked altogether. There appears to be substantial blockade of stress-induced decreases in hippocampal BDNF when animals are co-treated with antidepressants and, concomitantly, a less robust increase in NT3 in the locus coeruleus occurs during antidepressant co-treatment compared with that during the stressor alone.

These data raise a variety of possibilities about the long-term effects of antidepressants in pharmacoprophylaxis of recurrent unipolar depression. Long-term effective prophylaxis could have multiple benefits for the individual with recurrent depression. The relative decrease in depressive episodes that occurs with a phenomenal level of statistical significance ($p < 10^{-34}$; Davis *et al.*, 1993) could spare the patient from considerable morbidity, and potential mortality from the illness by suicide. In addition, if the episode sensitization model proves valid, such pharmacoprophylaxis could alter the long-term course of the illness in a more favourable direction. To the extent that these agents exert some clinically relevant anti-stress effects at the level of gene expression on neurotrophic factors such as BDNF, antidepressants could help to lessen the impact of stressors, either as precipitating events for a depressive episode or on the microstructure of the brain as affected by the ratio of apoptotic to neurotrophic factors.

POTENTIAL NEUROTROPHIC AND NEUROPROTECTIVE EFFECTS OF LITHIUM CARBONATE

The mechanisms of action of lithium carbonate in recurrent affective disorders remain uncertain, although a host of candidate mechanisms have been postulated, as reviewed elsewhere (Post *et al.*, 2000). The latest findings on the mechanisms of lithium are of particular interest in relation to this chapter (Table XVIII-11.1). Lithium appears to exert neuroprotective effects in both a variety of *in vitro* cell culture model systems and *in vivo* in several models. Chuang and colleagues have shown that treatment with lithium reduces both the degree of neurological defect and the size of a brain infarct by approximately 50% in an animal receiving a middle cerebral artery ligation (Nonaka and Chuang, 1998). Similarly, they found that lithium reduced pathological effects of quinolinic acid injection into the striatum, a useful model for the striatal losses of Huntington's disease (Chuang *et al.*, 1999).

The groups headed by Manji and Chuang have demonstrated that lithium treatment is associated with the induction of neuroprotective factors such as Bcl2 and BDNF and decrements in cell death factors such as Bax and p53 (Chen and Chuang, 1999; Chen *et al.*, 1999; Manji *et al.*, 2000). That these alterations could be clinically relevant is revealed by several lines of evidence in addition to the *in vivo* models noted above. The changes in cell culture and in animals occur at clinically relevant concentrations of lithium, and preliminary evidence suggests that three weeks of treatment with lithium is able to increase *N*-acetylaspartate (NAA) in human brain as measured by magnetic resonance spectroscopy (Moore *et al.*, 2000a). Moreover, Moore *et al.* (2000b) demonstrated an increase in grey matter volume (using magnetic resonance imaging) in those exposed to lithium treatment compared with baseline. Thus, it remains possible that even on the level of synaptic and cellular structure of the brain, *endogenous* adaptations and *exogenous*

Table XVIII-11.1 Lithium: anti-apoptotic effects; neuroprotection; antisuicide effects (summary of data from Chuang and colleagues and Manji and colleagues)

In vitro	*In vitro* (rodent)	*In vitro* (Human)
Prevention of apoptosis in cultured neurons: Cerebellar granule cells Hippocampal (DG) cells Cortical cells	↑ Neurogenesis ↓ Size and neurological dysfunction of stroke (ligation MCA)	↓ Clinical suicide (UP & BP) ↓ Excess medical mortality (UP & BP)
Induction of cell survival factors: ↑ BCl-2; ↑ BDNF	↓ Lesion size model Huntington's chorea (Quinolinic acid in striatum)	↑ Neural integrity NAA (MRS) with 3 weeks of lithium
Inhibition of cell death factors: ↓ BAX; ↓ P53	↓ AIDS model apoptosis	↑ Neuronal volume Grey matter (MRI)

neurochemical alterations may be significant factors of short-term, if not long-term, therapeutic value.

Among the psychotropic agents used in the treatment of the recurrent affective disorders, the evidence is best for the antisuicide effect of lithium in those remaining on the drug long term (Muller-Oerlinghausen *et al.*, 1992a, b). Moreover, such long-term lithium treatment also appears to normalize the increased medical mortality that accompanies the recurrent affective disorders (Ahrens *et al.*, 1995). The data on the stroke and Huntington's disease models noted previously raise the question of whether some of lithium's effects on longevity in patients with affective illness could be mediated through cardiovascular and neuroprotective mechanisms in man similar to those demonstrated preclinically.

CONCLUSIONS

Given the multiplicity of postulated genetic and experientially driven changes in gene expression to which we have briefly alluded, one can envision the eventual use of gene therapy in reversing or ameliorating some of the key neurobiological alterations underlying vulnerability to recurrent affective disorders. However, already, currently available approaches include inhibiting or ameliorating adverse environmental experiential effects on gene expression through preventive measures and psychotherapeutic treatment, and enhancing compensatory mechanisms and minimizing primary pathological mechanisms through appropriate pharmacotherapy.

Thus, the conceptual overview espoused here is ripe for both further preclinical experimental testing and exploratory clinical therapeutic interventions. Given the virtually unlimited potential of the human brain for neuroplasticity, we look forward to increasingly effective therapeutics targetted to both pathological and adaptive processes, and ultimately, to the elucidation of the most opportune targets for gene therapy. Even when the era of gene therapy for psychiatric illness arrives, however, a role for interpersonal support and specific psychotherapeutic interventions attuned to the unique needs of patients with recurrent affective disorders will still be crucial to the successful acute treatment and long-term prevention of these otherwise recurrent disorders.

REFERENCES

Ahrens, B., Grof, P., Moller, H.J., Muller-Oerlinghausen, B. and Wolf, T., 1995. Extended survival of patients on long-term lithium treatment. *Can. J. Psychiat.*, **40**, 241–6.

Altshuler, L.L., Bartzokis, G., Grieder, T., Curran, J. and Mintz, J., 1998. Amygdala enlargement in bipolar disorder and hippocampal reduction in schizophrenia: an MRI study demonstrating neuroanatomic specificity [letter]. *Arch. Gen. Psychiat.*, **55**, 663–4.

Anisman, H., Zaharia, M.D., Meaney, M.J. and Merali, Z., 1998. Do early-life events permanently alter behavioural and hormonal responses to stressors? *Int. J. Dev. Neurosci.*, **16**, 149–64.

Banki, C.M., Bissette, G., Arato, M. and Nemeroff, C.B., 1988. Elevation of immunoreactive CSF TRH in depressed patients. *Am. J. Psychiat.*, **145**, 1526–31.

Barrett, G.L., 2000. The p75 neurotrophin receptor and neuronal apoptosis. *Prog. Neurobiol.*, **61**, 205–29.

Beaulieu, S., Rousse, I., Gratton, A., Barden, N. and Rochford, J., 1994. Behavioural and endocrine impact of impaired type II glucocorticoid receptor function in a transgenic mouse model. *Ann. N. Y. Acad. Sci.*, **746**, 388–91.

Berman, K.F., Torrey, E.F., Daniel, D.G. and Weinberger, D.R., 1992. Regional cerebral blood flow in monozygotic twins discordant and concordant for schizophrenia. *Arch. Gen. Psychiat.*, **49**, 927–34.

Bifulco, A.T., Brown, G.W. and Harris, T.O., 1987. Childhood loss of parent, lack of adequate parental care and adult depression: a replication. *J. Affect. Disord.*, **12**, 115–28.

Bolshakov, V.Y. and Siegelbaum, S.A., 1994. Postsynaptic induction and presynaptic expression of hippocampal long-term depression. *Science*, **264**, 1148–52.

Breier, A., Kelsoe, J.R.J., Kirwin, P.D., Beller, S.A., Wolkowitz, O.M. and Pickar, D., 1988. Early parental loss and development of adult psychopathology. *Arch. Gen. Psychiat.*, **45**, 987–93.

Bremner, J.D., Narayan, M., Anderson, E.R., Staib, L.H., Miller, H.L. and Charney, D.S., 2000. Hippocampal volume reduction in major depression. *Am. J. Psychiat.*, **157**, 115–18.

Bremner, J.D., Randall, P., Scott, T.M., Bronen, R.A., Seibyl, J.P., Southwick, S.M., Delaney, R.C., McCarthy, G., Charney, D.S. and Innis, R.B., 1995. MRI-based measurement of hippocampal volume in patients with combat-related posttraumatic stress disorder. *Am. J. Psychiat.*, **152**, 973–81.

Bremner, J.D., Randall, P., Vermetten, E., Staib, L., Bronen, R.A., Mazure, C., Capelli, S., McCarthy, G., Innis, R.B. and Charney, D.S., 1997. Magnetic resonance imaging-based measurement of hippocampal volume in posttraumatic stress disorder related to childhood physical and sexual abuse—a preliminary report. *Biol. Psychiat.*, **41**, 23–32.

Bremner, J.D., Southwick, S.M., Johnson, D.R., Yehuda, R. and Charney, D.S., 1993. Childhood physical abuse and combat-related posttraumatic stress disorder in Vietnam veterans. *Am. J. Psychiat.*, **150**, 235–9.

Breslau, N., Chilcoat, H.D., Kessler, R.C. and Davis, G.C., 1999. Previous exposure to trauma and PTSD effects of subsequent trauma: results from the Detroit Area Survey of Trauma. *Am. J. Psychiat.*, **156**, 902–7.

Brown, G.W., Harris, T.O. and Peto, J., 1973b. Life events and psychiatric disorders Part 2: Nature of causal link. *Psychol. Med.*, **3**, 159–76.

Brown, G.W., Sklair, F., Harris, T.O. and Birley, J.L.T., 1973a. Life events and psychiatric disorders Part 1: Some methodological issues. *Psychol. Med.*, **3**, 74–87.

Cameron, H.A. and McKay, R.D., 2001. Adult neurogenesis produces a large pool of new granule cells in the dentate gyrus. *J. Comp Neurol.*, **435**, 406–417.

Chen, G., Zeng, W.Z., Yuan, P.X., Huang, L.D., Jiang, Y.M., Zhao, Z.H. and Manji, H.K., 1999. The mood-stabilizing agents lithium and valproate robustly increase the levels of the neuroprotective protein bcl-2 in the CNS. *J. Neurochem.*, **72**, 879–82.

Chen, R.W. and Chuang, D.M., 1999. Long term lithium treatment suppresses p53 and Bax expression but increases Bcl-2 expression. A prominent role in neuroprotection against excitotoxicity. *J. Biol. Chem.*, **274**, 6039–42.

Chuang, D.M., Wei, H., Qin, Z., Wei, W., Wang, Y. and Qian, Y., 1999. Lithium inhibits striatal damage in an animal model of Huntington's disease. *Soc. Neurosci. Abstr.*, **25**, 600.

Davis, J.M., Wang, Z. and Janicak, P.G., 1993. A quantitative analysis of clinical drug trials for the treatment of affective disorders. *Psychopharmacol. Bull.*, **29**, 175–81.

Drevets, W.C., Ongur, D. and Price, J.L., 1998. Neuroimaging abnormalities in the subgenual prefrontal cortex: implications for the pathophysiology of familial mood disorders. *Molec. Psychiat.*, **3**, 220–1.

Duman, R.S., 1998. Novel therapeutic approaches beyond the serotonin receptor. *Biol. Psychiat.*, **44**, 324–35.

Duman, R.S., Heninger, G.R. and Nestler, E.J., 1997. A molecular and cellular theory of depression. *Arch. Gen. Psychiat.*, **54**, 597–606.

Emde, R.N., Polak, P.R. and Spitz, R.A., 1965. Anaclitic depression in an infant raised in an institution. *J. Am. Acad. Child Psychiat.*, **4**, 545–53.

Field, T.M., Schanberg, S.M., Scafidi, F., Bauer, C.R., Vega-Lahr, N., Garcia, R., Nystrom, J. and Kuhn, C.M., 1986. Tactile/kinesthetic stimulation effects on preterm neonates. *Pediatrics*, **77**, 654–8.

Francis, D., Diorio, J., Liu, D. and Meaney, M.J., 1999. Nongenomic transmission across generations of maternal behaviour and stress responses in the rat. *Science*, **286**, 1155–8.

Gould, E. and Tanapat, P., 1999. Stress and hippocampal neurogenesis. *Biol. Psychiat.*, **46**, 1472–9.

Gryfe, R., Swallow, C., Bapat, B., Redston, M., Gallinger, S. and Couture, J., 1997. Molecular biology of colorectal cancer. *Curr. Probl. Cancer*, **21**, 233–300.

Gurvits, T.V., Shenton, M.E., Hokama, H., Ohta, H., Lasko, N.B., Gilbertson, M.W., Orr, S.P., Kikinis, R., Jolesz, F.A., McCarley, R.W. and Pitman, R.K., 1996. Magnetic resonance imaging study of hippocampal volume in chronic, combat-related posttraumatic stress disorder. *Biol. Psychiat.*, **40**, 1091–9.

Hammen, C. and Gitlin, M., 1997. Stress reactivity in bipolar patients and its relation to prior history of disorder. *Am. J. Psychiat.*, **154**, 856–7.

Harlow, H.F., Dodsworth, R.O. and Harlow, M.K., 1965. Total social isolation in monkeys. *Proc. Natl Acad. Sci. USA*, **54**, 90–7.

Harmon, R.J., Wagonfeld, S. and Emde, R.N., 1982. Anaclitic depression. A follow-up from infancy to puberty. *Psychoanal. Study Child*, **37**, 67–94.

Harris, T., Brown, G.W. and Bifulco, A., 1986. Loss of parent in childhood and adult psychiatric disorder: the role of lack of adequate parental care. *Psychol. Med.*, **16**, 641–59.

Harris, T., Brown, G.W. and Bifulco, A., 1987. Loss of parent in childhood and adult psychiatric disorder: the role of social class position and premarital pregnancy. *Psychol. Med.*, **17**, 163–83.

Hauser, P., Matochik, J., Altshuler, L.L., Denicoff, K.D., Conrad, A., Li, X. and Post, R.M., 2000. MRI-based measurements of temporal lobe and ventricular structures in patients with bipolar I and bipolar II disorders. *J. Affect. Disord.*, **60**, 25–32.

Hubel, D.H. and Wiesel, T.N., 1979. Brain mechanisms of vision. *Sci. Am.*, **241**, 150–62.

Hubel, D.H. and Wiesel, T.N., 1998. Early exploration of the visual cortex. *Neuron*, **20**, 401–12.

Huot, R.L., Thrivikraman, K.V., Meaney, M.J. and Plotsky, P.M., 2001. Development of adult ethanol preference and anxiety as a consequence of neonatal maternal separation in Long Evans rats and reversal with antidepressant treatment. *Psychopharmacol (Berl)*, **158**, 366–373.

Kempermann, G., Kuhn, H.G. and Gage, F.H., 1998. Experience-induced neurogenesis in the senescent dentate gyrus. *J. Neurosci.*, **18**, 3206–12.

Kendler, K.S., Kessler, R.C., Neale, M.C., Heath, A.C. and Eaves, L.J., 1993. The prediction of major depression in women: toward an integrated etiologic model. *Am. J. Psychiat.*, **150**, 1139–48.

Kessing, L.V., 1998. Recurrence in affective disorder. II. Effect of age and gender. *Br. J. Psychiat.*, **172**, 29–34.

Kessing, L.V., Andersen, P.K., Mortensen, P.B. and Bolwig, T.G., 1998. Recurrence in affective disorder. I. Case register study. *Br. J. Psychiat.*, **172**, 23–8.

Knable, M.B., 1999. Schizophrenia and bipolar disorder: findings from studies of the Stanley Foundation Brain Collection. *Schizophrenia Res.*, **39**, 149–52.

Korte, M., Kang, H., Bonhoeffer, T. and Schuman, E., 1998. A role for BDNF in the late-phase of hippocampal long-term potentiation. *Neuropharmacology*, **37**, 553–9.

Korte, M., Staiger, V., Griesbeck, O., Thoenen, H. and Bonhoeffer, T., 1996. The involvement of brain-derived neurotrophic factor in hippocampal long-term potentiation revealed by gene targeting experiments. *J. Physiol. Paris*, **90**, 157–64.

Kraepelin, E., 1921. *Manic-Depressive Insanity and Paranoia*. E.S. Livingstone, Edinburgh.

Kuhn, C.M., Butler, S.R. and Schanberg, S.M., 1978. Selective depression of serum growth hormone during maternal deprivation in rat pups. *Science*, **201**, 1034–6.

Ladd, C.O., Huot, R.L., Thrivikraman, K.V., Nemeroff, C.B., Meaney, M.J. and Plotsky, P.M., 2000. Long-term behavioural and neuroendocrine adaptations to adverse early experience. *Prog. Brain Res.*, **122**, 81–103.

Lawrie, S.M. and Abukmeil, S.S., 1998. Brain abnormality in schizophrenia. A systematic and quantitative review of volumetric magnetic resonance imaging studies. *Br. J. Psychiat.*, **172**, 110–20.

Leverich, G.S., McElroy, S.L., Suppes, T., Keck, P.E., Jr, Denicoff, K.D., Nolen, W.A., Altshuler, L.L., Rush, A.J., Kupka, R., Frye, M., Autio, K. and Post, R.M., 2002a. Early physical and sexual abuse associated with an adverse course of bipolar illness. *Biol. Psychiat.*, **51**, 288–97.

Leverich, G.S., Altshuler, L.L., Frye, M.A., Suppes, T., Keck, P.E., Jr., McElroy, S., Denicoff, K.D., Obrocea, G., Nolen, W.A., Kupka, R., Walden, J., Grunze, H., Perez, S., Luckenbaugh, D. and Post, R.M., 2002b. Factors associated with suicide attempts in 648 patients with bipolar disorder in the Stanley Foundation Bipolar Network. Manuscript submitted for publication.

Levine, S., Huchton, D.M., Wiener, S.G. and Rosenfeld, P., 1991. Time course of the effect of maternal deprivation on the hypothalamic–pituitary–adrenal axis in the infant rat. *Dev. Psychobiol.*, **24**, 547–58.

Liu, D., Diorio, J., Tannenbaum, B., Caldji, C., Francis, D., Freedman, A., Sharma, S., Pearson, D., Plotsky, P.M. and Meaney, M.J., 1997. Maternal care, hippocampal glucocorticoid receptors, and hypothalamic-pituitary-adrenal responses to stress. *Science*, **277**, 1659–62.

Loosen, P.T. and Prange, A.J., Jr., 1982. Serum thyrotropin response to thyrotropin-releasing hormone in psychiatric patients: a review. *Am. J. Psychiat.*, **139**, 405–16.

Malenka, R.C., Kauer, J.A., Perkel, D.J. and Nicoll, R.A., 1989. The impact of postsynaptic calcium on synaptic transmission — its role in long-term potentiation. *Trends Neurosci.*, **12**, 444–50.

Malenka, R.C. and Nicoll, R.A., 1999. Long-term potentiation — a decade of progress? *Science*, **285**, 1870–4.

Manji, H.K., Moore, G.J., Rajkowska, G. and Chen, G., 2000. Neuroplasticity and cellular resilience in mood disorders. *Molec. Psychiat.*, **5**, 578–93.

Marangell, L.B., George, M.S., Callahan, A.M., Ketter, T.A., Pazzaglia, P.J., L'Herrou, T.A., Leverich, G.S. and Post, R.M., 1997. Effects of intrathecal thyrotropin-releasing hormone (protirelin) in refractory depressed patients. *Arch. Gen. Psychiat.*, **54**, 214–22.

Meaney, M.J., Brake, W. and Gratton, A., 2002. Environmental regulation of the development of mesolimbic dopamine systems: a neurobiological mechanism for vulnerability to drug abuse? *Psychoneuroendocrinol*, **27**, 127–138.

Moore, G.J., Bebchuk, J.M., Hasanat, K., Chen, G., Seraji-Bozorgzad, N., Wilds, I.B., Faulk, M.W., Koch, S., Glitz, D.A., Jolkovsky, L. and Manji, H.K., 2000a. Lithium increases *N*-acetyl-aspartate in the human brain: *in vivo* evidence in support of bcl-2's neurotrophic effects? *Biol. Psychiat.*, **48**, 1–8.

Moore, G.J., Bebchuk, J.M., Wilds, I.B., Chen, G. and Manji, H.K., 2000b. Lithium-induced increase in human brain grey matter. *Lancet*, **356**, 1241–2.

Muller-Oerlinghausen, B., Ahrens, B., Grof, E., Grof, P., Lenz, G., Schou, M., Simhandl, C., Thau, K., Volk, J. and Wolf, R., 1992b. The effect of long-term lithium treatment on the mortality of patients with manic-depressive and schizoaffective illness. *Acta Psychiatr. Scand.*, **86**, 218–22.

Muller-Oerlinghausen, B., Muser-Causemann, B. and Volk, J., 1992a. Suicides and parasuicides in a high-risk patient group on and off lithium long-term medication. *J. Affect. Disord.*, **25**, 261–9.

Nibuya, M., Morinobu, S. and Duman, R.S., 1995. Regulation of BDNF and trkB mRNA in rat brain by chronic electroconvulsive seizure and antidepressant drug treatments. *J. Neurosci.*, **15**, 7539–47.

Nonaka, S. and Chuang, D.M., 1998. Neuroprotective effects of chronic lithium on focal cerebral ischemia in rats. *Neuroreport*, **9**, 2081–4.

Ongur, D., Drevets, W.C. and Price, J.L., 1998. Glial reduction in the subgenual prefrontal cortex in mood disorders. *Proc. Natl. Acad. Sci. USA*, **95**, 13290–5.

Pauk, J., Kuhn, C.M., Field, T.M. and Schanberg, S.M., 1986. Positive effects of tactile versus kinesthetic or vestibular stimulation on neuroendocrine and ODC activity in maternally-deprived rat pups. *Life Sci.*, **39**, 2081–7.

Pearlson, G.D., Barta, P.E., Powers, R.E., Menon, R.R., Richards, S.S., Aylward, E.H., Federman, E.B., Chase, G.A., Petty, R.G. and Tien, A.Y., 1997. Ziskind–Somerfeld Research Award 1996. Medial and superior temporal gyral volumes and cerebral asymmetry in schizophrenia versus bipolar disorder. *Biol. Psychiat.*, **41**, 1–14.

Pepin, M.C., Pothier, F. and Barden, N., 1992. Impaired type II glucocorticoid-receptor function in mice bearing antisense RNA transgene. *Nature*, **355**, 725–8.

Plotsky, P.M. and Meaney, M.J., 1993. Early, postnatal experience alters hypothalamic corticotropin-releasing factor (CRF) mRNA, median eminence CRF content and stress-induced release in adult rats. *Molec. Brain Res.*, **18**, 195–200.

Post, R.M., 1992. Transduction of psychosocial stress into the neurobiology of recurrent affective disorder. *Am. J. Psychiat.*, **149**, 999–1010.

Post, R.M. and Weiss, S.R., 1992. Ziskind–Somerfeld Research Award 1992. Endogenous biochemical abnormalities in affective illness: therapeutic versus pathogenic. *Biol. Psychiat.*, **32**, 469–84.

Post, R.M. and Weiss, S.R.B., 1996. A speculative model of affective illness cyclicity based on patterns of drug tolerance observed in amygdala-kindled seizures. *Molec. Neurobiol.*, **13**, 33–60.

Post, R.M., Weiss, S.R.B., Clark, M., Chuang, D.M., Hough, C. and Li, H., 2000. Lithium, carbamazepine and valproate in affective illness: biochemical and neurobiological mechanisms. In: Manji, H., Bowden, C.L. and Belmaker, R.H. (eds), *Bipolar Medications: Mechanisms of Action*, pp. 219–48. American Psychiatric Press, Washington, DC.

Powell, G.F., Brasel, J.A. and Blizzard, R.M., 1967. Emotional deprivation and growth retardation simulating idiopathic hypopituitarism. I. Clinical evaluation of the syndrome. *N. Engl. J. Med.*, **276**, 1271–8.

Prange, A.J., Jr, Lara, P.P., Wilson, I.C., Alltop, L.B. and Breese, G.R., 1972. Effects of thyrotropin-releasing hormone in depression. *Lancet*, **2**(7785), 999–1002.

Rajkowska, G., 2000. Postmortem studies in mood disorders indicate altered numbers of neurons and glial cells. *Biol. Psychiat.*, **48**, 766–77.

Rajkowska, G., Miguel-Hidalgo, J.J., Wei, J., Dilley, G., Pittman, S.D., Meltzer, H.Y., Overholser, J.C., Roth, B.L. and Stockmeier, C.A., 1999. Morphometric evidence for neuronal and glial prefrontal cell pathology in major depression. *Biol. Psychiat.*, **45**, 1085–98.

Rots, N.Y., De Jong, J., Workel, J.O., Levine, S., Cools, A.R. and De Kloet, E.R., 1996. Neonatal maternally deprived rats have as adults elevated basal pituitary-adrenal activity and enhanced susceptibility to apomorphine. *J. Neuroendocrinol.*, **8**, 501–6.

Selemon, L.D., Rajkowska, G. and Goldman-Rakic, P.S., 1995. Abnormally high neuronal density in the schizophrenic cortex. A morphometric analysis of prefrontal area 9 and occipital area 17. *Arch. Gen. Psychiat.*, **52**, 805–18; discussion 819-2.

Selemon, L.D., Rajkowska, G. and Goldman-Rakic, P.S., 1998. Elevated neuronal density in prefrontal area 46 in brains from schizophrenic patients: application of a three-dimensional, stereologic counting method. *J. Comp. Neurol.*, **392**, 402–12.

Seligman, M.E. and Maier, S.F., 1967. Failure to escape traumatic shock. *J. Exp. Psychol.*, **74**, 1–9.

Seligman, M.E., Weiss, J., Weinraub, M. and Schulman, A., 1980. Coping behaviour: learned helplessness, physiological change and learned inactivity. *Behav. Res. Ther.*, **18**, 459–512.

Sheline, Y.I., Wang, P.W., Gado, M.H., Csernansky, J.G. and Vannier, M.W., 1996. Hippocampal atrophy in recurrent major depression. *Proc. Natl Acad. Sci. USA*, **93**, 3908–13.

Silva, A.J., Stevens, C.F., Tonegawa, S. and Wang, Y., 1992. Deficient hippocampal long-term potentiation in alpha-calcium-calmodulin kinase II mutant mice. *Science*, **257**, 201–6.

Smith, M.A., Kim, S.Y., van Oers, H.J. and Levine, S., 1997. Maternal deprivation and stress induce immediate early genes in the infant rat brain. *Endocrinology*, **138**, 4622–8.

Smith, M.A., Makino, S., Altemus, M., Michelson, D., Hong, S.K., Kvetnansky, R. and Post, R.M., 1995b. Stress and antidepressants differentially regulate neurotrophin 3 mRNA expression in the locus coeruleus. *Proc. Natl Acad. Sci. USA*, **92**, 8788–92.

Smith, M.A., Makino, S., Kvetnansky, R. and Post, R.M., 1995a. Stress and glucocorticoids affect the expression of brain-derived neurotrophic factor and neurotrophin-3 mRNAs in the hippocampus. *J. Neurosci.*, **15**, 1768–77.

Stanton, M.E., Gutierrez, Y.R. and Levine, S., 1988. Maternal deprivation potentiates pituitary-adrenal stress responses in infant rats. *Behav. Neurosci.*, **102**, 692–700.

Stein, M.B., Koverola, C., Hanna, C., Torchia, M.G. and McClarty, B., 1997. Hippocampal volume in women victimized by childhood sexual abuse. *Psychol. Med.*, **27**, 951–9.

Strakowski, S.M., DelBello, M.P., Sax, K.W., Zimmerman, M.E., Shear, P.K., Hawkins, J.M. and Larson, E.R., 1999. Brain magnetic resonance imaging of structural abnormalities in bipolar disorder. *Arch. Gen. Psychiat.*, **56**, 254–60.

Suchecki, D., Mozaffarian, D., Gross, G., Rosenfeld, P. and Levine, S., 1993. Effects of maternal deprivation on the ACTH stress response in the infant rat. *Neuroendocrinology*, **57**, 204–12.

Suddath, R.L., Christison, G.W., Torrey, E.F., Casanova, M.F. and Weinberger, D.R., 1990. Anatomical abnormalities in the brains of monozygotic twins discordant for schizophrenia. *N. Engl J. Med.*, **322**, 789–94.

Suomi, S.J., Harlow, H.F. and Domek, C.J., 1970. Effect of repetitive infant–infant separation of young monkeys. *J. Abnorm. Psychol.*, **76**, 161–72.

Torrey, E.F., Taylor, E.H., Gottesman, I.I. and Bowler, A.E., 1995. *Schizophrenia and Manic-Depressive Disorder: The Biological Roots of Mental Illness as Revealed by the Landmark Study of Identical Twins*. Basic Books, New York.

Vakili, K., Pillay, S.S., Lafer, B., Fava, M., Renshaw, P.F., Bonello-Cintron, C.M. and Yurgelun-Todd, D.A., 2000. Hippocampal volume in primary unipolar major depression: a magnetic resonance imaging study. *Biol. Psychiat.*, **47**, 1087–90.

Wan, R.Q., Noguera, E.C. and Weiss, S.R., 1998. Anticonvulsant effects of intra-hippocampal injection of TRH in amygdala kindled rats. *Neuroreport*, **9**, 677–82.

Weinberger, D.R., Berman, K.F., Suddath, R. and Torrey, E.F., 1992. Evidence of dysfunction of a prefrontal-limbic network in schizophrenia: a magnetic resonance imaging and regional cerebral blood flow study of discordant monozygotic twins. *Am. J. Psychiat.*, **149**, 890–7.

Weiss, S.R., Clark, M., Rosen, J.B., Smith, M.A. and Post, R.M., 1995. Contingent tolerance to the anticonvulsant effects of carbamazepine: relationship to loss of endogenous adaptive mechanisms. *Brain Res. Brain Res. Rev.*, **20**, 305–25.

Wiesel, T.N. and Hubel, D.H., 1965. Comparison of the effects of unilateral and bilateral eye closure on cortical unit responses in kittens. *J. Neurophysiol.*, **28**, 1029–40.

Xing, G.Q., Smith, M.A., Levine, S., Yang, S.T., Post, R.M. and Zhang, L.X., 1998. Suppression of CaMKII and nitric oxide synthase by maternal deprivation in the brain of rat pups. *Soc. Neurosci.*, **24**, 452.

Xing, G.Q., Russell, S., Hough, C., O'Grady, J., Zhang, L., Yang, S., Zhang, L.X. and Post, R.M., 2002. *NeuroReport*, **13**, 501–505.

Yehuda, R., Kahana, B., Schmeidler, J., Southwick, S.M., Wilson, S. and Giller, E.L., 1995. Impact of cumulative lifetime trauma and recent stress on current posttraumatic stress disorder symptoms in holocaust survivors. *Am. J. Psychiat.*, **152**, 1815–18.

Young, L.D., Suomi, S.S., Harlow, H.F. and McKinney, W.T., Jr., 1973. Early stress and later response to separation in rhesus monkeys. *Am. J. Psychiat.*, **130**, 400–5.

Zhang, L.X., Xing, G.Q., Levine, S., Post, R.M. and Smith, M.A., 1998. Effects of maternal deprivation on neurotrophic factors and apoptosis-related genes in rat pups. *Soc. Neurosci. Abstr.*, **24**, 451.

Zhang, L.X., Levine, S., Dent, G., Zhan, Y., Xing, G., Okimoto, D., Kathleen, G.M., Post, R.M. and Smith, M.A., 2002. *Brain Res. Dev. Brain Res.*, **133**, 1–11.

XVIII-12

Female-Specific Mood Disorders

Meir Steiner, Edward Dunn, Leslie Born

The lifetime prevalence of mood disorders in women is approximately twice that of men. This higher incidence of depression in women is primarily seen from puberty on and is less marked in the years after menopause (Weissman and Olfson, 1995), with the exception of an additional perimenopausal blip (Kessler *et al.*, 1993). The underlying causality of this gender difference in mood-related disorders is not clear at this time. Since mood disorders occur in both men and women it is assumed that a unified basis for the development of these diseases exists. The principal constituent of this unified theory is believed to be related to genetic predisposition. Multiple environmental stressful events cause biochemical changes in a host of neuroendocrine systems and neuroanatomical areas. The genetic predisposition, which is multi-factorial, determines how stressful life events are interpreted and predicts the response, which can lead to the development of mood disorders (Heim and Nemeroff, 2001).

Notwithstanding, marked variations in the presentation of depression, comorbidity and treatment point to meaningful underlying sex differences. Women are about twice as likely as men to suffer from major depression or dysthymia (Kessler *et al.*, 1994; Weissman *et al.*, 1991). Women are prone to depressive episodes triggered by hormonal fluctuations related to reproductive events, such as during the premenstrual period, during pregnancy or the post-partum period, and around the menopause. Clinically, women present with a notably different depression symptom profile and more often develop a seasonal pattern to their depression (Ernst and Angst, 1992; Frank *et al.*, 1988; Leibenluft *et al.*, 1995; Moldin *et al.*, 1993; Whybrow, 1995). The burden of illness in women with chronic depression is profound (Kornstein *et al.*, 2000), while men may be more likely to 'forget' depressive episodes over time, a phenomenon which in turn may serve to protect them against recurrence (Ernst and Angst, 1992; Nolen-Hoeksema, 1987). Sex differences in the efficacy and tolerability of antidepressant medications is suggested by placebo-controlled and comparative studies (Kornstein, 1997, 2001; Kornstein and Wojcik, 2000). Moreover, there are marked differences between men and women in the pharmacokinetic and pharmacodynamic parameters of a number of psychotropic agents, including antidepressants (Kornstein and Wojcik, 2000; Yonkers *et al.*, 1992).

Collectively, the literature points to a higher prevalence of mood disorders in women related to an increased genetic predisposition, an increased vulnerability/exposure to stressful life events, modulation of the neuroendocrine system by fluctuating gonadal hormones, or a combination of any or all of these factors.

A biological susceptibility hypothesis has been previously proposed, to account for gender differences in the prevalence of mood disorders based on the idea that there is a disturbance in the interaction between the hypothalamic–pituitary–gonadal (HPG) axis and other neuromodulators in women (Dunn and Steiner, 2000; Meller *et al.*, 2001; Steiner and Dunn, 1996; Young *et al.*, 2000). According to this hypothesis, the neuroendocrine rhythmicity related to female reproduction is vulnerable to change and is sensitive to psychosocial, environmental and physiological factors. Thus, premenstrual dysphoric disorder (PMDD), depression with post-partum onset (PPD), and mood disorders associated with the perimenopause or with menopause may all be related to hormone-modulated changes in neurotransmitter function.

Control of mood and behaviour involves many different neurotransmitter systems, including glutamate, gamma aminobutyric acid (GABA), acetylcholine (ACh), serotonin (5-HT), dopamine (DA), noradrenalin (NA) and neuropeptides. Given the observation that prevalence and symptomatology of mood disorders is often different between males and females, it is presumed that gonadal steroid hormones are somehow involved. For example, declining levels of oestrogen in women have been associated with post-natal depression and postmenopausal depression, and the cyclical variations of oestrogens and progesterone are probably the trigger of premenstrual complaints in women with premenstrual syndrome (Fink *et al.*, 1996). The interaction between neurotransmitters and steroid hormones is extremely complex and delicately balanced. Each system appears to have a modulatory function on the other, and changes in one system may have dramatic effect on the other systems.

Glucocorticoid and gonadal steroid receptors are abundant in different areas of the brain. Gonadal steroid receptors are found in the amygdala, hippocampus, basal forebrain, cortex, cerebellum, locus ceruleus, midbrain raphe nuclei, pituitary gland and hypothalamus (Stomati *et al.*, 1998). Oestrogen receptors are also located in the preoptic area and amygdala (McEwen, 1988) and in the ventromedial nucleus and arcuate nucleus of the hypothalamus (Herbison *et al.*, 1995).

Activation of cholinergic, dopaminergic or adrenergic neurotransmitter systems can alter concentrations of cytosolic hypothalamic oestrogen receptors. Muscarinic agonists and antagonists can increase oestrogen-binding sites in the female rat hypothalamus (Lauber and Whalen, 1988). Oestrogen, progesterone and glucocorticoid receptors can also be activated by insulin-like growth factor 1 (IGF-1), epidermal growth factor (EGF), transforming growth factor alpha (TGF-alpha), cyclic AMP (cAMP), protein kinase activators and by various neurotransmitters (Culig *et al.*, 1995). Thus activation of neurotransmitter systems can have a direct modulatory effect on binding of gonadal hormones in the central nervous system (CNS).

Conversely, steroid hormones can modulate neuronal transmission by a variety of mechanisms. They may affect the synthesis and/or release of neurotransmitters, as well as the expression of receptors, membrane plasticity and permeability. It has been suggested that steroid hormone receptors function as general transcription factors to achieve integration of neural information in the CNS (Mani *et al.*, 1997; Stahl, 2001a). Steroids are believed to act primarily by classical genomic mechanisms through intracellular receptors to modulate transcription and protein synthesis. This

Biological Psychiatry: Edited by H. D'haenen, J.A. den Boer and P. Willner. ISBN 0-471-49198-5

mechanism involves the binding of the steroid to a cytoplasmic or nuclear receptor. The hormone–receptor complex then binds to DNA to trigger RNA-dependent protein synthesis. The response time for this mechanism is on the order of several minutes, hours or days. It has also been shown that steroids can also produce rapid effects on electrical excitability and synaptic function through direct membrane mechanisms, such as ligand-gated ion channels, G-proteins and neurotransmitter transporters (Sumner and Fink, 1998; Wong *et al.*, 1996). These short-term (seconds to minutes) effects of steroids may occur through binding to the cell membrane, binding to membrane receptors, modulation of ion channels, direct activation of second messenger systems (Moss *et al.*, 1997) or activation of receptors by factors such as cytokines and dopamine (Brann *et al.*, 1995). Topical application of oestrogen or progesterone to nervous tissue has been shown to result in a rapid change in membrane potential, and sex steroids can affect membrane fluidity by modifying ion transport or receptor function (Maggi and Perez, 1985).

The role and potential relevance of oestrogen and other sex steroids to psychiatric disorders is the focus of current scientific attention. Oestrogen has been described as a 5-HT, NA, and ACh agonist, and it also modulates DA/D_2 receptors. Likewise, oestrogen may also alter the action of drugs that work on target neurotransmitters. The antidepressant properties of oestradiol have recently been demonstrated in a placebo-controlled trial of perimenopausal women with major depression (Soares *et al.*, 2001). Indeed, oestrogen is regarded by some as the 'new frontier' of potential therapeutic action in the treatment of women with mood disorders (Stahl, 2001b).

In this chapter, mood disorders across the reproductive life cycle in women will be briefly reviewed with particular attention to the impact of hormonal fluctuations during menarche, the premenstruum, pregnancy and post-partum, and the perimenopause.

MENARCHE AND MOOD DISORDERS IN ADOLESCENCE

Epidemiological studies consistently show that beginning at menarche, mood disorders are at least twice as common in women than in men. Why these gender differences exist and why they start at puberty is perhaps one of the most intriguing and least understood phenomena in clinical psychiatry (Lewinsohn *et al.*, 1998).

Prior to adolescence, the rates of depression are similar in girls and boys (or are slightly higher in boys), yet with the onset of puberty, the gender proportion of depression dramatically shifts to a 2 : 1 female to male ratio (Kessler and Walters, 1998; Lewinsohn *et al.*, 1998). In the US general population, the lifetime prevalence of major depression (MD) in adolescents and young adults (15–24 years of age) has been reported as 20.6% for females and 10.5% for males (Kessler and Walters, 1998). Lifetime rates of MD in early- as well as late-maturing girls were even higher (30% versus 22% and 34% versus 22%, respectively) when compared to 'on-time' girls.

There is conflicting opinion regarding the age at which gender differences in rates of MD emerge: researchers are divided between the 12–14 and the 15–19 year age brackets (Cohen *et al.*, 1993; Hankin *et al.*, 1998; Lewinsohn *et al.*, 1998).

An integrative theory of depression in adolescents has been introduced (Lewinsohn *et al.*, 1998), although a persuasive explanation of the sharp rise in the prevalence of depression in females after menarche has yet to be elucidated.

The onset of puberty is heralded by a growth spurt, which begins with rapid growth in height and weight typically between 7.5 and 11.5 years of age. Following this initial burst, physical growth continues at a slow pace for several years. The first sign of sexual maturation in girls is breast budding at about 10.5 years, followed by growth of pubic hair, which begins at about 11.5 years, growth of the uterus and vagina, and the enlargement of the labia and clitoris. Menstruation begins after these changes occur. Finally, axillary hair appears, hips broaden, and fat deposits increase. On average, these changes take 4–5 years; however, considerable variation exists in the sequence and tempo of these events.

In North America and Europe, the age of menarche has declined about 4 months per decade since 1850; in North America, menarche now occurs around 12.5 years of age on average (Tanner, 1968). This dramatic decline in the age at which girls reach puberty is one of the strongest examples of environmental factors that affect hormonal responses. The search to isolate the particular environmental factors involved in this acceleration, however, has been only marginally helpful. It has been suggested that urbanization has a major role in this change, as well as improvements in general health, nutrition and other sociocultural factors. But other environmental factors also seem to be implicated in the timing of menarche. Girls who are blind with some perception of light reach menarche earlier than normally sighted girls, and totally blind girls with no light perception reach puberty even earlier (Zacharias and Wurtman, 1964). Moreover, fewer girls start to menstruate during spring and summer time as compared to during seasons of reduced amounts of daylight (autumn and winter) (Bojlen and Bentzon, 1974).

The relationship between psychosocial development and physical maturation has been widely examined. Girls undergoing pubertal change are thought to experience greater distress and to be more vulnerable to stress than pre- or postpubertal girls (Caspi and Moffitt, 1991). Two parameters of pubertal change in particular have received much attention: pubertal status and pubertal timing. *Pubertal status* is defined as the current level of physical development of an adolescent relative to the overall process of pubertal change (a biological factor), usually denoted by a series of stages from prepubertal (stage I) to adult (stage V) according to Tanner (Tanner, 1962). *Pubertal timing*, on the other hand, is defined as the maturation of an adolescent relative to her peers (a psychosocial factor).

There appears to be a relatively sharp demarcated period in mid-puberty when girls become more vulnerable to depression than boys. In a recent report on 1073 US children aged 9–13 years, the depression rates in girls rose significantly in mid-puberty, i.e., with the transition to Tanner stage III. In contrast, the prevalence of depression in boys *declines* from Tanner stage II (Angold *et al.*, 1998). Further, it has been determined that in girls, pubertal status (versus the age at puberty) better predicted the emergence of the sex ratio in depression rates. Thus, the onset of menarche may signal an increased but latent biological vulnerability to mood dysregulation in women (Nolen-Hoeksema and Girgus, 1994).

Although changes in affect, mood and behaviour are considered to be related to cyclic hormonal changes, studies of female adolescents and premenstrual syndrome (PMS) are inconclusive, with one study reporting no relationship between menstrual cycle phase and negative affect (Golub and Harrington, 1981) and others showing that PMS is associated with other distress factors in this age group (Freeman *et al.*, 1993; Raja *et al.*, 1992). Notwithstanding, relationships between changes in pubertal hormones and negative affect in female adolescents have been observed. For example, investigators have found that negative affect was significantly related to a rapid increase in oestradiol levels (Warren and Brooks-Gunn, 1989). Negative affect in healthy girls was also associated with higher levels of testosterone and cortisol, and lower levels of dehydroepiandrosterone sulphate (Susman *et al.*, 1991).

There is both direct and indirect — albeit limited — evidence of the involvement of the serotonergic system in the aetiology of depressive disorders in child and adolescent depression. In a comparative study of psychiatric inpatients and normal controls (aged 7–17 years), levels of whole-blood 5-HT were lowest inpatients with mood disorders (Hughes *et al.*, 1996). There is some indication of the responsiveness of children and adolescents with

MD to serotonergic but not noradrenergic agents; researchers have hypothesized that, in childhood, the serotonergic systems may mature at an earlier rate than the noradrenergic systems (Ryan and Varma, 1998). Gonadal hormones affect the production of 5-HT receptors at the transcriptional level, and the altered distribution or function of 5-HT receptor subtypes brought on by changes in the hormonal milieu at menarche may increase vulnerability to mood disorders.

It is nevertheless still unclear how the dramatic changes in the hormonal milieu associated with menarche and a host of psychosocial stressors combine to produce depressive symptoms. One possible unifying hypothesis suggests that disruption of biological rhythms, such as disturbed sleep patterns (Armitage *et al.*, 2001) or irregular menstrual cycles, together with psychosocial losses causing the disruption of social rhythms (also known as 'social zeitgebers') could trigger the onset of a major depressive episode in vulnerable individuals (Ehlers *et al.*, 1988). Another complementary theory emphasizes the neurobiology of stress and the dysregulation of affect during female biological transitions such as menarche, a transition which may be associated with changes in the reactivity of the stress system (Dorn and Chrousos, 1997). The newly fluctuating levels of gonadal hormones as well as gonadotropins, which mark the onset of menarche and the establishment of menstrual cycles, introduce a major change in the hormonal milieu to which the rest of the system has to adjust. This is the period during which the hypothalamic–pituitary–adrenal (HPA) axis has to mature and be sensitized to a variety of new feedback mechanisms. This is also the time during which the HPA axis may be more vulnerable to external psychosocial stressors, to sleep deprivation as well as to the influences of nicotine, alcohol and other drugs, resulting in a higher incidence of HPA axis dysregulation and mood instability.

Taken together, it is suggested that pubertal and other hormonal changes should be monitored prospectively along with individual, genetic, constitutional and psychological characteristics in our efforts to predict the development of negative affect during puberty (Steiner *et al.*, 2000).

PREMENSTRUAL DYSPHORIA

The inclusion of research diagnostic criteria for PMDD in the *Diagnostic and Statistical Manual of Mental Disorders*, 4th edn (DSM-IV) recognizes that some women in their reproductive years have extremely distressing emotional and behavioural symptoms premenstrually (American Psychiatric Association, 1994 pp. 717–18). Through the use of these criteria, PMDD can be differentiated from *premenstrual syndrome* (PMS) which has milder physical symptoms, i.e., breast tenderness, bloating, headache and minor mood changes (World Health Organization, 1996a). PMDD can also be differentiated from *premenstrual magnification* (concurrent diagnoses of PMS or PMDD *and* a major psychiatric or an unstable medical condition) and from *premenstrual exacerbation* of a current psychiatric disorder or medical condition (Steiner and Wilkins, 1996).

Epidemiological surveys have estimated that as many as 75% of women with regular menstrual cycles experience some symptoms of premenstrual syndrome (Johnson, 1987). PMDD, on the other hand, is much less common. It affects only 3–8% of women in this group (Angst *et al.*, 2001; Johnson *et al.*, 1988; Ramcharan *et al.*, 1992), but it is more severe and exerts a much greater psychological toll. These women report premenstrual symptoms that seriously interfere with their lifestyle and relationships (Freeman *et al.*, 1985; O'Brien *et al.*, 1995).

The aetiology of PMS and PMDD is still largely unknown. That PMS and PMDD are biological phenomena (as opposed to psychological or psychosocial events) is primarily underscored by recent, convincing evidence of the heritability of premenstrual symptoms (Kendler *et al.*, 1998) and the elimination of premenstrual complaints with suppression of ovarian activity (Schmidt *et al.*, 1998) or surgical menopause (Casson *et al.*, 1990). In women with PMDD, the ovarian axis is apparently functioning normally with normal oestrogen and progesterone levels (Schmidt *et al.*, 1998). The current consensus seems to be that normal ovarian function rather than simple hormone imbalance is the cyclic trigger for biochemical events within the central nervous system and other target tissues which unleash premenstrual symptoms in vulnerable women (Roca *et al.*, 1996). This viewpoint is attractive in that it encourages investigation of the neuroendocrine-modulated central neurotransmitters and the role of the HPG axis in PMDD.

There is increasing attention to the metabolite of progesterone, allopregnanolone, in the manifestation of premenstrual symptomatology. Current evidence suggests that progesterone and progestogens are not likely to be effective in the treatment of premenstrual syndromes (Wyatt *et al.*, 2001). Allopregnanolone, on the other hand, is thought to modulate GABA receptor functioning and produce an anxiolytic effect (Rapkin *et al.*, 1997); quantitative differences in progesterone and allopregnanolone levels between PMS subjects and controls have been examined. The findings to date, however, are contradictory (Bicikova *et al.*, 1998; Girdler *et al.*, 2001; Monteleone *et al.*, 2000; Rapkin *et al.*, 1997; Schmidt *et al.*, 1994; Wang *et al.*, 1996). A recent study using an animal model, though, is more promising. In a progesterone-withdrawal paradigm designed to mimic PMS and post-partum depression in female rats, Smith and colleagues have found that decreased levels of allopregnanolone lead to increased production of the $\alpha 4$ subunit of the $GABA_A$ receptor. This changes the sensitivity of the $GABA_A$ receptor to endogenous ligands, resulting in symptoms associated with PMS (Smith *et al.*, 1998).

The role of the female sex hormones in premenstrual symptomatology has been considered of central importance. Notwithstanding, attention by some has shifted from a focus on oestrogen and progesterone to the role of androgens in premenstrual dysphoria.

Early investigations of androgens have suggested that women with PMS or PMDD have elevated levels of serum testosterone in the luteal phase compared with controls (but still within the normal range), which may contribute primarily to the symptom of irritability (Dunn *et al.*, 2001; Eriksson *et al.*, 1992). This hypothesis of increased androgenicity is backed by both animal and human studies of androgens and irritability and/or aggression. Androgens promote sexual drive in humans, and also have been tentatively linked with mood (e.g. depression and premenstrual irritability) and impulsive behaviour (e.g. compulsions and binge eating). Enhanced serotonin availability (e.g. with the use of selective serotonin reuptake inhibitors; SSRIs), on the other hand, is associated with reduction in irritability, depression and impulsive behaviour, as well as reduced libido. An inverse relationship between serotonin and androgens, and their effects on human behaviour has been proposed; the behavioural effects of androgens may be therefore partly mediated by a reduction in serotonin activity (Eriksson *et al.*, 2000).

Reduction of premenstrual dysphoria with androgen antagonists in women with PMS who showed higher mean levels of total testosterone in the late luteal phase also lends support to the idea of increased androgenicity (Burnet *et al.*, 1991; Rowe and Sasse, 1986). Others, however, have not observed differences in plasma testosterone in comparisons of women with or without PMS (Dougherty *et al.*, 1997), and one study has reported significantly *lower* total and free testosterone plasma levels in a sample of 10 women with PMS (Bloch *et al.*, 1998). Further comparative studies of women with PMS and PMDD are therefore required.

An alternative strategy to measuring various hormone plasma levels in an attempt to discern the aetiology of PMDD has been to search for endocrine abnormalities that have been repeatedly associated with various other forms of psychopathology. The main advantage of this approach is its potential to help further our understanding of PMDD as well as its relation to other psychiatric disorders. The current literature suggests that thyroid dysfunction may be found in a small group of women with premenstrual symptoms but that PMDD should not be viewed as a masked form of hypothyroidism (Korzekwa *et al.*, 1996; Schmidt *et al.*, 1993).

Of the neurotransmitters studied to date, increasing evidence suggests that 5-HT may be important in the pathogenesis of PMDD (Steiner *et al.*, 1997; Rapkin, 1992). PMDD shares many features of other mood and anxiety disorders linked to serotonergic dysfunction. In addition, reduction in brain 5-HT neurotransmission is thought to lead to poor impulse control, depressed mood, irritability and increased carbohydrate craving — all mood and behavioural symptoms associated with PMDD.

The serotonergic system is in close reciprocal relationship with gonadal hormones. In the hypothalamus, oestrogen induces a diurnal fluctuation in 5-HT (Cohen and Wise, 1988), whereas progesterone increases the turnover rate of 5-HT (Ladisich, 1977).

More recently, several studies concluded that 5-HT *function* may also be altered in women with PMDD. Some studies used models of neuronal function (such as whole-blood 5-HT levels, platelet uptake of 5-HT, and platelet tritiated imipramine binding) and found altered 5-HT function during all phases of the menstrual cycle (Ashby *et al.*, 1988; Bixo *et al.*, 2001; Rapkin, 1992; Steege *et al.*, 1992). Other studies that used challenge tests (with L-tryptophan, fenfluramine, buspirone, *m*-chlorophenylpiperazine) suggested abnormal serotonin function in symptomatic women but differed in their findings as to whether the response to 5-HT is blunted or heightened (Bancroft and Cook 1995; Bancroft *et al.*, 1991; FitzGerald *et al.*, 1997; Rasgon *et al.*, 2001; Su *et al.*, 1997; Steiner *et al.*, 1999). Acute tryptophan depletion (suppressing brain 5-HT synthesis) was significantly associated with exacerbation of premenstrual symptoms, in particular irritability (Menkes *et al.*, 1994). Additional evidence suggesting the involvement (although not necessarily aetiological) of the serotonergic system has emerged from treatment studies: drugs facilitating serotonergic transmission, such as SSRIs, are very effective in reducing premenstrual symptoms. These studies imply, at least in part, a possible change in 5-HT transporter/receptor sensitivity in women with premenstrual dysphoria (Steiner and Born, 2000).

The current consensus is that women with premenstrual dysphoria may be behaviourally or biochemically sub- or supersensitive to biological challenges of the serotonergic system. It is not yet clear whether these women present with a trait or state marker (alternatively, both conditions could be possible) of premenstrual syndromes.

The reciprocal relationship between the serotonergic system and the gonadal hormones has been identified as the most plausible target for interventions. This notion has recently gained further support in a very elegant study showing that an SSRI (fluoxetine) reduces sex-steroid-related aggression in female rats in a paradigm which is proposed as an animal model of premenstrual dysphoria/irritability (Ho *et al.*, 2001). Thus, beyond the conservative treatment options such as lifestyle and stress management, and the more extreme interventions that eliminate ovulation altogether, the SSRIs are emerging as the most effective treatment option for this population (Steiner and Born, 2000).

POST-PARTUM DEPRESSION

The specific link and the uniqueness of psychiatric disorders precipitated or triggered by pregnancy or childbirth have recently been acknowledged by the American Psychiatric Association (1994, pp. 386–7). Based primarily on the work of the Task Force on DSM-IV (Purnine and Frank, 1996) the manual now has a course-specific designation 'post-partum onset', which can be applied to both psychotic and non-psychotic post-partum mental disorders. Thus, major depressive disorders, bipolar disorders (manic and depressed), schizoaffective disorders, and psychotic disorders (not otherwise specified) will have the qualifier 'with post-partum onset'.

Post-partum 'blues' is considered the most mild of the post-partum mood disturbances; its prevalence has been reported to be 26–85%, depending on the diagnostic criteria used (Stein *et al.*, 1981). The symptoms of this syndrome typically begin within the first week following childbirth, peak on the fifth day and resolve by the twelfth day post-partum. Symptoms include dysphoria, mood lability, crying, anxiety, insomnia, poor appetite and irritability. The mood disturbance characterizing post-partum blues is considered transient and insufficient in and of itself to cause serious impairment of a woman's functioning (O'Hara *et al.*, 1991). In some women, however, the disturbance may persist beyond the initial post-partum period, leading to more serious PPD (Cox *et al.*, 1993).

Epidemiological studies of the nature, prevalence and course of an episode of major PPD have found that 10–15% of women exhibit depressive symptoms in the first weeks following delivery (Carothers and Murray, 1990; Pop *et al.*, 1993), and that the great majority of these depressive episodes resolve spontaneously within three to six months (Cooper and Murray, 1995; Cox *et al.*, 1993). The symptom profile of PPD resembles that of a major depressive episode experienced at other times in life, but it is unique in its timing and in that it always involves at least the mother–baby dyad and in most cases an entire family unit.

Post-partum psychosis is much more rare and more severe than either depression or the blues. It has a prevalence of approximately 1 in 500–1000 births, and a rapid onset within the first few days to two weeks post-partum (Brockington *et al.*, 1982). Post-partum psychosis, believed to be in most cases an episodic presentation of a manic-depressive illness, severely impairs the affected woman's ability to function. In the most extreme cases, the risks of suicide or infanticide are high (Millis and Kornblith, 1992), requiring admission to a psychiatric hospital (Kendell *et al.*, 1987).

Pregnancy and childbirth have an enormous combined psychological, physiologic and endocrine effect on a woman's body and mind. Since the changes in mood coincide with these profound changes in hormones and other humoral agents related to pregnancy and childbirth, a causal link has been supposed probable (Steiner, 1998). In the animal kingdom, maternal behaviour is mediated by hormonal and neurochemical changes associated with reproduction (Rosenblatt *et al.*, 1988). In animals, it has been suggested that the various neuromodulators be divided into groups which define their proposed role in maternal response: primers — most important during late pregnancy (e.g. steroid hormones and prolactin); triggers — released during parturition (e.g. oxytocin); and modifiers — of oxytocin release (e.g. beta-endorphins, other neurotransmitters) (Keverne and Kendrick, 1994). There is, of course, considerable scope for interactions between these changes and varying repertoires of maternal behaviour across different species (Fleming and Corter, 1988) and the relevance to human behaviour is as yet unclear.

The peak in mood disturbance during the blues at around the fifth day post-partum coincides with extreme hormonal fluctuations that are a natural consequence of parturition. These hormones act within the central nervous system at a variety of limbic sites known to be involved in emotional responses, arousal and reinforcement. Only a handful of studies have attempted to measure these changes, especially in gonadal hormones and prolactin. To date, most of the results do not seem to correlate strongly with changes in mood and are inconsistent. Serum allopregnanolone levels were shown to be lower in women experiencing post-partum blues (Nappi *et al.*, 2001), whereas serum testosterone levels have been weakly correlated with depression and anger in the first post-partum days (Hohlagschwandter *et al.*, 2001). A rapid fall in progesterone showed a weak but significant relationship to the development of the blues in one study (Harris *et al.*, 1994) but not in another (Heidrich *et al.*, 1994).

Similarly, increased plasma cortisol levels correlated with the blues and with PPD in one study (Okano and Nomura, 1992) but not in others (O'Hara *et al.*, 1991; Smith *et al.*, 1990). Preliminary results suggest that natural-killer-cell activity is lower in post-partum dysphorics and that this decrease is related to higher levels of cortisol (Pedersen *et al.*, 1993a). In contrast, negative or false-positive results with the dexamethasone suppression test do not correlate with mood changes, indicating that the HPA axis is physiologically hyperactive post-partum ('ceiling effect') and measurements along this axis as an indicator for depression in this population are probably invalid (O'Hara *et al.*, 1991; Smith *et al.*, 1990; Steiner *et al.*, 1986). The HPA, rather than the HPG, axis may in fact play a unique role in human maternal behaviour. Euthymic new mothers with positive maternal attitudes and high levels of cortisol post-partum exhibit the highest level of post-partum maternal approach behaviour (Fleming *et al.*, 1987). None of the other hormones measured (oestradiol, progesterone, testosterone and thyroid indices) were correlated with any of the maternal behaviours measured (Fleming *et al.*, 1987, 1995). These results suggest that cortisol does not induce maternal behaviour directly but it probably facilitates maternal attitudes, which may then be expressed as emotions and/or behaviour.

Thyroid dysfunction has been implicated in mood disorders and it has been suggested that transient thyroid dysfunction following childbirth is associated with PPD (Pederson *et al.*, 1993b). In some women, pregnancy and the post-partum period are associated with pathological changes in thyroid function. A review of the literature in this area clearly indicates the possibility that a subgroup of women with PPD have a basis for the depressed mood in thyroid disorder. More specifically, in some women depressive symptoms are associated with positive thyroid antibody status during the post-partum period (Harris *et al.*, 1992). It is believed that 1% of all post-partum women will show a mood disorder associated with transient thyroid dysfunction, and treatment of the thyroid condition must be part of the management.

The direct and/or indirect effect of the rate of the post-partum withdrawal of some of the other major hormones and neuromodulators involved is nevertheless still intriguing. It has been suggested that women who experience a more rapid beta-endorphin withdrawal are more prone to mood changes (Smith *et al.*, 1990). A sharp fall in circulating oestrogen concentrations after delivery has been associated with acute onset of post-partum psychosis (Wieck *et al.*, 1991). These changes are believed to be the triggers to a cascade of changes at central and peripheral monoamine centres. Very preliminary data suggest an increased sensitivity of dopamine receptors in acute post-partum psychosis (Wieck *et al.*, 1991) and an abnormality in $alpha_2$ adrenoceptor sensitivity associated with the blues (Best *et al.*, 1988). Changes in sensitivities of serotonergic receptors have been documented in PPD (Hannah *et al.*, 1992), but not in women with the blues (Katona *et al.*, 1985).

More recently it has been hypothesized that PPD may be caused by transient hypothalamic corticotropin-releasing hormone (CRH) suppression (Magiakou *et al.*, 1996). The HPA axis is progressively hyperactive throughout pregnancy, with increasing levels of circulating CRH of placental origin and decreasing levels of CRH-binding protein. Both these phenomena, together with the elevated levels of oestradiol of pregnancy, which also stimulate the HPA axis, particularly during the third trimester, contribute to the elevated levels of CRH, ACTH and cortisol (Cizza *et al.*, 1997). After parturition the source of placental CRH is removed, and together with the post-partum oestrogen withdrawal, which is further prolonged by breastfeeding (Kim *et al.*, 2000), may lead to a prolonged state of HPA axis hypoactivity. Indeed, it has been demonstrated that in a subgroup of women with PPD, the suppression of the HPA axis was more severe and lasted longer than that of women who had no post-partum mood instability (Magiakou *et al.*, 1996).

CRH has been associated with the neurobiology of stress and depression (Chrousos and Gold, 1992). PPD also appears to be a state of central CRH dysregulation. With the additional established evidence of direct oestrogenic regulation of the CRH gene expression (Vamvakopoulos and Chrousos, 1993) it is therefore not surprising that oestrogen has been proposed as a treatment for PPD (Ahokas *et al.*, 2001; Gregoire *et al.*, 1996; Sichel *et al.*, 1995). In the only double-blind, placebo-controlled study published to date, a 3-month course of 200 μg per day of 17ß-oestradiol significantly improved the clinical symptoms of severely depressed women post-partum (Gregoire *et al.*, 1996). Unfortunately further research on the role of oestrogen therapy for PPD has not yet emerged. Similarly, progesterone has been widely used for the treatment of post-natal depression but without controlled trials (O'Brien and Pitt, 1994).

The role of hormone replacement therapy is of interest beyond the realm of the post-partum period and, as discussed in the next section, is of major relevance during the perimenopausal and menopausal years and beyond.

The reciprocal relationship between the serotonergic system and gonadal hormones has not as yet been studied during pregnancy or in post-partum women. However, preliminary results from studies in post-partum rats indicate that 5-HT receptor changes in the limbic area are negatively correlated with progesterone levels (Glaser *et al.*, 1990). It is argued that post-partum withdrawal of gonadal hormones may cause changes along the serotonergic cascade, which may lead to a mood disorder in vulnerable or genetically predisposed women. (It should therefore be possible to treat the disturbance by 'adjusting' the levels of the hormone (the trigger) (Henderson *et al.*, 1991) or by reversing the sensitivity (predisposition). Results from some preliminary studies on preventative interventions with lithium prophylaxis (Cohen *et al.*, 1995; Stewart *et al.*, 1991) and with SSRIs (Appleby *et al.*, 1997; Stowe *et al.*, 1995) are very encouraging. Since mood disorders associated with childbearing have different times of onset in different women and are heterogenous in their presentation, concomitant measurements of the changes over time in gonadal hormones and the biochemical changes in the monoamine system are crucial.

Further evidence of a biological component of post-partum mood disorders comes from family and family history studies. It has been suggested that women with a history of post-partum depression are differentially sensitized to mood-destabilizing effects of gonadal steroids (Bloch *et al.*, 2000). A study of women with post-partum mood disturbances and their first-degree relatives found that at least one family member met criteria for a past or present psychiatric disorder in 71% of the cases for which the information was available. Positive histories for MD and alcoholism were found in 48% and 30% of these families, respectively (Steiner and Tam, 1999). Further analysis of these data revealed an interesting gender distribution of psychiatric disorders in the first-degree relatives of the post-partum women. A female : male ratio greater than 2 : 1 was found in relatives with a past or present diagnosis of MD; in the case of alcoholism, a male : female ratio of 4 : 1 was evident. This lifetime prevalence of mood-related disorders in the first-degree relatives of women presenting with post-partum mood disorders is much higher than in the population at large and may indicate potential genetic or familial components of the disorders.

Despite the fact that most animals share the same physiological events at parturition, the differences in behavioural response between humans (as well as other primates) and non-primate mammals are remarkable. The differences between primates and non-primates are mainly in the organization of social structures, the complex influences of the family unit, and the constant exposure of all members of a group to the young. It is therefore easy to assume that, in humans, even thinking about children may be sufficient to stimulate maternal responsiveness. The psychosocial literature to date has advanced several psychological and social stress factors as potential aetiological theories of primary non-psychotic PPD. These factors include lack of social support, negative life events, occupational instability, lack of prior experience with children, unplanned pregnancy and antenatal 'pessimism', dissatisfaction with the marital relationship (or being unmarried), and a poor relationship between the affected woman and her own mother (Murray *et al.*, 1995; Paykel *et al.*, 1980).

In summarizing these studies, no unifying conclusion can be reached, and it is impossible at this stage to translate any of these results into predictive, diagnostic, therapeutic, prognostic or preventative applications. It seems more likely that an intrinsic abnormal reaction to some of the hormonal changes, rather than the changes themselves, is responsible for the disorder. If the psychobiological factors (or their interactions) responsible for the emotional disorders associated with childbearing could be elucidated, our understanding of the aetiology not only of PPD but also of a wider range of psychiatric disorders might be enhanced.

PERIMENOPAUSE, MENOPAUSE AND BEYOND

The transition into menopause is a major hormonal event and is associated in many women with both physical and psychosocial symptoms. The term perimenopause describes the period immediately before the menopause — from the time when the hormonal and clinical features of approaching menopause commence until the end of the first year after menopause (World Health Organization, 1996b).

The physiological hallmark of the transition into menopause is gradual oestrogen depletion. In the 1960s and 1970s 'depletion' was equated with 'deficiency' and menopause, representing a state of oestrogen deficiency, was therefore considered a medical disorder warranting treatment. A famous quotation from that era highlights this approach: 'It sometimes seems as if the only thing worse than being subjected to the raging hormonal influences of the female cycle is to have those influences subside' (Parlee, 1976). The notion of universal hormone replacement for *all* menopausal women was so rampant that the WHO convened a special session and eventually came out with a consensus statement to counter the above, which read: 'Menopause is part of the normal aging process which in itself does not require therapeutic intervention. The health status of women during this period is not recognized as being a simple endocrine-deficiency state which could or should be corrected by attempting to create for each woman a premenopausal normal environment' (WHO, 1981).

Changes most commonly associated with oestrogen depletion (and/or unpredictable fluctuations) include vasomotor symptoms such as hot flushes and night sweats (Freedman, 2000; Guthrie *et al.*, 1996), urogenital dryness/atrophy causing dyspareunia as well as an increased risk over time of osteoporosis and cardiovascular disease (Mitchell and Woods, 1996). The relationship between the perimenopause/menopause and mood disorders is less well understood. Epidemiological data indicates that the majority of postmenopausal women do not experience prominent symptoms of depression, but a higher than expected prevalence of depressive-like symptoms has been observed in peri- and postmenopausal women attending gynaecological clinics (Avis and McKinlay, 1991; Schmidt and Rubinow, 1991).

It is unclear as to whether there is decline in new-onset episodes of major depression in females of this age group, as suggested by the Epidemiologic Catchment Area study, a finding not supported by data from the National Comorbidity Survey. The role of sociocultural factors and demographic differences have been the focus of much study but the results are controversial (Anderson *et al.*, 1987; Hay *et al.*, 1994).

Some cross-cultural differences are nevertheless noteworthy: Japanese women experience very few physical as well as emotional symptoms around menopause. It has been proposed that these findings are indicative not only of cultural and demographic differences but also reflect the influence of biological, genetic and nutritional/dietary factors (Lock, 1994; Nagata *et al.*, 1998).

The most prevalent mood symptoms during the perimenopause include irritability, tearfulness, anxiety, depressed/labile mood, lack of motivation/energy, poor concentration and interrupted sleep. These symptoms have been linked to predictable fluctuations in oestradiol, especially abrupt withdrawal from very high erratic levels, rather than to times when levels are slowly and gradually declining (Prior, 1998).

Several lines of evidence point to the link between oestrogen depletion/deficiency and mood disorders in vulnerable or predisposed women. Oestrogen has direct effects on the CNS in areas which are not strictly relevant to reproduction. For example, oestrogen regulates synaptogenesis, has a general trophic effect on cholinergic neurons and stimulates a significant increase in 5-HT_{2A} binding sites in areas which are involved in regulating both mood and cognition. It is therefore not surprising that oestrogen has been shown to improve psychological functioning and well-being in nondepressed postmenopausal women (Ditkoff *et al.*, 1991; Palinkas and Barret-Connor, 1992) and that oestrogen replacement therapy (ERT) has a positive effect on mood states (Zweifel and O'Brien, 1997). The ability of oestrogen to act as a 5-HT agonist/modulator is of particular significance. Oestrogen not only increases the number of 5-HT_{2A} receptor binding sites but also increases 5-HT synthesis, uptake and 3H-imipramine binding; it decreases 5-HT_1 receptor binding sites and 5-HT transporter mRNA and increases the prolactin response to 5-HT agonists — all in line with antidepressant-like action (Biegon and McEwen, 1982; Fink *et al.*, 1996; Halbreich *et al.*, 1995; Pecins-Thompson *et al.*, 1998; van Amelsvoort *et al.*, 2001). The clinical relevance of these effects to the pathophysiology of women-specific mood and anxiety disorders remains to be determined.

The strongest evidence to date for oestrogen's ability to improve mood and cognitive functioning comes from studies in young surgically menopausal women treated with ERT (Sherwin, 1988; Sherwin and Suranyi-Cadotte, 1990). It is encouraging to note that several very preliminary studies seem to indicate the beneficial effects of combining ERT with SSRIs in the treatment of postmenopausal depressed women (Schneider *et al.*, 1997). Preliminary evidence also indicates the efficacy of transdermal 17ß-oestradiol alone in the treatment of perimenopausal women with major and minor depression (Schmidt *et al.*, 2000; Soares *et al.*, 2001).

Oestrogen specifically maintains verbal memory in women and may prevent or forestall the deterioration in short- and long-term memory that occurs with age (Sherwin, 1999a). There is also evidence that oestrogen may have a role in the prevention and treatment of Alzheimer's disease (AD). Theoretically, oestrogen could be the perfect anti-Alzheimer's treatment (Garcia-Segura *et al.*, 2001). Oestrogen has the properties of an antioxidant, can modify inflammatory response, increases growth of ACh neurons, can affect amyloid precursor protein cleavage, inhibits ApoE levels, stimulates glucocorticoid levels, increases glucose utilization and increase cerebral blood flow. Unfortunately the clinical data to date are somewhat mixed: the estimated risk of AD decreases significantly in women who have been on long-term ERT (Kawas *et al.*, 1997; Paganini-Hill and Henderson, 1994) but others have reported only 50% reduction in incidence (Waring *et al.*, 1999), with some benefit in early-onset AD only and some protection against further deterioration (Costa *et al.*, 1999) whereas others have seen no beneficial effect at all (Mulnard *et al.*, 2000).

The use of ERT continues to be controversial, with the risk of breast and endometrial cancer in long-term users still looming. At the same time, the search for the perfect selective oestrogen receptor modulator (SERM) is ongoing. The 'ideal' SERM would have negative receptor activity on breast and endometrial cells and positive receptor activity on bone, cardiovascular and brain. So far there is evidence that raloxifene is effective in preventing osteoporosis and has protective cardiovascular properties and also seems to reduce the risk for breast cancer (Cauley *et al.*, 2001; Delmas *et al.*, 1997) but its effect on cognitive function in humans has not been established. There is some indication that it may lower the risk of decline in attention and memory (Yaffe *et al.*, 2001) and in animals there is some indication that raloxifene plus oestradiol induces neurite outgrowth to a greater extent than raloxifene or oestradiol alone (Nilsen *et al.*, 1998).

Progesterone, which in the past has been promoted by some as an antidepressant, by itself can not only cause depression but seems also to reverse the oestrogen-induced receptor expression. Progestogens also have potent anaesthetic properties and dampen brain excitability; they also increase the concentration of monoamine oxidase, the enzyme that catabolizes 5-HT in the brain, whereas oestrogen decreases the enzyme, thereby increasing the concentration of 5-HT (Luine *et al.*, 1975; Sherwin, 1999b).

Testosterone is also an extremely important psychoactive compound and its relevance to women's well-being is just beginning to be recognized (Tuiten *et al.*, 2000).

While we are awaiting results of the ongoing long-term prospective studies with ERT and SERM, it is important to recognize that depressive symptoms are a significant risk factor for mortality in older women (Whooley and Browner, 1998). Whether depressive symptoms are a marker for, or a cause of, life-threatening conditions remains to be determined. Nevertheless, treatment for depression may not only enhance the quality of life but may also reduce mortality in this population.

CONCLUSION

The complex integration of the neurotransmitter and steroid hormone systems implies that circulating steroid hormones from peripheral endocrine glands can directly regulate brain function and modulate behaviour. Regulation occurs through a variety of mechanisms, including, for example, direct interaction with or upregulation of specific receptors on neuronal cells. Thus, the hormonal milieu surrounding a neuronal cell will, in part, determine the response of that cell to various stimuli.

Adrenal and gonadal steroids regulate the transcription of most of the major neurotransmitter systems.

Steroid hormones also have direct effects on neuronal cell function by non-genomic mechanisms influencing the sensitivity and responsiveness of the neurons.

Levels of oestrogen and progesterone vary significantly across the female lifespan. At puberty there is an increase in oestrogen and initiation of cyclic and diurnal variation in oestrogen production. The sudden appearance of higher levels of oestrogen in puberty alters the sensitivity of the neurotransmitter systems. Behaviours such as moodiness, irritability and conflicts with parents around this time may in part reflect this increased sensitivity. The constant flux of oestrogen and progesterone levels continues throughout the reproductive years. The neurotransmitter systems are thus constantly being attenuated or amplified. PMS and PMDD may be the result of an altered activity (or sensitivity) of certain neurotransmitter systems. Pregnancy and delivery produce dramatic changes in oestrogen and progesterone levels as well as significant suppression along the HPA axis, possibly increasing vulnerability to depression. Finally, at menopause, oestrogen levels decline while pituitary LH and FSH levels increase. The loss of modulating effects of oestrogen and progesterone may underlie the development of perimenopausal mood disorders in vulnerable women.

Since these hormonal changes occur in all women, it seems safe to speculate that the development of mood disorders requires more than just fluctuating levels of hormones, but also a genetic predisposition. These as yet unidentified genetic 'defects' probably relate to subtle alterations in number and function of various receptors and enzymes and to subtle structural and anatomical differences in the CNS. These differences caused by genetic polymorphism, combined with the flux in the hormonal milieu, determine how the system reacts to multiple environmental stresses and predicts the development of mood disorders. Further research into this complex system is needed to identify specific genetic markers which might help us better understand how the balance between oestrogen, progesterone, testosterone and other steroid hormones affects neurotransmitter function.

REFERENCES

Ahokas, A., Kaukoranta, J., Wahlbeck, K. and Aito, M., 2001. Estrogen deficiency in post-partum depression: successful treatment with sublingual physiologic 17ß-estradiol: a preliminary study. *Journal of Clinical Psychiatry*, **62**, 332–6.

American Psychiatric Association, 1994. *DSM-IV: Diagnostic and Statistical Manual of Mental Disorders*, 4th edn. American Psychiatric Association, Washington, DC.

Anderson, E., Hamburger, S., Liu, J.H. and Rebar, R.W., 1987. Characteristics of menopausal women seeking assistance. *American Journal of Obstetrics and Gynecology*, **156**, 428–33.

Angold, A., Costello, E.J. and Worthman, C.M., 1998. Puberty and depression: the roles of age, pubertal status and pubertal timing. *Psychological Medicine*, **28**, 51–61.

Angst, J., Sellaro, R., Merikangas, K.R. and Endicott, J., 2001. The epidemiology of perimenstrual psychological symptoms. *Acta Psychiatrica Scandinavica*, **104**, 110–6.

Appleby, L., Warner, R., Whitton, A. and Faragher, B., 1997. A controlled study of fluoxetine and cognitive-behavioural counselling in the treatment of postnatal depression. *British Medical Journal*, **314**, 932–6.

Armitage, R., Emslie, G.J., Hoffmann, R.F., Rintelmann, J. and Rush, J.A., 2001. Delta sleep EEG in depressed adolescent females and healthy controls. *Journal of Affective Disorders*, **63**, 139–48.

Ashby, C.R., Jr, Carr, L.A., Cook, C.L., Steptoe, M.M. and Franks, D.D., 1988. Alteration of platelet serotonergic mechanisms and monoamine oxidase activity on premenstrual syndrome. *Biological Psychiatry*, **24**, 225–33.

Avis, N.E. and McKinlay, S.M., 1991. A longitudinal analysis of women's attitudes toward the menopause: results from the Massachusetts Women's Health Study. *Maturitas*, **13**, 65–79.

Bancroft, J. and Cook, A., 1995. The neuroendocrine response to d-fenfluramine in women with premenstrual depression. *Journal of Affective Disorders*, **36**, 57–64.

Bancroft, J., Cook, A., Davidson, D., Bennie, J. and Goodwin, G., 1991. Blunting of neuroendocrine responses to infusion of L-tryptophan in women with perimenstrual mood change. *Psychological Medicine*, **21**, 305–12.

Best, N.R., Wiley, M., Stump, K., Elliott, J.M. and Cowen, P.J., 1988. Binding of tritiated yohimbine to platelets in women with maternity blues. *Psychological Medicine*, **18**, 837–42.

Bicikova, M., Dibbelt, L., Hill, M., Hampl, R. and Starka, L., 1998. Allopregnanolone in women with premenstrual syndrome. *Hormone and Metabolic Research*, **30**, 227–30.

Biegon, A. and McEwen, B.S., 1982. Modulation by estradiol of serotonin receptors in brain. *Journal of Neuroscience*, **2**, 199–205.

Bixo, M., Allard, P., Backstrom, T., Mjorndal, T., Nyberg, S., Spigset, O. and Sundstrom-Poromaa, I., 2001. Binding of [3H]paroxetine to serotonin uptake sites and of [3H]lysergic acid diethylamide to 5-HT2A receptors in platelets from women with premenstrual dysphoric disorder during gonadotropin releasing hormone treatment. *Psychoneuroendocrinology*, **26**, 551–64.

Bloch, M., Schmidt, P., Danaceau, M., Murphy, J., Nieman, L. and Rubinow, D.R., 2000. Effects of gonadal steroids in women with a history of post-partum depression. *American Journal of Psychiatry*, **157**, 924–30.

Bloch, M., Schmidt, P.J., Su, T.P., Tobin, M.B. and Rubinow, D.R., 1998. Pituitary-adrenal hormones and testosterone across the menstrual cycle in women with premenstrual syndrome and controls. *Biological Psychiatry*, **43**, 897–903.

Bojlen, K. and Bentzen, M.W., 1974. Seasonal variation in the occurrence of menarche. *Danish Medical Bulletin*, **21**, 161–8.

Brann, D.W., Hendry, L.B. and Mahesh, V.B., 1995. Emerging diversities in the mechanism of action of steroid hormones. *Journal of Steroid Biochemistry and Molecular Biology*, **52**, 113–33.

Brockington, I.F., Winokur, G. and Dean, C., 1982. Puerperal psychosis. In: Brockington, I.F. and Kumar, R. (eds), *Motherhood and Mental Illness*, pp. 37–69. Academic Press, London.

Burnet, R.B., Radden, H.S., Easterbrook, E.G. and McKinnon, R.A., 1991. Premenstrual syndrome and spironolactone. *Australia and New Zealand Journal of Obstetrics and Gynaecology*, **31**, 366–9.

Carothers, A.D. and Murray, L., 1990. Estimating psychiatric morbidity by logistic regression: application to post-natal depression in a community sample. *Psychological Medicine*, **20**, 695–702.

Caspi, A. and Moffitt, T.E., 1991. Individual differences are accentuated during periods of social change: the sample case of girls at puberty. *Journal of Personality and Social Psychology*, **61**, 157–68.

Casson, P., Hahn, P.M., Van Vugt, D.A. and Reid, R.L., 1990. Lasting response to ovariectomy in severe intractable premenstrual syndrome. *American Journal of Obstetrics and Gynecology*, **162**, 99–105.

Cauley, J.A., Norton, L., Lippman, M.E., Eckert, S., Krueger, K.A., Purdie, D.W., Farrerons, J., Karasik, A., Mellstrom, D., Ng, K.W., Stepan, J.J., Powles, T.J., Morrow, M., Costa, A., Silfen, S.L., Walls, E.L., Schmitt, H., Muchmore, D.B., Jordan, V.C. and Ste-Marie, L.G., 2001. Continued breast cancer risk reduction in postmenopausal women treated with raloxifene: 4-year results from the MORE trial. Multiple outcomes of raloxifene evaluation. *Breast Cancer Research and Treatment*, **65**, 125–34.

Chrousos, G.P. and Gold, P.W., 1992. The concepts of stress and stress system disorders: overview of physical and behavioral homeostasis. *Journal of the American Medical Association*, **267**, 1244–52.

Cizza, G., Gold, P.W. and Chrousos, G.P., 1997. High dose transdermal estrogen corticotropin-releasing hormone and postnatal depression. *Journal of Clinical Endocrinology Metabolism*, **82**, 704.

Cohen, I.R. and Wise, P.M., 1988. Effects of estradiol on the diurnal rhythm of serotonin activity in microdissected brain areas of ovariectomized rats. *Endocrinology*, **122**, 2619–25.

Cohen, L.S., Sichel, D.A., Robertson, L.M., Heckscher, E. and Rosenbaum, J.F., 1995. Post-partum prophylaxis for women with bipolar disorder. *American Journal of Psychiatry*, **152**, 1641–5.

Cohen, P., Cohen, J., Kasen, S., Velez, C.N., Hartmark, C., Johnson, J.R., Rojas, M., Brook, J. and Streuning, E.L., 1993. An epidemiological study of disorders in late childhood and adolescence — I: Age- and gender-specific prevalence. *Journal of Child Psychology and Psychiatry*, **34**, 851–67.

Cooper, P.J. and Murray, L., 1995. Course and recurrence of postnatal depression. Evidence for the specificity of the diagnostic concept. *British Journal of Psychiatry*, **166**, 191–5.

Costa, M.M., Reus, V.I., Wolkowitz, O.M., Manfredi, F. and Lieberman, M., 1999. Estrogen replacement therapy and cognitive decline in memory-impaired post-menopausal women. *Biological Psychiatry*, **46**, 182–8.

Cox, J.L., Murray, D. and Chapman, G., 1993. A controlled study of the onset, duration and prevalence of postnatal depression. *British Journal of Psychiatry*, **163**, 27–31.

Culig, Z., Hobisch, A., Cronauer, M.V., Hittmair, A., Radmayr, C., Bartsch, G. and Klocker, H., 1995. Activation of the androgen receptor by polypeptide growth factors and cellular regulators. *World Journal of Urology*, **13**, 285–9.

Delmas, P.D., Bjarnason, N.H., Mitlak, B.H., Ravoux, A.C., Shah, A.S., Huster, W.J., Draper, M. and Christiansen, C., 1997. Effects of raloxifene on bone mineral density serum cholesterol concentrations and uterine endometrium in postmenopausal women. *New England Journal of Medicine*, **337**, 1641–7.

Ditkoff, E.C., Crary, W.G., Cristo, M. and Lobo, R.A., 1991. Estrogen improves psychological function in asymptomatic postmenopausal women. *Obstetrics and Gynecology*, **78**, 991–5.

Dorn, L.D. and Chrousos, G.P., 1997. The neurobiology of stress: understanding regulation of affect during female biological transitions. *Seminars in Reproductive Endocrinology*, **15**, 19–35.

Dougherty, D.M., Bjork, J.M., Moeller, F.G. and Swann, A.C., 1997. The influence of menstrual-cycle phase on the relationship between testosterone and aggression. *Physiological Behaviours*, **62**, 431–5.

Dunn, E.J. and Steiner, M., 2000. The functional neurochemistry of mood disorders in women. In: Steiner, M., Yonkers, K.A. and Eriksson, E. (eds), *Mood Disorders in Women*, pp. 71–82. Martin Dunitz, London.

Dunn, E., Macdougall, M., Coote, M. and Steiner, M., 2001. Biochemical correlates of symptoms associated with premenstrual dysphoric disorder. *Archives of Women's Mental Health*, **3**(suppl 2), 1.

Ehlers, C.L., Frank, E. and Kupfer, D.J., 1988. Social zeitgebers and biological rhythms. *Archives of General Psychiatry*, **45**, 948–52.

Eriksson, E., Sundblad, C., Lisjo, P., Modigh, K. and Andersch, B., 1992. Serum levels of androgens are higher in women with premenstrual irritability and dysphoria than in controls. *Psychoneuroendocrinology*, **17**, 195–204.

Eriksson, E., Sundblad, C., Landen, M. and Steiner, M., 2000. Behavioural effects of androgens in women. In: Steiner, M., Yonkers, K.A. and Eriksson, E. (eds), *Mood Disorders in Women*, pp. 233–46. Martin Dunitz, London.

Ernst, C. and Angst, J., 1992. The Zurich Study. XII. Sex differences in depression. Evidence from longitudinal epidemiological data. *European Archives of Psychiatry and Clinical Neurosciences*, **241**, 222–30.

Fink, G., Sumner, B.E., Rosie, R., Grace, O. and Quinn, J.P., 1996. Estrogen control of central neurotransmission: effect on mood, mental state, and memory. *Cellular and Molecular Neurobiology*, **16**, 325–44.

FitzGerald, M., Malone, K.M., Li, S., Harrison, W.M., McBride, P.A., Endicott, J., Cooper, T. and Mann, J.J., 1997. Blunted serotonin response to fenfluramine challenge in premenstrual dysphoric disorder. *American Journal of Psychiatry*, **154**, 556–8.

Fleming, A.S. and Corter, C., 1988. Factors influencing maternal responsiveness in humans: usefulness of an animal model. *Psychoneuroendocrinology*, **13**, 189–212.

Fleming, A.S., Steiner, M. and Anderson, V., 1987. Hormonal and attitudinal correlates of maternal behaviour during the early post-partum period in first-time mothers. *Journal of Reproductive and Infant Psychology*, **5**, 193–205.

Fleming, A.S., Corter, C. and Steiner, M., 1995. Sensory and hormonal control of maternal behavior in rat and human mothers. In: Pryce, C.R., Martin, R.D. and Skuse, D. (eds), *Motherhood in Human and Nonhuman Primates*, pp. 106–14. Karger, Basel.

Frank, E., Carpenter, L.L. and Kupfer, D.J., 1988. Sex differences in recurrent depression: are there any that are significant? *American Journal of Psychiatry*, **145**, 41–5.

Freedman, R.R., 2000. Hot flashes revisited. *Menopause*, **7**, 3–4.

Freeman, E.W., Sondheimer, K., Weinbaum, P.J. and Rickels, K., 1985. Evaluating premenstrual symptoms in medical practice. *Obstetrics and Gynecology*, **65**, 500–5.

Freeman, E.W., Rickels, K. and Sondheimer, S.J., 1993. Premenstrual symptoms and dysmenorrhea in relation to emotional distress factors in adolescents. *Journal of Psychosomatic Obstetrics and Gynaecology*, **14**, 41–50.

Garcia-Segura, L.M., Azcoitia, I. and DonCarlos, L.L., 2001. Neuroprotection by estradiol. *Progress in Neurobiology*, **63**, 29–60.

Girdler, S.S., Straneva, P.A., Light, K.C., Pedersen, C.A. and Morrow, A.L., 2001. Allopregnanolone levels and reactivity to mental stress in premenstrual dysphoric disorder. *Biological Psychiatry*, **49**, 788–97.

Glaser, J., Russell, V.A., de Villiers, A.S., Searson, J.A. and Taljaard, J.J., 1990. Rat brain monoamine and serotonin S2 receptor changes during pregnancy. *Neurochemical Research*, **15**, 949–56.

Golub, S. and Harrington, D.M., 1981. Premenstrual and menstrual mood changes in adolescent women. *Journal of Personality and Social Psychology*, **41**, 961–5.

Gregoire, A.J., Kumar, R., Everitt, B., Henderson, A.F. and Studd, J.W., 1996. Transdermal oestrogen for treatment of severe postnatal depression. *Lancet*, **347**, 930–3.

Guthrie, J.R., Dennerstein, L., Hopper, J.L. and Burger, H.G., 1996. Hot flushes, menstrual status and hormone levels in a population-based sample of midlife women. *Obstetrics and Gynecology*, **88**, 437–42.

Halbreich, U., Rojansky, N., Palter, S., Tworek, H., Hissen, P. and Wang, K., 1995. Estrogen augments serotonergic activity in postmenopausal women. *Biological Psychiatry*, **37**, 434–41.

Hankin, B.L., Abramson, L.Y., Moffitt, T.E., Silva, P.A., McGee, R. and Angell, K.E., 1998. Development of depression from preadolescence to young adulthood: emerging gender differences in a 10-year longitudinal study. *Journal of Abnormal Psychology*, **107**, 128–40.

Hannah, P., Adams, D., Glover, V. and Sandler, M., 1992. Abnormal platelet 5-hydroxytryptamine uptake and imipramine binding in postnatal dysphoria. *Journal of Psychiatry Research*, **26**, 69–75.

Harris, B., Othman, S., Davies, J.A., Weppner, G.J., Richards, C.J., Newcombe, R.G., Lazarus, J.H., Parkes, A.B., Hall, R. and Phillips, D.I., 1992. Association between post-partum thyroid dysfunction and thyroid antibodies and depression. *British Medical Journal*, **305**, 152–6.

Harris, B., Lovett, L., Newcombe, R.G., Read, G.F., Walker, R. and Riad-Fahmy, D., 1994. Maternity blues and major endocrine changes: Cardiff puerperal mood and hormone study II. *British Medical Journal*, **308**, 949–53.

Hay, A.G., Bancroft, J. and Johnstone, E.C., 1994. Affective symptoms in women attending a menopause clinic. *British Journal of Psychiatry*, **164**, 513–6.

Heidrich, A., Schleyer, M., Spingler, H., Albert, P., Knoche, M., Fritze, J. and Lanczik, M., 1994. Post-partum blues: relationship between not-protein bound steroid hormones in plasma and post-partum mood changes. *Journal of Affective Disorders*, **30**, 93–8.

Heim, C. and Nemeroff, C.B., 2001. The role of childhood trauma in the neurobiology of mood and anxiety disorders: preclinical and clinical studies. *Biological Psychiatry*, **49**, 1023–39.

Henderson, A.F., Gregoire, A.J., Kumar, R.D. and Studd, J.W., 1991. Treatment of severe postnatal depression with estradiol skin patches. *Lancet*, **338**, 816–7.

Herbison, A.E., Horvath, T.L., Naftolin, F. and Leranth, C., 1995. Distribution of estrogen receptor-immunoreactive cells in monkey hypothalamus: relationship to neurones containing luteinizing hormone-releasing hormone and tyrosine hydroxylase. *Neuroendocrinology*, **61**, 1–10.

Ho, H., Olsson, M., Westberg, L., Melke, J. and Eriksson, E., 2001. The serotonin reuptake inhibitor fluoxetine reduces sex steroid-related aggression in female rats: an animal model of premenstrual irritability? *Neuropsychopharmacology*, **24**, 502–10.

Hohlagschwandtner, M., Husslein, P., Klier, C. and Ulm, B., 2001. Correlation between serum testosterone levels and peripartal mood states. *Acta Obstetricia Gynecologica Scandinavica*, **80**, 326–30.

Hughes, C.W., Petty, F., Sheikha, S. and Kramer, G.L., 1996. Whole-blood serotonin in children and adolescents with mood and behavior disorders. *Psychiatry Research*, **65**, 79–95.

Johnson, S.R., 1987. The epidemiology and social impact of premenstrual symptoms. *Clinical Obstetrics and Gynecology*, **30**, 367–76.

Johnson, S.R., McChesney, C. and Bean, J.A., 1988. Epidemiology of premenstrual symptoms in a nonclinical sample. I Prevalence, natural history and help-seeking behaviour. *Journal of Reproductive Medicine*, **33**, 340–6.

Katona, C.L.E., Theodorou, A.E., Missouris, C.G., Bourke, M.P., Horton, R.W., Moncrieff, D., Paykel, E.S. and Kelly, J.S., 1985. Platelet ^{3}H-imipramine binding in pregnancy and the puerperium. *Psychiatry Research*, **14**, 33–7.

Kawas, C., Resnick, S., Morrison, A., Brookmeyer, R., Corrada, M., Zonderman, A., Bacal, C., Lingle, D.D. and Metter, E., 1997. A prospective study of estrogen replacement therapy and the risk of developing Alzheimer's disease: the Baltimore Longitudinal Study of Aging. *Neurology*, **48**, 1517–21.

Kendell, R.E., Chalmers, J.C. and Platz, C., 1987. Epidemiology of puerperal psychoses. *British Journal of Psychiatry*, **150**, 662–73.

Kendler, K.S., Karkowski, L.M., Corey, L.A. and Neale, M.C., 1998. Longitudinal population-based twin study of retrospectively reported premenstrual symptoms and lifetime major depression. *American Journal of Psychiatry*, **155**, 1234–40.

Kessler, R.C. and Walters, E.E., 1998. Epidemiology of DSM-III-R major depression and minor depression among adolescents and young adults in the National Comorbidity Survey. *Depression and Anxiety*, **7**, 3–14.

Kessler, R.C., McGonagle, K.A., Swartz, M., Blazer, D.G. and Nelson, C.B., 1993. Sex and depression in the national comorbidity survey I: lifetime prevalence chronicity and recurrence. *Journal of Affective Disorders*, **29**, 85–96.

Kessler, R.C., McGonagle, K.A., Nelson, C.B., Hughes, M., Swartz, M. and Blazer, D.G., 1994. Sex and depression in the National Comorbidity Survey. II: Cohort effects. *Journal of Affective Disorders*, **30**, 15–26.

Keverne, E.B. and Kendrick, K.M., 1994. Maternal behaviour in sheep and its neuroendocrine regulation. *Acta Paediatrica Supplement*, **397**, 47–56.

Kim, J., Alexander, C., Korst, L. and Agarwal, S., 2000. Effects of breast-feeding on hypoestrogenic symptoms in post-partum women. *Obstetrics and Gynecology*, **95**(suppl 4), 65S.

Kornstein, S.G., 1997. Gender differences in depression: implications for treatment. *Journal of Clinical Psychiatry*, **58**(suppl 15), 12–18.

Kornstein, S.G., 2001. The evaluation and management of depression in women across the life span. *Journal of Clinical Psychiatry*, **62**(suppl 24), 11–17.

Kornstein, S.G. and Wojcik, B.A., 2000. Gender effects in the treatment of depression. *Psychiatric Clinics of North America*, **7**, 23–57.

Kornstein, S.G., Schatzberg, A.F., Thase, M.E., Yonkers, K.A., McCullough, J.P., Keitner, G.I., Gelenberg, A.J., Ryan, C.E., Hess, A.L., Harrison, W., Davis, S.M. and Keller, M.B., 2000. Gender differences in chronic major and double depression. *Journal of Affective Disorders*, **60**, 1–11.

Korzekwa, M.I., Lamont, J.A. and Steiner, M., 1996. Late luteal phase dysphoric disorder and the thyroid axis revisited. *Journal of Clinical Endocrinology and Metabolism*, **81**, 2280–4.

Ladisich, W., 1977. Influence of progesterone on serotonin metabolism: a possible causal factor for mood changes. *Psychoneuroendocrinology*, **2**, 257–66.

Lauber, A.H. and Whalen, R.E., 1988. Muscarinic cholinergic modulation of hypothalamic estrogen binding sites. *Brain Research*, **443**, 21–6.

Leibenluft, E., Hardin, T.A. and Rosenthal, N.E., 1995. Gender differences in seasonal affective disorder. *Depression*, **3**, 13–19.

Lewinsohn, P.M., Rhode, P. and Seeley, J.R., 1998. Major depressive disorder in older adolescents: prevalence risk factors and clinical implications. *Clinical Psychology Review*, **18**, 765–94.

Lock, M., 1994. Menopause in cultural context. *Experimental Gerontology*, **29**, 307–17.

Luine, V.N., Khylchevskaya, R.I. and McEwen, B.S., 1975. Effect of gonadal steroids on activities of monoamine oxidase and choline acetylase in rat brain. *Brain Research*, **86**, 293–306.

Maggi, A. and Perez, J., 1985. Role of female gonadal hormones in the CNS: clinical and experimental aspects. *Life Sciences*, **37**, 893–906.

Magiakou, M.A., Mastorakos, G., Rabin, D., Dubbert, B., Gold, P.W. and Chrousos, G.P., 1996. Hypothalamic corticotropin-releasing hormone suppression during the postpartum period: implications for the increase in psychiatric manifestations at this time. *Journal of Clinical Endocrinology and Metabolism*, **81**, 1912–17.

Mani, S.K., Blaustein, J.D. and O'Malley, B.W., 1997. Progesterone receptor function from a behavioral perspective. *Hormones and Behavior*, **31**, 244–55.

McEwen, B.S., 1988. Genomic regulation of sexual behavior. *Journal of Steroid Biochemistry*, **30**, 179–83.

Meller, W.H., Grambsch, P.L., Bingham, C. and Tagatz, G.E., 2001. Hypothalamic pituitary gonadal axis dysregulation in depressed women. *Psychoneuroendocrinology*, **26**, 253–9.

Menkes, D.B., Coates, D.C. and Fawcett, J.P., 1994. Acute tryptophan depletion aggravates premenstrual syndrome. *Journal of Affective Disorders*, **32**, 37–44.

Millis, J.B. and Kornblith, P.R., 1992. Fragile beginnings: identification and treatment of post-partum disorders. *Health and Social Work*, **17**, 192–9.

Mitchell, E.S. and Woods, N.F., 1996. Symptom experiences of midlife women: observations from the Seattle Midlife Women's Health Study. *Maturitas*, **25**, 1–10.

Moldin, S.O., Scheftner, W.A., Rice, J.P., Nelson, E., Knesevich, M.A. and Akiskal, H., 1993. Association between major depressive disorder and physical illness. *Psychological Medicine*, **23**, 755–61.

Monteleone, P., Luisi, S., Tonetti, A., Bernardi, F., Genazzani, A.D., Luisi, M. and Petraglia, F., 2000. Allopregnanolone concentrations and premenstrual syndrome. *European Journal of Endocrinology*, **142**, 269–73.

Moss, R.L., Gu, Q. and Wong, M., 1997. Estrogen: nontranscriptional signaling pathway. *Recent Progress in Hormone Research*, **52**, 33–69.

Mulnard, R.A., Cotman, C.W., Kawas, C., van Dyck, C.H., Sano, M., Doody, R., Koss, E., Pfeiffer, E., Jin, S., Gamst, A., Grundman, M., Thomas, R. and Thal, L.J., 2000. Estrogen replacement therapy for treatment of mild to moderate Alzheimer disease. *Journal of the American Medical Association*, **283**, 1007–15.

Murray, D., Cox, J.L., Chapman, G. and Jones, P., 1995. Childbirth: life event or start of a long-term difficulty? Further data from the Stoke-on-Trent controlled study of postnatal depression. *British Journal of Psychiatry*, **166**, 595–600.

Nagata, C., Takatsuka, N., Inaba, S., Kawakami, N. and Shimizu, H., 1998. Association of diet and other lifestyle with onset of menopause in Japanese women. *Maturitas*, **29**, 105–13.

Nappi, R.E., Petraglia, F., Luisi, S., Polatti, F., Farina, C. and Genazzani, A.R., 2001. Serum allopregnanolone in women with post-partum 'blues'. *Obstetrics and Gynecology*, **97**, 77–80.

Nilsen, J., Mor, G. and Naftolin, F., 1998. Raloxifene induces neurite outgrowth in estrogen receptor positive PC 12 cells. *Menopause*, **5**, 211–16.

Nolen-Hoeksema, S., 1987. Sex differences in unipolar depression: evidence and theory. *Psychological Bulletin*, **101**, 259–82.

Nolen-Hoeksema, S. and Girgus, J.S., 1994. The emergence of gender differences in depression during adolescence. *Psychological Bulletin*, **115**, 424–43.

O'Brien, P.M.S. and Pitt, B., 1994. Hormonal theories and therapy for postnatal depression. In: Cox, J.L. and Holden, J. (eds), *Perinatal Psychiatry: Use and Misuse of the Edinburgh Postnatal Depression Scale*, pp. 103–11. Gaskell, London.

O'Brien, P.M.S., Abukhalil, I.E.H. and Henshaw, C., 1995. Premenstrual syndrome. *Current Obstetrics and Gynecology*, **5**, 30–7.

O'Hara, M.W., Schlechte, J.A., Lewis, D.A. and Wright, E.J., 1991. Prospective study of post-partum blues: biologic and psychosocial factors. *Archives of General Psychiatry*, **48**, 801–6.

Okano, T. and Nomura, J., 1992. Endocrine study of the maternity blues. *Progress in Neuropsychopharmacology and Biological Psychiatry*, **16**, 921–32.

Paganini-Hill, A. and Henderson, V.W., 1994. Estrogen deficiency and risk of Alzheimer's disease in women. *American Journal of Epidemiology*, **140**, 256–61.

Palinkas, L.A. and Barrett-Connor, E., 1992. Estrogen use and depressive symptoms in postmenopausal women. *Obstetrics and Gynecology*, **80**, 30–6.

Parlee, M.B., 1976. Social factors in the psychology of menstruation, birth, and menopause. *Primary Care*, **3**, 477–90.

Paykel, E.S., Emms, E.M., Fletcher, J. and Rassaby, E.S., 1980. Life events and social support in puerperal depression. *British Journal of Psychiatry*, **136**, 339–46.

Pecins-Thompson, M., Brown, N.A. and Bethea, C.L., 1998. Regulation of serotonin re-uptake transporter mRNA expression by ovarian steroids in rhesus macaques. *Molecular Brain Research*, **53**, 120–9.

Pedersen, C.A., Stern, R.A., Evans, D.L., Pate, J., Jamison, C. and Ozer, H., 1993a. Natural killer cell activity is lower in post-partum dysphorics. *Biological Psychiatry*, **33**, 85A.

Pederson, C.A., Stern, R.A., Pate, J., Senger, M.A., Bowes, W.A. and Mason, G.A., 1993b. Thyroid and adrenal measures during late pregnancy and the puerperium in women who have been major depressed or who become dysphoric post-partum. *Journal of Affective Disorders*, **29**, 201–11.

Pop, V.J.M., Essed, G.G., de Geus, C.A., vanSon, M.M. and Komproe, I.H., 1993. Prevalence of post partum depression — or is it post-puerperium depression? *Acta Obstetricia Gynecologica Scandinavica*, **72**, 354–8.

Prior, J.C., 1998. Perimenopause: the complex endocrinology of the menopausal transition. *Endocrinology Review*, **19**, 397–428.

Purnine, D. and Frank, E., 1996. Should post-partum mood disorders be given a more prominent or distinctive place in DSM-IV? In: Widiger, T.A., Frances, A.J., Pincus, H.A., Ross, R., First, M.B. and Davis, W.W. (eds), *DSM-IV Sourcebook*, vol. 2, pp. 261–79. American Psychiatric Association, Washington, DC.

Raja, S.N., Feehan, M., Stanton, W.R. and McGee, R., 1992. Prevalence and correlates of the premenstrual syndrome in adolescence. *Journal of the American Academy of Child and Adolescent Psychiatry*, **31**, 783–9.

Ramcharan, S., Love, E.J., Fick, G.H. and Goldfien, A., 1992. The epidemiology of premenstrual symptoms in a population based sample of 2650 urban women. *Journal of Clinical Epidemiology*, **45**, 377–92.

Rapkin, A.J., 1992. The role of serotonin in premenstrual syndrome. *Clinical Obstetrics and Gynecology*, **35**, 629–36.

Rapkin, A.J., Morgan, M., Goldman, L., Brann, D.W., Simone, D. and Mahesh, V.B., 1997. Progesterone metabolite allopregnanolone in women with premenstrual syndrome. *Obstetrics and Gynecology*, **90**, 709–14.

Rasgon, N., Serra, M., Biggio, G., Pisu, M.G., Fairbanks, L., Tanavoli, S. and Rapkin, A., 2001. Neuroactive steroid–serotonergic interaction: responses to an intravenous L-tryptophan challenge in women with premenstrual syndrome. *European Journal of Endocrinology*, **145**, 25–33.

Roca, C.A., Schmidt, P.J., Bloch, M. and Rubinow, D.R., 1996. Implications of endocrine studies of premenstrual syndrome. *Psychiatric Annals*, **26**, 576–80.

Rosenblatt, J.S., Mayer, A.D. and Giordano, A.L., 1988. Hormonal basis during pregnancy for the onset of maternal behaviour in the rat. *Psychoneuroendocrinology*, **13**, 29–46.

Rowe, T. and Sasse, V., 1986. Androgens and premenstrual symptoms — the response to therapy. In: Dennerstein, L. and Frazer, I. (eds), *Hormones and Behaviour*, pp. 160–5. Elsevier Science, New York.

Ryan, N.D. and Varma, D. (1998) Child and adolescent mood disorders — experience with serotonin-based therapies. *Biological Psychiatry*, **44**, 336–40.

Schmidt, P.J. and Rubinow, D.R., 1991. Menopause-related affective disorders: a justification for further study. *American Journal of Psychiatry*, **148**, 844–52.

Schmidt, P.J., Grover, G.N., Roy-Byrne, P.P. and Rubinow, D.R., 1993. Thyroid function in women with premenstrual syndrome. *Journal of Clinical Endocrinology and Metabolism*, **76**, 671–4.

Schmidt, P.J., Purdy, R.H., Moore, P.H., Jr, Paul, S.M. and Rubinow, D.R., 1994). Circulating levels of anxiolytic steroids in the luteal phase in women with premenstrual syndrome and in control subjects. *Journal of Clinical Endocrinology and Metabolism*, **79**, 1256–60.

Schmidt, P.J., Nieman, L.K., Danaceau, M.A., Adams, L.F. and Rubinow, D.R., 1998. Differential behavioral effects of gonadal steroids in women with and in those without premenstrual syndrome. *New England Journal of Medicine*, **338**, 209–16.

Schmidt, P.J., Neiman, L., Danaceau, M.A., Tobin, M.B., Roca, C.A., Murphy, J.H. and Rubinow, D.R., 2000. Estrogen replacement in perimenopause-related depression: a preliminary report. *American Journal of Obstetrics and Gynecology*, **183**, 414–20.

Schneider, L.S., Small, G.W., Hamilton, S.H., Bystritsky, A., Nemeroff, C.B. and Meyers, B.S., 1997. Estrogen replacement and response to fluoxetine in a multicenter geriatric depression trial. *American Journal of Geriatric Psychiatry*, **5**, 97–106.

Sherwin, B.B., 1988. Affective changes with estrogen and androgen replacement therapy in surgically menopausal women. *Journal of Affective Disorders*, **14**, 177–87.

Sherwin, B.B., 1999a. Can estrogen keep you smart? Evidence from clinical studies. *Journal of Psychiatry and Neuroscience*, **24**, 315–21.

Sherwin, B.B., 1999b. Progestogens used in menopause. Side effects, mood and quality of life. *Journal of Reproductive Medicine*, **44**(Suppl. 2), 227–32.

Sherwin, B.B. and Suranyi-Cadotte, B.E., 1990. Up-regulatory effect of estrogen on platelet 3H-imipramine binding sites in surgically menopausal women. *Biological Psychiatry*, **28**, 339–48.

Sichel, D.A., Cohen, L.S., Robertson, L.M., Ruttenberg, A. and Rosenbaum, J.F., 1995. Prophylactic estrogen in recurrent post-partum affective disorder. *Biological Psychiatry*, **38**, 814–18.

Smith, R., Cubis, J., Brinsmead, M., Lewin, T., Singh, B., Owens, P., Chan, E.C., Hall, C., Alder, R., Lovelock, M., Hurt, D., Rowley, M. and Nolan, M., 1990. Mood changes, obstetric experience and alterations in plasma cortisol; beta-endorphin and CRH during pregnancy and the puerperium. *Journal of Psychosomatic Research*, **34**, 53–69.

Smith, S.S., Gong, Q.H., Hsu, F.-C., Markowitz, R.S., French-Mullen, J.M. and Li, X., 1998. $GABA_A$ receptor $\alpha4$ subunit suppression prevents withdrawal properties of an endogenous steroid. *Nature*, **392**, 926–30.

Soares, C., Almeida, O.P., Joffe, H. and Cohen, L.S., 2001. Efficacy of estradiol for the treatment of depressive disorders in perimenopausal women: a double blind randomized placebo-controlled trial. *Archives of General Psychiatry*, **58**, 529–34.

Stahl, S.M., 2001a. Why drugs and hormones may interact in psychiatric disorders. *Journal of Clinical Psychiatry*, **62**, 225–6.

Stahl, S.M., 2001b. Sex and psychopharmacology: is natural estrogen a psychotropic drug in women? *Archives of General Psychiatry*, **58**, 537–8.

Steege, J.F., Stout, A.L., Knight, D.L. and Nemeroff, C.B., 1992. Reduced platelet tritium-labeled imipramine binding sites in women with premenstrual syndrome. *American Journal of Obstetrics and Gynecology*, **167**, 168–72.

Stein, G., Marsh, A. and Morton, J., 1981. Mental symptoms, weight changes and electrolyte excretion in the first post partum week. *Journal of Psychosomatic Research*, **25**, 395–408.

Steiner, M., 1998. Perinatal mood disorders: position paper. *Psychopharmacology Bulletin*, **34**, 301–6.

Steiner, M. and Born, L., 2000. Advances in the diagnosis and treatment of premenstrual dysphoria. *CNS Drugs*, **13**, 286–304.

Steiner, M. and Dunn, E.J., 1996. The psychobiology of female-specific mood disorders. *Infertility and Reproductive Medicine Clinics of North America*, **7**, 297–313.

Steiner, M. and Tam, W.Y.K., 1999. Post-partum depression in relation to other psychiatric disorders. In: Miller, L.J. (ed.), *Post-partum Mood Disorders*, pp. 47–63. American Psychiatric Press, Washington, DC.

Steiner, M. and Wilkins, A., 1996. Diagnosis and assessment of premenstrual dysphoria. *Psychiatric Annals*, **26**, 571–5.

Steiner, M., Fleming, A.S., Anderson, V.N., Monkhouse, E. and Boulter, G.E., 1986. A psychoneuroendocrine profile for post-partum blues? In: Dennerstein, L. and Fraser, I. (eds), *Hormones and Behaviour*, pp. 327–35. Elsevier Science, Amsterdam.

Steiner, M., LePage, P. and Dunn, E., 1997. Serotonin and gender specific psychiatric disorders. *International Journal of Psychiatry in Clinical Practice*, **1**, 3–13.

Steiner, M., Yatham, L.N., Coote, M., Wilkins, A. and Lepage, P., 1999. Serotonergic dysfunction in women with pure premenstrual dysphoric disorder: is the fenfluramine challenge test still relevant? *Psychiatry Research*, **87**, 107–15.

Steiner, M., Born, L. and Marton, P., 2000. Menarche and mood disorders in adolescence. In: Steiner, M., Yonkers, K.A. and Eriksson, E. (eds), *Mood Disorders in Women*, pp. 247–68. Martin Dunitz, London.

Stewart, D.E., Klompenhouwer, J.L., Kendell, R.E. and van Hulst, A.M., 1991. Prophylactic lithium in puerperal psychosis. *British Journal of Psychiatry*, **158**, 393–7.

Stomati, M., Genazzani, A.D., Petraglia, F. and Genazzani, A.R., 1998. Contraception as prevention and therapy: sex steroids and the brain. *European Journal of Contraception and Reproductive Health Care*, **3**, 21–8.

Stowe, Z.N., Cassarella, J., Landry, J. and Nemeroff, C.B., 1995. Sertraline in the treatment of women with post-partum major depression. *Depression*, **3**, 49–55.

Su, T.P., Schmidt, P.J., Danaceau, M., Murphy, D.L. and Rubinow, D.R., 1997. Effect of menstrual cycle phase on neuroendocrine and behavioral responses to the serotonin agonist *m*-chlorophenylpiperazine in women with premenstrual syndrome and controls. *Journal of Clinical Endocrinology and Metabolism*, **82**, 1220–8.

Sumner, B.E. and Fink, G., 1998. Testosterone as well as estrogen increases serotonin2A receptor mRNA and binding site densities in the male rat brain. *Molecular Brain Research*, **59**, 205–14.

Susman, E.J., Dorn, L.D. and Chrousos, G.P., 1991. Negative affect and hormone levels in young adolescents: concurrent and predictive perspectives. *Journal of Adolescence*, **20**, 167–90.

Tanner, J.M., 1962. *Growth at Adolescence*, 2nd edn. Blackwell, Oxford.

Tanner, J.M., 1968. Earlier maturation in man. *Scientific American*, **218**, 21–7.

Tuiten, A., Van Honk, J., Koppeschaar, H., Bernaards, C., Thijssen, J. and Verbaten, R., 2000. Time course of effects of testosterone administration on sexual arousal in women. *Archives of General Psychiatry*, **57**, 149–53.

Vamvakopoulos, N.C. and Chrousos, G.P., 1993. Evidence of direct estrogenic regulation of human corticotropin-releasing hormone gene expression. *Journal of Clinical Investigation*, **92**, 1896–1902.

van Amelsvoort, T.A., Abel, K.M., Robertson, D.M., Daly, E., Critchley, H., Whitehead, M. and Murphy, D.G., 2001. Prolactin response to d-fenfluramine in postmenopausal women on and off ERT: comparison with young women. *Psychoneuroendocrinology*, **26**, 493–502.

Wang, M., Seippel, L., Purdy, R.H. and Bäckström, T., 1996. Relationship between symptom severity and steroid variation in women with premenstrual syndrome: study on serum pregnenolone, pregnenolone sulfate, 5α-pregnane-3,20-dione and 3α-hydroxy-5-α-pregnan-20-one. *Journal of Clinical Endocrinology and Metabolism*, **81**, 1076–82.

Waring, S.C., Rocca, W.A., Petersen, R.C., O'Brien, P.C., Tangalos, E.G. and Kokmen, E., 1999. Postmenopausal estrogen replacement therapy and risk of AD: a population-based study. *Neurology*, **52**, 965–70.

Warren, M.P. and Brooks-Gunn, J., 1989. Mood and behavior at adolescence: evidence for hormonal factors. *Journal of Clinical Endocrinology and Metabolism*, **69**, 77–83.

Weissman, M.M. and Olfson, M., 1995. Depression in women: implications for health care research. *Science*, **269**, 799–801.

Weissman, M.M., Livingston, B.M., Leaf, P.J., Florio, L.P. and Holzer, C., 1991. Affective disorders. In: Robins, L.N. and Regier, D.A. (eds), *Psychiatric Disorders in America*, pp. 53–80. Free Press, New York.

Whooley, M.A. and Browner, W.S., 1998. Association between depressive symptoms and mortality in older women. *Archives of Internal Medicine*, **158**, 2129–35.

Whybrow, P.C., 1995. Sex differences in thyroid axis function: relevance to affective disorder and its treatment. *Depression*, **3**, 33–42.

Wieck, A., Kumar, R., Hirst, A.D., Marks, M.N., Campbell, I.C. and Checkley, S.A., 1991. Increased sensitivity of dopamine receptors and recurrence of affective psychosis after childbirth. *British Medical Journal*, **303**, 613–6.

Wong, M., Thompson, T.L. and Moss, R.L., 1996. Nongenomic actions of estrogen in the brain: physiological significance and cellular mechanisms. *Critical Reviews in Neurobiology*, **10**, 189–203.

World Health Organization, 1981. Research on the menopause. *World Health Organization Technical Report Series*, **670**, 3–120.

World Health Organization, 1996a. Mental behavioral and developmental disorders. In: *Tenth Revision of the International Classification of Diseases (ICD-10)*. World Health Organization, Geneva.

World Health Organization, 1996b. Research on the menopause in the 1990s. *World Health Organization Technical Report Series*, **866**, 1–79.

Wyatt, K., Dimmock, P., Jones, P., Obhrai, M. and O'Brien, S., 2001. Efficacy of progesterone and progestogens in management of premenstrual syndrome: systematic review. *British Medical Journal*, **323**, 776–80.

Yaffe, K., Krueger, K., Sarkar, S., Grady, D., Barrett-Connor, E., Cox, D.A. and Nickelsen, T., 2001. Cognitive function in postmenopausal women treated with raloxifene. *New England Journal of Medicine*, **344**, 1207–13.

Yonkers, K.A., Kando, J.C., Cole, J.O. and Blumenthal, S., 1992. Gender differences in pharmacokinetics and pharmacodynamics of psychotropic medication. *American Journal of Psychiatry*, **149**, 587–95.

Young, E.A., Midgley, A.R., Carlson, N.E. and Brown, M.B., 2000. Alteration in the hypothalamic–pituitary–ovarian axis in depressed women. *Archives of General Psychiatry*, **57**, 1157–62.

Zacharias, L. and Wurtman, R.J., 1964. Blindness: its relation to age of menarche. *Science*, **144**, 1154–5.

Zweifel, J.E. and O'Brien, W.H., 1997. A meta-analysis of the effect of hormone replacement therapy upon depressed mood. *Psychoneuroendocrinology*, **22**, 189–212.

XVIII-13

Therapeutic Armamentarium

Robert H. Howland and Michael E. Thase

INTRODUCTION

Currently, a wide variety of therapies are available for the treatment of mood disorders. These therapies have been studied mainly in major depressive disorder and bipolar I disorder, although they also are commonly used in clinical practice for the treatment of such related mood disorders as dysthymia, minor depression, cyclothymia and bipolar II disorder (Howland, 1991; Howland and Thase, 1993). The diversity of the many antidepressant and antimanic therapies that are effective likely reflects the underlying pathophysiological heterogeneity that exists among the mood disorders (Howland and Thase, 1999b), although seemingly different therapies also may share common therapeutic mechanisms of action. For a significant proportion of mood disorder patients, the available standard antidepressant and antimanic therapies are not entirely effective, contributing to the development and clinical use of novel treatments. In this chapter we review standard antidepressant and antimanic therapies for mood disorders. We also review novel pharmacological and non-pharmacological therapies that are being studied and sometimes used for the treatment of major depressive and bipolar disorders.

TREATMENT OF DEPRESSION

Antidepressant Drugs

During the 1950s, the clinical effects of tricyclic antidepressant (TCA) and monoamine oxidase inhibiting (MAOI) drugs were first discovered (Crane, 1957; Kuhn, 1958). Since the 1980s, numerous antidepressant drugs unrelated to the TCAs and MAOIs have been developed and studied for the treatment of depression (Kent, 2000; Sampson, 2001).

Tricyclic Antidepressants (TCAs)

After their discovery, the TCAs were the cornerstone of pharmacotherapy for depression for nearly three decades (Nelson, 2000). The most commonly used TCAs, so called because of their cyclic chemical structure, include imipramine, desipramine, amitriptyline and nortriptyline. Doxepin, trimipramine and protriptyline are less commonly used. Clomipramine is approved for use in the United States only for the treatment of obsessive-compulsive disorder, but it is a highly effective antidepressant. The antidepressant effects of the TCAs are believed to be primarily due to their inhibition of the reuptake of the neurotransmitters norepinephrine and serotonin (Richelson, 2001), although they and other antidepressant drugs also directly or indirectly affect second-messenger systems (Popoli *et al.*, 2000; Vaidya and Duman, 2001) that are implicated in the neurobiology of depression (Duman *et al.*, 1997). Aside from clomipramine, the TCAs are more active on noradrenergic reuptake inhibition. They also potently block several important postsynaptic neurochemical receptors, which account for most of their typical side effects. Dry mouth, constipation, blurred vision, sinus tachycardia, urinary retention and memory dysfunction are due to cholinergic receptor blockade. Sedation and weight gain are primarily related to histaminic receptor blockade, although serotonergic and anticholinergic effects may also contribute to the weight gain associated with the TCAs and other types of antidepressant drugs (Fava *et al.*, 2000). Dizziness, hypotension and reflex tachycardia are caused by their blockade of α-1 adrenergic receptors. The TCAs also have quinidine-like effects on cardiac conduction, which can cause serious cardiotoxic effects, including arrhythmias and conduction abnormalities, and can be fatal with an overdose as small as 7–10 times a daily therapeutic dose.

As a group, the TCAs do not differ significantly in their relative antidepressant efficacy (Thase, 1997). Two TCAs, nortriptyline and desipramine, are secondary amine metabolites of amitriptyline and imipramine, respectively, and they are often preferred because of less pronounced anticholinergic side effects. Placebo-controlled studies have found TCAs to be effective in adult and geriatric patients, but not in younger age groups (Brent *et al.*, 1995). Interestingly, compared to men and to postmenopausal women, there is evidence that premenopausal women respond less well to TCAs than to other antidepressant drugs (Kornstein *et al.*, 2000; Thase *et al.*, 2000a). Higher TCA doses are often associated with greater therapeutic benefit, but this is limited by their greater side effect burden. Measuring plasma levels of imipramine, amitriptyline, desipramine and nortriptyline is clinically useful for achieving a therapeutic response (Bernstein, 1995). Because of their side effects and potential lethality, the use of TCAs has been gradually supplanted by newer generation antidepressants. The TCAs, however, can be quite effective in treating patients who do not respond to other drugs, and they remain especially effective treatments for more severe melancholic depressions (Thase and Rush, 1995).

Monoamine Oxidase Inhibitors (MAOIs)

The pharmacology and presumed mechanism of action of the MAOIs is distinctly different from all other antidepressants (Kennedy *et al.*, 2000). The MAOIs phenelzine, tranylcypromine and isocarboxazid irreversibly and non-selectively inhibit the enzyme monoamine oxidase (MAO), which degrades norepinephrine, serotonin and dopamine, thereby increasing the availability of these neurotransmitters and likely contributing to their antidepressant effects (Richelson, 2001), although they may also directly or indirectly affect second-messenger systems (Popoli *et al.*, 2000; Vaidya and Duman, 2001) that are implicated in the neurobiology of depression (Duman *et al.*, 1997). Typical side

Biological Psychiatry: Edited by H. D'haenen, J.A. den Boer and P. Willner. ISBN 0-471-49198-5

effects of the MAOIs include hypotension, dizziness, sedation, weight gain, dry mouth and sexual dysfunction. Phenelzine is more often associated with these side effects than is tranylcypromine, whereas tranylcypromine may be more likely to cause insomnia. Because the MAOIs inhibit MAO in the gut, severe hypertension can occur when foods containing the amino acid tyramine (which stimulates the release of norepinephrine) are ingested. As a result, patients treated with MAOIs must follow a tyramine-free diet. In addition, use of the MAOIs is associated with potentially severe and fatal interactions with various other drugs, including antidepressants, narcotics and sympathomimetics.

Because of their side effect profile and dietary restrictions, the MAOIs are not commonly used in clinical practice. However, comparative studies have found the MAOIs to be more effective than the TCAs and other antidepressants in the treatment of atypical depression (Jarrett *et al.*, 1999; McGrath *et al.*, 2000) and bipolar depression (Thase and Sachs, 2000). In addition, the MAOIs have consistently been found to be effective in 40–60% of patients who do not respond to other antidepressants (Thase *et al.*, 1995). Like the TCAs, higher doses (within the therapeutic range) also are associated with a greater antidepressant effect if tolerable.

Some MAOIs are relatively selective for the Type A or Type B subforms of MAO (Lotufo-Neto *et al.*, 1999). Selegiline is a selective inhibitor of MAO-B at low doses, but there is little evidence that it has antidepressant effects at these doses. At higher doses, however, selegiline loses its selectivity and has greater antidepressant effects. A selegiline transdermal application system is currently being developed, which avoids peripheral MAO-A inhibition in the gut and permits greater systemic selegiline levels without the risk of a tyramine reaction, potentially making it a more viable antidepressant therapy (Barrett *et al.*, 1997; Mahmood 1997; Sacktor *et al.*, 2000). By contrast, moclobemide and brofaromine are reversible inhibitors of MAO-A (RIMAs). The RIMAs have demonstrated antidepressant effects, are much better tolerated than the TCAs and older MAOIs, and do not require any dietary restrictions, although there is some evidence that they may be slightly less effective compared to TCAs and older MAOIs (Amrein *et al.*, 1997; Lotufo-Neto *et al.*, 1999; Parker *et al.*, 2001; Philipp *et al.*, 2000).

Heterocyclic Antidepressants

Problems with the tolerability and safety of the TCAs and MAOIs led to interest in developing alternative antidepressant drugs (Bernstein, 1995). These pharmacologically diverse drugs include amoxapine, maprotiline and trazodone (Richelson, 2001). Amoxapine is a TCA-like compound that is related to the antipsychotic drug loxapine, and can have similar extrapyramidal side effects (e.g. dystonia, akathesia, parkinsonian symptoms, and possibly tardive dyskinesia). As a result, it has not been a commonly used antidepressant, although it is sometimes used as a 'monotherapy' for the treatment of psychotic depression (Wheeler Vega *et al.*, 2000). Maprotiline is a tetracyclic drug that primarily blocks the reuptake of norepinephrine, but is rarely used because of a higher risk of seizures and cardiac toxicity compared to other antidepressants. Trazodone is a phenylpiperazine compound that has weak effects on monoamine reuptake, but does block postsynaptic serotonin (5-HT2) receptors. Trazodone has been used almost exclusively in lower doses as a safe and effective non-habit forming hypnotic, often in combination with other antidepressants. Higher doses are usually needed to treat severe depression and have been associated with severe hypotension and, rarely, the development of priapism.

Serotonin Reuptake Inhibitors (SRIs)

The SRIs have become the most commonly used class of antidepressants for the treatment of depression around much of the world (Gram, 1994). These drugs include fluoxetine, paroxetine, sertraline and citalopram (Sampson, 2001). A fifth SRI, fluvoxamine, is approved in the United States as a treatment for obsessive-compulsive disorder, but also is an effective antidepressant. As a class, the SRIs are chemically dissimilar, which accounts for various pharmacologic differences (e.g. different half-lives, active metabolites and hepatic enzyme inhibitory effects). Despite the pharmacologic differences, these drugs have a similar mechanism of action, which is their potent and specific inhibition of serotonin reuptake (Richelson, 2001), although they also directly or indirectly affect second-messenger systems (Popoli *et al.*, 2000; Vaidya and Duman, 2001) that are implicated in the neurobiology of depression (Duman *et al.*, 1997). Typical side effects of the SRIs include nausea, diarrhoea, insomnia, nervousness, headache and sexual dysfunction. Additional clinical experience with the SRIs also suggests that some patients may complain of sweating, fatigue and weight gain (Fava *et al.*, 2000). They do not have significant cardiac effects, and are much safer than the TCAs and MAOIs in overdose. Several of the SRIs also can inhibit various hepatic enzymes, which are important for drug metabolism and can lead to clinically significant drug interactions, but this limitation has not lessened the utility of the SRIs (Thase, 1997).

As a group, the SRIs do not differ significantly in their relative efficacy or typical side effect profiles, although there may be subtle differences in the degree of certain side effects (Kelsey and Nemeroff, 2000). There is some evidence that patients who do not respond to or cannot tolerate one SRI may do better after switching to an alternative SRI (Howland and Thase, 1999a). Comparative studies with the TCAs have generally found similar efficacy rates, although indices of tolerability usually favour the SRIs. There continues to be debate about whether the TCAs are more effective among patients with more severe melancholic depressions (Perry, 1996; Thase and Rush, 1995). Unlike the TCAs, placebo-controlled studies have found the SRIs to be effective in treating depression in adolescents (Emslie *et al.*, 1997). Moreover, compared to men and to postmenopausal women, premenopausal women may respond relatively better to SRIs than to other antidepressant drugs (Kornstein *et al.*, 2000; Thase *et al.*, 2000a). The SRIs are generally considered to be safe for use during pregnancy (Ericson *et al.*, 1999).

Atypical Antidepressants

The term 'atypical antidepressants' is used to group the remaining antidepressant drugs (bupropion, venlafaxine, nefazodone, mirtazapine and reboxetine), which are chemically unrelated to each other and to the TCAs, MAOIs or SRIs (Preskorn, 1995; Kent, 2000).

Bupropion

Bupropion is a novel antidepressant that belongs to the aminoketone class of drugs (Golden and Nicholas, 2000). Its mechanism of action is uncertain, although bupropion appears to facilitate or modulate the effects of norepinephrine and dopamine. Bupropion has virtually no effect on serotonergic, cholinergic, histaminic or other adrenergic systems (Richelson, 2001). As a result, it lacks the usual side effects seen with the TCAs, MAOIs or SRIs. Typical side effects include restlessness, insomnia, nausea, headache, constipation and tremors. Bupropion is not associated with sexual dysfunction or weight gain and does not have significant cardiac effects. Bupropion is a modest inhibitor of the hepatic isoenzyme CYP450 2D6, but is not notorious for clinically significant drug interactions. High doses (greater than 450 mg per day) are associated with an increased risk of seizures, but within the manufacturer's recommended dose range the rate of seizures does not differ from other antidepressant drugs.

Comparative studies of bupropion and other antidepressants in depression have not found any significant differences in efficacy, but it has a different tolerability profile (especially with regard to sexual and weight effects) (Spier, 1998). It is sometimes combined with SRIs to lessen sexual dysfunction or augment antidepressant effects (Howland and Thase, 1999a). Bupropion may not be as effective in the treatment of severe anxiety states associated with depression (e.g. obsessive-compulsive or panic anxiety), but might be especially useful in anergic, atypical, seasonal or bipolar depressions (Sachs *et al.*, 1994; Thase, 1997).

Venlafaxine

Venlafaxine is a novel antidepressant belonging to the phenylethylamine class of drugs (Beauclair *et al.*, 2000). The primary mechanism of action is the inhibition of serotonin and, at higher doses, norepinephrine reuptake (Richelson, 2001). Typical side effects include nausea, headache, dizziness, dry mouth, constipation, loss of appetite, nervousness and insomnia (Kent, 2000). Some patients may complain of fatigue, sweating and sexual dysfunction. A small proportion of patients may develop increased blood pressure at high doses, but it does not have any other significant cardiac effects. It also does not have any clinically significant effect on hepatic metabolic enzymes and appears to be relatively safe in an overdose.

Some studies directly comparing venlafaxine to several different SRIs have found it to be more effective and more likely to lead to a full remission, especially at higher doses (Thase *et al.*, 2001a). There also is some evidence that venlafaxine may have a more rapid onset of action compared to other antidepressants, but this has not been well studied (Thase *et al.*, 2001c). In addition, other studies have found it effective in the treatment of refractory depression, including patients who had not responded to various antidepressants from different classes (Thase *et al.*, 2000b).

Nefazodone

Nefazodone is a novel antidepressant that, like trazodone, belongs to the phenylpiperazine class of drugs (Garlow *et al.*, 2000). Its primary mechanism of action may be blockade of postsynaptic serotonin-2 receptors. It has very weak inhibitory effects on reuptake of norepinephrine and serotonin (Richelson, 2001). Typical side effects include sedation, dry mouth, nausea, headache, constipation and dizziness (Kent, 2000). Compared to SRIs and TCAs, it is not associated with sexual dysfunction or weight gain (Ferguson *et al.*, 2001; Sussman *et al.*, 2001). Although nefazodone is a chemical analogue of the antidepressant trazodone, it is much less sedating initially and has not been found to cause priapism. Hypotension may occur rarely at high doses and rare cases of hypatotoxicity have been reported, but it does not have any other significant cardiac effects and seems to be relatively safe in an overdose. Nefazodone can inhibit the hepatic isoenzyme CYP450 3A4, which has some potential for drug–drug interactions (Thase, 1997).

Comparative studies have not found any significant difference in efficacy between nefazodone and SRIs or TCAs in the treatment of depression (Feighner *et al.*, 1998). Across 6–8 weeks of treatment, nefazodone appears to have more beneficial effects (than SRIs) on insomnia associated with depression. Nefazodone is effective in treating anxiety symptoms in depression, and its side effect profile (especially its sexual and weight effects) may be preferable for some patients compared to the SRIs (Sajatovic *et al.*, 1999).

Mirtazapine

Mirtazapine is a novel tetracyclic antidepressant belonging to the piperazinoazepine class of drugs (Claghorn, 2000). It has a very complicated presumed mechanism of action, involving blockade of several different adrenergic and serotonergic receptors, with the net effect of increasing serotonin and norepinephrine transmission (Richelson, 2001). It also blocks postsynaptic histamine receptors, which contributes to its most common side effects (i.e. sedation and weight gain). Compared to the SRIs, it is less likely to cause nausea, headache and sexual dysfunction (Kent, 2000). In some patients, it can cause dry mouth, constipation and dizziness. It does not have significant cardiac effects, or any clinically significant drug interactions, and it appears to be relatively safe in an overdose.

Comparative studies with other antidepressants generally have not found any significant differences in efficacy (Fawcett and Barkin, 1998; Guelfi *et al.*, 2001), although several recent studies found mirtazapine to have a more rapid onset of action compared to SRIs (Thase *et al.*, 2001c). Its advantage over the SRIs with respect to gastrointestinal and sexual effects must be counterbalanced against its greater degree of sedation and weight gain. However, it may have more rapid and beneficial effects on sleep and anxiety in many patients, compared to the clinical effects of other antidepressants.

Reboxetine

Reboxetine is a novel antidepressant compound, not yet approved for use in the United States, that is unrelated to the TCAs, MAOIs, SRIs or other atypical antidepressant drugs (Healy and Healy, 1998). It is a potent and selective norepinephrine reuptake inhibitor and does not bind to serotonin, dopamine, cholinergic or histamine receptors (Richelson, 2001). As a result, reboxetine is not associated with sedation, weight gain or sexual dysfunction (Kent, 2000). Typical side effects include dry mouth, constipation, insomnia, increased heart rate and urinary hesitancy/retention (in men). It does not have significant cardiac effects, does not have any clinically significant effect on hepatic metabolic enzymes, and appears to be relatively safe in an overdose. Comparative studies with other antidepressants generally have not found any significant differences in efficacy, although the side effect profile differs (Massana, 1998; Versiani *et al.*, 2000).

Antidepressant Psychotherapies

Historically, before the discovery of effective antidepressant compounds, long-term psychodynamic therapy was considered the treatment of choice for non-psychotic depressions. This approach, although helpful to patients in many ways, was never studied to determine if it is effective in treating the core symptoms of depression. During the past 30 years, psychological models of depression have been used to develop short-term highly-structured forms of psychotherapy specifically for treating depression (Wells and Giannetti, 1990). Compared to traditional forms of psychotherapy, several of these depression-focused psychotherapies have been studied in clinical trials and found to be as effective as pharmacotherapy for the treatment of depressed outpatients (Persons *et al.*, 1996; Rush and Thase, 1999). Depression-focused psychotherapies should not be considered for treatment of psychotic or bipolar forms of depression without concomitant pharmacotherapy, although there is developing evidence that the use of specific psychosocial interventions together with pharmacotherapy may lead to a better outcome in bipolar disorder (Frank *et al.*, 2000; Miklowitz *et al.*, 2000).

Interpersonal psychotherapy (IPT) is a time-limited form of psychotherapy that focuses on difficulties in the patient's intimate and vocational relationships (Klerman *et al.*, 1984). IPT has been shown to be an effective and easily used intervention in the treatment of depression (Klerman and Weissman, 1993; Markowitz, 1998). Some studies have found it to be as effective as medication among outpatients with mild to moderate levels of depression (Persons *et al.*, 1996; Weissman and Markowitz, 1994). Interestingly, a recent functional brain imaging study of patients with major depression treated with paroxetine or IPT found that regional brain metabolic abnormalities tended to normalize with either treatment (Brody *et al.*, 2001). There also is developing evidence that IPT may be beneficial for the depressive phase of bipolar disorder (Swartz and Frank, 2001).

Various behavioural therapy (BT) approaches have been developed and studied in the treatment of depression, such as activity scheduling, self-control techniques and social skills training (Becker *et al.*, 1987; Rush and Thase, 1999). A number of controlled studies have found BT to be effective among outpatients with depression. Some evidence suggests that BT may be as effective as antidepressant medications in depression (Hersen *et al.*, 1984; Rush and Thase, 1999).

Cognitive behavioural therapy (CBT) is another time-limited form of psychotherapy that is based on the theory that depression is invariably associated with automatic negative thoughts about oneself, the world and the future (Beck *et al.*, 1979; Clark and Fairburn, 1997). CBT is the best studied form of psychotherapy for major depression and dysthymia (Howland, 1996a; Persons *et al.*, 1996). Many studies have found it to be as effective a treatment for major depression as TCAs (Hollon *et al.*, 1992). Several controlled studies have found that the efficacy of CBT may be limited in more severe depressions, but this finding has not been observed by a number of other studies (Rush and Thase, 1999). Cognitive Behavioural Analysis System of Psychotherapy (CBASP) is a modified form of CBT that incorporates some principles of IPT (McCullough, 2000). CBASP was recently found to be as effective as nefazodone in the treatment of chronic depression (Keller *et al.*, 2000). There also is some evidence that CBT may be helpful for depression in bipolar disorder, but this deserves further study (Patelis-Siotis, 2001).

Other Standard Drug Therapies for Depression

Despite the availability and effectiveness of a large number and variety of antidepressant drugs, some important problems exist in the treatment of depression (Howland and Thase, 1997). First, all antidepressants have a delayed onset of action. Second, a significant minority of patients do not respond to an initial choice of drug, and the majority of patients who do respond show only a partial improvement in their depression. Third, a large proportion of patients who have an initially good response to an antidepressant will suffer a subsequent relapse or recurrence despite adequate ongoing treatment. Finally, many patients who respond to an antidepressant drug will have intolerable side effects. As a result, many different drugs have been studied and/or used in clinical practice to accelerate the antidepressant response, improve partial- or non-responders, treat depressive relapses or recurrences, or alleviate noxious side effects (Howland and Thase, 1999a).

Lithium, buspirone (a 5-HT1A receptor agonist), pindolol (a beta-adrenergic receptor antagonist that also blocks presynaptic 5-HT1A receptors) and stimulant drugs have been used to accelerate the response to antidepressants (Howland and Thase, 1999a). With the exception of pindolol, which has been shown to be effective in some placebo-controlled studies (Bordet *et al.*, 1998), these approaches have not been adequately studied under controlled conditions.

Lithium is the most extensively studied and best established augmentation strategy for treatment-resistant depression (Bauer and Dopfmer, 1999; Baumann *et al.*, 1996). Augmentation with many other drugs is commonly done, but has little empirical support (Thase *et al.*, 1998). These include the use of buspirone, pindolol, anticonvulsants such as valproate, atypical antipsychotics such as risperidone and olanzapine, the analgesic tramadol (which also inhibits the reuptake of serotonin and norepinephrine), the opioid buprenorphine, and psychostimulants such as methylphenidate, pemoline and modafanil (Bodkin *et al.*, 1995; Howland and Thase, 1999a; Menza *et al.*, 2000; Shelton *et al.*, 2001b). Combining different antidepressants (e.g. SRIs with TCAs, bupropion, mirtazapine or nefazodone) also has been a common clinical practice for treatment-resistant depression. Psychotic depression does not respond well to antidepressant monotherapy (with the exception of amoxapine), and combining antidepressants and antipsychotics is considered the treatment of choice (Wheeler Vega *et al.*, 2000). Many of these augmentation strategies or drug combinations have been employed in the management of patients who have depressive relapses or recurrences while taking antidepressants, but none have been sufficiently studied to clearly demonstrate their efficacy (Howland and Thase, 1999a).

Psychostimulant drugs, because they affect dopamine and norepinephrine transmission, may be useful in treating the apathy and sexual dysfunction that sometimes occur during antidepressant treatment, especially with the SRIs, but have not been well studied for this indication (Howland and Thase, 1999a). These drugs include modafanil, methylphenidate, pemoline, amphetamine, amantadine, bromocriptine, pramipexole, ropinirole and pergolide (Zajecka, 2001). Other drugs that have been used for treating antidepressant-associated sexual dysfunction include cyproheptadine, yohimbine, buspirone, bethanechol, bupropion, mirtazapine and nefazodone (Ferguson *et al.*, 2001).

Novel Drug Therapies for Depression

Abnormal regulation of the hypothalamic–pituitary–adrenal (HPA) axis, leading to persistent elevations in cortisol levels, has been implicated in the pathophysiology of depression (Reus *et al.*, 1997). A number of open-label and controlled studies of drugs that suppress or inhibit HPA axis function, such as dexamethasone, aminoglutethimide, metyrapone, ketoconazole and mifepristone, have shown promise in the treatment of major depression, including refractory depression (Belanoff *et al.*, 2001; Brown *et al.*, 2001; Murphy *et al.*, 1993, 1998; Thakore and Dinan 1995; Wolkowitz *et al.*, 1999). Other drugs acting on the HPA axis (e.g. CRH or glucocorticoid receptor antagonists) are currently being developed for study in depression and other psychiatric disorders (McQuade and Young, 2000).

Several lines of evidence have suggested an important role for gonadal and adrenal steroid hormones in mood regulation. Women are especially vulnerable to mood disturbances during premenstrual, post-partum and perimenopausal periods (Epperson *et al.*, 1999). There also is evidence that mood disturbances may be associated with decreased steroid hormone levels in men (Margolese, 2000; Seidman and Walsh, 1999). In addition, steroid hormones act on specific receptors in the brain and affect neuronal function and neurotransmission. Considerable evidence suggests that oestrogen may improve mild mood symptoms in perimenopausal women (Epperson *et al.*, 1999; Joffe and Cohen, 1998), but there is less consistent evidence that oestrogen is an effective monotherapy for major depression (Halbreich, 1997; Morrison and Tweedy, 2000; Saletu *et al.*, 1995). There also is inconsistent evidence of the antidepressant effects of testosterone in men (Grinspoon *et al.*, 2000; Seidman *et al.*, 2001). Several recent placebo-controlled studies, however, found that oestradiol was effective for post-partum and perimenopausal major depression, suggesting important mood differences among oestrogen preparations (Ahokas *et al.*, 2001; De Novaes-Soares *et al.*, 2001). Some, but not all, studies have found that oestrogen or testosterone may augment the effects of antidepressant drugs in major depression (Amsterdam *et al.*, 1999; Schneider *et al.*, 1997; Seidman and Rabkin, 1998; Shapira *et al.*, 1985). Finally, there is developing evidence that adrenal steroid hormones such as dehydroepiandrosterone (DHEA) have significant antidepressant effects in older men and women (Bloch *et al.*, 1999).

Thyroid hormone also has been studied and used in the treatment of depression, especially as an augmentation strategy in refractory depression (usually triiodothyronine; T3) (Thase *et al.*, 1998).

The antidepressant use of thyroid hormone is based on the known association between depression and hypothyroidism as well as evidence that the hypothalamic–pituitary–thyroid axis affects neuronal function and neurotransmission in the brain (Howland, 1993). Thyroid augmentation has been studied almost exclusively in TCA non-responders, and these studies have suggested that it may be more effective in women, perhaps because of their higher risk for thyroid disease (Howland and Thase, 1999a).

Melatonin is a pineal gland hormone that regulates circadian sleep cycles. Although melatonin has not been adequately investigated in controlled trials of major depression, some evidence suggests that it has antidepressant effects (Wetterberg, 1998). Moreover, it also may be a clinically useful adjunct together with antidepressants, because of its potentially beneficial effects on disturbed circadian sleep–wake rhythms found in mood disorders (Wirz-Justice, 1995).

Although most psychotropic drugs have direct effects on neurotransmitter reuptake sites or neurotransmitter receptors, they may also have direct or indirect effects on second-messenger signal transduction systems, which ultimately mediate the synthesis of various protein products that lead to their therapeutic benefit (Chen *et al.*, 1999; Vaidya and Duman, 2001). Inositol, a precursor of the phosphatidyl-inositol second-messenger system, has been found effective in unipolar and bipolar depression in some, but not all, studies (Chengappa *et al.*, 2000; Levine *et al.*, 1995, 1999; Nemets *et al.*, 1999). Omega-3 fatty acids, which have an inhibitory effect on neuronal signal transduction systems, have been studied as a mood stabilizer in bipolar disorder. One recent study found that they had relatively greater antidepressant than antimanic effects (Stoll *et al.*, 1999).

Numerous herbs and plant extracts are known to have psychotropic effects, and historically many have been used therapeutically for the treatment of depression, anxiety and other emotional maladies (Fugh-Berman and Cott, 1999). Indeed, the use of herbs, nutritional supplements and other unorthodox homeopathic therapies has increased tremendously in recent years, but unfortunately many of these products have not been well studied with respect to their safety or efficacy. Two exceptions to this are studies of St John's wort and S-adenosylmethionine (SAMe) in the treatment of major depression. St John's wort (*Hypericum perforatum*), a wild flowering plant, has been used since ancient times to treat a variety of nervous conditions, and has become a very commonly used contemporary treatment for depression and anxiety. The most common adverse effects of St John's wort include photosensitivity, headache, dry mouth, dizziness, constipation and other gastrointestinal problems. St John's wort also is a potent inducer of hepatic metabolic enzyme systems, which may lead to decreased levels of various drugs (especially protease inhibitors, cyclosporine, theophylline, warfarin, digoxin and oral contraceptives). A meta-analysis of randomized trials in outpatients with mild to moderate levels of depression concluded that St John's wort was significantly superior to placebo and comparably effective to standard antidepressant drugs, although many of these trials were considered to have serious methodological flaws (Linde *et al.*, 1996). A recent large multicentre randomized study in patients with more severe and chronic symptoms of major depression did not find any difference between St John's wort and placebo (Shelton *et al.*, 2001a). Results from another large randomized study did not find any significant difference among St John's wort, sertraline, or placebo (Hypericum Depression Trial Study Group, 2002). The dietary supplement SAMe is an amino acid compound that is essential for methylation processes in the nervous system, which are important for neurotransmitter synthesis and second-messenger system function (Reynolds and Stramentinoli, 1983). The most common adverse effects are insomnia, nervousness, headaches and mild gastrointestinal problems, and it is not known to interact adversely with other drugs (Fava *et al.*, 1995). A meta-analysis of randomized trials in depressed outpatients found that SAMe was more effective than placebo and as effective as TCAs (Bressa, 1994), but it has not been compared to newer generation antidepressants and it has not been well studied in more severe forms of depression (Echols *et al.*, 2000).

Other Somatic Therapies for Depression

Electroconvulsive Therapy (ECT)

Historically, ECT has been considered the most effective treatment for major depression, and has also been shown to be highly effective for the treatment of severe melancholia, psychotic depression, bipolar depression, catatonia associated with mood disorders and treatment-resistant depression (Swartz *et al.*, 2001; Thase and Rush, 1995; Thase and Sachs, 2000; Wheeler Vega *et al.*, 2000). Because of its relative effectiveness, tolerability and safety, ECT is considered to be especially appropriate for geriatric patients and pregnant women, who might otherwise be at risk for adverse pharmacological effects (Kelly and Zisselman, 2000). ECT involves the passage of a brief electrical current through the brain to induce a generalized seizure lasting about 30–90 seconds, and is performed under general anaesthesia and muscle relaxation using short-acting drugs. A typical course of ECT consists of 6–12 treatments given three times weekly, although some patients might require a greater number of treatments. One of two electrode placements are used for ECT: unilateral non-dominant hemisphere placement or bilateral placement. Most patients are treated initially with unilateral ECT. Bilateral ECT usually is reserved for patients who have shown a minimal response after six unilateral treatments, or for patients with a history of a poor response to prior courses of unilateral ECT, a history of a positive prior bilateral ECT response, or extremely severe symptoms (Bailine *et al.*, 2000). Aside from the potential adverse effects and risks associated with general anaesthesia, the most common adverse effects of ECT include transient changes in heart rate and blood pressure, postictal and postanaesthetic confusion, memory impairment, muscle soreness, nausea and headaches. There is no convincing evidence that acute or long-term treatment with ECT causes brain damage. Increased efficacy and side effects of ECT are correlated with higher intensities of the electrical current, and efficacy and side effects are also somewhat greater with bilateral ECT (McCall *et al.*, 2000; Sackeim *et al.*, 2000). The acute clinical benefits of ECT are usually time-limited. For this reason, patients at risk for a depressive relapse should receive longer-term continuation treatment with pharmacotherapy or ECT after completing a course of acute ECT (Sackeim *et al.*, 2001a). However, patients who failed to respond to adequate trials of antidepressant medication prior to ECT have a higher risk of relapsing with pharmacotherapy after successful ECT and therefore should preferentially receive continuation treatment with ECT (Sackeim, 1994). Moreover, there is some evidence that continuation ECT is more effective than medications alone in preventing relapse and recurrence in depression (Gagne *et al.*, 2000).

Repetitive Transcranial Magnetic Stimulation (rTMS)

By contrast with ECT, rTMS is a novel non-invasive method for causing focal non-electrical stimulation of the brain (George *et al.*, 1999). In rTMS, a high-intensity electrical current is passed through an electromagnetic coil on the scalp. Rapidly turning the current on and off generates repetitive pulses of a magnetic field that can be focused on particular regions of the brain. Slow frequency stimulation with rTMS tends to inhibit neurons, whereas fast stimulation is excitatory. The most common adverse effect is headache, but seizures have been reported. Adverse cognitive effects of rTMS also are uncommon. Short-term placebo-controlled (using sham rTMS) studies of fast rTMS focused on the left dorsolateral prefrontal cortex have found it effective in major depression (George *et al.*, 1997, 2000a), although there is evidence that slow rTMS focused on the right prefrontal cortex also is effective (Klein *et al.*, 1999). The results from studies using rTMS in treatment-resistant depression are mixed (Berman *et al.*, 2000; Loo *et al.*, 1999). A recent open study found that ECT may be somewhat more effective than rTMS, especially among patients with psychotic depression (Grunhaus *et al.*, 2000). Unfortunately, the long-term clinical efficacy, tolerability and safety of rTMS in mood disorders is unknown.

Vagus Nerve Stimulation (VNS)

The vagus nerve (cranial nerve X) is a parasympathetic nerve composed of afferent (carrying sensory information from the viscera) and efferent (regulating parasympathetic autonomic function) fibres. Animal studies found that VNS has behavioural and anticonvulsant effects, which led to the study and approved clinical use of VNS as a treatment for refractory partial-onset seizures in epilepsy (George *et al.*, 2000b). VNS involves the surgical implantation of a pacemaker-like programmable pulse generator, which is connected to and intermittently stimulates the left cervical vagus nerve. Studies in epilepsy patients also found that VNS had positive effects on mood symptoms. Brain imaging and neurochemical studies have shown that VNS activates various limbic regions and affects various neurotransmitters. This work led to interest in studying VNS in depression. An open-label pilot study using VNS in a group of very chronic and highly treatment-resistant patients with major depression reported a response rate of approximately 40% (Rush *et al.*, 2000). VNS was very safe and generally well tolerated, similar to its safety and side effect profile in epilepsy (Sackeim *et al.*, 2001b). Longer-term follow-up of these patients has found that the antidepressant response to VNS increases over time and continues to be well tolerated (Marangell *et al.*, 2002). Results of a recently completed large multicentre randomized controlled study of VNS in treatment-resistant major depression have not yet been reported.

Acupuncture

Acupuncture, like other complementary and alternative therapies, is becoming a more popular medical treatment for depression (Ulett *et al.*, 1998). Several controlled studies comparing 'active' acupuncture to 'sham' acupuncture and/or to antidepressant medication have reported some antidepressant benefit (Allen *et al.*, 1998; Luo *et al.*, 1998; Roschke *et al.*, 2000). Although these studies suffer from various methodological problems, the results suggest that acupuncture might be considered a safe and well tolerated alternative treatment for some depressed patients that warrants further study. More research clearly is needed to establish the safety and efficacy of acupuncture in major depression and other mood disorders. Moreover, because different procedures are used in the application of acupuncture, additional work is needed to determine the most effective acupuncture procedure in depression.

Psychosurgery

In the absence of effective pharmacological therapies, psychosurgery was widely accepted and commonly practised during the 1940s and 1950s for the treatment of schizophrenia, mood disorders and anxiety disorders. Although somewhat effective, the early surgical procedures were rather primitive (i.e. the prefrontal lobotomy crudely severed white matter connections between the prefrontal cortex and the rest of the brain) and had significant complications (e.g. bleeding, seizures, frontal lobe syndrome and death). However, the refinement of stereotactic neurosurgical methods, together with a better understanding of the neuroanatomical pathophysiology of psychiatric disorders, has led to more selective interventions with improved clinical outcomes and reduced morbidity and mortality. The most common currently performed neurosurgical procedures are anterior cingulotomy, subcaudate tractotomy, limbic leukotomy and anterior capsulotomy, which involve selective lesioning of particular brain regions using magnetic resonance imaging-guided stereotactic techniques. Psychosurgery is considered a treatment of last resort, for patients with chronic, severe and debilitating illnesses that have not responded to any available treatment. Short-term and long-term studies have found that one-third to two-thirds of patients with intractable depression show clinically significant improvement after psychosurgery, with low rates of surgical and neurological complications and minimal adverse effects on intellectual, personality and behavioural functioning (Binder and Iskandar, 2000; Spangler *et al.*, 1996).

Non-Somatic Therapies for Depression

Mood disorders are commonly characterized by clinical and EEG sleep disturbances. Hence, disturbed sleep is not only a symptom of depression, but may also reflect abnormal underlying biological processes that regulate sleep–wake cycles and are relevant to the pathophysiology of mood disorders (Wirz-Justice, 1995). Approximately 30–50% of depressed patients have a significant but transient antidepressant effect from total sleep deprivation, but this positive benefit is often lost with a full night of sleep (Wu *et al.*, 1999). Serial partial sleep deprivation, whereby patients stay awake daily from 2 a.m. to 10 p.m., has been used to achieve a more sustained antidepressant response, but this has not been especially effective. Sleep deprivation followed by pharmacotherapy may be more effective (Benedetti *et al.*, 1999; Smeraldi *et al.*, 1999). In addition, some evidence suggests that sleep deprivation may accelerate the response to antidepressant drugs and may be a useful augmentation strategy for antidepressant partial responders (Thase and Rush, 1995). Patients with seasonal depression or bipolar depression may be somewhat more sensitive to the antidepressant effects of sleep deprivation. Indeed, sleep deprivation may precipitate mania in patients with bipolar disorder.

Phototherapy (bright light therapy) was studied and introduced as a treatment for seasonal affective disorder, primarily winter depressions (Wirz-Justice, 1995). Phototherapy typically involves the daily morning use of 1–2 hours of bright light (2000 lux or more) (Terman *et al.*, 2001). The most common adverse effects are irritability and headache. Phototherapy also may be beneficial for patients with non-seasonal depression or bipolar depression (sometimes precipitating hypomania or mania), and has been used to accelerate or augment the effects of antidepressant drugs (Kripke, 1998; Thase and Rush, 1995). A positive response to sleep deprivation predicts a positive response to phototherapy, and the combination has been used to obtain a more sustained antidepressant effect (Colombo *et al.*, 2000; Fritzsche *et al.*, 2001). An alternative form of phototherapy is dawn simulation, which uses a low intensity light that gradually increases in illuminance before the subject awakens. This has been found to be as or more effective than bright light therapy in some studies (Avery *et al.*, 2001).

A novel approach in the treatment of winter depression is the use of a negative ion generator as an antidepressant therapy (Terman and Terman, 1995). In this method, an electronic negative ion generator is used to produce negative ions in the ambient air. Patients use the device at home for approximately 30 minutes. A controlled trial comparing low-density and high-density negative ion generation found a greater antidepressant effect with the high-density treatment. This method is currently being compared to phototherapy and dawn simulation in a randomized trial of winter depression.

Clinical Issues in the Treatment of Depression

Given the availability of a wide variety of effective antidepressant therapies, how does one choose among these treatments? Because of the delay in onset of action of treatment, adherence to treatment is very important. Hence, patient preference is important to consider. Patients who strongly favour medication or psychotherapy should be offered treatment as such. The choice of psychotherapy will depend, of course, on the availability of a therapist trained in the use of a particular therapy model. The choice of medication also will depend on such factors as patient preference, past treatment history, family treatment history, clinical symptoms, health and side effect profile (Thase, 1997).

The goal of antidepressant treatment should be an optimal outcome; that is, the absence of any depressive symptoms along with a complete recovery of psychosocial function. This type of outcome is referred to as remission. About 50% of patients will have a significant response to the first-choice treatment, which is defined as a 50% or greater decrease in their symptoms of depression. Of these responders, however, only about one-half to one-third attain a full remission. Hence, a significant number of depressed patients are left with residual or persistent symptoms despite adequate antidepressant treatment (Rush and Trivedi, 1995). For these patients, switching to an alternative antidepressant drug or therapy, or combining different antidepressant treatments (e.g. pharmacotherapy and psychotherapy) may lead to a full remission.

The treatment of depression, whether with pharmacotherapy or psychotherapy, is now provided in three phases, each having different therapeutic goals (Thase and Kupfer, 1996). The acute phase, which typically lasts 6–12 weeks, refers to the initial treatment period, where the treatment is administered with the goal of full symptom remission. The continuation phase, which typically lasts 4–9 months, follows acute phase treatment and is recommended for all patients. The goal of continuation phase treatment is to prevent early relapse and to allow further symptomatic and psychosocial functional improvement. The goal of maintenance phase treatment is to prevent further recurrences of depression among patients who have a high risk of developing depression again. Such risk factors include three or more previous episodes of major depression, chronic depression, residual or persistent symptoms despite adequate treatment, and severe or disabling episodes of depression. The length of maintenance treatment will depend on the number of risk factors, and may range from a year to even life-long treatment.

For patients who do not have a satisfactory response to their initial antidepressant treatment, various strategies have been advocated (Thase and Rush, 1995). Switching to a different treatment (e.g. an alternative antidepressant drug or psychotherapy) is recommended for patients who have shown no response at all or for those who have intolerable side effects (Howland and Thase, 1999a). Augmentation (the strategy of adding a second medication to an antidepressant drug) may be most useful in patients who have shown a partial response to treatment (Thase *et al.*, 1998). Although combining pharmacotherapy and psychotherapy is commonly recommended, there is no clear evidence that the combination is more effective than either modality alone in the treatment of uncomplicated depressions (Thase *et al.*, 1997). Complicated depressions (e.g. very severe depression, treatment-resistant depression, chronic forms of depression, and partially remitted depression), however, may respond better to the combination of psychotherapy and pharmacotherapy (Fava *et al.*, 1997; Keller *et al.*, 2000; Paykel *et al.*, 1999; Thase *et al.*, 2001b).

TREATMENT OF BIPOLAR DISORDER

Antimanic Drugs

Lithium

Compared to other antimanic therapies (McElroy and Keck, 2000; Sachs and Thase, 2000), lithium is the best studied short-term and long-term treatment for bipolar disorder in adults (Baldessarini and Tondo, 2000; Maj, 2000) and in children and adolescents (Kowatch *et al.*, 2000). There is some evidence that patients with mixed episodes (mania together with depression) or a rapid-cycling pattern of illness may be less responsive to lithium (Montgomery *et al.*, 2000; Post *et al.*, 2000), but this has not been definitively proven (Baldessarini *et al.*, 2000). Although its antimanic effects are relatively greater than its antidepressant effects, it is the best studied and established pharmacological treatment for bipolar depression (Nemeroff *et al.*, 2001; Zornberg and Pope, 1993), and is less likely than antidepressants to be associated with the development of hypomania, mania, mixed states or rapid-cycling (Montgomery *et al.*, 2000; Post *et al.*, 2001; Thase and Sachs, 2000). There also is clear evidence that long-term treatment with lithium is associated with a reduced risk of suicide in bipolar and unipolar disorders (Coppen, 2000; Tondo and Baldessarini, 2000), an effect that has not been demonstrated with other antimanic therapies (Goodwin, 1999).

Although lithium has been used clinically for more than three decades, its precise mechanism of action is uncertain. Developing evidence, however, strongly suggests that lithium has direct and indirect effects on various components of second-messenger signal transduction systems, including G proteins, adenylyl cyclases, protein kinase C and the phosphoinositide cycle, which have been implicated in the neurobiology of bipolar disorder (Manji *et al.*, 1995, 1999). Typical adverse effects of lithium include gastrointestinal irritation, sedation, tremors, polyuria, polydipsia, oedema, acne, psoriasis and weight gain (Watson and Young, 2001). Careful serum level monitoring is required, as lithium toxicity can be serious (affecting cardiac, renal and central nervous system function) and potentially life threatening. Chronic lithium therapy is associated with the development of hypothyroidism, which is easily treated with thyroid hormone replacement. Lithium treatment is associated with teratogenic effects (i.e. cardiac anomalies). With careful clinical monitoring, lithium can be used safely with anticonvulsants, antipsychotics and antidepressants, but adverse interactions can occur with drugs that affect renal functioning (e.g. diuretics, non-steroidal anti-inflammatory drugs, calcium channel antagonists and ACE inhibitors).

Anticonvulsant Drugs

Lithium has been the standard treatment for bipolar disorder for nearly 30 years, but a significant proportion of patients do not respond to or cannot tolerate it (Watson and Young, 2001). As a result, various anticonvulsant drugs have been actively investigated and are increasingly used in clinical practice in the treatment of bipolar disorder (Dunn *et al.*, 1998; Keck *et al.*, 2000; Sachs *et al.*, 2000). There is now abundant evidence of the effectiveness of two anticonvulsants, divalproex and carbamazepine (Dunn *et al.*, 1998; McElroy and Keck, 2000). Divalproex is now considered by many physicians to be the most appropriate first-line treatment. For other patients, these anticonvulsants are useful second-line or adjunctive treatments for patients who are intolerant of or do not respond to lithium (e.g. those with rapid-cycling or mixed states). Long-term treatment with anticonvulsants has not been as well studied as lithium in adults (Bowden *et al.*, 2000b; Sachs and Thase, 2000) or in children and adolescents (Kowatch *et al.*, 2000). More recently, a variety of newer anticonvulsant drugs have become available for clinical use, including lamotrigine, topiramate, gabapentin, oxcarbazepine, tiagabine, zonisamide and levetiracetam (Tatum *et al.*, 2000). Among these, lamotrigine, topiramate and gabapentin have been of particular clinical and research interest as potentially promising treatments for bipolar disorder (Dunn *et al.*, 1998). Surprisingly, oxcarbazepine, which is a better tolerated pharmacological analogue of carbamazepine, has been studied more extensively than many other anticonvulsants in the treatment of bipolar disorder, but is not yet commonly used in clinical practice (Dunn *et al.*, 1998; Teitelbaum, 2001). Tiagabine, zonisamide and levetiracetam, structurally and pharmacologically novel drugs unrelated to other anticonvulsants, have not been systematically investigated in bipolar disorder (Dunn *et al.*, 1998; McElroy and Keck, 2000; Tatum *et al.*, 2000). Like lithium, the therapeutic mechanism of action of anticonvulsants in bipolar disorder is uncertain. Recent studies, however, have suggested that carbamazepine, divalproex and perhaps other anticonvulsant drugs have direct and indirect effects on various components of second-messenger signal transduction systems (Chang *et al.*, 2001; Manji *et al.*, 1996, 1999).

Divalproex has been intensively studied in the treatment of bipolar disorder. Double-blind placebo-controlled studies have found it to be as effective as lithium in acute mania (Bowden *et al.*, 1994). Divalproex has not been as well studied in the long-term treatment of bipolar disorder, but there is evidence from a number of open studies that it has prophylactic benefits (Bowden *et al.*, 2000b; Sachs and Thase, 2000). The results from a recently completed double-blind placebo-controlled study suggested that it was somewhat more effective than lithium on some clinical measures, especially with regard to depressive symptoms, but there were no overall significant differences in outcome among patients treated with divalproex, lithium or placebo (Bowden *et al.*, 2000a). Open-label studies have shown it to be effective in bipolar depression, although it likely has relatively greater antimanic than antidepressant effects and is less likely than antidepressants to be associated with the development of hypomania, mania, mixed states or rapid-cycling (Montgomery *et al.*, 2000; Thase and Sachs, 2000; Young *et al.*, 2000). Mixed states, rapid-cycling and a poor lithium response tend to predict a positive response to divalproex (Swann *et al.*, 1997). The most common dose-dependent side effects are nausea, sedation and tremor. Transient hair loss can occur, and weight gain is common with long-term use. Blood dyscrasias, typically thrombocytopaenia, are rare. Mild transient hepatic enzyme elevations may occur, but hepatotoxicity is rare. Reports of severe hepatitis have been described primarily among young children with epilepsy taking valproic acid together with other anticonvulsants. There is some concern that women treated with divalproex may be at risk for developing polycystic ovarian syndrome, based on studies in epilepsy, but this has not been clearly demonstrated in mood disorder patients. Divalproex treatment is associated with teratogenic effects (i.e. neural tube defects) (Ferrier, 2001). In general, divalproex appears to be better tolerated than lithium or carbamazepine. Drug interactions are less common with divalproex compared to carbamazepine, because it is a weak inhibitor of hepatic enzymes, but it can increase serum levels of carbamazepine, lamotrigine and TCAs. Aspirin and naproxen can increase levels of divalproex, whereas carbamazepine can decrease its levels. Therefore, use of these drugs together with divalproex may require dose adjustments. Divalproex also can be used safely and effectively in combination with lithium, other anticonvulsants, antipsychotics and antidepressants.

Carbamazepine has been the most extensively studied anticonvulsant in bipolar disorder, although it has not been formally approved for this indication (McElroy and Keck, 2000). Double-blind placebo-controlled studies have found it to be effective in the acute and prophylactic treatment of mania (Keck *et al.*, 2000). Most controlled comparative studies have found that carbamazepine is as effective as lithium, though some have found it slightly less effective (Bowden *et al.*, 2000b). The results from controlled studies also have shown that it is effective in bipolar depression (Thase and Sachs, 2000). Similar to lithium, however, it may be relatively more effective in mania than in depression (Sachs *et al.*, 2000). Patients with mixed mania, rapid-cycling or a poor response to lithium often respond well to carbamazepine (Montgomery *et al.*, 2000). Because carbamazepine induces its own metabolism, periodic dose increases may be needed during treatment. Serum levels may therefore be especially useful to assess compliance, distinguish between poor and rapid drug metabolizers, and maintain patients at a steady-state level during long-term treatment. Sedation, dizziness, ataxia and diplopia are the most common dose-dependent side effects; weight gain frequently occurs during long-term use. Many patients develop benign skin rashes, mild leukopaenia or transient hepatic enzyme elevations, but the Stevens–Johnson syndrome, agranulocytosis, aplastic anaemia and hepatitis are rare complications. Although monitoring blood counts is recommended, this is not needed as frequently as has been suggested in the past. Carbamazepine treatment is associated with teratogenic effects (Ferrier, 2001). Because carbamazepine induces hepatic enzymes, drug interactions are common. It can significantly decrease levels of other anticonvulsants (including divalproex and lamotrigine), antipsychotics, benzodiazepines, TCAs and oral contraceptives. Erythromycin, cimetidine, divalproex, fluoxetine, fluvoxamine and calcium channel antagonists can increase carbamazepine levels. Therefore, concurrent use of these drugs with carbamazepine may require dose adjustments. Carbamazepine has been found to be relatively safe and often effective when combined with lithium or valproate, although the combinations are more likely to cause side effects than monotherapy with any of these drugs alone.

Lamotrigine has pharmacological effects that are very different from those of divalproex and carbamazepine (McElroy and Keck, 2000). The published literature on the use of lamotrigine in bipolar disorder is limited compared to divalproex and carbamazepine, but is very promising. Open-label reports have found that lamotrigine is effective alone or in combination with other antimanic drugs in patients with bipolar disorder, including many who were treatment-resistant or had rapid-cycling (Calabrese *et al.*, 1999a). Double-blind placebo-controlled studies have also found it effective in bipolar disorder (Frye *et al.*, 2000), especially in bipolar depression (Calabrese *et al.*, 1999b) and rapid-cycling (Calabrese *et al.*, 2000). The most common adverse effects are nausea, headache, dizziness, ataxia and diplopia. A benign rash occurs in approximately 10% of patients, and more severe rashes occur in 0.5–1.0%; the Stevens–Johnson syndrome also has been reported. Rashes tend to occur more commonly when higher starting doses are used or the dose is rapidly increased, and when it is used together with divalproex (which inhibits its metabolism). Lamotrigine does not affect hepatic metabolism. Carbamazepine can increase its metabolism, while divalproex decreases it.

Topiramate is a structurally and pharmacologically novel drug unrelated to other anticonvulsants (McElroy and Keck, 2000). The published literature on the use of lamotrigine in bipolar disorder is very limited compared to divalproex, carbamazepine and lamotrigine. Open-label reports have found that lamotrigine may be effective in combination with other antimanic drugs in patients with bipolar disorder, including many who were treatment-resistant (Chengappa *et al.*, 1999; Marcotte, 1998; McElroy, *et al.*, 2000). Unfortunately, the results from one double-blind placebo-controlled study reported only limited benefit with topiramate in mania

(Chengappa *et al.*, 2001). The most common adverse effects are somnolence, dizziness, anxiety, ataxia, speech difficulties, cognitive impairment, anorexia and weight loss.

Gabapentin also has pharmacological effects that differ from all other anticonvulsants. The published literature on the use of gabapentin in bipolar disorder is limited to case reports, uncontrolled open-label studies and two placebo-controlled trials. The open-label reports found that gabapentin was effective alone or in combination with other mood stabilizers in about 60–90% of patients, including those with treatment-resistant or rapid-cycling bipolar disorder (Ghaemi and Goodwin, 2001; McElroy and Keck, 2000). However, the double-blind studies did not find a significant drug–placebo difference (Frye *et al.*, 2000; McElroy and Keck, 2000). Sedation, dizziness and ataxia are the most common adverse effects. Gabapentin is not metabolized, does not affect hepatic metabolism, does not have significant drug interactions, and is not associated with hepatic or haematologic abnormalities. Because it is renally excreted, lower doses may be required in patients with renal disease, but serious toxicity in such patients is unlikely compared to lithium. The combination of gabapentin and other psychotropic drugs is generally well tolerated.

Antipsychotic Drugs

Typical Antipsychotics

For many years, the use of the older typical antipsychotic drugs has been a common clinical practice for the treatment of acute mania and psychotic mania (Keck *et al.*, 2000; Sachs and Thase, 2000). These drugs have a relatively rapid effect on manic and psychotic symptoms, psychomotor agitation and sleep. Most controlled studies have been conducted using chlorpromazine or haloperidol, which had antimanic effects comparable to lithium, divalproex and carbamazepine (McElroy and Keck, 2000). Typical antipsychotics are associated with parkinsonian side effects, akathesia and tardive dyskinesia. They also may be associated with the development of depression in some patients. One advantage of typical antipsychotics is that they are generally considered to be safe for use during pregnancy, and would be an appropriate treatment alternative to lithium or anticonvulsants in pregnant women with bipolar disorder. Another potential advantage is that two of the typical antipsychotics (haloperidol and fluphenazine) have long-acting depot formulations, which may be useful for maintaining compliance during long-term treatment for some patients (Sachs and Thase, 2000).

Atypical Antipsychotics

Because of their clinical effects and side effect profile, atypical antipsychotics have gradually supplanted use of the typical antipsychotics, even in the treatment of bipolar disorder (Sachs *et al.*, 2000). They are less likely to cause extrapyramidal side effects or tardive dyskinesia, and they appear to have more positive effects on mood (Dunayevich and McElroy, 2000; Ghaemi and Goodwin, 1999; Guille *et al.*, 2000). Olanzapine is the best studied and most established atypical antipsychotic for the acute treatment of mania (Bhana and Perry, 2001), and also may be effective for mixed states and rapid-cycling (Meehan *et al.*, 2001; Tohen *et al.*, 1999, 2000). There is evidence from controlled trials that risperidone is effective in the acute treatment of mania when added to ongoing antimanic drugs, but it has not been studied as a monotherapy in placebo-controlled trials (McElroy and Keck, 2000; Sachs *et al.*, 2000). Small open-label reports have suggested some benefit for quetiapine in treatment-resistant bipolar disorder, but there are no controlled studies (Dunayevich and Strakowski, 2000; Ghaemi and Katzow, 1999; Zarate *et al.*, 2000). One randomized double-blind placebo-controlled study of ziprasidone found it effective in bipolar patients with mania or mixed episodes (McElroy and Keck 2000). Clozapine has been reported in open-label studies to be effective in bipolar disorder, especially in treatment-resistant cases, but has not been studied in controlled trials (Dunayevich and McElroy, 2000; Ghaemi and Goodwin, 1999; Guille *et al.*, 2000). The clinical use of clozapine is limited, however, by its side effect profile and the risk of agranulocytosis. Compared to lithium and some anticonvulsants, none of the atypical antipsychotics has been well studied for long-term treatment (Bowden *et al.*, 2000b; Sachs and Thase, 2000; Vieta *et al.*, 2001). Sedation and weight gain are a problem with some of these drugs (e.g. olanzapine, quetiapine and clozapine), although ziprasidone is associated with weight loss. These drugs also are generally well tolerated when combined with other psychotropic drugs.

Novel Drug Therapies for Bipolar Disorder

Considerable evidence suggests that lithium and anticonvulsant drugs have direct and indirect effects on various components of second-messenger signal transduction systems, which may underlie their therapeutic mechanism of action (Chen *et al.*, 1999). As a result, other drugs that affect second-messenger systems have been studied in bipolar disorder. Calcium channel antagonists, which affect intracellular calcium metabolism, have been studied in bipolar disorder (Hollister and Garza Trevino, 1999; Post *et al.*, 2000), with some evidence of efficacy using nimodipine in rapid-cycling (Pazzaglia *et al.*, 1998), but mixed results with verapamil (Dose *et al.*, 1986; Janicak *et al.*, 1998). Omega-3 fatty acid, which has an inhibitory effect on neuronal signal transduction systems, has been studied as a mood stabilizer in bipolar disorder, but may have relatively greater antidepressant than antimanic effects (Stoll *et al.*, 1999). A small open-label study of the protein kinase C inhibitor tamoxifen showed a significant antimanic effect (Bebchuk *et al.*, 2000).

Various cholinomimetic drugs, which stimulate cholinergic pathways (Cummings, 2000), have been found in small open-label studies to have antimanic effects, including physostigmine, RS 86, and donepezil (Burt *et al.*, 1999; Davis *et al.*, 1978; Krieg and Berger, 1986). Other studies using choline or phosphatidylcholine, which are precursors of acetylcholine, also have suggested some antimanic effects (Leiva, 1990; Stoll *et al.*, 1996). These approaches may work in the treatment of mania by readjusting the hypothesized 'adrenergic-cholinergic imbalance'. Alternatively, these drugs may work by inhibiting phosphatidylcholine second-messenger systems (Chen *et al.*, 1999).

A number of reports have suggested that the adjunctive use of high doses of thyroid hormone may be effective in treatment-resistant bipolar disorder, including rapid-cycling, refractory mania and intractable depression (Bauer and Whybrow 1990; Bauer *et al.*, 1998; Baumgartner *et al.*, 1994).

Other Somatic Therapies for Bipolar Disorder

As discussed previously, ECT and rTMS have demonstrated efficacy in the treatment of major depression, including bipolar depression. Surprisingly, there is some evidence that these treatments also are effective in the treatment of mania. A double-blind controlled trial of right versus left prefrontal cortex fast rTMS found greater antimanic effects with right-sided stimulation, which would be consistent with the known antidepressant effects of left-sided stimulation (Grisaru *et al.*, 1998). ECT also has been used in the treatment of refractory mixed states and rapid-cycling, as well as catatonia associated with bipolar disorder (Keck *et al.*, 2000; Mukherjee *et al.*, 1994). Finally, sleep deprivation and phototherapy have been used as adjunctive therapies for rapid-cycling (Sachs *et al.*, 2000).

Clinical Issues in the Treatment of Bipolar Disorder

Bipolar disorder is a chronically recurrent phasic illness. As a result, acute treatments often are phase-specific (Sachs *et al.*, 2000). For acute bipolar mania, lithium, anticonvulsants and antipsychotics are clearly effective. High-potency benzodiazepines (such as lorazepam or clonazepam) or low-potency sedating antipsychotics (such as chlorpromazine or thioridazine) can be used adjunctively to promote sleep, which will have an additional therapeutic antimanic effect. For refractory mania, antimanic drug combinations, atypical antipsychotics, novel anticonvulsants, calcium channel antagonists, cholinomimetics, omega-3 fatty acids, thyroid hormone and ECT can be useful.

For bipolar depression, lithium and anticonvulsants can have antidepressant effects. They are the preferred initial treatment because they are less often associated with the development of hypomania, mania, mixed states or rapid-cycling. Antidepressant drugs can be effective, but may induce hypomania, mania, psychosis, mixed states or rapid-cycling (Altshuler *et al.*, 1995). Although there is some clinical evidence that the risk of antidepressant-induced mania may differ among antidepressant drugs, this has not been clearly established (Boerlin *et al.*, 1998; Howland, 1996b). The dose and/or serum level of antimanic drugs should be optimized if antidepressants are used. For treatment-resistant bipolar depression, atypical antipsychotics, dopamine agonist drugs, sleep deprivation, phototherapy and ECT are potentially effective alternatives. Mixed states and rapid-cycling, which are more common in women than in men, predict a poorer response to most treatments and a poorer long-term prognosis (Montgomery *et al.*, 2000). In these situations, anticonvulsants, atypical antipsychotics, thyroid hormone, calcium channel antagonists, sleep deprivation, phototherapy and ECT may be effective, along with minimizing or avoiding the use of antidepressants.

Virtually all patients with bipolar disorder will require longer-term continuation and maintenance therapy to prevent relapse or recurrence of mood episodes (Sachs and Thase, 2000). For many patients, it is prudent to continue acute treatments indefinitely if their tolerability and efficacy are acceptable. Changes in symptoms (such as depression, hypomania or psychosis) during long-term therapy can usually be effectively managed by careful titration of ongoing antimanic, antipsychotic and/or antidepressant treatments. Significant symptoms unresponsive to titration of current therapies can be treated by adding an appropriate symptom-specific therapy. Because of the inherent mood instability in bipolar disorder, however, medication changes or additions should be done gradually while closely monitoring the patient's clinical condition. For example, adding or discontinuing antidepressant drugs are both associated with the development of mania (Goldstein *et al.*, 1999). Therefore, adjusting the antidepressant dose (rather than abruptly stopping the drug) while maximizing the antimanic drug dose and/or serum level would be an appropriate strategy for managing antidepressant-associated mania.

REFERENCES

Ahokas, A., Kaukoranta, J., Wahlbeck, K. and Aito, M., 2001. Estrogen deficiency in severe postpartum depression: successful treatment with sublingual physiologic 17beta-estradiol: a preliminary study. *Journal of Clinical Psychiatry*, **62**(5), 332–6.

Allen, J.J.B., Schnyer, R.N. and Hitt, S.K., 1998. The efficacy of acupuncture in the treatment of major depression in women. *Psychological Science*, **4**, 397–401.

Altshuler, L.L., Post, R.M., Leverich, G.S., Mikalauskas, K., Rosoff, A. and Ackerman, L., 1995. Antidepressant-induced mania and cycle acceleration: a controversy revisited. *American Journal of Psychiatry*, **152**, 1130–8.

Amrein, R., Stabl, M., Henauer, S., Affolter, E. and Jonkanski, I., 1997. Efficacy and tolerability of moclobemide in comparison with placebo, tricyclic antidepressants, and selective serotonin reuptake inhibitors in elderly depressed patients: a clinical overview. *Canadian Journal of Psychiatry*, **42**, 1043–50.

Amsterdam, J., Garcia-Espana, F., Fawcett, J., Quitkin, F., Reimherr, F., Rosenbaum, J. and Beasley, C., 1999. Fluoxetine efficacy in menopausal women with and without estrogen replacement. *Journal of Affective Disorders*, **55**(1), 11–17.

Avery, D.H., Eder, D.N., Bolte, M.A., Hellekson, C.J., Dunner, D.L., Vitiello, M.V. and Prinz, P.N., 2001. Dawn simulation and bright light in the treatment of SAD: a controlled study. *Biological Psychiatry*, **50**, 205–16.

Bailine, S.H., Rifkin, A., Kayne, E., Selzer, J.A., Vital-Herne, J., Blieka, M. and Pollack, S., 2000. Comparison of bifrontal and bitemporal ECT for major depression. *American Journal of Psychiatry*, **157**(1), 121–3.

Baldessarini, R.J. and Tondo, L., 2000. Does lithium treatment still work? Evidence of stable responses over three decades. *Archives of General Psychiatry*, **57**, 187–90.

Baldessarini, R.J., Tondo, L., Floris, G. and Hennen, J., 2000. Effects of rapid cycling on response to lithium maintenance treatment in 360 bipolar I and II disorder patients. *Journal of Affective Disorders*, **61**, 13–22.

Barrett, J.S., Hochadel, T.J., Morales, R.J., Rohatagi, S., DeWitt, K.E., Watson, S.K., Darnow, J., Azzaro, A.J. and DiSanto, A.R., 1997. Pressor response to tyramine after single 24-hour application of selegiline transdermal system in healthy males. *Journal of Clinical Pharmacology*, **37**(3), 238–47.

Bauer, M.S. and Whybrow, P.C., 1990. Rapid cycling bipolar affective disorder: II. Treatment of refractory rapid cycling with high-dose levothyroxine: a preliminary study. *Archives of General Psychiatry*, **47**, 435–40.

Bauer, M. and Dopfmer, S., 1999. Lithium augmentation in treatment-resistant depression: meta-analysis of placebo-controlled studies. *Journal of Clinical Psychopharmacology*, **19**, 427–34.

Bauer, M., Hellweg, R., Graf, K.J. and Baumgartner, A., 1998. Treatment of refractory depression with high-dose thyroxine. *Neuropsychopharmacology*, **18**(6), 444–55.

Baumann, P., Nil, R., Souche, A., Montaldi, S., Baettig, D., Lambert, S., Uehlinger, C., Kasas, A., Amey, M. and Jonzier-Perey, M., 1996. A double-blind, placebo-controlled study of citalopram with and without lithium in treatment of therapy-resistant depressive patients: a clinical, pharmacokinetic, and pharmacogenetic investigation. *Journal of Clinical Psychopharmacology*, **16**, 307–14.

Baumgartner, A., Bauer, M. and Hellweg, R., 1994. Treatment of intractable non-rapid cycling bipolar affective disorder with high-dose thyroxine: an open clinical trial. *Neuropsychopharmacology*, **10**(3), 183–9.

Beauclair, L., Radoi-Andraous, D. and Chouinard, G., 2000. Selective serotonin-noradrenaline reuptake inhibitors. In: Sadock, B.J. and Sadock, V.A. (eds), *Comprehensive Textbook of Psychiatry*, 7th edn, pp. 2427–32. Lippincott Williams & Wilkins, Philadelphia, PA.

Bebchuk, J.M., Arfken, C.L., Dolan-Manji, S., Murphy, J., Hasanat, K. and Manji, H.K., 2000. A preliminary investigation of a protein kinase c inhibitor in the treatment of acute mania. *Archives of General Psychiatry*, **57**, 95–7.

Beck, A.T., Rush, A.J., Shaw, B.F. and Emery, G., 1979. *Cognitive Therapy of Depression*. Guilford Press, New York.

Becker, R.E., Heimberg, R.G. and Bellack, A.S., 1987. *Social Skills Training Treatment for Depression*. Pergamon Press, New York.

Belanoff, J.K., Flores, B.H., Kalezhan, M., Sund, B. and Schatzberg, A.F., 2001. Rapid reversal of psychotic depression using mifepristone. *Journal of Clinical Psychopharmacology*, **21**, 516–21.

Benedetti, F., Colombo, C., Barbini, B., Campori, E. and Smeraldi, E., 1999. Ongoing lithium treatment prevents relapse after total sleep deprivation. *Journal of Clinical Psychopharmacology*, **19**(3), 240–5.

Berman, R.M., Narasimhan, M., Sanacora, G., Miano, A.P., Hoffman, R.E., Hu, X.S., Charney, D.S. and Boutros, N.N., 2000. A randomized clinical trial of repetitive transcranial magnetic stimulation in the treatment of major depression. *Biological Psychiatry*, **47**, 332–7.

Bernstein, J.G., 1995. *Handbook of Drug Therapy in Psychiatry*, 3rd edn, Mosby, St Louis, MO.

Bhana, N. and Perry, C.M., 2001. Olanzapine: a review of its use in the treatment of bipolar I disorder. *CNS Drugs*, **15**, 871–904.

Binder, D.K. and Iskandar, B.J., 2000. Modern neurosurgery for psychiatric disorders. *Neurosurgery*, **47**, 9–23.

Bloch, M., Schmidt, P.J., Danaceau, M.A., Adams, L.F. and Rubinow, D.R., 1999. Dehydroepiandrosterone treatment of midlife dysthymia. *Biological Psychiatry*, **45**, 1533–41.

Bodkin, J.A., Zornberg, G.L., Lukas, S.E. and Cole, J.O., 1995. Buprenorphine treatment of refractory depression. *Journal of Clinical Psychopharmacology*, **15**(1), 49–57.

Boerlin, H.L., Gitlin, M.J., Zoellner, L.A. and Hammen, C.L., 1998. Bipolar depression and antidepressant-induced mania: a naturalistic study. *Journal of Clinical Psychiatry*, **59**, 374–9.

Bordet, R., Thomas, P. and Dupuis, B., 1998. Effect of pindolol on onset of action of paroxetine in the treatment of major depression: intermediate analysis of a double-blind, placebo-controlled trial. *American Journal of Psychiatry*, **155**, 1346–51.

Bowden, C.L., Brugger, A.M., Swann, A.C., Calabrese, J.R., Janicak, P.G., Petty, F., Dilsaver, S.C., Davies, J.M., Rush, A.J., Small, J., Garza-Trevino, E.S., Risch, S.C., Goodnick, P.J. and Morris, D.D., 1994. Efficacy of divalproex vs lithium and placebo in the treatment of mania. *JAMA*, **271**(12), 918–24.

Bowden, C.L., Calabrese, J.R. and McElroy, S.L., 2000a. A randomized, placebo-controlled 12-month trial of divalproex and lithium in treatment of outpatients with bipolar I disorder. *Archives of General Psychiatry*, **57**, 481–9.

Bowden, C.L., Lecrubier, Y., Bauer, M., Goodwin, G., Greil, W., Sachs, G. and von Knorring, L., 2000b. Maintenance therapies for classic and other forms of bipolar disorder. *Journal of Affective Disorders*, **59**, S57–S67.

Brent, D.A., Ryan, N., Dahl, R. and Birmaher, B., 1995. Early-onset mood disorder. In: Bloom, F.E. and Kupfer, D.J. (eds), *Psychopharmacology: The Fourth Generation of Progress*, pp. 1631–42. Raven Press, New York.

Bressa, G.M., 1994. S-adenosyl-l-methionine (SAMe) as antidepressant: meta-analysis of clinical studies. *Acta Neurological Scandinavica*, **89**(suppl 154), 7–14.

Brody, A.L., Saxena, S., Stoessel, P., Gillies, L.A., Fairbanks, L.A., Alborzian, S., Phelps, M.E., Huang, S.C., Wu, H.M., Ho, M.L., Ho, M.K., Au, S.C., Maidment, K. and Baxter, L.R., 2001. Regional brain metabolic changes in patients with major depression treated with either paroxetine or interpersonal therapy: preliminary findings. *Archives of General Psychiatry*, **58**, 631–40.

Brown, E.S., Bobadilla, L. and Rush, A.J., 2001. Ketoconazole in bipolar patients with depressive symptoms: a case series and literature review. *Bipolar Disorder*, **3**, 23–9.

Burt, T., Sachs, G.S. and Demopulos, C., 1999. Donepezil in treatment-resistant bipolar disorder. *Biological Psychiatry*, **45**, 959–64.

Calabrese, J.R., Bowden, C.L., McElroy, S.L., Cookson, J., Andersen, J., Keck, P.E., Rhodes, L., Bolden-Watson, C., Zhou, J. and Ascher, J.A., 1999a. Spectrum of activity of lamotrigine in treatment-refractory bipolar disorder. *American Journal of Psychiatry*, **156**(7), 1019–23.

Calabrese, J.R., Bowden, C.L., Sachs, G.S., Ascher, J.A., Monaghan, E. and Rudd, G.D., 1999b. A double-blind placebo-controlled study of lamotrigine monotherapy in outpatients with bipolar I depression. *Journal of Clinical Psychiatry*, **60**, 79–88.

Calabrese, J.R., Suppes, T., Bowden, C.L., Sachs, G.S., Swann, A.C., McElroy, S.L., Kusumakar, V., Ascher, J.A., Earl, N.L., Greene, P.L. and Monaghan, E.T., 2000. A double-blind, placebo-controlled, prophylaxis study of lamotrigine in rapid-cycling bipolar disorder. *Journal of Clinical Psychiatry*, **61**(11), 841–50.

Chang, M.C.J., Contreras, M.A., Rosenberger, T.A., Rintala, J.J.O., Bell, J.M. and Rapoport, S.I., 2001. Chronic valproate treatment decreases the *in vivo* turnover of arachidonic acid in brain phospholipids: a possible common effect of mood stabilizers. *Journal of Neurochemistry*, **77**, 796–803.

Chen, G., Hasanat, K.A., Bebchuk, J.M., Moore, G.J., Glitz, D. and Manji, H.K., 1999. Regulation of signal transduction pathways and gene expression by mood stabilizers and antidepressants. *Psychosomatic Medicine*, **61**, 599–609.

Chengappa, K.N.R., Rathore, D., Levine, J., Atzert, R., Solai, L., Parepally, H., Levin, H., Moffa, N., Delaney, J. and Brar, J.S., 1999. Topiramate as add-on treatment for patients with bipolar mania. *Bipolar Disorders*, **1**, 42–53.

Chengappa, K.N., Levine, J., Gershon, S., Mallinger, A.G., Hardan, A., Vagnucci, A., Pollock, B., Luther, J., Buttenfield, J., Verfaille, S. and Kupfer, D.J., 2000. Inositol as an add-on treatment for bipolar depression. *Bipolar Disorders*, **2**(1), 47–55.

Chengappa, K.N.R., Gershon, S. and Levine, J., 2001. The evolving role of topiramate among other mood stabilizers in the management of bipolar disorder. *Bipolar Disorders*, **3**, 215–32.

Claghorn, J.L., 2000. Mirtazapine. In: Sadock, B.J. and Sadock, V.A. (eds), *Comprehensive Textbook of Psychiatry*, 7th edn, pp. 2390–7. Lippincott Williams & Wilkins, Philadelphia, PA.

Clark, D.M. and Fairburn, C.G., 1997. *Science and Practice of Cognitive Behaviour Therapy*. Oxford University Press, New York.

Colombo, C., Lucca, A., Benedetti, F., Barbini, B., Campori, E. and Smeraldi, E., 2000. Total sleep deprivation combined with lithium and light therapy in the treatment of bipolar depression: replication of main effects and interaction. *Psychiatry Research*, **95**(1), 43–53.

Coppen, A., 2000. Lithium in unipolar depression and the prevention of suicide. *Journal of Clinical Psychiatry*, **61**, 52–6.

Crane, G.E., 1957. Iproniazid (Marsilid) phosphate, a therapeutic agent for mental disorders and debilitating disease. *Psychiatric Research Reports*, **8**, 142–52.

Cummings, J.L., 2000. Cholinesterase inhibitors: a new class of psychotropic compounds. *American Journal of Psychiatry*, **157**, 4–15.

Davis, K.L., Berger, P.A., Hollister, L.E. and Defraites, E., 1978. Physostigmine in mania. *Archives of General Psychiatry*, **35**, 119–22.

De Novaes-Soares, C., Almeida, O.P., Joffe, H. and Cohen, L.S., 2001. Efficacy of estradiol for the treatment of depressive disorders in perimenopausal women: a double-blind, randomized, placebo-controlled trial. *Archives of General Psychiatry*, **58**(6), 529–34.

Dose, M., Emrich, H.M., Cording-Toemmel, C. and von Zerssen, D., 1986. Use of calcium antagonists in mania. *Psychoneuroendocrinology*, **11**, 241–3.

Duman, R.S., Heninger, G.R. and Nestler, E.J., 1997. A molecular and cellular theory of depression. *Archives of General Psychiatry*, **54**, 597–606.

Dunayevich, E. and McElroy, S.L., 2000. Atypical antipsychotics in the treatment of bipolar disorder: pharmacological and clinical effects. *CNS Drugs*, **13**, 433–41.

Dunayevich, E. and Strakowski, S.M., 2000. Quetiapine for treatment-resistant mania. *American Journal of Psychiatry*, **157**, 1341.

Dunn, R.T., Frye, M.S., Kimbrell, T.A., Denicoff, K.D., Leverich, G.S. and Post, R.M., 1998. The efficacy and use of anticonvulsants in mood disorders. *Clinical Neuropharmacology*, **21**, 215–35.

Echols, J.C., Naidoo, U. and Salzman, C., 2000. SAMe (S-adenosylmethionine). *Harvard Review of Psychiatry*, **8**(2), 84–90.

Emslie, G.J., Rush, A.J., Weinberg, W.A., Kowatch, R.A., Hughes, C.W., Carmody, T. and Rintelmann, J., 1997. A double-blind, randomized, placebo-controlled trial of fluoxetine in children and adolescents with depression. *Archives of General Psychiatry*, **54**(11), 1031–7.

Epperson, C., Neill, M.D., Wisner, K.L. and Yamamoto, B., 1999. Gonadal steroids in the treatment of mood disorders. *Psychosomatic Medicine*, **61**(5), 676.

Ericson, A., Kallen, B. and Wiholm, B.E., 1999. Delivery outcome after the use of antidepressants in early pregnancy. *European Journal of Clinical Pharmacology*, **55**, 503–8.

Fava, M., Giannelli, A., Rapisarda, V. and Patralia, A., 1995. Rapidity of onset of the antidepressant effect of parenteral *S*-adenosyl-L-methionine. *Psychiatry Research*, **56**(3), 295–7.

Fava, G.A., Savron, G., Grandi, S. and Rafanelli, C., 1997. Cognitive-behavioral management of drug-resistant major depressive disorder. *Journal of Clinical Psychiatry*, **58**, 278–82.

Fava, M., Rajinder, J., Hoog, S.L., Nilsson, M.E. and Koke, S.C., 2000. Fluoxetine versus sertraline and paroxetine in major depressive disorder: changes in weight with long-term treatment. *Journal of Clinical Psychiatry*, **61**, 863–7.

Fawcett, J. and Barkin, R.L., 1998. A meta-analysis of eight randomized, double-blind, controlled clinical trials of mirtazapine for the treatment of patients with major depression and symptoms of anxiety. *Journal of Clinical Psychiatry*, **59**, 123–7.

Feighner, J., Targum, S.D., Bennett, M.E., Roberts, D.L., Kensler, T.T., D'Amico, M.F. and Hardy, S.A., 1998. A double-blind, placebo-controlled trial of nefazodone in the treatment of patients hospitalized for major depression. *Journal of Clinical Psychiatry*, **59**, 246–53.

Ferguson, J.M., Shrivastava, R.K., Stahl, S.M., Hartford, J.T., Borian, F., Ieni, J., McQuade, R.D. and Jody, D., 2001. Reemergence of sexual dysfunction in patients with major depressive disorder: double-blind comparison of nefazodone and sertraline. *Journal of Clinical Psychiatry*, **62**, 24–9.

Ferrier, I.N., 2001. Developments in mood stabilizers. *British Medical Bulletin*, **57**, 179–92.

Frank, E., Swartz, H.A. and Kupfer, D.J., 2000. Interpersonal and social rhythm therapy: managing the chaos of bipolar disorder. *Biological Psychiatry*, **48**, 593–604.

Fritzsche, M., Heller, R., Hill, H. and Kick, H., 2001. Sleep deprivation as a predictor of response to light therapy in major depression. *Journal of Affective Disorders*, **62**(3), 207–15.

Frye, M.A., Ketter, T.A., Kimbrell, T.A., Dunn, R.T., Speer, A.M., Osuch, E.A., Luckenbaugh, D.A., Cora-Locatelli, G., Leverich, G.S. and Post, R.M., 2000. A placebo-controlled study of lamotrigine and gabapentin monotherapy in refractory mood disorders. *Journal of Clinical Psychopharmacology*, **20**, 607–14.

Fugh-Berman, A. and Cott, J.M., 1999. Dietary supplements and natural products as psychotherapeutic agents. *Psychosomatic Medicine*, **61**, 712–22.

Gagne, G.G., Furman, M.J., Carpenter, L.L. and Price, L.H., 2000. Efficacy of continuation ECT and antidepressant drugs compared to long-term antidepressants alone in depressed patients. *American Journal of Psychiatry*, **157**(12), 1960–5.

Garlow, S.J., Owens, M.J. and Nemeroff, C.B., 2000. Nefazodone. In: Sadock, B.J. and Sadock, A.V. (eds), *Comprehensive Textbook of Psychiatry*, 7th edn, pp. 2412–19. Lippincott Williams & Wilkins, Philadelphia, PA.

George, M.S., Wassermann, E., Kimbrell, T.A., Little, J.T., Williams, W.E., Danielson, A.L., Greenberg, B.D., Hallett, M. and Post, R.M., 1997. Mood improvement following daily left prefrontal repetitive transcranial magnetic stimulation in patients with depression: a placebo-controlled crossover trial. *American Journal of Psychiatry*, **154**(12), 1752–6.

George, M.S., Lisanby, S. and Sackeim, H.A., 1999. Transcranial magnetic stimulation: applications in neuropsychiatry. *Archives of General Psychiatry*, **56**(4), 300–11.

George, M.S., Nahas, Z., Molloy, M., Speer, A.M., Oliver, N.C., Li, X.-B., Arana, G.W., Risch, S.C. and Ballenger, J.C., 2000a. A controlled trial of daily left prefrontal cortex TMS for treating depression. *Biological Psychiatry*, **48**, 962–70.

George, M.S., Sackeim, H.A., Rush, A.J., Marangell, L.B., Nahas, Z., Husain, M.M., Lisanby, S., Burt, T., Goldman, J. and Ballenger, J.C., 2000b. Vagus nerve stimulation: a new tool for brain research and therapy. *Biological Psychiatry*, **47**, 287–95.

Ghaemi, S.N. and Goodwin, F.K., 1999. Use of atypical antipsychotic agents in bipolar and schizoaffective disorders: review of the empirical literature. *Journal of Clinical Psychopharmacology*, **19**, 354–61.

Ghaemi, S.N. and Goodwin, F.K., 2001. Gabapentin treatment of the non-refractory bipolar spectrum: an open case series. *Journal of Affective Disorders*, **65**, 167–71.

Ghaemi, S.N. and Katzow, J.J., 1999. The use of quetiapine for treatment-resistant bipolar disorder: a case series. *Annals of Clinical Psychiatry*, **11**, 137–40.

Golden, R.N. and Nicholas, L.M., 2000. Bupropion. In: Sadock, B.J. and Sadock, A.V. (eds), *Comprehensive Textbook of Psychiatry*, 7th edn, pp. 2324–9. Lippincott Williams & Wilkins, Philadelphia, PA.

Goldstein, T.R., Frye, M.A., Denicoff, K.D., Smith-Jackson, E., Leverich, G.S., Bryan, A.L., Ali, S.O. and Post, R.M., 1999. Antidepressant discontinuation-related mania: critical prospective observation and theoretical implications in bipolar disorder. *Journal of Clinical Psychiatry*, **60**, 568–9.

Goodwin, F.K., 1999. Anticonvulsant therapy and suicide risk in affective disorders. *Journal of Clinical Psychiatry*, **60**, 89–93.

Gram, L.F., 1994. Fluoxetine. *New England Journal of Medicine*, **331**, 1354–61.

Grinspoon, S., Corcoran, C., Stanley, T., Baaj, A., Basgoz, N. and Klibanski, A., 2000. Effects of hypogonadism and testosterone administration on depression indices in HIV-infected men. *Journal of Clinical Endocrinology and Metabolism*, **85**(1), 60–5.

Grisaru, N., Chudakov, B., Yaroslavsky, Y. and Belmaker, R.H., 1998. Transcranial magnetic stimulation in mania: a controlled study. *American Journal of Psychiatry*, **155**, 1608–10.

Grunhaus, L., Dannon, P.N., Schreiber, S., Dolberg, O.H., Amiaz, R., Ziv, R. and Lefkifker, E., 2000. Repetitive transcranial magnetic stimulation is as effective as electroconvulsive therapy in treatment of nondelusional major depressive disorder: an open study. *Biological Psychiatry*, **47**, 314–24.

Guelfi, J.D., Ansseau, M., Timmerman, L., Korsgaard, S. and the Mirtazapine-Venlafaxine Study Group, 2001. Mirtazapine versus venlafaxine in hospitalized severely depressed patients with melancholic features. *Journal of Clinical Psychopharmacology*, **21**, 425–31.

Guille, C., Sachs, G.S. and Ghaemi, S.N., 2000. A naturalistic comparison of clozapine, risperidone, and olanzapine in the treatment of bipolar disorder. *Journal of Clinical Psychiatry*, **61**, 638–42.

Halbreich, U., 1997. Role of estrogen in postmenopausal depression. *Neurology*, **48**(5, suppl 7), 16–20.

Healy, D. and Healy, H., 1998. The clinical pharmacologic profile of reboxetine: does it involve the putative neurobiological substrates of wellbeing? *Journal of Affective Disorders*, **51**, 313–22.

Hersen, M., Bellack, A.S., Himmelhoch, J.M. and Thase, M.E., 1984. Effects of social skills training, amitriptyline, and psychotherapy in unipolar depressed women. *Behavior Therapy*, **15**, 21–40.

Hollister, L.E. and Garza Trevino, E.S., 1999. Calcium channel blockers in psychiatric disorders: a review of the literature. *Canadian Journal of Psychiatry*, **44**, 658–64.

Hollon, S.D., DeRubeis, R.J., Evans, M.D., Wiemer, J.J., Garvey, J.G., Grove, W.M. and Tuason, V.B., 1992. Cognitive therapy and pharmacotherapy for depression: singly and in combination. *Archives of General Psychiatry*, **49**, 774–81.

Howland, R.H., 1991. Pharmacotherapy of dysthymia: a review. *Journal of Clinical Psychopharmacology*, **11**(2), 83–92.

Howland, R.H., 1993. Thyroid dysfunction in refractory depression: implications for pathophysiology and treatment. *Journal of Clinical Psychiatry*, **54**(2), 47–54.

Howland, R.H., 1996a. Psychosocial therapies for dysthymia. In: *The Hatherleigh Guide to Managing Depression*, pp. 225–41. Hatherleigh Press, New York.

Howland, R.H., 1996b. Induction of mania with serotonin reuptake inhibitors. *Journal of Clinical Psychopharmacology*, **16**, 425–7.

Howland, R.H. and Thase, M.E., 1993. A comprehensive review of cyclothymic disorder. *Journal of Nervous and Mental Disease*, **181**(8), 485–93.

Howland, R.H. and Thase, M.E., 1997. Switching strategies for the treatment of unipolar major depression. In: Rush, A.J. (ed.), *Mood Disorders: Systematic Medication Management. Modern Problems of Pharmacopsychiatry*, pp. 56–65. Karger, Basel.

Howland, R.H. and Thase, M.E., 1999a. what to do with SSRI nonresponders? *Journal of Practical Psychiatry and Behavioral Health*, **5**(4), 216–23.

Howland, R.H. and Thase, M.E., 1999b. Affective disorders: biological aspects. In: Millen, T., Blaney, P.H. and Davis, R.D. (eds), *Oxford Textbook of Psychopathology*, pp. 166–202. Oxford University Press, New York.

Hypericum Depression Trial Study Group, 2002. Effect of Hypericum perforatum (St John's Wort) in major depressive disorder: a randomized controlled trial. *JAMA*, **287**(14), 1807–1814.

Janicak, P.G., Sharma, R.P., Pandey, G. and Davis, J.M., 1998. Verapamil for the treatment of acute mania: a double-blind, placebo-controlled trial. *American Journal of Psychiatry*, **155**, 972–3.

Jarrett, R.B., Schaffer, M., McIntire, D., Witt-Browder, A., Kraft, D. and Risser, R.C., 1999. Treatment of atypical depression with cognitive therapy or phenelzine: a double-blind, placebo-controlled trial. *Archives of General Psychiatry*, **56**(5), 431–7.

Joffe, H. and Cohen, L.S., 1998. Estrogen, serotonin, and mood disturbance: where is the therapeutic bridge? *Biological Psychiatry*, **44**(9), 798–811.

Keck, P.E., Mendlwicz, J., Calabrese, J.R., Fawcett, J., Suppes, T., Vestergaard, P.A. and Carbonell, C., 2000. A review of randomized, controlled clinical trials in acute mania. *Journal of Affective Disorders*, **59**, S31–S37.

Keller, M.B., McCullough, J.P., Klein, D.N., Arnow, B., Dunner, D.L., Gelenberg, A.J., Markowitz, J.C., Nemeroff, C.B., Russell, J.M., Thase, M.E., Trivedi, M.H. and Zajecka, J., 2000. A comparison of nefazodone, the cognitive behavioral-analysis system of psychotherapy, and their combination for the treatment of chronic depression. *New England Journal of Medicine*, **342**, 1462–70.

Kelly, K.G. and Zisselman, M., 2000. Update on electroconvulsive therapy (ECT) in older adults. *Journal of the American Geriatrics Society*, **48**, 560–6.

Kelsey, J.E. and Nemeroff, C.B., 2000. Selective serotonin reuptake inhibitors. In: Sadock, B.J. and Sadock, V.A. (eds), *Comprehensive Textbook of Psychiatry*, 7th edn, pp. 2432–55. Lippincott Williams & Wilkins, Philadelphia, PA.

Kennedy, S.H., McKenna, K.F. and Baker, G.B., 2000. Monoamine oxidase inhibitors. In: Sadock, B.J. and Sadock, V.A. (eds), *Comprehensive*

Textbook of Psychiatry, 7th edn, pp. 2397–407. Lippincott Williams & Wilkins, Philadelphia, PA.

Kent, J.M., 2000. SnaRIs, NaSSAs, and NaRIs: new agents for the treatment of depression. *Lancet*, **355**, 911–18.

Klein, E., Kreinin, I., Chistyakov, A., Koren, D., Mecz, L., Marmur, S., Ben-Shachar, D. and Feinsod, M., 1999. Therapeutic efficacy of right prefrontal slow repetitive transcranial magnetic stimulation in major depression: a double-blind controlled study. *Archives of General Psychiatry*, **56**(4), 315–20.

Klerman, G.L. and Weissman, M.M., 1993. *New Applications of Interpersonal Psychotherapy*. American Psychiatric Press, Washington, DC.

Klerman, G.L., Weissman, M.M., Rounsaville, B.J. and Chevron, E.S., 1984. *Interpersonal Psychotherapy of Depression*. Basic Books, New York.

Kornstein, S.G., Schatzberg, A.F., Thase, M.E., Yonkers, K.A., McCullough, J.P., Keitner, G.I., Gelenberg, A.J., Davis, S.M., Harrison, W.M. and Keller, M.B., 2000. Gender differences in treatment response to sertraline versus imipramine in chronic depression. *American Journal of Psychiatry*, **157**(9), 1445–52.

Kowatch, R.A., Suppes, T., Carmody, T.J., Bucci, J.P., Hume, J.H., Kromelis, M.R., Emslie, G.J., Weinberg, W.A. and Rush, A.J., 2000. Effect size of lithium, divalproex sodium, and carbamazepine in children and adolescents with bipolar disorder. *Journal of the American Academy of Child and Adolescent Psychiatry*, **36**(9), 713–20.

Krieg, J.C. and Berger, M., 1986. Treatment of mania with the cholinomimetic agent RS 86. *British Journal of Psychiatry,* **148**, 613.

Kripke, D.F., 1998. Light treatment for nonsensical major depression: are we ready? In: Lam, R.W. (ed.), *Seasonal Affective Disorder and Beyond*, pp. 159–72. American Psychiatric Press, Washington, DC.

Kuhn, R., 1958. The treatment of depressive states with G-22355 (imipramine hydrochloride). *American Journal of Psychiatry*, **115**, 459–64.

Leiva, D.B., 1990. The neurochemistry of mania: a hypothesis of etiology and rationale for treatment. *Neuro-Psychopharmacology and Biological Psychiatry*, **14**(3), 423–9.

Levine, J., Barak, Y., Gonzalves, M., Szor, H., Elizur, A., Kofman, O. and Belmaker, R.H., 1995. Double-blind, controlled trial of inositol treatment of depression. *American Journal of Psychiatry*, **152**(5), 792–4.

Levine, J., Mishori, A., Susnosky, M., Martin, M. and Belmaker, R.H., 1999. Combination of inositol and serotonin reuptake inhibitors in the treatment of depression. *Biological Psychiatry*, **45**(3), 270–3.

Linde, K., Ramirez, G., Mulrow, C.D., Pauls, A., Weidenhammer, W. and Melchart, D., 1996. St John's wort for depression: an overview and meta-analysis of randomized clinical trials. *British Medical Journal*, **313**, 253–8.

Loo, C., Mitchell, P., Sachdev, P., McDarmont, B., Parker, G. and Gandevia, S., 1999. Double-blind controlled investigation of transcranial magnetic stimulation for the treatment of resistant major depression. *American Journal of Psychiatry*, **156**(6), 946–8.

Lotufo-Neto, F., Trivedi, M. and Thase, M.E., 1999. Meta-analysis of the reversible inhibitors of monoamine oxidase type A moclobemide and brofaromine for the treatment of depression. *Neuropsychopharmacology*, **20**, 226–47.

Luo, H., Meng, F., Jia, Y. and Zhao, X., 1998. Clinical research on the therapeutic effect of the electro-acupuncture treatment in patients with depression. *Psychiatry Clinical Neuroscience*, **52**, S338–340.

Mahmood, I., 1997. Clinical pharmacokinetics and pharmacodynamics of selegiline: an update. *Clinical Pharmacokinetics*, **33**(2), 91–102.

Maj, M., 2000. The impact of lithium prophylaxis on the course of bipolar disorder: a review of the research evidence. *Bipolar Disorders*, **2**, 93–101.

Manji, H.K., Potter, W.Z. and Lenox, R.H., 1995. Signal transduction pathways: molecular targets for lithium's actions. *Archives of General Psychiatry*, **52**, 531–43.

Manji, H.K., Chen, G., Hsiao, J.K., Risby, E.D., Masana, M.I. and Potter, W.Z., 1996. Regulation of signal transduction pathways by mood-stabilizing agents: implications for the delayed onset of therapeutic efficacy. *Journal of Clinical Psychiatry*, **57**(suppl 13), 34–46.

Manji, H.K., Bebchuk, J.M., Moore, G.J., Glitz, D., Hasanat, K.A. and Chen, G., 1999. Modulation of CNS signal transduction pathways and gene expression by mood-stabilizing agents: therapeutic implications. *Journal of Clinical Psychiatry*, **60**(suppl 2), 27–39.

Marangell, L.B., Rush, A.J., George, M.S., Sackeim, H.A., Johnson, C.R., Husain, M.M., Nahas, Z. and Lisanby, S.H., 2002. Vagus nerve stimulation (VNS) for major depressive episodes: one year outcomes. *Biological Psychiatry*, **51**, 280–287.

Marcotte, D., 1998. Use of topiramate, a new anti-epileptic as a mood stabilizer. *Journal of Affective Disorders*, **50**, 245–51.

Margolese, H.C., 2000. The male menopause and mood: testosterone decline and depression in the aging male — is there a link? *Journal of Geriatric Psychiatry and Neurology*, **13**(2), 93–101.

Markowitz, J.C., 1998. *Interpersonal Psychotherapy for Dysthymic Disorder*. American Psychiatric Press, Washington, DC.

Massana, J., 1998. Reboxetine versus fluoxetine: an overview of efficacy and tolerability. *Journal of Clinical Psychiatry*, **59**(suppl 14), 8–10.

McCall, W., Vaughn, M.S., Reboussin, D.M., Weiner, R.D. and Sackeim, H.A., 2000. Titrated moderately suprathreshold vs. fixed high-dose right unilateral electroconvulsive therapy: acute antidepressant and cognitive effects. *Archives of General Psychiatry*, **57**(5), 438–44.

McCullough, J.P., 2000. *Treatment for Chronic Depression: Cognitive Behavioral Analysis System of Psychotherapy*. Guilford Press, New York.

McElroy, S.L. and Keck, P.E., 2000. Pharmacologic agents for the treatment of acute bipolar mania. *Biological Psychiatry*, **48**, 539–57.

McElroy, S.L., Suppes, T., Keck, P.E., Frye, M.A., Denicoff, K.D., Altshuler, L.L., Brown, E.S., Nolen, W.A., Kupka, R.W., Rochussen, J., Leverich, G.S. and Post, R.M., 2000. Open-label adjunctive topiramate in the treatment of bipolar disorders. *Biological Psychiatry*, **47**, 1025–33.

McGrath, P.J., Stewart, J.W., Janal, M.N., Petkova, E., Quitkin, R.M. and Klein, D.F., 2000. A placebo-controlled study of fluoxetine versus imipramine in the acute treatment of atypical depression. *American Journal of Psychiatry*, **157**(3), 344–50.

McQuade, R. and Young, A.H., 2000. Future therapeutic targets in mood disorders: the glucocorticoid receptor. *British Journal of Psychiatry*, **177**, 390–5.

Meehan, K., Zhang, F., David, S., Tohen, M., Janicak, P., Small, J., Koch, K., Rizk, R., Walker, D., Tran, P. and Breier, A., 2001. A double-blind, randomized comparison of the efficacy and safety of intramuscular injections of olanzapine, lorazepam, or placebo in treating acutely agitated patients diagnosed with bipolar mania. *Journal of Clinical Psychopharmacology*, **21**, 389–97.

Menza, M.A., Kaufman, K.R. and Castellanos, A., 2000. Modafinil augmentation of antidepressant treatment in depression. *Journal of Clinical Psychiatry*, **61**, 378–81.

Miklowitz, D.J., Simoneau, T.L., George, E.L., Richards, J.A., Kalbag, A., Sachs-Ericsson, N. and Suddath, R., 2000. Family-focused treatment of bipolar disorder: 1-year effects of psychoeducational programme in conjunction with pharmacotherapy. *Biological Psychiatry*, **48**, 582–92.

Montgomery, S.A., Schatzberg, A.F., Guelfi, J.D., Kasper, S., Nemeroff, C., Swann, A. and Zajecka, J., 2000. Pharmacotherapy of depression and mixed states in bipolar disorder. *Journal of Affective Disorders*, **59**, S39–S56.

Morrison, M.F. and Tweedy, K., 2000. Effects of estrogen on mood and cognition in aging women. *Psychiatric Annals*, **30**(2), 113–19.

Mukherjee, S., Sackeim, H.A. and Schnur, D.B., 1994. Electroconvulsive therapy of acute manic episodes: a review of 50 years' experience. *American Journal of Psychiatry*, **151**, 169–76.

Murphy, B.E.P., Filipini, D. and Ghadirian, A.M., 1993. Possible use of glucocorticoid receptor antagonists in the treatment of major depression: preliminary results using RU 486. *Journal of Psychiatry and Neuroscience,* **18**(5), 209–13.

Murphy, B.E.P., Ghadirian, A.M. and Dhar, V., 1998. Neuroendocrine responses to inhibitors of steroid biosynthesis in patient with major depression resistant to antidepressant therapy. *Canadian Journal of Psychiatry*, **43**, 279–86.

Nelson, J.C., 2000. Tricyclics and tetracyclics. In: Sadock, B.J. and Sadock, A.V. (eds), *Comprehensive Textbook of Psychiatry*, 7th edn, pp. 2491–502. Lippincott Williams & Wilkins, Philadelphia, PA.

Nemeroff, C.B., Evans, D.L., Gyulai, L., Sachs, G.S., Bowden, C.L., Gergel, I.P., Oakes, R. and Pitts, C.D., 2001. Double-blind, placebo-controlled comparison of imipramine and paroxetine in the treatment of bipolar depression. *American Journal of Psychiatry*, **158**, 906–12.

Nemets, B., Mishory, A., Levine, J. and Belmaker, R.H., 1999. Inositol addition does not improve depression in SSRI treatment failures. *Journal of Neural Transmission*, **106**, 795–8.

Parker, G., Roy, K., Wilhelm, K. and Mitchell, P., 2001. Assessing the comparative effectiveness of antidepressant therapies: a prospective clinical practice study. *Journal of Clinical Psychiatry*, **62**(2), 117–25.

Patelis-Siotis, I., 2001. Cognitive-behavioral therapy: applications for the management of bipolar disorder. *Bipolar Disorders*, **3**, 1–10.

Paykel, E.S., Scott, J., Teasdale, J.D., Johnson, A.L., Garland, A., Moore, R., Jenaway, A., Cornwall, P.L., Hayhurst, H., Abbott, R. and

Pope, M., 1999. Prevention of relapse in residual depression by cognitive therapy: a controlled trial. *Archives of General Psychiatry*, **56**, 829–35.

Pazzaglia, P.J., Post, R.M., Ketter, T.A., Callahan, A.M., Marangell, L.B., Frye, M.A., George, M.S., Kimbrell, T.A., Leverich, G.S., Cora-Locatelli, G. and Luckenbaugh, D., 1998. Nimodipine monotherapy and carbamazepine augmentation in patients with refractory recurrent affective illness. *Journal of Clinical Psychopharmacology*, **18**, 404–13.

Perry, P.J., 1996. Pharmacotherapy for major depression with melancholic features: relative efficacy of tricyclic versus selective serotonin reuptake inhibitor antidepressants. *Journal of Affective Disorders*, **39**, 1–6.

Persons, J.B., Thase, M.E. and Crits-Christoph, P., 1996. The role of psychotherapy in the treatment of depression. *Archives of General Psychiatry*, **53**, 283–90.

Philipp, M., Tiller, J.W.G., Baier, D. and Kohnen, R., 2000. Comparison of moclobemide with selective serotonin reuptake inhibitors (SSRIs) on sexual function in depressed adults. *European Neuropsychopharmacology*, **10**(5), 305–14.

Popoli, M., Brunello, N., Perez, J. and Racagni, G., 2000. Second messenger-regulated protein kinases in the brain: their functional role and the action of antidepressant drugs. *Journal of Neurochemistry*, **74**, 21–31.

Post, R.M., Frye, M.A., Denicoff, K.D., Leverich, G.S., Dunn, R.T., Osuch, E.A., Speer, A.M., Obrocea, G. and Jajodia, K., 2000. Emerging trends in the treatment of rapid cycling bipolar disorder: a selected review. *Bipolar Disorders*, **2**, 305–15.

Post, R.M., Altshuler, L.L., Frye, M.A., Suppes, T., Rush, A.J., Keck, P.E., McElroy, S.L., Denicoff, K.D., Leverich, G.S., Kupka, R. and Nolen, W.A., 2001. Rate of switch in bipolar patients prospectively treated with second-generation antidepressants as augmentation to mood stabilizers. *Bipolar Disorders*, **3**, 259–65.

Preskorn, S.H., 1995. Comparison of the tolerability of bupropion, fluoxetine, imipramine, nefazodone, paroxetine, sertraline, and venlafaxine. *Journal of Clinical Psychiatry*, **56**(suppl 6), 12–21.

Reus, B.I., Wolkowitz, O.M. and Frederick, S., 1997. Antiglucocorticoid treatments in psychiatry. *Psychoneuroendocrinology*, **22**(suppl 1), 121–4.

Reynolds, E.H. and Stramentinoli, G., 1983. Folic acid, S-adenosylmethionine and affective disorder. *Psychological Medicine*, **13**(4), 705–10.

Richelson, E., 2001. Pharmacology of antidepressants. *Mayo Clinic Proceedings*, **76**, 511–27.

Roschke, J., Wolf, C., Muller, P., Wagner, K., Mann, K., Grozinger, M. and Bech, S., 2000. The benefit from whole body acupuncture in major depression. *Journal of Affective Disorders*, **57**, 73–81.

Rush, A.J. and Thase, M.E., 1999. Psychotherapies for depressive disorders: a review. In: Maj, M. and Sartorius, N. (eds), *Evidence and Experience in Psychiatry*, vol. 1 *Depressive Disorders*, pp. 161–206. John Wiley & Sons, Chichester.

Rush, A.J. and Trivedi, M.H., 1995. Treating depression to remission. *Psychiatric Annals*, **25**, 704–9.

Rush, A.J., George, M.S., Sackeim, H.A., Marangell, L.B., Husain, M.M., Giller, C., Nahas, Z., Haines, S., Simpson, R.K. and Goodman, R., 2000. Vagus nerve stimulation (VNS) for treatment-resistant depressions: a multicenter study. *Biological Psychiatry*, **47**, 276–86.

Sachs, G.S. and Thase, M.E., 2000. Bipolar disorder therapeutics: maintenance treatment. *Biological Psychiatry*, **48**, 573–81.

Sachs, G.S., Lafer, B., Stoll, A.L. and Banov, M., 1994. A double-blind trial of bupropion versus desipramine for bipolar depression. *Journal of Clinical Psychiatry*, **55**, 391–3.

Sachs, G.S., Printz, D.J., Kahn, D.A., Carpenter, D. and Docherty, J.P., 2000. The expert consensus guideline series: medication treatment of bipolar disorder 2000. *Postgraduate Medicine Special Report*, April, 1–104.

Sackeim, H.A., 1994. Continuation therapy following ECT: directions for future research. *Psychopharmacology Bulletin*, **30**, 501–21.

Sackeim, H.A., Prudic, J., Devanand, D.P., Nobler, M.S., Lisanby, S.H., Peyser, S., Fitzsimons, L., Moody, B.J. and Clark, J., 2000. A prospective, randomized, double blind comparison of bilateral and right unilateral electroconvulsive therapy at different stimulus intensities. *Archives of General Psychiatry*, **57**(5), 425–434.

Sackeim, H.A., Haskett, R.F., Mulsant, B.H., Thase, M.E., Mann, J.J., Pettinati, H.M., Greenberg, R.M., Crowe, R.R., Cooper, T.B., Thomas, B. and Prudic, J., 2001a. Continuation pharmacotherapy in the prevention of relapse following electroconvulsive therapy: a randomized controlled trial. *JAMA*, **285**(10), 1299–1307.

Sackeim, H.A., Rush, A.J., George, M.S., Marangell, L.B., Husain, M.M., Nahas, Z., Johnson, C.R., Seidman, S., Giller, C., Haines, S., Simpson, R.K. and Goodman, R.R., 2001b. Vagus nerve stimulation (VNS) for treatment-resistant depression: efficacy, side effects, and predictors of outcome. *Neuropsychopharmacology*, **25**, 713–28.

Sacktor, N., Schifitto, G., McDermott, M.P., Marder, K., McArthur, J.C. and Kieburtz, K., 2000. Transdermal selegiline in HIV-associated cognitive impairment: pilot, placebo-controlled study. *Neurology*, **54**(1), 233–5.

Sajatovic, M., DiGiovanni, S., Fuller, M., Belton, J., DeVega, E., Marqua, S. and Liebling, D., 1999. Nefazodone therapy in patients with treatment-resistant or treatment-intolerant depression and high psychiatric comorbidity. *Clinical Therapeutics*, **21**, 733–40.

Saletu, B., Brandstaetter, N., Metka, M., Stamenkovic, M., Anderer, P., Semlitsch, H.V., Heytmanek, G., Huber, J., Gruenberger, J., Linzmayer, L., Kurz, C.h., Decker, K., Binder, G., Knogler, W. and Koll, B., 1995. Double-blind, placebo-controlled, hormonal, syndromal and EEG mapping studies with transdermal oestradiol therapy in menopausal depression. *Psychopharmacology*, **122**(4), 321–9.

Sampson, S.M., 2001. Treating depression with selective serotonin reuptake inhibitors: a practical approach. *Mayo Clinic Proceedings*, **76**, 739–44.

Schneider, L.S., Small, G.W., Hamilton, S.H., Bystritsky, A., Nemeroff, C.B. and Meyers, B.S., 1997. Estrogen replacement and response to fluoxetine in a multicenter geriatric depression trial. *American Journal of Geriatric Psychiatry*, **5**(2), 97–106.

Seidman, S.N. and Rabkin, J.G., 1998. Testosterone replacement therapy for hypogonadal men with SSRI-refractory depression. *Journal of Affective Disorders*, **48**, 157–61.

Seidman, S.N. and Walsh, B.T., 1999. Testosterone and depression in aging men. *American Journal of Geriatric Psychiatry*, **7**(1), 18–33.

Seidman, S.N., Spatz, E., Rizzo, C. and Roose, S.P., 2001. Testosterone replacement therapy for hypogonadal men with major depressive disorder: a randomized, placebo-controlled clinical trial. *Journal of Clinical Psychiatry*, **62**(6), 406–12.

Shapira, B., 1985. Lack of efficacy of estrogen supplementation to imipramine in resistant female depressives. *Biological Psychiatry*, **20**(5), 576–79.

Shelton, R.C., Keller, M.B., Gelenberg, A., Dunner, D.L., Hirshfield, R., Thase, M.E., Russell, J., Lydiard, R.B., Crits-Cristoph, P., Gallop, R., Todd, L., Hellerstein, D., Goodnick, P., Keitner, G., Stahl, S.M. and Halbreich, U., 2001a. Effectiveness of St John's Wort in major depression: a randomized controlled trial. *JAMA*, **285**(15), 1978–86.

Shelton, R.C., Tollefson, G.D., Tohen, M., Stahl, S., Gannon, K.S., Jacobs, T.C., Buras, W.R., Bymaster, F.P., Zhang, W., Spencer, K.A., Feldman, P.D. and Meltzer, H.Y., 2001b. A novel augmentation strategy for treating resistant major depression. *American Journal of Psychiatry*, **158**, 131–4.

Smeraldi, E., Benedetti, F., Barbini, B., Campori, E. and Colombo, C., 1999. Sustained antidepressant effect of sleep deprivation combined with pindolol in bipolar depression: a placebo-controlled trial. *Neuropsychopharmacology*, **20**(4), 380–5.

Spangler, W.J., Cosgrove, G.R., Ballantine, H.T., Cassem, E.H., Rauch, S.L., Nierenberg, A. and Price, B.H., 1996. Magnetic resonance image-guided stereotactic cingulotomy for intractable psychiatric disease. *Neurosurgery*, **38**, 1071–8.

Spier, S.A., 1998. Use of bupropion with SRIs and venlafaxine. *Depression and Anxiety*, **7**, 73–5.

Stoll, A.L., Sachs, G.S., Cohen, B.M., Lafer, B., Christensen, J.D. and Renshaw, P.F., 1996. Choline in the treatment of rapid-cycling bipolar disorder: clinical and neurochemical findings in lithium-treated patients. *Biological Psychiatry*, **40**, 382–8.

Stoll, A.L., Severus, W.E., Freeman, M.P., Rueter, S., Zboyan, H.A., Diamond, E., Cress, K.K. and Marangell, L.B., 1999. Omega3 fatty acids in bipolar disorder: a preliminary double-blind, placebo-controlled trial. *Archives of General Psychiatry*, **56**, 407–12.

Sussman, N., Ginsberg, D.L. and Bikoff, J., 2001. Effects of nefazodone on body weight: a pooled analysis of selective serotonin reuptake inhibitor- and imipramine-controlled trials. *Journal of Clinical Psychiatry*, **62**, 256–60.

Swann, A.C., Bowden, C.L., Morris, D., Calabrese, J.R., Petty, F., Small, J., Dilsaver, S.C. and Davis, J.M., 1997. Depression during mania: treatment response to lithium or divalproex. *Archives of General Psychiatry*, **54**(1), 37–42.

Swartz, H.A. and Frank, E., 2001. Psychotherapy for bipolar depression: a phase-specific treatment strategy? *Bipolar Disorders*, **3**, 11–22.

Swartz, C.M., Morrow, V., Surles, L. and James, J.F., 2001. Long-term outcome after ECT for catatonic depression. *Journal of ECT*, **17**(3), 180–3.

Tatum, W.O., Galvez, R., Benbadis, S. and Carrazana, E., 2000. New antiepileptic drugs: into the new millennium. *Archives of Family Medicine*, **9**, 1135–41.

Teitelbaum, M., 2001. Oxcarbazepine in bipolar disorder. *Journal of the American Academy of Child and Adolescent Psychiatry*, **40**, 993–94.

Terman, J.S., Terman, M., Lo, E.-S. and Copper, T., 2001. Circadian time of morning light administration and therapeutic response in winter depression. *Archives of General Psychiatry*, **58**(1), 69–75.

Terman, M. and Terman, J.S., 1995. Treatment of seasonal affective disorder with a high-output negative ionizer. *Journal of Alternative and Complementary Medicine*, **1**(1), 87–92.

Thakore, J.H. and Dinan, T.G., 1995. Cortisol synthesis inhibition: a new treatment strategy for the clinical and endocrine manifestations of depression. *Biological Psychiatry*, **37**(6), 364–8.

Thase, M.E., 1997. Do we really need all these new antidepressants? Weighing the options. *Journal of Practical Psychiatry and Behavioral Health*, **3**(1), 3–17.

Thase, M.E. and Kupfer, D.J., 1996. Recent developments in pharmacotherapy of mood disorders. *Journal of Consulting and Clinical Psychology*, **64**, 646–59.

Thase, M.E. and Rush, A.J., 1995. Treatment-resistant depression. In: Bloom, F.E. and Kupfer, D.J. (eds), *Psychopharmacology: The Fourth Generation of Progress*, pp. 1081–97. Raven Press, New York.

Thase, M.E. and Sachs, G.S., 2000. Bipolar depression: pharmacotherapy and related therapeutic strategies. *Biological Psychiatry*, **48**, 558–72.

Thase, M.E., Trivedi, M.H. and Rush, A.J., 1995. MAOIs in the contemporary treatment of depression. *Neuropsychopharmacology*, **12**, 185–219.

Thase, M.E., Greenhouse, J.B., Frank, E., Reynolds, C.F., Pilkonis, P.A., Hurley, K., Grochocinski, V. and Kupfer, D.J., 1997. Treatment of major depression with psychotherapy or psychotherapy–pharmacotherapy combinations. *Archives of General Psychiatry*, **54**, 1009–15.

Thase, M.E., Howland, R.H. and Friedman, E.S., 1998. Treating antidepressant nonresponders with augmentation strategies: an overview. *Journal of Clinical Psychiatry*, **59**(suppl 5), 5–15.

Thase, M.E., Frank, E., Kornstein, S.G. and Yonkers, K.A., 2000a. Gender differences in response to treatments of depression. In: Frank, E. (ed.), *Gender and its Effects on Psychopathology*, pp. 103–29. American Psychiatric Press, Washington, DC.

Thase, M.E., Friedman, E.S. and Howland, R.H., 2000b. Venlafaxine and treatment-resistant depression. *Depression and Anxiety*, **12**(suppl 1), 55–62.

Thase, M.E., Entsuah, A.R. and Rudolph, R.L., 2001a. Remission rates during treatment with venlafaxine or selective serotonin reuptake inhibitors. *British Journal of Psychiatry*, **178**, 234–41.

Thase, M.E., Friedman, E.S. and Howland, R.H., 2001b. Management of treatment-resistant depression: psychotherapeutic perspectives. *Journal of Clinical Psychiatry*, **62**(suppl 18), 18–24.

Thase, M.E., Howland, R.H. and Friedman, E.S., 2001c. Onset of action of selective and multi-action antidepressants. In: den Boer, J.A. and Westenberg, H.G.M. (eds), *Antidepressants: Selectivity or Multiplicity*, pp. 101–16. Benecke, Amsterdam.

Tohen, M., Anger, T.M., McElroy, S.L., Tollefson, G.D., Chengappa, K.N.R., Daniel, D.G., Petty, F., Centorrino, F., Wang, R., Grundy, S.L., Greaney, M.G., Jacobs, T.G., David, S.R. and Toma, V., 1999. Olanzapine versus placebo in the treatment of acute mania. *American Journal of Psychiatry*, **156**, 702–9.

Tohen, M., Jacobs, T.G., Grundy, S.L., McElroy, S.L., Banov, M.C., Janicak, P.G., Sanger, T., Risser, R., Zhang, F., Toma, V., Francis, J., Tollefson, G.D. and Breier, A., 2000. Efficacy of olanzapine in acute bipolar mania: a double-blind, placebo-controlled study. *Archives of General Psychiatry*, **57**, 841–9.

Tondo, L. and Baldessarini, R.J., 2000. Reduced suicide risk during lithium maintenance treatment. *Journal of Clinical Psychiatry*, **61**, 97–104.

Ulett, G.A., Han, S. and Han, J.-S., 1998. Electroacupuncture: mechanisms and clinical application. *Biological Psychiatry*, **44**, 129–8.

Vaidya, V.A. and Duman, R.S., 2001. Depression: emerging insights from neurobiology. *British Medical Bulletin*, **57**, 61–79.

Versiani, M., Amin, M. and Chouinard, G., 2000. Double-blind, placebo-controlled study with reboxetine in inpatients with severe major depressive disorder. *Journal of Clinical Psychopharmacology*, **20**(1), 28–34.

Vieta, E., Reinares, M., Corbella, B., Benabarre, A., Gilaberte, I., Colom, F., Martinez-Aran, A., Gasto, C. and Tohen, M., 2001. Olanzapine as long-term adjunctive therapy in treatment-resistant bipolar disorder. *Journal of Clinical Psychopharmacology*, **21**, 469–73.

Watson, S. and Young, A.H., 2001. The place of lithium salts in psychiatric practice 50 years on. *Current Opinion in Psychiatry*, **14**, 57–63.

Weissman, M.M. and Markowitz, J.C., 1994. Interpersonal psychotherapy: current status. *Archives of General Psychiatry*, **51**, 599–606.

Wells, R.A. and Giannetti, V.J., 1990. *Handbook of the Brief Psychotherapies*. Plenum Press, New York.

Wetterberg, L., 1998. Melatonin in adult depression. In: Shafii, M. (ed.), *Progress in Psychiatry: Melatonin in Psychiatric and Neoplastic Disorders*, pp. 43–79. American Psychiatric Press, Washington DC.

Wheeler Vega, J.A., Mortimer, A.M. and Tyson, P.J., 2000. Somatic treatment of psychotic depression: review and recommendations for practice. *Journal of Clinical Psychopharmacology*, **20**, 504–19.

Wirz-Justice, A., 1995. Biological rhythms in mood disorders. In: Bloom, F.E. and Kupfer, D.J. (eds), *Psychopharmacology: The Fourth Generation of Progress*, pp. 999–1017. Raven Press, New York.

Wolkowitz, O.M., Reus, V.I., Chan, T., Manfredi, F., Raum, W., Johnson, R. and Canick, J., 1999. Antiglucocorticoid treatment of depression: double-blind ketoconazole. *Biological Psychiatry*, **45**(8), 1070–4.

Wu, J., Buchsbaum, M.S., Gillin, J.C., Tang, C., Cadwell, S., Wiegand, M., Najafi, A., Klein, E., Hazen, K. and Bunney, W.E., 1999. Prediction of antidepressant effects of sleep deprivation by metabolic rates in the ventral anterior cingulate and medial prefrontal cortex. *American Journal of Psychiatry*, **156**(8), 1149–58.

Young, L.T., Joffe, R.T., Robb, J.C., MacQueen, G.M., Marriott, M. and Patelis-Siotis, I., 2000. Double-blind comparison of addition of a second mood stabilizer versus an antidepressant to an initial mood stabilizer for treatment of patients with bipolar depression. *American Journal of Psychiatry*, **157**, 124–6.

Zajecka, J., 2001. Strategies for the treatment of antidepressant-related sexual dysfunction. *Journal of Clinical Psychiatry*, **62**(suppl 3), 35–43.

Zarate, C.A., Rothschild, A., Fletcher, K.E., Madrid, A. and Zapatel, J., 2000. Clinical predictors of acute response with quetiapine in psychotic mood disorders. *Journal of Clinical Psychiatry*, **61**, 185–9.

Zornberg, G.L. and Pope, H.G., 1993. Treatment of depression in bipolar disorder: new directions for research. *Journal of Clinical Psychopharmacology*, **13**, 397–408.

XIX

Anxiety Disorders

XIX-1

Animal Models of Anxiety Disorders

Frederico G. Graeff and Hélio Zangrossi Jr

INTRODUCTION

The last decades have witnessed a growing interest in the use and development of animal models in psychiatry. The demand for these models has been motivated by the ethical, methodological and economical constraints that restrain the study of neurobiological processes in human subjects. It is undeniable that animal experimentation has contributed to advances in psychopharmacology and to our understanding of brain mechanisms involved in psychiatric disorders. Suffice to remember that benzodiazepine anxiolytics have been discovered because of the taming effect of chlordiazepoxide observed in *Cynomolgus* monkeys by Randall (Randall *et al.*, 1960). Also, hypotheses on the role of serotonin (5-HT) in anxiety were based on experimental work with conflict tests in rats and pigeons (Robichaud and Sledge, 1969; Graeff and Schoenfeld, 1970; Stein, Wise and Berger, 1973) as well as with aversive electrical stimulation of the rat dorsal periaqueductal grey matter (DPAG) (Kiser and Lebovitz, 1975; Schenberg and Graeff, 1978, Schütz, de Aguiar and Graeff, 1985).

Early animal models of anxiety were developed when behaviourism was the main conceptual framework within experimental psychology, and before classifications of psychiatric disorders split pathological anxiety into distinct nosological entities (see later). These animal models of anxiety rely on either inhibition of ongoing behaviour elicited by conditioned stimuli that predicted unavoidable electric shock or on suppression of rewarded responding by electric-shock punishment. The first type of model is based on principles of associative or Pavlovian conditioning, and the second on instrumental or operant conditioning. Punishment tests also suggest clinically derived constructs that emphasize the role of inner conflict in pathological anxiety, and this may be the reason why these tests became known as conflict models. Early pharmacological analysis showed conflict models to have a higher predictive value than conditioned suppression and, as a result, punishment tests became paradigmatic for assaying anti-anxiety drugs (Kelleher and Morse, 1968).

Surprisingly, classical conflict tests failed to consistently detect the anxiolytic action of drugs that act primarily on the neurotransmission mediated by serotonin (5-HT), such as buspirone and ritanserin (Handley *et al.*, 1993; Griebel, 1995). Such false-negative results undermined the general confidence in conflict models, although many arguments may be summoned to their defence, as for instance the time course of drug action. Unlike benzodiazepine anxiolytics, the newer drugs need several weeks of continuous administration to become clinically effective, initial doses being sometimes anxiogenic (Nutt, 1991). Why, then, should one expect single administration of these agents to be anxiolytic in animal models? In spite of this, it became generally accepted that conflict tests were good only for anxiolytics that acted primarily on the neurotransmission mediated by γ-aminobutyric acid (GABA), which is the case for barbiturates and benzodiazepines.

A theoretical shift from behaviourism to ethology has also contributed to the discredit of conflict models, which have been criticized because of their artificiality and the confounding influence of appetitive drives, such as hunger and thirst, and of pain (Treit, 1985). As a result, a search for ethologically based animal models of anxiety has begun. The most widely used animal model of anxiety resulting from this trend has been the elevated 'X' or 'plus' maze, which is based on the natural fear that rats have for elevated, open spaces, represented by the two open arms of the apparatus (Handley and Mithani, 1984; Pelow and File, 1986). Countless drugs have been assayed in this model, and the results obtained summarized in several comprehensive reviews (e.g., Handley *et al.*, 1993; Rodgers, 1994; Griebel, 1995). Disappointingly, this model also failed to detect non-benzodiazepine anxiolytics. To do this, ethological analysis of behavioural items shown by the animals while exploring the elevated plus-maze has been added to the procedure (Cruz, Frei and Graeff, 1994; Rodgers and Johnson, 1995). However, with this modification one of the main advantages of the test, which is simplicity, is lost.

As these developments were taking place in basic research, the split of anxiety disorders into distinct diagnostic categories, a trend that was initiated by the DSM III classification of psychiatric disorders (American Psychiatric Association, 1980), became accepted worldwide. Even though present-day psychiatric classifications cluster symptoms empirically, they constitute a necessary starting point for systematic research. It is hoped that the evidence thus obtained will either validate or modify the original categories.

The following categories from the DSM IV classification of psychiatric disorders (American Psychiatric Association, 1994) will be considered in the present analysis. (1) Generalized anxiety disorder (GAD), a state of excessive anxiety or apprehension lasting for more than six months. Neurovegetative symptoms are often present, but relatively minor. (2) Panic disorder (PD), characterized by recurrent panic attacks, either unexpected or associated with particular situations. Panic attacks are sudden surges of intense fear or terror, desire of fleeing and feeling of imminent death, going crazy or loosing control. These subjective symptoms are accompanied by major neurovegetative changes, such as palpitation, hypertension, dyspnoea, difficulty in deep breathing, sweating, urge to void the bladder and increased peristalsis. This leads to worry about the next attack or anticipatory anxiety, and avoidance of places where a panic attack would be embarrassing. Ultimately, generalized avoidance or agoraphobia may ensue. Nevertheless, agoraphobia sometimes occurs without panic attacks. (3) Obsessive–compulsive disorder (OCD) characterized by intrusive, distressing thoughts (obsessions) and/or stereotyped or ritualized behaviour (compulsions) that must be performed in order to alleviate intense anxiety. (4) Specific phobias, which are irrational fears of either objects (animals, blood, pointed instruments) or situations (heights, closed environments). (5) Social

Biological Psychiatry: Edited by H. D'haenen, J.A. den Boer and P. Willner. ISBN 0-471-49198-5

phobia, or marked anxiety experienced in social situations, such as speaking in public or going to parties or class rooms.

Given this background, it is no longer acceptable to look for animal models of anxiety, in general. Instead, models that represent specific anxiety disorders are due. Animal models of psychopathology have been evaluated according to criteria of predictability of drug response, analogy or face validity, and homology or theoretical construct validity (Treit, 1985; Willner, 1991). As Willner (1991) pointed out, 'Earlier attempts to develop criteria for validating animal models of human behaviour have tended to be concentrated largely on the assessment of face validity. The identification of two further categories reflects two ways in which the literature has developed in recent years. First, there has been a considerable expansion in the literature dealing with the pharmacological exploitation of animal models, much of which contributes to the assessment of predictive validity. Second, there has been significant growth in our understanding of the psychological mechanisms underlying psychopathological states, and examination of construct validity provides a convenient way of bringing animal models into contact with this very relevant literature'.

Indeed, the predictive criterion alone may be insufficient to characterize a test as an animal model of anxiety, since correlation between drug response in the model and in the clinics may happen, despite differences in brain mechanisms of pathophysiology and drug effect (e.g., drug-induced catalepsy and schizophrenia). The analogy criterion in itself may also be misleading, since in different species similar behaviours often serve different adaptive functions and, conversely, distinct behaviours may lead to the same goal. For instance, rat probe-burying behaviour is attenuated by anxiolytics (Treit, 1985), although it does not resemble any symptom of GAD. However, this behaviour is one of the defensive strategies of the rat's repertoire, and thus may be theoretically related to anxiety (see later).

It may be concluded that only homology qualifies animal models as representative of psychopathologies. Yet this conclusion does not look very promising, considering the (purposefully) non-theoretical stance of present-day psychiatric classifications and the scant knowledge available on how psychiatric symptoms are generated and on the neural events that underlie different animal models of anxiety. Nevertheless, we have to face the challenge or, otherwise, are bound to create theoretically shallow animal models, which are likely to generate more noise than information.

In order to assess homology, theories that encompass both pathophysiology and animal behaviour indexes have to be constructed. In this regard, evolutionary psychology and psychiatry provide a sound theoretical framework (see, e.g., McGuire and Troisi, 1998). Charles Darwin himself laid the ground for this line of thought in his book *The Expression of Emotions in Man and Animals* (Darwin, 1872) by advocating that behavioural, no less than physical, characteristics would be acquired as a result of selective pressure exerted by biological evolution. This view justifies the use of animals belonging to the phylogenetic line that resulted in humans to study the neurobiology of psychological phenomena, to the extent that brain properties be conserved along evolution. Since several environmental constraints are similar across species, or even genera and families, many adaptations are species-general, among which stand the basic emotions. Although emotional expression varies from one species to another, functional behavioural classes, such as escape and avoidance from danger or approach sources of food, remain the same and constitute the basis for the classification of basic emotions (Nesse, 1990). No wonder that the neural substrate of such emotions is conserved along biological evolution. On this basis, Panksepp proposed that basic emotions, such as rage, fear, panic and expectancy, are represented by inborn neural networks that co-ordinate behavioural strategies allowing animals to deal with enduring environmental (including social) challenges (Panksepp, 1982).

Fear and anxiety are emotional states with high adaptive value, rooted as they are in defensive reactions displayed in situations of threat to the physical integrity or survival of the organism. The sources of danger are manifold, including predators, environmental stimuli or situations, such as height, illumination, painful stimuli, novel places or objects, and confrontation or competition with animals from the same species. To deal with these challenges, animals generally use one of four basic defensive strategies, namely escape, immobilization, defensive attack and submission (Adams, 1979; Marks, 1987; Blanchard and Blanchard, 1988). The decision to choose one particular strategy takes into account several factors, such as the characteristics of the environment, distance from the threatening stimulus and previous experience with the stimulus and/or environment. Thus, in a highly discernible situation of threat, as in the confrontation with an approaching predator, the animal will preferentially escape, if an exit route is available. In turn, the animal will become tensely immobile (freezing) if the predator is not in close proximity and/or escape is impossible. In this case, being motionless decreases the probability of detection or attack by the predator. On the other hand, in a situation of close proximity or contact with the predator, vigorous flight or defensive threat and attack toward the predator may be more efficient in deflecting predatory action. Alternatively, certain species, including birds, fishes and some mammals, may display a state of tonic immobility, feigning death, by means of which the animals may decrease the predator's interest (Marks, 1987). Finally, submission postures are often observed in confrontation with conspecifics. By acting submissively, the individual may inhibit the attack by a socially dominant animal. However, submissive responses hardly ever inhibit predatory attack (Adams, 1979).

The evolutionary approach views anxiety disorders as pathologies of defence (Panksepp, 1982; Marks, 1987; Marks and Nesse, 1994; Graeff, 1994; Hofer, 1995; Stein and Bouwer, 1997; Gray and McNaughton, 2000; Blanchard *et al.*, 2001). For instance, specific phobias, GAD and PD may be related to predatory aggression. In this regard, the work carried out by Robert and Caroline Blanchard on predatory defence in rats and mice (Blanchard and Blanchard, 1988; Blanchard, Griebel and Blanchard, 1997) classified the behavioural strategies displayed according to the level of threat, namely potential or uncertain, distal and proximal. The first level evokes cautious exploration and hesitant behaviour aimed at risk assessment. The second induces either directed escape or immobility. Finally, when the predator is very close or in contact with the prey, either vigorous flight or defensive aggression occurs. To this ethoexperimental analysis, Gray and McNaughton (2000) have added elements of learning theory, including conditioned stimuli that signal either punishment or loss of an expected reward (frustration) as elicitors of anxiety (first level of defence). The same authors have also highlighted the importance of approach-avoidance conflict and of the direction of response to distinguish anxiety from fear. Thus, anxiety exists only when there is a tendency to approach the source of danger. When only the escape or avoidance component exists there is fear. Indeed, pharmacological data show that active avoidance and escape responses are remarkably resistant to anxiolytic drugs, in contrast to risk-assessment and punished suppressed responding (Gray and McNaughton, 2000).

In a synthesis of experimental evidence from several research fields, the above levels of defence have been related to different emotions and to distinct anxiety disorders (Graeff, 1994; Gray and McNaughton, 2000). Table XIX-1.1 summarizes this view, which provides the theoretical framework presently used to qualify an animal model as representative of GAD, PD and specific phobias, respectively.

Following the same evolutionary approach, social phobia has been related to submissive displays that are expressed by subordinates in social interaction with dominant animals of the same

Table XIX-1.1 Levels of defence, main neural substrate, related emotion and anxiety disorder, and their drug sensitivity

Danger	Defence reaction	Critical brain structures	Emotion	Disorder	Drug sensitivity
Potential (Conflict)	Risk-assessment/behavioural inhibition	Septo-hippocampal system/amygdala	Anxiety	GAD	Anxiolytics Antidepressants
Anticipated (CS)	Freezing	Amygdala VPAG	Anticipatory anxiety		
	Avoidance	Amygdala	Conditioned fear	Specific phobias	None
Distal (US)	Escape	Medial hypothalamus	Unconditioned fear	Specific phobias	None
Proximal (US)	Flight/freezing	DPAG	Panic	PD	Antidepressants

Key: CS, conditioned stimulus; US, unconditioned stimulus; VAPG, ventral periaqueductal grey; DPAG, dorsal periaqueductal grey; GAD, generalized anxiety disorder; PD, panic disorder (Modified from Graeff, 1994 and Gray and McNaughton, 2000).

species (Stein and Bouwer, 1997). Nevertheless, to our knowledge this hypothesis has not been explored to generate animal models of this disorder.

Finally, the most frequent compulsive behaviours found in OCD, washing and checking, have been related to self-grooming and territorial checking routines that many animal species perform to protect themselves against micro-organisms and intruders, respectively (Rapoport, 1991).

The subsequent sections will focus on pharmacological evidence that is relevant to the validation of selected models of each psychiatric disorder. Because the aim of this article is to relate animal models and psychiatric disorders, only drugs that have been evaluated in clinical assays will be considered. Whenever pertinent, there will be mention of evidence from studies using direct intervention on the brain.

MODELS OF GENERALIZED ANXIETY DISORDER

As pointed out earlier, the ethoexperimental analysis of defence strategies against predatory attack made by the Blanchards (Blanchard and Blanchard, 1988; Blanchard *et al.*, 1997) led them to relate GAD to behaviours that occur in response to potential threat, chiefly the so-called risk-assessment behaviour. Gray and McNaughton (2000) also view 'behaviours that occur in the context of potential threat as paradigmatic of anxiety'. But they suggest that 'the critical feature for such behaviours was the approach-avoidance conflict inherent in the "potential threat" situation rather than the potentiality of threat as such'. They also broadened the notion of potentially threatening stimuli to include 'novelty stimuli of certain kinds, signals of punishment, and signals of reward omission, in addition to the paradigmatic innate anxiety stimuli'. Gray and MacNaughton (2000) have further suggested that anxiety has a cognitive component — approach-avoidance conflict — managed by the septo-hippocampal system, and an affective component — aversion — accomplished by the uppermost structure of the brain defence ('fight/flight/freezing') system, the amygdala.

It follows that conflict tests would rank first in homology regarding GAD, since they would engage both the septo-hippocampal system and the amygdala (Gray and MacNaughton, 2000). Because of the shortcomings analysed in the introduction of this paper, classical conflict tests are seldom used for assessing anxiolytic drug action. However, a modification of the latter, inhibitory avoidance in the elevated T-maze (Graeff, Viana and Tomaz, 1993), eliminates most of the objections raised against punishment models, since animals are not deprived, and aversion for an open, elevated arm of the maze replaces electric foot-shock. Also, the light-dark transition model (Crawley and Goodwin, 1980), in which rats or mice are placed inside an experimental chamber divided into two compartments, one bright and another dark, may be viewed as a conflict test: the naïve animal tends to explore both compartments of the box, but the entrance to one of them is punished by exposure to bright light.

Also at the first level of homology are models that involve risk-assessment behaviour determined by potential threat from innate fear stimuli, such as in the anxiety/defence test battery (Blanchard and coworkers, 1993, 2001) and a component of the mouse defence test battery (Griebel, Blanchard and Blanchard, 1996a).

In anxiety models such as conditioned suppression (Estes and Skinner, 1941) and fear-potentiated startle (Davis, 1986) an exteroceptive stimulus predicts unavoidable foot-shock, causing, respectively, suppression of rewarded responding and increased amplitude of the acoustic startle response. Therefore, there is no approach-avoidance conflict and according to Gray and McNaughton (2000) the septo-hippocampal system is not involved. Therefore, the behavioural inhibition seen in these situations would rely entirely on the amygdala. Indeed both the amygdala and the ventral periaqueductal grey (VPAG) have been shown to be critical for the expression of conditioned freezing (Davis, 1992; Fanselow, 1991). Since these tests activate the affective, but not the cognitive component of anxiety (Gray and McNaughton, 2000), they only partially fulfil the theoretical requirements for a model of GAD. It is more likely that these models represent anticipatory anxiety, which like GAD is also sensitive to anxiolytic drugs (Table XIX-1.1). A remark about fear-potentiated startle is in order. Although the anxiety index is the enhancement of the startle response, this is directly proportional to the degree of freezing produced by the conditioned aversive stimulus (Leaton and Borszcz, 1985). Therefore, fear-potentiated startle may be viewed as behavioural inhibition in disguise.

There are also anxiety models that involve defensive aggression — usually threat — provoked by an approaching danger stimulus. A typical example is the primate defensive reaction evoked by the experimenter's gloved hand. Despite the historical importance of this model — in particular the discovery of the anxiolytic action of chlordiazepoxide (Randall *et al.*, 1960) — they are little used today, due to its high cost and low feasibility. Nevertheless, a rodent model that measures defensive behaviour against a conditioned aversive stimulus, the shock-probe-burying test (Pinel and Treit, 1978) deserves attention.

Social interaction in young rats has a pharmacological profile suggestive of GAD (File, 1995). Nevertheless, it seems to involve many variables, and the theoretical construct underlying the test has not been fully clarified. Therefore, this model will not be addressed here.

In the following subsections, the main models of GAD are discussed in detail. The mouse defence test battery and the elevated T-maze will be analysed in a separate section, because these tests are intended to model PD, in addition to GAD.

The Anxiety/Defence Test Battery

The anxiety/defence test battery (A/DTB) was developed in order to measure drug effects on risk-assessment behaviours (Blanchard and coworkers, 1993, 2001). In this model, measures of risk-assessment and inhibition of non-defensive behaviour are evaluated in rats submitted to three situations representing potential threat associated with a predator. In the first situation, the 'proxemics/activity test', the rat's location in the test chamber is measured after non-contact exposure to a cat. It has been shown that after a 5-minute encounter with the predator, rats avoid locations near the cat compartment. In the second condition, the 'eat/drinking test', the frequency and duration of two non-defensive behaviours, feeding and drinking, are measured during and after a 5-minute non-contact exposure to a cat. In the presence of the predator these behaviours are inhibited, being gradually resumed over time. Finally, in the 'cat odour test', the frequency and duration of risk assessment expressed towards an object saturated with cat odour are measured. The indexes used are flat-back approach and stretch-attend posture, as well as the frequency and time spent by rats in direct contact with the cat odour source (for further details on these tests see Blanchard and coworkers, 1990, 1993).

The effects of different classes of anxiolytics in the A/DTB are reviewed elsewhere (Blanchard and coworkers, 1993, 1997, 1998). Overall, benzodiazepines and buspirone-like drugs decrease avoidance from the area close to the cat compartment and counteract inhibition of feeding and/or drinking after cat exposure. These drugs interfere with the expression of risk-assessment behaviours in a bi-directional way. They increase risk assessment when the baseline expression of these behaviours in the control group is low or absent, due to enhanced freezing behaviour. However, they decrease risk assessment in less aversive situations, in which a considerable level of risk assessment is already being expressed by the animals. In both cases the drugs decrease reactivity to the threatening situation, thus moving the animal to a level of defensiveness where approach to the aversive stimulus is more likely to occur. The non-selective 5-HT_2 antagonist ritanserin failed to show the same anxiolytic profile. Chronic administration of the tricyclic antidepressant imipramine caused anxiolytic effects similar to that of diazepam and chlordiazepoxide, but the panicolytic benzodiazepine alprazolam, administered acutely, had no effect. The full pharmacological validation of this test awaits further analysis since neither the effect of anxiogenic drugs nor the selectivity of the model have been explored.

The Light/Dark Transition Model

The light/dark transition model was elaborated by Crawley and Goodwin (Crawley and Goodwin, 1980; Crawley, 1985), based on the exploratory behaviour of mice in a two-compartment box, where one chamber is brightly lit and the other dark. In such conditions, mice and rats have a clear preference for the dark side of the box and the number of transitions made by them between the two compartments and the time spent in the bright side have been used as indices of anxiety. Over the years several procedural modifications have been introduced in order to improve the feasibility of the test or its pharmacological predictability. These modifications include, among others, the introduction of a connecting tunnel between the two compartments (De Angelis, 1992), changes in the dimensions or spatial disposition of the compartments (Imaizumi, Miyazaki and Onodera, 1994; Shimada *et al.*, 1995), use of fully automated data collection (Onaivi and Martin, 1989; Young and Johnson, 1991b; Hascoët and Bourin, 1998) and analyses of additional behavioural indices of anxiety and locomotor activity (Chaouloff, Durand and Mormede, 1997; Smythe *et al.*, 1998; Hascoët and Bourin, 1998).

When interpreting the pharmacological results so far obtained with the light/dark transition model, one should keep in mind that what poses as a simple procedural modification may change the way animals respond to the aversive challenge. As discussed before, the type of defensive response determines the effect of anxiety-modulating drugs in the test. For instance, increasing the illumination of the bright compartment may decrease the amount of risk assessment made by the animal in the transition area between the two compartments of the apparatus. Although this alteration may not necessarily lead to changes in the absolute amount of time spent in the two compartments, it may interfere with the expression of an important set of GAD-related behaviours. Moreover, when comparing results of different studies it is important to notice that in this test, as in other anxiety models, uneven levels of basal anxiety are expressed by different strains of animals (Crawley and Davis, 1982; Hascoët and Bourin, 1998; Griebel *et al.*, 2000). Baseline anxiety also changes along the animal's life span (Hascoët, Colombel and Bourin, 1999). Discrepancies among studies on these and others parameters may be responsible for many of the reported conflicting drug effects found in the literature.

Despite the above caveats, drug results with anti-anxiety agents are remarkably consistent, using either the original protocol or modified versions of the test. Thus, reported results show that acute injection of benzodiazepines (e.g., diazepam, chlordiazepoxide and alprazolam) or buspirone-like drugs have anxiolytic effects in both mice and rats (Crawley, 1985; Pich and Samanin, 1989; Young and Johnson, 1991a; Shimada *et al.*, 1995; Sanchez, 1996; Griebel, Sanger and Perrault, 1996b; Hascoët and Bourin, 1998). Overall, the time spent in the bright compartment seems to be more reliable for assessing anxiety relief than the number of transitions (Hascoët and Bourin, 1998).

However, conflicting results (anxiolytic, anxiogenic or lack of effect) have been obtained with acute injection of the antidepressants imipramine (Pich and Samanin, 1989; Onaivi and Martin, 1989; Young and Johnson, 1991a; De Angelis, 1996), fluoxetine (Kshama *et al.*, 1990; De Angelis, 1996; Sanchez and Maier, 1997; Artaiz, Zazpe and Del Rio, 1998) and citalopram (Griebel *et al.*, 1994; Sanchez and Maier, 1997). Other SSRIs, such as paroxetine, sertraline and fluvoxamine, were ineffective in rats (Sanchez and Maier, 1997), but paroxetine exerted an anxiolytic effect in mice (Hascoët, Bourin and Nic Dhonnchadha, 2000). However, as none of these drugs has been evaluated after chronic administration, the pharmacological profile of the test is incomplete.

Some drugs known to increase anxiety in man and in rodents, such as mCPP and pentylenetetrazol (PTZ), also have an anxiogenic effect in the light/dark transition model (Onaivi and Martin, 1989; Griebel *et al.*, 1991; Bilkei-Gorzo, Gyertyan and Levay, 1998). However, other anxiogenic drugs, such as yohimbine and FG-7142, have shown either an anxiogenic or no effect in the test (Pich and Samanin, 1989; Singh *et al.*, 1991; Shimada *et al.*, 1995; Hascoët and Bourin, 1998; Bilkei-Gorzo, Gyertyan and Levay, 1998).

The selectivity of the light/dark transition model for anxiety-modulating drugs has been supported by findings that the neuroleptics, chlorpromazine, piperone, haloperidol and clozapine (Young and Johnson, 1991a; Costall and Naylor, 1995; Bilkei-Gorzo, Gyertyan and Levay, 1998) as well as the psychostimulant amphetamine (Young and Johnson, 1991a; Bilkei-Gorzo, Gyertyan and Levay, 1998) did not alter the classical anxiety indices. However, in the case of amphetamine and of another psychostimulant drug caffeine, evidences of anxiogenic effects are also reported (Onaivi and Martin, 1989; Imaizumi, Miyazaki and Onodera, 1994; Hascoët and Bourin, 1998).

Fear-Potentiated Startle

The fear-potentiated startle paradigm has been successfully used for studying the neurobiological basis of fear/anxiety conditioning, mostly by Davis and coworkers (Davis, 1986; Davis *et al.*, 1993; Walker *et al.*, 1997). This model, first described by Brown, Kalish and Faber (1951), is based on principles of Pavlovian classical conditioning and its performance involves two distinctive steps. Initially, the animals are trained to associate a neutral stimulus (the to-be-conditioned stimulus), generally a light, with an aversive stimulus such as an electric foot-shock. After training, the animals are submitted to an intense sound and the amplitude of their startle reflex to this unconditioned aversive stimulus is measured, either in the presence or in the absence of the conditioned stimulus (light). It has been shown that the amplitude of the acoustic startle reflex is higher when the eliciting acoustic stimulus occurs in the presence of the light. This potentiation of the startle response can be found even one month after the training session. Further evidence shows that maximum potentiated startle in the test session is achieved at the time after light onset which was followed by foot-shock presentation in training, that is, when shock is most expected. These results strengthen the view of fear-potentiated startle as a model of anticipatory anxiety (Davis *et al.*, 1993). Considering the above definition of fear, given by Gray and McNaughton (2000), a more appropriate denomination for this test would be 'conditioned anxiety-potentiated startle'. However, for sake of clarity the original name is preserved.

The effects of different classes of psychoactive drugs in rats submitted to the fear-potentiated startle are reviewed by Davis *et al.* (1993) and Hijzen *et al.* (1995).

A selective anxiolytic effect in this test is characterized by attenuation of fear-potentiated startle with no change in the baseline level of startle, that is, the startle response obtained in the absence of the conditioned stimulus. Decreases in both measures may indicate non-specific impairment of motor control. Overall, benzodiazepines, including alprazolam, as well as buspirone-like drugs decrease fear-potentiated startle, often without any change in baseline startle. However, it is interesting to notice that in some cases buspirone and ipsapirone, a similar 5-HT_{1A} agonist, *increase* baseline startle response, in addition to decreasing potentiated startle (Kehne, Cassella and Davis, 1988). These results suggest that these drugs may have differential effects on conditioned and unconditioned responses. In fact, the mechanisms by which 5-HT_{1A} drugs exert their effects seem to be complex, as attested by evidence showing that 5-HT_{1A} antagonists also have anxiolytic effects in this test (Joordens, Hijzen and Olivier, 1998).

As observed with acute injection of the antidepressants amitriptyline (Hijzen *et al.*, 1995) and fluvoxamine (Joordens *et al.*, 1996), administration of imipramine either acutely or chronically (3 weeks) did not affect either fear-potentiated or baseline startle. The lack of imipramine effect has led to the view that this test dissociates anticipatory anxiety from panic (Davis *et al.*, 1993). However, the effects of SSRIs, such as fluoxetine and citalopram, in the test are still unknown.

As expected, the anxiogenic drug yohimbine enhanced potentiated startle, but mCPP had no such effect. The selectivity of the test for anxiety-modulating drugs has been obscured by false positive results obtained with haloperidol (Hijzen *et al.*, 1995) and with the α_2-adrenergic agonist clonidine (Davis *et al.*, 1993). As in the light/dark transition model, amphetamine has been shown to be either anxiogenic (Borowski and Kokkinidis, 1998) or without effect (Hijzen *et al.*, 1995).

Defensive Burying

The conditioned defensive burying test was originally developed by Pinel and Treit (1978, 1979) and explores rodent's species-typical behaviour of burying objects that represent or are associated with aversive stimulation. In the original description of the test, the authors reported that rats shocked once by a probe mounted on the wall of the test box returned to the probe and buried it with bedding material from the floor of the box. They also showed that this behaviour was still observed even when the shock had been delivered 20 days before testing, supporting the role of aversive learning in this paradigm (for further details on the behavioural validation of this test see Treit (1985)). Later on, it was observed that anxiolytic drugs, like diazepam, chlordiazepoxide and pentobarbital, decreased the time spent by animals spraying and pushing bedding material towards the shock source in a way comparable to their relative potencies in clinical settings (Treit, Pinel and Fibiger, 1981). Other psychoactive drugs as picrotoxin, PTZ, d-amphetamine and morphine, injected in a single dose, were ineffective.

However, with the growing use of the test in other laboratories, conflicting results emerged (see Craft, Howard and Pollard, 1988). Soon it became clear that procedural changes, such as intensity and number of shocks delivered (Treit and Fundytus, 1988; Tsuda, Ida and Tanaka, 1988; Treit, 1990), previous habituation to the test box (Treit and Fundytus, 1988) as well as the animal's strain (Pare, 1992) and age (Lopes-Rubalcava, Fernandez-Guasti and Urba-Holmgren, 1996), may influence drug effects. Furthermore, by measuring only the time spent by rats burying the probe it was not possible to clearly separate the anxiolytic effect of the drug from its non-specific effects on general motor activity, due to sedation and/or ataxia. The latter problem still remains as one of the main drawbacks of the model. Nevertheless, the introduction of other indices of anxiety, such as the latency to initiate the defensive burying (Beardsley *et al.*, 1990) and the frequency of contact with a constant electrified probe (Treit and Fundytus, 1988), offered some gains in predictability of drug response. Yet the use of concurrent behavioural tasks for checking animals general activity, such as the rotarod or the arena, has been adopted to discriminate confounding drug effects (Sakamoto *et al.*, 1998; Fernandez-Guasti and Lopez-Rubalcava, 1998).

The conditioned defensive burying test consistently detects acute anxiolytic effects of benzodiazepines and buspirone-like drugs in both rats and mice (Treit, 1990; Fernandez-Guasti, Hong and Lopez-Rubalcava, 1992). Chronic treatment with the antidepressants imipramine, pargyline and desipramine had no effect on rats' burying behaviour (Beardsley *et al.*, 1990).

The pharmacological predictability of the test has been questioned because of failure in consistently detecting anxiogenic drug effects. Neither PTZ nor picrotoxin (Treit and coworkers, 1981, 1987, 1990) enhance burying behaviour and FG-7142, in fact, decreased its expression (Rohmer, Di Scalar and Sandner, 1990). Conflicting results have been obtained with yohimbine, since this drug is reported to be either anxiolytic (Tanaka *et al.*, 2000) or anxiogenic (Tsuda, Ida and Tanaka, 1988; Lopez-Rubalcava and Fernandez-Guasti, 1994) and even to have no effect (Treit, 1990). The selectivity of the test has also been undermined. Whereas the neuroleptic haloperidol had no effect (Sakamoto *et al.*, 1998), as would be expected, other agents ineffective on GAD, such as chlorpromazine (Treit, Pinel and Fibiger, 1981), clonidine and prazosin (Lopez-Rubalcava and Fernandez-Guasti, 1994) behaved as anxiolytics in the animal test (however, in the case of chlorpromazine, lack of effect on anxiety indices was observed with a modified conditioning protocol (Treit, 1990)).

MODELS OF PANIC DISORDER

The available models of panic disorder (PD) are based on two complementary hypotheses. The first considers panic to be related to the flight response induced by proximal threat (Blanchard and Blanchard, 1988), as discussed in the introduction to this paper. The second hypothesis suggests that panic attacks are due to activation of the medial hypothalamus and/or DPAG (Gentil, 1988; Graeff, 1988, 1991; Deakin and Graeff, 1991), which are brain structures that integrate escape and flight responses, respectively (Table XIX-1.1). The former hypothesis gave origin to the fear/defence test battery (Blanchard, Flannelly and Blanchard, 1986), the mouse defence test battery (Griebel, Blanchard and Blanchard, 1996a) and the one-way escape task in the elevated T-maze (Graeff, Viana and Tomaz, 1993). The second proposal led to animal models that use either electrical (Jenck, Moreau and Martin, 1995; Schenberg *et al.*, 2001) or chemical stimulation (Beckett *et al.*, 1992b) of the DPAG, as well as chemical stimulation of the dorso-medial hypothalamus (DMH) (Shekhar, 1994).

The experimental evidence implicating the DAPG in panic has been extensively discussed elsewhere (Graeff, 1988, 1991; Deakin and Graeff, 1991; Graeff *et al.*, 1996b). One of the main arguments in favour of this view is that electrical or chemical (by excitatory amino acids or anti-GABA agents) stimulation of the DPAG evokes abrupt and clumsy flight responses in experimental animals, reminiscent of a panic attack (Graeff, 1988, 1991). Similar results have been reported with infusion of $GABA_A$ antagonists into the DMH (Shekhar and Di Micco, 1987), although escape induced by $GABA_A$ antagonists or synthesis inhibitors injected into this brain area is more co-ordinated and well oriented toward environmental goals than that obtained in the DPAG (Schmitt *et al.*, 1986). Another argument is that electrical stimulation of the DPAG of patients undergoing neurosurgery produces neurovegetative changes and feelings of terror that are characteristic of clinical panic attacks (Nashold, Wilson and Slaughter, 1974; Amano *et al.*, 1978). Moreover, a PET study carried out by Reiman *et al.* (1989) showed that the midbrain tectum, which includes the DPAG was activated during lactate-induced panic attack.

Blanchard and colleagues (2001) have recently reviewed several of above models of PD. The following description is in large measure based on their account. We have added the version of DPAG electrical stimulation developed by Schenberg's group and the chemical stimulation of the DPAG model introduced by Marsden and coworkers. Because the mouse/defence test battery and the elevated T-maze address both to GAD and PD, they will be analysed separately.

Fear/Defence Test Battery

The fear/defence test battery measures defensive behaviours of wild rats (*Rattus rattus*), more specifically, freezing, flight, defensive sonic vocalization and defensive attack to an approaching/contacting predator, a human subject (Blanchard and coworkers, 1986, 1993). It has been shown that these responses are more evident in wild than in laboratory rats (Blanchard, Flannelly and Blanchard, 1986). Overall, benzodiazepines (diazepam, chlordiazepoxide and midazolam) and buspirone-like drugs did not affect the expression of freezing, avoidance and more importantly, flight responses, during confrontation with the predator. The lack of effect of these GAD-effective drugs on these defensive responses has supported analogies between the test and PD. These compounds do decrease defensive threat/attack reactions towards the predator (Blanchard *et al.*, 1993, 1997, 1998), but the reliability of these behaviours as indices of anxiety has been questioned (Blanchard *et al.*, 1997).

The complexity of this test, derived mainly from the use of wild animals, limits its widespread use in psychopharmacological analysis. This fact can be attested by the lack of studies on the effects in this test of panicolytic drugs such as alprazolam and antidepressants, or panicogens such as yohimbine, in animals submitted to this test.

Electrical Stimulation of the Dorsal Periaqueductal Grey

In the version of this model utilized by Jenck and coworkers, rats are trained to switch off DPAG electrical stimulation by jumping into the opposite compartment of a shuttle-box. Several drugs that affect PD were tested to assess predictive validity. As expected, the anti-panic agents alprazolam and clonazepam impaired switch-off behaviour dose-dependently, while the panicogenic agents caffeine, yohimbine and flesinoxan and CCKb agonists facilitated escape from DPAG electrical stimulation. Nevertheless, several results seem to be inconsistent with the hypothesis that DPAG stimulation models PD, such as the anti-aversive action of the panicogenic mCPP, and of single administration of the SSRIs fluvoxamine and fluoxetine. The latter drugs are known to aggravate PD in the initial phase of drug treatment (Saran and Halaris, 1989; Den Boer and Westenberg, 1990). In addition, there were false positive results, since the antipsychotic agent haloperidol and the CCK_B antagonist L365,260 had anti-aversive effects in the animal test, but do not improve PD (for primary references, see Blanchard, Griebel and Blanchard, 2001).

In the version of DPAG electrical stimulation developed by Schenberg and coworkers (Schenberg *et al.*, 1990; Sudré *et al.*, 1993), the rat is placed inside an arena and the intensity of the electrical current is gradually increased. In this way, a sequence of behavioural and neurovegetative changes is elicited, namely immobility, running, jumping, exophthalmus, micturition and defecation. Pharmacological analysis indicates that running and jumping seem to be correlated with panic. Thus, the threshold current intensity for eliciting these responses was markedly increased by chronic, but not acute, administration of the panicolytic drugs clomipramine and fluoxetine. Long-term administration of the anxiolytics diazepam and buspirone as well as of the selective NA reuptake inhibitor maprotiline was ineffective. Moreover, the panicogenic drug PTZ decreased running threshold (Schenberg *et al.*, 2001; Vargas and Schenberg, 2001). The latter study also showed that plasma levels of ACTH were not affected by DPAG electrical stimulation that induced panic-like behaviour. This finding further supports this test as a model of PD, in relation to claims that the hypothalamus–hypophysis–adrenal axis is not activated during panic attacks (Liebowitz *et al.*, 1985).

Chemical Stimulation of the Dorsal Periaqueductal Grey

In this model microinjection of the excitatory amino acid d,l-homocysteic acid (DLH) is made in both rostral and caudal DPAG, causing explosive motor behaviour characteristic of proximal defence. This behaviour is quantified in terms of response duration, arena revolutions and number of defensive jumps made by the rats inside an arena (Beckett, Marsden and Marshal, 1992a). In the automated version of the test, distance travelled is recorded with a computer-driven automated tracking system (Beckett and Marsden, 1995). As reported with electrical stimulation (Nogueira and Graeff, 1995), pre-treatment with 5-HT_{1A} agonists directly injected into the DPAG markedly attenuated the defence reaction elicited by DLH (Beckett *et al.*, 1992b; Beckett and Marsden, 1997). Conversely, systemic injection of the 5-HT_{1A} agonist 8-OH-DPAT enhanced the DLH effect (Beckett and Marsden, 1997), probably because stimulation of autosomic receptors in the dorsal raphe nucleus decreases inhibitory 5-HT input to the DPAG. Also, intra-DPAG injection of the 5-HT_2-receptor agonist mCPP intensified the defence reaction induced by DLH (Beckett, Marsden and Marshal, 1992a). Chronic (3 weeks), but not short-term (2–3 days) treatment with imipramine enhanced the 5-HT_{1A}-mediated inhibition of flight induced by intra-DPAG injection of DLH (Mongeau and Marsden, 1997a). The latter result supports the suggestion that the therapeutic effect of antidepressants on PD is due to enhancement of 5-HT inhibition of DPAG neurones commanding flight (Graeff, 1991). Finally, intracerebroventricular injection of the panicogen CCK-4 prolonged the tachycardia induced by intra-DPAG DLH, but failed to affect the flight response. The latter was potentiated by systemically injected butoxycarbonyl-CCK-4, indicating a peripheral site of action (Mongeau and Marsden, 1997b). Although only one panicolytic and one panicogenic drug have been used so far to validate this model, the above results testify to its importance for the study of the neurobiology of PD.

Chemical Stimulation of the Dorso-Medial Hypothalamus

Infusion of the $GABA_A$ receptor blockers bicuculline and picrotoxin into the DMH induces oriented escape response accompanied by hyperventilation and increases in arterial blood pressure and heart rate, reminiscent of a panic attack (Shekhar and Di Micco, 1987). The effects of bicuculline infusion have been abolished following chronic treatment with either imipramine or clonazepam (Shekhar, 1994). The same drug regimen is clinically effective on PD (Nutt, 1991). Also as expected, the panicogenic agents yohimbine and fenfluramine enhanced the behavioural and physiological effects of bicuculline in the DMH (Keim and Sekhar, 1999). However, because a comparative study has shown that escape from the hypothalamus is controlled by environmental stimuli whereas that from the DPAG is undirected (Schmitt *et al.*, 1986), the DMH model is less akin to panic attacks.

COMBINED MODELS OF GENERALIZED ANXIETY AND PANIC DISORDERS

The two animal models analysed below are intended to assess behaviours related to both GAD and PD in the same animal.

The Mouse Defence Test Battery

Based on their ethoexperimental analysis of defence (see the introduction of this paper), Blanchards' group elaborated a test battery to measure both risk assessment, related to GAD and predator-induced flight, related to PD. In the mouse defence test battery (MDTB) a mouse is placed inside an oval runway and a deeply anaesthetized rat, held by the experimenter's hand, is approached at a fixed speed. When the rat–mouse distance reaches about 1 m, the mouse generally flees, running in the alley until the threat is out of sight. This defence reaction is taken as an index related to panic (Griebel, Blanchard and Blanchard, 1996a). During the predator's approach, mice also express risk-assessment behaviour consisting of an abrupt movement arrest often followed by orientation toward the approaching rat. Risk-assessment behaviour (approach to/withdrawal from the rat) is also evidenced when the predator–prey interaction is carried out in a straight alley. These risk-assessment responses are taken as indexes related to GAD. The pharmacological profile of the MDTB evidences its high predictive validity. Thus, flight was reduced by two high-potency benzodiazepines that are clinically effective on PD, namely alprazolam and clonazepam, as well as by chronic administration of several antidepressants, including imipramine, fluoxetine, moclobemide and phenelzine. Whereas either acute or chronic alprazolam had no appreciable effect on risk-assessment responses, chronic administration of imipramine and fluoxetine decreased the expression of these behaviours. The results obtained with these two antidepressants are consonant with their anxiolytic effects on GAD symptoms (Nutt, 1991; Rickels *et al.*, 1993). In addition, panicogenic agents, such as yohimbine, flumazenil and cocaine, as well as therapeutic drugs like imipramine and fluoxetine, that nonetheless aggravate PD in the initial phase of treatment, facilitated flight in the MDTB test when injected acutely. Finally, drugs clinically ineffective on PD, such as the benzodiazepine anxiolytic chlordiazepoxide, the $5\text{-}HT_{1A}$ agonist buspirone and the $5\text{-}HT_2$ antagonist miaserin, did not affect the same flight response, but consistently reduced the GAD-related risk-assessment behaviours (for primary references, see Blanchard, Griebel and Blanchard (2001).

The Elevated T-maze

The elevated T-maze (ETM) is derived from a hypothesis about the role of 5-HT in GAD and PD. In an attempt to conciliate conflicting results on the role of 5-HT in anxiety, Deakin and Graeff (1991) have suggested that conditioned anxiety is related to GAD while unconditioned fear is associated to PD. The former would be facilitated whereas the latter would be inhibited by 5-HT released from fibres originated in the dorsal raphe nucleus (DRN). As a consequence, the ETM was intended to separate conditioned anxiety from unconditioned fear (Graeff, Viana and Tomaz, 1993; Viana, Tomaz and Graeff, 1994). The apparatus is derived from the elevated X- or plus-maze (Handley and Mithani, 1984; Pellow and File, 1986) by sealing the entrance to one of its enclosed arms. As a result, the ETM consists of three arms of equal dimension (50×12 cm) elevated 50 cm from the floor. One of these arms is enclosed by lateral walls (40 cm high) and stands perpendicular to the two opposite open arms. In the experimental session, the rat performs two consecutive tasks, inhibitory avoidance and one-way escape, supposed to represent conditioned anxiety and unconditioned fear, respectively. When placed at the end of the enclosed arm, the rat does not see the open arms until it pokes its head beyond the walls of the closed arm. Being on the open arm seems to be an aversive experience, since rats have an innate fear of height and openness (Treit, Menard and Royan, 1993). This would allow the animal to learn inhibitory avoidance if repeatedly placed inside the enclosed arm to explore the maze. On the other hand, when the rat is placed at the end of one of the open arms it can move towards the closed arm, presumably performing an escape response.

The ETM may also be viewed as a way to circumvent the ambiguities of the elevated plus-maze (see the introduction of this paper). According to Handley *et al.* (1993), the elevated plus-maze is a mixed model, leading to inconsistencies in drug response. To circumvent this shortcoming, systematic recording of behavioural items has been added. Some of these items are selectively affected by non-benzodiazepine anxiolytics, thus improving the predictive value of the test (e.g., Rodgers and Johnson, 1995). However, this strategy is time consuming and strips the elevated plus-maze of its main advantage, which is simplicity. Also, critical behavioural items, such as risk assessment may be more easily observed in contexts different from the elevated plus-maze. An alternative to ethological analysis is the separation of functional categories of behaviour through experimental analysis, which is accomplished by the ETM.

A series of experiments has been performed to validate the ETM behaviourally (Zangrossi and Graeff, 1997). The results obtained showed that restraining the animals at the end of the enclosed arm for 30 s did not change the first (baseline) withdrawal latency, indicating that rats are not escaping from the experimenter's hand. In addition, rats trained in a T-maze with the three arms enclosed did not show the usual increase in withdrawal latency along three consecutive trials. Therefore, open arm experience seems to be critical for inhibitory avoidance learning. The same experiment also showed that the latency to leave the open arm did not undergo habituation over five consecutive trials, evidencing the aversive motivation of this response.

For pharmacological validation, drugs that are known to either decrease or increase clinical anxiety have been used (Graeff *et al.*, 1998). Table XIX-1.2 summarizes the results obtained. As may be seen, the anxiolytics diazepam, buspirone, ipsapirone and ritanserin impaired inhibitory avoidance while leaving one-way escape unchanged. This selective effect on avoidance correlates with the clinical effectiveness of these drugs on GAD, as opposed to their inefficacy on PD (Nutt, 1991). It is worth mentioning that several additional drugs that had anxiolytic-like effects in other animal models of anxiety also selectively impaired avoidance in the ETM (Graeff, Ferreira Netto and Zangrossi, 1998). However, since these drugs have not been assayed in humans, clinical correlation cannot be assessed.

Also as predicted by Deakin and Graeff's hypothesis, the anxiogenic agents yohimbine, TFPP and mCPP facilitated inhibitory avoidance in the ETM. However, the two last drugs attenuated escape, a result that contrasts with clinical reports on aggravation of PD by the same drugs. It may be argued that in these clinical studies anticipatory anxiety rather than panic was enhanced, since mCPP also enhances anxiety in normal subjects (Charney *et al.*, 1987). Moreover, Deakin and Graeff (1991) have further hypothesized that the brain mechanisms that underlie anxiety and panic interact, the former exerting inhibitory influence on the latter. Thus, drugs that facilitate avoidance could indirectly decrease escape. Against this argument, however, stand the results obtained with yohimbine, which facilitated avoidance without impairing escape in the ETM. Another caveat is that in these studies rats had not been pre-exposed to the open arm before the test (see later).

Tricyclic antidepressants usually aggravate anxiety earlier in treatment, the therapeutic effect appearing only following several days of repeated administration (Johnson, Lydiard and Ballenger, 1995). This correlates with the anxiogenic-like effect of clomipramine and imipramine on inhibitory avoidance following single injection (Table XIX-1.2). More important, an anxiolytic effect of imipramine on avoidance developed after chronic administration, and escape from the open arm was simultaneously impaired, which correlates well with the clinical effectiveness of this drug regime on both GAD and PD (Rickels *et al.*, 1993; Johnson, Lydiard and Ballenger, 1995). Nevertheless, the interpretation of the drug effects on escape is not as straightforward as on avoidance. As expected, this behaviour was unaffected by acute clomipramine. Yet, it was impaired by a single injection of imipramine. This inconsistency reminds one of the above-discussed differences between yohimbine, on one hand, and mCPP and TFPP, on the other.

Table XIX-1.2 Effect of clinically assayed drugs on the tasks performed in the elevated T-maze

Drug class	Compound	Avoidance	Escape
Anxiolytic			
	Diazepam	−	0
	Buspirone	−	0
	Ipsapirone	−	0
	Ritanserin	−	0
Anxiogenic			
	Yohimbine	+	0
	MCPP	+	−
	TFMPP	+	−
Antidepressant			
	Clomipramine	+	0
	Imipramine	+	−[p,2]
	Imipramine[c]	−	−[p,2]
5-HT releaser			
	d-Fenfluramine	+	−

Key: + Facilitation; − impairment; 0 no change; [c]chronic administration; [p]pre-exposure to the open arm; [2]two trials.

In addition, there was what appears to be a critical methodological difference, namely the rats used in the imipramine study had been pre-exposed to the open arm for 30 min before the test, and one additional measure of escape latency was taken. This procedure had two consequences: (1) the first escape response became significantly faster and (2) the anti-escape effect of chronic imipramine became statistically significant (Teixeira, Zangrossi and Graeff, 2000). Further comparisons with intracerebral drug injection led to the conclusion that pre-exposure to the open arm renders the escape task more sensitive and reliable to the effect of different brain manipulations. This is probably due to the habituation of behavioural reactions to novelty (exploration, behavioural inhibition), which are likely to interfere with one-way escape.

The 5-HT releaser and uptake inhibitor fenfluramine has been reported to induce attacks in panic patients (Targum and Marshall, 1989). Thus, the impairment of escape that was found with this drug (Table XIX-1.2) was quite unexpected. Nevertheless, Targum and Marshall (1989) themselves point out that, unlike the sudden surge of natural panic attacks, fenfluramine induced a slow wave of anxiety, more like an enhancement of anticipatory anxiety. Accordingly, d-fenfluramine has been shown to facilitate inhibitory avoidance in the ETM (Table XIX-1.2). Results obtained with two human models of anxiety seem to correlate with the opposite effects of d-fenfluramine on the two tasks of the ETM. Thus, the same drug tended to enhance conditioning of skin conductance responses in healthy volunteers, whereas markedly reducing the rise in anxiety induced by simulation of public speaking, a model of anxiety that has been associated with panic (Hetem *et al.*, 1996). Furthermore, a recent study showed that pre-treatment with d-fenfluramine enhanced anticipatory anxiety in PD patients following CO_2 inhalation. In contrast, the intensity of the CO_2-induced panic attack was decreased by the same drug treatment (Mortimore and Anderson, 2000). From these results, d-fenfluramine is expected to have anti-panic properties. Indeed, an open study (Solyom, 1994) as well as a case history (Hetem, 1995) provide suggestive clinical evidence supporting this view. Unfortunately, clinical investigation had to be interrupted because d-fenfluramine was withdrawn from the market due to cardiovascular untoward effects (Curzon and Gibson, 1999). In any case, the results obtained are enough to show that what at first seemed to be a major flaw of the ETM model turned out to strengthen the predictive value of escape in regard to PD.

Taking into account the above discussion on models of GAD, the drug profile of ETM avoidance comes as no surprise. Indeed, inhibitory avoidance of the open arm of the ETM is not unlike classical conflict tests. However, the present version has the advantages of not involving hunger or thirst, which are increased by some anxiolytic drugs (e.g., Berridge and Pecina, 1995). Moreover, the unconditioned aversive stimulus is neither painful nor artificial, like electric foot-shock. Another point that deserves some comment is the similarity of the motor performance in both tasks performed by the rat in the ETM. This serves as a control for non-specific drug effects on motor activity, particularly when the withdrawal latencies for the enclosed arm and the open arm are changed to opposite directions by the treatment. However, whenever the latencies are similarly increased or decreased, there is need for independent assessment of motor effects. Measuring motor activity inside an arena fulfils this requirement (Teixeira, Zangrossi and Graeff, 2000), albeit adding further complexity to the model.

The results of experiments with intracerebral drug injection (Graeff, Viana and Mora 1996a, 1997) and of a recent c-Fos study (Silveira *et al.*, 2001) indicate that the neural substrate of inhibitory avoidance is different from that of one-way escape.

MODELS OF SPECIFIC PHOBIAS

Specific phobias have been attributed to traumatic learning experiences. The classical conditioning of animal phobia in a boy by Watson and Rayner (1920) typifies this approach. Nevertheless, reports of traumatic experiences are lacking in most histories of phobic patients (Barlow, 1988). In addition, despite current dangers in civilized societies including, for example, electricity plugs or approaching cars, practically no exaggerated fears for such objects occur in the clinic. Instead, the most frequent phobic objects belong to certain categories that are constant through history and among different cultures, such as heights (acrophobia), closed environments (claustrophobia), the sight of blood (erythrophobia) or poisonous animals. This led to the alternative view that specific phobias are an exaggeration of ancestral fears, evoked by objects or situations that threatened survival of our hominid ancestors (Marks 1987; Marks and Nesse, 1994). A place for learning is kept in these theories of specific phobia, but learning prepared by evolution, such as in the experiments carried out by Ohman, Erixon and Loftberg (1975) showing that aversive conditioning to images of spiders was far easier and stronger than to pictures of flowers.

From this theoretical perspective, animal models of specific phobia should explore defence reaction against species-specific fears. Examples are the primate fear reaction to snakes (Mineka, 1985) and rats' avoidance response to cat odour (Zangrossi and File, 1992a). Whereas both tests have been used for analysing the behavioural characteristics of fear reactions and aspects of fear habituation/extinction, only the latter has been employed in pharmacological investigations.

The cat odour test developed by Zangrossi and File (1992a, 1992b) is based on the studies of Blanchards' group on the A/DTB discussed above. In this test, rats are exposed to a cloth impregnated with cat odour while in their single home-cage. These rats spend a greater amount of time hiding underneath the shelter formed by the water and food compartment of the home-cage and make fewer contacts with the cloth, compared to animals exposed to a neutral odour cloth. The benzodiazepine chlordiazepoxide has only a weak effect on rats' avoidance reactions; $5\,\text{mg}\,\text{kg}^{-1}$ of the drug increased the time spent in contact with the cloth, but did not decreased the time spent sheltering. On the other hand, this drug was fully effective in counteracting the anxiogenic effect of cat odour detected by the elevated plus-maze and social interaction tests (Zangrossi and File, 1992b). Acute or chronic (21 days) treatment with other anxiety-modulating drugs, such as buspirone, imipramine and the MAO inhibitor phenelzine, also failed to consistently decrease rats avoidance response to cat odour (File, 1995). Based on evidence showing that human-specific phobias are resistant to treatment with the drugs currently used to alleviate anxiety disorders (Marks, 1987), Zangrossi and File (1992b) have suggested that rats' avoidance to cat odour reflects the development of a phobic-like state. However, the generality of this proposal has been recently questioned by reported results showing that under a different test condition (use of a specific test-cage, different strain of rats and way of presenting the cat odour), benzodiazepine drugs can inhibit the avoidance response to cat odour (Dielenberg, Arnold and McGregor, 1999; McGregor and Dielenberg, 1999). Therefore, more studies are necessary to characterize this test as a model of specific phobia.

Although the homology argument is less strong, the suggestion has also been made that second exposure to the elevated plus-maze generates an emotional state that is akin to phobia (File *et al.*, 1993; File, 1993, 1995). This idea comes from evidence showing that benzodiazepines and barbiturates have either a weak or no anxiolytic effect in rats or mice previously exposed to the elevated plus-maze (File, 1990, 1993). This contrasts with the marked anxiolytic effect of these compounds on the first trial (see Rodgers, 1994). This phenomenon, called one-trial tolerance (OTT), has been observed even when the second trial is performed 2 weeks after the first, and is independent of drug state (either drugged or non-drugged) in the first trial. These results suggest that in the first experience with the plus-maze the animals are acquiring a different anxiety state that is insensitive to benzodiazepines. This idea is supported by findings showing that in a factorial analysis study, plus-maze scores of anxiety taken on the first and the second trials load on different factors. Interestingly, increasing the total time of testing on both trials from the usual 5 to 10 mins, abolishes the phenomenon of OTT. This result has been interpreted in terms of fear extinction after prolonged exposure to the aversive stimuli generated by the elevated plus-maze (File *et al.*, 1993). Based on knowledge that specific phobias respond favourably to exposure to the feared object/situation (Marks, 1987; Barlow, 1988), File *et al.* (1993) proposed that the trial second (trial-two) in the elevated plus-maze represents phobia. This trial-two phobic state would be different from that generated by exposure to cat odour in the sense that, whereas the former is acquired by a learning process, the latter is innate. Recent studies have explored the neural substrate involved in trial-two fear conditioning, revealing the participation of the basolateral amygdala (File, Gonzalez and Gallant, 1998) and dorso-medial hypothalamus (File, Gonzalez and Gallant, 1999) in this process. Further studies have shown that benzodiazepines and buspirone-like drugs exert differential effects on plus-maze trial-one and trial-two anxiety scores after microinjection in brain areas as the DRN (Gonzalez and File, 1997), dorsal hippocampus and lateral septum (Cheeta, Kenny and File, 2000).

MODELS OF OBSESSIVE–COMPULSIVE DISORDER

Clinical observation has shown that hand-washing and checking whether windows or doors are locked are the prevailing compulsive rituals. Rapoport (1991) suggested that these rituals may be related to animal behavioural routines of self-grooming and checking territorial borders, respectively. The adaptive function of grooming is to protect the animal against diseases caused by micro-organisms or parasites, while checking prevents invasion of the territory needed for reproduction and feeding by animals of the same or alien species. Neuroethological research has implicated the striatum in the control of these behavioural routines. Thus, an indirect support to Rapoport's ideas came from functional neuro-imaging studies showing hyperactivation of the nucleus caudatum of symptomatic obsessive–compulsive disorder (OCD) patients, which faded following successful treatment with either fluoxetine or cognitive behavioural therapy (Baxter *et al.*, 1996).

Acral Lick Dermatitis

Based on the preceding argument, Rapoport has looked for repetitive behaviours in animals that resemble compulsive symptoms, and found acral lick dermatitis in dogs the most appealing. Since OCD is responsive to clomipramine (Zohar *et al.*, 1988), similar treatment for the dog's disease was suggested, and indeed was effective (Goldberger and Rapoport, 1991). On this basis, acral lick dermatitis became a candidate for an animal model of OCD (Rapoport, Ryland and Kriete, 1992). The efficacy of clomipramine on canine compulsive disorder was confirmed by a double-blind, placebo-controlled study (Hewson *et al.*, 1998). Like human OCD, acral lick dermatitis is improved by SSRIs, such as fluoxetine (Wynchank and Berk, 1998) and citalopram (Stein *et al.*, 1998). However, acral lick dermatitis is not a true experimental model, in the sense that the conditions cannot be reproduced at will in the laboratory, but rather an animal analogue of OCD. Also, the use of a large and expensive subject such as dogs, and particularly sick dogs, detracts from its feasibility.

Adjunctive Behaviour Models

Some attempts to model OCD in laboratory animals have been made. Earlier operant behaviour studies have shown that when rats are given food reinforcement under fixed interval schedules, several collateral (adjunctive) behaviours are generated during the post-reinforcement period, among which are compulsive drinking or polydipsia (Falk, 1961). Woods and coworkers (1993) have shown that schedule-induced polydipsia was attenuated by chronic administration of the anti-obsessional drugs clomipramine, fluoxetine and fluvoxamine, and not affected by desipramine, haloperidol and diazepam, all of which are ineffective on OCD. These results qualify schedule-induced polydipsia as a potential animal model of OCD.

Another possible model of OCD is food-restriction-induced hyperactivity. Rats fed for 90 min per day lose some weight and then stabilize. If given access to a running wheel, these animals run excessively, loose weight, and often die. A pharmacological study has shown that chronic administration of fluoxetine decreased running and weight loss. Conversely, depleting 5-HT stores with para-chlorophenylalanine potentiated the effects of food restriction. Imipramine, which is ineffective on OCD, was also devoid of any action in this model (Altemus *et al.*, 1996).

Other Potential Models

Further repetitive behaviours that have been considered as potential models of OCD are the spontaneous alternation of food-deprived rats in a T-maze (Yadin, Friedman and Bridger, 1991) and marble burying in mice (Ichimaru, Egawa and Sawa, 1995). Both were responsive to SSRIs.

Pharmacological models for OCD have also been suggested. One of those is chronic treatment with the dopamine agonist quinpirole, inducing stereotyped behaviour in rats interpreted as compulsive checking. This would provide face validity to the model. This behaviour is attenuated by clomipramine, and its mechanism seems to involve sensitization of dopaminergic neurotransmission in the striatum, implicating this neurotransmitter in OCD (Szechtman, Culver and Eilam, 1999).

There is high comorbidity between OCD and Tourette's syndrome (see, e.g., Frankel *et al.*, 1986). From this background, a transgenic mouse model of comorbid Tourette's syndrome and OCD was created by expressing a neuropotentiating cholera toxin transgene in a subset of dopamine D_1 receptor-expressing neurones thought to enhance cortical and amygdalar output to the striatum. These animals manifest episodes of perseveration and repetitive behaviour, as in OCD, and repeated climbing/leaping and tics, as in Tourette's syndrome (McGrath *et al.*, 2000). Although of interest for the study of the role of glutamate in these conditions, this model lacks pharmacological validation.

CONCLUDING REMARKS

In the preceding sections several potential models of specific anxiety disorder were analysed. These tests have been selected mainly according to the criterion of construct validity or homology. For that, a theoretical stance based on the evolutionary paradigm has been taken.

Since present-day psychiatric classification is based on phenomenology, it may not be a suitable basis for establishing the neurobiological correlates of anxiety disorders. As pointed out by Gray and McNaughton (2000), genetic studies indicate that there is no specific inheritance for diagnostic categories, because what is inheritable is a general vulnerability for anxiety disorders. In this regard, dimensional approaches of personality may qualify as an alternative approach to provide better psychological correlates of biological markers.

Table XIX-1.3 presents an attempt to evaluate comparatively the models of GAD and PD, which have been more systematically explored than the models for other diagnostic categories. From the traditional criteria of model validation, the criterion of analogy was omitted, as it makes little sense within the comparative approach adopted here. In addition, the criterion of feasibility was added, because it often determines the extent to which a given animal model will be used.

Drug response remains the cornerstone for empirical validation, but under the precedence of homology the correlation between drug response in the model and in the clinic is viewed as a test for hypotheses about the model and the disorder rather than a separate criterion. Nevertheless, some critical remarks are due, concerning the interpretation of pharmacological correlation. With regard to models of GAD, non-benzodiazepine agents, such as buspirone and ritanserin, have anxiolytic-like effects after single administration in several models of GAD. However, these drugs improve clinical anxiety only after weeks of continuous administration (Nutt, 1991; Johnson, Lydiard and Ballenger, 1995). Therefore, the question of whether the effects in the animal models reflect reduced anxiety or merely behavioural disinhibition (Thiébot, Bizot and Soubrié, 1991) remains. Against the latter view are the results showing that buspirone-like drugs decrease probe burying as well as attenuate potentiated startle (see earlier). In these tests, the anxiolytic effect is expressed as decreased, rather than increased, motor activity. Yet, the case of potentiated startle is weakened by the demonstrated correlation between the intensity of startle potentiation and the degree of freezing (Leaton and Borszcz, 1985). Thus, it may still be argued that anxiolytic drugs reduce potentiated startle because they decrease behavioural inhibition.

Another instance is the effect of chronically administered antidepressants in models of GAD. In some cases a lack of effect of these treatments is suggested to support the specificity of the model. However, clinical studies have shown that prolonged administration of these drugs improves GAD, in addition to

Table XIX-1.3 Comparison among animal models of GAD and PD

Disorder	Animal model	Homology	Predictability	Feasibility
GAD				
	Light–dark transition	+++	+++	+++
	ETM avoidance	+++	+++	+++
	ADTB	+++	+++	++
	MDTB	+++	+++	++
	Potentiated startle	++	++	+
	Shock-probe burying	++	++	++
PD				
	FDTB	+++	++	+
	MDTB	+++	+++	++
	ETM escape	+++	++	+++
	DPAG electrical stimulation	+++	++	+
	DPAG chemical stimulation	+++	+	+
	DMH chemical stimulation	++	+	+

Key: ETM, elevated T-maze; ADTM, anxiety defence test battery; MDTB, mouse defence test battery; FDTB, fear/anxiety test battery; DPAG, dorsal periaqueductal grey matter; DMH, dorso-medial hypothalamus.

other anxiety disorders (Nutt, 1991; Rickels *et al.*, 1993). In the same way, psychostimulants, such as caffeine, cocaine and amphetamine, are often ineffective in GAD models, and this is taken as evidence for their drug selectivity. Yet, human studies show that these drugs may increase anxiety (Mitchell, Laurent and de Wit, 1996; Nehlig, Daval and Debry, 1992). Such instances undoubtedly blur the pharmacological validation of GAD models.

Similar restrictions can be made with respect to panic models. All the animal models of PD analysed show a reduction of the panic index after treatment with at least one clinically effective antipanic agent. This is indeed a necessary condition for a test to be classified as a model of panic disorder. Yet, it is not sufficient, since the same drug treatments also alleviate GAD (Nutt, 1991; Rickels *et al.*, 1993). Another criterion is the increase of the behavioural index of panic by drugs that induce panic attacks. Once more the interpretation of the results obtained is not straightforward. Some of these agents are specific, in the sense that they induce panic attacks only in panic patients. Among these are sodium lactate and inhalation of CO_2. Others, like cocaine, mCPP, yohimbine, caffeine and d-fenfluramine, induce anxiety in normal subjects as well, although panic patients may be particularly sensitive to these drugs. Therefore, it is difficult to ascertain whether the latter drugs induce a true panic attack or otherwise enhance anticipatory anxiety (Bourin, Baker and Bradwejn, 1998).

The above caveats expose the fragility of the current animal models. Only the capacity for detecting new, clinically useful drugs or behavioural therapies will ultimately validate any animal test, and warrant the approach advocated here of developing animal models theoretically oriented to specific anxiety disorders.

ACKNOWLEDGEMENTS

Frederico G. Graeff and Hélio Zangrossi Jr. are supported by research fellowships from FAEPA–HCFMRP and CNPq, respectively.

REFERENCES

Adams, D.B., 1979. Brain mechanisms for offense, defense, and submission. *The Behavioral and Brain Sciences*, **2**, 201–241.

Altemus, M., Glowa, J.R., Galliven, E., Leong, Y.-M. and Murphy, D., 1996. Effects of serotonergic agents on food-restriction-induced hyperactivity. *Pharmacology Biochemistry and Behavior*, **53**, 123–131.

Amano, K., Tanikawa, T., Iseki, H., Notani, M., Kawamura, H. and Kitamura, K., 1978. Single neuron analysis of the human midbrain tegmentum. *Applied Neurophysiology*, **41**, 66–78.

American Psychiatry Association, 1980. *Diagnostic and Statistical Manual of Mental Disorders*, 1st edn. APA Press, Washington DC.

American Psychiatry Association, 1994. *Diagnostic and Statistical Manual of Mental Disorders*, 4th edn, revised. APA Press, Washington DC.

Artaiz, I., Zazpe, A. and Del Rio, J., 1998. Characterization of serotonergic mechanisms involved in the behavioural inhibition induced by 5-hydroxytryptophan in a modified light-dark test in mice. *Behavioural Pharmacology*, **9**, 103–112.

Barlow, D.H., 1988. Simple phobia. In: *Anxiety and Its Disorders*, pp. 475–498. The Guilford Press, New York.

Baxter, L.R., Jr, Saxena, S., Brody, A.L., Ackermann, R.F., Colgan, M., Schwartz, J.M., Allen-Martinez, Z., Fuster, J.M. and Phelps, M.E., 1996. Brain mediation of obsessive-compulsive disorder symptoms: evidence from functional brain imaging studies in the human and nonhuman primate. *Seminars of Clinical Neuropsychiatry*, **1**, 32–47.

Beardsley, S.L., Papdakis, E., Fontana, D.J. and Comissaris, R.L., 1990. Antipanic drug treatments: failure to exhibit anxiolytic-like effects on defensive burying behavior. *Pharmacology Biochemistry and Behavior*, **35**, 451–455.

Beckett, S. and Marsden, C.A., 1995. Computer analysis and quantification of periaqueductal grey-induced defence behaviour. *Journal of Neuroscience Methods*, **58**, 157–161.

Beckett, S. and Marsden, C.A., 1997. The effect of central and systemic injection of the 5-HT1A receptor agonist 8-OHDPAT and the 5-HT1A receptors antagonist WAY 100635 on periaqueductal grey-induced defence behaviour. *Journal of Psychopharmacology*, **11**, 35–40.

Beckett, S.R.G., Marsden, C.A. and Marshal, P.W., 1992a. Intra periaqueductal grey administration of mCPP potentiates a chemically induced defence response. *British Journal of Pharmacology*, **107**, 8P.

Beckett, S.R.G., Lawrence, A.J., Marsden, C.A. and Marshal, P.W., 1992b. Attenuation of chemically induced defence response by $5\text{-}HT_1$ receptor agonists administered into the periaqueductal gray. *Psychopharmacology*, **108**, 110–114.

Berridge, K.C. and Pecina, S., 1995. Benzodiazepines, appetite, and taste palatability. *Neuroscience and Biobehavioral Reviews*, **19**, 121–131.

Bilkei-Gorzo, A., Gyertyan, I. and Levay, G., 1998. mCPP-induced anxiety in the light–dark box in rats: a new method for screening anxiolytic activity. *Psychopharmacology*, **136**, 291–298.

Blanchard, D.C. and Blanchard, R.J., 1988. Ethoexperimental approaches to the biology of emotion. *Annual Reviews of Psychology*, **39**, 43–68.

Blanchard, D.C., Griebel, G. and Blanchard, R.J., 2001. Mouse defensive behaviors: pharmacological and behavioral assays for anxiety and panic. *Neuroscience and Biobehavioral Reviews*, **25**, 205–218.

Blanchard, D.C., Blanchard, R.J., Tom, P. and Rodgers, R.J., 1990. Diazepam changes risk assessment in an anxiety/defense test battery. *Psychopharmacology*, **101**, 511–518.

Blanchard, D.C., Griebel, G., Rodgers, R.J. and Blanchard, R.J., 1998. Benzodiazepine and serotonergic modulation of antipredator and conspecific defense. *Neuroscience Biobehavioral Reviews*, **22**, 597–612.

Blanchard, R.J., Flannelly, K.J. and Blanchard, D.C., 1986. Defensive behaviors of laboratory and wild *Rattus Norvegicus*. *Journal of Comparative Psychology*, **100**, 101–107.

Blanchard, R.J., Griebel, G., Henrie, J.A. and Blanchard, D.C., 1997. Differentiation of anxiolytic and panicolytic drugs by effects on rat and mouse defense test batteries. *Neuroscience Biobehavioral Reviews*, **21**, 783–789.

Blanchard, R.J., Yudko, E.B., Rodgers, R.J. and Blanchard, D.C., 1993. Defense system psychopharmacology: an ethological approach to the pharmacology of fear and anxiety. *Behavioural Brain Research*, **58**, 155–165.

Borowski, T.B. and Kokkinidis, L., 1998. The effects of cocaine, amphetamine and the dopamine D1 receptor agonist SKF 38393 on fear extinction as measured with potentiated startle: implications for psychomotor stimulant psychosis. *Behavioral Neuroscience*, **112**, 952–965.

Bourin, M., Baker, G.B. and Bradwejn, J., 1998. Neurobiology of panic disorder. *Journal of Psychosomatic Research*, **44**, 163–180.

Brown, J.S., Kalish, J.W. and Faber, I.E., 1951. Conditioned fear as revealed by magnitude of startle response to an auditory stimulus. *Journal of Experimental Psychology*, **41**, 317–328.

Chaouloff, F., Durand, M. and Mormede, P., 1997. Anxiety- and activity-related effects of diazepam and chlordiazepoxide in the rat light/dark and dark/light tests. *Behavioural Brain Research*, **85**, 27–35.

Cheeta, S., Kenny, P.J. and File, S.E., 2000. Hippocampal and septal injections of nicotine and 8-OH-DPAT distinguish among differential animal tests of anxiety. *Progress in Neuropsychopharmacology and Biological Psychiatry*, **24**, 1053–1067.

Charney, D.S., Woods, S.W., Goodman, W.K. and Henninger, G.R., 1987. Serotonin function in anxiety. II. Effects of the serotonin agonist MCPP in panic disorder patients and healthy subjects. *Psychopharmacology*, **92**, 14–24.

Costall, B. and Naylor, R.J., 1995. Behavioural interactions between 5-hydroxytryptophan, neuroleptic agents and 5-HT receptor antagonists in modifying rodent responding to aversive situations. *British Journal of Pharmacology*, **116**, 2989–2999.

Craft, R.M., Howard, J.L. and Pollard, G.T., 1988. Conditioned defensive burying as a model for identifying anxiolytics. *Pharmacology Biochemistry and Behavior*, **30**, 775–780.

Crawley, J.N., 1985. Exploratory behavior models of anxiety in mice. *Neuroscience Biobehavioral Reviews*, **9**, 37–44.

Crawley, J.N. and Davis, L.G., 1982. Baseline exploratory activity predicts anxiolytic responsiveness to diazepam in five mouse strains. *Brain Research Bulletin*, **8**, 609–612.

Crawley, J.N. and Goodwin, F.K., 1980. Preliminary report of a single animal behavior model for the anxiolytic effects of benzodiazepines. *Pharmacology Biochemistry and Behavior*, **13**, 167–170.

Cruz, A.P.M., Frei, F. and Graeff, F.G., 1994. Ethopharmacological analysis of rat behavior on the elevated plus-maze. *Pharmacology Biochemistry and Behaviour*, **49**, 171–176.

Curzon, G. and Gibson, E.L., 1999. The serotonergic appetite suppressant fenfluramine. Reappraisal and rejection. *Advances in Experimental Medicine and Biology*, **467**, 95–100.

Darwin, C., 1872. *The Expression of Emotions in Man and Animals*, (reprint 1985). Philosophical Library, New York.

Davis, M., 1986. Pharmacological and anatomical analysis of fear conditioning using the fear-potentiated startle paradigm. *Behavioral Neuroscience*, **100**, 814–824.

Davis, M., 1992. The role of the amygdala in fear and anxiety. *Annual Reviews of Neuroscience*, **15**, 353–375.

Davis, M., Fall, W.A., Campeau, S. and Kim, M., 1993. Fear-potentiated startle: a neural and pharmacological analysis. *Behavioural Brain Research*, **58**, 175–198.

Deakin, J.F.W. and Graeff, F.G., 1991. 5-HT and mechanisms of defence. *Journal of Psychopharmacology*, **5**, 305–315.

De Angelis, L., 1992. The anxiogenic-like effects of pentylenetetrazol in mice treated chronically with carbamazepine or valproate. *Methods and Findings in Experimental and Clinical Pharmacology*, **14**, 767–771.

De Angelis, L., 1996. Experimental anxiety and antidepressant drugs: the effects of moclobemide, a selective reversible MAO-A inhibitor, fluoxetine and imipramine in mice. *Naunyn Schmiedebergs Archives of Pharmacology*, **354**, 379–383.

Den Boer, J.A. and Westenberg, H.G.M., 1990. Serotonin function in panic disorder: a double blind placebo controlled study with fluvoxamine and ritanserin. *Psychopharmacology*, **102**, 85–94.

Dielenberg, R.A., Arnold, J.C. and McGregor, I.S., 1999. Low-dose midazolam attenuates predatory odor avoidance in rats. *Pharmacology Biochemistry and Behavior*, **62**, 197–201.

Estes, W.K. and Skinner, F.B., 1941. Some quantitative properties of anxiety. *Journal of Experimental Psychology*, **29**, 390–400.

Falk, J.L., 1961. Production of polydipsia in normal rats by an intermittent food schedule. *Science*, **133**, 195–196.

Fanselow, M.S., 1991. The midbrain periaqueductal gray as a coordinator of action in response to fear and anxiety. In: De Paulis, A. and Bandler, R. (eds), *The Midbrain Periaqueductal Gray Matter*, pp. 151–173. Plenum Press, New York.

Fernandez-Guasti, A. and Lopez-Rubalcava, C., 1998. Modification of the anxiolytic action of 5-HT1A compounds by GABA-benzodiazepines agents in rats. *Pharmacology Biochemistry and Behavior*, **60**, 27–32.

Fernandez-Guasti, A., Hong, E. and Lopez-Rubalcava, C., 1992. Species differences in the mechanism through which the serotonergic agonists indorenate and ipsapirone produce their anxiolytic action. *Psychopharmacology*, **107**, 61–68.

File, S.E., 1990. One-trial tolerance to the anxiolytic effects of chlordiazepoxide in the plus-maze. *Psychopharmacology*, **100**, 281–282.

File, S.E., 1993. The interplay of learning and anxiety in the elevated plus-maze. *Behavioural Brain Research*, **58**, 199–202.

File, S.E., 1995. Animal models of different anxiety states. In: Biggio, G., Sanna, E., Serra, M. and Costa, E. (eds), *$GABA_A$ Receptors and Anxiety—From Neurobiology to Treatment*, pp. 93–113. Raven Press, New York.

File, S.E., Gonzalez, L.E. and Gallant, R., 1998. Role of the basolateral nucleus of the amygdala in the formation of a phobia. *Neuropsychopharmacology*, **19**, 397–405.

File, S.E., Gonzalez, L.E. and Gallant, R., 1999. Role of the dorsomedial hypothalamus in mediating the response to benzodiazepine on trial 2 in the elevate plus-maze test of anxiety. *Neuropsychopharmacology*, **21**, 312–320.

File, S.E., Zangrossi, Jr, H., Viana, M. and Graeff, F.G., 1993. Trial 2 in the elevated plus-maze: a different form of fear? *Psychopharmacology*, **111**, 381–388.

Frankel, M., Cummings, J.L., Robertson, M.M., Trimble, M.R., Hill, M.A. and Benson, D.F., 1986. Obsessions and compulsions in Gilles de la Tourette's syndrome. *Neurology*, **36**, 378–382.

Gentil, V., 1988. The aversive system, 5-HT and panic attacks. In: Simon, P., Soubrié, P. and Widlocher, D. (eds), *Animal Models of Psychiatry, Vol. 2: Selected Models of Anxiety, Depression and Psychosis*, pp. 142–145. Karger, Basel.

Goldberger, E. and Rapoport, J.L., 1991. Canine acral lick dermatitis: response to the anti-obsessional drug clomipramine. *Journal of the American Animal Hospital Association*, **27**, 179–182.

Gonzalez, L.E. and File, S.E., 1997. A five minute experience in the elevated plus-maze alters the state of the benzodiazepine receptor in the dorsal raphe nucleus. *Journal of Neuroscience*, **17**, 1505–1511.

Graeff, F.G., 1988. Animal models of aversion. In: Simon, P., Soubrié, P. and Widlocher, D. (eds), *Animal Models of Psychiatry, Vol. 2: Selected Models of Anxiety, Depression and Psychosis*, pp. 115–141. Karger, Basel.

Graeff, F.G., 1991. Neurotransmitters in the dorsal periaqueductal gray and animal models of panic anxiety. In: Briley, M. and File, S.E. (eds), *New Concepts in Anxiety*, pp. 288–312. MacMillan Press, London.

Graeff, F.G., 1994. Neuroanatomy and neurotransmitter regulation of defensive behaviors and related emotions in mammals. *Brazilian Journal of Medical and Biological Research*, **27**, 811–829.

Graeff, F.G. and Schoenfeld, R.I., 1970. Tryptaminergic mechanisms in punished and nonpunished behavior. *Journal of Pharmacology and Experimental Therapeutics*, **173**, 277–283.

Graeff, F.G., Ferreira Netto, C. and Zangrossi, Jr, H., 1998. The elevated T-maze as an experimental model of anxiety. *Neuroscience and Biobehavioral Reviews*, **23**, 237–246.

Graeff, F.G., Viana, M.B. and Mora, P.O., 1996a. Opposed regulation by dorsal raphe nucleus 5-HT pathways of two types of fear in the elevated T-maze. *Pharmacology Biochemistry and Behavior*, **53**, 171–177.

Graeff, F.G., Viana, M.B. and Mora, P., 1997. Dual role of 5-HT in defense and anxiety. *Neuroscience and Biobehavioral Reviews*, **21**, 791–799.

Graeff, F.G., Viana, M.B. and Tomaz, C., 1993. The elevated T maze, a new experimental model of anxiety and memory: Effect of diazepam. *Brazilian Journal of Medical and Biological Research*, **26**, 67–70.

Graeff, F.G., Guimarães, F.S., De Andrade, T.G.C.S. and Deakin, J.F.W., 1996b. Role of 5-HT in stress, anxiety and depression. *Pharmacology Biochemistry and Behavior*, **54**, 129–141.

Gray, J.A. and McNaughton, N., 2000. *The Neuropsychology of Anxiety*. Oxford University Press, Oxford.

Griebel, G., 1995. 5-Hydroxytryptamine-interacting drugs in animal models of anxiety disorders: more than 30 years of research. *Pharmacology and Therapeutics*, **65**, 319–395.

Griebel, G., Blanchard, D.C. and Blanchard, R.J., 1996a. Predator elicited flight responses in the Swiss Webster mice: an experimental model of panic attacks. *Progress in Neuropsychology and Biological Psychiatry*, **20**, 185–205.

Griebel, G., Sanger, D.J. and Perrault, G., 1996b. Further evidence for differences between non-selective and BZ-1 (omega 1) selective benzodiazepine receptor ligands in murine models of 'state' and 'trait' anxiety. *Neuropharmacology*, **35**, 1081–1091.

Griebel, G., Belzung, C., Perrault, G. and Sanger, D.J., 2000. Differences in anxiety-related behaviours and in sensitivity to diazepam in inbred and outbred strains of mice. *Psychopharmacology*, **148**, 164–170.

Griebel, G., Misslin, R., Pawlowski, M. and Vogel, E., 1991. m-Chorophenylpiperazine enhances neophobic and anxious behaviour in mice. *Neuroreport*, **2**, 627–629.

Griebel, G., Moreau, J.L., Jenck, F., Mutel, V., Martin, J.R. and Misslin, R., 1994. Evidence that tolerance to the anxiogenic-like effects of mCPP does not involve alteration in the function of 5-HT(2C) receptors in the rat choroid plexus. *Behavioural Pharmacology*, **5**, 642–645.

Handley, S.L., McBlane, J.W., Critchley, M.A.E. and Njung'e, K., 1993. Multiple serotonin mechanisms in animal models of anxiety: environmental, emotional and cognitive factors. *Behavioral Brain Research*, **58**, 203–210.

Handley, S.L. and Mithani, S., 1984. Effects of alpha-adrenoceptor agonists in a maze-exploration model of 'fear'-motivated behaviour. *Naunyn-Schmiedeberg's Archives of Pharmacology*, **327**, 1–5.

Hascoët, M. and Bourin, M., 1998. A new approach to the light/dark test procedure in mice. *Pharmacology Biochemistry and Behavior*, **60**, 645–653.

Hascoët, M., Bourin, M. and Nic Dhonnchadha, B.A., 2000. The influence of buspirone, and its metabolite 1-PP, on the activity of paroxetine in the mouse light/dark paradigm and four plate test. *Pharmacology Biochemistry and Behavior*, **67**, 45–53.

Hascoët, M., Colombel, M.C. and Bourin, M., 1999. Influence of age on behavioural response in the light/dark paradigm. *Physiology and Behavior*, **66**, 567–570.

Hetem, L.A.B., 1995. Addition of d-fenfluramine to benzodiazepines produced a marked improvement in refractory panic disorder — a case report. *Journal of Clinical Psychopharmacology*, **16**, 77–78.

Hetem, L.A.B., Souza, C.J., Guimarães, F.S., Zuardi, A.W. and Graeff, F.G., 1996. Effect of d-fenfluramine on human experimental anxiety. *Psychopharmacology*, **127**, 276–282.

Hewson, C.J., Lueschener, U.A., Parent, J.M., Conlon, P.D. and Ball, R.O., 1998. Efficacy of clomipramine in the treatment of canine compulsive disorder: a randomized, placebo-controlled, double-blind clinical trial. *Journal of the American Veterinary Medicine Association*, **213**, 1760–1766.

Hijzen, T.H., Houtzager, S.W.J., Joordens, R.J.E., Olivier, B. and Slangen, J.L., 1995. Predictive validity of the potentiated startle response as behavioral model of anxiolytic drugs. *Psychopharmacology*, **118**, 150–154.

Hofer, M.A., 1995. An evolutionary perspective on anxiety. In: Roose, S.P. and Glick, R.A. (eds), *Anxiety as Symptom and Signal*. Analytic Press, Hillsdale, NJ.

Ichimaru, Y., Egawa, T. and Sawa, A., 1995. 5-HT_{1A}-receptor subtype mediates the effect of fluvoxamine, a selective serotonin reuptake inhibitor, on marble-burying behavior in mice. *Japanese Journal of Pharmacology*, **68**, 65–70.

Imaizumi, M., Miyazaki, S. and Onodera, K., 1994. Effects of xantines derivatives in a light/dark test in mice and contribution of adenosine receptors. *Methods and Findings in Experimental and Clinical Pharmacology*, **16**, 639–644.

Jenck, F., Moreau, J.L. and Martin, J.R., 1995. Dorsal periaqueductal gray induced aversion as a simulation of panic anxiety: elements of face and predictive validity. *Psychiatry Research*, **57**, 181–191.

Johnson, M.R., Lydiard, R.B. and Ballenger, J.C., 1995. Panic disorder: Pathophysiology and drug treatment. *Drugs*, **49**, 328–344.

Joordens, R.J.E., Hijzen, T.H. and Olivier, B., 1998. The effects of 5-HT1A receptor agonists, 5-HT1A receptor antagonists and their interaction on the fear-potentiated startle response. *Psychopharmacology*, **139**, 383–390.

Joordens, R.J.E., Hijzen, T.H., Peeters, B.W.M.M. and Olivier, B., 1996. Fear-potentiated startle response is remarkably similar in two laboratories. *Psychopharmacology*, **126**, 104–109.

Kehne, J.H., Cassella, J.V. and Davis, M., 1988. Anxiolytic effects of buspirone and gepirone in the fear-potentiated startle paradigm. *Psychopharmacology*, **94**, 8–13.

Keim, S.R. and Sekhar, A., 1999. NE and 5HT receptors involved in eliciting panic-like responses following i.v. infusions of yohimbine and fenfluramine. *Society of Neuroscience Abstracts*, **25**, 2139.

Kelleher, R.T. and Morse, W.H., 1968. Determinants of the specificity of behavioral effects of drugs. *Ergebnisse der Physiologie*, **60**, 1–56.

Kiser Jr, R.S. and Lebovitz, R.M., 1975. Monoaminergic mechanisms in aversive brain stimulation. *Physiology and Behavior*, **15**, 47–53.

Kshama, D., Hrishikeshavan, H.J., Shanbhogue, R. and Munonyedi, U.S., 1990. Modulation of baseline behavior in rats by putative serotonergic agents in three ethoexperimental paradigms. *Behavioral and Neural Biology*, **54**, 234–253.

Leaton, R.N. and Borszcz, G.S., 1985. Potentiated startle: its relation to freezing and shock intensity in rats. *Journal of Experimental Psychology. Animal Behavior Processes*, **11**, 421–428.

Liebowitz, M.R., Gorman, J.M., Dillon, Levy, G., Appleby, I.L., Anderson, S., Palij, M., Davies, S.O. and Klein, D.F., 1985. Lactate provocation of panic attacks. II. Biochemical and physiological findings. *Archives of General Psychiatry*, **42**, 709–719.

Lopez-Rubalcava, C. and Fernandez-Guasti, A., 1994. Noradrelanine–serotonin interactions in the anxiolytic effects of 5-HT(1A) agonists. *Behavioural Pharmacology*, **5**, 42–51.

Lopez-Rubalcava, C., Fernandez-Guasti, A. and Urba-Holmgren, R., 1996. Age-dependent differences in the rat's conditioned defensive burying behavior: effect of 5-HT1A compounds. *Developmental Psychobiology*, **29**, 157–169.

Marks, I.M. and Nesse, R.M., 1994. Fear and fitness: An evolutionary analysis of anxiety disorders. *Ethology and Sociobiology*, **15**, 247–261.

Marks, I.M., 1987. *Fears, Phobias and Rituals: Panic, Anxiety and their Disorders*. Oxford University Press, New York.

McGrath, M.J., Campbell, K.M., Parks III, C.R. and Burton, F.H., 2000. Glutamatergic drugs exacerbate symptomatic behavior in a transgenic model of comorbid Tourette's syndrome and obsessive–compulsive disorder. *Brain Research*, **877**, 23–30.

McGregor, I.S. and Dielenberg, R.A., 1999. Differential anxiolytic efficacy of a benzodiazepine on first versus second exposure to a predatory odor in rats. *Psychopharmacology*, **147**, 174–181.

McGuire, M. and Troisi, A., 1998. *Darwinian Psychiatry*. Oxford University Press, Oxford.

Mineka, S., 1985. Animal models of anxiety based disorders: Their usefulness and limitations. In: Tuma, A.H. and Maser, J.D. (eds), *Anxiety and the Anxiety Disorders*, pp. 199–244. Lawrence Erlbaum Associated Publishers, Hillsdale, New Jersey.

Mitchell, S.H., Laurent, C.L. and de Wit, H., 1996. Interaction of expectancy and the pharmacological effects of d-amphetamine: subjective effects and self-administration. *Psychopharmacology*, **125**, 371–378.

Mongeau, R. and Marsden, C.A., 1997a. Effect of imipramine treatments on the 5-HT1A-receptor-mediated inhibition of panic-like behaviours in rats. *Psychopharmacology*, **131**, 321–328.

Mongeau, R. and Marsden, C.A., 1997b. Effect of central and peripheral administrations of cholecystokinin-tetrapeptide on panic-like reactions induced by stimulation of the dorsal periaqueductal grey area in the rat. *Biological Psychiatry*, **42**, 335–344.

Mortimore, C. and Anderson, I.M., 2000. *d*-Fenfluramine in panic disorder: a dual role for 5-hydroxytryptamine. *Psychopharmacology*, **149**, 251–258.

Nashold, Jr, B.S., Wilson, N.P. and Slaughter, G.S., 1974. The midbrain and pain. In: Bonica, J.J. (ed.), *Advances in Neurology, Volume 4: International Symposium on Pain*, pp. 191–196. Raven Press, New York.

Nehlig, A., Daval, J.L. and Debry, G., 1992. Caffeine and the central nervous system: mechanisms of action, biochemical, metabolic and psychostimulant effects. *Brain Research Reviews*, **17**, 139–170.

Nesse, R.M., 1990. Evolutionary explanation of emotions. *Human Nature*, **1**, 261–289.

Nogueira, R.L. and Graeff, F.G., 1995. Role of 5-HT receptor subtypes in the modulation of aversion generated in the dorsal periaqueductal gray. *Pharmacology Biochemistry and Behavior*, **52**, 1–6.

Nutt, D.J., 1991. Anxiety and its therapy: today and tomorrow. In: Briley, M. and File, S.E. (eds), *New Concepts in Anxiety*, pp. 1–12. MacMillan Press, London.

Ohman, A., Erixon, G. and Lofberg, I., 1975. Phobias and preparedness: phobic versus neutral pictures as conditioned stimuli for human autonomic responses. *Journal of Abnormal Psychology*, **1**, 41–45.

Onaivi, E.S. and Martin, B.R., 1989. Neuropharmacological and physiological validation of a computer-controlled two-compartment black and white box for the assessment of anxiety. *Progress in Neuropsychopharmacology and Biological Psychiatry*, **13**, 967–976.

Panksepp, J., 1982. Toward a general psychobiological theory of emotions. *Behavioural and Brain Sciences*, **5**, 407–467.

Pare, W.P., 1992. The performance of WKY rats on three tests of emotional behavior. *Physiology and Behavior*, **51**, 1051–1056.

Pellow, S. and File, S.E., 1986. Anxiolytic and anxiogenic drug effects on exploratory activity in an elevated plus-maze: a novel test of anxiety in the rat. *Pharmacology Biochemistry and Behavior*, **24**, 525–529.

Pich, M. and Samanin, R., 1989. A two-compartment exploratory model to study anxiolytic/anxiogenic effects of drug in the rat. *Pharmacological Research*, **21**, 595–602.

Pinel, J.P.J. and Treit, D., 1978. Burying as a defensive response in rats. *Journal of Comparative Physiology and Psychology*, **92**, 708–712.

Pinel, J.P.J. and Treit, D., 1979. Conditioned defensive burying in rats: availability of burying materials. *Animal Learning and Behavior*, **7**, 392–396.

Randall, L.O., Schallek, W., Heise, G.A., Keith, E.F. and Bagdon, R.E., 1960. The psychosedative properties of methaminodiazepoxide. *Journal of Pharmacology and Experimental Therapeutics*, **129**, 163–161.

Rapoport, J.L., 1991. Recent advances in obsessive–compulsive disorder. *Neuropsychopharmacology*, **5**, 1–10.

Rapoport, J.L., Ryland, D.H. and Kriete, M., 1992. Drug treatment of canine acral lick. An animal model of obsessive–compulsive disorder. *Archives of General Psychiatry*, **49**, 517–521.

Reiman, E.M., Reichle, M.E., Robins, E., Mintun, M.A., Fusselman, M.J., Fox, P.T., Price, J.L. and Hackman, K.A., 1989. Neuroanatomical correlates of a lactate-induced anxiety attack. *Archives of General Psychiatry*, **46**, 493–500.

Rickels, K., Downing, R., Schweizer, E. and Hassman, H., 1993. Antidepressants for the treatment of generalized anxiety disorder. A placebo-controlled comparison of imipramine, trazodone, and diazepam. *Archives of General Psychiatry*, **50**, 884–895.

Robichaud, R.C. and Sledge, K.L., 1969. The effects of p-chlorophenylalanine on experimentally induced conflict in the rat. *Life Sciences*, **8**, 965–969.

Rodgers, R.J., 1994. The elevated plus-maze: pharmacology, methodology and ethology. In: Cooper, S.J. and Endrie, C.A. (eds), *Ethology and Psychopharmacology*, pp. 9–44. John Wiley & Sons, Chichester.

Rodgers, R.J. and Johnson, N.J.T., 1995. Factor analysis of spatio temporal and ethological measures in the murine elevated plus-maze. *Pharmacology Biochemistry and Behavior*, **49**, 297–303.

Rohmer, J.G., Di Scala, G. and Sandner, G., 1990. Behavioral analysis of the presence of benzodiazepine receptor ligands in the conditioned burying paradigm. *Behavioural Brain Research*, **38**, 45–54.

Sakamoto, H., Matsumoto, K., Ohno, Y. and Nakamura, M., 1998. Anxiolytic-like effects of perospirone, a novel serotonin-2 and dopamine-2 antagonists (SDA)-type antipsychotic agent. *Pharmacology Biochemistry Behavior*, **60**, 873–878.

Sanchez, C., 1996. 5-HT1A receptors play an important role in modulation of behavior of rats in a two-compartment black and white box. *Behavioural Pharmacology*, **7**, 788–797.

Sanchez, C. and Maier, E., 1997. Behavioral profiles of SSRIs in animal models of depression, anxiety and aggression. Are they alike? *Psychopharmacology*, **129**, 197–205.

Saran, A. and Halaris, A., 1989. Panic attack precipitated by fluoxetine. *Journal of Neuropsychiatry and Clinical Neuroscience*, **1**, 219–220.

Schenberg, L.C. and Graeff, F.G., 1978. Role of periaqueductal gray substance in the antianxiety action of benzodiazepines. *Pharmacology Biochemistry and Behavior*, **9**, 287–295.

Schenberg, L.C., Costa, M.B., Borges, P.C.L. and Castro, F.S., 1990. Logistic analysis of the defense reaction induced by electrical stimulation of the rat mesencephalic tectum. *Neuroscience and Biobehavioral Reviews*, **14**, 473–479.

Schenberg, L.C., Vargas, L.C., Silva, S.R., Reis, A.M. and Tufik, S., 2001. Modeling panic attacks. *Neuroscience and Biobehavioral Reviews*, **25**, 647–659.

Schmitt, P., Carrive, P., Di Scala, G., Jenck, F., Brandão, M.L., Bagri, A., Moreau, J.L. and Sandner, G., 1986. A neuropharmacological study of the periventricular neural substrate involved in flight. *Behavioral Brain Research*, **22**, 181–190.

Schütz, M.T.B., de Aguiar, J.C. and Graeff, F.G., 1985. Anti-aversive role of serotonin in the dorsal periaqueductal grey matter. *Psychopharmacology*, **85**, 340–345.

Shekhar, A., 1994. Effects of treatment with imipramine and clonazepam on an animal model of panic disorder. *Biological Psychiatry*, **36**, 748–758.

Shekhar, A. and Di Micco, J.A., 1987. Defense reaction elicited by injection of GABA antagonists and synthesis inhibitors into the posterior hypothalamus in rats. *Neuropharmacology*, **26**, 407–417.

Shimada, T., Matsumoto, K., Osanai, M., Matsuda, H., Terasawa, K. and Watanabe, H., 1995. The modified light/dark transition test in mice: evaluation of classic and putative anxiolytic and anxiogenic drugs. *General Pharmacology*, **26**, 205–210.

Silveira, M.C.L., Zangrossi, Jr, H., Viana, M.B., Silveira, R. and Graeff, F.G., 2001. Differential expression of Fos protein in the rat brain induced by performance of avoidance or escape in the elevated T-maze. *Behavioral Brain Research*, **126**, 13–21.

Singh, L., Field, M.J., Hughes, J., Menzies, R., Oles, R.J., Vass, C.A. and Woodruff, G.N., 1991. The behavioural properties of CI-988, a selective cholecystokininB receptor antagonist. *British Journal of Pharmacology*, **104**, 239–245.

Smythe, J.W., Bhatnagar, S., Murphy, D., Timothy, C. and Costall, B., 1998. The effects of intrahippocampal scopolamine infusions on anxiety in rats as measured by the black–white box test. *Brain Research Bulletin*, **45**, 89–93.

Solyom, L., 1994. Controlling panic attacks with fenfluramine. *American Journal of Psychiatry*, **151**, 621–622.

Stein, D.J. and Bouwer, C., 1997. A neuro-evolutionary approach to the anxiety disorders. *Journal of Anxiety Disorders*, **4**, 409–429.

Stein, D.J., Mendelsohn, I., Ptocnik, F., Van Kradenberg, J. and Wessels, C., 1998. Use of the selective serotonin reuptake inhibitor citalopram in a possible animal analogue of obsessive–compulsive disorder. *Depression and Anxiety*, **8**, 39–42.

Stein, L., Wise, C.D. and Berger, B.D., 1973. Anti-anxiety action of benzodiazepines: Decrease in activity of serotonin neurons in the punishment system. In: Garattini, S., Mussini, E. and Randall, L.O. (eds), *Benzodiazepines*, pp. 299–326. Raven Press, New York.

Sudré, E.C.M., de Barros, M.R., Sudré, G.N. and Schenberg, L.C., 1993. Thresholds of electrically induced defence reaction of the rat: short- and long-term adaptation mechanisms. *Behavioural Brain Research*, **58**, 141–154.

Szechtman, H., Culver, K. and Eilam, D., 1999. Role of dopamine systems in obsessive–compulsive disorder (OCD): implications form a novel psychostimulant-induced animal model. *Polish Journal of Pharmacology*, **51**, 55–61.

Tanaka, M., Yoshida, M., Emoto, H. and Ishii, H., 2000. Noradrenaline system in the hypothalamus, amygdala and locus coeruleus are involved in the provocation of anxiety: basic studies. *European Journal of Pharmacology*, **405**, 397–406.

Targum, S.D. and Marshall, L.E., 1989. Fenfluramine provocation of anxiety in patients with panic disorder. *Psychiatry Research*, **28**, 295–306.

Teixeira, R.C., Zangrossi, Jr, H. and Graeff, F.G., 2000. Behavioral effects of acute and chronic imipramine in the elevated T-maze model of anxiety. *Pharmacology Biochemistry and Behavior*, **65**, 571–576.

Thiébot, M.H., Bizot, J.C. and Soubrié, P., 1991. Waiting capacity in animals. A behavioral component crossing nosologic boundaries of anxiety and depression? In: Soubrié, P. (ed.), *Animal Models in Psychiatric Disorders, Vol. 3: Anxiety, Depression and Mania*, pp. 48–67. Karger, Basel.

Treit, D., 1985. Animal models for the study of anti-anxiety agents: A review. *Neuroscience and Biobehavioral Reviews*, **9**, 203–222.

Treit, D., 1987. Ro-15-1788, CGS 8216, picrotoxin, and pentylenetetrazol: do they antagonize anxiolytic drug effects through an anxiogenic action? *Brain Research Bulletin*, **19**, 401–405.

Treit, D., 1990. A comparison of anxiolytic and nonanxiolytic agents in the shock-probe/burying test for anxiolytics. *Pharmacology Biochemistry Behavior*, **36**, 203–205.

Treit, D. and Fundytus, M., 1988. A comparison of buspirone and chlordiazepoxide in the shock-probe/burying test for anxiolytics. *Pharmacology Biochemistry Behavior*, **30**, 1071–1075.

Treit, D., Menard, J. and Royan, C., 1993. Anxiogenic stimuli in the elevated plus-maze. *Pharmacology Biochemistry and Behavior*, **44**, 463–469.

Treit, D., Pinel, J.P. and Fibiger, H.C., 1981. Conditioned defensive burying: a new paradigm for the study of anxiolytic agents. *Pharmacology Biochemistry and Behavior*, **15**, 619–626.

Tsuda, A., Ida, Y. and Tanaka, M., 1988. The constrating effects of diazepam and yohimbine on conditioned defensive burying in rats. *Psychobiology*, **16**, 213–217.

Vargas, L.C. and Schenberg, L.C., 2001. Long-term effects of clomipramine and fluoxetine on dorsal periaqueductal grey-evoked innate defensive behaviours of the rat. *Psychopharmacology*, **155**, 260–268.

Viana, M.B., Tomaz, C. and Graeff, F.G., 1994. The elevated T-maze: a new animal model of anxiety and memory. *Pharmacology Biochemistry and Behavior*, **49**, 549–554.

Walker, D.L., Cassella, J.V., Lee, Y., de Lima, T.C.M. and Davis, M., 1997. Opposing roles of the amygdala and dorsolateral periaqueductal gray in fear-potentiated startle. *Neuroscience and Biobehavioral Reviews*, **21**, 743–753.

Watson, J. and Rayner, R., 1920. Conditioned emotional reactions. *Journal of Genetic Psychology*, **37**, 394–419.

Willner, P., 1991. Behavioural models in psychopharmacology. In: Willner, P. (ed.), *Behavioural Models in Psychopharmacology: Theoretical, Industrial and Clinical Perspectives*, pp. 3–18. Cambridge University Press, Cambridge.

Woods, A., Smith, C., Szewczak, M., Dunn, R.W., Cornfeldt, M. and Corbett, R., 1993. Selective serotonin re-uptake inhibitors decrease schedule-induced polydipsia in rats: a potential model for obsessive compulsive disorder. *Psychopharmacology*, **112**, 195–198.

Wynchank, D. and Berk, M., 1998. Fluoxetine treatment of acral lick dermatitis in dogs: a placebo-controlled randomized double blind trial. *Depression and Anxiety*, **8**, 21–23.

Yadin, E., Friedman, E. and Bridger, W.H., 1991. Spontaneous alternation behavior: an animal model for obsessive–compulsive disorder. *Pharmacology Biochemistry and Behavior*, **40**, 311–315.

Young, R. and Johnson, D.N., 1991a. A fully automated light/dark apparatus useful for comparing anxiolytic agents. *Pharmacology Biochemistry and Behavior*, **40**, 739–743.

Young, R. and Johnson, D.N., 1991b. Comparison of routes of administration and time course effects of zacopride and buspirone in mice using an automated light/dark test. *Pharmacology Biochemistry and Behavior*, **40**, 733–737.

Zangrossi, Jr, H. and File, S.E., 1992a. Behavioral consequences in animal tests of anxiety and exploration of exposure to cat odor. *Brain Research Bulletin*, **29**, 381–388.

Zangrossi, Jr, H. and File, S.E., 1992b. Chlordiazepoxide reduces the generalised anxiety, but not the direct responses, of rats exposed to cat odor. *Pharmacology Biochemistry and Behavior*, **43**, 1195–1200.

Zangrossi, Jr, H. and Graeff, F.G., 1997. Behavioral validation of the elevated T-maze, a new animal model of anxiety. *Brain Research Bulletin*, **44**, 1–5.

Zohar, J., Insel, T.R., Zohar-Kadouch, R.C. and Murphy, D.L., 1988. Serotonergic responsivity in obsessive–compulsive disorder: effects of clomipramine treatment. *Archives of General Psychiatry*, **45**, 167–172.

XIX-2

Aminergic Transmitter Systems

Neil McNaughton

INTRODUCTION

A fundamental goal of biological psychiatry should be the separation of symptoms from syndromes. It is clear, for example, that 'headache' is not an appropriate diagnostic category. You cannot use it to define the treatment of the underlying disorder giving rise to the symptom. Nor is the regular decrease in headache symptoms produced by aspirin or paracetamol evidence for common aetiology of the causes of headache or for an 'analgesic insufficiency' as the primary cause of headache.

This problem is particularly acute with mood disorders. In the case of depression, which at first blush seems more coherent as an entity than the spectrum of 'anxiety disorders',

> 'in the DSM-III the "choice principle" was introduced. For the diagnosis of a particular syndrome the presence of X out of a list of Y symptoms suffices, no matter which ones. Hence the various disorders that are distinguished are symptomatologically ill defined. In fact, many different syndromes carry the same designation: major depression and dysthymia.... The utility of the ... discrete diagnostic entities characterized by multiple criteria ... is questionable. Our studies at least have failed to validate them.... Another fundamental shortcoming ... is the lack of an aetiological axis [since] with today's methodologies, one can arrive at an aetiological hypothesis with no less reliability as one can regarding the presence or absence and severity of particular psychopathological symptoms.... Another [problem] is that of [classification in the presence of] comorbidity ... For the diagnosis of major depression, psychotic and organic conditions have to be ruled out. The diagnosis of generalized anxiety disorder cannot be made in the presence of a mood disorder.
>
> This principle is not applicable in biological psychiatry. One can and should not simply discart [*sic*] the possibility that a biological variable observed in a psychotic condition is linked to a concurrent depression, or one found in depression is in fact related to an anxiety disorder....
>
> For [these] reasons I consider these concepts unsuited for [mood disorder] research, particularly biological research, requiring as it does well-defined and assessable diagnostic concepts.'
>
> Van Praag (1995, p. 270)

The problem of comorbidity may be even more acute in the diagnosis of anxiety disorders. For example, panic and obsession, *as disorders*, may well have no necessary connection to anxiety as such. Rather, each may be an indirect cause of, essentially 'normal', anxiety when they occur (as unexpected, uncontrollable and bizarre events) in someone with a pre-existing sensitivity to threatening events. Conversely, both panic and obsession can occur as a simple, non-pathological, consequence of high levels of anxiety. Even this anxiety need not be pathological — consider the obsessive behaviour of a parent with a young and extremely mobile child at an airport.

Syndrome identification faces two additional problems. First, is a lack of connection between cause and treatment. A purely cognitively mediated post-traumatic stress disorder can nonetheless result in brain damage and require pharmacological treatment. Panic attacks resulting from a neural disturbance may be best treated psychologically — resolving the anxiety-related problems engendered by the panic attacks without completely eliminating the latter (Franklin, 1990). Other exclusion criteria, such as the exclusion by 'DSM-III-R [of] persons with socially phobic symptoms secondary to axis III conditions ... [such as] disfiguring or disabling conditions [can lack] empirical basis.... [and cause] a patient group [to be] overlooked with regard to treatment options' (Oberlander, Schneier and Liebowitz, 1994).

A final problem for diagnosis is that the grouping of 'anxiety disorders' as a single class in DSM-III, DSM-IIR and DSM-IV seems inappropriate from the point of view of pharmacology or preclinical analysis of brain systems. These suggest that the different symptomatologies and therapeutic responses of patients presenting with 'anxiety disorders' reflects a confusion of diagnostic categories. Diagnoses should, but currently do not, reflect the primary brain systems that are dysfunctional in any particular case. Symptomatology must often reflect the brain systems, whether functional or dysfunctional, that have extremes of activity. For both these reasons, brains systems will be the focus of the next section.

The most significant aminergic neurotransmitter systems for anxiety and the conventional grouping of anxiety disorders are the monoamines serotonin and noradrenaline. As discussed in the section entitled 'The Neuropsychology of the aminergic systems' basic research implicates them as modulators of the entire defense system with a clear contribution to anxiety — in the sense that this can be distinguished from fear (Blanchard *et al.*, 1988, 1991, 1997). Drugs that manipulate them have therapeutic effects that usually span several of the different types of anxiety disorder (den Boer *et al.*, Chapter XIX-13). Finally, disturbances of their metabolism appear to play a significant role in the generation of anxiety disorders (see below). A weaker case can, also, be made for dopamine. The preclinical review below will also include consideration of acetylcholine because, although not a monoamine, it shares many of the anatomical and functional features of the monoamines.

The primary conclusion is that the success or failure of treatment with a particular drug is likely to reflect the secondary impact of alteration in monoamines on primary brain systems more often than an original disturbance of monoamines was the primary basis of the symptomatology.

THE NEUROPSYCHOLOGY OF ANXIETY

The view of the neuropsychology of anxiety disorders in this chapter is justified at great length in Gray and McNaughton

Biological Psychiatry: Edited by H. D'haenen, J.A. den Boer and P. Willner. ISBN 0-471-49198-5

(Gray and McNaughton, 2000) and in its appendices available at http://www.oup.co.uk/academic/medicine/medical_updates/neuropsych_anxiety/ (see also Mohanty and Heller, Chapter XVIII-7).

The most important point to note is that, for each anxiety disorder or symptom recognized by the DSM and ICD classifications, there appears to be a distinct pharmacological specificity (Table XIX-2.1). This specificity is demonstrated by dissociations produced by particular drugs (e.g., buspirone affects anxiety and depression but not panic) and can be obscured in the clinical setting by the fact that a number of drugs can have concurrent but distinct effects on different 'anxiety disorders'. Indeed, clinicians will tend to prefer less specific drugs as a means of protecting against incorrect diagnosis.

Together with much other data (Gray and McNaughton, 2000), this allows us to allocate each symptom and/or syndrome to a specific portion of a hierarchically organized defense system (Figure XIX-2.1). However, this allocation does not allow us to assign a particular symptomatology to pathology in a particular area and so use it to define a particular syndrome. For example, a primary panic disorder (arising, say, from paroxysmal activity in the periaqueductal gray) could result in panic attacks. Given the effects of arousal on panic, full blown attacks are more likely to occur in a public place. Any particular place occasioning the first attack will condition anticipatory anxiety and so an increased probability of panic. The resultant increased general arousal would increase the probability of panic in other locations. Thus conditioning would produce agoraphobia as a symptom not a cause. But this would be likely to be diagnosed as agoraphobia proper. Panic attacks would then be both a primary cause of anxiety *and* a secondary consequence. Conversely, a primary anxiety disorder (conceivably presenting as agoraphobia) could result in panic attacks as a symptom of extreme anxiety (Goisman *et al.*, 1995; Marks, 1987). Indeed, a pure primary 'panic disorder' might not be diagnosed as such unless it was accompanied by additional symptoms resulting from its interaction with a neurotic personality and its resultant production of symptoms of anxiety (Holt, 1990; Gray and McNaughton, 2000).

Table XIX-2.1 Various classes of drugs effective in treating neurotic disorders and their relative effects on different neurotic syndromes and the extent to which they share classical anxiolytic side effects (muscle relaxant; anticonvulsant, sedative, addictive). Exceptional effects of individual members of a class are ignored (e.g., the antidepressant and panicolytic actions of benzodiazepines such as alprazolam). It should be noted that antidepressant monoamine oxidase inhibitors (MAOI), in particular phenelzine, are unlike novel anxiolytics (novel) such as buspirone and tricyclic drugs such as imipramine (IMI) that have separate anxiolytic and antidepressant action. They treat depression but also appear particularly effective in treating atypical depression (in which many symptoms overlap anxiety disorders but are resistant to anxiolytic drugs). They have not been reported to be effective in generalized anxiety

	Class	Novel	IMI	CMI	MAOI	SSRI
Phobia	0	?	?	?	?	?
Generalized Anxiety	–	–	–	–	0?	–
Panic Attacks	0	0	–	—	–	–
Obsessions/Compulsions	0	?	(–)	—	(–)	—
Atypical Depression	0	?	(–)	?	–	?
Unipolar Depression	0	–	–	–	–	–
Classical Anxiolytic Side Effects	=	#	0	0	0	(#)

Class, classical anxiolytics such as benzodiazepines, barbiturates and meprobamate; CMI, Clomipramine; 0, no effect; –, reduction; —, extensive reduction; +, increase; ( ), small or discrepant effects; =, same as classical anxiolytics; #, opposite to classical anxiolytics. Adapted from Gray and McNaughton (2000), see also den Boer *et al.* Chapter XIX-13.

THE NEUROPSYCHOLOGY OF THE AMINERGIC SYSTEMS[1]

The general form of the anatomy of the different aminergic systems is very similar (see also previous chapter). This is shown in cartoon form in Figure XIX-2.2. For example, serotonergic cell bodies are located in the raphe nuclei of the brainstem. From there, they send projections forward making collateral connections with many structures before innervating the cortex fairly diffusely. 'Early studies that used older tracing techniques reported exceedingly few [descending] projections from the dorsal raphe (DR) to the brainstem.... [However, there are] moderate to dense projections from the DR [to] pontomesencephalic central gray, mesencephalic reticular nucleus pontis oralis, nucleus pontis caudalis, locus coeruleus, laterodorsal tegmental nucleus, and raphe nuclei, including the central linear nucleus, median raphe nucleus, and raphe pontis' (Vertes and Kocsis, 1994, p. 340). Of particular interest in relation to anxiety disorders, there is serotonergic input to the periaqueductal gray, the hypothalamus, the amygdala, the septo-hippocampal system and the frontal and cingulate cortex (see e.g., Handley, 1995, Fig. 1). As can be seen from Figure XIX-2.1, these structures essentially represent the entirety of the defense system and collectively are involved in the entire spectrum of clinical anxiety disorder.

This anatomy suggests that the aminergic systems are modulatory of other structures in a very general sense. They originate in very small, often caudally placed, nuclei and then innervate huge areas of the forebrain via multiple collaterals. Their fibres, as a group, follow three basic paths (Gaykema *et al.*, 1990; Jacobs and Azmitia, 1992) which 'appear to have remained remarkably stable across phylogeny' (Jacobs and Azmitia, 1992, p. 179). The most ventral innervation of the telencephalon usually involves fibres that send collaterals into the amygdala *en passage* to the temporal portion of the hippocampus. Next there are fibres that pass through the septal area in the medial forebrain bundle and then run in the fornix/fimbria, just under the corpus callosum (the light grey band in Figure XIX-2.2) to innervate the septal portion of the hippocampus. The third path is taken by fibres primarily destined for the cortex. They pass over the corpus callosum peeling off progressively from the cingulum bundle to innervate the neocortex. At its most caudal extent the cingulum bundle provides some fibres that innervate the septal parts of the hippocampus, retrosplenially (Azmitia and Segal, 1978). The dopaminergic system is the most rostral and least diffuse of these systems.

In the case of the noradrenergic system conventional synapses are formed only in the dentate gyrus (Koda, Schulman and Bloom, 1978) and the lack of specialization of the bulk of terminals suggests release of noradrenaline is more neurohormonal than as a neurotransmitter (Descarries, Watkins and Lapierre, 1977; Shimizu *et al.*, 1979).

Nonetheless, there appears to be differentiation of cells even in the locus coeruleus with respect to targets (McNaughton and Mason, 1980). For the other aminergic systems there are discrete components, originating in different nuclei that then have both distinct and overlapping projections compared to other aminergic nuclei.

The amine systems are very similar in anatomy to the ascending cholinergic system. Their similarity to it in function will also be discussed below and, although this does not appear particularly significant for clinical pathology, the amine systems and cholinergic systems have extensive reciprocal interactions with each other. The cholinergic system has a basically similar anatomy to the amine systems but there is better evidence that its connections to the

[1] This section (except for 'Dopaminergic Systems') is a summary of the relevant portions of Appendix 10 of Gray and McNaughton (2000). Many of the ideas are either those of J.A. Gray or arose in discussion with him. Where no reference is given for a statement it can be found at http://www.oup.co.uk/academic/medicine/medical_updates/neuropsych_anxiety/app10/.

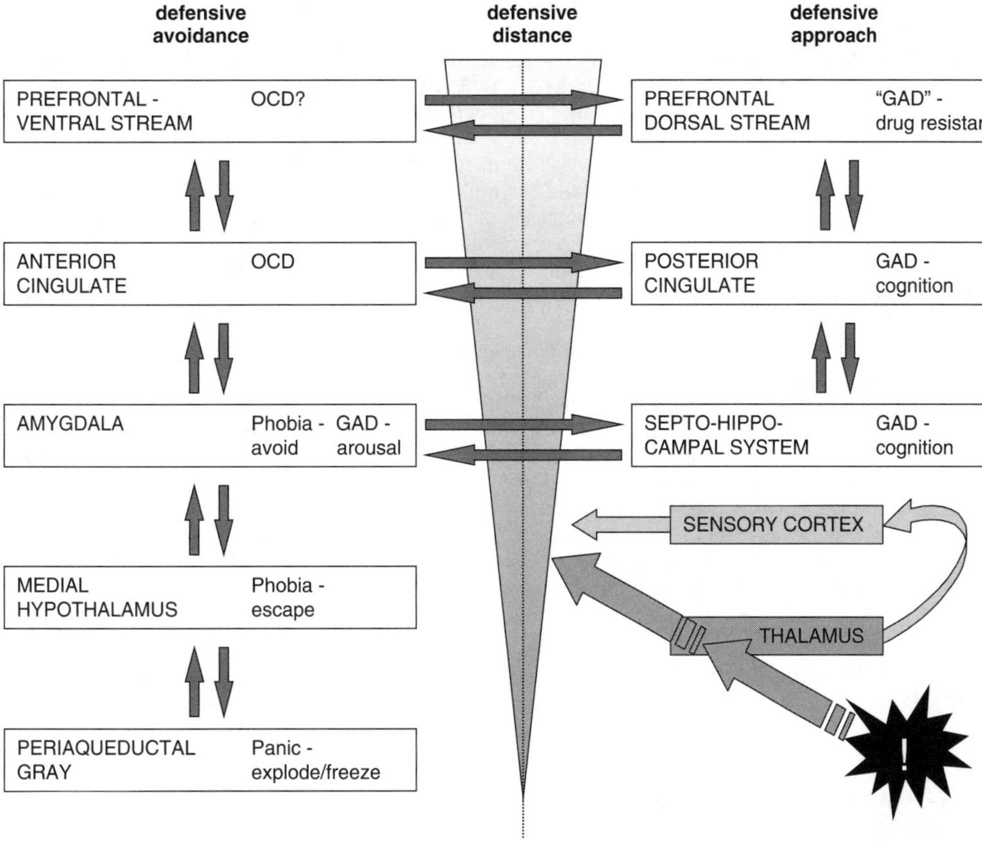

Figure XIX-2.1 A two-dimensional view of the neural systems controlling defense and their relation to neurotic disorders. There is a hierarchy of reciprocally connected neural systems (Graeff, 1994) in which control of behaviour is exerted by the lowest levels when danger is most immediate with control passing to progressively higher levels as the danger becomes less immediate (see also Table XIX-2.3, Figure XIX-2.3). This reflects a dimension of 'defensive distance' (Blanchard and Blanchard, 1989, 1990). In addition there is an essentially orthogonal dimension of defensive direction (Gray and McNaughton, 2000). Avoidance of a dangerous situation and approach into a dangerous situation are controlled by distinct sets of structures. The perception of defensive distance and direction depends on processing by sensory systems that can also be viewed as hierarchical. Signals of danger (!) activate a 'quick and dirty' route through the thalamus that can initiate immediate action if a crude assessment of the situation suggests this is necessary and also activate, in parallel, slower and more sophisticated cortical processing that can confirm or cancel the action or inaction resulting from the crude assessment (LeDoux, 1994, 1998). Figure adapted from Gray and McNaughton (2000), Figures 1.8 and 11.1

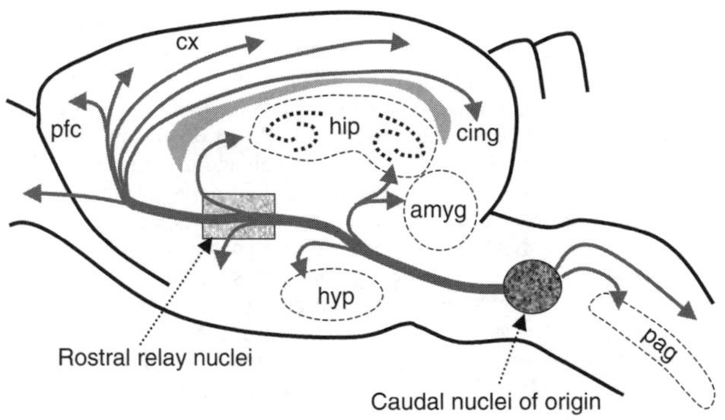

Figure XIX-2.2 A schematic overview of the general anatomy of the aminergic and cholinergic systems. In general, nuclei of origin are relatively caudal and then may relay more rostrally. There tend to be few cells with many collaterals providing diffuse innervation of much of the forebrain. There appears to be some topographic anatomical organization of the systems but relatively little functional differentiation between the parts. The dopamine system is the most rostral, most differentiated, and least diffuse. The cholinergic system originates most caudally, appears functionally least differentiated (see text), and is most diffuse. For the detailed anatomy of each system, see Gray and McNaughton (2000) Figures 6.5, 6.6 and 6.7

forebrain are highly topographically organized (Gaykema *et al.*, 1990, 1992; Zaborszky *et al.*, 1997). The cholinergic system is different from the amine systems in having the most caudally placed nuclei of origin and, possibly as a consequence, having extensive relay nuclei in the basal forebrain. However, functionally, the superficially more differentiated cholinergic nuclei and pathways appear to be part of a coherent, diffuse system originating in the pons (McNaughton *et al.*, 1997, 2001; Swain-Campbell and McNaughton, 2001).

For all the aminergic systems, and the cholinergic system, there is evidence both for a general modulatory role and some capacity of the systems to select subsets of targets of that modulation. The preclinical data on each of these systems is summarized below in alphabetical order followed by an overview of them as contributing to a common general modulation of higher systems. This preclinical summary provides a skeleton for the body of interpretation of the clinically oriented data in the section entitled 'Aminergic involvement in clinical anxiety'.

Cholinergic Systems

Neither anti- nor pro-cholinergic drugs are generally used clinically as anxiolytics. However, systemic or specific intracranial anticholinergic dysfunctions have not only similar behavioural effects to noradrenergic and serotonergic dysfunction, but also similar neural effects. They all change the signal-to-noise ratio in targets such as the hippocampus and amygdala. Yet, in man, the anticholinergics are amnestic rather than anxiolytic; and some pro-cholinergic drugs may even be anxiolytic (see Brioni *et al.*, 1994; Garvey *et al.*, 1994).

The similar behavioural profiles of nominally 'anxiolytic' and nominally 'amnestic' treatments may reflect a partial overlap in functions. Benzodiazepines block the release of acetylcholine onto cortical targets and this could underlie some but not all of their behavioural effects (Anglade *et al.*, 1994; Sarter and Bruno, 1994). Anticholinergic drugs, by contrast, probably do not produce their amnestic effects via release of endogenous benzodiazepine ligands and there are definite cases where cholinergic dysfunction produces neural effects quite unlike those of anxiolytics (Gray and McNaughton, 2000, Appendix 10).

There are few reports of the effects of specific cholinergic lesions on behaviour. The effects of systemic anticholinergic (usually antimuscarinic) drugs have been well studied (Bignami, 1976; Aigner, 1995) and a superficial resemblance to the behavioural profile of anxiolytic drugs can be seen in the general release of behavioural inhibition they produce (Carlton, 1969). However, they differ from anxiolytics in that they impair some learning tasks in which there is no behavioural inhibition and, consistent with this, acetylcholine is released when simple learning is occurring (Orsetti, Casamenti and Pepeu, 1996).

> 'While there is little doubt that manipulation of cholinergic function can rather specifically alter offensive behaviour in a variety of species, evidence also supports a role for central muscarinic receptors in defensive responding.... Antimuscarinics have ... been reported to inhibit shock-induced defensive fighting in rats and mice ... Under more naturalistic test conditions ... scopolamine reduced fear reactions in laboratory rats confronted with a cat ... reduced fear was indicated by consummatory behaviour in the presence of the cat, more approaches to the cat enclosure and less freezing'.
>
> Rodgers *et al.* (1990, p. 575)

More detailed ethological analysis of the role of anticholinergics in fear and anxiety, respectively suggests they do not alter 'avoidance, freezing, defensive threat or attack in wild *Rattus rattus* confronted by the experimenter and other threat-related stimuli ... During cat exposure, however, [they] ... increased the amount of time spent in the vicinity of the cat, increased scanning and rearing, and reduced grooming behaviour. Although reliable, the latter effects were not pronounced' (Rodgers *et al.*, 1990, p. 575). Rather than a genuinely anxiolytic effect this suggests 'a situation- and response-dependent alteration in mechanisms of selective attention' (op. cit. p. 581). However, even in the 'ethological' form of the elevated-plus-maze test of anxiety anticholinergics are anxiogenic (Rodgers and Cole, 1995). Likewise, anticholinergics can reduce fear conditioning to a tone while leaving conditioning to context intact. Hippocampal lesions have the opposite effect, while amygdala lesions affect both (Young, Bohenek and Fanselow, 1995).

Overall then, while the cholinergic system may influence anxiety in a variety of ways these appear to be both anxiolytic and anxiogenic depending on other factors. Like peripheral injections of adrenaline or the partial pressure of carbon dioxide, then, it appears to be able to influence central systems controlling anxiety without being a fundamental component of such systems.

Dopaminergic Systems

There are two main dopaminergic systems innervating the forebrain that only partially conform to the picture of Figure XIX-2.2. 'A dorsal tier of dopamine neurons receive input from the ventral (limbic-related) striatum and from the amygdala and [largely as the mesolimbic system] project widely throughout cortex. A more ventrally located group of dopamine cells receives input from both the limbic and association areas of striatum and projects widely [largely as the nigro-striatal system] throughout the striatum, including the sensorimotor region. Through these projections the limbic system has an enormous influence on dopamine output and can therefore affect the emotional and motivational "colouring" of a wide range of behaviours' (Haber and Fudge, 1997). We will focus here on the more ventrally coursing mesolimbic system and, in particular, its projections to prefrontal cortex (PFC). While strongly implicated in schizophrenia, this input to prefrontal cortex appears also to be involved in anxiety and depression.

The initial component of the ventral system is the dopaminergic input from the ventral tegmental area (VTA) to the nucleus accumbens (or more fully nucleus accumbens septi, NAS). This system is presented in texts as being a 'reward pathway'. However,

> 'Stress consistently has been found to activate peripheral and central catecholamine systems. Dopamine turnover in the prefrontal cortex is especially sensitive to stress produced by relatively mild footshock, conditioned fear or exposure to a novel cage.... electrolytic lesions of the central nucleus of the amygdala significantly attenuated the increase in DA turnover in the prefrontal cortex normally seen after mild stress.... Dopamine neurons in the ventral tegmental area receive direct input from the central nucleus of the amygdala ... Stress may activate ... the central nucleus of the amygdala. In turn this could activate dopamine cells in the ventral tegmental area that project to prefrontal cortex and thereby increase dopamine turnover in this brain area.'
>
> Davis *et al.* (1994)

We will deal later with the peculiarity that stress increases PFC dopamine by double the amount of NAS dopamine (which in turn is about double the amount of striatal dopamine release) in contrast to the fact that 'the noradrenergic projections to forebrain appear to respond to stress in a uniform manner' (Abercrombie *et al.*, 1989). What is needed at this point is

> 'a unifying interpretation that can account for the functions of NAS DA in a variety of behavioural contexts: (1) its role in appetitive behavioural arousal, (2) its role as a facilitator as well as an induced of reward processes, and (3) its presently undefined role in aversive contexts.... NAS DA [appears to] facilitate flexible approach responses.... Fixed instrumental approach responses (habits) ... involve the nigro-striatal system more.... NAS DA [operates] in two stages: unconditioned behavioural invigoration effects and incentive learning effects. (1) When organisms are presented with salient stimuli (e.g., novel stimuli and incentive stimuli), NAS DA is released and invigorates flexible approach responses. (2) When proximal exteroceptive receptors are stimulated by unconditioned stimuli, NAS DA is released and enables stimulus representations to acquire incentive properties with specific environmental context [*sic*].... Both conditioned and unconditioned aversive stimuli stimulate DA release in the NAS [because] NAS DA invigorates *approach responses* toward 'safety'. Moreover, NAS DA modulates incentive properties of the environment so that organisms emit *approach responses* toward 'safety' (i.e. avoidance responses) when animals later encounter similar environmental contexts.'
>
> Ikemoto and Panksepp (1999) [my italics]

In this view, dopamine release is not a sign of aversion even in aversive paradigms. Indeed 'brief aversive foot shock delivered for the first time does not increase NAS DA, but NAS DA levels increase more and more as,... with succeeding trials, animals develop more effective approach to safety strategies' (op. cit.). The increase in dopamine release during avoidance learning to some extent parallels that of corticosterone — which ceases to be released as avoidance becomes perfect, and so shock is no longer delivered (Coover, Ursin and Levine, 1973). However, with repeated inescapable stress, dopamine is not released during the stress but only after it. In this, 'the activation of the mesolimbic dopaminergic system induced by aversive stimuli adapts to repeated experiences differently from that produced by pleasurable events' (Imperato *et al.*, 1992). It also contrasts with both noradrenaline and corticosterone. Like dopamine, they are not released by shock initially. But unlike dopamine they continue to be released in response to conditioned fear (Brady, 1975a, 1975b).

Thus, in aversive paradigms the release of dopamine appears to equate with 'relieving non-punishment'. It is released by the omission of an expected punisher. Such omission can been equated functionally with reward (Gray, 1975) since stimuli associated with either will elicit approach and are functionally antagonistic to aversive events. In this view the 'anxiolytic' effects of D2 agonists (Bartoszyk, 1998) may reflect the antagonistic relationship between punishers and rewards when these are associated — an antagonism that is not affected by conventional anxiolytic drugs (McNaughton and Gray, 1983). Conversely, desensitization of these receptors by, for example, repeated methamphetamine administration could have the inverse effect (Tsuchiya, Inoue and Koyama, 1996).

The peculiarities of the PFC dopaminergic input remain to be dealt with. As noted above this often shows a greater release of dopamine to aversive stimuli than does the NAS. More surprisingly, unstressed rats can show a DA increase in PFC to both appetitive and aversive stimulation at times when the NAS shows an increase to appetitive but a decrease to aversive stimuli (Di Chiara, Loddo and Tanda, 1999). After chronic mild stress, the responses to appetitive stimuli decreased and to aversive stimuli increased in both areas — with the NAS response to aversive stimuli reversing to the increase commonly observed.

> 'We have proposed that NAS shell DA is involved in associative learning and in the acquisition of motivation, whereas PFC DA is involved in its motor expression. ... [It is through] phasic DA transmission in the NAS shell ... [that] stimuli are attributed a motivational value that reflects the biological value of the stimulus ... [hence] D_1 antagonists ... impair the acquisition of conditioned place preference and place aversion. ... This hypothesis interprets the symptoms of anhedonia, lack of interest, and loss of self esteem that are typical of depression as the result of blunting of appetitive motivation; it interprets feelings of worthlessness and guilt ... as the result of enhancement of aversive motivation. ... [These] changes in DA responsiveness are [likely to be] secondary to a primary dysfunction of tonic noradrenergic transmission. ... The relative ineffectiveness of dopamine agonists as antidepressants [is because] increase of tonic DA transmission by a DA agonist would not correct the dysfunction in phasic DA responsiveness that takes place in depression.'
>
> Di Chiara *et al.* (1999)

Thus, at least part of the distinctive dopamine release in PFC would be due to increased noradrenaline release acting on dopaminergic terminals presynaptically. Increased noradrenaline release in PFC increases dopamine levels and decreased noradrenaline release decreases dopamine levels, suggesting a tonic modulation (Gresch *et al.*, 1995). Further, an initial brief experience of stress can release noradrenaline without dopamine or serotonin, with the latter released in addition on a second experience (Jordan *et al.*, 1994). Release of noradrenaline may then produce sensitization of dopaminergic and serotonergic terminals. However, part could also be due to selective activation of a small pool of VTA and NAS cells projecting only to PFC, as occurs with purely cognitively mediated stress in the absence of concurrent release of noradrenaline or serotonin (Kaneyuki *et al.*, 1991). These authors even suggest that inhibition of VTA DA neurons may be 'implicated in the specific anxiolytic action of benzodiazepines'. Certainly, very large doses of benzodiazepines reduce stress-induced dopamine release in PFC (Feenstra, Botterblom and Van Uum, 1995) and, like the anxiolytic effects of benzodiazepines, this does not show tolerance (Hegarty and Vogel, 1995). But chronic stress eliminates the effect (Finlay, Zigmond and Abercrombie, 1995).

There are three main reasons for rejecting this point of view. First, is the fact that prefrontal lesions are effective in treating anxiety that is resistant to conventional anxiolytic drugs. Anxiolytic action on prefrontal dopamine could be a component of their effects — but prefrontal cortex clearly contains additional anxiety-related mechanisms. Second, rapid sampling of extracellular dopamine in the rat prefrontal cortex during food consumption, handling and exposure to novelty found the response was graded to the general intensity rather than valence of stimuli with 'emotional arousal [being] a common denominator'. Interestingly, in this study dopamine release outlasted, e.g., eating by 10–20 min (Feenstra and Botterblom, 1996). Third, data (Espejo, 1997) that suggest that PFC DA 'activation reflects either heightened attention or activation of cognitive processes [that is] a general phenomenon in various adaptive situations'. PFC DA depletion *increased* + maze anxiety while decreasing motility. 'The findings confirm that prefrontocortical dopamine activation is necessary for coping with an anxiogenic challenge, allowing the animal to display adaptive exploratory responses in a fear-inducing environment' (op. cit.).

Thus, for prefrontal dopamine we seem justified in borrowing the conclusion of Ikemoto and Panksepp for NAS dopamine. 'Both conditioned and unconditioned aversive stimuli stimulate DA release [to] invigorate approach responses toward "safety" [and] modulate incentive properties of the environment so that organisms emit approach responses toward "safety" (i.e. avoidance responses) when animals later encounter similar environmental contexts.'

Noradrenergic Systems

The locus coeruleus is the nucleus of origin of ascending noradrenergic fibres that has been most clearly implicated in the control of anxiety. Further, receptors for the benzodiazepine-GABA complex exist in the locus coeruleus and probably mediate some part of the action of classical anxiolytics (Iversen and Schon, 1973). A major output from the locus coeruleus travels in the dorsal noradrenergic bundle (DANB) and follows the general plan of Figure XIX-2.2, reaching frontal cortex, cingulate cortex, pyriform cortex, hippocampal formation, amygdala, thalamus, hypothalamus and basal forebrain. A second output, the ventral noradrenergic bundle travels more ventrally and innervates more ventral structures including an innervation of the hypothalamus and septum that overlaps that of the dorsal bundle (Moore and Bloom, 1979; Owen *et al.*, 1982). The ventral bundle also carries fibres from other noradrenergic nuclei.

The anatomy of the ascending noradrenergic system limits its possible functions. There are only about 1500 cells in the locus coeruleus of the rat and these innervate huge regions of the brain, including the olfactory bulb, much of the neocortex, the hippocampus, septal area and amygdala, some thalamic and hypothalamic nuclei, the geniculate bodies, the cerebellum, and the spinal cord. Although there is some topographic organization, each cell projects to multiple areas (Olson and Fuxe, 1971; Pickel, Krebs and Bloom, 1973). The system cannot, therefore, carry large volumes of data and is likely to be generally modulatory.

Consistent with this, noradrenergic activity increases throughout the brain in response to aversive stimuli (Segal, 1978) and stress, and specifically to increases in corticotropin-releasing hormone (Valentino, Foote and Page, 1993; Smagin, Swiergiel and Dunn, 1995), with a significant part of this being due to outflow from the locus coeruleus (Corrodi *et al.*, 1971). This increase may be a significant component of stress-induced anxiety since it is blocked by classical anxiolytics. Novel anxiolytics tend to increase locus coeruleus firing (Trulson and Henderson, 1984; Wilkinson *et al.*, 1987) but this appears to be an effect of feedback from presynaptic blockade of noradrenergic terminals by $5HT_{1A}$ agonists. So, all classes of anxiolytic drug appear to block the release of central noradrenaline.

However, novel stimuli and reward can also release noradrenaline. Like dopamine, then, it seems less specifically concerned with aversion than generally related to arousal in the sense of activation of the ascending reticular activating system or the regulation of attention or vigilance (Aston-Jones, Chiang and Alexinsky, 1991).

A role in vigilance would account for changes in noradrenergic output in relation to sleep phases without a role for noradrenaline in the control of sleep itself and for the release of noradrenaline by unconditioned stimuli and 'by stimuli which are not themselves intense or conspicuous, but are salient to the animal by virtue of conditioning' (Aston-Jones *et al.*, 1994, p. 4468). Thus, when the significance of stimuli is changed, noradrenergic cell firing shifts to the new target stimulus (Aston-Jones *et al.*, 1994; see also Rajkowski, Kubiak and Aston-Jones, 1994).

Detailed comparison of the effects of anxiolytic drugs with lesions of the DANB (Table XIX-2.2) shows some interesting parallels and dissociations. Where anxiolytics are without effect so too are DANB lesions. Likewise, where DANB lesions have an effect it is essentially the same as those of anxiolytics drugs, in size as well as nature. However, there are a substantial number of anxiolytic-sensitive tasks where DANB lesions are totally without effect. A review of the electrophysiological evidence suggests that inhibition of release of noradrenaline by anxiolytic drugs (acting at cell bodies in the case of classical anxiolytics and at terminals in the case of novel anxiolytics) accounts for part of the behavioural profile of the anxiolytics. This could include the slight pro-convulsant effect of buspirone and anxiolytic SSRIs (Ferraro *et al.*, 1994; Kokaia *et al.*, 1994).

Table XIX-2.2 Comparison of the common effects of classical and novel anxiolytics (Anx), common effects of lesions of the septum and hippocampus (S = H), lesions of the amygdala (Amyg), lesions of the dorsal ascending noradrenergic bundle (NA), lesions of the ascending serotonergic system (5HT) and systemic blockade of muscarinic cholinergic systems (ACh). Adapted from Gray and McNaughton (2000)

	Anx	S = H	Amyg	NA	5HT	ACh
Simple rewarded learning	0	0	0	0	0	–
Simultaneous spatial discrimination	0	0	?	0	?	?
Defecation	0	0	?	0	?	?
Escape	0	0	–	0	0	?
Frustration	0	0	–	0	?	?
1-way avoid	0	0	–	0	?	0
Aggression	+	–	–	0	–	?
Fixed Interval	–	–	0	0	?	0
Water maze	–	–	0	0	?	–
Reversal	(–)	–	0/–	0	?	?
DRL	–	–	–	0	–	–
Social Interaction	–	–?	–	0	–	?
Passive avoidance	–	–	–	0/–	–	–
Non-spatial Avoidance	+	+	?	0	?	+
2-way avoidance	+	+	–	0/+	?	+
PREE	–	–	0	–	?	?
Rearing	–	–	+	–	–	–
Conditioned freezing	–	–	–	–	?	?
Extinction	–	–	–	–	–/0	–
Successive discrimination	–	–	–	–	0	–
Single alternation	–	?	–	–	?	?
Spontaneous alternation	–	–	–	–	?	–
Conditioned suppression on baseline	–	0	–	–	–	?

A partial involvement of noradrenaline in the effects of anxiolytic drugs and, by implication, the control of anxiety is understandable if it is a quite general arousing system similar in function to the old idea of the reticular activating system (Magoun, 1963). Such arousal, in aversive situations, would normally be termed alarm and even, in some meanings of the word, 'anxiety'. Thus, release of noradrenaline, centrally, is like activation of the sympathetic system peripherally (Aston-Jones, Chiang and Alexinsky, 1991; Van Bockstaele and Aston-Jones, 1995; Haller, Makara and Kruk, 1998).

On the other hand, noradrenergic cells 'decreased tonic discharge ... during certain high arousal behaviours (grooming and consumption) when attention (vigilance) was low.... The most effective and reliable stimuli for eliciting LC responses were those that disrupted behaviour and evoked orienting responses' (Aston-Jones, Chiang and Alexinsky, 1991, pp. 501). So, 'LC cells respond to novelty or change in incoming information, but do not have a sustained response to stimuli, even when these have a high level of biological significance' (Sara, Vankov and Hervé, 1994). Central release of noradrenaline would, then, increase vigilance to external events consistent with the fact that it increases the neural signal-to-noise ratio (Gray & McNaughton, 2000, Appendix 10).

The effect of noradrenaline is not limited to stimulus processing. Its release also increases the vigour of ongoing behaviour (Aston-Jones *et al.*, 1994), another echo of the effects of dopamine. The noradrenergic system, then, appears important for general vigilance and reactivity to stimuli (including, of course, aversive stimuli) but does not equate with arousal in the sense that this can be high when external stimuli are being ignored.

Of particular relevance to clinical anxiety and its relation to depression is the specific case of such effects of noradrenaline on aggressive behaviour.

> 'Hormonal catecholamines (adrenaline and noradrenaline) appear to be involved in metabolic preparations for the prospective fight; the sympathetic system ensures appropriate cardiovascular reaction, while the CNS noradrenergic system prepares the animal for the prospective fight. Indirect CNS effects include: the shift of attention towards socially relevant stimuli; the enhancement of olfaction...; the decrease in pain sensitivity; and the enhancement of memory (an aggressive encounter is very relevant to the future of the animal).... [However, while] a slight activation of the central noradrenergic systems stimulates aggression, a strong activation decreases fight readiness. This biphasic effect may allow the animal to engage or to avoid the conflict, depending on the strength of social challenge.'
>
> Haller, Makara and Kruk (1998)

Serotonergic Systems

Central serotonin has previously been postulated to be involved in anxiety (Iversen, 1984) and in specifically anxiolytic action (Moon *et al.*, 1994) but also appears implicated in many other psychiatric disorders (Swerdlow, 1995; Boulenguez *et al.*, 1998; Collier *et al.*, 1996; De Oliveira *et al.*, 1998; Dean *et al.*, 1995; Gobert *et al.*, 2000; Gurevich and Joyce, 1997; Laruelle *et al.*, 1993; Leonard, 1996; Naylor *et al.*, 1996; Sumiyoshi *et al.*, 1996). The serotonergic system conforms to the general plan of Figure XIX-2.2. However, there is noticeable anatomical differentiation within it that is significant for the possible role of different areas in the causes of anxiety. This differentiation cuts across the differentiation of receptor subtypes that is significant for the treatment of anxiety.

'The median raphe supplies the dorsal hippocampus and medial septum, the proposed origins of the Behaviour Inhibition System, while the dorsal raphe nucleus innervates the lateral septum and ventral hippocampus, the possible origin of safety signalling. The amygdala, the "head nucleus" of the Defence System, is almost entirely supplied by the dorsal raphe nucleus.'

Handley (1995, p. 108–109)

This differentiation is not complete, as there are minor contributions of, e.g., the dorsal raphe to the septo-hippocampal system. In particular, the dorsal raphe sends projections (which may well be collaterals of the same source cells and hence carry the same information} to the periaqueductal gray (5HT2/1C receptors); ... the amygdala (5HT1A receptors), the ventral striatum (5HT1D receptors), the hippocampus (5HT1A receptors), and the frontal cortex (5HT2 receptors). It can therefore have widespread effects on the defense system.

The dorsal raphe does not appear totally committed to defense, however, since it seems 'to play a role in modulating circadian rhythms ... [and] these modulations may be, in part, mediated by the [direct] retinal projection to the periaqueductal gray and serotonin neurons in the dorsal raphe nucleus' (Shen and Semba, 1994, p. 166; see also review by Morin, 1994). Although there are fewer data on central serotonergic lesions than noradrenergic there are enough to reinforce this conclusion. Inspection of Table XIX-2.2, shows that to a large extent, like noradrenergic lesions, serotonergic lesions have no effect when anxiolytics have an effect and that when serotonergic lesions have an effect so do anxiolytics. Also, as with noradrenergic lesions, there are many cases where anxiolytics have an effect but serotonergic lesions do not. Strikingly, these blanks in the serotonergic and noradrenergic profiles appear to complement each other so that the effects of anxiolytics could, perhaps, be accounted for by concurrent suppression of central noradrenergic and serotonergic function. If this is true then neither system can, by itself, be the basis for anxiety.

Table XIX-2.3 Levels of threat processing and related levels of neural integration. Adapted by Gray and McNaughton (2000) from Graeff (1994)

Level of processing	Behaviour	Neural substrate
Potential danger (to approach)	Risk assessment and Behavioural Inhibition	Posterior Cingulate Septo-Hippocampal System
Potential danger (to avoid)	Avoidance	Anterior Cingulate Amygdala
Distal danger	Escape Inhibition of Aggression	Medial Hypothalamus
Proximal danger	Freezing Flight Fight	Periaqueductal grey

Graeff (1993) (see also Graeff *et al.*, 1996; Graeff and Zangrossi, Chapter XIX-1) provides a detailed analysis of the role of serotonin in the defense system. His starting point is a unidimensional hierarchical view of threat processing which in a slightly modified form (Table XIX-2.3) is the foundation on which the two-dimensional Figure XIX-2.1 was constructed and a further dimension of avoidability could also be added (Figure XIX-2.4). Figure XIX-2.3 shows his picture of how serotonin (5HT) interacts with the lower levels of the defense system.

The key point is that the periaqueductal gray, medial hypothalamus and amygdala will often be activated together by threatening stimuli. But, explosive undirected escape or aggression (periaqueductal gray) is inappropriate if avoidance (amygdala) or directed escape (medial hypothalamus) is possible. As indicated in

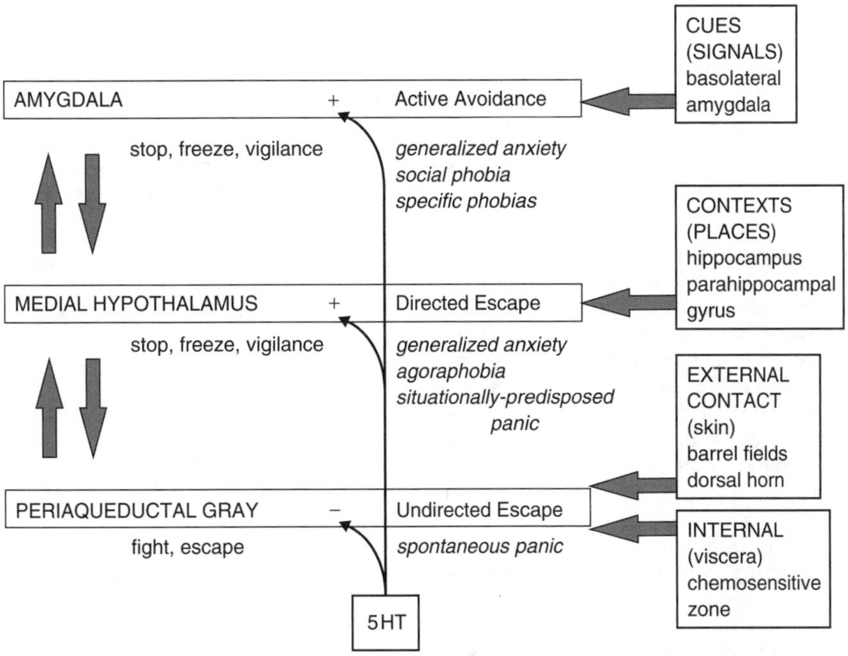

Figure XIX-2.3 The role of serotonin (5HT) in the control of anxiety as proposed by Deakin and Graeff (1991). The opposing effects of input to PAG, compared to structures higher in the defense hierarchy, provides an explanation of the paradoxical effects of some treatments and for phenomena such as panic associated with relaxation or sleep. Note that Deakin and Graeff localize generalized anxiety to the amygdala and hypothalamus and view the hippocampus as a purely sensory structure. This is essentially the same as the view of LeDoux (1994) but differs from Figure XIX-2.1. However, these differences of detail do not have major consequences for the predictions to be derived from the Deakin and Graeff model or for the general principles of operation they attribute to the serotonin system

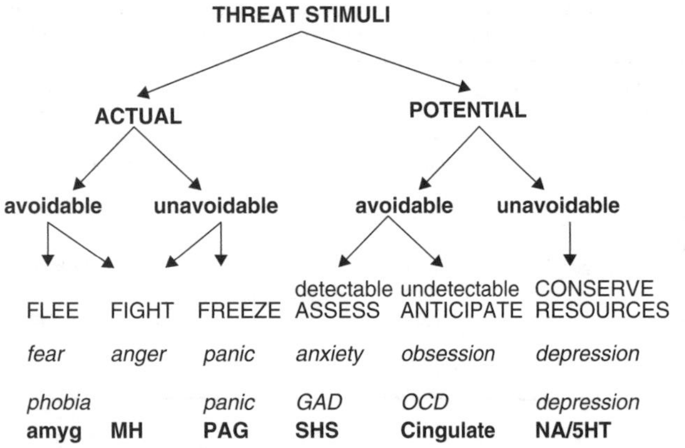

Figure XIX-2.4 The functional differentiation of threat stimuli and its likely relation to neural systems. The stimuli are categorized into different functional classes in the top three rows. The specific functional output required by each class is shown in the fourth row (capitals) and its relation to nominal emotions in the fifth row (small italics). It should be noted that these emotions are presumed to be usually functionally adaptive. The related psychological disorders are given in the sixth row (large italics) and the principle neural system involved in pathology or symptomatology as well as normal function is indicated in the last row. Amyg, amygdala; MH, medial hypothalamus; SHS, septo-hippocampal system; NA/5HT changes in the balance between the monoamine systems. From Gray and McNaughton (2000), Figure 11.2

the figure, (see also Deakin and Graeff, 1991) serotonin shifts the balance between the structures. It 'facilitates defensive behaviour elicited by potential or distal danger signals ... by acting on the amygdala, but, in the periventricular system, inhibits the expression of fight/flight responses that are adaptive only when the threat stimulus is proximal to the animal' (Graeff, 1993). In humans also, 'measures that are believed to represent conditioned anxiety were increased by D-fenfluramine, ... a drug that seems to release 5HT selectively from terminals of the dorsal raphe, ... whereas those thought to reflect unconditioned fear were attenuated' (Graeff, Viana and Mora, 1997). This idea of antagonism between anxiety and panic (at least at low levels of anxiety) also accounts for such paradoxical phenomena as relaxation-related panic attacks (Graeff, 1994).

A similar differential effect, coupled to receptor- or channel-linked polymorphisms may underlie the occasional paradoxical effects of SSRIs. These are usually beneficial in patients with panic. However, fluoxetine can occasionally exacerbate pre-existing panic and Altshuler (Altshuler, 1994) reported two cases where fluoxetine induced panic *de novo* that continued as non-remitting spontaneous panic attacks (see discussion of kindling below) in two patients with no prior history of panic. He noted that 'in the two cases presented, the timing of the onset of the panic attacks (within 10 days of medication) is certainly earlier than the time of onset of the [usual therapeutic] action'. Thus, variation in differential effects across the defense system could result from different rates of receptor adaptation and/or sensitization in different parts of the defense system to serotonin released from collaterals of the same neurons onto different receptor subtypes.

The release of serotonin (and the firing of raphe cells) seems to prime tonic or repetitive motor circuits while suppressing phasic, orienting, startle, and related circuits. This priming also has major effects on circuits (primarily in the septo-hippocampal system) whose business is to *inhibit* ongoing, tonic motor circuits. Thus, the firing of serotonin cells will often be functionally silent; and the effects of serotonin on behavioural inhibition, for example, will become functionally evident only when other conditions are fulfilled. One way to look at this is to view the serotonin signal as increasing 'motor attention', an effect that will have obvious behavioural consequences only when an event occurs to interrupt the motor programme.

Despite their involvement in the processing of threat, then, serotonin systems (like dopamine and noradrenaline) cannot be seen as threat promoting or threat inhibiting as such.

The situation is rendered even more complex by the effects of drugs active at different serotonin receptors. The receptor subtypes cut across the distinct neural systems we have been discussing so far and so select out only part of the action of serotonin with respect to each system while having effects general to all systems. This problem is particularly acute with $5HT_{1A}$ receptors. These are the principal targets of novel anxiolytics such as buspirone and the SSRIs. The drugs act as serotonin agonists in the sense of acting on the $5HT_{1A}$ receptor in the same way as serotonin but, in a number of areas, these receptors are autoreceptors involved in inhibitory feedback and so have an inhibitory effect on overall serotonergic output. Agonists at other serotonin receptors tend to have opposite effects to $5HT_{1A}$ agonists (Aprison and Ferster, 1961; Graeff and Schoenfeld, 1970; Stein, Wise and Berger, 1973). An important point for understanding possible genetic differences in vulnerability to anxiety disorders is that each receptor is a potential target of genetic modulation or deletion and that disorder may result as much from a disruption of normal balance between components of the serotonin system as from loss of a specific receptor-mediated action. A brief summary of the receptors is given in Table XIX-2.4.

Table XIX-2.4 Serotonin (5HT) receptor subtypes. For reviews see Griebel (1995), Saxena (1995), Zifa and Fillion (1992), Wilkinson and Dourish (1991), Uphouse (1997) and Meneses (1999)

5HT-1A	Anxiolytic at low doses. Action both at autoreceptors (dorsal and median raphe) and presynaptically (septum, hippocampus, amygdala). This results in a combination of functional 5HT-agonist-like and functional 5HT-antagonist-like actions.
5HT-1B	Occur in rodents but not humans.
5HT-1C	Now reclassified as part of the 5HT2 family, see 5HT2C.
5HT-1D	Likely to be a homologue of 5HT-1B. High density in the basal ganglia, lower in the hippocampus, neocortex and raphe nuclei. Function unknown. Peripherally involved in vasodilation. Antagonists useful in migraine.
5HT-2A	May be separate receptor or a separate state of the 5HT2B (q.v.).
5HT-2B	(and 5HT-2A) are distinct from 5HT2C. Highest density in the hippocampal formation, frontal cortex, cingulate cortex, nucleus accumbens, hypothalamus and mammillary bodies. Moderate density in the basal ganglia. The mixed 5HT2/1C antagonist, ritanserin, improves generalised anxiety disorder but worsens panic (see Graeff, 1993; see also Figure XIX-2.3 and Griebel, 1995, p. 374). 5HT2 receptors are also involved in the regulation of sleep, temperature and some aspects of motor control.
5HT-2C	(originally 5HT-1C). Highest density in the choroid plexus. Function unknown (but see Zifa and Fillion, 1992, p. 432).
5HT3	Highest density in the area postrema. Low, but detectable levels in septum, hippocampal formation, frontal cortex, cingulate cortex, nucleus accumbens, amygdala, thalamus and hypothalamus. Antagonists initially suggested to be anxiolytic but main current regular use is as anti-emetics (Saxena, 1995).
5HT-4	Agonists have effects on gastric motility.
5HT5+	for 5HT-n with $n > 4$ there is virtually no current evidence of function but they may be involved in learning and memory, possibly via modulation of cholinergic function (Meneses, 1999).

Neural sites are not identifiable with specific receptor subtypes. 5-HT_{1A}, 5-HT_2, and 5-HT_3 occur in the septo-hippocampal system, in the amygdala (5-HT_{1A}, 5-HT_3); in the frontal and cingulate cortex and in the nucleus accumbens, and hypothalamus (5-HT_2, 5-HT_3). Except for 5-HT_{1A} and 5-HT_3, most types are found in the basal ganglia. It seems unlikely that specific ligands will have specific, coherent functions (see also Griebel, 1995).

Under normal conditions, indeed, different levels and patterns of activation of relatively diffuse serotonergic projections could have fairly specific effects on particular areas. They could also affect particular functions within areas through the differences among receptor subtypes. The receptors can differ in their affinity (allowing, e.g., opposite effects to different concentrations of transmitter); in their transduction pathways (targeting different second messenger systems or rates of change); in their amount of desensitization/downregulation (allowing differential changes in response to acute as opposed to chronic serotonin release); and in their reaction to the cellular environment, including interaction with other serotonin receptors (Uphouse, 1997).

Like the cholinergic, dopaminergic and noradrenergic system, then, the serotonergic system is in a position to modulate the function of limbic structures and to influence the processing of threatening stimuli and the motor output resulting from them. Of all the systems we have considered so far it has the closest involvement in fear and anxiety. However, also like the noradrenergic system, there is no reason to see the serotonergic system as having a function specifically dedicated to defense as such — although specific receptor ligands could, in principle, have much more selective targets. Conversely, some selective ligands may have more influence on learning and memory than anxiety (Meneses, 1999).

Interactions of the Systems

The neuroanatomy and primary physiological effect (an increase in signal-to-noise ratio) of the systems we have considered is very similar. They may, then, each discharge an essentially similar function, but triggered by different environmental conditions.

In many cases the critical conditions may partially overlap and the systems act synergistically as with spatial learning (Decker and Gallagher, 1987). In some, there is evidence that noradrenaline produces its effects by releasing acetylcholine (Dalmaz, Introini-Collison and McGaugh, 1993) or that acetylcholine acts to increase the release of noradrenaline (Engberg and Hajos, 1994). Likewise, there are synergistic interactions between central serotonergic and cholinergic systems (Riekkinen, Sirvio and Riekkinen, 1990) and many 'histological, electrophysiological, pharmacological and behavioural data suggesting that serotonin is able to modulate central cholinergic function and that this modulation may have, in some respects, cognitive implications' (review by Cassel and Jeltsch, 1995, p. 31). Indeed, one study that recorded from putative cholinergic, noradrenergic and serotonergic neurons concluded 'the rapid cholinergic system controls the general condition of the brain (including sleep and wakefulness), cooperating with the "slow" noradrenergic and serotonergic systems. The three systems, which may interact mutually, may share the function of "the ascending reticular activating system"' (Koyama, Jodo and Kayama, 1994, p. 1030). We also noted, in the section 'Dopaminergic Systems', interactions between the systems that were often quite local (e.g., presynaptic effects of noradrenaline on dopaminergic cells in PFC).

This is not to say that these systems or their interactions are solely concerned with sudden changes of state of the sort that would characterize normal anxiety in response to ecologically valid threatening stimuli. As is extensively dealt with elsewhere in this book, both serotonin and noradrenaline have important separate involvements in responses to stress, which may underlie the therapeutic effects of their specific re-uptake inhibitors in depression. There may also be important interactions between them in determining the behaviour of depressed people, for example, 'the expression of tyrosine hydroxylase [which controls noradrenaline synthesis] in locus coeruleus may be relevant in the pathophysiology of suicide' (Ordway, Smith and Haycock, 1994, p. 680).

Preclinical Overview of the Aminergic Systems

Combining all of the preclinical data reviewed in this section, we can arrive at a relatively simple picture of the aminergic systems as a whole (and of the similar cholinergic system) — despite the complexities of each of their component parts. Taken together, they appear to function to prime sensory-motor systems for action. At the neural level this represents an increase in signal-to-noise ratio, decreasing the effectiveness of ongoing background processing while increasing the response to any higher level upcoming input. Importantly, their activity, on this view, will only have major functional effects if there is such an upcoming signal to process. Much of the time changes in aminergic or cholinergic activity may be functionally silent.

The systems differ in the circumstances under which they produce such priming. Cholinergic systems act on a short time scale to increase the acuity of the processing of the sensory stimuli (and their associations/'memories') likely to be crucial for upcoming action. Dopaminergic systems act to increase the vigor of current approach responses and increase the probability of future approach responses (including, in both cases, approach to safety). Noradrenergic systems act, like a central 'sympathetic nervous system', to prime systems for upcoming sudden, unexpected action, in particular orienting responses. This priming involves an increase both in acuity of processing and in the vigor of upcoming motor output. Serotonergic systems are most strongly associated with motor output as opposed to sensory processing and prime systems for upcoming actions that cope with common repeated requirements.

To put this another way:

> 'The serotonergic system will be more concerned to prevent the dominant motor programme (e.g., avoidance) from being interrupted by concurrent activation of some other motor programme (e.g., escape); the noradrenergic system will be more concerned to prevent the dominant controlling stimulus from having its control of behaviour interrupted by other concurrent stimuli; and the cholinergic system will be more concerned to prevent the current-to-be-associated stimulus from having its associative connections interrupted by other concurrently activated associations (Vinogradova *et al.*, 1993). These increases in signal-to-noise ratio will have functional effects only if the target structure is processing a signal and if the result of that processing is a functional output.
>
> In achieving these different effects, we can assume that the aminergic systems produce largely similar direct neural effects, but produce their different patterns of response through requiring different adequate stimuli for their activation. We can also assume that the fundamental effect of release of transmitter by the systems is not only similar between them but very simple. The apparent complexities of the effects of drugs and lesions are then attributed to the complexities of the functions of the various target areas.'
>
> Gray and McNaughton (2000, Appendix 10)

AMINERGIC INVOLVEMENT IN CLINICAL ANXIETY

Determining the functional role of aminergic transmitter systems in anxiety disorders is complicated by at least six methodological issues.

First, is the problem of localization of action. This can be exemplified by panic. Related compounds, such as adrenaline (epinephrine) when present in the blood stream can induce high levels of arousal and hence panic (Veltman *et al.*, 1996, 1998) while the state of platelet adrenergic receptors can influence panic (Gurguis *et al.*, 1999). Likewise, peripheral physiological challenges such as an increased partial pressure of CO_2 can induce panic. Interpretation of the effects of any pharmacological manipulation or state-related biochemical marker on any aspect of any anxiety disorder must therefore allow for the fact that a non-specific peripheral change rather than a specific central change may be the basis of observed effects. Likewise, even if a central action can be demonstrated, it may be as non-specific as a peripheral challenge.

Second, the three monoamine transmitters share a common enzyme that destroys them in the synapse and so renders them ineffective: monoamine oxidase (MAO). Any pharmacological changes (produced by monoamine oxidase inhibitors, MAOI) or effects of genetic differences in MAO-related systems (Deckert *et al.*, 1999) can be due to changes in any or all of the monoamine systems. Of course, MAO itself is a perfectly respectable aetiological candidate — and will be considered separately from the individual monoamines below, as will catechol-0-methyl transferase (COMT) an enzyme that breaks down dopamine and noradrenaline but not serotonin.

Third, dopamine is a precursor to noradrenaline. Treatments that affect dopamine synthesis (e.g., α-methyl-p-tyrosine) will therefore affect noradrenaline synthesis as well. Demonstration of specificity to one or the other transmitter will therefore require additional manipulations (e.g., administration of di-hydroxy-phenylserine that acts as a precursor for noradrenaline but not dopamine).

Fourth, as discussed in the section 'Interactions of the system', there are clear neural interactions between the systems. This is a particular problem in assessing drugs that act presynaptically. Not only may, for example, a $5HT_{1A}$ agonist have the primary effect of releasing noradrenaline but, concurrently, in a different part of the brain it could act to inhibit the release of noradrenaline or one of the other aminergic systems or the cholinergic system.

Fifth, such a presynaptic agonist may, again as exemplified by $5HT_{1A}$, be a functional antagonist of its parent system by acting at autoreceptors. An effect of a nominal agonist (i.e. a compound that has an effect at a receptor like the transmitter) at one receptor may be the equivalent of an antagonist at a different receptor type or of a synthesis blocker. Indeed, where there are high and low affinity receptors, low affinity receptors frequently have an opposite effect to high. The former provide the endogenous ligand with a form of negative feedback that can prevent overdriving of the system.

Sixth, there is a therapeutic lag in the clinical effects of specific serotonergic re-uptake inhibitors (SSRI), specific noradrenergic re-uptake inhibitors, $5HT_{1A}$ binding drugs and even benzodiazepines (e.g., Wheatley, 1990, Figure 14.2). This can lead one to ask whether an abnormality in any system that is involved in these therapeutic approaches to anxiety reflects anxiety disorder itself. They may rather be non-specifically involved as critical components of feedback loops maintaining symptoms.

These problems exist for each symptom or syndrome being studied and are rendered even more problematic by the diagnostic problems of the DSM scheme detailed at the beginning of this chapter. In understanding the role of the aminergic systems in anxiety two simplifying strategies can be used. The first is to base the analysis on the dissection of the anxiety disorders provided by the preclinical data. The second is to focus most attention on acute challenge studies in non-clinical populations (where results are not confounded by pre-existing disorder, but may of course be non-specific) and on genetic analysis of clinical populations (where the detected differences between probands and controls must have existed before the onset of the disorder).

Specific Dopaminergic Involvement

The bulk of attempts to address this question have focussed on changes in plasma or urinary levels of noradrenaline or its metabolites. A review of the data up to 1990 (Norman, Judd and Burrows, 1990) found 'a number of studies are suggestive of a role of catecholamines in the aetiology of anxiety states, particularly panic disorder'. Let us focus on the words 'catecholamines' and 'suggestive'. Why do they not draw specific conclusion about dopamine? Why are their conclusions not definite?

Dopamine presents major problems for attempts to claim specificity. It has, as a major metabolite, noradrenaline and so treatments that alter its synthesis also change noradrenaline. Further, it shares both MAO and COMT with noradrenaline as breakdown enzymes. In essence, this means we must rely on the preclinical data for our assessment of its role in anxiety and anxiety-related disorders. These did not suggest any major involvement. Likewise, genetic polymorphisms of the D4 receptor and dopamine transporter do not appear to be strongly linked to panic (Hamilton *et al.*, 2000).

Even if we ignore specificity to dopamine, why can we not make definite claims about the two catecholamines, lumped together?

> 'Evidence ... has been sought in the measurement of epinephrine, norepinephrine and [its metabolite MHPG] in the periphery.... Interpretation of the findings in relation to changes in brain adrenergic function is, of course, problematic, as indeed is the relationship for other peripheral markers. This question has been addressed for the use of plasma-free MHPG concentrations. In brain "free" or unconjugated MHPG is the major metabolite of norepinephrine and its measurement provides a good estimate of turnover. Evidence from animal studies suggest [*sic*] a direct correlation between MHPG concentrations in noradrenergic-containing brain regions and CSF and plasma in untreated animals or in those treated with drugs that increase or decrease activity. A similar situation pertains in humans where positive correlations between CSF and plasma MHPG concentrations have been observed. Furthermore, the effects of administration of some drugs on plasma MHPG in humans are consistent with their effects on brain MHPG in primates. [However,] the contribution of brain MHPG to plasma concentrations has been estimated as [only] 20–65%. [But], despite [these] significant contributions from outside the brain, is thought to be under central control. [Unfortunately,] numerous other factors such as motor activity, temperature, exercises, sexual arousal, mental tasks requiring concentration and diet may all influence catecholaminergic function.
>
> [Thus, there can be] a highly significant correlation between change in anxiety score and change in urinary MHPG output, but urinary MHPG excretion at baseline and state anxiety score did not covary significantly. Baseline anxiety cannot be used to predict baseline MHPG and vice versa.... Urinary MHPG does not appear to be a useful marker to study comparison with normal control groups. On the other hand within subject designs (i.e. pre- and post-treatment) may be more useful for assessing individual changes of adrenergic function in anxiety disorders.'
>
> Norman, Judd and Burrows (1990, pp. 226–228)

An important negative conclusion, here, is that there is no evidence for a general baseline increase in catecholamines as a cause of excessive anxiety responses. Much more likely, given the preclinical data, is that anxiety-induced arousal results in changes in catecholaminergic output as a non-specific symptom.

Attempts to alter dopamine in normal subjects have been no more conclusive.

> 'Decreased dopaminergic function can be elicited experimentally using low doses of apomorphine, which are thought to act as a presynaptic agonist. However, problems with apomorphine include concern about its specificity for the presynaptic rather than postsynaptic receptor, and side effects.... Repeated administration of α-methyl-p-tyrosine [reduces noradrenaline and dopamine and]

produces primarily fatigue and sedation [while] administration of the catecholamine ... precursor, tyrosine, attenuates mood lowering and cognitive deficits associated with stressful environmental challenges.... Reducing catecholamine neurotransmission by means of acute phenylalanine/tyrosine depletion ... were similar to those reported to occur in response to other used to decrease catecholamine neurotransmission in humans ... [It] lowered mood, energy, and calmness, but only the mood-lowering effect ... after an aversive psychological challenge (public speaking and mental arithmetic) ... was statistically significant.'

Leyton *et al.* (2000, pp. 52–59)

These effects, then, could have been due to changes in noradrenaline as well as dopamine and appeared to relate more to depression than anxiety. It should also be noted that they are in the opposite direction to the effects that would be predicted if release of catecholamines by stress were producing anxiety but are in the same direction as would be predicted from the therapeutic effects of noradrenergic re-uptake blockers and monoamine oxidase inhibitors.

Specific Noradrenergic Involvement

The evidence of the previous section is as relevant, or irrelevant, to assessment of central noradrenaline function as it was to dopamine. In this section we will consider studies that have attempted to exclude dopamine when assessing the effects of noradrenaline. Noradrenaline has a much longer and closer association with anxiety than dopamine.

'In humans electrical stimulation in the region of the locus ceruleus [*sic*] has been reported to produce feelings of fear and imminent death. Coupled with the anxiolytic effects in humans of drugs that decrease locus ceruleus noradrenergic activity and the anxiogenic properties of drugs that increase it, Redmond and Huang suggest[ed] a role for this nucleus in human anxiety states.'

Norman, Judd and Burrows (1990, p. 224)

Our preclinical analysis of the noradrenergic system should make us wary of accepting this suggestion too restrictively, especially in its more specific form that noradrenergic systems are critical for panic disorder. Clearly a pathological increase in 'arousal' could engender anxiety — but only in the non-specific way of other disturbances of the body. However, all anxiolytic drugs so far tested do appear to reduce the outflow of forebrain noradrenaline (although as noted above, buspirone increases rather than decreases locus coeruleus firing as a result of its presynaptic inhibition of outflow). But the same drugs alter other systems, particularly serotonin, in the same way and specific noradrenergic lesions appear to be only partially anxiolytic (Table XIX-2.2). A hard-line equation of noradrenaline release with anxiety does not square with these facts. Equally, as emphasized at the beginning of this chapter a role for a compound in the amelioration of symptoms of a state does not necessarily implicate the systems on which the compound acts in the aetiology of the disorder giving rise to that state.

We are left with the looser question of whether disorders of the noradrenergic system can induce, or increase the likelihood, of anxiety disorders. Certainly, drugs like yohimbine, that increase locus coeruleus firing, can increase panic attacks. But, as emphasised in Section 2 panic and anxiety should be kept distinct and 'the list of "successful" and presumably "biological" challenges has grown quite long over the past few years. It now includes lactate infusion, carbon dioxide inhalation, and hyperventilation as well as oral or intravenous yohimbine, isoproterenol, (nor)epinephrine, caffeine, beta-carboline ligands ... and GABA.... [However,] the effects of [such] panic challenges can be strongly altered by manipulating expectancy experimentally' (Margraf and Ehlers, 1990). This is reminiscent of the older work on the effects of adrenaline challenge in normal subjects. 'The differences in the results of [different] workers are explicable in retrospect by the presence or absence of anxiety-provoking environmental cues. In a neutral setting, the injection of epinephrine (adrenaline) produced no emotional changes, "cold emotion", or "as if" emotion.... In an anxiety-provoking setting, intentionally or accidentally created by the experimenters, subjects showed more evidence of anxiety and in a minority of cases panic attacks were elicited' (Lader and Tyrer, 1975). These data all suggest that increased central or peripheral noradrenaline, like peripheral adrenaline, may increase the effect of existing external or (in the case of panic) internal anxiogenic stimuli but are not anxiety provoking in and of themselves. In this we echo the conclusion of our preclinical analysis that central noradrenaline increase vigilance to and vigor of response to stimuli and the conclusion is nonetheless consistent with the view that these effects need not be limited to aversive stimuli. A final point to note, here, is that apparently selective effects of drugs like yohimbine on patients with panic disorder as compared to controls — which can occur with startle as well as panic (Morgan, III *et al.*, 1995) — may reflect no more than a pre-existing heightened sensitivity to stimuli in such patients. Certainly, carbon dioxide inhalation produces more panic in persons with panic disorder than it does in controls (Gorman *et al.*, 1994).

Surprisingly, there is better evidence for the involvement of noradrenaline in depression, and even in the effects of serotonergic antidepressants, than there is for its involvement in anxiety. For example, in depressed patients treated with tricyclic, SSRI or MAOI antidepressants, plasma MHPG (the metabolite of noradrenaline) was reduced as were both anxiety and depression. But the change in MHPG correlated with the change in depression and not the change in anxiety (Karege *et al.*, 1993). Plasma noradrenaline is also high in depressives, independent of the type of depression, and its level has no relation to the level of anxiety (Kelly and Cooper, 1998). Likewise, in post-traumatic stress disorder there appears to be a general change in the 5HT transporter, which is accompanied by $\alpha 2$ adrenergic receptor changes only in those cases with major depression. Conversely, $\alpha 2$ density prior to treatment of panic disorder predicts the efficacy of that treatment without being changed by it. There is, then, no evidence for $\alpha 2$ involvement in the production of anxiety but 'increased ... density and abnormal coupling may represent an adaptive mechanism ... in Panic Disorder' (Gurguis *et al.*, 1999). Nor is there good evidence that polymorphism of the receptor genes relates to differences in panic (Ohara *et al.*, 2000).

Finally, social phobia (arguably a disorder involving anxiety if not caused by it) in the absence of depression does not appear to be accompanied by peripheral signs of catecholaminergic abnormality (Stein, Asmundson and Chartier, 1994; Stein, Walker and Forde, 1994).

Overall, then, we can be happy with the idea that noradrenergic systems can modulate anxiety. However, it seems clear that increased noradrenergic outflow, as such, need not be linked to anxiety. High levels accompany anxiety states in some cases and can exacerbate panic, but increased outflow is also a common action of all anxiolytic drugs. One way of resolving this apparent paradox (consistent with the fact that anxiolytic drugs, including buspirone, do not alter panic) is to suggest that noradrenaline can increase the probability of panic (as can many other agents) while contributing to decreases in anxiety as such. For noradrenaline, this is speculative. However, we noted earlier Graeff's model of the interaction of serotonin with the defence system where (see Figure XIX-2.3) he postulated an opposite effect on the periaqueductal gray (reducing spontaneous panic) to that on higher levels of the system (increasing avoidance).

Specific Serotonergic Involvement

Serotonergic systems have achieved prominence because of their role in antidepressant action. However, it is clear that they are also involved in specifically anxiolytic action. Disentangling causes and effects is difficult here. But it has been suggested that for some types of depression, the depression is secondary to changes in anxiety and aggression that are in turn secondary to 5HT dysfunction. Specifically, a deficient serotonin system would decrease coping ability and hence increase vulnerability to stress. The stress would activate anxiety and aggression and failure to cope with these would precipitate a depressive episode. Importantly, 'the two subgroups — the one in which anxiety/aggression heralds the depression and the other in which anxiety/aggression are first to respond to antidepressants — coincide to a large extent' (Van Praag, 1996).

'A [single] serotonergic deficit, interacting with different pathophysiological mechanisms, could underlie a component of the vulnerability to [and] recurrence or exacerbation of ... [progressing] panic anxiety disorder, [post-traumatic stress disorder (PTSD)] and OCD.... [In particular, it could underlie the] decreasing well-interval between episodes, and a transition from episodes that were precipitated by losses and related psychosocial stressors to those that occurred more spontaneously' via a kindling-like phenomenon (Post and Weiss, 1998) (Kindling is the gradual development and then increase in severity of seizures to repeated electrical stimulation that does not initially generate seizures). Consistent with this, $5HT_{1A}$ agonists decrease kindling and $5HT_{2A}$ agonists increase it, in line with the relation of these receptors to anxiolytic (and antidepressant) action (Post and Weiss, 1998).

> 'Remarkably, in the restraint stress paradigm, antidepressants with activity at either noradrenergic or serotonergic synapses are sufficient to oppose and block some of the effects of stress on neurotrophic factor gene expression.... Whereas the benefit of not having recurrent depressive episodes based on adequate pharmacoprophylaxis is substantial in itself, it is also possible that antidepressants could impact the course of illness, both by removing the sensitizing effect of episodes on subsequent vulnerability to recurrence and by ameliorating the potential acute and concomitant long-term impact of the stressor.... [Serotonergic vulnerability] could be set either by an inherited genetic mechanism or by an experience-dependent, stressor-mediated impact on gene expression ... or by both mechanisms in combination, providing a "double hit" like that required in the development of some cancers.'
>
> Post and Weiss (1998)

The link with kindling may be even tighter than this. Partial electrical kindling of the limbic system in animals results in increased anxiety-like behaviour that has been explicitly suggested as a model of PTSD and there are many other links between kindling and anxiety in preclinical data (Adamec, 1997).

The idea that serotonin-related changes in depression may be at least in part secondary to changes in anxiety is consistent with results from healthy human subjects subjected to a psychological challenge. Relative to the effects of acute lowering of noradrenaline, acute lowering of serotonin had about twice as big an effect on anxious mood as on depressed mood. Of particular interest relative to van Praag's hypothesis (above) is the fact that, unlike noradrenaline depletion, serotonin depletion increased hostility (Leyton *et al.*, 2000) and that no change was observed in mood in the absence of psychological challenge (making a speech). A similar lack of effect in the absence of challenge has been observed in remitted panic disorder patients (Goddard *et al.*, 1994) and in numerous other studies in healthy subjects (Klaassen *et al.*, 1998). In healthy human subjects submitted to a carbon dioxide challenge serotonin depletion appears to produce a highly variable increase in reported anxiety and produces a significant increase in neurovegetative symptoms of panic (Klaassen *et al.*, 1998). These results are also consistent with van Praag's hypothesis that serotonin deficiency creates a vulnerability to anxiety that is only expressed in response to challenge. However, worsening of symptoms has been observed in remitted OCD patients (Barr *et al.*, 1994 — cited by Goddard *et al.*, 1994).

While a general depletion of 5HT may produce general effects, as with treatment, receptor-specific challenge can produce more specific effects — and even opposite effects. Thus, a $5HT_{2c}$ agonist, while being panicogenic like many other non-specific agents, can increase symptoms in OCD patients in a way that other panicogenic agents do not (Bagdy, 1998). This selectivity mirrors the fact that anti-obsessional agents tend to be panicolytic, but not necessarily vice versa. Likewise 'patients with OCD who also had a family history of OCD had significantly higher whole blood 5-HT levels than either patients with OCD without a family history of OCD or normal control subjects (Hanna *et al.*, 1991)' (Cook, Jr. *et al.*, 1994). The idea that there is a subgroup in which a high (rather than low) level of serotonin (in the blood not necessarily in the brain) is linked to OCD might seem to be supported by the fact that those parents of autistic children who have a high whole blood serotonin have a tendency to higher OCD scores than those with normal whole blood serotonin. However, in their case, hyperserotonemia is much more clearly related to higher depression scores than OCD scores (Cook, Jr. *et al.*, 1994). Unfortunately, Cook *et al.*, did not measure anxiety as opposed to obsession. It is possible, then, that the link with depression was mediated by a change in anxiety.

Support both for this idea, and for a link to central as opposed to peripheral serotonin is provided by studies on blood platelets. These have a serotonin uptake mechanism that appears similar to the central one in that it is blocked by SSRIs. Genetic or environmental changes in this transporter system are likely to occur similarly in platelets and in the brain and are likely to be one of the factors controlling whole blood serotonin levels. Assessment of the serotonin re-uptake mechanism via 'paroxetine binding was negatively correlated with both state and trait anxiety, as well as with depressive and overall PTSD symptoms. However, ... [it did not differ] as a function of comorbid psychiatric diagnoses including major depression, other anxiety disorders, and substance abuse' (Fichtner *et al.*, 1995). 'Arora *et al.* (1993) [also] reported ... a negative correlation ... with state-dependent anxiety score. Unlike patients with PTSD, no significant alterations in platelet ... binding ... could be found in major depression. These negative findings in major depression are in agreement with our results that there were no significant differences in ... binding ... between PTSD patients with and without major depression' (Maes *et al.*, 1999).

It might seem peculiar that, on the one hand, a $5HT_{2c}$ agonist or increased blood serotonin levels or decreased serotonin transporter levels should be positively related to neurotic disorder while, on the other hand, challenges that deplete serotonin should increase symptoms related to those same disorders. The difficulty of interpreting such studies (and one of the reasons for this chapter having an extensive preclinical review) is highlighted by the fact that the 'hyperserotonemia' reported in whole blood may be due to 'increased platelet 5-HT uptake.... [such] increased 5-HT uptake may predispose ... to depression' (Cook, Jr. *et al.*, 1994). That is, increased measured whole blood serotonin, if it is inside platelets, would correspond to increased serotonin inside presynaptic terminals and so *decreased* serotonin in the synaptic cleft and so decreased postsynaptic effects. Similarly with the $5HT_{2c}$ agonist, the effects could be the opposite of systemic changes in serotonin if the net effect of the systemic increase on the specific terminals of interest was a decrease of release either through presynaptic or autoreceptors. With the serotonin transporter 'binding correlates highly with tissue 5-HT content' (Fichtner *et al.*,

1995), i.e. the more 5-HT there is around the more transporters there are to transport it. So, while high levels of transporter, all other things being equal, should lead to lower levels of serotonin in the cleft it is likely that high measured levels of transporter indicate that all other things are not equal. It is a higher functionality of the serotonin system that is likely to have produced a feedback increase in number of transporters.

Despite the strong link between the platelet serotonin transporter and anxiety in PTSD, it does not seem to be a basis for anxiety disorder in general. Both social phobics and panic disorder patients have normal binding (Stein *et al.*, 1995). This could be because these are distinct entities from anxiety proper (in which GAD patients would be expected to have low binding) or it may be that transporter changes are related more to aetiology than symptomatology—and are a marker of the means of acquisition of PTSD, or simply of the levels of stress previously experienced.

A causal role for the transporter itself (rather than a role as a marker) is suggested by the linkage of polymorphisms in its genes with anxiety (Evans *et al.*, 1997; Ohara *et al.*, 1998a, 1998b; Katsuragi *et al.*, 1999; Melke *et al.*, 2001). There may be a similar causal role for genetic differences in serotonin synthesis (Du, Bakish and Hrdina, 2001) and these could, of course, combine with transporter differences to produce synergistic (or antagonistic) effects. However, as emphasized earlier, genetic control of the serotonin system is likely to reflect increased vulnerability to stressors rather than a direct and specific promotion of PTSD in general or anxiety in particular.

Given the possible opposite functional effects of different receptor subtypes it is of interest that, as with '"knock-out" mice lacking the gene that regulates the expression of the 5-HT_{1A} receptor [which] display greater anxiety ... in the open-field and the elevated-plus-maze tests, ... [with] regional 5-HT_{1A} [in] ... healthy volunteers ... there was a significant negative correlation between 5-HT_{1A} binding potential and anxiety in [all of] four regions: the dorsolateral prefrontal cortex, anterior cingulate cortex, parietal cortex, and occipital cortex' (Tauscher *et al.*, 2001).

Aminergic Interactions

There has been much less analysis of the possible interactions of the amine systems at the clinical than preclinical level. Given the difficulty of connecting a particular measure of aminergic activity with functional effect for a single amine (previous sections), we cannot expect too much from studies of more than one amine at a time. The critical feature of such studies will be to partial out the effects of the different systems. For example, we already concluded that anxiety, but not depression, in PTSD is linked to the serotonin transporter. There was also evidence that the serotonin transporter was not linked to depression in cases of depressive disorder as opposed to PTSD. And yet depression itself is a major feature of PTSD and can be treated with specific serotonin agents. Interestingly, in PTSD the presence of major depression is associated with a down regulation of $\alpha 2$ receptors. Decreased serotonergic traffic, then (whether as a result of acute or chronic trauma or genetic polymorphism), could increase the risk of anxiety and/or aggression to stressful events. Combination of this with a decrease in noradrenergic presynaptic autoinhibitory receptors could result in depression, which would also be characterized by increased autonomic activity (Maes *et al.*, 1999). The effectiveness of SSRIs in such cases could then be due to the elimination of one of two necessary or, at least, synergistic changes. If specific noradrenergic re-uptake inhibitors are proved to be effective in PTSD patients with depression, this could result from overcoming decreased autoinhibitory function.

A similar interactive relationship is suggested in generalized anxiety disorder by the pattern of plasma metabolites. Urinary output of serotonergic and noradrenergic metabolites is positively correlated in GAD patients, with 50% common shared variance (Garvey *et al.*, 1995a, 1995b). Apparently the same patient group (Garvey *et al.*, 1995a, 1995b), although there is no cross reference between the papers, showed a weaker[2] relationship (tension being the best with 25% variance accounted for) between a multiple regression function including both these measures and a subset of, mostly somatic, items in the Hamilton Anxiety Scale. The critical point is that the partial correlations of the serotonergic and noradrenergic measures were opposite in sign from each other both within and across items. As with PTSD data, and with the preclinical data, this suggests a complex partially synergistic interaction between the two monoamines in determining anxiety and/or its symptoms and comorbidities.

Conversely, there are 'recent studies of depressed patients where the NE and 5HT neurotransmitter systems have been suggested to produce distinguishable contributions to therapeutic efficacy.... Dietary depletion of 5-HT pre-cursors leads to clinical relapse in depressed patients who have been successfully treated with SSRIs, but not those treated with NE selective uptake inhibitors, and that blockade of NE synthesis has complementary effects' (Detke, Rickels and Lucki, 1995, p. 71).

Involvement of Monoaminoxidase and COMT

Synergy between the aminergic systems and differences in the balances between different parts of the defense system would account for the wide variations in treatment sensitivity across symptomatologically similar patients. They would also account for the cases where specific noradrenergic agents appear as effective as specific serotonin agents.

The enzyme COMT breaks down both dopamine and noradrenaline and MAO breaks down dopamine, noradrenaline and serotonin. Given synergy between the amines we would expect significant effects on clinical anxiety of disruption of these non-specific amine breakdown systems. It should be noted here that, while tricyclic drugs can be non-specific in their effect on re-uptake systems, genetic polymorphisms are much more likely to be system specific. Polymorphisms affecting the breakdown enzymes will, of course, be more general in their effects. We might, then, expect changes in COMT and MAO to be more significant aetiologically since they would allow synergy. However, for aminergic transmitters, re-uptake is more important for inactivation than breakdown. This said, MAO inhibitors are at least as effective clinically as tricyclic drugs and this appears to remain true for the reversible inhibitors selective for the A form of MAO (MAO-A). These interact much less with tyramine and so are much less toxic (Buller, 1995). Indeed MAO inhibitors can be effective in patients resistant to other antidepressant drugs (Modigh, 1987). They also appear more effective in treating endogenous anxiety than do tricyclic drugs (Sheehan, Ballenger and Jacobson, 1981).

The preclinical data also suggest a potential involvement of MAO-A in anxiety disorders. Mice mutants lacking MAO-A show increased noradrenaline and serotonin in the forebrain (including theoretically important areas such as hippocampus and prefrontal cortex). They show increased fear conditioning to both simple stimuli and environmental context and increased passive avoidance (suggesting effects on both fear and anxiety, see above). However, simple eye blink conditioning is normal suggesting a relatively specific emotional effect (Kim *et al.*, 1997). Interestingly, a polymorphism that would lead to higher levels of MAO activity is found

[2] Some of the weakness in the observed correlations is likely to have been due to compression of the scale scores as a result of the exclusion criteria used rather than reflecting a weak underlying relationship in the normal population.

more in male OCD patients than in either female OCD patients or controls (Camarena *et al.*, 2001).

Polymorphism of genes controlling human COMT can result in as much as a four-fold variation in the activity of the enzyme (Lachman *et al.*, 1996). This might be thought to provide a basis for considerable psychological impact but no marked effects have been reported. It may be significant in OCD but does not appear to be relevant to other anxiety disorders (Ohara *et al.*, 1998a, 1998b).

AMINERGIC INVOLVEMENT IN PERSONALITY

There is a common theme linking the preclinical data, the delayed effects of therapeutic drugs, and the development of disorder later in life linked to polymorphisms present from conception. They all imply that aminergic systems are modulatory of the defense system as a whole. Disorder, then, appears to result from the combination of the presence of long-term general aminergic modulatory risk factors with more specific genetic and environmental factors. 'Modulatory risk factors', in this sense, are best seen as an element of personality.

This is not to imply that personality itself is unmodifiable by events. Even in Australian fire fighters (arguably pre-selected to be relatively insensitive to danger) exposure to a major stressor[3] generated post-traumatic stress disorder in about a third of them and the PTSD appeared to remain chronic (McFarlane, 1989). Thus, rather than being a disorder proper, PTSD may better be thought of as an extreme change in the same personality dimension that controls the risk of anxiety disorder normally (Pitman, Orr and Shalev, 1993). Consistent with this, brief extreme activation of brain defense systems with either anxiogenic chemicals or electrical stimulation can produce increases in reactivity of the defense system that are very long lasting and have been seen as animal models of PTSD (Adamec, 1998a, 1998b, 1998c).

A major contributor to personality, however, is likely to be genes. The tendency to anxiety disorder in current populations has about a 30% contribution from genetic factors and this is true of the tendency to generalised anxiety even when it is comorbid with other conditions, including depression (Kendler *et al.*, 1992a, 1992b, 1992c). This genetic vulnerability appears general to 'neurotic disorders' (including depression) and does not appear selective for individual 'anxiety disorders' (Andrews *et al.*, 1990). With respect to comorbidity, it is interesting that depression and anxiety appear to be the 'result of the same genetic factors. Environmental risk factors that predispose to "pure" GAD episodes may be relatively distinct from those that increase risk for major depression'. By contrast, GAD and panic share only about half of their genetic control, each having a distinct other half (Scherrer *et al.*, 2000). In the case of panic, for example, genetic influences on anxiety, via polymorphisms of aminergic systems, could operate in parallel with panic susceptibility, via polymorphism of CCK systems (Wang *et al.*, 1998a, 1998b). This suggests a tight linking of anxiety with depression but (as argued earlier) a weaker link with panic. The latter is a distinct entity that can be both a cause and a symptom of anxiety, but can occur alone.

The dimensional analysis of personality (Eysenck and Eysenck, 1969; Watson, Clark and Harkness, 1994) suggests that psychiatric patients are simply located near the extreme pole of one or more dimensions of normal personality (Eysenck, 1960). This is analogous to the clustering of disorders such as stroke in those who are at one extreme of the normal distribution of blood pressure. This dimensional approach is becoming increasingly accepted in psychiatry (e.g., Cloninger, Svrakic and Przybecky, 1993). The blood pressure analogy is exact here as personality dimensions reflect liability to disorder not presentation. Prevalence of cases is strongly correlated with mean symptom scores in the normal range, even when diagnosed cases are excluded (Rose and Day, 1990); and there is a high frequency of subthreshold disorders (Goldberg and Huxley, 1992).

In terms of Eysenck's Personality Inventory (Eysenck and Eysenck, 1969; Eysenck and Eysenck, 1976; Costa and McCrae, 1985) those prone to anxiety are neurotic introverts. These people can be viewed as having a 'trait anxiety' that loads about 0.7 on neuroticism and 0.3 on introversion. It should be noted, here, that the risk of specific phobias of items such as snakes (unlike other 'anxiety disorders') is not related to this factor (Marks, 1969) and, consistent with this, such phobias are not relieved by anxiolytic drugs (Fredrikson and Öhman, 1979; Sartory, MacDonald and Gray, 1990). It should also be emphasized that 'trait anxiety' represents a risk for 'state anxiety' and neurotic disorder but is not identical to them. Thus, in the fire fighters mentioned earlier, the traumatic event was required to generate PTSD but, even in this selected population and with this single specific traumatic event, the tendency to neurotic personality predicted the disorder better than the extent of exposure to the event (McFarlane, 1989). Consistent with the heritability of neurotic disorder, the Eysenck dimensions are controlled almost equally by genes and environment (Floderus-Myhred, Pedersen and Rasmuson, 1980).

Factor analysis determines the number of dimensions of personality but not their nature. Although Eysenck's personality inventory is used very extensively it has been argued (Gray, 1970, 1981) that the axes representing the dimensions of neuroticism and extraversion should be rotated resulting in a dimension (0.7 neuroticism, −0.3 extraversion) corresponding to the 'trait anxiety' extracted by others (Cattell, 1965; Taylor, 1953) and an orthogonal dimension of 'impulsivity'. This dimension of 'trait anxiety' is what appears to be changed by the lesions of cingulate and prefrontal cortex used to treat drug-resistant anxiety (Powell, 1979).

There is evidence that 'emotionality' in rats is a homologue of neuroticism or trait anxiety (Broadhurst, 1960; Gray, 1987). It has a major genetic component (Hall, 1951; see review by Gray, 1987) and selective breeding has resulted in the Maudsley Reactive and Maudsley Non-reactive strains of rat.

The two Maudsley strains differ on a huge range of items (for reviews, see Broadhurst, 1975; Blizard, 1981; Gray, 1987). The bulk of these can be interpreted as showing a greater response to fear-provoking stimuli in general rather than to anxiety in particular. Note that this is an increased emotional response rather than an increased sensory response since they do not differ in pain sensitivity (Commissaris *et al.*, 1992) nor in rate of learning as such (Commissaris *et al.*, 1986). They also differ in an animal model of depression (Abel, Altman and Commissaris, 1992; Viglinskaya *et al.*, 1995). and this effect shows a strong linkage between changes in scores on an anxiety test with those on the depression test (Commissaris *et al.*, 1996). Just like 'trait anxiety', then, they appear to influence susceptibility to the full spectrum of neurotic reactions.

I have discussed this issue in such detail because analysis of aminergic systems has been carried out on the Maudsely strains at a depth currently impossible with people with trait anxiety. The Maudsley reactive strain (MR) has an increased response of locus coeruleus neurons to stress (Buda *et al.*, 1994; Blizard and Liang, 1979), need a higher dose of $\alpha 2$ agonist for the same effect and have lower $\alpha 2$ binding in LC, suggesting a less effective autoinhibition[4] (Sara, Devauges and Biegon, 1993). A primary involvement of autoinhibition could well underlie the paradoxical

[3] A bush fire, which comes within the ICD-10 definition of a traumatic situation, i.e. one 'of an exceptionally threatening or catastrophic nature, which is likely to cause pervasive distress in almost anyone (e.g., natural or manmade disaster, combat, serious accident, witnessing the violent death of others, or being a victim of torture, terrorism, rape, or other crime' (World Health Organization, 1992, p. 147).

[4] But note that an opposite pattern appears to be obtained under urethane anaesthesia (Verbanac *et al.*, 1994).

increase in the difference between the two strains on a conflict task after administration of a peripheral noradrenergic neurotoxin (Verbanac *et al.*, 1993). This only reduced central noradrenaline by 30%, whereas over 95% depletion is normally needed for behavioural effects (McNaughton and Mason, 1980) and may have been selectively affecting autoinhibition thus increasing rather than decreasing overall noradrenergic function.

Maudsley reactive rats have also been reported to have higher levels of serotonin in the limbic system (Maas, 1963) and in the brainstem, but the difference in the brainstem does not appear to be a reliable finding (Blizard and Liang, 1979) and, under urethane, neither dorsal raphe discharge rates nor sensitivity of 5HT1A autoreceptors is different (Verbanac *et al.*, 1995). Unfortunately, the sensitivity of presynaptic 5HT1A receptors in the limbic system (on which drugs like buspirone are likely to have their major action) has not been reported. A lack of difference in 5HT levels would be expected if the main difference between the strains, as with healthy humans (Tauscher *et al.*, 2001), is in binding and hence postsynaptic effect of the serotonin released.

Overall, then, we have a picture of polygenetic effects on the efficacy of both the noradrenergic and serotonergic systems that, through synergistic interactions (both within and between the amine systems) contributes to a normal personality factor that can be viewed clinically also as a risk factor for high levels of anxiety and hence anxiety disorder. Additional genetic and particularly specific environmental factors would then increase the risk of, or precipitate, particular disorders. These would then be specific instantiations within a 'trait diathesis common to all anxiety disorders' (Zinbarg and Barlow, 1996; Brown, Chorpita and Barlow, 1998).

CONCLUSIONS

There appears little question that the aminergic systems play a role in adaptive responses to stressors and that their general state of reactivity, set by genes and (often early) experience, contributes to a personality factor of 'trait anxiety' that can be largely equated with neuroticism. However, specific neurotic disorders do not appear to equate with disorder of the aminergic systems as such. They reflect distortions of activity in particular brain centres. The selectivity of therapeutic agents (and receptor-linked genes) then reflects postsynaptic differences in particular terminal areas. The lack of selectivity of trait anxiety for specific disorders reflects changes in synthesis and breakdown that are not only general to many terminal areas but also can be general to several aminergic systems (monoamine oxidase being particularly indiscriminate). The complex effects of kindling, opposite effects of normal and autoinhibitory receptors and direct interactions between terminals of the different amine systems render analysis of the clinical situation difficult. However, there is no reason to suppose that anxiety disorders cannot be viewed as extremes of normal psychological variation or that the component parts of the systems of interest (including their genetic control) cannot be studied, one at a time, in animal models. Highly efficient future treatments are likely if we can understand the different roles of different aspects of monoamine function in anxiety and obtain reliable markers that can reliably indicate specific treatment modalities for specific patients.

REFERENCES

Abel, E.L., Altman, H.J. and Commissaris, R.L., 1992. Maudsley reactive and nonreactive rats in the forced swim test: comparison in fresh water and soiled water. *Physiol. Behav.*, **52**, 1117–1119.

Abercrombie, E.D., Keefe, K.A., DiFrischia, D.S. and Zigmond, M.J., 1989. Differential effect of stress on *in vivo* dopamine release in striatum, nucleus accumbens, and medial frontal cortex. *J. Neurochem.*, **52**(5), 1655–1658.

Adamec, R., 1997. Transmitter systems involved in neural plasticity underlying increased anxiety and defense — implications for understanding anxiety following traumatic stress. *Neurosci. Biobehav. Rev.*, **21**, 755–765.

Adamec, R.E., 1998a. Evidence that NMDA-dependent limbic neural plasticity in the right hemisphere mediates pharmacological stressor (FG-7142)-induced lasting increases in anxiety-like behavior — Study 1 — Role of NMDA receptors in efferent transmission from the cat amygdala. *J. Psychopharmacol.*, **12**, 122–128.

Adamec, R.E., 1998b. Evidence that NMDA-dependent limbic neural plasticity in the right hemisphere mediates pharmacological stressor (FG-7142)-induced lasting increases in anxiety-like behavior — Study 2 — The effects on behavior of block of NMDA receptors prior to injection of FG-7142. *J. Psychopharmacol.*, **12**, 129–136.

Adamec, R.E., 1998c. Evidence that NMDA-dependent limbic neural plasticity in the right hemisphere mediates pharmacological stressor (FG-7142)-induced lasting increases in anxiety-like behavior. Study 3 — The effects on amygdala efferent physiology of block of NMDA receptors prior to injection of FG-7142 and its relationship to behavioral change. *J. Psychopharmacol.*, **12**, 227–238.

Aigner, T.G., 1995. Pharmacology of memory: Cholinergic-glutamatergic interactions. *Curr. Opin. Neurobiol.*, **5**, 155–160.

Altshuler, L.L., 1994. Fluoxetine-associated panic attacks. *J. Clin. Psychopharmacol.*, **14**, 433–434.

Anglade, F., Bizot, J.-C., Dodd, R.H., Baudoin, C. and Chapouthier, G., 1994. Opposite effects of cholinergic agents and benzodiazepine receptor ligands in a passive avoidance task in rats. *Neurosci. Lett.*, **182**, 247–250.

Andrews, G., Stewart, G., Morris-Yates, A., Holt, P. and Henderson, S., 1990. Evidence for a general neurotic syndrome. *Br. J. Psychiatr.*, **157**, 6–12.

Aprison, M.H. and Ferster, C.B., 1961. Neurochemical correlates of behavior: II. Correlation of brain monoamine oxidase activity with behavioral changes after iproniazid and 5-hydroxytryptophan. *J. Neurochem.*, **6**, 350–357.

Aston-Jones, G., Chiang, C. and Alexinsky, T., 1991. Discharge of noradrenergic locus coeruleus neurons in behaving rats and monkeys suggests a role in vigilance. *Prog. Brain Res.*, **88**, 501–520.

Aston-Jones, G., Rajkowski, J., Kubiak, P. and Alexinsky, T., 1994. Locus coeruleus neurons in monkey are selectively activated by attended cues in a vigilance task. *J. Neurosci.*, **14**, 4467–4480.

Azmitia, E.C. and Segal, M., 1978. An autoradiographic analysis of the differential ascending projections of the dorsal and median raphe nuclei in the rat. *J. Comp. Neurol.*, **179**, 641–667.

Bagdy, G., 1998. Serotonin, anxiety, and stress hormones — Focus on 5-HT receptor subtypes, species and gender differences. *Ann. N. Y. Acad. Sci.*, **851**, 357–363.

Bartoszyk, G.D., 1998. Anxiolytic effects of dopamine receptor ligands: I. Involvement of dopamine autoreceptors. *Life Sci.*, **62**, 649–663.

Bignami, G., 1976. Nonassociative explanations of behavioural changes induced by central cholinergic drugs. *Acta Neurobiol. Exp.*, **36**, 5–90.

Blanchard, D.C. and Blanchard, R.J., 1988. Ethoexperimental approaches to the biology of emotion. *Annu. Rev. Psychol.*, **39**, 43–68.

Blanchard, D.C., Blanchard, R.J. and Rodgers, R.J., 1991. *Animal Models in Psychopharmacology: Advances in Pharmacological Sciences*. Birkhauser Verlag, Basel.

Blanchard, R.J. and Blanchard, D.C., 1989. Antipredator defensive behaviors in a visible burrow system. *J. Comp. Psychol.*, **103**(1), 70–82.

Blanchard, R.J. and Blanchard, D.C., 1990. An ethoexperimental analysis of defense, fear and anxiety. In: McNaughton, N. and Andrews, G. (eds), *Anxiety*, pp. 124–133. Otago University Press, Dunedin.

Blanchard, R.J., Griebel, G., Henrie, J.A. and Blanchard, D.C., 1997. Differentiation of anxiolytic and panicolytic drugs by effects on rat and mouse defense test batteries. *Neurosci. Biobehav. Rev.*, **21**, 783–789.

Blizard, D.A., 1981. The Maudsley reactive and nonreactive strains: a North American perspective. *Behav. Genet.*, **11**, 469–489.

Blizard, D.A. and Liang, B., 1979. Plasma catecholamines under basal and stressful conditions in rat strains selectively bred for differences in response to stress. In: Usdin, E., Kopin, I.J. and Bachas, J. (eds), *Catecholamines: Basic and Clinical Frontiers*, pp. 1795–1797. Pergamon, New York.

Boulenguez, P., Peters, S.L., Mitchell, S.N., Chauveau, J., Gray, J.A. and Joseph, M.H., 1998. Dopamine release in the nucleus accumbens and latent inhibition in the rat following microinjections of a 5-HT_{1B} agonist into the dorsal subiculum: implications for schizophrenia. *J. Psychopharmacol.*, **12**, 258–267.

Brady, J.V., 1975a. Conditioning and emotion. In: Levi, L. (ed.), *Emotions: Their Parameters and Measurement*, pp. 309–340. Raven Press, New York.

Brady, J.V., 1975b. Toward a behavioural biology of emotion. In: Levi, L. (ed.), *Emotions: Their Parameters and Measurement*, pp. 17–46. Raven Press, New York.

Brioni, J.D., O'Neill, A.B., Kim, D.J.B., Buckley, M.J., Decker, M.W. and Arneric, S.P., 1994. Anxiolytic-like effects of the novel cholinergic channel activator ABT-418. *J. Pharmacol. Exp. Ther.*, **271**, 353–361.

Broadhurst, P.L., 1960. Applications of biometrical genetics to the inheritance of behaviour. In: Eysenck, H.J. (ed.), *Experiments in Personality, Vol. 1 Psychogenetics and Psychopharmacology*, pp. 1–102. Routledge Kegan Paul, London.

Broadhurst, P.L., 1975. The Maudsley reactive and nonreactive strains of rats: a survey. *Behav. Genet.*, **5**, 299–319.

Brown, T.A., Chorpita, B.F. and Barlow, D.H., 1998. Structural relationships among dimensions of the DSM-IV anxiety and mood disorders and dimensions of negative affect, positive affect, and autonomic arousal. *J. Abnorm. Psychol.*, **107**, 179–192.

Buda, M., Lachuer, J., Devauges, V., Barbagli, B., Blizard, D. and Sara, S.J., 1994. Central noradrenergic reactivity to stress in Maudsley rat strains. *Neurosci. Lett.*, **167**, 33–36.

Buller, R., 1995. Reversible inhibitors of monoamine oxidase A in anxiety disorders. *Clin. Neuropharmacol.*, **18**(Suppl. 2), S38–S44.

Camarena, B., Rinetti, G., Cruz, C., Goméz, A., De la Fuente, J.R. and Nicolini, H., 2001. Additional evidence that genetic variation of MAO-A gene supports a gender subtype in obsessive–compulsive disorder. *Am. J. Med. Genet.*, **105**, 279–282.

Carlton, P.L., 1969. Brain acetylcholine and inhibition. In: Tapp, J. (ed.), *Reinforcement and Behaviour*, pp. 286–327. Academic Press, New York.

Cassel, J.-C. and Jeltsch, H., 1995. Serotonergic modulation of cholinergic function in the central nervous system: Cognitive implications. *Neuroscience*, **69**, 1–41.

Cattell, R.B., 1965. *The Scientific Analysis of Personality*. Pelican, Harmondsworth.

Cloninger, C.R., Svrakic, D.M. and Przybecky, T.R., 1993. A psychobiological model of temperament and character. *Arch. Gen. Psychiatr.*, **50**, 975–990.

Collier, D.A., Arranz, M.J., Sham, P., Battersby, S., Vallada, H., Gill, P., Aitchison, K.J., Sodhi, M., Li, T., Roberts, G.W., Smith, B., Morton, J., Murray, R.M., Smith, D. and Kirov, G., 1996. The serotonin transporter is a potential susceptibility factor for bipolar affective disorder. *Neuroreport*, **7**, 1675–1679.

Commissaris, R.L., Franklin, L., Verbanac, J.S. and Altman, H.J., 1992. Maudsley reactive (MR/Har) and non-reactive (MNRA/Har) rats: performance in an operant conflict paradigm. *Physiol. Behav.*, **52**, 873–878.

Commissaris, R.L., Harrington, G.M., Ortiz, A.M. and Altman, H.J., 1986. Maudsley reactive and non-reactive rat strains: differential performance in a conflict task. *Physiol. Behav.*, **38**, 291–294.

Commissaris, R.L., Verbanac, J.S., Markovska, V.L., Altman, H.J. and Hill, T.J., 1996. Anxiety-like and depression-like behavior in Maudsley reactive (MR) and non-reactive (MNRA) rats. *Prog. Neuropsychopharmacol. Biol. Psychiatry*, **20**, 491–501.

Cook, E.H., Jr., Charak, D.A., Arida, J., Spohn, J.A., Roizen, N.J.M. and Leventhal, B.L., 1994. Depressive and obsessive-compulsive symptoms in hyperserotonemic parents of children with autistic disorder. *Psychiatr. Res.*, **52**, 25–33.

Coover, G.D., Ursin, H. and Levine, S., 1973. Plasma corticosterone levels during active avoidance learning in rats. *J. Comp. Physiol. Psychol.*, **82**, 170–174.

Corrodi, H., Fuxe, K., Lidbrink, P. and Olson, L., 1971. Minor tranquilizers, stress, and central catecholamine neurons. *Brain Res.*, **29**, 1–16.

Costa, P.T. and McCrae, R.R., 1985. *The NEO Personality Inventory Manual*. Psychological Assessment Resources, Odessa, FL.

Dalmaz, C., Introini-Collison, I.B. and McGaugh, J.L., 1993. Noradrenergic and cholinergic interactions in the amygdala and the modulation of memory storage. *Behav. Brain Res.*, **58**, 167–174.

Davis, M., Hitchcock, J.M., Bowers, M.B., Berridge, C.W., Melia, K.R. and Roth, R.H., 1994. Stress-induced activation of prefrontal cortex dopamine turnover: Blockade by lesions of the amygdala. *Brain Res.*, **664**, 207–210.

De Oliveira, J.R.M., Otto, P.A., Vallada, H., Lauriano, V., Elkis, H., Lafer, B., Vasquez, L., Gentil, V., Passos-Bueno, M.R. and Zatz, M., 1998. Analysis of a novel functional polymorphism within the promoter region of the serotonin transporter gene (5-HTT) in Brazilian patients affected by bipolar disorder and schizophrenia. *Am. J. Med. Genet.*, **81**, 225–227.

Deakin, J.F.W. and Graeff, F.G., 1991. 5-HT and mechanisms of defence. *J. Psychopharmacol.*, **5**, 305–315.

Dean, B., Hayes, W., Opeskin, K., Naylor, L., Pavey, G., Hill, C., Keks, N. and Copolov, D.L., 1995. Serotonin$_2$ receptors and the serotonin transporter in the schizophrenic brain. *Behav. Brain Res.*, **73**, 169–175.

Decker, M.W. and Gallagher, M., 1987. Scopolamine-disruption of radial arm maze performance: modification by noradrenergic depletion. *Brain Res.*, **417**, 59–69.

Deckert, J., Catalano, M., Syagailo, Y.V., Bosi, M., Okladnova, O., Di Bella, D., Nöthen, M.M., Maffei, P., Franke, P., Fritze, J., Maier, W., Propping, P., Beckmann, H., Bellodi, L. and Lesch, K.P., 1999. Excess of high activity monoamine oxidase A gene promoter alleles in female patients with panic disorder. *Hum. Mol. Genet.*, **8**, 621–624.

Descarries, L., Watkins, K.C. and Lapierre, Y., 1977. Noradrenergic axon terminals in the cerebral cortex of rat: III. Topometric ultrastructural analysis. *Brain Res.*, **133**, 197–222.

Detke, M.J., Rickels, M. and Lucki, I., 1995. Active behaviors in the rat forced swimming test differentially produced by serotonergic and noradrenergic antidepressants. *Psychopharmacol. (Berl)*, **121**, 66–72.

Di Chiara, G., Loddo, P. and Tanda, G., 1999. Reciprocal changes in prefrontal and limbic dopamine responsiveness to aversive and rewarding stimuli after chronic mild stress: Implications for the psychobiology of depression. *Biol. Psychiatry*, **46**, 1624–1633.

Du, L., Bakish, D. and Hrdina, P.D., 2001. Tryptophan hydroxylase gene 218A/C polymorphism is associated with somatic anxiety in major depressive disorder. *J. Affect. Disord.*, **65**, 37–44.

Engberg, G. and Hajos, M., 1994. Nicotine-induced activation of locus coeruleus neurons — An analysis of peripheral versus central induction. *Naunyn Schmiedebergs Arch. Pharmacol.*, **349**, 443–446.

Espejo, E.F., 1997. Selective dopamine depletion within the medial prefrontal cortex induces anxiogenic-like effects in rats placed on the elevated plus maze. *Brain Res.*, **762**, 281–284.

Evans, J., Battersby, S., Ogilvie, A.D., Smith, C.A.D., Harmar, A.J., Nutt, D.J. and Goodwin, G.M., 1997. Association of short alleles of a VNTR of the serotonin transporter gene with anxiety symptoms in patients presenting after deliberate self harm. *Neuropharmacol.*, **36**, 439–443.

Eysenck, H.J., 1960. Classification and the problem of diagnosis. In: Eysenck, H.J. (ed.), *Handbook of Abnormal Psychology*, pp. 1–31. Pitman, London.

Eysenck, H.J. and Eysenck, S.B.G., 1969. *The Structure and Measurement of Personality*. Routledge and Kegan Paul, London.

Eysenck, H.J. and Eysenck, S.B.G., 1976. *Psychoticism as a Dimension of Personality*. Hodder and Stoughton, London.

Feenstra, M.G.P. and Botterblom, M.H.A., 1996. Rapid sampling of extracellular dopamine in the rat prefrontal cortex during food consumption, handling and exposure to novelty. *Brain Res.*, **742**, 17–24.

Feenstra, M.G.P., Botterblom, M.H.A. and Van Uum, J.F.M., 1995. Novelty-induced increase in dopamine release in the rat prefrontal cortex *in vivo*: Inhibition by diazepam. *Neurosci. Lett.*, **189**, 81–84.

Ferraro, G., Sardo, P., Sabatino, M., Caravaglios, G. and La Grutta, V., 1994. Anticonvulsant activity of the noradrenergic locus coeruleus system: Role of beta mediation. *Neurosci. Lett.*, **169**, 93–96.

Fichtner, C.G., O'Connor, F.L., Yeoh, H.C., Arora, R.C. and Crayton, J.W., 1995. Hypodensity of platelet serotonin uptake sites in posttraumatic stress disorder: Associated clinical features. *Life Sci.*, **57**, PL37–PL44.

Finlay, J.M., Zigmond, M.J. and Abercrombie, E.D., 1995. Increased dopamine and norepinephrine release in medial prefrontal cortex induced by acute and chronic stress: Effects of diazepam. *Neuroscience*, **64**, 619–628.

Floderus-Myhred, B., Pedersen, N. and Rasmuson, I., 1980. Assessment of heritability for personality, based on a short-form of the Eysenck Personality Inventory: a study of 12,898 twin pairs. *Behav. Genet.*, **10**, 153–162.

Franklin, J.A., 1990. Behavioural treatment for panic disorder. In: McNaughton, N. and Andrews, G. (eds), *Anxiety*, pp. 84–91. University of Otago, Dunedin.

Fredrikson, M. and Öhman, A., 1979. Cardiovascular and electrodermal responses conditioned to fear-relevant stimuli. *Psychophysiol.*, **16**, 1–7.

Garvey, M.J., Noyes, R., Jr., Woodman, C. and Laukes, C., 1995a. Relationship of generalized anxiety symptoms to urinary 5-hydroxyindoleacetic acid and vanillylmandelic acid. *Psychiatr. Res.*, **57**, 1–5.

Garvey, M.J., Noyes, R., Jr., Woodman, C. and Laukes, C., 1995b. The association of urinary 5-hydroxyindoleacetic acid and vanillylmandelic acid in patients with generalized anxiety. *Neuropsychobiol.*, **31**, 6–9.

Garvey, D.S., Wasicak, J.T., Decker, M.W., Brioni, J.D., Buckley, M.J., Sullivan, J.P., Carrera, G.M., Holladay, M.W., Arneric, S.P. and Williams, M., 1994. Novel isoxazoles which interact with brain cholinergic channel receptors have intrinsic cognitive enhancing and anxiolytic activities. *J. Med. Chem.*, **37**, 1055–1059.

Gaykema, R.P.A., 1992. The Basal Forebrain Cholinergic System: Organization of Connections and Long-Term Effects of Lesions in the Rat. PhD Thesis, University of Groningen, pp. 1–185.

Gaykema, R.P.A., Luiten, P.G.M., Nyakas, C. and Traber, J., 1990. Cortical projection patterns of the medial septum-diagonal band complex. *J. Comp. Neurol.*, **293**, 103–124.

Gobert, A., Rivet, J.M., Lejeune, F., Newman-Tancredi, A., Adhumeau-Auclair, A., Nicolas, J.P., Cistarelli, L., Melon, C. and Millan, M.J., 2000. Serotonin$_{2C}$ receptors tonically suppress the activity of mesocortical dopaminergic and adrenergic, but not serotonergic, pathways: A combined dialysis and electrophysiological analysis in the rat. *Synapse*, **36**, 205–221.

Goddard, A.W., Sholomskas, D.E., Walton, K.E., Augeri, F.M., Charney, D.S., Heninger, G.R., Goodman, W.K. and Price, L.H., 1994. Effects of tryptophan depletion in panic disorder. *Biol. Psychiatry*, **36**, 775–777.

Goisman, R.M., Warshaw, M.G., Steketee, G.S., Fierman, E.J., Rogers, M.P., Goldenberg, I., Weinshenker, N.J., Vasile, R.G. and Keller, M.B., 1995. DSM-IV and the disappearance of agoraphobia without a history of panic disorder: New data on a controversial diagnosis. *Am. J. Psychiatry*, **152**, 1438–1443.

Goldberg, D.P. and Huxley, P., 1992. *Common Mental Disorders: A Biosocial Model*. Routledge, London.

Gorman, J.M., Papp, L.A., Coplan, J.D., Martinez, J.M., Lennon, S., Goetz, R.R., Ross, D. and Klein, D.F., 1994. Anxiogenic effects of CO_2 and hyperventilation in patients with panic disorder. *Am. J. Psychiatry*, **151**, 547–553.

Graeff, F.G., 1993. Role of 5-HT in defensive behaviour and anxiety. *Rev. Neurosci.*, **4**, 181–211.

Graeff, F.G., 1994. Neuroanatomy and neurotransmitter regulation of defensive behaviors and related emotions in mammals. *Braz. J. Med. Biol. Res.*, **27**, 811–829.

Graeff, F.G., Guimaraes, F.S., De Andrade, T.G.C.S. and Deakin, J.F.W., 1996. Role of 5-HT in stress, anxiety, and depression. *Pharmacol. Biochem. Behav.*, **54**, 129–141.

Graeff, F.G. and Schoenfeld, R.I., 1970. Tryptaminergic mechanisms in punished and nonpunished behavior. *J. Pharmacol. Exp. Ther.*, **173**, 277–283.

Graeff, F.G., Viana, M.B. and Mora, P.O., 1997. Dual role of 5-HT in defense and anxiety. *Neurosci. Biobehav. Rev.*, **21**, 791–799.

Gray, J.A., 1970. The psychophysiological basis of introversion–extraversion. *Behav. Res. Ther.*, **8**, 249–266.

Gray, J.A., 1975. *Elements of a Two-Process Theory of Learning*. Academic Press, London.

Gray, J.A., 1981. A critique of Eysenck's theory of personality. In: Eysenck, H.J. (ed.), *A Model for Personality*, pp. 246–276. Springer, New York.

Gray, J.A., 1987. Interactions between drugs and behaviour therapy. In: Eysenck, H.J. and Martin, I. (eds), *Theoretical Foundations of Behaviour Therapy*. Plenum Press, New York.

Gray, J.A. and McNaughton, N., 2000. *The Neuropsychology of Anxiety: An Enquiry into the Functions of the Septo-Hippocampal System*, 2 edn. Oxford University Press, Oxford.

Gresch, P.J., Sved, A.F., Zigmond, M.J. and Finlay, J.M., 1995. Local influence of endogenous norepinephrine on extracellular dopamine in rat medial prefrontal cortex. *J. Neurochem.*, **65**, 111–116.

Griebel, G., 1995. 5-hydroxytryptamine-interacting drugs in animal models of anxiety disorders: More than 30 years of research. *Pharmacol. Ther.*, **65**, 319–395.

Gurevich, E.V. and Joyce, J.N., 1997. Alterations in the cortical serotonergic system in schizophrenia: A postmortem study. *Biol. Psychiatry*, **42**, 529–545.

Gurguis, G.N.M., Antai-Otong, D., Vo, S.P., Blakeley, J.E., Orsulak, P.J., Petty, F. and Rush, A.J., 1999. Adrenergic receptor function in panic disorder — I. Platelet α_2 receptors: G_i protein coupling, effects of imipramine, and relationship to treatment outcome. *Neuropsychopharm.*, **20**, 162–176.

Haber, S.N. and Fudge, J.L., 1997. The interface between dopamine neurons and the amygdala: Implications for schizophrenia. *Schizophr. Bull.*, **23**, 471–482.

Hall, C.S., 1951. The genetics of behavior. In: Stevens, S.S. (ed.), *Handbook of Experimental Psychology*, pp. 304–329. Wiley, New York.

Haller, J., Makara, G.B. and Kruk, M.R., 1998. Catecholaminergic involvement in the control of aggression: hormones, the peripheral sympathetic, and central noradrenergic systems. *Neurosci. Biobehav. Rev.*, **22**, 85–97.

Hamilton, S.P., Haghighi, F., Heiman, G.A., Klein, D.F., Hodge, S.E., Fyer, A.J., Weissman, M.M. and Knowles, J.A., 2000. Investigation of dopamine receptor (*DRD4*) and dopamine transporter (*DAT*) polymorphisms for genetic linkage or association to panic disorder. *Am. J. Med. Genet.*, **96**, 324–330.

Handley, S.L., 1995. 5-hydroxytryptamine pathways in anxiety and its treatment. *Pharmacol. Ther.*, **66**, 103–148.

Hegarty, A.A. and Vogel, W.H., 1995. The effect of acute and chronic diazepam treatment on stress-induced changes in cortical dopamine in the rat. *Pharmacol. Biochem. Behav.*, **52**, 771–778.

Holt, P., 1990. Panic disorder: some historical trends. In: McNaughton, N. and Andrews, G. (eds), *Anxiety*, pp. 54–65. University of Otago Press, Dunedin.

Imperato, A., Angelucci, L., Casolini, P., Zocchi, A. and Puglisi-Allegra, S., 1992. Repeated stressful experiences differently affect limbic dopamine release during and following stress. *Brain Res.*, **577**, 194–199.

Iversen, L.L. and Schon, F., 1973. The use of radioautographic techniques for the identification and mapping of transmitter-specific neurons in CNS. In: Mandell, A. and Segal, D. (eds), *New Concepts of Transmitter Regulation*, pp. 153–193. Plenum Press, New York.

Iversen, S.D., 1984. 5-HT and anxiety. *Neuropharmacol.*, **23**, 1553–1560.

Jacobs, B.L. and Azmitia, E.C., 1992. Structure and function of the brain serotonin system. *Physiol. Rev.*, **72**, 165–229.

Jordan, S., Kramer, G.L., Zukas, P.K. and Petty, F., 1994. Previous stress increases *in vivo* biogenic amine response to swim stress. *Neurochem. Res.*, **19**, 1521–1525.

Kaneyuki, H., Yokoo, H., Tsuda, A., Yoshida, M., Mizuki, Y., Yamada, M. and Tanaka, M., 1991. Psychological stress increases dopamine turnover selectively in mesoprefrontal dopamine neurons of rats: Reversal by diazepam. *Brain Res.*, **557**, 154–161.

Karege, F., Bovier, P., Hilleret, H. and Gaillard, J.-M., 1993. Lack of effect of anxiety on total plasma MHPG in depressed patients. *J. Affect. Disord.*, **28**, 211–217.

Katsuragi, S., Kunugi, H., Sano, A., Tsutsumi, T., Isogawa, K., Nanko, S. and Akiyoshi, J., 1999. Association between serotonin transporter gene polymorphism and anxiety-related traits. *Biol. Psychiatry*, **45**, 368–370.

Kelly, C.B. and Cooper, S.J., 1998. Differences and variability in plasma noradrenaline between depressive and anxiety disorders. *J. Psychopharmacol.*, **12**, 161–167.

Kendler, K.S., Neale, M.C., Kessler, R.C., Heath, A.C. and Eaves, L.J., 1992a. Generalized anxiety disorder in women: a population-based twin study. *Arch. Gen. Psychiatr.*, **49**, 267–272.

Kendler, K.S., Neale, M.C., Kessler, R.C., Heath, A.C. and Eaves, L.J., 1992b. Major depression and generalized anxiety disorder. Same genes, (partly) different environments? *Arch. Gen. Psychiatr.*, **49**, 716–722.

Kendler, K.S., Neale, M.C., Kessler, R.C., Heath, A.C. and Eaves, L.J., 1992c. The genetic epidemiology of phobias in women: the interrelationship of agoraphobia, social phobia, situational phobia and simple phobia. *Arch. Gen. Psychiatr.*, **49**, 273–281.

Kim, J.J., Shih, J.C., Chen, K., Chen, L., Bao, S.W., Maren, S., Anagnostaras, S.G., Fanselow, M.S., De Maeyer, E., Seif, I. and Thompson, R.F., 1997. Selective enhancement of emotional, but not motor, learning in monoamine oxidase A-deficient mice. *Proc. Natl. Acad. Sci. USA*, **94**, 5929–5933.

Klaassen, T., Klumperbeek, J., Deutz, N.E.P., Van Praag, H.M. and Griez, E., 1998. Effects of tryptophan depletion on anxiety and on panic provoked by carbon dioxide challenge. *Psychiatr. Res.*, **77**, 167–174.

Kocsis, B., Thinschmidt, J.S., Kinney, G.G. and Vertes, R.P., 1994. Separation of hippocampal theta dipoles by partial coherence analysis in the rat. *Brain Res.*, **660**, 341–345.

Koda, L.Y., Schulman, J.A. and Bloom, F.E., 1978. Ultrastructural identification of noradrenergic terminals in rat hippocampus: Unilateral destruction of the locus coeruleus with 6-hydroxydopamine. *Brain Res.*, **145**, 190–195.

Kokaia, M., Cenci, M.A., Elmér, E., Nilsson, O.G., Kokaia, Z., Bengzon, J., Björklund, A. and Lindvall, O., 1994. Seizure development and noradrenaline release in kindling epilepsy after noradrenergic reinnervation of the subcortically deafferented hippocampus by superior cervical ganglion or fetal locus coeruleus grafts. *Exp. Neurol.*, **130**, 351–361.

Koyama, Y., Jodo, E. and Kayama, Y., 1994. Sensory responsiveness of "broad-spike" neurons in the laterodorsal tegmental nucleus, locus coeruleus and dorsal raphe of awake rats: Implications for cholinergic and monoaminergic neuron-specific responses. *Neuroscience*, **63**, 1021–1031.

Lachman, H.M., Papolos, D.F., Saito, T., Yu, Y.-M., Szumlanski, C.L. and Weinshilboum, R.M., 1996. Human catechol-*O*-methyltransferase pharmacogenetics: Description of a functional polymorphism and its potential application to neuropsychiatric disorders. *Pharmacogenetics*, **6**, 243–250.

Lader, M., 1990. Introduction: use and abuse. In: Wheatley, D. (ed.), *In the Anxiolytic Jungle: Where Next?*, pp. 3–7. John Wiley & Sons, Chichester.

Lader, M. and Tyrer, P., 1975. Vegetative system and emotion. In: Levi, L. (ed.), *Emotions: Their Parameters and Measurement*. Raven Press, New York.

Laruelle, M., Abi-Dargham, A., Casanova, M.F., Toti, R., Weinberger, D.R. and Kleinman, J.E., 1993. Selective abnormalities of prefrontal serotonergic receptors in schizophrenia: A postmortem study. *Arch. Gen. Psychiatr.*, **50**, 810–818.

LeDoux, J., 1998. Fear and the brain: Where have we been, and where are we going? *Biol. Psychiatry*, **44**, 1229–1238.

LeDoux, J.E., 1994. Emotion, memory and the brain. *Sci. Am.*, **270**, 50–59.

Leonard, B.E., 1996. Serotonin receptors and their function in sleep, anxiety disorders and depression. *Psychother. Psychosom.*, **65**, 66–75.

Leyton, M., Young, S.N., Pihl, R.O., Etezadi, S., Lauze, C., Blier, P., Baker, G.B. and Benkelfat, C., 2000. Effects on mood of acute phenylalanine/tyrosine depletion in healthy women. *Neuropsychopharm.*, **22**, 52–63.

Maas, J.W., 1963. Neurochemical differences between two strains of mice. *Nature*, **197**, 255–257.

Maes, M., Lin, A.H., Verkerk, R., Delmeire, L., Van Gastel, A., Van der Planken, M. and Scharpé, S., 1999. Serotonergic and noradrenergic markers of post-traumatic stress disorder with and without major depression. *Neuropsychopharm.*, **20**, 188–197.

Magoun, H.W., 1963. *The Waking Brain*, 2 edn. Thomas, Springfield, IL.

Margraf, J. and Ehlers, A., 1990. Biological models of panic disorder and agorophobia: theory and evidence. In: Burrows, G.D., Roth, M. and Noyes, R. (eds), *Handbook of Anxiety*, pp. 79–139. Elsevier Science Publishers, Oxford.

Marks, I., 1987. Agoraphobia, panic disorder and related conditions in the DSM-IIIR and ICD-10. *J. Psychopharmacol.*, **1**, 6–12.

Marks, I.M., 1969. *Fears and Phobias*. Heinemann, London.

McFarlane, A.C., 1989. The aetiology of post-traumatic morbidity: predisposing, precipitating and perpetuating factors. *Br. J. Psychiatr.*, **154**, 221–228.

McNaughton, N., Forster, G.L., Swain-Campbell, N.R. and Ripandelli, F.M., 1997. Cholinergic relays in superior colliculus, substantia nigra and amygdala co-operate to gate theta activity. *Soc. Neurosci. Abstr.*, **23**, 487.

McNaughton, N. and Gray, J.A., 1983. Pavlovian counterconditioning is unchanged by chlordiazepoxide or by septal lesions. *Q. J. Exp. Psychol.*, **35B**, 221–233.

McNaughton, N. and Mason, S.T., 1980. The neuropsychology and neuropharmacology of the dorsal ascending noradrenergic bundle — a review. *Prog. Neurobiol.*, **14**, 157–219.

McNaughton, N., Ripandelli, N. and Swain-Campbell, N.R., 2001. Confirmation from the amygdala of the disrupted cholinergic network gating hippocampal theta activity. *Int. J. Neurosci.*

Melke, J., Landén, M., Baghei, F., Rosmond, R., Holm, G., Björntorp, P., Westberg, L., Hellstrand, M. and Eriksson, E., 2001. Serotonin transporter gene polymorphisms are associated with anxiety-related personality traits in women. *Am. J. Med. Genet.*, **105**, 458–463.

Meneses, A., 1999. 5-HT system and cognition. *Neurosci. Biobehav. Rev.*, **23**, 1111–1125.

Modigh, K., 1987. Antidepressant drugs in anxiety disorders. *Acta Psychiatr. Scand.*, **76**, 57–71.

Moon, C.A.L., Jago, W., Wood, K. and Doogan, D.P., 1994. A double-blind comparison of sertraline and clomipramine in the treatment of major depressive disorder and associated anxiety in general practice. *J. Psychopharmacol.*, **8**, 171–176.

Moore, R.Y. and Bloom, F.E., 1979. Central catecholamine neuron systems: anatomy and physiology of the norepinephrine and epinephrine systems. *Annu. Rev. Neurosci.*, **2**, 113–167.

Morgan, C.A., III, Grillon, C., Southwick, S.M., Nagy, L.M., Davis, M., Krystal, J.H. and Charney, D.S., 1995. Yohimbine facilitated acoustic startle in combat veterans with post-traumatic stress disorder. *Psychopharmacol. (Berl)*, **117**, 466–471.

Morin, L.P., 1994. The circadian visual system. *Brain Res. Rev.*, **67**, 102–127.

Naylor, L., Dean, B., Opeskin, K., Pavey, G., Hill, C., Keks, N. and Copolov, D., 1996. Changes in the serotonin transporter in the hippocampus of subjects with schizophrenia identified using [^{3}H]paroxetine. *J. Neural Transm.*, **103**, 749–757.

Norman, T.R., Judd, F.K. and Burrows, G.D., 1990. Catecholamines and anxiety. In: Burrows, G.D., Roth, M. and Noyes, R., Jr. (eds), *Handbook of Anxiety, Vol. 3: The Neurobiology of Anxiety*, pp. 223–241. Elsevier, Amsterdam.

Oberlander, E.L., Schneier, F.R. and Liebowitz, M.R., 1994. Physical disability and social phobia. *J. Clin. Psychopharmacol.*, **14**, 136–143.

Ohara, K., Nagai, M., Suzuki, Y. and Ochiai, M., 1998a. Association between anxiety disorders and a functional polymorphism in the serotonin transporter gene. *Psychiatr. Res.*, **81**, 277–279.

Ohara, K., Nagai, M., Suzuki, Y. and Ochiai, M., 1998b. No association between anxiety disorders and catechol-*O*-methyltransferase polymorphism. *Psychiatr. Res.*, **80**, 145–148.

Ohara, K., Suzuki, Y., Ochiai, M. and Terada, H., 2000. Polymorphism in the promoter region of the alpha$_{2A}$-adrenergic receptor gene and panic disorders. *Psychiatr. Res.*, **93**, 79–82.

Olson, L. and Fuxe, K., 1971. On the projections from the locus coeruleus noradrenaline neurons: the cerebellar innervation. *Brain Res.*, **28**, 165–171.

Ordway, G.A., Smith, K.S. and Haycock, J.W., 1994. Elevated tyrosine hydroxylase in the locus coeruleus of suicide victims. *J. Neurochem.*, **62**, 680–685.

Orsetti, M., Casamenti, F. and Pepeu, G., 1996. Enhanced acetylcholine release in the hippocampus and cortex during acquisition of an operant behavior. *Brain Res.*, **724**, 89–96.

Owen, S., Boarder, M.R., Gray, J.A. and Fillenz, M., 1982. Acquisition and extinction of continuously and partially reinforced running in rats with lesions of the dorsal noradrenergic bundle. *Behav. Brain Res.*, **5**, 11–41.

Pickel, V.M., Krebs, H. and Bloom, F.E., 1973. Proliferation of norepinephrine-containing axons in rat cerebellar cortex after peduncle lesions. *Brain Res.*, **59**, 169–179.

Pitman, R.K., Orr, S.P. and Shalev, A.Y., 1993. Once bitten, twice shy: beyond the conditioning model of PTSD. *Biol. Psychiatry*, **33**, 145–146.

Post, R.M. and Weiss, S.R.B., 1998. Sensitization and kindling phenomena in mood, anxiety, and obsessive–compulsive disorders: The role of serotonergic mechanisms in illness progression. *Biol. Psychiatry*, **44**, 193–206.

Powell, G.E., 1979. *Brain and Personality*. Saxon House, London.

Rajkowski, J., Kubiak, P. and Aston-Jones, G., 1994. Locus coeruleus activity in monkey: Phasic and tonic changes are associated with altered vigilance. *Brain Res. Bull.*, **35**, 607–616.

Redmond, D.E., Jr., 1979. New and old evidence for the involvement of a brain norepinephrine system in anxiety. In: Fann, W.G., Karacan, I., Pokorny, A.D. and Williams, R.L. (eds), *Phenomenology and Treatment of Anxiety*, pp. 153–203. Spectrum, New York.

Riekkinen, P., Sirvio, J. and Riekkinen, P., Jr., 1990. Interaction between raphe dorsalis and nucleus basalis magnocellularis in spatial learning. *Brain Res.*, **527**, 342–345.

Rodgers, R.J., Blanchard, D.C., Wong, L.K. and Blanchard, R.J., 1990. Effects of scopolamine on antipredator defense reactions in wild and laboratory rats. *Pharmacol. Biochem. Behav.*, **36**, 575–583.

Rodgers, R.J. and Cole, J.C., 1995. Effects of scopolamine and its quaternary analogue in the murine elevated plus-maze test of anxiety. *Behav. Pharmacol.*, **6**, 283–289.

Rose, G. and Day, S., 1990. The population mean predicts the number of deviant individuals. *Br. Med. J.*, **391**, 1031–1034.

Sara, S.J., Devauges, V. and Biegon, A., 1993. Maudsley rat strains, selected for differences in emotional responses, differ in behavioral response to clonidine and in [^{125}I]clonidine binding in the locus coeruleus. *Behav. Brain Res.*, **57**, 101–104.

Sara, S.J., Vankov, A. and Hervé, A., 1994. Locus coeruleus-evoked responses in behaving rats: A clue to the role of noradrenaline in memory. *Brain Res. Bull.*, **35**, 457–465.

Sarter, M.F. and Bruno, J.P., 1994. Cognitive functions of cortical Ach: Lessons from studies on trans-synaptic modulation of activated efflux. *TINS*, **17**, 217–221.

Sartory, G., MacDonald, R. and Gray, J.A., 1990. Effects of diazepam on approach, self-reported fear and psychophysiological responses in snake phobics. *Behav. Res. Ther.*, **28**, 273–282.

Saxena, P.R., 1995. Serotonin receptors: Subtypes, functional responses and therapeutic relevance. *Pharmacol. Ther.*, **66**, 339–368.

Scherrer, J.F., True, W.R., Xian, H., Lyons, M.J., Eisen, S.A., Goldberg, J., Lin, N. and Tsuang, M.T., 2000. Evidence for genetic influences common and specific to symptoms of generalized anxiety and panic. *J. Affect. Disord.*, **57**, 25–35.

Segal, M., 1978. Serotonergic innervation of the locus coeruleus from the dorsal raphe. *J. Physiol. (Lond.)*, **286**, 401–415.

Sheehan, D.V., Ballenger, J. and Jacobson, G., 1981. Relative efficacy of monoamine oxidase inhibitors and tricyclic antidepressants in the treatment of endogenous anxiety. In: Klein, D.F. and Rabkin, J. (eds), *Anxiety New Research and Changing Concepts*, pp. 47–67. Raven Press, New York.

Shen, H. and Semba, K., 1994. A direct retinal projection to the dorsal raphe nucleus in the rat. *Brain Res.*, **635**, 159–168.

Shimizu, N., Katoh, Y., Hida, T. and Satoh, K., 1979. The fine structural organization of the locus coeruleus in the rat with reference to noradrenaline contents. *Exp. Brain Res.*, **37**, 139–148.

Smagin, G.N., Swiergiel, A.H. and Dunn, A.J., 1995. Corticotropin-releasing factor administered into the locus coeruleus, but not the parabrachial nucleus, stimulates norepinephrine release in the prefrontal cortex. *Brain Res. Bull.*, **36**, 71–76.

Stein, L., Wise, C.D. and Berger, B.D., 1973. Anti-anxiety action of benzodiazepines: decrease in activity of serotonin neurons in the punishment system. In: Garattini, S., Mussini, E. and Randall, L.O. (eds), *The Benzodiazepines*, pp. 299–326. Raven Press, New York.

Stein, M.B., Asmundson, G.J.G. and Chartier, M., 1994. Autonomic responsivity in generalized social phobia. *J. Affect. Disord.*, **31**, 211–221.

Stein, M.B., Delaney, S.M., Chartier, M.J., Kroft, C.D.L. and Hazen, A.L., 1995. [^{3}H]paroxetine binding to platelets of patients with social phobia: Comparison to patients with panic disorder and healthy volunteers. *Biol. Psychiatry*, **37**, 224–228.

Stein, M.B., Walker, J.R. and Forde, D.R., 1994. Setting diagnostic thresholds for social phobia: Considerations from a community survey of social anxiety. *Am. J. Psychiatry*, **151**, 408–412.

Sumiyoshi, T., Stockmeier, C.A., Overholser, J.C., Dilley, G.E. and Meltzer, H.Y., 1996. Serotonin$_{1A}$ receptors are increased in postmortem prefrontal cortex in schizophrenia. *Brain Res.*, **708**, 209–214.

Swain-Campbell, N.R. and McNaughton, N., 2001. Pedunculopontine control of hippocampal theta rhythm: mapping in the region of the supramammillary nucleus. *Int. J. Neurosci.*

Swerdlow, N.R., 1995. Serotonin, obsessive compulsive disorder and the basal ganglia. Special issue: Serotonin receptor subtypes in psychiatry. *Int. Rev. Psychiatr.*, **7**, 115–129.

Tauscher, J., Bagby, R.M., Javanmard, M., Christensen, B.K., Kasper, S. and Kapur, S., 2001. Inverse relationship between serotonin 5-HT$_{1A}$ receptor binding and anxiety: a [^{11}C]WAY-100635 PET investigation in healthy volunteers. *Am. J. Psychiatry*, **158**, 1326–1328.

Taylor, J.A., 1953. A personality scale of manifest anxiety. *J. Abnorm. Soc. Psychol.*, **48**, 285–290.

Trulson, M.E. and Henderson, L.J., 1984. Buspirone increases locus coeruleus noradrenergic neuronal activity *in vitro*. *Eur. J. Pharmacol.*, **106**, 195–198.

Tsuchiya, K., Inoue, T. and Koyama, T., 1996. Effect of repeated methamphetamine pretreatment on freezing behavior induced by conditioned fear stress. *Pharmacol. Biochem. Behav.*, **54**, 687–691.

Uphouse, L., 1997. Multiple serotonin receptors: Too many, not enough, or just the right number? *Neurosci. Biobehav. Rev.*, **21**, 679–698.

Valentino, R.J., Foote, S.L. and Page, M.E., 1993. The locus coeruleus as a site for integrating corticotropin-releasing factor and noradrenergic mediation of stress responses. *Ann. N. Y. Acad. Sci.*, **697**, 173–188.

Van Bockstaele, E.J. and Aston-Jones, G., 1995. Integration in the ventral medulla and coordination of sympathetic, pain and arousal functions. *Clin. Exp. Hypertens.*, **17**, 153–165.

Van Praag, H.M., 1995. Concerns about depression. *Eur. Psychiatr.*, **10**, 269–275.

Van Praag, H.M., 1996. Serotonin-related, anxiety/aggression-driven, stressor-precipitated depression. A psycho-biological hypothesis. *Eur. Psychiatr.*, **11**, 57–67.

Veltman, D.J., Van Zijderveld, G., Tilders, F.J.H. and Van Dyck, R., 1996. Epinephrine and fear of bodily sensations in panic disorder and social phobia. *J. Psychopharmacol.*, **10**, 259–265.

Veltman, D.J., Van Zijderveld, G.A., Van Dyck, R. and Bakker, A., 1998. Predictability, controllability, and fear of symptoms of anxiety in epinephrine-induced panic. *Biol. Psychiatry*, **44**, 1017–1026.

Verbanac, J.S., Altman, H.J., Dhingra, P., Harrington, G.M. and Commissaris, R.L., 1993. Conflict behavior in Maudsley reactive and nonreactive rats: effects of noradrenergic neuronal destruction. *Pharmacol. Biochem. Behav.*, **45**, 429–438.

Verbanac, J.S., Commissaris, R.L., Altman, H.J. and Pitts, D.K., 1994. Electrophysiological characteristics of locus coeruleus neurons in the Maudsley reactive (MR) and non-reactive (MNRA) rat strains. *Neurosci. Lett.*, **179**, 137–140.

Verbanac, J.S., Commissaris, R.L. and Pitts, D.K., 1995. An electrophysiological evaluation of serotonergic dorsal raphe neurons in Maudsley rats. *Life Sci.*, **58**, 245–250.

Vertes, R.P. and Kocsis, B., 1994. Projections of the dorsal raphe nucleus to the brainstem: PHA-L analysis in the rat. *J. Comp. Neurol.*, **340**, 11–26.

Viglinskaya, I.V., Overstreet, D.H., Kashevskaya, O.P., Badishtov, B.A., Kampov-Polevoy, A.B., Seredenin, S.B. and Halikas, J.A., 1995. To drink or not to drink: Tests of anxiety and immobility in alcohol-preferring and alcohol-non-preferring rat strains. *Physiol. Behav.*, **57**, 987–991.

Vinogradova, O.S., Brazhnik, E.S., Kitchigina, V.F. and Stafekhina, V.S., 1993. Acetylcholine, theta-rhythm and activity of hippocampal neurons in the rabbit — IV. Sensory stimulation. *Neuroscience*, **53**, 993–1007.

Wang, Z., Valdes, J., Noyes, R., Zoega, T. and Crowe, R.R., 1998a. Possible association of a cholecystokinin promotor polymorphism (CCK$_{-36CT}$) with panic disorder. *Am. J. Med. Genet.*, **81**, 228–234.

Wang, Z.W., Valdes, J., Noyes, R., Zoega, T. and Crowe, R.R., 1998b. Possible association of a cholecystokinin promotor polymorphism (CCK$_{-36CT}$) with panic disorder. *Am. J. Med. Genet.*, **81**, 228–234.

Watson, D., Clark, L.A. and Harkness, A.R., 1994. Structures of personality and their relevance to psychopathology. *J. Abnorm. Psychol.*, **103**, 18–31.

Wheatley, D., 1990. The new alternatives. In: Wheatley, D. (ed.), *In the Anxiolytic Jungle: Where Next?*, pp. 163–184. Wiley, Chichester.

Wilkinson, L.O., Abercrombie, E.D., Rasmussen, K. and Jacobs, B.L., 1987. Effect of buspirone on single unit activity in locus coeruleus and dorsal raphe nucleus in behaving cats. *Eur. J. Pharmacol.*, **136**, 123–127.

Wilkinson, L.O. and Dourish, C.T., 1991. Serotonin and Animal Behavior. In: Venter, J.C. and Harrison, L.C. (eds), *Receptor Biochemistry and Methodology*, 15 edn, pp. 147–210. Wiley-Liss Inc., New York.

World Health Organization, 1992. *The ICD-10 Classification of Mental and Behavioural Disorders*. World Health Organization, Geneva.

Young, S.L., Bohenek, D.L. and Fanselow, M.S., 1995. Scopolamine impairs acquisition and facilitates consolidation of fear conditioning: Differential effects for tone vs context conditioning. *Neurobiol. Learn. Mem.*, **63**, 174–180.

Zaborszky, L., Gaykema, R.P., Swanson, D.J. and Cullinan, W.E., 1997. Cortical input to the basal forebrain. *Neuroscience*, **79**, 1051–1078.

Zifa, E. and Fillion, G., 1992. 5-Hydroxytryptamine receptors. *Pharmac. Rev.*, **44**(3), 401–458.

Zinbarg, R.E. and Barlow, D.H., 1996. Structure of anxiety and the anxiety disorders: a hierarchical model. *J. Abnorm. Psychol.*, **105**, 181–193.

XIX-3

Amino Acid Transmitter Systems

Catherine Belzung, Guy Griebel, Florence Dubois-Carmagnat and Jean Michel Darves-Bornoz

INTRODUCTION

Amino acids correspond to a wide range of compounds, including precursors of catecholamine and serotonin synthesis (tyrosin and tryptophan respectively) as well as neurotransmitter systems such as the excitatory amino acids glutamate and aspartate and the inhibitory amino acids γ-aminobutyric acid (GABA) and glycine. As few studies revealed anxiolytics acting on excitatory amino acids via the N-methyl-D-aspartate (NMDA) complex and/or the metabotropic glutamate (mGlu) receptors, only a short paragraph will be devoted to such agents. Furthermore, data suggesting abnormalities in excitatory amino acid systems in some anxiety disorders will be mentioned. On the other hand, we will focus on anxiolytic drugs acting on GABAergic neurotransmission, as most anxiolytics act via GABA-related mechanisms, first focusing on the mechanisms underlying the anxiolytic action of some anti-anxiety agents such as benzodiazepines (BZs) and second describing the use of such compounds in the clinic, in an attempt to link the pharmacology with neurochemical changes that have been observed in these disorders.

ANXIOLYTIC AGENTS ACTING ON EXCITATORY AMINO ACID NEUROTRANSMISSION

The anti-anxiety-like action of compounds acting on excitatory amino acid neurotransmission has mainly been investigated in pre-clinical studies, using animal models of anxiety. Indeed, because of multiple side effects of such compounds (ataxia, myorelaxation, impairment of learning and memory), such agents cannot be proposed as potential anxiolytic drugs in the clinic.

Glutamate and aspartate bind to two types of receptors: the ionotropic receptors (AMPA, kainite and NMDA receptors) and the metabotropic glutamate receptor. Among the ionotropic receptors, solely the NMDA receptor has been proposed as a potential target for anxiolytic agents in pre-clinical studies.

Ligands of the NMDA Receptor

The NMDA complex consists of various binding sites, including a glutamate recognition site, a polyamine site, a glycine site, a phencyclidine site (channel site) and a Zn^{2+} site. Low doses of the non-competitive NMDA antagonist MK-801 or of the competitive NMDA antagonists AP5, AP7 and CPP elicited anxiolytic behaviour in several animal tests (see Chojnacka-Wójcik and Klodzinska (2001) for a recent review). Similar effects were observed with antagonists (7-CIKYN and 5,7-CIKYN) and partial agonists (HA-966, ACPC and D-cycloserine) of the Glycine_B receptors; however, none of these agents crosses the blood–brain barrier. Finally, discrepant results were obtained with antagonists of the polyamine site (ifenprodil and eliprodil) as these compounds are endowed with anxiolytic properties in some, but not all animal models of anxiety.

Ligands of the Metabotropic Glutamate Receptor

The mGlu receptors are a family of eight receptors designated mGlu1 through mGlu8, which can be divided in three groups based on the similarity of the amino acid sequence, pharmacology and second messenger coupling. The first group, which consists of mGlu1 and mGlu5, is positively coupled with phospholipase C and is sensitive to *trans*-ACPD as well as quisqualate. The second group, which includes mGlu2 and mGlu3, is negatively coupled to adenylate cyclase and is sensitive to *trans*-ACPD but not quisqualate. The third group, consisting of mGlu4, mGlu6, mGlu7 and mGlu8, is negatively coupled to adenylate cyclase and does not respond to *trans*-ACPD and quisqualate but rather binds specific compounds. Antagonists of Group I mGlu receptors such as S-4C3HPG or (S)-4CPG, as well as an antagonist of the mGlu1 (CPCCOEt) or of the mGlu5 (MPEP) elicited anxiolytic effects in pre-clinical models. Furthermore, LY-354740, an agonist of Group II mGlu receptors, displayed anxiolytic activity in several models of anxiety. In fact, as Group II mGlu receptors are localized presynaptically, their receptor agonists may inhibit glutamate release, so that they are parallel to the effects of Group I mGlu receptors antagonists. Finally, regarding Group II mGlu receptors ligands, the issue remains to be clarified as discrepant results have been obtained.

ANXIOLYTIC AGENTS ACTING ON GABAERGIC NEUROTRANSMISSION

Early Anxiolytics Acting via a GABAergic Mechanism

Ethanol

There is evidence suggesting that ethanol, a compound usually termed as alcohol, has been used in prehistoric times. It can therefore be considered as the first anxiolytic compound. Mead, a fermentation product of honey, is considered as the oldest alcoholic beverage; it seems that it existed in the paleolithic age, about 8000 B.C. Alcoholic beverages are known to produce relaxation, elevation of mood, anxiolysis and disinhibition in response to social constraints. At higher doses it induces sedation. Most alcohol users drink occasionally (75% of the population of the USA). However, 15% of users are considered alcoholics. This highlights the great abuse potential of this compound.

Biological Psychiatry: Edited by H. D'haenen, J.A. den Boer and P. Willner. ISBN 0-471-49198-5

Barbiturates

In 1864, Adolph von Baeyer synthesized barbituric acid (malonylurea). The name of this drug is said to be linked to the presence, on the day of the experiment, of Baeyer in a tavern in which officers were celebrating the Day of St. Barbara, their patron saint. Barbituric acid was devoid of clinical potency but it led to the development of barbiturates after 1903, the date of the synthesis of barbital that became rapidly popular. These compounds rapidly took a dominant place because they facilitated sleep and produced relaxation. However, the bioavailability of barbital was rather low because of the poor solubility in lipids of that drug. Furthermore, it was metabolized slowly so that the effects on drowsiness extended over 36 hours. Consequently, new drugs with short duration of action (amobarbital, pentobarbital, secobarbital) and later, in the 1930s, ultra-short duration of action (hexobarbital, thiopental, methohexital) were introduced into therapeutics. These drugs, termed barbiturates, are widely used as anaesthetics but they also have an excellent efficacy in alleviating anxiety. For example, pentobarbital (Figure XIX-3.1) is effective in most rodent models of anxiety. However, their development in the treatment of anxiety has been spurred by their high abuse potential. This has been shown in animal as well as human studies. Furthermore, it also elicited lethal effects (1500 deaths per year), principally due to accidental poisoning in drug abusers and to suicide.

Carbamates

As in many other cases, the starting point of the use of carbamates in the treatment of anxiety had nothing to do with their action in the central nervous system. In the 1940s, the Wallace Laboratories were developing new antibacterial agents and therefore chemists attempted to improve the potency of phenoxetol, a compound used as disinfectant, by lengthening the carbon chain. When testing the toxicity of that newly synthesized compound, termed mephenesin, they observed that it produced muscle relaxation and a sleeping-like condition in animals. They described this action as 'quieting influence on the demeanor of the animal', an effect that was named in 1946 'tranquillization'. The drug was marketed in 1947 as a short-action muscle relaxant but in 1949 several authors proposed that it may alleviate anxiety. However, mephenesin had several drawbacks, including a very short duration of action. Therefore, researchers attempted to alter the chemical structure of mephenesin to overcome these shortcomings: the result was meprobamate (Figure XIX-3.2), a compound whose duration of action was eight times that of mephenesin. In the early 1950s, Berger demonstrated that meprobamate possessed anxiolytic properties. This was shown in monkeys whose fear was reduced in threatening environmental situations, and in rats, in which meprobamate was effective in disinhibiting behaviour that was suppressed by punishment (Geller–Seifter test). Berger claimed that unlike alcohol or barbiturates, the anxiolytic effects of meprobamate were not associated with impairment of intellectual or physical performance. He explained these effects by an action on 'those specific areas in the brain as the thalamus and the limbic system, that represent the biological substrate of anxiety'. Consequently, between 1950 and 1960, meprobamate was one of the most commonly used drugs for the treatment of anxiety worldwide. Later, however, the image of meprobamate was tarnished by numerous reports of lethal overdoses. Moreover, the anxiolytic effect was accompanied by drowsiness and ataxia.

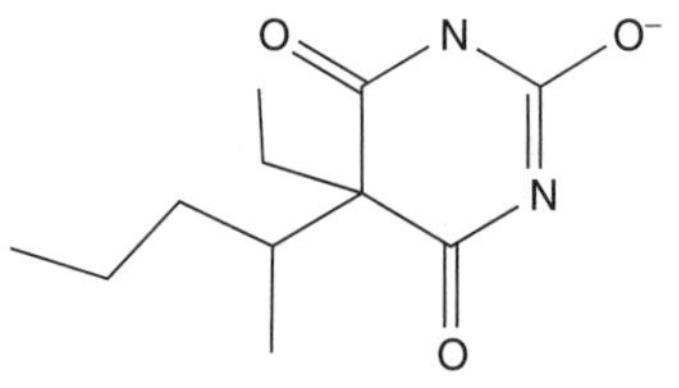

Figure XIX-3.1 The structure of pentobarbital

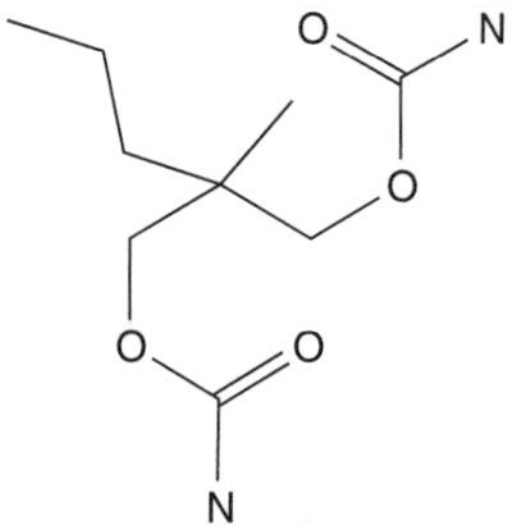

Figure XIX-3.2 The structure of meprobamate

As will be discussed later, these three categories of compounds interfere with GABAergic neurotransmission, which is the principal inhibitory neurotransmitter within the central nervous system.

The Discovery of Benzodiazepines

The Discovery of Chlordiazepoxide

At the end of the 1950s, pharmaceutical companies started to become interested in the field of psychopharmacology. This was related to the commercial success of meprobamate and other psychoactive agents such as chlorpromazine. In this context, a team at Hoffman–La Roche, led by Leo Sternbach, started to study some heptoxdiazines that Sternbach synthesized in the early 1920s when he was a postdoctoral student at the university of Cracow, looking for dyestuffs. In fact, these compounds had no interesting properties as dyes, and no evidence existed in favour of an action of these compounds on the central nervous system. Sternbach decided to study them only because they were unexplored and convenient to test because of their chemical versatility that allowed many transformations. First Sternbach discovered that these compounds were not heptoxdiazines but quinazolone 3-oxides. He then synthesized 40 derivatives and found that all of them, except one that was not tested, were biologically inactive. The last one, labelled RO 5-0690, was disregarded, mainly because of other research priorities. In May 1957, during a cleanup of the laboratory, one of the collaborators of Sternbach found this drug and suggested that it may be tested. Therefore RO 5-0690 was given to the team led by Randall for animal testing. Six tests were used for the screening: a test for sedation and muscle relaxation, a foot-shock test to measure 'taming' effects, another test for muscle relaxation and three tests for anticonvulsant activity. The drug was compared to phenobarbital, chlorpromazine and meprobamate. It was superior to the latter compounds in all tests and therefore Randall announced in 1960 that chlordiazepoxide (the new name of RO 5-0690) may have potent sedative, muscle relaxant, taming and anticonvulsant activity. It was introduced into pharmacotherapy under the tradename 'Librium' (from 'Equilibrium') in 1960, only two-and-a-half years after the first pre-clinical tests. It was then shown that this compound also elicited anti-anxiety effects.

Synthesis of other BZs

A more potent analogue, diazepam, was synthesized in 1961 and, later, 50 other BZs were marketed throughout the world.

Table XIX-3.1 Half-life of major BZs

BZ	Duration of action (h)*
Chlordiazepoxide	55 +/− 35
Diazepam	55 +/− 35
Oxazepam	17 +/− 11
Lorazepam	16 +/− 8
Alprazolam	11 +/− 5

*Including active metabolite

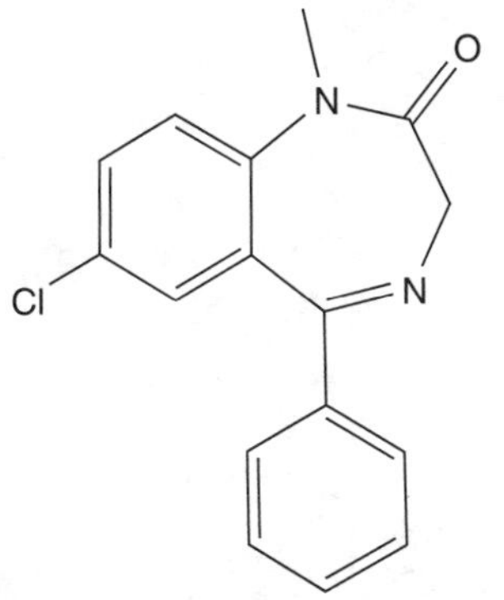

Figure XIX-3.3 Chemical structure of diazepam. The figure shows the core structure made up of the benzene ring (left ring) fused to a diazepine ring (right part, top). The third ring is an aryl substituent ring (bottom, right part)

These new compounds include oxazepam (1965), nitrazepam (1965), clorazepate (marketed in 1968), lorazepam (marketed in 1973), bromazepam (1974), clobazam (1975) and flunitrazepam (1978). The need for new compounds was mainly related to the necessity to develop compounds with a shorter half-life than chlordiazepoxide and diazepam (see Table XIX-3.1 for more details).

BZs are metabolized extensively, generating active metabolites. Some of these metabolites are biotransformed more slowly than the parent compound so that there is no clear relationship between the half-life of a BZ and its duration of action. It should also be noted that BZs display metabolic inter-relationship with common active metabolites. For example, chlordiazepoxide, clorazepate, prazepam, diazepam as well as demozepam are all metabolized in desmethyldiazepam. Some BZs (prazepam, flurazepam) reach the systemic circulation only in the form of active metabolites. All these compounds have a rather close chemical structure. In fact, the name BZ is derived from the benzene ring fused to the diazepine ring (Figure XIX-3.3). They all share common pharmacological properties as they are all sedative–hypnotic, muscle relaxant, anxiolytic and anticonvulsant. Unfortunately, they also display unwanted side effects: they induce anterograde amnesia, tolerance and dependence. However, when compared to the early anxiolytic agents (barbiturates and meprobamate), they displayed a high therapeutic index so that they became rapidly and widely prescribed and very popular, in particular in the treatment of anxiety. In 1972, chlordiazepoxide and diazepam accounted for half of all psychoactive prescriptions in the USA. This led to increasing concerns about their over-use, so that some countries such as the UK introduced a limited prescription list of these compounds in the mid 1980s. However, the prevalence of BZ use is still very high.

Mechanisms of Action

Mechanisms of Action: First Discoveries

The mechanism of action of BZs remained a mystery until a key observation was made in the unravelling of this knot. Indeed, in 1967, electrophysiological studies on the cat spinal cord revealed that diazepam could potentiate the dorsal root potential. The significance of this observation was, however, not realized until the discovery that the dorsal root potential was associated with the activation of local inhibitory neurotransmission using GABA. In fact, the effects of BZs on the dorsal root potential requires an intact GABA system within the spinal cord. It was later observed that the ability of BZs to potentiate GABAergic neurotransmission was a ubiquitous phenomenon, present in many brain areas. This evidence originates not only from electrophysiological studies but also from a biochemical study. The major type of GABA receptor in the brain, termed $GABA_A$ receptor, is associated with an ionophoric postsynaptic Cl^- channel that mediates inhibitory neurotransmission in the brain regulating Cl^- permeability. BZs do not bind to the $GABA_A$ receptor but they potentiate the action of GABA on the $GABA_A$ receptors. Therefore, they require the presence of GABA to express their pharmacological actions.

BZ Receptors

The next milestone in the understanding of the mechanism of action of BZs was the discovery in membrane preparation of high affinity binding sites for [^{3}H]-diazepam that were saturable and stereospecific. This was first reported in 1977 by two independent teams (Braestrup and Squires in Copenhagen, and Möhler and Okada in Basle). One year later, similar binding sites were identified in the human brain, using another ligand, [^{3}H]-flunitrazepam. BZ receptors are located on dendrites, nerve cell bodies and nerve terminals. Autoradiographic studies showed that BZ binding sites are widely distributed within the central nervous system, with the highest concentrations in the cerebral cortex, intermediate concentrations in the limbic system and the cerebellum, and lowest in the pons-medulla and spinal cord (Figure XIX-3.4).

The clinical efficacy of BZs has been attributed to their ability to bind BZ receptors. Indeed, there is a positive correlation between the Ki values for the inhibition of [^{3}H]-diazepam binding by various BZs and their average therapeutic recommended doses (Figure XIX-3.5).

It is important to emphasize that BZs not only bind to BZ receptors. For example, they have also nanomolar affinity for adenosine receptors. However, this is often forgotten so that their psychoactive effects are always attributed to their binding to BZ receptors.

Binding sites are also found in certain peripheral tissues, and represent the so-called mitochondrial BZ binding site. They were first discovered in the kidney, and later they were found in other peripheral tissues such as the adrenal glands and the testes. Such sites also exist in the central nervous system, where they are mainly found on glial cells. These sites are not associated with the $GABA_A$ receptor. The binding site is different from the brain BZ receptor, since it does not recognize all psychoactive BZs (for example clonazepam) and binds some compounds such as the isoquinoline, PK 11195, with nanomolar affinity. They are located subcellularly on the outer membrane of the mitochondria, rather than on the cell membrane. Their function is not well known in all cell types, but it has been suggested that in steroid hormone-producing organs (adrenal glands, testes), they are involved in the transport of cholesterol from the outer to the inner mitochondrial membrane. In the brain, it has been proposed that these receptors may be involved in neurosteroidogenesis.

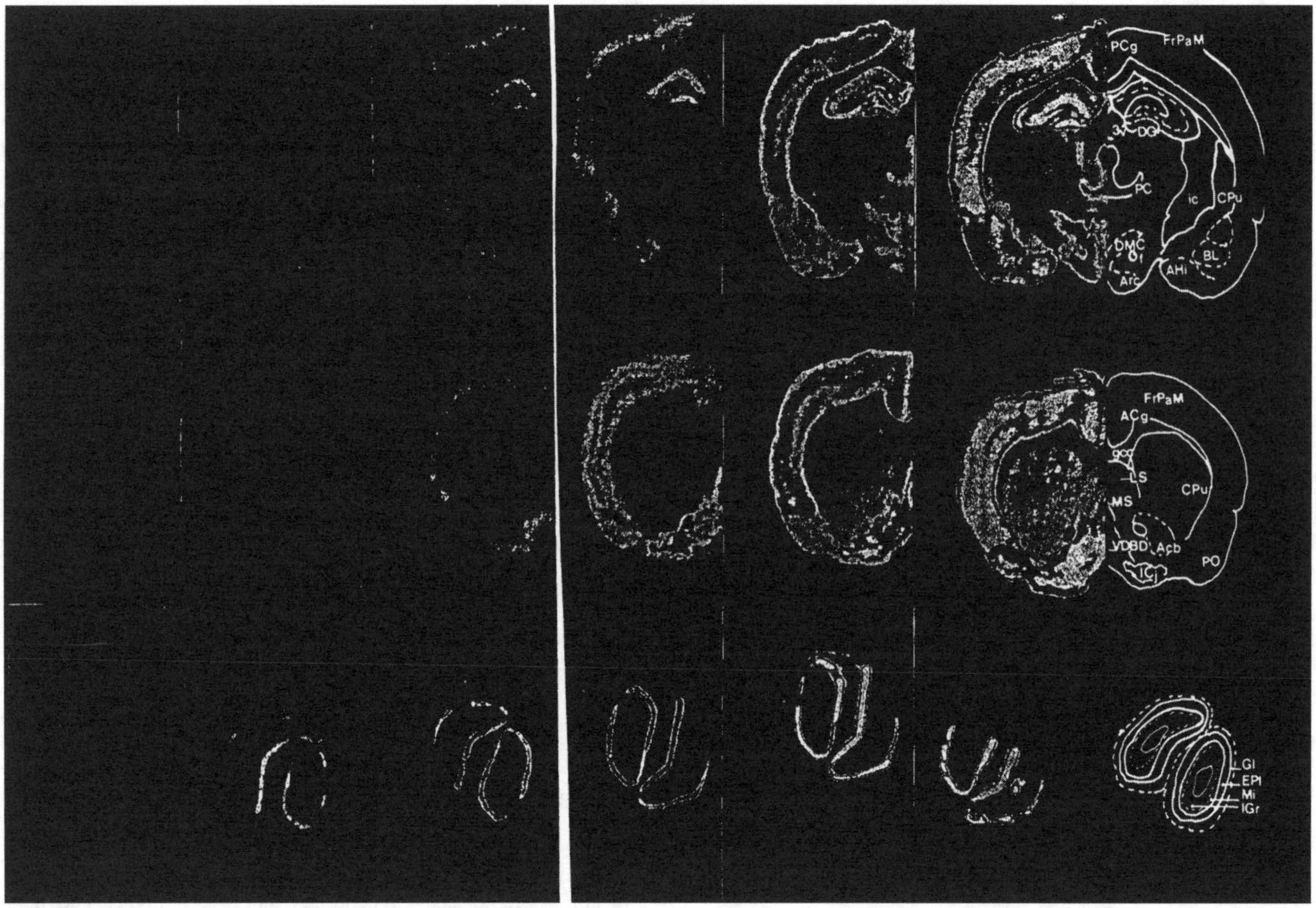

Figure XIX-3.4 Autoradiography of ^{3}H-Flunitrazepam binding sites in the rat brain. PCg: Posterior cingulated cortex; FrPaM: Frontoparietal cortex, motor area; 3v: third ventricle; DG: Dentate Gyrus; PC: Posterior Cingulate; iC: Internal capsule; Cpu: Caudate Putamen; BL: Basolateral amygdaloid nucleus; Ahi: Amygdalohippocampal area; Arc: Arcuate hypothalamus nucleus; f: fornix; Acg: anterior cingulate cortex; gcc: genu corpus callosum; LS: Lateral septum; MS: Medial septum; VDBD: Nucleus Vertical limb, diagonal band, dorsal part; Acb: Accumbens nucleus; PO: Primary olfactory cortex, Icj: Island of Calleja; EPI: external plexiform layer of the olfactory bulb. Reproduced from photostat by permission from Marcel, D., Weissmann-Nanopoulos, D., Mach, E. and Pujol, J.F., 1986. Benzodiazepine binding sites: localization and characterization in the limbic system of the rat brain. *Brain Research Bulletin*, **16**, 573–596

Ligands of BZ Receptors

Up until the early 1980s, it was widely admitted that the chemical structure of BZs was a prerequisite for the binding to the BZ receptor. However, this view was challenged by the discovery that some chemically unrelated drugs (Figure XIX-3.6) such as cyclopyrrolones (zopiclone, suriclone), triazolopyridazines (CL 218,872), phenyl-imidazo-pyridine acetamides (alpidem, zolpidem), quinolines (PK 8165) and pyrazoloquinolines (CGS 8216, CGS 9896) bind to the same site as BZs, sometimes with dissociation constants in the low picomolar range, thus equalling the affinities of the most potent BZs. They act on the BZ receptor in a similar way to BZs.

However, not all compounds that bind with high affinity to the BZ receptor exhibit the same pharmacological profile as BZs. Indeed, compounds have been described that do not have any intrinsic activity when injected alone, but they block the pharmacological action of BZs. These compounds have therefore been termed antagonists of which the first to be identified was flumazenil, also called RO 15-1788 (Figure XIX-3.7). Indeed, this drug has antagonistic properties both *in vitro* and *in vivo*; it is able to block the anxiolytic, anticonvulsant, amnesic, myorelaxant and sedative effects of BZs. Flumazenil is used therapeutically to control BZ anesthesia. Furthermore, other pharmacological agents that bind to the BZ receptor, such as ethyl-β-carboline-3-carboxylate (β-CCE), have been described, but they induce a pharmacological profile opposite to the one induced by BZs. Indeed, they produce anxiogenic, proconvulsant and promnesic effects. They have therefore been termed inverse agonists. Not all inverse agonists have the same potency. For example, compounds such as DMCM and β-CCM (Figure XIX-3.7) are convulsant, while others such as β-CCE or FG 7142 cannot trigger seizures *per se*, but will sensitize animals to the convulsant effects of other pharmacological agents (proconvulsant effects): the first category has been termed full inverse agonists while the second is called partial inverse agonists.

In fact, subsequent studies have revealed compounds that span the complete efficacy spectrum from full agonists to full inverse agonists, including partial agonists such as bretazenil. Antagonists are able to block the effects of agonists and also the effects of inverse agonists or of partial agonists. See Table XIX-3.2

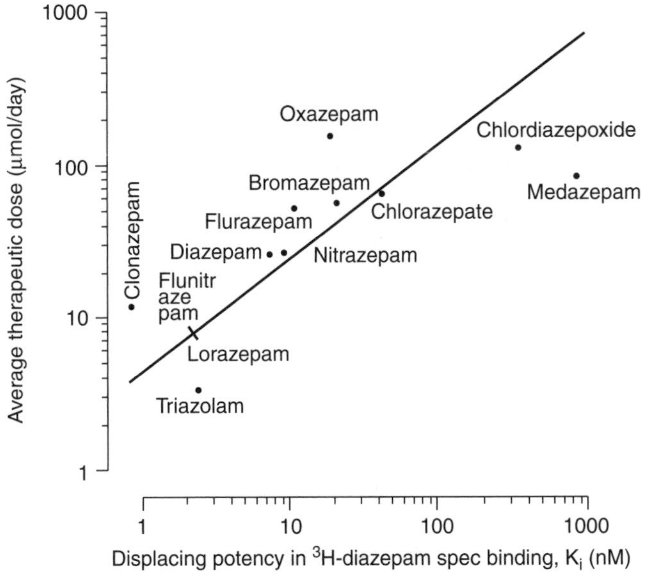

Figure XIX-3.5 Correlation between BZ K_i and mean therapeutical dose recommended. Reproduced by permission from Möhler, H. and Okada, T., 1978. The benzodiazepine receptor in normal and pathological human brain. *British Journal of Psychiatry*, **133**, 261–268

Table XIX-3.2 Properties of the various types of BZ receptor ligands

Different types of ligands	Example of compounds	Pharmacological action
Full agonist	Classical BZ (chlordiazepoxide, diazepam, oxazepam, flunitrazepam, etc.)	Sedative Anxiolytic Anticonvulsant Amnesic Myorelaxant
Partial agonist	Bretazenil	Anxiolytic
Antagonist	Flumazenil	No effect
Partial inverse agonist	β-CCE, FG 7142, RO 15-4513	Anxiogenic Proconvulsant
Inverse agonist	DMCM, β-CCM	Anxiogenic Convulsant Promnesic

A great amount of data exists showing that higher doses of a full agonist are required to produce sedative/myorelaxant effects than to produce anticonvulsant/anxiolytic effects. For example in mice, the dose to induce sedation is twice the minimal effective dose for anxiolytic activity. By combining this approach with *in vivo* binding studies, it is possible to assign a level of receptor occupancy to a given pharmacological effect. This type of analysis demonstrates that for full agonists such as diazepam, between 20 and 40 percent of receptor occupancy is required to produce anxiolytic or anticonvulsant effects. For the same compound, the receptor occupancy must be higher than 60% to elicit sedation or myorelaxant effects (Figure XIX-3.8). This idea has led to the development of partial agonists as anxiolytic agents devoid of sedative side effects. Indeed, partial agonists are not able to activate all the receptors they occupy, so that the dose eliciting sedation may be considerably larger than that inducing anxiolysis (Doble and Martin, 1996).

Endogenous Ligand of BZ Receptors

The presence of BZ receptors has provided some support for the notion that some natural BZ receptor ligands may exist in the central nervous system. Therefore, some research began in the early 1980s that aimed at finding an endogenous ligand for BZ receptors. Such a compound must be present in the organism, bind to the BZ receptors with high affinity and elicit behavioural effects. Diazepam Binding Inhibitor (DBI) is an 86 amino acid peptide that was initially isolated from rat brain on the basis of its ability to displace diazepam from BZ receptors. Splicing of DBI generates several biologically active fragments including the triakontatetraneuropeptide DBI_{17-50} (TTN) and the octadecaneuropeptide DBI_{33-50} (ODN) which are designated by the generic term endozepines. Intracerebroventricular injections of endozepines in rodents elicit anxiogenic effects (Garcia de Mateos-Verchere *et al.*, 1998) and block the anxiolytic action of diazepam. Evidence from *in vitro* and *in vivo* studies indicates that these compounds may act as inverse agonists at the BZ receptor, thus negatively modulating the $GABA_A$ receptor function. Subsequently, it was also observed that endozepines interact with peripheral BZ receptors and stimulate cholesterol transport in the mitochondria, thus participating in the biosynthesis of neurosteroids by brain tissues. It is to be noted here that neurosteroids also modulate the $GABA_A$ receptor function. *In situ* hybridization experiments showed strong DBI mRNA expression in the vicinity of the third ventricle, the hypothalamus and the cerebellum. Long-term isolation in mice, which is a rather stressful procedure in this species, has been shown to induce a decrease in mRNA expression for DBI in the hypothalamus, further suggesting that these peptides may have a biological function related to anxiety and/or stress (Dong *et al.*, 1999).

Interaction with GABA

As mentioned above, BZs potentiate the action of GABA on the $GABA_A$ receptors. Interestingly, the ability of anxiolytic compounds to act on GABAergic neurotransmission is shared by other anti-anxiety agents, such as barbiturates, meprobamate and ethanol. For example, barbiturates such as pentobarbital increase the affinity of $GABA_A$ receptors to GABA and increase the duration of the opening of GABA-activated Cl^- ionophoric channels. Moreover, at high doses, this compound is able to directly open Cl^- channels, even in the absence of GABA. This action is exerted via a specific binding site, termed the barbiturate binding site. As to the mechanism of action of carbamates, recent data suggest that meprobamate may also act at the barbiturate binding site of the $GABA_A$ receptor (Rho, Donevan and Rogawski, 1997). However, the enigma of the mechanism of action of meprobamate is not completely resolved, because meprobamate does not always have the same effects as barbiturates (Haefely *et al.*, 1981). Finally, ethanol is also able to interact with the GABAergic neurotransmission. Indeed, ethanol activates the $GABA_A$ receptor-coupled Cl^- channel, thereby increasing Cl^- conductance and mimicking the action of GABA. Although some effects of ethanol are also mediated via other molecular targets such as the NMDA and the $5\text{-}HT_3$ receptors, one may suggest that its anxiolytic effects are mediated via $GABA_A$ receptors. Indeed, BZ antagonists such as flumazenil or BZ inverse agonists such as RO 15-4513 are able to block the anxiolytic effects of ethanol in rodents at doses where they do not have any intrinsic activity.

Present knowledge proposes a model in which the $GABA_A$ receptor may in fact be allosterically modulated by compounds binding to at least six different sites (for a review, see Hevers and Lüddens (1998)): the BZ receptors; a binding site for barbiturates; a site for neurosteroids; a site for the convulsant drugs picrotoxine and TBPS; one for flurosemide and one for loreclezole. Binding

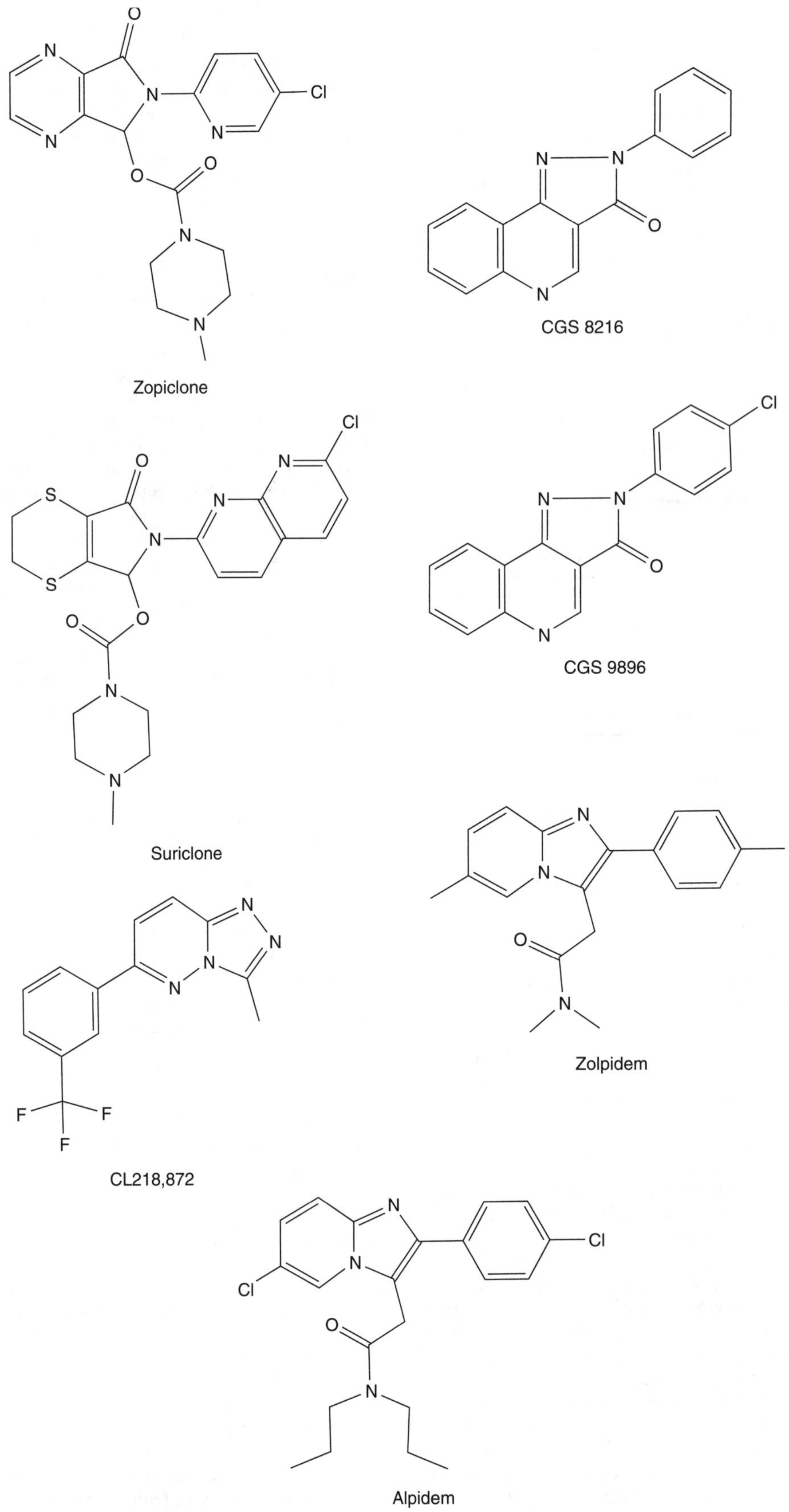

Figure XIX-3.6 Chemical structure of zopiclone, suriclone, CL 218,872, alpidem, zolpidem, CGS 9896 and CGS 8216

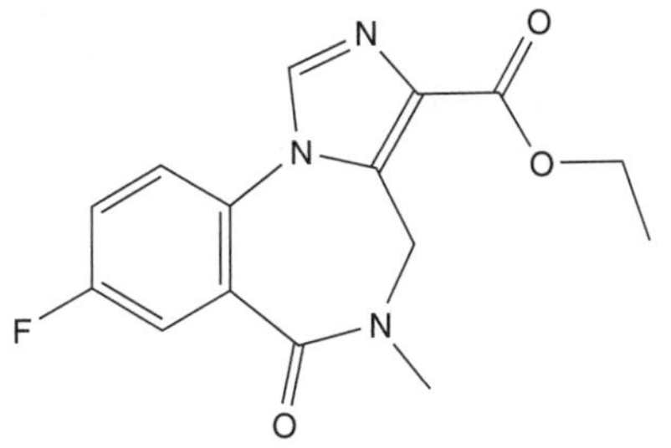

Flumazenil

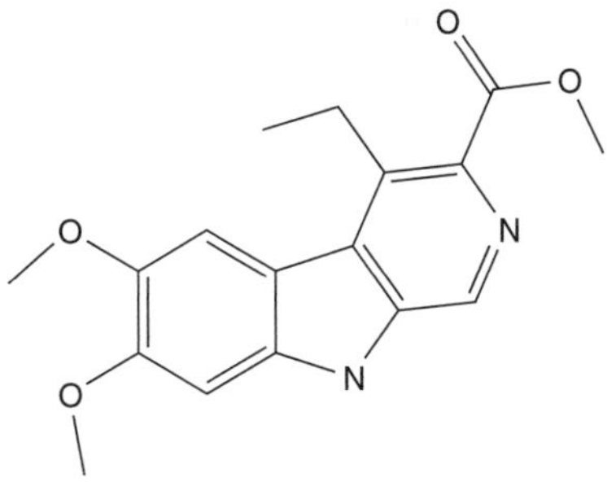

DMCM

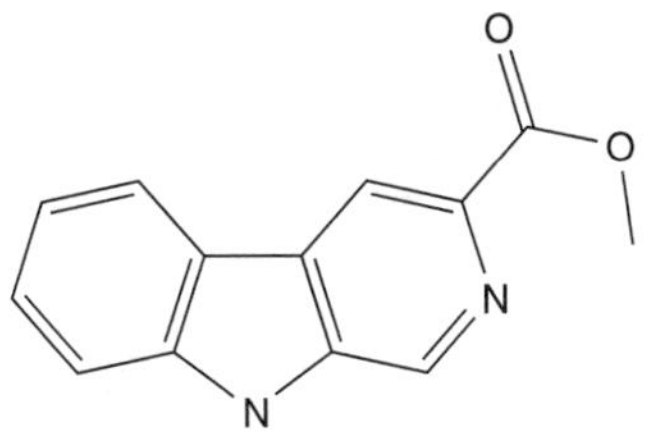

β-CCM

Figure XIX-3.7 Chemical structure of the BZ antagonist flumazenil and of the BZ inverse agonists DMCM and β-CCM

of BZs to the BZ receptors, of barbiturates to the barbiturate binding site, of steroids such as metabolites of progesterone to the neurosteroid site, or of loreclezole to the loreclezole site, are all associated with an anticonvulsant effect underlined by a positive modulation of GABAergic neurotransmission, that is an increase in GABA function. By contrast, binding of picrotoxin to the picrotoxin site induces convulsions, an effect related to the ability of this compound to block GABA-evoked Cl^- conductance. Furosemide, a loop diuretic, inhibits GABA function in some (for example in the cerebellum) but not all neuronal population (for example not in hippocampal neurons) via a mechanism independent of the other allosteric sites.

None of these sites are associated with anxiolytic or anxiogenic effects. As mentioned above, BZs and barbiturates are potent anxiolytics. Antagonists of the picrotoxin site such as etifoxin also induce anxiolysis: this effect is not blocked by flumazenil, thereby indicating that it is not linked to an action at BZ receptors. Some endogenous steroids such as progesterone and its 3α-reduced metabolite produce a dose-dependent anxiolytic response in animal models of anxiety. However, negative modulators of the neurosteroid site, such as pregnenolone sulphate have not been shown to induce the opposite effect in a consistent manner. Finally, some data suggested that loreclezole may induce anxiolytic effects in the rat: these effects are not blocked by flumazenil, suggesting that they are not related to the BZ site. To our knowledge, no data have shown any effect of ligands at the furosemide binding site on anxiety. Moreover, facilitation of GABAergic neurotransmission by the $GABA_A$ receptor agonist THIP or the GABA transaminase inhibitor γ-acetylene GABA (a compound that increases GABA function by inhibiting the degradation enzyme of GABA) does not elicit anxiolytic effects in the rat while drugs that have the opposite action, such as GABA synthesis inhibitors or $GABA_A$ receptor antagonists fail to induce anxiogenic effects (Ågmo *et al.*, 1991).

Molecular Biology of GABAergic Pentamer

The findings mentioned in the precedent chapter can appear contradictory as GABA mimetic drugs are not able to elicit an anxiolytic effect, while the positive modulation of allosteric sites linked to this receptor induce anxiolysis. An explanation of this apparent discrepancy is related to the molecular structure of the $GABA_A$ receptor complex. Indeed, molecular biology has revealed that the GABA receptor is composed of five subunits that co-assemble. Six classes of subunits have been described : $\alpha, \beta, \gamma, \delta, \varepsilon$ and ρ (for a review, see Hevers and Lüddens, 1998). Within each type of subunit, several isoforms are possible: in mammals, these are $\alpha 1-6$, $\beta 1-3$, $\gamma 1-3$, δ, ε and $\rho 1-3$. The $\rho 1-3$ subunits do not seem to co-assemble with α or β subunits within $GABA_A$ receptors and are mainly described in the retina. As to the ε subunit, little information is available because it has only been recently described. The most frequent stochiometric combination

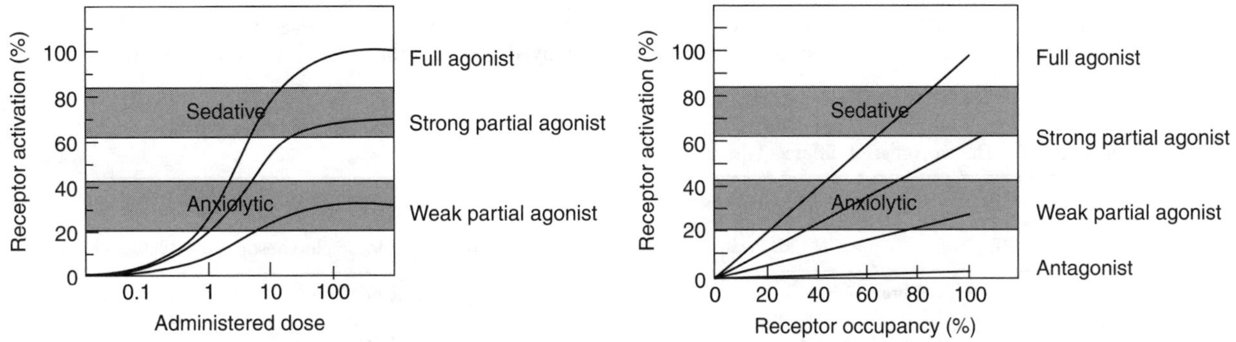

Figure XIX-3.8 Receptor occupancy–activity relationships for full and partial agonists. Left: receptor activation as a function of receptor occupation. Right: receptor activation as a function of dose administered. Reproduced by permission from Doble, A. and Martin, I.L., 1996. The $GABA_A$/Benzodiazepine Receptor as a Target for Psychoactive Drugs. Springer

includes 2 αi, 1 βj and 2 γk as well as 2 αi, 2 βj and 1 γk (with $i = 1$–6, $j = 1$–3 and $k = 1$–3). However, other stoichiometries have been described, such as 3 αi, 1 βj and 1 γk. Thus, the number of possible isoforms of the $GABA_A$ receptor may exceed 100 000. However, not all of the possible isoforms have been described within the central nervous system and approximately 20 isoforms seem to represent the most abundant ones.

Among the $\alpha 1$–6 subunits, the $\alpha 1$ is the most frequent and it has been described in almost all brain areas. It is often co-localized with $\beta 2$ and $\gamma 2$. Clustering is characteristic of GABA-A receptor genes on human chromosomes. In humans, the $\alpha 1$ subunit maps on Chr5q34-q35, in a cluster including the gene for the $\gamma 2$ and the $\alpha 6$ subunit. The human gene for $\alpha 1$ does not appear to have any mutations associated with disease entities. The $\alpha 2$ subunit is mainly localized in the cortex, in limbic areas and in the striatum (where it represents the only α subunit reported). None are found in the cerebellum. It often co-localizes with $\beta 3$ subunits. $\alpha 2$ (with $\alpha 4$ and $\gamma 2$) is expressed at low levels during early development, with a significant increase about one week after birth. However, the biological importance of that is not well understood for the moment. The $\alpha 2$ and the $\beta 1$ subunits map close together Ch4 p13-p12. The human gene for this subunit does not appear to have any mutations associated with anxiety disorders or other diseases. The $\alpha 3$ subunit is mainly localized in the monoaminergic nuclei, particularly on serotoninergic cell bodies in the raphe nuclei, as well as on cholinergic neurons of the basal forebrain. The gene coding for the $\alpha 3$ subunit is located in the central region of chromosome X and has been suggested as a candidate for X-linked manic depression, a psychiatric disease that has some comorbidity with anxiety disorders. The $\alpha 4$ subunit is localized in the hippocampus and the thalamus and the gene encoding for this subunit is located on chromosome 4 in humans. The $\alpha 5$ subunit is located quasi exclusively in the hippocampus and the gene encoding for this subunit is located on human chromosome 15, in the region of the Angelman and Prader–Willi syndromes. In fact, a single paternal allele of this gene is found in cases of Angelman syndrome, and a single maternal allele in cases of Prader–Willi syndrome. However, evidence of abnormal anxiety in these disorders is scarce. Finally, the $\alpha 6$ subunit is located mainly in the cerebellar granule cells and the cochlear nuclei. The gene encoding for this subunit forms a cluster on chromosome 5 with the genes encoding for the $\gamma 2$ and $\alpha 1$ subunits. All these data are summarized in Table XIX-3.3.

Interestingly, the α subunits seem to determine the ability of the BZ receptors to respond to BZ. Indeed, receptors containing $\alpha 4$ or $\alpha 6$ subunits lack the modulation by classical BZs. Classical BZs such as chlordiazepoxide interact indiscriminately with receptors containing $\alpha 1$, $\alpha 2$, $\alpha 3$ or $\alpha 5$ subunits, that are termed benzodiazepine-sensitive. These receptors have a histidine at a conserved position ($\alpha 1$-H101, $\alpha 2$-H101, $\alpha 3$-H126 and $\alpha 5$-H105) while the benzodiazepine insensitive receptors containing $\alpha 4$ or $\alpha 6$ subunit have an arginine in the corresponding position. Therefore, diazepam-sensitive receptors can be rendered insensitive by replacing this histidine by an arginine while the regulation of this receptor by GABA is preserved. Recent data show that replacement of histidine by arginine at the 101 position of the gene encoding for the murine $\alpha 1$ subunit gene has rendered the $\alpha 1$-type $GABA_A$ receptors insensitive to diazepam ($\alpha 1$-knock-in mice). These $\alpha 1$-knock-in mice display no overt change in spontaneous behaviour and bred normally but they failed to show the sedative, amnesic and anticonvulsant action of diazepam. By contrast, the anti-anxiety and myorelaxant properties of the BZ are fully retained (Rudolph *et al.*, 1999). A similar point-mutation technique has been used to render $\alpha 2$ and $\alpha 3$ insensitive to BZs. As for the $\alpha 1$-knock-in mice, no obvious modification of basal behaviour was observed. However, pharmacological challenge with diazepam failed to induce anxiolysis in the $\alpha 2$-knock-in mice (Low *et al.*, 2000). No similar modification could be found with the $\alpha 3$-knock-in mice. These observations point to new strategies for drug design, as one can imagine drugs of the future acting specifically on some α-subunit subtypes, that is on BZ receptors within a particular brain area. For example, drug acting in an agonistic way specifically on $\alpha 2$-type $GABA_A$ may elicit an anxiolysis not accompanied by sedation or amnesic effects (see below).

As to the β subunits, they seem to have little influence on the action of BZ receptor ligands. Indeed, *in vitro* studies showed that the type of β isoform did not modify the ability of diazepam to increase GABA-activated Cl^- currents. In fact, they seem to be involved in brain development as they are all expressed in the developing mouse cerebellum, the $\beta 2$ and $\beta 3$ subunits being present at birth, and displaying spatial correspondence with areas of GABAergic synapses. The $\beta 1$ subunit mRNA does not appear until the second week after birth, and may be associated with Bergmann glia or basket cells.

More data suggest that the γ subunits may be involved in the action of BZ. When compared to the $\gamma 2$ isoform, the $\gamma 3$ isoforms displays a marked decrease in affinity for the BZ antagonist flumazenil or the inverse agonist DMCM while replacement of the $\gamma 2$ isoform with a $\gamma 1$ isoform results in an agonistic affinity of DMCM. By using targeted mutation, $\gamma 2$ knock-out mice have been generated ($\gamma 2$ −/−). These mice display severe growth retardation, sensorimotor abnormalities and a reduced life span as survival was never superior to 17 days of postnatal life. They are insensitive to BZs, indicating that this subunit is critical for BZ sensitivity. As no behavioural studies could be undertaken in such young mice, features of anxiety-related disorders have been investigated in $\gamma 2$ +/− mice. These mice exhibited a region-specific reduction of BZ receptors. This decrease was more pronounced in some areas of the hippocampus (reduction of 35% in CA1 and 28% in CA3), in the cingulate cortex (−25%), in the frontal cortex (−23%), in the piriform cortex (−25%) and in the lateral septum (−30%) than in other brain areas such as the striatum (−6%), the globus pallidus (−13%) or the amygdala. These mice exhibited enhanced state and trait anxiety that was reversed by diazepam. Furthermore, they displayed a bias for threat cues, resulting in an increased sensitivity

Table XIX-3.3 The properties of different types of α subunits

Type of α subunit	Ability to bind BZ	CNS localization	Human chromosome	Mouse chromosome	Cluster
$\alpha 1$	Yes	All brain areas	Chr 5q34-q35	Chr 11	$\gamma 2$ and $\alpha 6$
$\alpha 2$	Yes	Cortex, limbic areas, striatum	Chr 4p13-p12	Chr 5	$\beta 1$
$\alpha 3$	Yes	Raphe nuclei Basal forebrain	X q28	Central part of X	No
$\alpha 4$	No	Hippocampus, thalamus	Chr 15 p14-q12	Chr 5	No
$\alpha 5$	Yes	Hippocampus	Chr 15q11–q15	Chr 7	$\beta 3$ and $\gamma 3$
$\alpha 6$	No	Cerebellar granule cells, cochlear nuclei	Chr 5q31.1-q35	Chr 11	$\gamma 2$ and $\alpha 1$

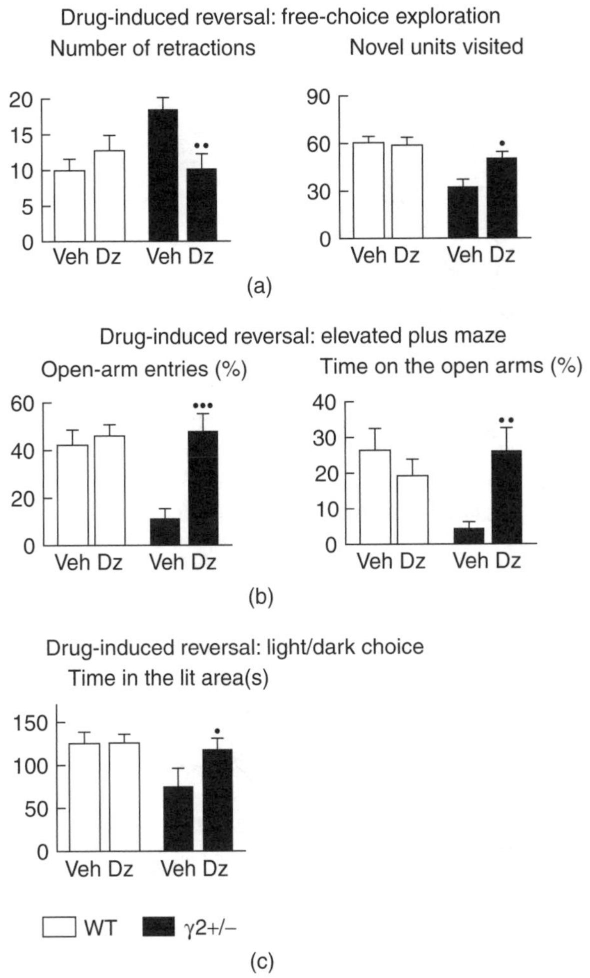

Figure XIX-3.9 Behaviour of wildtype (WT) and $\gamma 2$ +/− mice subjected to three tests of anxiety ((a) the free exploratory test; (b) the elevated plus maze; (c) the light/dark choice test) and treated either with vehicle or diazepam (0.3 mg kg^{-1}, i.p.). Results show that $\gamma 2$ +/− mice display increased anxiety when compared to wildtype mice as they exhibit an increased number of retraction, a decrease in novel units visited, a decrease of entries and time spent on the open arms and a decreased time spent in the lit box. At the dose used, diazepam did not elicit anxiolysis in vehicle-treated WT while it reversed the anxiogenic pattern observed in $\gamma 2$ +/− mice. Reproduced by permission from Crestani, F., Lorez, M., Baer, K., Essrich, C., Benke, D., Laurent, J.P., Belzung, C., Fritschy, J.M., Luscher, B. and Mohler, H., 1999. Decreased $GABA_A$-receptor clustering results in enhanced anxiety and a bias for threat cues. *Nature Neuroscience*, **2**, 833–839

to negative associations (Figure XIX-3.9) (Crestani *et al.*, 1999). Alternate RNA splicing produces two alternative forms of the $\gamma 2$ subunit (γ2L and γ2S) that are expressed in different brain regions, more γ2L being found in the cerebellum, while γ2S is in the ascendant in the cerebral cortex. Moreover, γ2S is expressed at a more or less constant level throughout brain development, while γ2L production increases with maturation. Mice lacking γ2L (γ2L −/−) display increased sensitivity to BZ agonists associated with a decreased sensitivity to BZ inverse agonists, indicating a possible shift of the BZ receptor from an inverse agonist, leaning towards an agonist preferring configuration (Quinlan, Firestone and Homanics, 2000). However, in that case, one might expect a decrease of anxiety levels in those mice, while the contrary was observed. Surprisingly, $\gamma 2$ over-expression did not elicit any changes in several animal models of anxiety (Wick *et al.*, 2000).

Little information is available concerning the relevance of the δ subunit in the $GABA_A$ receptor in relation to anxiety. A $GABA_A\delta$ null mutant (δ −/−) mouse has been described that did not exhibit any modification of anxiety in animal models. However, the neuroactive steroid ganaxolone was unable to elicit anxiolytic action in the knock-out mice, as it does in wildtype mice suggesting a possible involvement of this subunit in the anti-anxiety-like effect modulators of the neurosteroid site of the $GABA_A$ receptor.

Drugs of the Future Acting at the $GABA_A$ Receptor Subtypes

The search for compounds chemically unrelated to the BZs with more specific therapeutic actions and without their concomitant unwanted effects has led to the development of drugs that selectively bind to a specific $GABA_A$ receptor subtype, display low efficacies at each $GABA_A$ receptor subtype, or combine selective affinity and differential intrinsic activity at these receptors (Griebel, Perrault and Sanger, 2000).

While there are $GABA_A$ receptor ligands claimed in patents or shown to bind selectively for all BZ-sensitive $GABA_A$ receptor subtypes, only compounds selective for the α_1 subtype have been studied extensively. These latter include compounds with greatly varying chemical structures. The most widely studied selective α_1 subtype ligands include the imidazopyridine zolpidem (see Figure XIX-3.6), the β-carboline abecarnil (Figure XIX-3.10) and the pyrazolopyrimidine zaleplon. These compounds are either marketed (zolpidem, zaleplon) or pre-registrated (abecarnil). In animal studies, zolpidem and abecarnil were found to produce sedative activity at much lower doses than those producing ataxia and myorelaxation, and after repeated treatment, did not produce tolerance and physical dependence as was observed with most BZs. However, selective $GABA_A$ α_1 subtype agonists are generally found to display weaker (if any) anxiolytic-like activity in animals than non-selective agents, thereby confirming the findings with α_1 knock-in mice which showed that this subtype is not primarily involved in the anxiolytic effects of $GABA_A$ receptor agonists (Rudolph *et al.*, 1999).

Unlike selective $GABA_A$ α_1 subtype agonists, non-selective $GABA_A$ receptor partial agonists such as bretazenil, imidazenil and Y-23684 (Figure XIX-3.10) were found to display comparable or even greater efficacy in anxiety models than BZs. In addition, they had lower liabilities for sedation and muscle relaxation compared to conventional BZs.

Based on the findings from experiments using mice with point-mutated diazepam-insensitive $GABA_A$ receptor subtypes, that the anxiolytic effects of $GABA_A$ receptor agonists are mediated by the α_2 $GABA_A$ receptor, research for anxioselective compounds acting at the $GABA_A$ receptor subtypes has focused on the development of ligands that display functionally selective agonist activity at the α_2 $GABA_A$ receptor subtype. The recently discovered pyridoindole derivative, SL651498 fulfils this criterion. Although the drug has also high affinities for the α_1 and α_3 subtypes, it displays higher intrinsic efficacy at the α_2 subtype as compared to the other $GABA_A$ receptor subtypes. In animal experiments, SL651498 elicited anxiolytic-like activity qualitatively and quantitatively similar to that of BZs, but unlike these latter, it induced central depressant effects at doses much higher than those producing anxiolytic-like activity. Moreover, in contrast to BZs, SL651498 did not produce tolerance to its anticonvulsant activity or physical dependence, and was much less active than BZs in potentiating the depressant effects of ethanol. The 'anxioselective' profile of SL651498 is in agreement with the idea that $GABA_A$ α_2 subtype plays a major role in regulating anxiety, and suggests that targeting selectively $GABA_A$ receptor subtypes can lead to drugs with increased clinical specificity (Low *et al.*, 2000).

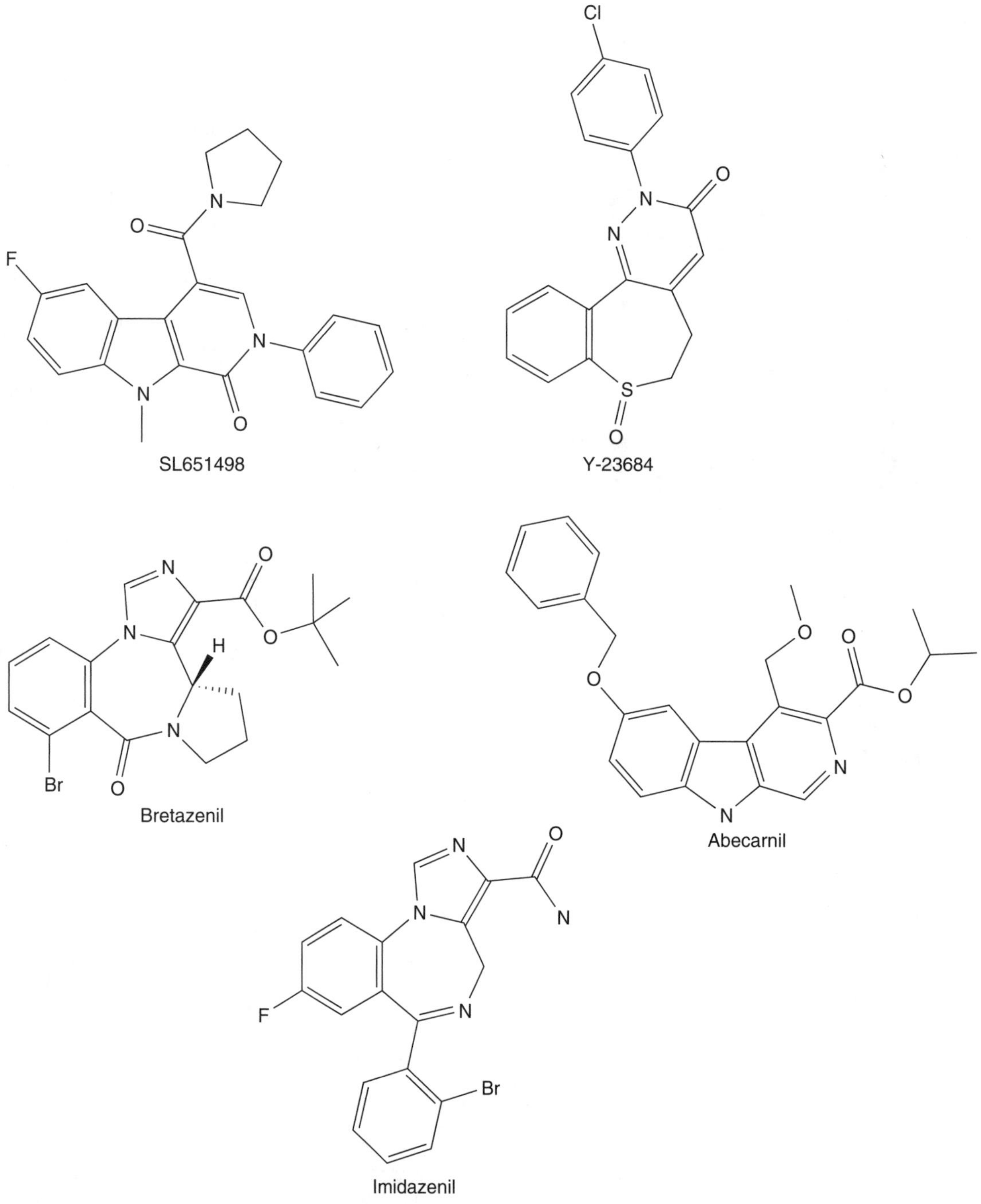

Figure XIX-3.10 Drugs of the future. Chemical structure of the partial agonists bretazenil, imidazenil and Y-23684, of the $\alpha 1$ selective agent abecarnil and of the $\alpha 2$ selective compound SL 651498

AMINO ACID NEUROTRANSMITTER SYSTEM IN ANXIETY DISORDERS

Anxiety Disorders

Anxiety can be considered as an everyday life emotion that ones experiences when subjected to threatening or stressful situations. However, in certain cases anxiety can become excessive, as in anxiety disorders. Anxiety disorders have a lifetime incidence of 16% (Walley, Beebe and Clark, 1994) and it is considered that in any six-month period, 9% of Americans are affected by such an affliction. Anxiety disorders include generalized anxiety disorder (GAD), panic disorder, obsessive–compulsive disorders, phobias and post-traumatic stress disorder (PTSD). In this chapter, we shall not consider dissociative and somatoform disorders as they are studied in further chapters of this book.

Generalized Anxiety Disorder (GAD)

GAD is considered to be a constant state of anxiety, worries occurring for almost any ordinary event. It frequently has other associated disorders accompanied by apprehension, increased tension and hyperalertness. Even if it is the most common anxiety disorder, (14.80% worldwide incidence), little research has been carried out on investigating the underlying psychobiological features of that affliction. It has been shown that platelet and lymphocyte BZ receptors have low binding in GAD. As for cerebral BZ receptor binding in subjects with GAD, the findings are contradictory. Some have found a decrease (Tiihonen *et al.*, 1997), while others did not see any difference (Abadie *et al.*, 1999).

BZs are largely prescribed in the treatment of GAD (Hoehn-Saric and McLeod, 1991). Patients are generally treated with BZ having long elimination half-life, so that they do not have to take the treatment several times a day to prevent rebound anxiety. The main risk is linked to the ability of BZs to elicit tolerance and to have abuse potential. As patients need long-term medication, there is a high risk to elicit withdrawal symptoms when the treatment is discontinued. It should be noted that these compounds do not only relieve anxiety, but they are also effective in reducing hyperalertness, insomnia, tension and some somatic symptoms. However, one has to keep in mind the fact that some symptoms of GAD, such as tension, somatic modifications or hyperalertness may in fact contribute to the increase in anxiety, as suggested by some emotion theoricians. In that case, neither anxiety nor other symptom of GAD can be suppressed by compounds that are not acting on the somato-visceral perception.

Panic Disorder and Conditioned Fears

Though the delineation of panic disorder as a specific category had heuristic value, it has also left other fruitful conceptions in the dark (Marks, 1987), which are now implicitly coming back when categorizing panic disorder as a fear-conditioned disorder (Gorman *et al.*, 2000). Indeed, in order to understand the onset of panic disorder (characterized by episodic paroxystic anxiety states, phobic fears, and several autonomic- and endocrine-related symptoms) beside heritable aetiological factors, environmental disruption is needed. Several studies have shown an association between disruptions of early attachment to parents and the development of panic disorder (Tweed *et al.*, 1989; Stein *et al.*, 1996).

When the term 'panic attacks' was introduced in the DSM-III in 1980, the prevalent view was that the anxiety disorder characterized by severe spontaneous panic attacks was mainly alleviated by tricyclic antidepressants, while the anxiety disorder corresponding to the absence of such acute crisis (GAD) was treated by BZs. This was the rationale for splitting anxiety neurosis in two different anxiety disorders in the DSM-III. This historical background led to the prejudice that BZs may be ineffective in panic attacks. This view was reinforced by the observation that imipramine was more effective than chlordiazepoxide in panic attacks (McNair and Kahn, 1981). However, the dose of chlordiazepoxide used in that study was rather low. More recently, the contribution of amino acids in panic disorders has been evoked by the demonstration of the efficacy of higher doses of BZs in blocking panic attacks. The prototypical BZs used in the treatment of panic are alprazolam and clonazepam, even if other BZs are also effective agents. Clonazepam has a longer half-life than alprazolam, which allows a decrease in the number of daily administrations and thus avoids interdose rebound anxiety. However, many clinicians continued to claim that BZs had weak antipanic efficacy when compared with antidepressants. This prompted some researchers to compare the potency of alprazolam with imipramine and placebo in a double-bind study (Sheehan and Raj, 1990). Results showed that alprazolam was as effective as imipramine (except for the depressive symptoms that are often co-morbid with panic disorder, which were only treated by imipramine), both compounds being superior to placebo. Alprazolam was also effective in attenuating lactate-induced panic attacks. The common problem is related to the abuse potential observed with BZs. Therefore, these compounds are often prescribed for their short-term effects and then dosage is rapidly tapered and antidepressant treatment initiated. BZ are not the sole treatment of panic attack involving increase in GABA function. Indeed, when patients do not respond to BZ or to antidepressants, a medication with valproic acid can be prescribed. Valproic acid increases GABA function by stimulating the activity of glutamic acid decarboxylase, the enzyme responsible for GABA synthesis, and by inhibiting GABA degradation enzymes such as GABA transaminase. Three studies show that valproic acid was superior to placebo on various components of panic attacks and was able to block lactate-induced panic attacks.

Moreover, psychobiological data have also revealed some abnormalities in GABA neurotransmission in patients with panic disorder, suggesting that pharmacological treatments with BZs or valproic acid may in fact act on these abnormalities. For example, patients with panic disorder have been shown less sensitive to BZs on several psychophysiological measures (Roy-Byrne *et al.*, 1996). Furthermore, pre-clinical findings suggested that a decrease of GABA transmission in a network centred in the amygdala — and involving hippocampus and prefrontal cortex — with projections to midbrain central grey and hypothalamus, leads to paroxystic anxiety responses (LeDoux *et al.*, 1988; Davis, 1992). Finally, intravenous lactate, which induces panic attacks, produces a decrease in circulating plasma GABA levels.

However, most studies of binding at the BZ-$GABA_A$ receptor are contradictory. Indeed, some findings suggest global reduction of binding (Malizia *et al.*, 1998); other findings affirm only local or state-related panic anxiety reduction (Bremner *et al.*, 2000); and further studies found no peculiarity or increase in BZ receptor density in association with up-regulation hypotheses (Brandt *et al.*, 1998; Abadie *et al.*, 1999). The idea that in this disorder the subject has difficulty in protecting himself in a state of stress could bring forward new hypotheses (Kellner and Yehuda, 1999; Strohle *et al.*, 1999).

Obsessive Compulsive Disorder (OCD)

OCD is characterized by repetitive thoughts or behaviour that are felt by the subject and are difficult to prevent. Most of the time the behaviour or thoughts are absurd, and consume so much time that they alter social functioning of the subject.

The psychobiological approach accumulates arguments — including those from lesional models (Laplane *et al.*, 1989) — for abnormalities associated with obsessive and compulsive manifestations in frontocortico-striatal-thalamic networks. Indeed, a hyperactivity of this axis has been shown within orbito-frontal and anterior cingulate cortex, as well as caudate nucleus and thalamus, and a decrease of N-Acetyl-Aspartate (NAA), a putative marker of neuron viability, within striatal areas — which could be sites of primary pathology — and thalamus, a site of integration and relay, especially involved in compulsions (Fitzgerald *et al.*, 2000).

Functional neuroimaging studies in OCD patients during symptom provocation suggests increased glutamatergic activity. Current psychobiological research on OCD puts forward that *basal ganglia* dysfunctions could contribute to the aetiology of the symptoms. Indeed, it has been suggested through functional imaging techniques on subjects with OCD, before and after treatment by Selective Serotonin Reuptake Inhibitors (SSRIs), (substances known for their positive effect on OCD symptomatology) that *caudate nucleus* seems primarily involved in the medication's efficacy on OCD (Baxter, Schwartz and Bergmam, 1992). The interrelations of amino acids such as γ*-aminobutyric acid* (GABA) or *glutamate* with serotonin (5-HT) pathways could be enlightened by some findings. First, the 5-HT_{2a} stimulation on GABA neurons opposes the glutamate action on the striatum, an area known for being rich in neurons with serotonin synthesis (Chugani *et al.*, 1998). Second, the prefrontal cortex highly innervates the caudate nucleus (Modell *et al.*, 1989) by glutamatergic projections. Third, glutamate can decrease the release of 5-HT in the caudate nucleus in humans (Becquet, Faudon and Hery, 1990) and be at the same time affected in its action by serotonin neurons (Edwards *et al.*, 1996).

As BZs are effective in the treatment of anxiety, their efficacy in OCD has also been evaluated. In fact, BZs are devoid of anti-obsessive–compulsive effect *per se* but they can alleviate the high anxiety or insomnia that are in some case associated with OCD. In this way they can be considered as a symptomatic treatment of OCD. They can also provide a short-term relief for the distress of the patients, before the anti-obsessive–compulsive effects of serotonin reuptake inhibitors can be observed, or before a cognitive therapy can be undertaken. It should be noted that this observation is not true for all BZs. In fact, there is an exception as the BZ clonazepam has been shown significantly more effective as a monotherapy than some antidepressant after 3-week treatment (Hewlett, Vinogradov and Agras, 1992). A proposed explanation as to the superiority of clonazepam over other BZs in the treatment of OCD is related to the fact that this drug may have specific effects on the serotoninergic system.

Post-Traumatic Stress Disorder

Post-traumatic stress disorder (PTSD) is a condition specified by repetition in thoughts, nightmares, physical and mental re-experiencing of the traumatic experience. It is associated with a negative semiology, such as numbing or amnesia, related to the dissociative field. Preclinical data put forward that stress induces cortico-limbic release of glutamate. Clinical observations suggest that N-methyl-D-aspartate antagonists may also induce glutamate release while provoking dissociative-like symptoms. Some authors then hypothesized that hyperglutamatergic states could contribute to acute and chronic consequences of trauma (Chambers *et al.*, 1999).

Among the psychobiological alterations observed in PTSD, the neuroendocrinological peculiarities in the hypothalamic-pituitary-adrenal axis, including cortisol decrease and reactivity alterations are documented the most. Specificities of GABA function have been studied in subjects with PTSD. The failure of the benzodiazepine antagonist flumanezil to produce flashbacks in PTSD suggest a weak role of attention deficit in the chronic disorder. The background of this topic includes the fact that $GABA_A$ receptors inhibit meso-prefrontal dopamine neurons, that BZs and neurosteroids enhance $GABA_A$ inhibition, that altered BZ receptors or a diminution of an endogenous ligand may decrease GABA inhibition and lead to excessive anxiety, and that PTSD may deplete an endogenous ligand and produce receptor alteration.

Morris and his colleagues (Morris *et al.*, 2000) presented an interesting positron emission tomography (PET) study to estimate the binding potential (BP) of $GABA_A$ benzodiazepine receptors *in vivo* using the BZ receptor antagonist radioligand C^{11}-flumanezil, comparing 13 subjects with PTSD and 13 without disorder. B_{max} was the same for subjects both with and without PTSD; K_d was lower in PTSD cases, and the B_p constant of the BZ receptor was higher in PTSD cases, especially in cerebellar, latero-temporal, occipital and prefrontal areas.

BZ medication in PTSD is still controversial. A study has shown that alprazolam induces a slight improvement in anxiety on the Hamilton scale in PTSD patients but there is no superiority of alprazolam over placebo on the PTSD scale. Moreover, alprazolam and clonazepam have positive effects on hyperarousal, as does valproic acid. The GABA transaminase vigabatrin has also been shown to ameliorate the exaggerated startle response that is found in PTSD. These observations suggest that increasing the GABA function may be a treatment of some symptoms of PTSD such as anxiety, increased startle or hypervigilance, rather than a treatment of PTSD *per se*. Furthermore, PTSD is co-morbid with other anxiety disorders such as GAD so that BZ may in fact alleviate some symptoms related to GAD, rather than treat PTSD.

Phobias

The main characteristic of phobias is marked and persistent fear of some specific situations (for example enclosed spaces) or objects/animals (small animals such as mice). Here we may emphasize on a particular type of phobia — social phobia — which is characterized by fear of social situations in which embarrassment may occur, as some arguments suggesting an involvement of the GABAergic system have been proposed. Indeed, compounds potentiating the action of GABA such as benzodiazepines and conventional anticonvulsants have been evaluated as treatments for social phobia. Among the benzodiazepines, clonazepam is the best studied, and showed efficacy in several studies. Among the anticonvulsants, gabapentin and pregabalin, which are analogues of GABA, have been shown to be more effective than placebo in double-blind studies. Furthermore, subjects with social phobia showed abnormalities in peripheral benzodiazepine receptors, which suggests that these receptors may play a role in the pathophysiology of this disorder.

BZ and Anxiety Disorders

With the exception of GAD and, to a lesser extent panic attack, it is noteworthy that BZs or drugs that increase GABA transmission may alleviate some symptoms associated with anxiety disorders (including anxiety, insomnia, tension, startle), rather than treat anxiety disorders *per se*. In these disorders, anxiety is often a symptom subsequent to a core semiology resulting mainly from cognitive activations, for instance 're-experiencing' in PTSD or 'obsession' in OCD, rather than a primary autonomic dysregulation and first rank therapeutic target. This is the reason why the ICD-10 classification of the World Health Organization (WHO) preferred to call the chapter from the DSM-IV 'Somatoform, stress-related and neurotic disorders' rather than 'Anxiety disorders'.

REFERENCES

Abadie, P., Boulenger, J.P., Benali, K., Barré, L., Zarifian, E. and Baron, J.C., 1999. Relationships between trait and state anxiety and the central benzodiazepine receptor: a PET study. *European Journal of Neurosciences*, **11**, 1470–1478.

Ågmo, A., Pruneda, R., Guzman, M. and Gutierrez, M., 1991. GABAergic drugs and conflict behavior in the rat: lack of similarities with the actions of benzodiazepines. *Naunyn-Schmiedeberg's Archives of Pharmacology*, **344**, 314–322.

Baxter, L.R., Schwartz, J.M. and Bergman, K.S., 1992. Caudate glucose metabolic rate changes with both drug and behavior therapy for obsessive compulsive disorder. *Archives of General Psychiatry*, **49**, 681–689.

Becquet, D., Faudon, M. and Hery, F., 1990. *In vivo* evidence for an inhibitory glutamatergic control of serotonin release in the cat caudate nucleus: involvement of GABA neurons. *Brain Research*, **519**, 82–88.

Brandt, C.A., Meller, J., Keweloh, L., Höschel, K., Staedt, J., Munz, D. and Stoppe, G., 1998. Increased benzodiazepine receptor density in the prefrontal cortex in patients with panic disorder. *Journal of Neural Transmission*, **105**, 1325–1333.

Bremner, J.D., Innis, R.B., White, T., Fujita, M., Silbersweig, D., Goddard, A.W., Staib, L., Stern, E., Cappiello, A., Woods, S., Baldwin, R. and Charney, D.S., 2000. SPECT [I-123] iomazenil measurement of the benzodiazepine receptor in panic disorder. *Biological Psychiatry*, **47**, 96–106.

Chambers, R.A., Bremner, J.D., Moghaddam, B., Southwick, S.M., Charney, D.S. and Krystal, J.H., 1999. Glutamate and post-traumatic stress disorder: toward a psychobiology of dissociation. *Seminars in Clinical Neuropsychiatry*, **4**, 274–281.

Chojnacka-Wójcik, E., Klodzinska, A. and Pilc, A., 2001. Glutamate receptor ligands as anxiolytics. *Current Opinion in Investigational Drugs*, **2**, 1112–1119.

Chugani, D.C., Muzik, O., Chakraborry, P., Mangner, T. and Chugani, H.A.T., 1998. Human brain serotonin synthesis capacity measured *in vivo* with alpha-[C11]methyl-L-tryptophan. *Synapse*, **28**, 33–43.

Crestani, F., Lorez, M., Baer, K., Essrich, C., Benke, D., Laurent, J.P., Belzung, C., Fritschy, J.M., Luscher, B. and Mohler, H., 1999. Decreased GABAA-receptor clustering results in enhanced anxiety and a bias for threat cues. *Nature Neuroscience*, **2**, 833–839.

Davis, M., 1992. The role of amygdala in fear and anxiety. *Annual Review of Neuroscience*, **15**, 353–375.

Doble, A. and Martin, A.L., 1996. *The $GABA_A$/Benzodiazepine Receptor as a Target for Psychoactive Drugs*. Springer, New York.

Dong, E., Matsumoto, K., Tohda, M., Kaneko, Y. and Watanabe, H., 1999. Diazepam binding inhibitor (DBI) gene expression in the brains of socially isolated and group-housed mice. *Neuroscience Research*, **33**, 171–177.

Edwards, E., Hampton, E., Ashby, C.R., Zhang, J. and Wang, R.Y., 1996. $5\text{-}HT_3$-like receptors in the rat medial prefrontal cortex: further pharmacological characterization. *Brain Research*, **733**, 21–30.

Fitzgerald, K.D., Moore, G.J., Paulson, L.A., Stewart, C.M. and Rosenberg, D.R., 2000. Proton spectroscopy imaging of the thalamus in treatment-naïve pediatric obsessive compulsive disorder. *Biological Psychiatry*, **47**, 174–182.

Garcia de Mateos-Verchere, J., Leprince, J., Tonon, M.C., Vaudry, H. and Costentin, J., 1998. The octadecaneuropeptide ODN induces anxiety in rodents: possible involvement of a shorter biologically active fragment. *Peptides*, **19**, 841–848.

Gorman, J.M., Kent, J.M., Sullivan, G.M. and Coplan, J.D., 2000. Neuroanatomical hypothesis of panic disorder, revised. *American Journal of Psychiatry*, **157**, 493–505.

Griebel, G., Perrault, G. and Sanger, D.J., 2000. *Subtype-selective benzodiazepine receptor ligands.* In: Briley, M. and Nutt, D. (eds), *Anxiolytics*, pp. 77–94. Birkhäuser, Basel.

Hevers, W. and Lüddens, H., 1998. The diversity of $GABA_A$ receptors. *Molecular Neurobiology*, **18**, 35–86.

Hewlett, W.A., Vinogradov, S. and Agras, W.S., 1992. Clomipramine, clonazepam and clonidine treatment of obsessive–compulsive disorder. *Journal of Clinical Psychopharmacology*, **12**, 420–430.

Haefely, W., Schaffner, P., Polc, P. and Pieri, L., 1981. General pharmacology and neuropharmacology of propanediol carbamates. *Handbook of Experimental Pharmacology*, **55**, 263–283.

Hoehn-Saric, R. and McLeod, D.R., 1991. Clinical management of generalized anxiety disorder? In: Coryell, W. and Winokur, G. (eds), *The Clinical Management of Anxiety Disorders*, pp. 79–100. Oxford University Press, New York.

Kellner, M. and Yehuda, R., 1999. Do panic disorder and posttraumatic stress disorder share a common psychoneuroendocrinology? *Psychoneuroendocrinology*, **24**, 485–504.

Laplane, D., Levasseur, M., Pillon, B., Dubois, B., Baulac, M. and Mazoyer, B., 1989. Obsessive compulsive and other behavioural changes with bilateral basal ganglia lesions. A neuropsychological, magnetic resonance imaging and positron tomography study. *Brain*, **112**(3), 699–725.

LeDoux, J.E., Iwata, J., Cicchetti, P. and Reis, D.J., 1988. Different projections of the central amygdaloid nucleus mediate autonomic and behavioral correlates of conditioned fear. *Journal of Neuroscience*, **8**, 2517–2519.

Low, K., Crestani, F., Keist, R., Benke, D., Brunig, I., Benson, J.A., Fritschy, J.M., Rulicke, T., Bluethmann, H., Mohler, H. and Rudolph, U., 2000. Molecular and neuronal substrate for the selective attenuation of anxiety. *Science*, **290**, 131–134.

Malizia, A.L., Cunningham, V.J., Bell, C.J., Liddle, P.F., Jones, T. and Nutt, D.J., 1998. Decreased brain $GABA_A$-benzodiazepine receptor binding in panic disorder. *Archives of General Psychiatry*, **55**, 715–720.

Marks, I.M., 1987. *Fears, Phobias and Rituals*. Oxford University Press, Oxford.

McNair, D.M. and Kahn, R.J., 1981. Imipramine compared with a benzodiazepine for agoraphobia. In: Klein, D.F. and Rabkin, J. (eds), *Anxiety: New Research and Changing Concepts*, pp. 69–79. Raven Press, New York.

Modell, J.G., Mountx, J.M., Curtis, G.C. and Greden, J.F., 1989. Neurophysiologic dysfunction in basal ganglia/limbic striatal and thalamocortical circuits as a pathogenic mechanism of obsessive compulsive disorder. *Journal of Neuropsychiatry*, **1**, 27–36.

Morris, P., Ellen, S., Olver, J., Constant, E., Burrows, J., Tochon-Danguy, H., McFarlane, A., Ignatiadis, S., Reutins, D., Norman, T., Hopwood, M. and Egan, G., 2000. A positron emission tomography study of benzodiazepine receptors in post-traumatic stress disorder. In: *Proceedings of the 16th Annual Meeting of the International Society for Traumatic Stress Studies*, San Antonio, 16–19 November 2000.

Quinlan, J.J., Firestone, L.L. and Homanics, G.E., 2000. Mice lacking the long splice variant of the $\gamma 2$ subunit of the $GABA_A$ receptor are more sensitive to benzodiazepines. *Pharmacology, Biochemistry and Behavior*, **66**, 371–374.

Rho, J.M., Donevan, S.D. and Rogawski, M.A., 1997. Barbiturate-like action of propanediol dicarbamates felbamate and meprobamate. *Journal of Pharmacology and Experimental Therapeutics*, **280**, 1383–1391.

Roy-Byrne, P., Wingerson, D.K., Radant, A., Greenblatt, D.J. and Cowley, D.S., 1996. Reduced benzodiazepine sensitivity in patients with panic disorder: comparison with patients with obsessive compulsive disorder and normal subjects. *American Journal of Psychiatry*, **153**, 1444–1449.

Rudolph, U., Crestani, F., Benke, D., Brunig, I., Benson, J.A., Fritschy, J.M., Martin, J.R., Bluethmann, H. and Mohler, H., 1999. Benzodiazepine actions mediated by specific γ-aminobutyric $acid_A$ receptor subtypes. *Nature*, **401**, 796–800.

Sheehan, D.V. and Raj, A., 1990. Benzodiazepine treatment of panic disorder. In: Noyes, R., Roth, M. and Burrows, G.D. (eds), *Handbook of Anxiety, Vol. 4: The Treatment of Anxiety*, pp. 169–206. Elsevier Science, Oxford.

Stein, M.B., Walker, J.R., Anderson, G., Hazen, A.L., Ross, C.A., Eldridge, G. and Forde, D.R., 1996. Childhood physical and sexual abuse in patients with anxiety disorders in a community sample. *American Journal of Psychiatry*, **153**, 275–277.

Strohle, A., Kellner, M., Holsboer, F. and Wiedemann, K., 1999. Behavioral, neuroendocrine, and cardiovascular response to flumanezil: no evidence for an altered benzodiazepine receptor sensitivity in panic disorder. *Biological Psychiatry*, **45**, 321–326.

Tiihonen, J., KUIkka, J., Rasanen, P., Lepola, U., Koponen, H., Liuska, A., Lehmusvaara, A., Vaino, P., Kononen, M., Bergstrom, K., Yu, M., Kinnunen, I., Akerman, K. and Kahru, J., 1997. Cerebral benzodiazepine receptor binding and distribution in generalized anxiety disorder: a fractal analysis. *Molecular Psychiatry*, **2**, 463–471.

Tweed, J.L., Schoenbach, V.J., George, L.K. and Blazer, D.G., 1989. The effects of childhood parental death and divorce on six-month history of anxiety disorders. *British Journal of Psychiatry*, **154**, 823–828.

Walley, E.J., Beebe, D.K. and Clark, J.L., 1994. Management of common anxiety disorders. *American Family Physician*, **50**, 1745–1753.

Wick, M.J., Radcliffe, R.A., Bowers, B.J., Mascia, M.P., Lüscher, B., Harris, R.A. and Wehner, J.M., 2000. Behavioral changes produced by transgenic overexpression of γ2L and γ2S subunits of the $GABA_A$ receptor. *European Journal of Neuroscience*, **12**, 2634–2638.

XIX-4

Peptidergic Transmitter System and Anxiety Disorders

Michel Bourin, Martine Hascoët, Denis David and Bríd Áine Nic Dhonnchadha

INTRODUCTION

Since their introduction in the beginning of the 1960s benzodiazepines (BZD) have been mainly used in treating anxiety disorders. With the exception of general anxiety disorder (GAD) the identity of the specific anxiety disorder for which each drug is most effective has been hindered by early clinical trials and psychiatric classification. Few proficient drugs have been launched since, the exception being buspirone a 5-HT_{1A} partial agonist. The recent utilization of 5-HT reuptake inhibitors is mainly in the field of panic disorder, social phobia, post-traumatic stress disorder and possibly GAD. Nevertheless, the treatment of anxiety disorders remains a very active field of research and there are some promising results in animal research with neuroactive peptides in the modulation of anxiety behaviours. This section reviews the literature on the potential effects of cholecystokinin (CCK), corticotrophin-releasing factor (CRF), neuropeptide Y (NPY), substance P (SP) and neurokinin (NK) and natriuretic peptides (NP) in anxiety disorders in various animal and human models.

CHOLECYSTOKININ AND ANXIETY

Cholecystokinin (CCK) is synthesized *de novo* in the brain (Goltermann, Rehfeld and Roigaard-Petersen, 1980). CCK has been shown to induce excitation of central neurons. However, inhibitory postsynaptic effects have been also recorded (Dodd and Kelly, 1981; Mac Vicar, Kerrin and Davison, 1987). CCK receptors have now been classified as CCK1 and CCK2 independent of their localization replacing CCK-A and CCK-B. CCK receptors are widely distributed throughout the CNS, with high densities in the striatum and nucleus accumbens (Hill *et al.*, 1987).

Animal Models

Evidence suggests that CCK is implicated in the regulation of anxiety. The peripheral administration of CCK agonists induces anxiety in various animal species, including mouse, rat, cat and monkey (Bourin *et al.*, 1996; Shlik, Vasar and Bradwejn, 1997). This effect is apparently mediated via CCK-2 receptors (previously named CCK-B) since the selective CCK-2 receptor agonists (CCK-4 and pentagastrin) are effective. Moreover, the anxiogenic action of CCK agonists is reversed by preferential CCK-2 receptor antagonists (L-365,260, Cl-988). It should be noted that CCK is active in ethological, but not in conditioned, models of anxiety. However, several studies were unable to reveal the anxiogenic action of CCK agonists in ethological models either. The anxiolytic action of CCK-2 receptor antagonists is even more doubtful since recent studies did not establish any significant action when CCK-2 receptor antagonists were given as single treatments (Dawson *et al.*, 1995).

Some evidence exists that CCK-induced anxiety may be dependent on the level of pre-experimental stress in animals (Koks *et al.*, in press). Therefore, an attempt was made to reveal the significance of pre-experimental stress on CCK-induced anxiety in the elevated plus-maze. Male Wistar rats were divided into four different groups. Two groups of rats were handled in the experimental room for three consecutive days before the experiment. The other two groups of animals were brought to the experimental room immediately before the beginning of the experiment. The handled and non-handled rats were divided into two groups after the injection of caerulein ($5\,\mu g\,kg^{-1}$), a CCK receptor agonist. Half of the animals were isolated after the injection, whereas the other half were returned to their home cage. The anxiogenic action of caerulein was strongest in the rats brought to the experimental room immediately before the plus-maze exposure and kept isolated after the injection of CCK agonist. By contrast, caerulein did not cause any anxiety in the handling habituated and non-isolated rats. Accordingly, the anxiogenic action of caerulein was dependent on the level of pre-experimental stress in rats. The anxiogenic action of caerulein in the stressed rats was dose-dependently reversed by L-365,260 ($1-100\,mg\,kg^{-1}$), a CCK-B receptor antagonist.

In another study the behavioural and neurochemical effects of long-term treatment with L-365,260, a CCK-B receptor antagonist, were investigated. L-365,260 ($100\,mg\,kg^{-1}$) was administered twice daily for 14 days. The repeated treatment with L-365,260 did not change locomotor activity, but it did reduce the exploratory behaviour of rats in the elevated plus-maze test (Koks *et al.*, in press). The neurochemical studies performed demonstrated that L-365,260 induced a sufficient blockade of CCK-B receptors in the brain. Namely, the density of CCK receptors was increased in the frontal cortex and the serum levels of thyrotrophin were reduced due to the repeated administration of L-365,260. Collectively, it is unlikely that CCK is directly involved in the neural networks mediating anxiety. The anxiogenic effect of CCK is rather mediated via other neurotransmitter systems like CRF, GABA, 5-hydroxytryptamine, noradrenaline and nitric oxide.

Human Studies

The starting point for human studies was in 1984 with the electrophysiological experiment of Bradwejn and de Montigny (1984), which demonstrated that benzodiazepine receptor agonists selectively and specifically antagonized sulphated CCK-8-induced excitation of hippocampal pyramidal neurons in rats. These studies provided evidence that anxiolytic benzodiazepines could antagonize the central action of a neuropeptide and it was proposed that benzodiazepine-mediated antagonism of CCK-induced excitation might be an important mechanism by which benzodiazepines exert

Biological Psychiatry: Edited by H. D'haenen, J.A. den Boer and P. Willner. ISBN 0-471-49198-5

their clinically relevant action. More importantly, the observation that an anxiolytic drug could block the excitatory action of CCK raised questions about whether CCK might be an endogenous anxiogenic compound.

De Montigny first reported that exogenous CCK-4 produced panic-like attacks in healthy volunteers and that these effects could be attenuated by pretreatment with lorazepam (de Montigny, 1989). Bradwejn and co-workers (1990) administered CCK-4 to patients with a current-point diagnosis of panic disorder using a double-blind placebo-controlled methodology. Bolus injections of CCK-4 (50 mg) precipitated a panic attack, as defined by DSM-III criteria and patient self-report, within one minute following administration in 11 trial patients studied, whereas none of the patients panicked following placebo. CCK-4 treatment elicited an average of 12 symptoms per patient, the most common symptoms being dyspnoea, palpitations/rapid heart, chest pain/discomfort, faintness, dizziness, paresthesia, hot flushes/cold chills, nausea/abdominal distress, anxiety/fear/apprehension and fear of losing control. It has been found that response to CCK-4 reliably differentiates panic disorder patients from healthy controls with no personal or family history of panic attacks. In a double-blind placebo control study, the patients with panic disorder experienced a greater number of symptoms and more intense symptoms following challenge with two doses of CCK-4 (25 and 50 mg) (Bradwejn, Koszycki and Shriqui, 1991). In addition, the incidence of panic attacks was markedly higher in patients than controls following injection of 25 mg (91% vs 17%) and 50 mg (100% vs 47%) of the peptide. Interestingly, the number and intensity of symptoms as well as the symptom profile were remarkably similar in both patients and normal subjects who panicked with the 50 mg dose of CCK-4, suggesting that the enhanced response in patients could not be readily attributed to a tendency to overendorse symptoms. These results are corroborated by studies of Abelson and colleagues (1991) and by van Megen and colleagues (1994) who used pentagastrin, a CCK agonist which incorporates the identical 4-amino acid sequence of CCK-4. Moreover, patients with panic disorder have been shown to have decreased concentrations of CCK-8s in the cerebrospinal fluid relative to control subjects (Lydiard *et al.*, 1992). Concentrations of CCK-8 in lymphocytes were also significantly reduced in patients with panic disorder compared to healthy controls (Brambilla *et al.*, 1993). These findings are also in favour of anomalies in the CCK system due to panic disorder. It is also likely that systemic administration of CCK-4 produces prominent respiratory and cardiovascular alterations in humans through a direct action on the brainstem (Bradwejn *et al.*, 1994).

Antipanic drugs and not other compounds, block the effect of CCK-4 (Bradwejn, 1995). Recently, it was demonstrated that the panic-induced effects of CCK-4 can be antagonized by chronic treatment with imipramine (Bradwejn and Koszycki, 1994). In one study, the pretreatment of patients with the selective CCK-B receptor antagonist L-365,260 dose-dependently blocked CCK-4-induced panic attacks (Bradwejn *et al.*, 1994). In a different study, the action of another CCK-B receptor antagonist Cl-988 was evaluated. There was a significant decrease in sum intensity scores and panic attack frequency following Cl-988 treatment (Bradwejn, 1995). These data apparently support the role of CCK-B receptors in the mediation of panicogenic-like action of CCK-4. Nevertheless, a placebo-controlled trial of L-365,260 did not result in any clinically significant improvement in patients with panic disorder (Kramer *et al.*, 1995). The possible reasons for lack of effect with L-365,260 are not clear, but the poor pharmacokinetic properties of the drug is the most plausible explanation.

A comparison of the neuronal responses to cholecystokinin tetrapeptide between younger and older patients was examined by Flint and colleagues (2000). In both age groups, maximum increase in prolactin Adrenocorticotrophic hormone ACTH and cortisol was significantly greater with CCK-4 than with placebo. Following administration of CCK-4, younger and older groups did not significantly differ in maximum increase in prolactin, ACTH or cortisol; older subjects had a statistically significant smaller increase in Growth Hormone GH compared with younger subjects but the magnitude of the difference was small and of doubtful clinical relevance. Older subjects who had a panic attack had significantly greater elevations of all hormones compared with those who did not panic, and younger panickers had a significantly greater elevation of GH compared with young non-panickers. For the most part, maximum changes in hormonal levels were not correlated with symptom severity, suggesting that other factors may have contributed to the differential effect of panic on the hypothalamic-pituitary-adrenal (HPA) axis.

More recently, the role of the HPA system in panic disorder was investigated (Ströhle, Holsboer and Rupprecht, 2000). Twenty-four patients with panic disorder were given injections of CCK-4 (25 µg). Panic attacks, psychological changes as well as ACTH and cortisol secretion were recorded. Fifteen of the 24 patients experienced a panic attack after CCK-4. ACTH secretion was significantly higher in the patients with CCK-4-induced panic attacks than in those without such attacks. The patients without CCK-4-induced attacks had a brief but less pronounced increase in ACTH concentrations. Cortisol concentrations were not significantly increased after CCK-4 administration. The increased ACTH concentrations suggest that the activation of the HPA system in CCK-4-induced panic attacks plays a physiological role. Corticotrophin-releasing factor (CRF) may be involved in experimentally and perhaps, naturally occurring panic attacks as well (see section on CRF). Several studies have found that the incidence and prevalence of panic disorder decline in later life (Flint, Cook and Rabins, 1996). The reason for this decline is unknown, but it has been hypothesized that age-related changes in brain neurotransmitter function may contribute.

CORTICOTROPHIN-RELEASING FACTOR AND ANXIETY

Corticotrophin-releasing factor (CRF) is a neuropeptide that plays a prominent role in the endocrine, autonomic, behavioural and immune responses to stress, through its action on the major physiological regulator of the HPA axis (Arborelius *et al.*, 2000). In response to stress, CRF released from the paraventricular nucleus (PVN) of the hypothalamus activates CRF receptors on anterior pituitary corticoreceptors, resulting in release of ACTH into the bloodstream. CRF induces various behavioural changes related to adaptation to stress, including food intake suppression, increase in locomotor activity and grooming in familiar environments, induction of aggression and enhancement of arousal.

CRF is widely distributed in the brain, with highest concentrations found in the hypothalamus. Moderate and low levels of CRF are also found in cortical and limbic structures. The amygdala is densely innervated by CRF neurons, which exert excitatory influences on various fear-circuit brain nuclei, including the locus coerulus (Coplan and Lydiard, 1998; Le Doux, 1998).

The effects of CRF are mediated by two specific G-protein receptors called CRF_1 and CRF_2. Tissue distribution analysis showed that CRF_1 receptor expression is most abundant in neocortical, cerebellar and limbic structures, whereas CRF_2 receptor expression is generally localized in subcortical structures, notably in the later septum and various hypothalamic areas (Chalmers, Lovenberg and De Souza, 1995). The CRF_1 receptor displays a high affinity for CRF, while the CRF_2 receptor shows a lower affinity (Grigoriadis, Lovenberg and De Souza, 1996; Radulovic *et al.*, 1999). This anatomical information provides a basis for functional hypotheses related to CRF receptor subtypes, suggesting that CRF may contribute significantly both to behavioural responses to stress and to emotional behaviour itself.

Animal Models

The hypothesis that CRF plays a role in the pathophysiology of anxiety disorders derives mainly from preclinical findings (Arborelius *et al.*, 1999). There are several studies supporting the hypothesis that hypersecretion of CRF is a crucial factor in anxiety disorders (Nemeroff *et al.*, 1984). A number of researchers showed that when CRF was injected into the brain of rats, it produced many of the signs and symptoms seen in patients with anxiety disorders (Arborelius *et al.*, 1999; Koob and Heinrichs, 1999).

A vast literature indicates that intracerebroventricular (i.c.v.) administration of CRF, which presumably increases the concentrations of CRF in the central nervous system, produces physiological and behavioural alterations virtually identical to those obtained in laboratory animals in response to stress, including changes in heart rate and mean arterial pressure, changes in gastrointestinal function, suppression of exploratory behaviour, induction of grooming, reduction of feeding and food intake and disruption of reproductive behaviour. Further actions of centrally administered CRF include the potentiation of acoustic startle responses, the facilitation of fear conditioning and the enhancement of shock-induced freezing and fighting behaviour. These actions of CRF are indicated not to involve the activation of the pituitary-adrenal axis but are mediated by CRF receptors present in the CNS (Griebel, 1999). Micro-injected of CRF directly into the locus coerulus of rats has been found to produce defensive withdrawal responses from a novel environment (Butler *et al.*, 1990) and to reduce drinking behaviour in a brightly illuminated area (Weiss *et al.*, 1994). Similarly, intra-amygdala infusion of CRF has been reported to produce anxiogenic-like behaviour in the open-field test and increase grooming in rats (Liang and Lee, 1988; Lee and Tsai, 1989; Elkabir *et al.*, 1990).

Several peptide and non-peptide CRF receptor antagonists have been studied extensively in experimental models of anxiety. Treatment with antagonists that selectively block CRF_1 receptor action was shown to promote anxiolytic responses in the elevated plus-maze, the light–dark box, the mouse defense test battery and the fear-potentiated startle test (Lundkvist *et al.*, 1996; Schulz *et al.*, 1996; Griebel, Perralut and Sanger, 1998; Okuyama *et al.*, 1999). Alpha-helical CRF, a non-specific CRF receptor antagonist, reduced anxiety-like behaviour in the elevated plus-maze whereas astressin, an antagonist with a higher *in vitro* potency, did not (Brauns *et al.*, 2001). Administration of CP-154,526, a specific CRF_1 receptor antagonist, to rats blocked both the acquisition and expression of conditioned fear, thus suggesting that the CRF_1 receptor might be related to anxiety (Hikichi *et al.*, 2000). The acute administration of CP-154,526, or its analogue antalarmin was demonstrated as blocking CRF- and stress-induced elevations in plasma adrenocorticotrophin and to possess anxiolytic activity in the elevated plus-maze (Lundkvist *et al.*, 1996; Deak *et al.*, 1999), in the light/dark test and the mouse defensive test battery, but not in conflict tests (Griebel, Perralut and Sanger, 1998). After 9 to 10 days of chronic treatment with CP-154,526 ($3.2\,mg\,kg^{-1}$), defensive withdrawal behaviour was also significantly decreased, indicating anxiolytic activity (Arborelius *et al.*, 2000). CP-154,526 was also shown to reduce separation-induced vocalization in rat pups (Kehne *et al.*, 2000).

Antagonism of CRF_2 receptors produces a consistent anxiolytic-like behavioural profile in a number of different animal models. Antisauvagine-30 (anti-SVG-30), a high affinity CRF_2 peptide antagonist was found to produce a dose dependant reduction in the duration of conditioned freezing, increase the level of open-arm exploration and increase the time spent in an open field in rats (Takahashi *et al.*, 2001).

It has been demonstrated that central administration of CRF increases anxiety-like behaviour in rodents and that transgenic mice that overexpress CRF exhibit anxiogenic behaviour. Two recent studies using CRF transgenic mouse lines overexpressing CRF further emphasized the anxiogenic properties of CRF, since these mice exhibited a behavioural state resembling that produced by anxiety (Stenzel-Poore *et al.*, 1996; Koob and Gold, 1997). Studies using CRF_1 receptor knockout mice have revealed that the anxiogenic effects of CRF appears to be mediated by the CRF_1 receptor subtype (Heinrichs *et al.*, 1997; Smith *et al.*, 1998; Timpli *et al.*, 1998). CRF_1 knockout mice show increased anxiolytic-like activity in the elevated plus-maze and a tendency to enter the illuminated region of a light–dark box (Smith *et al.*, 1998; Timpli *et al.*, 1998). Varying results have been observed with CRF_2 knockout mice. Using open-field exploration as a measure, one study reported that CRF_2 knockout mice showed increased centre activity (Kishimoto *et al.*, 2000), another found a decrease in centre scores (Bale *et al.*, 2000) and a third study found no effects of CRF_2 knockout on anxiety behaviour (Coste *et al.*, 2000). In another model of anxiety a decrease in open-arm exploration, suggesting an increase in anxiety was reported (Bale *et al.*, 2000; Kishimoto *et al.*, 2000).

There is considerable evidence that CRF is involved in the anxiogenic and aversive effects of withdrawal from abuse drugs such as cocaine (Basso *et al.*, 1999). Since CRF is suggested to play a critical role in the development of stress and because anxiety is recognized as an important result of cessation of chronic drug administration, it is possible to postulate that brain CRF modulates the neurobiological mechanisms that underlie the anxiety and stress associated with drug withdrawal (Lu, Liu and Ceng, 2001). Lu and colleagues (2001) have suggested that the CRF_1 receptor, but not type 2, mediated the stress-induced reactivation of cocaine-conditioned place preference, as only the CRF_1 antagonist CP-154,526 but not the CRF_2 antagonist, AS-30 was capable of the reactivation.

Suggestions of an inverse relationship between the CRF_1 and CRF_2 receptor systems have been reported using an anxiety model based on adverse early-life experience (Skelton *et al.*, 2000). Thus CRF neuronal systems may be comprised of two separate, but interrelated, subdivisions that can be coordinately and inversely regulated by stress, anxiety or anxiolytic drugs.

Human Studies

Although there is no direct evidence that CRF or CRF receptor ligands may modulate anxiety in humans, clinical data suggesting a role for CRF in anxiety disorders have been accumulating over recent years. Clinical studies have not revealed any consistent changes in cerebrospinal fluid (CSF) CRF concentrations in patients with anxiety disorders; however preclinical findings strongly implicate a role for CRF in the pathophysiology of certain anxiety disorders (Arborelius *et al.*, 1999). CSF levels of CRF have been shown to be elevated in patients suffering from obsessive compulsive disorder (Altemus *et al.*, 1994), post-traumatic stress (Stout, Kilts and Nemeroff, 1995; Holsboer, 1999) but not panic disorder (Jolkkonen *et al.*, 1993). Fossey *et al.* (1996) examined the CSF concentrations of CRF in a group of patients with anxiety disorders and found no difference between four diagnostic categories: panic disorder, generalized anxiety disorder, obsessive compulsive disorder and normal comparison subjects.

The findings that CRF stimulation increases anxiety-related behaviours in a variety of animal models suggest that agents acting at CRF receptors may have therapeutic effects in anxiety- or stress-related disorders. CRF receptor antagonists may represent a new option for pharmacotherapy of stress-related disorders and some of these CRF receptor antagonists are currently undergoing clinical trials to determine their efficacy and tolerability in patients with anxiety disorders as well as testing of the hypothesis that CRF hypersecretion is responsible for certain features of anxiety disorders.

NEUROPEPTIDE Y AND ANXIETY

Neuropeptide Y (NPY) is widely distributed throughout the peripheral and central nervous system. In the brain high concentrations of NPY are found in most cerebral regions including the cerebral cortex, hippocampus, thalamus and brainstem. However, regarding NPY receptors designated Y1, Y2, Y3, Y4, Y5 and Y6 (Gehlert *et al.*, 2001), the distribution varies. Y1 receptors are essentially present in high density in the cerebral cortex, thalamus and in some parts of the amygdala. Y2 receptors are found in the hippocampus, substantia nigralateralis, hypothalamus and brainstem. The so-called Y3 receptors may only be present in the brainstem but are not well characterized and have not as yet been cloned (Lee and Miller, 1998), and so far their existence remains controversial (Ingenhoven and Beck-Sickinger, 1999). Y4 receptor mRNA is mainly expressed in the peripheral nervous system, in the colon, small intestine and prostate (Michel *et al.*, 1998). Both the human and rat Y5 receptor have been cloned and with its mouse analogue, the Y6 receptor, form the latest members of the neuropeptide Y receptor family. Y5 receptor mRNA has been found in a number of brain regions implicated in the regulation of emotion (Nichol *et al.*, 1999) including hypothalamic nuclei, lateral septum, locus coeruleus and the amygdala.

The presence of NPY receptors in many regions implicated in the regulation of stress and the anxiolysis process provides the hypothesis of the implication of NPY in such mechanisms, leading to studies in animal models of anxiety.

Animals Models

Exogenous neuropeptide Y (NPY) reduces experimental anxiety in a wide range of valid animal models. The i.c.v. administration of NPY induces anxiolytic-like effects in various animal models of anxiety including ethological models such as the elevated plus-maze and social interaction test, models based on fear suppression of behaviour, including non-operant punished drinking, i.e. the Vogel's test (see Griebel (1999) for review), and operant food reinforced paradigm, as well as fear-potentiated startle. Heiling *et al.* (1989) have demonstrated using two rat models of anxiety, namely the Montgomery's conflict and the Vogel's drinking conflict test that NPY (0.4 to 2 nmol i.c.v.) induced anxiolytic-like effects with sedation and ataxia at higher doses. Increased plasma levels of immunoreactive NPY are observed following multiple aversive stimuli such as cold stress and handling (Zukowska-Grojec *et al.*, 1991), hypoxia (Cheng *et al.*, 1992) and emotional stress (Castagne *et al.*, 1987). NPY has an anticonflict effect when micro-injected into the amygdala (Heiling *et al.*, 1993). Micro-injected of NPY into the basolateral nucleus of the amygdala produced an increase in social interaction time in rats (Sajdyk, Vandergriff and Gehlert, 1999). The discovery and use of specific NPY agonists have demonstrated that the Y1 receptors are likely to be involved in the anxiolytic action of NPY (Broqua *et al.*, 1995). In this study the central administration of NPY increased the time spent in the open arms of an elevated plus-maze in the rat. Furthermore the administration of the NPY agonists, NPY_{2-36} and [Leu^{31}, Pro^{34}] NPY was found to increase the percentage of time spent in the open arms of the maze, while the Y2 receptor agonist NYP_{13-36} failed to do so. In the fear-potentiated startle model, a conditioned paradigm which is totally different from the precedent model, NPY, PYY and the agonists NPY_{2-36} or [Leu^{31}, Pro^{34}] NPY had similar effects to those of conventional anxiolytic drugs such as diazepam or even buspirone. Taken together these results are in agreement with the hypothesis that the antianxiety effects of NPY are mediated through Y1 receptors. The use of specific antagonists could help in understanding the involvement of endogenous NPY in the regulation of anxiety in animals. A highly selective, non-peptide NPY1 receptor antagonist, BIBP3226 induced an anxiogenic-like effect in the elevated plus-maze at a dose of 0.5 µg i.c.v. (Kask, Rago and Harro, 1996). This supports the hypothesis that endogenous NPY could reduce anxiety and/or neophobia through Y1 receptors. The anxiolytic-like effect of NPY in the rat social interaction test was antagonized by the specific Y1 receptor antagonist, ((R)-N-[[4-(aminocarbonylaminomethyl)phenyl]methyl]-N2-(diphenylacetyl)-argininamide trifluoroacetate) 3304 (Sajdyk, Vandergriff and Gehlert, 1999). In order to confirm the participation of endogenous NPY in regulating anxiety, Wahlestedt *et al.* (1993) synthesized an antisense 18-base-oligodeoxynucleotide on the basis of the sequence of the rat Y1 receptor. The i.c.v. administration of this antisense via chronic implanted guide cannulas (injection of 50 µg, four times over 2 days) produced an anxiogenic-like effect in the rat elevated plus-maze with more than 60% decrease in the activity in open arms, with no difference in overall locomotor activity. After testing, rats were killed and binding was performed on cortical and striatum tissue. The Y1-type binding site was decreased by almost 60%.

On the other hand, BIBP3226-induced anxiogenic effects is counteracted by the administration of 0.5 $\mu g\,mg^{-1}$ of the benzodiazepine diazepam (Kask, Rago and Harro, 1996). This suggests that the neuropeptidic Y neurotransmission is connected to the GABAergic system. However, Britton *et al.* (1997) have demonstrated that flumazenil, a benzodiazepine receptor antagonist and picrotoxin, a GABA receptor antagonist, failed to alter NPY-induced punished responding in a rat conflict paradigm. These results confirm that the anxiolytic action of NPY is independent of a direct implication of the GABA/benzodiazepine receptor complex. On the other hand, the hypothesis that the opioid system may interact with NPY, is supported by the fact that naloxone (0.25 to 2 $mg\,kg^{-1}$) antagonized the effects of NPY in a conflict test and that central administration of the selective mu opiate antagonist CTAP partially blocked NPY-induced conflict responding (Britton and Southerland, 2001). Furthermore, concerning NPY neurotransmission interaction with other systems, a study reported that the anxiogenic effect of a selective Y1 receptor was prevented by the blockade of CRF receptors, suggesting antagonistic effects of endogenous NPY and CRF in shaping the response to novelty (Kask, Rago and Harro, 1997; Britton *et al.*, 2000).

A recent study, (Kask, Rago and Harro, 1998) reported new data on the mechanism of action of NPY. In fact, NPY has an anticonflict effect when micro-injected into the central nucleus of the amygdala but NPY is also found in other brain structures including the locus coeruleus. Interestingly, the anxiolytic-like effect of NPY in the vicinity of the locus coeruleus may involve the Y2 receptor subtype instead of Y1, as the Y2 agonist NPY_{13-36} was active and the Y1 agonist [Leu^{13}, Pro^{34}] was without effect. One explanation is that NPY transmission in the locus coeruleus modulates noradrenergic transmission via Y2 receptors in response to stress or novelty. Neuropeptide Y_{13-36} was found to be a mixed Y2/Y5 receptor agonist. Taken together these data suggest that the anxiolytic-like effect of NPY is not mediated via the single Y1 receptor subtype and that other receptors such as Y2 and Y5 may be involved. Using the Y5 receptor antagonist CGP71683A, Criscione *et al.* (1998) have shown that high doses of this compound induce conditioned taste aversion suggesting that Y5 receptor antagonism may cause anxiety or sickness behaviour. Recently, Kask *et al.* (2001) have demonstrated that CGP71683A failed to induce anxiogenic-like effects in the elevated plus-maze or decrease social interaction under testing conditions that were appropriate to detect anxiogenic-like effects of the drug. Nevertheless, rats stressed by prior exposure to an elevated plus-maze test session have shown increased anxiety in the open-field test (Kask *et al.*, 2001). It is suggested that Y1 receptor mediates tonic NPY-induced anxiolysis and that the Y5 receptor contributes to adaptive changes that occur after stress exposure.

A role for endogenous NPY in the control of anxiety and stress is suggested by the fact that acute restraint stress suppresses NPY mRNA and peptide levels, within the cortex and the amygdala (Möller *et al.*, 1997). In the same way, repeated exposure to the same stressor chronically for 10 days leads to behavioural habituation and to an upregulation of amygdala NPY expression. One hypothesis is that endogenous NPY may contribute to the behavioural adaptation of stress. The use of NPY-transgenic (NPYtr) rats in a model of anxiety has provided an important tool in understanding the role of NPY in anxiety. Centrally injected exogenous NPY produced anxiolytic-like effects in the elevated plus-maze; the same effect was found with NPYtr rats only when the elevated plus-maze session was preceded by a stressor (Thorsell *et al.*, 2000). This presumes that neuronal activation may be needed for endogenous release of NPY.

Human Studies

Neuropeptide Y attenuates the action of CRF and other stress-released peptides. Preliminary trials with military personnel undergoing arduous basic training have shown that those individuals with the highest NPY levels tolerated excessive stress better than those with low levels (Morgan *et al.*, 2000). These findings suggest that it could be possible to treat post-traumatic stress disorder (PTSD) with a pharmacological agent promoting higher NPY levels (Friedman, 2000).

SUBSTANCE P AND NEUROKININS

The mammalian Tachykinin TKs are a group of neuropeptides comprised of substance P (SP), Neurokinin A (NK-A), and Neurokinin B (NK-B). These three endogenous peptides bind to G-protein coupled receptors, designated NK1, NK2 and NK3 respectively, to mediate their effects (Regoli, Boudon and Fauchere, 1994). The NK receptors are located in the central nervous system (CNS). NK1 and NK3 are widely distributed in the CNS (septum, striatum, amygdala, periaqueductal grey matter) whereas NK2 is distributed with lower levels in the CNS (Otsuka and Yoshioka, 1993; Maggi, 1995).

Animals Studies

Data suggests that SP may play a physiological role in the modulation of anxiety as this peptide is released after aversive environmental stimuli. The behavioural effects of SP have been investigated in animal models of anxiety (e.g. elevated plus-maze, social interaction). The effect of SP in anxiety models may be dependent on dose and specific brain regions (Griebel, 1999). Indeed, the administration of SP into various brain areas (the lateral ventricles, the region of the nucleus basalis magnocellularis, the bed nucleus of stria terminalis or the basolateral nucleus of the amygdala), produces anxiogenic-like effects in the elevated plus-maze in rodents (rats or mice) (De Lima and Ribeiro, 1996; Jentiens *et al.*, 1996; Teixeira *et al.*, 1996) whereas 1 mg of SP administered in the nucleus basalis magnocellularis showed anxiolytic-like properties in the rat social interaction test (Hasenöhrl *et al.*, 1996; Jentiens *et al.*, 1996).

The effect of NK2 agonists in animal models of anxiety show an anxiogenic-like profile. The endogenous ligand for NK2 receptors (NK-A) or the selective NK2 receptor agonist [β-Ala^8]NK-A-(4-10), a fragment of NK-A have been reported to produce anxiogenic-like effects in the mouse elevated plus-maze (De Lima *et al.*, 1995; Teixeira *et al.*, 1996). Studies are still lacking concerning the effects of NK-B on NK3 receptors, but De Lima *et al.* (1995) showed that senktide (a NK-B analogue) produces an anxiolytic-like effect in the elevated plus-maze, suggesting that NK3 receptors could play a modulatory role in anxiety (Griebel, 1999).

The potential of NK receptor antagonists as a novel treatment for anxiety and depression has been investigated (Kramer *et al.*, 1998). During 6 weeks, in a double-blind placebo-controlled study in patients with major depression, the NK1 antagonist MK 869 (300 mg per day), produced a positive outcome as measured by both the Hamilton depression (HAM-D21) and anxiety (HAM-A) scales.

There is clinical evidence that TK NK1 receptor antagonists may represent an important advance in the search for novel treatments of anxiety (Nutt, 1998). A wide range of chemically diverse SP receptor antagonists have now been synthesized, but vary markedly in their ability to cross the blood–brain barrier. Poor brain penetrant compounds include SR 14033, LY 303870, RPR 100893 and CGP 49823, while good brain penetrant compounds include the piperidines CP 99,994 and GR 203040, the piperidine ether L-733,060, and morpholines such as L-742,694 (Rupniak *et al.*, 1996, 1997; Kramer *et al.*, 1998). L-733,060 also exhibits a long duration of central NK1 receptor binding ($t_{1/2} > 6$ h), compared with the piperidine CP 99,994, making it particularly suitable for chronic administration studies in appropriate species (Rupniak *et al.*, 1996).

In preclinical studies evidence has been limited by the prevalence of tests utilizing rats and mice, whose NK1 receptor pharmacology differs to that of the human receptor (Beresford *et al.*, 1991; Gitter *et al.*, 1991). The majority of NK1 antagonist compounds display only low affinity for the rat receptor whereas they have high affinity for the human NK1 receptor. For example, L-733,060 in species that possess the human-like NK1 receptor (notably gerbils and guinea pigs), displays sub-nanomolar affinity while it does not possess affinity for the rat NK1 receptor (IC50nM) (Rupniak *et al.*, 1993). A small number of compounds have been described that possess nanomolar affinity for the rat receptor (RP 67580 and SR 140333), but their utility for *in vivo* studies is severely limited by their short half-life and poor brain penetration (Rupniak *et al.*, 1997). Nonetheless, data show an anxiolytic-like profile of the TK receptor antagonist in rodents. MK-869 reduces vocalization in guinea pig pups after maternal separation, suggesting an involvement in the integration of emotional responses to stress by amygdala or related brain areas (Saria, 1999). (±)-CP-96,345 has been reported to increase the time spent in the more aversive light compartment in the mouse light/dark test, albeit at high doses which caused sedation and motor impairment (Zernig, Troger and Saria, 1993). File (1997) also reported the anxiolytic activity of the TK NK1 antagonist, CGP 49823, in the rat social interaction test.

However, the picture is less clear with other selective NK1 receptor antagonists such as FK 888. Although the drug produced anxiolytic-like activity in the mouse elevated plus-maze (De Lima *et al.*, 1995; Teixeira *et al.*, 1996), these effects were not confirmed in a subsequent experiment in rats (De Lima and Ribeiro, 1996). Only at non-consecutive doses and only on one index of anxiety (time on open arms) was there an anxiolytic-like activity found after FK 888 administration in studies. Chronic treatment of NK1 antagonists were also studied in animal models of anxiety (File, 2000). After NKP608 administration, rats were tested in various conditions of the social interaction test. NKP608 administration had significant anxiolytic effects at 0.01, 0.03 and 0.01 mg kg^{-1} (p.o.) in an unfamiliar arena lit by both high and low light test conditions, but was without effect in the familiar arena under low light illumination. The anxiolytic effect of $0.03\,mg\,kg^{-1}$ remained after 3 weeks of chronic treatment and there was no anxiogenic effect after 24 h of drug withdrawal. At 6 weeks tolerance had developed, but no anxiogenic withdrawal effect was seen 24 h after the last dose.

Foot taping may be elicited in gerbils (a species whose NK1 receptor resembles that of the human (Beresford *et al.*, 1991; Gitter *et al.*, 1991)), by an aversive stimulus, i.e. electroshock and notably by cues paired with unconditioned stimulus. Recently, data supported the view that shock-induced foot taping in the gerbil is robustly inhibited by two NK1 antagonists. MK-869 ($0.3–3\,mg\,kg^{-1}$, i.p.) dose-dependently blocked this foot tapping response and CP-99,994 ($3\,mg\,kg^{-1}$, i.p.) inhibited foot tapping whereas its less active enantiomer (CP-100,263) had no effect (Ballard, Sänger and Higgins, 2001).

In contrast with NK1 studies, which can have contradictory results, NK2 antagonist studies show more reliable results. However, all results were obtained in exploration and social investigation procedures, but not conflict tests. Indeed, NK2 antagonists could possess antianxiety activity. The selective NK2 antagonist, SR 48968, increased the time spent in open arms and also increased the frequency of entries into the open arms in the mouse elevated plus-maze (Teixeira *et al.*, 1996). GR 159897, another non-peptide NK2 receptor antagonist was evaluated in two models of anxiety (the mouse light–dark box and the marmoset human intruder response test) and demonstrated in both rodent and primate species the ability to restore behaviour which had been suppressed by novel aversive environments (Walsh *et al.*, 1995). The effects of GR 159897 ($0.0005–50\,\mu g\,kg^{-1}$, s.c.) are similar to SR 48968 ($0.0005–50\,\mu g\,kg^{-1}$, s.c.) and diazepam ($1–1.75\,mg\,kg^{-1}$, s.c.), as the three molecules increased time spent in the light compartment, without affecting locomotor activity. In the marmoset human intruder response, GR 159897 ($0.2–50\,\mu g\,kg^{-1}$, s.c.), SR 48968 ($10–50\,\mu g\,kg^{-1}$, s.c.) and chlordiazepoxide ($0.3–3.0\,mg\,kg^{-1}$, s.c.) significantly increased the amount of time marmosets spent at the front of the cage during confrontation with humans. In fact, GR 159897 and SR 48968 produced similar effects to the classical antianxiety agents diazepam or chlordiazepoxide, but these two molecules produced positive effects over a wide dose range, with minimum dose levels in the microgram range. Another compound tested in the light–dark paradigm, GR 100679 ($0.02–200\,\mu g\,kg^{-1}$, s.c.) which dose-dependently increased the time mice spent in the light side of the light–dark paradigm, had a similar effect to diazepam (Stratton *et al.*, 1993).

The present review suggests that centrally acting NK antagonists may have clinical utility in a number of psychiatric disorders that are currently treated with benzodiazepines and 5-HT1A agonists. The variable effects produced by NK1 receptor ligands in various anxiety models requires further investigation. The use of NK1 receptor knockout mice could be an alternative for this investigation.

Humans Studies

Investigators in a study undertaken by Merck Research Laboratories, studying 213 patients over 6 weeks, reported antidepressant effects for MK-869, a selective NK-1 antagonist, in the first week. By contrast, the study by California Clinical Trials, which took place also over a similar period, reported that statistically significant antidepressant activity of MK-869 was initially observed at week 4 and was maintained at week 6. The Californian trial formed part of a multicentre study comparing MK-869 to placebo in patients with Major Depressive Disorder (Hung, 2000).

NATRIURETIC PEPTIDES AND ANXIETY

There are at least three peptides constituting the natriuretic peptides (NP) system, namely the atrial natriuretic peptide (ANP), the brain natriuretic peptide (BNP) and the C-type natriuretic peptide (CNP). These peptides are natriuretic factors in the periphery and have a role in regulation of homeostasis of body fluid electrolytic balance and blood pressure in the CNS (Nicholls, 1994). The corresponding natriuretic peptide receptors NPR-A, NPR-B and NPR-C have been identified in the brain (Imura, Nakao and Itoh, 1992). In the CNS of rodents NPR-A is found mainly in the cortex and hippocampus, whereas NPR-B is present in the amygdala and several brainstem regulatory sites. NPR-C is found widely within the CNS, i.e. in the neocortex, limbic cortex, the hippocampal area and the amygdala. These peptides and their receptors represent an important neuromodulatory system within the CNS which is involved not only in the regulation of fluid homeostasis but also directly influences emotional behaviour such as anxiety and arousal.

Animal Models

Strohle *et al.* (1997) studied the effects of the central and peripheral administration of atriopeptin II, an aminoacid residue peptide of atrial natriuretic peptide (Ser103-Arg125), on anxiety-related behaviour and locomotor activity. Its behaviour on the elevated plus-maze after social deficit stress indicated that i.c.v. (2.5 and $5\,\mu g$) and i.p. ($50\,\mu g$) administration of atriopeptin II produced anxiolysis. A low dose of $0.25\,\mu g$ atriopeptin II administered bilaterally into the central nucleus of amygdala was also found to be anxiolytic.

The anxiolytic effects observed after central and peripheral administration support the hypothesis that atrial natriuretic peptide, which is increased in panic anxiety, may be involved in the tapering of anxiety-related behaviour. In contrast, ANP failed to diminish punished responses in the Geller–Sefter conflict test in rats (Heilig *et al.*, 1992). It was previously found that i.c.v. administration of ANP, PNP and CNP increased the exploratory activity of rats in the elevated plus-maze (Biro, Toth and Telegdy, 1995, 1996; Bhattacharya *et al.*, 1996). ANP-induced anxiolysis was also observed in the open field, social interaction and novelty-induced feeding suppression tests in rats (Bhattacharya *et al.*, 1996).

Isatin is an endogenous indole which has been shown to counteract some of the effects of ANP both *in vitro* and *in vivo*. Given intraperitoneally isatin reduced the effects of both BNP and CNP in a model of passive-avoidance learning in rats (Telegdy, Adamik and Glover, 2000) and the anxiolytic effect of ANP in the elevated plus-maze (Bhattacharya *et al.*, 1996). On the other hand small amounts of isatin are anxiogenic in rodent models. Furthermore, isatin has a wide spectrum of biological properties: a marker of stress and anxiety, an antiseizure agent, an inhibitor of benzodiazepine receptors and ANP binding to its receptors (Hamaue, 2000).

Human Studies

It has been suggested that ANP receptor modulation may have antipanic activity in patients with panic disorder. A double-blind placebo-controlled study was conducted in nine patients presenting with panic disorder and nine healthy control subjects. After pretreatment with an infusion of $150\,\mu g$ ANP or placebo in random order, each subject received $50\,\mu g$ CCK-4 (Wiedemann *et al.*, 2001). After pretreatment with ANP, the number of CCK-4-induced panic attacks decreased from eight to six in patients and from five to two in controls. Infusion of ANP significantly curtailed the CCK-4-induced release of corticotrophin in patients. ANP exerts anxiolytic-like effects on patients with panic disorder. These results are supported by another study (Strohle *et al.*, 2001) using 25 μg CCK-4 in 10 panic disorder patients. These two studies support the antipanic activity of ANP, however it is possible that non-peptidergic ANP receptor ligands may be ultimately used to treat anxiety disorders.

CONCLUSION

The pharmacological, behavioural and molecular investigations of neuropeptides has advanced remarkably the knowledge of the peptidergic transmitter system in recent years. This knowledge has led to the development of new compounds with potential clinical interest and development has reached clinical studies in some examples of anxiety disorders. Although there is little clinical evidence so far of peptidergic involvement in human anxiety, the results from animal studies are encouraging. However, much research is required to address the hypotheses that neuropeptides may represent a new option for pharmacotherapy of stress-related disorders.

REFERENCES

Abelson, J.L., Nesse, R.M. and Vinik, A., 1991. Stimulation of corticotrophin release by pentagastrin in normal subjects and patients with panic disorder. *Biol. Psychiatry*, **29**, 1220–1223.

Altemus, M., Swedo, S.E., Leonard, H.L., Richter, D., Rubinow, D.R., Potter, W.Z. and Rapoport, J.L., 1994. Changes in cerebrospinal fluid neurochemistry during treatment of obsessive–compulsive disorder with clomipramine. *Arch. Gen. Psychiat*, **51**, 794–803.

Arborelius, L., Owens, M.J., Bissette, G., Plotsky, P.M. and Nemeroff, CB., 1999. The role of corticotrophin-releasing factor in depression and anxiety. *J. Endocrinol.*, **160**(1), 1–12.

Arborelius, L., Skelton, K.H., Thrivikraman, K.V., Plotsky, P.M., Schulz, D.W. and Owens, M.J., 2000. Chronic administration of the selective corticotrophin-releasing factor 1 receptor antagonist CP-154,526: behavioural, endocrine and neurochemical effects in the rat. *J. Pharmacol. Exp. Ther.*, **294**(2), 588–597.

Bale, T.L., Contarino, A., Smith, G.W., Chan, R., Gold, L.H., Sawchenko, P.E., Koob, G.F., Vale, W.W. and Lee, K.-F., 2000. Mice deficient for corticotrophin-releasing hormone receptor-2 display anxiety-like behaviour and are hypersensitive to stress. *Nat. Genet.*, **24**, 410–414.

Ballard, T.M., Sänger, S. and Higgins, G.A., 2001. Inhibition of shock-induced foot taping behaviour in the gerbil by a tachykinin NK1 receptor antagonist. *Eur. J. Pharmacol.*, **412**, 255–264.

Basso, A.M., Spina, M., Rivier, J., Vale, W. and Koob, G.F., 1999. Corticotrophin-releasing factor antagonist attenuates the "anxiogenic-like" effect in the defensive burying paradigm but not in the elevated plus maze following chronic cocaine in rats. *Psychopharmacology*, **145**, 21–30.

Bersesford, I.J.M., Birch, P.J., Hagan, R.M. and Ireland, S.J., 1991. Investigation into species variants in tachykinin NK1 receptors by use of the non-peptide antagonist, CP-96,345. *Br. J. Pharmacol.*, **104**, 292–293.

Bhattacharya, S.K., Chakrabarti, A., Sandler, M. and Glover, V., 1996. Anxiolytic activity of intraventricularly administered atrial natriuretic peptide in the rat. *Neuropsychopharmacology*, **15**, 199–206.

Biro, E., Toth, G. and Telegdy, G., 1995. Involvement of neurotransmitters inn the anxiolytic like action of atrial natriuretic peptide in rats. *Neuropeptides*, **29**, 215–220.

Biro, E., Toth, G. and Telegdy, G., 1996. Effect of receptor blockers on brain natriuretic peptide and C-type natriuretic peptide caused anxiolytic state in rats. *Neuropeptides*, **30**, 59–65.

Bourin, M., Malinge, M., Vasar, E. and Bradwejn, J., 1996. Two faces of cholecystokinin: anxiety and schizophrenia. *Fundam. Clin. Pharmacol.*, **10**, 116–120.

Bradwejn, J. and de Montigny, C., 1984. Benzodiazepines antagonize cholecystokinin-induced activation of rat hippocampal neurons. *Nature*, **312**, 363–364.

Bradwejn, J. and Koszycki, D., 1994. Imipramine antagonizes the panicogenic effects of CCK-4 in panic disorder patients. *Am. J. Psychiat.*, **1511**, 261–263.

Bradwejn, J., Koszycki, D. and Meterissian, G., 1990. Cholecystokinin-tetrapeptide in panic disorder. *Can. J. Psychiat.*, **35**, 83–85.

Bradwejn, J., Koszycki, D. and Shriqui, C., 1991. Enhanced sensitivity to cholecystokinin tetrapeptide in panic disorder. *Arch. Gen. Psychiatry*, **48**, 603–610.

Bradwejn, J., Koszycki, D., Couëtoux du Tertre, A., van Megen, H., Den Boer, J., Westenberg, H. and Annable, L., 1994. The panicogenic effects of cholecystokinin tetrapeptide are antagonized by L-365.260, a central cholecystokinin receptor antagonist, in patients with panic disorder. *Arch. Gen. Psychiat.*, **51**, 486–493.

Bradwejn, J., 1995. Cholecystokinin and panic disorder. In: Bradwejn, J. and Vasar, E. (eds), *Cholecystokinin and Anxiety: from Neuron to Behavior*, pp. 73–86. RG Landes, Austin.

Brambilla, F., Bellodi, L., Perna, G., Garberi, A. and Sacerdote, P., 1993. Lymphocyte cholecystokinin concentrations in panic disorder. *Am. J. Psychiat.*, **150**, 1111–1113.

Brauns, O., Liepold, T., Radulovic, J. and Spiess, J., 2001. Pharmacological and chemical properties of astressin, antisauvagine-30 and alpha-helCRF: significance for behavioural experiments. *Neuropharmacology*, **41**(4), 507–516.

Britton, K.T., Southerland, S., Van Uden, E., Kirby, D., Rivier, J. and Koob, G., 1997. Anxiolytic activity of NPY receptor agonists in the conflict test. *Psychopharmacology*, **132**, 6–13.

Britton, K.T. and Southerland, S., 2001. Naloxone blocks anxiolytic effects of neuropeptide Y. *Peptides*, **22**, 607–612.

Britton, K.T., Akwa, Y., Spina, M.G. and Koob, G.F., 2000. Neuropeptide Y blocks anxiogenic-like behavioural action of corticotrophin-releasing factor in an operant conflict test and elevated plus maze. *Peptides*, **1**, 37–44.

Broqua, P., Wettstein, J.G., Rocher, M.N., Gauthier-Martin, B. and Junien, J.L., 1995. Behavioural effects of neuropeptide Y agonists in the elevated plus maze and fear-potentiated startle procedures. *Behav. Pharmacol.*, **6**, 215–222.

Butler, P.D., Weiss, J.M., Stout, J.C. and Nemeroff, C.B., 1990. Corticotrophin-releasing factor produces fear-enhancing and behavioural activating effects following infusion into the locus coeruleus. *J. Neurosci.*, **10**, 176–183.

Castagne, V., Corder, R., Gaillard, R. and Mormede, P., 1987. Stress induced changes in circulating neuropeptide Y in the rat: comparison with catecholamines. *Reg. Peptides*, **19**, 55–63.

Chalmers, D.T., Lovenberg, T.W. and De Souza, E.B., 1995. Localisation of novel corticotrophin-releasing factor receptor (CRF2) mRNA expression to specific subcortical nuclei in rat brain: comparison with CRF1 receptor mRNA expression. *J. Neurosci.*, **15**, 6340–6350.

Cheng, J.T., Chen, C.F., Shum, A., Wang, J.Y. and Chen, H., 1992. Increase of plasma neuropeptideY-like immuno-reactivity following chronic hypoxia with catecholamine. *Neurosci. Lett.*, **140**, 211–214.

Coplan, J. and Lydiard, R.B., 1998. Brain circuits in panic disorder. *Biol. Psychiatry*, **44**, 1264–1276.

Coste, S.C., Kesterson, R.A., Heldwein, K.A., Stevens, S.L., Heard, A.D., Hollis, J.H., Murray, S.E., Hill, J.K., Pantely, G.A., Hohimer, A.R., Hatton, D.C., Phillips, T.J., Finn, D.A., Low, M.J., Rittenber, M.B., Stenzel, P. and Stenzel-Poore, M.P., 2000. Abnormal adaptations to stress and impaired cardiovascular function in mice lacking corticotrophin-releasing hormone receptor-2. *Nat. Genet.*, **24**, 403–409.

Criscione, L., Rigollier, P., Batzl-Hartmann, C., Rueger, H., Stricker-Krongrad, A., Wyss, P., Brunner, L., Whitebread, S., Yamagushi, W., Hofbauer, K.G. and Levens, N., 1998. Food intake in free-feeding and energy deprived lean rats is mediated by the neuropeptide Y5 receptor. *J. Clin. Invest.*, **102**, 2136–2145.

Dawson, G.R., Rupniak, N.M.J., Iversen, S.D., Curnow, R., Tye, S., Stanhope, K.J. and Trickleband, M.D., 1995. Lack of effect of CCK-B receptor antagonists in ethological and conditioned animal screens for anxiolytic drugs. *Psychopharmacology*, **121**, 109–117.

De Lima, T.C.M. and Ribeiro, S.J., 1996. Central effects of tachykinin NK receptor agonists and antagonists on the plus-maze behaviour in rats. *Soc. Neurosci. Abstr.*, **22**, 1154.

De Lima, T.C.M., Teixiera, R.M., Santos, A.R.S, Rae, G.A. and Calixto, J.B., 1995. Behavioural effect of substance P in mice in the elevated plus-maze. *Soc. Neurosci. Abstr.*, **23**, 1859.

De Montigny, C., 1989. Cholecystokinin tetrapeptide induces panic-like attacks in healthy volunteers. *Arch. Gen. Psychiat.*, **46**, 511–517.

Deak, T., Nguyen, K.T., Ehrlich, A.L., Watkins, L.R., Spencer, P.L., Maier, S.F., Licinio, J., Wong, M.-L., Chrousos, G.P., Webster, E. and Gold, P.W., 1999. The impact of the nonpeptide corticotrophin-releasing hormone antagonist antalarmin on behavioural and endocrine responses to stress. *Endocrinology*, **140**, 79–86.

Dodd, J. and Kelly, J.S., 1981. The actions of cholecystokinin and related peptides on pyramidal neurons of the mammalian hippocampus. *Brain Res.*, **205**, 337–350.

Elkabir, D.R., Wyatt, M.E., Vellucci, S.V. and Herbert, J., 1990. The effects of separate or combined infusions of corticotropin-releasing factor and vasopressin either intraventricularly or into the amygdala on aggressive and investigative behaviour in the rat. *Regul. Pept.*, **28**, 199–214.

File, S.E., 1997. Anxiolytic action of a neurokinin1 receptor antagonist in the social interaction test. *Pharmacol. Biochem. Behav.*, **58**, 747–752.

File, S.E., 2000. NKP608, an NK1 receptor antagonist, has an anxiolytic action in the social interaction test in rats. *Psychopharmacology*, **152**, 105–109.

Flint, A.J., Cook, J.M. and Rabins, P.V., 1996. Why is panic disorder less frequent in late life? *Am. J. Ger. Psychiat.*, **4**, 96–109.

Flint, A.J., Koszycki, D., Bradwejn, J. and Vaccarino, F.J., 2000. Neurohormonal responses to cholecystokinin tetrapeptide: a comparison of younger and older healthy subjects. *Psychoneuroendocrinology*, **25**, 633–647.

Fossey, M.D., Lydiard, R.B., Ballenger, J.C., Laraia, M.T., Bissette, G. and Nemeroff, C.B., 1996. Cerebrospinal fluid corticotrophin-releasing factor concentrations in patients with anxiety disorders and normal comparison subjects. *Biol. Psychiatry*, **39**(8), 703–707.

Friedman, M.J., 2000. What might the psychobiology of post-traumatic stress disorder teach us about future approaches to pharmacotherapy. *J. Clin. Psychiatry*, **61**, 44–51.

Gehlert, D.R., Yang, P., George, C., Wang, Y., Schober, D., Gackenheimer, S., Johnson, D., Beavers, L.S., Gadski, R.A. and Baez, M., 2001. Cloning and characterisation of rhesus monkey neuropeptide Y receptor subtypes. *Peptides*, **3**, 343–345.

Gitter, B.D., Waters, D.C., Bruns, R.F., Mason, N.R., Nixon, J.A. and Howbert, J.J., 1991. Species differences in affinities of non-peptide antagonists for substance P receptors. *Eur. J. Pharmacol.*, **197**, 237–238.

Goltermann, N.R., Rehfeld, J.F. and Roigaard-Petersen, H., 1980. *In vivo* biosynthesis of cholecystokinin in rat cerebral cortex. *J. Biol. Chem.*, **255**, 6181–6185.

Griebel, G., Perralut, G. and Sanger, D.J., 1998. Characterisation of the behavioural profile of the non-peptide CRF receptor antagonist CP-154,526 in anxiety models in rodents: comparison with diazepam and buspirone. *Psychopharmacology*, **138**, 55–66.

Griebel, G., 1999. Is there a future for neuropeptide receptor ligands in the treatment of anxiety disorder? *Pharmacol. Ther.*, **82**, 1–61.

Grigoriadis, D.E., Lovenberg, T.W. and De Souza, E.B., 1996. Characterisation of corticotrophin-releasing factor receptor subtypes. *Ann. N. Y. Acad. Sci.*, **780**, 60–80.

Hamaue, N., 2000. Pharmacological role of isatin, an endogenous MAO inhibitor. *Yakugaku Zasshi*, **120**, 352–362.

Hasenöhrl, R.U., Jentiens, O., De Souza Silva, M.A., Tomaz, C. and Huston, J.P., 1996. Anxiolytic action of substance P administered systemically or into the basal forebrain. *Soc. Neurosci. Abstr.*, **22**, 1152.

Heilig, M., McLeod, S., Koob, G.K. and Britton, K.T., 1992. Anxiolytic-like effect of neuropeptide Y (NPY), but not other peptides in an operant conflict test. *Regul. Pept.*, **41**, 61–69.

Heiling, M., McLeod, S., Brost, M., Heinrichs, S.C., Menzaghi, F., Koob, G.F. and Britton, K.T., 1993. Anxiolytic like action of neuropeptide Y: mediation by Y1 receptors in amygdala and dissociation from food intake effects. *Neuropsychopharmacology*, **8**, 357–363.

Heiling, M., Söderpalm, B., Engel, J.A. and Widerlöv, E., 1989. Centrally administered neuropeptide Y (NPY) produces anxiolytic-like effects in animal anxiety models. *Psychopharmacology*, **98**, 524–529.

Heinrichs, S.C., Lapsansky, J., Lovenberg, T.W., De Souza, E.B. and Chalmers, D.T., 1997. Corticotrophin-releasing factor CRF1, but not CRF2 receptors mediate anxiogenic-like behaviour. *Regul. Pept.*, **71**, 15–21.

Hikichi, T., Akiyoshi, J., Yamammoto, Y., Tsutsummmi, T., Isogawa, K. and Nagayama, H., 2000. Suppression of conditioned fear by administration of CRF receptor antagonist CP-154,526. *Pharmacopsychiatry*, **33**, 189–193.

Hill, D.R., Campbell, N.J., Shaw, T.M. and Woodruff, G.N., 1987. Autoradioographic localization and biochemical characterization of peripherical type CCK receptors in rat CNS using highly selective non-peptide CCK agonists. *J. Neurosci.*, **7**, 2967–2976.

Holsboer, F., 1999. Clinical neuroendocrinology. In: Charney, D.S., Nestler, E.J. and Bunney, B.S. (eds), *Neurobiology of Mental Illness*, pp. 149–161. Oxford University Press, New York.

Hung, M., 2000. Substance P antagonists represent new approach to antidepressant therapy. *XXIInd Congress of the Collegium Internationale Neuro-Psychopharmacologicum*, 9, July.

Imura, H., Nakao, K. and Itoh, H., 1992. The natriuretic peptide system in the brain: implications in the central control of cardiovascular and neuroendocrines functions. *Front. Neuroendocrinol.*, **13**, 217–249.

Ingenhoven, N. and Beck-Sickinger, A.G., 1999. Molecular characterisation of the ligand-receptor interaction of neuropeptide. *Y. Curr. Med. Chem.*, **11**, 1055–1066.

Jentiens, O., Hasenöhrl, R.U., de Souza Siva, M.A., Toma, C. and Huston, J.P., 1996. Anxiolytic-like effect of injecting neurokinin substance P systematically or into the basal forebrain. *2nd Meeting of European Neuroscience*, Strasbourg, p. 197.

Jolkkonen, J., Lepola, U., Bissette, G., Nemeroff, C. and Riekkinen, P., 1993. CRF corticotrophin-releasing factor is not affected in panic disorder. *Biol. Psychiatry*, **33**, 136–138.

Kask, A., Rago, L. and Harro, J., 1997. Alpha-helical CRF(9-14) prevents anxiogenic-like effect of NPY Y1 receptor antagonist BIBP3226 in rats. *Neuroreport*, **8**, 3645–3647.

Kask, A., Rago, L. and Harro, J., 1996. Anxiogenic-like effect of the neuropeptide YY1receptor antagonist BIBP3226: antagonism with diazepam. *Eur. J. Pharmacol.*, **317**, R3–R4.

Kask, A., Rago, L. and Harro, J., 1998. Anxiolytic-like effect of neuropeptide Y (NPY) and NPY_{13-36} microinjected into vicinity of locus coeruleus in rats. *Brain Res.*, **788**, 345–348.

Kask, A., Vasar, E., Heidmets, L.T., Allikmets, L. and Wikberg, J.E.S., 2001. Neuropeptide YY5 receptor antagonist CGP71683A: the effects on food intake and anxiety related behaviour. *Eur. J. Pharmacol.*, **414**, 215–224.

Kehne, J.H., Coverdale, S., McCloskey, T.C., Hoffman, D.C. and Cassella, J.V., 2000. Effects of the CRF(1) receptor antagonist, CP-154,526, in the separation-induced vocalisation anxiolytic test in rat pups. *Neuropharmacology*, **39**(8), 1357–1367.

Kishimoto, T., Radulovic, J., Radulovic, M., Lin, C.R., Schrick, C., Hooshman, F., Hermanson, O., Rosenfeld, M.G. and Spiess, J., 2000. Deletion of CRHR2 reveals anxiolytic role for corticotropin-releasing hormone receptor-2. *Nat. Genet.*, **24**, 415–419.

Koks, S., Volke, V., Soosar, A., Lang, A., Männisto, P.T., Bourin, M. and Vasar, E. Repeated treatment with cholecystokinin antagonists devazepide and L-365.260 does not cause anxiolytic-like action in rats. *Eur. Neuropsychopharm.*, (in press).

Koob, G.F. and Gold, L.H., 1997. Molecular biological approaches in the pharmacology of anxiety and depression. *Behav. Pharmacol.*, **8**, 652.

Koob, G.F. and Heinrichs, S.C., 1999. A role for corticotrophin releasing factor and urocortin in behavioural responses to stressors. *Brain Res.*, **848**(1–2), 141–145.

Kramer, M.S., Cutler, N.R., Ballenger, J.C., Patterson, W.M., Mendels, J., Chenault, A., Shirastava, R., Matzurawolfe, D., Lines, C. and Reines, S., 1995. A placebo-controlled trial of L-365.260, a CCK-B antagonist, in panic disorder. *Biol. Psychiatry*, **37**, 162–166.

Kramer, M.S., Cutler, N.R., Feighner, J., Shrivastava, R., Carman, J., Sramek, J.J., Reines, S.A., Liu, G., Snavely, D., Wyatt-Knowles, E., Hale, J.J., Mills, S.G., MacCoss, M., Swain, C.J., Harrison, T., Hill, R.G., Hefti, F., Scolnick, E.M., Cascieri, M.A., Chicchi, G.G., Sadowski, S., Williams, A.R., Hewson, L., Smith, D., Carlson, E.J., Hargreaves, R.J. and Rupniak, N.M., 1998. Distinct mechanism for antidepressant activity by blockade of central substance P receptors. *Science*, **281**, 1640–1645.

Le Doux, J., 1998. Fear and the brain: where have we been, and where are we going? *Biol. Psychiat.*, **44**, 1229–1238.

Lee, C.C. and Miller, R.J., 1998. Is there really an NPY receptor? *Regul. Pept.*, **75**, 71–78.

Lee, E.H. and Tsai, M.J., 1989. The hippocampus and amygdala mediate the locomotor stimulating effects of corticotrophin-releasing factor in mice. *Behav. Neural. Biol.*, **51**, 412–423.

Liang, K.C. and Lee, E.H., 1988. Intra-amygdala injections of corticotrophin releasing factor facilitate inhibitory avoidance learning and reduce exploratory behaviour in rats. *Psychopharmacology*, **96**, 232–236.

Lu, L., Liu, D. and Ceng, X., 2001. Corticotropin-releasing factor receptor type 1 mediates stress-induced relapse to cocaine-conditioned place preference in rats. *Eur. J. Pharmacol.*, **415**, 203–208.

Lundkvist, J., Chai, Z., Teheranian, R., Hasanvan, H., Bartfai, T., Jenck, F., Widmer, U. and Moreau, J.-L., 1996. A non-peptide corticotrophin releasing factor receptor antagonist attenuates fever and exhibits anxiolytic-like activity. *Eur. J. Pharmacol.*, **309**, 195–200.

Lydiard, R.B., Ballenger, J.C., Laraia, M.T., Fossey, M.D. and Beinfeld, M.C., 1992. CSF cholecystokinin concentrations in patients with panic disorder and in normal comparison subjects. *Am. J. Psychiat.*, **149**, 691–693.

Mac Vicar, B.A., Kerrin, J.P. and Davison, J.S., 1987. Inhibition of synaptic transmission in the dorsal hippocampus by cholecystokinin (CCK) and its antagonism by a CCK analog (CCK 27-33). *Brain Res.*, **406**, 130–135.

Maggi, C.A., 1995. The mammalian tachykinin receptors. *Gen. Pharmacol.*, **26**, 911–944.

Michel, M.C., Beck-Sickinger, A., Cox, H., Doods, H.N., Herzog, H., Larhammar, D., Quirion, R., Schwartz, T. and Westfall, T., 1998. XVI international union of pharmacology recommendation for the nomenclature of neuropeptide Y, peptide YY and pancreatic polypeptide receptors. *Pharmacol. Rev.*, **50**, 143–150.

Möller, C., Wiklund, L., Sommer, W., Thorsell, A. and Heilig, M., 1997. Decreased experimental anxiety and voluntary consumption in rats following central but not basolateral amygdala lesions. *Brain Res.*, **760**, 94–101.

Morgan, C.A., Wang, S., Southwick, S.M., Ramusson, A., Hazlett, G., Hauger, R.L. and Charney, D.S., 2000. Plasma neuropeptide-Y concentration in humans exposed to military survival training. *Biol. Psychiatry*, **47**, 902–909.

Nemeroff, C.B., Widerlov, E., Bissette, G., Walleus, H., Karlsson, I., Eklund, K., Kilts, C.D., Loosen, P.T. and Vale, W., 1984. Elevated concentrations of CSF corticotrophin-releasing factor-like immunoreactivity in depressed patients. *Science*, **226**(4680), 1342–1344.

Nichol, K.A., Morey, A., Couzens, M.H., Shine, J. and Herzog, H., 1999. Conservation of expression of neuropeptide Y5 receptor between human and rat hypothalamus and limbic regions suggests an integral role in central neuroendocrine control. *J. Neurosci.*, **19**, 10 295–10 304.

Nicholls, M.G., 1994. Minisymposium: the natriuretic peptide hormones. Introduction. Editorial and historical review. *J. Intern. Med.*, **235**, 507–514.

Nutt, D., 1998. Substance-P antagonists: a new treatment for depression? *Lancet*, **352**, 1644–1646.

Okuyama, S., Chaki, S., Kawashima, N., Yoshiko, S., Ogawa, S.-I., Nakazato, A., Kumagi, T., Okubo, T. and Tomisawa, K., 1999. Receptor binding, behavioural and electrophysiological profiles of non-peptide corticotrophin-releasing factor subtype 1 receptor antagonist CRA100 and CRF1001. *J. Pharmacol. Exp. Ther.*, **289**, 926–935.

Otsuka, M. and Yoshioka, K., 1993. Neurotransmitter functions of mammalian tachykinins. *Physiol. Rev.*, **73**, 229–308.

Radulovic, J., Ruhmann, A., Liepoid, T. and Speiss, J., 1999. Modulation of learning and anxiety by corticotrophin-releasing factor and stress: differential role of CRF receptors. *J. Neurosci.*, **19**, 5025–5616.

Regoli, D., Boudon, A. and Fauchere, J.L., 1994. Receptors and antagonists for substance P and related peptides. *Pharmacol. Rev.*, **46**, 551–599.

Rupniak, N.M.J., Boyce, S., Williams, A.R., Cook, G., Longmore, J., Seabrook, G.R., Caeser, M., Iversen, S.D. and Hill, R.G., 1993. Antinociceptive activity of NK1 receptor antagonists: non-specific effects of racemic RP67580. *Br. J. Pharmacol.*, **110**, 1607–1613.

Rupniak, N.M.J., Carlson, E., Boyce, S., Webb, J.K. and Hill, R.G., 1996. Enantioselective inhibition of the formalin paw late phase by the NK1 receptor antagonist L-733,060 in gerbils. *Pain*, **67**, 189–195.

Rupniak, N.M.J., Tattersall, F.D., Williams, A.R., Rycroft, W., Carlson, E.J., Cascieri, M.A., Saowski, S., Ber, E., Hale, J.J., Mills, S.G., MacCoss, M., Seward, E., Huscroft, I., Owen, S., Swain, C.J., Hill, R.G. and Hargreaves, R.J., 1997. *In vitro* and *in vivo* predictors of the antiemetic activity of tachykinin NK1 receptor antagonists. *Eur. J. Pharmacol.*, **326**, 201–209.

Sajdyk, T., Vandergriff, M.G. and Gehlert, D.R., 1999. Amygdalar neuropeptide YY1 receptors mediate the anxiolytic-like actions of neuropeptide Y in the social interaction test. *Eur. J. Pharmacol.*, **368**, 143–147.

Saria, A., 1999. The tachykinin NK1 receptor in the brain: pharmacology and putative functions. *Eur. J. Pharmacol.*, **375**, 51–60.

Schulz, D.W., Mansbach, R.S., Sprouse, J., Braselton, J.P., Collins, J., Corman, M., Dunaiskis, A., Farach, S., Schmidt, A.W., Seeger, T., Seymour, P., Tingley III, F.D., Winston, E.N., Chen, Y.L. and Heym, J., 1996. CP-154,526: a potent and selective non-peptide antagonist of corticotrophin-releasing factor receptors. *Proc. Natl. Acad. Sci. USA*, **96**, 10 477–10 482.

Shlik, J., Vasar, E. and Bradwejn, J., 1997. Cholecystokinin and psychiatric disorders: role in aetiology and potential of receptor antagonist in therapy. *CNS Drugs*, **8**, 134–152.

Skelton, K.H., nemeroff, C.B., Knight, D.L. and Owens, M.J., 2000. Chronic administration of the triazolobenzadiazepine alprazolam produces opposite effects on corticotrophin-releasing factor and urocortin neuronal systems. *J. Neurosci.*, **20**(3), 1240–1248.

Smith, G.W., Aubry, J.-M., Dellu, F., Contarino, L.M., Bilezikjian, L.H., Gold, R., Chen, Y., Marchulk, C., Hauser, C.A., Bentley, P.E., Sawchenko, G.F., Koop, W., Vale, K.-F. and Lee, E.H., 1998. Corticotrophin releasing factor receptor 1-deficient mice display decreased anxiety, impaired stress response and aberrant neuroendocrine development. *Neuron*, **20**, 1093–1102.

Stenzel-Poore, M.P., Duncan, J.E., Rittenberg, M.B., Bakke, A.C. and Heinrichs, S.C., 1996. CRF overproduction in transgenic mice: behavioural and immune system modulation. *Ann. NY Acad. Sci.*, **780**, 36–48.

Stout, S.C., Kilts, C.D. and Nemeroff, C.B., 1995. Neuropeptides and stress: preclinical findings and implications for pathophysiology. In: Friedman, M.J., Charney, S. and Deutch, A.Y. (eds), *Neurobiological and Clinical Consequences of Stress: From Normal Adaptation to Post-traumatic Stress Disorder*, pp. 103–123. Lippencott-Raven, Philadelphia.

Stratton, S.C., Beresford, I.J., Harvey, F.J., Turpin, M.P., Hagan, R.M. and Tyers, M.B., 1993. Anxiolytic activity of tachykinin NK2 receptor antagonists in the mouse light-dark box. *Eur. J. Pharmacol.*, **250**, R11–R12.

Ströhle, A., Holsboer, F. and Rupprecht, R., 2000. Increased ACTH concentrations associated with cholecystokinin tetrapeptide-induced panic attacks in patients with panic disorder. *Neuropsychopharmacology*, **22**(3), 251–256.

Ströhle, A., Jahn, H., Montkowskin, A., Liebsch, G., Boll, E., Landgraf, R., Holsboer, F. and Wiedemann, K., 1997. Central and peripheral administration of atriopeptin is anxiolytic in rats. *Neuroendocrinology*, **65**, 210–215.

Ströhle, A., Kellner, M., Holsboer, F. and Wiedemann, K., 2001. Anxiolytic activity of atrial natriuretic in patients with panic disorder. *Am. J. Psychiatry*, **158**, 1514–1516.

Takahashi, L.K., Ho, S.P., Livanov, V., Graciani, N. and Arneic, S.P., 2001. Antagonism of CRF2 receptors produces anxiolytic behaviour in animal models of anxiety. *Brain Res.*, **902**, 135–142.

Teixeira, R.M., Santos, A.R.S., Ribeiro, S.J., Calixto, J.B., Rae, G.A. and De Lima, T.C.M., 1996. Effects of central administration of tachykinin receptor agonists and antagonists on plus-maze behaviour in mice. *Eur. J. Pharmacol.*, **311**, 7–14.

Telegdy, G., Adamik, A. and Glover, 2000. The action of isatin (2,3-dioxoindole) an endogenous indole on brain natriuretic and C-type natriuretic peptide-induced facilitation of memory consolidation in passive-avoidance learning in rats. *Brain Res. Bull.*, **53**, 367–370.

Thorsell, A., Michalkiewicz, M., Dumont, Y., Quirion, R., Cabertto, L., Rimondini, R., Mathé, A.A. and Heiling, M., 2000. Behavioral insensitivity to restraint stress, absent fear suppression of behaviour and impaired spatial learning in transgenic rats with hippocampal neuropeptide Y over expression. *Proc. Natl. Acad. Sci.*, **97**, 12 852–12 857.

Timpli, P., Spangel, R., Sillaber, I., Kresse, A., Reul, J.M.H.M., Stalla, G.K., Blanquet, V., Steckler, T., Holsboer, F. and Wurst, W., 1998. Impaired stress response and reduced anxiety in mice lacking a functional corticotrophin-releasing hormone receptor 1. *Nat. Genet.*, **19**, 162–166.

van Megen, H.J.G.M., Westenberg, H.G.M., Den Boer, J.A., Haigh, J.R.M. and Traub, M., 1994. Pentagastrin induced panic attacks: enhanced sensitivity in panic disorder patients. *Psychopharmacology*, **114**, 1021–1033.

Wahlestedt, C., Pich, E.M., Koob, G.F., Yee, F. and Heilig, M., 1993. Modulation of anxiety and neuropeptide Y-Y1 receptors by antisense oligodeoxynucleotides. *Science*, **259**, 528–531.

Walsh, D.M., Stratton, S.C., Harvey, F.J., Beresford, I.J. and Hagan, R.M., 1995. The anxiolytic-like activity of GR159897, a non peptide NK2 receptor antagonist, in rodent and primate models of anxiety. *Psychopharmacology*, **121**, 186–191.

Weiss, J.M., Stout, J.C., Aaron, M.F., Quan, N., Owens, M.J., Butler, P.D. and Nemeroff, C.B., 1994. Depression and anxiety: role of the locus coeruleus and corticotrophin-releasing factor. *Brain Res. Bull.*, **35**, 561–572.

Wiedemann, K., Jahn, H., Yassouridis, A. and Kellner, M., 2001. Anxiolytic-like effect of atrial natriuretic peptide on cholecystokinin tetrapeptide-induced panic attacks: preliminary findings. *Arch. Gen. Psychiatry*, **58**, 371–377.

Zernig, G., Troger, J. and Saria, A., 1993. Different profiles of the non-peptide substance P (NK1) antagonist CP-96,345 and RP 67580 in Swiss albino mice in the black-and-white box. *Neurosci. Lett.*, **151**, 64–66.

Zukowska-Grojec, Z., Shen, Z., Capraro, P. and Vaz, C., 1991. Cardiovascular, neuropeptide Y and adrenergic responses to stress are sexually differentiated. *Physiol. Behav.*, **49**, 771–777.

XIX-5

Neuroendocrinology of Anxiety Disorders: Post-traumatic Stress Disorder

W.S. de Loos

INTRODUCTION

History of Neuroendocrinology

The General Adaptation Syndrome

Endocrinology has strongly been linked to stress since Hans Selye formulated his concept of the 'general adaptation syndrome' (GAS) in his initial description of 'A syndrome produced by diverse nocuous agents' in *Nature* in 1936 (Selye, 1936a). He connected the initial response under the name 'alarm reaction' to the stage of resistance during continued exposure to the stressor and the subsequent stage of exhaustion ultimately followed by death. Shortly thereafter, he put the word 'stress' on stage as a concept of 'the nonspecific response of the body to any demand made upon it'. He drew the attention to the hypertrophic response of the adrenal glands, especially their cortical layers, and named the hormonal substances derived from them 'corticoids', such as 'cortisone'. Ever since, the glucocorticoids (cortisol/hydrocortisone and, in rodents, corticosterone) have figured as the stress hormones *in optima forma* and taken a role as the biological parameters or 'proof' of the stress response. Selye did not deny the role of the adrenal medulla and its main product adrenaline/epinephrine (EP) but the scientific community became very much focused on cortisol as the hallmark of the stress response.

Interestingly, Selye's attention was primarily drawn by physical causes of stress such as injuries, cold, restraint, hunger and numerous chemical substances (atropine, morphine, formaldehyde, epinephrine) (Selye, 1936b). Already in this and a further publication, he outlined the role of the pituitary gland in exerting the effect on the adrenal (cortical) hypertrophy marking the road to our present-day interest in the hypothalamo-pituitary-adrenocortical (HPA) axis in psychoneuroendocrinology (Selye and Collip, 1936). He also made the link to the immune system in his observations on thymicolymphatic atrophy laying the base for modern psychoneuroimmunology.

The Defence Reaction

Selye's original focus at physical causes of the GAS is of great value as it draws our attention to the unconditional stimuli that provoke it. Twenty-five years earlier, Walter B. Cannon had already described the physical (= unconditional) and psychological (= conditional) stimuli for adrenomedullary activation (Cannon and de la Paz, 1911; Cannon and Hoskins, 1911). He extended his observations to a concept of the emergency response of the individual by changes that are 'directly serviceable in making the organism more efficient in the struggle which fear or rage or pain may involve' (Cannon, 1914). His description of the 'Bodily Changes in Pain, Hunger, Fear and Rage' (Cannon, 1915) has become classical as the immediate response to the perception of threat mediated by epinephrine which is *sensori strictu* as much a hormone as cortisol. He described these changes here as 'The organic preparation for action ... in fight or conflict — either one requiring perhaps the utmost struggle'. This emergency response has later been named the 'defence reaction' (Hess and Brügger, 1943) and has its organizational centre in the amygdala (LeDoux, 1998).

The defence reaction consists of both behavioural and physiological components. The behavioural components are species specific; the physiological ones are more general, such as: pupillodilation; pilo-erection; increase of muscle tone, ventilation, cardiac output, oxygen consumption and muscle blood flow; decrease of blood flow in the skin, intestine and kidneys; bladder and bowel emptying; and many others like neurohumoral, hormonal, immunological and haemostatic changes. Understanding of the ethology and comparative physiology of the defence reaction permits excellent understanding of the psychophysiology of alarm and anxiety in humans, both under normal and pathological conditions.

The other important survival response is the above-described GAS which is characterized by behavioural inhibition when active ways of surviving a challenge have been blocked off. It can be compared to the psychodynamic concept of unsolvable conflict or to Seligman's behavioural model of learned helplessness (Abramson, Seligman and Teasdale, 1978), while Henry described it from a comparative physiological and ethological point of view as conservation-withdrawal expressing subordinate behaviour (Henry, 1992). The corresponding neuroanatomy has important organizing centres in the septum and hippocampus and has every right to be acronymized as the LHPA axis, for limbic-hypothalamo-pituitary-adrenocortical (Sapolsky, Zola-Morgan and Squire, 1991; López, Akil and Watson, 1999), including important physiological outflow through the vagal motor system. The effect of chronic mild stress on the HPA axis is organized in the hippocampus by modulation of hippocampal inhibition on the paraventricular nucleus (PVN) of the hypothalamus (Bratt *et al.*, 2001).

The emergency, or alarm, or defence reaction and the general adaptation, or conservation-withdrawal, or inhibition syndrome have been renamed 'allostasis' (Charles Kahn, see Sterling and Eyer (1988). Allostatic responses are temporary encroachments on homeostasis, a term we owe to Walter B. Cannon.

Looking back on almost a century of stress hormone research (EP and cortisol), we conclude that EP is a hormone that increases energy expenditure acutely and mobilizes quickly available resources (glucose, free fatty acids). It generates a metabolic response that can only last for a rather short time and should be followed by recuperation under better circumstances. Cortisol,

Biological Psychiatry: Edited by H. D'haenen, J.A. den Boer and P. Willner. ISBN 0-471-49198-5

however, is a hormone that becomes useful under prolonged circumstances of adversity and generates a slowly catabolic response of long duration which can be used by the organism to consume its own structure as a resource for energy. It causes slow but general breakdown of the entire organism ultimately leading to death.

Syndromal Versus Matrix Diagnosis

Biological Parameters

Although challenging and even inspiring, the parallels between animal models and human disorders are defective. It remains to be seen, however, whether the clinical diagnosis of human psychiatric disorder is so much superior to ethological observation of animal behaviour or the biological responses referred to in the previous paragraph. Certainly, at group level interesting biological properties of psychiatric syndromes have been discovered, one of them the escape from dexamethasone feedback suppression of the HPA axis in major depressive disorder (MDD), a well-known phenomenon nowadays (see Gutman and Nemeroff in this book; Mitchell, 1998). Still, at the individual level this has not given us a tool to 'prove' whether a patient is suffering from MDD or not. We are far from using biological parameters to support psychiatric clinical diagnosis. Often, confusing findings have been reported, even at a group level (*vide infra*), which makes us doubt, at times, the validity of syndromal diagnosis. Biological parameters seem not to parallel the syndromal level and syndromal diagnoses inadequately predict the success of therapeutic strategies, as one of the founders of biological psychiatry, Herman M. van Praag, has pointed out (van Praag *et al.*, 1987). It is even highly questionable what the relevance is of the syndromal diagnostic constructs we use to work with. They seem to be based on a nineteenth century disease model that has been derived mainly from the paradigm of infectious diseases, a one pathogen — one disease model that is not valid any more in a world where this model of syndromal diagnosis is becoming less effective with the growth of our physiological, biochemical and genetic insights. In many cases we should speak, in fact, of common final pathways or end points with heterogeneous aetiologies or initiators. Concerning common final pathways, we know that different mutations within a single gene will often cause the same genetic defect. Different genetic defects may still lead to similar phenotypical disease expressions. Diseases that have been known for ages under a single name, had to be split into sub-groups with significant differences.

Co-morbidity

Another artifact of modern diagnostic classification is that of co-morbidity suggesting that psychiatric diagnoses can simply be added up like we do with somatic pathology, e.g. juvenile diabetes plus hypothyroidism plus Addison's disease, or hypertension plus osteoarthritis plus colorectal cancer. Not without reason van Praag again — 'rebel with a cause' — writes about 'classificatory inflation', a nosological doctrine hanging around psychiatry's neck as an albatross (van Praag, 2000). It seems more fruitful to follow a system of developmental elements as they have emerged during phylogeny and ontogeny, the natural history of biology, to form the basis of nosological diagnosis (de Loos, 2001). A matrix of relevant elements would form a diagnostic matrix that is less sensitive to unvalidated constructs and taxonomic changes.

A Diagnostic Matrix

- Dimension I: the genetic code, the set of unchangeable biological properties is at the basis of this system. It includes not only the structural floorplan and homeostatic regulatory mechanisms but also the inborn psychophysiological responses initially described by Cannon and Selye (*vide supra*). Such responses cannot be learnt or suppressed voluntarily; they can be enhanced by conditioning.
- Dimension II: acquired automated mechanisms (organizing effects, imprinting, long-term potentiation/depression, pruning and dendrite plasticity, association). Imprinting and learning are processes directly based on the genetic make-up of an individual. Imprinting is the creation of read-only-memories (ROMs), a biological parallel of computer 'firmware', and happens at a developmental stage when the nervous system is receptive for information that fulfils certain specifications. It is a process that occurs under circumstances created by the first dimension.
- Dimension III: the declarative faculty (reflexive consciousness, emotional declaration). From a heuristic point of view it seems logical to separate linguistic development from the second dimension considering the phylogeny of homo sapiens. Reflexive consciousness and the development of emotional expression are representations of the declarative faculty including aspects of relational behaviour, literature, etc.
- Dimension IV: complex language-dependent systems (science, logic, mathematics, philosophy and political systems). They can be seen as the present ultimate development of phylogeny and ontogeny. They constitute what we use to call human 'civilization' including structures based on semantically explicit cognition. Although scientific theory development requires economy in calling in assumptions or abstractions, it seems appropriate and efficacious to categorize this level of development in a separate dimension.

Construction of an individual matrix for every patient may seem tedious at first glance but respects individual variability more than our present-day system of syndromes and co-morbidity. Modern DNA technology is unravelling genetic codes of adaptive (healthy) polymorphisms and maladaptive mutations. Although still costly at present, DNA diagnostics are becoming available at the individual patient's level and may fill in Dimension I at a certain time. Dimension II can already be filled in with traits like hypervigilance, increased startle, increased impulsiveness, dissociation, sympatho-adrenomedullary activation, (L)HPA activation, intrusive memory, etc. For many of these we have knowledge about neural circuits, transmitters and neuromodulators that are involved and drugs that can or cannot interfere.

Changes or disturbances in the regulation of the HPA axis (Dimension II) do not parallel the classificatory division between mood and anxiety disorders (for an overview see Heim and Nemeroff (1999) Table 1). Within the group of anxiety disorders differences are found between panic disorder (PD) and post-traumatic stress disorder (PTSD) (*vide infra*) while somatoform disorders like chronic fatigue syndrome (Demitrack *et al.*, 1991) and fibromyalgia (Griep, Boersma and De Kloet, 1993) resemble PTSD in the down-regulation of HPA axis activity (Heim, Ehlert and Hellhammer, 2000; Altemus *et al.*, 2001). Chronic fatigue syndrome overlaps with major depressive disorder (MDD) but shows opposite HPA axis regulation (Demitrack, 1997). It would thus be more helpful to assess and value HPA axis regulation as a dimensional feature as it seriously confounds syndromal diagnosis.

Dimension II of the matrix is also the domain of interaction between developmental conditions and the influence of environmental factors on adult outcome. What this implies for rodents, especially the responsiveness of the HPA axis, has been reviewed by numerous authors. The HPA axis of developing rats is, in part, regulated by maternal factors like feeding, licking and grooming the pup after a separation, which all seem to act in concert to limit and prevent the so-called stress hormones and more specifically corticosterone from exceeding some optimal level. The pattern of ACTH releasing factors is affected, not only corticotrophin releasing hormone (CRH) gene (hnRNA and mRNA) and AVP gene activation, but also immediate early genes (the transcription factor c-*fos* and the growth factor NGF-1a) in a differentiated way demonstrating a significant plasticity of the system (Levine, 2001). Differences between mothers are fairly stable over subsequent litters and are transmitted to the next generation by environmental as well as genetic factors. Environment can thus alter the genetic trajectory demonstrating the adaptive value of plasticity (Francis *et al.*, 1999). Numerous retrospective studies in humans support these animal studies with consistent results suggesting sensitization of the neuroendocrine stress responses after early life stress in humans. Differences found between childhood versus adulthood stress on the results in adulthood underscore the interaction with the developmental stage (Heim and Nemeroff, 2001).

General Principles of Endocrine Regulatory Systems

Classical and Clinical Endocrinology

Base line values of hormonal secretions have limited value in endocrinology as they may be confounded by many factors such as inter-individual variability of normal values while intra-individual variability is much smaller in general. Base line values can be more dependent on unrecognized environmental or intra-individual circumstances than is generally acknowledged. This is known, for instance, for 'normal' morning cortisol values taken from outpatients in hospital surroundings and considerable variation has been recorded in studies with 'base line' 24-hour urine cortisol in patients with PTSD (*vide infra*).

Other problems are met with the difference in analogous (continuous) versus digital (pulse frequency) regulation of end-organ function. Releasing hormones from the hypothalamus and pituitary hormones generally are of the latter type, steroid hormones have properties of both while thyroid hormone may be the most continuous in level. An important role is being played by hormone binding proteins. They strongly dampen the oscillations in total hormone concentrations found but this can be unmasked by measuring free hormone levels in plasma or saliva. Only the free hormone can act biologically.

Understanding of hormone function and assessment of normality of function is often better achieved by stimulation or blocking (feedback sensitivity) tests. The difficulty with the tests generally applied is, however, that at least in clinical endocrinology they are of a pharmacological kind using doses far exceeding physiological levels. This may have value in detecting organ failure in autoimmune or post-operative endocrine disease, or of endocrine tumors but is of very limited value in detecting changes in set point of a regulatory system, or even in so-called subclinical thyroid disease. Modifications have been found by applying 1 in stead of 250 μg of i.v. $ACTH_{1-24}$ for adrenal stimulation and 0.5 or 0.25 instead of 1.0 mg of dexamethasone for the 'overnight' suppression test.

Many problems arise from the existence of pre- and pre-prohormones and from split products that may be biologically active or inactive. Examples are pro-opio-melano-corticotropin (POMC), the endorphins and enkephalins and, the endocrinologist's nightmare, parathyroid hormone. Laboratory assays may not find the difference and local transformation may mask the 'visibility' of the substance, e.g. of tri-iodothyronine (T_3) in brain tissue where it is being transformed from its biologically almost inactive precursor L-thyroxine (T_4). Also, the sensitivity of assays may be a serious problem in the range of normal function as it has been with thyroid stimulation hormone or thyrotropin (TSH) until the third generation assay became available. The transformation of pro-hormones may be regulated at multiple levels and differently in different tissues as is the case with thyroid hormone of which only 20% is readily produced in its active form T_3 in the thyroid gland itself. Deiodination from T_4 to T_3 occurs intracellularly in many tissues while especially the liver exports T_3 to the general circulation. Half-life of these substances varies considerably, in the case of T_4 and T_3 from 7 days to a few hours only.

The classical hormones are defined by their signal function transported through the general circulation. The releasing hormones and the intra-cerebral and intra-medullary peptides can hardly be found in the peripheral circulation and even in the cerebrospinal fluid the levels found must be considered as spillover from tissue to the gutter of the brain which helps to clear this organ from products that have not been degraded locally or removed by presynaptic re-uptake. Lastly, psychoneuroimmunological research has shown that peptide hormones like CRH and the cytokines are being secreted by lymphocytes at the femtomolar level (10^{-15} mol l^{-1}) where they have a paracrine function and still can influence the brain that way by uptake through the blood–brain barrier at specific sites and connection to specific neuronal circuits (Breder, Dinarello and Saper, 1988).

Neuroendocrinology

Still, when we have taken into account all these technical points, we must realize that by studying a few substances we are only looking to a few links in a long chain of events. In classical ('clinical') endocrinology, hormone systems are described as separate domains. In neuroendocrinology the limitations of this way of thinking become obvious: there are important connections with other neurochemical and neurophysiological systems. The classical hormone concept is also too limited. CRH, for instance, has endocrine, autonomic, behavioural and immune effects. It acts as a classical hormone in the hypothalamo-pituitary portal system, as a neuromodulator in widespread areas of the central nervous system (CNS) confirming David de Wied's neuropeptide concept (de Wied and Jolles, 1982) and paracrine in the immune system.

POST-TRAUMATIC STRESS DISORDER

Neuroendocrinology, Psychophysiology and Post-Traumatic Symptoms

Early Biological Predictors

Peri-traumatic dissociation has been found to be a good predictor of the development of PTSD, better and stronger than depression, anxiety and intrusive symptoms (Shalev *et al.*, 1996). Heart rate in the peri-traumatic phase, i.e. in the emergency room after traffic accidents etc., was also positively correlated to the development of PTSD (Shalev *et al.*, 1998a). In an extension of the study, again peri-traumatic dissociation and heart rate predicted the development of PTSD and were associated with more intrusive symptoms and exaggerated startle (Shalev *et al.*, 1998b). Heart rate is controlled by two extracardial mechanisms. EP increases it and the vagal nerve lowers it. The sympathetic innervation only influences electrical conductance (induction of arrhythmia's), stroke volume and coronary artery blood flow. No acute studies, in the emergency room, have been done on EP production, but assessment after one and six months after an accident has shown elevated EP production rates in men with PTSD symptoms. Catecholamine rates were also associated with intrusive thoughts at one month and avoidance at six months. In this study urinary cortisol production rates were elevated in men at one month and normal at six months. Both in men and women, greater emotional numbing predicted a lower cortisol production rate at six months (Hawk *et al.*, 2000). This is a finding that seems to be confirmed by Mason *et al.* (2001) who linked lower cortisol levels with disengagement defence mechanisms (numbing) in combat veterans with PTSD.

A negative correlation between serum cortisol immediately after traumatization and the development of PTSD was found in two different settings, namely sexual assault and motor vehicle accidents (Resnick *et al.*, 1995; McFarlane, Atchison and Yehuda, 1997). Significantly lowered urinary cortisol over 15 hours at acute assessment in the emergency room predicted PTSD at one month and especially the occurrence of intrusive and avoidant thoughts (Delahanty, Raimonde and Spoonster, 2000). These psychophysiological factors raise the issue of pre-traumatic vulnerability in the development of PTSD (Yehuda *et al.*, 1998).

Acute stress disorder (ASD) is characterized by dissociation and strongly predicts the development of PTSD (Brewin *et al.*, 1999; Koren, Arnon and Klein, 1999). No specific neuroendocrine research focused on ASD *per se* has been done. Studies on initial cortisol responses predicting development of PTSD may be seen as relevant to ASD as such. When combining the elements of dissociation and stress-induced analgesia with the known effects of opioids, it is suggestive to infer a central opioid effect as a core mechanism in the initiation of this disorder (*vide infra*).

Psychophysiological Testing: Heart Rate and Epinephrine

Reference has been made to increased EP production at early stages after traumatic accidents. Analysis of heart rate variability by means of power spectrum analysis in PTSD patients many years after traumatization again showed higher heart rates and lower heart rate variability at rest. This was interpreted as an indication for lower cardiac parasympathetic (vagal) tone and elevated sympathetic activity (Cohen *et al.*, 1997).

In laboratory settings cardiovascular and other psychophysiological responses, mainly galvanic skin response (GSR) and electromyography (EMG), to stimuli of various kind have been studied extensively. Many studies have demonstrated strong specific responses of blood pressure and especially heart rate to startling unspecific noises and to individually significant sensory input in subjects with PTSD, combat veterans from various war theatres (Pallmeyer, Blanchard and Kolb, 1986; Pitman, Orr and Steketee, 1989; Blanchard *et al.*, 1990, 1991a), and in other populations of trauma survivors (Shalev *et al.*, 1993, 1997). Also in Rorschach testing the projection of traumatic content elicited significant increases in skin conductance (sympathetic activation) and heart rate (Goldfinger, Amdur and Liberzon, 1998).

Yohimbine, an α_2-adrenergic receptor antagonist that activates noradrenergic neurons, e.g. in the locus coeruleus, hippocampus and amygdala, increased systolic blood pressure significantly more in PTSD subjects than in healthy controls, especially when they had a flashback and/or a panic reaction after administration of this drug. The same occurred with heart rate which showed no significant response in the controls (Southwick *et al.*, 1993). None of these studies discriminates between sympathetic mediated decrease of vagal tone versus EP mediated cardioacceleration. A role of the latter can only be inferred by the above-mentioned study by Hawk *et al.* (2000). But all these point to a strongly increased sympatho-adrenomedullary activation in PTSD.

Vasopressin and Oxytocin

Vasopressin and oxytocin are two hormones of the central nervous system (neuropeptides) that are of special importance in memory processing. Behavioural and cardiovascular conditioning in animals has shown that vasopressin increases the retention of both appetitive and aversive memory while oxytocin in low doses has the opposite effect (Bohus, Kovacs and De Wied, 1978; Wan *et al.*, 1992). Similar results have been demonstrated in humans with PTSD with respect to psychophysiological parameters in relation to personal traumatic imagery, most specifically exerted by vasopressin on EMG (Pitman, Orr and Lasko, 1993).

Opioids

'Addiction' to the trauma, a strong need to return to memories, memorials and other symbols of the trauma, is a clinical phenomenon in many PTSD patients that was poorly understood until the role of the opioid peptides was discovered. It may also be related to novelty/sensation seeking or risk taking behaviour (Van der Kolk *et al.*, 1985). Pain-induced analgesia was known as an experimental model in pharmacology for a considerable time and has been extended, later, to stress-induced analgesia. In animal experiments it has been connected to learned helplessness (*vide supra*) and shown to be dependent on μ-opioid mechanisms at the time of initial uncontrollable footshock (Hemingway and Reigle, 1987). It can be blocked with the classical morfine antagonist naloxone. These mechanisms have been associated with post-traumatic symptoms, such as numbing (Van der Kolk and Saporta, 1991; Glover, 1992). There are indications that flashbacks and other dissociative phenomena in PTSD patients and also emotional numbing are opioid mediated phenomena that can be blocked by naloxone (Van der Kolk *et al.*, 1989; Pitman *et al.*, 1990). Improvement of many PTSD symptoms has been reported after the administration of nalmefene (Glover, 1993), a relative pure opioid μ-receptor antagonist more potent than naloxone (Reisine and Pasternak, 1996). It is possible although speculative at this moment that clinical phenomena like dissociation, auto-mutilation and conditioned or self-induced analgesia like the fakir syndrome are mental states in which the opioids play an important role. A puzzling finding is that plasma levels of β-endorphin, both in the morning and the evening, were found in one study to be lower than in controls (Hoffman *et al.*, 1989). In this same study morning cortisol levels in PTSD subjects were higher than in controls which is at variance with most later findings (see below). The above reported opioid responses to traumatic flashbacks were not accompanied in that study by detectable changes of opioids in the general circulation (B.A. van der Kolk, personal communication). The effects are confined to the CNS compartment exclusively as was shown in a study in which subarachnoid cerebrospinal fluid (CSF) sampling was compared to peripheral plasma. It was shown that PTSD patients have significantly increased CSF levels of β-endorphin and that higher levels corresponded with less intrusive and avoidance symptoms (Baker *et al.*, 1999). Also, the connection to the hypothalamic-pituitary-adrenal axis is to be considered in the light of its inhibition by opioids at the hypothalamic level (Hockings *et al.*, 1994).

The HPA Axis

Interaction with the Sympatho-Adrenal System

Many studies have addressed the complex interplay between the sympatho-adrenomedullary system and the hypothalamic-pituitary-adrenocortical (HPA) axis. In most studies PTSD is characterized by increased norepinephrine (NE) spillover (Kosten *et al.*, 1987; Blanchard *et al.*, 1991b) on one hand but decreased total daily cortisol production (Mason *et al.*, 1986; Yehuda *et al.*, 1990a, 1995b) and decreased circulating cortisol levels on the other (Yehuda *et al.*, 1996a; Boscarino, 1996; Kanter *et al.*, 2001). Urinary cortisol was also found to be lower in adult offspring from Holocaust survivors with PTSD while offspring with parental PTSD and own lifetime PTSD had the lowest levels (Yehuda *et al.*, 2000).

Daily free cortisol excretion was found to be normal at group level but to correlate inversely with intrusive PTSD symptoms in one study (Baker *et al.*, 1999) while it was increased similarly to patients with major depression and without any correlation to symptoms in another (Maes *et al.*, 1998). One difference between the last study and the previous ones is that it was done on civilians with a majority of females without control for menstrual cycle phase while most of the previous studies were done on male combat veterans. The study by Hawk *et al.* (2000) has the same limitation mainly due to the set-up, namely emergency room assessment of accident victims. A study that did control for menstrual cycle phase showed no effect of phase on total urinary-free cortisol output, and no effect of PTSD although there was a trend towards an increased cortisol output in PTSD (Rasmusson *et al.*, 2001). It was also argued that single traumatic events might cause an increased HPA axis response while repetitive and prolonged trauma might do the opposite. Some support for this view can be found in other research but this problem has not been solved satisfactorily.

In concordance to the release rates reported above, α_2-adrenergic receptors are down-regulated (Perry, Giller and Southwick, 1987; Yehuda *et al.*, 1990b) and glucocorticoid receptors (GRs) are up-regulated (Yehuda *et al.*, 1991, 1995c). Norepinephrine release and the up-regulation of GRs correlate with the severity of PTSD symptomatology (Kellner, Baker and Yehuda, 1997). A significant negative correlation between 24-hour urinary-free cortisol and PTSD symptoms reported in another study confirmed this (Baker *et al.*, 1999).

Feedback Systems

In PTSD the efficacy of glucocorticoid feedback is increased as demonstrated by a significantly enhanced dexamethasone suppression in comparison to normals (Kudler *et al.*, 1987; Yehuda *et al.*, 1993; Stein *et al.*, 1997b; Heim *et al.*, 1998) and it is opposite to depression which is known for its dexamethasone non-suppression. One would even conclude that PTSD and biological depression as defined in this neuroendocrine way exclude one another. Yet, many studies describe co-morbidity of PTSD and major depressive disorder (MDD) (Shalev *et al.*, 1998b), not merely dysthymia. It should be kept in mind that a biological definition of depression is not by itself concordant with a psychological one. Individuals with PTSD and co-morbid depression are still better than normal suppressors, but less than having PTSD alone (Yehuda *et al.*, 1993). The enhanced negative feedback of dexamethasone is not reflected by lower levels of circulating adrenocorticotropic hormone (ACTH) but the pituitary capacity to release ACTH is markedly enhanced which excludes pituitary insufficiency and confirms the increased feedback sensitivity (Yehuda *et al.*, 1996b).

The high levels of NE in PTSD are interpreted as to reflect high sympathetic activity which corresponds with many findings on cardiovascular stimulation and galvanic skin response (GSR) reactivity. A positive correlation between intrusive PTSD symptoms and urinary excretion of the catecholamines dopamine and EP points in the same direction (Yehuda *et al.*, 1992). Thus, PTSD with or without accompanying symptoms of depression seems to be characterized, on one hand, by sympatho-adrenal arousal which is reflected by increased cardiovascular responsiveness and sweat gland activation as signs of the defence reaction, the paradigm of active survival strategy; on the other hand, it is characterized by a turn-down of the conservation-withdrawal response and its catabolic survival hormone cortisol that induces the organism to consume its intrinsic resources while waiting for a better time.

CRH, the 'Stress Superhormone'

CRH Testing

The response of ACTH to CRH has been found to be blunted in male PTSD patients as in depression and to result in slightly but not significantly lower cortisol responses (Smith *et al.*, 1989) while in panic disorder (PD) enhanced and blunted responses have been reported (Heim and Nemeroff, 1999). In PTSD this cannot be understood as a feedback effect of functional hypercortisolism, as in the case of depression (Gold, Goodwin and Chrousos, 1988). In premenopausal women ACTH response to CRH was increased and slightly prolonged with an increased and prolonged cortisol response. Cortisol response to $ACTH_{1-24}$ was tested in the follicular phase (high progesterone) and also showed an increased response. The cortisol responses correlated to each other and to 24-hour urinary cortisol excretion (Rasmusson *et al.*, 2001). It demonstrates once more the importance of accounting for sex and, as we will see, age.

Children: CRH Testing and Urine Sampling

The neuroendocrine pattern in children has not been investigated as intensively as in adults. In one study CRH testing was performed in children of 7–15 years old who were living in a stable and safe environment but who had been sexually abused 1–12 years earlier. Some of them had concurrent dysthymia and suicidal ideation and had attempted suicide but none of them was reported to have PTSD. They showed smaller than normal ACTH responses but nonetheless normal cortisol responses to this (De Bellis *et al.*, 1994), which resembles the result found in male adults.

A very different finding is the increased ACTH response to CRH in abused children who experienced ongoing chronic adversity and were rated as depressed. They differed from abused depressive children living in a stable environment, depressive non-abused controls and healthy children who all showed the same ACTH response. The increased ACTH response in the first group was not followed by an increased cortisol response which thereby was the same in all four groups (Kaufman *et al.*, 1997).

A group of children of the same age (8–13) with PTSD was compared to normal controls and children with overanxious disorder. Childhood PTSD was associated with greater co-morbid psychopathology including depressive and dissociative symptoms, lower global assessment of functioning and increased suicidal ideation and suicide attempts. The children in this group excreted significantly greater amounts of urinary dopamine and norepinephrine per day than in both comparison groups. Their free cortisol excretion was equal to that of the overanxious group but exceeded the controls. Catecholamine and cortisol excretion was correlated to the duration of traumatization and to PTSD symptoms (De Bellis *et al.*, 1999).

It is unclear what the discrepancies between these studies and the results found in adults imply. One of the possibilities is that the psychobiological development stage is a critical factor. Also in a broader sense, age may be a factor influencing the HPA axis response to challenge (Seeman and Robbins, 1994). Repetition or perseverance of traumatization is likely to influence the neurohumoral response to it as has been observed in rape victims (Resnick *et al.*, 1995). Other possibilities accounting for the discrepancies are that the studies were done on non-patients and patients with different diagnoses (diagnosing PTSD in young children poses its own difficulties), sample sizes, time of the day and baseline values.

Systems Integration

No convincing correlations have been found between HPA axis activity in the morning, when it is as high in PTSD patients as in controls, and circulating catecholamines or psychophysiologic parameters like GSR (which reflects sympathetic activity), heart rate or frontalis EMG (Liberzon *et al.*, 1999). The conclusion was drawn, then, that no integrated, multisystem stress response occurred in PTSD and this conclusion is supported by other findings when the HPA axis response was studied in connection with CNS noradrenergic activity as represented by 3-methoxy-4-hydroxyphenylglycol (MHPG or MOPEG) spillover (Goenjian *et al.*, 1996; Yehuda *et al.*, 1998) which can be considered a metabolic parameter of central NE turnover reflecting spillover from the CSF compartment into the systemic circulation (Webster, 1989). This may seem, but is not necessarily, at variance with the above-described findings on the HPA axis and catecholamine activity. It means that within an individual these systems are not being coupled per single event. This conclusion is in concordance with the insight that the sympatho-adrenal response system and the HPA axis are not connected to each other through the activation of CRH, as this neurohormone or neuromodulator acts at different locations in the CNS independently, in different circuits and functions (Schulkin, Gold and McEwen, 1998). CRH gene expression in the central nucleus of the amygdala and the bed nucleus of the stria terminalis (BNST) is dissociated from that of the paraventricular nucleus of the hypothalamus which is the classical top of the HPA axis organization. Direct application of CRH by infusion into the third ventricle induces multiple physiological stress responses like increase of plasma epinephrine, norepinephrine, glucose and glucagon, of mean arterial blood pressure and heart rate, and inhibition of gastric acid production, all by autonomic nervous system activation (Lenz *et al.*, 1987). The gastric inhibition could, in part, be inhibited by naloxone or a vasopressin antagonist. This implies involvement of an opioid neuropeptide as a neuromodulator, e.g. a pro-opiomelanocortin (POMC)-derived endorphin (De Wied, 1999). The possibility of a relation with dissociation and flashback-related analgesia is intriguing within this context (Pitman *et al.*, 1990). The role of vasopressin is interesting from the viewpoint of its role in the consolidation of memory (Bohus, Korac and De Wied, 1978; Chepkova *et al.*, 1995), including the psychophysiologic concomitants of emotional memory (Bohus *et al.*, 1983; Pitman, Orr and Lasko, 1993) and its role in the potentiation of CRH-induced ACTH release (Scott, Medbak and Dinan, 1999).

The Role of CRH

The question of the specificity of CRH activity in the CNS is of special importance in the case of PTSD as higher levels of this neurohormone have been found in the cerebrospinal fluid of patients compared to controls, which may seem paradoxical at first sight given the increased feedback sensitivity of the system (Bremner *et al.*, 1997b; Baker *et al.*, 1999). CRH in the CSF is mainly of extrahypothalamic origin, not related to HPA axis activity (Garrick *et al.*, 1987). Interestingly, this was accompanied in patients, but not in controls, by positively correlated CSF levels of somatostatin which often acts as an inhibitory hormone or neuromodulator both in the CNS and peripherally, but its role in these particular circumstances remained unclear. It is also unclear, at this point, what actually causes the increased feedback sensitivity within the HPA axis and whether stimulation of this axis at the level of CRH production by the paraventricular nucleus (PVN) of the hypothalamus is decreased. As mentioned above, the elevated CRH levels in the cerebrospinal fluid are not likely to be generated by the PVN but to be due to spillover from the central amygdala, the bed nucleus of the stria terminalis and the locus coeruleus. The latter three nuclei have important roles in organizing or mediating vigilance, arousal and anxiety reactions and they activate both the central norepinephric system and the sympathetic nervous system (Lenz *et al.*, 1987). Central norepinephric system activation has not systematically been demonstrated (Yehuda *et al.*, 1998). However, frequently repeated activation of the sympathetic nervous system is a general feature of chronic PTSD. Similarly to PTSD symptoms, of panic and flashbacks, yohimbine challenge has indeed produced increases in systolic blood pressure and heart rate, but also MHPG spillover as a putative parameter of central norepinephrine activation (Southwick *et al.*, 1993).

Hippocampal Glucocorticoid Receptors

One of the options for increased HPA feedback sensitivity is increased GR function in the hippocampus which is an important centre for control over the HPA axis function (Meaney *et al.*, 1989). The hippocampus with its dense population of GRs is now broadly recognized as the top of the system by exerting inhibitory control over hypothalamic CRH production (Jacobson and Sapolsky, 1991). GRs may have been up-regulated conforming to a theory derived from the model of neonatal handling in rats in which attenuation of stress responses in adulthood has been observed (Levine, 1957; Denenberg, 1964). This model has been differentiated by more recent studies showing that individual differences in caring behaviour by the mother animal after separation from the litter are responsible for differential effects of such handling. The better the caring attention of the mother after replacement of the pup into the litter, the higher the GR density in the hippocampus and the more efficacious the feedback of circulating glucocorticoid hormone (Liu *et al.*, 1997; Sapolsky, 1997). This process is thought to have a protective effect on the hippocampus against later damage by high glucocorticoid responses under environmental stress or allostasis. The hippocampal atrophy found in PTSD, like in depression and Cushing's disease (Sapolsky, 1996), is not compatible with such protection if, indeed, the damage is due to high glucocorticoid responses under traumatic circumstances.

Hippocampal GRs may respond differently to cortisol than to dexamethasone. This has been shown in an intravenous cortisol inhibition study in PTSD patients in whom adrenal cortisol synthesis was partly blocked with metyrapone. Its precursor, 11-deoxycortisol, can be measured as a parameter of ACTH stimulation of the adrenal cortex. No significant difference in ACTH response to cortisol was found in the PTSD subjects who had lower baseline cortisol and 11-deoxycortisol conforming to the expected HPA axis down-regulation. The PTSD subjects showed no increased feedback sensitivity to cortisol, contrary to expectations from the dexamethasone studies (Kanter *et al.*, 2001). This difference could be based on the lack of effect of dexamethasone on the hippocampus and the PVN as it does not penetrate into the CNS. It implies that the enhanced feedback sensitivity is not present at the level of hippocampal or PVN GR. Other mechanisms must be responsible for the HPA axis down-regulation.

Atrophy of the Hippocampus

A smaller volume of the hippocampus found in several PTSD studies (Bremner *et al.*, 1995, 1997a, 1997b; Stein *et al.*, 1997a), which is enigmatic in the light of the atrophy found in MDD and Cushing's disease with their increased levels of cortisol (Sapolsky, 2000), is the opposite of what is thought to be happening in PTSD. The finding has been confirmed with more sensitive neurochemical methods independent of gross neuroanatomical morphology (Schuff *et al.*, 2001). There is not much doubt about the potential harm of glucocorticoids for the hippocampus, especially the granulosa cells and the dendritic outgrowths and sprouting of the pyramidal cells (McEwen, Gould and Sakai, 1992; Gould and Tanapat, 1999). It has been postulated that the impact of the initial adversive experience may trigger damaging levels of glucocorticoid release thus causing the observed atrophy in PTSD (Bremner, 1999). Other causes for neuronal damage are excitatory amino acid neurotransmitters, especially glutamate, via its N-methyl-D-aspartate (NMDA) receptor and possibly also its kanainate-type feedforward autoreceptor, and serotonin which may also potentiate the NMDA receptor (McEwen and Magariños, 1997; Gould and Tanapat, 1999). Neuroprotection by GABA-ergic inhibition or by neurotrophins (NT) such as brain-derived neurotrophic factor (BDNF) and NT-3 may decrease under certain stressful circumstances.

A postulated consequence of hippocampal atrophy with respect to the striking down-tuning of the HPA axis is the putative disinhibition of CRH release from the PVN which, then, should result in CRH receptor down-regulation in the pituitary and thereby cause a decrease of ACTH stimulation. From the viewpoint of classical endocrinology, however, it seems improbable that this would result in an absolute decrease of ACTH release from the pituitary, instead of an attenuated increase, and hence produce a decrease of cortisol release from the adrenal and, lastly, an enhanced glucocorticoid feedback effect. Continuous hormonal overstimulation at a pharmacological level produces receptor down-regulation and a sharp and almost complete decline of end-organ activity. This is applied in the treatment of prostatic cancer by the use of a long-acting gonadotropin-releasing hormone agonist that down-regulates testosterone production to almost zero, but in physiological circumstances it is not known to occur and the neuroendocrinology of major depression with its increased activity of the HPA axis does not confirm this either. Moreover, experiments in primates examining the effects of lesions of the hippocampus and other related structures produced chronic glucocorticoid hypersecretion lasting 6 to 15 months (Sapolsky, Zola-Morgan and Squire, 1991).

Vasopressin, Somatostatin and the HPA Axis

Thus, there must be other reasons for the opposite characteristics of PTSD and MDD with respect to the HPA axis. Vasopressin is one candidate for discriminating between PTSD and MDD although this may be part of a very complex pattern of interaction. Vasopressin potentiates the release of ACTH (Antoni, 1993; Aguilera, 1998) and it has been shown to co-occur with CRH in the median eminence in a way modulated by neonatal handling and stress (Bhatnagar and Meaney, 1995). It also has an important role in the consolidation of memory (De Wied, 1999) and could play a role in the conditioned physiologic responses found in PTSD (Pitman, Orr and Lasko, 1993). Arginine vasopressin (AVP) is secreted into the median eminence where it enters the portal blood circulation that brings it to the pituitary. Experiments in rats have shown that this is controlled indepently from CRH by axonal transport through AVP-containing versus AVP-deficient CRH neurons, and that under conditions of chronic or repeated stress plastic changes in hypothalamic CRH neurons evolve resulting in increased AVP stores and co-localization in CRH nerve terminals (De Goeij *et al.*, 1991). Also under conditions of chronic or intermittent stressful stimulation, a shift in hypothalamic signals for ACTH release in favour of AVP may ensue as it has been found in rats (De Goeij, Binnekade and Tilders, 1992). Experimental analysis in rats at the level of CRH and AVP responses in the PVN measured by primary transcript (heteronuclear) RNA and messenger RNA has confirmed that there is a desensitization of CRH, but not AVP transcription responses to repeated restraint stress. It has also been demonstrated that animals that adapted to a chronic homotypic stress show a greater response of CRH and AVP gene transcription in the parvocellular PVN after a novel, heterotypic stress. The hypothalamus clearly has the flexibility to adapt to homotypic stress while at the same time maintaining its ability to respond to novel stressors (Ma, Lightman and Aguilera, 1999). These experiments show that, with regard to the responses of the HPA axis, vasopressin is a mediator for the discrimination between chronic (homotypic) and acute (heterotypic) stressors, which can to some extent be controlled independently from CRH. In human depression not only an increase in CRH expressing neurones in the PVN was found, but also an increased co-expression of AVP and of AVP *per se* (Hoogendijk *et al.*, 2000). If PTSD is indeed the mirror image of depression it seems to be, the feedback of cortisol on the hypothalamus should be enhanced through parallel inhibition by another central mechanism.

CSF levels of the inhibitory neuropeptide somatostatin have been found to be elevated and to be correlated with the elevated CRH levels in PTSD patients but not in controls (Bremner *et al.*, 1997b). Somatostatin is known to inhibit the release of both CRH and ACTH (Richardson and Schonbrunn, 1981; Heisler *et al.*, 1982; Brown, Rivier and Vale, 1984). This points to the possibility that somatostatin is a pivotal link in the down-regulation of the LHPA axis.

The question that remains unanswered is what the advantage for survival of these lowered cortisol responses could be. The answer may be given by the fact that CRH gene expression in the brain is differentially stimulated by glucocorticoids. In the parvocellular region of the PVN, CRH gene expression is inhibited but in the central nucleus of the amygdala and in the lateral bed nucleus of the stria terminalis it is elevated. The elevation of CRH gene expression in these two nuclei may underlie a number of fear/anxiety or pathological states (Schulkin, Gold and McEwen, 1998). This is clearly applicable to PTSD, as we have seen, and it is almost too attractive as an explanation to presume that the organism has found a way to contain this limbic CRH fly-wheel by counter-regulation in order to protect the amygdala from unlimited positive feedback.

Glucocorticoid Receptor Gene Polymorphism

A possibility that has not been considered by researchers in the field of the psychobiology of PTSD until now, is the existence of a receptor polymorphism accounting for lower than expected circulating levels of cortisol and increased dexamethasone feedback sensitivity. In an epidemiological field study of an elderly population a close relationship was found between basal cortisol levels and the feedback sensitivity of the HPA axis to a low dose of dexamethasone, lower cortisol corresponding with higher feedback effect which looks the same, so far, as in PTSD. This suggested a genetic influence on the set point of the HPA axis. Over a two-and-a-half year follow-up period, individual characteristics remained fairly constant denying an effect of ageing on HPA activity or feedback sensitivity (Huizenga *et al.*, 1998a). Among 216 elderly people 13 heterozygotes for the N363S GR gene polymorphism (codon 363) were identified as showing increased cortisol suppression to 0.25 mg dexamethasone but no differences in GR number or ligand binding affinity on peripheral mononuclear leucocytes (Huizenga *et al.*, 1998b). In PTSD patients increased receptor numbers on lymphocytes have been found and a correlation with specific symptomatology which suggests that this is indeed a disease-specific phenomenon (Yehuda *et al.*, 1991). Nevertheless, this finding calls for control of receptor polymorphism in studies on the HPA axis of PTSD patients.

Overall View of HPA Axis Regulatory Abnormalities in PTSD

- The enhanced sensitivity of HPA feedback at the pituitary level and a down-regulation of the set point seem to be consistent.
- The anxiety-related CRH system which is intimately connected to central noradrenergic neurotransmission, is activated and is probably driven by the amygdala.
- The limbic-HPA down-regulation may be mediated by somatostatin and may serve as a counter-regulation to protect the amygdala from too much CRH gene expression by cortisol stimulation.

The Hypothalamo-Pituitary-Thyroid Axis

Much less work has been done on thyroid function in PTSD compared to the HPA axis. The first publication that is relevant to cite in this work is from John W. Mason's group, which has accumulated the work on this topic so far (Mason *et al.*, 1994, 1995). Mason and his collaborators have substantiated their initial findings in several subsequent studies of which the highlights are that PTSD is accompanied by an increased level of free T_3 which is the biologically active form of thyroid hormone (*vide supra*). It was also correlated with hyperarousal (Wang *et al.*, 1995) and with novelty/sensation seeking and this finding coincided with positive correlations with urinary total NE and NE/cortisol ratio while it correlated negatively with urinary total cortisol (Wang *et al.*, 1997). It was not restricted to the population of American Vietnam veterans but was also found in Israeli veterans (Mason *et al.*, 1996) and older Second World War veterans who had suffered from PTSD over decades (Wang and Mason, 1999). The latter finding was accompanied by slightly, although not statistically significant, higher levels of TSH. The long duration of the psychiatric disorder made it unlikely that it was men with this pattern of thyroid axis hormones that were especially vulnerable to PTSD. Probably these changes are the result of the disorder, or part of the process (Prange, 1999).

In conjunction with the above discussion on CRH and hippocampal function in PTSD it is relevant to note that thyroid hormone causes long-lasting increases in hippocampal GR numbers through intermediate serotonergic projections (Sapolsky, 1997). On the other hand, there is an intricate relationship of thyroid function with noradrenergic neurotransmission which thus seems to support the arousal response and confirms the catecholamine findings by Mason's group. It is suggested that the excess of free T_3 is produced in the thyroid gland itself by direct sympathetic nervous control (Prange, 1999) but an increase of de-iodination by any of the multiple mechanisms that control it, such as transmembrane transport and tissue-specific de-iodinase, cannot be excluded. Free T_3 production has been reported to follow rapidly on the TSH surge after thyrotropin-releasing hormone administration before T_4 responds, which makes it indeed functional as an emergency response hormone.

GENERAL CONCLUSION

PTSD is one of the most extensively studied of the anxiety disorders concerning their psychoneuroendocrine properties. It consists of response patterns that are pathological in the sense that they continue and even may manifest themselves long after the initial stimulus has occurred. They show all features of the emergency response and these are detectable at all levels of neurobehavioural and metabolic regulation. The response patterns have become fixed like fossil imprints in stone although they may not be continuous but many of them phasic in nature. The marker hormones do not always act as we would have expected and this forces us to differentiate our understanding of these substances and their dynamics. The study of PTSD has enriched our knowledge substantially in this respect. It is highly probable that this will also lead to therapeutic innovations of which the CRH antagonists are among the most promising given the central role this neuromodulator plays in the congealed emergency response of post-traumatic stress disorder.

REFERENCES

Abramson, L.Y., Seligman, M.E.P. and Teasdale, J.D., 1978. Learned helplessness in humans: critique and reformulation. *Journal of Abnormal Psychology*, **87**, 49–74.

Aguilera, G., 1998. Corticotropin releasing hormone, receptor regulation and the stress response. *Trends in Endocrinology and Metabolism*, **9**, 329–336.

Altemus, M., Dale, J.K., Michelson, D., Demitrack, M.A., Gold, P.W. and Straus, S.E., 2001. Abnormalities in response to vasopressin in chronic fatigue syndrome. *Psychoneuroendocrinology*, **26**, 175–188.

Antoni, F.A., 1993. Vasopressinergic control of pituitary adrenocorticotropin secretion comes of age. *Frontiers in Neuroendocrinology*, **14**, 76–122.

Baker, D.G., West, S.A., Nicholson, W.E., Ekhator, N.N., Kasckow, J.W., Hill, K.K., Bruce, A.B., Orth, D.N. and Geracioti, T.D., 1999. Serial CSF corticotropin-releasing hormone levels and adrenocortical activity in combat veterans with posttraumatic stress disorder. *American Journal of Psychiatry*, **156**, 585–588.

Bhatnagar, S. and Meaney, M.J., 1995. Hypothalamic-pituitary-adrenal function in chronic intermittently cold-stressed neonatally handled and non handled rats. *Journal of Neuroendocrinology*, **7**, 97–108.

Blanchard, E.B., 1990. Elevated basal levels of cardiovascular responses in Vietnam veterans with PTSD: a health problem in the making? *Journal of Anxiety Disorders*, **4**, 233–237.

Blanchard, E.B., Kolb, L.C. and Prins, A., 1991a. Psychophysiologic responses in the diagnosis of posttraumatic stress disorder in Vietnam veterans. *Journal of Nervous and Mental Diseases*, **179**, 97–101.

Blanchard, E.B., Kolb, L.C., Prins, A., Gates, S. and McCoy, G.C., 1991b. Changes in plasma norepinephrine to combat-related stimuli among Vietnam veterans with posttraumatic stress disorder. *Journal of Nervous and Mental Diseases*, **179**, 371–373.

Bohus, B., Kovacs, G.L. and De Wied, D., 1978. Oxytocin, vasopressin and memory: opposite effects on consolidation and retrieval processes. *Brain Research*, **157**, 414–417.

Bohus, B., De Jong, W., Hagan, J.J., De Loos, W.S., Maas, C.M. and Versteeg, C.A.M., 1983. Neuropeptides and steroid hormones in adaptive autonomic processes: implications for psychosomatic disorders. In: Endröczi, E., De Wied, D., Angelucci, L. and Scapagnini, U. (eds), *Integrative Neurohumoral Mechanisms: Developments in Neuroscience*, Vol. 16, pp. 35–49. Elsevier Biomedical Press, Amsterdam.

Boscarino, J.A., 1996. Posttraumatic stress disorder, exposure to combat, and lower plasma cortisol among Vietnam veterans: findings and implications. *Journal of Consultative and Clinical Psychology*, **64**, 191–201.

Bratt, A.M., Kelly, S.P., Knowles, J.P., Barrett, J., Davis, K. and Mittleman, G., 2001. Long term modulation of the HPA axis by the hippocampus. Behavioral, biochemical and immunological endpoints in rats exposed to chronic mild stress. *Psychoneuroendocrinology*, **26**, 121–145.

Breder, C.D., Dinarello, C.A. and Saper, C.B., 1988. Interleukin-1 immunoreactive innervation of the human hypothalamus. *Science*, **240**, 321–324.

Bremner, J.D., 1999. Does stress damage the brain? *Biological Psychiatry*, **45**, 797–805.

Bremner, J.D., Licinio, J., Darnell, A., Krystal, J.H., Owens, M.J., Southwick, S.M., Nemeroff, C.B. and Charney, D.S., 1997b. Elevated CSF corticotropin-releasing factor concentrations in posttraumatic stress disorder. *American Journal of Psychiatry*, **154**, 624–629.

Bremner, D., Randall, P., Scott, T.M., Bronen, R.A., Seibyl, J.P., Southwick, S.M., Delaney, R.C., McCarthy, G., Charney, D.S. and Innis, R.B., 1995. MRI-based measurement of hippocampal volume in patients with combat-related posttraumatic stress disorder. *American Journal of Psychiatry*, **152**, 973–981.

Bremner, J.D., Randall, P., Vermetten, E., Staib, L., Bronen, R.A., Mazure, C., Capelli, S., McCarthy, G., Innis, R.B. and Charney, D., 1997a. Magnetic resonance imaging-based measurement of hippocampal volume in posttraumatic stress disorder related to childhood physical and sexual abuse—A preliminary report. *Biological Psychiatry*, **41**, 23–32.

Brewin, C.R., Andrews, B., Rose, S. and Kirk, M., 1999. Acute stress disorder and posttraumatic stress disorder in victims of violent crime. *American Journal of Psychiatry*, **156**, 360–366.

Brown, M.R., Rivier, C. and Vale, W., 1984. Central nervous system regulation of adrenocorticotropin secretion: role of somatostatins. *Endocrinology*, **114**, 1546–1549.

Cannon, W.B., 1914. The emergency function of the adrenal medulla in pain and the major emotions. *American Journal of Physiology*, **33**, 356–372.

Cannon, W.B., 1915. *Bodily Changes in Pain, Hunger, Fear and Rage: An Account of Recent Researches Into the Function of Emotional Excitement*. D. Appleton and Company, New York and London.

Cannon, W.B. and de la Paz, D., 1911. Emotional stimulation of adrenal secretion. *American Journal of Physiology*, **28**, 64–70.

Cannon, W.B. and Hoskins, R.G., 1911. The effects of asphyxia, hyperpnea, and sensory stimulation on adrenal secretion. *American Journal of Physiology*, **29**, 274–279.

Chepkova, A.N., French, P., De Wied, D., Ontskul, A.H., Ramakers, G.M.J., Skrebitski, V.G., Gispen, W.H. and Urban, I.J.A., 1995. Long-lasting enhancement of synaptic excitability of CA1/subiculum neurons of rat ventral hippocampus by vasopressin and vasopressin(4–8). *Brain Research*, **701**, 255–266.

Cohen, H., Kotler, M., Matar, M.A., Kaplan, Z., Miodownik, H. and Cassuto, Y., 1997. Power spectral analysis of heart rate variability in posttraumatic stress disorder patients. *Biological Psychiatry*, **41**, 627–629.

De Bellis, M.D., Baum, A.S., Birmaher, B., Keshavan, M.S., Eccard, C.H., Boring, A.M., Jenkins, F.J. and Ryan, N.D., 1999. Developmental traumatology part I: Biological stress systems. *Biological Psychiatry*, **45**, 1259–1270.

De Bellis, M.D., Chrousos, G.P., Dorn, L.H., Burke, L., Helmers, K., Kling, M.A., Trickett, P.K. and Putnam, F.W., 1994. Hypothalamic-pituitary-adrenal axis dysregulation in sexually abused girls. *Journal of Clinical Endocrinology and Metabolism*, **78**, 249–255.

De Goeij, D.C.E., Binnekade, R. and Tilders, F.J.H., 1992. Chronic stress enhances vasopressin but not corticotropin-releasing factor secretion during hypoglycemia. *American Journal of Physiology*, **263**, E394–399.

De Goeij, D.C.E., Kvetnansky, R., Whitnall, M.H., Jezova, D., Berkenbosch, F. and Tilders, F.J.H., 1991. Repeated stress-induced activation of corticotropin-releasing factor neurons enhances vasopressin stores and colocalization with corticotropin-releasing factor in the median eminence of rats. *Neuroendocrinology*, **53**, 150–159.

De Loos, W.S., 2001. Post-traumatic syndromes: comparative biology and psychology. In: Griez, E.J.L., Favarelli, C., Nutt, D. and Zohar, J. (eds), *Anxiety Disorders: An Introduction to Clinical Management and Research*, pp. 205–221. John Wiley & Sons, Chichester.

De Wied, D., 1999. Behavioral pharmacology of neuropeptides related to melanocortins and the neurohypophyseal hormones. *European Journal of Pharmacology*, **375**, 1–11.

De Wied, D. and Jolles, J., 1982. Neuropeptides derived from pro-opiocortin: behavioral, physiological and neurochemical effects. *Physiological Reviews*, **62**, 976–1059.

Delahanty, D.L., Raimonde, A.J. and Spoonster, E., 2000. Initial posttraumatic urinary cortisol levels predict subsequent PTSD symptoms in motor vehicle accident victims. *Biological Psychiatry*, **48**, 940–947.

Demitrack, M.A., 1997. Neuroendocrine correlates of chronic fatigue syndrome: a brief review. *Journal of Psychiatric Research*, **31**, 69–82.

Demitrack, M.A., Dale, J.K., Straus, S.E., Laue, L., Listwak, S.J., Kruesi, M.J.P., Chrousos, G.P. and Gold, P.W., 1991. Evidence for impaired activation of the hypothalamic-pituitary-adrenal axis in patients with chronic fatigue syndrome. *Journal of Clinical Endocrinology and Metabolism*, **73**, 1224–1234.

Denenberg, V.H., 1964. Critical periods, stimulus input, and emotional reactivity: a theory of infantile stimulation. *Psychological Reviews*, **71**, 335–351.

Francis, D.D., Caldji, C., Champagne, F., Plotsky, P.M. and Meany, M.J., 1999. The role of corticotropin-releasing factor–norepinephrine systems in mediating the effects of early experience on the development of behavioral and endocrine responses to stress. *Biological Psychiatry*, **46**, 1153–1166.

Garrick, N.A., Hill, J.L., Szele, F.G., Tomai, T.P., Gold, P.W. and Murphy, D.L., 1987. Corticotropin-releasing factor: a marked circadian rhythm in primate cerebrospinal fluid peaks in the evening and is inversely related to the cortisol circadian rhythm. *Endocrinology*, **121**, 1329–1334.

Glover, H., 1992. Emotional numbing: a possible endorphin-mediated phenomenon associated with post-traumatic stress disorders and other allied psychopathological states. *Journal of Traumatic Stress*, **5**, 643–675.

Glover, H., 1993. A preliminary trial of nalmefene for the treatment of emotional numbing in combat veterans with post-traumatic stress disorder. *Israelean Journal of Psychiatry and Related Sciences*, **30**, 255–263.

Goenjian, A.K., Yehuda, R., Pynoos, R.S., Steinberg, A.M., Tashjian, M., Yang, R.K., Najarian, L.M. and Fairbanks, L.A., 1996. Basal cortisol, dexamethasone suppression of cortisol, and MHPG in adolescents after the 1988 earthquake in Armenia. *American Journal of Psychiatry*, **153**, 929–934.

Gold, P.W., Goodwin, F.K. and Chrousos, G.P., 1988. Clinical and biochemical manifestations of depression. Relation to the neurobiology of stress. Part II. *New England Journal of Medicine*, **319**, 413–420.

Goldfinger, D.A., Amdur, R.L. and Liberzon, I., 1998. Psychophysiologic responses to the Rorschach in PTSD patients, noncombat and combat controls. *Depression and Anxiety*, **8**, 112–120.

Gould, E. and Tanapat, R., 1999. Stress and hippocampal neurogenesis. *Biological Psychiatry*, **46**, 1472–1479.

Griep, E.N., Boersma, J.W. and De Kloet, E.R., 1993. Altered reactivity of the hypothalamic-pituitary-adrenal axis in the primary fibromyalgia syndrome. *Journal of Rheumatology*, **20**, 469–474.

Hawk, L.W., Dougall, A.L., Ursano, R.J. and Baum, A., 2000. Urinary catecholamines and cortisol in recent-onset posttraumatic stress disorder after motor vehicle accidents. *Psychosomatic Medicine*, **62**, 423–434.

Heim, C. and Nemeroff, C.B., 2001. The role of childhood trauma in the neurobiology of mood and anxiety disorders: preclinical and clinical studies. *Biological Psychiatry*, **49**, 1023–1039.

Heim, C. and Nemeroff, C.B., 1999. The impact of early adverse experiences on brain systems involved in the pathophysiology of anxiety and affective disorders. *Biological Psychiatry*, **46**, 1509–1522.

Heim, C., Ehlert, U. and Hellhammer, D.H., 2000. The potential role of hypocortisolism in the pathophysiology of stress-related bodily disorders. *Psychoneuroendocrinology*, **25**, 1–35.

Heim, C., Ehlert, U., Hanker, J.P. and Hellhammer, D.H., 1998. Abuse-related posttraumatic stress disorder and alterations of the hypothalamic-pituitary-adrenal axis in women with chronic pelvic pain. *Psychosomatic Medicine*, **60**, 309–318.

Heisler, S., Reisine, T.D., Hook, V.Y. and Axelrod, J., 1982. Somatostatin inhibits multireceptor stimulation of cyclic AMP formation and corticotropin secretion in mouse pituitary tumor cells. *Proceedings of the National Academy of Sciences of the United States of America*, **79**, 6502–6506.

Hemingway, R.B. and Reigle, T.G., 1987. The involvement of endogenous opiate systems in learned helplessness and stress-induced analgesia. *Psychopharmacology*, **93**, 353–357.

Henry, J.P., 1992. Biological basis of the stress response. *Integrated Physiological and Behavioural Sciences*, **27**, 66–83.

Hess, W.R. and Brügger, M., 1943. Das subkortikale Zentrum der affektiven Abwehrreaktion. *Helvetica Physiologica et Pharmacologica Acta*, **1**, 33–52.

Hockings, G.I., Jackson, R.V., Grice, J.E., Ward, W.K. and Jensen, G.R., 1994. Cell-mediated immunity in combat veterans with post-traumatic stress disorder. *Medical Journal of Australia*, **161**, 287–288.

Hoffman, L., Burges Watson, P., Wilson, G. and Montgomery, J., 1989. Low plasma β-endorphin in posttraumatic stress disorder. *Australian and New Zealand Journal of Psychiatry*, **23**, 269–273.

Hoogendijk, W.J.G., Meynen, G., Eikelenboom, P. and Swaab, D.F., 2000. Brain alterations in depression. *Acta Neuropsychiatrica*, **12**, 54–58.

Huizenga, N.A.T.M., Koper, J.W., De Lange, P., Pols, H.A.P., Stolk, R.P., Grobbee, D.E., De Jong, F.H. and Lamberts, S.W.J., 1998a. Interperson variability but intraperson stability of baseline plasma cortisol concentrations, and its relation to feedback sensitivity of the hypothalamo-pituitary-adrenal axis to a low dose of dexamethasone in elderly individuals. *Journal of Clinical Endocrinology and Metabolism*, **83**, 47–54.

Huizenga, N.A.T.M., Koper, J.W., De Lange, P., Pols, H.A.P., Stolk, R.P., Burger, H., Grobbee, D.E., Brinkmann, A.O., De Jong, F.H. and Lamberts, S.W.J., 1998b. A polymorphism in the GR gene may be associated with an increased sensitivity to glucocorticoids *in vivo*. *Journal of Clinical Endocrinology and Metabolism*, **83**, 144–151.

Jacobson, L. and Sapolsky, R., 1991. The role of the hippocampus in feedback regulation of the hypothalamic-pituitary-adrenocortical axis. *Endocrine Reviews*, **12**, 118–134.

Kanter, E.D., Wilkinson, C.W., Radant, A.D., Petrie, E.C., Dobie, D.J., McFall, M.E., Peskind, E.R. and Raskind, M.A., 2001. Glucocorticoid feedback sensitivity and adrenocortical responsiveness in posttraumatic stress disorder. *Biological Psychiatry*, **50**, 238–245.

Kaufman, J., Birmaher, B., Perel, J., Dahl, R.E., Moreci, P., Nelson, B., Wells, W. and Ryan, N.D., 1997. The corticotropin-releasing hormone challenge in depressed abused, depressed nonabused, and normal control children. *Biological Psychiatry*, **42**, 669–679.

Kellner, M., Baker, D.G. and Yehuda, R., 1997. Salivary cortisol in operation desert storm returnees. *Biological Psychiatry*, **42**, 849–850.

Koren, D., Arnon, I. and Klein, E., 1999. Acute stress response and posttraumatic stress disorder in traffic accident victims: a one-year prospective, follow-up study. *American Journal of Psychiatry*, **156**, 367–373.

Kosten, T.R., Mason, J.W., Giller, E.L., Ostroff, R.B. and Harkness, L., 1987. Sustained urinary norepinephrine and epinephrine elevation in post-traumatic stress disorder. *Psychoneuroendocrinology*, **12**, 13–20.

Kudler, H., Davidson, J., Mendor, K., Lipper, S. and Ely, T., 1987. The DST and posttraumatic stress disorder. *American Journal of Psychiatry*, **144**, 1068–1071.

LeDoux, J., 1998. Fear and the brain: where have we been, and where are we going? *Biological Psychiatry*, **44**, 1229–1238.

Lenz, H.J., Raedler, A., Greten, H. and Brown, M.R., 1987. CRF initiates biological actions within the brain that are observed in response to stress. *American Journal of Physiology*, **252**, R34–39.

Levine, S., 1957. Infantile experience and resistance to physiological stress. *Science*, **126**, 405–406.

Levine, S., 2001. Primary social relationships influence the development of the hypothalamic-pituitary-adrenal axis in the rat. *Physiology and Behaviour*, **73**, 255–260.

Liberzon, I., Krstov, M. and Young, E.A., 1997. Stress-restress: effects on ACTH and fast feedback. *Psychoneuroendocrinology*, **22**, 443–453.

Liberzon, I., Abelson, J.L., Flagel, S.B., Raz, J. and Young, E.A., 1999. Neuroendocrine and psychophysiologic responses in PTSD: a symptom provocation study. *Neuropsychopharmacology*, **21**, 40–50.

Liu, D., Diorio, J., Tannenbaum, B., Caldji, C., Francis, D., Freedman, A., Sharma, S., Pearson, D., Plotsky, P.M. and Meaney, M.J., 1997. Maternal care, hippocampal glucocorticoid receptors, and hypothalamic-pituitary-adrenal responses to stress. *Science*, **277**, 1659–1662.

López, J.F., Akil, H. and Watson, S.J., 1999. Neural circuits mediating stress. *Biological Psychiatry*, **46**, 1461–1471.

Ma, X.M., Lightman, S. and Aguilera, G., 1999. Vasopressin and corticotropin-releasing hormone gene responses to novel stress in rats adapted to repeated restraint. *Endocrinology*, **140**, 3623–3632.

Maes, M., Lin, A., Bonaccorso, S., van Hunsel, F., van Gastwel, A., Delmeire, L., Biondi, M., Bosmans, E., Kenis, G. and Scharpé, S., 1998. Increased 24-hour urinary cortisol excretion in patients with posttraumatic stress disorder and patients with major depression, but not in patients with fibromyalgia. *Acta Psychiatrica Scandinavica*, **98**, 328–335.

Mason, J.W., Giller, E.L., Kosten, T.R., Ostroff, R.B. and Podd, L., 1986. Urinary free-cortisol levels in posttraumatic stress disorder patients. *Journal of Nervous and Mental Diseases*, **174**, 145–149.

Mason, J.W., Wang, S., Yehuda, R., Riney, S., Charney, D.S. and Southwick, S.M., 2001. Psychogenic lowering of urinary cortisol levels linked to increased emotional numbing in combat related posttraumatic stress disorder. *Psychosomatic Medicine*, **63**, 387–401.

Mason, J., Weizman, R., Laor, N., Wang, S., Schujovitsky, A., Abramovitz-Schneider, P., Feiler, D. and Charney, D., 1996. Serum triiodothyronine elevation in Israeli combat veterans with posttraumatic stress disorder: a cross-cultural study. *Biological Psychiatry*, **39**, 835–838.

Mason, J.W., Wang, S., Yehuda, R., Bremner, J.D., Riney, S.J., Lubin, H., Johnson, D.R., Southwick, S.M. and Charney, D.S., 1995. Some approaches to the study of the clinical implications of thyroid alterations in post-traumatic stress disorder. In: Friedman, M.J., Charney, D.S. and Deutch, A.Y. (eds), *Neurobiological and Clinical Consequences of Stress: From Normal Adaptation to PTSD*, pp. 367–379. Lippincott-Raven Publishers, Philadelphia.

Mason, J., Southwick, S., Yehuda, R., Wang, S., Riney, S., Bremner, D., Johnson, D., Lubin, H., Blake, D., Zhou, G., Gusman, F. and Charney, D., 1994. Elevations of serum free triiodothyronine, total triiodothyronine, thyroxine-binding globulin, and total thyroxine levels in combat-related posttraumatic stress disorder. *Archives of General Psychiatry*, **51**, 629–641.

McEwen, B.S., 1998. Protective and damaging effects of stress mediators. *New England Journal of Medicine*, **338**, 171–179.

McEwen, B.S. and Magariños, M., 1997. Stress effects on morphology and function of the hippocampus. In: Yehuda, R. and McFarlane, A.C. (eds), Psychobiology of posttraumatic stress disorder. *Annals of the New York Academy of Sciences*, **821**, 271–284.

McEwen, B.S., Gould, E.A. and Sakai, R.R., 1992. The vulnerability of the hippocampus to protective and destructive effects of glucocorticoids in relation to stress. *British Journal of Psychiatry*, **160**, 18–24.

McFarlane, A.C., Atchison, M. and Yehuda, R., 1997. The acute stress response following motor vehicle accidents and its relation to PTSD. In: Yehuda, R. and McFarlane, A.C. (eds), Psychobiology of posttraumatic stress disorder. *Annals of the New York Academy of Sciences*, **821**, 437–441.

Meaney, M.J., Aitken, D.H., Viau, V., Sharma, S. and Sarrieau, A., 1989. Neonatal handling alters adrenocortical negative feedback sensitivity and hippocampal type II glucocorticoid receptor binding in the rat. *Neuroendocrinology*, **50**, 597–604.

Mitchell, A.J., 1998. The role of corticotropin releasing factor in depressive illness: a critical review. *Neuroscience and Biobehavioral Reviews*, **22**, 635–661.

Pallmeyer, T.P., Blanchard, E.B. and Kolb, L.C., 1986. The psychophysiology of combat-induced post-traumatic stress disorder in Vietnam veterans. *Behaviour Research and Therapy*, **24**, 645–652.

Perry, B.D., Giller, E.L. and Southwick, S.M., 1987. Altered platelet alpha2-adrenergic binding sites in posttraumatic stress disorder. *American Journal of Psychiatry*, **144**, 1511–1512.

Pitman, R.K., Orr, S.P. and Lasko, N.B., 1993. Effects of intranasal vasopressin and oxytocin on physiologic responding during personal combat imagery in Vietnam veterans with posttraumatic stress disorder. *Psychiatry Research*, **48**, 107–117.

Pitman, R.K., Orr, S.P. and Steketee, G.S., 1989. Psychophysiological investigations of posttraumatic stress disorder imagery. *Psychopharmacolical Bulletin*, **25**, 426–431.

Pitman, R.K., Van der Kolk, B.A., Orr, S.P. and Greenberg, M.S., 1990. Naloxone-reversible analgesic response to combat related stimuli in posttraumatic stress disorder. *Archives of General Psychiatry*, **47**, 541–544.

Prange, A.J., 1999. Thyroid axis sustaining hypothesis of posttraumatic stress disorder. *Psychosomatic Medicine*, **61**, 139–140.

Rasmusson, A.M., Lipschitz, D.S., Wang, S., Hu, S., Vojvoda, D., Bremner, J.D., Southwicj, S.M. and Charney, D.S., 2001. Increased pituitary and adrenal activity on premenopausal women with posttraumatic stress disorder. *Biological Psychiatry*, **50**, 965–977.

Reisine, T. and Pasternak, G., 1996. Opioid analgesics and antagonists. In: Hardman, J.G., Limbird, L.E., Molinoff, P.B., Ruddon, R.W. and Gilman, A.G. (eds), *Goodman & Gilman's the Pharmacological Basis of Therapeutics*, 9th edn, pp. 521–555. MacGraw–Hill, New York.

Resnick, H.S., Yehuda, R., Pitman, R.K. and Foy, D.W., 1995. Effect of previous trauma on acute plasma cortisol level following rape. *American Journal of Psychiatry*, **152**, 1675–1677.

Richardson, U.I. and Schonbrunn, A., 1981. Inhibition of adrenocorticotropin secretion by somatostatin in pituitary cells in culture. *Endocrinology*, **108**, 281–290.

Sapolsky, R.M., 1996. Why stress is bad for your brain. *Science*, **273**, 749–750.

Sapolsky, R.M., 1997. The importance of a well-groomed child. *Science*, **277**, 1620–1621.

Sapolsky, R.M., 2000. Glucocorticoids and hippocampal atrophy in neuropsychiatric disorders. *Archives of General Psychiatry*, **57**, 925–935.

Sapolsky, R.M., Zola-Morgan, S. and Squire, L.R., 1991. Inhibition of glucocorticoid secretion by the hippocampal formation in the primate. *Journal of Neuroscience*, **11**, 3695–3704.

Schuff, N., neylan, T.C., Lenoci, M.A., Du, A.-T., Weiss, D.S., Marmar, C.R. and Weiner, M.W., 2001. Decreased hippocampal *N*-acetylaspartate in the absence of atrophy in posttraumatic stress disorder. *Biological Psychiatry*, **50**, 952–959.

Schulkin, J., Gold, P.W. and McEwen, B.S., 1998. Induction of corticotropin-releasing hormone gene expression by glucocorticoids: implications for understanding the states of fear and anxiety and allostatic load. *Psychoneuroendocrinology*, **23**, 219–243.

Scott, L.V., Medbak, S. and Dinan, T.G., 1999. Desmopressin augments pituitary-adrenal responsivity to corticotropin-releasing hormone in subjects with chronic fatigue syndrome and in healthy volunteers. *Biological Psychiatry*, **45**, 1447–1454.

Seeman, T.E. and Robbins, R.J., 1994. Ageing and hypothalamic-pituitary-adrenal response to challenge in humans. *Endocrine Reviews*, **15**, 233–260.

Selye, H., 1936a. A syndrome produced by diverse nocuous agents. *Nature*, **138**, 32.

Selye, H. and 1936b. Thymus and adrenals in the response of the organism to injuries and intoxications. *British Journal of Experimental Pathology*, **17**, 234–248.

Selye, H. and Collip, J.B., 1936. Fundamental factors in the interpretation of stimuli influencing endocrine glands. *Endocrinology*, **20**, 667–672.

Shalev, A.Y., Bonne, O.B. and Peri, T., 1996. Auditory startle response during exposure to war stress. *Comprehensive Psychiatry*, **37**, 134–138.

Shalev, A.Y., Orr, S.P. and Pitman, R.K., 1993. Psychophysiologic assessment of traumatic imagery in Israeli civilian patients with posttraumatic stress disorder. *American Journal of Psychiatry*, **150**, 620–624.

Shalev, A.Y., Peri, T., Canettti, L. and Schreiber, S., 1996. Predictors of PTSD in injured trauma survivors: a prospective study. *American Journal of Psychiatry*, **153**, 219–225.

Shalev, A.Y., Peri, T., Gelpin, E., Orr, S.P. and Pitman, R.K., 1997. Psychophysiologic assessment of mental imagery of stressful events in Israeli civilian posttraumatic stress disorder patients. *Comprehensive Psychiatry*, **38**, 269–273.

Shalev, A.Y., Freedman, S., Peri, T., Brandes, D., Sahar, T., Orr, S.P. and Pitman, R.K., 1998b. Prospective study of posttraumatic stress disorder and depression following trauma. *American Journal of Psychiatry*, **155**, 630–637.

Shalev, A.Y., Sahar, T., Freedman, S., Peri, T., Glick, N., Brandes, D., Orr, S.P. and Pittman, R.K., 1998a. A prospective study of heart rate response following trauma and the subsequent development of posttraumatic stress disorder. *Archives General Psychiatry*, **55**, 553–559.

Smith, M.A., Davidson, J., Ritchie, J.C., Kudler, H., Lipper, S., Chappell, P. and Nemeroff, C.B., 1989. The corticotropin-releasing hormone test in patients with posttraumatic stress disorder. *Biological Psychiatry*, **26**, 349–355.

Southwict, S.M., Krystal, J.H., Morgan, C.A., Johnson, D., Nagy, L.M., Nicolaou, A., Heninger, G.R. and Charney, D.S., 1993. Abnormal noradrenergic function in posttraumatic stress disorder. *Archives of General Psychiatry*, **50**, 266–274.

Stein, M.B., Koverola, C., Hanna, C., Torchia, M.G. and McClarty, B., 1997a. Hippocampal volume in women victimized by childhood sexual abuse. *Psychological Medicine*, **27**, 951–959.

Stein, M.B., Yehuda, R., Koverola, C. and Hanna, C., 1997b. Enhanced dexamethasone suppression of plasma cortisol in adult women traumatized by childhood sexual abuse. *Biological Psychiatry*, **42**, 680–686.

Sterling, P. and Eyer, J., 1988. Allostasis: a new paradigm to explain arousal pathology. In: Fisher, S. and Reason, J. (eds), *Handbook of Life Stress, Cognition and Health*, pp. 629–649. John Wiley & Sons, Chichester.

Van der Kolk, B.A. and Saporta, S., 1991. The biological response to psychic trauma: mechanisms and treatment of intrusion and numbing. *Anxiety Research*, **4**, 199–212.

Van der Kolk, B.A., Greenberg, M., Boyd, H. and Krystal, J., 1985. Inescapable shock, neurotransmitters, and addiction to trauma: toward a psychobiology of posttraumatic stress. *Biological Psychiatry*, **20**, 314–325

Van der Kolk, B.A., Greenberg, M.S., Orr, S.P. and Pitman, R.K., 1989. Endogenous opioids and stress induced analgesia in post-traumatic stress disorder. *Psychopharmacological Bulletin*, **25**, 108–112.

Van Praag, H.M., 2000. Nosologomania: a disorder of psychiatry. *World Journal of Biological Psychiatry*, **1**, 151–158.

Van Praag, H.M., Kahn, R.S., Asnis, G.M., Wetzler, S., Brown, S.L., Bleich, A. and Korn, M.L., 1987. Denosologisation of biological psychiatry or the specificity of 5-HT disturbances in psychiatric disorders. *Journal of Affective Disorders*, **13**, 1–8.

Wan, R., Diamant, M., De Jong, W. and De Wied, D., 1992. Differential effects of ACTH4-10, DG-AVP, and DG-OXT on heart rate and passive avoidance behaviour in rats. *Physiology and Behavior*, **51**, 507–513.

Wang, S. and Mason, J., 1999. Elevations of serum T3 levels and their association with symptoms in World War II veterans with combat-related posttraumatic stress disorder: replication of findings in Vietnam combat veterans. *Psychosomatic Medicine*, **61**, 131–138.

Wang, S., Mason, J.W., Charney, D.S., Yehuda, R., Riney, S. and Southwick, S., 1997. Relationships between hormonal profile and novelty seeking in combat-related posttraumatic stress disorder. *Biological Psychiatry*, **41**, 145–151.

Wang, S., Mason, J., Southwick, S., Johnson, D., Lubin, H. and Charney, D., 1995. Relationships between thyroid hormones and symptoms in combat-related posttraumatic stress disorder. *Psychosomatic Medicine*, **57**, 398–402.

Webster, R.A., 1989. The catecholamines (noradrenaline and dopamine). In: Webster, R.A. and Jordan, C.C. (eds), *Neurotransmitters, Drugs and Disease*, pp. 95–125. Blackwell Scientific Publications, Oxford.

Wolkowitz, O.M., Epel, E.S. and Reus, V.I., 2001. Stress hormone-related psychopathology: pathophysiological and treatment implications. *World Journal of Biological Psychiatry*, **2**, 115–143.

Yehuda, R., Bierer, L.M., Schmeidler, J., Aferiat, D.H., Breslau, I. and Dolan, S., 2000. Low cortisol and risk for PTSD in adult offspring of holocaust survivors. *American Journal of Psychiatry*, **157**, 1252–1259.

Yehuda, R., Keefe, R.S.E., Harvey, P.D., Levengood, R.A., Gerber, D.K., Geni, J. and Siever, L.J., 1995a. Learning and memory in combat veterans with posttraumatic stress disorder. *American Journal of Psychiatry*, **152**, 137–139.

Yehuda, R., Kahana, B., Binder-Brynes, K., Southwick, S.M., Mason, J.W. and Giller, E.L., 1995b. Low urinary cortisol in holocaust survivors with posttraumatic stress disorder. *American Journal of Psychiatry*, **152**, 982–986.

Yehuda, R., Boisoneau, D., Lowy, M.T. and Giller, E.L., 1995c. Dose response changes in plasma cortisol and lymphocyte glucocorticoid receptors following dexamethasone administration in combat veterans with and without posttraumatic stress disorder. *Archives of General Psychiatry*, **52**, 583–593.

Yehuda, R., Teicher, M.H., Trestman, R.L., Levengood, R.A. and Siever, L.J., 1996a. Cortisol regulation in posttraumatic stress disorder and major depression: a chronobiological analysis. *Biological Psychiatry*, **40**, 79–88.

Yehuda, R., Levengood, R.A., Schmeidler, J., Wilson, S., Ling Song Guo and Gerber, D., 1996b. Increased pituitary activation following metyrapone administration in post-traumatic stress disorder. *Psychoneuroendocrinology*, **21**, 1–16.

Yehuda, R., Lowy, M.T., Southwick, S.M., Shaffer, D. and Giller, E.L., 1991. Lymphocyte glucocorticoid receptor number in posttraumatic stress disorder. *American Journal of Psychiatry*, **148**, 499–504.

Yehuda, R., Southwick, S.M., Nussbaum, G., Wahby, V., Giller, E.L. and Mason, J.W., 1990a. Low urinary cortisol excretion in patients with posttraumatic stress disorder. *Journal of Nervous and Mental Diseases*, **178**, 366–369.

Yehuda, R., Perry, B.D., Southwick, S.M. and Giller, E.L., 1990b. Platelet alpha2-receptor binding in PTSD, generalized anxiety disorder, and major depressive disorder. *New Research Abstracts*, **143**, NR286.

Yehuda, R., Resnick, H.S., Schmeidler, J., Yang, R.-K. and Pitman, R.K., 1998. Predictors of cortisol and 3-methoxy-4-hydroxyphenylglycol responses in the acute aftermath of rape. *Biological Psychiatry*, **43**, 855–859.

Yehuda, R., Southwick, S.M., Giller, E.L., Ma, X. and Mason, J.W., 1992. Urinary catecholamine excretion and severity of PTSD symptoms in Vietnam combat veterans. *Journal of Nervous and Mental Diseases*, **180**, 321–325.

Yehuda, R., Southwick, S.M., Krystal, J.H., Bremner, D., Charney, D.S. and Mason, J.W., 1993. Enhanced suppression of cortisol following dexamethasone admission in posttraumatic stress disorder. *American Journal of Psychiatry*, **150**, 83–86.

XIX-6

Neuroimmunology of Anxiety Disorders

Palmiero Monteleone

INTRODUCTION

There is unequivocal evidence that stress is both causally related and a concomitant of most psychiatric disorders, including anxiety syndromes. For example, the post-traumatic stress disorder typically arises after unusual stress life experiences. Panic disorder is a syndrome with anxiety as the core of the disease and panic attacks possibly representing repeatedly recurring stress episodes. The obsessive–compulsive disorder involves recurrent thoughts (obsessions), that are experienced as intrusive and senseless, and/or repetitive seemingly purposeful behaviours (compulsions); both obsessions and compulsions cause marked distress. In phobic disorders, the phobic fear is a potent stressor.

There is agreement in the literature that stress profoundly affects immune function. Therefore, since patients with anxiety disorders endure considerable stress, it is plausible to expect alterations of immune competence in these subjects. On the other hand, it has been demonstrated that immune elements, namely some cytokines, are able to induce 'ansiogenic-like' and/or 'depressive-like' effects in the animal (Anisman *et al.*, 1998; Dantzer *et al.*, 1998); hence, it is likely that changes in immune parameters following real-life stress may be involved in the aetiopathology of anxiety syndromes and/or symptoms. Conversely, one would expect that if alterations of immunity occur in anxiety disorder patients, treatments aiming to alleviate anxiety symptoms should restore immune parameters.

The purpose of this review is to first consider the effects of stress on immune function; then, the changes in immune system that are associated with different anxiety syndromes will be discussed; finally, the effects of both pharmacological treatments and psychotherapeutic interventions on immune parameters will be analysed.

STRESS AND IMMUNE FUNCTION

Early evidence for an association between stress and immune function in humans came from the demonstration that human susceptibility to infections was increased by stress events. Kissen (1958) suggested a link between recent loss of a love object and the morbidity and mortality of pulmonary tuberculosis. Other authors suggested that hypnotically induced stress reactivates herpes simplex infection in susceptible individuals (Ullman, 1947), whereas hypnosis itself was found to be able to reverse both immediate-type and delayed-type hypersensitivity to tuberculin (Black, 1963; Black, Humphrey and Niven, 1963).

There is a large body of literature showing that stress has a significant impact on immune function. Initially, human studies examining the effects of experimental (speech task and mental arithmetic task) and real-life stressors (academic examination stress, bereavement, unemployment, divorce, caring for patients with chronic diseases) suggested that stress is associated with reduced immune responsiveness, and therefore it may compromise immune function (Dantzer and Mormede, 1995). However, there is now agreement in the literature that stress may even enhance immune activity.

In bereaved widows and widowers, a suppression of mitogen-induced lymphocyte proliferation was noted (Schleifer *et al.*, 1983); similarly, divorce, separation and unemployment were reported to decrease lymphocyte mitogen reactivity (Arnetz *et al.*, 1987; Kiecolt-Glaser *et al.*, 1987). A blunted unstimulated proliferation of peripheral blood mononuclear cells (PBMC) was observed in Israeli civilians during the period of Scud missile attacks (Weiss *et al.*, 1996), while recently released prisoners of war in Bosnia showed altered immune functions with reduced number of natural killer (NK) cells (Dekaris *et al.*, 1993).

Subacute or chronic real-life stressors were shown to decrease the number or the percentage of T-helper ($CD4^+$) cells, the T-helper/T-suppressor ($CD4^+/CD8^+$) cell ratio, and the number of NK cells in peripheral blood (Glaser *et al.*, 1985; Bachen *et al.*, 1992). To the contrary, acute laboratory and naturalistic stressors were reported to transiently elevate the number of total T and B lymphocytes, $CD8^+$ cells and the NK cells in the peripheral blood of healthy subjects (Fittshen *et al.*, 1990; Brosschot *et al.*, 1992). Moreover, Maes *et al.* (1999a) reported that students who responded to academic examination stress with a strong psychological reaction showed an increased number of activated T cell leukocyte subset profile. Furthermore, in those students, modifications of immune profile were positively and significantly associated with the stress-induced increase in self-rated severity of perceived stress and negative emotions.

Similarly to what occurs in cell-mediated immunity, increases or decreases in humoral immune parameters were reported after stress experiences. Some authors found increased salivary levels of immunoglobulin (Ig) A, while others reported reduced salivary concentrations of these Igs after exposure to acute or subacute stressors (Jemmott and Magloire, 1988; Bosch *et al.*, 1996). Increased concentrations of serum IgA, IgM and IgG were found by Maes *et al.* (1997a) in students with high levels of stress perception following academic examination, but not in those with low stress perception. Moreover, academic examination stress significantly increased serum levels of the C3 complement factor as well as those of the acute phase (AP) protein α_2-macroglobulin. Furthermore, students with high stress perception had a trend toward significant increases in serum levels of the complement C4 factor and AP proteins haptoglobin and α_1-acid glycoprotein, whereas students with low stress perception exhibited a reduction of these immune parameters (Maes *et al.*, 1997a).

Several studies assessed the effects of stress on cytokine production in humans. Early reports showed that psychological stress did not affect plasma interleukin-1 (IL-1) or interleukin-6 (IL-6) concentrations (Dugué *et al.*, 1993) or decreased the production of interferon-γ (IFγ) or increased that of IL-1β (Dobbin *et al.*,

Biological Psychiatry: Edited by H. D'haenen, J.A. den Boer and P. Willner. ISBN 0-471-49198-5

1991). Maes *et al.* (1998) and Song *et al.* (1999) found that academic examination stress significantly enhanced the production of proinflammatory cytokines, such as IL-6, tumour necrosis factor-α (TNFα) and IFγ, but decreased that of the 16kd Clara cell (CC-16) protein, a natural anti-inflammatory secretory protein. These data support the idea that the immune response to psychological stressors resembles that of organic stressors (injury, infection, necrosis), being characterized by the secretion of proinflammatory cytokines (IL-1, IL-6, TNFα) which, in turn, activate an AP response in order to cope with stress and minimize its impact on the homeostasis of the organism.

In sum, this brief review emphasizes that stress may suppress or enhance immune function depending on a number of variables, including the acute or chronic nature of stressors, the severity of the triggered stress response, the immune variable under consideration, the individual's perception of the stressor, the personality characteristics of the subject, and the nature of the stress-induced affective states.

SUBCLINICAL ANXIETY AND IMMUNE FUNCTION

Studies examining the relationships between subclinical anxiety and immunity are sparse. Linn, Lin and Jensen (1981) reported a negative correlation between anxiety and lymphocyte responses to mitogens in hospitalized patients. Decreased levels of salivary IgA were found in nurses with subclinical anxiety as compared to those without anxiety (Graham *et al.*, 1988); similar results were reported in dental students (Jemmott, Borysenko and Chapman, 1983). Moreover, healthy male students with high levels of subclinical anxiety had a significantly lower lymphocyte proliferative response to concanavalin A (ConA) as well as lower levels of circulating IL-1β (Zorrilla, Redel and DeRubeis, 1994). Among women undergoing adjuvant chemotherapy for breast cancer, those with high trait anxiety evidenced a reduced number of monocytes and $CD4^+/CD8^+$ T cell ratio, and a compromised activity of NK cells (Fredrikson *et al.*, 1993). Finally, a decreased lymphocyte proliferative response to phytohaemoagglutinin (PHA) was observed in healthy students with high anxiety scores independently from a previous history of life events (Gonzales-Quijano *et al.*, 1998).

On the contrary, a few studies suggested that subclinical anxiety may increase immune function. Indeed, a positive correlation was found between NK cell activity, IL-2 production and scores on the SCL-90-R anxiety subscale during an examination period in medical college students (Koh, 1996, 1997).

GENERALIZED ANXIETY DISORDER

La Via, Workman and Lydiard (1992) first reported that subjects with generalized anxiety disorder (GAD) and/or panic disorder (PD) had a significantly higher frequency of upper respiratory infections as compared with normal controls, which suggests a decrease of the immune defences in these individuals. Moreover, the same group of investigators (La Via *et al.*, 1996) showed that a 72-hour stimulation of peripheral lymphocytes with anti-$CD3^+$ induced a significantly lower expression of $CD25^+$ cell subtype in GAD patients with respect to healthy subjects.

Castilla-Cortazar, Castilla and Gurpegui (1998) investigated several immune parameters in 16 patients with GAD and five patients with obsessive–compulsive disorder (OCD). As compared to a control group, anxiety disorder patients showed increased number of monocytes and $CD13^+$ cells, normal counts of T lymphocytes, $CD4^+$ and $CD8^+$ T cell subtypes, and decreased number and activity of $CD16^+$ (NK) cells with a blunted lymphoproliferative response to PHA, and a normal *in vitro* production of IFγ from peripheral blood mononuclear cells (PBMC). Moreover, patients with anxiety displayed an anergy to candidin and tuberculin, alterations in the expression of both monocyte surface HLA-DR molecules (involved in the mechanisms of antigen presentation) and membrane CR1 receptors (important in phagocytosis of opsonized particles and microrganisms) as well as a reduced number of monocytes expressing cytoplasmic vimentin filaments, which are implicated in the cytoskeletal organization. Incubation *in vitro* of these monocytes with naloxone normalized the number of cells expressing vimentin filaments and their ability to ingest *Candida albicans*. These findings suggest that at least some immune alterations detected in patients with GAD may be dependent on an increased opioid tonus. Indeed, plasma levels of β-endorphins were found to be elevated in those patients.

Koh and Lee (1998) investigated cell-mediated immunity in a cohort of 31 patients, 20 with GAD and 11 with PD, and 31 healthy subjects. They found that both GAD patients and subjects with PD had reduced blastogenic responses to PHA and decreased PHA-induced IL-2 production. No significant differences were found in NK cell activity between the two patient groups and healthy subjects.

SIMPLE PHOBIA

It has been recently shown that phobic fear is a potent stressor, which results in increases of autonomic activity, NK cell percentages and cytotoxicity (Gerritsen *et al.*, 1996). These immune effects, however, seem to be influenced by the individual's level of worry. Indeed, people with spider or snake phobia who experienced high levels of trait worry showed a blunted increase in the number of peripheral NK cells after exposure to the phobic stimulus, whereas those with normal levels of worry showed a marked increase in this immune parameter (Segerstrom *et al.*, 1999).

One study reported that patients with agoraphobia had normal counts of peripheral $CD3^+$, $CD4^+$, $CD8^+$ and $CD57^+$ cells, normal value of the $CD4^+/CD8^+$ ratio and an increased frequency of $CD14^+$ cell types (monocytes) (Covelli *et al.*, 1990). Moreover, *in vitro* phagocytosis and killing of *Candida albicans* exerted by polymorphonuclear cells and monocytes were reduced in those patients. After an 8-week treatment with the synthetic thymic hormone, thymopoietin, the phagocytic capacity of monocytes significantly increased, whereas that of polymorphonuclear cells remained unchanged. Moreover, treatment with the thymic hormone led to a significant recovery of polymorphonuclear and monocyte killing capacity, even if values remained below the normal range (Covelli *et al.*, 1990).

SOCIAL PHOBIA

A limited number of studies investigated immune function in people with social phobia.

Rapaport and Stein (1994a) found normal levels of serum IL-2 and soluble IL-2 receptor (sIL-2R) in 15 patients with generalized social phobia, and suggested that these patients do not have evidence of T-lymphocyte activation. This hypothesis was supported by the findings of a subsequent study, in which patients with social phobia exhibited normal values of peripheral $CD3^+$, $CD4^+$, $CD8^+$, $CD19^+$, $CD25^+$ lymphocyte subtypes and B cells expressing HLA-DR molecules, with only a slight increase in the number of NK ($CD16^+$) cells (Rapaport, 1998).

PANIC DISORDER

The studies of circulating lymphocyte phenotypes in patients with PD have provided conflicting results. In particular, no difference in total lymphocytes, leukocytes, T cells and B cells or decreased total lymphocytes and increased total T cells have been reported in PD patients (Schleifer *et al.*, 1990; Ramesh *et al.*, 1991; Andreoli *et al.*, 1992; Marazziti *et al.*, 1992). The number of $CD4^+$ and $CD8^+$ cell subtypes and the $CD4^+/CD8^+$ ratio were found to be normal in three studies (Schleifer *et al.*, 1990; Perini *et al.*, 1995; Rapaport, 1998), but decreased in another study (Marazziti *et al.*, 1992). The peripheral NK cell number has been reported to be mostly normal, with only one study reporting an increased value (Schleifer *et al.*, 1990; Marazziti *et al.*, 1992; Perini *et al.*, 1995; Koh and Lee, 1998; Rapaport, 1998). Two groups of investigators found increased values of $CD19^+$ B cells and lymphocytes expressing the HLA-DR antigen (Perini *et al.*, 1995; Rapaport, 1998), whereas Marazziti *et al.* (1992) detected normal values of these cells. Similarly, the $CD57^+$ cell number was reported to be normal in two studies (Marazziti *et al.*, 1992; Rapaport, 1998), but was decreased by another study (Perini *et al.*, 1995). Finally, $CD56^+$ cells and lymphocytes expressing the CD25 molecule, which is the surface receptor for IL-2, were not increased in patients with PD (Perini *et al.*, 1995; Rapaport, 1998).

The *in vitro* mitogen response of lymphocytes from PD patients has been found to vary within a wide range. Two studies reported normal blastogenic responses to PHA (Surman *et al.*, 1986; Brambilla *et al.*, 1992), two others found a reduced proliferative responses to ConA, Pokeweed mitogen (PWM) and PHA (Schleifer *et al.*, 1990; Koh and Lee, 1998), and one found increased blastogenic responses to PHA and ConA (Andreoli *et al.*, 1992).

Serum levels of immunoglobulins were investigated by Ramesh *et al.* (1991) who found increased concentrations of IgA, but normal values of IgM, IgG and IgE in PD patients as compared to normal controls. Brambilla *et al.* (1994) detected increased plasma concentrations of IL-1β in PD patients both before and after successful alprazolam therapy, whereas Rapaport and Stein (1994b) found normal serum levels of IL-1β, IL-1α and sIL-2R, with a slight but not significant increase in serum IL-2 levels. The finding of normal serum sIL-2R is consistent with the normal values of $CD25^+$ lymphocytes reported in these patients (Rapaport, 1998). Moreover, blood levels of TNFα in people with PD were reported to be the same as those from normal controls (Brambilla, Bellodi and Perna, 1999). Finally, *in vitro* experiments have shown a decreased production of PHA-induced IL-2 and a normal unstimulated synthesis of IL-2 and IL-3 from PBMC of panic patients (Koh and Lee, 1998; Weizman *et al.*, 1999).

The patient selection is likely the most relevant factor accounting for this discrepancy. Indeed, studies widely differed in the patient populations since they included subjects with or without agoraphobia, previous histories of major depression, and concomitant depressive disorders.

OBSESSIVE–COMPULSIVE DISORDER

Several lines of evidence suggest that some cases of children-onset obsessive–compulsive disorder (OCD) may have an autoimmune aetiology. Swedo *et al.* (1989, 1998) reported an increased incidence of OCD in paediatric patients with Sydenham's chorea, an autoimmune disease of the basal ganglia. These investigators showed that some children may develop obsessive–compulsive symptoms with motor and/or vocal tics in the aftermath of group A beta-haemolytic streptococcal infection, presumably on the basis of antineuronal antibodies, and introduced the term of paediatric autoimmune neuropsychiatric disorders associated with streptococcal infection (PANDAS) to characterize these patients. As in Sydenham's chorea, the pathogenesis of PANDAS is thought to be autoimmune. This idea is supported by the following: (a) autoimmune antibodies reactive with nuclei of the basal ganglia have been detected in some of these patients (Black, Lamke and Walikonis, 1998); (b) a temporal link between symptom exacerbation and streptococcal infection has been described (Allen, Leonard and Swedo, 1995); (c) a progressive clinical improvement has been observed in those patients undergoing antibiotic prophylaxis at dosages effective in preventing recurrent streptococcal infections (Leonard and Swedo, 2001). Furthermore, Murphy *et al.* (1997) found that the B lymphocyte antigen D8/17, a marker of vulnerability to rheumatic fever, was more common in patients with childhood-onset OCD than in comparison subjects, despite the absence of documented Sydenham's chorea or rheumatic fever.

Very recently, a case of a 25-year-old man who developed OCD after a severe antibiotic-responsive pharyngitis and exhibited increased levels of antibodies to group A beta-haemolytic streptococci has been described (Bodner, Morshed and Peterson, 2001). This subject had elevated serum D8/17 lymphocytes, positive antistriatal antibodies and positive anticytoskeletal antibodies. This case report suggests that post-streptococcal OCD may occur also in adult individuals.

Similarly to patients with major depression who produce antibodies against β-endorphin and somatostatin-14 (Roy *et al.*, 1988), patients with OCD have been shown to exhibit high circulating levels of antibodies for somatostatin-14 and prodynorphin 209–240, although the pathophysiological significance of these immune changes has not been clarified (Roy *et al.*, 1994). Finally, Khanna *et al.* (1990, 1997) documented higher levels of IgG in the blood and increased antibodies to herpes virus type-1 in the cerebrospinal fluid of subjects with OCD.

Investigations of cell-mediated and humoral immunity in people with OCD have provided conflicting results. Plasma levels of IL-1β have been reported to be normal by both Maes, Meltzer and Bosmans (1994) and our group (Monteleone *et al.*, 1998), but decreased by Brambilla *et al.* (1997). Serum levels of IL-6, sIL-2R, soluble IL-6 receptor (sIL-6R) and transferrin, an AP protein, have been found to be unchanged (Maes, Meltzer and Bosmans, 1994; Monteleone *et al.*, 1998), whereas plasma concentrations of TNFα have been detected to be reduced (Brambilla *et al.*, 1997; Monteleone *et al.*, 1998). *In vitro* assessment of IL-1β, IL-2 and IL-3 production from unstimulated PBMC of OCD patients did not display any alteration (Weizman *et al.*, 1996). Finally, Barber *et al.* (1996) did not find any change in T-lymphocyte subsets in a small sample of obsessive–compulsive patients, whereas Marazziti *et al.* (1999), in a study involving a larger group of adult patients with OCD, reported a significant increase in $CD8^+$ and a decrease in $CD4^+$ lymphocytes.

POST-TRAUMATIC STRESS DISORDER

Among the anxiety syndromes, post-traumatic stress disorder (PTSD) may be considered the prototype of stress-induced diseases. In fact, by definition, PTSD occurs in response to unusually stressful life events (extreme and catastrophic stresses). Given the above-mentioned relationships between stress events and immune activity, one would expect dramatic changes in immune parameters in people with PTSD.

Watson *et al.* (1993) first reported that Vietnam combat veterans with chronic PTSD, compared with healthy control subjects, had enhanced cell-mediated immunity, as assessed by means of delayed skin responsivity to a panel of antigens (CMI multitest). Ironson *et al.* (1997), instead, found that NK cell cytoxicity, $CD4^+$ and $CD8^+$ cell counts were significantly lower in PTSD patients, while the number of white blood cells was positively and significantly related to the severity of PTSD symptoms. Normal counts of $CD2^+$, $CD4^+$, $CD8^+$, $CD16^+$, $CD20^+$ and $CD56^+$ cell subtypes, and increased activity of NK cell activity were detected by Laudenslager *et al.* (1998) in combat veterans with long-term PTSD. Finally, significantly increased counts of total leukocytes, total lymphocytes,

T cells, $CD4^+$ and $CD8^+$ cell subtypes were reported by Boscarino and Chang (1999) in Vietnam veterans with current PTSD; moreover, in this study, patients exhibited a delayed cutaneous hypersensitivity, as assessed by the CMI multitest. This finding confirmed the occurrence of a delayed skin hypersensitivity in PTSD patients, previously reported by Watson *et al.* (1993). Recently, a normal lymphoproliferative response to PHA, but a reduced blastogenic response to tetanus toxoid (a specific recall antigen recognized by memory T cells) has been found in Gulf War veterans with a diagnosis of PTSD (Everson, Kotler and Blackburn, 1999).

With regard to humoral immunity, increased levels of serum IL-1β and normal values of sIL-2R have been detected in Israeli male veterans with PTSD (Spivak *et al.*, 1997). In this study, serum levels of IL-1β were positively correlated with the duration of the illness. Finally, Maes *et al.* (1999b) reported normal plasma levels of soluble IL-1 receptor antagonist, CC-16, glycoprotein 130 (gp130) and soluble CD8 antigen, but increased concentrations of IL-6 and sIL-6R in subjects with PTSD following accidental man-made traumatic events. Since serum sIL-6R mediates IL-6 signals, while serum gp130 has the potential to inhibit IL-6 signalling, the findings of Maes and coworkers suggest an increased IL-6 signal transducing and, consequently, an activation of the inflammatory response system in PTSD. These results, together with the above-reported observation of increased production of IL-1β in war veterans with PTSD (Spivak *et al.*, 1997), support the idea that proinflammatory cytokines may play a role in the development of anxiety subsequent to stressful traumatic events.

ANTIANXIETY TREATMENTS AND IMMUNE FUNCTION

Drug Treatments

Although several pharmacological agents are commonly used in the treatment of anxiety syndromes, we will focus exclusively on the immune effects of benzodiazepines (BDZs) and selective serotonin reuptake inhibitors (SSRIs), that are actually the most widely prescribed drugs for these disorders.

Benzodiazepines

Evidence that BDZs influence immune function emerged from studies showing the presence of BDZ receptors on immune cells. Peripheral-type BDZ receptors have been detected on immune cells of the experimental animal (Zavala, Haumont and Lenfant, 1984) and on human monocytes, polymorphonuclear neutrophils, B cells, NK cells, $CD4^+$ and $CD8^+$ cells (Canat *et al.*, 1992). It has been shown that activation of these receptors stimulates chemotaxis of human monocytes (Ruff *et al.*, 1985), enhances the production of reactive oxygen species (an essential step in oxygen-dependent phagocytic defence against pathogens) (Zavala and Lenfant, 1988), and modulates the production of proinflammatory cytokines such as IL-1β, TNFα, IL-6, IL-8 and granulocyte/macrophage-colony stimulating factor (Taupin *et al.*, 1991; Zavala *et al.*, 1991). Moreover, peripheral-type BDZ receptors have been detected also on microglial cells, which are considered the resident macrophages of the brain (Bender and Hertz, 1985), and their activation has been shown to enhance the production of IL-1, TNFα and IL-6 in the rat cortex after a fluid percussion trauma (Taupin *et al.*, 1993).

A number of studies suggest that anxiolytic BDZs reverse or attenuate the stress-induced immunosuppression. For example, chronic treatment with alprazolam, diazepam or imidazolam protects mice against the stress-induced decreases in thymus cellularity and weight, blastic response to ConA and NK cell activity (Freire-Garabal *et al.*, 1991a, 1991b). Partially consistent with animal data, Lechin *et al.* (1994) recently reported that chronic BDZ users without psychotic or depressive symptoms had lower-than-normal $CD3^+$, $CD4^+$ and $CD16^+ + CD56^+$ (NK) cell counts with a reduced $CD4^+/CD8^+$ ratio, and enhanced NK cell activity and $CD57^+$ cell number. After 15 days of BDZ discontinuation, some of these immune parameters ($CD3^+$, $CD4^+$ cell counts and NK cell activity) returned to normal values, others ($CD16^+$ cell number) persisted significantly lower than controls, while $CD4^+/CD8^+$ ratio and $CD56^+$ cell number exceeded normal values.

Selective Serotonin Reuptake Inhibitors

There are some indications that both acute and chronic administration of SSRIs may compromise cellular immune responses in the animal. For instance, fluoxetine administration has been reported to increase tumour growth and tumour formation following tumour transplantation and exposure to chemical carcinogens in rodents (Brandes *et al.*, 1992). In addition, acute fluoxetine has been shown to decrease immune cell infiltration and inflammation in rats following exposure to irritants (Bianchi *et al.*, 1995). Finally, either fluoxetine or sertraline have been shown to decrease NK cell cytolytic activity and lymphocyte proliferative responses (Pellegrino and Bayer, 1998; Pellegrino and Bayer, 2000).

Other studies, however, point to an immunopotentiating effect of prolonged administration of SSRIs to experimental animals. Indeed, chronic administration of sertraline has been shown to increase the percentage of neutrophils and enhance the proliferative activity of T-lymphocytes (Song and Leonard, 1994), while chronic treatment with fluoxetine has been reported to inhibit the growth of induced and spontaneous neoplasms in rodents (Bendele *et al.*, 1992; Abdul, Logothetis and Hoosein, 1995). It has been suggested that, at least in animals, SSRIs may exhibit both immunoenhancing and immunosuppressive effects depending on the type of drug and the duration of its administration (Kubera *et al.*, 2000).

With regard to human studies, although a direct assessment of the immune effects of SSRIs in people with anxiety disorders is lacking, there are some data *in vitro* and in depressed patients that support an immunosuppressive action of these drugs. For example, *in vitro* studies have shown that SSRIs decreased splenic lymphocyte proliferation (Berkeley *et al.*, 1994), while coincubation of mitogen-stimulated human immunocytes with fluoxetine, sertraline or citalopram significantly reduced the production of proinflammatory cytokines IL-1β, IL-6, IFNγ and TNFα and/or increased the production of IL-10, an anti-inflammatory cytokine, with a consequent decrease of the IFNγ/IL-10 ratio (Xia, DePierre and Nassberger, 1996; Maes *et al.*, 1999c). Moreover, it has been reported that some patients receiving fluoxetine for the treatment of a depressive condition experienced a reactivation of a herpes simplex infection or developed cutaneous pseudolymphoma lesions, that promptly reverted when the drug was discontinued (Reed and Glick, 1991; Crowson and Magro, 1995). In patients chronically treated with SSRIs, a significant reduction in the number of leukocytes and neutrophils, but no significant changes in the absolute number of PBMC and $CD4^+/CD8^+$ cell ratio have been reported (Maes *et al.*, 1997b; Kubera, Van Bockstaele and Maes, 1999). Moreover, subchronic treatment with fluoxetine has been shown to normalize the pathologically elevated blood levels of IL-6, α_1-acid glycoprotein and IL-2R in major depression (Maes *et al.*, 1995; Sluzewska *et al.*, 1995). To the contrary, a 12-week treatment with sertraline has been reported to not affect the abnormally increased plasma concentrations of IL-1β in dysthymic subjects (Anisman *et al.*, 1999), while both fluoxetine and fluvoxamine, administered for 3 months, did not influence plasma levels of IL-1β, IL-6 and TNFα in people with eating disorders (Brambilla *et al.*, 1998).

The exact mechanisms by which SSRIs exert their activity on immune functions are still unknown. It has been suggested that the immune effects of SSRIs are mediated by endogenously released serotonin (5-HT). Indeed, in animals depleted of endogenous 5-HT stores, the administration of both fluoxetine and sertraline was not able to reduce lymphocyte proliferative responses (Pellegrino and Bayer, 2000). Moreover, it has been shown that T-lymphocytes constitutively express 5-HT receptors as well as the high-affinity 5-HT transporter system (Aune, Golden and McGrath, 1994; Faraj, Olkowski and Jackson, 1994).

Psychotherapeutic Interventions

Further to initial reports of immune effects of hypnosis (Ullman, 1947; Black, 1963; Black, Humphrey and Niven, 1963), the effects of psychotherapeutic interventions on immune function have been assessed in two categories of subjects: (a) patients dealing with different types of cancer; (b) healthy subjects exposed to different kinds of stressors.

The effects of short-term (6 weeks) structured cognitive-behavioural therapy on immune parameters were evaluated by Fawzy *et al.* (1990) in patients with post-surgical malignant melanoma. At the sixth-month evaluation point, along with a reduction in levels of psychological distress and greater use of active coping methods, patients in the intervention group exhibited significant increases in the percent of large granular lymphocytes and NK cells along with an increase in NK cytotoxic activity and a small decrease in the percent of $CD4^+$ cells. In post-surgical early-stage breast cancer patients, a 10-week cognitive-behavioural intervention programme induced a significant increase in the number of circulating lymphocytes (Schedlowski *et al.*, 1994). Finally, in the study of van der Pompe *et al.* (1997), cancer patients who had been treated for early-stage breast cancer and were diagnosed with either positive axillary lymph nodes or distant metastases, were assigned to a 13-week experimental–existential group psychotherapy (EEGP) or to a waiting list control condition (WLC). EEGP patients with a higher percentage of $CD4^+$, $CD8^+$ and $CD16^+/56^+$ T-lymphocytes at baseline had lower post-treatment percentages than their counterparts in the WLC with similar initial levels. Similarly, those EEGP patients with the highest lymphoproliferative response to PWM at baseline had smaller post-treatment responses than patients in the WLC. These authors, on the basis of literature suggestions showing that lower percentages of NK and $CD8^+$ cells were associated with a better prognosis in cancer patients, speculated that EEGP by normalizing increased immune parameters may positively affect the outcome of these patients.

Several groups have studied the effects of psychotherapeutic interventions on stress-induced immune changes. After a 1-month intervention period, geriatric patients who received relaxation training reported a decrease in distress symptoms coupled with increased NK cell cytotoxicity and decreased antibody titres to latent herpes simplex virus (Kiecolt-Glaser *et al.*, 1985). In a study by Peavy, Lawlis and Goven (1985), in subjects with high life stress scores coupled with poor phagocytic capacity, a biofeedback-assisted relaxation training significantly enhanced neutrophil activation capacity, suggesting a qualitative improvement of phagocytic ability. In a subsequent study (Green and Green, 1987) a single 20-minute relaxation session resulted in a significant increase in salivary IgA concentrations. Finally, in males at high risk for HIV-1 infection, significant positive correlations were found between the frequency of relaxation procedures and the number of $CD4^+$, $CD8^+$, NK cells and the $CD4^+/CD8^+$ ratio during the high stress week of serostatus determination (Antoni *et al.*, 1990).

Two studies examined the effects of self-hypnosis/relaxation intervention on immune changes induced by academic examination stress in medical students. The first one (Kiecolt-Glaser *et al.*, 1986) showed that the hypnosis/relaxation programme prevented exam-related increases in distress symptoms, but did not influence immune parameters. Indeed, both the intervention and control groups showed significant decreases in the percentages of $CD4^+$ lymphocytes and NK cell activity at the examination time; however, the frequency of the relaxation procedures was a good predictor of the increases in the $CD4^+/CD8^+$ cell ratio during the exam period. The second study (Whitehouse *et al.*, 1996) demonstrated that significant increases in the number of B lymphocytes, activated T-lymphocytes, PHA-induced and PWM-induced blastogenesis and NK cytotoxicity occurred during the examination period in both students assigned to a self-hypnosis/relaxation intervention and in those assigned to the control group. Nevertheless, within the self-hypnosis group, the quality of relaxation exercises predicted both the number of NK cells and their cytotoxicity.

Finally, it has been very recently reported that, in medical students undergoing academic examination, massage therapy induced a significant increase in the total number of white blood cells with a decrease in the percentage of T cells, no significant changes in the lymphocyte responses to mitogens and a significant increase in the killing activity of NK cells (Zeitlin *et al.*, 2000).

CONCLUSIONS

The existing literature is highly controversial and fraught with several methodological problems. The diagnostic heterogeneity of the subject samples is certainly one of the most relevant factors contributing to the inconsistency of the results. Indeed, in some studies patients were suffering from pure anxiety disorders, in others patients had concomitant major depressive disorder or positive histories of previous depressive episodes. Moreover, most of the studies did not include healthy controls matched to patients on age and gender; as there may be age-dependent alterations (Weksler, 1983) and gender-specific differences (Oyeyinka, 1984) in immune function, these factors must be taken into account in this kind of research. Furthermore, patients differed on the duration and/or severity of the illness, personality characteristics and treatment status. This last variable is particularly relevant in light of the immune effects of both BZD and psychotherapeutic techniques. Differences in both methodology (e.g., evaluation of absolute number of lymphocytes versus lymphocyte percentages, assay techniques) and/or immune parameters investigated may also add to the variability of results. Finally, smoking, excessive drinking, disturbed sleep and poor nutrition are known to affect immune function (Locke and Gorman, 1989), hence variations of these behaviours may further explain controversies among the studies.

All these factors limit the interpretation and generalization of the findings. Notwithstanding, there is unequivocal evidence that immune changes do occur in anxiety disorders, with the majority of studies suggesting an impairment of the immune function in these syndromes. Only PTSD seems to be associated with an immune enhancement rather than immunosuppression. It has been suggested that the increase in immune activity in patients with PTSD may have a pathogenetic role (Spivak *et al.*, 1997; Maes *et al.*, 1999b). Moreover, there is consistent evidence that at least some cases of childhood-onset OCD may have an autoimmune aetiology, possibly linked to the streptococcal infection and rheumatic fever. Finally, it has been almost uniformly reported that psychotherapeutic interventions aiming to alleviate anxiety symptoms potentiate immune functions, whereas antianxiety drugs may have both immunoenhancing and immunosuppressive effects.

In conclusion, whether in anxiety disorders immune changes occur as a consequence of the psychological distress or are primitive and aetiopathogenetically linked to the disorders themselves, it becomes more evident every day that they are part of the biological substrate of these syndromes and, as such, they are worthy of every effort by both clinicians and researchers in order to better understand their implications in the course and the treatment of anxiety disorders.

REFERENCES

Abdul, M., Logothetis, C.J. and Hoosein, N.M., 1995. Growth-inhibitory effects of serotonin uptake inhibitors on human prostate carcinoma cell lines. *Journal of Urology*, **131**, 925–929.

Allen, A.J., Leonard, H.L. and Swedo, S.E., 1995. Case study: A new infection-triggered, autoimmune subtype of pediatric OCD and Tourette's Syndrome. *Journal of the American Academy of Child and Adolescent Psychiatry*, **34**, 307–311.

Andreoli, A., Keller, S.E., Rabaeus, M., Zaugg, L., Garrone, G. and Taban, C., 1992. Immunity, major depression, and panic disorder comorbidity. *Biological Psychiatry*, **31**, 896–908.

Anisman, H., Kokkinidis, L., Borowski, T. and Merali, Z., 1998. Differential effects of interleukin (IL)-1beta, IL-2 and IL-6 on responding for rewarding lateral hypothalamic stimulation. *Brain Research*, **779**, 177–187.

Anisman, H., Ravindran, A.V., Griffiths, J. and Merali, Z., 1999. Interleukin-1β production in dysthymia before and after pharmacotherapy. *Biological Psychiatry*, **46**, 1649–1655.

Antoni, M.H., August, S.M., LaPerriere, A., Baggett, H.L., Klimas, N., Ironson, G., Shneiderman, N. and Fletcher, M.A., 1990. Psychological and neuroendocrine measures related to functional immune changes in anticipation of HIV-1 serostatus notification. *Psychosomatic Medicine*, **52**, 496–510.

Arnetz, B.B., Wasserman, J., Petrini, B., Brenner, O., Levi, L., Eneroth, P., Salovaara, H., Hielm, R., Salovaara, L., Theorell, T. and Petterson, L., 1987. Immune function in unemployed women. *Psychosomatic Medicine*, **49**, 3–12.

Aune, T.M., Golden, H.W. and McGrath, K.M., 1994. Inhibitors of serotonin synthesis and antagonists of serotonin 1A receptors inhibit T lymphocyte function *in vitro* and cell-mediated immunity *in vivo*. *Journal of Immunology*, **153**, 489–498.

Bachen, E.A., Manuck, S.B., Marsland, A.L., Cohen, S., Malkoff, S.B., Muldoon, M.F. and Rabin, B.S., 1992. Lymphocyte subset and cellular immune responses to a brief experimental stressor. *Psychosomatic Medicine*, **54**, 673–679.

Barber, Y., Toren, P., Achiron, A., Noy, S., Wolmer, L., Weizman, R. and Laor, N., 1996. T cell subsets in obsessive–compulsive disorder. *Neuropsychobiology*, **34**, 63–66.

Bendele, R.A., Adams, E.R., Hoffman, W.P., Gries, C.L. and Morton, D.M., 1992. Carcinogenicity studies of fluoxetine hydrochloride in rats and mice. *Cancer Research*, **52**, 6931–6935.

Bender, A.S. and Hertz, L., 1985. Pharmacological evidence that the non-neural diazepam binding site in primary cultures of glial cells is associated with a calcium channel. *European Journal of Pharmacology*, **110**, 287–288.

Berkeley, M.B., Daussin, S., Hernandez, M.C. and Bayer, B.M., 1994. *In vitro* effects of cocaine, lidocaine, and monoamine uptake inhibitors on lymphocyte proliferative responses. *Immunopharmacology and Immunotoxicology*, **16**, 165–178.

Bianchi, M., Rossini, G., Sacerdote, P., Panerai, A.E. and Berti, F., 1995. Effects of chlormipramine and fluoxetine in subcutaneous carrageenin-induced inflammation in the rat. *Inflammation Research*, **66**, 466–469.

Black, S., 1963. Inhibition of immediate-type hypersensitivity by direct suggestion under hypnosis. *British Medical Journal*, **1**, 925–928.

Black, S., Humphrey, J.H. and Niven, J., 1963. Inhibition of the Mantoux reaction by direct suggestion under hypnosis. *British Medical Journal*, **1**, 1649.

Black, J.L., Lamke, G.T. and Walikonis, J.E., 1998. Serologic survey of adult patients with obsessive–compulsive disorder for neuron-specific and other antibodies. *Psychiatry Research*, **81**, 371–380.

Bodner, S.M., Morshed, S.A. and Peterson, B.S., 2001. The question of PANDAS in adults. *Biological Psychiatry*, **49**, 807–810.

Boscarino, J. and Chang, J., 1999. Higher abnormal leukocyte and lymphocyte counts 20 years after exposure to severe stress: research and clinical implications. *Psychosomatic Medicine*, **61**, 378–386.

Bosch, J.A., Brand, H.S., Ligtenberg, T.J.M., Bermond, B., Hoogstraten, J. and Nieuw Amerongen, A.V., 1996. Psychological stress as a determinant of protein levels and salivary-induced aggregation of streptococcus gordonii in human whole saliva. *Psychological Medicine*, **58**, 374–382.

Brambilla, F., Bellodi, L. and Perna, G., 1999. Plasma levels of tumor necrosis factor-alpha in patients with panic disorder: effect of alprazolam therapy. *Psychiatry Research*, **89**, 21–27.

Brambilla, F., Bellodi, L., Brunetta, M. and Perna, G., 1998. Plasma concentrations of interleukin-1β, interleukin-6 and tumor necrosis factor-α in anorexia and bulimia nervosa. *Psychoneuroendocrinology*, **23**, 439–447.

Brambilla, F., Bellodi, L., Perna, G., Bertani, A., Panerai, A. and Sacerdote, P., 1994. Plasma interleukin-1 beta concentrations in panic disorder. *Psychiatry Research*, **54**, 135–142.

Brambilla, F., Perna, G., Bellodi, L., Arancio, C., Bertani, A., Perini, G., Carraro, C. and Gava, F., 1997. Plasma interleukin-1beta and tumor necrosis factor concentrations in obsessive-compulsive disorders. *Biological Psychiatry*, **42**, 976–981.

Brambilla, F., Bellodi, L., Perna, G., Battaglia, M., Sciuto, G., Diaferia, G., Petraglia, F., Panerai, A. and Sacerdote, P., 1992. Psychoimmunoendocrine aspects of panic disorder. *Neuropsychobiology*, **26**, 12–22.

Brandes, L.J., Arron, R.J., Bogdanevic, R.P., Tong, J., Zaborniak, C.L., Hogg, G.R., Warrington, R.C., Fang, W. and Labella, F.S., 1992. Stimulation of malignant growth in rodents by antidepressant drugs at clinically relevant doses. *Cancer Research*, **52**, 3796–3800.

Brosschot, J.F., Benshop, R.J., Godaert, G.L.R., Olff, M., de Smet, M., Heijnen, C.J. and Ballieux, R.E., 1992. Effects of experimental psychological stress on distribution and function of peripheral blood cells. *Psychosomatic Medicine*, **54**, 394–406.

Canat, X., Carayon, P., Bouaboula, M., Cahard, D., Shire, D., Roque, C., Le Fur, G. and Casellas, P., 1992. Distribution profile and properties of peripheral-type benzodiazepine receptors on human hemopoietic cells. *Life Sciences*, **52**, 107–118.

Castilla-Cortazar, I., Castilla, A. and Gurpegui, M., 1998. Opioid peptides and immunodysfunction in patients with major depression and anxiety disorders. *Journal of Physiology and Biochemistry*, **54**, 203–216.

Covelli, V., Munno, I., Altamura, M., Pellegrino, N.M., Decandia, P. and Jirillo, E., 1990. Administration of thymopentin to patients with phobic disorders improves depressed phagocytic functions. *Immunopharmacology and Immunotoxicology*, **12**, 619–631.

Crowson, A.N. and Magro, C.M., 1995. Antidepressant therapy: a possible cause of atypical cutaneous lymphoid hyperplasia. *Archives of Dermatology*, **131**, 925–929.

Dantzer, R. and Mormede, P., 1995. Psychoneuroimmunology of stress. In: Leonard, B.E. and Miller, K. (eds), *Stress, the Immune System and Psychiatry*, pp. 48–83. Wiley, Chichester.

Dantzer, R., Bluthé, R.M., Laye, S., Gret-Dibat, J.L., Parnet, P. and Kelley, K.W., 1998. Cytokines and sickness behaviour. *Annals of New York Academy of Sciences*, **840**, 586–590.

Dekaris, D., Sabioncello, A., Mazuran, R., Rabatic, S., Svoboda-Beusan, I., Racunika, N.L. and Tomasic, J., 1993. Multiple changes of immunological parameters in prisoners of war. *Journal of the American Medical Association*, **270**, 595–599.

Dobbin, J.P., Harth, M., McCain, G.A., Martin, R.A. and Cousin, K., 1991. Cytokine production and lymphocyte transformation during stress. *Brain Behaviour and Immunity*, **5**, 339–348.

Dugué, B., Lappanen, E.A., Teppo, A.M., Fyrquist, F. and Grasbeck, R., 1993. Effects of psychological stress on plasma interleukins-1 and beta and 6, C-reactive protein, tumor necrosis factor alpha, anti-diuretic hormone and serum cortisol. *Scandinavian Journal of Clinical and Laboratory Investigation*, **56**, 555–561.

Everson, M.P., Kotler, S. and Blackburn, W.D., 1999. Stress and immune dysfunction in Gulf war veterans. In: Cutolo, M., Masi, A.T., Bijlsma, J.W., Chikanza, I.C., Bradlow, H.L. and Castagnetta, L. (eds), *Neuroendocrine Immune Basis of the Rheumatic Diseases*, pp. 413–418. The New York Academy of Sciences, New York.

Faraj, B.A., Olkowski, Z.L. and Jackson, R.T., 1994. Expression of a high-affinity serotonin transporter in human lymphocytes. *International Journal of Immunopharmacology*, **16**, 561–567.

Fawzy, F.I., Kemeny, M.E., Fawzy, N.W., Elashoff, R., Morton, D., Cousins, N. and Fahey, J.L., 1990. A structured psychiatric intervention for cancer patients. *Archives of General Psychiatry*, **47**, 729–735.

Fittschen, B., Schulz, K.-H., Schulz, H., Raedler, A. and Kerekjarto, M., 1990. Changes of immunological parameters in healthy subjects under examination stress. *International Journal of Neuroscience*, **51**, 241–242.

Fredrikson, M., Furst, C.J., Lekander, M., Rotstein, S. and Blomgren, H., 1993. Trait anxiety and anticipatory immune reactions in women receiving adjuvant chemotherapy for breast cancer. *Brain Behavior and Immunity*, **7**, 79–90.

Freire-Garabal, M., Belmonte, A., Orallo, F., Couceiro, J. and Nunez, M.J., 1991a. Effects of alprazolam on T-cell immunosuppressive response to surgical stress in mice. *Cancer Letters*, **58**, 183–187.

Freire-Garabal, M., Couceiro, J., Balboa, J.L., Nunez, M.J., Fernandez-Rial, J.C., Cimadevila, B., Gutierrez, C., Loza, M.I. and Belmonte, A., 1991b. Effects of diazepam on the resistance, on the development of immunity and on the passive transfer of immunity to *Listeria* monocytogenes in mice submitted to surgical stress. *Acta Therapeutica*, **17**, 355–362.

Gerritsen, W., Heijnen, C.J., Wiegant, V.M., Bermond, B. and Frijda, N.H., 1996. Experimental social fear: immunological, hormonal and autonomic concomitants. *Psychosomatic Medicine*, **58**, 273–286.

Glaser, R., Kiecolt-Glaser, J.K., Stout, J.C., Tarr, K.L., Speicher, C.E. and Holliday, J.E., 1985. Stress-induced impairments in cellular immunity. *Psychiatry Research*, **16**, 233–239.

Gonzales-Quijano, M.I., Martin, M., Millàn, S. and Lòpez-Calderòn, A., 1998. Lymphocyte response to mitogens: influence of life events and personality. *Neuropsychobiology*, **38**, 90–96.

Graham, N., Bartohlomeuse, R., Taboonpong, N. and Labrody, T., 1988. Does anxiety reduce the secretion rate of secretory IgA in saliva? *Medical Journal of Australia*, **148**, 131–133.

Green, R.G. and Green, M.L., 1987. Relaxation increases salivary immunoglobulin A. *Psychology of Reproduction*, **61**, 623–629.

Ironson, G., Wynings, C., Schneiderman, N., Baum, A., Rodriguez, M., Greenwood, D., Benight, C., Antoni, M., LaPerriere, A., Huang, H., Klimas, N. and Fletcher, M.A., 1997. Posttraumatic stress symptoms, intrusive thoughts, loss, and immune function after hurricane Andrew. *Psychosomatic Medicine*, **59**, 128–141.

Jemmott, J., Borysenko, M. and Chapman, R., 1983. Academic stress, power motivation and decrease in secretion rate of salivary secretory immunoglobulin A. *Lancet*, **i**, 1400–1402.

Jemmott, J.B. and Magloire, K., 1988. Academic stress, social support, and secretory immunoglobulin A. *Journal of Personality and Social Psychology*, **55**, 803–810.

Khanna, S., Ravi, V., Shenoy, P.K., Chandramuki, A. and Channabasavanna, S.M., 1997. Cerebrospinal fluid viral antibodies in obsessive–compulsive disorder in an Indian population. *Biological Psychiatry*, **41**, 883–890.

Kiecolt-Glaser, J.K., Fisher, L.D., Ogrocki, P., Stout, J.C., Speicher, C.E. and Glaser, R., 1987. Marital quality, marital disruption, and immune function. *Psychosomatic Medicine*, **49**, 13–34.

Kiecolt-Glaser, J.K., Glaser, R., Strain, E.C., Stout, J.C., Tarr, K.L., Holliday, J.E. and Speicher, C.E., 1986. Modulation of cellular immunity in medical students. *Journal of Behavioral Medicine*, **9**, 5–21.

Kiecolt-Glaser, J.K., Glaser, R., Williger, D., Stout, J., Messick, G., Sheppard, S., Ricker, D., Romisher, S.C., Briner, W. and Bonnell, G., 1985. Psychosocial enhancement of immunocompetence in a geriatric population. *Healthy Psychology*, **4**, 25–41.

Kissen, D.M., 1958. *Emotional Factors in Pulmonary Tuberculosis*. Tavistok, London.

Koh, K.B., 1993. The relationship between stress and natural killer-cell activity in medical college students. *Korean Journal of Psychosomatic Medicine*, **3**, 3–10.

Koh, K.B., 1997. Exam stress enhances lymphocyte proliferation. 14th World Congress of Psychosomatic Medicine (abstract).

Koh, K.B., 1998. Emotion and immunity. *Journal of Psychosomatic Research*, **45**, 107–115.

Koh, K.B. and Lee, B.K., 1998. Reduced lymphocyte proliferation and interleukin-2 production in anxiety disorders. *Psychosomatic Medicine*, **60**, 479–483.

Kubera, M., Van Bockstaele, D. and Maes, M., 1999. Leukocyte subsets in treatment resistant major depression. *Polish Journal of Pharmacology*, **51**, 547–549.

Kubera, M., Simbirtsev, A., Mathison, R. and Maes, M., 2000. Effects of repeated fluoxetine and citalopram administration on cytokine release in C57BL/6 mice. *Psychiatry Research*, **96**, 255–266.

La Via, M.F., Workman, E.W. and Lydiard, R.B., 1992. Subtype response to stress-induced immunodepression. *Functional Neurology*, **7**(Suppl. 3), 19–22.

La Via, M.F., Munno, I., Lydiard, R.B., Workman, E.W., Hubbard, J.R., Michel, Y. and Paulling, E., 1996. The influence of stress intrusion on immunodepression in generalized anxiety disorder patients and controls. *Psychosomatic Medicine*, **58**, 138–142.

Laudenslager, M.L., Aasal, R., Adler, L., Berger, C.L., Montgomery, P.T., Sandberg, E., Wahlberg, L.J., Wilkins, R.T., Zweig, L. and Reite, M.L., 1998. Elevated cytotoxicity in combat veterans with long-term post-traumatic stress disorder: preliminary observations. *Brain Behavior and Immunity*, **12**, 74–79.

Lechin, F., van der Dijs, B., Vitelli-Flores, G., Benarez, S., Lechin, M.E., Lechin, A.E., Orozco, B., Rada, I., Leòn, G. and Jimenez, V., 1994. Peripheral blood immunological parameters in long-term benzodiazepine users. *Clinical Neuropharmacology*, **17**, 63–72.

Leonard, H.L. and Swedo, S.E., 2001. Pediatric autoimmune neuropsychiatric disorders associated with streptococcal infection (PANDAS). *International Journal of Neuropsychopharmacology*, **4**, 191–198.

Linn, B.S., Linn, M.W. and Jensen, J., 1981. Anxiety and immune responsiveness. *Psychological Reports*, **49**, 969–970.

Locke, S.E. and Gorman, J.R., 1989. Behavior and immunity. In: Kaplan, H.I. and Sadock, B.J. (eds), *Comprehensive Textbook of Psychiatry*, pp. 1240–1249. Williams & Wilkins, Baltimore, Maryland.

Maes, M., Meltzer, H.Y. and Bosmans, E., 1994. Psychoimmune investigation in obsessive–compulsive disorder: assays of plasma transferrin, IL-2 and IL-6 receptor, and IL-1beta and IL-6 concentrations. *Neuropsychobiology*, **30**, 57–60.

Maes, M., Meltzer, H.Y., Bosmans, E., Bergmans, R., Vandoolaeghe, E., Ranjan, R. and Desnyder, R., 1995. Increased plasma concentrations of interleukin-6, soluble interleukin-6, soluble interleukin-2 and transferrin receptor in major depression. *Journal of Affective Disorders*, **34**, 301–309.

Maes, M., Hendriks, D., Van Gastel, A., Demedts, P., Wauters, A., Neels, H., Janca, A. and Scharp, S., 1997a. Effects of psychological stress on serum immunoglobulin, complement and acute phase protein concentrations in normal volunteers. *Psychoneuroendocrinology*, **22**, 397–409.

Maes, M., Vandoolaeghe, E., Van Hunsel, F., Bril, T., Demedts, P., Wauters, A. and Neels, H., 1997b. Immune disturbances in treatment-resistant depression: modulation by antidepressive treatment. *Human Psychopharmacology*, **12**, 153–162.

Maes, M., Song, C., Lin, A., DeJongh, R., Van Gastel, A., Kenis, G., Bosman, E., De Meester, I., Benoy, I., Neels, H., Demedts, P., Ianca, A., Scharpé, S. and Smith, R.S., 1998. The effects of psychological stress on humans: increased production of proinflammatory cytokines and a Th1-like response in stress-induced anxiety. *Cytokine*, **10**, 310–318.

Maes, M., Van Bockstaele, D., Van Gastel, A., Van Hunsel, F., Neels, H., DeMeester, I., Scharpé, S. and Janca, A., 1999a. Influence of psychological stress on leukocyte subset distribution in normal humans: evidence for interrelated immunosuppression and T cell activation. *Neuropsychobiology*, **39**, 1–9.

Maes, M., Lin, A., Delmeire, L., Van Gastel, A., Kenis, G., De Jongh, R. and Bosmans, E., 1999b. Elevated serum interleukin-6 (IL-6) and IL-6 receptor concentrations in posttraumatic stress disorder following accidental man-made traumatic events. *Biological Psychiatry*, **45**, 833–839.

Maes, M., Song, C., Lin, A.-H., Bonaccorso, S., Kenis, G., De Jongh, R., Bosmans, E. and Scharpé, S., 1999c. Negative immunoregulatory effects of antidepressants: inhibition of interferon-γ and stimulation of interleukin-10 secretion. *Neuropsychopharmacology*, **20**, 370–379.

Marazziti, D., Ambrogi, F., Vanacore, R., Mignani, V., Savino, M., Palego, L., Cassano, G.B. and Akiskal, H.S., 1992. Immune cell imbalance in major depressive and panic disorders. *Neuropsychobiology*, **26**, 23–26.

Marazziti, D., Presta, S., Pfanner, C., Gemignani, A., Rossi, A., Sbrana, S., Rocchi, V., Ambrogi, F. and Cassano, G.B., 1999. Immunological alterations in adult obsessive–compulsive disorder. *Biological Psychiatry*, **46**, 810–814.

Monteleone, P., Catapano, F., Fabrazzo, M., Tortorella, A. and Maj, M., 1998. Decreased blood levels of tumor necrosis factor-alpha in patients with obsessive-compulsive disorder. *Neuropsychobiology*, **37**, 182–185.

Murphy, T.K., Goodman, W.K., Fudge, M.W., Williams, R.C., Ayoub, E.M., Dalal, M., Lewis, M.K. and Zabriskie, J.B., 1997. B Lymphocyte antigen D8/17: a peripheral marker for childhood-onset obsessive–compulsive disorder and Tourrette's Syndrome? *American Journal of Psychiatry*, **154**, 402–407.

Oyeyinka, G.O., 1984. Age and sex difference in immunocompetence. *Gerontology*, **30**, 188–195.

Peavy, B.S., Lawlis, G.F. and Goven, A., 1985. Biofeedback assisted relaxation: effect on phagocytic capacity. *Biofeedback Self Regulation*, **10**, 33–47.

Pellegrino, T.C. and Bayer, B.M., 1998. Modulation of immune cell function following fluoxetine administration in rats. *Pharmacology, Biochemistry and Behavior*, **59**, 151–157.

Pellegrino, T.C. and Bayer, B.M., 2000. Specific serotonin reuptake inhibitor-induced decreases in lymphocyte activity require endogenous serotonin release. *Neuroimmunomodulation*, **8**, 179–187.

Perini, G.I., Zara, M., Carraro, C., Tosin, C., Gava, F., Santucci, M.G., Valverde, S. and De Franchis, G., 1995. Psychoimmunoendocrine aspects of panic disorders. *Human Psychopharmacology*, **10**, 461–465.

Ramesh, C., Yeragani, V.K., Balon, R. and Pohl, R., 1991. A comparative study of immune status in panic disorder patients and controls. *Acta Psychiatrica Scandinava*, **84**, 396–197.

Rapaport, M.H., 1998. Circulating lymphocyte phenotypic surface markers in anxiety disorder patients and normal volunteers. *Biological Psychiatry*, **43**, 458–463.

Rapaport, M.H. and Stein, M.B., 1994a. Serum interleukin-2 and soluble interleukin-2 receptor levels in generalized social phobia. *Anxiety*, **1**, 50–53.

Rapaport, M.H. and Stein, M.B., 1994b. Serum cytokine and soluble interleukin-2 receptors in patients with panic disorder. *Anxiety*, **1**, 22–25.

Reed, S.M. and Glick, J.W., 1991. Fluoxetine and reactivation of the herpes simplex virus. *American Journal of Psychiatry*, **148**, 949–950.

Roy, B.F., Rose, J.W., Sunderland, T., Morihisa, J.M. and Murphy, D.L., 1988. Anti-somatostatin immunoglobulin G in major depressive disorder: a preliminary study with implications for an autoimmune mechanism of depression. *Archives of General Psychiatry*, **45**, 924–928.

Roy, B.F., Benkelfat, C., Hill, J.L., Pierce, P.F., Dauphin, M.M., Kelly, T.M., Sunderland, T., Weinberger, D.R. and Breslin, N., 1994. Serum antibody for somatostatin-14 and prodynorphin 209–240 in patients with obsessive–compulsive disorder, schizophrenia, Alzheimer's disease, multiple sclerosis, and advanced HIV infection. *Biological Psychiatry*, **35**, 335–344.

Ruff, M.R., Pert, C.B., Weber, R.J., Wahl, L.M., Wahl, S.M. and Paul, S.M., 1985. Benzodiazepine receptor-mediated chemotaxis of human monocytes. *Science*, **229**, 1281–1283.

Schedlowski, M., Jung, C., Schimanski, G., Tewes, U. and Schmoll, H.J., 1994. Effects of behavioral intervention on plasma cortisol and lymphocytes in breast cancer patients: an exploratory study. *Psychooncology*, **3**, 181–187.

Schleifer, S.J., Keller, S.E., Scott, B.J. and Vecchione, J., 1990. Lymphocyte function in panic disorder. *Biological Psychiatry*, **27**(Suppl. 9A), 66A.

Schleifer, S.J., Keller, S.E., Camerino, M., Thornton, J.C. and Stein, M., 1983. Suppression of lymphocyte stimulation following bereavement. *Journal of the American Medical Association*, **250**, 374–377.

Segerstrom, S.C., Glover, D.A., Craske, M.G. and Fahey, J.L., 1999. Worry affects the immune response to phobic fear. *Brain Behaviour and Immunity*, **13**, 80–92.

Sluzewska, A., Rybakowski, J.K., Laciak, M., Mackiewicz, A., Sobieska, M. and Wiktorowiz, K., 1995. Interleukin-6 serum levels in depressed patients before and after treatment with fluoxetine. *Annals of New York Academy of Sciences*, **762**, 474–476.

Song, C. and Leonard, B.E., 1994. An acute phase protein response in the olfactory bulbectomized rat: effect of sertraline treatment. *Medical Science Research*, **22**, 313–314.

Song, C., Kenis, G., Van Gastel, A., Bosmans, E., Lin, A., De Jong, R., Neels, H., Scharp, S., Janca, A., Yasukawa, K. and Maes, M., 1999. Influence of psychological stress on immune-inflammatory variables in normal humans. Part II. Altered serum concentrations of natural anti-inflammatory agents and soluble membrane antigens of monocytes and T-lymphocytes. *Psychiatry Research*, **85**, 293–303.

Spivak, B., Shohat, B., Mester, R., Avraham, S., Gil-Ad, I., Bleich, A., Valevski, A. and Weizman, A., 1997. Elevated levels of serum interleukin-1beta in combat-related posttraumatic stress disorder. *Biological Psychiatry*, **42**, 345–348.

Surman, O.S., Williams, J., Sheean, D.V., Strom, T.B., Jones, K.J. and Coleman, J., 1986. Immunological Response to stress in agoraphobia and panic attacks. *Biological Psychiatry*, **21**, 768–774.

Swedo, S.E., Rapoport, J.L., Cheslow, D.L., Leonard, H.L., Ayoub, E.M., Hosier, D.M. and Wald, E.R., 1989. High prevalence of obsessive–compulsive symptoms in patients with Sydehnam's Chorea. *American Journal of Psychiatry*, **146**, 246–249.

Swedo, S.E., Leonard, H.L., Garvey, M., Mittleman, B., Allen, A.J., Perlmutter, S., Lougee, L., Dow, S., Zamkoff, J. and Dubbert, B.K., 1998. Pediatric autoimmune neuropsychiatric disorders associated with streptococcal infections: clinical description of the first 50 cases. *American Journal of Psychiatry*, **155**, 264–271.

Taupin, V., Toulmond, S., Serrano, A., Benavides, J. and Zavala, F., 1993. Increase in IL-6, IL-1 and TNF levels in rat brain following traumatic lesion: influence of pre- and posttraumatic treatment with Ro54864, a peripheral type (p site) benzodiazepine ligand. *Journal of Neuroimmunology*, **42**, 177–185.

Taupin, V., Jayais, P., Descamps-Latscha, B., Cazalaa, J.B., Barrier, G., Bach, J.F. and Zavala, F., 1991. Benzodiazepine anaesthesia in humans modulates the interleukin-1 beta, tumor necrosis factor-alpha and interleukin-6 responses of blood monocytes. *Journal of Neuroimmunology*, **35**, 13–19.

Ullman, M., 1947. Herpes simplex and second degree burn induced under hypnosis. *American Journal of Psychiatry*, **103**, 828–830.

Van der Pompe, G., Duivenvoorden, H.J., Antoni, M.H., Visser, A. and Heljnen, C.J., 1997. Effectiveness of a short-term group psychotherapy program on endocrine and immune function in breast cancer patients: an exploratory study. *Journal of Psychosomatic Research*, **42**, 453–466.

Watson, I.P.B., Muller, H.K., Jones, I.H. and Bradley, A.J., 1993. Cell-mediated immunity in combat veterans with post-traumatic stress disorder. *Medical Journal of Australia*, **159**, 513–516.

Weiss, D.W., Hirt, R., Tarcic, N., Berzon, Y., Ben-Zur, H., Breznitz, S., Glaser, B., Grover, N.B., Baras, M. and O'Dorisio, T.M., 1996. Studies in psychoneuroimmunology: psychological, immunological, and neuroendocrinological parameters in Israeli civilians during and after a period of Scud missile attack. *Behavioral Medicine*, **22**, 5–14.

Weizman, R., Laor, N., Wiener, Z., Wolmer, N. and Bessler, H., 1999. Cytokine production in panic disorder patients. *Clinical Neuropharmacology*, **22**, 107–109.

Weizman, R., Laor, N., Barber, Y., Hermesh, H., Notti, I., Djaldetti, M. and Bessler, H., 1996. Cytokine production in obsessive–compulsive disorder. *Biological Psychiatry*, **40**, 908–912.

Weksler, M.E., 1983. Senescence of the immune system. *Medical Clinic of North America*, **67**, 263–272.

Whitehouse, W.G., Dinges, D.F., Orne, E.C., Keller, S.E., Bates, B.L., Bauer, N.K., Morahan, P., Haupt, B.A., Carlin, M.M., Bloom, P.B., Zaugg, L. and Orne, M.T., 1996. Psychosocial and immune effects of self-hypnosis training for stress management throughout the first semester of the medical school. *Psychosomatic Medicine*, **58**, 249–263.

Xia, Z., DePierre, J.W. and Nassberger, L., 1996. Tricyclic antidepressants inhibit IL-6, IL-1β and TNF-α release in human blood monocytes and IL-2 and interferon-γ in T cells. *Immunopharmacology*, **34**, 27–37.

Zavala, F. and Lenfant, M., 1988. Peripheral benzodiazepines enhance the respiratory burst of macrophage-like P388D1 cells stimulated by arachidonic acid. *International Journal of Immunopharmacology*, **9**, 269–274.

Zavala, F., Haumont, J. and Lenfant, M., 1984. Interaction of benzodiazepines with mouse macrophages. *European Journal of Pharmacology*, **106**, 561–566.

Zavala, F., Masson, A., Brys, L., de Baerselier, P. and Descamps-Latscha, B., 1991. A monoclonal antibody against peripheral benzodiazepine receptor activates the human neutrophil NADPH-oxidase. *Biochemical and Biophysical Research Communication*, **176**, 1577–1583.

Zeitlin, D., Keller, S.E., Shiflett, S.C., Schleifer, S.J. and Bartlett, J.A., 2000. Immunological effects of massage therapy during academic stress. *Psychosomatic Medicine*, **62**, 83–87.

Zorrilla, E.P., Redel, E. and DeRubeis, R.J., 1994. Reduced cytokine levels and T-cell function in healthy males: relation to individual differences in subclinical anxiety. *Brain Behavior and Immunity*, **8**, 293–312.

XIX-7

Psychophysiology of Anxiety Disorders

G. Wiedemann and A. Mühlberger

INTRODUCTION

The use of psychophysiological methods in the assessment of a condition and the evaluation of treatment can be separated from research on mechanisms in the aetiology of fear (see also Hugdahl, 1989). In the following section, we will focus on condition assessment and treatment evaluation. For an extended discussion of experimental research on the mechanisms of fear, we refer you to the corresponding section in this book or to the *Handbook of Psychophysiology* (Bradley, 2000; Öhman, Hamm and Hugdahl, 2000).

The investigation of anxiety in psychophysiological research has a long history and is based on the dualistic view of emotions as consisting of both a cognitive and a somatic component (James, 1884). Obvious changes in different physiological systems, such as pounding of the heart, sweaty palms, and trembling hands upon confrontation with fear-eliciting stimuli, indicate the importance of physiological assessments, especially in anxiety disorders. The physiological reactions may tell us not only about the intensity of fear, but also about the quality of fear responses. In current psychophysiology research, a three-system concept of fear and emotion (Lang, 1968; Foa and Kozak, 1993) is widely accepted. The phobic reaction is seen as consisting of three loosely coupled components: psychophysiological responses, cognitive reports, and avoidance behaviour (Lang, 1971). As the three systems do not always react to the same extent or in the same temporal course (e.g. Rachman, 1977), the assessment of fear responses in all three component levels is recommended (e.g. Hugdahl, 1989). Many of the issues arising regarding one anxiety disorder may be equally applicable to other anxiety disorders. Research on panic disorder, for instance, may be difficult because of diagnostic co-morbidity, particularly with depression. On the other hand, the issue of the nature of the stimuli used to elicit physiological responses is illustrated by disorders such as post-traumatic stress disorder.

This paper is subdivided according to the Diagnostic and Statistical Manual (DSM-IV, American Psychiatric Association, 1994) diagnoses of the different anxiety disorders: (1) phobias; (2) panic disorder (PD); (3) generalized anxiety disorder (GAD); (4) post-traumatic stress disorder (PTSD); and (5) obsessive–compulsive disorder (OCD).

PHOBIAS

Phobias are subdivided into three subcategories: specific phobia; social phobia and agoraphobia.

Specific Phobia

No evidence of abnormal reactions of subjects (Ss) with specific phobia was found if no phobic context was present (Klorman, Weissberg and Wiesenfeld, 1977; Lang, Cuthbert and Bradley, 1998b). However, there is clear evidence for differences during exposure to phobic stimuli. The most established paradigm is to compare phobic Ss with control Ss in their reactions to phobic stimuli (e.g. spider pictures) in contrast to neutral, pleasant, or unpleasant stimuli. Early investigations focused on responses of the autonomic nervous system (ANS, e.g. heart rate (HR), skin conductance (SC) and respiration). More recently, focus was drawn to protective reflexes (e.g. startle response (SR), measured by corrugator electromyography (EMG) upon exposure to electric shocks or loud noise) and direct central nervous system (CNS) parameters, e.g. EEG/EP (evoked potentials). Spontaneous EMG measures were most frequently used to measure frontalis or forearm extensor muscle activity. The results were inconsistent (see e.g. review by Sartory and Lader (1981). Hamm *et al.*, (1997) found no significant group-specific differences in corrugator EMG in animal and mutilation phobic Ss during perception of phobic or neutral pictures. This seems to reflect heterogeneity of EMG reactions among subjects. This would be confirmed by subjective evaluations. Phobic Ss quite commonly experience mixed feelings of muscles becoming weak or tense (Hugdahl and Öst, 1985).

Many studies dealing with specific phobias investigated selected fearful, but non-clinical Ss. Since these Ss were comparable to diagnosed phobic Ss in many measures, selected investigations including analogous samples will be included in this section. Fearful samples without a clinical diagnosis are described as fearful Ss whereas diagnosed samples are described as phobic Ss.

According to the DSM IV, phobias can be subdivided in five types: animal type; natural environment type; blood-injection-injury type; situational type and other type. Most research was done on the animal type, the blood/injection/injury type and the situational type (e.g. flight phobia). The following sections will deal with these three types only.

Animal Type Specific Phobia

The autonomic system activity profile is dominated by a strong activation of the sympathetic branch. SC level (SCL) is considered a good candidate for measuring sympathetic activation, because the electrodermal system is thought to be controlled exclusively by the sympathetic part of the autonomic nervous system (Bradley, 2000). Nevertheless, there are some drawbacks. Firstly, sweat gland activity relies on a cholinergic mechanism rather than an adrenergic mechanism like most other sympathetic actions. Secondly, it is assumed that there are different types of sweating (e.g. Dawson, Schell and Filion, 2000). It is possible, for example, that sweating of the palms, which is most commonly measured, is an effect of parasympathetic regulation (Guyton and Hall, 1996). Nevertheless, SC reaction (SCR) is reliably modulated by emotional arousal in perception, anticipation and imagination (Bradley, 2000) and

Biological Psychiatry: Edited by H. D'haenen, J.A. den Boer and P. Willner. ISBN 0-471-49198-5

many publications used SCL as an index of sympathetic activation (Sartory, 1983; Hugdahl, 1989; Bradley, 2000). In laboratory settings, the SCR upon presentation of emotional (e.g. phobic) pictures is widely investigated. Geer (1966) showed an increased SCL for spider phobic Ss compared to control Ss during the perception of spider pictures. Wilson (1967) was able to show the same effects when pictures were presented tachistoscopically. This suggests that conscious perception is not necessary for this type of reaction.

Special focus was drawn to the underlying mechanism of these autonomic responses. Öhman and Soares (1994) exposed selected snake- and spider-fearful Ss to masked- and non-masked phobic and control pictures in a backward masking paradigm. SCR of phobic Ss was enhanced in the unmasked as well as the masked condition only upon exposure to their phobic stimuli (snakes or spiders). Further, snake phobic Ss rated snakes as more arousing and more negative in valence (with similar results for spider phobic Ss upon exposure to spider stimuli). This suggests that SCRs are individual rather than evolutionally prepared. Guided by these results, Öhman and Soares (1994) proposed a pre-attentive perceptual analysis of physical stimuli characteristics by a supposed *'physical feature detector'*. This feature detector can activate the arousal system. Van den Hout and co-workers (2000) tested the hypothesis of the *'physical feature detector'* (Öhman and Soares, 1994) by exposing spider phobic Ss (DSM-IV) to words (fear-related, general threat and neutral) instead of pictures. Control Ss were not included. As expected, the researchers found the strongest reaction of phobic Ss to phobia-related words, followed by progressively milder reactions to common threat words and neutral words during unmasked presentation. In the masked condition, spider phobic Ss reacted more strongly to general threat words and phobia-related words than to neutral words, but reactions did not differ between spider words and threat words. It was concluded that pictures are processed as words semantically, that the hypothetical significance evaluator (Öhman and Soares, 1994) directly influences the arousal system and that for this process, no conscious perception is required (Van den Hout, De Jong and Kindt, 2000).

Additionally, cardiovascular measures verify the sympathetic dominance in animal phobic Ss during anticipation or perception of phobic pictures. Spider or snake phobic Ss show strong HR acceleration, whereas control Ss show HR deceleration (e.g. Klorman, Weissberg and Wiesenfeld, 1977; Cook *et al.*, 1988). The HR acceleration in phobic subjects is accompanied by an increase in peripheral resistance in skin blood vessels (vasoconstriction measured by a decrease in digit pulse amplitude) and a decrease in peripheral resistance in muscle blood vessels (vasodilatation, measured by an increase of forearm blood volume) (e.g. Kelly, 1980). Furthermore, an increase in average blood pressure was found (Hamm *et al.*, 1997). To summarize, cardiovascular responses and SCR suggest that confrontation with phobic stimuli results in a defensive reaction (DR) (Sokolov, 1963) in phobic Ss, but an orientation reaction (OR) Sokolov, 1963) in non-phobic comparison Ss. For a review of the OR/DR literature see for example Öhman and co-workers (2000). According to the idea that the phobic reaction is a DR and includes the activation of a fight–flight system (Lang, 1968), not only the sympathetic nervous system should be activated, but also behavioural avoidance as well as protective reflexes (e.g. acoustic SR (ASR)) should be facilitated (Lang, Bradley and Cuthbert, 1990). To test this hypothesis, Hamm *et al.* (1997) assessed blood pressure (BP), HR, and eyeblink reflex (ASR, measured by orbicularis occuli EMG reaction to sudden, loud noise) during the perception of spider/snake pictures. In a second part of the experiment, subjects were able to stop the presentation themselves. An increased ASR during the perception of phobic stimuli was found only in animal fearful Ss, but not in control Ss. No differences between groups were found for neutral, pleasant or unpleasant pictures. Additionally, fearful Ss showed a strong avoidance reaction. While control Ss looked at spider/snake pictures and neutral pleasant/unpleasant pictures for the same length of time, fearful Ss stopped examining spider/snake pictures after a few seconds. Globisch *et al.* (1999) studied the temporal course of ASR potentiation. The researchers found a *relative* potentiation of the ASR beginning 300 ms after the onset of phobic pictures in animal fearful Ss. Furthermore, increased SCR, HR and average BP reaction were found. Similar results were observed when pictures were shown only for 150 ms, with the exception of the blood pressure (BP) reaction. Further research is necessary to differentiate whether this fast onset of relative startle potentiation is a result of reduced pre-pulse inhibition due to rapid encoding of the threat cue, or due to the fast onset of fear-potentiated startle response (Globisch *et al.*, 1999).

Central nervous measurements of phobic responses focus on alpha activity (8–13 Hz) and different features of Event-Related Potentials (ERPs). Within the ERPs, the Contingent Negative Variation (CNV), which occurs between signal stimulus, and target stimulus, e.g. in conditioning paradigms, and the P300 after stimulus presentation were investigated. Unfortunately, results are inconsistent. Larger (more negative) CNVs were observed in phobic subjects anticipating phobic stimuli compared to subjects awaiting neutral stimuli (e.g. Dubrovsky, Solyom and Barbas, 1978); however, smaller (less negative) CNVs have also been observed under these conditions (e.g. Lumsden, Howard and Fenton, 1986). To summarize, it seems that smaller CNVs may be associated with phobic fear states (Hugdahl, 1989).

Not only the perception of phobic stimuli results in physiological reactions. Memory retrieval or imagery of phobic stimuli (spiders/snakes) in animal phobic Ss results in sympathetic activation. Imagery is typically realized by presenting a script to the subject with instructions to imagine the presented situation. Scripts can be standardized or created with respect to individual fear stimuli (Cuthbert and Lang, 1989). Different investigations showed that even very short scripts of a few seconds in duration can induce subjective anxiety as well as physiological activation (e.g. Vrana, Cuthbert and Lang, 1986; Bradley, Land and Cuthbert, 1991).

Lang and co-workers (1970) showed accelerated HR in snake phobic Ss during imagery. This acceleration was linearly correlated with subjective fear, and could be enhanced by including more extensive use and description of text portions describing a reaction to stimuli in the imagery script (Lang *et al.*, 1980, 1983). In addition to this HR acceleration, Watson and Marks (1971) and Marks and co-workers (1971) verified an acceleration of spontaneous SC fluctuations (SCF) correlated with the extent of reaction-describing material in imagery scripts. Hamm *et al.* (1992) showed increased HR along with enhanced ASR in spider/snake phobic Ss during presentation of short, 12-second scripts. Compared to control Ss and neutral scripts, this increase was even higher during a period of imagery following the script presentation. This study also involved presentation of different picture categories (e.g. phobic, neutral). No differences between perception and imagination were found.

Another important application of psychophysiology is the evaluation of treatment outcome. As the presentation of real spiders within the laboratory is relatively inexpensive, *in vivo* confrontation as well as Behaviour Avoidance Tests (BAT) have been quite thoroughly investigated. Öst (1996) compared the effects of small and large therapy groups in a one-session exposure treatment of spider phobia. Significant time effects, but no group differences were found in any variable. Self-rating anxiety, assessor's rating of anxiety severity and BAT performance as well as systolic BP (SBP), diastolic BP (DBP) and HR during the BAT were improved after the therapy. The improvements were maintained up to a 6-month follow-up.

Watts, Trezise and Sharrock (1986) compared treated and untreated spider phobic Ss in a modified Stroop Test (Stroop, 1938). In this reaction time paradigm, they presented spider-related and control words in different colours. The Ss' task was to name the colour while ignoring the semantic word. Untreated Ss were severely retarded in naming the colour only for spider-related words (see also Mathews and MacLeod, 1985), while treated Ss were not. This effect probably is suppressed when measured directly before or during exposure treatment (Armir *et al.*, 1996). This paradigm allows the investigation of attentional aspects through psychophysiological methods. De Jong *et al.* (1992) additionally showed that the amount of covariation bias (Tomarken, Mineka and Cook, 1989), which is found in untreated spider phobic Ss, has decreased in treated Ss. The covariation bias seems to measure cognitive changes and may be used in outcome or relapse prediction (De Jong *et al.*, 1992). Another noteworthy predictor of treatment success is the initial HR response during perception of phobic pictures, as found by Lang (Lang, Bradley and Cuthbert, 1998a).

Blood/Injection/Injury Type Specific Phobia

Symptoms such as weakness, dizziness, and fainting or near-fainting while being confronted with phobic stimuli are more common in blood/injury phobia than in any other type of phobia. This very different type of reaction is also shown in psychophysiological measures. Enhanced sweat gland activity, measured by SC, was not found in blood/injury phobic Ss as compared to control Ss (e.g. Hamm *et al.*, 1997). Furthermore, no HR accelerations were found, as had been observed in other phobia types. However, after a short acceleration phase, strong HR decelerations were found, accompanied by a drop in mean BP (e.g. Hamm *et al.*, 1997). Blood/injury fearful subjects do not respond with a relative enhancement of sympathetic activation when exposed to their fear-relevant pictures, as do other phobic Ss. Interestingly, enhanced ASR was also found in blood/injury phobic Ss (e.g. Hamm *et al.*, 1997). Therefore, Hamm *et al.* (1997) concluded that the startle probe methodology provides important information for the clinical assessment and the evaluation of treatment outcome in phobias.

Situational Type Specific Phobia

We would like to present flight phobia as one prevalent and specific situational phobia. In the investigation of flight phobia, excellent ambulatory psychophysiological studies have been recently conducted by Wilhelm and Roth at Stanford University.

One study investigated the effect of benzodiazepine (alprazolam) on acute subjective and physiological responses during and following real flights in 28 flight phobic women (Wilhelm and Roth, 1997). Interestingly, alprazolam reduced self-reported anxiety and symptoms more than placebo, but induced an increase of HR and respiratory rate. In a second flight two weeks later, none of the Ss received alprazolam. However, subjects who had received alprazolam before the first flight indicated more anxiety, experienced panic attacks more often, and showed further increased HR during the second flight, compared to the placebo group. Wilhelm and Roth concluded that alprazolam increases physiological activation during acute stress situations and hinders therapeutic effects of exposure.

Another goal was to establish valid measures of HR response due to emotional activation. Therefore, the ability to distinguish whether HR increases are due to exercise or due to emotional response is necessary. This is especially important in ambulatory settings, where body movements or speech behaviour cannot be prevented. These sources of potential artefacts (e.g. walking, speaking) are essential to realize a natural setting. An early attempt to discriminate emotionally induced from exercise-induced HR increases involved an estimate of exercise-induced HR increases by measurement of oxygen consumption (Blix, Stromme and Ursin, 1974). By regression analysis, this source of variance was excluded and the resulting *additional* HR was attributed to emotional activation. Wilhelm and Roth (1998b) substituted the estimation of exercise due to oxygen consumption for practical reasons with a measurement of respiratory minute ventilation. Twenty-eight flight phobics and 15 control Ss were examined in different situations before and during a real flight. Previously, Ss completed different exercise tasks in the laboratory to obtain a function for the estimation of exercise-induced HR increases. The computed additional HR could be used to distinguish the phobic group from the control group during the walk to the airplane, which was not possible by examining HR or HR difference. During the flight, there were no differences, because exercise variation was negligible. One shortcoming of this technique is that anxiety-induced hyperventilation may distort the results. In another article, Wilhelm and Roth (1998a) described different physiological measures that were recorded in flight phobics and control Ss before, during and after a real flight. They were able to distinguish flight phobics from control Ss by measuring increased additional HR, more SC fluctuations, and less respiratory sinus arrhythmia during flight. By using the additional HR measure, they were able to classify 90% of flight phobics correctly. No differences between groups were found when respiratory rate or minute ventilation was recorded. For comparison, Sartory, Roth and Kopell (1992) also found encouraging results while investigating ambulatory assessment of driving phobia. They compared driving phobic Ss (e.g. avoidance of freeway drives for more than one year) with control Ss while performing different driving-related tasks within a BAT. Increased HR and respiratory minute volume were observed, but no differences in T-wave amplitude, respiratory sinus arrhythmia or respiratory rate were observed.

A new tool for the investigation and treatment of phobias is virtual reality. Virtual reality makes it possible to investigate states of phobic anxiety within a naturalistic, but highly controllable and repeatable setting. Mühlberger *et al.* (2001) compared the effect of repeated exposure to flights in virtual reality (VR) on flight phobics with effects resulting from relaxation training (RT). To test the effects, fear reports and physiological response were assessed during additional short virtual flights before and after the treatment. A decrease in subjective fear, SCL and HR reaction was found in both groups, but SCL and fear reports in the VR group were reduced compared to the RT group. Furthermore, a stronger initial HR response correlated highly with post-treatment fear of flying reduction at least up until a 3-month follow-up. Substantial correlations were only found in the VR group, and not in the RT group (Mühlberger, 1997). This may be in part due to the smaller changes within this group. However, it may also be the case that the predictive value of initial HR response is especially high in exposure-based treatments.

Social Phobia

An overview of earlier research on psychophysiology in social phobia is given by Öst (1989). Typically, giving a speech (e.g. in the paradigm of public speaking) or having a conversation with an unknown person (especially of opposite sex) is used as an anxiety-provoking stimulus in laboratory settings. Turner, Beidel and Larkin (1986) compared 26 socially anxious Ss and 26 non-socially anxious Ss with a clinical sample of 17 social phobics. During an impromptu speech, both the anxious and phobic group had higher SBP than the non-socially anxious Ss. DBP and HR did not differ between groups. In selected socially anxious and non-socially anxious students, Panayiotou and Vrana (1998) found no HR differences due to self-focus instructions while performing a digit rehearsal task, and an increased ASR only in socially anxious Ss. Lang (1993) compared speech fearful Ss with spider-fearful Ss during an impromptu speech *in vivo* as well as *in sensu*. Increased HR was found in speech fearful Ss and also in spider-fearful Ss, with no difference between the two groups. McNeil *et al.* (1993) were able to verify these results in a clinical sample. They found an increase in HR during the imagination of a scene most fearful for the individual being tested, but observed no difference in HR increase compared to dental phobic Ss. In a second analysis, Ss were divided based on questionnaires into two subgroups: a fear group and an avoidance group. The fear group (14% assigned) showed a strong increase in HR correlating with their subjective fear, whereas the avoidance group (71% assigned) showed only a small increase. However, both groups subjectively stated experiencing strong anxiety and vivid imaginations. Turner and Beidel (1985) also found a high correlation between strong physiological reactions (BP) and subjective fear as major symptom after splitting their sample into high and low physiological responders. Similar results were described by Heimberg *et al.* (1990). They found stronger HR accelerations but less subjective fear in speech fearful Ss giving a talk or interacting socially than in Ss with a diagnosis of social phobia of the *generalized type* (Specifier of DSM-IV diagnosis). Levin *et al.* (1993) replicated these results by comparing specific social phobics and generalized social phobics. Hofmann *et al.* (1995) compared social phobics with and without avoidance personality structure and control Ss. Phobics without personality disorder reacted with a stronger HR increase than the other two groups, whereas phobics with additional personality disorder reacted with more subjective anxiety than the other two groups while presenting a public speech.

In treatment outcome studies, usually a decrease in physiological response, but no differences in treatment comparison tests were found. Jerremalm, Jansson and Öst (1986) divided 38 patients into physiological or cognitive reactors and assigned them either to applied relaxation (AR), self-instructional training (SIT), or waiting list (WL) group. They found a reduced HR reaction during a conversation test after AR and SIT compared to the WL group in physiological reactors, but no treatment group differences.

One major challenge in research involving social phobia or agoraphobia is the confusion of cognitive demand or motor exercise with emotional activation. One strategy for dealing with this difficulty is to disentangle these two sources of variance by manipulating the anxiety (e.g. Ss are observed by authorities or not) or the demand parameters (e.g. known or unknown speech topic (e.g. Erdmann and Baumann, 1996). Another strategy is to simply use the anticipatory anxiety, measuring the physiological states during expectation of giving an impromptu talk (e.g. Davidson *et al.*, 2000). Recently, Davidson *et al.* (2000) published an interesting article comparing the ANS responses and spontaneous EEG alpha power values of 18 social phobics with those of 10 control Ss. HR was elevated among phobics in most conditions. Furthermore, a marked increase in right-side activation of the anterior temporal and lateral prefrontal brain regions was found in social phobics. These EEG and HR measures explained more than 48% of the variance of the negative affect during speech anticipation. Like the results of Wilhelm and Roth, this indicates that when using physiological parameters within the correct paradigm, subjective anxiety can be predicted very well.

The results indicate that based on the phobic reaction, social phobia can be divided into two subgroups, simple phobia-like and generalized or agoraphobia-like. The two subgroups seem to reflect the different diagnoses in social phobia. One subgroup may reflect the simple diagnosis social phobia, the other one the diagnosis social phobia with specifier *generalized* (or even the additional diagnosis of a personality disorder). These promising results in distinguishing different types of social phobia might prompt a broader use of psychophysiology in further research of social phobia.

Agoraphobia

An overview of the earlier research on the psychophysiology in agoraphobia is given by Öst (1990). In some laboratory assessments, a general increased ANS activation without anxiety-eliciting stimulation could be found (Öst, 1990). This increase is accompanied by reduced habituation. Interestingly, the reactions to phobic stimuli or imagery tend to be less intensive than in specific phobia. Cook *et al.* (1988) compared the reaction of specific phobic, social phobic and agoraphobic (with PD) patients during imagery of phobic scripts describing their most feared scene. It was found that all three groups of patients rated their subjective fear-related cues as very arousing and highly unpleasant. However, when ANS responses were examined, simple phobics showed the largest and agoraphobics the smallest overall reactivity (HR and SCL changes). Specific phobics also showed a strong correlation between subjective anxiety and physiological reactions, whereas agoraphobic Ss did not. Cuthbert *et al.* (1994) replicated these results and found in addition a general increased level of ASR reactions during phobic and neutral imagery as well as between imageries, but the modulation of the ASR by emotional content as in social or specific phobics was not found (see Figure XIX-7.1, adapted by permission of the author). The presentation of external stimuli led to the same results as *in vivo* exposure (e.g. Fisher and Wilson, 1985). Unfortunately, like in social phobia, *in vivo* exposure or ambulatory assessments are often confounded by motor exercise. For instance, having a walk is a common paradigm in the assessment of agoraphobia. As discussed above, it is difficult to disentangle the different sources of physiological changes. It is not possible to state whether the HR acceleration during *in vivo* exposition (e.g. having a walk) commonly found not only in agoraphobics but also in control Ss is due to artefacts or the lack of differences between these groups. Therefore, the use of different physiological measurements (e.g. including respiratory) and methodological improvements in ambulatory measurements (see e.g. Wilhelm and Roth, 1998b) is strongly recommended in the assessment of agoraphobia.

In treatment studies, an overall HR reduction during different tasks was found (see Öst, 1990). Öst, Jerremalm and Jansson (1984) found a reduction of HR reactivity through both exposure and relaxation training. Bonn, Readhead and Timmons (1984) found (upon follow-up measurement) *in vivo* exposition combined with breathing retraining to be superior to *in vivo* exposition alone. Michelson *et al.* (1990) compared paradoxical intervention (PI), graduated exposure (GE) and relaxation training (RT). Only RT and

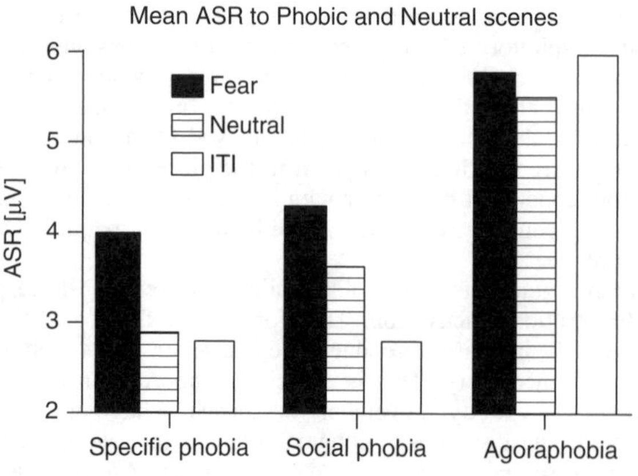

Figure XIX-7.1 Average acoustic startle responses (ASR) during the imagery of phobic or neutral scenes and during the Inter-Stimulus-Interval (ITI) for patients of these phobias. Adapted by permission from Cuthbert *et al.*, © 1994 by B. Cuthbert

GE led to substantial reductions in HR reactivity. No correlation between pre-treatment physiological reactivity and therapy outcome was observed. Additionally, the authors categorized persons with improvements across all three systems of phobic reactions (physiology, behaviour, self-report; see e.g. Lang, 1968) as synchronizers. Ss that exhibited discrepant patterns of improvement and worsening were classified as desynchronizers. Treatment outcome of synchronizers (e.g. Michelson *et al.*, 1990) was found to be superior to that of desynchronizers (e.g. Michelson *et al.*, 1990) in all but the physiological (HR) measures. In a comparison of behavioural and pharmacological (imipramine) treatment, Michelson, Mavissakalian and Marchione (1985) observed substantial decreases in HR through the behavioural treatment. Conversely, HR increases in imipramine-treated Ss were found.

Interestingly, in some investigations a substantial correlation of pre-treatment HR and post-treatment as well as follow-up treatment response was found (e.g. Craske, Sanderson and Barlow, 1987; Roth *et al.*, 1988), but also contrary results were reported (see Michelson *et al.*, 1990).

To summarize, strong evidence has been found that psychophysiological measures in agoraphobia are important. Nevertheless, there is still a dearth of investigations using psychophysiological measures in assessment or outcome prediction.

Direct Comparison of Phobias

Some studies were able to show in direct comparisons that different phobias are related to different physiological reactivity (Cook *et al.*, 1988; Cuthbert *et al.* 1994; Lang, Bradley and Cuthbert, 1998a). *Specific phobia* is generally characterized by a marked sympathetic activation and potentiated protective reflexes (e.g. ASR) during presentation or imagination of phobic stimuli. This was attributed to the activation of a DR (Lang, Bradley and Cuthbert, 1997), which protects against potentially dangerous stimuli. The phobic reactions were very reliable and accompanied by strong avoidance tendencies. However, no abnormal signs have been found in baseline reactions. Also, in *social phobia*, no abnormal ANS or ASR baseline reactivity was found (Lang, Bradley and Cuthbert, 1998a). Reactions upon phobic cues were somehow less salient than in simple phobia. In *agoraphobia*, more baseline ANS activation and enhanced ASR accompanied by smaller reactions during the presentation or the imagery of phobic stimuli was discovered (see Figure XIX-7.1, adapted by permission of the author) (Lang, Bradley and Cuthbert, 1998a).

Recent findings in animal research led to the conclusion that different neurophysiological pathways are involved in fear behaviour under different paradigms. It was assumed that fear can be divided into cue-explicit fear and more generalized context-related fear (Lang, Bradley and Cuthbert, 1998a). This implies that object-related phobias (e.g. snakes, spiders phobia) differ fundamentally from more general phobias (e.g. agoraphobia). They differ not only in a quantitative matter, i.e. in amount of subjective, physiological and behavioural reactions, but also in a qualitative matter, in the underlying mechanisms of fear processing. This would imply that very different therapy strategies may be effective for different types of anxiety disorders.

PANIC DISORDER WITH OR WITHOUT AGORAPHOBIA

Discrepant Findings in Resting Heart Rate as an Example for Different Explanations

Many studies of panic disorder (PD) have found higher resting heart rates (HR) among patients in comparison to healthy control participants (Freedman *et al.*, 1984; Liebowitz *et al.*, 1985; Ehlers *et al.*, 1986; Castellani *et al.*, 1988; Aronson *et al.*, 1989; Nutt, 1989; Uhde *et al.*, 1989; Yeragani *et al.*, 1990; Hoehn-Saric, McLeod and Zimmerli, 1991; Stein, Tancer and Uhde, 1992). However, several other authors did not find such differences (Charney, Heninger and Breier, 1984; Cowley *et al.*, 1987; Villacres *et al.*, 1987; Gaffney *et al.*, 1988; Stein and Uhde, 1991; Stein, Tancer and Uhde, 1992; Gurguis, Vitton and Uhde, 1997). Some authors claim underlying physiological differences are responsible (Stein and Uhde, 1998; Ballenger, 1990), others suggest that these discrepant findings may result from anticipatory anxiety in response to the experimental environment (Margraf, Ehlers and Roth, 1986; McNally, 1994). Ambulatory monitoring studies have found that the resting HR of patients with PD did not differ from those of healthy control individuals (Freedman *et al.*, 1985; Cameron *et al.*, 1987; Taylor *et al.*, 1987; Pauli *et al.*, 1991). Therefore, Larson *et al.* (1998) compared the resting HR of patients with PD, social phobia, and healthy control participants during two consecutive laboratory sessions. The authors found no significant differences in resting HR between groups on either day. Patients with PD had significantly higher mean resting HR during their first laboratory session, which may be due to elevated anticipatory anxiety in these patients. This study highlights a potential confounding factor in many studies. It suggests that anticipatory anxiety and its effect on baseline physiological reactivity in patients with PD may be reduced by pre-exposing them to the experimental environment.

Theoretical Models for the Development of Panic Disorder and Psychophysiological Response Patterns

A uniform theoretical model for the development of panic disorder and/or phobia has not yet been established, but according to research thus far, two important theories have emerged: a learning-theory based conditioning model and a cognitive model. Classic conditioning processes and dysfunctional cognitions are thought to be vulnerability factors for the development of panic disorders with or without agoraphobia (Beck, Emery and Greenberg, 1985; Ehlers *et al.*, 1986; Clark, 1988; Carr, Lehrer and Hochron, 1992).

Mowrer (1939) developed a two-factor theory. Firstly, common and naturally triggering factors for an anxiety response become linked to neutral stimuli by spatial and temporal association. Thus, these neutral situations are able to set into action an anxiety reaction without necessitating the presence of a 'natural' trigger (classical conditioning). Secondly, avoidance behaviour is developed, which prevents the learned anxiety reaction from becoming habituated. According to operant conditioning models, this avoidance behaviour acts as negative reinforcement and thus maintains the pathological anxiety response. In fact, retrospective assessments of agoraphobia cases point to conditioning experiences as triggering factors (Öst and Hugdahl, 1983).

Ehlers *et al.* (1986) were able to show that patients with a panic disorder exhibit altered perception of their normal interoceptive stimuli, such as heart beat. This selective focusing on bodily reactions did not correspond to a real improvement in their ability to appraise such changes (Rapee *et al.*, 1992), but this readiness to appraise physical experiences as anxiety-provoking events leads to fears which themselves provoke psychophysiological changes, such as even further accelerated heart beat or hyperventilation. These observations again confirm the original fear and act as reinforcement. Thus, a vicious circle has been established, which ultimately leads to a panic attack. These theories are based on studies examining psychophysiological response patterns in patients with panic disorders compared to healthy, depressive, or somatically ill control participants (e.g. Hoehn-Saric, McLeod and Zimmerli, 1991; Yeragani *et al.*, 1993; Klein *et al.*, 1995).

Respiratory Psychophysiology and its Explanatory Capacity in Panic Disorder

In the context of respiratory psychophysiology, Ley outlined a dyspnoea/suffocation-fear theory of panic which later led to a tripartite categorization of panic attacks (Hibbert and Pilsbury, 1988; Ley, 1989; Sanderson, Rapee and Barlow, 1989; Craske and Barlow, 1990; Ley, 1994a, 1994b). In contrast, Klein's false suffocation alarm theory hypothesizes a deranged suffocation monitor, which is assumed to trigger a hypothetical suffocation alarm (Klein, 1993; Taylor and Rachman, 1994; McNally, Hornig and Donnell, 1995; Stein *et al.*, 1995). This hypothesis relies on the physiological mechanism whereby potential suffocation is detected by increasing P_{CO_2} and brain lactate.

In his critique of Klein's theory, Ley emphasizes the distinction between dyspnoea, the sensation of difficulties in breathing, and suffocation, the condition that may give rise to dyspnoea (Ley, 1998).

Asmundson and Stein (1994) found an association between a measure of pulmonary function, the forced expiratory flow rate, and the severity of panic symptoms in patients with PD. Thus, they provided relatively strong support for the dyspnoea/suffocation-fear theory, stating that uncontrollable dyspnoea is the source of panic fear. On the contrary, Spinhoven, Onstein and Sterk (1995) did not succeed in replicating these findings; however, this study was criticized by Ley as containing flawed methodology and statistical anomalies. Although the significant findings of Asmundson and co-workers might be subject to type I error, the study of Spinhoven and co-workers cannot be seen as proof for this.

Papp *et al.* (1997) challenged patients with PD and healthy individuals with 5% and 7% CO_2 inhalation and hyperventilation of room air. Patients were more sensitive to the anxiogenic effects of CO_2 compared to healthy participants. Furthermore, CO_2 was a more potent panic stimulus than hyperventilation. The authors identified several respiratory abnormalities, and concluded that patients with PD are behaviourally and physiologically more sensitive to CO_2 inhalation. Panic attacks are explained by inefficient compensatory mechanisms of respiratory rate.

In summation, many studies have shown that patients with PD have a greater propensity to experience increased anxiety and more panic attacks during inhalation of CO_2 compared to healthy participants (Griez *et al.*, 1987; Sanderson and Wetzler, 1990; Perna *et al.*, 1994; Gorman *et al.*, 1994, 1997). In patients with PD, rates of panic during CO_2 inhalation decrease after successful treatment of the disorder (Sanderson, Wetzler and Asnis, 1994; Perna *et al.*, 1997; Bocola *et al.*, 1998). Some authors even claim that CO_2-induced panic is specific to patients with PD (Griez *et al.*, 1990; Perna *et al.*, 1995a, 1995b), but others could show that other patients are also susceptible, e.g. in social phobia (Caldirola *et al.*, 1997) or premenstrual dysphoric disorder (Harrison *et al.*, 1989).

CO_2 sensitivity is increased even in clinically asymptomatic, first-degree relatives of patients with PD (Perna *et al.*, 1995c; Coryell and Arndt, 1999). This could represent a specific abnormality in the afferent neural pathways that respond to increased levels of CO_2 (Klein, 1993). Others argue that the non-specific somatic distress produced by CO_2 inhalation triggers the panic attack (Roth *et al.*, 1992), but studies that addressed this controversy led to conflicting results (Gorman *et al.*, 1988; Pain, Biddle and Tilter, 1988; Papp *et al.*, 1995, 1997). As a result, the mechanism of action is still a matter of intense debate.

Therefore, Gorman *et al.* (2001) investigated differences in respiratory response to CO_2 breathing by comparing patients with PD, healthy control participants, patients with major depression (MD), and patients with premenstrual dysphoric disorder (PMDD). Both latter groups had no co-morbidity with panic disorder. Patients with MD generally do not respond to panic-producing agents such as CO_2, whereas patients with PMDD do.

In sum, patients with PD exhibit higher rates of panic attacks during CO_2 inhalation than other groups, but have no fundamental abnormality in their ventilatory physiology. The exaggerated respiratory responses are more a function if a panic attack occurs than the diagnostic group. The panic response to CO_2 involves a generalized fear response that is not specific to PD. These results are compatible with preclinical fear conditioning models.

These CO_2 studies have pointed the way for neuroimaging studies of cortical and subcortical sites.

Is Regional Brain Asymmetry Associated with (Different) Anxiety Disorders?

Evidence has accumulated from non-psychiatric and psychiatric populations, that individual differences in electroencephalogram (EEG) resting frontal brain asymmetry are associated with differences in basic dimensions of emotion, i.e. in dispositional mood and temperament (see Davidson, 1992; for review, Schaffer, Davidson and Saron, 1983; Henriques and Davidson, 1990; Tomarken *et al.*, 1990; Henriques and Davidson, 1991; Wheeler, Davidson and Tomarken, 1993; Heller, Etienne and Miller, 1995). In particular, increased relative activation of right hemisphere anterior regions is linked to negative affects, such as depressive or sad emotions. In contrast, relatively higher activation of the left frontal area is associated with positive affects, i.e. cheerful emotions. Davidson (1992) has conceptualized this frontal brain asymmetry as reflecting specialized systems in the right hemisphere for withdrawal behaviour coupled with negative emotions and in the left frontal region for approach behaviour associated with positive affects. Much of the data supporting this relationship comes from studies measuring EEG alpha activity during different emotional states (Davidson *et al.*, 1990; Tomarken *et al.*, 1992).

Hemisphere Asymmetry and General Negative Emotional Dispositions

Davidson found that sub-clinically as well as clinically depressed individuals have significantly higher right frontal hemispheric activation than non-depressed subjects (Schaffer, Davidson and Saron, 1983; Henriques and Davidson, 1991, 1992). This difference did not depend on the acute phase of the disorder. Also, remitted depressives that were upon examination normothymic showed increased right frontal activation (Henriques and Davidson, 1990). Thus, this seems to be a trait marker of individuals reacting with negative affect.

Hemisphere Asymmetry and Negative Emotional States

However, individuals differ dramatically in their affective responses to emotional provocations, as they do in their propensity to approach or withdraw from unfamiliar situations. These differences in action have been linked with corresponding differences in emotional reactivity. Therefore, in response to elicitors of dimensions of positive emotion, there should be more intense positive affect and less intense negative affect in subjects with strong left-sided frontal activation. The opposite pattern of reactivity should occur in individuals with stronger right frontal activation. So, increased right frontal hemisphere activation is not only a trait marker for depressives, but also a state marker in conditions predominated by negative affect.

Laterality Findings in Anxiety Disorders

Tucker and co-workers found that anxiety-producing conditions in healthy volunteers were linked to significantly more left than right lateral eye movements (Tucker *et al.*, 1977) and resulted specifically in decreased performance in the right visual field (Tucker *et al.*, 1978). Tucker *et al.* (1978) also showed that high trait-anxious subjects reported tones at the right ear as significantly louder compared to low trait-anxious people with the same tone in quantity and quality (Tucker *et al.*, 1978). Moreover, high trait-anxious individuals showed reduced left lateral eye movements. So, Tucker and co-workers argue that anxiety is associated with greater left-hemisphere activation. Therefore, left-hemisphere tasks are more poorly performed, as there is a concomitant processing overload. In contrast, further studies with imaging techniques during anxious states revealed more right than left activation in parietotemporal regions (Buchsbaum and Wu, 1987; Naveteur *et al.*, 1992), while others found no asymmetry (Fredrikson *et al.*, 1993). One EEG study even showed increased left brain activation (Carter, Johnson and Borkovec, 1986).

These patterns of hemisphere activation therefore also vary as a function of anxious mood. The findings, however, have been inconsistent (Heller, Etienne and Miller, 1995), and this variability has made generalizations difficult. According to reviews by Heller (1990, 1993), this could be due to the possibility that anxiety and depression may be linked to opposite patterns of activation in the cerebral hemispheres. Depressive mood might be associated with right-hemisphere activation and anxiety with left-hemisphere activation. In populations with much co-morbidity of anxiety and depression, these patterns might suppress each other. Such opposing tendencies could account for the variable patterns in different studies, depending on the ratio of these two emotional states in the particular sample. Because studies of anxiety-depressive conditions and depression studies do not account for anxiety, this might have led to confounded effects. More so, because the co-morbidity of depression and anxiety is high: 40% to 80% of patients with panic disorder have had an episode of major depression (Katon and Roy-Byrne, 1991). However, the overlap between symptoms of anxiety and depression decreases, as the severity of symptoms increases (Hiller, Zaudig and von Bose, 1989).

Heller and co-workers (1995) classified more than 1000 subjects as either high- or low-depressive and high- or low-anxious, and gave a face-processing task that elicits left hemispatial bias (chimeric faces task, CFT). High-depressed probands showed smaller left hemispatial biases than low-depressed ones (corresponding to lower right hemisphere activation), whereas high-anxious subjects had larger left hemispatial biases than low-anxious individuals (corresponding to higher right hemisphere activation). As there was no interaction effect, the number of depressive symptoms cannot be made responsible for the right or left hemispheric asymmetry of anxiety.

Consequently, Heller and co-workers (1995) hypothesize that different kinds of anxiety might be associated with different patterns of hemispheric asymmetry. Left-hemisphere functions may be linked to experiences of worry involving verbal rumination, i.e. cognitive and anticipatory anxiety (Öhman, 1993), whereas right hemisphere activation may be associated with fear or panic responses, i.e. more autonomic and physiological changes (Spence, Shapiro and Zaidel, 1996). These subtypings have been based primarily on behavioural data from lateralized tasks and on lateralized EEG findings. Beyond Heller and colleagues, this distinction has not yet been systematically assessed.

Right frontal brain activation seems to represent an activation of an avoidance–withdrawal system and appears to be associated with negative emotions. Since panic patients are characterized by negative emotions and by avoidance behaviour, this hemispheric asymmetry might be expected. Therefore, Wiedemann *et al.* (1999) compared the spontaneous EEG of 23 panic patients and 25 healthy control subjects during resting phases and while being confronted with neutral, panic-relevant, anxiety-relevant but panic-irrelevant, or anxiety-irrelevant but emotionally relevant stimuli, or when performing a motor task. This study showed that in the spontaneous electroencephalogram of panic patients there are asymmetries in frontal hemispheric activation during resting phases (see Figure XIX-7.2, adapted by permission of the author) and when being confronted with anxiety-relevant stimuli (see Figure XIX-7.3, adapted by permission of the author).

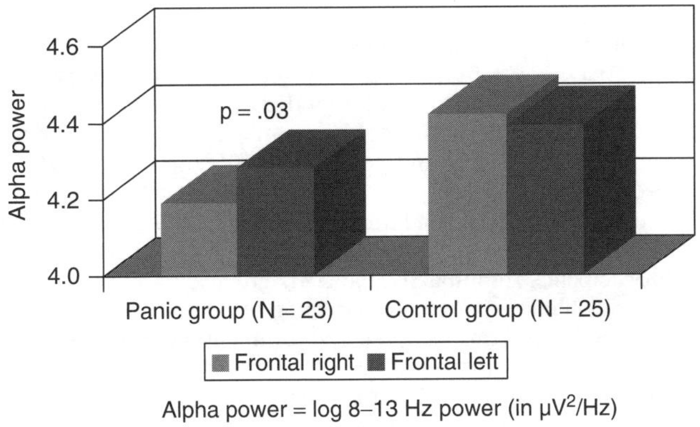

Figure XIX-7.2 Frontal alpha power during resting phases in patients with panic disorder. Adapted by permission

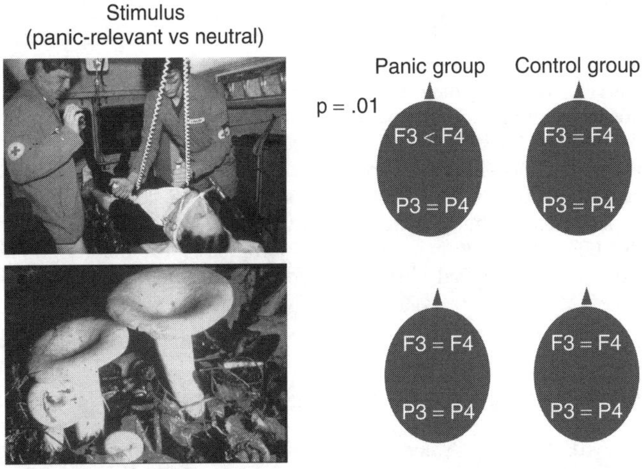

Figure XIX-7.3 Frontal and parietal hemispheric activation in patients with panic disorder when being confronted with panic-relevant and neutral stimuli. Adapted by permission

The right frontal alpha power was significantly decreased in these patients compared to that of the left side, while control subjects did not show a frontal asymmetry during these phases.

There was no frontal asymmetry when patients observed an emotionally neutral picture or while performing a motor task. Thus, panic patients were characterized by greater activation of a right frontal avoidance–withdrawal system in negatively valenced situations.

Studies that investigate both central and autonomic measures are warranted to further develop the theory of distinct, psychophysiologically defined subtypes of anxiety disorders.

GENERALIZED ANXIETY DISORDER

In generalized anxiety disorder (GAD), persistent, uncontrollable worry represents the central defining feature. This state of apprehension is maintained by defensive attentional mechanisms such as pre-attentive bias for threat information and poor habituation to novel stimuli (Mathews, 1990). The persistent cognitive anxiety of GAD may be based on an adaptive coping strategy gone awry. Thayer *et al.* (2000) tried to bridge the attentional and physiological underpinnings of GAD by examining phasic heart period responses to cued threat and non-threat word stimuli in an S1–S2 procedure. The GAD group showed HR acceleration in response to threat stimuli, and a conditioned anticipatory HR deceleration to threat stimuli over repeated trials, in comparison to healthy control participants. Additionally, the GAD group showed smaller and impaired habituation of cardiac orienting responses to neutral stimuli. These findings are interpreted as a diminished global adaptive variability in GAD patients.

Although it is reasonable to assume that patients with GAD exhibit physiological hyperarousal at rest and heightened responses to stressors, this is not the case. Patients with GAD show increased muscle tension (Hoehn-Saric, McLeod and Zimmerli, 1989; Hazlett, McLeod and Hoehn, 1994), but not autonomic hyperarousal. Interestingly, GAD patients under stress show less efficient and more rigid but not higher autonomic responses compared to healthy individuals (Hoehn-Saric, 1998). This physiological rigidity may result from a physiological adaptation to chronic arousal, or represent a constitutional predisposition. On the other hand, a patient with GAD may not be aware of stressful situations that are not incorporated into his pathological preoccupations. Furthermore, the relationship between physiological changes and their perception is weak. This inconsistency may be due to alterations of body sensations by psychological factors. Excessive attention to and expectation of body states may exaggerate body sensations on the one hand, but may on a long-term basis (in the long run) lead to a perceptual distortion and to a disregard of the body states.

POST-TRAUMATIC STRESS DISORDER (PTSD)

According to the American Psychiatric Association's Diagnostic and Statistical Manual of Mental Disorders (DSM-IV) symptoms of PTSD include irritability, hypervigilance, exaggerated startle response, and intense physiological reactivity upon re-exposure to events that symbolize or resemble an aspect of the traumatic event (American Psychiatric Association, 1994). In a series of studies, heart rate (HR), blood pressure (BP), skin conductance (SC), and electromyogram (EMG) have been used as outcome measures. The paradigms differed in the nature of the stimulus used to elicit physiological responses: external stimuli reminiscent of the trauma, internal (mental) imagery of the trauma, and intense but neutral stimulations, e.g. auditory startle stimulus (Shalev, Orr and Pitman, 1993a). Following this subdivision, the corresponding studies will be described.

Psychophysiological Responses to External Stimuli

World War II veterans with ($n = 8$) and without ($n = 13$) decompensated combat neurosis and student control individuals ($n = 10$) were exposed to a tape of artillery barrage, small arms fire, and aerial bombardment sounds (Dobbs and Wilson, 1960). While only one of the student control subjects showed a moderate or marked increase in pulse rate, eight of the healthy veterans did so, and five of the decompensated veterans even asked that the tape be turned off. Vietnam veterans with PTSD and non-veteran control individuals underwent mental arithmetic and combat sounds from an audiotape (Blanchard *et al.*, 1982). The mental arithmetic aroused both groups (heart rate, electromyogram, and blood pressure responses), whereas the combat sounds did so only in the PTSD group. However, this study did not differentiate the effect of combat from that of PTSD, as there was no control group with combat exposure.

Therefore, Malloy, Fairbank and Keane (1983) compared the physiological responses of Vietnam veterans with PTSD, psychiatric inpatients, and veterans without PTSD. The audio-visual presentation of combat sounds resulted in significantly greater heart rate and skin conductance responses to combat scenes in the group with PTSD only.

The methodology was further refined by comparing Vietnam veterans with PTSD, veterans with other psychiatric disorders, veterans with combat experience, Vietnam-era veterans, and non-veterans patients with anxiety disorders (Pallmeyer, Blanchard and Kolb, 1986). Physiological responses (HR, BP, SC) were compared during rest, mental arithmetic, and combat sounds. Larger HR responses to combat sounds were found in the PTSD group compared to all other groups. McFall *et al.* (1990) used additional outcome measures by comparing the group's (Vietnam veterans with and without PTSD) HR, BP, subjective responses, and plasma epinephrine upon viewing of combat and non-combat stress films. Greater increases in all outcome measures were found in the PTSD group during the combat films.

Blanchard *et al.* (1991) tested the reliability of the psychophysiological measures. They compared HR and BP responses to combat sounds in two large samples ($n = 104$ and 96, respectively) of Vietnam veterans with and without PTSD. The cumulative difference in HR and BP response to combat sounds correctly classified 80% in the first and 83% in the second sample of testees as individuals with or without PTSD.

These studies resulted in a neuropsychological hypothesis explaining PTSD (Kolb, 1987). The disorder was defined as a conditioned emotional response to overwhelming stressful exposure. Excessive stimulation was thought to result in permanent neuronal changes. These might lead to impairment of learning, habituation, and stimulus discrimination. Thus, the disorder results from strong associative learning. Originally, individuals react to a traumatic event (unconditioned stimulus, UCS) with arousal and fear (unconditioned response, UCR). Associative learning implies that finally, individuals show the same response to external cues associated with the stressful experience. By then, these cues have become conditioned stimuli (CS). The physiological response generated by these cues represents the equivalent of a conditioned response (CR).

However, combat is only one condition capable of provoking PTSD. Rape, motor vehicle accidents, torture, natural disasters etc., are other conditions considered to be potential stimuli.

Psychophysiological Responses to Mental Imagery

Brende (1982) found that hypnotically induced imagery of past traumatic events in PTSD patients was associated with increased electrodermal response of the left side of the body. According to Brende, this lateralization might be explained by the preferential processing of images by the right brain hemisphere.

Pitman hypothesized that in PTSD, there is a pathological emotional network, which can be provoked by mental imagery, resulting in physiological and other responses (Pitman, 1988). Lang and co-workers had shown that emotionally loaded imagery correlates with HR, SC, and EMG responses in general (Lang *et al.*, 1983). According to their theory, emotional memories are stored as an associative network. These networks consist of memory traces of the sensory input, the meaning derived from this input, and the physiological response.

Following this theoretical approach, Pitman and co-workers conducted a series of studies. Vietnam veterans with and without PTSD listened to recorded scripts describing traumatic events. Some of these were standardized, others were based on the individual's own experience. Imagery of the personal events resulted in strong HR, SC, and EMG responses in PTSD patients only (Pitman *et al.*, 1987). In a further study, Pitman and co-workers compared Vietnam veterans with PTSD and Vietnam veterans with other anxiety disorders (Pitman *et al.*, 1990). The response to combat imagery was specific to PTSD. Shalev and co-workers assessed the psychophysiological response to traumatic imagery in Israeli trauma survivors. These subjects were of both sexes with PTSD of different origin, i.e. rape, road accidents, terrorist acts (Shalev and Rogel-Fuchs, 1993b). In subjects whose disorder was the result of non-military events, increases in HR and EMG in response to traumatic imagery were observed compared with the response of survivors without PTSD, the same trend seen in the studies of Pitman *et al.*

Response to mental imagery was also used as a measure of treatment outcome. Keane and Kaloupek (1982) treated a Vietnam veteran suffering from PTSD with imaginal flooding. The heart rate response to imaginal scenes of combat memories was reduced after therapy. Similarly, Fairbank and Keane (1982) showed that imaginal flooding reduced heart rate and skin conductance response to combat-related imaginal scenes in PTSD patients. Boudewyns and Heyr (1990) compared direct therapeutic exposure and counselling in Vietnam veterans with PTSD. Regardless of treatment protocol, clinical improvement as an outcome measure is correlated with decreases in physiological responses to combat imagery. However, Shalev *et al.* (1992) also showed that such reductions might not generalize to recollections of other traumatic events, although their treatment of desensitization of the specific trauma resulted in a decrease of HR, SC, and EMG responses to that trauma.

In a further study, Shalev (1997) explored the physiological responses of PTSD patients to reminders of a significant stressor that had preceded the onset of the disorder and was not related to its cause. They compared outpatients with PTSD, survivors of traumatic events who had not developed PTSD, panic disorder patients, and mentally healthy individuals with no history of trauma. PTSD individuals showed higher SC and EMG responses than the other groups. The authors concluded that PTSD patients may acquire and maintain prolonged conditioned responses to various stressors during their lifetime or become sensitized to reminders of past traumata following the onset of their illness. Heightened susceptibility to acquire conditioned responses or an inability to extinguish such responses may be expressed before the trauma in individuals who are liable to develop PTSD.

In a recent study, Orr *et al.* (2000) found evidence that individuals with PTSD show greater conditionability than those without. This stronger conditionability could reflect pre-trauma vulnerability to developing PTSD.

Keane *et al.* (1998) were able to show that more severe PTSD symptomatology is associated with greater physiological responsivity to trauma-related cues.

Blanchard *et al.* (1996) found that higher physiological responsivity to imagery one-to-four months after a motor vehicle accident predicted the persistence of chronic PTSD after one year.

In a recent study, Orr *et al.* (1998) showed that PTSD and non-PTSD groups do not differ in the magnitude of their physiological responsivity to standard stressors (mental arithmetic, postural challenge).

The consistency of the results across various studies suggests that the method of using responses to mental imagery represents a good measurement of the traumatic experiences. Mental representations of the trauma may constitute a mental network of recollections, verbal representations and images. These may be able to reinforce learning and conditioning even in the absence of external reinforcement. Thus, cogitations and nightmares of recollections may result in endless sequences of self-induced reinforcement of the conditioned emotional response.

Psychophysiological Responses to Intense but Neutral Stimulation (Auditory Startle)

The acoustic startle response (ASR) consists of a characteristic sequence of muscular and autonomic responses to sudden, intense stimuli. It is measured as the magnitude of the eyeblink reflexes.

The ASR is modified by non-startling effects that precede the startling stimulus. Such warning stimuli may facilitate or inhibit the magnitude of the ASR. If such a stimulus had previously been paired with a shock, the presence of such a cue augmented the amplitude of the ASR. Conditioning of this type is called fear-potentiated startle effect.

Affective valence and arousal can be induced by background information. Lang and co-workers (1990) studied the extent to which this modulates the acoustic startle response. They found that the ASR is associated with affective valence, whereas the skin conductance response is reflective of arousal.

Increased ASR is one of the cardinal features of PTSD.

Ornitz and Guthrie (1989) found impaired pre-pulse modulation, i.e. a significant loss of normal inhibitory modulation of the ASR by warning stimuli, in children with PTSD compared to age-matched, healthy control children.

In a group of Vietnam veterans with combat-related PTSD, Butler *et al.* (1990) found a higher eyeblink EMG response to an acoustic stimulus of intermediate intensity compared to a group of Vietnam veterans without PTSD. Paige *et al.* (1990) found larger HR responses to ASR in Vietnam veteran PTSD patients. Ross *et al.* (1989), however, found no difference in habituation of the ASR to a series of 100 dB tones between PTSD patients and healthy volunteers.

A study by Morgan *et al.* (1995) showed that infusion of yohimbine, which stimulates noradrenaline transmission in the brain, facilitated the acoustic startle response in combat veterans with PTSD. Another study by Grillon *et al.* (1997) found that darkness facilitated the acoustic startle reflex in combat veterans both with and without PTSD in comparison to non-combat control individuals. There seem to be important influences of contextual fear on the startle response.

Shalev *et al.* (1992) compared autonomic (ANS)- and central nervous system (CNS)-mediated responses to ASR in Israeli PTSD patients, patients with other anxiety disorders, healthy individuals with past traumatic experiences, and healthy individuals having experienced no traumatic event. They found a larger HR and SC response, and an impaired habituation of the SC response to the consecutive presentation of auditory stimuli in the PTSD patients compared to all other groups.

In a recent study, Shalev *et al.* (2000) showed that patients showed differential effects after a psychologically traumatic event. Patients who developed PTSD showed increased HR responses and slower habituation of SC responses to startling stimuli one and four months after the trauma. However, these responses were not seen one week after the trauma. These results suggest a progressive sensitization of the autonomic response to startling stimuli. These studies of ASR in PTSD have some characteristics which differentiate them from the previously mentioned studies. Firstly, the startle reflex represents an elementary stimulus, which is not associated with the traumatic experience and for which previous conditioning is unlikely. Secondly, ASR studies do not require deliberate mental activity by the individual. Thus, confounding by (un)conscious manipulations is less likely. Thirdly, it reflects impairments in structures such as the amygdala and other mesocortical areas, which are responsible for evaluation of the stimulus, memory, and arousal. Therefore, these studies suggest that in PTSD, there is an alteration of the responsiveness of the central nervous system to elementary stimuli. In addition, the capacity to effectively appraise intensive but redundant stimuli and to regulate the arousal response seems to be impaired, as habituation of the SC response is slow.

Summary

The studies using external stimuli support the associative learning paradigm, studies using the imagery technique extend the conditioning paradigm to mental representations of traumatic experiences, and studies of intense but neutral stimulations (ASR) show the abnormal responsiveness to elementary stimuli in PTSD patients.

Event-Related Electroencephalographic Potentials (ERPs)

The latency and amplitude of ERP components index specific aspects of stimulus and information processing. In contrast to responses by the autonomic nervous system, which occur within seconds, those of the central nervous system occur within milliseconds. The studies of Paige *et al.* (1990) and Lewine *et al.* (1997) showed an augmentation–reduction of P2 responses. Increases in acoustic stimulus intensity are normally directly correlated to increasing P2 amplitude responses. In contrast to such an augmenting response pattern, PTSD combat veterans showed a decreasing response pattern, i.e. decreasing P2 amplitudes. Such a pattern reflects a protectively tuned sensory system that dampens increased stimulation. Similar to findings in other diseases (schizophrenia, cocaine abusers), combat veterans with PTSD exhibited less habituation of the P50 potential to the second click in comparison to control individuals (Gillette *et al.*, 1997). This auditory P50 habituation was inversely correlated with re-experiencing symptoms within the PTSD group.

In the auditory oddball paradigm, PTSD patients were exposed to a series of high-frequency non-target tones, low-frequency distractor tones, and low-frequency target tones. PTSD patients showed longer reaction times, delayed N2, and attenuated P3 amplitudes to target and distractor stimuli (McFarlane *et al.*, 1993; Charles *et al.*, 1995; Metzger *et al.*, 1997a, 1997b). It is unclear whether this response abnormality is secondary to a motivational deficit or reflects a higher order cognitive impairment.

In summation, ERP findings provide evidence for increased cortical inhibition in response to high-intensity stimuli, auditory gating deficits, impairments in memory and concentration, and increased selective attention to trauma-related stimuli.

This psychophysiological research into PTSD supports the validity of the diagnostic entity, but more work needs to be done to test the robustness of the various results. Some of the stimulus presentation techniques are now being incorporated into neuroimaging symptom provocation studies. These are described elsewhere in this book.

OBSESSIVE–COMPULSIVE DISORDER (OCD)

Two loosely related goals have been pursued in the research of OCD. Firstly, the search for the biological basis of OCD led to an intense investigation of the EEG properties of OCD sufferers. Secondly, ANS measures were used in the assessment of OCD and in the treatment evaluation. An overview of the earlier research on psychophysiology in OCD is given by Sartory (1989).

EEG Studies

In OCD patients, some abnormalities in sleep EEG have been found. OCD patients have longer Stage 1 sleep and reduced Stage 3 and 4 sleep, which is indicated by the amount of delta activity (review by Sartory, 1989). However, these findings are not disorder-specific and have been found in depression and schizophrenia as well.

Furthermore, awake resting EEG measurements are variable and conflicting (Sartory, 1989; Towey *et al.*, 1994; Simpson *et al.*, 2000). One possible reason is that different subgroups of OCD patients exist. All show the symptoms of OCD, but perhaps differ in psychophysiological measures. Prichep *et al.* (1993) assumed two distinct groups of OCD patients. One group of patients is thought to be characterized by an excess in relative theta power and a second group by increased relative alpha power. By dividing 27 patients into two groups according to this classification, the response to treatment with serotonin reuptake inhibitors (fluvoxamine, fluoxetine, or clomipramine) could be predicted. Eighty percent of patients characterized by increased theta power were non-responders, whereas 82% of patients characterized by increased alpha power were responders. Interestingly, this result is consistent with the finding that serotonin reuptake inhibitors decrease alpha activity, but increase slow and fast activity (Prichep *et al.*, 1993). It might be helpful to follow-up on such a differentiation, in order to ensure more validity in further research results. Once established, such psychophysiological measures may be for use in clinical treatment assignment and the prediction of treatment response.

Symptom provocation studies constitute a further area of research. Possibly the first symptom provocation study including EEG measures was done by Simpson *et al.* (2000). Significant changes in alpha activity during live exposure were found. Unfortunately, only six patients and no control group were investigated so, as yet, no concrete evidence for specific EEG changes has been given. Future research is necessary to identify potential differences in power bands and to specify activated brain regions during sensitive stimulation.

In the investigation of event-related potentials (ERPs), consistent results were found for some components. Different studies found reduced latencies of the N200 and the P300 components (see Sartory, 1989; Towey *et al.*, 1990, 1994). The increase in N200 and P300 latency as a function of task difficulty, which is found in control Ss, was not found in OCD patients (Sartory, 1989; Towey *et al.*, 1990). These results are interesting, since other psychiatric disorders (depression, schizophrenia) are not accompanied by reduced, but rather by increased, ERP latencies. The reduced ERP latencies are interpreted as indicators of cortical hyperarousal. Towey *et al.* (1994) also found that attention-related processing negativity (PN) began earlier, lasted longer and was increased in OCD patients compared to control Ss. This may be interpreted as overfocused attention in OCD patients (Towey *et al.*, 1994). Another well-established finding is the enhanced contingent negative variation (CNV) during preparation of a (motor) response. This enhanced CNV also seems to be specific for OCD patients (Sartory, 1989). Sartory and Master (1984) found that with an interval of 5 s between warning and imperative stimulus, only the late, but not the early component of the CNV was affected. They proposed that this is due to the uncertainty of the situation and that this reflects the doubts of OCD patients regarding the requirements made of them.

ANS Activity

Emotional arousal or anxiety is a common observation in OCD during exposure to obsession-related stimuli, prevention of ritual behaviour, or while experiencing obsessive thoughts. The most effective therapy for OCD is exposure with response prevention, as is effective in severe phobias (Foa and Kozak, 1985). Therefore, the relevance for investigation of ANS responses is obvious.

One hypothesis was that OCD patients are in a state of abnormal arousal which, in the end, results in a failure to adapt to unwanted thoughts (Beech, Ciesielski and Gordon, 1983). This should lead to elevated baseline ANS activation, or at least to an elevated responsiveness to stressful stimuli. Although earlier studies found a generally increased ANS activation (e.g. Kelly, 1980; Insel, Zahn and Murphy, 1985), more recent studies were not able to confirm the hypothesis of a general hyperactivation (Berg *et al.*, 1986; Hoehn-Saric *et al.*, 1995; Zahn *et al.*, 1996). The hypothesis of a general hyper-responsiveness of OCD patients to stress was investigated during stressful mental activity. Despite some positive results (e.g. Insel, Zahn and Murphy, 1985), this hypothesis remains empirically unconfirmed (Kelly, 1980; Zahn *et al.*, 1996). On the contrary, patients with OCD react with less physiological flexibility to general stressful tasks (Hoehn-Saric, McLeod and Hipsley, 1995), but this is not specific for OCD patients, having also been found in other anxiety disorders (Hoehn-Saric, McLeod and Hipsley, 1995). Nevertheless, a significant positive correlation between symptom severity and general ANS reactivity was found in children and adolescents with OCD (Zahn *et al.*, 1996).

However, disorder-specific stimuli as well as obsessive thoughts increase ANS activity (SCF, SCL, HR) in OCD patients (Rabavilas and Boulougouris, 1974; Boulougouris, Rabavilas and Stefanis, 1977; Haines *et al.*, 1998). Patients with obsessional ruminations react with HR accelerations during the presentation of sensitive words in the same way as phobic Ss do (Eves and Tata, 1989). Words that are used to neutralize the obsessions evoked no HR reactions, whereas neutral words resulted in an HR deceleration (OR) (Eves and Tata, 1989).

A few studies investigated the effect of psychological treatment on ANS responses. A substantially greater reduction of HR and SCF was found for long-duration *in vivo* exposition compared to short-duration *in vivo* exposition (Boulougouris, Rabavilas and Stefanis, 1977). A study by Grayson, Foa and Steketee, (1982) focused on the investigation of the treatment process. A group of patients with washing compulsions performed *in vivo* exposure with focused attention, while a second group was distracted during exposure by playing a video game. Interestingly, HR reactions were attenuated during exposure in both conditions. The improvement was maintained in the focusing condition, but not in the distraction condition between the sessions (Grayson, Foa and Steketee, 1982).

Recent studies focused on the changes occurring during a pharmacological treatment. One major challenge in these studies was to disentangle disorder-independent drug effects from clinical changes, as psychoactive substances are known to induce changes in the ANS. In one study, clomipramine (a tricyclic antidepressant and serotonin reuptake inhibitor) effectively decreased symptoms in patients with OCD (Hoehn-Saric *et al.*, 1993). But tricyclic antidepressants are also known to generally induce HR accelerations (Sartory 1989). Zahn, Insel and Murphy, (1984) were able to demonstrate more clinical benefits and a marked reduction of SCL in clomipramine compared to placebo or clogyline (a monoamine oxidase (MAO) inhibitor) treatment time periods (crossover design). The number of non-specific SCR was reduced after clomipramine and clogyline compared to placebo periods. This was found during rest and during a threshold discrimination task. Additionally, after clomipramine periods, the OR (measured in amplitude of SCR) to startle-like loud noise was reduced and habituation was hastened. In contrast to the reduction in SC activity, a substantial increase of HR was found after treatment with clomipramine (12 beats per minute) and clogyline (six beats per minute), compared to placebo periods. In another study, Hoehn-Saric *et al.* (1993) found no effects of clomipramine during rest in a broad range of ANS measures. The only exception was the HR, which increased during clomipramine treatment and decreased during placebo treatment. However, the ANS reactivity to non-specific and to pathology-specific stressful stimuli compared to placebo was reduced. The conclusion was that the ANS effect of clomipramine is not disorder-specific. The effect might reflect a generally heightened indifference to psychological stressors.

It would be interesting to observe whether ANS reactivity differences can be found in subgroups of OCD patients (with groups divided, e.g. according to EEG power).

In summary, the hypotheses of a general hyperactivity or a general hyper-reactivity in OCD patients were not confirmed. Future research may focus on symptom provocation studies, to determine differences in OCD patient reactions to obsessive cues compared to control Ss and Ss suffering from other anxiety disorders. Especially interesting will be the investigation of EEG differences within symptom provocation studies. ANS measures may be valuable for complete assessment of OCD and evaluation of treatment outcome.

REFERENCES

American Psychiatric Association, 1994. *Diagnostic and Statistical Manual of Mental Disorders: DSM-IV*. American Psychiatric Association, Washington, DC.

Armir, N., McNally, R.J., Rieman, B.C., Burns, J., Lorenz, M. and Mullen, J.T., 1996. Suppression of the emotional stroop effect by increased anxiety in patients with social phobia. *Behaviour Research and Therapy*, **34**, 945–948.

Aronson, T.A., Carasiti, I., McBane, D. and Whitaker, A.P., 1989. Biological correlates of lactate sensitivity in panic disorder. *Biological Psychiatry*, **26**, 463–477.

Asmundson, G.J. and Stein, M.B., 1994. A preliminary analysis of pulmonary function in panic disorder: Implications for the dyspnea-fear theory. *Journal of Anxiety Disorders*, **8**, 63–69.

Ballenger, J.C., 1990. *Neurobiology of Panic Disorder*. Wiley-Liss, New York.

Beck, A.T., Emery, G. and Greenberg, R.L., 1985. *Anxiety Disorders and Phobias—A Cognitive Perspective*. Basic Books, New York.

Beech, H.R., Ciesielski, K.T. and Gordon, P.K., 1983. Further observations of evoked potentials in obsessional patients. *British Journal of Psychiatry*, **142**, 605–609.

Berg, C.J., Zahn, T.P., Behar, D. and Rapoport, J.L., 1986. Childhood obsessive–compulsive disorder: an anxiety disorder? In: Gittelman, R. (ed.), *Anxiety Disorder of Childhood*, pp. 126–135. Guilford Press, New York.

Blanchard, E.B., Kolb, L.C., Pallmeyer, T.P. and Gerardi, R.J., 1982. A psychophysiological study of post traumatic stress disorder in Vietnam veterans. *The Psychiatric Quarterly*, **54**, 220–229.

Blanchard, E.B., Kolb, L.C., Prins, A., Gates, S. and McCoy, G.C., 1991. Changes in plasma norepinephrine to combat-related stimuli among Vietnam veterans with posttraumatic stress disorder. *The Journal of Nervous and Mental Disease*, **179**, 371–373.

Blanchard, E.B., Hickling, E.J., Buckley, T.C., Taylor, A.E., Vollmer, A. and Loos, W.R., 1996. Psychophysiology of posttraumatic stress disorder related to motor vehicle accidents: replication and extension. *Journal of Consulting and Clinical Psychology*, **64**, 742–751.

Blix, A.S., Stromme, S.B. and Ursin, H., 1974. Additional heart rate: An indicator of psychological activation. *Aerospace Medicine*, **45**, 1219–1222.

Bocola, V., Trecco, M.D., Fabbrini, G., Paladini, C., Sollecito, A. and Martucci, N., 1998. Antipanic effect of fluoxetine measured by CO_2 challenge test. *Biological Psychiatry*, **43**, 612–615.

Bonn, J.A., Readhead, C.P.A. and Timmons, B.H., 1984. Enhanced adaptive behavioural response in agoraphobic patients pretreated with breathing retraining. *Lancet*, **1**, 665–669.

Boudewyns, P.A. and Heyr, L., 1990. Physiological to combat memories and preliminary treatment outcome in Vietnam veterans PTSD patients treated with direct therapeutic exposure. *Behavior Therapy*, **21**, 63–87.

Boulougouris, J.C., Rabavilas, A.D. and Stefanis, C., 1977. Psychophysiological responses in obsessional–compulsive patients. *Behaviour Research and Therapy*, **15**, 221–230.

Bradley, M.M., 2000. Emotion and motivation. In: Cacioppo, J.T., Tassinary, L.G. and Berntson, G.G. (eds), *Handbook of Psychophysiology*, pp. 602–642. Cambridge University Press, Cambridge.

Bradley, M.M., Lang, P.J. and Cuthbert, B.N., 1991. The Gainesville murders: Imagining the worst. *Psychophysiology*, **28**, S14 (Abstract).

Brende, J.O., 1982. Electrodermal responses in post-traumatic stress syndromes: A pilot study of cerebral hemisphere functioning in Vietnam veterans. *Journal of Nervous and Mental Disease*, **170**, 352–361.

Buchsbaum, M.S. and Wu, J.C., 1987. Hypofrontality in schizophrenia as assessed by PET. *American Journal of Psychiatry*, **144**, 122–122.

Butler, R.W., Braff, D.L., Rausch, J.L., Jenkins, M.A., Sprock, J. and Geyer, M.A., 1990. Physiological evidence of exaggerated startle response in a subgroup of Vietnam veterans with combat-related PTSD. *American Journal of Psychiatry*, **147**, 1308–1312.

Caldirola, D., Perna, G., Arancio, C., Bertani, A. and Bellodi, L., 1997. The 35% CO_2 challenge test in patients with social phobia. *Psychiatry Research*, **71**, 41–48.

Cameron, O.G., Lee, M.A., Curtis, G.C. and McCann, D.S., 1987. Endocrine and physiological changes during "spontaneous" panic attacks. *Psychoneuroendocrinology*, **12**, 321–331.

Carr, R.E., Lehrer, P.M. and Hochron, S.M., 1992. Panic symptoms in asthma and panic disorder: a preliminary test of the dyspnea-fear theory. *Behavior Research and Therapy*, **30**, 251–261.

Carter, W.R., Johnson, M.C. and Borkovec, T.D., 1986. Worry: An electrocortical analysis. *Advances in Behavioural Research and Therapy*, **8**, 193–204.

Castellani, S., Quillen, M.A., Vaughan, D.A., Hund, M.A., Ho, L., Ziegler, M.G. and Le-Vine, W.R., 1988. TSH and catecholamine response to TRH in panic disorder. *Biological Psychiatry*, **24**, 87–90.

Charles, G., Hansenne, M., Ansseau, M., Pitchot, W., Machowski, R., Schittecatte, M. and Wilmotte, J., 1995. P300 in posttraumatic stress disorder. *Neuropsychobiology*, **32**, 72–74.

Charney, D.S., Heninger, G.R. and Breier, A., 1984. Noradrenergic function in panic anxiety. Effects of yohimbine in healthy subjects and patients with agoraphobia and panic disorder. *Archives of General Psychiatry*, **41**, 751–763.

Clark, D.M., 1988. A cognitive model of panic attacks. In: Rachman, S. and Maser, T.J. (eds), *Panic: Psychological Perspectives*, p. 71. Lawrence Erlbaum, New Jersey.

Cook, E.W., Melamed, B.G., Cuthbert, B.N., McNeil, D.W. and Lang, P.J., 1988. Emotional imagery and the differential diagnosis of anxiety. *Journal of Consulting and Clinical Psychology*, **56**, 734–740.

Coryell, W. and Arndt, S., 1999. The 35% CO_2 inhalation procedure: test–retest reliability. *Biological Psychiatry*, **45**, 923–927.

Cowley, D.S., Hyde, T.S., Dager, S.R. and Dunner, D.L., 1987. Lactate infusions: the role of baseline anxiety. *Psychiatry Research*, **21**, 169–179.

Craske, M. and Barlow, D., 1990. Nocturnal panic: Response to hyperventilation and carbon dioxide challenges. *Journal of Abnormal Psychology*, **99**, 302–307.

Craske, M.G., Sanderson, W.C. and Barlow, D.H., 1987. How do desynchronous response systems relate to the treatment of agoraphobia: A follow-up evaluation. *Behaviour Research and Therapy*, **25**, 117–122.

Cuthbert, B.N. and Lang, P.J., 1989. Imagery, memory, and emotion: a psychophysiological analysis of clinical anxiety. In: Turpin, G. (eds), *Handbook of Clinical Psychophysiology*, pp. 105–134. Wiley, New York.

Cuthbert, B.N., Drobes, D., Patrick, C.J. and Lang, P.J., 1994. Autonomic and startle responding during affective imagery among anxious patients. *Psychophysiology*, **31**, S37 (Abstract).

Davidson, R.J., 1992. Emotion and affective style: Hemispheric substrates. *Psychological Science*, **3**, 39–43.

Davidson, R.J., Marshall, J.R., Tomarken, A.J. and Henriques, J.B., 2000. While a phobic waits: Regional brain electrical and autonomic activity in social phobics during anticipation of public speaking. *Biological Psychiatry*, **47**, 85–95.

Davidson, R.J., Ekman, P., Saron, C., Senulis, J.A. and Friesen, W.V., 1990. Approach-withdrawal and cerebral asymmetry: Emotional expression and brain physiology I. *Journal of Personality and Social Psychology*, **58**, 330–341.

Dawson, M.E., Schell, A.M. and Filion, D.L., 2000. The electrodermal system. In: Cacioppo, J.T., Tassinary, L.G. and Berntson, G.G. (eds), *Handbook of Psychophysiology*, pp. 200–223. Cambridge University Press, Cambridge.

De Jong, P.J., Merckelbach, H., Arntz, A. and Nijman, H., 1992. Covariation detection in treated and untreated spider phobics. *Journal of Abnormal Psychology*, **101**, 724–727.

Dobbs, D. and Wilson, W.P., 1960. Observations on the persistence of war neurosis. *Diseases of Nervous System*, **21**, 40–46.

Dubrovsky, B., Solyom, L. and Barbas, H., 1978. Characteristics of the contingent negative variation in patients suffering from specific phobias. *Biological Psychiatry*, **13**, 531–540.

Ehlers, A., Margraf, J., Roth, W.T., Taylor, C.B., Maddock, R.J., Sheikh, J., Kopell, M.L., McClenahan, K.L., Gossard, D., Blowers, G.H. and Agras, W.S.K.B.S., 1986. Lactate infusions and panic attacks: do patients and controls respond differently? *Psychiatry Research*, **17**, 295–308.

Erdmann, G. and Baumann, S., 1996. Sind psychophysiologische Veränderungen im Paradigma "Öffentliches Sprechen" Ausdruck emotionaler Belastung? *Zeitschrift für experimentelle Psychologie*, **XLIII**, 224-255.

Eves, F. and Tata, P., 1989. Phasis cardiac and electrodermal reactions to idiographic stimuli in obsessional subjects. *Behavioral Psychotherapy*, **17**, 71–83.

Fairbank, J.A. and Keane, T.M., 1982. Flooding for combat-related stress disorder: assessment of anxiety reduction across traumatic memories. *Behavior Therapy*, **13**, 499–510.

Fisher, L.M. and Wilson, G.T., 1985. A study of the psychology of agoraphobia. *Behaviour Research and Therapy*, **23**, 97–107.

Foa, E.B. and Kozak, M.J., 1985. Treatment of anxiety disorders: implications for psychopathology. In: Tuma, A.H. and Maser, J. (eds), *Anxiety and Anxiety Disorders*, pp. 421–452. Lawrence Erlbaum, Hillsdale, NJ.

Foa, E.B. and Kozak, M.J., 1993. Pathological anxiety: The meaning and the structure of fear. In: Birbaumer, N. and Öhman, A. (eds), *The Structure of Emotion*, pp. 110–121. Hogrefe & Huber, Seattle.

Fredrikson, M., Wik, G., Greitz, T., Eriksson, L., Stone Elander S, Ericson, K. and Sedvall, G., 1993. Regional cerebral blood flow during experimental phobic fear. *Psychophysiology*, **30**, 126–130.

Freedman, R.R., Ianni, P., Ettedgui, E. and Puthezhath, N., 1985. Ambulatory monitoring of panic disorder. *Archives of General Psychiatry*, **42**, 244–248.

Freedman, R.R., Ianni, P., Ettedgui, E., Pohl, R. and Rainey, J.M., 1984. Psychophysiological factors in panic disorders. *Psychopathology*, **17**, 66–73.

Gaffney, F.A., Fenton, B.J., Lane, L.D. and Lake, C.R., 1988. Hemodynamic, ventilatory, and biochemical responses of panic patients and normal controls with sodium lactate infusion and spontaneous panic attacks. *Archives of General Psychiatry*, **45**, 53–60.

Geer, J.H., 1966. Fear and autonomic arousal. *Journal of Abnormal Psychology*, **71**, 253–255.

Gillette, G.M., Skinner, R.D., Rasco, L.M., Fielstein, E.M., Davis, D.H., Pawelak, J.E., Freeman, T.W., Karson, C.N., Boop, F.A. and Garcia, R.E., 1997. Combat veterans with posttraumatic stress disorder exhibit decreased habituation of the P1 midlatency auditory evoked potential. *Life Sciences*, **61**, 1421–1434.

Globisch, J., Hamm, A.O., Esteves, F. and Öhman, A., 1999. Fear appears fast: Temporal course of startle reflex potentiation in animal fearful subjects. *Psychophysiology*, **36**, 66–75.

Gorman, J.M., Browne, S.T., Papp, L.A., Martinez, J., Welkowitz, L., Coplan, J.D., Goetz, R.R., Kent, J. and Klein, D.F., 1997. Effect of antipanic treatment on response to carbon dioxide. *Biological Psychiatry*, **42**, 982–991.

Gorman, J.M., Fyer, M.R., Goetz, R., Askanazi, J., Liebowitz, M.R., Fyer, A.J., Kinney, J. and Klein, D.F., 1988. Ventilatory physiology of patients with panic disorder. *Archives of General Psychiatry*, **45**, 31–39.

Gorman, J.M., Kent, J., Martinez, J., Browne, S., Coplan, J. and Papp, L.A., 2001. Physiological changes during carbon dioxide inhalation in patients with panic disorder, major depression, and premenstrual dysphoric disorder. *Archives of General Psychiatry*, **58**, 125–131.

Gorman, J.M., Papp, L.A., Coplan, J.D., Martinez, J.M., Lennon, S., Goetz, R.R., Ross, D. and Klein, D.F., 1994. Anxiogenic effects of CO_2 and hyperventilation in patients with panic disorder. *American Journal of Psychiatry*, **151**, 547–553.

Grayson, J.B., Foa, E.B. and Steketee, G., 1982. Habituation during exposure treatment: Distraction vs. attention-focussing. *Behavior Research and Therapy*, **20**, 323–328.

Griez, E., de-Loof, C., Pols, H., Zandbergen, J. and Lousberg, H., 1990. Specific sensitivity of patients with panic attacks to carbon dioxide inhalation. *Psychiatry Research*, **31**, 193–199.

Griez, E.J., Lousberg, H., van-den-Hout, M.A. and van-der-Molen G.M., 1987. CO_2 vulnerability in panic disorder. *Psychiatry Research*, **20**, 87–95.

Grillon, C., Pellowski, M., Merikangas, K.R. and Davis, M., 1997. Darkness facilitates the acoustic startle reflex in humans. *Biological Psychiatry*, **42**, 453–460.

Gurguis, G.N., Vitton, B.J. and Uhde, T.W., 1997. Behavioral, sympathetic and adrenocortical responses to yohimbine in panic disorder patients and normal controls. *Psychiatry Research*, **71**, 27–39.

Guyton, A.C. and Hall, J.E., 1996. *Textbook of Medical Physiology*. Saunders, Philadelphia.

Haines, J., Josephs, S., Williams, C.L. and Wells, J.H., 1998. The psychophysiology of obsessive–compulsive disorder. *Behaviour Change*, **15**, 244–254.

Hamm, A.O., Cuthbert, B.N., Globisch, J. and Vaitl, D., 1997. Fear and the startle reflex: Blink modulation and autonomic response patterns in animal and mutilation fearful subjects. *Psychophysiology*, **34**, 97–107.

Hamm, A.O., Gerlach, M., Globisch, J. and Vaitl, D., 1992. Phobia specific startle reflex modulation during affective imagery and slide viewing. *Psychophysiology*, **29**, S36 (Abstract).

Harrison, W.M., Sandberg, D., Gorman, J.M., Fyer, M., Nee, J., Uy, J. and Endicott, J., 1989. Provocation of panic with carbon dioxide inhalation in patients with premenstrual dysphoria. *Psychiatry Research*, **27**, 183–192.

Hazlett, R.L., McLeod, D.R. and Hoehn, S.R., 1994. Muscle tension in generalized anxiety disorder: elevated muscle tonus or agitated movement? *Psychophysiology*, **31**, 189–195.

Heimberg, R.G., Hope, D.A., Dodge, C.S. and Becker, R.E., 1990. DSM-III subtypes of social phobia. *The Journal of Nervous and Mental Disease*, **178**, 172–179.

Heller, W., 1990. The neuropsychology of emotion: Developmental patterns and implications for psychopathology. In: Stein, N., Leventhal, B.L. and Trabasso, T. (eds), *Psychological and Biological Approaches to Emotion*, pp. 167–211. Erlbaum, Hillsdale, NJ.

Heller, W., 1993. Neuropsychological mechanisms of individual differences in emotion, personality, and arousal. *Neuropsychology*, **7**, 476–489.

Heller, W., Etienne, M.A. and, Miller, G.A., 1995. Patterns of perceptual asymmetry in depression and anxiety: Implications for neuropsychological models of emotion and psychopathology. *Journal of Abnormal Psychology*, **104**, 327–333.

Henriques, J.B. and Davidson, R.J., 1990. Regional brain electrical asymmetries discriminate between previously depressed and healthy control subjects. *Journal of Abnormal Psychology*, **99**, 22–31.

Henriques, J.B. and Davidson, R.J., 1991. Left frontal hypoactivation in depression. *Journal of Abnormal Psychology*, **100**, 535–545.

Hibbert, G. and Pilsbury, D., 1988. Hyperventilation in panic attacks. Ambulant monitoring of transcutaneous carbon dioxide. *British Journal of Psychiatry*, **153**, 76–80.

Hiller, W., Zaudig, M. and von Bose, M. 1989. The overlap between depression and anxiety on different levels of psychopathology. *Journal of Affective Disorders*, **16**, 223–231.

Hoehn-Saric, R., 1998. Psychic and somatic anxiety: worries, somatic symptoms and physiological changes. *Acta Psychiatrica Scandinavica*, **98**, 32–38.

Hoehn-Saric, R., McCleod, D.R. and Zimmerli, W.D., 1989. Somatic manifestations in women with generalized anxiety disorder. *Archives of General Psychiatry*, **46**, 1113–1119.

Hoehn-Saric, R., McLeod, D.R. and Hipsley, P.A., 1995. Is hyperarousal essential to obsessive–compulsive disorder? *Archives of General Psychiatry*, **52**, 688–693.

Hoehn-Saric, R., McLeod, D.R. and Zimmerli, W.D., 1991. Psychophysiological response patterns in panic disorder. *Acta Psychiatrica Scandinavica*, **83**, 4–11.

Hoehn-Saric, R., McLeod, D.R., Zimmerli, W.D. and Hipsley, P.A., 1993. Symptoms and physiologic manifestations in obsessive compulsive patients before and after treatment with clomipramine. *Journal of Clinical Psychiatry*, **54**, 272–276.

Hofmann, S.G., Newmark, M., Ehlers, A. and Roth, W.T., 1995. Psychophysiological differences between subgroups of social phobia. *Journal of Abnormal Psychology*, **104**, 224–231.

Hugdahl, K., 1989. Simple phobias. In: Turpin, G. (eds), *Handbook of Clinical Psychophysiology*, pp. 283–308. Wiley, New York.

Hugdahl, K. and Öst, L.-G., 1985. Subjectively rated physiological and cognitive symptoms in six different clinical phobias. *Personality and Individual Differences*, **6**, 175–188.

Insel, T.R., Zahn, T.P. and Murphy, D.L., 1985. Obsessive–compulsive disorder: an anxiety disorder? In: Tuma, A.H. and Maser, J. (eds), *Anxiety and the Anxiety Disorders*, pp. 577–590. Lawrence Erlbaum Associates, Hillside, NJ.

James, W., 1884. What is emotion? *Mind*, **19**, 188–205.

Jerremalm, A., Jansson, L. and Öst, L.-G., 1986. Cognitive and physiological reactivity and the effects of different behavioral methods in the treatment of social phobia. *Behaviour Research and Therapy*, **24**, 171–180.

Katon, W. and Roy-Byrne, P.P., 1991. Mixed anxiety and depression. *Journal of Abnormal Psychology*, **100**, 337–345.

Keane, T.M. and Kaloupek, D.G., 1982. Imaginal flooding in the treatment of post traumatic stress disorder. *Journal of Consulting and Clinical Psychology*, **50**, 138–140.

Keane, T.M., Kolb, L.C., Kaloupek, D.G., Orr, S.P., Blanchard, E.B., Thomas, R.G., Hsieh, F.Y. and Lavori, P.W., 1998. Utility of psychophysiological measurement in the diagnosis of posttraumatic stress disorder: results from a Department of Veterans Affairs Cooperative Study. *Journal of Consulting and Clinical Psychology*, **66**, 914–923.

Kelly, D., 1980. *Anxiety and Emotions*. Charles C. Thomas, Springfield.

Klein, D.F., 1993. False suffocation alarms, spontaneous panics, and related conditions. An integrative hypothesis. *Archives of General Psychiatry*, **50**, 306–317.

Klein, E., Cnaani, E., Harel, T., Braun, S. and Ben-Haim, S.A., 1995. Altered heart rate variability in panic disorder patients. *Biological Psychiatry*, **37**, 18–24.

Klorman, R., Weissberg, R.P. and Wiesenfeld, A.R., 1977. Individual differences in fear and autonomic reactions to affective stimulation. *Psychophysiology*, **17**, 513–523.

Kolb, L.C., 1987. A neuropsychological hypothesis explaining the post-traumatic stress disorder. *American Journal of Psychiatry*, **144**, 989–995.

Lang, P.J., 1968. Fear reduction and fear behavior: Problems in treating a construct. In: Shlien, J.M. (ed.), *Research in Psychotherapy*, pp. 90–103. American Psychological Association, Washington DC.

Lang, P.J., 1971. The application of psychophysiological methods in the study of psychotherapy and behavior modification. In: Bergin, A.E. and Garfield, S.L. (eds), *Handbook of Psychotherapy and Behavior Modification*, pp. 75–125. Wiley, New York.

Lang, P.J., 1993. The three-system approach to emotion. In: Birbaumer, N. and Öhman, A. (eds), *The Structure of Emotion*, pp. 18–30. Hogrefe & Huber, Seattle.

Lang, P.J., Bradley, M.M. and Cuthbert, B.N., 1990. Emotion, attention, and the startle reflex. *Psychological Review*, **97**, 377–398.

Lang, P.J., Bradley, M.M. and Cuthbert, B.N., 1997. Motivated attention: affect, activation, and action. In: Lang, P.J., Simons, R.F. and Balban, M.T. (eds), *Attention and Orienting: Sensory and Motivational Processes*, pp. 97–133. Lawrence Erlbaum Associates, New Jersey, London.

Lang, P.J., Bradley, M.M. and Cuthbert, B.N., 1998a. Emotion, motivation, and anxiety: brain mechanisms and psychophysiology. *Society of Biological Psychiatry*, **44**, 1248–1263.

Lang, P.J., Cuthbert, B.N. and Bradley, M.M., 1998b. Measuring emotion in therapy: Imagery, activation, and feeling. *Behavior Therapy*, **29**, 655–674.

Lang, P.J., Kozak, M.J., Miller, G.A., Levin, D.N. and McLean, A., 1980. Emotional imagery: Conceptual structure and pattern of somato-visceral response. *Psychophysiology*, **17**, 179–192.

Lang, P.J., Levin, D.N., Miller, G.A. and Kozak, M.J., 1983. Fear behavior, fear imagery, and the psychophysiology of emotion: The problem of affective response integration. *The Journal of Abnormal Psychology*, **92**, 276–306.

Lang, P.J., Melamed, B.G. and Hart, J., 1970. A psychophysiological analysis of fear modification using an automated desensitization procedure. *Journal of Abnormal Psychology*, **76**, 220–234.

Larson, C.L., Davidson, R.J., Abercrombie, H.C., Ward, R.T., Schaefer, S.M., Jackson, D.C., Holden, J.E. and Perlman, S.B., 1998. Relations between PET-derived measures of thalamic glucose metabolism and EEG alpha power. *Psychophysiology*, **35**, 162–169.

Levin, A.P., Saoud, J.B., Strauman, T., Gorman, J.M., Fyer, A., Crawford, R. and Liebowitz, M.R., 1993. Responses of "generalized" and "discrete" social phobics during public speaking. *Journal of Anxiety Disorders*, **7**, 207–221.

Lewine, J.D., Canive, J.M., Orrison, W.W.J., Edgar, C.J., Provencal, S.L., Davis, J.T., Paulson, K., Graeber, D., Roberts, B., Escalona, P.R. and Calais, L., 1997. Electrophysiological abnormalities in PTSD. *Annals of the New York Academy of Sciences*, **821**, 508–511.

Ley, R., 1989. Dyspneic-fear and catastrophic cognitions in hyperventilatory panic attacks. *Behavior Research and Therapy*, **27**, 549–554.

Ley, R., 1994a. Breathing and the psychology of emotion, cognition, and behavior. In: Timmons, B. and Ley, R. (eds), *Behavioral and Psychological Approaches to Breathing Disorders*. Plenum, New York.

Ley, R., 1994b. The "suffocation alarm" theory of panic attacks: a critical commentary. *Journal of Behavior Therapy and Experimental Psychiatry*, **25**, 269–273.

Ley, R., 1998. Pulmonary function and dyspnea/suffocation theory of panic. *Journal of Behavior Therapy and Experimental Psychiatry*, **29**, 1–11.

Liebowitz, M.R., Gorman, J.M., Fyer, A.J., Levitt, M., Dillon, D., Levy, G., Appleby, I.L., Anderson, S., Palij, M., Davies, S.O. *et al.*, 1985. Lactate provocation of panic attacks. II. Biochemical and physiological findings. *Archives of General Psychiatry*, **42**, 709–719.

Lumsden, J., Howard, R.C. and Fenton, G.W., 1986. The contingent negative variation (CNV) to fear-related stimuli in acquisition and extinction. *International Journal of Psychophysiology*, **3**, 253–261.

Malloy, P.F., Fairbank, J.A. and Keane, T.M., 1983. Validation of a multimethod assessment of posttraumatic stress disorders in Vietnam veterans. *Journal of Consulting and Clinical Psychology*, **51**, 488–494.

Margraf, J., Ehlers, A. and Roth, W.T., 1986. Sodium lactate infusions and panic attacks: a review and critique. *Psychosomatic Medicine*, **48**, 23–51.

Marks, I., Boulougouris, J. and Marset, P., 1971. Flooding versus desensitization in the treatment of phobic patients: A crossover study. *British Journal of Psychiatry*, **119**, 353–375.

Mathews, A., 1990. Why worry? The cognitive function of anxiety. *Behaviour Research and Therapy*, **28**, 455–468.

Mathews, A. and MacLeod, C., 1985. Selective processing of threat cues in anxiety states. *Behaviour Research and Therapy*, **23**, 563–569.

McFall, M.E., Murburg, M.M., Ko, G.N. and Veith, R.C., 1990. Autonomic responses to stress in Vietnam combat veterans with posttraumatic stress disorder. *Biological Psychiatry*, **27**, 1165–1175.

McFarlane, W.R., Dunne, E., Lukens, E., Newmark, M., McLaughlin, T.J., Deakins, S. and Horen, B., 1993. From research to clinical practice: dissemination of New York State's family psychoeducation project. *Hospital and Community Psychiatry*, **44**, 265–270.

McNally, R.J., 1994. *Panic Disorder: A Critical Analysis*. Guilford, New York.

McNally, R.J., Hornig, C.D. and Donnell, C.D., 1995. Clinical versus nonclinical panic: A test of suffocation false alarm theory. *Behavior Research and Therapy*, **33**, 127–131.

McNeil, D.W., Vrana, S.R., Melamed, B.G., Cuthbert, B.N. and Lang, P.J., 1993. Emotional imagery in simple and social phobia: Fear versus anxiety. *Journal of Abnormal Psychology*, **102**, 212–225.

Metzger, L.J., Orr, S.P., Lasko, N.B., Berry, N.J. and Pitman, R.K., 1997a. Evidence for diminished P3 amplitudes in PTSD. *Annals of the New York Academy of Sciences*, **821**, 499–503.

Metzger, L.J., Orr, S.P., Lasko, N.B. and Pitman, R.K., 1997b. Auditory event-related potentials to tone stimuli in combat-related posttraumatic stress disorder. *Biological Psychiatry*, **42**, 1006–1015.

Michelson, L., Mavissakalian, M. and Marchione, K., 1985. Cognitive and behavioral treatments of agoraphobia: clinical, behavioral, and psychophysiological outcomes. *Journal of Consulting and Clinical Psychology*, **53**, 913–925.

Michelson, L., Mavissakalian, M., Marchione, K., Ulrich, R.F., Marchione, N. and Testa, S., 1990. Psychophysiological outcome of cognitive, behavioral and psychophysiologically-based treatments of agoraphobia. *Behaviour Research and Therapy*, **28**, 127–139.

Morgan, C.A., Grillon, C., Southwick, S.M., Nagy, L.M., Davis, M., Krystal, J.H. and Charney, D.S., 1995. Yohimbine facilitated acoustic startle in combat veterans with post-traumatic stress disorder. *Psychopharmacology*, **117**, 466–471.

Mowrer, O.H., 1939. A stimulus-response analysis of anxiety and its role as a reinforcement agent. *Psychological Review*, **46**, 553–556.

Mühlberger, A., 1997. *Exposition in virtuellen Welten zur Therapie von Flugangst. Prozeßanalyse*. Unveröffentlichte Diplomarbeit: Universität Würzburg, Würzburg.

Mühlberger, A., Herrmann, M., Wiedemann, G., Ellgring, H. and Pauli, P., 2001. Repeated exposure of flight phobics to flights in virtual reality. *Behaviour Research and Therapy*, **39**, 1033–1050.

Naveteur, J., Roy, J.C., Ovelac, E. and Steinling, M., 1992. Anxiety, emotion and cerebral blood flow. *International Journal of Psychophysiology*, **13**, 137–146.

Nutt, D.J., 1989. Altered central alpha 2-adrenoceptor sensitivity in panic disorder. *Archives of General Psychiatry*, **46**, 165–169.

Ornitz, E.M. and Guthrie, D., 1989. Long-term habituation and sensitization of the acoustic startle response in the normal adult human [published erratum appears in *Psychophysiology* 1989 Sep; **26**(5), 602]. *Psychophysiology*, **26**, 166–173.

Orr, S.P., Meyerhoff, J.L., Edwards, J.V. and Pitman, R.K., 1998. Heart rate and blood pressure resting levels and responses to generic stressors in Vietnam veterans with posttraumatic stress disorder. *Journal of Traumatic Stress*, **11**, 155–164.

Orr, S.P., Metzger, L.J., Lasko, N.B., Macklin, M.L., Peri, T. and Pitman, R.K., 2000. De novo conditioning in trauma-exposed individuals with and without posttraumatic stress disorder. *Journal of Abnormal Psychology*, **109**, 290–298.

Öhman, A., 1993. Fear and anxiety as emotional phenomena: Clinical phenomenology, evolutionary perspectives, and information-processing mechanisms. In: Lewis, M. and Haviland, M. (eds), *Handbook of Emotions*, pp. 511–536. Guilford Press, New York.

Öhman, A. and Soares, J.J.F., 1994. "Unconscious anxiety": Phobic responses to masked stimuli. *Journal of Abnormal Psychology*, **103**, 231–240.

Öhman, A., Hamm, A.O. and Hugdahl, K., 2000. Cognition and the autonomic nervous system: orienting, anticipation, and conditioning. In: Cacioppo, J.T., Tassinary, L.G. and Berntson, G.G. (eds), *Handbook of Psychophysiology*, pp. 533–575. Cambridge University Press, Cambridge.

Öst, L.G., 1989. Panic disorder, agoraphobia, and social phobia. In: Turpin, G. (ed.), *Handbook of Clinical Psychophysiology*, pp. 309–327. John Wiley & Sons, New York.

Öst, L.G., 1990. Psychophysiological assessment of agoraphobia. *Journal of Psychophysiology*, **4**, 315–319.

Öst, L.G., 1996. One-session group treatment of spider phobia. *Behavior Research and Therapy*, **34**, 707–715.

Öst, L.G. and Hugdahl, K., 1983. Acquisition of agoraphobia, mode of onset and anxiety response patterns. *Behavior Research and Therapy*, **21**, 623–631.

Öst, L.G., Jerremalm, A. and Jansson, L., 1984. Individual response patterns and the effects of different behavioral methods in the treatment of agoraphobia. *Behavior Research and Therapy*, **22**, 697–707.

Paige, S.R., Reid, G.M., Allen, M.G. and Newton, J.E., 1990. Psychophysiological correlates of posttraumatic stress disorder in Vietnam veterans. *Biological Psychiatry*, **27**, 419–430.

Pain, M.C., Biddle, N. and Tiller, J.W., 1988. Panic disorder, the ventilatory response to carbon dioxide and respiratory variables. *Psychosomatic Medicine*, **50**, 541–548.

Pallmeyer, T.P., Blanchard, E.B. and Kolb, L.C., 1986. The psychophysiology of combat-induced post traumatic stress disorder in Vietnam veterans. *Behavior Research and Therapy*, **24**, 645–652.

Panayiotou, G. and Vrana, S.R., 1998. Effect of self-focused attention on the startle reflex, heart rate, and memory performance among socially anxious and nonanxious individuals. *Psychophysiology*, **35**, 328–336.

Papp, L.A., Martinez, J.M., Klein, D.F., Coplan, J.D. and Gorman, J.M., 1995. Rebreathing tests in panic disorder. *Biological Psychiatry*, **38**, 240–245.

Papp, L.A., Martinez, J.M., Klein, D.F., Coplan, J.D., Norman, R.G., Cole, R., de-Jesus, M.J., Ross, D., Goetz, R. and Gorman, J.M., 1997. Respiratory psychophysiology of panic disorder: three respiratory challenges in 98 subjects [see comments]. *American Journal of Psychiatry*, **154**, 1557–1565.

Pauli, P., Marquardt, C., Hartl, L., Nutzinger, D.O., Holzl, R. and Strian, F., 1991. Anxiety induced by cardiac perceptions in patients with panic attacks: a field study. *Behavior Research and Therapy*, **29**, 137–145.

Perna, G., Barbini, B., Cocchi, S., Bertani, A. and Gasperini, M., 1995a. 35% CO_2 challenge in panic and mood disorders. *Journal of Affective Disorders*, **33**, 189–194.

Perna, G., Bertani, A., Arancio, C., Ronchi, P. and Bellodi, L., 1995b. Laboratory response of patients with panic and Obsessive–compulsive disorders to 35% CO_2 challenges. *American Journal of Psychiatry*, **152**, 85–89.

Perna, G., Battaglia, M., Garberi, A., Arancio, C., Bertani, A. and Bellodi, L., 1994. Carbon dioxide/oxygen challenge test in panic disorder. *Psychiatry Research*, **52**, 159–171.

Perna, G., Cocchi, S., Bertani, A., Arancio, C. and Bellodi, L., 1995c. Sensitivity to 35% CO_2 in healthy first-degree relatives of patients with panic disorder. *American Journal of Psychiatry*, **152**, 623–625.

Perna, G., Bertani, A., Gabriele, A., Politi, E. and Bellodi, L., 1997. Modification of 35% carbon dioxide hypersensitivity across one week of treatment with clomipramine and fluvoxamine: a double-blind, randomized, placebo-controlled study. *Journal of Clinical Psychopharmacology*, **17**, 173–178.

Pitman, R.K., 1988. Post-traumatic stress disorder, conditioning, and network theory. *Psychiatric Annals*, **18**, 182–189.

Pitman, R.K., Orr, S.P., Forgue, D.F., Altman, B. and Jong, J.B.D., 1990. Psychophysiologic responses to combat imagery of Vietnam veterans with posttraumatic stress disorder versus other anxiety disorders. *The Journal of Abnormal Psychology*, **99**, 49–54.

Pitman, R.K., Orr, S.P., Forgue, D.F., de-Jong, J.B. and Claiborn, J.M., 1987. Psychophysiologic assessment of posttraumatic stress disorder imagery in Vietnam combat veterans. *Archives of General Psychiatry*, **44**, 970–975.

Prichep, L.S., Mas, F., Hollander, E., Liebowitz, M., John, E.R., Almas, M., DeCaria, C.M. and Levine, R.H., 1993. Quantitative electroencephalographic subtyping of obsessive–compulsive disorder. *Psychiatry Research: Neuroimaging*, **50**, 25–32.

Rabavilas, A.D. and Boulougouris, J.C., 1974. Physiological accompaniments of ruminations, flooding and thought-stopping in obsessive patients. *Behavior Research and Therapy*, **12**, 239–243.

Rachman, S., 1977. The conditioning theory of fear-acquisition: a critical examination. *Behavior Research and Therapy*, **14**, 333–338.

Rapee, R.M., Brown, T.A., Antony, M.M. and Barlow, D.H., 1992. Response to hyperventilation and inhalation of 5.5% carbon dioxide-enriched air across the DSM-III-R anxiety disorders. *Journal of Abnormal Psychology*, **101**, 538–552.

Ross, R.J., Ball, W.A., Cohen, M.E., Silver, S.M., Morrison, A.R. and Dinges, D.F., 1989. Habituation of the startle reflex in posttraumatic stress disorder. *Journal of Neuropsychiatry and Clinical Neuroscience*, **1**, 305–307.

Roth, W.T., Telch, M.J., Taylor, C.B. and Agras, W.S., 1988. Autonomic changes after treatment of agoraphobia with panic attacks. *Psychiatry Research*, **24**, 95–107.

Roth, W.T., Margraf, J., Ehlers, A., Taylor, C.B., Maddock, R.J., Davies, S. and Agras, W.S., 1992. Stress test reactivity in panic disorder. *Archives of General Psychiatry*, **49**, 301–310.

Sanderson, W.C. and Wetzler, S., 1990. Five percent carbon dioxide challenge: valid analogue and marker of panic disorder? *Biological Psychiatry*, **27**, 689–701.

Sanderson, W.C., Rapee, R.M. and Barlow, D.H., 1989. The influence of an illusion of control on panic attacks induced via inhalation of 5.5% carbon dioxide-enriched air. *Archives of General Psychiatry*, **46**, 157–162.

Sanderson, W.C., Wetzler, S. and Asnis, G.M., 1994. Alprazolam blockade of CO_2-provoked panic in patients with panic disorder. *American Journal of Psychiatry*, **151**, 1220–1222.

Sartory, G., 1983. The orienting response and psychopathology: Anxiety and phobias. In: Siddle D.A.T. (ed.), *Orienting and Habituation: Perspectives in Human Research*, pp. 449–474. Wiley, New York.

Sartory, G., 1989. Obsessional–compulsive disorder. In: Turpin, G. (eds), *Handbook of Clinical Psychophysiology*, pp. 329–356. John Wiley & Sons, New York.

Sartory, G. and Lader, M.H., 1981. Psychophysiology and drugs in anxiety and phobias. In: Christie, M.I. and Mellett, P. (eds), *Foundations of Psychosomatics*, pp. 169–191. Wiley, Chichester.

Sartory, G. and Master, D., 1984. Contingent negative variation in obsessional–compulsive patients. *Biological Psychology*, **18**, 253–267.

Sartory, G., Roth, W.T. and Kopell, M.L., 1992. Psychophysiological assessment of driving phobia. *Journal of Psychology*, **6**, 311–320.

Schaffer, C.E., Davidson, R.J. and Saron, C., 1983. Frontal and parietal EEG asymmetries in depressed and non-depressed subjects. *Biological Psychiatry*, **46**, 753–762.

Shalev, A.Y., 1997. Discussion: treatment of prolonged posttraumatic stress disorder–learning from experience [comment]. *Journal of Traumatic Stress*, **10**, 415–423.

Shalev, A., Orr, S.P. and Pitman, R.K., 1993a. Psychophysiologic assessment of traumatic imagery in Israeli trauma survivors with post-traumatic stress disorder. *American Journal of Psychiatry*, **50**, 620–624.

Shalev, A.Y. and Rogel-Fuchs, Y., 1993b. Psychophysiology of the posttraumatic stress disorder: From sulfur fumes to behavioral genetics. *Psychosomatic Medicine*, **55**, 413–423.

Shalev, A.Y., Orr, S.P., Peri, T., Schreiber, S. and Pitman, R.K., 1992. Physiologic responses to loud tones in Israeli patients with posttraumatic stress disorder. *Archives of General Psychiatry*, **49**, 870–875.

Shalev, A.Y., Peri, T., Brandes, D., Freedman, S., Orr, S.P. and Pitman, R.K., 2000. Auditory startle response in trauma survivors with posttraumatic stress disorder: a prospective study. *American Journal of Psychiatry*, **157**, 255–261.

Simpson, H.B., Tenke, C.E., Towey, J.B., Liebowitz, M. and Bruder, G.E., 2000. Symptom provocation alters behavioral ratings and brain electrical activity in Obsessive–compulsive disorder: a preliminary study. *Psychiatry Research*, **95**, 149–155.

Sokolov, E.N., 1963. *Perception and the Conditioned Reflex*. Pergamon, Oxford.

Spence, S., Shapiro, D. and Zaidel, E., 1996. The role of the right hemisphere in the physiological and cognitive components of emotional processing. *Psychophysiology*, **33**, 112–122.

Spinhoven, P., Onstein, E.J. and Sterk, P.J., 1995. Pulmonary function in panic disorder: evidence against the dyspnea-fear theory. *Behaviour Research and Therapy*, **33**, 457–460.

Stein, M.B. and Uhde, T.W., 1991. Endocrine, cardiovascular, and behavioral effects of intravenous protirelin in patients with panic disorder. *Archives of General Psychiatry*, **48**, 148–156.

Stein, M.B. and Uhde, T.W., 1998. The biology of anxiety disorders. In: Nemeroff, C.B. and Schatzberg, A.F. (eds), *American Psychiatric Press Textbook of Psychopharmacology*, pp. 609–628. American Psychiatric Press, Washington, DC.

Stein, M.B., Tancer, M.E. and Uhde, T.W., 1992. Heart rate and plasma norepinephrine responsivity to orthostatic challenge in anxiety disorders. Comparison of patients with panic disorder and social phobia and normal control subjects. *Archives of General Psychiatry*, **49**, 311–317.

Stein, M., Millar, T., Larsen, D.K. and Kryger, M., 1995. Irregular breathing during sleep in patients with panic disorder. *American Journal of Psychiatry*, **152**, 1168–1173.

Stroop, J.R., 1938. Factors affecting speed in serial verbal reactions. *Psychological Monographs*, **50**, 38–48.

Taylor, S. and Rachman, S., 1994. Klein's suffocation theory of panic [letter; comment]. *Archives of General Psychiatry*, **51**, 505–506.

Taylor, C.B., King, R., Ehlers, A., Margraf, J., Clark, D., Hayward, C., Roth, W.T. and Agras, S., 1987. Treadmill exercise test and ambulatory measures in panic attacks. *American Journal of Cardiology*, **60**, 48J–52J.

Thayer, J.F., Friedman, B.H., Borkovec, T.D., Johnsen, B.H. and Molina, S., 2000. Phasic heart period reactions to cued threat and non-threat stimuli in generalized anxiety disorder. *Psychophysiology*, **37**, 361–368.

Tomarken, A.J., Davidson, R.J. and Henriques, J.B., 1990. Resting frontal brain asymmetry predicts affective responses to films. *Journal of Personality and Social Psychology*, **59**, 791–801.

Tomarken, A.J., Mineka, S. and Cook, M., 1989. Fear-relevant selective associations and covariation bias. *Journal of Abnormal Psychology*, **98**, 381–394.

Tomarken, A.J., Davidson, R.J., Wheeler, R.E. and Doss, R.C., 1992. Individual differences in anterior brain asymmetry and fundamental dimensions of emotion. *Journal of Personality and Social Psychology*, **62**, 676–687.

Towey, J.P., Tenke, C.E., Bruder, G.E., Leite, P., Friedman, D., Liebowitz, M. and Hollander, E., 1994. Brain event-related potential correlates of overfocused attention in Obsessive–compulsive disorder. *Psychophysiology*, **31**, 535–543.

Towey, J., Bruder, G., Hollander, E., Friedman, D., Erhan, H., Liebowitz, M. and Sutton, S., 1990. Endogenous event-related potentials in Obsessive–compulsive disorder. *Biological Psychiatry*, **28**, 92–98.

Tucker, D.M., Antes, J.R., Stenslie, C.E. and Barnhardt, T.M., 1978. Anxiety and lateral cerebral function. *Journal of Abnormal Psychology*, **87**, 380–383.

Tucker, D.M., Roth, R.S., Arneson, B.A. and Buckingham, V., 1977. Right hemisphere activation during stress. *Neuropsychologia*, **15**, 697–700.

Turner, S.M. and Beidel, D.C., 1985. Empirically derived subtypes of social anxiety. *Behavior Therapy*, **16**, 384–392.

Turner, S.M., Beidel, D.C. and Larkin, K.T., 1986. Situational determinants of social anxiety in clinic and nonclinic samples: Physiological and cognitive correlates. *Journal of Consulting and Clinical Psychology*, **54**, 523–527.

Uhde, T.W., Stein, M.B., Vittone, B.J., Siever, L.J., Boulenger, J.P., Klein, E. and Mellman, T.A., 1989. Behavioral and physiologic effects of short-term and long-term administration of clonidine in panic disorder. *Archives of General Psychiatry*, **46**, 170–177.

Van den Hout, M.A., De Jong, P. and Kindt, M., 2000. Masked fear words produce increased SCRs: An anomaly for Öhman's theory of pre-attentive processing in anxiety. *Psychophysiology*, **37**, 283–288.

Villacres, E.C., Hollifield, M., Katon, W.J., Wilkinson, C.W. and Veith, R.C., 1987. Sympathetic nervous system activity in panic disorder. *Psychiatry Research*, **21**, 313–321.

Vrana, S.R., Cuthbert, B.N. and Lang, P.J., 1986. Fear imagery and text processing. *Psychophysiology*, **23**, 247–353.

Watson, J.P. and Marks, I.M., 1971. Relevant and irrelevant fear in flooding—a crossover study of phobic patients. *Behavior Therapy*, **2**, 275–293.

Watts, F.N., Trezise, L. and Sharrock, R., 1986. Processing of phobic stimuli. *British Journal of Clinical Psychology*, **25**, 253–259.

Wheeler, R.E., Davidson, R.J. and Tomarken, A.J., 1993. Frontal brain asymmetry and emotional reactivity: A biological substrate of affective style. *Psychophysiology*, **30**, 82–89.

Wiedemann, G., Pauli, P., Dengler, W., Lutzenberger, W., Birbaumer, N. and Buchkremer, G., 1999. Frontal brain asymmetry as a biological substrate of emotions in patients with panic disorders. *Archives of General Psychiatry*, **56**, 78–84.

Wilhelm, F.H. and Roth, W.T., 1997. Acute and delayed effects of Alprazolam on flight phobics during exposure. *Behaviour Research and Therapy*, **35**, 831–841.

Wilhelm, F.H. and Roth, W.T., 1998a. Taking the laboratory to the skies: Ambulatory assessment of self-report, autonomic, and respiratory responses in flying phobia. *Psychophysiology*, **35**, 596–606.

Wilhelm, F.H. and Roth, W.T., 1998b. Using minute ventilation for ambulatory estimation of additional heart rate. *Biological Psychology*, **49**, 137–150.

Wilson, G.D., 1967. GSR responses to fear related stimuli. *Perceptual and Motor Skills*, **24**, 401–402.

Yeragani, V.K., Balon, R., Pohl, R., Ramesh, C., Glitz, D., Weinberg, P. and Merlos, B., 1990. Decreased R-R variance in panic disorder patients. *Acta Psychiatrica Scandinavica*, **81**, 554–559.

Yeragani, V.K., Pohl, R., Berger, R., Balon, R., Ramesh, C., Glitz, D., Srinivasan, K. and Weinberg, P., 1993. Decreased heart rate variability in panic disorder patients: a study of power-spectral analysis of heart rate. *Psychiatry Research*, **46**, 89–103.

Zahn, T.P., Insel, T.R. and Murphy, D.L., 1984. Psychophysiological treatment of patients with Obsessive–compulsive disorder. *British Journal of Psychology*, **145**, 39–44.

Zahn, T.P., Leonard, H.L., Swedo, S.E. and Rapoport, J.L., 1996. Autonomic activity in children and adolescents with Obsessive–compulsive disorder. *Psychiatry Research*, **60**, 67–76.

XIX-8

The Neuropsychology of Anxiety Disorders: Affect, Cognition, and Neural Circuitry

Jack B. Nitschke and Wendy Heller

INTRODUCTION

In attempting to construct a neuropsychology of anxiety, findings can be drawn from several related, yet often perceived as separate, domains of research, including cognitive science and neuroscience. The relatively new fields of cognitive neuroscience and affective neuroscience are concerned with very similar questions regarding brain–behaviour relationships as were fundamental to the older field of neuropsychology, and the neuroimaging tools central to those disciplines are no less pertinent to neuropsychology than are traditional neuropsychological test batteries or cognitive/behavioural paradigms. Thus, this review of the neuropsychological findings in anxiety disorders covers a wide array of methods that together inform knowledge of the brain mechanisms involved in the circuitry governing pathological forms of anxiety.

Although often overlooked by neuroscientists studying brain function in anxiety, cognitive research over the past two decades has contributed substantially to knowledge about brain function in anxiety. A large body of work demonstrates that anxiety disorders are characterized by cognitive biases, indicating a heightened response to the possibility of threat (for review, see McNally, 1998). Attentional biases have been elicited very reliably across a variety of paradigms in which potentially threatening information is associated with greater attentional capture in individuals with anxiety disorders than in controls. The interference of this attentional capture with other cognitive processing serves as the operationalization of this bias in research studies. Furthermore, attentional biases have been found to disappear upon remission (for review, see McNally, 1998), suggesting that such biases are state-dependent. Cognitive biases have also been observed in the form of interpretation and memory biases. Across a number of different paradigms involving ambiguous stimuli that can be interpreted as threatening or neutral, anxious people choose the threatening meaning. Accruing evidence suggests that anxiety disorders are also accompanied by enhanced memory for negative or threatening information under certain conditions. These cognitive data suggest dysfunctional activation of a right hemisphere system involved in threat perception (for review, see Nitschke, Heller and Miller, 2000; see also Compton *et al.*, 2000, 2002).

In addition to these cognitive biases, cognitive deficits have been documented in anxiety disorders. One is a tendency to do poorly on tasks that require selective attention and concentration. This deficit has been suggested to reflect a general problem of preoccupation and distraction due to worry or rumination that interferes with other mental processes (for review, see Nitschke, Heller and Miller, 2000). Compromised visual–spatial functioning has also been reported. In addition, individuals with posttraumatic stress disorder often exhibit deficits in explicit memory. Taken together, these cognitive deficits suggest aberrant frontal, anterior cingulate, right parietal, and hippocampal functioning. Building on this cognitive research as well as on behavioural and electroencephalographic (EEG) findings (for review, see Nitschke, Heller and Miller, 2000) and an extensive literature in non-human animals examining fear and anxiety (for reviews, see LeDoux, 1996; Davis and Lee, 1998), haemodynamic neuroimaging research has implicated a number of the suggested regions.

Although emotional, cognitive, and neural commonalities are apparent, the diversity of findings also warrants the importance of respecting unique patterns and heterogeneity both among and within the various anxiety disorders. An observation that has become increasingly salient in the burgeoning neuropsychological literature on anxiety and its disorders is the lack of clarity and specificity about what anxiety is. Views of anxiety range from its usage in contemporary clinical research as a rubric term that encompasses fear, panic, worry, and all the anxiety disorders listed in the DSM-IV to its very specific operationalization referring to context conditioning and long-term sensitization (e.g., Davis and Lee, 1998) to a more generic personality dimension closely linked to neuroticism (e.g., Gray, 1982). Further, the heterogeneity within each of the different anxiety disorders has become increasingly apparent and represents a major problem for investigators attempting to uncover the neurobiological correlates of individual anxiety disorders. Inconsistencies across studies may be explained by the fact that anxiety is not a unitary phenomenon and that different types and symptoms of anxiety are associated with particular cognitive patterns (Heller and Nitschke, 1998; Nitschke, Heller and Miller, 2000). An important mission of neuroscience research in this area is to help unravel the inchoate notions of anxiety that currently exist. Thus, although it is important to look for generalizations regarding the neural mechanisms of anxiety, it is also necessary to consider the possibility of heterogeneity by being as specific as possible regarding the disorder or type of anxiety under investigation.

The aim of this chapter is to assess what is known about the neuropsychology and neural circuitry of anxiety disorders by examining the relevant cognitive research. Structural and functional neuroimaging data will also be reviewed, including morphometric magnetic resonance imaging (MRI), functional MRI (fMRI), positron emission tomography (PET) using various radiotracers such as $[^{18}F]$fluorodeoxyglucose (FDG) for glucose metabolism and ^{15}O-labelled water for blood flow, single-photon emission computed tomography (SPECT) with $^{133}Xenon$ or ^{99m}Tc-HMPAO, and scalp-recorded EEG. This review of the cognitive and neuroscience literatures reveals that the anxiety disorders engage brain regions involved in threat perception (e.g., right hemisphere

Biological Psychiatry: Edited by H. D'haenen, J.A. den Boer and P. Willner. ISBN 0-471-49198-5

regions; Compton *et al.*, 2000, 2002; Nitschke, Heller and Miller, 2000), anxious arousal (right posterior regions; Nitschke, Heller and Miller, 2000), fear (e.g., amygdala; LeDoux, 1996), vigilance for motivationally salient events (e.g., amygdala; Whalen *et al.*, 1998; Davis and Whalen, 2001), decoding of motivationally relevant emotional information such as the reward and punishment value of a stimulus [e.g., orbital frontal cortex (OFC); Rolls, 1999], worry (e.g., left-hemisphere regions; Nitschke, Heller and Miller, 2000), response conflict [e.g., anterior cingulate cortex (ACC); Carter *et al.*, 1999, 2000; Davidson *et al.*, 2002], and memory (e.g., hippocampus; Squire, 1992). The aforementioned heterogeneity should also lead to some diverse findings for the different anxiety disorders. The focus here is on the anxiety disorders as defined by the *Diagnostic and Statistical Manual of Mental Disorders* (DSM-IV) although consistent patterns have emerged in studies using nonclinical and brain-lesioned human populations (for review, see Nitschke, Heller and Miller, 2000).

OBSESSIVE–COMPULSIVE DISORDER

The most widely investigated anxiety disorder from a neuropsychological perspective has been obsessive–compulsive disorder (OCD). The emphasis on obsessions and compulsions in connection with the experienced anxiety and distress reported by individuals suffering from OCD is unique among the anxiety disorders and can be linked to a number of neuropsychological abnormalities.

Cognitive Studies

An extensive cognitive literature on OCD points most strongly to non-verbal memory and other visual–spatial deficits (e.g., Boone *et al.*, 1991; Zielinski, Taylor and Juzwin, 1991; Christensen *et al.*, 1992; Cohen *et al.*, 1996; Purcell *et al.*, 1998; Savage *et al.*, 1996, 1999; see also McNally and Kohlbeck, 1993; Constans *et al.*, 1995). No evidence of a verbal memory deficit has been found (Foa *et al.*, 1997). There is also ample documentation of impaired executive functions (e.g., Head, Bolton and Hymas, 1989; Veale, Owen and Marks, 1996; Abbruzzese, Ferri and Scarone, 1997; Purcell *et al.*, 1998), with trends reported by Cohen *et al.* (1996) for several neuropsychological tests. It is possible that problems in executive function could account for at least some of the visual–spatial deficits found. For example, Savage *et al.* (1999) found that poor organizational strategies for copying a figure mediated the non-verbal memory deficit for reproducing a figure among OCD patients. Morphometric data for OCD subjects by the same group suggests that larger right prefrontal volumes are associated with worse non-verbal memory using the same task (Grachev *et al.*, 1998). Should this finding be replicated, one possible explanation is that the heightened threat perception and negative affect accompanying OCD occupy the resources in the right prefrontal cortex (PFC) that are normally dedicated to non-verbal memory and also lead to structural changes.

Of additional relevance to cognitive functioning in OCD, Foa *et al.* (1993) documented that the attentional bias toward threat-related material seen across all the anxiety disorders for the emotional Stroop paradigm also emerges in OCD. In this paradigm, subjects are asked to name the colour of words varying in emotional content while ignoring their meanings. Foa *et al.* (1993) found that OCD patients with washing rituals took longer to name the colour for contamination words than for neutral words, suggesting that the threatening nature of the contamination words interfered with the task of naming the colour. They also had longer response latencies to contamination words than did OCD non-washers or non-psychiatric controls. On the other hand, OCD non-washers had longer latencies to negative than neutral words, whereas the opposite pattern was seen in controls. In a similar study in which the contamination words did not reflect the primary concerns of the OCD patients, no interference effects were observed (McNally *et al.*, 1990). These attentional findings implicate the involvement of right hemisphere regions important for threat perception (Compton *et al.*, 2000, 2002; Nitschke, Heller and Miller, 2000).

With regard to memory biases, Foa *et al.* (1997) found no bias for contamination sentences for either explicit or implicit memory. However, they did replicate the finding that OCD patients are less confident than non-psychiatric controls about memory-related judgements (McNally and Kohlbeck, 1993; Constans *et al.*, 1995). Thus, the cognitive literature is fairly conclusive in demonstrating that the memory concerns frequently voiced by OCD patients (e.g., 'Did I lock the door?') are not the result of a memory deficit or a memory bias but rather a lack of confidence in their memory. This lack of confidence is likely to be related to the characteristic fear of forgetting some activity that has become a target for compulsive behaviour, and thus is a reflection of the underlying anxiety in OCD. As such, the degree to which confidence is lacking might correlate with activity in neural structures associated with fear and other anxiety-related features.

Neuroimaging Studies

The most common finding to emerge in morphometric MRI studies to date is a reduction in caudate volume (Robinson *et al.*, 1995; Rosenberg *et al.*, 1997), with a trend also reported by Jenike *et al.* (1996). However, Aylward *et al.* (1996) found no caudate differences, and Scarone *et al.* (1992) reported an increase in right caudate volume (see Table XIX-9.3A in Martis *et al.*, Chapter XIX-9). Similar inconsistencies for the caudate have emerged in functional imaging studies examining resting states using PET and SPECT to measure glucose metabolism and blood flow. Increases were reported in three samples (Baxter *et al.*, 1987, 1988; Rubin *et al.*, 1992), with Perani *et al.* (1995) reporting a trend in the same direction. However, Lucey *et al.* (1997a, 1997b) found a reduction, and others observed no differences from non-psychiatric controls (e.g., Swedo *et al.*, 1989). In contrast, symptom provocation paradigms employing PET (McGuire *et al.*, 1994; Rauch, Jenike and Alpert, 1994) and fMRI (Breiter *et al.*, 1996) have consistently shown caudate activation.

The cortico-striatal model of OCD proposed by Rauch *et al.* (1998) posits that pathology within the caudate results in OFC and ACC hyperactivity via inefficient thalamic gating. An OFC-caudate loop may comprise much of the neural circuitry associated with the repetitive and perseverative nature of obsessions and compulsions (see also Alexander, Crutcher and DeLong, 1991). Further pursuing the evidence of caudate abnormalities, Rauch and colleagues employed PET and fMRI while OCD patients performed an implicit learning task shown to be dependent on striatal function in non-psychiatric volunteers (Rauch *et al.*, 1995b, 1997c). As noted by Martis *et al.* (Chapter XIX-9), the striatum was not activated in OCD subjects (Rauch *et al.*, 1997a), suggesting that OCD symptoms pertinent to perseveration occupy the resources normally allocated to implicit learning. The caudate activation observed in the symptom provocation studies suggests that inconsistencies in other reported findings may be due to heterogeneity in the degree of symptom severity among OCD patient samples. Taken together, these data suggest that augmented caudate activation is associated with the perseverative nature of obsessions and compulsions, which also may serve to enlarge that structure.

Haemodynamic studies of OCD have implicated a number of other regions, most consistently OFC and ventral ACC, areas of the brain frequently found to be involved in aspects of emotion and attention. PET and SPECT studies using protocols not involving a task have revealed that patients with OCD have more blood flow or glucose metabolism than non-psychiatric controls in OFC (Baxter *et al.*, 1987, 1988; Swedo *et al.*, 1989; Rubin *et al.*, 1992; but see Machlin *et al.*, 1991; Busatto *et al.*, 2001) and ventral ACC (Machlin *et al.*, 1991; Perani *et al.*, 1995; but see Busatto *et al.*, 2001; see Table XIX-9.3B in Martis *et al.*, Chapter XIX-9).

Similar findings for the OFC were also observed during an auditory continuous performance task in a PET study measuring glucose metabolism (Nordahl *et al.*, 1989). OFC and ventral ACC activations have also been reported in fMRI (Breiter *et al.*, 1996; Adler *et al.*, 2000) and PET (Rauch, Jenike and Alpert, 1994) studies employing symptom provocation paradigms with actual obsessional stimuli. In another study employing symptom provocation via presentation of individually specified contaminants in OCD patients, McGuire *et al.* (1994) found symptom intensity to be correlated with right inferior frontal/OFC but not ACC activation. Busatto *et al.* (2001) also found that obsessive–compulsive symptoms correlated positively with left OFC blood flow. A less potent experimental elicitation of symptoms via auditory presentation of obsessional material did not induce blood flow changes in these areas using PET (Cottraux *et al.*, 1996).

With the amygdala often highlighted in models of the neural circuitry of fear, anxiety and emotion (e.g., LeDoux, 1996; Charney, Grillon and Bremner, 1998), it is worth noting that amygdala activation has been documented in only one study examining OCD, that conducted by Breiter *et al.* (1996), who exposed 10 OCD subjects to stimuli highly relevant to their obsessions. One of the subjects studied by McGuire *et al.* (1994) also showed amygdala activation, as did two of the seven OCD patients examined by Adler *et al.* (2000). Further evidence of frontal and ACC dysfunction in OCD can be inferred from two EEG studies examining event-related potentials (ERPs) in a Go–NoGo task (Malloy *et al.*, 1989) and a selective attention task (Towey *et al.*, 1994).

Treatment studies further inform the neural circuitry characterizing OCD (see also Martis *et al.*, Chapter XIX-9). Both cognitive-behavioural and pharmacological therapies have been associated with normalized (i.e., decreased) glucose metabolism in the caudate nucleus (Benkelfat *et al.*, 1990; Baxter *et al.*, 1992; Schwartz *et al.*, 1996; Saxena *et al.*, 1999; but see Baxter *et al.*, 1987; Swedo *et al.*, 1992), OFC (Benkelfat *et al.*, 1990; Swedo *et al.*, 1992; Saxena *et al.*, 1999; but see Baxter *et al.*, 1987, 1992; Schwartz *et al.*, 1996), and ventral ACC (Perani *et al.*, 1995; marginally significant in Baxter *et al.*, 1992, and Swedo *et al.*, 1992). Similar findings have emerged for blood flow measured by SPECT in the OFC (Rubin *et al.*, 1995) and ventral ACC (Hoehn-Saric *et al.*, 1991). Baxter and colleagues have reported that pre-treatment correlations between caudate and orbital regions ranging from 0.44 to 0.74 decreased significantly after effective treatment (Baxter *et al.*, 1992; Schwartz *et al.*, 1996). In addition, lower pre-treatment OFC glucose metabolism may be associated with better response to medications, whereas the converse may be true for psychotherapy (Swedo *et al.*, 1989; Brody *et al.*, 1998; Saxena *et al.*, 1999). Response to pharmacotherapy has also been predicted by glucose metabolic reductions in the ACC (Swedo *et al.*, 1989) and left caudate (Benkelfat *et al.*, 1990); however, Brody *et al.* (1998) did not replicate those findings Saxena *et al.*, 1999, only reported conducting tests for the OFC). Overall, treatment studies further implicate the caudate, OFC, and ACC in OCD. They suggest that the hyperactivity of these structures in OCD is state-dependent and that pre-treatment levels of activity may have prognostic value. The inconsistencies in findings remain to be addressed in further research.

The cognitive data implicating right hemisphere regions suggest the importance of threat perception and evaluation in OCD. The functional significance of the caudate, OFC, and ACC hyperactivity often reported prior to treatment are consistent with their roles in the perseverative nature of obsessions and compulsions, in decoding reward and punishment values of perceived and real events (c.f. Rauch, in press), and in response conflict about whether to perform some mental activity or compulsive behaviour. As noted above, the cognitive data suggest the engagement of right hemisphere regions involved in threat perception. The absence of more right-sided effects in the imaging data should be interpreted with caution, as it may be due to the difficulty of conducting adequate tests of asymmetry (Davidson and Irwin, 1999).

A final important consideration is the high level of comorbid depression in people with OCD. Visual–spatial (including non-verbal memory) and executive deficits in depression are well established and are congruent with the reduced activity in right parietal and bilateral frontal regions often reported for depression (Heller and Nitschke, 1997, 1998). The extent to which the non-verbal memory and executive deficits in OCD can be attributed to depression, anxiety, obsessions, or compulsions has not been determined, in part because the co-occurrence of these various symptoms makes disentangling their effects exceedingly difficult. Furthermore, the pronounced brain abnormalities accompanying depression (for reviews, see Davidson *et al.*, 2002; Mohanty and Heller, 2002, Chapter XVIII-7) certainly have consequences for the neuropsychology of OCD. For example, Martinot *et al.* (1990) reported a bilateral diminution of PFC glucose metabolism in 16 OCD patients as compared to eight non-psychiatric controls and no effects for OFC; however, despite not meeting criteria for DSM-III current major depressive episode, these patients were characterized by significantly higher levels of depression than the controls.

POSTTRAUMATIC STRESS DISORDER

The past decade has witnessed an explosion of research examining the neurobiological mechanisms and neuropsychological, behavioural, and cognitive concomitants of posttraumatic stress disorder (PTSD). The diagnostic requirement of exposure to a traumatic event makes this disorder an ideal candidate for testing aetiological hypotheses based on the rich conditioning literature, including classical cue conditioning, operant conditioning, and context conditioning. However, the array of re-experiencing, avoidance, and arousal symptoms and the common comorbidity with depression (and substance abuse in war veterans) add layers of complexity that make unraveling the neural circuitry of PTSD seem an intractable enterprise. Moreover, classification of PTSD remains a highly controversial topic, not only with regard to prototypic symptoms and subtyping but also with regard to whether it should be considered an anxiety disorder at all. Despite these obstacles, the emerging body of research is contributing to understanding this elusive condition.

Cognitive Studies

As with OCD, a commonly reported cognitive abnormality in PTSD is an attentional bias towards threat-related stimuli on tasks such as the emotional Stroop test. This effect has been reported for rape victims (e.g., Foa *et al.*, 1991), combat veterans (e.g., McNally *et al.*, 1990, 1993, 1996; Kips *et al.*, 1995; Vrana, Roodman and Beckham, 1995), motor vehicle accident victims (Bryant and Harvey, 1995), and people involved in a ferry disaster (Thrasher, Dalgleish and Yule, 1994). Recovery from PTSD has been shown to eliminate the attentional bias (Foa *et al.*, 1991), whereas PTSD patients who have not recovered continue to show the bias toward threat cues when retested (McNally and Kohlbeck, 1993). A memory bias toward trauma-relevant material has also been found in PTSD patients for explicit memory (Vrana, Roodman and Beckham, 1995) and conceptual implicit memory (Amir, McNally and Wiegartz, 1996c), suggesting a more pervasive proclivity towards threat-related material that is not confined to the frequently reported attentional effect. No bias was found on an implicit-memory task that depended more on physical, perceptual features of the words than on their meaning (McNally and Amir, 1996). Consistent with these cognitive data, a recent ERP study using threat words as the low-probability stimulus type in an oddball paradigm reported that PTSD patients had larger P3 amplitudes than non-psychiatric controls for trauma-relevant but not trauma-irrelevant threat words (Stanford *et al.*, 2001). The oddball paradigm is comprised of frequent presentations of one stimulus type and infrequent presentations of a second stimulus type, which typically elicits an enlarged ERP component known as P3 or P300. Taken together, these data are suggestive of right hemisphere abnormalities pertinent to threat perception.

The other salient cognitive finding in PTSD is an explicit memory deficit. Compromised memory performance has been observed in combat veterans (e.g., Bremner *et al.*, 1993; Uddo *et al.*, 1993; McNally *et al.*, 1994, 1995; Yehuda *et al.*, 1995), rape victims (Jenkins *et al.*, 1998), and adult survivors of childhood abuse (e.g., Bremner *et al.*, 1995b; but see Stein *et al.*, 1997). These data corroborate the reports of reduced hippocampal volume in PTSD to be reviewed next.

Neuroimaging Studies

As covered by Martis *et al.* (Chapter XIX-9), the handful of studies examining structural abnormalities in PTSD consistently implicate the hippocampi, with reduced volume ranging from 8% to 30% (Bremner *et al.*, 1995a, 1997; Gurvits *et al.*, 1996). A 5% reduction in the left hippocampus was observed by Stein *et al.* (1997) in 21 adult survivors of childhood abuse, 15 of whom met DSM-IV criteria for PTSD. Schuff *et al.* (1997) also reported a trend for a 6% right hippocampal reduction in combat veterans. It is not known whether this smaller hippocampal size is due to cell loss, cell atrophy, or to some other cause (Rajkowska, 2000; Sapolsky, 2000; Sheline, 2000). Controversy persists with regard to the role of cortisol as a causative factor in the hippocampal reductions observed in PTSD (Yehuda, 1997). Regardless of this, these hippocampal data are clearly linked to the aforementioned explicit memory deficit in PTSD. Indeed, Bremner *et al.* (1995a) reported a strong correlation ($r = 0.64$) between verbal memory and right hippocampal volume in combat veterans with PTSD.

In contrast to the above morphometric data, functional neuroimaging studies examining PTSD have implicated a host of structures (see Table XIX-9.1B in Martis *et al.*, Chapter XIX-9). Two recent symptom provocation studies used script-driven imagery in conjunction with PET in adult female victims of childhood sexual abuse with and without PTSD (Bremner *et al.*, 1999a; Shin *et al.*, 1999). Bremner *et al.* (1999a) found that personalized traumatic scripts were associated with less blood flow in the right hippocampus and more blood flow in ventral ACC, PFC, insula, posterior cingulate, and motor cortex for women with PTSD than those without. Shin *et al.* (1999) reported more blood flow in the ventral ACC, OFC, and insula for childhood abuse victims with PTSD than those without. Two studies reported activation of the ventral ACC in combat veterans with PTSD as well as in combat controls without PTSD (Bremner *et al.*, 1999b; Liberzon *et al.*, 1999). Using SPECT, Liberzon and coworkers observed activation of the ventral ACC/medial PFC in non-psychiatric controls as well. Another report from this group indicated that only PTSD subjects showed more blood flow in the medial PFC, whereas both PTSD subjects and non-psychiatric controls showed a trend for increased blood flow in the ventral ACC (Zubieta *et al.*, 1999). Using PET, Bremner *et al.* (1999b) also found PTSD to be associated with increased blood flow in parietal, posterior cingulate, and motor areas. It remains to be seen whether activation in some of these regions (e.g., ventral ACC) is specific to PTSD, or has more to do with task demands or other phenomena (e.g., mood, comorbid depression, the presence of other types of anxiety).

Several symptom provocation studies of PTSD have found amygdala activation (Rauch *et al.*, 1996; Shin *et al.*, 1997; Liberzon *et al.*, 1999). Other areas implicated by Rauch *et al.* (1996) in a PET study using script-driven imagery were the ventral ACC and right OFC, insula, and temporal cortex. The same group also found increased blood flow in the ventral ACC in another sample of combat veterans for a paradigm involving combat, negative, and neutral pictures (Shin *et al.*, 1997a, 1997b). Both those studies also reported a blood flow decrease in Broca's area (see also Fischer, Wik and Fredrikson, 1996), perhaps indicative of downregulation of this verbal generation region in the service of more effective recruitment of phylogenetically older structures more appropriate for the extreme fear and horrific traumas experienced by people who go on to develop PTSD.

The importance of the amygdala and OFC for the circuitry implicated in PTSD is further underscored by research not targeting symptom-related stimuli. Using fMRI and a backward masking paradigm previously shown to activate the amygdala in non-psychiatric volunteers (Whalen *et al.*, 1998), Rauch *et al.* (2000) found that combat veterans with PTSD had larger right amygdala responses to fearful faces masked by neutral faces than did combat controls without PTSD. These responses to fear expressions are consistent with cognitive biases toward threat discussed above for PTSD patients. An older study conducted by Semple *et al.* (1993) reported more OFC blood flow as measured by PET during an auditory continuous performance task and a word generation task in combat veterans with PTSD and substance abuse than non-psychiatric controls. Less parietal blood flow during the continuous performance task was also observed (Semple *et al.*, 1996). A newer study from that group found that a similar sample of PTSD patients had more right amygdalar and left parahippocampal blood flow during the same continuous performance task than non-psychiatric controls (Semple *et al.*, 2000), adding further support to the symptom provocation findings above.

In sum, both cognitive and neuroimaging findings suggest the engagement of several right hemisphere regions, consistent with evidence that these areas are differentially involved in responding to threat. In addition, the neuroimaging data highlight a distributed array of structures not clearly lateralized, including the OFC, ACC, amygdala, and hippocampus, regions associated with decoding motivationally salient material, response conflict, fear and vigilance for motivationally salient events, and memory. As with OCD, the OFC and ventral ACC appear to be involved in the brain circuitry associated with the pathogenesis and expression of PTSD. Important points of divergence between the two disorders emerge in the subcortex, with the caudate specific to OCD and the amygdala and hippocampus implicated in numerous studies examining PTSD. It is unclear whether the decrease in Broca's area is unique to PTSD, in part because deactivations often are not reported. As with OCD, the rates of depressive disorders in PTSD populations is extremely high, which again warrants attention to the known cognitive and neurobiological correlates of depression in any discussion of the brain circuitry central to PTSD.

PANIC DISORDER

Characterized by recurrent unexpected panic attacks that share many features with basic fear responses, panic disorder has been viewed as the pre-eminent candidate condition for postulating dysfunction of the fear circuitry identified in research with non-human animals. However, the literature has shown this to be a disappointing enterprise, and the neural machinery involved remains largely a mystery. It is important to note that even in the majority of individuals experiencing frequent panic attacks (once or more per day), more time is spent worrying about having future attacks or about the implications of those attacks than having actual attacks. For obvious reasons, animal models are not particularly conducive to tracking the circuitry associated with worry, although research on context conditioning, long-term sensitization, and anticipatory anxiety is certainly relevant (e.g., Davis and Lee, 1998; Nitschke *et al.*, 2001). The various neuropsychological research tools now available with humans may hold the most promise for identifying the circuitry affected in panic disorder.

Cognitive Studies

Cognitive reports in the literature on panic disorder have been more sparse than for OCD or for PTSD. The most common finding is a bias for panic-relevant words on implicit and explicit memory tasks (e.g., McNally, Foa and Donnell, 1989; Cloitre and Liebowitz, 1991; Cloitre *et al.*, 1994; Amir *et al.*, 1996b; Becker *et al.*, 1994, 1999), although negative findings have been reported (Otto *et al.*, 1994; Rapee, *et al.*, 1994). Perceptual asymmetry on a dichotic listening task suggestive of more left than right hemisphere activity was associated with better memory for threat words in panic disorder patients but not in non-psychiatric controls (Otto *et al.*, 1994). These results suggest a pattern of brain activity akin to that found for generalized anxiety disorder (see below), anxious apprehension, and worry (for review, see Nitschke, Heller and Miller, 2000). There is also evidence of a bias towards threatening words in a priming task involving lexical and non-lexical word pairs, one presented above the other (McNally *et al.*, 1997). Panic patients showed faster reaction times in naming the threat targets following the threat prime but only when the target was in the bottom position. Emotional Stroop interference has also been observed in panic disorder patients (Ehlers *et al.*, 1988; McNally *et al.*, 1990, 1994). These cognitive biases again point to the involvement of right hemisphere systems corresponding to threat, with dichotic listening data suggesting left-hemisphere engagement, perhaps reflecting anxious apprehension.

Neuroimaging Studies

The one known quantitative morphometric study found that panic disorder patients had smaller temporal lobes than non-psychiatric controls but no hippocampal differences (Vythilingam *et al.*, 2000). Evidence for temporal lobe aberrations has also been documented using qualitative grading methods (Fontaine *et al.*, 1990). Eleven patients exhibited abnormal signal activity in the temporal lobes, which was most prominent at the interface of the right medial temporal lobe and parahippocampal cortex (see Table XIX-9.2A in Martis *et al.*, Chapter XIX-9).

Consistent with these data, haemodynamic imaging studies have repeatedly implicated abnormalities in hippocampal and parahippocampal regions. The first report was a PET study finding more right than left parahippocampal blood flow in panic disorder patients who responded to lactate infusion (Reiman *et al.*, 1984). This finding held for the full sample, with right-sided parahippocampal asymmetries also observed for blood volume and oxygen metabolism (Reiman *et al.*, 1986). Differential hippocampal asymmetries in the same direction were found for glucose metabolism in panic disorder patients while engaged in an auditory continuous performance task (Nordahl *et al.*, 1990, 1998; see Table XIX-9.2B in Martis *et al.*, Chapter XIX-9). In the first study, patients also exhibited more right frontal and occipital metabolism and less left parietal metabolism than non-psychiatric controls. An inferior frontal asymmetry with more right than left metabolism was observed in both patient samples. Similar group differences in inferior PFC asymmetry (right > left), right frontal (marginally significant), and occipital cortex were reported in a SPECT study conducted by De Cristofaro *et al.* (1993). There were no differences in hippocampal asymmetry, but rather patients showed bilateral decreases.

Consistent with the reports of hippocampal and parahippocampal asymmetries, Bisaga *et al.* (1998) found that panic disorder patients exhibited more glucose metabolism in the left hippocampus and parahippocampal area than non-psychiatric controls. Those patients also had less metabolism in right inferior parietal and right superior temporal regions, which could be due to comorbid depression (Heller and Nitschke, 1998). In light of hippocampal involvement in explicit memory, these findings suggest that hippocampal and parahippocampal asymmetries may play a role in the explicit memory bias toward threat emerging in the cognitive literature.

The first quantitative EEG study on panic disorder documented abnormal patterns of asymmetry in both frontal and parietal regions, with patients exhibiting relatively more right-sided activity than non-psychiatric controls (Wiedemann *et al.*, 1999). More right than left frontal activity was documented for the patients but not the controls, whereas the patients did not exhibit the parietal left > right asymmetry observed in controls. Furthermore, the same frontal asymmetry was also present while the patients viewed a spider, an erotic, and an emergency picture, but not a mushroom.

Symptom provocation studies of panic disorder employing haemodynamic methods have assumed the form of pharmacological challenges. Using SPECT during sodium lactate infusion that induced global blood flow increases, Stewart *et al.* (1988) found that patients who panicked following infusion exhibited larger occipital increases, especially on the right, than non-panicking subjects, whereas the non-panicking subjects showed larger global increases, especially over the left hemisphere. In a PET study, Reiman *et al.* (1989) found no blood flow increases following sodium lactate infusion among non-panicking subjects, whereas the panic disorder patients who had panic attacks exhibited increased blood flow in anterior temporal, insula/claustrum/putamen, superior colliculus/periacquenductal grey, and cerebellar vermis regions (see also Table XIX-9.2C in Martis *et al.*, Chapter XIX-9). Of note, the anterior temporal findings may be an artifact of muscular contraction of the jaw (Drevets, Videen and MacLeod, 1992; Benkelfat *et al.*, 1995), such that recent imaging studies on anxiety often employ teeth-clenching control conditions (e.g., Rauch *et al.*, 1996; Reiman, 1997; Javanmard *et al.*, 1999).

The parallel between the most frequently observed cognitive and neuroimaging findings is noteworthy. As the only anxiety disorder with a memory bias toward threat just as reliable as an attentional bias, if not more so, panic disorder also is unique with regard to the consistent hippocampal findings across several functional imaging studies. With the hippocampus known to be the critical structure for explicit memory function, these findings suggest that the commitment of certain right hemisphere regions to threat may extend to the hippocampus. Consistent with the argument forwarded for OCD and PTSD, the involvement of broader right hemisphere systems encompassing various territories governing threat perception corresponds to findings of memory and attentional biases. The PFC asymmetry observed in three studies using different technologies is in concordance with that position. The OFC, ACC, and caudate regions highlighted in the above sections for OCD and PTSD have not emerged with any consistency in research on patients with panic disorder.

Again, the issue of comorbidity with depression deserves mention, because the explicit memory bias and the PFC asymmetry are commonly seen in depression. However, evidence reviewed above suggests that increases in right PFC activity are driving this asymmetry in panic disorder, whereas the preponderance of literature on major depressive disorder indicates that decreased left PFC activity likely contributes to that asymmetry in depression.

SPECIFIC PHOBIA (SIMPLE PHOBIA)

Characterized by a persistent, excessive, and unreasonable fear of a specific object or situation, this disorder is very amenable to research investigation both with regard to experimental designs (e.g., presenting subjects with phobic stimuli) and subject sampling due to the prevalence of specific phobias and the relatively low rates of comorbidity with other mental disorders. However, studies with phobics are few, perhaps due to minimal public health interest in specific phobias because they generally do not compromise the occupational or social functioning of affected individuals to the same extent as other anxiety disorders. The preponderance of physiological research to date has focused on peripheral psychophysiological measures such as skin conductance, cardiovascular, and neuroendocrine activity (for review, see Fyer, 1998). No structural imaging data are available for specific phobias, and other neuropsychological research has been quite limited.

Cognitive Studies

The handful of studies investigating cognitive function in phobic individuals has documented the presence of an attentional bias but no memory bias. In women with spider phobia, Van den Hout *et al.* (1997) documented interference for both masked and unmasked words associated with spiders on a modified Stroop task similar to those employed in the OCD, PTSD, and panic disorder studies above. Using Stroop tests involving spider, general negative, and neutral words, Watts *et al.* (1986) and Lavy, Van den Hout and Arntz (1993) found larger interference for the spider words in spider phobics than matched non-anxious controls. No Stroop interference effects were observed in driving phobics for motor vehicle accident words; however, the words did not reflect their primary concerns but rather were designed for accident victims who developed PTSD (Bryant and Harvey, 1995). Evidence of a memory bias in spider phobia has not been reported (Watts and Coyle, 1993).

Neuroimaging Studies

Consistent with the conclusion drawn by Martis *et al.* (Chapter XIX-9), functional neuroimaging data have been inconsistent across studies. When small animal phobics were exposed to containers housing the feared animal, Rauch *et al.* (1995a) found blood flow increases using PET in a number of regions implicated in the above studies for OCD and PTSD (see Rauch *et al.*, 1997b), including the right ACC, left insular cortex, and left OFC. Conversely, two earlier PET studies by Fredrikson and colleagues using film clips of the feared stimuli with snake and spider phobics did not find blood flow increases in any region except the secondary visual cortex (Fredrikson *et al.*, 1993, 1995; Wik *et al.*, 1993). The only other PET study conducted with specific phobics found that confronting animal phobics with their feared animal did not elicit blood flow changes in any region of the brain although significant cardiovascular and self-reported anxiety changes were observed (Mountz *et al.*, 1989). They also reported no resting baseline differences between the phobics and non-psychiatric controls. In a SPECT study of women with spider phobia, those reporting panic while watching a video of spiders exhibited less frontal blood flow, especially on the right side, than during a neutral film (Johanson *et al.*, 1998). The remaining phobic women who reported anxiety but did not panic showed more right frontal blood flow to the spider film (although significance level was not reported). The sole published EEG study of specific phobia found more right than left parietal activity to be associated with higher pre-treatment spider phobia scores, whereas frontal activity was not related to pre-treatment or post-treatment clinical measures (Merckelbach *et al.*, 1998). There have been no published findings of amygdala activation in specific phobia despite the clear relevance of that structure for the fear response evoked by confronting phobic stimuli.

Due to the dearth of cognitive and neuroimaging research investigating specific phobias, little is known about the neuropsychology accompanying such intense, long-standing fear of an object that is often harmless. The attentional bias suggests the involvement of right hemisphere regions oriented towards threat; however, the imaging data are inconsistent. Although the structures implicated in the study by Rauch *et al.* (1995a, 1997b) suggest some commonality with other anxiety disorders, those findings have not been supported by the other studies examining specific phobia. It may be that the circuitry implicated is much less pronounced or complex than appears to be the case for the other anxiety disorders, just as the impact on everyday functioning is on average far less than for the others.

SOCIAL PHOBIA (SOCIAL ANXIETY DISORDER)

Now often referred to as social anxiety disorder, social phobia can be viewed as a variant of specific phobia that pertains to social or performance situations. Individuals suffering from social phobia fear that they will act in a humiliating or embarrassing way when in the presence of other people. Recent epidemiological studies have identified it as the third largest psychological disorder in the United States, after depression and alcoholism. Accordingly, the past five years has witnessed an explosion of research interest in the disorder, with efforts to identify the affected neural circuitry very much in their infancy.

Cognitive Studies

Cognitive research has implicated a number of abnormalities in social phobia, the majority of which are consistent with the information processing biases described in other anxiety disorders. The numerous studies examining attention, interpretation, and memory biases in social phobia have recently been reviewed (Heinrichs and Hofmann, 2001). This literature abounds in evidence of attention and interpretation biases towards social threat across multiple different paradigms.

One relevant study not reviewed by Heinrichs and Hofmann (2001) examined attention bias for facial expressions in generalized social phobia (Gilboa-Schechtman, Foa and Amir, 1999). Consistent with the dot probe and Stroop studies reviewed, phobic subjects showed an attentional bias toward angry faces as measured via several metrics using the face-in-the-crowd paradigm, whereas non-anxious controls did not. Moreover, successful treatment has resulted in the attenuation of attention (e.g., Mattia, Heimberg and Hope, 1993) and interpretation (e.g., Foa *et al.*, 1996) biases.

In other findings, Amir *et al.* (1996a) found suppression of Stroop interference to social-threat words in social phobics but not non-psychiatric controls prior to giving a speech (see Mathews and Sebastian, 1993, for comparable findings in snake-fearful subjects when in the presence of a snake they are told they will have to approach upon completion of the Stroop task). The authors suggested that subjects might increase their efforts when anxious, thereby compensating for the interference. Another possibility is that the right hemisphere resources devoted to threat might all be allocated to the situation surrounding the impending social performance, such that the threat words no longer are perceived as threatening (relative to the impending speech) to the same degree as they are under non-anxious experimental conditions.

Research eliciting anticipatory anxiety in interpretation/judgement bias paradigms is needed to determine if this phenomenon extends to other domains of information processing.

Until very recently, it was widely accepted that social phobia was not accompanied by a memory bias (e.g., Rapee *et al.*, 1994). However, recent evidence suggests otherwise (Amir *et al.*, 2000, 2001). Two reports using face stimuli provide further evidence for an explicit memory bias in social phobia. Lündh and Öst (1996) first documented the effect in a paradigm where social phobics and non-psychiatric controls were asked to judge faces as either critical or accepting. Unlike the controls, the phobics showed a memory bias for faces they had previously judged as critical. In two elegant experiments following up the seminal report by Lündh and Öst (1996), Foa *et al.* (2000) found that social phobics recognized more angry and disgust faces than happy or neutral ones, whereas no differences were observed for non-anxious controls. The same pattern was seen for reaction time data, with social phobics showing longer latencies in making a decision about the negative than the non-negative facial expressions. Furthermore, phobic subjects had longer latencies for angry than disgust faces, whereas controls did not. Similar specificity was observed in the attentional paradigm employing faces mentioned above, with social phobics detecting anger faces faster than disgust ones, whereas controls showed no difference (Gilboa-Schechtman, Foa and Amir, 1999). Taken together, data from these face paradigms suggest a general negativity bias (e.g., all negative emotion expressions) that is amplified by faces connoting threat (e.g., anger expressions), again implying that the right hemisphere regions involved in threat perception should be involved.

Consistent with cognitive findings for OCD, visual–spatial impairment including non-verbal memory deficits has been documented in social phobia (Cohen *et al.*, 1996; Hollander *et al.*, 1996), as has executive dysfunction (Cohen *et al.*, 1996). Along with other findings of left-sided neurological soft signs (Hollander *et al.*, 1996), these visual–spatial deficits are consistent with right hemisphere dysfunction in social phobia. Possibly, these deficits are produced by the augmented engagement of the right hemisphere in threat perception with a consequent lack of resources for other processes lateralized to the right hemisphere such as visual–spatial functions.

Neuroimaging Studies

Structural abnormalities of the brain have not been observed in social phobics (Potts *et al.*, 1994); however, a set of recent functional neuroimaging studies point to several critical regions. Surveying EEG at the scalp, Davidson *et al.* (2000) found that social phobics exhibited a larger anterior temporal right > left asymmetry (marginally significant for lateral frontal and parietal sites) during anticipation of making a public speech than non-psychiatric controls. Using PET to measure blood flow in social phobics, Reiman (1997) reported that singing in front of observers activated a number of cortical and subcortical regions, including lateral PFC, anterior temporal, and posterior cingulate regions, with trends noted in the ACC, medial PFC, amygdala, and hippocampus. In another PET study, Tillfors *et al.* (2001) found that social phobics exhibited larger blood flow increases than non-psychiatric controls in the right amygdaloid complex (extending into the hippocampus) while speaking in front of an audience. On the other hand, controls had larger increases in right parietal, restrosplenial, and right secondary visual cortices than social phobics did.

An fMRI study found that social phobics showed greater amygdala activation bilaterally to neutral faces than did non-psychiatric controls despite no differences in subjective ratings of the faces, whereas both groups showed the expected activation of the amygdala to aversive odors (Birbaumer *et al.*, 1998). However, it appears that this effect for the amygdala did not maintain for the full sample (Schneider *et al.*, 1999), with social phobics only exhibiting greater amygdalar and hippocampal activation than controls when the neutral faces were paired with the aversive odors (see Table XIX-9.4A in Martis *et al.*, Chapter XIX-9). Three additional neuroimaging reports presented pilot or preliminary data with mixed results for the structures implicated in the above studies on social phobia (Stein and Leslie, 1996; Van Ameringen *et al.*, 1998; Van der Linden *et al.*, 2000).

Overall, these cognitive and neuroimaging data point most strongly to the right cortical regions and the amygdala, especially in paradigms involving methods that are ecologically relevant to social phobia such as face stimuli and social performance. The concordance of the cognitive findings with the right-sided brain activation reported by Davidson *et al.* (2000) suggests that the circuitry of social phobia includes right hemisphere regions involved in threat perception. The involvement of the amygdala in fear and in vigilance for motivationally salient events is certainly applicable for the paradigms involving anticipatory anxiety and social performance.

GENERALIZED ANXIETY DISORDER

The salience of worry and verbal rumination in generalized anxiety disorder (GAD) suggests the involvement of left-hemisphere structures dedicated to language. In contrast to the other anxiety disorders which may involve varying degrees of worry about disorder-specific content, worry is the hallmark of GAD. Although worry about everyday problems is not pathological in itself, the person with GAD worries excessively, has difficulty controlling the worry, and experiences significant distress and impaired social and occupational functioning as a result. The exceedingly high rates of comorbidity with depression have made it very difficult to isolate brain abnormalities in GAD. Both cognitive and neuroimaging studies have therefore often been quite compromised in terms of diagnostic specificity.

Cognitive Studies

As with the other anxiety disorders covered above, GAD is characterized by an attentional bias towards threat in Stroop (Mathews and MacLeod, 1985; Mogg *et al.*, 1987, 1993; Martin, Williams and Clark, 1991; Bradley *et al.*, 1995; Mathews *et al.*, 1995), dot probe (MacLeod, Mathews and Lata, 1986), distractor (Mathews *et al.*, 1990, 1995), and dichotic listening (Mathews and MacLeod, 1986) paradigms. Consistent findings have emerged in two newer paradigms using emotional faces. Using a variant of the dot probe task, Bradley *et al.* (1999) reported that GAD patients had slower reaction times for threatening than neutral faces, compared to controls. Using a similar probe detection task, Mogg, Miller and Bradley (2000) measured eye movements and found that GAD subjects showed a bias toward threat faces for the two eye-movement metrics employed, but they did not replicate the reaction time differences documented by Bradley *et al.* (1999). Several of these studies reported the absence of an attentional bias in comparison groups with clinical depression (Mogg *et al.*, 1993, 2000) or with comorbid GAD and depression (Bradley *et al.*, 1995). Evidence for general rather than threat-specific distractibility has also been found (Bradley *et al.*, 1999; see also Mathews *et al.*, 1990, 1995), although even these studies found results for threat conditions to be more robust than for non-threat conditions. Despite earlier evidence to the contrary (Mathews *et al.*, 1990), recovery from GAD does not appear to be accompanied by a residual attentional bias (Mathews *et al.*, 1995; see also Mogg, Mathews and Eysenck, 1992), consistent with findings reviewed above for other anxiety disorders.

Findings of a memory bias in GAD have been mixed. A bias towards threat has generally not been observed for explicit memory tasks (Mogg, Mathews and Weinman, 1987; Mathews *et al.*, 1989a; Otto *et al.*, 1994; MacLeod and McLaughlin, 1995; Becker *et al.*, 1999). However, Friedman, Thayer and Borkovec (2000) found an explicit memory bias in two separate GAD samples with extremely low rates of comorbid depression (although comorbidity with social phobia was 60%). Several important methodological differences from earlier studies (e.g., incidental learning task, no imagery instructions, longer stimulus exposure) suggest the presence of an explicit memory bias in GAD under conditions optimal for detecting memory biases in clinical anxiety (see Becker *et al.*, 1999). In addition, Otto *et al.* (1994) documented the same relationship between auditory perceptual asymmetry and memory bias toward threat discussed above for panic disorder in a sample of GAD patients. The inferred pattern of more left than right hemisphere activity was associated with better memory for threat words, consistent with left-sided neuroimaging findings for GAD reviewed below.

Implicit-memory bias has emerged for GAD under some conditions (MacLeod and McLaughlin, 1995; Mathews *et al.*, 1989a) but not others (Mathews *et al.*, 1995), a discrepancy that cannot be explained by the type of implicit-memory tested (see above discussion contrasting conceptual and perceptual implicit-memory in PTSD). There is also evidence that GAD patients have a bias to interpret ambiguous stimuli as threatening (Mathews, Richards and Eysenck, 1989b; Eysenck *et al.*, 1991). Recovered patients do not show implicit memory or interpretive biases (Mathews, Richards and Eysenck, 1989b; Eysenck *et al.*, 1991). Again, the cognitive bias literature suggests state-dependent recruitment of right hemisphere regions involved in threat perception, perhaps superimposed upon the left-sided perceptual asymmetry and neuroimaging findings also observed in GAD patients.

There is some indication of mild cognitive deficits in GAD that are consistent with the notion that worry occupies cognitive resources that otherwise might be deployed for various experimental tasks and everyday functions. Wolski and Maj (1998) documented performance deficits on a modified Sternberg memory task in a group of 87 anxiety patients, 77 of whom had GAD. The general distractibility effects reviewed above (e.g., Bradley *et al.*, 1999) provide further support for this position. However, overall performance deficits are generally not seen on attention and memory tasks (e.g., Mathews *et al.*, 1990; Otto *et al.*, 1994).

Neuroimaging Studies

The one published morphometric MRI study on GAD was conducted with children and adolescents (De Bellis *et al.*, 2000). The right amygdala was larger in patients than in matched non-psychiatric controls. No differences were found in the temporal lobe, hippocampi, corpus callosum, or basal ganglia or for total intracranial or total cerebral volumes.

In contrast to the other anxiety disorders covered here, functional neuroimaging studies are older, with no work published in the past decade. Wu *et al.* (1991) found that patients had less glucose metabolism in the basal ganglia (comprised of caudate, putamen, and globus pallidus) and more in left inferior frontal, left inferior occipital, right posterior temporal, and right precentral regions than non-psychiatric controls during a passive viewing task. The left inferior frontal finding and concomitant greater left than right frontal metabolism are in line with the hypothesis that language centres involved in worry (e.g., Broca's area) are activated. During a visual continuous performance task using degraded stimuli performed only by the patients, basal ganglia and right parietal metabolism increased, whereas decreases were seen in right temporal and occipital lobes. Consistent with their earlier report (Buchsbaum *et al.*, 1987), which they claimed was on the same GAD sample (the gender breakdown was slightly different), benzodiazepine therapy resulted in decreased occipital, basal ganglia, and limbic system (comprised of the amygdala, hippocampus, and cingulate) metabolism. In a SPECT study, GAD patients showed increased left orbital frontal blood flow when asked to freely associate about threatening pictures presented prior to rCBF measurement (Johanson *et al.*, 1992). The specificity of the effects to GAD in the latter two studies is not clear because neither one included a control group.

Involvement of different brain areas in GAD can also be gleaned from several EEG studies. EEG topography from 32 sites revealed no baseline differences between GAD patients and non-psychiatric controls (Grillon and Buchsbaum, 1987). When presented with neutral lights in a basic orienting response paradigm, patients showed less alpha suppression (presumably reflecting decreased mental activity) than controls, especially over the occipital lobe, perhaps reflecting a diminution of attention to external stimulation because of competing processes devoted to worry. An earlier EEG study by the same group examined benzodiazepine treatment effects in patients with random assignment to placebo or drug group and in non-psychiatric controls (Buchsbaum *et al.*, 1985). Using 16 midline and left-hemisphere sites, they found that patients had less delta and alpha (more activity) than controls, especially over left posterior temporal cortex. Drug effects were seen in different bands across several regions of the brain but were of limited utility in isolating patterns of brain activity critical for GAD because only four of the nine patients administered benzodiazepines showed clinical improvement as measured by the Hamilton Anxiety Scale (none of the 11 patients taking placebo improved). However, correlational analyses revealed that increased left frontal alpha (decreased activity) was associated with clinical improvement for patients in the drug group, consistent with above findings of left frontal involvement in GAD and worry.

Of relevance to imaging research despite only recording from three midline electrodes, a recent treatment study of GAD explored frontal midline theta activity, which is thought to reflect reduction of anxiety during task performance (Suetsugi *et al.*, 2000). Criteria for frontal midline theta at the midfrontal site were not met for any of the 28 patients at the initial visit. The 26 patients for whom frontal midline theta appeared following psychotherapy or pharmacotherapy showed dramatic clinical improvement, whereas the remaining two individuals continued to exhibit high levels of anxiety. Although these data are certainly preliminary, they again implicate the frontal cortex and suggest that worry interferes with the production of frontal midline theta.

The dearth of recent neuroimaging data for GAD — also noted by Martis *et al.* (Chapter XIX-9) — is striking when compared to the proliferation of such research conducted with the other five anxiety disorders covered in this review. The few studies conducted, along with the more extensive cognitive science literature examining GAD, point to several brain regions deserving further investigation. Based on the cognitive deficit and left-sided neuroimaging findings, the circuitry involved in worry and the structures overlapping with attention and working memory (e.g., PFC, parietal regions, particularly left hemisphere) are conspicuous candidates for uncovering brain aberrations in GAD. In addition, the right hemisphere territories implicated by the cognitive biases accompanying GAD are also likely constituents of the brain circuitry involved in the pathophysiology of GAD.

DISCUSSION

Across the many cognitive and neuroimaging studies reviewed here, cognitive biases toward threat is the one attribute common to all six anxiety disorders covered. Attentional biases have been observed in all disorders, whereas data for explicit and implicit-memory biases have been mixed. Findings of a memory bias have been replicated most consistently for panic disorder, with substantial evidence also reported for PTSD, social phobia, and GAD. On the other hand, no studies have found a memory bias in OCD or specific phobia. Interpretation (i.e., judgement) biases have not been extensively examined among clinical populations, although there is ample evidence of such a bias in OCD, social phobia, and GAD. This orientation towards threat in anxiety disorder populations suggests the involvement of particular anterior and posterior right hemisphere regions (for reviews, see Compton *et al.*, 2000, 2001; Nitschke, Heller and Miller, 2000). As described by Nitschke and coworkers (2000), these biases may be related to an emotion surveillance system of the right hemisphere designed to evaluate the presence of a threat in the external environment. This right hemisphere system may correspond to the cortical processes that McNally (1998) postulated to accompany a subcortical circuit involved in attentional biases toward threat. The hyperactivation of this right hemisphere system may interfere with visual–spatial functions for which right posterior regions are specialized, as seen in OCD and social phobia. The right-sided increases in activation reported in many of the neuroimaging studies examining anxiety disorders — with the notable exception of GAD, which likely invokes left-hemisphere regions devoted to verbal processes needed for worry — may be a manifestation of the heightened reliance on this emotional surveillance system governing threat perception and evaluation.

The anxiety disorders covered here are further characterized by a number of divergent neuropsychological patterns. In contrast to the morphometric and functional studies on OCD, the caudate nucleus is not implicated in any other anxiety disorders. PTSD is the only disorder to be accompanied by memory deficits and by reduced hippocampal volume. Findings of hippocampal asymmetries have been reported exclusively for panic disorder. Unlike the other disorders, the preponderance of imaging findings for GAD implicates left-hemisphere regions. Amygdala activation has not been observed with any inconsistency, except in PTSD and social phobia. OFC and ventral ACC activations have been reliably found only in OCD and PTSD. Finally, visual–spatial deficits have been observed for OCD and social phobia but not the others. This summary of the findings points to the substantial heterogeneity among the anxiety disorders.

Although anxiety is often referred to as a homogenous construct, neuropsychological data clearly indicate the importance of noting distinctions and variable symptom expression both across and within diagnoses. Several useful neurobiological models have been proposed, including one proposed by Rauch *et al.* (1998) on OCD and another proposed by Charney, Grillon and Bremner (1998) concentrating primarily on PTSD. We have proposed a neuropsychological framework positing a distinction between two types of anxiety (e.g., Nitschke *et al.*, 2000). Anxious apprehension is characterized primarily by worry and relies on left-hemisphere processes, whereas anxious arousal is characterized by immediate fear and panic symptoms and closely aligned with the emotion surveillance system of the right hemisphere. In general, GAD is characterized more strongly by anxious apprehension than are the other disorders, whereas panic disorder is likely accompanied by the highest levels of anxious arousal. However, it is important to note that these two forms of anxiety are not mutually exclusive and likely exist in all individuals with anxiety disorders to varying degrees. Pronounced individual differences within a disorder in the expression of both forms of anxiety are also likely, as are intra-individual differences across time. Although several models explain some of the variability in the neuropsychological findings, no current formulation can account for all the heterogeneity.

Attending to psychological and biological mechanisms should inform this heterogeneity that impedes attempts to unravel the neuropsychology and neural circuitry of clinical anxiety. One means of accomplishing this is research with clinical populations that rigorously examines the brain correlates of specific anxiety symptoms, such as worry, contamination obsessions, and avoidance of feared objects or situations. Another approach is to appeal to knowledge about which brain regions govern specific functions relevant to anxiety pathology (see Davidson *et al.*, 2002). Basic research with humans and non-human animals has uncovered some of the circuitry involved in those psychological phenomena central to anxiety disorders and showcased in this review (e.g., threat evaluation, fear, response conflict). This emphasis on mechanisms is also promising for research examining the interface with other neurobiological systems shown to be critical for the expression of fear and to manifest irregularities in anxiety disorders, such as cortisol, corticotropin-releasing factor (CRF), cholecystokinin (CCK), tachykinins, neuropeptide-Y, serotonin, norepinephrine, gamma-aminobutyric acid (GABA), and *N*-methyl-D-aspartate (NMDA). These are some of the areas that await synthesis with the neuropsychological concomitants of anxiety that have been identified in the large corpus of cognitive and neuroimaging research examining anxiety disorders.

ACKNOWLEDGEMENTS

We gratefully acknowledge the assistance of Kristen Mackiewicz with the preparation of this chapter.

REFERENCES

Abbruzzese, M., Ferri, S. and Scarone, S., 1997. The selective breakdown of frontal functions in patients with obsessive–compulsive disorder and in patients with schizophrenia: A double dissociation experimental finding. *Neuropsychologia*, **35**, 907–912.

Adler, C.M., McDonough-Ryan, P., Sax, K.W., Holland, S.K., Arndt, S. and Strakowski, S.M., 2000. fMRI of neuronal activation with symptom provocation in unmedicated patients with obsessive–compulsive disorder. *Journal of Psychiatric Research*, **34**, 317–324.

Alexander, G.E., Crutcher, M.D. and DeLong, M.R., 1991. Basal ganglia-thalamocortical circuits: Parallel substrates for motor, oculomotor, "prefrontal" and "limbic" functions. *Progress in Brain Research*, **85**, 119–146.

Amir, N., McNally, R.J., Riemann, B.C., Burns, J., Lorenz, M. and Mullen, J.T., 1996a. Suppression of the emotional Stroop effect by increased anxiety in patients with social phobia. *Behaviour Research & Therapy*, **34**, 945–948.

Amir, N., McNally, R.J., Riemann, B.C. and Clements, C., 1996b. Implicit memory bias for threat in panic disorder: Application of the 'white noise' paradigm. *Behaviour Research & Therapy*, **34**, 157–162.

Amir, N., McNally, R.J. and Wiegartz, P.S., 1996c. Implicit memory bias for threat in posttraumatic stress disorder. *Cognitive Therapy and Research*, **20**, 625–635.

Amir, N., Foa, E.B. and Coles, M.E., 2000. Implicit memory bias for threat-relevant information in individuals with generalized social phobia. *Journal of Abnormal Psychology*, **109**, 713–720.

Amir, N., Coles, M.E., Brigidi, B. and Foa, E.B., 2001. The effect of practice on recall of emotional information in individuals with generalized social phobia. *Journal of Abnormal Psychology*, **110**, 76–82.

Aylward, E.H., Harris, G.J., Hoehn-Saric, R., Barta, P.E., Machlin, S.R. and Pearlson, G.D., 1996. Normal caudate nucleus in obsessive–compulsive disorder assessed by quantitative neuroimaging. *Archives of General Psychiatry*, **53**, 577–584.

Baxter, L.R., Jr., Phelps, M.E., Mazziotta, J.C., Guze, B.H., Schwartz, J.M. and Selin, C.E., 1987. Local cerebral glucose metabolic rates in obsessive–compulsive disorder. A comparison with rates in unipolar depression and in normal controls. *Archives of General Psychiatry*, **44**, 211–218.

Baxter, L.R., Jr., Schwartz, J.M., Mazziotta, J.C., Phelps, M.E., Pahl, J.J., Guze, B.H. and Fairbanks, L., 1988. Cerebral glucose metabolic rates in nondepressed patients with obsessive–compulsive disorder. *American Journal of Psychiatry*, **145**, 1560–1563.

Baxter, L.R., Jr., Schwartz, J.M., Bergman, K.S., Szuba, M.P., Guze, B.H., Mazziotta, J.C., Alazraki, A., Selin, C.E., Ferng, H.K. and Munford, P., 1992. Caudate glucose metabolic rate changes with both drug and behaviour therapy for obsessive–compulsive disorder. *Archives of General Psychiatry*, **49**, 681–689.

Becker, E., Rinck, M. and Margraf, J., 1994. Memory bias in panic disorder. *Journal of Abnormal Psychology*, **103**, 396–399.

Becker, E.S., Roth, W.T., Andrich, M. and Margraf, J., 1999. Explicit memory bias in anxiety disorders. *Journal of Abnormal Psychology*, **108**, 153–163.

Benkelfat, C., Nordahl, T.E., Semple, W.E., King, A.C., Murphy, D.L. and Cohen, R.M., 1990. Local cerebral glucose metabolic rates in obsessive–compulsive disorder. Patients treated with clomipramine. *Archives of General Psychiatry*, **47**, 840–848.

Benkelfat, C., Bradwejn, J., Meyer, E., Ellenbogen, M., Milot, S., Gjedde, A. and Evans, A., 1995. Functional neuroanatomy of CCK_4-induced anxiety in normal healthy volunteers. *American Journal of Psychiatry*, **152**, 1180–1184.

Birbaumer, N., Grodd, W., Diedrich, O., Klose, U., Erb, M., Lotze, M., Schneider, F., Weiss, U. and Flor, H., 1998. fMRI reveals amygdala activation to human faces in social phobics. *Neuroreport*, **9**, 1223–1226.

Bisaga, A., Katz, J.L., Antonini, A., Wright, C.E., Margouleff, C., Gorman, J.M. and Eidelberg, D., 1998. Cerebral glucose metabolism in women with panic disorder. *American Journal of Psychiatry*, **155**, 1178–1183.

Boone, K.B., Ananth, J., Philpott, L., Kaur, A. and Djenderedjian, A., 1991. Neuropsychological characteristics of nondepressed adults with obsessive–compulsive disorder. *Neuropsychiatry, Neuropsychology, and Behavioural Neurology*, **4**, 96–109.

Bradley, B.P., Mogg, K., Millar, N. and White, J., 1995. Selective processing of negative information: Effects of clinical anxiety, concurrent depression, and awareness. *Journal of Abnormal Psychology*, **104**, 532–536.

Bradley, B.P., Mogg, K., White, J., Groom, C. and de Bono, J., 1999. Attentional bias for emotional faces in generalized anxiety disorder. *British Journal of Clinical Psychology*, **38**, 267–278.

Breiter, H.C., Rauch, S.L., Kwong, K.K., Baker, J.R., Weisskoff, R.M., Kennedy, D.N., Kendrick, A.D., Davis, T.L., Jiang, A., Cohen, M.S., Stern, C.E., Belliveau, J.W., Baer, L., O'Sullivan, R.L., Savage, C.R., Jenike, M.A. and Rosen, B.R., 1996. Functional magnetic resonance imaging of symptom provocation in obsessive–compulsive disorder. *Archives of General Psychiatry*, **53**, 595–606.

Bremner, J.D., Randall, P., Scott, T.M., Bronen, R.A., Seibyl, J.P., Southwick, S.M., Delaney, R.C., McCarthy, G., Charney, D.S. and Innis, R.B., 1995a. MRI-based measurement of hippocampal volume in patients with combat-related posttraumatic stress disorder. *American Journal of Psychiatry*, **152**, 973–981.

Bremner, J.D., Randall, P., Scott, T.M., Capelli, S., Delaney, R., McCarthy, G. and Charney, D.S., 1995b. Deficits in short-term memory in adult survivors of childhood abuse. *Psychiatry Research*, **59**, 97–107.

Bremner, J.D., Randall, P., Vermetten, E., Staib, L., Bronen, R.A., Mazure, C., Capelli, S., McCarthy, G., Innis, R.B. and Charney, D.S., 1997. Magnetic resonance imaging-based measurement of hippocampal volume in posttraumatic stress disorder related to childhood physical and sexual abuse — a preliminary report. *Biological Psychiatry*, **41**, 23–32.

Bremner, J.D., Scott, T.M., Delaney, R.C., Southwick, S.M., Mason, J.W., Johnson, D.R., Innis, R.B., McCarthy, G. and Charney, D.S., 1993. Deficits in short-term memory in posttraumatic stress disorder. *American Journal of Psychiatry*, **150**, 1015–1019.

Bremner, J.D., Narayan, M., Staib, L.H., Southwick, S.M., McGlashan, T. and Charney, D.S., 1999a. Neural correlates of memories of childhood sexual abuse in women with and without posttraumatic stress disorder. *American Journal of Psychiatry*, **156**, 1787–1795.

Bremner, J.D., Staib, L.H., Kaloupek, D., Southwick, S.M., Soufer, R. and Charney, D.S., 1999b. Neural correlates of exposure to traumatic pictures and sound in Vietnam combat veterans with and without posttraumatic stress disorder: A positron emission tomography study. *Biological Psychiatry*, **45**, 806–816.

Brody, A.L., Saxena, S., Schwartz, J.M., Stoessel, P.W., Maidment, K., Phelps, M.E. and Baxter, L.R., Jr., 1998. FDG-PET predictors of response to behavioural therapy and pharmacotherapy in obsessive–compulsive disorder. *Psychiatry Research: Neuroimaging*, **84**, 1–6.

Bryant, R.A. and Harvey, A.G., 1995. Processing threatening information in posttraumatic stress disorder. *Journal of Abnormal Psychology*, **104**, 537–541.

Buchsbaum, M.S., Hazlett, E., Sicotte, N., Stein, M., Wu, J. and Zetin, M., 1985. Topographic EEG changes with benzodiazepine administration in generalized anxiety disorder. *Biological Psychiatry*, **20**, 832–842.

Buchsbaum, M.S., Wu, J., Haier, R., Hazlett, E., Ball, R., Katz, M., Sokoloski, K., Lagunas-Solar, M. and Langer, D., 1987. Positron emission tomography assessment of effects of benzodiazepines on regional glucose metabolic rate in patients with anxiety disorder. *Life Sciences*, **40**, 2393–2440.

Busatto, G.F., Buchpiguel, C.A., Zamignani, D.R., Garrido, G.E., Glabus, M.F., Rosario-Campos, M.C., Castro, C.C., Maia, A., Rocha, E.T., McGuire, P.K. and Miguel, E.C., 2001. Regional cerebral blood flow abnormalities in early-onset obsessive–compulsive disorder: An exploratory SPECT study. *Journal of the American Academy of Child & Adolescent Psychiatry*, **40**, 347–354.

Carter, C.S., Botvinick, M.M. and Cohen, J.D., 1999. The contribution of the anterior cingulate cortex to executive processes in cognition. *Reviews in the Neurosciences*, **10**, 49–57.

Carter, C.S., Macdonald, A.M., Botvinick, M., Ross, L.L., Stenger, V.A., Noll, D. and Cohen, J.D., 2000. Parsing executive processes: Strategic vs. evaluative functions of the anterior cingulate cortex. *Proceedings of the National Academy of Sciences*, **97**, 1994–1998.

Charney, D.S., Grillon, C.C.G. and Bremner, J.D., 1998. The neurobiological basis of anxiety and fear: Circuits, mechanisms, and neurochemical interactions (Part 1). *Neuroscientist*, **4**, 35–44.

Christensen, K.J., Kim, S.W., Dysken, M.W. and Hoover, K.M., 1992. Neuropsychological performance in obsessive–compulsive disorder. *Biological Psychiatry*, **31**, 4–18.

Cloitre, M. and Liebowitz, M.R., 1991. Memory bias in panic disorder: An investigation of the cognitive avoidance hypothesis. *Cognitive Therapy and Research*, **15**, 371–386.

Cloitre, M., Shear, M.K., Cancienne, J. and Zeitlin, S.B., 1994. Implicit and explicit memory for catastrophic associations to bodily sensation words in panic disorder. *Cognitive Therapy and Research*, **18**, 225–240.

Cohen, L.J., Hollander, E., DeCaria, C.M., Stein, D.J., Simeon, D., Liebowitz, M.R. and Aronowitz, B.R., 1996. Specificity of neuropsychological impairment in obsessive–compulsive disorder: A comparison with social phobic and normal control subjects. *Journal of Neuropsychiatry & Clinical Neurosciences*, **8**, 82–85.

Compton, R.J., Heller, W., Banich, M.T., Palmieri, P.A. and Miller, G.A., 2000. Responding to threat: Effects of hemispheric asymmetry and interhemispheric division of input. *Neuropsychology*, **14**, 254–264.

Compton, R.J., Banich, M.T., Mohanty, A., Milham, M.P., Miller, G.A., Scalf, P.E. and Heller, W., 2002. Paying attention to emotion: An fMRI investigation of cognitive and emotional Stroop tasks. Submitted for publication.

Constans, J.I., Foa, E.B., Franklin, M.E. and Mathews, A., 1995. Memory for actual and imagined events in OC checkers. *Behaviour Research & Therapy*, **33**, 665–671.

Cottraux, J., Gerard, D., Cinotti, L., Froment, J.C., Deiber, M.P., Le Bars, D., Galy, G., Millet, P., Labbe, C., Lavenne, F., Bouvard, M. and Mauguiere, F., 1996. A controlled positron emission tomography study of obsessive and neutral auditory stimulation in obsessive–compulsive disorder with checking rituals. *Psychiatry Research*, **60**, 101–112.

Davidson, R.J. and Irwin, W., 1999. The functional neuroanatomy of emotion and affective style. *Trends in Cognitive Sciences*, **3**, 11–21.

Davidson, R.J., Marshall, J.R., Tomarken, A.J. and Henriques, J.B., 2000. While a phobic waits: Regional brain electrical and autonomic activity in social phobics during anticipation of public speaking. *Biological Psychiatry*, **47**, 85–95.

Davidson, R.J., Pizzagalli, D., Nitschke, J.B. and Putnam, K., 2002. Depression: Perspectives from affective neuroscience. *Annual Review of Psychology*, **53**, 545–574.

Davis, M. and Lee, Y., 1998. Fear and anxiety: Possible roles of the amygdala and bed nucleus of the stria terminalis. *Cognition and Emotion*, **12**, 277–305.

Davis, M. and Whalen, P.J., 2001. The amygdala: Vigilance and emotion. *Molecular Psychiatry*, **6**, 13–34.

De Bellis, M.D., Casey, B.J., Dahl, R.E., Birmaher, B., Williamson, D.E., Thomas, K.M., Axelson, D.A., Frustaci, K., Boring, A.M., Hall, J. and Ryan, N.D., 2000. A pilot study of amygdala volumes in pediatric generalized anxiety disorder. *Biological Psychiatry*, **48**, 51–57.

De Cristofaro, M.T., Sessarego, A., Pupi, A., Biondi, F. and Faravelli, C., 1993. Brain perfusion abnormalities in drug-naive, lactate-sensitive panic patients: A SPECT study. *Biological Psychiatry*, **33**, 505–512.

Drevets, W.C., Videen, T.O. and MacLeod, A.K., 1992. PET images of blood flow changes during anxiety: A correction. *Science*, **256**, 1696.

Ehlers, A., Margraf, J., Davies, S. and Roth, W.T., 1988. Selective processing of threat cues in subjects with panic attacks. *Cognition and Emotion*, **2**, 201–219.

Eysenck, M.W., 1992. *Anxiety: The Cognitive Perspective*. Lawrence Erlbaum Associates Ltd., Hove, UK.

Eysenck, M.W., Mogg, K., May, J., Richards, A. and Mathews, A., 1991. Bias in interpretation of ambiguous sentences related to threat in anxiety. *Journal of Abnormal Psychology*, **100**, 144–150.

Fischer, H., Wik, G. and Fredrikson, M., 1996. Functional neuroanatomy of robbery re-experience: Affective memories studied with PET. *Neuroreport*, **7**, 2081–2086.

Foa, E.B., Feske, U., Murdock, T.B., Kozak, M.J. and McCarthy, P.R., 1991. Processing of threat-related information in rape victims. *Journal of Abnormal Psychology*, **100**, 156–162.

Foa, E.B., Ilai, D., McCarthy, P.R., Shoyer, B. and Murdock, T.B., 1993. Information processing in obsessive–compulsive disorder. *Cognitive Therapy and Research*, **17**, 173–189.

Foa, E.B., Franklin, M.E., Perry, K.J. and Herbert, J.D., 1996. Cognitive biases in generalized social phobia. *Journal of Abnormal Psychology*, **105**, 433–439.

Foa, E.B., Amir, N., Gershuny, B., Molnar, C. and Kozak, M.J., 1997. Implicit and explicit memory in obsessive–compulsive disorder. *Journal of Anxiety Disorders*, **11**, 119–129.

Foa, E.B., Gilboa-Schechtman, E., Amir, N. and Freshman, M., 2000. Memory bias in generalized social phobia: Remembering negative emotional expressions. *Journal of Anxiety Disorders*, **14**, 501–519.

Fontaine, R., Breton, G., Dery, R., Fontaine, S. and Elie, R., 1990. Temporal lobe abnormalities in panic disorder: An MRI study. *Biological Psychiatry*, **27**, 304–310.

Fredrikson, M., Wik, G., Greitz, T., Eriksson, L., Stone-Elander, S., Ericson, K. and Sedvall, G., 1993. Regional cerebral blood flow during experimental phobic fear. *Psychophysiology*, **30**, 126–130.

Fredrikson, M., Wik, G., Annas, P., Ericson, K. and Stone-Elander, S., 1995. Functional neuroanatomy of visually elicited simple phobic fear: Additional data and theoretical analysis. *Psychophysiology*, **32**, 43–48.

Friedman, B.H., Thayer, J.F. and Borkovec, T.D., 2000. Explicit memory bias for threat words in generalized anxiety disorder. *Behaviour Therapy*, **31**, 745–756.

Fyer, A.J., 1998. Current approaches to etiology and pathophysiology of specific phobia. *Biological Psychiatry*, **44**, 1295–1304.

Gilboa-Schechtman, E., Foa, E.B. and Amir, N., 1999. Attentional bias for facial expressions in social phobia: The face-in-the-crowd paradigm. *Cognition and Emotion*, **13**, 305–318.

Grachev, I.D., Breiter, H.C., Rauch, S.L., Savage, C.R., Baer, L., Shera, D.M., Kennedy, D.N., Makris, N., Caviness, V.S. and Jenike, M.A., 1998. Structural abnormalities of frontal neocortex in obsessive–compulsive disorder. *Archives of General Psychiatry*, **55**, 181–182.

Gray, J.A., 1982. *The Neuropsychology of Anxiety: An Enquiry into the Functions of the Septo-Hippocampal System*. Oxford University Press, Oxford, UK.

Grillon, C. and Buchsbaum, M.S., 1987. EEG topography of response to visual stimuli in generalized anxiety disorder. *Electroencephalography and Clinical Neurophysiology*, **66**, 337–348.

Gurvits, T.V., Shenton, M.E., Hokama, H., Ohta, H., Lasko, N.B., Gilbertson, M.W., Orr, S.P., Kikinis, R., Jolesz, F.A., McCarley, R.W. and Pitman, R.K., 1996. Magnetic resonance imaging study of hippocampal volume in chronic, combat-related posttraumatic stress disorder. *Biological Psychiatry*, **40**, 1091–1099.

Head, D., Bolton, D. and Hymas, N., 1989. Deficit in cognitive shifting ability in patients with obsessive–compulsive disorder. *Biological Psychiatry*, **25**, 929–937.

Heinrichs, N. and Hofmann, S.G., 2001. Information processing in social phobia: A critical review. *Clinical Psychology Review*, **21**, 751–770.

Heller, W., 1990. The neuropsychology of emotion: Developmental patterns and implications for psychopathology. In: Stein, N., Leventhal, B.L. and Trabasso, T. (eds), pp. 167–211. *Psychological and Biological Approaches*. Lawrence Erlbaum, Hillsdale, NJ.

Heller, W. and Nitschke, J.B., 1997. Regional brain activity in emotion: A framework for understanding cognition in depression. *Cognition and Emotion*, **11**, 637–661.

Heller, W. and Nitschke, J.B., 1998. The puzzle of regional brain activity in depression and anxiety: The importance of subtypes and comorbidity. *Cognition and Emotion*, **12**, 421–447.

Hoehn-Saric, R., Pearlson, G.D., Harris, G.J., Machlin, S.R. and Camargo, E.E., 1991. Effects of fluoxetine on regional cerebral blood flow in obsessive–compulsive patients. *American Journal of Psychiatry*, **148**, 1243–1245.

Hollander, E., Weiller, F., Cohen, L.J., Kwon, J.H., DeCaria, C.M., Liebowitz, M.R. and Stein, D.J., 1996. Neurological soft signs in social phobia. *Neuropsychiatry, Neuropsychology, and Behavioural Neurology*, **9**, 182–185.

Javanmard, M., Shlik, J., Kennedy, S.H., Vaccarino, F.J., Houle, S. and Bradwejn, J., 1999. Neuroanatomic correlates of CCK-4-induced panic attacks in healthy humans: A comparison of two time points. *Biological Psychiatry*, **45**, 872–882.

Jenike, M.A., Breiter, H.C., Baer, L., Kennedy, D.N., Savage, C.R., Olivares, M.J., O'Sullivan, R.L., Shera, D.M., Rauch, S.L., Keuthen, N., Rosen, B.R., Caviness, V.S. and Filipek, P.A., 1996. Cerebral structural abnormalities in obsessive–compulsive disorder: A quantitative morphometric magnetic resonance imaging study. *Archives of General Psychiatry*, **53**, 625–632.

Jenkins, M.A., Langlais, P.J., Delis, D. and Cohen, R., 1998. Learning and memory in rape victims with posttraumatic stress disorder. *American Journal of Psychiatry*, **155**, 278–279.

Johanson, A.M., Smith, G., Risberg, J., Silfverskiöld, P. and Tucker, D., 1992. Left orbital frontal activation in pathological anxiety. *Anxiety, Stress, and Coping*, **5**, 313–328.

Johanson, A., Gustafson, L., Passant, U., Risberg, J., Smith, G., Warkentin, S. and Tucker, D., 1998. Brain function in spider phobia. *Psychiatry Research: Neuroimaging*, **84**, 101–111.

Kaspi, S.P., McNally, R.J. and Amir, N., 1995. Cognitive processing of emotional information in posttraumatic stress disorder. *Cognitive Therapy and Research*, **19**, 433–444.

Lavy, E., van den Hout, M. and Arntz, A., 1993. Attentional bias and spider phobia: Conceptual and clinical issues. *Behaviour Research & Therapy*, **31**, 17–24.

LeDoux, J.E., 1996. *The Emotional Brain*. Simon and Schuster, New York.

Lepola, U., Nousiainen, U., Puranen, M., Riekkinen, P. and Rimon, R., 1990. EEG and CT findings in patients with panic disorder. *Biological Psychiatry*, **28**, 721–727.

Liberzon, I., Taylor, S.F., Amdur, R., Jung, T.D., Chamberlain, K.R., Minoshima, S., Koeppe, R.A. and Fig, L.M., 1999. Brain activation in PTSD in response to trauma-related stimuli. *Biological Psychiatry*, **45**, 817–826.

Lucey, J.V., Costa, D.C., Adshead, G., Deahl, M., Busatto, G., Gacinovic, S., Travis, M., Pilowsky, L., Ell, P.J., Marks, I.M. and Kerwin, R.W., 1997a. Brain blood flow in anxiety disorders, OCD, panic disorder with agoraphobia, and post-traumatic stress disorder on 99m TcHMPAO single photon emission tomography (SPET). *British Journal of Psychiatry*, **171**, 346–350.

Lucey, J.V., Costa, D.C., Busatto, G., Pilowsky, L.S., Marks, I.M., Ell, P.J. and Kerwin, R.W., 1997b. Caudate regional cerebral blood flow in obsessive–compulsive disorder, panic disorder and healthy controls on single photon emission computerised tomography. *Psychiatry Research: Neuroimaging*, **74**, 25–33.

Lündh, L.G. and Öst, L.G., 1996. Recognition bias for critical faces in social phobics. *Behaviour Research & Therapy*, **34**, 787–794.

Machlin, S.R., Harris, G.J., Pearlson, G.D., Hoehn-Saric, R., Jeffery, P. and Camargo, E.E., 1991. Elevated medial-frontal cerebral blood flow in obsessive–compulsive patients: A SPECT study. *American Journal of Psychiatry*, **148**, 1240–1242.

MacLeod, C., 1990. Mood disorders and cognition. In: Eysenck, M.W. (ed.), pp. 9–56. *Cognitive Psychology: An International Review*. Wiley, Chichester, UK.

MacLeod, C. and Hagan, R., 1992. Individual differences in the selective processing of threatening information, and emotional responses to a stressful life event. *Behaviour Research & Therapy*, **30**, 151–161.

MacLeod, C. and McLaughlin, K., 1995. Implicit and explicit memory bias in anxiety: A conceptual replication. *Behaviour Research & Therapy*, **33**, 1–14.

MacLeod, C. and Rutherford, E.M., 1992. Anxiety and the selective processing of emotional information: Mediating roles of awareness, trait and state variables, and personal relevance of stimulus material. *Behaviour Research & Therapy*, **30**, 479–491.

MacLeod, C., Mathews, A. and Tata, P., 1986. Attentional bias in emotional disorders. *Journal of Abnormal Psychology*, **95**, 15–20.
Malloy, P., Rasmussen, S., Braden, W. and Haier, R.J., 1989. Topographic evoked potential mapping in obsessive–compulsive disorder: Evidence of frontal lobe dysfunction. *Psychiatry Research*, **28**, 63–71.
Martin, M., Williams, R. and Clark, D.M., 1991. Does anxiety lead to selective processing of threat-related information? *Behaviour Research & Therapy*, **29**, 147–160.
Martinot, J.L., Allilaire, J.F., Mazoyer, B.M., Hantouche, E., Huret, J.D., Legaut-Demare, F., Deslauriers, A.G., Hardy, P., Pappata, S. and Baron, J.C., 1990. Obsessive–compulsive disorder: A clinical, neuropsychological and positron emission tomography study. *Acta Psychiatrica Scandinavica*, **82**, 233–242.
Martis, B., Malizia, A. and Rauch, S.L., 2002. Functional Neuroanatomy of Anxiety Disorders. In: D'Haenen, H., den Boer, J.A. and Wilner, P. (eds), *Textbook of Biological Psychiatry*. John Wiley & Sons, Chichester.
Mathews, A., 1984. Cognitive processes in generalised anxiety. Paper presented at the meeting of the European Association for Behaviour Therapy, Brussels.
Mathews, A. and MacLeod, C., 1985. Selective processing of threat cues in anxiety states. *Behaviour Research & Therapy*, **23**, 563–569.
Mathews, A. and MacLeod, C., 1986. Discrimination of threat cues without awareness in anxiety states. *Journal of Abnormal Psychology*, **95**, 131–138.
Mathews, A. and MacLeod, C., 1994. Cognitive approaches to emotion and emotional disorders. *Annual Review of Psychology*, **45**, 25–50.
Mathews, A. and Sebastian, S., 1993. Suppression of emotional Stroop effects by fear-arousal. *Cognition and Emotion*, **7**, 517–530.
Mathews, A., Mogg, K., May, J. and Eysenck, M., 1989a. Implicit and explicit memory bias in anxiety. *Journal of Abnormal Psychology*, **98**, 236–240.
Mathews, A., Richards, A. and Eysenck, M., 1989b. Interpretation of homophones related to threat in anxiety states. *Journal of Abnormal Psychology*, **98**, 31–34.
Mathews, A., May, J., Mogg, K. and Eysenck, M., 1990. Attentional bias in anxiety: Selective search or defective filtering? *Journal of Abnormal Psychology*, **99**, 166–173.
Mathews, A., Mogg, K., Kentish, J. and Eysenck, M., 1995. Effect of psychological treatment on cognitive bias in generalized anxiety disorder. *Behaviour Research & Therapy*, **33**, 293–303.
Mattia, J.I., Heimberg, R.G. and Hope, D.A., 1993. The revised Stroop color-naming task in social phobics. *Behaviour Research & Therapy*, **31**, 305–313.
McGuire, P.K., Bench, C.J., Frith, C.D., Marks, I.M., Frackowiak, R.S. and Dolan, R.J., 1994. Functional anatomy of obsessive–compulsive phenomena. *British Journal of Psychiatry*, **164**, 459–468.
McNally, R.J., 1998. Information-processing abnormalities in anxiety disorders: Implications for cognitive neuroscience. *Cognition and Emotion*, **12**, 479–495.
McNally, R.J. and Amir, N., 1996. Perceptual implicit memory for trauma-related information in post-traumatic stress disorder. *Cognition and Emotion*, **10**, 551–556.
McNally, R.J. and Kohlbeck, P.A., 1993. Reality monitoring in obsessive–compulsive disorder. *Behaviour Research & Therapy*, **31**, 249–253.
McNally, R.J., Foa, E.B. and Donnell, C.D., 1989. Memory bias for anxiety information in patients with panic disorder. *Cognition and Emotion*, **3**, 27–44.
McNally, R.J., Kaspi, S.P., Riemann, B.C. and Zeitlin, S.B., 1990. Selective processing of threat cues in posttraumatic stress disorder. *Journal of Abnormal Psychology*, **99**, 398–402.
McNally, R.J., Amir, N., Louro, C.E., Lukach, B.M., Riemann, B.C. and Calamari, J.E., 1994. Cognitive processing of idiographic emotional information in panic disorder. *Behaviour Research & Therapy*, **32**, 119–122.
McNally, R.J., Amir, N. and Lipke, H.J., 1996. Subliminal processing of threat cues in posttraumatic stress disorder? *Journal of Anxiety Disorders*, **10**, 115–128.
McNally, R.J., Hornig, C.D., Otto, M.W. and Pollack, M.H., 1997. Selective encoding of threat in panic disorder: Application of a dual priming paradigm. *Behaviour Research & Therapy*, **35**, 543–549.
Merckelbach, H., Muris, P., Pool, K. and de Jong, P.J., 1998. Resting EEG asymmetry and spider phobia. *Anxiety, Stress, and Coping*, **11**, 213–223.
Mogg, K., Mathews, A. and Weinman, J., 1987. Memory bias in clinical anxiety. *Journal of Abnormal Psychology*, **96**, 94–98.
Mogg, K., Mathews, A. and Eysenck, M., 1992. Attentional bias to threat in clinical anxiety states. *Cognition and Emotion*, **6**, 149–159.
Mogg, K., Bradley, B.P., Williams, R. and Mathews, A., 1993. Subliminal processing of emotional information in anxiety and depression. *Journal of Abnormal Psychology*, **102**, 304–311.
Mogg, K., Millar, N. and Bradley, B.P., 2000. Biases in eye movements to threatening facial expressions in generalized anxiety disorder and depressive disorder. *Journal of Abnormal Psychology*, **109**, 695–704.
Mohanty, A. and Heller, W., 2002. The neuropsychology of mood disorders. In: D'Haenen, H., den Boer, J.A. and Wilner, P. (eds), *Textbook of Biological Psychiatry*. John Wiley & Sons, Chichester.
Mountz, J.M., Modell, J.G., Wilson, M.W., Curtis, G.C., Lee, M.A., Schmaltz, S. and Kuhl, D.E., 1989. Positron emission tomographic evaluation of cerebral blood flow during state anxiety in simple phobia. *Archives of General Psychiatry*, **46**, 501–504.
Nitschke, J.B., Heller, W. and Miller, G.A., 2000. Anxiety, stress, and cortical brain function. In: Borod, J.C. (ed.), pp. 298–319. *The Neuropsychology of Emotion*. Oxford University Press, New York.
Nitschke, J.B., Schaefer, H.S., Mackiewicz, K.L., Skinner, B.T., Lee, H., Oakes, T.R., Anderle, M.J., Ihde-Scholl, T., Tartleton, L.C., Marler, C., Pederson, A.J.C., Ferber, K.L. and Davidson, R.J., 2001. Disentangling the anticipation of and response to aversive pictures: An event-related fMRI study. *Neuroscience Abstracts*, **27**, 840.
Nordahl, T.E., Benkelfat, C., Semple, W.E., Gross, M., King, A.C. and Cohen, R.M., 1989. Cerebral glucose metabolic rates in obsessive–compulsive disorder. *Neuropsychopharmacology*, **2**, 23–28.
Nordahl, T.E., Semple, W.E., Gross, M., Mellman, T.A., Stein, M.B., Goyer, P., King, A.C., Uhde, T.W. and Cohen, R.M., 1990. Cerebral glucose metabolic differences in patients with panic disorder. *Neuropsychopharmacology*, **3**, 261–272.
Nordahl, T.E., Stein, M.B. and Benkelfat, C., 1998. Regional cerebral metabolic asymmetries replicated in an independent group of patients with panic disorders. *Biological Psychiatry*, **44**, 998–1006.
Nugent, K. and Mineka, S., 1994. The effect of high and low trait anxiety on implicit and explicit memory tasks. *Cognition and Emotion*, **8**, 147–163.
Otto, M.W., McNally, R.J., Pollack, M.H., Chen, E. and Rosenbaum, J.F., 1994. Hemispheric laterality and memory bias for threat in anxiety disorders. *Journal of Abnormal Psychology*, **103**, 828–831.
Perani, D., Colombo, C., Bressi, S., Bonfanti, A., Grassi, F., Scarone, S., Bellodi, L., Smeraldi, E. and Fazio, F., 1995. [^{18}F] FDG PET study in obsessive–compulsive disorder: A clinical/metabolic correlation study after treatment. *British Journal of Psychiatry*, **166**, 244–250.
Potts, N.L., Davidson, J.R., Krishnan, K.R. and Doraiswamy, P.M., 1994. Magnetic resonance imaging in social phobia. *Psychiatry Research*, **52**, 35–42.
Purcell, R., Maruff, P., Kyrios, M. and Pantelis, C., 1998. Neuropsychological deficits in obsessive–compulsive disorder: A comparison with unipolar depression, panic disorder, and normal controls. *Archives of General Psychiatry*, **55**, 415–423.
Rajkowska, G., 2000. Postmortem studies in mood disorders indicate altered numbers of neurons and glial cells. *Biological Psychiatry*, **48**, 766–777.
Rapee, R.M., McCallum, S.L., Melville, L.F., Ravenscroft, H. and Rodney, J.M., 1994. Memory bias in social phobia. *Behaviour Research & Therapy*, **32**, 89–99.
Rauch, S.L. (in press). Neuroimaging and the neurobiology of anxiety disorders. In: Davidson, R.J., Scherer, K. and Goldsmith, H.H. (eds), *Handbook of Affective Sciences*.
Rauch, S.L., Jenike, M.A. and Alpert, N.M., 1994. Regional cerebral blood flow measured during symptom provocation in obsessive–compulsive disorder using oxygen 15-labeled carbon dioxide and positron emission tomography. *Archives of General Psychiatry*, **51**, 62–70.
Rauch, S.L., Savage, C.R., Alpert, N.M., Miguel, E.C., Baer, L., Breiter, H.C., Fischman, A.J., Manzo, P.A., Moretti, C. and Jenike, M.A., 1995a. A positron emission tomographic study of simple phobic symptom provocation. *Archives of General Psychiatry*, **52**, 20–28.
Rauch, S.L., Savage, C.R. and Brown, H.D., 1995b. A PET investigation of implicit and explicit sequence learning. *Human Brain Mapping*, **3**, 271–286.
Rauch, S.L., van der Kolk, B.A., Fisler, R.E., Alpert, N.M., Orr, S.P., Savage, C.R., Fischman, A.J., Jenike, M.A. and Pitman, R.K., 1996. A symptom provocation study of posttraumatic stress disorder using positron emission tomography and script-driven imagery. *Archives of General Psychiatry*, **53**, 380–387.
Rauch, S.L., Savage, C.R., Alpert, N.M., Dougherty, D., Kendrick, A., Curran, T., Brown, H.D., Manzo, P., Fischman, A.J. and Jenike, M.A.,

1997a. Probing striatal function in obsessive–compulsive disorder: A PET study of implicit sequence learning. *Journal of Neuropsychiatry & Clinical Neurosciences*, **9**, 568–573.

Rauch, S.L., Savage, C.R., Alpert, N.M., Fischman, A.J. and Jenike, M.A., 1997b. The functional neuroanatomy of anxiety: A study of three disorders using positron emission tomography and symptom provocation. *Biological Psychiatry*, **42**, 446–452.

Rauch, S.L., Whalen, P.J., Savage, C.R., Curran, T., Kendrick, A., Brown, H.D., Bush, G., Breiter, H.C. and Rosen, B.R., 1997c. Striatal recruitment during an implicit sequence learning task as measured by functional magnetic resonance imaging. *Human Brain Mapping*, **5**, 124–132.

Rauch, S.L., Whalen, P.J., Dougherty, D.D. and Jenike, M.A., 1998. Neurobiological models of obsessive–compulsive disorders. In: Jenike, M.A., Baer, L. and Minichiello, W.E. (eds), pp. 222–253. *Obsessive–Compulsive Disorders: Practical Management*. Moby, Boston.

Rauch, S.L., Whalen, P.J., Shin, L.M., McInerney, S.C., Macklin, M.L., Lasko, N.B., Orr, S.P. and Pitman, R.K., 2000. Exaggerated amygdala response to masked facial stimuli in posttraumatic stress disorder: A functional MRI study. *Biological Psychiatry*, **47**, 769–776.

Reiman, E.M., 1997. The application of positron emission tomography to the study of normal and pathologic emotions. *Journal of Clinical Psychiatry*, **58**, S4–S12.

Reiman, E.M., Raichle, M.E., Butler, F.K., Herscovitch, P. and Robins, E., 1984. A focal brain abnormality in panic disorder, a severe form of anxiety. *Nature*, **310**, 683–685.

Reiman, E.M., Raichle, M.E., Robins, E., Butler, F.K., Herscovitch, P., Fox, P. and Perlmutter, J., 1986. The application of positron emission tomography to the study of panic disorder. *American Journal of Psychiatry*, **143**, 469–477.

Reiman, E.M., Raichle, M.E., Robins, E., Mintun, M.A., Fusselman, M.J., Fox, P.T., Price, J.L. and Hackman, K.A., 1989. Neuroanatomical correlates of a lactate-induced anxiety attack. *Archives of General Psychiatry*, **46**, 493–500.

Robinson, D., Wu, H., Munne, R.A., Ashtari, M., Alvir, J.M., Lerner, G., Koreen, A., Cole, K. and Bogerts, B., 1995. Reduced caudate nucleus volume in obsessive–compulsive disorder. *Archives of General Psychiatry*, **52**, 393–398.

Rolls, E.T., 1999. The functions of the orbitofrontal cortex. *Neurocase: Case Studies in Neuropsychology, Neuropsychiatry, and Behavioural Neurology*, **5**, 301–312.

Rosenberg, D.R., Keshavan, M.S., O'Hearn, K.M., Dick, E.L., Bagwell, W.W., Seymour, A.B., Montrose, D.M., Pierri, J.N. and Birmaher, B., 1997. Frontostriatal measurement in treatment — naive children with obsessive–compulsive disorder. *Archives of General Psychiatry*, **54**, 824–830.

Rubin, R.T., Villanueva-Meyer, J., Ananth, J., Trajmar, P.G. and Mena, I., 1992. Regional xenon 133 cerebral blood flow and cerebral technetium 99m HMPAO uptake in unmedicated patients with obsessive–compulsive disorder and matched normal control subjects: Determination by high-resolution single-photon emission computed tomography. *Archives of General Psychiatry*, **49**, 695–702.

Rubin, R.T., Anath, J., Villanueva-Meyer, J., Trajmar, P.G. and Mena, I., 1995. Regional ^{133}xenon cerebral blood flow and cerebral ^{99m}Tc-HMPAO uptake in patients with obsessive–compulsive disorder before and during treatment. *Biological Psychiatry*, **38**, 429–437.

Sapolsky, R.M., 2000. Glucocorticoids and hippocampal atrophy in neuropsychiatric disorders. *Archives of General Psychiatry*, **57**, 925–935.

Savage, C.R., Keuthen, N.J. and Jenike, M.A., 1996. Recall and recognition memory in obsessive–compulsive disorder. *Journal of Neuropsychiatry & Clinical Neurosciences*, **8**, 99–103.

Savage, C.R., Baer, L., Keuthen, N.J., Brown, H.D., Rauch, S.L. and Jenike, M.A., 1999. Organizational strategies mediate nonverbal memory impairment in obsessive–compulsive disorder. *Biological Psychiatry*, **45**, 905–916.

Saxena, S., Brody, A.L., Maidment, K.M., Dunkin, J.J., Colgan, M., Alborzian, S., Phelps, M.E. and Baxter, L.R., Jr., 1999. Localized orbitofrontal and subcortical metabolic changes and predictors of response to paroxetine treatment in obsessive–compulsive disorder. *Neuropsychopharmacology*, **21**, 683–693.

Scarone, S., Colombo, C., Livian, S., Abbruzzese, M., Ronchi, P., Locatelli, M., Scotti, G. and Smeraldi, E., 1992. Increased right caudate nucleus size in obsessive–compulsive disorder: Detection with magnetic resonance imaging. *Psychiatry Research*, **45**, 115–121.

Schneider, F., Weiss, U., Kessler, C., Muller-Gartner, H.W., Posse, S., Salloum, J.B., Grodd, W., Himmelmann, F., Gaebel, W. and Birbaumer, N., 1999. Subcortical correlates of differential classical conditioning of aversive emotional reactions in social phobia. *Biological Psychiatry*, **45**, 863–871.

Schuff, N., Marmar, C.R., Weiss, D.S., Neylan, T.C., Schoenfold, F., Fein, G. and Weiner, M.W., 1997. Reduced hippocampal volume and N-acetyl aspartate in posttraumatic stress disorder. *Annals of the New York Academy of Sciences*, **821**, 516–520.

Schwartz, J.M., Stoessel, P.W., Baxter, L.R., Jr., Martin, K.M. and Phelps, M.E., 1996. Systematic changes in cerebral glucose metabolic rate after successful behaviour modification treatment of obsessive–compulsive disorder. *Archives of General Psychiatry*, **53**, 109–113.

Semple, W.E., Goyer, P., McCormick, R., Morris, E., Compton, B., Muswick, G., Nelson, D., Donovan, B., Leisure, G. and Berridge, M., 1993. Preliminary report: Brain blood flow using PET in patients with posttraumatic stress disorder and substance-abuse histories. *Biological Psychiatry*, **34**, 115–118.

Semple, W.E., Goyer, P.F., McCormick, R., Compton-Toth, B., Morris, E., Donovan, B., Muswick, G., Nelson, D., Garnett, M.L., Sharkoff, J., Leisure, G., Miraldi, F. and Schulz, S.C., 1996. Attention and regional cerebral blood flow in posttraumatic stress disorder patients with substance abuse histories. *Psychiatry Research: Neuroimaging*, **67**, 17–28.

Semple, W.E., Goyer, P.F., McCormick, R., Donovan, B., Muzic, R.F., Jr., Rugle, L., McCutcheon, K., Lewis, C., Liebling, D., Kowaliw, S., Vapenik, K., Semple, M.A., Flener, C.R. and Schulz, S.C., 2000. Higher brain blood flow at amygdala and lower frontal cortex blood flow in PTSD patients with comorbid cocaine and alcohol abuse compared with normals. *Psychiatry*, **63**, 65–74.

Sheline, Y.I., 2000. 3D MRI studies of neuroanatomic changes in unipolar major depression: The role of stress and medical comorbidity. *Biological Psychiatry*, **48**, 791–800.

Shin, L.M., Kosslyn, S.M., McNally, R.J., Alpert, N.M., Thompson, W.L., Rauch, S.L., Macklin, M.L. and Pitman, R.K., 1997a. Visual imagery and perception in posttraumatic stress disorder: A positron emission tomographic investigation. *Archives of General Psychiatry*, **54**, 233–241.

Shin, L.M., McNally, R.J., Kosslyn, S.M., Thompson, W.L., Rauch, S.L., Alpert, N.M., Metzger, L.J., Lasko, N.B., Orr, S.P. and Pitman, R.K., 1997b. A positron emission tomographic study of symptom provocation in PTSD. *Annals of the New York Academy of Sciences*, **821**, 1521–1523.

Shin, L.M., McNally, R.J., Kosslyn, S.M., Thompson, W.L., Rauch, S.L., Alpert, N.M., Metzger, R.L., Lasko, H.B., Orr, S.P. and Pitman, R.K., 1999. Regional cerebral blood flow during script-driven imagery in childhood sexual abuse-related PTSD: A PET investigation. *American Journal of Psychiatry*, **156**, 575–584.

Squire, L.R., 1992. Memory and the hippocampus: A synthesis from findings with rats, monkeys, and humans. *Psychological Review*, **99**, 195–231.

Stanford, M.S., Vasterling, J.J., Mathias, C.W., Constans, J.I. and Houston, R.J., 2001. Impact of threat relevance on P3 event-related potentials in combat-related post-traumatic stress disorder. *Psychiatry Research*, **102**, 125–137.

Stein, M.B. and Leslie, W.D., 1996. A brain single photon-emission computed tomography (SPECT) study of generalized social phobia. *Biological Psychiatry*, **39**, 825–828.

Stein, M.B. and Uhde, T.W., 1989. Infrequent occurrence of EEG abnormalities in panic disorder. *American Journal of Psychiatry*, **146**, 517–520.

Stein, M.B., Koverola, C., Hanna, C., Torchia, M.G. and McClarty, B., 1997. Hippocampal volume in women victimized by childhood sexual abuse. *Psychological Medicine*, **27**, 951–959.

Stewart, R.S., Devous, M.D.S., Rush, A.J., Lane, L. and Bonte, F.J., 1988. Cerebral blood flow changes during sodium-lactate-induced panic attacks. *American Journal of Psychiatry*, **145**, 442–449.

Suetsugi, M., Mizuki, Y., Ushijima, I., Kobayashi, T., Tsuchiya, K., Aoki, T. and Watanabe, Y., 2000. Appearance of frontal midline theta activity in patients with generalized anxiety disorder. *Neuropsychobiology*, **41**, 108–112.

Swedo, S.E., Schapiro, M.B., Grady, C.L., Cheslow, D.L., Leonard, H.L., Kumar, A., Friedland, R., Rapoport, S.I. and Rapoport, J.L., 1989. Cerebral glucose metabolism in childhood-onset obsessive–compulsive disorder. *Archives of General Psychiatry*, **46**, 518–523.

Swedo, S.E., Pietrini, P., Leonard, H.L., Schapiro, M.B., Rettew, D.C., Goldberger, E.L., Rapoport, S.I., Rapoport, J.L. and Grady, C.L., 1992. Cerebral glucose metabolism in childhood-onset obsessive–compulsive disorder: Revisualization during pharmacotherapy. *Archives of General Psychiatry*, **49**, 690–694.

Thrasher, S.M., Dalgleish, T. and Yule, W., 1994. Information processing in posttraumatic stress disorder. *Behaviour Research & Therapy*, **32**, 247–254.

Towey, J.P., Tenke, C.E., Bruder, G.E., Leite, P., Friedman, D., Liebowitz, M. and Hollander, E., 1994. Brain event-related potential correlates of over focused attention in obsessive–compulsive disorder. *Psychophysiology*, **31**, 535–543.

Trandel, D.V. and McNally, R.J., 1987. Perception of threat cues in post-traumatic stress disorder: Semantic processing without awareness? *Behaviour Research & Therapy*, **25**, 469–476.

Uddo, M., Vasterling, J.J., Brailey, K. and Sutker, P.B., 1993. Memory and attention in combat-related post-traumatic stress disorder (PTSD). *Journal of Psychopathology and Behavioural Assessment*, **15**, 43–51.

Van Ameringen, M., Mancini, C., Oakman, J.M., Kamath, M., Nahmias, C. and Szechtman, H., 1998. A pilot study of PET in social phobia. *Biological Psychiatry*, **43**, 31S.

Van den Hout, M., Tenney, N., Huygens, K. and de Jong, P., 1997. Preconscious processing bias in specific phobia. *Behaviour Research & Therapy*, **35**, 29–34.

Van der Linden, G., van Heerden, B., Warwick, J., Wessels, C., van Kradenburg, J., Zungu-Dirwayi, N. and Stein, D.J., 2000. Functional brain imaging and pharmacotherapy in social phobia: Single photon emission computed tomography before and after treatment with the selective serotonin reuptake inhibitor citalopram. *Progress in Neuro-Psychopharmacology & Biological Psychiatry*, **24**, 419–438.

Veale, D.M., Owen, A.M. and Marks, I.M., 1996. Specific cognitive deficits in tests sensitive to frontal lobe dysfunction in obsessive–compulsive disorder. *Psychological Medicine*, **26**, 1261–1269.

Vrana, S.R., Roodman, A. and Beckham, J.C., 1995. Selective processing of trauma-related words in posttraumatic stress disorder. *Journal of Anxiety Disorders*, **9**, 515–530.

Vythilingam, M., Anderson, E.R., Goddard, A., Woods, S.W., Staib, L.H., Charney, D.S. and Bremner, J.D., 2000. Temporal lobe volume in panic disorder — a quantitative magnetic resonance imaging study. *Psychiatry Research: Neuroimaging*, **99**, 75–82.

Watts, F.N., McKenna, F.P., Sharrock, R. and Trezise, L., 1986. Colour naming of phobia-related words. *British Journal of Psychology*, **77**, 97–108.

Watts, F.N. and Coyle, K., 1993. Phobics show poor recall of anxiety words. *British Journal of Psychology*, **66**, 373–382.

Whalen, P.J., Bush, G., McNally, R.J., Wilhelm, S., McInerney, S.C., Jenike, M.A. and Rauch, S.L., 1998. The emotional counting Stroop paradigm: A functional magnetic resonance imaging probe of the anterior cingulate affective division. *Biological Psychiatry*, **44**, 1219–1228.

Wiedemann, G., Pauli, P., Dengler, W., Lutzenberger, W., Birbaumer, N. and Buchkremer, G., 1999. Frontal brain asymmetry as a biological substrate of emotions in patients with panic disorders. *Archives of General Psychiatry*, **56**, 78–84.

Wik, G., Fredrikson, M., Ericson, K., Eriksson, L., Stone-Elander, S. and Greitz, T., 1993. A functional cerebral response to frightening visual stimulation. *Psychiatry Research*, **50**, 15–24.

Williams, J.M.G., Watts, F.N., MacLeod, C. and Mathews, A., 1988. *Cognitive Psychology and Emotional Disorders*. Wiley, Chichester, UK.

Wolski, P. and Maj, S., 1998. Performance of clinical anxiety group on Sternberg memory scanning task: Possible cognitive and affective effects of worry. *Polish Psychological Bulletin*, **29**, 47–56.

Wu, J.C., Buchsbaum, M.S., Hershey, T.G., Hazlett, E., Sicotte, N. and Johnson, J.C., 1991. PET in generalized anxiety disorder. *Biological Psychiatry*, **29**, 1181–1199.

Yehuda, R., Keefe, R.S., Harvey, P.D., Levengood, R.A., Gerber, D.K., Geni, J. and Siever, L.J., 1995. Learning and memory in combat veterans with posttraumatic stress disorder. *American Journal of Psychiatry*, **152**, 137–139.

Yehuda, R., 1997. Sensitization of the hypothalamic–pituitary–adrenal axis in posttraumatic stress disorder. *Annals of the New York Academy of Sciences*, **821**, 57–75.

Zielinski, C.M., Taylor, M.A. and Juzwin, K.R., 1991. Neuropsychological deficits in obsessive–compulsive disorder. *Neuropsychiatry, Neuropsychology, and Behavioural Neurology*, **4**, 110–126.

Zubieta, J.K., Chinitz, J.A., Lombardi, U., Fig, L.M., Cameron, O.G. and Liberzon, I., 1999. Medial frontal cortex involvement in PTSD symptoms: A SPECT study. *Journal of Psychiatric Research*, **33**, 259–264.

XIX-9

Functional Neuroanatomy of Anxiety Disorders

Brian Martis, Andrea Malizia and Scott L. Rauch

INTRODUCTION

In this chapter, current hypotheses regarding the functional neuroanatomy of anxiety disorders are examined. Initially, the concepts of anxiety and stress as well as anxiety disorders are discussed. Next, relevant research on animal fear conditioning as well as human anxiety studies are briefly reviewed. This provides the necessary foundation for the ensuing coverage of human data on anxiety disorders and related contemporary neurobiological models.

Anxiety and Fear

In humans, anxiety is a normal unpleasant affective state with experiential, cognitive, autonomic, neuroendocrine and behavioural components. Fear behaviour is the response to specific environmental stimuli that are perceived as potentially dangerous. Though details are still debated, fear behaviour refers to a stimulus-bound response while anxiety is understood as a state of anticipatory apprehension and dread in humans (Davis, 1998; Nitschke, Heller and Miller, 2000). Fear processes are innate and mediated by rapid-response neurobiological systems in animals and humans. It is appealing to consider that these adaptive mechanisms have evolved to enable harm avoidance and enhance chances of survival. Animal research findings suggest that the fear system is a dynamic, integrated network of neural circuits, comprised of processing nodes (specific brain areas), that detects and responds to danger (LeDoux, 2000a). Given the wealth of behavioural and neurobiological similarities between fear responses in animals and humans, animal research in this area plays an important role in guiding anxiety research in humans. However, the conscious and cognitive aspects of human anxiety are undeniably complex and unique, thereby warranting caution when extrapolating from fear research in animals to the neurobiology of anxiety in humans. Similarly, there are substantial inferential leaps to be acknowledged when moving from theories regarding normal human anxiety to the anxiety disorders, which are complex, multifactorially determined syndromes.

Stress

Stress is generally defined as a circumstance that disturbs the normal physiological or psychological functioning of an individual, as well as the disturbed state that results (derived from The Oxford English Dictionary, Second Edition, 1989). Physiological stress responses are coordinated, multisystem (e.g. autonomic, neuroendocrine and immune) adaptive changes in organisms. Stress inducing stimuli or 'stressors' can be positive or adverse. Stress research in humans is particularly challenging due to the convergent and less well described effects of psychological, social and cultural stressors on biological systems. Excessive stress in humans contributes to increased morbidity and mortality and is a significant predictor of adverse outcomes in many medical and psychiatric disorders, e.g. ischaemic heart disease and major depression (Chrousos and Gold, 1998; O'Connor, Gurbel and Serebrauny, 2000; Monroe *et al.*, 2001). Stress responses are closely related to anxiety disorders; this being inferred mainly from overt exposure to stressful life events or trauma. The effects of chronic low level stress are less well established in relation to psychiatric disorders. In the current Diagnostic and Statistical Manual of Mental Disorders (DSM-IV; APA, 1994), two disorders, Acute Stress Disorder and Post-Traumatic Stress Disorder, specifically require exposure to overt traumatic stress as a diagnostic criterion.

Anxiety Disorders

Anxiety disorders, (DSM-IV, (APA, 1994); ICD 10, under 'neurotic, stress-related and somatoform disorders', Chapter V (F), WHO, 1992), are characterized by exaggerated anxiety and fear responses occurring either spontaneously or to relatively innocuous stimuli. Additional hallmarks of these disorders include hypervigilance, hyperarousal, ritualized avoidance and subjective distress. When severe, these manifestations can be disabling. Sufferers tend to display attention and interpretation biases resulting in hypervigilance and overestimation of risk (Nitschke, Heller and Miller, 2000). Psychiatric comorbidity is common among individuals who suffer from an anxiety disorder; the most prevalent comorbid conditions include another anxiety disorder, depression, and substance use disorders. People with anxiety disorders are also at increased risk of suicide and exhibit increased medical service utilization (Regier *et al.*, 1998; Dunner, 2001). Discrete anxiety disorder diagnoses in the DSM-IV include: panic disorder (with and without agoraphobia), acute stress and post traumatic stress disorder, specific and social phobias (social anxiety disorder), generalized anxiety disorder and obsessive compulsive disorder (APA, 1994). Emerging neurobiological evidence provides an opportunity to critically review and refine these nosological constructs, though making sense of inconsistent evidence from studies that involve different modalities and paradigms in heterogeneous populations is a challenge.

FUNCTIONAL NEUROANATOMY OF FEAR AND ANXIETY

Fear Conditioning: Animal Research

The fear-conditioning behavioural paradigm has been a centrepiece for advancing science in this domain via hypothesis-driven research in both animals and humans. Fear conditioning involves the temporal pairing of a neutral stimulus (known as a conditioned stimulus (CS); e.g. a tone), with an aversive stimulus (the unconditioned stimulus (US); e.g. a shock) that can innately elicit fear responses.

Biological Psychiatry: Edited by H. D'haenen, J.A. den Boer and P. Willner. ISBN 0-471-49198-5

After one or several paired presentations, the CS alone can trigger the fear responses. This process can be shown to habituate (i.e. repeated presentations cause decremental intensity in the response). Moreover, if the CS is subsequently repeatedly presented without the paired US, the fear responses decline and cease, a process referred to as 'extinction'. These phenomena and pathways subserving them have been reliably demonstrated in multiple animal species as well as in humans (LeDoux, 2000a).

Evidence accumulated from neuroanatomical tract tracing, ablation, and unit-recording studies of animal fear conditioning implicates the amygdala as central in the 'fear network'. The critical role of the amygdala is further supported by evidence of its abundant reciprocal connections with other brain areas (e.g. sensory thalamus, primary somatosensory cortex, prefrontal cortex, striatum, and brain stem) that comprise the fear network, subserving the various elements of the characteristic fear response (see below).

The amygdala also houses an internal circuitry, involving its various nuclei. Based on animal findings (best mapped out in the context of auditory CS in rats), sensory information from the sensory thalamus is rapidly conveyed to the lateral nucleus of the amygdala (LA). Further transmission occurs from the LA to the central nucleus of the amygdala (CeA), both directly and via the accessory basal (abA) and basal (bA) amygdalar nuclei. The CeA has projections to multiple output areas which subserve the characteristic components of the conditioned fear response such as autonomic activity (subserved by the brainstem autonomic centres including the locus caeruleus), the stress neuroendocrine response (lateral hypothalamic nuclei), attentional processes and response choice (the anterior cingulate cortex) as well as templates of action tendency and overt response behaviour (periaqueductal gray, the striatum) (Kapp *et al.*, 1992; Maren and Fanselow, 1996; LeDoux, 2000b; Davis, 2000).

Animals thus conditioned also express similar responses to the context in which the conditioning occurred. This phenomenon, called 'contextual fear conditioning' is evidenced when the same characteristic fear responses can be elicited following fear conditioning, simply by exposing the subject to the situation where conditioning occurred, even in the absence of re-exposure to a discrete CS. Lesion studies have demonstrated the crucial role of the hippocampal projections to the amygdala in contextual fear conditioning (Maren and Fanselow, 1995).

The neurobiology of fear conditioning has been further elucidated by studies that assess changes occurring at the cellular and molecular levels within the amygdala, hippocampus and other relevant structures. Plasticity has been studied via cell recordings in various amygdalar nuclei as well as at other nodes within the fear-conditioning network. Long-term potentiation (LTP) has been demonstrated in the amygdalo-hippocampal pathways in fear conditioning though these results are mixed and less well characterized. Specifically, the NMDA receptor activation is implicated in the mediation of LTP in some subnuclei of the amygdala (Chapman and Chattarji, 2000). The amygdala is considered to be essential in fear-related learning and thus may have an important role in decision making (by emotional weighting) and in the early stages of memory formation for emotionally salient events. However, much remains to be understood about the role of the amygdala and relevant neural pathways in fear learning and memory in humans.

The orbitofrontal cortex (OFC) is implicated in the extinction of conditioned fear response. There is evidence for a dynamic interaction between the OFC and the amygdala with regard to processing of fear-conditioning responses. When the potentially threatening nature of a particular stimulus diminishes, the OFC is purported to attenuate responses to that stimulus via projections to the amygdala. Thus prefrontal connections of the amygdala are believed to modulate threat-related information (Wilson and Rolls, 1990; Morgan, Romanski and LeDoux, 1993; Morgan and LeDoux, 1995), conferring flexibility and adaptability needed to successfully navigate a rapidly changing environment.

Primate Studies

Extending fear-conditioning work in rats to primates could be viewed as an essential intermediate step in the understanding of human anxiety and fear. The seminal work of Kluver and Bucy (1939) in describing the behavioural effects of bilateral anterior temporal lobectomy in monkeys set the stage for more detailed investigations into amygdala involvement in fear behaviour. It is important to note that subsequent studies, involving more selective lesions of the amygdala, have shown the ensuing deficits to share some but not all features of the Kluver–Bucy syndrome, confirming that some of the features were due to lesions in the adjacent brain regions. Contemporary data from primates has, however, strengthened the argument that the amygdala is critically involved in stimulus–affect association (i.e. in the elicitation of learned emotional responses; see Baxter and Murray (2000) for a detailed review of these newer studies).

Much of the work on fear conditioning in rodents with specific reference to the role of the amygdala in stimulus-reinforcer associations has been extended in primates. The amygdala neurons have been shown to respond to primary reinforcers (e.g. taste), visual stimuli previously paired with rewarding primary reinforcer, novel stimuli and faces (Rolls, 1999). The interactions between the OFC and amygdala have been demonstrated to similarly contribute to acquisition and extinction of fear conditioning. However, more recent studies highlight the anticipated difficulty in making inferential leaps across different species towards human brain functioning. For example, Kalin *et al.* (2001) reported that rhesus monkeys with previously characterized 'anxious temperament' endophenotype, demonstrated blunted acute unconditioned fear responses in the face of >70% bilateral amygdalar destruction, but were unchanged on unconditioned trait-like anxiety-fear responses in the face of >95% bilateral amygdala destruction. Thus, caution must be exercised while using findings from animal research to hypothesize about human anxiety and its disorders.

Studies of Humans with Brain Lesions

Brain lesions that arise in humans are rarely neuroanatomically configured to involve only the entirety of a brain region of interest. Furthermore, the capacity of spared regions to compensate for lost structures complicates meaningful interpretation of regional function. Nevertheless, the study of humans with discrete brain lesions offers valuable clues to functional neuroanatomy.

Adolphs *et al.* (1994, 1995) reported studies with a single subject (SM), a 32-year-old lady with a rare heritable disorder of primarily epithelial tissue, the Urbach–Wiethe syndrome, characterized by avascular/atrophic mineralizations of medial temporal tissue including the amygdala. SM was reported to have selective, complete and stable bilateral amygdalar damage (as well as minor damage to anterior entorhinal cortices) by magnetic resonance imaging (MRI). Extensive testing on SM revealed a persistent deficit in recognition of fear expression despite the cognitive ability to describe fear and what it entailed. This has been replicated in subsequent studies on humans with bilateral amygdala damage (Calder *et al.*, 1996; Broks *et al.*, 1998; Adolphs *et al.*, 1999b). In humans with discrete lesions of the amygdala or more extensive temporal lobe lesions that include the amygdala, deficits have also been demonstrated involving fear conditioning (Bechara *et al.*, 1995; LaBar *et al.*, 1998). The few studies in subjects with varying amounts of amygdala damage using a task of emotional prosody recognition have yielded mixed results: impairment (Scott *et al.*, 1997) vs no deficits (Anderson and Phelps, 1998; Adolphs *et al.*, 1999a). Thus, taken together, human lesion studies have extended the research in animals, by demonstrating amygdala involvement in the recognition of facial expressions of negative emotions including but not limited to, fear.

Based on these findings it has been hypothesized that the amygdala is an important component in a specialized human neural system that detects and responds to danger-related stimuli (with or without a social context). The role of the amygdala in this system is to detect the emotional relevance of stimuli and help trigger rapid behavioural responses and conscious awareness of aversive stimuli through its subcortical and cortical connections (Adolphs and Tranel, 2000).

Human brain lesion studies involving other regions germane to the purported fear network, provide further information to guide contemporary circuitry models of anxiety disorders. For instance, OFC lesions are associated with disruption in the rapid flexible response to changes in rule set. This may parallel the established role of the OFC in dynamic response attenuation when stimulus salience has changed (i.e. extinction). This is consistent with a broad role for the OFC in top-down control over subcortical structures in fear processing. Thus, OFC dysfunction in top-down control may lead to an inflexible persistence of fear responses, manifesting as pervasive cognitive misinterpretation of danger even in the face of relatively innocuous stimuli (or conversely a lack of recognition of danger).

Neuroimaging Studies of Anxiety in Healthy Subjects

It is important to understand the neural processing of normal anxiety to gain insight into anxiety disorders where this mechanism is presumably dysfunctional. Recent positron emission tomography (PET) and functional magnetic resonance imaging (fMRI) studies have attempted to map the mediating neuroanatomy associated with perception of threat-related or emotionally valenced stimuli (mainly faces) as well as behaviourally or pharmacologically induced anxiety (see Rauch and Shin, 2002 for review). Such studies of anxiety in healthy volunteers have demonstrated relatively consistent patterns of brain activation in the anterior paralimbic cortical structures (i.e. posterior medial orbitofrontal, anterior temporal, anterior cingulate, and insular cortex) and the amygdala.

Much of the work in this area has involved mapping brain activity in healthy volunteers when presented with emotionally expressive faces (fear, happy, angry and disgust). Perception of fearful faces has been reported to be associated with amygdala activation both when the stimulus was overtly (Breiter *et al.*, 1996a; Morris *et al.*, 1996, 1998a; Phillips *et al.*, 1997) or covertly presented with a backward masking technique (Whalen *et al.*, 1998). Extending this work, Morris, Öhman and Dolan (1998b, 1999) demonstrated significant correlation of right amygdala neural activity (to masked fear-conditioned faces) with activity in visual structures implicated in non conscious processing (pulvinar nucleus of thalamus and superior colliculus). Based on this the authors suggest that processing of behaviourally relevant unseen visual stimuli may be subserved by a right-sided subcortical pathway in parallel to a cortical route necessary for conscious identification.

Habituation in the brain represents an adaptive mechanism by which resources can be preferentially allocated to survival-relevant (e.g. threat-related) stimuli by rapid attenuation of response to stimuli that are no longer salient. Lack of habituation may help to explain some symptoms of anxiety such as persisting anxiety beyond the point of stimulus relevance. Investigators have attempted to demonstrate habituation in fMRI studies of healthy subjects by showing response decrements in various brain areas activated by emotionally relevant stimuli (e.g. faces bearing emotional expressions) (Breiter *et al.*, 1996a; Whalen *et al.*, 1998; Fischer *et al.*, 2000a, 2000b). Although preliminary there seem to be lateralized differences in habituation of amygdala responses (significant signal decrement over time in right but not left amygdala) and differential habituation to emotional valence in the left prefrontal cortex (greater signal decrement to positive vs negatively valenced stimuli) (Wright *et al.*, 2000, 2001).

The phenomena of fear conditioning and extinction are relevant to models of anxiety disorders. Innovative functional neuroimaging paradigms have been employed to study the neural substrates of fear conditioning in humans. Morris *et al.* (1997, 1998a, 1998b) reported association of the fear-conditioned state with increased activity in bilateral amygdala, right thalamus and OFC, further demonstrating lateralized amygdala activation based on subjects' awareness of the fear-related stimuli (right-sided with covert stimuli and left-sided with overt stimuli). Other groups using different conditioning paradigms, have demonstrated anterior paralimbic activation and habituation of conditioning-related signals in the amygdala and hippocampal region (Büchel *et al.*, 1998, 1999; LaBar *et al.*, 1998).

ANXIETY DISORDERS

Overview

The anxiety disorders share many common core features (hypervigilance, excessive anxiety, and avoidance); yet, they are also distinguishable from one another clinically (e.g. spontaneous attacks of terrifying anxiety in panic disorders versus a pervasive state of anxiety in GAD). It is appealing to consider that common neurobiological substrates may underlie the spectrum of anxiety disorders, while unique pathophysiological mechanisms exist that distinguish among them. Investigators have developed tentative models regarding the neurobiology of anxiety disorders drawing from animal research and human imaging data as outlined above.

Currently, neurobiological and neuroanatomical hypotheses for some of these disorders (e.g. PTSD, OCD and PD) are more coherent than for others (e.g. GAD, phobias). A logical starting point is to identify core characteristics of specific anxiety disorders and based on animal and human research findings, test hypotheses of regional dysfunction in specific disorders. Advances in neuroimaging have accelerated this effort. Structural as well as neutral state and symptom provocation functional neuroimaging studies are giving way to more sophisticated cognitive, pharmacological and multimodal paradigms.

In the following section, research findings and current hypotheses pertaining to the functional neuroanatomy of specific anxiety disorders will be discussed. Note that a comprehensive model requires an integration between neurocircuitry and relevant neurochemistry/neuropharmacology of the implicated brain pathways. For clarity of organization, these complementary topics have been addressed in a separate chapter in this volume (Malizia *et al.*, Chapter XIX-10).

POST-TRAUMATIC STRESS DISORDER (PTSD)

PTSD is characterized by a triad of symptom clusters that occur in the aftermath of a precipitating traumatic event: (1) recurrent intrusive 're-experiencing' of the trauma (2) hypervigilance/hyperarousal and (3) emotional numbing/avoidance (DSM-IV; APA, 1994). Neurobiological research in PTSD has mostly involved patients with combat or childhood abuse related PTSD. In fact, there are a wide variety of types of trauma that can cause PTSD, and it is not clear whether different characteristics of the trauma history are reflected in different neurobiological subtypes of the disorder. For instance, the trauma can be a single event, or a series of multiple events; it can occur over a brief time or chronically; the exposure can occur in childhood or adulthood; and it can be perpetrated by humans or not. Regardless of the aetiology of the PTSD, patients are prone to comorbidities such as mood and substance-abuse disorders. Despite these numerous sources of heterogeneity in PTSD, findings from human studies seem to converge with data from animal research in certain areas discussed below.

Stress, Glucocorticoids/HPA Axis and the Hippocampus in Animals and Humans

Rodent and non-human primate studies have demonstrated neural damage such as apical dendrite atrophy (CA3 neurons), degeneration of CA3 hippocampal neurons, and decreased hippocampal blood flow in response to a variety of chronic stressors (social, restraint, physical) (Uno *et al.*, 1989; Watanabe, Gould and McEwen, 1992; Endo *et al.*, 1999). These effects appear to be a consequence of stress-related excessive glucocorticoid (GC) secretion which in part seems to be mediated by an excess of excitatory amino acids (EAA's) such as glutamate, producing NMDA receptor mediated excitotoxic effects (Sapolsky, Krey and McEwen, 1985; Woolley, Gould and McEwen, 1990; Gould and Tanapat, 1999).

Smaller hippocampal volumes have also been demonstrated in human subjects with PTSD, due to combat as well as childhood sexual abuse (in both sexes, ranging from 5–26%) (see Table XIX-9.1A for structural studies in PTSD) with the exception of one study involving children/adolescent subjects with PTSD (De Bellis *et al.*, 1999). Bremner *et al.* (1995), reported smaller right hippocampal volumes in 26 veterans with PTSD (vs 22 civilian controls without PTSD). In the PTSD subjects, lower percent retention scores on a standard test of verbal memory were associated with lower right hippocampal volumes. Gurvits *et al.* (1996) found smaller bilateral hippocampal volumes in seven Vietnam combat veterans with PTSD (vs seven Vietnam combat veterans without and eight civilians without PTSD). The hippocampal volumes across the 14 veterans were inversely correlated with the extent of combat exposure and PTSD symptom severity. This raises the question of the specificity of the volumetric reductions to the PTSD process. Thus the basis for these volumetric differences is still unclear. Several possibilities exist including volume loss being the effect of the traumatic exposure vs sequelae of the development of the PTSD symptoms, or that people with smaller hippocampi are predisposed to developing PTSD following trauma (Pitman, 2001).

Clinical research has revealed decreased hippocampal volumes and elevated cortisol levels in Cushing's syndrome, which was reversed with treatment (Starkman *et al.*, 1992, 1999). Smaller hippocampal volumes and high cortisol levels have also been reported in major depressive disorder (for review see Brown, Rush and McEwen, 1999). The hippocampus is also involved in the modulation of the hypothalamic-pituitary-adrenal (HPA) axis, and lesions of the hippocampus appear to increase the release of glucocorticoids during stress which in turn may further damage the hippocampus (Feldman and Conforti, 1980; Sapolsky, Krey and McEwen, 1986; Herman *et al.*, 1989). However, hypo and not hypercortisolaemia has been frequently reported in patients with PTSD (Newport and Nemeroff, 2000), which is harder to reconcile with the GC mediated hippocampal volume loss theory. One hypothesis that attempts to explain this apparent disparity suggests GC hypersensitivity in PTSD patients resulting in hypocortisolaemia (due to feedback inhibition) and reduced hippocampal volumes (Yehuda, 1998).

Fear Conditioning, PTSD Symptoms and Functional Neuroimaging Studies in PTSD

The fear-conditioning paradigm seems relevant to the understanding of some PTSD symptomatology. For example, certain aspects of the response to environmental triggers of past trauma strongly resemble the animal fear-conditioning response. However, the indelibility of the trauma-related memory and resistance to extinction of the fear response in PTSD is distinct from normal fear conditioning in animal studies. Simple experimental noxious stimuli currently used in animal research provide a suboptimal comparison to the real life complexity of the human post-traumatic stress response. Thus, one of the challenges in PTSD research is to disentangle pre-existing neurobiological factors that might predispose to developing PTSD in the face of trauma exposure (i.e. risk factors) from fundamental pathophysiological elements of the disease process as well as non-specific consequences of traumatic exposure.

According to the 'amygdalocentric' model of PTSD, hyperresponsivity within the amygdala to threat-related stimuli, in the face of disrupted functional connectivity between the OFC, amygdala and hippocampal regions may explain some of the cognitive, affective and psychomotor manifestations of PTSD (Rauch and Baxter, 1998; Rauch and Shin, 2002). According to this theory the hyperresponsivity of the amygdala results in characteristic symptoms of hyperarousal. Dysfunctional governance of the amygdala by the prefrontal cortex (specifically the affective division of the anterior cingulate cortex) is implicated in the inappropriate assessment of and response to threat and the persistence of this beyond the relevant period (i.e. inflexibility and dysfunctional 'extinction'). Hippocampal dysfunction may contribute to contextual avoidance, difficulty in identifying safe contexts and explicit memory deficits

Table XIX-9.1A Structural neuroimaging studies in PTSD

Authors	Subjects	Methods	Findings
Bremner *et al.*, 1995	26 Vet-PTSD vs 22 healthy civilians	MRI morphometry	R-hippo. volumes 8% ↓ in vets vs controls. ↓ scores on a standard measure of verbal mem. correlated directly with ↓ R-hippo. volumes.
Gurvits *et al.*, 1996	7 Vietnam vets with PTSD; 7 Vets. and 8 nonvet. controls without PTSD	MRI morphometry	Significantly ↓ B/L-hippo. volumes in PTSD vs both control groups. Hippo. volume inversely correlated with extent of exposure (14 vets.)
Bremner *et al.*, 1997a	17 adults with PTSD (childhood abuse) vs 21 non abused controls	MRI morphometry	12% ↓ L-hippocampal volumes.
Stein *et al.*, 1997	21 adults with PTSD vs 21 non abused controls	MRI morphometry	5% smaller L-hippo. volumes in abused subjects. Total hippo. volumes ↓ in abused with ↑ PTSD symptom severity than those with ↓ severity.
DeBellis *et al.*, 1999	44 maltreated children and adolescents vs 61 healthy controls	MRI morphometry	No differences in hippocampal volumes PTSD group had ↓ intracranial and cerebral volumes.

Table XIX-9.1B Functional neuroimaging studies in PTSD

Authors	Subjects	Methods	Findings
Semple *et al.*, 1993	6 combat PTSD and substance abuse vs 7 normal controls	PET-Auditory CPT and word generation	PTSD group exhibited ↑ rCBF in orbitofrontal cortex during auditory CPT and word generation.
Rauch *et al.*, 1996	Mixed gender, 8 PTSD subjects	PET-Symptom provocation with script-driven imagery	Provoked vs control: ↑ rCBF in ACC, R-OFC, insula, Ant. Temp. and visual cortex and right amygdala. ↓ rCBF decreases in L Brocas and L middle temporal cortex. No comparison group.
Shin *et al.*, 1999	8 F with PTSD (childhood sexual abuse) vs 8 trauma controls with out PTSD	PET-Symptom provocation with script-driven imagery	Trauma tic vs neutral contrast: Anterior paralimbic activation in both groups. Group by condition interaction: PTSD group showed significantly > rCBF increases within ant. temp. and OFC. > rCBF increase within ACC in controls than PTSD group.
Bremner *et al.*, 1999a	10 F with PTSD (childhood sexual abuse) vs 12 trauma controls without PTSD	PET-Symptom provocation with script-driven imagery	↓ recruitment of ACC in PTSD group.
Bremner *et al.*, 1999b	10 Vietnam vets. with PTSD vs 10 Vietnam vets. without	PET-Responses to trauma-related pictures and sounds	PTSD group showed ↑ rCBF in medial PFC (subcallosal gyrus) and ACC.
Liberzon *et al.*, 1999	14 Viet. Vets. With PTSD, 11 vet controls, 14 healthy nonvets	SPECT-Study	Combat sound vs. white noise: All three groups showed activation of ACC/MPFC. PTSD group showed activation in L amygdaloid region.
Bremner *et al.*, 1997b	10 combat vets. With PTSD vs 10 nonvets, no PTSD	PET-Yohimbine (Y) challenge	Y administration associated with increased anxiety and panic symptoms and widespread decreased ↓ CBF in PTSD group.
Shin *et al.*, 1997	7 vets. With combat PTSD and 7 matched trauma exposed vets. without	PET-Cognitive activation: neutral, negative, combat pictures perception and imagery	Combat imagery vs control: PTSD group showed ↑ rCBF in R-amygdala and ventral ACG and ↓ rCBF in L-Inf. frontal gyrus (Brocas).
Rauch *et al.*, 2000	8 combat vets. with PTSD vs 8 control combat vets	fMRI-Study Fearful and happy faces masked temporally by neutral faces	> amygdala activation in PTSD group than control. Magnitude of activation correlated with PTSD severity.

(especially for the traumatic event/s). Conscious appreciation of trigger stimuli may not be necessary to trigger symptomatology. Rauch *et al.* (2000) have previously demonstrated that subjects with PTSD have hyperactive amygdalar responses to emotional facial expression even when subjects were unaware of seeing them (using a backward masking technique).

Functional neuroimaging studies in PTSD have involved symptom provocation studies and neurocognitive probes of specific areas implicated in the pathophysiology of PTSD. Upon exposure to reminders of their traumatic event (script-driven imagery or trauma-related pictures and sounds), patients with PTSD have been shown to exhibit abnormal activity in the anterior paralimbic areas (OFC, ACC) as well as subcortical circuitry involving the amygdala (Rauch *et al.*, 1996; Shin *et al.*, 1999; Bremner *et al.*, 1999b; see Table XIX-9.1B for other functional neuroimaging studies in PTSD).

Semple *et al.* (1993) using an auditory continuous performance test (CPT) and word generation task with PET, reported increased rCBF in the orbitofrontal cortex in six veterans with combat PTSD and substance abuse (vs seven healthy controls). Using a Yohimbine challenge PET study Bremner *et al.* (1997b), reported increased anxiety and panic symptoms and widespread decreased rCBF in 10 combat vets with PTSD (vs 10 healthy controls). Rauch *et al.* (2000), probing amygdala function using fearful and happy faces masked by neutral faces, found greater amygdala activity in the PTSD subjects (vs controls) to masked fearful faces. In this study, the magnitude of amygdala activation correlating with PTSD severity.

Thus some of these studies provide positive evidence for the amygdalocentric hypothesis in the genesis/maintenance of PTSD symptoms. Neuroimaging advances provide an attractive method of testing hypotheses regarding other brain structures in PTSD.

PANIC DISORDER (PD)

PD is one of the most extensively studied of the anxiety disorders, in part due to occurrence of discrete characteristic symptoms, familial segregation, response to specific pharmacological agents and demonstration of the panicogenic effects of specific agents. PD is characterized by mostly spontaneous discrete attacks of terrifying anxiety with cognitive, affective and autonomic hyperarousal. In between attacks, the patient often experiences significant anxious apprehension, in anticipation of the next attack. Contextual avoidance completes the picture and contributes to most of the disability. A comprehensive theory of PD should explain the genesis of spontaneous recurrent panic attacks and associated symptom states such as anticipatory anxiety, agoraphobia and avoidance behaviour.

Panic disorder could be viewed as a result of a normal threat-related system being repeatedly inappropriately triggered/governed by a dysfunctional threat detection system, or a threat response system gone awry, responding excessively to minor or innocuous stimuli. An attractive hypothesis of the genesis of spontaneous panic attacks, is the possibility of subconscious processing of threat-related stimuli by a hyperresponsive amygdalar system, resulting in a full blown panic attack. There is evidence in healthy subjects for amygdalar recruitment while viewing fear-related stimuli (Whalen *et al.*, 1998) and hyperresponsivity to masked fearful stimuli has been demonstrated in subjects with PTSD (Rauch *et al.*, 2000). According to this model, one of the major processes in PD may be hyperresponsivity of the amygdala circuitry to environmental cues processed without consciousness, resulting in the characteristic panic response without an apparent context (Rauch and Shin, 2002). This remains to be demonstrated in panic disorder.

Phenomenological similarities between panic symptoms and fear-conditioned responses in animals have drawn attention to analogous brain pathways in humans. A deficit in the relay and coordination of upstream (cortical) and downstream (brainstem) sensory information is hypothesized in PD (Gorman *et al.*, 2000). This may result in a hypersensitive amygdalar network, which could inappropriately trigger the brainstem and hypothalamic autonomic and stress neuroendocrine centres causing the characteristic acute panic symptoms (akin to the fear-conditioned response in rats). Cognitive misattribution and contextual fear may result from the involvement of the OFC and hippocampus respectively. The therapeutic effects of serotonergic medications may be explained by their general transmission damping effect in the subcortical and brain stem areas while cognitive therapies may work by enhancing the top-down control of the OFC over the amygdala and related subcortical structures (Gorman *et al.*, 1989, 2000).

Neuroimaging research in subjects with PD has employed diverse modalities. In one qualitative MRI study, the frequency of gross structural abnormalities has been reported to be greater in the PD group (40%) than in the control group (10%; Fontaine *et al.*, 1990; see Table XIX-9.2A). Resting state neuroimaging studies in patients with PD (including those vulnerable to lactate-induced panic), have suggested abnormal hippocampal activity (Reiman *et al.*, 1986; and Table XIX-9.2B), One group has reported post clomipramine treatment normalization of abnormally low left/right asymmetry in hippocampal activity in subjects with PD (Nordahl *et al.*, 1990, 1998). Symptom provocation studies (with pharmacological challenges) have revealed reduced activity in widespread cortical regions, including the prefrontal cortex, during symptomatic states (Reiman *et al.*, 1989; and Table XIX-9.2C). Magnetic resonance spectroscopy studies have reported greater brain lactate levels in response to hyperventilation and lactate infusions (Dager *et al.*, 1995, 1999).

Table XIX-9.2A Structural neuroimaging studies in panic disorder

Authors	Subjects	Methods	Findings
Fontaine *et al.*, 1990	31 patients with PD vs 20 matched controls	Qualitative MRI study	Frequency of gross structural abnormalities: PD group (40%) > control group (10%).
Vythilingam *et al.*, 2000	13 with PD vs 14 control subjects	Quantitative volumetric methods	Sig. smaller mean vols. of L and R-temporal lobes in PD vs controls (normal hippo. volumes).

Table XIX-9.2B Functional neuroimaging studies in panic disorder (PD)

Authors	Subjects	Methods	Findings
Reiman *et al.*, 1986	16 patients with PD and 25 controls	PET-Neutral state study	In patients vulnerable to lactate-induced panic ($N = 8$), abnormally low left/right ratios of parahippo. blood flow.
DeCristofaro *et al.*, 1993	7 treatment-naive with PD vs 5 age-matched controls	SPECT-rCBF at rest	PD (vs control) group showed ↑ rCBF in L-occipital cortex, and ↓ rCBF in the B/L-hippo. areas.
Nordahl *et al.*, 1990	12 PD patients vs 30 controls	PET-FDG while engaged in an auditory CPT	PD group exhibited a lower left/right hippo. rCMRGlu ratio.
Nordahl *et al.*, 1998	IMI-treated subjects with panic disorder	PET-FDG Follow-up study (1990): same methods	R-shift in rCMRglu symmetry within hippo. and post. inf. frontal cortex. IMI-treated group showed ↓ rCMRglu in post. OFC.
Bisaga *et al.*, 1998	6 F with PD and 6 matched controls	PET-FDG	PD subjects showed ↓ rCMRglu in the L-hippo. and parahippo. area.

Table XIX-9.2C Symptom provocation studies in panic disorder

Authors	Subjects	Methods	Findings
Stewart *et al.*, 1988	10 with PD vs 5 controls	SPECT-xenon inhalation r CBF during lactate infusion	PD subjects who had lactate-induced panic attacks ($n = 6$) displayed global cortical CBF ↓.
Woods *et al.*, 1988	6 patients with PD vs 6 controls	SPECT-Yohimbine (Y) infusions	PD group: Y administration increased anxiety and decreased rCBF in bilateral frontal cortex.
Reiman *et al.*, 1989	17 patients with PD vs 15 controls	PET-rCBF during lactate infusions	Patients who had lactate-induced panic ($n = 8$) had ↑ rCBF in B/L temporopolar cortex and B/L insula/claustrum/putamen. Controls and PD patients without lactate-induced panic did not display these changes.
Fischer *et al.*, 1998	Case report	Spontaneous panic attack	↓ rCBF R-orbitofrontal, prelimbic (area 25) ant. cingulate, and ant. temp. cortex.

Consistent with prevailing neurobiological models of PD, it is possible that fundamental abnormalities in monoaminergic neurotransmitter systems, originating in the brain stem, underlie the abnormalities of metabolism, haemodynamics, and chemistry found in widespread territories of cortex. Further, regional abnormalities within the medial temporal lobes provide some support for theories regarding hippocampal or amygdala dysfunction in PD.

OBSESSIVE COMPULSIVE DISORDER (OCD)

The cardinal manifestations of OCD are recurrent, intrusive, egodystonic thoughts, images and urges portending adverse consequences leading to feelings of anxious dread. Patients therefore engage in mental and motor compulsions (repetitive ritualized thoughts or acts) in an attempt to 'neutralize' the obsession/adverse consequence. They often spend many hours a day engaged in these symptoms, leading to significant distress and potential disability. OCD is considered a group of heterogeneous neuropsychiatric disorders. Characteristic neuropsychological dysfunction on tests of organizational strategy and memory, purportedly subserved by the OFC, has been described in OCD patients (Savage *et al.*, 2000). This may explain symptoms of doubt as well as cognitive inflexibility especially related to risk assessment often seen in OCD.

Current animal models are unsatisfactory and have proved of limited value in elucidating OCD pathophysiology. Much of our understanding of functional neuroanatomy implicated in OCD comes from neuroimaging evidence (Rauch and Baxter, 1998). The results of several morphometric MRI (mMRI) studies done in OCD have suggested abnormalities in the volume of the caudate nucleus, though findings between studies have been inconsistent (Scarone *et al.*, 1992; see Table XIX-9.3A for mMRI studies in OCD). Neutral state PET and SPECT paradigms have most consistently reported increased activity in the OFC and ACC areas in OCD subjects versus controls (Baxter *et al.*, 1988; Swedo *et al.*, 1989; see Table XIX-9.3B for other neutral state studies in OCD). Importantly, pre/post treatment studies have reported a treatment-related decrease of activity in the OFC, ACC and CN, regardless of treatment modality (i.e. both for pharmacotherapy with serotonergic reuptake inhibitors, and cognitive behaviour therapy) (e.g. Baxter *et al.*, 1992; Schwartz *et al.*, 1996; and Table XIX-9.3B). Studies designed to investigate predictors of treatment response have yielded impressively consistent results: lower activity within OFC at the pretreatment time point is associated with a positive response to treatment with SRIs while higher left OFC activity predicted a better response in the behavioural therapy responders (Swedo *et al.*, 1989; Brody *et al.*, 1998; Saxena *et al.*, 1999). PET and fMRI symptom provocation studies have shown increased activity in the anterior/lateral OFC, ACC and CN during the provoked state (Rauch *et al.*, 1994; Breiter *et al.*, 1996b). More recently investigators have used neurocognitive probes to study brain areas implicated in OCD. One such task used is the serial reaction task, which leads to implicit or procedural learning demonstrated by shortening reaction times without the subjects' conscious knowledge. Implicit/procedural learning has been shown to be subserved by the striatum, while the medial temporal lobes have been demonstrated to be preferentially involved in explicit or conscious learning. Rauch *et al.* (1997) in a PET study of implicit sequence learning, reported failure of OCD subjects to normally recruit striatum like healthy controls, instead recruiting the medial temporal lobes typically associated with explicit processing (see Table XIX-9.3B for summary of the various functional studies in OCD).

On the basis of evidence from neuropsychiatric disorders effecting the basal ganglia, together with brain imaging data, contemporary models of OCD focus on medial orbitofrontal-striatal-thalamo-cortical circuits (Rauch and Baxter, 1998). According to this scheme striatal dysfunction leads to inefficient thalamic gating, resulting in hyperactivity within the OFC and cingulate cortex. This could result in the intrusive cognitive phenomena and the associated anxiety. Extending this line of thought, compulsions could be conceptualized as repetitive mental and motor behaviours performed to recruit the striatum so as to ultimately achieve thalamic gating (ultimately transiently neutralizing the anxiety and thoughts; Rauch and Shin, 2002).

OCD also provides a more direct approach to investigating functional neuroanatomy, through study of patients undergoing specific neurosurgical lesions for refractory OCD. Rauch *et al.*, (2001) reported a hypermetabolic focus in the posterior cingulate (PET-FDG) to predict better response in refractory OCD patients undergoing stereotactic MRI guided cingulotomy. Ongoing Deep Brain Stimulation studies in OCD (Greenberg, personal communication), involving indwelling electrodes in the anterior limb of the internal capsule, may yield crucial functional neuroanatomic information.

SOCIAL PHOBIA (SoP) AND SPECIFIC PHOBIAS (SpP)

The phobic syndromes involve an excessive, irrational fear of relatively innocuous and usually non-threatening stimuli. Two subtypes of social phobia (also known as social anxiety disorder) are generally recognized, namely, the generalized type and performance-related type. In the generalized subtype, patients experience excessive and irrational fear of negative social scrutiny in most unfamiliar social situations. In the performance subtype the

Table XIX-9.3A Structural neuroimaging studies in OCD

Authors	Subjects	Methods	Findings
Scarone *et al.*, 1992	20 patients with OCD (mixed gender) vs 16 matched controls	MRI morphometry	↑ right caudate volume in OCD group.
Robinson *et al.*, 1995	26 patients with OCD (mixed gender) vs 26 matched controls	MRI morphometry	B/L ↓ caudate volumes in the OCD group.
Jenike *et al.*, 1996	10 F patients with OCD vs matched controls	MRI morphometry	Trends toward a R-shift in caudate volume ($p = 0.06$) as well as overall ↓ caudate volume ($p = 0.10$) in OCD group.
Aylward *et al.*, 1996	24 patients with OCD (mixed gender) vs 21 matched controls	MRI morphometry	No significant differences in striatal volumes.
Rosenberg *et al.*, 1997	19 treatment-naive children with OCD vs 19 matched controls	MRI morphometry	↓ striatal volumes in the OCD group, and inverse correlation between striatal volume and OCD symptom severity.

Table XIX-9.3B Functional neuroimaging studies in OCD

Authors	Subjects	Methods	Findings
Neutral State			
Baxter *et al.*, 1987	14 OCD vs 14 controls and 14 MDD	PET-FDG	OCD: metabolic rates were significantly ↓ in the L-orbital gyrus and B/L in the caudate nuclei. ↑ C/H ratio B/L in treatment responders.
Baxter *et al.*, 1988	10 OCD vs 10 age and sex matched controls	PET-FDG	↑ rCMRGlu in whole cerebral hemispheres, heads of caudate, OG and O/H ratio similar to previous study.
Machlin *et al.*, 1991	10 OCD vs 8 controls	SPECT	OCD group had higher medial-frontal/whole cortex ratio, negatively correlated with anxiety.
Nordahl *et al.*, 1989	8 OCD vs 30 controls	PET-FDG	Higher norm. rCMRGlu in R-OFC and L-ant. OFC in OCD vs controls.
Rubin *et al.*, 1992	10 OCD (adult males) vs 10 age-matched controls	SPECT Xe-133 rCBF and 99mTc-HMPAO	No difference in rCBF with Xe-133. OCD group had ↑ 99mTc uptake in B/L parietal and OFC and L-posterofrontal regions.
Swedo *et al.*, 1989	18 adults with OCD (childhood onset) vs matched controls	PET-FDG	OCD group had ↑ rCMRglu in the L-OF, R-sensorimotor, and B/L prefrontal and ACC. Significant correlation between CMRGlu and OCD severity.
Pre/post Rx			
Baxter *et al.*, 1992		PET-FDG	R-C/H ratio significantly ↓ post Rx (Fluoxetine and CBT).
Benkelfat *et al.*, 1990	8 OCD subjects before and on CMI	PET-rCMRGlu	Significant ↓ in L-caudate rCMRglu in responders vs non responders.
Hoehn-Saric *et al.*, 1991	6 drug free OCD subjects before and during fluoxetine	SPECT	Rx. significantly ↓. symptoms and associated with ↓ medial-frontal/whole brain ratio.
Perani *et al.*, 1995	11 OCD subjects before and after SSRI; 15 age-matched controls	PET [18F]FDG	rCMRGlu significantly ↑ in CC, thalamus and basal ganglia. Post Rx YBOCS improvements associated with B/L ↓ rCMRGlu in CC.
Schwartz *et al.*, 1996	9 OCD before and after 10 weeks of ERP	PET-rCMRGlu	Significant ↓ in B/L-caudate rCMRGlu in ERP responders.
Swedo *et al.*, 1992	Repeat scans in 13 OCD subjects (10 on meds. at least ×1 year)	PET-FDG	Significant ↓ in norm. rCMRGlu in B/L-OF areas. R-OFC rCMRGlu partially correlated with symptom improvement.
Predictors of response			
Brody *et al.*, 1998	27 OCD Before and after 10 ± 2 wks. of BT ($n = 18$) or fluoxetine (F) ($n = 9$)	PET-FDG	↑ norm. rCMRGlu in L-OFC predicted better treatment response in BT group but worse outcome in F group.
Saxena *et al.*, 1999	20 OCD before and after 8–12 weeks of paroxetine (P) 40 mg per day^{-1}	PET-FDG	Paroxetine responders had significant ↓ in rCMRGlu in R-ant. Lat. OFC and caudate. Lower B/L-OFC rCMRglu predicted better improvement in OCD Sx.
Swedo *et al.*, 1989	18 adults with OCD (child onset) and matched controls	PET-FDG	OCD group had ↑ rCMRglu in L-OF, R-SM, and B/L PF and ACC. Significant correlation between rCMRGlu and OCD severity.
Symptom provocation			
McGuire *et al.*, 1994	4 OCD patients	PET H2 15 O	Significant correlation between Sx. severity and rCBF in R-IFG, caudate, parietal, globus pallidus and thalamus and L-hippo and PCG. Also neg. correlation in R-sup. PFC and T/P junction.
Rauch *et al.*, 1994	8 OCD	PET O 15 CO_2 rest and provoked	Sig. ↑ in rCBF during OCD state vs rest in R-caudate, B/L-OFC and L-ACC.
Breiter *et al.*, 1996b	10 OCD and 5 controls	fMRI/control and provoked	Most OCD subjects showed activations in OFC, ACC, insula, caudate and amygdala.
Cognitive activation			
Rauch *et al.*, 1997	OCD vs normal	PET-FDG: Serial Reaction Time task	Both groups showed implicit learning. However OCD group recruited B/L medial temporal areas rather than ventral striatum (seen in controls).

R = Right, L = Left, B/L = Bilateral, M = Male, F = Female, OFC = orbitofrontal cortex, mPFC = medial prefrontal cortex, OG = orbital gyri, O/H = orbital/hemispheric ratio, PCG = posterior cingulate gyrus, T/P = Temporo-parietal, C/H = caudate/hemispheric ratio, ACC = anterior cingulate cortex, Hippo. = hippocampus, PET = Positron Emission Tomography, fMRI = functional Magnetic Resonance Imaging, SPECT = Single Photon Emission Computed Tomography, rCBF = regional cerebral blood flow, rCMRglu = regional cerebral metabolic rate (glucose), Norm. rCMRglu = Normalized regional cerebral metabolic rate (glucose).

phobic symptoms are circumscribed around performance in specific social situations such as public speaking. In specific phobias, the feared object could be animate or inanimate (APA, 1994). Symptoms of anticipatory anxious apprehension, anxiety and panic symptoms and avoidance of triggering situations are common to both disorders. The subtype of blood injury phobia, differs in part from the other phobias, due to a vasovagal syncopal response to blood exposure (Marks, 1988).

Currently, there are no cohesive functional neuroanatomically based models for the phobias (Stein, 1998). Phobias could be viewed as learned aversive responses to specific stimuli or situations, resembling fear conditioning in animals. From a

Table XIX-9.4A Neuroimaging studies in social phobia (SoP)

Authors	Subjects	Methods	Findings
Potts *et al.*, 1994	22 SoP subjects and 22 matched controls	MRI morphometry: Total cerebral, caudate, putaminal and thalamic volumes	The groups did not significantly differ on any of these measures.
Stein *et al.*, 1996	SoP subjects and healthy controls	SPECT-study Neutral state	No significant between-group differences in rCBF.
Birbaumer *et al.*, 1998	7 SoP subjects and 5 controls	fMRI: exposure to neutral human faces or aversive odours	Compared to controls, the SoP group exhibited human face specific amygdalar hyperresponsivity.
Schneider *et al.*, 1999	12 SoP subjects and 12 controls	fMRI classical conditioning paradigm: neutral faces (CS) paired with negative odour and odourless air (US) s	In response to conditioned stimuli associated with the negative odour, the SoP group displayed signal ↑ within amygdala and hippo., whereas controls displayed signal ↓ in these regions.

Table XIX-9.4B Neuroimaging studies in specific phobias (SpP)

Authors	Subjects	Methods	Findings
Mountz *et al.*, 1989	7 small-animal phobics vs 8 controls	PET	Phobics exhibited increased HR, RR and subjective anxiety during exposure to phobic stimuli. No changes in rCBF measurements were observed.
Wik *et al.*, 1993	6 patients with snake phobias	PET exposure to neutral, generally aversive, and snake-related scenes (videotapes)	Phobic condition was associated with significantly ↑ rCBF in secondary visual cortex and ↓ rCBF in prefrontal, post. cingulate and ant. temporopolar cortex, and hippocampus.
Rauch *et al.*, 1995	7 subjects with a variety of small-animal phobias	PET *in vivo* exposure	Provoked vs control condition: ↑ rCBF within multiple ant. paralimbic territories (R-ant. cingulate, R-ant. temporal pole, L-post. orbitofrontal and L-insular cortex), L-somatosensory cortex, and L-thalamus.

neuroanatomical perspective, phobias could represent the product of dysregulated threat detection systems for detecting potentially threatening stimuli or situations. Ongoing studies are actively investigating such hypotheses (Rauch and Shin, 2002).

More recently, contribution from animal research on attachment and affiliative behaviour, social subordination stress and environmental rearing have provided a partial yet useful framework to investigate social phobia (for reviews see Stein, 1998; Mathew, Coplan and Gorman, 2001). Surprisingly few neuroimaging studies exist in this area (see Table XIX-9.4A). In the only morphometric study published to date, Potts *et al.* (1994) compared the total cerebral, caudate, putaminal and thalamic volumes in 22 subjects with SoP vs 22 matched controls and found no differences. More recently Birbaumer *et al.* (1998), used fMRI to study seven SoP subjects and five healthy controls while they were exposed to slides of neutral human faces or aversive odours. The SoP group showed human face specific amygdalar hyperresponsivity compared to the control group. In another fMRI study, Schneider *et al.* (1999) presented 12 subjects with SoP and 12 healthy controls with paired conditioned (CS; neutral facial expressions) and unconditioned stimuli (US; negative odour vs unmanipulated air). The SoP group showed signal increases within the amygdalar and hippocampal in response to the CS paired with the negative odour while controls showed signal decreases in these regions. These findings, while in need of replication, suggest that hyperresponsivity of the medial temporal lobes may be one of the candidate neural substrates for SoP.

It is appealing to try to understand specific phobias from the viewpoint of conditioned fear studies in animals. This is supported by the fact that behavioural therapy for the phobias involving exposure and desensitization (akin to 'extinction') has been used to effectively treat many patients. While this perspective clearly does not explain aetiology or pathophysiology, the resemblance of components of these disorders to animal fear conditioning should trigger a closer look at analogous brain circuits. In a PET-symptom provocation study, Rauch *et al.* (1995) reported increased activity in prefrontal, posterior cingulate, anterior temporopolar, hippocampal and secondary visual areas as well as in multiple anterior paralimbic territories in seven subjects with small-animal phobias. These findings may reflect a hypersensitive threat detection and response network (therefore triggered by relatively innocuous stimuli). However, as is evident in Table XIX-9.4B, the few symptom provocation studies in SpP report inconsistent findings and are hard to meaningfully interpret. More work is clearly needed in this area.

GENERALIZED ANXIETY DISORDER (GAD)

GAD is, in some sense, the prototypical anxiety disorder. Patients usually have pervasive anxiety symptoms pertaining to, but not confined to, two or more life areas for at least a 6 month period. However, 'free-floating' anxiety and pervasive anxious dread is harder to characterize objectively. Perhaps consequently, genetic evidence and biological evidence in GAD is less compelling.

Rodent experiments involving the fear potentiated acoustic startle response (fear-like; conditioning dependent, shows 'extinction') vs the light-enhanced startle response (anxiety-like; unconditioned, slow onset and rate of decay, reduced by anxiolytics) show that these processes are subserved by different neural systems. Based on these findings, it is hypothesized that the bed nucleus of the stria terminalis (BNST) may subserve the anxiety-like phenomena, while the CeA subserves fear phenomena and may not contribute directly to anxiety. Stress (fear)-induced phasic release of CRH by the neurons in the CeA may lead to long-term activation of the BNST (Davis, 1998). Thus by extension, hypersensitivity of the BNST pathway may be manifested by a state of chronic generalized anxiety with generalization to many innocuous stimuli (internal and external). This remains to be tested in humans with GAD. Neuroimaging evidence is scant and preliminary at this stage. In a recent MRI volumetric study in 12 children with GAD (compared with 24 matched controls), De Bellis *et al.* (2000) reported that the right and total amygdala volumes were significantly larger in those with GAD, all other volumes not differing significantly. The implications of these findings are currently unclear.

Thus no coherent neurocircuitry model exists currently for GAD. Chronic hyperactivity of the danger assessment and response circuits may underlie GAD. However, it is not known if this may be common to all anxiety disorders or could be a process specifically related to GAD.

DISCUSSION AND FUTURE DIRECTIONS

Anxiety disorders are common and are associated with considerable comorbidity (Regier *et al.*, 1998). A better understanding of the neural mechanisms of adaptive as well as pathological anxiety and fear promises to enhance the development of more effective preventive and therapeutic strategies. Advances in animal fear research provide a springboard to related research in humans. The advent of sophisticated neuroimaging techniques promises to accelerate progress in this field, by providing a means for probing human functional anatomy non-invasively.

Based on animal research, the subnuclei of the amygdala have emerged as the central component of the early, rapid processing of danger-related stimuli. The rich connections between the subnuclei of the amygdala and the sensory thalamus, the orbitofrontal and sensory cortices, the hypothalamus and brainstem areas as well as the striatum have been shown to subserve the various characteristic components of the fear response. The amygdala is a crucial component in stimulus-reinforcer association learning and possible modulation of other relevant brain areas. The cellular and molecular basis of fear conditioning and emotional learning and memory are being vigorously investigated. Of specific interest are the processes of plasticity, kindling, LTP and at a cellular level, NMDA receptor and voltage gated calcium channel mediated signal transduction (LeDoux, 2000b).

In healthy human volunteers, induced transient states of anxiety and fear are associated with increased activity in anterior paralimbic regions and decreased activity in heteromodal association cortex (Rauch and Shin, 2002). These findings are in need of further refinement given that other experimentally induced emotions (such as anger and guilt) also activate overlapping pathways (Dougherty *et al.*, 1999; Shin *et al.*, 2000). The processes of habituation and extinction of fear responses, explored via novel functional neuroimaging paradigms, are relevant to the understanding of normal and pathological anxiety, as well as therapies that rely on desensitization.

Functional neuroimaging studies, combined with specific human brain lesions, implicate the amygdala and associated structures in the innate processing of fear-related faces. The medial frontal and OFC are implicated in the top-down governance of the amygdala and related structures. The anterior cingulate cortex is important in attention and choice making, the brain stem nuclei and lateral hypothalamus in the control of the somatic reactions to stress and anxiety, and the striatal regions in mediating automated response routines, as well as influencing gating at the level of the thalamus (Rauch and Shin, 2002). The insular cortex, which has rich connections with the amygdala, is commonly activated in anxiety-related studies. However, most work has implicated the insula in functions related to taste, including the perception of disgust (Phillips *et al.*, 1997, 1998). Its role in fear and anxiety is less clear.

The convergence of different modes and fields of inquiry are enabling growth from simple to more complex models befitting the nature of human anxiety/fear mechanisms. This increased sophistication also reflects an integration of data across scales — from the systems level to the molecular level. In the area of PTSD, evidence from animal fear conditioning and stress research, clinical traumatology as well as innovative neuroimaging paradigms in patients have helped to increase our understanding of the PTSD syndrome. Thus, the amygdala in functional connectivity with the OFC, hippocampus, the hypothalamus as well as brainstem regions, are thought to mediate the characteristic symptoms of the disorder. The contemporary neurocircuitry model of OCD has been derived from the neuropsychiatry of the basal ganglia as well as from neuroimaging studies (Rauch and Savage, 1997; Saxena and Rauch, 2000). Abnormal activity in the orbitofrontal-thalamo-striato-cortical circuits has been shown to normalize with clinical response to both drug and behavioural treatments. With the emergence of deep brain stimulation as an experimental treatment modality for OCD, there is the potential for learning much about the implicated circuitry in human subjects. In PD, panic attacks accompanied by anticipatory anxiety and avoidance suggest involvement of the amygdala, the medial temporal lobes (specifically hippocampus) and functional connections with the OFC and brainstem areas (Gorman *et al.*, 2000). Currently, neurocircuitry models for the phobic disorders and GAD are less coherent, although preliminary, contemporary neurocircuitry models of anxiety disorders facilitate hypothesis-driven research in this domain. While delineating the functional neuroanatomy of psychiatric diseases is extremely important, these neural substrates must be understood in the context of interdigitating environmental influences. The interactions between genetic/temperamental predisposition of individual neural systems with environmental events (e.g. trauma during early neurodevelopment, stressful life events) are important in the development and maintenance of anxiety disorders.

Further research across modes of inquiry and across scales is required to understand the neural substrates of normal relevant brain functions as well as the pathophysiology of anxiety disorders. An integrated approach combining animal studies, molecular biology, genetics, clinical psychiatry, behavioural neurology, cognitive neuroscience, and neuroimaging is essential to make meaningful progress in this field. Ultimately, the hope is for better preventive and therapeutic options to help people who might otherwise suffer from anxiety disorders.

REFERENCES

Adolphs, R., Damasio, H., Tranel, D. and Damasio, A.R., 1996. Cortical systems for the recognition of emotion in facial expressions. *J. Neurosci.*, **16**(23), 7678–7687.

Adolphs, R., Tranel, D., Damasio, H. and Damasio, A., 1994. Impaired recognition of emotion in facial expressions following bilateral damage to the human amygdala. *Nature*, **15**(372), 669–672.

Adolphs, R., Tranel, D., Damasio, H. and Damasio, A.R., 1995. Fear and the human amygdala. *J. Neurosci.*, **15**(9), 5879–5891.

Adolphs, R. and Tranel, D., 1999a. Intact recognition of emotional prosody following amygdala damage. *Neuropsychologia*, **37**(11), 1285–1292.

Adolphs, R., Tranel, D., Hamann, S., Young, A.W., Calder, A.J., Phelps, E.A., Anderson, A., Lee, G.P. and Damasio, A.R., 1999b. Recognition of facial emotion in nine individuals with bilateral amygdala damage. *Neuropsychologia*, **37**(10), 1111–1117.

Adolphs, R. and Tranel, D., 2000. Emotion recognition and the human amygdala. In: Aggleton, J.P. (ed.), *The Amygdala: A Functional Analysis*, second edition, pp. 587–630. Oxford University Press Inc., New York.

American Psychiatric Association, 1994. *Diagnostic and Statistical Manual of Mental Disorders*, fourth edition, pp. 393–444. American Psychiatric Association, Washington DC.

Anderson, A.K. and Phelps, E.A., 1998. Intact recognition of vocal expressions of fear following bilateral lesions of the human amygdala. *Neuroreport*, **9**(16), 3607–3613.

Aylward, E.H., Harris, G.J., Hoehn-Saric, R., Barta, P.E., Machlin, S.R. and Pearlson, G.D., 1996. Normal caudate nucleus in obsessive compulsive disorder assessed by quantitative neuroimaging. *Arch. Gen. Psychiatry*, **53**(7), 577–584.

Baxter, L.R., Jr, Schwartz, J.M., Mazziotta, J.C., Phelps, M.E., Pahl, J.J., Guze, B.H. and Fairbanks, L., 1988. Cerebral glucose metabolic rates in nondepressed patients with obsessive–compulsive disorder. *Am. J. Psychiatry*, **145**, 1560–1563.

Baxter, L.R., Jr, Schwartz, J.M., Bergman, K.S., Szuba, M.P., Guze, B.H., Mazziotta, J.C., Alazraki, A., Selin, C.E., Ferng, H.K., Munford, P. *et al.*, 1992. Caudate glucose metabolic rate changes with both drug and behavior therapy for obsessive–compulsive disorder. *Arch. Gen. Psychiatry*, **49**(9), 681–689.

Baxter, L.R., Jr, Phelps, M.E., Mazziotta, J.C., Guze, B.H., Schwartz, J.M. and Selin, C.E., 1987. Local cerebral glucose metabolic rates in obsessive compulsive disorder: A comparison with rates in unipolar depression and in normal controls. *Arch. Gen. Psychiatry*, **44**(3), 211–218.

Baxter, M.G. and Murray, E.A., 2000. Reinterpreting the behavioral effects of amygdala lesions in non-human primates. In: Aggleton, J.P. (ed.), *The Amygdala. A Functional Analysis*, second edition, pp. 545–568. Oxford University Press, New York.

Bechara, A., Tranel, D., Damasio, H., Adolphs, R., Rockland, C. and Damasio, A.R., 1995. Double dissociation of conditioning and declarative knowledge relative to the amygdala and hippocampus in humans. *Science*, **25**(269), 1115–1118.

Benkelfat, C., Nordahl, T.E., Semple, W.E., King, A.C., Murphy, D.L. and Cohen, R.M., 1990. Local cerebral glucose metabolic rates in obsessive–compulsive disorder. Patients treated with clomipramine. *Arch. Gen. Psychiatry*, **47**(9), 840–848.

Birbaumer, N., Grodd, W., Diedrich, O., Klose, U., Erb, M., Lotze, M., Schneider, F., Weiss, U. and Flor, H., 1998. fMRI reveals amygdala activation to human faces in social phobics. *Neuroreport*, **9**(6), 1223–1226.

Bisaga, A., Katz, J.L., Antonini, A., Wright, C.E., Margouleff, C., Gorman, J.M. and Eidelberg, D., 1998. Cerebral glucose metabolism in women with panic disorder. *Am J Psychiatry*, **155**(9), 1178–1183.

Breiter, H.C., Etcoff, N.L., Whalen, P.J., Kennedy, W.A., Rauch, S.L., Buckner, R.L., Strauss, M.M., Hyman, S.E. and Rosen, B.R., 1996a. Response and habituation of the human amygdala during visual processing of facial expression. *Neuron*, **17**(5), 875–887.

Breiter, H.C., Rauch, S.L., Kwong, K.K., Baker, J.R., Weisskoff, R.M., Kennedy, D.N., Kendrick, A.D., Davis, T.L., Jiang, A., Cohen, M.S., Stern, C.E., Belliveau, J.W., Baer, L., O'Sullivan, R.L., Savage, C.R., Jenike, M.A. and Rosen, B.R., 1996b. Functional magnetic resonance imaging of symptom provocation in obsessive compulsive disorder. *Arch. Gen. Psychiatry*, **53**(7), 595–606.

Bremner, J.D., Innis, R.B., Ng, C.K., Staib, L.H., Salomon, R.M., Bronen, R.A., Duncan, J., Southwick, S.M., Krystal, J.H., Rich, D., Zubal, G., Dey, H., Soufer, R. and Charney, D.S., 1997b. Positron emission tomography measurement of cerebral metabolic correlates of yohimbine administration in combat-related posttraumatic stress disorder. *Arch. Gen. Psychiatry*, **54**(3), 246–254.

Bremner, J.D., Narayan, M., Staib, L.H., Southwick, S.M., McGlashan, T. and Charney, D.S., 1999a. Neural correlates of memories of childhood sexual abuse in women with and without posttraumatic stress disorder. *Am. J. Psychiatry*, **156**, 1787–1795.

Bremner, J.D., Randall, P., Scott, T.M., Bronen, R.A., Seibyl, J.P., Southwick, S.M., Delaney, R.C., McCarthy, G., Charney, D.S. and Innis, R.B., 1995. MRI-based measurement of hippocampal volume in patients with combat-related posttraumatic stress disorder. *Am. J. Psychiatry*, **152**(7), 973–981.

Bremner, J.D., Randall, P., Vermetten, E., Staib, L., Bronen, R.A., Mazure, C., Capelli, S., McCarthy, G., Innis, R.B. and Charney, D.S., 1997a. Magnetic resonance imaging-based measurement of hippocampal volume in posttraumatic stress disorder related to childhood physical and sexual abuse — A preliminary report. *Biol. Psychiatry*, **41**, 23–32.

Bremner, J.D., Staib, L.H., Kaloupek, D., Southwick, S.M., Soufer, R. and Charney, D.S., 1999b. Neural correlates of exposure to traumatic pictures and sound in Vietnam combat veterans with and without posttraumatic stress disorder: a positron emission tomography study. *Biol. Psychiatry*, **45**(7), 806–816.

Brody, A.L., Saxena, S., Schwartz, J.M., Stoessel, P.W., Maidment, K., Phelps, M.E. and Baxter, L.R., Jr, 1998. FDG-PET predictors of response to behavioral therapy versus pharmacotherapy in obsessive–compulsive disorder. *Psychiatry Res.: Neuroimaging*, **84**(1), 1–6.

Broks, P., Young, A.W., Maratos, E.J., Coffey, P.J., Calder, A.J., Isaac, C.L., Mayes, A.R., Hodges, J.R., Montaldi, D., Cezayirli, E., Roberts, N. and Hadley, D., 1998. Face processing impairments after encephalitis: amygdala damage and recognition of fear. *Neuropsychologia*, **36**(1), 59–70.

Brown, E.S., Rush, A.J. and McEwen, B.S., 1999. Hippocampal remodeling and damage by corticosteroids: Implications for mood disorders. *Neuropsychopharm.*, **21**, 474–484.

Büchel, C., Dolan, R.J., Armony, J.L. and Friston, K.J., 1999. Amygdala-hippocampal involvement in human aversive trace conditioning revealed through event-related functional magnetic resonance imaging. *J. Neurosci.*, **19**, 10869–10876.

Büchel, C., Morris, J., Dolan, R.J. and Friston, K.J., 1998. Brain systems mediating aversive conditioning: an event-related fMRI study. *Neuron*, **20**, 947–957.

Calder, A.J., Young, A.W., Rowland, D., Perrett, D.I., Hodges, J.R. and Etcoff, N.L., 1996. Facial emotion recognition after bilateral amygdala damage: Differentially severe impairment of fear. *Cognitive Neuropsychology*, **13**, 699–745.

Chapman, P.F. and Chattarji, S., 2000. Synaptic plasticity in the amygdala. In: Aggleton, J.P. (ed.), *The Amygdala. A Functional Analysis*, second edition, pp. 117–153. Oxford University Press, New York.

Chrousos, G.P. and Gold, P.W., 1998. A healthy body in a healthy mind — and vice versa — the damaging power of "uncontrollable" stress. *J. Clin. Endocrinol. Metab.*, **83**, 1842–1845.

Dager, S.R., Strauss, W.L., Marro, K.I., Richards, T.L., Metzger, G.D. and Artru, A.A., 1995. Proton magnetic resonance spectroscopy investigation of hyperventilation in subjects with panic disorder and comparison subjects. *Am. J. Psychiatry*, **152**(5), 666–672.

Dager, S.R., Friedman, S.D., Heide, A., Layton, M.E., Richards, T., Artru, A., Strauss, W., Hayes, C. and Posse, S., 1999. Two-dimensional proton echo-planar spectroscopic imaging of brain metabolic changes during lactate-induced panic. *Arch. Gen. Psychiatry*, **56**(1), 70–77.

Davis, M., 2000. The role of the amygdala in conditioned and unconditioned fear and anxiety. In: Aggleton, J.P. (ed.), *The Amygdala. A Functional Analysis*, second edition, pp. 213–287. Oxford University Press, New York.

Davis, M., 1998. Are different parts of the extended amygdala involved in fear versus anxiety? *Biol. Psychiatry*, **44**(12), 1239–1247.

Davis, M., 1992. The role of the amygdala in fear and anxiety. *Annu. Rev. Neurosci.*, **15**, 353–375.

De Bellis, M.D., Casey, B.J., Dahl, R.E., Birmaher, B., Williamson, D.E., Thomas, K.M., Axelson, D.A., Frustaci, K., Boring, A.M., Hall, J. and Ryan, N.D., 2000. A pilot study of amygdala volumes in pediatric generalized anxiety disorder. *Biol. Psychiatry*, **48**(1), 51–57.

De Bellis, M.D., Keshavan, M.S., Clark, D.B., Casey, B.J., Giedd, J.N., Boring, A.M., Frustaci, K. and Ryan, N.D., 1999. Developmental traumatology part II: Brain development. *Biol. Psychiatry*, **45**, 1271–1284.

De Cristofaro, M.T., Sessarego, A., Pupi, A., Biondi, F. and Faravelli, C., 1993. Brain perfusion abnormalities in drug-naive, lactate-sensitive panic patients: a SPECT study. *Biol. Psychiatry*, **33**(7), 505–512.

Dougherty, D.D., Shin, L.M., Alpert, N.M. *et al.*, 1999. Anger in healthy men: A PET study using script-driven imagery. *Biol. Psychiatry*, **46**, 466–472.

Dunner, D.L., 2001. Management of anxiety disorders: the added challenge of comorbidity. *Depress Anxiety*, **13**(2), 57–71.

Endo, Y., Nishimura, J.-I., Kobayashi, S. and Kimura, F., 1999. Chronic stress exposure influences local cerebral blood flow in the rat hippocampus. *Neuroscience*, **93**, 551–555.

Feldman, S. and Conforti, N., 1980. Participation of the dorsal hippocampus in the glucocorticoid feedback effect on adrenocortical activity. *Neuroendocrinol.* **30**, 52–55.

Fischer, H., Andersson, J.L., Furmark, T. and Fredrikson, M., 1998. Brain correlates of an unexpected panic attack: a human positron emission tomographic study. *Neurosci. Lett.*, **251**(2), 137–140.

Fischer, H., Furmark, T., Wik, G. and Fredrikson, M., 2000a. Brain representation of habituation to repeated complex visual stimulation studied with PET. *NeuroReport*, **11**, 123–126.

Fischer, H., Wright, C.I., Whalen, P.J., McInerney, S.C., Shin, L.M. and Rauch, S.L., 2000b. Effects of repeated presentations of facial stimuli on human brain function: An fMRI study. *NeuroImage*, **11**, S250.

Fontaine, R., Breton, G., Dery, R., Fontaine, S. and Elie, R., 1990. Temporal lobe abnormalities in panic disorder: an MRI study. *Biol. Psychiatry*, **27**(3), 304–310.

Fyer, A.J., 1998. Current approaches to etiology and pathophysiology of specific phobia. *Biol. Psychiatry*, **44**, 1295–1304.

Gorman, J.M., Kent, J.M., Sullivan, G.M. and Coplan, J.D., 2000. Neuroanatomical hypothesis of panic disorder, revised. *Am. J. Psychiatry*, **157**(4), 493–505.

Gorman, J.M., Liebowitz, M.R., Fyer, A.J. and Stein, J., 1989. A neuroanatomical hypothesis for panic disorder. *Am. J. Psychiatry*, **146**(2), 148–161.

Gould, E. and Tanapat, P., 1999. Stress and hippocampal neurogenesis. *Biol. Psychiatry*, **46**, 1472–1479.

Gurvits, T.V., Shenton, M.E., Hokama, H., Ohta, H., Lasko, N.B., Gilbertson, M.W., Orr, S.P., Kikinis, R., Jolesz, F.A., McCarley, R.W. and Pitman, R.K., 1996. Magnetic resonance imaging study of hippocampal volume in chronic, combat-related posttraumatic stress disorder. *Biol. Psychiatry*, **40**(11), 1091–1099.

Herman, J.P., Schafer, M.K., Young, E.A., Thompson, R., Douglass, J., Akil, H. and Watson, S.J., 1989. Evidence for hippocampal regulation of neuroendocrine neurons of hypothalamo-pituitary-adrenocortical axis. *J. Neurosci.*, **9**, 3072–3082.

Hoehn-Saric, R., Pearlson, G.D., Harris, G.J., Machlin, S.R. and Camargo, E.E., 1991. Effects of fluoxetine on regional cerebral blood flow in obsessive–compulsive patients. *Am. J. Psychiatry*, **148**(9), 1243–1245.

The ICD-10 Classification of Mental and Behavioral Disorders, 1992. Clinical descriptions and diagnostic guidelines. World Health Organization, Geneva.

Jenike, M.A., Breiter, H.C., Baer, L., Kennedy, D.N., Savage, C.R., Olivares, M.J., O'Sullivan, R.L., Shera, D.M., Rauch, S.L., Keuthen, N., Rosen, B.R., Caviness, V.S. and Filipek, P.A., 1996. Cerebral structural abnormalities in obsessive–compulsive disorder: a quantitative morphometric magnetic resonance imaging study. *Arch. Gen. Psychiatry*, **53**(7), 625–632.

Kalin, N.H., Shelton, S.E., Davidson, R.J. and Kelley, A.E., 2001. The primate amygdala mediates acute fear but not the behavioral and physiological components of anxious temperament. *J. Neurosci.*, **21**(6), 2067–2074.

Kapp, B.S., Whalen, P.J., Supple, W.F. and Pascoe, J.P., 1992. Amygdaloid contributions to conditioned arousal and sensory information processing. In: Aggleton, J.P. (ed.), *The Amygdala*, pp. 229–254. Wiley-Liss, New York.

Kluver, H. and Bucy, P.C., 1939. Preliminary analysis of functions of the temporal lobes in monkeys. *Archives of Neurology and Psychiatry*, **42**, 979–1000 (classical article). *Int. J. Neuropsychiatry Clin. Neurosci.* (1997) **9**, 606–620.

LaBar, K.S., Gatenby, C., Gore, J.C., LeDoux, J.E. and Phelps, E.A., 1998. Human amygdala activation during conditioned fear acquisition and extinction: A mixed-trial fMRI study. *Neuron*, **20**, 937–945.

LeDoux, J.E., 2000a. Emotion circuits in the brain. *Annu. Rev. Neurosci.*, **23**, 155–184.

LeDoux, J.E., 2000b. The amygdala and emotion: a view through fear. In: Aggleton, J.P. (ed.), *The Amygdala. A Functional Analysis*, second edition, pp. 289–310. Oxford University Press, New York.

LeDoux, J.E., Iwata, J., Cicchetti, P. and Reis, D.J., 1988. Different projections of the central amygdaloid nucleus mediate autonomic and behavioral correlates of conditioned fear. *J. Neurosci.*, **8**(7), 2517–2529.

Liberzon, I., Taylor, S.F., Amdur, R., Jung, T.D., Chamberlain, K.R., Minoshima, S., Koeppe, R.A. and Fig, L.M., 1999. Brain activation in PTSD in response to trauma-related stimuli. *Biol. Psychiatry*, **45**, 817–826.

Machlin, S.R., Harris, G.J., Pearlson, G.D., Hoehn-Saric, R., Jeffery, P. and Camargo, E.E., 1991. Elevated medial-frontal cerebral blood flow in obsessive–compulsive patients: A SPECT study. *Am. J. Psychiatry*, **148**, 1240–1242.

Maren, S. and Fanselow, M.S., 1995. Synaptic plasticity in the basolateral amygdala induced by hippocampal formation stimulation *in vivo*. *J. Neurosci.*, **15**(11), 7548–7564.

Maren, S. and Fanselow, M.S., 1996. The amygdala and fear conditioning: has the nut been cracked? *Neuron*, **16**(2), 237–240.

Marks, I., 1988. Blood-injury phobia: a review. *Am. J. Psychiatry*, **145**(10), 1207–1213.

Mathew, S.J., Coplan, J.D. and Gorman, J.M., 2001. Neurobiological mechanisms of social anxiety disorder. *Am. J. Psychiatry*, **158**(10), 1558–1567.

McGuire, P.K., Bench, C.J., Frith, C.D., Marks, I.M., Frackowiak, R.S. and Dolan, R.J., 1994. Functional anatomy of obsessive–compulsive phenomena. *Br. J. Psychiatry*, **164**, 459–468.

Monroe, S.M., Harkness, K., Simons, A.D. and Thase, M.E., 2001. Life stress and the symptoms of major depression. *J. Nerv. Ment. Dis.*, **189**(3), 168–175.

Morgan, M.A. and LeDoux, J.E., 1995. Differential contribution of dorsal and ventral medial prefrontal cortex to the acquisition and extinction of conditioned fear in rats. *Behav. Neurosci.*, **109**(4), 681–688.

Morgan, M.A., Romanski, L.M. and LeDoux, J.E., 1993. Extinction of emotional learning: contribution of medial prefrontal cortex. *Neurosci. Lett.*, **163**, 109–113.

Morris, J.S., Friston, K.J., Buchel, C., Frith, C.D., Young, A.W., Calder, A.J. and Dolan, R.J., 1998a. A neuromodulatory role for the human amygdala in processing emotional facial expressions. *Brain*, **121**(1), 47–57.

Morris, J.S., Friston, K.J. and Dolan, R.J., 1997. Neural responses to salient visual stimuli. *Proc. R. Soc. Lond. B.*, **264**, 769–775.

Morris, J.S., Frith, C.D., Perrett, D.I., Rowland, D., Young, A.W., Calder, A.J. and Dolan, R.J., 1996. A differential neural response in the human amygdala to fearful and happy facial expressions. *Nature*, **383**(6603), 812–815.

Morris, J.S., Öhman, A. and Dolan, R.J., 1998b. Conscious and unconscious emotional learning in the human amygdala. *Nature*, **393**, 467–470.

Morris, J.S., Ohman, A. and Dolan, R.J., 1999. A subcortical pathway to the right amygdala mediating "unseen" fear. *Proc. Natl. Acad. Sci. USA*, **96**(4), 1680–1685.

Mountz, J.M., Modell, J.G., Wilson, M.W., Curtis, G.C., Lee, M.A., Schmaltz, S. and Kuhl, D.E., 1989. Positron emission tomographic evaluation of cerebral blood flow during state anxiety in simple phobia. *Arch. Gen. Psychiatry*, **46**, 501–504.

Newport, D.J. and Nemeroff, C.B., 2000. Neurobiology of posttraumatic stress disorder. *Curr. Opin. Neurobiol.*, **10**(2), 211–218.

Nitschke, J.B., Heller, W. and Miller, G.A., 2000. Anxiety, stress, and cortical brain function. In: Borod, J.C. (ed.), *The Neuropsychology of Emotion*, Series in Affective Science, pp. 298–319. Oxford University Press, New York.

Nordahl, T.E., Benkelfat, C., Semple, W.E., Gross, M., King, A.C. and Cohen, R.M., 1989. Cerebral glucose metabolic rates in obsessive–compulsive disorder. *Neuropsychopharmacology*, **2**, 23–28.

Nordahl, T.E., Semple, W.E., Gross, M., Mellman, T.A., Stein, M.B., Goyer, P., King, A.C., Uhde, T.W. and Cohen, R.M., 1990. Cerebral glucose metabolic differences in patients with panic disorder. *Neuropsychopharmacology*, **3**(4), 261–272.

Nordahl, T.E., Stein, M.B., Benkelfat, C., Semple, W.E., Andreason, P., Zametkin, A., Uhde, T.W. and Cohen, R.M., 1998. Regional cerebral metabolic asymmetries replicated in an independent group of patients with panic disorders. *Biol. Psychiatry*, **44**(10), 998–1006.

O'Connor, C.M., Gurbel, P.A. and Serebruany, V.L., 2000. Depression and ischemic heart disease. *Am. Heart J.*, **140**(4 Suppl), 63–69.

Simpson, J. and Weiner, E. (eds), 1989. *The Oxford English Dictionary*, second edition. The Oxford University Press, Oxford, UK.

Perani, D., Colombo, C., Bressi, S., Bonfanti, A., Grassi, F., Scarone, S., Bellodi, L., Smeraldi, E. and Fazio, F., 1995. FDG PET study in obsessive–compulsive disorder: A clinical metabolic correlation study after treatment. *Br. J. Psychiatry*, **166**, 244–250.

Phillips, M.L., Young, A.W., Senior, C., Brammer, M., Andrew, C., Calder, A.J., Bullmore, E.T., Perrett, D.I., Rowland, D., Williams, S.C., Gray, J.A. and David, A.S., 1997. A specific neural substrate for perceiving facial expressions of disgust. *Nature*, **389**(6650), 495–498.

Phillips, M.L., Young, A.W., Scott, S.K., Calder, A.J., Andrew, C., Giampietro, V., Williams, S.C., Bullmore, E.T., Brammer, M. and Gray, J.A., 1998. Neural responses to facial and vocal expressions of fear and disgust. *Proc. R. Soc. Lond. B. Biol. Sci.*, **265**(1408), 1809–1817.

Pitman, R.K., 2001. Hippocampal diminution in PTSD: more (or less?) than meets the eye. *Hippocampus*, **11**(2), 73–74.

Potts, N.L., Davidson, J.R., Krishnan, K.R. and Doraiswamy, P.M., 1994. Magnetic resonance imaging in social phobia. *Psychiatry Res.*, **52**(1), 35–42.

Rauch, S.L., Dougherty, D.D., Cosgrove, G.R., Cassem, E.H., Alpert, N.M., Price, B.H., Nierenberg, A.A., Mayberg, H.S., Baer, L., Jenike, M.A. and Fischman, A.J., 2001. Cerebral metabolic correlates as potential predictors of response to anterior cingulotomy for obsessive compulsive disorder. *Biol. Psychiatry*, **50**(9), 659–667.

Rauch, S.L. and Shin, L.M., 2002. Structural and functional imaging of anxiety and stress disorders. In: Davis, K., Charney, D., Coyle, J.T. and Nemeroff, C. (eds), *Neuropsychopharmacology: The Fifth Generation of Progress*, pp. 953–966. Lippincott Williams and Wilkins, New York.

Rauch, S.L. and Baxter, L.R., Jr, 1998. Neuroimaging in obsessive–compulsive disorder and related disorders. In: Jenike, M.A., Baer, L. and Minichiello, W.E. (eds), *Obsessive–Compulsive Disorders Practical Management*, 3rd edition, pp. 289–317. St. Louis, Mosby.

Rauch, S.L., Jenike, M.A., Alpert, N.M., Baer, L., Breiter, H.C., Savage, C.R. and Fischman, A.J., 1994. Regional cerebral blood flow measured during symptom provocation in obsessive–compulsive disorder using ^{15}O-labeled CO_2 and positron emission tomography. *Arch. Gen. Psychiatry*, **51**(1), 62–70.

Rauch, S.L., Savage, C.R., Alpert, N.M., Dougherty, D., Kendrick, A., Curran, T., Brown, H.D., Manzo, P., Fischman, A.J. and Jenike, M.A., 1997. Probing striatal function in obsessive compulsive disorder: A PET study of implicit sequence learning. *J. Neuropsychiatry Clin. Neurosci.*, **9**(4), 568–573.

Rauch, S.L., Savage, C.R., Alpert, N.M., Miguel, E.C., Baer, L., Breiter, H.C., Fischman, A.J., Manzo, P.A., Moretti, C. and Jenike, M.A., 1995. A positron emission tomographic study of simple phobic symptom provocation. *Arch. Gen. Psychiatry*, **52**(1), 20–28.

Rauch, S.L. and Savage, C.R., 1997. Neuroimaging and neuropsychology of the striatum. Bridging basic science and clinical practice. *Psychiatr. Clin. North Am.*, **20**(4), 741–768.

Rauch, S.L., van der Kolk, B.A., Fisler, R.E., Alpert, N.M., Orr, S.P., Savage, C.R., Fischman, A.J., Jenike, M.A. and Pitman, R.K., 1996. A symptom provocation study of posttraumatic stress disorder using positron emission tomography and script-driven imagery. *Arch. Gen. Psychiatry*, **53**(5), 380–387.

Rauch, S.L., Whalen, P.J., Shin, L.M., McInerney, S.C., Macklin, M.L., Lasko, N.B., Orr, S.P. and Pitman, R.K., 2000. Exaggerated amygdala response to masked fearful vs. happy facial stimuli in post-traumatic stress disorder: A functional MRI study. *Biol. Psychiatry*, **47**, 769–776.

Regier, D.A., Rae, D.S., Narrow, W.E., Kaelber, C.T. and Schatzberg, A.F., 1998. Prevalence of anxiety disorders and their comorbidity with mood and addictive disorders. *Br. J. Psychiatry Suppl.*, **34**, 24–28.

Reiman, E.M., Raichle, M.E., Robins, E., Mintun, M.A., Fusselman, M.J., Fox, P.T., Price, J.L. and Hackman, K.A., 1989. Neuroanatomical correlates of a lactate-induced anxiety attack. *Arch. Gen. Psychiatry*, **46**(6), 493–500.

Reiman, E.M., Raichle, M.E., Robins, E., Butler, F.K., Herscovitch, P., Fox, P. and Perlmutter, J., 1986. The application of positron emission tomography to the study of panic disorder. *Am. J. Psychiatry*, **143**(4), 469–477.

Robinson, D., Wu, H., Munne, R.A., Ashtari, M., Alvir, J.M., Lerner, G., Koreen, A., Cole, K. and Bogerts, B., 1995. Reduced caudate nucleus volume in obsessive–compulsive disorder. *Arch. Gen. Psychiatry*, **52**(5), 393–398.

Rolls, E.T., 1999. *The Brain and Emotion*, pp. 94–138. Oxford University Press, Oxford.

Rosenberg, D.R., Keshavan, M.S., O'Hearn, K.M., Dick, E.L., Bagwell, W.W., Seymour, A.B., Montrose, D.M., Pierri, J.N. and Birmaher, B., 1997. Frontostriatal measurement in treatment—naive children with obsessive–compulsive disorder. *Arch. Gen. Psychiatry*, **54**(9), 824–830.

Rubin, R.T., Villanueva-Meyer, J., Ananth, J., Trajmar, P.G. and Mena, I., 1992. Regional xenon-133 cerebral blood flow and cerebral Technetium 99 m HMPAO uptake in unmedicated patients with obsessive–compulsive disorder and matched normal control subjects. Determination by high-resolution single-photon emission computed tomography. *Arch. Gen. Psychiatry*, **49**(9), 695–702.

Sapolsky, R.M., Krey, L.C. and McEwen, B.S., 1985. Prolonged glucocorticoid exposure reduces hippocampal neuron number: implications for aging. *J. Neurosci.*, **5**, 1222–1227.

Sapolsky, R.M., Krey, L.C. and McEwen, B.S., 1986. The neuroendocrinology of stress and aging: The glucocorticoid cascade hypothesis. *Endocr. Rev.*, **7**, 284–301.

Savage, C.R., Deckersbach, T., Wilhelm, S., Rauch, S.L., Baer, L., Reid, T. and Jenike, M.A., 2000. Strategic processing and episodic memory impairment in obsessive compulsive disorder. *Neuropsychology*, **14**(1), 141–151.

Saxena, S., Brody, A.L., Maidment, K.M., Dunkin, J.J., Colgan, M., Alborzian, S., Phelps, M.E. and Baxter, L.R., Jr, 1999. Localized orbitofrontal and subcortical metabolic changes and predictors of response to paroxetine treatment in obsessive–compulsive disorder. *Neuropsychopharmacology*, **21**(6), 683–693.

Saxena, S. and Rauch, S.L., 2000. Functional neuroimaging and the neuroanatomy of obsessive–compulsive disorder. *Psychiatr. Clin. North Am.*, **23**(3), 563–586.

Scarone, S., Colombo, C., Livian, S., Abbruzzese, M., Ronchi, P., Locatelli, M., Scotti, G. and Smeraldi, E., 1992. Increased right caudate nucleus size in obsessive compulsive disorder: detection with magnetic resonance imaging. *Psychiatry Res.*, **45**(2), 115–121.

Schneider, F., Weiss, U., Kessler, C., Muller-Gartner, H.W., Posse, S., Salloum, J.B., Grodd, W., Himmelmann, F., Gaebel, W. and Birbaumer, N., 1999. Subcortical correlates of differential classical conditioning of aversive emotional reactions in social phobia. *Biol. Psychiatry*, **45**(7), 863–871.

Schwartz, J.M., Stoessel, P.W., Baxter, L.R., Jr, Martin, K.M. and Phelps, M.E., 1996. Systematic changes in cerebral glucose metabolic rate after successful behavior modification of obsessive compulsive disorder. *Arch. Gen. Psychiatry*, **53**(2), 109–113.

Scott, S.K., Young, A.W., Calder, A.J., Hellawell, D.J., Aggleton, J.P. and Johnson, M., 1997. Impaired auditory recognition of fear and anger following bilateral amygdala lesions. *Nature*, **385**(6613), 254–257.

Semple, W.E., Goyer, P., McCormick, R., Morris, E., Compton, B., Muswick, G., Nelson, D., Donovan, B., Leisure, G. and Berridge, M., 1993. Preliminary report: Brain blood flow using PET in patients with posttraumatic stress disorder and substance-abuse histories. *Biol. Psychiatry*, **34**(1–2), 115–118.

Shin, L.M., Dougherty, D., Macklin, M.L., Orr, S.P., Pitman, R.K. and Rauch, S.L., 2000. Activation of anterior paralimbic structures during guilt-related script-driven imagery. *Biol. Psychiatry*, **48**, 43–50.

Shin, L.M., Kosslyn, S.M., McNally, R.J., Alpert, N.M., Thompson, W.L., Rauch, S.L., Macklin, M.L. and Pitman, R.K., 1997. Visual imagery and perception in posttraumatic stress disorder: A positron emission tomographic investigation. *Arch. Gen. Psychiatry*, **54**(3), 233–241.

Shin, L.M., McNally, R.J., Kosslyn, S.M., Thompson, W.L., Rauch, S.L., Alpert, N.M., Metzger, L.J., Lasko, N.B., Orr, S.P. and Pitman, R.K., 1999. Regional cerebral blood flow during script-driven imagery in childhood sexual abuse-related posttraumatic stress disorder: a PET investigation. *Am. J. Psychiatry*, **156**(4), 575–584.

Starkman, M.N., Gebarski, S.S., Berent, S. and Schteingart, D.E., 1992. Hippocampal formation volume, memory dysfunction, and cortisol levels in patients with Cushing's syndrome. *Biol. Psychiatry*, **32**, 756–765.

Starkman, M.N., Giordani, B., Gebarski, S.S., Berent, S., Schork, M.A. and Schteingart, D.E., 1999. Decrease in cortisol reverses human hippocampal atrophy following treatment of Cushing's disease. *Biol. Psychiatry*, **46**, 1595–1602.

Stein, M.B., Koverola, C., Hanna, C., Torchia, M.G. and McClarty, B., 1997. Hippocampal volume in women victimized by childhood sexual abuse. *Psychol. Med.*, **27**(4), 951–960.

Stein, M.B. and Leslie, W.D., 1996. A brain SPECT study of generalized social phobia. *Biol. Psychiatry*, **39**, 825–828.

Stein, M.B., 1998. Neurobiological perspectives on social phobia: from affiliation to zoology. *Biol. Psychiatry*, **44**, 1277–1285.

Stewart, R.S., Devous, M.D. Sr, Rush, A.J., Lane, L. and Bonte, F.J., 1988. Cerebral blood flow changes during sodium-lactate-induced panic attacks. *Am. J. Psychiatry*, **145**(4), 442–449.

Swedo, S.E., Pietrini, P., Leonard, H.L., Schapiro, M.B., Rettew, D.C., Goldberger, E.L., Rapoport, S.I., Rapoport, J.L. and Grady, C.L., 1992. Cerebral glucose metabolism in childhood-onset obsessive–compulsive disorder: revisualization during pharmacotherapy. *Arch. Gen. Psychiatry*, **49**(9), 690–694.

Swedo, S.E., Schapiro, M.B., Grady, C.L., Cheslow, D.L., Leonard, H.L., Kumar, A., Friedland, R., Rapoport, S.I. and Rapoport, J.L., 1989. Cerebral glucose metabolism in childhood-onset obsessive–compulsive disorder. *Arch. Gen. Psychiatry*, **46**(6), 518–523.

Uno, H., Tarara, R., Else, J., Suleman, M. and Sapolsky, R.M., 1989. Hippocampal damage associated with prolonged and fatal stress in primates. *J. Neurosci.*, **9**, 1705–1711.

Vythilingam, M., Anderson, E.R., Goddard, A., Woods, S.W., Staib, L.H., Charney, D.S. and Bremner, J.D., 2000. Temporal lobe volume in panic disorder—a quantitative magnetic resonance imaging study. *Psychiatry Res.*, **99**(2), 75–82.

Watanabe, Y., Gould, E. and McEwen, B.S., 1992. Stress induces atrophy of apical dendrites of hippocampal CA3 pyramidal neurons. *Brain Res.*, **588**, 341–345.

Whalen, P.J., Rauch, S.L., Etcoff, N.L., McInerney, S., Lee, M.B. and Jenike, M.A., 1998. Masked presentations of emotional facial expressions modulate amygdala activity without explicit knowledge. *J. Neurosci.*, **18**, 411–418.

Wik, G., Fredrikson, M., Ericson, K., Eriksson, L., Stone-Elander, S. and Greitz, T., 1993. A functional cerebral response to frightening visual stimulation. *Psychiatry Res.*, **50**(1), 15–24.

Wilson, F.A. and Rolls, E.T., 1990. Learning and memory is reflected in the responses of reinforcement-related neurons in the primate basal forebrain. *J. Neurosci.*, **10**(4), 1254–1267.

Woods, S.W., Koster, K., Krystal, J.K., Smith, E.O., Zubal, I.G., Hoffer, P.B. and Charney, D.S., 1988. Yohimbine alters regional cerebral blood flow in panic disorder. *The Lancet*, **2**(8612), 678.

Woolley, C.S., Gould, E. and McEwen, B.S., 1990. Exposure to excess glucocorticoids alters dendritic morphology of adult hippocampal pyramidal neurons. *Brain Res.*, **531**, 225–231.

Wright, C.I., Fischer, H., Whalen, P.J., McInerney, S.C., Shin, L.M. and Rauch, S.L., 2000. Suppression of human brain activity by repeatedly presented emotional facial expressions. *NeuroImage*, **11**, S252.

Wright, C.I., Fischer, H., Whalen, P.J., McInnerney, S.I., Shin, L.M. and Rauch, S.L., 2001. Differential prefrontal cortex and amygdala habituation to repeatedly presented emotional stimuli. *Neuroreport*, **12**(2), 379–383.

Yehuda, R., 1998. Neuroendocrinology of trauma and posttraumatic stress disorder. In: Yehuda, R. (ed.), *Psychological Trauma*, pp. 97–131. American Psychiatric Press, Inc., Washington, DC.

XIX-10

In Vivo Functional Neurochemistry of Anxiety Disorders

Andrea L. Malizia, Brian Martis and Scott L. Rauch

INTRODUCTION

Human anxiety disorders are the most prevalent psychiatric conditions affecting at least two fifths of the population in their lifetime. About one in 20 of the population has enduring or recurrent anxiety disorders and therefore these conditions are responsible for the highest societal global (medical and social) costs of any psychiatric condition. For instance, out of 92 million working days lost in the UK. due to mental illness in 1993 (18% of all lost days), 49% were due to anxiety or stress representing a cost of over £3 billion (approximately ∈/$ 4.5 billion).

In order to understand the aetiology of these disorders, possibly leading to better treatments, research has been carried out on the biological basis of healthy and pathological anxiety. Compared with other emotions and other psychiatric conditions, anxiety and fear (as defined in Martis *et al.*, Chapter XIX-9) are constructs which have a reasonable mapping between animals and man. Therefore, the study of anxiety and fear in preclinical experiments can provide leads for human research. Animal experiments have generated two overlapping sets of information. One set describes the sufficient or necessary neuroanatomical structures underlying the expression of these emotions (whether innate or conditioned) in animals and the other the neurochemical changes which predispose to or accompany the behavioural changes. However, despite the similarities in anxiety expression between man and other animals, data from preclinical experiments are not sufficient to understand the biology of human anxiety or anxiety disorders.

Direct human experimentation has also contributed to increase our knowledge about brain function and anxiety. Yet, the traditional investigation of human brain processes *in vivo* has many constraints related to the inaccessibility of the tissue under study and to functional complexity whereby understanding of individual modules from lesion studies, pharmacological challenges and electrophysiological recordings cannot provide sufficiently comprehensive hypotheses of system architecture. Indeed, up to the late 1980s, the most informative experimental strategies employed in clinical psychopharmacology recorded behavioural, physiological and cognitive responses to pharmacological probes where the aim was to characterize the central neurochemical changes underlying particular processes or diseases based on preclinical knowledge. These challenges were, and are, limited by their intrinsic inability to characterize neural networks in detail and by the fact that ligand binding and neurotransmitter release cannot be quantified *ex vivo* or by microdialysis in man (except recently in very selected samples of neurosurgical patients). These limitations prevent the conduct of any quantitative human research which aims to relate changes in physiology or behaviour to synaptic parameters. Further, many of the probes used to selectively affect one system or one subset of receptors have often subsequently been discovered to be relatively less selective than originally postulated.

Since the late 1980s, human imaging (Table XIX-10.1) has been used to describe the functional anatomy (discussed in Chapter XIX-9), pharmacology and functional neurochemistry (this chapter) of human anxiety and anxiety disorders with macroanatomical (up to about 1 cm) brain resolution. The use of these technological advances is still in its infancy as novel paradigms and analytical methods are developed; however, the vision for the future is that their utilization should lead to a more robust understanding of the brain mechanisms underlying disease and response to treatments.

This chapter has two aims: a brief commentary on the technical issues related to pharmacological imaging and a review of the current human psychopharmacology imaging knowledge regarding anxiety and anxiety disorders, including some preliminary data.

PHARMACOLOGICAL IMAGING

Two strategies can be employed to detect drug effects on the brain: detection of changes in brain metabolism or activation induced by pharmacological agents and radioligand assay of binding to receptors, transporters, enzymes and of tracer kinetics of precursor pools.

Changes in Brain Metabolism or Activation

The paradigms used here depend on the detection of changes in regional brain metabolism or blood flow following the administration of pharmaceuticals. The principles are as follows.

- Changes in local brain metabolism are mostly induced by changes in neuronal activity; while there is debate on the cellular location of the metabolic changes (i.e., neurons or glia), energy is mostly expended at synaptic sites.
- Changes in local metabolism are tightly linked to changes in local blood perfusion, which overcompensates for the increases in oxygen demands by delivering an excess of deoxyhaemoglobin.
- Imaging techniques can measure changes in local metabolism ([^{11}C] glucose PET or ^{18}fluorodeoxyglucose (FDG) PET), in local perfusion ($H_2{}^{15}0$ PET or $C^{15}O_2$ PET or [^{11}C]butanol PET; ^{99}Tc HMPAO SPECT; ASL (arterial spin labelling) or gadolinium MRI), in local deoxyhaemoglobin concentration (fMRI), in oxygen extraction ($^{15}O_2$ PET) or in local blood volume ($C^{15}O$ PET).

One complicating factor in the interpretation of these techniques is the fact that pharmacological manipulations have effects not only on the brain processes of interest but also on other neuronal or

Biological Psychiatry: Edited by H. D'haenen, J.A. den Boer and P. Willner. ISBN 0-471-49198-5

Table XIX-10.1 Types of human imaging used for investigating *in vivo* neurochemical processes in the human brain. Note that the significant parameters are derived from the primary measures by using mathematical and statistical models

Imaging modality	Technique	Primary measure	Deduction/physiological significance
MRI	Functional MRI	Deoxyhaemoglobin signal	Change in perfusion.
	Spectroscopy	Specific spectral signal	Total concentration of molecule of interest (GABA, lactate) in whole brain.
PET	Water, butanol	Radioactive counts	Perfusion or change in perfusion.
	Fluorodeoxyglucose (FDG)	Radioactive counts	Regional integrated (over time) glucose analogue transport into brain tissue.
	Receptor binding	Radioactive counts	Binding potential or volume of distribution (related to B_{max}/K_d).
	Labelled precursor	Radioactive counts	Local brain transport of precursors. Relationship with transmitter synthesis unproven.
	Enzyme binding	Radioactive counts	Regional enzyme concentration.
	Transporter binding/uptake	Radioactive counts	Regional transporter availability.
SPET	HMPAO	Radioactive counts	Change in perfusion.
	Receptor binding Transporter binding	Radioactive counts	Relative binding potential or volume of distribution. (related to B_{max}/K_d) or transporter availability.

glial processes and on the innervation to the cerebral vasculature (adventitia). Further, the signal associated with pharmacological modulation of specific brain activations is often very small and the statistical techniques needed to detect these changes have to be more sensitive than ones often employed in simple activation experiments. Newer strategies will improve the quality of data generated. These include the following.

- Comprehensive evaluation of the cerebral effects of the drugs under study using more than one imaging modality and detailing a number of the physiological responses. This strategy would measure changes in regional metabolism as well as in perfusion, or measure changes in magnitude and distribution of activation with control tasks as well as with tasks of interest or compare metabolic maps with maps of changes in radioligand binding. In the few occasions where such combinations of data have been acquired in the past, important differences between changes in regional metabolism and regional perfusion have been detected.
- The inclusion of other measured physiological responses in the analysis, thus allowing detection of the relationship between changes in regional brain activity and another physiological parameter of interest such as saccadic eye movement parameters.
- Use of statistical methods such as path or network analysis which are more sensitive to small predicted changes in activity.

Measure of Radioligand Binding

The principle of these studies is that a ligand is administered which is labelled with a radioactive nucleus. The time course of the distribution of radioactivity in the tissue of interest is recorded with SPET or PET cameras and the data is analysed with an appropriate mathematical model (Gunn, Gunn and Cunningham, 2001) in order to obtain the parameters of interest. Since the signal recorded is a tomographic, time dependent measure of radioactivity in a particular image segment or voxel, it is made up of a number of components (Figure XIX-10.1) comprising free and bound ligand and metabolites in the blood and tissue of interest. Thus the identifiability of the measure of interest depends on a number of factors (Table XIX-10.2) mostly related to radioligand properties. These factors explain why there are very few PET/SPET radioligands that can be successfully used to measure brain chemistry *in vivo* in man despite the fact that thousands have been developed.

Radioligand binding can be used to measure a number of processes.

- Receptor density and affinity. Often a composite measure of these is used such as binding potential or volume of distribution. These are proportional to B_{max}/K_d. Composite parameters are used because a measure can be obtained by doing only one scan and without the injection of significant amounts of cold ligand (Mintun *et al.*, 1983). A number of receptors have thus been measured including dopamine D1 and D2, serotonin 1A, 2 and 2A, $GABA_A$ benzodiazepine, substance P (NK1) and opiate.
- Changes in neurotransmitter concentration. This is deduced by measuring the change in binding potential as receptor availability increases or decreases with changes in neurotransmitter release. So far this strategy has only been successful in measuring dopamine and possibly opiate release.
- Precursor pools — this method has been used to measure the concentration of radiolabelled fluoroDOPA and alpha-methyl-L-tryptophan in the brain. The interest in these measures is that they are thought to relate to precursor pool and rate of synthesis of derivative neurotransmitters such as dopamine and serotonin. The demonstration that they are more likely to be measuring local brain uptake than any other process (Shoaf *et al.*, 2000) recommends caution in the interpretation of results obtained when using these techniques.
- Transporter density. This technique has been used successfully to measure dopamine (Laruelle *et al.*, 1997) and to a lesser extent serotonin reuptake sites.
- Enzyme concentrations. So far this technique has been used to measure MAO in the brain.
- Occupancy or inhibition of any of the above.

NEUROCHEMISTRY OF ANXIETY DISORDERS *IN VIVO* IN MAN

Studies in this area have been scarce to date with most of the effort being concentrated on the $GABA_A$ benzodiazepine receptor. In the receptor binding arena, this has been in part due to practical issues related to the availability of good radiotracers. Preclinical work indicates that investigation of the ascending monoaminergic systems (dopamine, serotonin, noradrenaline), of some peptidergic transmitters such as substance P and the NK1 receptor and CCK, of adenosine receptors and of benzodiazepine-GABAergic activity

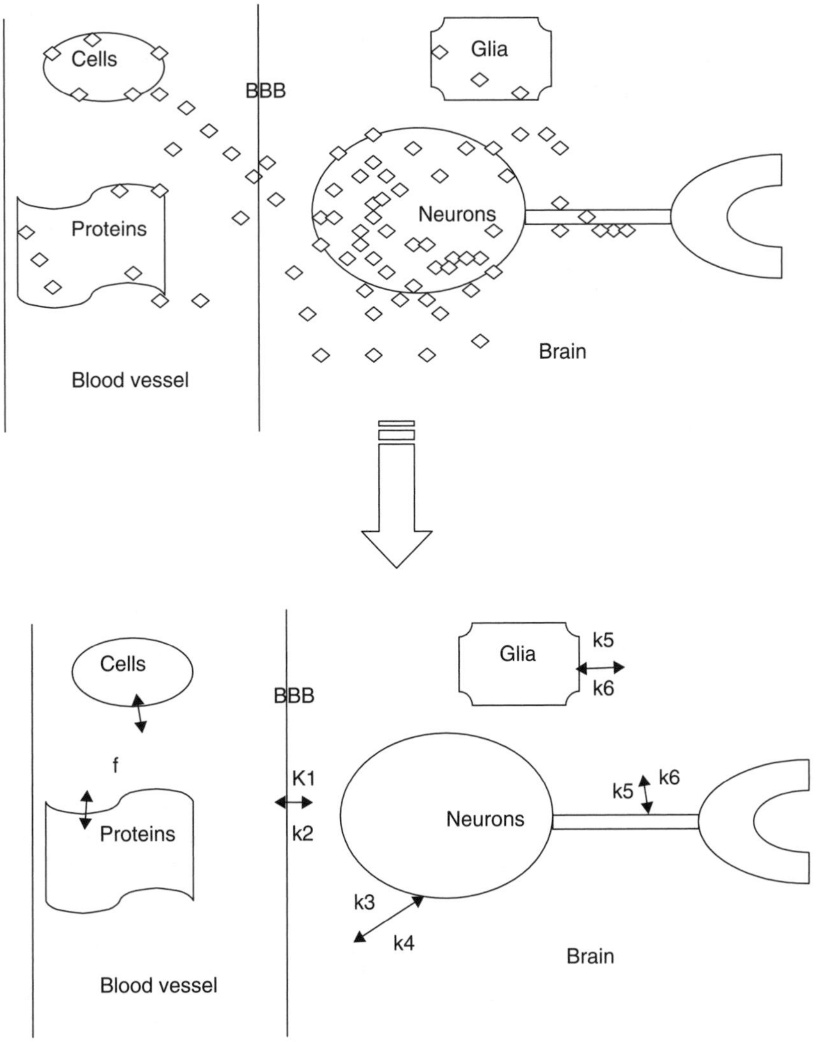

Figure XIX-10.1 (Upper panel) Schematic representation of radioligand (◇) topography. In the vasculature the radioligand is partly bound to cells and proteins. Once it crosses the blood–brain barrier (BBB) it may bind to specific sites on the neurons and sometimes glia and to non-specific sites on neurons and glia. In addition it can exist in the interstitial spaces. (Lower panel) The same scheme with processes as described by common symbols. f is the free fraction in plasma. K1/k2 represents the constants characterizing movement to and from tissue, k3/k4 describes the rate constants for specific binding and k5/k6 the rate constants for non-specific binding

Table XIX-10.2 Necessary characteristics of radioligands for pharmacological imaging in the brain. The essential feature is that the signal recorded is from the whole of the tissue and vasculature *in vivo* and therefore the radioligand characteristics are stringent in order to make it interpretable

Essential and desirable characteristics	Significance
Radioligand crosses blood–brain barrier easily	Allows measurement of total brain concentration of radioligand.
Radioligand specific binding is at least 3× non-specific binding	Allows measurement of specific binding and changes in specific binding.
Radioligand has no radioactive metabolites **OR** *Radioactive metabolites do not cross blood–brain barrier*	Signal becomes very difficult to model mathematically if radioactive metabolites are present in the tissue.
Radioligand has no metabolites which also bind to receptor of interest	*Avoids potential for displacement by metabolite.*
Radioligand has high affinity (low K_d)	*Mean transit time in tissue has to be of same order of magnitude as timing of imaging.*
Radioligand binds to one receptor only **OR** If to multiple receptors, these have distinct anatomical distribution	Resolution of signal specific to one site of specific binding is otherwise not possible.
Radioligand has no physiological actions at injected concentrations	Pharmacodynamic effects may affect pharmacokinetic parameters.
Radioligand has high specific (radio) activity	Must inject tracer doses of radioligand (<2% occupancy) for tracer kinetics to apply.
Appropriate reference activity can be obtained from plasma or tissue	Separation of parameters depends on being able to account for signal which is not specific.

would be the most relevant for human anxiety disorders. However, only some of the above can be currently explored in terms of receptor binding. This section of the chapter will examine the extant data, organized by neurotransmitter system and disease.

$GABA_A$ BENZODIAZEPINE

Benzodiazepines, first discovered in the 1950s, were found in the 1970s and 1980s to act by modulating GABA chloride ionophores, thus increasing the effectiveness of local neuronal inhibition. Benzodiazepines and GABA potentiation are known to have an immediate effect on anxiety in man and therefore investigation of their binding in the brain is a field of interest (Nutt and Malizia, 2001). The $GABA_A$ ionophore is a structure made up of five subunits; benzodiazepines in clinical practice bind to receptors expressing $\alpha 1$, $\alpha 2$, $\alpha 3$, and $\alpha 5$ subunits. This includes iomazenil and flumazenil, two benzodiazepine antagonists routinely used to image these receptors in man with SPET and PET respectively. Further, other agents that bind at these sites are being developed, which have differential affinity for some of the subtypes (e.g., Ro 15-4513 which has higher affinity for $\alpha 5$-containing receptors). In addition, GABA concentrations can now be measured with MR spectroscopy. Three conditions have been investigated: Panic Disorder, Generalized Anxiety Disorder and Post Traumatic Stress Disorder.

Panic Disorder

Benzodiazepine Binding

The separation of Panic Disorder (PD) from other anxiety disorder followed the observation that PD patients did not respond clinically to benzodiazepines but were treated by adequate courses of tricyclic antidepressants. It is now known that higher doses of benzodiazepines or compounds with higher potency at the $GABA_A$ benzodiazepine site are effective at treating PD; however, the original findings were an indication that PD patients have a lower sensitivity to these compounds. Further experimental evidence was produced, showing that PD patients are less sensitive to benzodiazepines on a number of psychophysiological measures, such as saccadic eye movements to target and suppression of noradrenaline appearance rate (Roy Byrne *et al.*, 1989). These findings, coupled with the observation that FG 7142 (a benzodiazepine site exogenous inverse agonist) is panicogenic in man and the discovery of putative endogenous inverse agonists in man (DBI (Elsworth *et al.*, 1986) and tribulin (Corda *et al.*, 1984)) led to theories which postulated that panic attacks were precipitated by the pathological production of a putative endogenous inverse agonist. However, Nutt and colleagues (1990) discovered that flumazenil, a benzodiazepine site antagonist, which has neutral anxiety effects in control subjects, provokes panic attacks in patients with PD. This disproved the putative benzodiazepine receptor inverse agonist theory and two possible explanations were put forward. The first is that fundamental changes at the $GABA_A$ benzodiazepine receptor result in changed receptor binding/function which alter the effects of flumazenil so that it behaves like an inverse agonist. The second is that flumazenil blocks a putative endogenous agonist which is present in a compensatory function in anxiety disorders and that this endogenous ligand is, however, insufficient to prevent the emergence of panic attacks. Following these leads, a number of investigators have sought to determine benzodiazepine receptor density using Iomazenil SPECT or Flumazenil PET. Many of these studies have considerable methodological shortcomings that prevent the formation of robust conclusions. In particular, early scanning after injection of iomazenil (thus contaminating the data with effects due to brain delivery), inappropriate control groups (for example patients with epilepsy who may themselves have alterations at the benzodiazepine site), comorbidity with other affective conditions and the study of patients who have been treated with benzodiazepines (thus inducing changes in regulation of the site) are the most common problems.

Schlegel *et al.* (1994) were the first to report decreased benzodiazepine receptor binding in panic disorder using Iomazenil SPECT comparing, at 90–110 min post-injection, 10 patients with PD with 10 patients with epilepsy on carbamazepine. The decreases were significant in the occipital and frontal lobes and maximal in the temporal lobes. Kaschka, Feistel and Ebert (1995) studied nine medicated patients with PD *and* comorbid depression with a matched group of medicated patients with dysthymia using Iomazenil SPECT (2 h). Decreases in binding were seen in the inferior temporal lobes both medially and laterally and in the inferior frontal lobes. These changes were already detectable at 10 min post-injection reflecting changes dominated by delivery effects. All participants were on antidepressants. Tokunaga *et al.* (1997) published an elegant technical study, having followed a very rigorous scanning methodology. However, their demonstration of reduced benzodiazepine binding in anxiety patients is limited by the uncertainty associated with the fact that he did not use a standard psychiatric classification. On the other hand, Kuikka *et al.* (1995) using two different SPECT cameras (at 90 min post-injection) studied 17 unmedicated patients with PD and 17 healthy age and sex matched controls using Iomazenil and found an increase in Iomazenil signal bilaterally in the temporal cortex and in the right middle/inferior lateral frontal gyrus, while Brandt *et al.* (1998) showed that patients with PD have a significant increase of benzodiazepine receptor binding in the right supraorbital cortex and a trend to an increased uptake in the right temporal cortex. Both these studies are however also likely to be contaminated by ligand delivery issues. Finally, Bremner *et al.* (2000a) showed a relative decrease in measures of benzodiazepine receptor binding in left hippocampus and precuneus in panic disorder patients relative to controls. The group further observed that panic disorder patients who had a panic attack compared with patients who did not have a panic attack at the time of the scan also had a decrease in benzodiazepine receptor binding in prefrontal cortex. They also reported an increase in benzodiazepine binding in the right caudate, in the occipital lobes, in the middle temporal and in the middle frontal cortex. Although patients were drug free at the time of the scan none of them were benzodiazepine naïve.

In summary, most SPECT studies demonstrate decreases in benzodiazepine binding in panic disorder. However, the direction and location of these changes is not consistent across all studies, probably due to methodological issues.

In the only fully quantitative study of benzodiazepine naïve subjects, Malizia *et al.* (1998) employed [^{11}C]flumazenil PET and found a global decrease in binding in benzodiazepine naive, drug-free patients with PD who had no comorbid conditions and did not abuse alcohol (Colour Plate XIX-10.2). These changes were maximal in ventral basal ganglia, orbitofrontal and temporal cortex. Having corrected for the global decrease in binding, PD patients showed a further statistically significant regional decrease in binding in the inferior parietal temporo-occipital areas which was maximal in the lateral posterior temporal lobes as well as decreases in orbitofrontal cortex and ventral striatum. Decreased binding in thalamus, dorso-lateral and medial prefrontal, medial temporal and cerebellar cortex and vermis were accounted for by the global changes. Another PET study (Abadie *et al.*, 1999) compared patients with a number of anxiety disorders and healthy volunteers using flumazenil PET and a tissue reference technique which is semi-quantitative. The variance of the reference areas was such that the data had to be pooled across subjects in order to avoid dealing with negative binding in the pons. No significant differences were

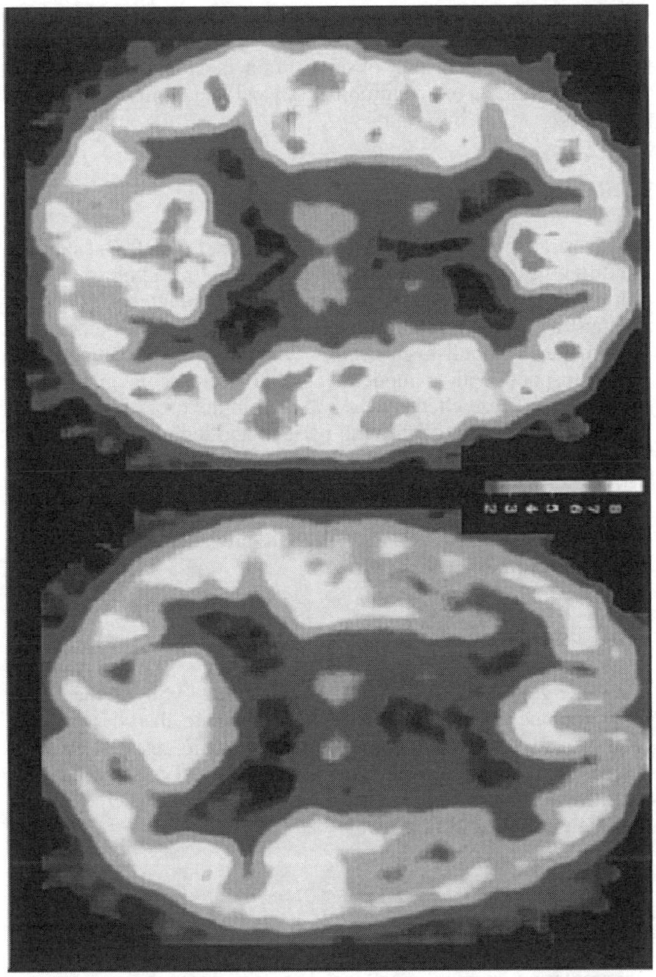

Figure XIX-10.2 A comparison of flumazenil binding between controls and panic disorder patients. The image shows a coloured scale of volume of distribution of flumazenil. The horizontal brain slice is through the middle of the brain showing occipital cortex (left) thalami amd basal ganglia (centre) temporal cortex (middle rim) and frontal cortex (right). A decrease in flumazenil binding is seen throughout the cortex and subcortical structures on the bottom which is the median map for panic disorder patients. The median map for controls is on the top (See Colour Plate XIX-10.2)

found between individual brain areas because of this large variance but for each area examined benzodiazepine receptor density was lower in patients with anxiety disorders.

Decreased benzodiazepine receptor binding is consistent with the idea that panic disorder is due to a deficiency in brain inhibition that leads to, or allows, paroxysmal elevations in anxiety during panic attacks. The peak decreases in benzodiazepine binding are in anatomical areas (e.g., orbitofrontal cortex and insula) thought to be involved in the experience of anxiety in man and could represent a primary pathology. The reduction in binding not only explains some of the known features of benzodiazepine receptor function in panic disorder but is also congruent with animal data showing that chronic stress decreases benzodiazepine binding (Inoue *et al.*, 1985; Weizman *et al.*, 1989, 1990) and that animals with genetically decreased flumazenil binding experience more anxiety (Crestani *et al.*, 1999). It is thus possible that this finding could be the result of experiencing repeated panic attacks or the consequence of one or more of the aetiological factors such as genetic predisposition or life events.

BRAIN GABA CONCENTRATIONS

One of the possible mechanisms by which benzodiazepine $GABA_A$ receptor subunit composition could be altered or downregulated is via a change in brain GABAergic activity. Goddard *et al.* (2001) have demonstrated that patients with panic disorder have a 22% reduction in total occipital cortex GABA concentration (GABA plus homocarnosine) compared with controls. GABA concentration was measured by using MR spectroscopy of occipital cortex *in vivo*; the selection of this area of the brain was dictated by current constraints in data acquisition using this method. This remarkable finding was present in 12 of the 14 patient–control pairs but there were no significant correlations between occipital cortex GABA levels and measures of illness or state anxiety. Clearly, further studies will be needed to determine what the GABA concentration is in areas more germane to the expression of anxiety, but these data provide an interesting model of pathophysiology in panic disorder which may be consistent with reduced flumazenil binding.

Post Traumatic Stress Disorder (PTSD)

Exposure to chronic stress decreases benzodiazepine binding which is maximal in the frontal cortex in some animal experiments (Weizmann *et al.*, 1989). The Yale group (Bremner *et al.*, 2000b) investigated Vietnam veterans with PTSD using Iomazenil SPECT and found that there was a significant decrease in the volume of distribution of benzodiazepine $GABA_A$ receptors in the frontal cortex of these patients in an area which corresponds to Brodmann Area 9. This finding may be of particular significance as this area is involved in extinction of conditioned responses, thus misfunction of local inhibitory circuits could be either a consequence or a predisposition to developing inappropriate responses to trauma.

Generalized Anxiety Disorder

Benzodiazepine binding was also investigated in Generalized Anxiety Disorder using ^{123}I NNC 13-8241 SPECT in Finland where Tiihonen *et al.* (1997) compared 10 patients with 10 age and sex matched healthy volunteers finding decreased benzodiazepine $GABA_A$ binding in the left temporal pole. In addition they found a difference in fractal dimensions of the binding parameters which the authors interpreted as a decrease in variation of cortical receptor density akin to the decrease variability of some heart rate parameters seen in cardiovascular disease. While intriguing, this interpretation is premature as the significance of changes in fractal parameters for binding have not been mapped to cellular or histological differences.

Two papers reported studies of changes in brain metabolism during a vigilance task in patients with generalized anxiety disorders before and after benzodiazepine or placebo administration (Buchsbaum *et al.*, 1987; Wu *et al.*, 1991). Reductions in anxiety could not be mapped to specific changes in cerebral metabolism for the drug group and the usual pattern of benzodiazepine-induced global reductions in metabolism emerged. These types of experiments, however, need to be repeated with more sophisticated analyses as it is likely that detection of the smaller specific modulatory signal is obscured by the global changes.

SEROTONIN (5HT)

Since the discovery of the anxiolytic therapeutic action of $5HT1_A$ agonists and selective serotonin reuptake inhibitors (SSRIs), changes in serotonergic function have been postulated in all anxiety disorders with some authors detailing possible differences in mechanisms between generalized anxiety and panic (Deakin and Graeff, 1991). Further, polymorphisms at the $5HT1_A$ site have been reported to contribute to variance in human anxiety disorders (Lesch *et al.*, 1992) and other receptor subtypes have been implicated in preclinical anxiety experiments. It may therefore seem surprising that the serotonergic system has been relatively underinvestigated.

Panic Disorder

Two sets of data are available in panic disorder. One relates to $5HT1_A$ binding and one to the effects of SSRI treatment on resting brain metabolism and on activations. $5HT1_A$ receptors are of particular interest as they have functional significance in decreasing raphe firing until functionally downregulated and are thought to mediate the cortical effects of increased serotonergic transmission.

[^{11}C]WAY100635 has been available as a useful PET radioligand to investigate $5HT1_A$ receptors. Following the demonstration of global decreases in benzodiazepine binding, global decreases in cortical and subcortical $5HT1_A$ binding in panic disorder patients when compared with controls have also been demonstrated by the same research group (Sargent *et al.*, 2000). These patients were, however, on active SSRI treatment when scanned and therefore the findings could be a consequence of the therapeutic interventions rather than a correlate of the psychopathology. In this light the findings of an inverse correlation between $5HT1_A$ binding and anxiety trait scores in healthy volunteers (Tauscher *et al.*, 2001) is however intriguing, as it may indicate that low $5HT1_A$ receptor density predisposes to anxiety in man.

The effect of serotonin transporter inhibition on brain metabolism in panic disorder was studied in nine patients successfully treated with imipramine by comparing their resting cerebral metabolism measured via ^{18}FDG PET with healthy volunteers and untreated panic disorder patients (Nordahl *et al.*, 1998). Compared with healthy volunteers, treated PD patients had lower Left/Right hippocampal and prefrontal metabolic ratios (but no difference with untreated PD patients). Lower posterior orbitofrontal metabolism was found in treated patients when compared with healthy volunteers or untreated patients and this effect was ascribed to antidepressant treatment since it was similar to effects observed with the tricyclic imipramine in OCD (Benkelfat *et al.*, 1990). *Post hoc* comparisons revealed that treated patients were no different from controls in the left parietal and left Rolandic areas which were however hypometabolic in untreated panic disorder patients.

Social Phobia

One leading group has employed [^{11}C]5hydroxy-L-tryptophan PET to investigate serotonergic basal metabolism in the brain of patients with social phobia (Marteinsdottir *et al.*, 2001) and has described decreases in signal in the basal ganglia and parts of the limbic system. However, signal with this ligand is closely linked to local transport into the brain (Shoaf *et al.*, 2000) and therefore the significance of these findings will have to be interpreted cautiously.

NORADRENALINE

While the status of noradrenergic manipulation as anxiogenic in preclinical experiments is much debated, there is a considerable body of evidence that $\alpha 2$ antagonists induce anxiety and $\alpha 2$ agonists decrease anxiety in patients with anxiety disorders. This has been mapped as noradrenaline release being anxiogenic while decreases are anxiolytic as activation of the $\alpha 2$ receptors in the locus coeruleus decreases firing. There are no viable noradrenergic ligands to study binding in the human brain *in vivo* but two experiments have been reported which observe brain metabolic changes after the administration of yohimbine (an $\alpha 2$ antagonist) in anxiety disorders.

PTSD

An investigation by the Yale group (Bremner *et al.*, 1997) examined the differences in regional metabolic rate after the administration of yohimbine to patients with PTSD and healthy volunteers. This study demonstrated that yohimbine generated a global small increase in grey matter metabolism in healthy volunteers, while patients with PTSD respond with a moderate global decrease in grey matter metabolism. These effects were maximal in the orbitofrontal cortex and significant in the prefrontal, parietal and temporal cortices and were accompanied by significant behavioural activation in PTSD patients. The authors interpreted this observation as evidence of increased sensitivity to the noradrenergic releasing properties of yohimbine in PTSD, in line with their previous pharmacological observations in this patient group.

Panic Disorder

The same group reported briefly (Woods *et al.*, 1988) on the effects of yohimbine on cerebral blood flow in panic disorder patients. In this study yohimbine provocation of panic resulted in large decreases in HMPAO-SPECT signal in the frontal cortex. The study has however not been described in more detail elsewhere so that a thorough critique is not possible.

DOPAMINE

Dopaminergic manipulation can alter the response to stress in animals and to some extent in man. The evidence for dopaminergic involvement in anxiety disorders is however scanty, both in the treatment and in the aetiology literatures. This may explain why few human imaging studies exist in this arena, despite the fact that there are some very robust dopaminergic radioligands for human work.

Social Phobia

Dopaminergic underactivity and social anxiety have been postulated to be related from animal models, human diseases such as Parkinson's and the effects of dopamine modulating agents (reviewed by Bell, Malizia and Nutt, 1999). Two studies have provided evidence for dopaminergic dysfunction in social phobia by measuring the density of dopamine transporters and D2 (mainly post synaptic) receptors in the basal ganglia of patients with this condition and controls, using SPET. The first study, using ^{123}I β CIT, demonstrated that 11 Finnish Social Phobia patients had decreased binding potential for the dopamine transporter in the striatum (Tiihonen *et al.*, 1997). This was followed by a study by Schneier *et al.* (2000) who demonstrated that 10 New York patients with Social Phobia had lower D2 binding potential than controls. These data suggest three possibilities:

- downregulation of both sites as a trait associated with possible dopaminergic hypofunction;
- increased dopaminergic tonic release, which would decrease the proportion of sites available for radioligand binding;
- mild atrophy of the basal ganglia.

PEPTIDES

CCK 4 and pentagastrin have been demonstrated to be powerful anxiogenic agents in patients with anxiety disorders and in particular with panic disorder. Imaging studies have demonstrated that induction of anxiety in volunteers using these agents activates brain areas thought to be germane to the experience of anxiety (Benkelfat *et al.*, 1995; Javanmard *et al.*, 1999). Further recent data suggests that SSRI treatment of PD patients modifies the brain activation pattern upon infusion of pentagastrin (Boshuisen *et al.*, 2001). These changes are most pronounced in frontal and limbic cortices, but to date it is not clear whether these changes are dominated by the change in anxiety experience after treatment.

SUMMARY AND CONCLUSION

Some human brain imaging techniques are mature and can be used to investigate a number of pharmacological systems in the human brain *in vivo*. While preclinical data have provided useful leads, some of the most striking results have come from investigating hypotheses suggested by observing human disorders. The demonstration of reduced benzodiazepine and $5HT1_A$ binding and reduced GABA concentrations in panic disorder and of dopaminergic dysfunction in the basal ganglia of patients with social phobia are the most notable examples.

It is increasingly important therefore that human imaging should be seen as able to provide leads which can be further validated and explored using preclinical methods. An intriguing example is the demonstration of reduced benzodiazepine binding in panic disorder which was almost immediately complemented by genetic experimentation in mice demonstrating that alterations in $\gamma 2$ and $\alpha 2$ subunits at the benzodiazepine receptors (Crestani *et al.*, 1999; Low *et al.*, 2000) can induce changes such as increased anxiety, decreased sensitivity to benzodiazepine agonists and decreased binding to flumazenil that are also observed in humans with anxiety disorders. Similarly, the demonstration that $5HT1_A$ knockout mice have increased anxiety and decreased flumazenil binding (Sibille *et al.*, 2000) also seems to link the reduced $5HT1_A$ binding seen in panic disorder to benzodiazepine site abnormalities in man and provides a link between the two systems which needs to be further explored.

It is therefore important that these techniques should be increasingly used in biological psychiatry research, as part of a strategy that aims to integrate preclinical and clinical data in a symbiotic cycle of enquiry. The responsibility that human brain imaging researchers face is to use methodology that is robust enough to allow appropriate interpretations of the studies.

ACKNOWLEDGEMENTS

ALM was in part supported from grants from the departments of psychopharmacology, old age medicine and clinical medicine of the University of Bristol while writing this chapter.

REFERENCES

Abadie, P., Boulenger, J.P., Benali, K., Barre, L., Zarifian, E. and Baron, J.C., 1999. Relationships between trait and state anxiety and the central benzodiazepine receptor: a PET study. *Eur. J. Neurosci.*, **11**, 1470–1478.

Bell, C.J., Malizia, A.L. and Nutt, D.J., 1999. The neurobiology of social phobia. *Eur. Arch. Psychiatry Clin. Neurosci.*, **249**(11), S11–8.

Benkelfat, C., Nordahl, T.E., Semple, W.E., King, A.C., Murphy, D.L. and Cohen, R.M., 1990. Local cerebral glucose metabolic rates in obsessive–compulsive disorder. Patients treated with clomipramine. *Archives of General Psychiatry*, **47**(9), 840–848.

Benkelfat, C., Bradwein, J., Meyer, E., Ellenbogen, B.A., Milot, S., Gjedde, A. and Evans, A., 1995. Functional neuroanatomy of CCK4-induced anxiety in normal healthy volunteers. *Am. J. Psychiatr.*, **152**, 1180–1184.

Boshuisen, M.L., Reinders, A., Paans, A.M. and den Boer, J.A., 2001. Changes in rCBF of panic disorder patients due to effective treatment with sertraline. *Neuroimage*, **13**(6), S1030.

Brandt, C.A., Meller, J., Keweloh, L., Hoschel, K., Staedt, J., Munz, D. and Stoppe, G., 1998. Increased benzodiazepine receptor density in the prefrontal cortex in patients with panic disorder. *Journal of Neural Transmission*, **105**(10–12), 1325–1333.

Bremner, J.D., Innis, R.B., Ng, C.K., Staib, L.H., Salomon, R.M., Bronen, R.A., Duncan, J., Southwick, S.M., Krystal, J.H., Rich, D., Zubal, G., Dey, H., Soufer, R. and Charney, D.S., 1997. Positron emission tomography measurement of cerebral metabolic correlates of yohimbine administration in combat-related posttraumatic stress disorder. *Archives of General Psychiatry*, **54**(3), 246–254.

Bremner, J.D., Innis, R.B., Southwick, S.M., Staib, L., Zoghbi, S. and Charney, D.S., 2000a. Decreased benzodiazepine receptor binding in prefrontal cortex in combat-related posttraumatic stress disorder. *American Journal of Psychiatry*, **157**(7), 1120–1126.

Bremner, J.D., Innis, R.B., White, T., Fujita, M., Silbersweig, D., Goddard, A.W., Staib, L., Stern, E., Cappiello, A., Woods, S., Baldwin, R. and Charney, D.S., 2000b. SPECT [I-123]iomazenil measurement of the benzodiazepine receptor in panic disorder. *Biological Psychiatry*, **47**(2), 96–106.

Buchsbaum, M.S., Wu, J., Haier, R., Hazlett, E., Ball, R., Katz, M., Sokolski, K., Lagunas-Solar, M. and Langer, D., 1987. Positron emission tomography assessment of effects of benzodiazepines on regional glucose metabolic rate in patients with anxiety disorder. *Life Sciences*, **40**(25), 2393–2400.

Corda, M.G., Ferrari, M., Guidotti, A., Konkel, D. and Costa, E., 1984. Isolation, purification and partial sequence of a neuropeptide (diazepam binding inhibitor) precursor of an anxiogenic putative ligand for benzodiazepine recognition site. *Neurosci. Lett.*, **47**, 319–324.

Crestani, F., Lorez, M., Baer, K. and Mohler, H., 1999. Decreased GABAA-receptor clustering results in enhanced anxiety and a bias for threat cues. *Nat. Neurosci.*, **2**, 833–839.

Deakin, J.F.W. and Graeff, F.G., 1991. Critique: 5-HT and mechanisms of defence. *Journal of Psychopharmacology*, **5**, 305–341.

Elsworth, J.D., Dewar, D., Glover, V., Goodwin, B.L., Clow, A. and Sandler, M., 1986. Purification and characterization of tribulin, and endogenous inhibitor of monoamine oxidase and of benzodiazepine receptor binding. *J. Neural Transm.*, **67**, 45–56.

Goddard, A.W., Mason, G.F., Almai, A., Rothman, D.L., Behar, K.L., Petroff, O.A., Charney, D.S. and Krystal, J.H., 2001. Reductions in occipital cortex GABA levels in panic disorder detected with 1h-magnetic resonance spectroscopy. *Archives of General Psychiatry*, **58**(6), 556–561.

Gunn, R.N., Gunn, S.R. and Cunningham, V.J., 2001. Positron emission tomography compartmental models. *Journal of Cerebral Blood Flow & Metabolism*, **21**(6), 635–652.

Inoue, O., Akimoto, Y., Hashimoto, K. and Yamasaki, T., 1985. Alterations in biodistribution of [3H]Ro 15 1788 in mice by acute stress: possible changes in *in vivo* binding availability of brain benzodiazepine receptor. *Int. J. Nucl. Med. Biol.*, **12**, 369–374.

Javanmard, M., Shlik, J., Kennedy, S.H., Vaccarino, F.J., Houle, S. and Bradwejn, J., 1999. Neuroanatomic correlates of CCK-4-induced panic attacks in healthy humans: a comparison of two time points. *Biological Psychiatry*, **45**(7), 872–882.

Kaschka, W., Feistel, H. and Ebert, D., 1995. Reduced benzodiazepine receptor binding in panic disorders measured by iomazenil SPECT. *J. Psychiatr. Res.*, **29**, 427–423.

Kuikka, J.T., Pitkanen, A., Lepola, U., Partanen, K., Vainio, P., Bergstrom, K.A., Wieler, H.J., Kaiser, K.P., Mittelbach, L. and Koponen, H., 1995. Abnormal regional benzodiazepine receptor uptake in the prefrontal cortex in patients with panic disorder. *Nucl. Med. Commun.*, **16**, 273–280.

Laruelle, M., Iyer, R.N., al Tikriti, M.S., Zea Ponce, Y., Malison, R., Zoghbi, S.S., Baldwin, R.M., Kung, H.F., Charney, D.S., Hoffer, P.B., Innis, R.B. and Bradberry, C.W., 1997. Microdialysis and SPECT measurements of amphetamine induced dopamine release in non-human primates. *Synapse*, **25**, 1–14.

Lesch, K.P., Wiesmann, M., Hoh, A., Muller, T., Disselkamp Tietze, J., Osterheider, M. and Schulte, H.M., 1992. 5-HT1A receptor effector system responsivity in panic disorder. *Psychopharmacology Berl.*, **106**, 111–117.

Low, K., Crestani, F., Keist, R., Benke, D., Brunig, I., Benson, J.A., Fritschy, J.M., Rulicke, T., Bluethmann, H., Mohler, H. and Rudolph, U., 2000. Molecular and neuronal substrate for the selective attenuation of anxiety. *Science*, **290**(5489), 131–134.

Malizia, A.L., Cunningham, V.J., Bell, C.J., Liddle, P.F., Jones, T. and Nutt, D.J., 1998. Decreased brain GABA(A)-benzodiazepine receptor binding in panic disorder: preliminary results from a quantitative PET study. *Archives of General Psychiatry*, **55**(8), 715–720.

Marteinsdottir, I., Furmark, T., Tillfors, M., Hartvig, P., Fredrikson, M., Fischer, H., Antoni, G. and Hagberg, G., 2001. Presynaptic serotonin imaging in social phobia using [3-11C]-5-hydroxy-L-tryptophan and PET. *Neuroimage*, **13**(6), S1070.

Mintun, M., Raichle, M., Kilbourn, M., Wooten, F. and Welch, M., 1983. A quantitative method for the *in vivo* assessment of drug binding sites with positron emission tomography. *Ann. Neurol.*, **15**, 217–227.

Nordahl, T.E., Stein, M.B., Benkelfat, C., Semple, W.E., Andreason, P., Zametkin, A., Uhde, T.W. and Cohen, R.M., 1998. Regional cerebral metabolic asymmetries replicated in an independent group of patients with panic disorders. *Biological Psychiatry*, **44**(10), 998–1006.

Nutt, D.J., Glue, P., Lawson, C. and Wilson, S., 1990. Flumazenil provocation of panic attacks. *Arch. Gen. Psych.*, **47**, 917–925.

Nutt, D.J. and Malizia, A.L., 2001. New insights into the role of the GABA(A)-benzodiazepine receptor in psychiatric disorder. *Br. J. Psychiatry*, **179**(5), 390–396.

Roy Byrne, P.P., Cowley, D.S., Greenblatt, D.J., Shader, R.I. and Hommer, D., 1990. Reduced benzodiazepine sensitivity in panic disorder. *Arch. Gen. Psychiatry*, **47**, 534–538.

Roy Byrne, P.P., Lewis, N., Villacres, E., Diem, H., Greenblatt, D.J., Shader, R.I. and Veith, R., 1989. Preliminary evidence of benzodiazepine subsensitivity in panic disorder. *Arch. Gen. Psychiatry*, **46**, 165–169.

Sargent, P.A., Nash, J., Hood, S., Rabiner, E., Messa, C., Cowen, P., Nutt, D.J. and Grasby, P., 2000. 5HT1A receptor binding in panic disorder: comparison with depressive disorder and healthy volunteers using PET and [11C] WAY 100635. *Neuroimage*, **11**(5), S189.

Schlegel, S., Steinert, H., Bockisch, A., Hahn, K., Schloesser, R. and Benkert, O., 1994. Decreased benzodiazepine receptor binding in panic disorder measured by Iomazenil SPECT. A preliminary report. *Eur. Arch. Psychiatry Clin. Neurosci.*, **244**, 49–51.

Schneier, F.R., Liebowitz, M.R., Abi-Dargham, A., Zea-Ponce, Y., Lin, S.H. and Laruelle, M., 2000. Low dopamine D(2) receptor binding potential in social phobia. *American Journal of Psychiatry*, **157**(3), 457–459.

Shoaf, S.E., Carson, R.E., Hommer, D., Williams, W.A., Higley, J.D., Schmall, B., Herscovitch, P., Eckelman, W.C. and Linnoila, M., 2000. The suitability of [11C]-alpha-methyl-L-tryptophan as a tracer for serotonin synthesis: studies with dual administration of [11C] and [14C] labeled tracer. *Journal of Cerebral Blood Flow & Metabolism*, **20**(2), 244–252.

Sibille, E., Pavlides, C., Benke, D. and Toth, M., 2000. Genetic inactivation of the Serotonin(1A) receptor in mice results in downregulation of major GABA(A) receptor alpha subunits, reduction of GABA(A) receptor binding, and benzodiazepine-resistant anxiety. *Journal of Neuroscience*, **20**(8), 2758–2765.

Tauscher, J., Bagby, R.M., Javanmard, M., Christensen, B.K., Kasper, S. and Kapur, S., 2001. Inverse relationship between serotonin 5-HT(1A) receptor binding and anxiety: a [(11)C]WAY-100635 PET investigation in healthy volunteers. *American Journal of Psychiatry*, **158**(8), 1326–1328.

Tiihonen, J., Kuikka, J., Bergstrom, K., Lepola, U., Koponen, H. and Leinonen, E., 1997. Dopamine reuptake site densities in patients with social phobia. *American Journal of Psychiatry*, **154**(2), 239–242.

Tiihonen, J., Kuikka, J., Rasanen, P., Lepola, U., Koponen, H., Liuska, A., Lehmusvaara, A., Vainio, P., Kononen, M., Bergstrom, K., Yu, M., Kinnunen, I., Akerman, K. and Karhu, J., 1997. Cerebral benzodiazepine receptor binding and distribution in generalized anxiety disorder: a fractal analysis. *Molecular Psychiatry*, **2**(6), 463–471.

Tokunaga, M., Ida, I., Higuchi, T. and Mikuni, M., 1997. Alterations of benzodiazepine receptor binding potential in anxiety and somatoform disorders measured by 123I-iomazenil SPECT. *Radiation Medicine*, **15**(3), 163–169.

Weizman, A., Weizman, R., Kook, K.A., Vocci, F., Deutsch, S.I. and Paul, S.M., 1990. Adrenalectomy prevents the stress induced decrease in *in vivo* [3H]Ro15 1788 binding to GABAA benzodiazepine receptors in the mouse. *Brain Res.*, **519**, 347–350.

Weizman, R., Weizman, A., Kook, K.A., Vocci, F., Deutsch, S.I. and Paul, S.M., 1989. Repeated swim stress alters brain benzodiazepine receptors measured *in vivo*. *J. Pharmacol. Exp. Ther.*, **249**, 701–707.

Woods, S.W., Koster, K., Krystal, J.K., Smith, E.O., Zubal, I.G., Hoffer, P.B. and Charney, D.S., 1988. Yohimbine alters regional cerebral blood flow in panic disorder [letter]. *Lancet*, **2**(8612), 678.

Wu, J.C., Buchsbaum, M.S., Hershey, T.G., Hazlett, E., Sicotte, N. and Johnson, J.C., 1991. PET in generalized anxiety disorder. *Biological Psychiatry*, **29**(12), 1181–1199.

XIX-11

Neurogenetics of Anxiety Disorders

Ronit Weizman and Abraham Weizman

INTRODUCTION

Family and twin studies show that distinct and/or common genetic factors may play a role in anxiety disorders, although the magnitude of the genetic effect in each of the anxiety disorders is as yet unclear. A genetic liability apparently underlies the phenotypic expression of some of them; however, like other mental disorders, anxiety disorders exhibit a complex inheritance. That is, their transmission most likely requires the interaction of several genes and environmental factors that may predispose individuals to the disorder but do not always lead to its full clinical expression. Anxiety disorders may share a common genetic background with depression, as evidenced by the frequent coexistence of depressive and anxiety symptoms and the response of the anxiety disorders to antidepressant agents. The advances in genetic molecular technology and genetic epidemiology may help researchers to identify the genes contributing to the predisposition to these disorders and to clarify the interaction between genetic and environmental factors. However, in addition to the common difficulties of the molecular genetics of complex diseases, namely, non-Mendelian inheritance patterns, incomplete penetrance, possibility of phenocopies, genetic heterogeneity, and variable expressivity (Lander and Schork, 1994), the major problem in the neurogenetic study of anxiety disorders is the definition of the heritable phenotype (Tsuang, Faraone and Lyons, 1993; Smoller and Tsuang, 1998).

PANIC DISORDER

Family Studies

Family studies have consistently shown that panic disorder (PD), with or without agoraphobia, is a familial phenotype (Tsuang, Faraone and Lyons, 1993; Vieland *et al.*, 1996). First-degree relatives of probands with PD show a 3- to 21-fold higher lifetime risk of the disorder than relatives of unaffected probands. Goldstein *et al.* (1997) found that the risks of PD in adult first-degree relatives of probands was 17-fold higher when the age of onset in the proband was 20 years or less, but only six-fold higher when onset was after age 20 years.

First-degree asymptomatic relatives of patients with PD have a tendency to be more reactive to the CO_2 challenge test (Perna *et al.*, 1996). Furthermore, Perna *et al.* (1996) showed that PD probands with CO_2 hypersensitivity accounted for most of the familial loading. It seems that CO_2 hypersensitivity may be due to a particular genetic dysfunction and individuate a genetically homogeneous subgroup of patients with PD (endophenotype).

Twin Studies

Twin and adoption studies serve as a powerful tool in genetic research. The comparison of concordance rates between monozygotic (MZ) and dizygotic (DZ) twins can help clinicians estimate heritability, which is an index of the contribution of genetic factors to vulnerability to a disorder.

An effect of genetic factors in PD was shown in an early study by Torgersen (1983) who found that PD and agoraphobia with panic attacks were five times as frequent in MZ than in same-sex DZ twins. Ten years later, Kendler *et al.* (1993) assessed 2163 women from a population-based twin registry and noted only a modest familial aggregation of PD on multifactorial-threshold analysis, the best estimates of the heritability of liability ranged from 30% to 40%. In a subsequent study, this team examined the structure of the genetic and environmental risk factors for six major psychiatric disorders (phobia, generalized anxiety disorder, panic disorder, bulimia, major depression, and alcoholism) in an epidemiologic sample of 1030 female–female twin pairs with known zygosity (Kendler *et al.*, 1995). The estimated heritability of PD was 44%. The twin concordancerate for PD was also studied by Bellodi *et al.* (1998) in a sample of 90 same-sex twin pairs. They found that the probandwise concordance rates for PD were significantly higher in the MZ than in the DZ pairs (67% vs 0%), as were the concordance rates for spontaneous panic attacks (71% vs 18%). For CO_2-induced PD, the rates were 55.6% and 12.5%, respectively. These data suggest a relevant role of genetic factors in CO_2-induced panic attacks. The marked differences indicate that the genetic relationship is complex and not simply additive.

Segregation Studies

Segregation analysis of pedigrees determines the mode of transmission of a disorder using mathematical methods. The inclusion of twin pairs or adoptive relatives enables quantification of the degree and nature of environmental effects. Pedigree analyses of PD have suggested that a single major locus contributes to the inheritance of the disorder, although the possibility of polygenic inheritance has not been completely ruled out. Pauls *et al.* (1980) analyzed 19 kindreds of PD patients and found that the disorder is transmitted as a Mendelian autosomal dominant trait with an allele frequency of 0.014, age-dependent penetrance, and average age of onset 21.9 years. Crowe *et al.* (1983), in a preliminary genetic analysis, tested the single major locus and multifactorial polygenic transmission models, and was unable to exclude either one. The best-fitting single-locus model predicted a disorder gene with an allele frequency of 0.05 and a penetrance of 45.5% in women and 24.6% in men. Vieland *et al.* (1996) performed a simple segregation analysis in 126 families of probands

Biological Psychiatry: Edited by H. D'haenen, J.A. den Boer and P. Willner. ISBN 0-471-49198-5

with DSM-III-R panic disorder and found comparable support for autosomal dominant and recessive models. The best-fitting dominant model predicted a disorder gene with an allele frequency of 0.01, a heterozygote penetrance of 50% and a phenocopy rate of 0.01. The best-fitting recessive model predicted a disorder gene with an allele frequency of 0.20, a homozygote penetrance of 70%, and a phenocopy rate of 0.01 among heterozygotes and normal homozygotes.

Finally, Cavallini and colleagues (1999b) performed a complex segregation analysis on a sample of 165 families of PD probands and on the subgroup homogeneous for CO_2 hypersensitivity. Their results fit a Mendelian hypothesis without distinction between different models of transmission. The analysis of the probands of 134 families found to be hypersensitive to CO_2 supported the existence of a single major locus model with a best fit for a dominant model.

Parent-of-Origin Effect

Since the lifetime risk of developing PD is higher in women than men (2 : 1), researchers have suggested it may be affected by the pattern of maternal vs paternal transmission. Using narrow and broad diagnostic models in a sample of 64 PD pedigrees, Haghighi *et al.* (1999) reported that the proportion of affected children born to a transmitting mother did not differ from the proportion born to a transmitting father, and there was no difference in the frequency of affected offspring from maternal or paternal transmission. However, when a subset of 'pure' pedigrees (including only maternal or paternal transmission of PD) was included under the broad diagnostic model, a significant difference was noted in the proportion of affected females and males from maternal (111 females and 23 males) and paternal (nine females and six males) transmissions. Furthermore, when affected and unaffected children were included in the analysis (excluding individuals with unknown status) the cumulative lifetime risk of PD for offspring of transmitting mothers was significantly higher than that of offspring of transmitting fathers. This finding may indicate that maternal transmission confers an increased susceptibility to PD on female offspring. Apparently, PD has a complex mode of inheritance, though further confirmation of the possibility of genomic imprinting or mitochondrial inheritance is still needed. By contrast, in a study of 38 families unlineally affected with PD and agoraphobia, Battaglia *et al.* (1999) noted no differences in sex distribution between offspring of transmitting mothers and offspring of transmitting fathers, nor was there a significant difference in the anticipation of age at onset of PD. The authors concluded that at least in their sample, there was no evidence of a parent-of-origin effect.

Molecular Genetics

Linkage Studies

As mentioned, some segregation analyses have suggested the involvement of a major gene in the aetiology of PD (Pauls *et al.*, 1980; Crowe *et al.*, 1983; Vieland *et al.*, 1996). These findings have prompted linkage analyses in families with multiple affected individuals. The aim of these studies is to pinpoint disease genes by showing that a genetic marker with a known genetic location tends to be transmitted along with the disease within families (Faraone, Tsuang and Tsuang, 1999).

Crowe *et al.* (1987b) studied 26 families segregating PD for linkage to 29 polymorphic blood group antigens and found a suggestion of linkage to the alpha-haptoglobin locus. However, this locus was later excluded by testing additional families with DNA markers (Crowe *et al.*, 1990). The candidate genes pro-opiomelanocortin (Crowe, Noyes and Persico, 1987a), tyrosine hydroxylase (Mutchler *et al.*, 1990), adrenergic receptor genes ($\alpha 1/\beta$ 2 pair on chromosome 5q32-q34, the $\alpha 2/\beta$ 1 pair on chromosome 10q24-q26, and a second $\alpha 2$ locus on chromosome 4) (Wang, Crowe and Noyes, 1992), Cys311 variant of dopamine receptor 2 (DRD2) (Crawford *et al.*, 1995), DRD4 and dopamine transporter (DAT) (Hamilton *et al.*, 2000a), the GABA-Aâl receptor (Schmidt, Zoega and Crowe, 1993) and GABA α1-5, β1, β3, γ2 (Crowe *et al.*, 1997) and the functional polymorphism in the promoter of the gene for serotonin transporter (5-HTT) (Hamilton *et al.*, 1999) have all been excluded.

Knowles *et al.* (1998) conducted a large-scale study on first-pass genomic screen for PD. They collected 23 multiplex families consisting of 368 individuals, of whom 269 were directly interviewed, and used 540 microsatellite DNA markers for genotyping. The data were analyzed with both a dominant and a recessive model. The authors failed to detect definitive evidence of linkage to PD (no lod scores exceed 2.0 for either dominant or recessive parametric model): they ruled out linkage over more than 95% of the genetic length of the autosomes under the homogeneous dominant model with reduced penetrance, and over 60% under the homogeneous recessive model with reduced penetrance. This team is currently trying to enlarge their sample size, refine the phenotype using an endophenotype (CO_2 sensitivity) (Perna *et al.*, 1996), and look for segregation of comorbid disorders. Since they failed to detect loci that contribute to the predisposition to develop PD in the genome-wide genetic screen, the authors concluded that the genetic structure of the disorder seems to be more complex than the simple autosomal and dominant recessive models. Crowe *et al.* (2001) performed a genome scan of 23 multiplex families of panic disorder, including 90 family members with PD and 23 members who had recurrent, spontaneous panic attacks that did not satisfy the full PD diagnostic criteria. Two-point lod scores were calculated with both a dominant and a recessive model, and maps of lod scores < -2.00, assuming genetic homogeneity, were constructed by using DSM-III-R panic disorder as the affected phenotype. The greatest lod score was 2.23 (theta $= 0.15$) at the D7S2846 locus, located at 57.8 cM on chromosome 7p.

A 10 cM linkage genome scan, in a set of 20 American pedigrees (153 subjects), ascertained through probands with panic disorder (PD), pointed towards two genomic regions which met criteria for suggestive linkage. One of these regions is on chromosome 1 (LOD score = 2.04) and the other (LOD score = 2.01) is located on chromosome 11p. For agoraphobia, the most promising potential linkage was on chromosome 3. The authors suggested that PD and agoraphobia are complex traits that share some, but not all, of their susceptibility loci (Gelernter *et al.*, 2001).

Association Studies: Candidate Genes

In this approach, candidate genes are selected on the basis of the biology of the disease, and molecular variants are sought. The distribution of different alleles of the candidate genes is compared between affected individuals and a non-related ethnically similar healthy population. If a particular allele is found to occur significantly more often among the affected persons, the researchers assume an association between the disease phenotype and a particular molecular variant of the gene. To overcome the pitfalls of case-control studies, some researchers perform family-based association studies wherein the control group is composed of the parents or siblings of affected individuals. In the haplotype relative risk (HRR) design, the untransmitted alleles of the parents serve as the ethnically matched controls (Stefanos, Dikeos and Papadimitrious, 1996) on the assumption that a variation in the distribution of alleles of the candidate genes can influence the expression of the genes or its properties. However, it is possible that this variation is not the actual cause of the biological expression but is in linkage disequilibrium with another molecular change (a mutation) which is the primary cause. While one advantage of association studies is their enhanced power to detect genes with small effects, their major disadvantage is the increased likelihood of false-positive results. One way to reduce the probability of first-order errors is to look for replication in an independent sample or verification in family-based internal controls allowing for linkage disequilibrium analysis using the HRR or transmission disequilibrium test (TDT).

Serotonin Transporter and Receptors

The serotonin transporter (5-HTT) regulates the sodium-dependent reuptake of serotonin into the presynaptic neuron. Platelet-binding studies have suggested a disruption in 5-HTT function in PD (Pecknold *et al.*, 1995). The 5-HTT is encoded by a gene (solute carrier six, member four; SLC6A4) on chromosome 17q11.1-q12 and is organized in 14 exons spanning about 13 kb. Recently, a functional deletion/insertion polymorphism was identified within the promoter of the 5-HTT gene (Heils *et al.*, 1996). *In vitro* research has shown that a polymorphism in the 5-HTT promoter region has an effect on gene expression wherein the long (L) allele of 5-HTT produces expression levels three times greater than the short (S) allele. Some researchers have claimed that this polymorphism (the S allele) may play a role in susceptibility to anxiety-related traits and affective disorders (Collier *et al.*, 1996; Lesch *et al.*, 1996). However, when the 5-HTT gene-linked promoter polymorphic region (5-HTTLPR) genotype and allele frequencies were compared between patients with PD and a control group, no differences were observed (Deckert *et al.*, 1997; Ishiguro *et al.*, 1997; Matsushita *et al.*, 1997). In a family-based study, 74 haplotype relative risk 'trios' were genotyped at the polymorphic locus, which consists of a 44 base pair deletion/insertion in the promoter region. There were no significant differences in allele frequencies or occurrence of genotypes within the triads (Hamilton *et al.*, 1999).

A challenge with m-chlorophenylpiperazine (mCPP), a non-selective 5-HT2C receptor agonist, is associated with emergence of panic attacks more frequently in PD patients as compared to normal controls (Germine *et al.*, 1994). Thus, 5-HT2C gene is a candidate genes for association studies in PD. The association between PD and two adjacent polymorphisms [(GT) 12-18 and (CT) 4-5] in the 5′-regulatory region of the X-chromosomal 5-HT2C was studied in German and an Italian sample (combined $n = 211$) of PD patients and compared it with allele frequencies in two ethnically matched control samples (combined $n = 226$) (Deckert *et al.*, 2000). In the German sample, a comparison of female genotypes containing the short polymorphism haplotype vs female genotypes containing only long haplotypes showed a significant difference ($p = 0.01$), However, such a difference could not be replicated in the Italian sample ($p = 0.54$). Thus it seems that these promoter-associated 5-HT2C receptor gene length polymorphisms do not have a major role in the genetics of PD.

Cholecystokinin

Cholecystokinin (CCK) is the most abundant neuropeptide in the mammalian brain and, in humans, it is expressed in significant quantities in all regions of the brain (Bradwejn and Koszychi, 1994a). The CCK receptors have been classified into two subtypes, CCK-A and CCK-B. A line of evidence suggests a possible role of the CCK system in the neurobiology of PD. The CCK receptor agonist CCK-tetrapeptide (CCK-4) has been found to provoke panic attacks in about half of all normal individuals and almost all patients with PD (Bradwejn, Koszycki and Shriqui, 1991). Furthermore, CCK-4-induced panic attacks can be blocked by imipramine (Bradwejn and Koszycki, 1994b), a tricyclic antidepressant which is efficacious in the treatment of PD. Patients with PD also show lower cerebrospinal fluid (CSF) and lymphocyte CCK concentrations than normal controls (Bradwejn, Koszycki and Shriqui, 1991). A search for mutations in the CCK gene in 30 probands of multiplex PD pedigrees was conducted by Wang *et al.* (1998). They identified a C $\rightarrow$ T transition at position-36 ($CCK_{-36C/T}$) in a GC box, a binding site for transcription factor Sp1, in the promoter region of the gene. However, a study on the function of the $CCK_{-36C/T}$ polymorphism in the human CCK gene promoter (Hansen, Rehfeld and Nielsen, 2000) showed that the C to T polymorphism does not affect CCK transcription or function, and therefore does not play a direct role in the pathogenesis of PD. The putative association of this polymorphism to PD is likely to be the result of co-segregation with a linked mutation. Another study of CCK polymorphism in 99 patients with PD compared to healthy controls matched for gender and ethnicity showed no significant differences in the CCK peptide gene or the CCK-A gene markers (Kennedy *et al.*, 1999). However, there was a significant association of a CCK-B polymorphism with PD, suggesting a role for this gene in the susceptibility to PD. A later study (Yamada *et al.*, 2001) including 91 unrelated Japanese patients and 100 matched controls did not find evidence for an association between PD and four confirmed polymorphic sites in the CCK-B receptor gene, i.e., three at exon 3 : 1550 G $\rightarrow$ A, 1962 T $\rightarrow$ C and 1985 G $\rightarrow$ A and one at intron 4 : 2491 C $\rightarrow$ A.

In a recent study (Hattori *et al.*, 2001) a polymorphic compound short tandem repeat (STR) stretch located in the 5′-upstream region of the cholecystokinin gene, approximately −2.2 to −1.8 kb from the cap site was identified. This STR was found to be with 10 different allele lengths. Dividing the STR alleles into three classes (Long: L, Medium: M, and Short: S) produced strong genotypic (MM) (nominal $P = 0.0014$) and allelic (M) (nominal $P = 0.0079$) associations with panic disorder. No such association was found with three single nucleotide polymorphisms (SNPs) in the CCK promoter region: −36C > T and −188A > G, and the rare −345G > C. Haplotypic distributions of the STR and SNPs −188 and −36 were significantly different between panic disorder patients and controls ($P = 0.0003$). The authors suggest that the novel STR or a nearby variant may confer susceptibility to the development of panic disorder.

Monoamine Oxidase-A

The monoamine oxidase-A (MAO-A) inhibitor moclobemide, like other antidepressants, has been reported to be effective in the treatment of PD (Tiller, Bouwer and Behnke, 1999). This makes the MAO-A gene, which is localized on chromosome X (Xp21-p11) (Ozelius *et al.*, 1988), a candidate gene for PD.

A possible association between a functional polymorphism in the MAO-A gene promoter and PD was investigated in two independent German ($n = 80$) (Sabol, Hu and Hamer, 1998) and Italian ($n = 129$) (Deckert *et al.*, 1999) samples. Four alleles [3, 3a, 4 and 5 30 base pair (bp) repeats] of the MAO-A gene promoter polymorphism were observed in both samples. The 3a allele contained three repeats plus 18 bp of the repeated motif. An additional rare fifth allele (two 30 bp repeats) was detected in the Italian sample. Functional characterization in a luciferase assay demonstrated that the longer alleles (3a, 4 and 5) were more active than allele 3. In both the German and Italian samples, the longer alleles were significantly more frequent in females with PD compared with female controls; no such significant difference was observed for males. The authors calculated that in females, homozygosity for the long alleles increases the relative risk over heterozygosity as well as homozygosity for the short alleles by factors of 1.4 and 1.8. They suggested that the discrepancy between the males and females may be related to the relatively smaller number of males, so that the statistical power to display significant differences of the magnitude found in females was very low (~14%). The discrepancy between the male and female patients with PD may also be related to gender differences in the genetic background of PD. The consistency of this finding in two independent samples from different geographic areas makes it unlikely that the association between long alleles of the MAO-A gene promoter polymorphism and PD was a false-positive finding. However, replicative studies as well as verification in haplotype relative risk samples with family-based internal controls are still required. Indeed in one recent family-based study including 620 individuals in 70 multiplex families and 81 triads consisting of proband (62 female and 19 male), mother and father, the authors failed to demonstrate a genetic linkage or association between the same functional promoter polymorphism in the MAO-A gene and PD (Hamilton *et al.*, 2000b). From the pathophysiological and pharmacological points of view, the association between genotype-related high MAO-A activity and PD symptoms (panic attacks, anticipatory anxiety or phobic avoidance) as well as the therapeutic response to MAO-A inhibitors merits further investigation.

α_2 Adrenergic Receptor

Three different genes coding for human α_2 receptor subtypes α_{2A}, α_{2B} and α_{2C} have been cloned and localized on chromosomes 10, 2 and 4, respectively (Bylund *et al.*, 1994). The α_{2A} receptor subtype is expressed in the central nervous system and peripheral tissues, the α_{2B} in the liver and kidneys, and the α_{2C} only in the brain (Lorenz *et al.*, 1990). Yohimbine, an α_2 adrenergic receptor antagonist, has been found to induce marked anxiety and panic attacks in patients with PD (Charney *et al.*, 1987). However, in a study of a polymorphism of the α_{2A} receptor gene in the promoter region at position −1291 in 55 patients with PD and 114 healthy control subjects, Ohara *et al.* (2000) reported no statistically significant difference between the groups in either genotype or allele frequency. These results are in accordance with the linkage study of Wang, Crowe and Noyes, (1992) which revealed no evidence to support the possibility that a genetic mutation at the α_{2A} and α_{2C} receptor loci is responsible for PD.

Adenosine Receptor

The rationale for searching for adenosine receptor gene mutations or polymorphisms in PD is based on the finding that the adenosine receptor antagonist caffeine can provoke panic attacks in patients with PD, and on the similarity between symptoms of caffeine intoxication and anxiety (Boulenger *et al.*, 1984). Deckert *et al.* (1998) screened 38 patients with PD for mutations in the coding sequence of the A_1 and A_{2a} adenosine receptor genes. One silent mutation (716T/G) in the A_1 receptor gene and two silent mutations (432C/T and 1083C/T) in the A_{2a} receptor gene were detected. Thereafter, an association study between the identified DNA sequence variants and PD was performed in an extended sample of 89 patients and matched controls, and it yielded a significant association between PD and the 1083T allele and 1083T/T genotype of the A_{2a} receptor gene. These findings support the hypothesis that the A_{2a} receptor gene, or a locus in linkage disequilibrium with it, confers susceptibility to PD. Yamada *et al.* (2001) in a case-control study in Japanese population did not find evidence for an association between the 1083C → T polymorphism in the A_{2a} receptor gene and PD. Hamilton *et al.* (2001) in a family-based design, employing 596 individuals in 70 panic disorder pedigrees, as well as 77 haplotype relative risk 'triads', examined any linkage or association between the single nucleotide polymorphism in the SP1 site of the CCK gene (in the promoter region) and a simple sequence repeat in the CCK-B receptor, and panic disorder. Employing a variety of diagnostic and genetic models, linkage analysis produced no significant lod scores at either locus. Family-based tests of association, the HRR statistic and the TDT, were likewise non-significant. These two recent studies provide little support for the role of these polymorphisms in CCK and CCK−B receptor in PD.

Dopamine Transporter and D4 Receptor

Challenge studies with dopaminergic agonists such as apomorphine (Pitchot *et al.*, 1992) and epidemiological data associating the use of the dopamine agonist cocaine with PD (Anthony, Tien and Petronis, 1989) provide modest evidence for the possible involvement of a dopaminergic component in PD. A family-based design, with 622 individuals in 70 families, as well as 82 HRR 'triad' families, was employed to detect a possible association between either dopamine transporter (DAT) or dopamine receptor 4 (DRD4) gene polymorphisms and PD (Hamilton *et al.*, 2000a). Three common polymorphisms were studied; two were in DRD4, a 12 bp insertion/deletion in exon 1 and a 48 bp repeat in exon 3, and one was a 40 bp repeat in the three untranslated regions of DAT. Alleles in the triad families were analyzed with the HRR method as well as the TDT statistic. There were no significant differences in allele frequencies or occurrence of genotypes within the triads for any of the three polymorphisms, indicating the absence of involvement of these polymorphisms in susceptibility to PD.

Table XIX-11.1 demonstrates the association studies reported in patients with PD.

PHOBIC DISORDERS

Family Studies

In a direct-interview study of first-degree relatives of probands with social phobia (SP) ($n = 83$) and never mentally ill controls ($n = 231$), Fyer *et al.* (1993) reported that the study group had a significantly increased risk of SP (16% vs 5%, relative risk = 3.12), but not of other anxiety disorders. In a subsequent study, the same authors assessed the rates of phobic disorders in first-degree relatives of four proband groups: simple phobia, SP, agoraphobia with panic attacks, and healthy controls (Fyer *et al.*, 1995). They found a moderate (two- to four-fold increased risk) but specific familial aggregation for each of the three phobic disorders (10% for agoraphobia, 15% for SP and 31% for simple phobia). The relative risk for agoraphobia was 2.7, for SP 3.1, and for simple phobia 3.3. The moderate elevations in familial risk indicate a familial contribution to each of the disorders. The mode of transmission is unknown and seems to be multifactorial complex.

In a direct-interview family study, Stein *et al.* (1998) assessed the familial liability for the discrete (performance-only), non-generalized [performance-only, limited-interactional-only (one or two socially interactive situations), or performance-plus-limited-interactional types of phobia], and generalized subtypes (DSM-IV criteria) of SP in 23 probands with generalized SP and their first-degree family relatives ($n = 106$) and 24 healthy subjects and their relatives ($n = 74$). The generalized subtype of SP was found to be present in 26.4% of the relatives of probands with generalized SP but only 2.7% of the relatives of probands in the comparison group. By contrast, the relative risks for discrete SP and non-generalized SP were not significantly different between the two groups. The authors concluded that only the generalized type (and its probable Axis II counterpart, avoidant personality disorder) occurs more often among the families of probands with generalized SP.

Twin Studies

The genetic epidemiology of phobias was studied in a population-based sample of 2163 female twins (Kendler *et al.*, 1992). The familial aggregation of agoraphobia, SP, situational phobia, and

Table XIX-11.1 Association studies in PD

Candidate gene	Polymorphism	Population	Analysis	Significance	Reference
Serotonin transporter	44-bp insertion/deletion (promoter)	Japanese	Case-control	NS	Ishiguro *et al.* (1997)
		German	Case-control	NS	Deckert *et al.* (1997)
		Japanese	Case-control	NS	Matushita *et al.* (1997)
Cholecystokinin	−36 C/T (promoter)	American	Case-control	$P < 0.05$	Wang *et al.* (1998)
		Canadian	Case-control	NS	Kennedy *et al.* (1999)
CCK-A receptor	New polymorphism	Canadian	Case-control	NS	Kennedy *et al.* (1999)
CCK-B receptor	Single nucleotide polymorphism	Canadian	Case-control	NS	Kennedy *et al.* (1999)
CCK-B receptor	CT repeats polymorphism (promoter)	Canadian	Case-control	$P < 0.004$	Kennedy *et al.* (1999)
Monoamine oxidase-A	30-bp repeats (promoter)	German and Italian	Case-control	Male: NS Female: $P = 0.001$	Deckert *et al.* (1999)
		American	Family-based	NS	Hamilton *et al.* (2000b)
α_{2A} adrenergic receptor	MspI, position — 1291 (promoter)	Japanese	Case-control	NS	Ohara *et al.* (2000)
A_2 adenosine receptor	1083 C/T allele (silent) in exon 2	German	Case-control	$P = 0.01$	Deckert *et al.* (1998)
		Japanese	Case-control	NS	Yamada *et al.* (2001)
Dopamine receptor 4	12-bp insertion/deletion in exon 1	American	Family-based	NS	Hamilton *et al.* (2000a)
	48-bp repeat in exon 3	American	Family-based	NS	Hamilton *et al.* (2000a)
Dopamine transporter	40-bp repeat in the 3 untranslated region	American	Family-based	NS	Hamilton *et al.* (2000a)

bp = base pair; CCK = cholecystokinin

simple phobia appeared to be due to genetic and not familial-environmental factors, with estimates of heritability of liability ranging from 30% to 40%. The authors concluded that the best-fitting multivariate genetic model indicates the existence of genetic and individual-specific environmental aetiologic factors. Nonspecific shared environmental experiences were most important for agoraphobia and SP, and unique environmental experiences for simple phobias. Genetic factors were most important in the predisposition to animal phobia and least important for agoraphobia. Thus, the simple phobias seem to result from the common effect of a modest genetic vulnerability and phobia-specific traumatic event in childhood, whereas agoraphobia and SP result from the combined effect of a more pronounced genetic influence and nonspecific environmental experiences.

Molecular Genetics

Linkage and Association Studies

A line of evidence from molecular genetics studies support the claim that SP, particularly the generalized form, is familial, and is frequently associated with at least one other anxiety disorder and with major depressive disorder. Furthermore, its apparent responsiveness to treatment with selective serotonin reuptake inhibitors (SSRIs) suggest the possible involvement of the serotonergic system in the genetic susceptibility to SP. Stein *et al.* (1998) excluded a possible genetic linkage of generalized SP to the serotonin transporter protein (promoter region) and $5HT_{2A}$ receptor genes. Seventeen multiplex families (122 subjects) were included in the study. In additional studies, the MspI silent T → C 102 polymorphism at the HTR2A gene (Warren *et al.*, 1993) and the insertion/deletion polymorphism in the promoter region of the serotonin transporter gene (Heils *et al.*, 1996) were genotyped, and LOD scores for pairwise analyses were calculated. Linkage studies to other 5-HT receptor subtypes as well as other regions of the genome were not performed as yet.

Gratacòs *et al.* (2001) identified a polymorphic interstitial duplication of human chromosome 15q24-26 (named DUP25), which is significantly associated with panic/agoraphobia/social phobia/joint laxity in families, and with panic disorder in non-familial cases. The authors proposed that DUP25, which is present in 7% control subjects, is a susceptibility factor for a clinical phenotype that includes panic and phobic disorders and joint laxity.

OBSESSIVE–COMPULSIVE DISORDER

The concept of a spectrum of OCD disorders has recently been suggested, including Tourette's syndrome, body dysmorphic disorder hypochondriasis, trichotillomania, pathological gambling, and other impulse control disorders (Hollander *et al.*, 1996). This broader definition of OCD poses problems in defining the phenotype of OCD in family and twin studies as well as in molecular genetic studies. Future research on age of onset, comorbidity, treatment, neuropsychological functioning, personality characteristics and neuroimaging will help to elucidate subsets of endophenotypes of the disorder, and these will broaden our understandings of its neurobiological and genetic mechanisms.

Family Studies

Lenane *et al.* (1990), who interviewed 145 first-degree relatives (89 parents and 56 siblings) of 46 children and adolescents with OCD, found that the familial rate of OCD was higher than the expected rate in the general population (30% of patients had at least one first-degree relative with OCD). Furthermore, there was a difference in the presenting symptoms of OCD in the probands and their relatives, indicating the possibility of genetic involvement rather than simple social or cultural transmission.

A possible aetiologic relationship between Tourette's disorder and OCD has been shown by several researchers. Leonard *et al.* (1992) re-evaluated 54 children with OCD, of whom 57% also had a lifetime history of tics, 2–7 years after the initial diagnosis of OCD. The presence or absence of tics and Tourette's disorder was also assessed in their first-degree relatives ($n = 171$). At follow-up, 59% ($n = 32$) of the probands were found to have a lifetime history of tics, including eight, all males, who met the criteria for Tourette's disorder. This subgroup had a younger age at onset of OCD. Tourette's disorder was noted in 1.8% of their relatives, and a tic disorder, in 14%. These results indicate that in some cases, OCD and Tourette's disorder may be alternative manifestations of the same underlying illness. In a similar study, Pauls *et al.* (1995) as well as Nestadt *et al.* (2000b) also demonstrated the heterogeneity of OCD, including familial tic-related OCD, familial tic-unrelated OCD, and sporadic OCD.

The familial relationship between OCD and other OCD spectrum disorders was investigated in 80 patients with OCD and their 343 first-degree relatives compared to 73 control probands and their 300 first-degree relatives (Bienvenu *et al.*, 2000). Body dysmorphic disorder, hypochondriasis, eating disorders, nail biting, skin picking, and trichotillomania all occurred more frequently in the case probands and their relatives, whether or not the case probands also had the same diagnosis. These data indicate that these conditions are part of the familial OCD spectrum. However, Black *et al.* (1994), in an earlier study, failed to find significant differences in the lifetime prevalences of anorexia nervosa, bulimia nervosa, or pathologic gambling between first-degree relatives of patients with OCD and first-degree relatives of control subjects.

Twin Studies

Inouye (1965) found an 80% concordance for OCD between pairs of MZ twins ($n = 10$) compared to 20% concordance between pairs of DZ twins ($n = 4$). Higher concordance rates in MZ than DZ twins were also reported by Carey and Gottesman (1981) (87% and 47%, respectively). In addition, the nature of the symptoms and response to treatment were more similar for the MZ twins (Kim, Dysken and Kline, 1990). Unfortunately, all these studies were performed in small samples and did not use blind methodology, so definite conclusions concerning the contribution of genetic factors cannot be made.

Segregation Studies

Cavallini *et al.* (1999a) performed a complex segregation analysis on a sample of 107 Italian families of OCD probands. Based on the hypothesis that OCD shares common underlying genetic factor(s) with Tourette's disorder (Pauls *et al.*, 1986), the authors applied two phenotypic definitions of affected subjects: OCD with and without Tourette's disorder/chronic motor tics. Analysis of the transmission of OCD alone (wherein relatives with Tourette's disorder or chronic motor tics were considered healthy) provided support for a major gene effect. However, when the phenotype was widened, the pattern of inheritance (dominant, recessive or additive) could not be established. Given the phenotypic heterogeneity observed in OCD, Alsobrook *et al.* (1999) studied inheritance patterns using symptom-based factor scores. Analyses limited to families with symmetry and ordering (high factor 3) probands led to a rejection of the polygenic model. Additionally, the relative risk of OCD or subclinical OCD was 1.7 for relatives of probands with a high factor 3 score compared with relatives of probands with a low factor 3 score. In this study patients were defined as having subclinical OCD if they met all DSM-III-R criteria for OCD except one of the following: their obsessions/compulsions consumed less than one hour per day, or they lacked insight into the unreasonable nature of their obsessions and compulsions. The authors suggested that these symptoms may constitute a genetically symptomatic subtype of OCD. In a recent large-scale study with a well-characterized sample, Nestadt *et al.* (2000a) analyzed 80 case families (423 subjects, including adult OCD probands and their first-degree relatives), and 73 control families (373 subjects, including probands and their first-degree relatives) for mode of inheritance. OCD was the only affected phenotype. The results provided further evidence of a Mendelian inheritance of a dominant allele. However, Mendelian factors alone could not fully explain the familial aggregation of this phenotype, and residual familial and sex effects probably play a role in the inheritance of the disorder. Thereafter, polygenic factors may also contribute to the aetiology of OCD. It is of note that this study included both case and control families; thus, the estimated disease frequencies and penetrances were likely less biased.

Molecular Genetics

The family, twin and segregation studies have consistently suggested that the underlying mechanisms of OCD involve genes of major effect. The recent progress in molecular genetic methods has encouraged the search for genes that confer susceptibility to complex diseases, including OCD.

Linkage Studies and Mutation Screening

In a study of a large British kindred multiply affected with Tourette's syndrome, chronic motor tics, and obsessive–compulsive behavior, Brett *et al.* (1995) reported no evidence to support the hypothesis that a genetic variation in the serotonin 5-HT1A receptor and tryptophan oxygenase genes causes susceptibility to Tourette's syndrome and chronic multiple tics.

Interaction between the glutamatergic and serotonergic systems within the striatum suggests the glutamate transporter protein as a functional candidate in OCD. The gene (SLC1A1) for this protein is localized in chromosome 9. Genomic organization of this gene and mutation screening was investigated in families of patients with early-onset OCD (Veenstra-VanderWeele *et al.*, 2001). No evidence was found for a functional mutation and capillary electrophoresis single-stranded conformational polymorphism (SSCP) analysis of a haplotype consisting of two common SNPs within this gene revealed no significant linkage disequilibrium.

Association Studies

The findings of the association studies in OCD are summarized in Table XIX-11.2.

The Serotonergic System

Pharmacological and neurochemical studies point to a dysregulation of the serotonergic system in OCD. SSRIs are effective in the treatment of OCD; exacerbations are common when SSRIs are discontinued (McDougle, Gordman and Price, 1993). Challenge with meta-chlorophenyl-piperazine (mCPP), a mainly serotonin 2C receptor agonist, can induce the emergence of symptoms in patients with OCD (Zohar *et al.*, 1987). Finally, OCD patients have lower platelet serotonin transporter (5-HTT) density than normal controls (Weizman *et al.*, 1986, 1992). It is of note that recent studies have reported an association between a polymorphism in the serotonin transporter gene regulatory region and anxiety-related

Table XIX-11.2 Association studies in OCD

Candidate gene	Polymorphism	Population	Analysis	Significance	Reference
Serotonin transporter	44-bp insertion/deletion (promoter)	European-American	TDT	$P < 0.03$	McDougle *et al.* (1998)
		Caucasian	Case-control	$P = 0.023$	Bengel *et al.* (1999)
		Canadian	Case-control	NS	Billet *et al.* (1997)
		Ashkenazi and Sephardic Jews	Case-control	NS	Frisch *et al.* (2000)
		Afrikaner	Case-control	NS	Kinnear *et al.* (2000)
	VNTR in the 2nd intron	Japanese	Case-control	0.032	Ohara *et al.* (1999)
Tryptophan hydroxylase (TPH)	BfaI	Ashkenazi and Sephardic Jews	Case-control	NS	Frisch *et al.* (2000)
Serotonin receptor 2A	T102C	Mexican	Case-control	NS	Nicolini *et al.* (1996)
	MspI	Ashkenazi and Sephardic Jews	Case-control	NS	Frisch *et al.* (2000)
Serotonin receptor 2C	Cys23Ser mutation	Italian	Case-control	NS	Cavallini *et al.* (1998)
		Ashkenazi and Sephardic Jews	Case-control	NS	Frisch *et al.* (2000)
Serotonin receptor 1Dβ	Silent G861C	Italy	TDT/ sub-TDT	$P < 0.006$	Mundo *et al.* (2000)
Dopamine receptor 2	TaqIA	Canadian	Case-control	NS	Billett *et al.* (1998)
Dopamine receptor 3	Msc I	Italian	Case-control	NS	Catalano *et al.* (1994)
		Canadian	Case-control	NS	Billett *et al.* (1998)
Dopamine receptor 4	48-bp repeat in exon 3	Canadian	Case-control	$P < 0.05$	Billett *et al.* (1998)
		Ashkenazi and Sephardic Jews	Case-control	NS	Frisch *et al.* (2000)
Dopamine transporter	40-bp VNTR	Ashkenazi and Sephardic Jews	Case-control	NS	Frisch *et al.* (2000)
Catechol-0-methyltransferase	G158A	American Caucasians	Case-control	$P = 0.0002$ in male OCD; NS in females	Karayiorgou *et al.* (1997)
		American Caucasians	TDT and HRR	$P = 0.0079$ and $P = 0.0079$ in male OCD; NS in females	Karayiorgou *et al.* (1999)
		American and Canadian	TDT and HRR	NS	Schindler *et al.* (2000)
		Afrikaner	Case-control	$P = 0.0017$	Niehaus *et al.* (2001)
	Promoter region	Afrikaner	Case-control	NS	Kinnear *et al.* (2001)
Monoamine oxidase-A	*Fnu*4H1 polymorphism in exon 8		TDT and HRR	$P = 0.0186$ and $P = 0.0129$ in male OCD; NS in females	Karayiorgou *et al.* (1999)
	EcoRV polymorphism	Mexican	HRR	$P < 0.05$ in female OCD;	Karayiorgou *et al.* (1999)

bp = base pairs; TDT = transmission disequilibrium test; VNTR = variable-number-tandem repeat; HRR = haplotype relative risk.

traits (Lesch *et al.*, 1996) as well as susceptibility to affective disorders (Collier *et al.*, 1996).

Serotonin Transporter

McDougle *et al.* (1998) found evidence of linkage disequilibrium between the serotonin transporter protein gene (SLC6A4) in the promoter region and OCD. The investigators used the TDT design, which examines linkage in the presence of association in affected probands and their biological parents and thereby controls for the stratification effect. The study included 34 European–American family trios, 30 unrelated and four extracted from an extended pedigree. Of the 35 heterozygous parents, 24 transmitted the long (L) allele and 11 transmitted the short (S) allele ($p < 0.03$) to the OCD probands. Separate analysis of the SRI non-responders ($n = 13$) yielded 10 parents who transmitted the L allele and three who transmitted the S allele ($p = 0.052$). Bengel *et al.* (1999) reported an association of a functional polymorphism in the 5-HTTLPR with OCD in a population-based study of 75 Caucasian patients with OCD and 397 ethnically matched individuals. The patients were found to be more likely to carry two copies of the long allele (L) (46.7% vs 32.3%: $\chi^2 = 5.19$, $p = 0.023$). However, this finding did not agree with the study of Billet *et al.* (1997) of 72 patients with OCD and 72 matched controls, which revealed no significant between-group difference in either genotype count or allele frequencies. Furthermore, no significant 5-HTT genetic difference was observed between the patients who responded to SSRIs and those who did not. The possible association of OCD with the insertion/deletion polymorphism in the promoter area of the serotonin transporter gene was also analyzed by Frisch *et al.* (2000) in 77 biologically unrelated OCD patients and ethnically matched controls (Ashkenazi and Sephardic Jews). There was no difference between patients and controls in the allelic distribution of the 5-HTT gene promoter region polymorphism. Similar negative results were reported also in a relatively genetically homogeneous Afrikaner population of South Africa (Kinnear *et al.*, 2000).

A case-control study of a possible association between 5-HTTLPR polymorphism and Tourette syndrome with and without OCD was carried out by Cavallini *et al.* (2000). The study included 52 patients (53.84% with OCD) and 63 healthy control subjects. No association was found, even when the study sample was divided by the presence or absence of OCD or family history of OCD or tics.

Ohara *et al.* (1999) compared the variable-number-tandem-repeat (VNTR) in the second intron of the 5-HTT gene between 103 patients with anxiety disorders and 106 controls. They found that the frequency of the allele containing 12 copies of the VNTR element (5-HTTin2.12) was significantly higher in the patients with OCD ($n = 15$) and that the presence of the 5-HTTin2.12 allele was significantly associated with the risk of OCD (odds ratio = 10.2, 95% CI 1.34-77.4).

Serotonin Receptors and Tryptophan Hydroxylase

Variants of the genes encoding the serotonin receptors 5-HT2A and 5-HT2C are not associated with OCD. Nicolini *et al.* (1996) studied 5HT2A gene polymorphisms in 67 OCD patients and 54 healthy controls and found no statistically significant between-group differences in either genotype or allele frequencies. Cavallini *et al.* (1998) investigated the role of the Cys23Ser mutation of the 5-HT2C receptor gene in OCD in a case-control study of comparing 109 OCD patients with 107 healthy control subjects. Again, no allelic or genotypic association was revealed. Furthermore, in a subsample of 39 patients with OCD who had previously undergone a challenge test with clomipramine, no association was noted between the 5-HT2C receptor gene mutation and the response to the test. This finding excludes any specific role for the Cys23Ser mutation of the 5-HT2C receptor gene in the aetiology of OCD.

The 5-HT1Dβ is a terminal autoreceptor, involved in the regulation of 5HT release, and it is expressed mostly in the limbic region and in the striatum. It is encoded by an intronless gene located on chromosome 6 (6q14-15) (Demchshyn *et al.* 1992). There are at least three polymorphisms known for this gene: the G861C, the T-261G, and the T371G (Lappalainen *et al.*, 1995; Mundo *et al.*, 2001). Gross *et al.* (1998) reported that acute administration of sumatriptan, a selective agonist of the 5-HT1Dβ receptor, was associated with acute worsening of obsessive–compulsive symptoms in patients with OCD. However, OCD patients resistant to conventional pharmacotherapy have shown improvements with chronic administration of sumatriptan (Stern *et al.*, 1998). Mundo *et al.* (2000) investigated the possibility of a linkage disequilibrium between the 5-HT1Dβ receptor gene G861C polymorphism and OCD using a combination of the TDT, which examines alleles preferentially transmitted from parents to affected offspring, with the sib-TDT, which compares the marker genotypes in affected and unaffected siblings. Sixty-seven OCD probands and their biological parents and siblings participated in the study. After genotyping, 32 families were found suitable for the TDT/sib-TDT procedure. Twenty-two were triads that showed heterozygosity at the marker, and 10 were sibships with one affected and one unaffected sibling. The authors found a significant linkage disequilibrium between the G861C variant of the 5-HT1Dβ receptor gene and OCD, with preferential transmission of the G allele to the affected subjects.

In a case-control study no association was found between OCD and polymorphism in the gene coding tryptophan hydroxylase (TPH), the key enzyme in the synthesis of 5-HT (Frisch *et al.*, 2000).

Dopamine Receptors and Transporter

The involvement of dopamine in the pathophysiology of OCD has been suggested by several pharmacological studies. Addition of dopamine receptor blockers seem to be effective in some SRI-resistant patients with OCD, especially those with comorbid tic disorder or psychotic features (McDougle, Goodman and Price, 1994). Accordingly, cocaine, which blocks the presynaptic dopamine transporter, can aggravate obsessive–compulsive symptoms in patients with OCD and induce such symptoms in subjects with a family history, but not a personal history, of OCD (Satel and McDougle, 1993).

Catalano *et al.* (1994) studied the D3 dopamine receptor gene polymorphisms in 97 patients with OCD and 97 control subjects. No statistically significant differences in allele or genotype frequencies were found. Negative results were reported also by Frisch *et al.* (2000) in a study of the possible association between OCD (75 patients and 172 controls), the D4 dopamine receptor gene and dopamine transporter gene.

In another case-control association study of 100 OCD patients and matched controls, Billett and his group (1998) examined a 40-base-pair repeat in the dopamine transporter gene; the TaqIA polymorphism and the serine/cysteine variation in the D2 dopamine receptor gene; the MscI polymorphism in the D3 dopamine receptor gene; and a 48-base-pair repeat in the D4 dopamine receptor gene. Significant differences in allele frequencies were found between patients and controls only for the D4 receptor gene.

Catechol-O-Methyltransferase

Catechol-O-methyltransferase (COMT) is an Mg^{2+}-dependent enzyme that catalyzes the transfer of methyl groups from S-adenosyl methionine to a hydroxyl group of a catecholic substrate. COMT is widely distributed in the mammalian brain. The gene for COMT, which is involved in the inactivation of catecholamines including the neurotransmitters dopamine and norepinephrine, has been mapped to the 22q11 region (Grossman, Emanuel and Budarf, 1992). In humans, a common functional polymorphism is associated with a three- to four-fold variation in COMT enzyme activity. This variation in activity is due to a GA transition at codon 158 of the COMT gene that results in a valine (high-activity allele, COMT*H)-to-methionine (low-activity allele, COMT*L) substitution (Lachman *et al.*, 1996).

Karayiorgou *et al.* (1997), in a study of 73 Caucasian patients with OCD (42 males and 31 females) and 148 ethnically matched and unrelated control subjects (75 males and 73 females), found that the COMT*L allele was significantly associated in a recessive manner with susceptibility to OCD, particularly in males. Furthermore, the COMT*L/COMT*L genotype was apparently a risk factor for OCD, with an estimated relative risk of 5.91 (95% CI: 2.40-14.53) versus the nonCOMT*L/COMT*L. These findings were later confirmed by the same group in a family-based study (Karayiorgou *et al.*, 1999) wherein the inheritance of the two functional variants of the COMT gene was investigated in 110 nuclear OCD families (affected proband and both biological parents). Both the TDT and HRR analyses revealed a preferential transmission of the low-activity COMT allele from the heterozygous parents of male (but not female) probands. This finding indicates a sexually dimorphic pattern of genetic susceptibility to OCD. Another family-based population study, in a group of 72 North American and Canadian OCD patient/parent trios, using the HRR TDT analyses, did not identify an association between a particular allele and OCD. Furthermore, no evidence was found to support the findings of a gender-based association for COMT. However, a genotype analysis demonstrated a tendency for association between homozygosity at the COMT locus and OCD (Schindler *et al.*, 2000). In contrast, a case-control study in Afrikaner community population found that heterozygosity (COMT*H/COMT*L genotype) was significantly more common than expected in OCD patients ($P = 0.0017$) (Niehaus *et al.*, 2001). No association was found between OCD and a novel polymorphism adjacent to the oestrogen response element (ERE 6) in the promoter region of the COMT gene (Kinnear *et al.*, 2001).

In a recent study by Cavallini *et al.* (2000) of 52 patients with Tourette disorder with or without OCD and 63 healthy control subjects, no association between the val-158-met substitution was noted in the COMT in any of the patients.

Monoamine Oxidase-A

Monoamine oxidases (MAOs) are flavin-containing enzymes that degrade a variety of biogenic amines, including the neurotransmitters norepinephrine, dopamine, and serotonin. Two forms of the enzyme, MAO-A and MAO-B, are encoded by two adjacent genes (Hsu *et al.*, 1989) located at the p11.23-11.4 region of the X chromosome. MAO inhibitors seem to have a beneficial effect in a subset of OCD patients (Liebowitz *et al.*, 1990). Karayiorgou *et al.* (1999), in their sample of 110 nuclear OCD families, found a sexual dimorphic association between OCD and an allele of the *MAO-A* gene (*MAO-A**297CGG allele of the *Fnu*4H1 marker), previously linked to high MAO-A enzymatic activity. This association was detected particularly among male OCD probands with comorbid major depression.

MAO-A/EcoRV polymorphism was examined in a sample of 122 Mexican OCD patients and 124 healthy subjects (Camarena *et al.*, 2001). An excess of allele 1 in OCD females with major depression disorder was confirmed as previously reported (Camarena *et al.*, 1998). This difference was more strongly associated with OCD females than males in the total sample. Additionally, an HRR analysis of the inheritance of the MAO-A variants was performed in a sample of 51 OCD trios. An allelic association between OCD and MAO-A gene was found in the female probands, i.e., 14 out of 19 transmitted the allele 1.

GENERALIZED ANXIETY DISORDER

Family Studies

A study by Noyes *et al.* (1987) demonstrated a higher frequency of GAD among first-degree relatives ($n = 123$) of GAD probands ($n = 20$) compared to first-degree relatives of control subjects ($n = 20$) and of PD ($n = 40$) and agoraphobia probands ($n = 40$). Among the relatives of GAD patients, more women (24.2%) than men (14%) had GAD. The categorization of GAD as a distinct entity was further confirmed by the distribution of anxiety disorders among the families.

Twin Studies

Kendler *et al.* (1995) addressed the possible interrelationship of genetic and environmental risk factors in six major psychiatric disorders (phobia, GAD, PD, bulimia, major depression and alcoholism). The study included 1030 female–female twin pairs with known zygosity, derived from the population-based Virginia Twin Registry. Major depression was found to be the most frequent comorbidity of GAD. On factor analysis, the authors found statistical evidence of two genetic factors: phobia, PD and bulimia loaded heavily on the first factor, and major depression and GAD on the second. A disorder-specific additive gene was present only for GAD and alcoholism. Individual-specific environmental influences on the risk of GAD and major depression were best explained by a single factor and played a strong aetiological role.

In a recent study, the genetic and environmental contributions to GAD and PD were investigated in 6724 MZ and DZ male–male twin pairs taken from the Vietnam Era Twin Registry (Scherrer *et al.*, 2000). The presence of a non-additive genetic factor specific to PD supports a distinction of PD from GAD. The authors suggested that the common genetic and unique environmental influences in GAD and PD may be partially responsible for the high lifetime co-occurrence of these disorders.

Association Studies: Candidate Genes

Serotonin Transporter

Ohara *et al.* (1999) studied the 5-HTTin2.12 polymorphism in 103 patients with anxiety and 106 control subjects. The frequency of the 5-HTTin2.12 allele was significantly higher compared with controls in both the whole group of anxious patients ($p = 0.027$; odds ratio = 2.06, 95% CI 1.09-3.90) and in the GAD patients separately ($p = 0.0123$; odds ratio = 3.61, 95% CI 1.23-10.6).

Serotonin Receptors

Fehr *et al.* (2000a), using a candidate gene approach, genotyped 50 patients with GAD, 209 patients with alcoholism, 108 patients with major depression, 32 patients with PD, 58 patients with narcolepsy, and 74 healthy volunteers for the serotonin HTR1B receptor gene 861G $\rightarrow$ C polymorphism. This common *Hinc*II polymorphism had been linked to antisocial alcoholism in a Finnish sample and a sample derived from an American-Indian tribe (Lappalainen *et al.*, 1998). A higher frequency of the HTR1B 861G allele was detected among the male alcohol-dependent patients, but not in the patients with other mental disorders, compared to the control subjects. The same group (Fehr *et al.*, 2000b) also genotyped patients with GAD, alcohol dependence, PD without agoraphobia, and narcolepsy and normal healthy volunteers ($n = 173$ females and 298 males) for the 5-HT2C Cys23Ser polymorphism, but no difference in frequencies and genotypes were found between patients and controls. No association was found between GAD and 5-HT2A receptor polymorphism (T102C), as well as the intron 7 TPH (A218C) polymorphism (Fehr *et al.*, 2001).

POST-TRAUMATIC STRESS DISORDER

Family Studies

Reich, Lyons and Cai (1996) investigated familial vulnerability factors to PTSD in male military veterans by examining family history of four proband groups: PTSD, mixed anxiety disorders, coexisting anxiety and depressive disorders, and screened normal controls. The pattern of psychopathology in the families of the PTSD probands most closely resembled that in the families of the coexisting anxiety and depressive disorders probands.

In a family history study of 36 patients with chronic post-traumatic stress disorder, Davidson *et al.* (1985) reported a positive history of familial psychopathology, mostly alcoholism, depression, and anxiety disorders, in 66% of the patients. Subsequently, these authors investigated the relationship between chronic PTSD and family psychiatric morbidity in first-degree relatives ($n = 285$) of 81 female rape survivors with or without lifetime PTSD, 31 major depressive disorder controls, 20 anxiety disorder controls, and 39 healthy controls (Davidson *et al.*, 1998). Information was also available by family history for 639 relatives. An increased risk of depression was noted in family members of PTSD probands with depression but not in relatives of PTSD probands without lifetime depression. The authors concluded that PTSD following rape seems to be associated with familial vulnerability to major depression, which may thus serve as a risk factor for PTSD.

Twin Studies

Male–male veteran MZ twin pairs ($n = 2092$) who were discordant for military service in southeast Asia were investigated to evaluate the impact of military service on PTSD (Goldberg *et al.*, 1990). The prevalence of PTSD was over three-fold higher in the twins who served in southeast Asia than in their co-twins who did not (16.8% vs 5.0%) and nine-fold higher in the twins who experienced high levels of combat (95% CI: 4.8-17.6). The same group (True *et al.*, 1993) also performed a twin study of genetic and environmental contributions to liability for PTSD. The sample included 4042 Vietnam-era veteran MZ and DZ male twin pairs. Quantitative genetic analysis revealed that inheritance had a substantial influence on liability for symptoms of re-experiencing the trauma (13%–30%), avoidance of stimuli related to the trauma (30%–34%), and increased arousal (28%–32%). The family environment did not have a significant effect on any of the variables. Another twin study by this group (Lyons *et al.*, 1993) on a similar sample ($n = 4029$) studied genetic and nongenetic factors that influence wartime exposure to traumatic events. Specific events examined were volunteering for service in Vietnam, actual service in southeast Asia, a composite index of 18 combat experiences, and awards for combat. Heritability estimates ranged from 35% to 47%. There was no evidence that shared environment had a significant effect on any of the variables.

Association Studies

The Dopaminergic System

Increased levels of 24-hour urine dopamine excretion have been reported in PTSD (Yehuda *et al.*, 1992), and higher than normal levels of 24-hour urine homovanillic acid have been found in sexually abused girls (Debellis *et al.*, 1994; Putnam and Trickett, 1997). Plasma dopamine was also found to be elevated in a small cohort of combat veterans compared to controls (Hamner and Diamond, 1993). Deutch and Young (1995) suggested that PTSD is associated with a dopamine dysregulation which limits the ability of patients to cope with trauma and increases their susceptibility to trauma-related contextual stimuli.

Using a case-control design, Comings *et al.* (1991) investigated the association of PTSD and the DRD2 TaqI polymorphism in 35 European–American patients with PTSD, all with drug or alcohol abuse. The control group was comprised of 314 subjects, 69 of them non-alcoholics. Among the total group of controls, 77 (24.5%) carried the A1 allele, whereas among the non-alcoholic controls, only 10 (14.5%) did so. An increased prevalence of the A1 allele (45.7%) was demonstrated in the PTSD patients compared to the controls. However, after correction for multiple comparisons, the statistical significance was lost. In a subsequent study (Comings, Muhleman and Gysin, 1996) of 56 combat-exposed subjects with ($n = 37$) and without ($n = 19$) PTSD who were hospitalized in an addiction treatment unit, the same authors noted an association between PTSD and the DRD2*A1 allele (59.5% vs 5.3%; $p < 0.0001$). Though this study has an advantage of the inclusion of both PTSD and non-PTSD subjects who were exposed to combat, its small sample size limits the conclusions. Further, a later case-control study conducted by Gelernter *et al.* (1999) failed to demonstrate such an association. The authors noted no allelic association between the DRD2 TaqI 'A1' as well as in the 'B' and 'D' alleles in 52 European-American PTSD patients. Furthermore, the DRD2 haplotype frequencies also did not differ between the patients with PTSD and healthy control subjects. The authors concluded that the DRD2 gene variants do not contribute significantly to the risk of PTSD.

CONCLUDING REMARKS

The pattern and repertoire of behaviors and emotions are determined by gene–environment interactions. Genomic and non-genomic factors influence the risk of emergence of anxiety disorders in individuals and across generations. In addition to the common difficulties in molecular genetics of complex diseases, namely, non-Mendelian inheritance patterns, incomplete penetrance, possibility of phenocopies, genetic heterogeneity, and variable expressivity (Lander and Schork, 1994), the neurogenetic study of anxiety disorders is hampered by the problem of defining the heritable phenotype, including subsets of endophenotypes of the disorders (Tsuang, Faraone and Lyons, 1993; Smoller and Tsuang, 1998). The human genome project, combined with other novel strategies, such as DNA microarrays (Watson *et al.*, 2000), functional magnetic resonance imaging (fMRI) (Rosenberg and Hanna, 2000), and identification of genes and proteins implicated in the brain neurocircuitry of anxiety and fear hold great promise in furthering our understanding of the cellular and molecular mechanisms involved in the pathogenesis of anxiety disorders and developing specific and efficient treatments.

REFERENCES

Alsobrook II, J.P., Leckman, J.F., Goodman, W.K., Rasmussen, S.A. and Pauls, D.L., 1999. Segregation analysis of obsessive–compulsive disorder using symptom-based factor scores. *American Journal of Medical Genetics*, **88**, 669–675.

Anthony, J.C., Tien, A.Y. and Petronis, K.R., 1989. Epidemiologic evidence on cocaine use and panic attacks. *American Journal of Epidemiology*, **129**, 543–549.

Battaglia, M., Bertella, S., Bajo, S., Binaghi, F., Ogliari, A. and Bellodi, L., 1999. Assessment of parent-of-origin effect in families unlineally affected with panic disorder-agoraphobia. *Journal of Psychiatry Research*, **33**, 37–39.

Bellodi, L., Perna, G., Caldirola, D., Arancio, C., Bertani, A. and Di Bella, D., 1998. CO_2-induced panic attacks: a twin study. *American Journal of Psychiatry*, **155**, 1184–1188.

Bengel, D., Greenberg, B.D., Cora-Locatelli, G., Altemus, M., Heils, A., Li, Q. and Murphy, D.L., 1999. Association of the serotonin transporter promoter regulatory region polymorphism and obsessive–compulsive disorder. *Molecular Psychiatry*, **4**, 436–463.

Bienvenu, O.J., Samuels, J.F., Riddle, M.A., Hoehn-Saric, R., Liang, K.Y., Cullen, B.A., Grados, M.A. and Nestadt, G., 2000. The relationship of obsessive–compulsive disorder to possible spectrum disorders: results from a family study. *Biological Psychiatry*, **48**, 287–293.

Billett, E.A., Richter, M.A., King, N., Heils, A., Lesch, K.P. and Kennedy, J.L., 1997. Obsessive compulsive disorder, response to serotonin reuptake inhibitors and the serotonin transporter gene. *Molecular Psychiatry*, **2**, 403–406.

Billett, E.A., Richter, M.A., Sam, F., Swinson, R.P., Dai, X.Y., King, N., Badri, F., Sasaki, T., Buchanan, J.A. and Kennedy, J.L., 1998. Investigation of dopamine system genes in obsessive–compulsive disorder. *Psychiatry Genetics*, **8**, 163–169.

Black, D.W., Goldstein, R.B., Noyes, R. and Blum, N., 1994. Compulsive behaviors and obsessive–compulsive disorder (OCD): Lack of a relationship between OCD, eating disorders, and gambling. *Comprehensive Psychiatry*, **35**, 145–148.

Boulenger, J.P., Uhde, T.W., Wolff, E.A. and Post, R.M., 1984. Increased sensitivity to caffeine in patients with panic disorders. Preliminary evidence. *Archives of General Psychiatry*, **41**, 1067–1071.

Bradwejn, J. and Koszycki, D., 1994a. The cholecystokinin hypothesis of anxiety and panic disorder. *Annals of the New York Academy of Science*, **713**, 273–282.

Bradwejn, J. and Koszycki, D., 1994b. Imipramine antagonism of the panicogenic effects of cholecystokinin tetrapeptide in panic disorder patients. *American Journal of Psychiatry*, **151**, 261–263.

Bradwejn, J., Koszycki, D. and Shriqui, C., 1991. Enhanced sensitivity to cholecystokinin tetrapeptide in panic disorder. Clinical and behavioral findings. *Archives of General Psychiatry*, **48**, 603–610.

Brett, P.M., Curtis, D., Robertson, M.M. and Gurling, H.M., 1995. Exclusion of the 5-HT1A serotonin neuroreceptor and tryptophan oxygenase genes in a large British kindred multiply affected with Tourette's syndrome, chronic motor tics, and obsessive–compulsive behavior. *American Journal of Psychiatry*, **152**, 437–440.

Bulbena, A., Duro, J.C., Porta, M. and Vallejo, J., 1988. Anxiety disorders in the joint hypermobility syndrome. *Lancet*, **2**, 694.

Bulbena, A., Duró, J.C., Porta, M., Martín-Santos, R., Mateo, A., Molina, L., Vallescar, R. and Vallejo, J., 1993. Anxiety disorder in the joint hypermobility syndrome. *Psychiatry Research*, **43**, 59–68.

Bylund, D.B., Eikenberg, D.C., Hieble, J.P., Langer, S.Z., Lefkowitz, R.J., Minneman, K.P., Molinoff, P.B., Ruffolo, R.R., Jr and Trendelenburg, U.,

1994. International Union of Pharmacology Nomenclature of Adrenoceptors. *Pharmacological Review*, **46**, 121–136.

Camarena, B., Cruz, C., de la Fuente, J.R. and Nicolini, H., 1998. A higher frequency of a low activity-related allele of the MAO-A gene in females with obsessive–compulsive disorder. *Psychiatric Genetics*, **8**, 255–257.

Camarena, B., Rinetti, G., Cruz, C., Gomez, A., de La Fuente, J.R. and Nicolini, H., 2001. Additional evidence that genetic variation of MAO-A gene supports a gender subtype in obsessive–compulsive disorder. *American Journal of Medical Genetics*, **105**, 279–282.

Carey, G. and Gottesman, I.I., 1981. Twin and family studies of anxiety, phobic, and obsessive disorders. In: Klein, D.F. and Rabkin, J.G. (eds), *Anxiety: New Research and Changing Concepts*, pp. 117–136. Raven Press, New York.

Catalano, M., Sciuto, G., Di Bella, D., Novelli, E., Nobile, M. and Bellodi, L., 1994. Lack of association between obsessive–compulsive disorder and the dopamine D3 receptor gene: some preliminary considerations. *American Journal of Medical Genetics*, **54**, 253–255.

Cavallini, M.C., Di Bella, D., Pasquale, L., Henin, M. and Bellodi, L., 1998. 5HT2C CYS23/SER23 polymorphism is not associated with obsessive–compulsive disorder. *Psychiatry Research*, **77**, 97–104.

Cavallini, M.C., Pasquale, L., Bellodi, L. and Smeraldi, E., 1999a. Complex segregation analysis for obsessive compulsive disorder and related disorders. *American Journal of Medical Genetics*, **88**, 38–43.

Cavallini, M.C., Perna, G., Caldirola, D. and Bellodi, L., 1999b. A segregation study of panic disorder in families of panic patients responsive to the 35% CO_2 challenge. *Biological Psychiatry*, **46**, 815–820.

Cavallini, M.C., Di Bella, D., Catalano, M. and Bellodi, L., 2000. An association study between 5-HTTLPR polymorphism, COMT polymorphism, and Tourette's syndrome. *Psychiatry Research*, **97**, 93–100.

Charney, D.S., Woods, S.W., Goodman, W.K. and Heninger, G.R., 1987. Neurobiological mechanisms of panic anxiety: biochemical and behavioral correlates of yohimbine-induced panic attacks. *American Journal of Psychiatry*, **144**, 1030–1036.

Collier, D.A., Stober, G., Li, T., Heils, A., Catalano, M., Di Bella, D., Arranz, M.J., Murray, R.M., Vallada, H.P., Bengel, D., Muller, C.R., Roberts, G.W., Smeraldi, E., Kirov, G., Sham, P. and Lesch, K.P., 1996. A novel functional polymorphism within the promoter of the serotonin transporter gene: possible role in susceptibility to affective disorders. *Molecular Psychiatry*, **1**, 453–460.

Comings, D.E., Comings, B.G., Muhleman, D., Dietz, G., Shahbahrami, B., Tast, D., Knell, E., Kocsis, P., Baumgarten, R., Kovacs, B.W., Levy, D.L., Smith, M., Kane, J.M., Lieberman, J.A., Klein, D.N., MacMurray, J., Tosk, J., Sverd, J., Gysin, R. and Flanagan, S., 1991. The dopamine D2 receptor locus as a modifying gene in neuropsychiatric disorders. *Journal of the American Medical Association*, **266**, 1793–1800.

Comings, D.E., Muhleman, D. and Gysin, R., 1996. Dopamine D2 receptor (DRD2) gene and susceptibility to posttraumatic stress disorder: A study and replication. *Biological Psychiatry*, **40**, 368–372.

Crawford, F., Hoyne, J., Diaz, P., Osborne, A., Dorotheo, J., Sheehan, D. and Mullan, M., 1995. Occurrence of the Cys311 DRD2 variant in a pedigree multiply affected with panic disorder. *American Journal of Medical Genetics*, **60**, 332–334.

Crowe, R.R., Noyes, R., Pauls, D.L. and Slymen, D., 1983. A family study of panic disorder. *Archives of General Psychiatry*, **40**, 1065–1069.

Crowe, R.R., Noyes, R., Jr and Persico, A.M., 1987a. Pro-opiomelanocortin (POMC) gene excluded as a cause of panic disorder in a large family. *Journal of Affective Disorders*, **12**, 23–27.

Crowe, R.R., Noyes, R., Jr, Wilson, A.F., Elston, R.C. and Ward, L.J., 1987b. A linkage study of panic disorder. *Archives of General Psychiatry*, **44**, 933–937.

Crowe, R.R., Noyes, R., Jr, Samuelson, S., Wesner, R. and Wilson, R., 1990. Close linkage between panic disorder and alpha-haptoglobin excluded in 10 families. *Archives of General Psychiatry*, **47**, 377–380.

Crowe, R.R., Wang, Z., Noyes, R., Jr, Albrecht, B.E., Darlison, M.G., Bailey, M.E., Johnson, K.J. and Zoega, T., 1997. Candidate gene study of eight GABAA receptor subunits in panic disorder. *American Journal of Psychiatry*, **154**, 1096–1100.

Crowe, R.R., Goedken, R., Samuelson, S., Wilson, R., Nelson, J. and Noyes, R., Jr, 2001. Genome-wide survey of panic disorder. *American Journal of Medical Genetics*, **105**, 105–109.

Davidson, J., Swartz, M., Storck, M., Krishnan, R.R. and Hammett, E., 1985. A diagnostic and family study of posttraumatic stress disorder. *American Journal of Psychiatry*, **142**, 90–93.

Davidson, J.R., Tupler, L.A., Wilson, W.H. and Connor, K.M., 1998. A family study of chronic post-traumatic stress disorder following rape trauma. *Journal of Psychiatric Research*, **32**, 301–309.

Debellis, D., Lefter, L., Trickett, P.K. and Putnam, F.W., 1994. Urinary catecholamine excretion in sexually abused girls. *Journal of the American Academy of Child and Adolescent Psychiatry*, **33**, 320–327.

Deckert, J., Catalano, M., Heils, A., Di Bella, D., Friess, F., Politi, E., Franke, P., Nothen, M.M., Maier, W., Bellodi, L. and Lesch, K.P., 1997. Functional promoter polymorphism of the human serotonin transporter: lack of association with panic disorder. *Psychiatry Genetics*, **7**, 45–47.

Deckert, J., Nothen, M.M., Franke, P., Delmo, C., Fritze, J., Knapp, M., Maier, W., Beckmann, H. and Propping, P., 1998. Systematic mutation screening and association study of the A1 and A2a adenosine receptor genes in panic disorder suggests a contribution of the A2a gene to the development of disease. *Molecular Psychiatry*, **3**, 81–85.

Deckert, J., Catalano, M., Syagailo, Y.V., Bosi, M., Okladnova, O., Di Bella, D., Nothen, M.M., Maffei, P., Franke, P., Fritze, J., Maier, W., Propping, P., Beckmann, H., Bellodi, L. and Lesch, K.P., 1999. Excess of high activity monoamine oxidase A gene promoter alleles in female patients with panic disorder. *Human Molecular Genetics*, **8**, 621–624.

Deckert, J., Meyer, J., Catalano, M., Bosi, M., Sand, P., DiBella, D., Ortega, G., Stober, G., Franke, P., Nothen, M.M., Fritze, J., Maier, W., Beckmann, H., Propping, P., Bellodi, L. and Lesch, K.P., 2000. Novel 5′-regulatory region polymorphisms of the 5-HT2C receptor gene: association study with panic disorder. *International Journal of Neuropsychopharmacology*, **3**, 321–325.

Demchshyn, L., Sunahara, R.K., Miller, K., Teitler, M., Hoffman, B.J., Kennedy, J.L., Seeman, P., Van Tol, H.H.M. and Niznik, H.B., 1992. A human serotonin 1D receptor variant (5HT1Dβ) encoded by an intronless gene on chromosome 6. *Proceeding of the National Academy of Sciences USA*, **89**, 5522–5526.

Deutch, A.Y. and Young, C.D., 1995. A model of the stress-induced activation of prefrontal cortical dopamine systems: Coping and the development of post-traumatic stress disorder. In: Friedman, M.J., Charney, D.S. and Deutch, A.Y. (eds), *Neurobiological and Clinical Consequences of Stress*, pp. 163–176. Lippincott-Raven Press, Philadelphia.

Faraone, S.V., Tsuang, M.T. and Tsuang, D.W., 1999. Molecular genetics and mental illness. In: *Genetics of Mental Disorders*, pp. 115–158. The Guilford Press, NY.

Fehr, C., Grintschuk, N., Szegedi, A., Anghelescu, I., Klawe, C., Singer, P., Hiemke, C. and Dahmen, N., 2000a. The HTR1B 861G $\rightarrow$ C receptor polymorphism among patients suffering from alcoholism, major depression, anxiety disorders and narcolepsy. *Psychiatry Research*, **97**, 1–10.

Fehr, C., Szegedi, A., Anghelescu, I., Klawe, C., Hiemke, C. and Dahmen, N., 2000b. Sex differences in allelic frequencies of the 5-HT2C Cys23Ser polymorphism in psychiatric patients and healthy volunteers: findings from an association study. *Psychiatry Genetics*, **10**, 59–65.

Fehr, C., Schleicher, A., Szegedi, A., Anghelescu, I., Klawe, C., Hiemke, C. and Dahmen, N., 2001. Serotonergic polymorphisms in patients suffering from alcoholism, anxiety disorders and narcolepsy. *Progress in Neuropsychopharmacology and Biological Psychiatry*, **25**, 965–982.

Frisch, A., Michaelovsky, E., Rockah, R., Amir, I., Hermesh, H., Laor, N., Fuchs, C., Zohar, J., Lerer, B., Buniak, S.F., Landa, S., Poyurovsky, M., Shapira, B. and Weizman, R., 2000. Association between obsessive–compulsive disorder and polymorphisms of genes encoding components of the serotonergic and dopaminergic pathways. *European Neuropsychopharmacology*, **10**, 205–209.

Fyer, A., Mannuzza, S., Chapman, T., Liebowitz, M. and Klein, D., 1993. A direct interview family study of social phobia. *Archives of General Psychiatry*, **50**, 286–293.

Fyer, A., Mannuzza, S., Chapman, T., Martin, L.Y. and Klein, D.F., 1995. Specificity in familial aggregation of phobic disorders. *Archives of General Psychiatry*, **52**, 564–573.

Gelernter, J., Southwick, S., Goodson, S., Morgan, A., Nagy, L. and Charney, D.S., 1999. No association between D2 dopamine receptor (DRD2) "A" system alleles, or DRD2 haplotypes, and posttraumatic stress disorder. *Biological Psychiatry*, **45**, 620–625.

Gelernter, J., Bonvicini, K., Page, G., Woods, S.W., Goddard, A.W., Kruger, S., Pauls, D.L. and Goodson, S., 2001. Linkage genome scan for loci predisposing to panic disorder or agoraphobia. *American Journal of Medical Genetics*, **105**, 548–557.

Germine, M., Goddard, A.W., Sholomskas, D.E., Woods, S.W., Charney, D.S. and Heninger, G.R., 1994. Response to meta-chlorophenylpiperazine in panic disorder patients and healthy subjects: influence of reduction in intravenous dosage. *Psychiatry Research*, **54**, 115–133.

Goldberg, J., True, W.R., Eisen, S.A. and Henderson, W.G., 1990. A twin study of the effects of the Vietnam War on posttraumatic stress disorder. *Journal of the American Medical Association*, **263**, 1227–1232.

Goldstein, R.B., Wickramaratne, P.J., Horwath, E. and Weissman, M.M., 1997. Familial aggregation and phenomenology of "early"-onset (at or before age 20 years) panic disorder. *Archives of General Psychiatry*, **54**, 271–278.

Gratacòs, M., Nadal, M., Martin-Santos, R., Pujana, M.A., Gago, J., Peral, B., Armengol, L., Ponsa, I., Miro, R., Bulbena, A. and Estivill, X., 2001. A polymorphic genomic duplication on human chromosome 15 is a susceptibility factor for panic and phobic disorders. *Cell*, **106**, 367–379.

Gross, R., Sasson, Y., Chopra, M. and Zohar, J., 1998. Biological models of obsessive–compulsive disorder: the serotonin hypothesis. In: Swinson, R.P., Antony, M.M., Rachman, S. and Richter, M.A. (eds), *Obsessive–Compulsive Disorder: Theory, Research, and Treatment*, pp. 141–153. Guilford, New York.

Grossman, M.H., Emanuel, B.S. and Budarf, M.L., 1992. Chromosomal mapping of the human catechol-O-methyltransferase gene to 22q11.1-q11.2. *Genomics*, **12**, 822–825.

Haghighi, F., Fyer, A.J., Weissman, M.M., Knowles, J.A. and Hodge, S.E., 1999. Parent-of-origin effect in panic disorder. *American Journal of Medical Genetics*, **88**, 131–135.

Hamilton, S.P., Heiman, G.A., Haghighi, F., Mick, S., Klein, D.F., Hodge, S.E., Weissman, M.M., Fyer, A.J. and Knowles, J.A., 1999. Lack of genetic linkage or association between a functional serotonin transporter polymorphism and panic disorder. *Psychiatric Genetics*, **9**, 1–6.

Hamilton, S.P., Haghighi, F., Heiman, G.A., Klein, D.F., Hodge, S.E., Fyer, A.J., Weissman, M.M. and Knowles, J.A., 2000a. Investigation of dopamine receptor (DRD4) and dopamine transporter (DAT) polymorphisms for genetic linkage or association to panic disorder. *American Journal of Medical Genetics*, **96**, 324–330.

Hamilton, S.P., Slager, S.L., Heiman, G.A., Haghighi, F., Klein, D.F., Hodge, S.E., Weissman, M.M., Fyer, A.J. and Knowles, J.A., 2000b. No genetic linkage or association between a functional promoter polymorphism in the monoamine oxidase-A gene and panic disorder. *Molecular Psychiatry*, **5**, 465–466.

Hamilton, S.P., Slager, S.L., Helleby, L., Heiman, G.A., Klein, D.F., Hodge, S.E., Weissman, M.M., Fyer, A.J. and Knowles, J.A., 2001. No association or linkage between polymorphisms in the genes encoding cholecystokinin and the cholecystokinin B receptor and panic disorder. *Molecular Psychiatry*, **6**, 59–65.

Hamner, M.B. and Diamond, B.L., 1993. Elevated plasma dopamine in posttraumatic stress disorder: A preliminary report. *Biological Psychiatry*, **33**, 304–306.

Hansen, T.V.O., Rehfeld, J.F. and Nielsen, F.C., 2000. Function of the C-36 to T polymorphism in the human cholecystokinin gene promoter. *Molecular Psychiatry*, **5**, 443–447.

Hattori, E., Ebihara, M., Yamada, K., Ohba, H., Shibuya, H. and Yoshikawa, T., 2001. Identification of a compound short tandem repeat stretch in the 5′-upstream region of the cholecystokinin gene, and its association with panic disorder but not with schizophrenia. *Molecular Psychiatry*, **6**, 465–470.

Heils, A., Teufel, A., Petri, S., Stober, G., Bengel, B. and Lesch, K.P., 1996. Allelic variation of human serotonin transporter gene expression. *Journal of Neurochemistry*, **6**, 2612–2624.

Hollander, E., Kwon, J.H., Stein, D.J., Broatch, J., Rowland, C.T. and Himelein, C.A., 1996. Obsessive–compulsive and spectrum disorders: overview and quality of life issues. *Journal of Clinical Psychiatry*, **57**(Suppl 8), 3–6.

Hsu, Y.P., Powell, J.F., Sims, K.B. and Breakefield, X.O., 1989. Molecular genetics of the monoamine oxidases. *Journal of Neurochemistry*, **53**, 12–18.

Inyoue, E., 1965. Similar and dissimilar manifestations of obsessive–compulsive neurosis in monozygotic twins. *American Journal of Psychiatry*, **121**, 1171–1175.

Ishiguro, H., Arinami, T., Yamada, K., Otsuka, Y., Toru, M. and Shibuya, H., 1997. An association study between a transcriptional polymorphism in the serotonin transporter gene and panic disorder in a Japanese population. *Psychiatry and Clinical Neurosciences*, **51**, 333–335.

Karayiorgou, M., Altemus, M., Galke, B.L., Goldman, D., Murphy, D.L., Ott, J. and Gogos, J.A., 1997. Genotype determining low catechol-O-methyltransferase activity as a risk factor for obsessive–compulsive disorder. *Proceedings of the National Academy of Sciences, USA*, **94**, 4572–4575.

Karayiorgou, M., Sobin, C., Blundell, M.L., Galke, B.L., Malinova, L., Goldberg, P., Ott, J. and Gogos, J.A., 1999. Family-based association studies support a sexually dimorphic effect of COMT and MAOA on genetic susceptibility to obsessive–compulsive disorder. *Biological Psychiatry*, **45**, 1178–1189.

Kendler, K.S., Neale, M.C., Kessler, R.C., Heath, A.C. and Eaves, L.J., 1992. The genetic epidemiology of phobias in women. The interrelationship of agoraphobia, social phobia, situational phobia, and simple phobia. *Archives of General Psychiatry*, **49**, 273–281.

Kendler, K.S., Neale, M.C., Kessler, R.C., Heath, A.C. and Eaves, L.J., 1993. Panic disorder in women: a population-based twin study. *Psychological Medicine*, **23**, 397–406.

Kendler, K.S., Walters, E.E., Neale, M.C., Kessler, R.C., Heath, A.C. and Eaves, L.J., 1995. The structure of the genetic and environmental risk factors for six major psychiatric disorders in women. *Archives of General Psychiatry*, **52**, 374–383.

Kennedy, J.L., Bradwejn, J., Koszycki, D., King, N., Crowe, R., Vincent, J. and Fourie, O., 1999. Investigation of cholecystokinin system genes in panic disorder. *Molecular Psychiatry*, **4**, 284–285.

Kim, S.W., Dysken, M.W. and Kline, M.D., 1990. Monozygotic twins with obsessive–compulsive disorder. *British Journal of Psychiatry*, **156**, 435–438.

Kinnear, C.J., Niehaus, D.J., Moolman-Smook, J.C., du Toit, P.L., van Kradenberg, J., Weyers, J.B., Potgieter, A., Marais, V., Emsley, R.A., Knowles, J.A., Corfield, V.A., Brink, P.A. and Stein, D.J., 2000. Obsessive–compulsive disorder and the promoter region polymorphism (5-HTTLPR) in the serotonin transporter gene (SLC6A4): a negative association study in the Afrikaner population. *International Journal of Neuropsychopharmacology*, **3**, 327–331.

Kinnear, C., Niehaus, D.J., Seedat, S., Moolman-Smook, J.C., Corfield, V.A., Malherbe, G., Potgieter, A., Lombard, C. and Stein, D.J., 2001. Obsessive–compulsive disorder and a novel polymorphism adjacent to the oestrogen response element (ERE 6) upstream from the COMT gene. *Psychiatric Genetics*, **11**, 85–87.

Knowles, J.A., Fyer, A.J., Vieland, V.J., Weissman, M.M., Hodge, S.E., Heiman, G.A., Haghighi, F., de Jesus, G.M., Rassnick, H., Preud'homme-Rivelli, X., Austin, T., Cunjak, J., Mick, S., Fine, L.D., Woodley, K.A., Das, K., Maier, W., Adams, P.B., Freimer, N.B., Klein, D.F and Gilliam, T.C., 1998. Results of a genome-wide genetic screen for panic disorder. *American Journal of Medical Genetics*, **28**(81), 139–147.

Lachman, H.M., Papolos, D.F., Saito, T., Yu, Y.M., Szumlanski, C.L. and Weinshilboum, R.M., 1996. Human catechol-O-methyltransferase pharmacogenetics: description of a functional polymorphism and its potential application to neuropsychiatric disorders. *Pharmacogenetics*, **6**, 243–250.

Lander, E.S. and Schork, N.J., 1994. Genetic dissection of complex traits. *Science*, **265**, 2037–2048.

Lappalainen, J., Dean, M., Charbonneau, L., Virkkunen, M., Linnoila, M. and Goldman, D., 1995. Mapping of the serotonin 5-HT1Dβ autoreceptor gene on chromosome 6 and direct analysis for sequence variants. *American Journal of Medical Genetics*, **60**, 157–161.

Lappalainen, J., Long, J.C., Eggert, M., Ozaki, N., Robin, R.W., Brown, G.L., Naukkarinen, H., Virkkunen, M., Linnoila, M. and Goldman, D., 1998. Linkage of antisocial alcoholism to the serotonin HTR1B receptor gene in 2 populations. *Archives of General Psychiatry*, **55**, 989–994.

Lenane, M.C., Swedo, S.E., Leonard, H., Pauls, D.L., Sceery, W. and Rapoport, J.L., 1990. Psychiatric disorders in first degree relatives of children and adolescents with obsessive compulsive disorder. *Journal of the American Academy of Child and Adolescent Psychiatry*, **29**, 407–412.

Leonard, H.L., Lenane, M.C., Swedo, S.E., Rettew, D.C., Gershon, E.S. and Rapoport, J.L., 1992. Tics and Tourette's disorder: a 2- to 7-year follow-up of 54 obsessive–compulsive children. *American Journal of Psychiatry*, **149**, 1244–1251.

Lesch, K.P., Bengel, D., Heils, A., Sabol, S.Z., Greenberg, B.D., Petri, S., Benjamin, J., Muller, C.R., Hamer, D.H. and Murphy, D.L., 1996. Association of anxiety-related traits with a polymorphism in the serotonin transporter gene regulatory region. *Science*, **274**, 1527–1531.

Lesch, K.P., Bengel, D., Heils, A., Sabol, S.Z., Greenberg, B.D., Petri, S., Benjamin, J., Muller, C.R., Hamer, D.H. and Murphy, D.L., 1996. Association of anxiety-related traits with a polymorphism in the serotonin transporter gene regulatory region. *Science*, **274**, 1527–1531.

Liebowitz, M.R., Hollander, E., Schneier, F., Campeas, R., Welkowitz, L., Hatterer, J. and Fallon, B., 1990. Reversible and irreversible monoamine oxidase inhibitors in other psychiatric disorders. *Acta Psychiatrica Scandinavica*, **360**(Suppl 1), 29–34.

Lorenz, W., Lomansney, J.W., Collins, S., Regan, J.W., Caron, M.G. and Lefkowitz, R.J., 1990. Expression of three alpha$_2$-adrenergic receptor subtypes in rat tissues: implication for alpha$_2$ receptor classification. *Molecular Pharmacology*, **38**, 599–603.

Lyons, M.J., Goldberg, J., Eisen, S.A., True, W., Tsuang, M.T., Meyer, J.M. and Henderson, W.G., 1993. Do genes influence exposure to trauma? A twin study of combat. *American Journal of Medical Genetics*, **48**, 22–27.

Martín-Santos, R., Bulbena, A., Porta, M., Gago, J., Molina, L. and Duro, J.C., 1998. Association between joint hypermobility syndrome and panic disorder. *American Journal of Psychiatry*, **155**, 1578–1583.

Matsushita, S., Muramatsu, T., Kimura, M., Shirakawa, O., Mita, T., Nakai, T. and Higuchi, S., 1997. Serotonin transporter gene regulatory region polymorphism and panic disorder. *Molecular Psychiatry*, **2**, 390–392.

McDougle, C.J., Gordman, W.K. and Price, L.H., 1993. The pharmacotherapy of obsessive–compulsive disorder. *Pharmacopsychiatry*, **26**(Suppl 1), 24–29.

McDougle, C.J., Goodman, W.K. and Price, L.H., 1994. Dopamine antagonist in tic-related and psychotic spectrum obsessive compulsive disorder. *Journal of Clinical Psychiatry*, **55**(Suppl 3), 24–31.

McDougle, C.J., Epperson, C.N., Price, L.H. and Gelernter, J., 1998. Evidence for linkage disequilibrium between serotonin transporter protein gene (SLC6A4) and obsessive compulsive disorder. *Molecular Psychiatry*, **3**, 270–273.

Mundo, E., Richter, M.A., Sam, F., Macciardi, F. and Kennedy, J.L., 2000. Is the 5-HT1Dβ receptor gene implicated in the pathogenesis of obsessive–compulsive disorder? *American Journal of Psychiatry*, **157**, 1160–1161.

Mundo, E., Zai, G., Lee, L., Parikh, S.V. and Kennedy, J.L., 2001. The 5-HT1Dβ receptor gene in bipolar disorder. A family-based association study. *Neuropsychopharmacology*, **25**, 608–613.

Mutchler, K., Crowe, R.R., Noyes, R., Jr and Wesner, R.W., 1990. Exclusion of the tyrosine hydroxylase gene in 14 panic disorder pedigrees. *American Journal of Psychiatry*, **147**, 1367–1369.

Nestadt, G., Lan, T., Samuels, J., Riddle, M., Bienvenu III, O.J., Liang, K.Y., Hoehn-Saric, R., Cullen, B., Grados, M., Beaty, T.H. and Shugart, Y.Y., 2000a. Complex segregation analysis provides compelling evidence for a major gene underlying obsessive–compulsive disorder and for heterogeneity by sex. *American Journal of Human Genetics*, **67**, 1611–1616.

Nestadt, G., Samuels, J., Riddle, M., Bienvenu III, O.J., Liang, K.-Y., LaBuda, M., Walkup, J., Grados, M. and Hoehn-Saric, R., 2000b. A family study of obsessive–compulsive disorder. *Archives of General Psychiatry*, **57**, 358–363.

Nicolini, H., Cruz, C., Camarena, B., Orozco, B., Kennedy, J.L., King, N., Weissbecker, K., de la Fuente, J.R. and Sidenberg, D., 1996. DRD2, DRD3 and 5HT2A receptor genes polymorphisms in obsessive–compulsive disorder. *Molecular Psychiatry*, **1**, 461–465.

Niehaus, D.J., Kinnear, C.J., Corfield, V.A., du Toit, P.L., van Kradenburg, J., Moolman-Smook, J.C., Weyers, J.B., Potgieter, A., Seedat, S., Emsley, R.A., Knowles, J.A., Brink, P.A. and Stein, D.J., 2001. Association between a catechol-o-methyltransferase polymorphism and obsessive–compulsive disorder in the Afrikaner population. *Journal of Affective Disorders*, **65**, 61–65.

Noyes, R., Jr, Clarkson, C., Crowe, R.R., Yates, W.R. and McChesney, C.M., 1987. A family study of generalized anxiety disorder. *American Journal of Psychiatry*, **144**, 1019–1024.

Ohara, K., Suzuki, Y., Ochiai, M., Tsukamoto, T., Tani, K. and Ohara, K., 1999. A variable-number-tandem-repeat of the serotonin transporter gene and anxiety disorders. *Progress in Neuropsychopharmacology and Biological Psychiatry*, **23**, 55–65.

Ohara, K., Suzuki, Y., Ochiai, M. and Terada, H., 2000. Polymorphism in the promoter region of the alpha(2A)-adrenergic receptor gene and panic disorders. *Psychiatry Research*, **93**, 79–82.

Ozelius, L., Hsu, Y.-P.P., Bruns, G., Powell, J.F., Chen, S., Weyler, W., Utterback, M., Zucker, D., Haines, J., Trofatter, J.A., Conneally, P.M., Gusella, J.F. and Breakefield, X.O., 1988. Human monoamine oxidase gene (MAOA): chromosome position (Xp21-p11) and DNA polymorphism. *Genomics*, **3**, 53–58.

Pauls, D.L., Bucher, K.D., Crowe, R.R. and Noyes, R., Jr, 1980. A genetic study of panic disorder pedigrees. *American Journal of Human Genetics*, **32**, 639–644.

Pauls, D.L., Towbin, K.E., Leckman, J.F., Zahner, G.E. and Cohen, D.J., 1986. Gilles de la Tourette's syndrome and obsessive–compulsive disorder. Evidence supporting a genetic relationship. *Archives of General Psychiatry*, **43**, 1180–1182.

Pauls, D.L., Alsobrook, J.P., Goodman, W., Rasmussen, S. and Leckman, J.F., 1995. A family study of obsessive–compulsive disorder. *American Journal of Psychiatry*, **152**, 76–84.

Pecknold, J.C., Luthe, L., Iny, L. and Ramdoyal, D., 1995. Fluoxetine in panic disorder: pharmacologic and tritiated platelet imipramine and paroxetine binding study. *Journal of Psychiatry and Neuroscience*, **20**, 193–198.

Perna, G., Bertani, A., Caldirola, D. and Bellodi, L., 1996. Family history of panic disorder and hypersensitivity to CO_2 in patients with panic disorder. *American Journal of Psychiatry*, **153**, 1060–1064.

Pitchot, W., Ansseau, M., Moreno, A.G., Hansenne, M. and von Frenckell, R., 1992. Dopaminergic function in panic disorder: comparison with major and minor depression. *Biological Psychiatry*, **32**, 1004–1011.

Putnam, F.W. and Trickett, P.K., 1997. Psychobiological effects of sexual abuse. A longitudinal study. *Annals of the New York Academy of Sciences*, **821**, 150–159.

Reich, J., Lyons, M. and Cai, B., 1996. Familial vulnerability factors to post-traumatic stress disorder in male military veterans. *Acta Psychiatrica Scandinavica*, **93**, 105–112.

Rosenberg, D.R. and Hanna, G.L., 2000. Genetic and imaging strategies in obsessive–compulsive disorder: Potential implications for treatment development. *Biological Psychiatry*, **48**, 1210–1222.

Sabol, S.Z., Hu, S. and Hamer, D., 1998. A functional polymorphism in the monoamine oxidase A gene promoter. *Human Genetics*, **103**, 273–279.

Satel, S.L. and McDougle, C.J., 1993. Obsessions and compulsions associated with cocaine abuse (Letter). *American Journal of Psychiatry*, **150**, 155–156.

Scherrer, J.F., True, W.R., Xian, H., Lyons, M.J., Eisen, S.A., Goldberg, J., Lin, N. and Tsuang, M.T., 2000. Evidence for genetic influences common and specific to symptoms of generalized anxiety and panic. *Journal of Affective Disorders*, **57**, 25–35.

Schindler, K.M., Richter, M.A., Kennedy, J.L., Pato, M.T. and Pato, C.N., 2000. Association between homozygosity at the COMT gene locus and obsessive compulsive disorder. *American Journal of Medical Genetics*, **96**, 721–724.

Schmidt, S.M., Zoega, T. and Crowe, R.R., 1993. Excluding linkage between panic disorder and the gamma-aminobutyric acid beta 1 receptor locus in five Icelandic pedigrees. *Acta Psychiatrica Scandinavica*, **88**, 225–228.

Smoller, J.W. and Tsuang, M.T., 1998. Panic and phobic anxiety: defining phenotypes for genetic studies. *American Journal of Psychiatry*, **155**, 1152–1162.

Stefanos, C.N., Dikeos, D.G. and Papadimitrious, G.N., 1996. Clinical strategies in genetic research. In: Weller, M.P.I. and van Kammen, D.P. (eds), *Balliere's Clinical Psychiatry, International Practice and Research: Genetics of Mental Disorders, Part I. Theoretical Aspects*, pp. 1–18. Balliere Tindall, London.

Stein, M.B., Chartier, M.J., Hazen, A.L., Kozak, M.V., Tancer, M.E., Lander, S., Furer, P., Chubaty, D. and Walker, R.J., 1998. A direct-interview family study of generalized social phobia. *American Journal of Psychiatry*, **155**, 90–97.

Stern, L., Zohar, J., Cohen, R. and Sasson, Y., 1998. Treatment of severe, drug resistant obsessive–compulsive disorder with the 5HT1D agonist sumatriptan. *European Neuropsychopharmacology*, **8**, 325–328.

Tiller, J.W., Bouwer, C. and Behnke, K., 1990. Moclobemide and fluoxetine for panic disorder. International Panic Disorder Study Group. *European Archives of Psychiatry and Clinical Neuroscience*, **249**(Suppl 1), S7–S10.

Torgersen, S., 1983. Genetic factors in anxiety disorders. *Archives of General Psychiatry*, **40**, 1085–1089.

True, W.R., Rice, J., Eisen, S.A., Heath, A.C., Goldberg, J., Lyons, M.J. and Nowak, J., 1993. A twin study of genetic and environmental contributions to liability for posttraumatic stress symptoms. *Archives of General Psychiatry*, **50**, 257–264.

Tsuang, M., Faraone, S. and Lyons, M., 1993. Identification of the phenotype in psychiatric genetics. *European Archives of Psychiatry and Clinical Neuroscience*, **243**, 131–142.

Veenstra-VanderWeele, J., Kim, S.J., Gonen, D., Hanna, G.L., Leventhal, B.L. and Cook, E.H., Jr, 2001. Genomic organization of the SLC1A1/EAAC1 gene and mutation screening in early-onset obsessive–compulsive disorder. *Molecular Psychiatry*, **6**, 160–167.

Vieland, V.J., Goodman, D., Chapman, T. and Fyer, A., 1996. New segregation analysis of panic disorder. *American Journal of Medical Genetics*, **67**, 147–153.

Wang, Z.W., Crowe, R.R. and Noyes, R., Jr, 1992. Adrenergic receptor genes as candidate genes for panic disorder: a linkage study. *American Journal of Psychiatry*, **149**, 470–474.

Wang, Z., Valdes, J., Noyes, R., Zoega, T. and Crowe, R.R., 1998. Possible association of a cholecystokinin promoter polymorphism (CCK-36CT) with panic disorder. *American Journal of Medical Genetics*, **81**, 228–234.

Watson, S.J., Meng, F., Thompson, R.C. and Akil, H., 2000. The "chip" as a specific genetic tool. *Biological Psychiatry*, **48**, 1147–1156.

Weizman, A., Carmi, M., Hermesh, H., Shahar, A., Apter, A., Tyano, S. and Rehavi, M., 1986. High-affinity imipramine binding and serotonin uptake in platelets of eight adolescent and ten adult obsessive–compulsive patients. *American Journal of Psychiatry*, **143**, 335–339.

Weizman, A., Mandel, A., Barber, Y., Weitz, R., Cohen, A., Mester, M. and Rehavi, M., 1992. Decreased platelet imipramine binding in Tourette patients with obsessive–compulsive disorder. *Biological Psychiatry*, **31**, 705–711.

Yamada, K., Hattori, E., Shimizu, M., Sugaya, A., Shibuya, H. and Yoshikawa, T., 2001. Association studies of the cholecystokinin B receptor and A2a adenosine receptor genes in panic disorder. *Journal of Neural Transmission*, **108**, 837–848.

Yehuda, R., Southwick, S., Giller, E.L., Xiaowan, M.A. and Mason, J.W., 1992. Urinary catecholamine excretion and severity of PTSD symptoms in Vietnam combat veterans. *Journal of Nervous and Mental Disorders*, **180**, 321–325.

Zohar, J., Muller, E.A., Insel, T.R., Zohar-Kadouch, R.C. and Murphy, D.L., 1987. Serotonergic responsivity in obsessive–compulsive disorder: Comparison of patient and healthy control. *Archives of General Psychiatry*, **44**, 946–951.

XIX-12

Gender Differences in Anxiety Disorders

Teresa A. Pigott and Lai T. Lac

ANXIETY DISORDERS: INTRODUCTION

Though rarely appreciated, anxiety disorders represent one of the most common psychiatric disorders. Nearly one out of four Americans will meet criteria for an anxiety disorder during their lifetime. Inexplicably, women are much more likely than men to develop anxiety disorders. In fact, lifetime prevalence estimates based on large-scale population surveys conducted within the US suggest that women are two to three times more likely than men to develop panic disorder (7.7% vs 2.9%), agoraphobia (9.0% vs 3.0%), simple phobia (13.9% vs 7.2%), or post-traumatic stress disorder (PTSD) (11.3% vs 6.0%). Lifetime prevalence estimates also suggest that women are 1.5 times more likely than men to develop obsessive–compulsive disorder (OCD) (3.1% vs 2.0%) or social anxiety disorder (16.4% vs 11.2%) (Robins *et al.*, 1984; Bourdon *et al.*, 1988; Breslau, Davis and Andreski, 1990; Regier, Narron and Rae, 1990; Kessler *et al.*, 1994; Leon, Portera and Weissman, 1995; Magee *et al.*, 1996; Yonkers and Ellison, 1996).

Results from the international epidemiological surveys also confirm that anxiety disorders are very common and that women have much higher prevalence rates than men. Although prevalence rates tend to decrease with advancing age, anxiety disorders remain more common in women throughout the life span (Krasucki, Howard and Mann, 1998). There is some evidence that the gender difference for anxiety disorders narrows after the age of 65. This finding, however, may represent an artifact from the combined effects of cumulative, anxiety-related mortality as well as the complex differentiation between anxiety and cognitive impairment. The narrowing of the gender difference may also result from the attenuation of hormonal factors that occurs with advancing age (Krasucki, Howard and Mann, 1998).

The presence of an anxiety disorder has important implications. A lifetime diagnosis of an anxiety disorder is associated with increased functional impairment, diminished educational and occupational opportunities, and elevated morbidity and mortality rates in comparison to the absence of an anxiety disorder. Elevated utilization rates for emergency medical and mental health care services are also linked to the presence of an anxiety disorder. Despite these adverse consequences, very few individuals with an anxiety disorder receive any type of psychiatric treatment (Lindal and Stefansson, 1993; Dick *et al.*, 1994a, 1994b; Kessler *et al.*, 1994, 1997; Weissman *et al.*, 1994; Leon, Portera and Weissman, 1995).

Low recognition rates for anxiety disorders represent a significant obstacle in delaying effective treatments. Somatic symptoms, a cardinal feature of excess anxiety, may effectively obscure their primary psychiatric basis. Most anxiety disorders initially present in a general medical rather than mental health setting. Unfortunately, results from numerous studies confirm that a primary anxiety disorder is unlikely to be considered in a primary care setting until the late stages of a routine diagnostic assessment (Hohmann, 1989; Kennedy and Schwab, 1997; Roy-Byrne and Katon, 1997; Bland, Newman and Orn, 1997b; Fleet *et al.*, 1998). Instead, anxiety is routinely relegated to the position of a diagnosis of exclusion. A number of studies have also suggested that gender differences in the presentation, attribution, and expression of anxiety symptoms may further delay the prompt recognition of anxiety disorders. Results from several studies also suggest that primary care physicians are more likely to attribute anxiety to a mood disorder, even when an anxiety disorder is primary (Rogers *et al.*, 1994).

Anxiety and mood disorders have extensive comorbidity. Lifetime prevalence estimates, in fact, suggest that more than two thirds of anxiety disorder patients will also develop a mood disorder, particularly depression (Kessler *et al.*, 1994). There is also substantial comorbidity between the anxiety disorders. For example, 40% of patients with OCD will also meet criteria for an additional anxiety disorder diagnosis during their lifetime (Rasmussen and Eisen, 1990; Pigott *et al.*, 1994; Hollander *et al.*, 1996a; Antony, Downie and Swinson, 1998). The frequent co-existence of mood and anxiety conditions may also further hinder the prompt and accurate diagnosis of anxiety disorders.

It remains unclear why anxiety disorders are so much more common in women than men. Genetic, biological, developmental, and environmental factors have all been implicated. Since anxiety and depression are both more prevalent in women than men, a shared or similar genetic basis may exist. Results from female twin studies provided some compelling support for a shared genetic diathesis between GAD and depression (Kendler *et al.*, 1992a, 1992b). However, available evidence suggests that the remaining anxiety disorders are characterized by less genetic homogeneity (Kendler *et al.*, 1992c, 1995).

Developmental and environmental factors are also likely to be important in the pathogenesis of anxiety disorders. Histories of childhood trauma or early separation anxiety increase the risk for both sexes that an anxiety disorder will subsequently occur (Young *et al.*, 1997; Stein *et al.*, 1998; Sutherland, Bybee and Sullivan, 1998). There is some intriguing evidence, however, that women may be differentially susceptible to the adverse consequences associated with childhood abuse. Breslau and colleagues have extensively investigated the impact of gender on PTSD. Their results suggest that when exposure rates are similar, women are more likely than men to develop PTSD after the occurrence of trauma. Moreover, a history of childhood trauma is a more reliable predictor in women than men that PTSD will be present as an adult (Breslau *et al.*, 1990, 1997a, 1997b). There is also evidence that gender differences exist in the type of anxiety disorder that may develop in response to chronic environmental stress. Galbaud and colleagues investigated the potential association in psychiatric diagnoses between spouses. They found that a diagnosis of depression, drug addiction, or antisocial personality disorder in one spouse increased the chances that the spouse would meet criteria for an anxiety disorder. However, a different anxiety disorder occurred in the women versus men spouses. That is,

Biological Psychiatry: Edited by H. D'haenen, J.A. den Boer and P. Willner. ISBN 0-471-49198-5

spouses with drug addiction or antisocial personality disorder were more likely to meet criteria for GAD if men, but PTSD if women (Galbaud-du-Fort *et al.*, 1998).

Although genetic and environmental factors are likely to be important in the development of anxiety disorders, the role of women gonadal hormones may be particularly critical in the pathogenesis of anxiety disorders. Women gonadal steroids, particularly oestrogen and progesterone, can elicit potent biological effects within the central nervous system. In addition, dramatic and cyclical fluctuations in gonadal hormone concentrations routinely occur throughout the female reproductive life span. These unique features may contribute to the finding that women have an increased risk for anxiety disorders. Despite the significant gender differences identified for prevalence rates, remarkably little research has focused on detecting any further gender differences in anxiety disorders. With these issues in mind, this chapter will provide a review of the available data concerning: (a) the potential impact of gender on the epidemiology, phenomenology, and clinical course of anxiety disorders; and (b) the impact of reproductive cycle events on the clinical course of anxiety disorders.

GENERALIZED ANXIETY DISORDER (GAD)

GAD is one of the most common of the anxiety disorders with most estimates suggesting a lifetime prevalence rate of between 5% and 6%. Women are two to three times more likely than men to meet lifetime criteria for GAD. The onset of GAD is typically during late adolescence or early adulthood and most studies suggest that a chronic, persistent course is most common (Boyd *et al.*, 1990; Kessler *et al.*, 1994; Wittchen *et al.*, 1994; Yonkers *et al.*, 1996; Woodman *et al.*, 1999). Although results from most population surveys suggest that anxiety disorders tend to decrease with increasing age, the prevalence rate for GAD remains at a constant rate throughout life (Krasucki, Howard and Mann, 1998).

GAD most commonly presents in the primary care setting (Woodman *et al.*, 1999). A diagnosis of GAD is associated with elevated rates of functional impairment. GAD is also linked to greater levels of medically unexplained symptoms and overutilization of health care resources. Roy-Byrne and Katon suggest that the increase in health care utilization reported with GAD does not occur by a direct path, but instead by acting as a catalyst that modifies the presentation of other psychiatric disorders that more directly affect health care costs (Roy-Byrne and Katon, 1997). Patients with GAD are also more likely to be prescribed psychotropic medication in comparison to patients without GAD (Wittchen *et al.*, 1994).

In addition to being associated with considerable disability and morbidity, remission rates with GAD are reported to be fairly low. For example, preliminary results from the large, prospective HARP Study indicate that after two years of follow-up only 8% of the patients with GAD were considered symptom-free (Yonkers *et al.*, 1996). A recent systematic comparison of GAD and panic patients revealed similarly dismal results. The GAD patients reported an earlier age of onset and a longer duration of illness. Moreover, significantly lower remission rates were noted in the patients with GAD (18%) than in the panic (45%) patients during the five-year study (Woodman *et al.*, 1999).

Gender Differences in GAD

More than 85% of patients with primary GAD will meet criteria for an additional lifetime psychiatric disorder (Boyd *et al.*, 1990; Kessler *et al.*, 1994; Wittchen *et al.*, 1994). Women with GAD are significantly more likely than men to meet criteria for an additional lifetime psychiatric condition (complicated GAD). Since results from population surveys and prospective studies suggest that complicated GAD has a worse prognosis and reduced chance of remission than GAD alone, this finding may help to explain why women with GAD are reported to have a more chronic course and greater symptom severity than men with GAD (Yonkers *et al.*, 1996). Women with GAD are also more likely than men with GAD to meet criteria for a depressive disorder, especially dysthymia (Wittchen *et al.*, 1994). This finding may also have important consequences since the presence of depression in patients with GAD has been associated with increased functional impairment and a greater risk of suicide in comparison to a diagnosis of GAD alone (Robins *et al.*, 1984; Wittchen *et al.*, 1994; Breslau, Schultz and Peterson, 1995; Bakish, 1999). Preliminary evidence also suggests that women with GAD are more likely to seek treatment with a health care professional than men, especially if comorbid diagnoses are also present (Bland, Newman and Orn, 1997a).

The finding that gender differences exist in GAD may have additional ramifications. The frequent co-occurrence of depression and GAD in women may also provide an important clue in understanding their underlying pathophysiology. That is, their common co-existence may reflect an enhanced vulnerability that is in part mediated by factors distinct to the women gender. While earlier investigations into the preponderance of anxiety disorders in women have tended to emphasize psychosocial and environmental factors, recent research has also investigated the potential role of genetic factors. Kendler and colleagues have investigated these issues by analysing data obtained from bivariate female twins. The female twin pair data provides compelling support for the role of genetic transmission as a primary mediating factor for GAD. The female twin data also suggests that GAD and depression may arise from the same genotype. That is, if a certain genotype is present within an individual, Kendler and colleagues hypothesize that either GAD or depression may develop as determined by a variety of environmental and biological influences (Kendler *et al.*, 1992a, 1992b, 1995).

The pathophysiology of GAD remains undetermined although serotonergic, noradrenergic, and GABAergic dysregulation are commonly implicated (Brawman-Mintzer and Lydiard, 1997). However, a neuroimaging study conducted in GAD patients demonstrated evidence of a more homogeneous distribution of benzodiazepine receptors throughout the cerebral hemispheres in the GAD patients versus control subjects. The reduced heterogeneity in cerebral blood flow associated with a diagnosis of GAD may be similar to the finding of reduced heterogeneity in myocardial blood flow associated with ischaemic heart disease (Tiihonen *et al.*, 1997). Unfortunately, the potential impact of gender on brain function in GAD has not been systematically assessed.

Medications reported to be effective for GAD include buspirone, benzodiazepines, venlafaxine and the SSRI antidepressants (Brawman-Mintzer and Lydiard, 1997). Data derived from animal models of anxiety suggest that response to anxiolytic medication, especially benzodiazepine anxiolytics, may be significantly influenced by gender as well as the phase of the oestrous cycle (Fernandez-Guasti and Picazo, 1990). While these results suggest that important gender differences in treatment response may occur in GAD, systematic data is not available. Unfortunately, the potential impact of gender on brain function in GAD has also not been systematically assessed.

There is some evidence that GAD symptoms become more severe during the premenstrual period in women with GAD and co-existing premenstrual syndrome (PMS). However, no change in symptom severity during the menstrual cycle was detected in the women with GAD who did not have co-existing PMS according to the same report (McLeod *et al.*, 1993). Further information about the impact of the menstrual cycle, pregnancy, or the menopause on the symptoms or course of GAD has not been reported at this time.

These findings indicate that important gender differences exist in the prevalence, clinical features, and comorbid conditions that may complicate GAD. There is some evidence that GAD symptom severity may be influenced by female reproductive hormone cycles but further information, especially about the potential impact of pregnancy and the post-partum period on GAD, is currently absent. Since preliminary evidence suggests that women with GAD have a more chronic course and a worse outcome, systematic data concerning gender differences in underlying pathophysiology and/or treatment response is clearly needed.

PANIC DISORDER

Estimates derived from large-scale community surveys suggest a 1.5%–2.0% lifetime prevalence rate for panic disorder. Women are two to three times more likely than men to meet lifetime criteria for panic disorder (Regier *et al.*, 1988, 1990; Eaton, Dryman and Weissman *et al.*, 1991; Kessler *et al.*, 1994; Dick, Bland and Newman, 1994b). Panic onset is typically during adolescence or early adulthood and is very rare after the age of 40. Men and women have a similar age of onset for panic disorder (Dick, Bland and Newman, 1994b). Despite substantial fluctuations in severity over time, most patients with panic disorder report a chronic clinical course (Joyce *et al.*, 1989; Keller and Hanks, 1993).

A diagnosis of panic disorder has been linked to a number of adverse consequences including increased utilization of medical and mental health services and elevated rates of suicidal behaviour (Weissman *et al.*, 1989; Katerndahl, 1990; Hollifield *et al.*, 1997; Katerndahl and Realini, 1997). Data from the largest prospective study of patients with anxiety disorders to date, the HARP study, confirm that 40% of panic patients will be in treatment at one year and 30%–40% are likely to require long-term, maintenance medication (Keller and Hanks, 1993).

Gender Differences in Panic Disorder

Several significant gender differences have been identified for panic disorder. As previously noted, panic is two to three times more common in women than in men. In addition, the occurrence of panic attacks even in the absence of meeting full criteria for panic disorder may represent a significant development, especially in women. For example, 63% of women and 40% of men that experienced panic attacks subsequently developed an additional psychiatric disorder in one report (Reed and Wittchen, 1998). Gender differences have also been identified in the phenomenology of panic disorder. Women with panic disorder report more individual panic symptoms and greater levels of phobic avoidance in comparison to men with panic disorder (Dick, Bland and Newman, 1994b). They are also more likely to report that leaving home alone or using public transportation triggers their panic attacks. Women with panic disorder are also more likely than men to report that they rely on family members to enter fearful situations. The apparently increased level of dependence on others endorsed by women with panic disorder may help to explain the finding that women with panic have a greater degree of functional impairment in comparison to men with panic (Weissman *et al.*, 1997; Starcevic *et al.*, 1998; Turgeon, Marchand and Dupuis, 1998).

Women with primary panic disorder are more likely than men to meet criteria for an additional lifetime psychiatric disorder (Yonkers *et al.*, 1998). Gender also appears to have a significant impact on the type of comorbid psychiatric diagnosis that will present during the course of panic disorder. Comorbid agoraphobia depression, GAD, simple phobia, and somatization disorder are more likely to complicate panic disorder in women than in men (Katerndahl, 1990; Andrade, Eaton and Chilcoat, 1996; Marshall, 1996; Yonkers *et al.*, 1996, 1998). In contrast, men with panic disorder have greater rates of comorbid alcohol abuse. Alcohol-related disorders are not uncommon in women with panic disorder, however, as illustrated by the finding that women with panic disorder are at an increased risk of developing alcohol abuse or dependence in comparison to women without panic disorder (Otto *et al.*, 1992; Cox *et al.*, 1993; Kessler *et al.*, 1994). Interestingly, preliminary evidence suggests that women with panic disorder may have an elevated rate of relatives with alcohol dependence. Although further research is needed, this and additional findings has resulted in considerable speculation concerning a possible genetic link between panic and alcohol abuse in women (Battaglia *et al.*, 1995; Kendler *et al.*, 1995).

The data suggesting that women with panic disorder have an elevated risk for comorbid psychiatric disorders in general and certain comorbid disorders in particular may have critical implications. The presence of agoraphobia in panic disorder is associated with a less favourable outcome than the presence of panic disorder alone. Since agoraphobia is more common in women than in men with panic disorder, women with panic disorder might be expected to have a worse prognosis. There is evidence supporting this finding. For example, women with panic disorder and agoraphobia report greater phobic avoidance, more catastrophic thoughts, and a heightened awareness of body sensations in comparison to men that have panic disorder with agoraphobia. Women with panic disorder complicated by agoraphobia are also more likely to meet criteria for social anxiety disorder and/or PTSD (Stein *et al.*, 1989; Turgeon, Marchand and Dupuis, 1998). The increased prevalence of agoraphobia in women with panic disorder may also contribute to the consistent finding of a more chronic and severe clinical course for panic disorder in women in comparison to men (Boyd *et al.*, 1990; Hollifield *et al.*, 1997; Katerndahl and Realini, 1997; Joyce *et al.*, 1989; Yonkers *et al.*, 1998). Recent prospective data also suggests that if a period of remission occurs during the course of panic disorder, women have an increased risk for recurrence of panic disorder (Yonkers *et al.*, 1998).

These findings indicate that a diagnosis of panic disorder in women in comparison to men is associated with a more complicated course and an overall poorer outcome. Since the aetiology of panic disorder remains obscure, it is difficult to explain why women have a greater risk and a more malevolent course for panic disorder than men. Numerous neurobiological and psychological theories have been proposed for panic disorder. Most psychological theories emphasize the importance of cognitive misinterpretation and ‘false threat alarms’ as the basis for the subsequent development of panic disorder (Windmann, 1998). Biological theories, in contrast, implicate altered brain function and an abnormal ventilatory response in the pathophysiology of panic (Klein, 1993; Bell and Nutt, 1998). Neural circuits within the amygdala and its ascending cortical pathways are most often speculated to represent the functional neuroanatomy of panic disorder. Altered dysregulation of the ventilatory response and associated neurovascular instability may also be important factors in the pathophysiology of panic disorder (Coplan and Lydiard, 1998). Both physiological (e.g., CO_2 sensitivity) and psychological (anxiety sensitivity) factors have been suggested as predisposing factors in the development of panic disorder (Coplan and Lydiard, 1998; Stein, Jang and Livesley, 1999). Despite the striking gender differences identified in the prevalence and clinical features associated with panic disorder, evidence of significant gender differences in the purported pathophysiology of panic disorder have not been detected.

Results from covariate female twin studies suggest that genetic or familial factors play a role in panic disorder, although their contribution is estimated to be relatively modest (Kendler *et al.*, 1993, 1995). There is some evidence that genetic factors may be particularly critical in determining risk for panic disorder in women. That is, the presence of a specific genetic polymorphism in women may convey an increased risk for panic disorder. Women with panic disorder are reported to have a higher occurrence of a novel repeat genetic polymorphism on chromosome X than control subjects. This genetic polymorphism is thought to mediate expression of monoamine oxidase A. Since monoamine-oxidase-inhibiting antidepressants are known to be effective anti-panic agents, this finding has been interpreted as evidence that altered monoamine oxidase A activity may be a risk factor for panic disorder, at least in women (Deckert *et al.*, 1999).

Important gender differences in the presentation, clinical features, and overall course of panic disorder have been identified. Women with panic disorder are more likely to have agoraphobia and other comorbid conditions than men with panic disorder. The elevated risk for comorbid conditions likely contributes to the poorer prognosis reported for women than men with panic disorder. However, the potential contribution of differential avoidance strategies and other clinical characteristics that may influence prognosis in panic disorder requires further study.

Panic Disorder and Female Reproductive Cycles

Oestrogen and progesterone have complex effects on the CNS. Oestrogen is generally considered a facilitator of neurotransmission via its ability to reduce MAO enzyme activity and enhance serotonergic tone. Oestrogen's biological actions are thought to convey some mood-enhancing or antidepressant effects. In contrast, progesterone increases MAO enzyme activity. Pregnanolone, a major metabolite of progesterone, enhances GABA tone via its effects as an allosteric modulator at the GABA-benzodiazepine receptor complex. Since GABA represents one of the major inhibitors of neurotransmission within the CNS, progesterone's biological effects may convey an anxiolytic action (Shear, 1997; Stahl, 1997; Warnock and Bundren, 1997).

The female reproductive cycle (menstruation, menopause, and pregnancy) is characterized by relatively dramatic fluctuations in oestrogen and progesterone concentrations. These hormonal fluctuations may have a role in determining the overall risk for panic disorder and may also have a substantial impact on the clinical course of panic disorder in women. The dramatic decline in oestrogen and progesterone levels that characterizes the mid-luteal phase of the menstrual cycle has been linked to the emergence or worsening of anxiety symptoms in women (Yonkers and Ellison, 1996). Several reports, primarily retrospective in nature, confirm that women with panic disorder report an increase in their anxiety and panic symptoms during the mid-luteal or premenstrual phase of the menstrual cycle (Cook *et al.*, 1990; Griez *et al.*, 1990). This finding, however, has not been replicated in studies conducted on a prospective basis. Instead, prospective studies reported to date have failed to detect any significant association between menstrual cycle phase and ratings of panic or anxiety symptoms in women with panic disorder (Stein *et al.*, 1989; Cook *et al.*, 1990).

In contrast, biological challenge paradigms conducted in women with panic disorder have detected some evidence of changes in anxiety sensitivity across the menstrual cycle. Acute ingestion of carbon dioxide (CO_2) is often used as a provocative challenge to precipitate anxiety and panic attacks in experimental conditions (Griez *et al.*, 1990). Women with panic disorder have been reported to demonstrate evidence of menstrual cycle phase (follicular vs luteal)-dependent changes in anxiety sensitivity in at least one report (Fishman *et al.*, 1994). In this report, women with panic disorder demonstrated elevated anxiety responses during the mid-luteal phase of the menstrual cycle in comparison to the earlier follicular phase when serially administered CO_2. The women control subjects did not demonstrate any significant relationship between CO_2-induced anxiety and phase of the menstrual cycle during the same study (Perna *et al.*, 1995). Interestingly, subsequent treatment of the same group of women with panic disorder with alprazolam was associated with apparent 'normalization' of the CO_2-induced anxiety response in the same report (Fishman *et al.*, 1994).

Precipitous oestrogen withdrawal, whether physiological or induced by medication or surgical intervention, has also been linked to the subsequent emergence of panic disorder. In a large study ($n = 390$) of peri-menopausal women with new-onset but 'ill-defined' psychological and somatic symptoms, 7% were found to meet criteria for panic disorder (Ushiroyama and Sugimoto, 1994). Moreover, results from another report indicate that a diagnosis of panic disorder should be considered in peri-menopausal women with hot flashes that fail to attenuate during hormone replacement therapy (van der Feltz-Cornelis, 1999). Medical interventions that have primary progesterone-like effects, such as birth control pills or Norplant implants, have also been associated with the acute development of panic disorder (Wagner and Berenson, 1994). Ovarian suppressants utilized for the treatment of endometriosis such as leuprolide may also elicit panic attacks and other psychiatric disturbances (Warnock and Bundren, 1997).

Pregnancy and the post-partum period are marked by particularly dramatic fluctuations in gonadal hormone concentrations. Pregnancy is characterized by 2–3-fold increases in oestrogen and a dramatic elevation (80–100 times) in progesterone concentration (Altshuler, Hendrick and Cohen, 1998). Progesterone is a potent stimulant for oxygen drive and as previously noted its metabolite, allopregnanolone, has GABA-enhancing effects. With these actions in mind, women with pre-existing panic disorder might be expected to experience a substantial attenuation or remission in panic during pregnancy. Available data, however, suggests a more variable course for pre-existing panic disorder during pregnancy. Summarizing available data, it appears that about half (40%–45%) will not have a significant change in their panic symptoms, whereas 30%–35% will experience improvement and a substantial worsening in panic will occur in 20%–30% of patients with pre-existing panic disorder during the course of pregnancy (Cohen *et al.*, 1994a, 1994b; Northcott and Stein, 1994). Interestingly, the course of panic disorder during successive pregnancies is often markedly different (Villeponteaux *et al.*, 1992; Cohen *et al.*, 1994a, 1994b; Northcott and Stein, 1994).

Post-partum worsening (35%–63%) is a much more consistent finding demonstrated in women with pre-existing panic disorder (Sholomskas *et al.*, 1993; Cohen *et al.*, 1994a, 1994b; Northcott and Stein, 1994; Beck, 1998). The post-partum period may also be associated with an increased risk for the onset of panic disorder. According to available data, 11%–29% of women with panic disorder report onset during the post-partum period (Sholomskas *et al.*, 1993; Wisner, Peindl and Hanusa, 1996). Since this rate is significantly greater than the expected age-corrected rate for panic onset in women, it is unlikely to represent a coincidental event (Sholomskas *et al.*, 1993). In patients with pre-existing panic disorder, pregnancy does not appear to increase the likelihood that medication for panic can be successfully discontinued (Cohen *et al.*, 1994a, 1994b). Instead, there is some rational for continuing or restarting pharmacotherapy during the latter part of pregnancy. Cohen and colleagues demonstrated that pregnant women with pre-existing panic disorder who receive anti-panic medication are significantly less likely to experience a post-partum exacerbation than those who did not receive treatment during pregnancy (Cohen *et al.*, 1994b).

Selective serotonin reuptake inhibitors (SSRI), monoamine oxidase inhibitors (MAOI), and tricyclic (TCA) antidepressants have all demonstrated efficacy in the treatment of panic disorder (Sheehan, 1999). High-potency benzodiazepine medications such as lorazepam, alprazolam, and clonazepam are also effective anti-panic agents. Each of the anti-panic medications (SSRI, MAOI, TCA, and benzodiazepines) is associated with a similar rate of improvement (60%–70%) in panic symptomatology. However, buspirone and other medications with primary serotonergic effects do not appear to be more effective than placebo for panic disorder (Bell and Nutt, 1998). Little information is available concerning the potential impact of gender on treatment response in panic disorder. Results from one study (Kalus *et al.*, 1991) suggest that the TCA, desipramine, may be less effective in men than in women with panic disorder.

These findings indicate that important gender differences exist in the prevalence, clinical features, and overall course of panic disorder. Women are more likely to have panic disorder with comorbid conditions, especially agoraphobia. They are also more likely than men to suffer a recurrence of panic symptoms after remission of panic disorder. Available data also suggests that the female reproductive cycle, especially pregnancy and the postpartum period, can have an important impact on the course of panic disorder. Moreover, declining female hormone levels associated with the ageing process or as a consequence of medical or surgical interventions can precipitate or elicit an exacerbation in panic disorder. Although preliminary evidence also suggests that treatment response may be different in men versus women with panic disorder, further studies that focus on this critical issue are clearly needed. The potential contribution of differential avoidance strategies and other clinical characteristics that may influence prognosis in panic disorder also requires further investigation.

SIMPLE PHOBIA

Results from large-scale population surveys confirm that simple phobias represent one of the most common psychiatric disorders. More than 20% of adults are estimated to meet criteria for simple phobia (Eaton, Dryman and Weissman, 1991; Kessler *et al.*, 1994). Simple phobias encompass a wide range of situations and 'feared' objects. Women are twice as likely as men to meet criteria for simple phobia (Bourdon *et al.*, 1988; Boyd *et al.*, 1990; Dick *et al.*, 1994a). Depression, substance abuse, and OCD are frequently comorbid with simple phobias (Bourdon *et al.*, 1988; Regier, Narron and Rae, 1990; Eaton, Dryman and Weissman, 1991; Kessler *et al.*, 1994; Magee *et al.*, 1996). Some authors have suggested that simple phobias can be sub-classified into three primary classes: (a) situational phobias (e.g., claustrophobia, acrophobia); (b) animal phobias (e.g., fear of spiders, insects, snakes, etc.); and (c) health-related phobias (e.g., fear of injections, blood, dental procedures, etc.). Using this schemata for simple phobia, situational phobias are most common, followed by animal and then health-related phobia, respectively. Women reportedly are two to three times more likely than men to meet criteria for situational and animal phobia, whereas health-related phobia appears to occur at a similar rate in women and men (Fredrikson *et al.*, 1996).

In addition to increased prevalence rates, women may also have an earlier age of onset for simple phobia than men (Dick *et al.*, 1994a). Although they tend to have a chronic course, the associated disability is generally reported as minimal and relatively few (20%–25%) people with simple phobias seek treatment (Boyd *et al.*, 1990; Lindal and Stefansson, 1993). Data derived from female twin studies suggest that environmental factors are more critical than genetic factors in the development of simple phobia (Kendler *et al.*, 1992c). Additional data concerning potential gender differences or the possible influence of reproductive cycles on simple phobia is currently lacking.

SOCIAL ANXIETY DISORDER

Although an initial population study reported that it was relatively rare, data from subsequent population surveys estimate that more than 13% of people will meet lifetime criteria for social anxiety disorder (Boyd *et al.*, 1990; Schneier *et al.*, 1992; Kessler *et al.*, 1994; Stein, Walker and Forde, 1994; Stein and Chavira, 1998). Women are slightly (1.5 times) more likely than men to meet criteria for social anxiety disorder (Kessler *et al.*, 1994; Dick *et al.*, 1994a). Two subtypes (generalized and discrete) of social anxiety disorder are generally recognized. The generalized subtype of social anxiety disorder is comprised of individuals with pervasive performance and interact ional fears in a broad range of social activities, whereas the discrete subtype is limited to anxiety in only certain, focal situations. The two subtypes of social anxiety disorder appear remarkably similar in terms of age of onset, family history, and certain socio-demographic correlates (Kessler *et al.*, 1994; Stein, Walker and Forde, 1994; Stein and Chavira, 1998). However, considerable differences have been identified between the subtypes in terms of clinical course and complications. Discrete social anxiety is associated with an episodic course and minimal functional impairment (Stein, Walker and Forde, 1994) In contrast, generalized social anxiety is more likely to be chronic, complicated by comorbid psychiatric conditions, and associated with substantial functional impairment (Kessler, Stein and Berglund, 1998). Despite the considerable disability associated with generalized social anxiety disorder, relatively few (20%–25%) patients enter treatment (Boyd *et al.*, 1990; Kessler *et al.*, 1994; Schneier *et al.*, 1994).

The low treatment rates reported may in part reflect the difficulties encountered in rapidly and accurately diagnosing social anxiety disorder. Most studies suggest that as many as 5% of patients evaluated in primary care meet criteria for social anxiety disorder, but very few are properly identified. Results from a recent primary care study illustrate the enormity of this problem. Their primary care physicians recognized less than half of the patients with social anxiety disorder as having 'a psychiatric illness'. Overall during the study, the physicians failed to identify 85% of the patients who met criteria for social anxiety disorder (Lecrubier and Weiller, 1997; Bisserbee *et al.*, 1996).

Comorbid disorders are extremely common and may help to obscure the primary diagnosis of social anxiety disorder. Since onset frequently occurs during adolescence, comorbid disorders generally develop after the emergence of social anxiety disorder (Schneier *et al.*, 1992; Stein and Chavira, 1998; Kessler, Stein and Berglund, 1998). Agoraphobia probably represents the most common comorbid psychiatric condition (odds ratio 10 : 4) in social anxiety disorder. Comorbid depression (60%–90%) and alcohol abuse (30%–40%) also frequently complicate generalized social anxiety disorder (Kessler *et al.*, 1994, 1998; Dick *et al.*, 1994a; Stein and Chavira, 1998). Patients with generalized social anxiety disorder have elevated rates of drug abuse including an increased risk for prescription drug abuse (Bisserbee *et al.*, 1996; Lecrubier and Weiller, 1997).

A considerable overlap in diagnostic criteria exists between avoidant personality and social anxiety disorder. It is not surprising, therefore, that 70%–90% of patients with generalized social anxiety have co-existing avoidant personality disorder. The co-occurrence of social anxiety disorder and avoidant personality disorder appears to convey an increased risk for depressive disorder as well as a greater degree of functional impairment in comparison to social anxiety alone (Alpert *et al.*, 1997).

Childhood behavioural inhibition is implicated as a non-specific risk factor for the development of an anxiety disorder in adults. However, social anxiety disorder, in particular, is most strongly associated with a history of behavioural inhibition during childhood (Mick and Telch, 1998). Childhood selective mutism may represent a precursor to the development of social anxiety disorder. In fact, 70% of the first-degree relatives of children with selective mutism were reported to have social anxiety disorder in one study (Black and Uhde, 1995).

The neurobiology of social anxiety disorder is poorly understood, although preliminary research has identified evidence of several different biological abnormalities. Challenge paradigms comparing social anxiety disorder patients and control subjects after acute administration of carbon dioxide, cholecystokinin, or caffeine have detected evidence of enhanced sensitivity and potential cardiovascular and adrenergic abnormalities in the social anxiety disorder patients. Serotonergic dysfunction is implicated by pharmacological challenge results as well as the efficacy of the SSRI antidepressants in the treatment of social anxiety disorder (Nutt, Bell and Malizia, 1998; Ballenger *et al.*, 1998; Davidson, 1998). Patients with social anxiety disorder administered serotonergic probes demonstrate evidence of altered neuroendocrine and behavioural responses in comparison to control subjects. Functional neuroimaging studies reveal evidence of altered dopaminergic function in social anxiety subjects. In particular, a significant reduction in striatal dopamine reuptake has been detected in social anxiety disorder patients versus control subjects (Nutt, Bell and Malizia, 1998).

A number of pharmacological treatments, including the MAOIs, reversible inhibitors of MAO-A, beta-blockers, high-potency benzodiazepines, and the SSRIs have all demonstrated efficacy in the treatment of social anxiety disorder (Ballenger *et al.*, 1998; Davidson, 1998; Pollack, 1999). In the largest multicentre, placebo-controlled trial reported to date, paroxetine was more effective than placebo in both moderate and severe social anxiety disorder (Stein *et al.*, 1998). According to the International Consensus Treatment Guidelines for Mood and Anxiety Disorders, SSRI antidepressants are considered first-line therapy for social anxiety disorder. These guidelines also advocate long-term (>12 months) treatment for patients with generalized social anxiety disorder that have: (a) persistent symptoms despite treatment; (b) a comorbid psychiatric condition; (c) a history of relapse after treatment discontinuation; or (d) a very early onset of social anxiety disorder (Ballenger *et al.*, 1998). However, little information is available concerning the potential impact of gender on treatment response in social anxiety disorder.

Gender Differences in SAD

Evidence of significant gender differences has been reported in patients with SAD. As previously noted, women (15.5%) have a slightly elevated risk for SAD than men (11.1%). Interestingly, men with SAD appear more likely to seek treatment than women with SAD (Weinstock, 1999). Turk and colleagues systematically assessed the potential impact of gender on SAD in a recent report. They failed to detect evidence of gender differences in the prevalence of SAD subtype, the occurrence of comorbid disorders such as additional anxiety disorders, mood disorders, or avoidant personality disorder, or in the clinical course of a group of patients with SAD. However, Turk and colleagues did identify some significant gender differences in the phenomenology of SAD. Women with SAD exhibited more severe social fears than men with GAD. In addition, data derived from self-report measures revealed that the SAD women endorsed more severe fear in a wide range of activities including talking to authority figures, acting/performing/speaking/working in front of others or while being observed, being the centre of attention, expressing disagreement or disapproval to people they do not know very well, or giving a party. Women were also more likely than men to report that going to a party was a trigger for SAD symptoms. In contrast, the men with SAD endorsed more severe symptoms in only two distinct situations: urinating in public bathrooms and returning goods to a store. Men more frequently reported fear of urinating in a public restroom than women in the same group of SAD patients (Turk *et al.*, 1998). Although no gender differences in comorbid conditions were detected in the report by Turk and Co-workers, results from two other studies (Dick *et al.*, 1994a; Lecrubier and Weiller, 1997) have that agoraphobia may be more frequent in women than in men with SAD.

Results from bivariate female twin studies and family studies provide support for the importance of genetic factors in the development of generalized SAD (Kendler *et al.*, 1992c; Stein *et al.*, 1998, 1999). Patients with generalized SAD are 10 times more likely to have relatives with SAD than control subjects (Stein *et al.*, 1998). Results from the Stein and Co-workers study (1998) also imparted strong support for the validity of separating SAD into generalized versus non-generalized groups for research purposes. Data derived during the same study failed to support the role of genetic or familial effects as primary factors in the transmission of the non-generalized form of SAD. Little information is available concerning the impact of female reproductive cycle events and SAD. However, since depression, panic, and substance abuse are frequent complications of untreated SAD, further research appears indicated (Weinstock, 1999).

These results suggest that women are slightly more likely to meet criteria for SAD during their lifetime and that the clinical features associated with SAD may be substantially influenced by gender. The presence of comorbid conditions in primary SAD may also be impacted by gender, although conflicting findings have been reported. Probably the largest vacuum in knowledge about SAD exists in the areas of treatment response and in the potential impact of reproductive hormone cycle events on the onset and/or clinical course of SAD in women. Given the significant psychosocial burden associated with a diagnosis of SAD, future research efforts should focus on these important issues.

OCD

Results from the ECA and the subsequent Cross-National OCD Collaborative Group Study confirm that the lifetime prevalence rate for OCD is between 2% and 3% worldwide. These studies also demonstrate that women are 1.5 times more likely than men to meet lifetime criteria for OCD (Karno *et al.*, 1988; Weissman *et al.*, 1994). The onset of OCD is generally during adolescence or young adulthood. Baer has demonstrated that OCD symptoms can be subdivided into three primary symptom factors: 'symmetry/hoarding', 'contamination/cleaning', and 'pure obsessions' (Baer, 1994). Sixty to seventy percent of patients with OCD endorse substantial psychosocial and occupational dysfunction (Koran, Thieneman and Davenport, 1996; Hollander *et al.*, 1998). An OCD diagnosis is also associated with elevated utilization of medical and mental health services (Kennedy and Schwab, 1997; Hollander *et al.*, 1998). The total annual cost of OCD-related impairment is estimated to exceed $8 billion dollars (Dupont *et al.*, 1995). Unfortunately, OCD remains vastly under-diagnosed and persistently under-treated. Moreover, results from a recently published survey of OCD patients suggest that the average time between symptom onset and initial treatment contact in OCD exceeds 10 years (Hollander *et al.*, 1998).

OCD has historically been considered to be chronic in course, but recent data suggests that the course may be more variable than previously appreciated. An episodic clinical course may occur in as much as 1/3 of OCD patients (Perugi *et al.*, 1998; Antony, Downie and Swinson, 1998; Steketee *et al.*, 1997; Thomsen and Mikkelsen, 1995). Factors reported to be associated with an episodic course of OCD include lower rates of checking rituals and an increased risk of relatives with mood disorders (Perugi *et al.*, 1998). Sustained remission, however, appears to be fairly rare in OCD with either an episodic or chronic clinical course (Hollander *et al.*, 1996b; Bland, Newman and Orn, 1997b; Perugi *et al.*, 1998).

Most patients with OCD will have comorbid psychiatric disorders. Major depressive disorder appears to be the most common comorbid diagnosis with a 60%–80% lifetime prevalence rate. Additional anxiety disorder diagnoses (40%) also frequently co-exist in OCD, especially panic disorder and social anxiety disorder (Rasmussen and Eisen, 1992; Pigott *et al.*, 1994; Weissman *et al.*, 1994; Antony, Downie and Swinson, 1998). Other conditions that frequently occur in OCD include substance abuse, schizophrenia, body dysmorphic disorder, hypochondriasis, Tourette's Syndrome, and anorexia nervosa (Rasmussen and Eisen, 1990, 1992; Pigott *et al.*, 1994; Weissman *et al.*, 1994; Antony, Downie and Swinson, 1998). Interestingly, the presence of comorbid mood or anxiety disorders does not appear to convey any additional burden in terms of the phenomenology, course, or prognosis of OCD (Demal *et al.*, 1993; Steketee *et al.*, 1997). In a systematic assessment of over 300 OCD patients, Perugi and colleagues found that 16% were comorbid for bipolar disorder. The OCD patients with co-existing bipolar disorder had a more gradual onset and a more episodic course. An elevated rate of sexual and religious obsessions was also associated with the presence of bipolar disorder in OCD (Perugi *et al.*, 1998).

Numerous challenge studies with serotonergic (5-HT) probes have revealed evidence of altered behavioural or neuroendocrine responses in OCD patients in comparison to control subjects. In contrast, OCD patients do not appear to exhibit evidence of altered noradrenergic and/or dopaminergic function in comparison to control subjects using various challenge paradigms (Zohar and Insel, 1987; Goodman *et al.*, 1990; Pigott, 1996). The preferential efficacy of serotonin-selective medications for OCD coupled with the evidence of selective serotonergic dysfunction in challenge studies provides fairly compelling evidence for the importance of serotonin in OCD.

Data from epidemiological and familial-genetic studies provide strong support for an important association between OCD and tic disorder/Tourette's syndrome (Karno *et al.*, 1988; Leonard *et al.*, 1992; Rasmussen and Eisen, 1992; Santangelo *et al.*, 1994). Tic disorder occurs in approximately 10%–15% of patients with OCD and patients with tic disorders have extremely high rates of comorbid OCD. In fact, most estimates suggest that 40%–60% of patients with TS or tic disorder will also have OCD. The considerable overlap in occurrence between OCD and tic disorders has elicited considerable interest. Several investigators have explored potential differences between patients with OCD and those with OCD and comorbid tic disorder (Pauls *et al.*, 1995). In terms of phenomenology, OCD patients with comorbid TS are more likely than OCD patients without TS to report obsessions involving non-violent images, excessive concern with appearance, and need for symmetry. Touching, blinking or staring, and counting compulsions are also reported to be more common in OCD patients with comorbid TS than in those with OCD alone. Preliminary evidence also suggests that a childhood history of ADHD is more common in OCD patients with tic disorder than in those without comorbid tic disorder (Petter, Richter and Sandor, 1998). In addition, OCD patients with co-existing TS have higher rates of bipolar disorder, social phobia, body dysmorphic disorder, attention deficit hyperactivity disorder (ADHD), and substance use disorders in comparison to those with OCD alone or TS alone (Coffey *et al.*, 1998). Family studies also provide support for the contention that OCD with comorbid tic disorder represents a distinct subtype of OCD. OCD is much more prevalent than tic disorder in the first-degree relatives of patients with OCD, whereas the risk for tic disorder is two times greater than the risk for OCD in the first-degree relatives of patients with OCD and tics (Yang and Liu, 1998).

These putative differences in clinical features have resulted in considerable speculation concerning potential differences in the underlying pathophysiology of OCD versus OCD with comorbid TS or tic disorder. In particular, OCD without tic disorder may arise primarily from serotonergic abnormalities, whereas dysfunction in the dopaminergic and serotonergic systems may occur in those with OCD comorbid for tic disorder (Petter, Richter and Sandor, 1998). Recent investigations using genetic association techniques have explored dopaminergic (D) function in OCD. Polymorphic variations have been identified in the genes that determine the expression of the D2, D3, and D4 receptors, respectively. Patients with OCD have been reported to have an increased frequency of the allele associated with a polymorphic variant of the D4 receptor; no differences were detected between the OCD and control subjects in the distribution of alleles in the genotypes for the D2 and D3 receptors (Billett *et al.*, 1998). However, results from another recent report suggest that future genetic association studies conducted in OCD should consider the presence of a comorbid tic disorder as a potential confounding factor. Patients with OCD and tic disorder were noted to have an increased frequency of the variant alleles identified for both the D2 and D4 receptor genes when compared to patients with OCD alone (Nicolini *et al.*, 1998). These findings provide further evidence that dopamine function may be altered in OCD, especially in OCD patients with comorbid tic disorder who may represent a genetically distinct subtype of OCD.

The SSRI antidepressants and the TCA, clomipramine, remain the cornerstone of the pharmacological treatment for OCD (Orloff *et al.*, 1994; Jefferson *et al.*, 1995; Stein, Spadaccini and Hollander, 1995). Although these medications effectively reduce OCD symptoms, the average improvement is fairly modest (30%–40%). Patients who developed OCD later in life had a better chance of response than do those who became ill earlier, independent of length of illness (Ackerman *et al.*, 1994). Re-analysis of data from the multicentre, placebo-controlled, fixed-dose trials of fluoxetine in OCD revealed that response rates and overall improvement were greatest for patients with histories of remission, lack of previous drug treatment, and more severe OCD (especially with greater interference and distress from obsessions) (Ackerman, Greenland and Bystritsky, 1998). Non-response to either clomipramine or fluoxetine treatment has been linked to the presence of: (a) concomitant schizotypal personality disorder; (b) prominent compulsions; and (c) a longer illness length (Ravizza *et al.*, 1995).

Gender Differences in OCD

The impact of gender has been extensively investigated in OCD in comparison to the other anxiety disorders. In addition to the gender difference noted in lifetime prevalence rates for OCD, results from community surveys have consistently demonstrated that the mean age of OCD onset is significantly earlier in men (20 years) than in women (25 years). Data from clinical samples also support the finding that OCD onset is earlier in males than in females, although the age of onset in clinical samples is typically during adolescence rather than young adulthood (Rasmussen and Eisen, 1990, 1992).

Children often manifest OCD-like behaviours as part of their normal development. For example, a standardized assessment for OCD symptoms was administered to a large community sample of children aged 9 to 15 years. The girls and the boys endorsed similar amounts of obsessive–compulsive behaviours during the study. The boys were more likely to admit to checking behaviours and cleaning behaviours were more common in the girls. OCD-like behaviours were more common in the 9- to 12-year-olds than in the 13–15-year-old children. Elevated anxiety levels were reported in the few subjects that continued to have persistent OCD behaviours during adolescence (Zohar and Bruno, 1997). These results suggest that OCD-like behaviours are common in elementary aged children, but persistence into adolescence is rare and may represent the initial symptoms of clinical OCD.

Childhood-onset OCD appears to have some unique features in comparison to adult-onset OCD. As previously noted, boys are two to three times more likely than girls to have OCD during childhood. Comorbid psychiatric disorders, especially ADHD and other developmental disorders, are very common in childhood-onset

OCD. Neuropsychological deficits and familial loading for OCD are also common in childhood-onset OCD. Long-term studies indicate that childhood-onset OCD may also be associated with a graver prognosis. Most reports suggest that patients with childhood-onset OCD rarely experience remission (Demal *et al.*, 1993; Thomsen and Mikkelsen, 1995; Hantouche and Lancrenon, 1996; Steketee *et al.*, 1997). In fact, Leonard and colleagues conducted one of the largest ($n = 54$) and longest (up to seven years) prospective follow-up study of children and adolescents with OCD. They reported that after an average of three years of follow-up, 81% of the patients treated with clomipramine were significantly improved, but only 6% of the subjects were considered to be in remission. Predictors of worse outcome for the childhood-onset OCD patients were: (a) more severe OCD symptoms score after 5 weeks of clomipramine therapy; (b) a lifetime history of a tic disorder; and (c) the presence of a parental Axis I psychiatric diagnosis (Leonard *et al.*, 1992).

As previously noted, men typically have an earlier onset of OCD than women. In fact, three times as many boys as girls meet diagnostic criteria for OCD. Recent investigations have identified a potential variant of OCD designated as early onset OCD. This variant is characterized by the onset of OCD before the age of 10, occurs predominantly in boys, and is strongly associated with tic disorder and a positive family history (Leonard *et al.*, 1992; Pauls *et al.*, 1995). The data concerning the potential link between OCD and tic disorder has already been reviewed; however, it is important to note that men are much more likely to have OCD with a comorbid tic disorder as well as an earlier onset of illness. This finding may also suggest that gender differences may exist in the pathophysiological mechanisms that underlie OCD. Dopamine dysregulation may be more prominent in men with OCD, whereas women gonadal steroid hormones and their complex interactions with serotonin may be more critical to the development of OCD in women. The dramatic shift that occurs in gender prevalence rates for OCD after the onset of puberty provides support for the importance of female reproductive hormones. Women begin to develop OCD at a much greater rate than men after menarche; the increase is sufficiently robust that the overall prevalence rate in OCD is greater for women (1.5 : 1.0) than men (Weissman *et al.*, 1994; Karno *et al.*, 1988).

Gender differences have also been identified in the phenomenology and clinical course of OCD. Aggressive obsessions and cleaning compulsions may occur more frequently in women with OCD (Noshirvani *et al.*, 1991; Castle, Deale and Marks, 1995; Lensi *et al.*, 1996). In a systematic assessment of adolescents with OCD, females endorsed a greater amount of compulsive rituals, whereas obsessions were more common in the males with OCD (Valleni-Basile *et al.*, 1994). Women with OCD may also have a more episodic clinical course and less severe symptoms (Thomsen and Mikkelsen, 1995; Hantouche and Lancrenon, 1996).

Women with OCD may also have a greater risk of certain comorbid conditions than men with OCD. Comorbid panic disorder and eating disorders such as anorexia nervosa or bulimia nervosa are reported to occur more frequently in women than men with OCD (Noshirvani *et al.*, 1991; Rubenstein *et al.*, 1992; Tamburrino, Kaufman and Hertzer, 1994; Castle, Deale and Marks, 1995; Kendler *et al.*, 1995; Yaryura-Tobias, Neziroglu and Kaplan, 1995; Lensi *et al.*, 1996). Since anorexia and bulimia nervosa are associated with marked alterations in female reproductive hormone function, the frequent association of OCD with eating disorders also provides indirect evidence for the importance of the female reproductive cycle in the course of OCD.

Gender differences may also exist in response to serotonergic probes during challenge studies conducted in OCD patients. Women with OCD administered the serotonergic probe fenfluramine have an attenuated cortisol response in comparison to men with OCD and control subjects (Monteleone *et al.*, 1997). Acute intravenous administration of clomipramine is also used as a probe of 5-HT function. Results from clomipramine challenge studies conducted in OCD also suggest gender differences in response. Men with OCD experienced an increase in symptoms during the clomipramine challenge, whereas no substantial change was detected in the OCD women. The OCD women also demonstrated a better antiobsessional response during a subsequent 10-week trial with either clomipramine or fluvoxamine. Interestingly, the gender difference detected in antiobsessional response was more pronounced after clomipramine than fluvoxamine treatment (Mundo *et al.*, 1999). Potential gender differences in treatment response have been explored from the data derived from the multicentre, placebo-controlled treatment trials of clomipramine and fluoxetine, respectively. Both analyses failed to detect any evidence of gender differences in medication response in OCD (Ackerman *et al.*, 1994, 1998). Given the differences highlighted between OCD and OCD with tic disorder, future studies should explore the potential relationship between distinct OCD subgroups and medication response.

OCD and Female Reproductive Cycle Events

There are numerous reports suggesting that the female reproductive cycle may have a substantial influence on OCD. The striking increase in prevalence rates for OCD that occurs in women after the onset of puberty has already been reviewed. Several reports suggest a relationship between menstrual cycle and OCD. Undergraduate women without demonstrable OCD have been reported to engage in more OCD-like behaviours such as 'excessive cleaning or cleaning of things not usually cleaned' during the luteal phase than at any other time during the menstrual cycle (Dillon and Brooks, 1992), Moreover, the premenstrual (late-luteal phase) period may be associated with an exacerbation in symptoms in women with OCD (Yaryura-Tobias, Neziroglu and Kaplan, 1995; Williams and Koran, 1997). In the largest study to date, the impact of the menstrual cycle on the course of their OCD symptoms was retrospectively examined in 57 women with OCD. Nearly half (42%) of the women reported premenstrual worsening in their OCD symptoms and a substantial number (21%) also noted premenstrual dysphoria (Williams and Koran, 1997).

Several case series suggest that a substantial portion (13%–36%) of women with OCD report the onset of their illness during pregnancy or the post-partum period (Buttolph and Holland, 1990; Sichel *et al.*, 1993; Neziroglu *et al.*, 1994; Williams and Koran, 1997; Altshuler, Hendrick and Cohen, 1998). A number of case reports suggest that women with pre-existing OCD will experience a worsening in symptomatology during pregnancy (Brandt and Mackenzie, 1987; Buttolph and Holland, 1990; Stein *et al.*, 1993; Neziroglu *et al.*, 1994; Weiss *et al.*, 1995; Chelmow and Halfin, 1997; Altshuler, Hendrick and Cohen, 1998). However, in the largest reported study to date concerning the impact of pregnancy on OCD, most of the women with pre-existing OCD (69%) reported no significant change in symptoms during pregnancy. Relatively few of the OCD patients reported a significant worsening (17%) or a substantial improvement (14%) in OCD symptoms during pregnancy. Relatively few (13%) of the women reported the onset of OCD during pregnancy. Substantial changes in OCD symptoms, however, were likely to occur during the post-partum period. Post-partum worsening of OCD (29%) and post-partum depression (37%) was a frequent finding in the OCD women (Williams and Koran, 1997). The exacerbation noted during the post-partum period is a fairly consistent finding in women with pre-existing OCD. Most studies have reported that 20%–30% of women with OCD will experience a significant post-partum worsening in OCD symptoms (Buttolph and Holland, 1990; Sichel *et al.*, 1993; Williams and Koran, 1997; Altshuler, Hendrick and Cohen, 1998).

These results provide further evidence that changes in female reproductive hormone concentrations can substantially influence the severity and course of OCD. Pregnancy and the post-partum period may represent a time of increased vulnerability for the initial emergence of OCD or for significant worsening in women with pre-existing OCD.

POST-TRAUMATIC STRESS DISORDER (PTSD)

Although many individuals are exposed to trauma, only one out of four will develop PTSD (Breslau, Davis and Andreski, 1990). Community surveys consistently report that the lifetime prevalence rate for PTSD is two times greater in women (12.5%) than men (6.2%) (Drummond, 1993). The most common cause of PTSD in men is combat exposure. In contrast, women are most likely to develop PTSD as a consequence of sexual assault, sexual molestation, or childhood physical abuse (Kessler *et al.*, 1995). PTSD is often complicated by comorbid conditions such as depression and alcohol abuse (Breslau *et al.*, 1997b). PTSD can occur at any age, but certain traumatic events are associated with an especially high risk of subsequent PTSD development. For example, Foa reported that 95% of rape victims and 75% of victims of non-sexual assaults develop PTSD symptoms within 2 weeks of the traumatic event (Foa, 1997).

Although exposure to life-threatening traumatic events is fairly common, a number of studies confirm that PTSD is poorly recognized in a variety of clinical settings. For example, Davidson *et al.* (1998) found that 81% of new patient referrals to an outpatient psychiatric clinic had a positive history of significant trauma. Although almost 30% of the patients with exposure to trauma met criteria for PTSD, only 8% were correctly diagnosed with PTSD. Unfortunately the low rates of recognition typically associated with PTSD can have catastrophic consequences. Comorbid conditions are extremely common in PTSD, especially mood and substance use disorders. In fact, the presence of PTSD has been associated with an elevated risk for major depression, dysthymia, and mania. According to the National Comorbidity Survey, comorbid alcohol and substance abuse occur twice as often in the presence of PTSD in comparison to patients without PTSD (Kessler *et al.*, 1995; Breslau *et al.*, 1997b).

Cumulative evidence indicates that the SSRI antidepressants constitute first-line pharmacotherapy for PTSD (Nagy *et al.*, 1993; Rothbaum, Ninan and Thomas, 1996; Marshall *et al.*, 1998; Davidson and Connor, 1999). TCA and MAOI antidepressants are also effective for PTSD and should be considered for patients with PTSD who fail to respond to SSRI treatment. The SSRI antidepressants appear to have a broad spectrum of activity in PTSD. Common PTSD symptoms such as anxiety, insomnia, and an exaggerated startle response are reported to improve during SSRI treatment. Moreover, SSRI treatment may also ameliorate PTSD symptoms such as intrusive trauma-related recollections, feelings of emotional numbing, and avoidance behaviours (Davidson and Connor, 1999). Pharmacotherapy for PTSD should be initiated at a relatively low dose and maintained for at least 12 months before discontinuation is considered.

Gender Differences in PTSD

The gender difference in prevalence rate for PTSD has been linked to a differential rate of exposure to trauma. However, this assumption appears to be incorrect. In a sample of over 1000 young adults, Breslau and colleagues found similar rates of exposure to traumatic events, but substantially more women than men met criteria for PTSD (Breslau *et al.*, 1997b). Potential confounding factors such as the increased prevalence of pre-existing anxiety or major depressive disorders in women were examined, but failed to account for the observed gender difference noted in the prevalence of PTSD. Instead, women appeared to have a markedly increased susceptibility for PTSD development, especially if the trauma occurred prior to age 15 (Breslau *et al.*, 1990, 1995, 1997b; Kessler *et al.*, 1994). Results from the National Comorbidity Survey also implicate multiple factors in the elevated risk of PTSD in women. However, there was substantial overlap between factors that predicted an increased risk for trauma exposure and development of PTSD. Once the overlapping risk factors are excluded, only one risk factor (history of affective disorder) predicted PTSD in women, whereas two (history of anxiety disorder and parental mental disorder) factors were associated with an increased risk of PTSD in men (Bromet, Sonnega and Kessler, 1998). These findings suggest that most variables identified as predictive of PTSD are actually more indicative of trauma exposure than PTSD.

Major depression and generalized anxiety disorder are common comorbid disorders in PTSD regardless of gender, whereas co-existing somatoform pain disorder is more common only in women with PTSD. Pre-existing depression appears to convey an increased risk for subsequent exposure to traumatic events as well as the development of PTSD once trauma occurs (Breslau *et al.*, 1997a, 1997b). Certain traumatic experiences are more likely to precipitate PTSD. Women who are victims of sexual assault have an extremely high risk of subsequent development of PTSD. For example, Foa and colleagues found that 3 months after the trauma, women rape victims were twice as likely as women victimized by non-sexual crimes (48% vs 25%) to have PTSD (Foa, 1997). Women may be particularly susceptible to the long-term complications of abuse that occurs during childhood. In fact, women with histories of childhood abuse are reported to have a level of functional impairment that is commensurate with that of women with recent abuse (McCauley *et al.*, 1997). Women victimized by domestic violence are more likely to develop anxiety symptoms as well as PTSD, whereas male victims of domestic violence are at greater risk of developing substance use disorders. An elevated risk of depression and an increased number of physical and psychological health problems have also been reported in women exposed to ongoing domestic violence. This finding appears to be independent of the severity of domestic violence or the presence of injuries sustained. That is, women who sustain severe injuries do not appear more likely to develop psychiatric symptoms or PTSD (Sutherland, Bybee and Sullivan, 1998). While this finding may seem counter-intuitive, it likely reflects the importance of 'perceived threat' in the formation of PTSD. That is, a victim's perception of danger or possibility of death during an assault or exposure to trauma may be more important subsequent risk for PTSD as compared to more objective or realistic assessments of life-threatening events. These findings suggest that sexual assault, childhood abuse, and individual assessment of threat during the occurrence of trauma may represent the strongest predictors of subsequent PTSD development in women.

These findings suggest that sexual assault and childhood sexual abuse represent significant risk factors for the development of PTSD in women. They also confirm that childhood abuse has particularly devastating complications that are likely to persist into adulthood in women. Certain factors appear to substantially increase the risk of development of PTSD and other complications in women. These factors include: (a) exposure to sexually related trauma or aggression; (b) occurrence of abuse or severe trauma during childhood or prior to the age of 15; and (c) perception within the victim that the traumatic event is life threatening or escape is unlikely. With these issues in mind, future research efforts should focus on identifying the biological correlates associated with childhood trauma and/or sexual abuse/assault.

Gender differences have also been identified in the biological alterations associated with PTSD. An elevated norepinephrine-to-cortisol ratio has been reported in men with PTSD, whereas women with PTSD have demonstrated significantly elevated levels of urinary norepinephrine, epinephrine, dopamine, and cortisol on a daily basis (Lemieux and Coe, 1995). The HPA axis has strong, multi-level inhibitory effects on the female reproductive hormones. Since HPA axis alterations are implicated in PTSD, the marked fluctuations in oestrogen and progesterone levels that characterize the female reproductive cycle may well have a significant impact on the course of PTSD. The relative hypercortisolism that occurs during the third trimester of pregnancy is speculated to cause a transient suppression of the adrenals during the post-partum period (Chrousos, Torpy and Gold, 1998). This finding suggests that women with pre-existing PTSD may experience substantial changes in symptomatology during pregnancy or the post-partum period. Unfortunately, very little systematic information is available concerning the potential impact of the reproductive cycle on PTSD.

SUMMARY

Women are much more likely than men to meet lifetime criteria for GAD, panic disorder, simple phobia, SAD, OCD, and/or PTSD. Potentially important gender differences have also been identified in the phenomenology and clinical course for each of the anxiety disorders. Women with GAD are more likely to meet criteria for a comorbid psychiatric disorder, seek treatment, and experience a more severe clinical course in comparison to men with GAD. Phobic avoidance, an elevated risk for comorbid conditions, and a less favourable clinical outcome are associated with female gender in patients with panic disorder. Women, in comparison to men, with simple phobia are more likely to have an earlier age of onset and a situational or animal-related simple phobia; men and women have a similar risk for developing health-related simple phobia. Men are more likely to seek treatment for SAD than women, but women with SAD endorse a wider range of activities that elicit severe anxiety and/or avoidance behaviours. Numerous gender differences have been identified in OCD including an earlier age of onset in males, gender-related symptom manifestations (cleaning compulsions more common in women, obsessions more common in men) and comorbid conditions (eating disorders common in women with OCD, tics more common in males with OCD), and a more episodic clinical course for women with OCD. Women appear to be more susceptible to the development of PTSD after the occurrence of severe trauma such as sexual assault or childhood abuse, whereas men are more likely to develop PTSD as a consequence of combat exposure.

The gender differences that have been identified are likely to arise from a variety of factors including genetic, environmental, and neurobiological influences. However, increasing evidence also suggests that the female reproductive hormone cycle may also have a substantial influence in the development and/or perpetuation of anxiety disorders in women. Despite the fact that the majority of people afflicted by anxiety disorders are women of childbearing potential, relatively little data is available concerning the impact of female reproductive hormone cycle events on the onset and/or clinical course of anxiety disorders. Much of the available information focuses on women with either panic disorder or OCD. Information concerning the impact of the menstrual cycle on panic disorder is somewhat mixed, but there is mounting evidence suggesting that the post-partum period, and perhaps the peri-menopause, are associated with exacerbations in panic symptomatology. Menarche appears to increase the prevalence of OCD in females and the post-partum period is often associated with an increased risk of OCD onset and/or symptom worsening in women with pre-existing OCD. While these results are intriguing, further research is clearly needed to further clarify these important relationships. Lastly, there is some evidence suggesting that gender differences may exist in the neurobiological and/or genetic basis of anxiety disorders. While preliminary in nature, these findings suggest that further research efforts should focus on delineating these potential gender differences as well as their subsequent impact on treatment response and functional outcome. Hopefully, such investigations will lead to improved prevention strategies and/or treatments that will eventually result in eliminating the finding that women afflicted with anxiety disorders often have a more severe clinical course and a worse overall outcome than men with anxiety disorders.

REFERENCES

Ackerman, D., Greenland, S., Bystritsky, A., Morgenstern, H. and Katz, R., 1994. Predictors of treatment response in obsessive–compulsive disorder: multivariate analyses from a multicenter trial of clomipramine. *Journal of Clinical Psychopharmacology*, **14**(4), 247–254.

Ackerman, D., Greenland, S. and Bystritsky, A., 1998. Clinical characteristics of response to fluoxetine treatment of obsessive–compulsive disorder. *Journal of Clinical Psychopharmacology*, **18**(3), 185–192.

Alpert, J.E., Uebelacker, L.A., McLean, N.E., Nierenberg, A.A., Pava, J.A., Worthington, J.J. III, Tedlow, J.R., Rosenbaum, J.F. and Fava, M., 1997. Social phobia, avoidant personality disorder and atypical depression: co-occurrence and clinical implications. *Psychological Medicine*, **27**(3), 627–633.

Altshuler, L., Hendrick, V. and Cohen, L.S., 1998. Course of mood and anxiety disorders during pregnancy and the postpartum period. *Journal of Clinical Psychiatry*, **2**, 29–33.

Andrade, L., Eaton, W.W. and Chilcoat, H.D., 1996. Lifetime co-morbidity of panic attacks and major depression in a population-based study: age of onset. *Psychological Medicine*, **26**, 991–996.

Antony, M., Downie, F. and Swinson, R., 1998. Diagnostic issues and epidemiology in OCD. In: Swinson, R., Antony, M., Rachman, S. and Richter, M. (eds), *OCD: Theory, Research, and Treatment*, pp. 3–32. The Guilford Press, New York.

Baer, L., 1994. Factor analysis of symptom subtypes of obsessive–compulsive disorder and their relation to personality and tic disorders. *Journal of Clinical Psychiatry*, **55**, 18–23.

Bakish, D., 1999. The patient with comorbid depression and anxiety: the unmet need. *Journal of Clinical Psychiatry*, **60**(6), 20–24.

Ballenger, J., Davidson, J., Lecrubier, Y., Nutt, D., Bobes, J., Beidel, D., Ono, Y. and Westenberg, H., 1998. Consensus statement on social anxiety disorder from the International Consensus Group on Depression and Anxiety. *Journal of Clinical Psychiatry*, **59**(17), 54–60.

Battaglia, M., Bernardeschi, L., Politi, E., Bertella, S. and Bellodi, L., 1995. Comorbidity of panic and somatization disorder: a genetic-epidemiological approach. *Comprehensive Psychiatry*, **36**(6), 411–420.

Beck, C., 1998. Postpartum onset of panic disorder. *Image Journal of Nursing School*, **30**(2), 131–135.

Bell, C. and Nutt, D., 1998. Serotonin and panic. *British Journal of Psychiatry*, **172**, 465–471.

Billett, E., Richter, M., Sam, F., Swinson, R., Daj, X., King, N., Badri, F., Sasaki, T., Buchanan, J. and Kennedy, J., 1998. Investigation of dopamine system genes in obsessive–compulsive disorder. *Psychiatry and Genetics*, **8**(3), 163–169.

Bisserbee, J.C., Weiller, E., Boyer, P., Lepine, J.P. and Lecrubier, Y., 1996. Social phobia in primary care: level of recognition and drug use. *International Journal of Clinical Psychopharmacology*, **3**, 25–28.

Black, B. and Uhde, T., 1995. Psychiatric characteristics of children with selective mutism: a pilot study. *Journal of American Academy of Child and Adolescent Psychiatry*, **34**(7), 847–856.

Bland, R., Newman, S. and Orn, H., 1997b. Age and remission of psychiatric disorders. *Canadian Journal of Psychiatry*, **42**(7), 722–729

Bland, R., Newman, S. and Orn, H., 1997a. Help-seeking for psychiatric disorders. *Canadian Journal of Psychiatry*, **42**(9), 935–942.

Bourdon, K., Boyd, J., Rae, D. *et al.*, 1988. Gender differences in phobias: results of the ECA community survey. *Journal of Anxiety Disorders*, **2**, 227–241.

Boyd, J.H., Rae, D.S., Thompson, J.W., Burns, B.J., Bourdon, K., Locke, B.Z. and Regier, D.A., 1990. Phobia: prevalence and risk factors. *Society of Psychiatry and Epidemiology*, **25**(6), 314–323.

Brandt, K.R. and Mackenzie, T.B., 1987. Obsessive–compulsive disorder exacerbated during pregnancy: a case report. *International Journal of Psychiatry and Medicine*, **17**(4), 361–366.

Brawman-Mintzer, O. and Lydiard, R., 1997. Biological basis of generalized anxiety disorder. *Journal of Clinical Psychiatry*, **58**(3), 16–25.

Breslau, N., Davis, G. and Andreski, P., 1990. Traumatic events and traumatic stress disorder in an urban population of young adults. *Archives of General Psychiatry*, **48**, 218–222.

Breslau, N., Davis, G.C., Andreski, P., Peterson, E.L. and Schultz, L.R., 1997a. Sex differences in posttraumatic stress disorder. *Archives of General Psychiatry*, **54**(11), 1044–1048.

Breslau, N., Davis, G.C., Peterson, E.L. and Schultz, L., 1997b. Psychiatric sequelae of posttraumatic stress disorder in women. *Archives of General Psychiatry*, **54**(1), 81–87.

Breslau, N., Schultz, L. and Peterson, E., 1995. Sex differences in depression: a role for pre-existing anxiety. *Psychiatry Research*, **58**, 1–12.

Bromet, E., Sonnega, A. and Kessler, R., 1998. Risk factors for DSM-III-R posttraumatic stress disorder: findings from the National Comorbidity Survey. *American Journal of Epidemiology*, **147**(4), 353–361.

Buttolph, M. and Holland, A., 1990. OCD in pregnancy and childbirth. In: Jenike, M., Baer, L. and Minichiello, W. (eds), *Obsessive–Compulsive Disorders: Theory and Management*, pp. 89–97. Year Book Medical, Chicago.

Castle, D.J., Deale, A. and Marks, I.M., 1995. Gender differences in obsessive compulsive disorder. *Australian and New Zealand Journal of Psychiatry*, **29**(1), 114–117.

Chelmow, D. and Halfin, V.P., 1997. Pregnancy complicated by obsessive–compulsive disorder. *Journal of Maternal and Fetal Medicine*, **6**(1), 31–34.

Chrousos, G.P., Torpy, D.J. and Gold, P.W., 1998. Interactions between the hypothalamic-pituitary-adrenal axis and the women reproductive system: clinical implications. *Annals of Internal Medicine*, **129**(3), 229–240.

Coffey, B., Miguel, E., Biederman, J., Baer, L., Rauch, S., O'Sullivan, R., Savage, C., Phillips, K., Borgman, A., Green-Leibovitz, M., Moore, E., Park, K. and Jenike, M.A., 1998. Tourette's disorder with and without obsessive–compulsive disorder in adults: are they different? *Journal of Nervous and Mental Disorders*, **186**(4), 201–206

Cohen, L.S., Sichel, D.A., Dimmock, J.A. and Rosenbaum, J.F., 1994a. Impact of pregnancy on panic disorder: a case series [see comments]. *Journal of Clinical Psychiatry*, **55**(7), 284–288.

Cohen, L.S., Sichel, D.A., Dimmock, J.A. and Rosenbaum, J.F., 1994b. Postpartum course in women with preexisting panic disorder [see comments]. *Journal of Clinical Psychiatry*, **55**(7), 289–292.

Cook, B., Noyes, R., Garvey, M., Beach, V., Sobotka, J. and Chaudhry, D., 1990. Anxiety and the menstrual cycle in panic disorder. *Journal of Affective Disorders*, **19**(3), 221–226.

Coplan, J. and Lydiard, R., 1998. Brain circuits in panic disorder. *Biological Psychiatry*, **44**(12), 1264–1276.

Cox, B.J., Swinson, R.P., Shulman, I.D., Kuch, K. and Reichman, J.T., 1993. Gender effects and alcohol use in panic disorder with agoraphobia. *Behavioral Research Therapy*, **31**(4), 413–416.

Davidson, J., 1998. Pharmacotherapy of social anxiety disorder. *Journal of Clinical Psychiatry*, **59**(17), 47–53.

Davidson, J.R. and Connor, K.M., 1999. Management of posttraumatic stress disorder: diagnostic and therapeutic issues. *J-Clin-Psychiatry*, **60**(18), 33–38.

Davidson, J.R., Rampes, H., Eisen, M., Fisher, P., Smith, R.D. and Malik, M., 1998. Psychiatric disorders in primary care patients receiving complementary medical treatments. *Compr-Psychiatry*, **39**(1), 16–20.

Deckert, J., Catalano, M., Syagailo, Y., Bosi, M., Okladnova, O., Di-Bella, D., Nothen, M., Maffei, P., Franke, P., Fritze, J., Maier, W., Propping, P., Beckmann, H., Bellodi, L. and Lesch, K., 1999. Excess of high activity monoamine oxidase A gene promoter alleles in women patients with panic disorder. *Human Molecular Genetics*, **8**(4), 621–624.

Demal, U., Lenz, G., Mayrhofer, A., Zapotoczky, H. and Zitterl, W., 1993. OCD and depression: a retrospective study on course and interaction. *Psychopathology*, **26**, 145–150.

Dick, C.L., Bland, R.C. and Newman, S.C., 1994b. Epidemiology of psychiatric disorders in Edmonton. Panic disorder. *Acta Psychiatrica Scandinavia Suppl*, **376**, 45–53.

Dick, C.L., Sowa, B., Bland, R.C. and Newman, S.C., 1994a. Epidemiology of psychiatric disorders in Edmonton. Phobic disorders. *Acta Psychiatrica Scandinavia Suppl*, **376**, 36–44.

Dillon, K. and Brooks, D., 1992. Unusual cleaning behavior in the luteal phase. *Psychological Reports*, **70**(1), 35–39.

Drummond, L.M., 1993. Behavioural approaches to anxiety disorders. *Postgrad-Med-J*, **69**(809), 222–226.

Dupont, R., Rice, D., Shiraki, S. and Rowland, C., 1995. Pharmacoeconomics: economic costs of obsessive–compulsive disorder. *Medical Interface*, **4**, 102–109.

Eaton, W., Dryman, A. and Weissman, M., 1991. Panic and phobia. In: Robins, L. and Regier, D. (eds), *Psychiatric Disorders in America: The Epidemiological Catchment Area Study*, pp. 53–80. Free Press, New York.

Fernandez-Guasti, A. and Picazo, O., 1990. The actions of diazepam and serotonergic anxiolytics vary according to the gender and the estrous cycle phase. *Pharmacology, Biochemistry, and Behavior*, **37**(1), 673–677.

Fishman, S., Carr, D., Beckett, A. and Rosenbaum, J., 1994. Hypercapneic ventilatory response in patients with panic disorder before and after alprazolam treatment and in pre- and postmenstrual women. *Journal of Psychiatry Research*, **28**(2), 165–170.

Fleet, R., Marchand, A., Dupuis, G., Kaczorowski, J. and Beitman, B., 1998. Comparing emergency department and psychiatric setting patients with panic disorder. *Psychosomatics*, **39**(6), 512–518.

Foa, E.B., 1997. Trauma and women: course, predictors, and treatment. *Journal of Clinical Psychiatry*, **9**, 25–28.

Fredrikson, M., Annas, P., Fischer, H. and Wik, G., 1996. Gender and age differences in the prevalence of specific fears and phobias. *Behavioral Research Therapy*, **34**(1), 33–39.

Galbaud-du-Fort, G., Bland, R., Newman, S. and Boothroyd, L., 1998. Spouse similarity for lifetime psychiatric history in the general population. *Psychological Medicine*, **28**(4), 789–802.

Goodman, W.K., McDougle, C., Price, L., Riddle, M., Pauls, D. and Leckman, J., 1990. Beyond the serotonin hypothesis: a role for dopamine in some forms of obsessive–compulsive disorder? *Journal of Clinical Psychiatry*, **51**(8), 36–43.

Griez, E., de Loof, C., Pols, H., Zandbergen, J. and Lousberg, H., 1990. Specific sensitivity of patients with panic attacks to carbon dioxide inhalation. *Psychiatric Research*, **31**(2), 193–199.

Hantouche, E.G. and Lancrenon, S., 1996. [Modern typology of symptoms and obsessive–compulsive syndromes: results of a large French study of 615 patients]. *Encephale*, (1), 9–21.

Hohmann, A.A., 1989. Gender bias in psychotropic drug prescribing in primary care. *Medical Care*, **27**(5), 478–490.

Hollander, E., Greenwald, S., Neville, D., Johnson, J., Hornig, C. and Weissman, M., 1996a. Uncomplicated and comorbid obsessive–compulsive disorder in an epidemiological sample. *Journal of Depression and Anxiety*, **4**(3), 111–119.

Hollander, E., Kwon, J.H., Stein, D.J., Broatch, J., Rowland, C.T. and Himelein, C.A., 1996b. Obsessive–compulsive and spectrum disorders: overview and quality of life issues. *Journal of Clinical Psychiatry*, **8**, 3–6.

Hollander, E., Stein, D., Kwon, J., Rowland, C., Wong, C., Broatch, J. and Himelein, C., 1998. Psychosocial function and economic costs of obsessive–compulsive disorder. *CNS Spectrums*, **3**(5), 48–58.

Hollifield, M., Katon, W., Skipper, B., Chapman, T., Ballenger, J.C., Mannuzza, S. and Fyer, A.J., 1997. Panic disorder and quality of life: variables predictive of functional impairment. *American Journal of Psychiatry*, **154**(6), 766–772.

Jefferson, J.W., Altemus, M., Jenike, M.A., Pigott, T.A., Stein, D.J. and Greist, J.H., 1995. Algorithm for the treatment of obsessive–compulsive disorder (OCD). *Psychopharmacology Bulletin*, **31**(3), 487–490.

Joyce, P.R., Bushnell, J.A., Oakley-Browne, M.A., Wells, J.E. and Hornblow, A.R., 1989. The epidemiology of panic symptomatology and agoraphobic avoidance. *Comprehensive Psychiatry*, **30**(4), 303–312.

Kalus, O., Asnis, G., Rubinson, E., Kahn, R., Friedman, J., Iqbal, N., Grosz, D., Van Praag, H. and Cahn, W., 1991. Desipramine treatment in panic disorder. *Journal of Affective Disorders*, **21**(4), 239–244.

Karno, M., Golding, J., Sorenson, S. and Burnam, M., 1988. The epidemiology of obsessive–compulsive disorder in five US communities. *Archives of General Psychiatry*, **45**, 1094–1099.

Katerndahl, D., 1990. Factors associated with persons with panic attacks seeking medical care. *Family Medicine*, **22**(6), 462–466.

Katerndahl, D.A. and Realini, J.P., 1997. Quality of life and panic-related work disability in subjects with infrequent panic and panic disorder. *Journal of Clinical Psychiatry*, **58**(4), 153–158.

Keller, M.B. and Hanks, D.L., 1993. Course and outcome in panic disorder. *Progress in Neuropsychopharmacology and Biological Psychiatry*, **17**(4), 551–570.

Kendler, K.S., Neale, M.C., Kessler, R.C., Heath, A.C. and Eaves, L.J., 1992a. Generalized anxiety disorder in women. A population-based twin study. *Archives of General Psychiatry*, **49**(4), 267–272.

Kendler, K.S., Neale, M.C., Kessler, R.C., Heath, A.C. and Eaves, L.J., 1992b. The genetic epidemiology of phobias in women. The interrelationship of agoraphobia, social phobia, situational phobia, and simple phobia. *Archives of General Psychiatry*, **49**(4), 273–281.

Kendler, K.S., Neale, M.C., Kessler, R.C., Heath, A.C. and Eaves, L.J., 1992c. Major depression and generalized anxiety disorder. Same genes, (partly) different environments? *Archives of General Psychiatry*, **49**(9), 716–722.

Kendler, K.S., Neale, M.C., Kessler, R.C., Heath, A.C. and Eaves, L.J., 1993. Panic disorder in women: a population-based twin study. *Psychological Medicine*, **23**(2), 397–406.

Kendler, K.S., Walters, E.E., Neale, M.C., Kessler, R.C., Heath, A.C. and Eaves, L.J., 1995. The structure of the genetic and environmental risk factors for six major psychiatric disorders in women. Phobia, generalized anxiety disorder, panic disorder, bulimia, major depression, and alcoholism. *Archives of General Psychiatry*, **52**(5), 374–383.

Kennedy, B. and Schwab, J., 1997. Utilization of medical specialists by anxiety disorder patients. *Psychosomatics*, **38**(2), 109–112.

Kessler, R., Berglund, P., Foster, C., Saunders, W., Stang, P. and Walters, E., 1997. Social consequences of psychiatric disorders II: Teenage parenthood. *American Journal of Psychiatry*, **154**(10), 1405–1411.

Kessler, R., McGonagle, K., Zhao, S., Nelson, C., Hughes, M., Eshleman, S., Wittchen, H.U. and Kendler, K., 1994. Lifetime and 12-month prevalence of DSM-III-R psychiatric disorders in the United States: results from the National Comorbidity Survey. *Archives of General Psychiatry*, **51**, 8–19.

Kessler, R.C., Sonnega, A., Bromet, E., Hughes, M. and Nelson, C.B., 1995. Posttraumatic stress disorder in the National Comorbidity Survey. *Archives of General Psychiatry*, **52**(12), 1048–1060.

Kessler, R.C., Stein, M.B. and Berglund, P., 1998. Social phobia subtypes in the National Comorbidity Survey. *American Journal of Psychiatry*, **155**(5), 613–619.

Klein, D., 1993. False suffocation alarms, spontaneous panics, and related conditions. An integrative hypothesis. *Archives of General Psychiatry*, **50**(4): 306–317.

Koran, L., Thieneman, M. and Davenport, R., 1996. Quality of life for patients with obsessive–compulsive disorder. *American Journal of Psychiatry*, **153**, 783–788.

Krasucki, C., Howard, R. and Mann, A., 1998. The relationship between anxiety disorders and age. *International Journal of Geriatric Psychiatry*, **13**(2), 79–99.

Lecrubier, Y. and Weiller, E., 1997. Comorbidities in social phobia. *International Journal of Clinical Psychopharmacology*, **12**(6), 0268–1315.

Lemieux, A. and Coe, C., 1995. Abuse-related posttraumatic stress disorder: evidence for chronic neuroendocrine activation in women. *Psychosomatic Medicine*, **57**(2), 105–115.

Lensi, P., Cassano, G., Correddu, G., Ravagli, S., Kunovac, J. and Akiskal, H.S., 1996. Obsessive–compulsive disorder. Familial-developmental history, symptomatology, comorbidity and course with special reference to gender-related differences. *British Journal of Psychiatry*, **169**(1), 101–107.

Leon, A., Portera, L. and Weissman, M., 1995. The social costs of anxiety disorders. *British Journal of Psychiatry*, **4**(27), 19–22.

Leonard, H., Lenane, M., Swedo, S., Rettew, D., Gershon, E. and Rapaport, J., 1992. Tics and Tourette's syndrome: a two to seven year follow-up of 54 OCD children. *American Journal of Psychiatry*, **149**, 1244–1251.

Lindal, E. and Stefansson, J.G., 1993. The lifetime prevalence of anxiety disorders in Iceland as estimated by the US National Institute of Mental Health Diagnostic Interview Schedule. *Acta Psychiatrica Scandinavia*, **88**(1), 29–34.

Magee, W., Eaton, W., Wittchen, H., McGonagle, K. and Kessler, R., 1996. Agoraphobia, simple phobia, and social phobia in the National Comorbidity Survey. *Archives of General Psychiatry*, **53**(2), 159–168.

Marshall, J.R., 1996. Comorbidity and its effects on panic disorder. *Bulletin of the Menninger Clinic*, **60**(2 Suppl A), 0025–9284.

Marshall, R.D., Schneier, F.R., Fallon, B.A., Knight, C.B., Abbate, L.A., Goetz, D., Campeas, R. and Liebowitz, M.R., 1998. An open trial of paroxetine in patients with noncombat-related, chronic posttraumatic stress disorder. *J-Clin-Psychopharmacol*, **18**(1), 10–18.

McCauley, J., Kern, D.E., Kolodner, K., Dill, L., Schroeder, A.F., DeChant, H.K., Ryden, J., Derogatis, L.R. and Bass, E.B., 1997. Clinical characteristics of women with a history of childhood abuse: unhealed wounds. *JAMA*, **277**(17), 1362–1368.

McLeod, D., Hoehn-Saric, R., Foster, G. and Hipsley, P., 1993. The influence of premenstrual syndrome on ratings of anxiety in women with generalized anxiety disorder. *Acta Psychiatrica Scandinavia*, **88**(4), 248–251.

Mick, M. and Telch, M., 1998. Social anxiety and history of behavioral inhibition in young adults. *Journal of Anxiety Disorders*, **12**(1), 1–20.

Monteleone, P., Catapano, F., Torttorella, A. and Maj, M., 1997. Cortisol response to d-fenfluramine in patients with obsessive–compulsive disorder and in healthy subjects: evidence for a gender-related effect. *Neuropsychobiology*, **36**(1), 8–12.

Mundo, E., Bareggi, S., Pirola, R. and Bellodi, L., 1999. Effect of acute intravenous clomipramine and antiobsessional response to proserotonergic drugs: is gender a predictive variable? *Biological Psychiatry*, **45**(3), 290–294.

Nagy, L.M., Morgan, C.A. III, Southwick, S.M. and Charney, D.S., 1993. Open prospective trial of fluoxetine for posttraumatic stress disorder. *J-Clin-Psychopharmacol*, **13**(2), 107–113.

Neziroglu, F., Yaryura-Tobias, J., Lemli, J. and Yaryura, R., 1994. Demographic study of obsessive compulsive disorder. *Acta Psiquiatr Psicol Am Lat*, **40**(3), 217–223.

Nicolini, H., Cruz, C., Paez, F. and Camarena, B., 1998. Dopamine D2 and D4 receptor genes distinguish the clinical presence of tics in obsessive–compulsive disorder. *Gac-Med-Mex*, **134**(5), 521–527.

Northcott, C.J. and Stein, M.B., 1994. Panic disorder in pregnancy. *Journal of Clinical Psychiatry*, **55**(12), 539–542.

Noshirvani, H., Kasvikis, Y., Marks, I., Tsakiris, F. and Monteiro, W., 1991. Gender-divergent aetiological factors in OCD. *British Journal of Psychiatry*, **158**, 260–263.

Nutt, D., Bell, C. and Malizia, A., 1998. Brain mechanisms of social anxiety disorder. *Journal of Clinical Psychiatry*, **59**(17), 4–11.

Orloff, L., Battle, M., Baer, L., Ivanjack, L., Pettit, A., Buttolph, M. and Jenike, M., 1994. Long-term follow-up of 85 patients with OCD. *American Journal of Psychiatry*, **151**, 441–442.

Otto, M.W., Pollack, M.H., Sachs, G.S., O'Neil, C.A. and Rosenbaum, J.F., 1992. Alcohol dependence in panic disorder patients. *Journal of Psychiatric Research*, **26**(1), 29–38.

Pauls, D., Alsobrook, J., Goodman, W.K., Rasmussen, S. and Leckman, J., 1995. A family study of obsessive–compulsive disorder. *American Journal of Psychiatry*, **152**, 76–84.

Perna, G., Brambilla, F., Arancio, C. and Bellodi, L., 1995. Carbon dioxide inhalation sensitivity in panic disorder: effect of menstrual cycle phase. *Biological Psychiatry*, **37**(8), 528–532.

Perugi, G., Akiskal, H., Gemignani, A., Pfanner, C., Presta, S., Milanfranchi, A., Lensi, P., Ravagli, S., Maremmani, I. and Cassano, G., 1998. Episodic course in obsessive–compulsive disorder. *European Archives of Psychiatry and Clinical Neuroscience*, **248**(5), 240–244.

Petter, T., Richter, M. and Sandor, P., 1998. Clinical features distinguishing patients with Tourette's syndrome and obsessive–compulsive disorder from patients with obsessive–compulsive disorder without tics. *Journal of Clinical Psychiatry*, **59**(9): 456–459.

Pigott, T.A., 1996. OCD: where the serotonin selectivity story begins. *Journal of Clinical Psychiatry*, **57**(Suppl 6), 11–20.

Pigott, T.A., L'Heureux, F., Dubbert, B., Bernstein, S. and Murphy, D., 1994. Obsessive–compulsive disorder: comorbid conditions. *Journal of Clinical Psychiatry*, **55**(10), 15–27.

Pollack, M., 1999. Social anxiety disorder: designing a pharmacologic treatment strategy. *Journal of Clinical Psychiatry*, **60**(9), 20–26.

Rasmussen, S. and Eisen, J., 1990. Epidemiology and clinical features of OCD. In Jenike, M., Baer, L. and Minichiello, W. (eds), *Obsessive–Compulsive Disorders: Theory and Management*, pp. 10–27. Mosby Year Book, St. Louis.

Rasmussen, S. and Eisen, J., 1992. The epidemiology and differential diagnosis of OCD. *Journal of Clinical Psychiatry*, **53**(s), 4–10.

Ravizza, L., Barzega, G., Bellino, S., Bogetto, F. and Maina, G., 1995. Predictors of drug treatment response in obsessive–compulsive disorder. *Journal of Clinical Psychiatry*, **56**(8), 368–373.

Reed, V. and Wittchen, H., 1998. DSM-IV panic attacks and panic disorder in a community sample of adolescents and young adults: how specific are panic attacks? *Journal of Psychiatric Research*, **32**(6), 335–345.

Regier, D., Boyd, J., Burke, J., Rae, D., Myers, J., Kramer, M., Robins, L., George, L., Karno, M. and Locke, B., 1988. One-month prevalence of mental disorders in the United States: Based on five Epidemiologic Catchment Area sites. *Archives of General Psychiatry*, **45**, 977–986.

Regier, D., Narron, W. and Rae, D., 1990. The epidemiology of anxiety disorders: the ECA experience. *Journal of Psychiatric Research*, **24**(2), 3–14.

Robins, L., Helzer, J., Weissman, M., Orvaschel, H., Gruenberg, E., Burke, J. and Regier, D., 1984. Lifetime prevalence of specific psychiatric disorders in three sites. *Arch Gen Psychiatry*, **41**, 949–958.

Rogers, M.P., White, K., Warshaw, M.G., Yonkers, K.A., Rodriguez-Villa, F., Chang, G. and Keller, M.B., 1994. Prevalence of medical illness in patients with anxiety disorders. *International Journal of Psychiatry and Medicine*, **24**(1), 83–96.

Rothbaum, B.O., Ninan, P.T. and Thomas, L., 1996. Sertraline in the treatment of rape victims with posttraumatic stress disorder. *J-Trauma-Stress*, **9**(4), 865–871.

Roy-Byrne, P. and Katon, W., 1997. Generalized anxiety disorder in primary care: the precursor/modifier pathway to increased health care utilization. *Journal of Clinical Psychiatry*, **58**(3), 34–38.

Rubenstein, C., Pigott, T.A., L'Heureux, F., Hill, J. and Murphy, D., 1992. A preliminary investigation of the lifetime prevalence rate of anorexia and bulimia nervosa in patients with OCD. *Journal of Clinical Psychiatry*, **53**(9), 309–314.

Santangelo, S.L., Pauls, D.L., Goldstein, J.M., Faraone, S.V., Tsuang, M.T. and Leckman, J.F., 1994. Tourette's syndrome: what are the influences of gender and comorbid obsessive–compulsive disorder? *Journal of American Academy of Child and Adolescent Psychiatry*, **33**(6), 795–804.

Schneier, F., Heckelman, L., Garfinkel, R., Campeas, R., Fallon, B., Gitow, A., Street, L., Del-Bene, D. and Liebowitz, M., 1994. Functional impairment in social phobia. *Journal of Clinical Psychiatry*, **55**(8), 322–331.

Schneier, F., Johnson, J., Hornig, C., Liebowitz, M. and Weissman, M., 1992. Social phobia: comorbidity and morbidity in an epidemiological sample. *Archives of General Psychiatry*, **49**, 282–291.

Shear, M.K., 1997. Anxiety disorders in women: gender-related modulation of neurobiology and behavior. *Seminars in Reproductive Endocrinology*, **15**(1), 69–76.

Sheehan, D., 1999. Current concepts in the treatment of panic disorder. *Journal of Clinical Psychiatry*, **60**(suppl 18), 16–21.

Sholomskas, D., Wickamaratne, P., Dogolo, L., O'Brien, D., Leaf, P. and Woods, S., 1993. Postpartum onset of panic disorder: a coincidental event? *Journal of Clinical Psychiatry*, **54**(12), 476–480.

Sichel, D., Cohen, L., Rosenbaum, J. and Driscoll, J., 1993. Postpartum onset of obsessive–compulsive disorder. *Psychosomatics*, **34**(3), 277–279.

Stahl, S., 1997. Reproductive hormones as adjuncts to psychotropic mediation in women. *Essential Psychopharmacology*, **2**(2), 147–164.

Starcevic, V., Djordjevic, A., Latas, M. and Bogojevic, G., 1998. Characteristics of agoraphobia in women and men with panic disorder with agoraphobia. *Depression and Anxiety*, **8**(1), 8–13.

Stein, D., Hollander, E., Simeon, D. *et al.*, 1993. Pregnancy and OCD. *American Journal of Psychiatry*, **150**, 1131–1132.

Stein, D.J., Spadaccini, E. and Hollander, E., 1995. Meta-analysis of pharmacotherapy trials for obsessive–compulsive disorder. *International Journal of Clinical Psychopharmacology*, **10**(1), 11–18.

Stein, M. and Chavira, D., 1998. Subtypes of social phobia and comorbidity with depression and other anxiety disorders. *Journal of Affective Disorders*, **50**(1), 11–16.

Stein, M., Jang, K. and Livesley, W., 1999. Heritability of anxiety sensitivity: a twin study. *American Journal of Psychiatry*, **156**(2), 246–251.

Stein, M., Liebowitz, M., Lydiard, R., Pitts, C., Bushnell, W. and Gergel, I., 1998. Paroxetine treatment of generalized social phobia: a randomized controlled trial. *Journal of American Medical Association*, **280**(8), 708–713.

Stein, M., Schmidt, P., Rubinow, D. and Uhde, T., 1989. Panic disorder and the menstrual cycle: panic disorder patients, healthy control subjects, and patients with premenstrual syndrome. *American Journal of Psychiatry*, **146**(10), 1299–1303.

Stein, M., Walker, J. and Forde, D., 1994. Setting diagnostic thresholds for social phobia: considerations from a community survey of social anxiety. *American Journal of Psychiatry*, **151**(3), 408–412.

Stein, M.B., Chartier, M.J., Hazen, A.L., Kozak, M.V., Tancer, M.E., Lander, S., Furer, P., Chubaty, D. and Walker, J.R., 1998. A direct-interview family study of generalized social phobia. *American Journal of Psychiatry*, **155**(1), 90–97.

Steketee, G., Eisen, J., Dyck, I., Warshaw, M. and Rasmussen, S., 1997. Course of Illness in OCD. In: Dickstein, L., Riba, M. and Oldham, J. (eds), *Review of Psychiatry Volume 16*, pp. 73–95. American Psychiatric Press, Inc, Washington, DC.

Sutherland, C., Bybee, D. and Sullivan, C., 1998. The long-term effects of battering on women's health. *Women's Health*, **4**(1), 41–70.

Tamburrino, M.B., Kaufman, R. and Hertzer, J., 1994. Eating disorder history in women with obsessive compulsive disorder. *J-Am-Med-Womens-Assoc*, **49**(1), 24–26.

Thomsen, P.H. and Mikkelsen, H.U., 1995. Course of obsessive–compulsive disorder in children and adolescents: a prospective follow-up study of 23 Danish cases. *Journal of American Academy of Child and Adolescent Psychiatry*, **34**(11), 1432–1440.

Tiihonen, J., Kuikka, J., Rasanen, P., Lepola, U., Koponen, H., Liuska, A., Lehmusvaara, A., Vainio, P., Kononen, M.B., Yu, M., Kinnunen, I., Akerman, K. and Karhu, J., 1997. Cerebral benzodiazepine receptor binding in GAD. *Molecular Psychiatry*, **2**(6), 463–471.

Turgeon, L., Marchand, A. and Dupuis, G., 1998. Clinical features in panic disorder with agoraphobia: a comparison of men and women. *Journal of Anxiety Disorders*, **12**(6), 539–553.

Turk, C., Heimberg, R., Orsillo, S., Holt, C., Gitow, A., Street, L., Schneier, F. and Liebowitz, M., 1998. An investigation of gender differences in social phobia. *Journal of Anxiety Disorders*, **12**(3), 209–223.

Ushiroyama, T. and Sugimoto, O., 1994. Correlation of ill-defined syndrome with depression in the climacterium. *Nippon Rinsho*, **52**(5), 1345–1349.

Valleni-Basile, L.A., Garrison, C.Z., Jackson, K.L., Waller, J.L., McKeown, R.E., Addy, C.L. and Cuffe, S.P., 1994. Frequency of obsessive–compulsive disorder in a community sample of young adolescents. *J-Am-Acad-Child-Adolesc-Psychiatry*, **33**(6), 782–791.

Villeponteaux, V., Lydiard, R., Laraia, M., Stuart, G. and Ballenger, J., 1992. The effects of pregnancy on preexisting panic disorder. *Journal of Clinical Psychiatry*, **53**(6), 201–203.

van der Feltz-Cornelis, C.M., 1999. Hot flashes resistant to hormone replacement in menopausal women: panic disorder? *Ned Tijdschr Geneeskd*, **143**(6), 281–284.

Wagner, K.D. and Berenson, A.B., 1994. Norplant-associated major depression and panic disorder. *Journal of Clinical Psychiatry*, **55**(11), 478–480.

Warnock, J. and Bundren, J., 1997. Anxiety and mood disorders associated with gonadotropin-releasing hormone agonist therapy. *Psychopharmacology Bulletin*, **33**(2), 311–316.

Weinstock, L., 1999. Gender differences in the presentation and management of social anxiety disorder. *Journal of Clinical Psychiatry*, **60**(9), 9–13.

Weiss, M., Baerg, E., Wisebord, S. and Temple, J., 1995. The influence of gonadal hormones on periodicity of obsessive–compulsive disorder. *Canadian Journal of Psychiatry*, **40**(4), 205–207.

Weissman, M., Bland, R., Canino, G., Greenwald, S., Hwu, H., Lee, C., Newman, S., Oakley-Browne, M., Rubio-Stipec, M., Wickramaratne, P., Wittchen, H. and Yeh, E., 1994. The cross national epidemiology of obsessive–compulsive disorder. *Journal of Clinical Psychiatry*, **55**, 5–10.

Weissman, M., Bland, R., Canino, G., Greenwald, S., Wittchen, H. and Lee, C., 1997. The cross-national epidemiology of panic disorder. *Archives of General Psychiatry*, **54**, 305–309.

Weissman, M., Klerman, G., Markowitz, J. and Ouellette, R., 1989. Suicidal ideation and suicide attempts in panic disorder and attacks. *New England Journal of Medicine*, **321**, 1209–1214.

Williams, K. and Koran, L., 1997. Obsessive–compulsive disorder in pregnancy, the puerperium, and the premenstruum. *Journal of Clinical Psychiatry*, **58**(7), 330–334.

Windmann, S., 1998. Panic disorder from a monistic perspective: integrating neurobiological and psychological approaches. *Journal of Anxiety Disorders*, **12**(5), 485–507.

Wisner, K.L., Peindl, K.S. and Hanusa, B.H., 1996. Effects of childbearing on the natural history of panic disorder with comorbid mood disorder. *Journal of Affective Disorders*, **41**(3), 173–180.

Wittchen, H.U., Zhao, S., Kessler, R.C. and Eaton, W.W., 1994. DSM-III-R generalized anxiety disorder in the National Comorbidity Survey. *Archives of General Psychiatry*, **51**(5), 355–364.

Woodman, C., Noyes, R., Black, D., Schlosser, S. and Yagla, S., 1999. A 5-year follow-up study of generalized anxiety disorder and panic disorder. *Journal of Nervous and Mental Diseases*, **187**(1), 3–9.

Yang, Y. and Liu, X., 1998. A family study of obsessive–compulsive disorder. *Chung-Hua-I-Hsueh-I-Chuan-Hsueh-Tsa-Chih*, **15**(5), 303–306.

Yaryura-Tobias, J.A., Neziroglu, F.A. and Kaplan, S., 1995. Self-mutilation, anorexia, and dysmenorrhea in obsessive compulsive disorder. *International Journal of Eating Disorders*, **17**(1), 33–38.

Yonkers, K. and Ellison, J., 1996. Anxiety disorders in women and their pharmacological treatment. In: Jensvold, M., Halbreich, U. and Hamilton, J. (eds), *Psychopharmacology and Women: Sex, Gender, and Hormones*, pp. 261–285. American Psychiatric Press, Inc, Washington, DC.

Yonkers, K.A., Warshaw, M.G., Massion, A.O. and Keller, M.B., 1996. Phenomenology and course of generalised anxiety disorder. *British Journal of Psychiatry*, **168**(3), 308–313.

Yonkers, K.A., Zlotnick, C., Allsworth, J., Warshaw, M., Shea, T. and Keller, M.B., 1998. Is the course of panic disorder the same in women and men? *American Journal of Psychiatry*, **155**(5), 596–602.

Young, E., Abelson, J., Curtis, G. and Nesse, R., 1997. Childhood adversity and vulnerability to mood and anxiety disorders. *Depression and Anxiety*, **5**(2), 66–72.

Zohar, A. and Bruno, R., 1997. Normative and pathological obsessive–compulsive behavior and ideation in childhood: a question of timing. *Journal of Child Psychology and Psychiatry*, **38**(8), 993–999.

Zohar, J. and Insel, T., 1987. Obsessive–compulsive disorder: psychobiological approaches to diagnosis, treatment, and pathophysiology. *Biological Psychiatry*, **22**, 667–687.

XIX-13

Therapeutic Armamentarium in Anxiety Disorders

J.A. den Boer, B.R. Slaap, G.J. ter Horst, T.I.F.H. Cremers and F.J. Bosker

INTRODUCTION

For decades benzodiazepines have been the mainstay in the treatment of anxiety disorders. It is only during the last decade that this situation has changed. With the introduction of serotonin reuptake inhibitors (SSRI's), 5-HT receptor-specific drugs like 5-HT_{1A} agonists and recently, dual action antidepressants, new possibilities have been created for the treatment of panic disorder, obsessive compulsive disorder, social phobia, generalized anxiety disorder and post-traumatic stress disorder. In this chapter the pharmacotherapeutic options for the treatment of these anxiety disorders will be reviewed. We will focus on new developments and not reiterate all the studies performed with old tricyclic antidepressants (TCAs) such as imipramine, as these studies have been mentioned and reviewed in many other textbooks and papers.

PANIC DISORDER

Panic disorder (PD) is a chronic and recurring syndrome which requires long-term treatment. The disorder encompasses five essential domains: the panic attacks themselves, the associated anticipatory anxiety, phobic avoidance, and the resultant functional impairment and effects on quality of life. However, the complete resolution of panic attacks, the signal feature of panic disorder, is clearly important to patients. Modern studies on the efficacy in PD should measure symptoms domains outlined above (Shear and Maser, 1994).

Originally, tricyclic antidepressants (TCAs) like imipramine and clomipramine were the first found to be beneficial in panic disorder. Imipramine originally played a role in the sixties in the pharmacological dissection of panic and anxiety, as it was discovered that in patients suffering from anxiety neurosis, panic attacks disappeared during treatment with imipramine. The efficacy of imipramine has been the subject of many studies and this drug was used as a reference drug for years. TCAs, in spite of their proven efficacy, have many drawbacks, including high rates of non-compliance due to anticholinergic side-effects, weight gain, daytime sedation, orthostatic hypotension, lethality in overdose and withdrawal reactions (Wolfe, 1997; Bennett *et al.*, 1998; den Boer, Bosker and Slaap, 2000). After six months treatment with imipramine dry mouth, constipation, sweating was still present as a substantial burden to patients (Mavissakalian and Perel, 2000). It is questionable whether by current standards, TCAs would be marketed if they were introduced today. Many studies have also been performed with BDZs in PD and there is a large database indicating that high potency BDZs such as clonazepam and alprazolam are efficacious in PD. Due to developments in psychopharmacology during the last decade it has, however, been questioned whether BDZs should be the first choice in the treatment of PD in view of their serious side-effects and withdrawal reactions.

Benzodiazepines in Panic Disorder

There are several placebo-controlled studies suggesting that clonazepam has therapeutic effects in PD. In one of the largest studies with clonazepam conducted so far, Rosenbaum and co-workers (1997) included 413 patients with PD in a fixed-dose placebo-controlled study in a 6-week study followed by a 7-week discontinuation phase. They used dosages ranging from 0.5 mg to 4.0 mg clonazepam daily and found that dosages of clonazepam of 1.0 mg were equally effective in reducing the number of panic attacks. During the discontinuation phase most patients worsened and reported increases in the number of panic attacks. Recently, Valenca *et al.* (2000) undertook a 6-week placebo-controlled study in 24 PD patients. They found that 11% of the placebo-treated patients were panic free after six weeks, whereas 62% of the clonazepam treated patients were panic free. Because treatment with BDZs has been associated with severe withdrawal reactions, Moroz and Rosenbaum (1999) treated PD patients with 0.25 up to 4.0 mg per day clonazepam for 6 weeks in a double-blind placebo controlled design, followed by a 7-week discontinuation phase during which the doses were gradually tapered. They observed no symptoms suggestive of withdrawal syndrome, nor evidence for rebound during the gradual tapering of clonazepam, but some patients did show worsening of symptomatology, most notably a recurrence of panic attacks. These data show that in the short-term clonazepam is efficacious but treatment in this study was probably too short to achieve full remission of panic attacks. On the other hand, a naturalistic follow-up study for 2 years in 204 patients showed that improvement in global severity of PD did not change during treatment with stable dosages of clonazepam, indicating that there was no development of tolerance (Worthington *et al.*, 1998). In spite of the fact that clonazepam has been marketed in the US for PD, the two pivotal studies did not fulfil all the criteria that were set forth by Shear and Maser (1994), moreover, there is evidence that the higher dosages that are required in many patients are associated with withdrawal symptoms (Davidson *et al.*, 1998).

Two large studies investigating the anxiolytic effects of alprazolam have been conducted in more than 1600 patients suffering from PD. The Cross-National Collaborative Panic Study and the Philadelphia study, which was a maintenance study (Ballenger *et al.*, 1988; Noyes *et al.*, 1988; Pecknold *et al.*, 1988; Rickels *et al.*, 1993; Schweizer *et al.*, 1993). The results of these studies suggested that alprazolam was an effective drug in reducing the number of panic attacks. In spite of these results, these studies were criticized for several points; there was a very high placebo drop-out rate and the average dose was high (mean dose at week 8: 5.6 to 5.8 mg per day). These are important issues as even lower dosages have been shown to lead to impaired recall and other cognitive disturbances (Pomara *et al.*, 1998). In addition, cessation of alprazolam treatment induces

Biological Psychiatry: Edited by H. D'haenen, J.A. den Boer and P. Willner. ISBN 0-471-49198-5

severe withdrawal reactions, for which PD patients appear to be very vulnerable compared to patients suffering from generalized anxiety disorder (Klein *et al.*, 1994). Cognitive-behavioural therapy (CBT), prescription of drugs such as trazodone, valproate and carbamazepine have all been shown to facilitate alprazolam discontinuation (Rickels *et al.*, 1999; Bruce, Spiegel and Hegel, 1999). In addition, there is a relapse rate of 44% to 56% after discontinuation of alprazolam (Spiegel, 1998).

One placebo-controlled study compared alprazolam with exposure and relaxation, either alone or in combination (Marks *et al.*, 1993). In this study, alprazolam plus exposure was more effective than alprazolam plus relaxation, although the number of panic-free patients did not differ between placebo (plus either relaxation of exposure) and alprazolam plus relaxation. There is evidence from placebo-controlled studies that diazepam could also be effective in the treatment of PD. However, in most studies conducted with diazepam very high dosages have been used. In a placebo-controlled 8-week study comparing diazepam with alprazolam, the mean dose of diazepam was 40 mg per day, which according to European standards is considered extremely high (Noyes *et al.*, 1996). Diazepam was found to be as effective as alprazolam in reducing the number of panic attacks, but throughout the study sedation was more severe for patients taking diazepam or alprazolam than for those taking placebo.

In sum, there is evidence that the high-potency BDZs clonazepam and alprazolam are effective in the treatment of PD. The onset of efficacy on BDZs in rapid, but due to the high number of side-effects and withdrawal reactions we would not consider them as first-line treatment of PD.

Table XIX-13.1 Percent of patients free from panic attacks at endpoint in placebo-controlled studies of SSRIs and clomipramine

Study	Duration (weeks)	*N*	Percent panic-free SSRI	Clomipramine	Placebo
Paroxetine					
Oehrberg *et al.*, 1995†	12	120	36%*	—	16%
Lecrubier *et al.*, 1997a	12	367	51%*	37%~	32%
Lecrubier *et al.*, 1997b	36	176	85%*	72%~	59%
Ballenger *et al.*, 1998	10	278	86%*	—	50%
Bakker *et al.*, 1999	12	131	75%	59%"	37%
Fluvoxamine					
Hoehn-Saric *et al.*, 1993	8	50	61%*	—	22%
Black *et al.*, 1993	8	75	73%*	—	25%
Citalopram					
Wade *et al.*, 1997	8	475	43–58%*	50%*	32%
Sertraline					
Pohl *et al.*, 1998	10	168	62%*	—	46%
Pollack *et al.*, 1998	10	176	57%~	—	47%
Londborg *et al.*, 1998	12	178	57%~	—	41%

*Significantly different from placebo; †one or zero panic attacks in a three week period; ~not significantly different from placebo; CT = cognitive therapy.

SELECTIVE SEROTONIN REUPTAKE INHIBITORS

Resolution of Panic Attacks

The SSRIs are effective in the treatment of panic disorder for which they are increasingly considered as first-line treatment. Comprehensive data has been published for SSRIs in particular, and the proportion of patients achieving panic-free rates have been reported in patients treated with paroxetine, fluvoxamine, citalopram, and sertraline in placebo-controlled studies (Table XIX-13.1).

Paroxetine

There is an extensive clinical database available for paroxetine — the largest data set among the SSRIs — which comprises data for over 700 patients with panic disorder treated with paroxetine for periods ranging from 10 to 36 weeks (Oehrberg *et al.*, 1995; Lecrubier and Judge, 1997; Lecrubier *et al.*, 1997; Ballenger *et al.*, 1998a). In a 12-week, double-blind, placebo-controlled comparison of paroxetine and clomipramine in 367 patients with panic disorder, paroxetine reduced the number of panic attacks to zero in 51% of patients, compared with 37% of patients treated with clomipramine and 32% of those on placebo (Lecrubier and Judge, 1997). In a two-centre study, Bakker *et al.* (1999) included 131 patients in a placebo-controlled double-blind study comparing paroxetine, clomipramine and cognitive therapy. They found that 37% of placebo treated patients were free from panic attacks in the last three week interval of this 12 weeks study. In the clomipramine and cognitive therapy group, this number was 17% and 54% and respectively. Interestingly, they reported a very low response-rate to clomipramine, in contrast to other studies. The highest response was found in the paroxetine treated patients: 75% from the patients were panic-free from week 10–12 or earlier. In this study, cognitive therapy did not differ from placebo on the pivotal measures.

Fluvoxamine

Fluvoxamine has been shown to reduce the number of panic attacks to zero in two, 8-week, placebo-controlled studies (125 patients in total): up to 73% of patients treated with fluvoxamine were panic free by the end of study, compared with approximately 25% of patients on placebo (Black, Uhde and Tancer, 1992; Hoehn-Saric *et al.*, 1993).

Citalopram

Citalopram has been compared with clomipramine in an 8-week, placebo-controlled study in 475 patients with panic disorder, with or without agoraphobia (Wade *et al.*, 1997). At the most effective citalopram dose (20–30 mg per day), approximately 58% of patients were panic-free compared with 50% of patients receiving clomipramine and 32% of placebo patients.

Sertraline

The results from a 12-week, double-blind, placebo-controlled, study of sertraline in 178 outpatients with panic disorder have recently been published (Londborg *et al.*, 1998). At study endpoint, 57% of the pooled sertraline sample were panic free compared with 41% of the placebo subjects; a non-significant difference. A large increase in the placebo response from week 9 onwards may have masked the treatment response. In a study with a similar design Pohl and associates (1998) found that significantly more sertraline-treated patients (62%) than placebo-treated patients were free of panic attacks at the end of treatment. From the analysis of the pooled results from these two studies it was concluded that the mean frequency of panic attacks was very high in this sample

(10 panic attacks per week), but this did not preclude superiority of sertraline over placebo, which was present in all dosages used (50 mg, 100 mg and 200 mg). In addition, analysis of the pooled data set showed that illness severity, chronicity or the presence of clinically relevant depressive symptomatology did not influence treatment results (Sheikh *et al.*, 2000). As yet there are no published comparative data for sertraline against other active treatments.

Fluoxetine

Fluoxetine was for a long time the least well-studied of the SSRIs in panic disorder, but a large multisite double-blind placebo-controlled study including 243 patients suffering from PD has now been published (Michelson *et al.*, 1998). In this study 10 and 20 mg per day were used in an acute 10 weeks treatment phase and responders to the acute phase were randomly assigned to a 24-week continuation-phase using the same double-blind design. Fluoxetine 20 mg appeared to be slightly superior to 10 mg, but both dosages led to statistically significant superior effects compared to placebo on the number of panic attacks, overall anxiety (20 mg better), phobic symptoms, depression and overall impairment.

Long-Term Efficacy

Of the SSRIs, only paroxetine, fluvoxamine and citalopram have demonstrated long-term efficacy in the treatment of panic disorder. A 9-month extension of an acute treatment study with paroxetine in 176 patients with panic disorder showed that, not only was the efficacy of paroxetine maintained, but the proportion of patients who became free of panic attacks continued to increase: after 9 months 85% of patients were panic-free compared with 72% of patients on clomipramine (Lecrubier *et al.*, 1997). Similarly, in a second study, 80 patients with panic disorder who responded to three months' maintenance treatment with paroxetine were randomized to paroxetine or placebo for a further 3 months (Judge and Steiner, 1996). Only 5% of those who continued to take paroxetine experienced a relapse compared with 30% of patients switched to placebo. Seventy-three patients with panic disorder underwent 12 months' further treatment with fluvoxamine in an open extension of two placebo-controlled studies (Holland *et al.*, 1994). Patients who had been transferred from placebo and those continuing on fluvoxamine continued to improve indicating that the effect of fluvoxamine in panic disorder is probably sustained in the long term. In a double-blind placebo-controlled long-term study lasting one year comparing citalopram (fixed dose ranges: 10 or 15 mg per day; 20 or 30 mg per day; 40 or 60 mg per day) vs clomipramine, it was found that all drug-treatment groups treatment outcome was better than placebo. Only the lowest dose of citalopram was less effective. In almost all patients remaining in the study ($N = 279$) panic attacks tended to disappear during active treatment (Lepola *et al.*, 1998).

Anxiety Levels

Reductions in global anxiety ratings with paroxetine, fluvoxamine, and citalopram have been reported in treatment studies in panic disorder (den Boer *et al.*, 1987, 1988; Black *et al.*, 1992; Hoehn-Saric *et al.*, 1993; Oehrberg *et al.*, 1995; Lecrubier and Judge, 1997; Lecrubier *et al.*, 1997; Wade *et al.*, 1997; Ballenger *et al.*, 1998a). All three SSRIs demonstrated comparable efficacy to clomipramine with respect to this endpoint measure (den Boer *et al.*, 1987; Lecrubier and Judge, 1997; Wade *et al.*, 1997).

Sertraline significantly reduced the time spent with anticipatory anxiety compared with placebo in a multicentre comparison in outpatients (Londborg *et al.*, 1998; Pohl, Wolkow and Clary, 1998), but in the study of Pollack *et al.* (1998) sertraline was not significantly different from placebo on measures for anticipatory anxiety. Limited data are available for the reduction of global anxiety in panic disorder with fluoxetine. It has been compared with desipramine in one small 10-week study where it was found to reduce anxiety levels (Bystritsky *et al.*, 1994). In the study by Michelson and co-workers (1998) it was found that fluoxetine 20 mg per day (but not 10 mg per day) significantly reduced global anxiety.

Phobic Avoidance

Paroxetine

Paroxetine produced a significant reduction in overall phobic score compared with placebo during a 12-week, placebo-controlled study in 367 patients (Lecrubier and Judge, 1997). The reduction was similar to that observed in patients on clomipramine. Further improvements in phobic avoidance were evident during the long-term extension phase of this study (Lecrubier *et al.*, 1997).

Fluvoxamine

Fluvoxamine was also found to be efficacious in the reduction of phobic avoidance in patients with panic disorder in several studies (den Boer *et al.*, 1987, 1988, 1990; van Vliet, Westenberg and den Boer, 1996). In all studies, although phobic avoidance was reduced, patients on fluvoxamine were still exhibiting signs of avoidance at study endpoint.

Fluoxetine and Citalopram

Fluoxetine reduced phobic avoidance in a small comparative study with desipramine (Bystrisky *et al.*, 1994). In the large double-blind study by Michelson *et al.* (1998) fluoxetine reduced phobic avoidance better than placebo. In the 12 months extension follow-up period of the study by Lepola *et al.* (1998) in which citalopram was compared to clomipramine and placebo, it was found that the reduction in total phobia score as assessed with the Phobia Scale was significantly greater in all patients receiving citalopram by month 9 and 12 compared to the group receiving placebo. Using the same scale, the group treated with clomipramine did not differ from placebo at month 12 (Leinonen *et al.*, 2000). In this study, however, no mention was made of the number of panic attacks, so that it is unclear whether clomipramine and citalopram showed comparable efficacy on this measure.

Overall Impairment

The effect of SSRIs on overall impairment in patients with panic disorder has been assessed in placebo-controlled clinical trials conducted with paroxetine (Lecrubier and Judge, 1997; Lecrubier *et al.*, 1997), fluvoxamine (Black, Uhde and Tancer, 1992; Hoehn-Saric *et al.*, 1993) sertraline (Pohl, Wolkow and Clary, 1998; Pollack *et al.*, 1998) and fluoxetine (Michelson *et al.*, 1998). Reductions in overall impairment, as assessed by the Sheehan Disability Scale in work, social and family life items, have been observed with both paroxetine, fluvoxamine and fluoxetine, whereas sertraline treated patients did significantly better than placebo on the Quality of Life Enjoyment and Satisfaction Questionnaire.

SSRI's Compared with Cognitive-Behavioural Therapy

There is limited data about the combination of cognitive therapy and pharmacotherapy in the short- and long-term treatment of PD. In order to evaluate whether drug therapy or psychosocial therapies are efficacious for PD, Barlow and co-workers conducted a double-blind placebo controlled study in 312 patients suffering from PD (Barlow *et al.*, 2000). Patients received imipramine (up to 300 mg per day), CBT only, placebo only, CBT plus imipramine, or CBT plus placebo. Patients were treated for 12 weeks, responders were seen monthly for 6 months. Both imipramine and CBT were found to be significantly superior to placebo in the acute phase (12 weeks) and during the 6 months continuation phase. Combining CBT with imipramine did not increase response rates in the acute phase, but by the end of maintenance (6 months) the combination led to more substantial advantage compared to either condition alone.

Two studies have compared the efficacy of fluvoxamine and cognitive-behavioural therapy (CBT) in PD (Black, Uhde and Tancer, 1992; Sharp, Power and Simpson, 1996). In dosages up to 300 mg per day for 8 weeks, fluvoxamine reduced anxiety levels significantly more effectively than CBT or placebo alone (Black, Uhde and Tancer, 1992). The percentage of patients who were panic free at the end of study was higher in patients receiving fluvoxamine than CBT of placebo alone. In usual dose-levels of 150 mg per day, fluvoxamine was not better than CBT, whereas an additive effect was seen when the two treatments were combined (Sharp, Power and Simpson, 1996). Although the number of studies combining exposure *in vivo* with pharmacotherapy was limited, van Balkom *et al.* (1997) concluded from a meta-analysis from studies pertaining to different treatment conditions, that in the short-term treatment of PD the combination is superior. De Beurs and co-workers (1995) compared fluvoxamine (150 mg per day) plus exposure therapy, placebo plus exposure, panic management plus exposure or exposure alone in a 12 week, double-blind study. They found that fluvoxamine plus exposure therapy reduced agoraphobic behaviour more than the other three treatment conditions. Also after a two-year follow-up study of patients from this study, it was found that the beneficial effects of combination therapy was maintained long term, although the differences between the treatment conditions were no longer significant (de Beurs *et al.*, 1999).

Dual Action Antidepressants in Panic Disorder

Although the aetiology of PD is unclear, it has been suggested that besides serotonergic dysfunction noradrenergic dysfunction is also associated with PD. Although SSRI's appear to be consistently effective in relieving the symptoms of PD the results of studies with selective noradrenergic agents are generally negative. Maprotiline (a selective noradrenergic agent) for example was found to be ineffective in PD (den Boer and Westenberg, 1988). On the other hand a small anxiolytic effect was seen during the use of the selective noradrenalin reuptake inhibitor reboxetine (Phillips *et al.*, 2000). In addition, a recent pilot study conducted in SSRI-resistant panic disorder found reboxetine to be efficacious in reducing the number of panic attacks (Dannon, Iancu and Grunhaus, 2001).

New drugs have been developed to combine noradrenergic and serotonergic sites of action. Mirtazapine is one of these drugs. It is an antidepressant with a different mode of action than the SSRI's and thus with a different side effect profile. The mechanism of action is enhancement of both noradrenergic and serotonergic neurotransmission without reuptake inhibition (den Boer *et al.*, 1994, 1995).

A number of placebo controlled studies have proven the efficacy of mirtazapine in major depressive disorder (Gorman, 1999; Thompson, 1999; Kent, 2000). Efficacy in moderate to severe depression is equivalent to that of TCAs and SSRIs. The tolerability and the safety profile of mirtazapine are more favourable than that of TCAs. The efficacy of mirtazapine in the treatment of anxiety symptoms has been described (Fawcett *et al.*, 1998; Connor *et al.*, 1999a, 1999b; Goodnick *et al.*, 1999; Nutt, 1998). So far, one open label study was published showing efficacy for mirtazapine in PD (Carpenter *et al.*, 1999). We recently completed a larger open-label study in 23 patients with PD according to DSM-IV (Boshuisen *et al.*, 2001). Patients were treated for 15 weeks including a three-week placebo run-in period. As primary efficacy measures we studied the decrease in the number of panic attacks and the number of patients being panic free in the last three weeks of the study. 73.6% were considered responders (decrease of at least 50% in panic attack frequency). The results of this open label study in panic disorder suggest that mirtazapine seems to be a fast and effective treatment in panic disorder with a different side effect profile from SSRI's. Double-blind studies with mirtazapine in PD are ongoing.

Experience with venlafaxine in PD is limited. Two open-label study reported complete cessation of panic attacks in patients suffering from PD (Geracioti, 1995; Papp *et al.*, 1998). In the only double-blind placebo-controlled study published so far, Pollack *et al.* (1996) evaluated the efficacy of immediate-release venlafaxine for the treatment of PD in an 8-week trial. In this small-scale study 25 outpatients suffering from PD were included. Based on endpoint analysis venlafaxine-treated patients showed significantly greater improvement than the placebo group on the CGI, whereas the difference in the mean number of panic attacks was not significant between the two treatment conditions.

5-HT RECEPTOR AGONISTS

Evidence regarding the efficacy of the partial $5\text{-}HT_{1A}$ receptor partial agonists, buspirone and gepirone in panic disorder has been conflicting. Buspirone has shown antipanic activity in two placebo-controlled trials (Robinson *et al.*, 1989; Sheehan *et al.*, 1993), but has not demonstrated superior efficacy to placebo on all outcome measures. Similarly, an 8-week placebo-controlled study of buspirone and imipramine in 52 patients with panic disorder showed that buspirone was not significantly superior to placebo in its anxiolytic effects (Sheehan *et al.*, 1990). There have been no reports supporting the ability of buspirone to reduce the number of panic attacks to zero in a population of patients with panic disorder. In contrast, 59% of patients ($n = 21$) on gepirone reached panic-free status by the end of a 6-week open trial (Pecknold *et al.*, 1993). However, the potent and selective $5\text{-}HT_{1A}$ agonist, flesinoxan did not reduce the number of panic attacks in two small pilot studies (20 patients in total) (van Vliet, Westenberg and den Boer, 1996). Furthermore, treatment with flesinoxan produced a profound increase in symptoms of anxiety in these patients.

Buspirone in combination with cognitive-behavioural therapy (CBT), has demonstrated greater efficacy than CBT and placebo, suggesting that buspirone may be an effective adjunct to CBT (Bouvard *et al.*, 1997), however, this effect was not maintained in the long term.

5-HT RECEPTOR ANTAGONISTS

Electrophysiological experiments in anaesthetized animals have highlighted the role of somatodendritic $5\text{-}HT_{1A}$ autoreceptors in the delayed onset of action of antidepressants (Blier, de Montigny and Chaput, 1987). Microdialysis experiments in conscious animals have shown that the increase in extracellular 5-HT following reuptake inhibition by SSRIs is counteracted by activation of these autoreceptors (Invernizzi, Belli and Samanin, 1992; Hjorth and Auerbach, 1994). Repeated administration of SSRIs is thought to desensitize the somatodendritic autoreceptors, resulting in an enhanced availability of serotonin (Chaput, de Montigny and Blier, 1991). Arguably, this desensitization process can be mimicked instantaneously by blockade of the autoreceptors with $5\text{-}HT_{1A}$

receptor antagonists. Consequently, coadministration of SSRIs with 5-HT_{1A} antagonists would hasten the therapeutic effect of SSRIs (Artigas, 1993). Several studies have indeed reported beneficial effects of this augmentation strategy with pindolol (e.g. Artigas, Perez and Alvarez, 1994; Blier and Bergeron, 1995) in major depression.

A preliminary report suggested that augmentation with pindolol is also effective in treatment resistant panic disorder (Dannon *et al.*, 1997). However, an augmentation study by van Vliet *et al.* (2001) with panic disorder patients was negative. In this open-label study patients were treated with either fluvoxamine and pindolol (7.5 mg daily) or fluvoxamine alone. The results of this study show that pindolol as add-on medication to fluvoxamine does not hasten the anxiolytic or antipanic effects of fluvoxamine. In a recent study 25 therapy-resistant PD patients received fluoxetine (20 mg per day) and additionally either placebo or pindolol (2.5 mg t.i.d.). Patients treated with the combination of pindolol and fluoxetine showed a significantly better treatment response over patients treated with fluoxetine plus placebo (Hirschmann *et al.*, 2000). Although preliminary in nature, this study is at odds with the findings with fluvoxamine. It is possible that pharmacological differences among the SSRI's could explain these differences, on the other hand it should be noted that there were differences in the inclusion criteria among the studies: in the study by van Vliet and co-workers treatment resistance was not a prerequisite for inclusion, whereas the other two studies did include only treatment resistant patients.

Preliminary open studies with the 5-HT_2 antagonists ritanserin and trazadone suggested that both agents may have antipanic and antiphobic activity (Griez, Pols and Lousberg, 1988; Charney *et al.*, 1986). However, placebo-controlled studies with a larger patient sample in which ritanserin was compared with fluvoxamine (den Boer and Westenberg, 1990), and trazodone with imipramine and alprazolam (Charney *et al.*, 1986) showed no reduction in panic attack frequency for either agent. Preliminary evidence has been reported for the efficacy of nefazodone in a small open, 8-week study of 14 patients with panic disorder and comorbid depression (DeMartinis, Schweizer and Rickels, 1996). Another open-label study reported beneficial effects of nefazodone in nine out of 10 patients (Bystritsky *et al.*, 1999). In spite of these promising open-label studies, these results have not been confirmed in well designed placebo controlled studies.

The 5-HT_3 antagonist ondansetron demonstrated only limited efficacy in a small pilot study of 31 patients with panic disorder and agoraphobia (Schneier *et al.*, 1996). The response rate of 48% was not beyond the upper limit of placebo response rates and, in the absence of a placebo control group, it was not possible to attribute the response rate to an improvement in panic attacks. As a result, the use of ondansetron in panic disorder is no longer being actively pursued.

Inositol

Inositol is a natural isomer of glucose and a precursor for the second-messenger phosphatidyl–inositol system. There is one recent double-blind comparative study versus fluvoxamine in which inositol has been investigated in panic disorder. In this study 20 patients were treated with inositol up to 18 mg per day for one month and the clinical outcome was compared to patients treated with fluvoxamine up to 150 mg per day (Palatnik *et al.*, 2001). The results of this preliminary study suggest similar efficacy for inositol and fluvoxamine in reducing the number of panic attacks. When replicated in larger studies treatment with inositol might offer an alternative for patients who are sensitive to the side-effects of SSRI's, as inositol is almost devoid of side-effects.

Conclusion

The only serotonergic agents which have clearly demonstrated efficacy as antipanic agents in both short and long-term investigations are the SSRIs. The SSRIs produce improvements in anticipatory anxiety and phobic avoidance. In addition, the SSRIs proven ability to enable patients with panic disorder to achieve panic-free status indicates that, as a first-line treatment in panic disorder, the SSRIs are a good therapeutic choice. In contrast, the 5-HT agonists and antagonists have demonstrated equivocal efficacy in panic disorder. Most of our judgements about the therapeutic efficacy of SSRIs (and other antidepressants) are based upon double-blind placebo controlled studies. To what extent the results of randomized clinical trials apply to everyday care cannot be judged without regular measurement of outcomes in daily practice. In a three-year naturalistic prospective study in PD, Toni *et al.* (2000) described the evolution of panic and agoraphoba in 326 DSM-IIIR PD patients. The main antidepressants used were paroxetine, imipramine and clomipramine. Although efficacy did not show major differences during the entire follow-up period, paroxetine-treated patients suffered significantly less from jitteriness and anticholinergic side-effects, thus reducing barriers to compliance for the SSRI treated patients. Preliminary results with inositol may appear promising, although the evidence for its efficacy is still circumstantial.

OBSESSIVE COMPULSIVE DISORDER

Introduction

The 'Serotonin Hypothesis of OCD' evolved from the speculation that the unique efficacy of the TCA, clomipramine, in OCD was due to its effects in facilitating 5-HT neurotransmission (Insel *et al.*, 1985; Zohar and Insel, 1987; Jenike *et al.*, 1989; Goodman *et al.*, 1990; Murphy and Pigott, 1990; Rasmussen, Elsen and Pato, 1993; Zohar *et al.*, 2000). Clomipramine was the first drug reported to be effective in OCD (Fernandez and Lopez-Ibor, 1967). The efficacy of clomipramine has been reviewed in many publications and will not be repeated here. OCD patients respond specifically to drugs that influence the serotonergic system; noradrenergic drugs like nortryptiline or drugs with weaker 5-HT reuptake inhibiting properties like imipramine and amitryptiline appear to be without effect on OCD symptomatology (Leonard *et al.*, 1989, 1991). The potential role of 5-HT in the pathogenesis of OCD has led to the investigation of other agents, in particular the SSRIs.

SSRIs in the Treatment of OCD

Paroxetine, fluvoxamine, sertraline and fluoxetine have all been investigated in large placebo-controlled trials and their efficacy as anti-obsessional agents is well established. A 12-week, fixed-dose study of paroxetine versus placebo in 263 patients with OCD demonstrated that paroxetine (40 and 60 mg per day) was significantly more effective than placebo in reducing OCD symptoms (mean reduction as assessed with the Yale–Brown Obsessive Compulsive Inventory (Y-BOCS), 25% and 29% versus 13% respectively) (Wheadon, Bushnell and Steiner, 1993).

Similarly, fluvoxamine was reported to be more effective than placebo in reducing OCD symptoms in a number of randomized double-blind studies (for review see Figgett and McClellan, 2000; Vythilingum, Cartwright and Hollander, 2000). In four placebo-controlled studies fluvoxamine at dosages of 100 to 300 mg per day was found to significantly reduce symptoms of OCD compared to placebo (Mallya, White and Waternaux, 1992; Greist, Jenike and Robinson, 1995a; Goodman *et al.*, 1996; Mundo, Bianchi and Bellodi, 1997). In most of these studies the response rate as measured with the Y-BOCS was in the range of 40–52%. As with the other SSRI's, the average dose for fluvoxamine in OCD is higher than in other anxiety disorders and depression and is in the range of 150–300 mg per day.

Greist and colleagues (1995b) reported the results of a 12-week, placebo-controlled, fixed-dose study of sertraline in 324 patients with OCD; the active treatment (50 and 200 mg per day) was significantly more effective than placebo in reducing OCD symptoms (mean Y-BOCS reduction, 24% and 28% versus 15%). In a follow-up study of 40 weeks duration Greist and colleagues (1995b) reported continued improvement of sertraline over time. Interestingly, the occurrence of side-effects subsided throughout the year of treatment. A recent double-blind placebo-controlled study using a flexible dose schedule of sertraline (50–200 mg per day) in 167 patients with OCD confirmed the anti-obsessional/compulsive effects of this SSRI (Kronig *et al.*, 1999). Also, in patients suffering from OCD who also met the criteria for major depression, sertraline was found to be more effective in reducing both OCD and depressed symptomatology compared to the noradrenaline reuptake inhibitor desipramine (Hoehn-Saric *et al.*, 2000).

In a double-blind, fixed-dose study 217 OCD patients were treated with fluoxetine (20, 40 or 60 mg) or placebo for 8 weeks (Montgomery *et al.*, 1993). Only the 40 and 60 mg dosages were found to be statistically superior to placebo, indicating that also with fluoxetine higher dosages are required. In a 13-week, multicentre, placebo-controlled, fixed-dose study of 355 patients with OCD, fluoxetine (20, 40 and 60 mg per day) was significantly more effective than placebo (mean Y-BOCS reduction, 20%, 22%, and 27% versus 3%) in reducing OCD symptoms (Tollefson *et al.*, 1994a). The trend may suggest greater efficacy with increasing dosage.

The efficacy of citalopram has been less well-studied in OCD than the other SSRIs. Recently, however, citalopram has also demonstrated efficacy in OCD in two open studies (Mundo, Bianchi and Bellodi, 1997; Koponen *et al.*, 1997). In one of these studies, a 24-week pilot study in 29 patients with OCD, 76% of patients showed alleviation of symptoms in comparison with baseline (Koponen *et al.*, 1997).

SSRIs vs Clomipramine

The efficacy of the SSRIs in the treatment of OCD has been compared with clomipramine, which for a long time was considered the gold-standard treatment for this anxiety disorder. Paroxetine, fluoxetine and fluvoxamine have been shown to be at least as effective as clomipramine in the treatment of patients with OCD, but better tolerated (Wheadon, Bushnell and Steiner, 1993; Zohar and Judge, 1996; Goodman *et al.*, 1997; Koran, Mueller and Maloney, 1996). The first multicentre, placebo-controlled study of an SSRI versus clomipramine, in 399 patients with OCD, was performed with paroxetine (Zohar and Judge, 1996). Both paroxetine and clomipramine were associated with similar efficacy at weeks 6, 8, and 12. Furthermore, during a multicentre, flexible dose, 10-week study in 66 patients with OCD, significant and similar reductions in OCD symptoms were seen for fluvoxamine and clomipramine (mean Y-BOCS reduction, 33% and 31%) (Freeman *et al.*, 1994). Similar results were obtained in a recent double-blind comparison of fluvoxamine and clomipramine in 133 patients suffering from OCD. In terms of efficacy as measured with the Y-BOCS, no statistically significant differences were found between the two treatment conditions but the side-effect profile was more favourable in the fluvoxamine treated patients (Mundo, Maina and Uslenghi, 2000).

In a 16-week comparative study of sertraline and clomipramine in 86 patients with OCD a significantly greater reduction in OCD symptoms was found for patients on sertraline compared with clomipramine (mean Y-BOCS reduction, 51% versus 43%; $p < 0.05$) (Bisserbe *et al.*, 1997). However, a fair comparison may have been precluded because of the greater number of clomipramine subjects who withdrew early in the study (18 clomipramine versus three sertraline within 28 days). When compared with clomipramine in a 26-week, double-blind, crossover study in 11 patients with OCD, fluoxetine was associated with significant reductions from baseline in OCD symptoms which were comparable with clomipramine (Pigott *et al.*, 1990). Similar results were observed in an 8-week double-blind comparative study of fluoxetine vs clomipramine in 55 OCD patients (Lopez-Ibor *et al.*, 1996). Interestingly, a 10-week, double-blind study comparing fluvoxamine, paroxetine and citalopram demonstrated that there were no significant differences between the three treatments in terms of efficacy (Mundo, Bianchi and Bellodi, 1997).

Despite the chronicity of OCD and the recommendation that pharmacotherapy should exceed 9–12 months' duration, there are comparatively few published data on the efficacy of SSRIs or clomipramine for periods longer than 20 weeks (Jenike *et al.*, 1990a, b; Rasmussen, Elsen and Pato, 1993). It has been demonstrated that OCD symptoms continued to improve for up to 6 months of paroxetine therapy. Furthermore, patients on placebo relapsed three times faster than those on paroxetine during the extension phase of one placebo-controlled study.

In terms of long-term efficacy, a two-year, open-label follow-up of responders to clomipramine and fluvoxamine, found both maintenance treatments to be significantly superior to placebo in preventing relapse in patients with OCD (Ravizza *et al.*, 1996). Seventy-six patients with OCD who responded to treatment with fluoxetine during an acute treatment study maintained symptom improvement during a 24-week continuation study (Tollefson *et al.*, 1994b). Similarly, in a two-year, open-label follow-up of responders to clomipramine and fluoxetine, both maintenance treatments were found to be significantly superior to placebo in preventing relapse (Ravizza *et al.*, 1996). There is no data available on the long-term efficacy of citalopram or sertraline in OCD.

Several meta-analyses have addressed the question of the differential efficacy of clompiramine and SSRI's in OCD (e.g. Picinelli *et al.*, 1995; Greist *et al.*, 1995c). The main conclusion of these meta-analyses was that clompiramine had a somewhat better effect on OCD-symptomatology than the SSRI's, although the side-effect profile of the SSRI's was superior to clomipramine. These findings stand in sharp contrast with the direct head-to-head comparative studies vs clomipramine reviewed above: in these studies similar efficacy of the SSRI's was found. We should, however, remain aware of the methodological problems encountered in meta-analyses. Variables such as study design, time period, chronology and site-specific factors, which may have impact on the results, cannot be considered in meta-analyses.

In sum, there is substantial evidence from head-to-head comparisons of paroxetine, fluoxetine, sertraline and fluvoxamine with clomipramine to conclude a similar efficacy and a lower incidence of side-effects with the SSRI (see also Pigott and Seay, 1999).

Anti-compulsive or Antidepressant Action?

Symptoms of depression often co-occur with OCD raising the possibility that non-specific antidepressant and anxiolytic effects may determine the success of SSRI's in OCD (e.g. Marks *et al.*, 1980). In subsequent studies discussed above it has been shown that initial depression was not predictive, nor related in any way to the degree of improvement in OCD (e.g. Price *et al.*, 1987). Moreover, if the anti-obsessional and anti-compulsive effects were in fact related to antidepressant efficacy, that other antidepressants such as nortryptiline should also be effective in the treatment of OCD, and this clearly is not the case.

5-HT RECEPTOR AGONISTS

The 5-HT_{1A} receptor agonist buspirone has demonstrated equivocal results in efficacy studies in patients with OCD. Buspirone was ineffective in a small, 8-week, open study in 14 patients with OCD (Jenike and Baer, 1988). However, Pato and colleagues (1991) demonstrated that buspirone and clomipramine produced significant improvements in symptoms in 18 patients with OCD; no differences were noted between the active treatments (Pato *et al.*, 1991). There is no published evidence of the efficacy of gepirone or ipsapirone in OCD.

Evidence for the augmenting effect of buspirone in SSRI treatment-refractory patients with OCD is also equivocal. In a 20-week, open study with fluoxetine, clinical response was enhanced in 50% of patients by addition of buspirone during the last 8 weeks of the study (Jenike, Baer and Greist, 1991). In contrast, however, in a double-blind study in which 13 fluoxetine-treated patients with OCD were given adjuvant buspirone or placebo for 4 weeks, there were no significant differences in improvement of OCD symptoms between the two treatment groups (Grady *et al.*, 1993).

5-HT RECEPTOR ANTAGONISTS AND TREATMENT REFRACTORY OCD

There is a paucity of data with respect to the treatment options in treatment refractory OCD. There is circumstantial evidence from open-label studies that adding another SSRI to ongoing treatment with clomipramine could lead to further improvement, but the evidence is not compelling (Pallanti *et al.*, 1999).

A small number of patients with SSRI treatment refractory OCD have been given open trials of risperidone (an atypical antipsychotic agent with potent dopaminergic and serotonergic antagonist activity) (Saxena *et al.*, 1996; Jacobsen, 1995). In the largest of these studies, 21 patients were treated openly with the combination of an SSRI (paroxetine, fluvoxamine, sertraline or fluoxetine) and risperidone (Saxena *et al.*, 1996). Sixteen patients tolerated the combined treatment and, of these, 87% had substantial reductions in OCD symptoms within 3 weeks. Similar results were reported in a recent open label study with risperidone as add-on to ongoing treatment with SSRIs (Pfanner *et al.*, 2000). In a recent double-blind placebo-controlled study it was found that adding risperidone for 6 weeks to ongoing therapy with SSRIs in treatment refractory patients led to a 50% response rate, which was not present in the placebo treated patients (McDougle *et al.*, 2000). There has also been a preliminary report that the $5\text{-HT}_{2A/2C}$ receptor antagonist ritanserin was effective as an adjunct to fluoxetine treatment in OCD patients with psychotic features (Bach, Aigner and Lenz, 1997).

Experience with other atypical antipsychotics in treatment refractory OCD is limited and studies are ongoing. There is one open-label study in which olanzapine (5 mg per day) was added to treatment with fluvoxamine (300 mg per day). It was found that this augmentation led to a significant decrease in the Y-BOCS (Bogetto *et al.*, 2000).

Open studies suggest that pindolol has shown some merit as an adjuvant to SSRIs (paroxetine, fluvoxamine, sertraline or fluoxetine) in OCD (Blier and Bergeron, 1995). In a recent study 14 patients who were nonresponders to previous treatment with two SSRIs and were currently unresponsive to treatment with paroxetine (60 mg per day) were included in a double-blind placebo-controlled pindolol (2.5 mg t.i.d.) augmentation study (Dannon *et al.*, 2000). As measured with the Y-BOCS, significant differences were noted in favour of pindolol compared to placebo, whereas no differences were present between placebo and pindolol on measures of anxiety and depression.

There is anecdotal evidence that treatment-refractory patients might respond to treatment with the 5-HT_{1D} agonist sumatriptan (Stern *et al.*, 1998). In a recent study, however, we were not able to show involvement of the 5-HT_{1D} receptor in OCD in a double-blind placebo controlled challenge study using the selective $5\text{-HT}_{1D/1B}$ receptor agonist zolmitriptan and therefore treating patients with 5-HT_{1D} agonists should not be encouraged before further clinical studies have been performed (Boshuisen and den Boer, 2000).

Finally, inositol augmentation to SSRI treatment did not lead to significant improvement in 10 OCD patients in an open-label study (Seedat and Stein, 1999).

THE LAST RESORT: PSYCHOSURGERY

In a small number of cases, OCD is refractory to irrespective which conventional treatment, and uncontrolled evidence suggests that such cases may respond to different types of psychosurgery. In spite of the fact that only a limited number of operations are performed, a variety of surgical techniques are used. They involve: capsulotomy, cingulotomy, subcaudate tractotomy, combined orbitofrontal/cingulate lesions.

During capsulotomy stereotactic lesions are produced in the anterior limb of the internal capsule. Cingulotomy involves stereotactic lesions of the anterior cingulate cortex. Subcaudate tractotomy involves placement of radioactive rods beneath and in front of the caudate nucleus.

All surgical treatments appear to be effective in approximately 30–40% of the patients, but no reliable clinical studies have been performed based upon which predictive indicators for good outcome can be defined. In addition, the site and size of the lesion remains to be established (for review, see Jenike, 1998). Cummings and co-workers (1995) studied 17 patients with OCD using a neuropsychological test battery after psychosurgery. The psychosurgery group appeared to perform more poorly only on the Wisconsin Card Sorting Test (WCST), indicating the impact of frontal lobe lesions on abilities mediating the formation and shifting of response sets. In another study 18 patients with intractable OCD who underwent cingulotomy participated in a follow-up study. In this small sample, 28% were responders, whereas 17% were partial responders (Baer *et al.*, 1995).

In one of the very rare studies investigating the effects of specific lesion sites in OCD, Irle *et al.* (1998) conducted a long-term follow-up of patients who underwent ventromedial frontal leukotomy during the seventies. Eight out of 11 subjects with lesions of the ventral striatum had developed substance dependence. Subjects with frontostriatal lesions showed most clinical improvement. In all patients, neuropsychological testing only revealed abnormalities on the WCST, whereas subjects with lesions of the dorsolateral frontal convexity showed other cognitive impairments such as attentional problems and memory problems.

In countries where psychosurgery is applied it is advised that an independent multidisciplinary legally constituted review board selects patients who apply for psychosurgery (Rosenfield and Lloyd, 1999).

Conclusion

The SSRIs have demonstrated efficacy in the treatment of OCD while the 5-HT agonists have shown equivocal results. Data from studies of the 5-HT antagonists in patients with OCD suggest that these agents may be useful as augmenting agents in treatment-refractory patients. However, drugs such as risperidone and olanzapine have mixed serotonergic and dopaminergic functions and the efficacy of these agents in OCD may be correlated with their action on more than one neurotransmitter.

Until recently, the placebo response in many studies using antidepressants in OCD has been very low (5–10%). In more recent studies, higher placebo responses were observed (up to 30%). The reason for this could be that patients who participated in the original clomipramine studies could distinguish placebo from clomipramine because of the severe side-effects. It is possible that the newer drugs can be less clearly distinguished from placebo thus yielding a greater placebo response. Lastly, it is conceivable that due to competing studies investigators may be inclined to include patients with mild OCD.

GENERALIZED ANXIETY DISORDER (GAD)

Introduction

Since 1968, the diagnostic and statistical manual, second edition (DSM-II) delineated anxiety neurosis. This category was abolished in the DSM-III from 1980, in which generalized anxiety disorder (GAD) and panic disorder were delineated. In the DSM-III GAD was considered a 'residual' mental disorder which was diagnosed by exclusion. In the DSM-III-R it was defined by the presence of excessive/unrealistic worry as the core symptoms plus additional associated anxiety symptoms. In the DSM-IV, GAD was redefined to include the A-criterion symptoms of excessive uncontrolled anxiety and worry for at least 6 months plus three or more additional somatic and psychological anxiety symptoms (which is consistent with ICD-10 criteria). These include among others: muscle tension, restlessness, fatigue, difficulty in concentrating, irritability, and sleep disturbance.

Usually GAD is considered to be a chronic disorder. The study by Yonkers *et al.* (1996) of 166 GAD patients reported a man duration of GAD of more than 20 years and a likelihood of GAD symptom remission of only 15% and 25% at 1 and 2 years, respectively. This chronicity is consistent with a previous study of a large group of anxiety disorder patients with different diagnoses which reported that GAD patients were symptomatic for 56% of their lives after onset compared with much lower proportions in anxiety disorders traditionally thought to be more severe (Roy-Byrne, 1996) (16% for panic and 29% for agoraphobia with panic).

Differences in Cognitions between GAD and PD: the Role of Worrying

McNally (1994) considered that the distinction between GAD and panic disorder in DSM-III-R was blurred in two ways. Firstly, eliminating the diagnostic hierarchies of DSM-III allowed for very high rates of comorbidity, and revealed that GAD was rarely diagnosed as a single disorder. Secondly, unexpected panic attacks often occur in GAD patients, but few of these patients suffer from panic disorder (Sanderson and Barlow, 1990). The most important worry for PD patients is focused on fear of having another panic attack, as opposed to any other worry (Adler *et al.*, 1989; McNally, 1992, 1994). Worry in GAD patients is usually associated with exaggerated predictions of external catastrophic events (Borkovec and Roemer, 1995; Lydiard, 2000).

In view of the high degree of comorbidity associated with GAD, it has been argued that GAD could be a trait-like 'platform' that sets the stage and confers the vulnerability for the development of major depression, panic and other anxiety disorders. Recent evidence, however, challenged this notion and suggests that initial concerns about extremely high degrees of comorbidity among patients with GAD are misplaced. Wittchen and co-workers showed that comorbidity is a high predictor of help-seeking behaviour in patients with GAD indicating that in earlier studies this sample was over-represented and constitutes a selection bias (Wittchen *et al.*, 1994). In a recent review Kessler (2000) concluded that GAD does not stand out in any particular way with respect to other disorders in predicting other anxiety or depressive disorders (see also Wittchen *et al.*, 2000). Therefore there is no reason to question the validity of GAD as a separate disorder, because this doubt should also apply to any other anxiety or mood disorder.

Benzodiazepines in GAD

Benzodiazepines (BDZs) are frequently prescribed for the treatment of GAD by general practioners. They are widely accepted by both patients and general practitioners because of their rapid onset of action and good tolerability. However, withdrawal symptoms hamper successful discontinuation after prolonged treatment and thus BDZs should not be recommended as first-line monotherapy for the long-term management of anxiety disorders. Interestingly, several studies have shown that BDZs are effective on specific GAD symptoms such as somatic/autonomic symptoms in contrast to the psychic symptoms cluster including apprehensive worry and irritability (for review see Connor and Davidson, 1998). Side-effects of BDZs include sedation, memory difficulties, additive effects on alcohol and severe withdrawal reactions. Several treatment strategies such as cognitive therapy (Otto *et al.*, 1993) and concomitant prescribing of pharmacological agents like carbamazepine (Schweizer *et al.*, 1991) have been employed to assist patients to overcome their severe withdrawal syndrome induced by tapering off BDZs. In a recent study Rickels *et al.* (2000a) studied 107 patients with GAD who were long-term BDZs users. They were enrolled in a BDZs withdrawal programme assessing the efficacy of concomitant imipramine (mean dose: 180 mg per day) vs buspirone (mean dose: 38 mg per day) in a double-blind placebo controlled study. The success of the taper was significantly higher for patients treated with imipramine (82.6%), compared to either buspirone (success rates of taper 67.9%) and placebo (success rate taper: 37.5%). There is also evidence that prior treatment with BDZs is a negative predictor for therapeutic effects of subsequent treatment with buspirone. In a recent study DeMartinis and co-workers (2000) found that clinical improvement with buspirone was similar to BDZs treatment in GAD if patients had no prior treatment of BDZs. When patients were recently treated with BDZs, the effects of buspirone could not be distinguished from placebo.

During the last few years many studies have been performed using SSRIs, dual action antidepressants, 5-HT_{1A} receptor agonists and mixed SSRI/5$HT_{2A/C}$ receptor antagonists like nefazodone in the treatment of GAD. Older antidepressants like imipramine have also been shown to reduce anxiety in patients with GAD, although few clinicians would favour imipramine due to its severe side-effect profile compared to modern antidepressants. Based upon a large review of the published randomized double-blind studies up to 1997, Casacalenda and Boulenger (1998) concluded that imipramine, trazodone and paroxetine displayed similar efficacy in the treatment of GAD. At that time there was, however, a paucity of data of the effects of SSRIs and dual action antidepressants in GAD.

In a recent study it was found that clinical improvement with imipramine in GAD was present in patients with the lowest plasma levels of desipramine. In addition, there was a strong relationship with desipramine and anticholinergic levels, indicating that imipramine may have properties that result in physiological states counteracting its therapeutic effects (McLeod *et al.*, 2000). In addition, there are tolerability limitations using TCAs like imipramine and clomipramine in the treatment of GAD (Wingerson, Nguyen and Roy-Byrne, 1992).

Selective Serotonin Reuptake Inhibitors

There have been few studies to date on the use of the SSRIs in the treatment of GAD. Rocca and colleagues investigated the efficacy of paroxetine, imipramine and 2′-chlordes-methyldiazepam in 81 patients with GAD (Rocca *et al.*, 1997). Both paroxetine and imipramine treatment resulted in more improvement than 2′-chlordes-methyldiazepam by the fourth week of treatment as measured by HAM-A and COVI Anxiety Rating Scale (CARS). At the end of the study, 68% of patients in the paroxetine group, 72% of those in the imipramine group, and 55% of those in the 2′-chlordes-methyldiazepam group showed a decrease of 50% or more on the HAM-A score. The efficacy of paroxetine in GAD (defined according to DSM-IV criteria) was evaluated in three other placebo-controlled 8-week studies and a long-term (32 week) relapse prevention study. In a multicentre study in 331 patients suffering from GAD paroxetine was found to be statistically superior to placebo on the HAM-A ($p < 0.01$). In addition, impairments in family and social life were beneficially influenced by paroxetine as assessed with the Sheehan disability Scale (McCafferty *et al.*, 2000). In a study in 566 GAD patients the results of treatment with placebo or paroxetine on the HAM-A and health related quality of life was investigated using the EuroQol (EQ)-5D questionnaire. This group reported that patients treated with 20 and 40 mg paroxetine not only showed significantly larger reductions in the HAM-A ($p < 0.001$), but also that improvement in GAD symptomatology is accompanied by improvement in health-related quality of life (Bellew *et al.*, 2000a, 2000b). The final multicentre study in 372 GAD patients treated with paroxetine or placebo provides supportive data for the efficacy of paroxetine in the treatment of GAD (SKB, data on file).

Stocchi and associates (2001) also studied the long-term efficacy of paroxetine (20–50 mg) in 652 patients with GAD. Patients received paroxetine (20–50 mg) for 8 weeks. Patients whose CGI scores had decreased by at least two points (to a score of three or less) at the week 8 visit were then randomized to double-blind treatment with either paroxetine ($n = 278$) or placebo ($n = 288$) for a period of 24 weeks. The results of this study showed that significantly fewer paroxetine- than placebo-treated patients (10.9% vs 39.9%, respectively, $p < 0.001$) relapsed during the 24 weeks of double-blind therapy indicating that anxiolytic efficacy in GAD is maintained during long-term treatment.

Dual Action Antidepressants in GAD

Venlafaxine

The therapeutic potential of venlafaxine extended release (XR) has been investigated in GAD and venlafaxine XR is the first antidepressant which has been registered for this indication. Three large placebo-controlled multicentre studies have been performed using venlafaxine XR in the treatment of GAD (for review see Hackett, 2000). A summary of these studies is shown in Table XIX-13.2.

The main conclusion of the 6-month flexible-dose study of Gelenberg and co-workers (2000) is that venlafaxine XR was significantly more effective than placebo on the main efficacy measures. Hackett, Parks and Salinas (1999a) performed a 24-weeks fixed-dose study of venlafaxine XR and found significant reductions of the HAM-A which were apparent after two weeks of treatment (for dosages and other details, see Table XIX-13.2). In a study with a similar design but a shorter study period Rickels *et al.* (2000b) found beneficial effects of venlafaxine XR in GAD. In addition there are two comparative studies with buspirone and diazepam as comparators (Davidson *et al.* 1999; Hackett, Desmet and Salinas, 1999b [the latter study is only available as a poster-presentation]).

In an 8-week randomized double-blind placebo-controlled multicentre study, venlafaxine XR (75 or 150 mg) was compared to buspirone 30 mg per day. At endpoint, there was a higher mean reduction in the main efficacy variable (HAM-A) in the venlafaxine-treated patients, but the difference with buspirone was not statistically significant (for detailed discussion, see Barman Balfourand and Jarvis, 2001). Reductions in psychic anxiety scores and score for anxious mood and tension were significantly lower for venlafaxine XR treated patients compared to placebo. The effects of buspirone on these measures, however, were not statistically different from placebo.

In sum, venlafaxine is the first antidepressant to be approved by the Food and Drug Administration of the USA and authorities in Europe for the treatment of GAD. It appears to be consistently better than placebo in the treatment for GAD in terms of inducing reductions of psychometric scales measuring severity of anxiety symptoms. There is substantial evidence from long-term studies that this improvement sustained over 6 months of treatment. Further studies are warranted to establish whether this improvement remains in time and contributes to improvements in the quality of life of these patients.

Mirtazapine

There is only one study in which mirtazapine was studied in GAD. In this open-label study patients with a DSM-IV diagnosis of major depressive disorder with comorbid GAD were prescribed mirtazapine for 8 weeks. In addition to its antidepressant effects, mirtazapine led to a significant reduction on the Hamilton Anxiety Rating Scale, indicating that mirtazapine could have potential value in the treatment of GAD (Goodnick *et al.*, 1999).

5-HT Agonists

Buspirone has been shown to be effective in the treatment of GAD in the short term. A 4-week single-blind study of 23 patients with GAD showed that, when titrated to a daily dose of 30 mg, buspirone provided effective anti-anxiety therapy as assessed by standard psychometric rating scales (Cohn, Wilcox and Meltzer, 1986). It needs to emphasized, however, that several of the studies of buspirone were conducted before proper criteria for GAD were defined, and therefore it cannot be stated that buspirone is effective in GAD according to DSM-IV criteria, because there simply are no studies of buspirone treatment in GAD according to DSM-IV criteria.

Concomitant depression occurs in at least 50% of patients with a primary diagnosis of GAD. A composite analysis of five placebo-controlled studies with buspirone in 382 patients with major depression and associated GAD showed significant improvements in anxiety (Robinson *et al.*, 1990). Interestingly, a 6-week, placebo-controlled efficacy study with buspirone in 121 patients with GAD and mild depression reported a significant reduction from baseline in anxiety and depression for patients on buspirone in comparison to those on placebo (Sramek *et al.*, 1996). In addition, a double-blind study in patients with GAD and depression showed that buspirone was equally effective as diazepam in reducing both anxiety and depression (Feighner *et al.*, 1982). These results suggest that buspirone may be suitable for the treatment of patients with GAD and comorbid depression. Furthermore, a meta-analysis of eight placebo-controlled studies in 520 patients with GAD demonstrated significant improvements over baseline for anxiety and depression for patients on buspirone in comparison with those on placebo (Gammans *et al.*, 1992). Similar results were also obtained when the efficacy of buspirone was assessed in comparison with clorazepate (Goldberg and Finnerty, 1982) and alprazolam (Enkelmann, 1991).

Gepirone is also effective in the treatment of GAD, however it has been suggested that the anxiolytic response to gepirone may be delayed: an 8-week, double-blind study in 198 patients

Table XIX-13.2 Efficacy of once-daily venlafaxine XR (VEN) in patients with generalized anxiety disorder without comorbid major depressive disorder in multicentre, randomized, double-blind, placebo-controlled studies

			Baseline scores		Results at endpoint (mean change from baseline)[a]						
Treatment mg per day	Duration (wk)	No. of pts	HAM-A total	HAM-A psychic anxiety	HAM-A total	HAM-A psychic anxiety	CGI-I	CGI-S	HAD	Response rate[b] (% of pts)	Discontinuations for unsatisfactory response(% of pts)
Gelenberg *et al.*, 2000 (flexible dose)											
VEN 75–225[c]	28	115	25	14	↓13.4***	↓7.4***	2.2***	↓2.1***		≥69***	8**
PL		123	25	14	↓8.7	↓4.2	3	↓1.1		42–46	22
Hackett *et al.*, 1999[d] (fixed dose)											
VEN 37.5	24	138	26.6	11.9	↓13.8*	↓7.6*			↓5.2*	61*[e]	17
VEN 75		130	26.3	11.6	↓15.5*	↓8.5*			↓6.3*	69**[e]	10
VEN 150		131	26.3	11.7	↓16.4*	↓9.2*†			↓7.1*†	75**[e]	2
PL		130	26.7	12.1	↓11.0	↓5.6			↓3.1	46[e]	21
Rickels *et al.* 2000 (fixed dose)											
VEN 75[f]	8	86	24.7	13.9	↓11.2	↓6.7	2.3	↓1.5	↓6.0*		5
VEN 150[f]		81	24.5	14.0	↓12.4	↓7.4*	2.3	↓1.7	↓6.2**		0
VEN 225[f]		86	23.6	13.4	↓11.5*	↓6.9**	2.2*	↓1.6**	↓6.2***		2
PL		96	24.1	13.9	↓9.5	↓5.6	2.6	↓1.3	↓4.2		5

[a]Last observation was carried forward for patients who withdrew from the study.
[b]Response rates were defined as 40 (Gelenberg *et al.*, 2000) or 50% (Hackett *et al.*, 1999) reductions from baseline in HAM-A total scores or a CGI-I score of 1 or 2 (Gelenberg *et al.*, 2000). Values presented from Gelenberg *et al.* (2000) pertain to weeks 6 through 28 of treatment.
[c]VEN dosage was started at 75 mg per day and increased at days 8 and 15 (to 150 and 225 mg per day, respectively) if required.
[d]The results of this study have not been published in full, but are available in a poster (Hackett *et al.*, 1999).
[e]Values estimated from a graph.
[f]VEN dosage was started at 75 mg per day and increased by 75 mg per day per week to the targetted dosage level.
CGI-I = Clinical Global Impression-Global Improvement; **CGI-S** = Clinical Global Impression-Severity of Illness; **HAD** = Hospital Anxiety and Depression Scale (anxiety subscale); **HAM-A** = Hamilton Rating Scale for Anxiety; **PL** = placebo; **pts** = patients; **XR** = extended release; ↓= decrease; * $p \leq 0.05$; ** $p \leq 0.01$; *** $p < 0.001$ vs PL;
† $p \leq 0.017$ vs VEN 37.5 mg per day
Reprinted with permission from Balfour and Jarvis (2000), *CNS Drugs (Adis International)* **15**(6), 494.

with GAD reported that clinical improvement was significant from week 6 for patients on gepirone compared with significant relief from week 1 onwards for patients on diazepam (Rickels *et al.*, 1997). A 5-week, placebo-controlled, dose-finding efficacy study in 267 patients with GAD has also suggested that ipsapirone represents a viable treatment option for GAD (Cutler, Hesselink and Sramek, 1994).

In a recent study weak anxiolytic effects were observed of the 5-HT_{1A} receptor agonist lesopitron in a double-blind placebo-controlled study vs lorazepam (Sramek *et al.*, 1996; Fresquet *et al.*, 2000). These findings need replication in larger trials.

In terms of long-term therapy, buspirone has been demonstrated to be effective as maintenance therapy: a 12-month, open study in 700 patients with GAD reported a significant reduction in anxiety in patients treated with buspirone (Feighner, 1987).

5-HT Antagonists

Early evidence with the 5-$HT_{2A/2C}$ receptor antagonist ritanserin indicated that it may be an effective anxiolytic agent: 24 patients with GAD treated for 6 weeks with ritanserin or lorazepam showed comparable improvements in symptoms (Bressa, Marini and Gregori, 1987). The efficacy of nefazodone was studied in an 8-week open trial in 21 patients with GAD. Fifteen of the patients completed the study, and of these 80% were rated as 'much' or 'very much' improved as measured by the CGI scale (Hedges *et al.*, 1996). Although promising, these results have not yet been substantiated in placebo-controlled, double-blind trials. Similarly, controlled data with the 5-HT_3 antagonist ondansetron are not yet available.

Conclusion

The 5-HT_{1A} agonists are the most studied of the serotonergic drugs in the treatment of GAD. It is questionable whether newly developed 5-HT1A receptor agonists like lepisetron will be able to conquer a niche in the treatment of GAD in view of the fact that several studies indicate that the efficacy of venlafaxine is better than buspirone. Evidence is also emerging for the efficacy of paroxetine in GAD, but further investigation is warranted for the SSRI drug class. Similarly, only preliminary data are available with the 5-$HT_{2/3}$ receptor antagonists.

SOCIAL ANXIETY DISORDER

Introduction

The majority of individuals will admit to recognizing an element of anticipatory anxiety on specific occasions when they are under public scrutiny, such as prior to giving a speech or playing a musical instrument; this has been called 'normal' social discomfort (Rosenbaum *et al.*, 1994). However, social anxiety disorder is the excessive fear harboured by some people that their performance or social interaction will be viewed as inadequate, to the point of causing them embarrassment or humiliation. These people experience extreme distress in, or will completely avoid, the feared social setting.

Social anxiety disorder is a common mental disorder, yet it is one of the least investigated and most misunderstood (Judd, 1994). Therefore, we will devote more attention in this introduction to diagnostic and epidemiological issues before we discuss the pharmacotherapeutic options. The avoidance of everyday social situations by patients with social anxiety disorder can cause considerable disruption to patients' work, relationships and normal functioning (Schneier *et al.*, 1992; den Boer, 1997; Lépine and Lellouch, 1995). Many patients with social anxiety disorder are single, divorced or separated (Magee *et al.*, 1996). In addition, they may have a lower educational attainment and a lower socioeconomic status; in an epidemiologic study, over 50% of patients with social anxiety disorder did not complete secondary school, more than 70% were in the lowest two quartiles in terms of socioeconomic status, and approximately 22% were receiving welfare payments, suggesting that they were unable to work (Schneier *et al.*, 1992). This level of functional disability imposes an economic burden on society, not only because of sufferers' financial dependency and lack of gainful productivity, but also because of the increased risk of suicide attempts, particularly if there is a comorbid disorder (Schneier *et al.*, 1992). This disabling condition therefore necessitates early recognition and treatment.

Defining and Diagnosing Social Anxiety Disorder

The updated DSM (DSM-IV) (APA, 1994) and the ICD-10 criteria can be used to define social anxiety disorder. Both criteria state that social anxiety disorder is a distinct disorder involving a marked fear or anxiety of behaving in an embarrassing or humiliating manner while under the gaze of other people, which then leads to avoidance of the situations that stimulate this fear (Lépine and Lellouch, 1995; den Boer, 1997). Two distinct subtypes of social anxiety disorder are recognized: non-generalized and generalized. Non-generalized social anxiety disorder involves one or two social or performance situations, such as public speaking, whereas individuals with generalized social anxiety disorder fear a multitude of social and performance situations (Heimberg *et al.*, 1990).

Other conditions from which social anxiety disorder should be distinguished are panic disorder, separation anxiety (in children), and atypical depression, although fear or avoidance of social or performance situations in a public setting should identify the patient with social anxiety disorder. Diagnoses of social anxiety disorder and avoidant personality disorder (APD) have arisen from different historical sources; however, the difference between these conditions has become indistinct with the introduction of the DSM-III-R criteria. Schneier *et al.* (1991) found that most (89%) of the patients with generalized social anxiety disorder were also diagnosed with APD. This co-occurrence of social anxiety disorder and APD may indicate a more severe form of social anxiety disorder (Holt, Heimberg and Hope, 1992).

Management Options

As the need for treatment of social anxiety disorder has been recognized only recently, optimum treatment strategies have not yet been defined. The SSRIs have been recommended as the pharmacologic treatment of choice (Ballenger *et al.*, 1998b) but the role of combined or sequential psychotherapeutic and pharmacologic treatment has still to be clarified (Heimberg, 1993). Drug treatment may relieve the symptoms of social anxiety disorder but habitual patterns of avoidant behaviour may take longer to respond; therefore, a combined strategy may be more effective than either alone (Marshall, 1992).

Pharmacological Approaches

Pharmacological treatment of social anxiety disorder has become established only in the past decade. The most recently investigated drug class is the SSRIs, for which there is growing support (Jefferson, 1995; van Ameringen, Mancini and Oakman, 1999a). Other explored drug classes include tricyclic antidepressants, monoamine oxidase inhibitors (MAOIs), benzodiazepines, and β-blockers (Davidson, 1998).

Table XIX-13.3 Summary of studies of SSRIs in patients with social anxiety disorder

Drug	Type of study	No. Patients	Outcome	Reference
Paroxetine	12 week, double-blind, placebo-controlled study	384	Relative to baseline, paroxetine produced significantly greater improvements than placebo in endpoint Leibowitz Social Anxiety Scale (LSAS) total scores ($p < 0.001$) for the 20 mg dose with similar degrees of improvement exhibited by the 40 mg and 60 mg doses. The proportion of responders CGI-I (score 1 or 2) was higher for paroxetine (20 mg 45%, 40 mg 47%, 60 mg 43%) than placebo (28%) with a statistically significant difference at the 40 mg dose.	Baldwin, 2000
Paroxetine	12-week, double-blind, placebo-controlled study	187	Relative to baseline, paroxetine produced significantly greater improvements than placebo in endpoint Liebowitz Social Anxiety Scale (LSAS) total scores ($p < 0.001$), subscale scores ($p < 0.001$), Social and Anxiety Distress Scale scores (SADS; $p < 0.001$) and Sheehan Disability Inventory social and work item scores (SDI; $p < 0.001$ and $p < 0.05$, respectively). The proportion of responders with paroxetine (55%) was significantly higher than with placebo (24%; $p < 0.001$) based on a CGI global improvement score of 1 or 2.	Stein *et al.*, 1998
	12-week, double-blind, placebo-controlled study	290	Patients receiving paroxetine experienced a significantly greater reduction in LSAS total score compared with placebo ($p \leq 0.001$). The proportion of responders (based on a CGI global improvement score of 1 or 2) in the paroxetine group was significantly greater than in the placebo group (65.7% vs 32.4%; $p < 0.001$). Paroxetine also produced significant improvements in social avoidance (as measured by the SADS) ($p < 0.032$) and in patients' family ($p < 0.001$), social ($p < 0.05$), and work ($p < 0.001$) lives (as measured by the SDI) compared with placebo.	Baldwin *et al.*, 1999
	Randomized, double-blind, placebo-controlled, 12-week trial	99	At week 12, 70.5% of paroxetine-treated patients and 8.3% of placebo-treated patients were responders ($p = 0.0001$). Paroxetine produced significantly greater improvements than placebo in endpoint LSAS total scores ($p = 0.0001$). Paroxetine was also significantly superior to placebo in terms of improvements in Brief Social Phobia Scale ($p = 0.0001$), Fear of Negative Evaluation Scale ($p = 0.0003$), and SDI work ($p = 0.0065$), social ($p = 0.0048$), and family life ($p = 0.0092$) scores.	Allgulander, 1999
	11-week, open study	36	23/30 patients (77%) were 'much' or 'very much' improved on the Clinical Global Impression scale. Baseline/Week 11 reductions on the Duke Social Phobia Scale and Liebowitz Social Phobia Scale were 36/20 ($p < 0.0005$) and 75/37 ($p < 0.0005$), respectively.	Stein *et al.*, 1996
	12-week, open study	18	Paroxetine produced an 83% response assessed by a moderate-to-marked symptomatic improvement on the Liebowitz Panic and Social Phobia disorders rating Scale.	Mancini and Ameringen, 1996
	12 week single-blind; 24 week double-blind	437	A significantly greater proportion of patients in the paroxetine group were 'much improved' or 'very much improved' (as assessed with the CGI) at the end of the study, and that significantly fewer patients relapsed with paroxetine (14%) compared to placebo (39%, $p < 0.001$) during the 24-week follow-up.	Hair *et al.*, 2000; Stein *et al.*, 2001
Sertraline	6-week, open study	24	After 4 and 6 weeks, sertraline produced significant improvements compared with baseline ($p < 0.05$) on the Davidson Brief Social Phobia Rating Scale and Clinical Global Impression Severity and Change scales. 58% responded to treatment.	Martins *et al.*, 1994
	12-week, open study	22	16/20 responded to treatment. All measures of social anxiety and functioning and depression significantly improved compared with baseline.	van Ameringen *et al.*, 1994
	20-week, randomized, double-blind, crossover study	12	Scores on the Liebowitz Social Anxiety Scale significantly improved with sertraline ($p = 0.001$) but not with placebo. 6/12 moderately or markedly improved while taking sertraline compared with 1/12 while taking placebo.	Katzelnick *et al.*, 1995
	12-week, open study	11	5/7 completers substantially responded to treatment.	Munjack *et al.*, 1994/95
Citalopram	12-week, open study	22	19 out of 22 were responders to treatment.	Bouwer and Stein, 1998

Table XIX-13.3 *(continued)*

Drug	Type of study	No. Patients	Outcome	Reference
Fluoxetine	12-week, open study	13	10 patients had a moderate-to-marked improvement independent of changes on the Beck Depression Inventory.	van Ameringen *et al.*, 1993
	6–40 weeks, open study	14	10 patients moderately or markedly improved.	Black *et al.*, 1992
	12 week, open study	20	13 out of 20 patients were responders.	Perugi *et al.*, 1995
Fluvoxamine	12-week, double-blind, placebo-controlled study with 12-week follow-up	30	Fluvoxamine significantly better than placebo on Symptom Checklist 90 ($p < 0.05$) and superior to placebo on social anxiety item of Social Phobia Scale. Further improvements observed during follow-up period.	van Vliet *et al.*, 1994
	Double-blind, randomized, placebo-controlled, 12-week trial	92	At week 12, 53.3% of the fluvoxamine group and 23.5% of the placebo group were responders ($p = 0.01$). Compared with placebo, fluvoxamine produced significantly greater improvements on the BSPS ($p < 0.05$), the Social Phobia Inventory (SPIN; $p < 0.05$), LSAS ($p < 0.05$), and the work and family life items of the SDI ($p < 0.05$).	Stein *et al.*, 1999

Serotonin-Selective Reuptake Inhibitors

Four large, double-blind, placebo-controlled 12-week trials and one long-term relapse prevention study have recently reported a significant improvement of patients with social anxiety disorder prescribed paroxetine compared with those given placebo (Allugander, 1999; Baldwin *et al.*, 1999; Stein *et al.*, 1999; Baldwin, 2000; Stein *et al.*, 2001). Two double-blind placebo-controlled trials of fluvoxamine have also demonstrated the efficacy of this SSRI against the symptoms of social anxiety disorder (Stein *et al.*, 1999; DeVane *et al.*, 1999). Data for other SSRIs are limited to mainly open and small scale trials. The results of open and double-blind studies using SSRIs to treat patients with social anxiety disorder are shown in Table XIX-13.3.

SSRIs also provide effective and well tolerated treatment for depression and panic disorder, both of which may be comorbid with social anxiety disorder. In a recent meta-analysis conducted along the methods set forth by the Cochrane Collaboration, van der Linden and co-workers (2000) concluded that SSRIs as a group were effective for the treatment of social phobia. In addition, SSRIs had a larger response-rate and effect-size compared to the reversible monoamine oxidase inhibitors. There is a paucity of data on the long-term pharmacotherapy of SAD. In order to study the effectiveness of long-term paroxetine treatment in the prevention of relapse in patients with SAD, Stein and co-workers (2001) studied 437 patients in a placebo-controlled, multicentre study. The study comprised a 12 week single-blind treatment phase (paroxetine 20–50 mg) with responders ($n = 323$) being randomized to double-blind treatment with paroxetine or placebo for a further 24 weeks. Stein and co-workers found that a significantly greater proportion of patients in the paroxetine group were 'much improved' or 'very much improved' (as assessed with the CGI) at the end of the study, and that significantly fewer patients relapsed with paroxetine (14%) compared to placebo (39%, $p < 0.001$) during the 24-week follow-up. This study lends support to the widely held belief that patients should at least be treated for a period of one year.

One study has recently been published on the efficacy of sertraline in SAD. In this study 204 patients suffering from SAD were randomly allocated to treatment with either placebo or sertraline (50–200 mg per day; van Ameringen *et al.*, 2001). As assessed with the social phobia subscale of the Marks Fear Questionnaire, 32.6% of the patients using sertraline and 10.8% using placebo were considered responders. The mean reductions of the score on the Brief Social Phobia Scale yielded statistical superiority of sertraline over placebo (34.3% and 18.6% respectively), indicating that also sertraline is an effective treatment for SAD.

There is hardly any information about the efficacy of dual action antidepressants in social phobia. In a 12-week open-label study in which the effects of mirtazapine were evaluated in 16 patients van Vliet and co-workers (2000) found significant reductions in social anxiety and avoidance. Further placebo-controlled studies are necessary to confirm these preliminary findings.

Tricyclic Agents

Studies published more than 20 years ago reported positive results for clomipramine in the treatment of phobic disorders (Beaumont, 1977; Gringras, 1977). However, these were open studies and the patient population was not well defined. A further small study found that clomipramine significantly improved some aspects of social anxiety disorder and agoraphobia compared with diazepam but the patient population was again ill-defined (Allsopp, Cooper and Poole, 1984). A recent small open trial of imipramine did not support its efficacy as a treatment for social anxiety disorder (Simpson *et al.*, 1998).

Monoamine Oxidase Inhibitors

Double-blind, placebo-controlled trials have shown that patients with social anxiety disorder respond better to phenelzine, an irreversible MAOI) than with alprazolam (Gelernter *et al.*, 1991) atenolol (Liebowitz *et al.*, 1992) or placebo (Gelernter *et al.*, 1991; Liebowitz *et al.*, 1992). Earlier studies also suggested that phenelzine was more effective than placebo but these studies suffered from methodologic problems, making interpretation of the results difficult (den Boer, van Vliet and Westenberg, 1995). However, the use of phenelzine is limited due to the potentiation of the tyramine pressor effect, which can lead to hypertensive crises.

Conflicting results have been obtained with reversible MAOIs, such as brofaromine and moclobemide, which do not exhibit the tyramine pressor effect. Brofaromine appeared to significantly improve the symptoms of social anxiety disorder compared with placebo (van Vliet, den Boer and Westenberg, 1992; Lott *et al.*, 1997) but is now no longer in development. Moclobemide also appeared to be statistically significantly more effective than placebo after 8 weeks' treatment in a small double-blind study (Versiani *et al.*, 1992) and a large ($n = 578$), 12-week trial in patients with social anxiety disorder (The International Multicenter Clinical Trial Group on Moclobemide in Social Phobia, 1997). However, a further large ($n = 583$), 12-week, double-blind, placebo-controlled trial in patients with social anxiety disorder failed to find a significant difference between moclobemide and placebo (Noyes *et al.*, 1997).

Benzodiazepines

Clonazepam and alprazolam have been evaluated in a few open studies and found to be effective in social anxiety disorder (Davidson, Tupler and Potts, 1994). Bromazepam was significantly superior to placebo in a 12-week double-blind study (Versiani *et al.*, 1997). In small controlled trials, clonazepam was significantly superior to placebo (Davidson *et al.*, 1993) while alprazolam was also superior to placebo, but inferior to phenelzine (Gelernter *et al.*, 1991). However, the putative efficacy of phenelzine in social anxiety disorder may partly be due to its sedative effect rather than due to true anxiolysis. Furthermore, since alcohol abuse is a common comorbid condition in social anxiety disorder, benzodiazepines should be avoided due to the risk of excessive sedation. Long-term use may also lead to dependency.

Beta-Blockers

Beta-blockers may alleviate anxiety as a secondary consequence of the reduction in autonomic symptoms (tremors, palpitations). These drugs have been effective in the short-term for performance anxiety (Laverdure and Boulenger, 1991; den Boer, van Vliet and Westenberg, 1994; Jefferson, 1996). Despite promising early work with atenolol, subsequent investigations have not established efficacy for β-blockers in generalized social anxiety disorder (den Boer, van Vliet and Westenberg, 1994).

Other Drugs

A recent randomized placebo-controlled trial involving 69 patients demonstrated the efficacy of the anticonvulsant, gabapentin, in the treatment of social anxiety disorder (Pande *et al.*, 1999). After 14 weeks of treatment, patients receiving gabapentin experienced a significant reduction in the symptoms of social anxiety disorder compared with those receiving placebo. In an open trial of nefazodone, 69% of patients ($n = 23$) showed moderate or marked improvement after 12 weeks of treatment (van Ameringen, Mancini and Oakman, 1999b). Venlafaxine has also produced improvements in social anxiety disorder symptoms in a small open study involving 12 patients (Altamura *et al.*, 1999). Larger placebo-controlled trials are required to fully determine the efficacy of these agents.

Non-Pharmacologic Approaches

Cognitive-Behavioural Therapy

Cognitive-behavioural treatment aims to help people to overcome anxiety reactions in social and performance situations and to alter the beliefs and responses that maintain this behaviour.

One type of treatment, cognitive-behavioural group therapy, is given in 12 weekly sessions, each lasting about two and a half hours. It has six elements: cognitive-behavioural explanation of social anxiety disorder; structured exercises to recognize maladaptive thinking; exposure to simulations of situations that provoke anxiety; cognitive restructuring sessions to teach patients to control maladaptive thoughts; homework assignments in preparation for real social situations; and a self-administered cognitive restructuring routine (Heimberg and Juster, 1994).

Cognitive-behavioural group therapy was associated with long-term benefit in moderately impaired patients, and compared well with pharmacologic treatment (phenelzine, alprazolam) (Heimberg, 1993). Group therapy has been shown to be an effective treatment of social anxiety disorder in comparison with control groups or pill placebo (Heimberg and Juster, 1994; Donohue, van Hasselt and Hersen, 1994).

Impact of Comorbidity on Treatment Strategies

Comorbidity may reflect a more severe psychopathology, with more disability and impaired functioning than in the absence of comorbidity. This may create the expectation of a more difficult treatment course and a less favourable outcome, resistance to treatment, the need to treat each disorder effectively, and extended or long-term maintenance treatment to prevent relapse (Rosenbaum and Pollock, 1994).

Empirically, there are four general principles for dealing with comorbid disorders: tailor treatment to individual patients; use monotherapy in preference to polypharmacy, provided that the chosen drug is effective in both disorders and the comorbid disorder is secondary to the social anxiety disorder; consider compatible drugs for some patients; and administer a combination of psychotherapy and pharmacotherapy (Rosenbaum and Pollock, 1994). Social anxiety disorder comorbid with alcoholism is a special case because of the risk of excessive sedation with concomitant medication (benzodiazepines, for example), and patients should be carefully questioned about their use of alcohol, as well as the amount and the pattern of intake (Marshall, 1994). Comorbidity affects the choice of treatment, as well as its efficacy. A treatment scheme for comorbid conditions is outlined in Table XIX-13.4 (Jefferson, 1995).

Table XIX-13.4 Treatment scheme for comorbid conditions

Disorder	Suggested treatment		
Social anxiety disorder and major depression	SSRI or MAOI		
Social anxiety disorder and panic disorder	SSRI, MAOI or benzodiazepine		
	One drug/both disorders	*One drug per disorder*	*Combined approach*
Social anxiety disorder and obsessive–compulsive disorder (OCD)	SSRI or MAOI	Clonazepam for social anxiety disorder, clomipramine for OCD	SSRI, clomipramine or MAOI and behaviour therapy
Social anxiety disorder and alcoholism	—	SSRI for social anxiety disorder, disulfiram for alcohol abuse	SSRI, disulfiram and Alcoholics Anonymous
Social anxiety disorder with *no* comorbidity	—	—	SSRI, MAOI or benzodiazepine (with or without cognitive-behavioural therapy)

Based on Rosenbaum and Pollock, 1994; Jefferson, 1995.

Conclusions

Social anxiety disorder was recognized as a condition separate from other phobias and panic disorders as recently as the 1960s (Marks and Gelder, 1966). Three decades later, there is still much to learn about the causes and treatment of the disorder.

While social anxiety disorder is common in the general population, it is probably under-reported in general practice because, by its very nature, patients are reluctant to seek treatment. The delay in seeking help for social anxiety disorder may lead to the development of other psychiatric disorders such as major depression, and consequently a greater disability and risk of suicide. In addition, the inability of the patient to function as a normal, productive member of the community places an economic burden on the sufferer and on society. Early diagnosis and treatment of social anxiety disorder may help to alleviate the burdens imposed by the condition.

Optimum treatment strategies for social anxiety disorder have not been clearly defined. However, no one would disagree that treatment should be aggressive in view of the potential disability caused by the disorder. SSRIs show the most promise for the treatment of social anxiety disorder.

POST-TRAUMATIC STRESS DISORDER

There is a sparse but expanding literature on treatment options for PTSD. Most studies in PTSD have been performed in combat-related trauma victims and other serious traumas including rape, sexual molestation and assault. Until recently, the role of pharmacotherapy in PTSD was more of an adjunctive therapy to alleviate depressive and other comorbid symptoms. During the last few years, however, several double-blind studies have been performed which studied the effects on core symptoms of PTSD.

There is a great need for better treatments in this disorder as a recent study has shown that in spite of consistent treatment efforts, more than 30% of patients with episodes of PTSD do not recover even after several years (Kessler *et al.*, 1995). It was recommended by the Expert Consensus Panel for PTSD that the first-line treatment should be psychotherapy, whereas in cases complicated by comorbid psychiatric conditions (which is often the case) a combination of psychotherapy and pharmacotherapy is recommended (The Expert Consensus Panel on PTSD, 1999). PTSD is characterized by different groups of symptoms: intrusive thoughts (recurrent flashbacks and nightmares), avoidance behaviour (active avoiding memories of the traumatic events, numbness) and hyperarousal (insomnia, concentration difficulties). These symptoms are rather specific for PTSD, but it should not be overlooked that many patients also report other symptoms not assessed by DSM-IV criteria such as feelings of shame and guilt and ruminations on existential fear (Wenzel *et al.*, 2000).

Together with the high degree of comorbidity there is the issue of symptom subtypes. If the different symptom-complexes are mediated by different underlying neurobiological systems, it is conceivable that they respond to different psychotropic drugs. Considering the limited number of studies in PTSD this question will be difficult to answer. In addition, we still do not know which scales are the most useful in establishing effective pharmacotherapy in PTSD.

Tricyclics and MAO-Inhibitors in PTSD

Older antidepressants like amitryptiline and desipramine have been shown to be only slightly better than placebo (Davidson *et al.*, 1990; Reist *et al.*, 1989). Only depressive symptoms associated with PTSD responded to treatment in these studies.

The irreversible and nonselective MAOI phenelzine was found to be effective in a number of studies. In comparative studies versus imipramine and placebo in male veterans, phenelzine led to significant improvements in intrusive thought and nightmares. Emotional numbing, however, was not affected (Frank *et al.*, 1988; Kosten *et al.*, 1991). Needless to say, the dietary restrictions posed upon patients during treatment with phenelzine are a disadvantage to this type of drug. The newer generation of MAO-A inhibitors, for which dietary restrictions are not necessary, has been scarcely investigated in PTSD. There are some controlled studies with brofaromine in PTSD with mixed results (e.g. Baker *et al.*, 1995), but since brofaromine has not been registered these studies will not be discussed. Moclobemide, another selective and reversible MAO-A inhibitor which has been marketed for depression was investigated in a 12-week open-label study in 20 patients suffering from PTSD (Neal, Shapland and Fox, 1997). Typical PTSD symptoms subsided and symptoms severity was diminished in most of the patients. Double-blind placebo controlled studies have, however, not been performed with moclobemide.

Benzodiazepines

The use of BDZs in PTSD has been described by several authors, but there are hardly any well designed studies. Clonazepam was found to reduce anxiety and depression in an open-label study (Lowenstein *et al.*, 1988). In a 5-week crossover trial, Braun *et al.* (1990) studied the efficacy of alprazolam in a mixed population ($N = 16$) of therapy-resistant combat-related and civilian PTSD patients. Alprazolam dosages were increased up to 6 mg per day. Although a modest anxiolytic effect (measured with the HAM-A) was described, alprazolam failed to improve typical PTSD symptoms.

SSRIs in the Treatment of PTSD

Fluvoxamine has been studied in three small studies in PTSD: two trials were conducted in war veterans and one in civilians; all studies used an open-label design and included only a small number of patients (Marmar *et al.*, 1996; Davidson *et al.*, 1998; de Boer *et al.*, 1992). The results of these studies suggest that fluvoxamine can diminish the severity of specific PTSD symptoms such as survival guilt, nightmares, insomnia, intrusive recollections and fear. Placebo-controlled studies of fluvoxamine in PTSD are warranted to evaluate the potential role of fluvoxamine in PTSD.

Fluoxetine has been more extensively investigated in PTSD. There are both open-label and double-blind placebo-controlled studies evaluating the effects of fluoxetine in PTSD. Here we will confine the discussion to the placebo-controlled studies. Van der Kolk and co-workers (1994) conducted a 5-week placebo-controlled study and found that fluoxetine was significantly more effective in both combat veterans and civilian casualties. They found the typical PTSD symptoms to respond to treatment with fluoxetine: numbing and arousal. Interestingly, the treatment effect was most robust in the civilian group who suffered from acute traumas, indicating that fluoxetine is perhaps less effective in chronic PTSD. In a more recent study Connor *et al.* (1999a) included 54 civilian PTSD patients (most notably females) and found that fluoxetine up to 60 mg per day had beneficial effects on all typical PTSD symptoms. In a reanalysis of the data it was found that fluoxetine has a broad spectrum effect on the symptomatology of PTSD. The symptoms who were found to be most responsive to treatment with fluoxetine were: being physically upset at reminders of the trauma, avoiding thoughts of the trauma, anhedonia, feeling distant and impaired concentration (Meltzer-Brody *et al.*, 2000). A recent small placebo-controlled study also reported improved quality of life as a result of fluoxetine treatment as assessed with the Short-Form Health Survey (SF-36; Malik *et al.*, 1999). In a small placebo-controlled study in severe PTSD male combat veterans fluoxetine could not be distinguished from placebo, indicating that severity or gender could influence treatment outcome (Hertzberg *et al.*, 2000).

Two open-label studies evaluated the effects of sertraline in PTSD and most of the core PTSD symptomatology showed a significant decrease (Brady, Sonne and Roberts, 1995; Rothbaum, Ninan and Thomas, 1996). In a 12-week double-blind placebo-controlled multicentre study Brady *et al.* (2000) studied the efficacy of sertraline (50–200 mg per day) in 187 outpatients suffering from non-combat-related PTSD. On three of the main efficacy parameters (Clinician Administered PTSD-scale; Clinical Global Impression Severity and Improvement Scales), sertraline showed a significantly better treatment effect compared to placebo. Around 53% of the patients were considered responders to treatment with sertraline and 32% responded to placebo. Significant efficacy was evident for sertraline on symptoms of avoidance/numbing, increased arousal, but not on re-experiencing traumatic events. Davidson and co-workers (2001) included 208 outpatients suffering from PTSD in a double-blind placebo controlled study. Although their study was not powered enough to evaluate clinical variables such as sex, type of trauma, duration of illness, or presence of comorbidity on treatment response, they reported a 60% response-rate for sertraline and a 38% response rate for placebo.

It has been argued that repeatedly responding to PTSD-related questions can possibly evoke an element of exposure and desensitization (Krakow, Hollifield and Warner, 2000). Thus, since there was a considerable placebo response in this study, this might have been achieved by covert cognitive-behavioural therapy. If this were true, then this reasoning should also apply to other syndromes for which CBT is an effective treatment (e.g. PD, OCD) and since many placebo-controlled studies have been performed yielding significant differences between active treatment and placebo it is almost impossible to disentangle the relative contribution of 'covert' CBT to the treatment. Nevertheless, in PTSD there is a need for studies exploring the interface between pharmacotherapy and psychotherapy.

Paroxetine was found to be effective in a small open-label study in chronic non-combat-related PTSD (Marshall *et al.*, 1998). All typical symptom clusters were improved and there were also beneficial effects of paroxetine on anxiety and depression-scores. Very recently, a number of placebo-controlled studies has been conducted with paroxetine in PTSD. Ruggiero and associates (2001) included 307 patients suffering form PTSD according to DSM-IV criteria in a flexible-dose study. As primary efficacy parameters they used the clinician administered PTSD scale (CAPS-2) and the Clinical Global Impression Scale. Their study showed that paroxetine in a dosage of 20–50 mg was more efficacious than placebo in reducing the symptom clusters of the CAPS-2 and in improving psychosocial functioning. In a 12-week double-blind fixed dose study in 550 outpatients with PTSD, Beebe and co-workers (2000) found paroxetine (20 and 40 mg) to be effective in reducing PTSD symptoms in all symptom domains including re-experiencing, avoidance, intrusion and hyperarousal. A further 12 week double-blind flexible-dose (20–50 mg per day) in 322 outpatients with PTSD showed similar efficacy (unpublished data). Interestingly, when PTSD patients were exposed to individual trauma scripts, another group found autonomic functioning (heart rate and blood-pressure) to be improved after treatment with paroxetine in a 10-week open-label study (Tucker *et al.*, 2000), indicating that a wide range of PTSD symptoms are affected by paroxetine.

In view of the repeatedly reported finding that PTSD patients often suffer from comorbid depression, Stein *et al.* (2001) pooled the data of the three mentioned double-blind placebo-controlled studies described here and found that both the depressed and the non-depressed subgroups showed a statistically significant improvement in the CAPS-total score and the CGI for paroxetine compared to placebo.

Dual Action Antidepressants in PTSD

There is only one small open-label study in which mirtazapine has been studied in PTSD. Six outpatients with chronic PTSD were treated with mirtazapine and three of them were responders (Connor *et al.*, 1999b). Due to the small sample any conclusion would be premature. One case study reported therapeutic effects of venlafaxine in a PTSD patient who did not respond to various serotonergic antidepressants (Hamner and Frueh, 1998).

Serotonin Receptor Antagonists in PTSD

There are a number of open studies in which therapeutic effects of trazodone and nefazodone in PTSD has been investigated. Trazodone was found to be effective in just one open-label study in six combat-related PTSD patients (Hertzberg *et al.*, 1996), but there are no published controlled studies of this compound. The therapeutic potential of nefazodone, an antidepressant which blocks 5-HT$_2$ receptors and 5-HT reuptake was studied in the beginning of the 1990s in six open-label studies (data pooled and reviewed by Hidalgo *et al.*, 1999). Both civilians and combat veterans were included in these studies, and results indicate beneficial effects on a broad range of typical PTSD symptoms. In chronic therapy-resistant Vietnam veterans, nefazone showed therapeutic effects in depression-scores and typical PTSD symptoms like intrusive recollection, avoidance and hyperarousal in an open-label study (Zisook *et al.*, 2000). Many patients with chronic combat-related PTSD also suffer from comorbid depression. Available evidence indicates that antidepressants affecting 5-HT reuptake are associated with a better outcome compared to compounds predominantly affecting noradrenalin reuptake (Dow and Kline, 1997).

A Role for Atypical Antipsychotics or Antiepileptics in PTSD?

In some cases of severe emotional turmoil in PTSD dopamine blockers can be prescribed and there are case reports indicating beneficial effects of atypical antipsychotics. Leyba and Wampler (1998) report therapeutic effects on nightmares and flashbacks in four cases of PTSD, and another case report describes the use of risperidone in the treatment of intrusive thoughts and subsequent emotional reactivity in combat-related PTSD (Krashin and Oates, 1999). Also in acute stress disorder after physical trauma, preliminary evidence indicates beneficial effects of risperidone on flashbacks (Eidelman, Seedat and Stein, 2000).

In view of the fact that symptoms of PTSD may point to sympathetic hyperarousal and hyperreactivity, it has been suggested that stress-induced limbic kindling could play a role. Consistent with this view is the reported efficacy in PTSD of carbamazepine and valproate. There are only a few open-label studies but all of them support the therapeutic efficacy of carbamazepine and valproate in this condition (Lipper, 1988; Wolf, Alavi and Mosnaim, 1988; Fesler, 1991; Looff *et al.*, 1995). More recently, Clark and co-workers (1999) studied divalproex in 16 combat-related PTSD patients and found reduced intrusion and diminished hyperarousal. Interestingly they also reported significant decreases in depression and anxiety.

Future Directions in the Treatment of PTSD

Based upon the studies described above there is evidence that rarely does a single medication benefit all symptom clusters equally or produce complete remission of the syndrome. Therefore it appears reasonable to further study the role of specific classes of drugs for particular symptom clusters.

As mentioned before, there is also a need for combination studies using pharmacotherapy and psychotherapy. A number of studies have shown that applying CBT and other psychotherapeutic techniques can reduce core PTSD symptoms in both acute stress disorder and PTSD (Bryant *et al.*, 1998; Devilly and Spence, 1999; Hembree and Foa, 2000). These additional therapeutic strategies probably have additive or synergistic effects on ongoing pharmacotherapy as they focus on the processing of traumatic events, emotional engagement of the traumatic memory, the organization of the trauma narrative and correction of dysfunctional cognitions that often follow traumatic experiences. Therefore, studies combining pharmacotherapy and CBT are clearly needed.

In depression, several studies have suggested potential therapeutic effects of augmentation strategies. The number of augmentation studies in PTSD is limited. One study suggested modest effects of clonidine augmentation to imipramine (Kinzie and Leung, 1989), another open-label study suggested additive effects of buspirone augmentation to SSRIs (and other antidepressants) in combat-related chronic PTSD (Hamner, Ulmer and Horne, 1997). In order to evaluate the therapeutic potential of these augmentation strategies, placebo-controlled studies are warranted.

There is a growing body of literature indicating that there exist dysfunctions in the regulation of the hypothalamic-pituitary axis (HPA) in PTSD (Baker *et al.*, 1999). Dysregulation of CRH is regarded the key component of the human stress response. Based upon a growing body of neurobiological studies it has been shown that other key components of the stress response include changes in the adrenergic system, serotonergic system, neuropeptide Y, opioid system and glutamatergic system. In addition, kindling/sensitization could play a role in developing PTSD. Based upon these findings it has been suggested that in addition to SSRIs future treatment possibilities for PTSD could include CRH antagonists, neuropeptide Y, β-adrenergic blockers, substance P, drugs that influence NMDA receptors and antiepileptics (Friedman, 2000).

If indeed developments in pharmacotherapy of PTSD and other anxiety disorders would be based upon the pathophysiology of the disorder this could lead to a more rational drug design which would greatly influence clinical practice and contribute to the well-being of our patients.

EPILOGUE

Serotonergic drugs have been developed and extensively investigated during the last decade in a range of depressive and anxiety disorders. As a result, a clinical database has been formed which allows us to view, and compare, their efficacy.

Of the serotonergic agents examined in this review, the SSRIs stand out with proven efficacy in the treatment of a wide spectrum of disorders including depression, panic disorder, OCD, PTSD and social anxiety disorder. Initial results with paroxetine have indicated that it may also be a suitable treatment for GAD.

The 5-HT_{1A} agonists have been used extensively in the treatment of GAD and depression, but reports of their efficacy in the treatment of panic disorder, OCD and social anxiety disorder have been equivocal, although they may prove useful in these anxiety disorders as augmenting agents for SSRI treatment-refractory patients.

The 5-HT antagonists are the least well-studied of the agents and have not yet been fully investigated in many of the psychiatric disorders discussed in this article. While they may have activity in the treatment of depression, the initial results in the treatment of panic disorder are disappointing. There are insufficient data concerning the 5-HT antagonists in GAD and social anxiety disorder to draw conclusions on their efficacy in these disorders, but preliminary reports have suggested that the drug class may be of use as adjuvants to the SSRIs in treatment refractory patients with OCD.

Large scale epidemiological studies such as the National Comorbidity Survey have clearly demonstrated that the rate of comorbidity between depression and anxiety disorders is high. Therefore, pharmacotherapy which is effective against a broad range of depressive and anxiety disorders could be of considerable utility to clinicians. The activity profile of the SSRIs in the treatment of depression and anxiety make this class of drug an attractive option for initial monotherapy in these disorders.

It should be stressed, that despite their attractive therapeutic profile, SSRIs have unwanted side effects and that response rates in clinical studies vary between 50% (e.g. OCD) and 70% (e.g. major depression and PD). Future research should focus on much overlooked items, such as pharmacokinetics, sex and ethnic differences and response prediction. Moreover, a sensible combination of clinical and preclinical research into the biological mechanisms is likely to provide information to further enhance (augment) pharmacotherapy of anxiety and depressive disorders.

REFERENCES

Adler, C.M., Craske, M.G., Kirshenbaum, S. and Barlow, D.H., 1989. 'Fear of panic': an investigation of its role in panic occurrence, phobic avoidance, and treatment outcome. *Behavior Research and Therapy*, **27**, 391–396.

Allgulander, C., 1999. Paroxetine in social anxiety disorder: a randomized placebo-controlled study. *Acta Psychiatrica Scandinavica*, **100**, 193–198.

Allsopp, L.F., Cooper, G.L. and Poole, P.H., 1984. Clomipramine and diazepam in the treatment of agoraphobia and social phobia in general practice. *Current Medical Research and Opinion*, **9**, 64–70.

Altamura, A.C., Pioli, R., Vitto, M. and Mannu, P., 1999. Venlafaxine in social phobia: a study in selective serotonin reuptake inhibitor non-responders. *International Clinical Psychopharmacology*, **14**, 239–245.

American Psychiatric Association, 1994. *Diagnostic and Statistical Manual of Mental Disorders*. American Psychiatric Association, Washington DC.

Artigas, F., 1993. 5-HT and antidepressants: new views from microdialysis studies. *Trends in Pharmacology Sciences*, **14**, 262.

Artigas, F., Perez, V. and Alvarez, E., 1994. Pindolol induces a rapid improvement of depressed patients treated with serotonin reuptake inhibitors. *Archives of General Psychiatry*, **51**, 248–251.

Assault survivors with PTSD: a preliminary report. *Journal of Traumatic Stress*, **13**, 589–609.

Bach, M., Aigner, M. and Lenz, G., 1997. Ritanserin as adjunct to fluoxetine treatment of OCD patients with psychotic features. *Pharmacopsychiatry*, **30**, 28–29.

Baer, L., Rauch, S.L., Ballantine, H.T., Martuza, R., Cosgrove, R., Cassem, E., Girinunas, I., Manzo, P.A., Dimino, C. and Jenike, M.A., 1995. Cingulotomy for intractable obsessive compulsive disorder. Prospective long-term follow-up of 18 patients. *Archives of General Psychiatry*, **52**(2), 384–392.

Baker, D.G., Diamond, B.I., Gillette, G., Hamner, M., Katzelnick, D., Keller, T., Mellman, T.A., Pontius, E., Rosenthal, M. and Tucker, P., 1995. A double-blind, randomized, placebo-controlled, multi-center study of brofaromine in the treatment of post-traumatic stress disorder. *Psychopharmacology (Berlin)*, **122**, 386–389.

Baker, D.G., West, S.A., Nicholson, W.E., Ekhator, N.N., Kasckow, J.W., Hill, K.K., Bruce, A.B., Orth, D.N. and Geracioti, T.D., 1999. Serial CSF corticotropin-releasing hormone levels and adrenocortical activity in combat veterans with posttraumatic stress disorder. *American Journal of Psychiatry*, **156**, 585–588.

Bakker, A., van Dyck, R., Spinhoven, P. and van Balkom, A.J., 1999. Paroxetine, clomipramine, and cognitive therapy in the treatment of panic disorder. *Journal of Clinical Psychiatry*, **60**, 831–838.

Baldwin, D., Bobes, J., Stein, D.J., Scharwachter, I. and Faure, M., 1999. Paroxetine in social phobia/social anxiety disorder. Randomised, double-blind, placebo-controlled study. Paroxetine Study Group. *British Journal of Psychiatry*, **175**, 120–126.

Baldwin, D.S., 2000. Clinical experience with paroxetine in social anxiety disorder. *International Clinical Psychopharmacology*, **15**, S19–S24.

Ballenger, J.C., Burrows, G.D., DuPont, R.L., Lesser, I.M., Noyes, R., Pecknold, J.C., Rifkin, A. and Swinson, R.P., 1988. Alprazolam in panic disorder and agoraphobia: results from a multicenter trial. I. Efficacy in short-term treatment. *Archives of General Psychiatry*, **45**, 413–422.

Ballenger, J.C., Davidson, J.R., Lecrubier, Y., Nutt, D.J., Bobes, J., Beidel, D.C., Ono, Y. and Westenberg, H.G.M., 1998b. Consensus statement on social anxiety disorder from the International Consensus Group on Depression and Anxiety. *Journal of Clinical Psychiatry*, **59**, 54–60.

Ballenger, J.C., Wheadon, D.E., Steiner, M., Bushnell, W. and Gergel, I.P., 1998a. Double-blind, fixed-dose, placebo-controlled study of paroxetine in the treatment of panic disorder. *American Journal of Psychiatry*, **155**, 36–42.

Barlow, D.H., Gorman, J.M., Shear, M.K. and Woods, S.W., 2000. Cognitive-behavioral therapy, imipramine, or their combination for panic disorder: A randomized controlled trial. *Journal of the American Medical Association*, **283**, 2529–2536.

Barman Balfourand, J.A. and Jarvis, B., 2001. Venlafaxine extended-release. A review of its clinical potential in the management of generalised anxiety disorder. *CNS Drugs*, **14**, 483–503.

Beaumont, G., 1977. A large open multicentre trial of clomipramine (Anafranil) in the management of phobic disorders. *Journal of Internal Medical Research*, **5**, 116–123.

Beebe, K.L., Pitts, C.D., Fuggerio, L., Ramming, S.R., Oldham, M. and Zaninelli, R., 2000. Paroxetine in the treatment of PTSD: a 12-week, placebo-controlled, multicenter study. Abstract presented at the 16th international Society for Traumatic Stress Studies, San Antonio, TX.

Bellew, K.M., McCafferty, J.P. and Zaninelli, R., 2000a. Paroxetine improves quality of life in patients with generalized anxiety disorder. Presented as an abstract at the CINP, Brussels.

Bellew, K.M., McCafferty, J.P., Iyengar, M. and Zaninelli, R., 2000b. Paroxetine for the treatment of generalized anxiety disorder: a double blind placebo controlled trial. Presented as an abstract at the APA, Chicago.

Bennett, J.A., Moioffer, M., Stanton, S.P., Dwight, M. and Keck, P.E., 1998. A risk-benefit assessment of pharmacological treatments for panic disorder. *Drug Safety*, **18**, 419–430.

Bisserbe, J.-C., Lane, R.M., Flament, M.F. and the Franco-Belgian OCD Study Group, 1997. A double-blind comparison of sertraline and clomipramine in outpatients with obsessive-compulsive disorder. *European Psychiatry*, **12**, 82–93.

Black, B., Uhde, T.W. and Tancer, M.E., 1992. Fluoxetine for the treatment of social phobia. *Journal of Clinical Psychopharmacology*, **12**, 293–295.

Blier, P. and Bergeron, R., 1995. Effectiveness of pindolol with selected antidepressant drugs in the treatment of major depression. *Journal of Clinical Psychopharmacology*, **15**, 217–222.

Blier, P., de Montigny, C. and Chaput, Y., 1987. Modifications of the serotonin system by antidepressant treatments: implications for the therapeutic response in major depression. *Journal of Clinical Psychopharmacology*, **7**, 24S–35S.

Bogetto, F., Bellino, S., Vaschetto, P. and Ziero, S., 2000. Olanzapine augmentation of fluvoxamine-refractory obsessive-compulsive disorder (OCD): a 12-week open trial. *Psychiatry Research*, **96**, 91–98.

Borkovec, T.D. and Roemer, L., 1995. Perceived functions of worry among generalized anxiety disorder subjects: distraction from more emotionally distressing topics? *Journal of Behavior Therapy and Experimental Psychiatry*, **26**, 25–30.

Boshuisen, M.L. and den Boer, J.A., 2000. Zolmitriptan (a 5-HT1B/1D receptor agonist with central action) does not increase symptoms in obsessive compulsive disorder. *Psychopharmacology (Berlin)*, **152**, 74–79.

Boshuisen, M.L., Slaap, B.R., Vester-Blokland, E.D. and den Boer, J.A., 2001. The effect of mirtazapine in panic disorder, an open label pilot study with a single blind placebo run in period, submitted.

Bouvard, M., Mollard, E., Guerin, J. and Cottraux, J., 1997. Study and course of the psychological profile in 77 patients expressing panic disorder with agoraphobia after cognitive behaviour therapy with or without buspirone. *Psychotherapy and Psychosomatics*, **66**, 27–32.

Brady, K., Pearlstein, T., Asnis, G.M., Baker, D., Rothbaum, B., Sikes, C.R. and Farfel, G.M., 2000. Efficacy and safety of sertraline treatment of posttraumatic stress disorder: a randomized controlled trial. *Journal of the American Medical Association*, **283**, 1837–1844.

Brady, K.T., Sonne, S.C. and Roberts, J.M., 1995. Sertraline treatment of comorbid posttraumatic stress disorder and alcohol dependence. *Journal of Clinical Psychiatry*, **56**, 502–505.

Bressa, G.M., Marini, S. and Gregori, S., 1987. Serotonin S2 receptors blockage and generalized anxiety disorders. A double-blind study on ritanserin and lorazepam. *International Journal of Clinical Pharmacology Research*, **7**, 111–119.

Bruce, T.J., Spiegel, D.A. and Hegel, M.T., 1999. Cognitive-behavioral therapy helps prevent relapse and recurrence of panic disorder following alprazolam discontinuation: a long-term follow- up of the Peoria and Dartmouth studies. *Journal of Consulting and Clinical Psychiatry*, **67**, 151–156.

Bryant, R.A., Harvey, A.G., Dang, S.T., Sackville, T. and Basten, C., 1998. Treatment of acute stress disorder: a comparison of cognitive-behavioral therapy and supportive counseling. *Journal of Consulting and Clinical Psychiatry*, **66**, 862–866.

Bystritsky, A., Rosen, R., Suri, R. and Vapnik, T., 1999. Pilot open-label study of nefazodone in panic disorder. *Depression and Anxiety*, **10**, 137–139.

Bystritsky, A., Rosen, R.M., Murphy, K.J., Bohn, P., Keys, S.A. and Vapnik, T., 1994. Double-blind pilot trial of desipramine versus fluoxetine in panic patients. *Anxiety*, **1**, 287–290.

Carpenter, L.L., Leon, Z., Yasmin, S. and Price, L.H., 1999. Clinical experience with mirtazapine in the treatment of panic disorder. *Annals of Clinical Psychiatry*, **11**, 81–86.

Casacalenda, N. and Boulenger, J.P., 1998. Pharmacologic treatments effective in both generalized anxiety disorder and major depressive disorder: clinical and theoretical implications. *Canadian Journal of Psychiatry*, **43**, 722–730.

Chaput, Y., de Montigny, C. and Blier, P., 1991. Presynaptic and postsynaptic modifications of the serotonin system by long-term administration of antidepressant treatments. An *in vivo* electrophysiologic study in the rat. *Neuropsychopharmacology*, **5**, 219–229.

Charney, D.S., Woods, S.W., Goodman, W.K., Rifkin, B., Kinch, M., Aiken, B., Quadrino, L.M. and Heninger, G.R., 1986. Drug treatment of panic disorder: the comparative efficacy of imipramine, alprazolam, and trazodone. *Journal of Clinical Psychiatry*, **47**, 580–586.

Clark, R.D., Canive, J.M., Calais, L.A., Qualls, C.R. and Tuason, V.B., 1999. Divalproex in posttraumatic stress disorder: an open-label clinical trial. *Journal of Traumatic Stress*, **12**, 395–401.

Cohn, J.B., Wilcox, C.S. and Meltzer, H.Y., 1986. Neuroendocrine effects of buspirone in patients with generalized anxiety disorder. *American Journal of Medicine*, **80**, 36–40.

Connor, K.M. and Davidson, J.R., 1998. Generalized anxiety disorder: neurobiological and pharmacotherapeutic perspectives. *Biological Psychiatry*, **44**, 1286–1294.

Connor, K.M., Davidson, J.R., Weisler, R.H. and Ahearn, E., 1999b. A pilot study of mirtazapine in post-traumatic stress disorder. *International Clinical Psychopharmacology*, **14**, 29–31.

Connor, K.M., Sutherland, S.M., Tupler, L.A., Malik, M.L. and Davidson, J.R., 1999a. Fluoxetine in post-traumatic stress disorder. Randomised, double-blind study. *British Journal of Psychiatry*, **175**, 17–22.

Cummings, S., Hay, P., Lee, T. and Sachdev, P., 1995. Neuropsychological outcome from psychosurgery for obsessive compulsive disorder. *Austr N ZJ Psychiatry*, **29**(2), 293–298.

Cutler, N.R., Hesselink, J.M. and Sramek, J.J., 1994. A phase II multicenter dose-finding, efficacy and safety trial of ipsapirone in outpatients with generalized anxiety disorder. *Progress in Neuropsychopharmacology and Biological Psychiatry*, **18**, 447–463.

Dannon, P.N., Hirschmann, S., Kindler, S., Iancu, T., Dolberg, O.T. and Grunhaus, L.J., 1997. Pindolol augmentation in the treatment of resistant panic disorder: a double-blind placebo-controlled trial. *P 3 013, Vienna, ENCP*.

Dannon, P.N., Iancu, I. and Grunhaus, L., 2001. Efficacy of reboxetine in the treatment of SSRI-resistant panic disorder. Presented at the APA meeting, Washington DC.

Dannon, P.N., Sasson, Y., Hirschmann, S., Iancu, I., Grunhaus, L.J. and Zohar, J., 2000. Pindolol augmentation in treatment-resistant obsessive compulsive disorder: a double-blind placebo controlled trial. *European Neuropsychopharmacology*, **10**, 165–169.

Davidson, J., Kudler, H., Smith, R., Mahorney, S.L., Lipper, S., Hammett, E., Saunders, W.B. and Cavenar, J.O., 1990. Treatment of posttraumatic stress disorder with amitriptyline and placebo. *Archives of General Psychiatry*, **47**, 259–266.

Davidson, J.R., 1998. Pharmacotherapy of social anxiety disorder. *Journal of Clinical Psychiatry*, **59**, 47–53.

Davidson, J.R., DuPont, R.L., Hedges, D. and Haskins, J.T., 1999. Efficacy, safety, and tolerability of venlafaxine extended release and buspirone in outpatients with generalized anxiety disorder. *Journal of Clinical Psychiatry*, **60**, 528–535.

Davidson, J.R., Potts, N., Richichi, E., Krishnan, R., Ford, S.M., Smith, R. and Wilson, W.H., 1993. Treatment of social phobia with clonazepam and placebo. *Journal of Clinical Psychopharmacology*, **13**, 423–428.

Davidson, J.R., Tupler, L.A. and Potts, N.L., 1994. Treatment of social phobia with benzodiazepines. *Journal of Clinical Psychiatry*, **55**, 28–32.

Davidson, J.R., Rothbaum, B.O., van der Kolk, B.A., Sikes, C.R. and Farfel, G.M., 2001. Multicentre double blind comparison of sertraline and placebo in the treatment of posttraumatic stress disorder. *Archives of General Psychiatry*, **58**, 485–492.

Davidson, J.R., Weisler, R.H., Malik, M. and Tupler, L.A., 1998. Fluvoxamine in civilians with posttraumatic stress disorder. *Journal of Clinical Psychopharmacology*, **18**, 93–95.

de Beurs, E., van Balkom, A.J., Lange, A., Koele, P. and van Dyck, R., 1995. Treatment of panic disorder with agoraphobia: comparison of fluvoxamine, placebo, and psychological panic management combined with exposure and of exposure *in vivo* alone. *American Journal of Psychiatry*, **152**, 683–691.

de Beurs, E., van Balkom, A.J., van Dyck, R. and Lange, A., 1999. Long-term outcome of pharmacological and psychological treatment for panic disorder with agoraphobia: a 2-year naturalistic follow-up. *Acta Psychiatrica Scandinavica*, **99**, 59–67.

de Boer, M., Op, D.V., Falger, P.J., Hovens, J.E., De Groen, J.H. and van Duijn, H., 1992. Fluvoxamine treatment for chronic PTSD: a pilot study. *Psychotherapy and Psychosomatics*, **57**, 158–163.

DeMartinis, N., Rynn, M., Rickels, K. and Mandos, L., 2000. Prior benzodiazepine use and buspirone response in the treatment of generalized anxiety disorder. *Journal of Clinical Psychiatry*, **61**, 91–94.

DeMartinis, N.A., Schweizer, E. and Rickels, K., 1996. An open-label trial of nefazodone in high comorbidity panic disorder. *Journal of Clinical Psychiatry*, **57**, 245–248.

den Boer, J.A., 1997. Social phobia: epidemiology, recognition, and treatment. *British Medical Journal*, **315**, 796–800.

den Boer, J.A. and Westenberg, H.G.M., 1988. Effect of a serotonin and noradrenaline uptake inhibitor in panic disorder; a double-blind comparative study with fluvoxamine and maprotiline. *International Clinical Psychopharmacology*, **3**, 59–74.

den Boer, J.A. and Westenberg, H.G.M., 1990. Serotonin function in panic disorder: a double blind placebo controlled study with fluvoxamine and ritanserin. *Psychopharmacology (Berlin)*, **102**, 85–94.

den Boer, J.A., Bosker, F.J. and Slaap, B.R., 2000. Serotonergic drugs in the treatment of depressive and anxiety disorders. *Human Psychopharmacology*, **15**, 315–336.

den Boer, J.A., van Vliet, I.M. and Westenberg, H.G.M., 1994. Recent advances in the psychopharmacology of social phobia. *Progress in Neuropsychopharmacology and Biological Psychiatry*, **18**, 625–645.

den Boer, J.A., van Vliet, I.M. and Westenberg, H.G.M., 1995. Recent developments in the psychopharmacology of social phobia. *European Archives of Psychiatry and Clinical Neuroscience*, **244**, 309–316.

den Boer, J.A., Westenberg, H.G.M., Kamerbeek, W.D., Verhoeven, W.M. and Kahn, R.S., 1987. Effect of serotonin uptake inhibitors in anxiety disorders; a double- blind comparison of clomipramine and fluvoxamine. *International Clinical Psychopharmacology*, **2**, 21–32.

DeVane, C.L., Ware, M.R., Emmanuel, N.P., Brawman-Mintzer, O., Morton, W.A., Villarreal, G. and Lydiard, R.B., 1999. Evaluation of the efficacy, safety and physiological effects of fluvoxamine in social phobia. *International Clinical Psychopharmacology*, **14**, 345–351.

Devilly, G.J. and Spence, S.H., 1999. The relative efficacy and treatment distress of EMDR and a cognitive-behavior trauma treatment protocol in the amelioration of posttraumatic stress disorder. *Journal of Anxiety Disorders*, **13**, 131–157.

Donohue, B.C., van Hasselt, V.B. and Hersen, M., 1994. Behavioral assessment and treatment of social phobia. An evaluative review. *Behavior Modification*, **18**, 262–288.

Dow, B. and Kline, N., 1997. Antidepressant treatment of posttraumatic stress disorder and major depression in veterans. *Annals of Clinical Psychiatry*, **9**, 1–5.

Eidelman, I., Seedat, S. and Stein, D.J., 2000. Risperidone in the treatment of acute stress disorder in physically traumatized in-patients. *Depression and Anxiety*, **11**, 187–188.

Enkelmann, R., 1991. Alprazolam versus buspirone in the treatment of outpatients with generalized anxiety disorder. *Psychopharmacology (Berlin)*, **105**, 428–432.

Feighner, J.P., 1987. Buspirone in the long-term treatment of generalized anxiety disorder. *Journal of Clinical Psychiatry*, **48**, 3–6.

Feighner, J.P., Merideth, C.H. and Hendrickson, G.A., 1982. A double-blind comparison of buspirone and diazepam in outpatients with generalized anxiety disorder. *Journal of Clinical Psychiatry*, **43**, 103–108.

Fernandez, C.E. and Lopez-Ibor, J.J., 1967. Monochlorimipramine in the treatment of psychiatric patients resistant to other therapies. *Actas Luso Esp Neurol Psiquitar Cienc Afines*, **26**, 119–147.

Fesler, F.A., 1991. Valproate in combat-related posttraumatic stress disorder. *Journal of Clinical Psychiatry*, **52**, 361–364.

Figgitt, D.P. and McClellan, K.J., 2000. Fluvoxamine. An updated review of its use in the management of adults with anxiety disorders. *Drugs*, **60**, 925–954.

Frank, J.B., Kosten, T.R., Giller, E.L. and Dan, E., 1988. A randomized clinical trial of phenelzine and imipramine for posttraumatic stress disorder. *American Journal of Psychiatry*, **145**, 1289–1291.

Freeman, C.P., Trimble, M.R., Deakin, J.F., Stokes, T.M. and Ashford, J.J., 1994. Fluvoxamine versus clomipramine in the treatment of obsessive compulsive disorder: a multicenter, randomized, double-blind, parallel group comparison. *Journal of Clinical Psychiatry*, **55**, 301–305.

Fresquet, A., Sust, M., Lloret, A., Murphy, M.F., Carter, F.J., Campbell, G.M. and Marion-Landais, G., 2000. Efficacy and safety of lesopitron in outpatients with generalized anxiety disorder. *Annals of Pharmacotherapy*, **34**, 147–153.

Friedman, M.J., 2000. What might the psychobiology of posttraumatic stress disorder teach us about future approaches to pharmacotherapy? *Journal of Clinical Psychiatry*, **61**, 44–51.

Gammans, R.E., Stringfellow, J.C., Hvizdos, A.J., Seidehamel, R.J., Cohn, J.B., Wilcox, C.S., Fabre, L.F., Pecknold, J.C., Smith, W.T. and Rickels, K., 1992. Use of buspirone in patients with generalized anxiety disorder and coexisting depressive symptoms. A meta-analysis of eight randomized, controlled studies. *Neuropsychobiology*, **25**, 193–201.

Gelenberg, A.J., Lydiard, R.B., Rudolph, R.L., Aguiar, L., Haskins, J.T. and Salinas, E., 2000. Efficacy of venlafaxine extended-release capsules in nondepressed outpatients with generalized anxiety disorder: A 6-month randomized controlled trial. *Journal of the American Medical Association*, **283**, 3082–3088.

Gelernter, C.S., Uhde, T.W., Cimbolic, P., Arnkoff, D.B., Vittone, B.J., Tancer, M.E. and Bartko, J.J., 1991. Cognitive-behavioral and pharmacological treatments of social phobia. A controlled study. *Archives of General Psychiatry*, **48**, 938–945.

Geracioti, T.D., Jr., 1995. Venlafaxine treatment of panic disorder: a case series. *Journal of Clinical Psychiatry*, **56**, 408–410.

Goldberg, H.L. and Finnerty, R., 1982. Comparison of buspirone in two separate studies. *Journal of Clinical Psychiatry*, **43**, 87–91.

Goodman, W.K., Kozak, M.J., Liebowitz, M. and White, K.L., 1996. Treatment of obsessive-compulsive disorder with fluvoxamine: a multicentre, double-blind, placebo-controlled trial. *International Clinical Psychopharmacology*, **11**, 21–29.

Goodman, W.K., Price, L.H., Delgado, P.L., Palumbo, J., Krystal, J.H., Nagy, L.M., Rasmussen, S.A., Heninger, G.R. and Charney, D.S., 1990. Specificity of serotonin reuptake inhibitors in the treatment of obsessive–compulsive disorder. Comparison of fluvoxamine and desipramine. *Archives of General Psychiatry*, **47**, 577–585.

Goodman, W.K., Ward, H., Kablinger, A. and Murphy, T., 1997. Fluvoxamine in the treatment of obsessive–compulsive disorder and related conditions. *Journal of Clinical Psychiatry*, **58**, 32–49.

Goodnick, P.J., Puig, A., DeVane, C.L. and Freund, B.V., 1999. Mirtazapine in major depression with comorbid generalized anxiety disorder. *Journal of Clinical Psychiatry*, **60**, 446–448.

Gorman, J.M., 1999. Mirtazapine: clinical overview. *Journal of Clinical Psychiatry*, **60**, 9–13.

Grady, T.A., Pigott, T.A., L'Heureux, F., Hill, J.L., Bernstein, S.E. and Murphy, D.L., 1993. Double-blind study of adjuvant buspirone for fluoxetine-treated patients with obsessive-compulsive disorder. *American Journal of Psychiatry*, **150**, 819–821.

Greist, J.H., Jefferson, J.W., Kobak, K.A., Chouinard, G., DuBoff, E., Halaris, A., Kim, S.W., Koran, L., Liebowtiz, M.R. and Lydiard, B., 1995b. A 1 year double-blind placebo-controlled fixed dose study of sertraline in the treatment of obsessive-compulsive disorder. *International Clinical Psychopharmacology*, **10**, 57–65.

Greist, J.H., Jefferson, J.W., Kobak, K.A., Katzelnick, D.J. and Serlin, R.C., 1995c. Efficacy and tolerability of serotonin transport inhibitors in obsessive-compulsive disorder. A meta-analysis. *Archives of General Psychiatry*, **52**, 53–60.

Greist, J.H., Jenike, M.A. and Robinson, D., 1995a. Efficacy of fluvoxamine in obsessive–compulsive disorder: results of a multicentre, double blind, placebo-controlled trial. *European Journal of Clinical Research*, **7**, 195–204.

Griez, E., Pols, H. and Lousberg, H., 1988. Serotonin antagonism in panic disorder: an open trial with ritanserin. *Acta Psychiatrica Belgica*, **88**, 372–377.

Gringras, M., 1977. An uncontrolled trial of clomipramine (Anafranil) in the treatment of phobic and obsessional states in general practice. *Journal of Internal Medical Research*, **5**, 111–115.

Hackett, D., 2000. Venlafaxine XR in the treatment of anxiety. *Acta Psychiatrica Scandinavica Supplement*, 30–35.

Hackett, D., Desmet, A. and Salinas, E.O., 1999b. Dose-response efficacy of venlafaxine XR in GAD. *11th World Congress of Psychiatry*.

Hackett, D., Parks, V. and Salinas, E., 1999a. A 6-Month Evaluation of 3 Dose Levels of Venlafaxine Extended-Release in Non-Depressed Outpatients With Generalized Anxiety Disorders. Poster presented at the ADAA, San Diego 26 March.

Hamner, M., Ulmer, H. and Horne, D., 1997. Buspirone potentiation of antidepressants in the treatment of PTSD. *Depression and Anxiety*, **5**, 137–139.

Hamner, M.B. and Frueh, B.C., 1998. Response to venlafaxine in a previously antidepressant treatment- resistant combat veteran with post-traumatic stress disorder. *International Clinical Psychopharmacology*, **13**, 233–234.

Hedges, D.W., Reimherr, F.W., Strong, R.E., Halls, C.H. and Rust, C., 1996. An open trial of nefazodone in adult patients with generalized anxiety disorder. *Psychopharmacology Bulletin*, **32**, 671–676.

Heimberg, R.G., 1993. Specific issues in the cognitive-behavioral treatment of social phobia. *Journal of Clinical Psychiatry*, **54**, 36–45.

Heimberg, R.G. and Juster, H.R., 1994. Treatment of social phobia in cognitive-behavioral groups. *Journal of Clinical Psychiatry*, **55**, 38–46.

Heimberg, R.G., Hope, D.A., Dodge, C.S. and Becker, R.E., 1990. DSM-III-R subtypes of social phobia. Comparison of generalized social phobics and public speaking phobics. *Journal of Nervous and Mental Disease*, **178**, 172–179.

Hembree, E.A. and Foa, E.B., 2000. Posttraumatic stress disorder: psychological factors and psychosocial interventions. *Journal of Clinical Psychiatry*, **61**, 33–39.

Hertzberg, M.A., Feldman, M.E., Beckham, J.C. and Davidson, J.R., 1996. Trial of trazodone for posttraumatic stress disorder using a multiple baseline group design. *Journal of Clinical Psychopharmacology*, **16**, 294–298.

Hertzberg, M.A., Feldman, M.E., Beckham, J.C., Kudler, H.S. and Davidson, J.R., 2000. Lack of efficacy for fluoxetine in PTSD: a placebo controlled trial in combat veterans. *Annals of Clinical Psychiatry*, **12**, 101–105.

Hidalgo, R., Hertzberg, M.A., Mellman, T., Petty, F., Tucker, P., Weisler, R., Zisook, S., Chen, S., Churchill, E. and Davidson, J., 1999. Nefazodone in post-traumatic stress disorder: results from six open- label trials. *International Clinical Psychopharmacology*, **14**, 61–68.

Hirschmann, S., Dannon, P.N., Iancu, I., Dolberg, O.T., Zohar, J. and Grunhaus, L., 2000. Pindolol augmentation in patients with treatment-resistant panic disorder: A double-blind, placebo-controlled trial. *Journal of Clinical Psychopharmacology*, **20**, 556–559.

Hjorth, S. and Auerbach, S.B., 1994. Further evidence for the importance of 5-HT1A autoreceptors in the action of selective serotonin reuptake inhibitors. *European Journal of Pharmacology*, **260**, 251–255.

Hoehn-Saric, R., Fawcett, J., Munjack, D.J. and Roy-Byrne, P.P., 1993. A multicentre, double-blind, placebo-controlled study of fluvoxamine in the treatment of panic disorder. *Neuropsychopharmacology*, **10**, 58–63.

Hoehn-Saric, R., Ninan, P., Black, D.W., Stahl, S., Greist, J.H., Lydiard, B., McElroy, S., Zajecka, J., Chapman, D., Clary, C. and Harrison, W., 2000. Multicenter double-blind comparison of sertraline and desipramine for concurrent obsessive-compulsive and major depressive disorders. *Archives of General Psychiatry*, **57**, 76–82.

Holland, R.L., Fawcett, J., Hoehn-Saric, R., Munjack, D.J. and Roy-Byrne, P.P., 1994. Long-term treatment of panic disorder with fluvoxamine in outpatients who had complete double-blind studies. *Neuropsychopharmacology*, **10**, 102.

Holt, C.S., Heimberg, R.G. and Hope, D.A., 1992. Avoidant personality disorder and the generalized subtype of social phobia. *Journal of Abnormal Psychology*, **101**, 318–325.

Insel, T.R., Mueller, E.A., Alterman, I., Linnoila, M. and Murphy, D.L., 1985. Obsessive–compulsive disorder and serotonin: is there a connection? *Biological Psychiatry*, **20**, 1174–1188.

Invernizzi, R., Belli, S. and Samanin, R., 1992. Citalopram's ability to increase the extracellular concentrations of serotonin in the dorsal raphe prevents the drug's effect in the frontal cortex. *Brain Research*, **584**, 322–324.

Irle, E., Exner, C., Thielen, K., Weniger, G. and Ruther, E., 1998. Obsessive compulsive disorder and ventromedial frontal lesions: clinical and neuropsychological findings. *American Journal of Psychiatry*, **155**, 255–263.

Jacobsen, F.M., 1995. Risperidone in the treatment of affective illness and obsessive–compulsive disorder. *Journal of Clinical Psychiatry*, **56**, 423–429.

Jefferson, J.W., 1995. Social phobia: a pharmacologic treatment overview. *Journal of Clinical Psychiatry*, **56**, 18–24.

Jefferson, J.W., 1996. Social phobia: everyone's disorder? *Journal of Clinical Psychiatry*, **57**, 28–32.

Jenike, M.A. and Baer, L., 1988. An open trial of buspirone in obsessive–compulsive disorder. *American Journal of Psychiatry*, **145**, 1285–1286.

Jenike, M.A., Baer, L. and Buttolph, L., 1991. Buspirone augmentation of fluoxetine in patients with obsessive compulsive disorder. *Journal of Clinical Psychiatry*, **52**, 13–14.

Jenike, M.A., Baer, L. and Greist, J.H., 1990a. Clomipramine versus fluoxetine in obsessive–compulsive disorder: a retrospective comparison of side effects and efficacy. *Journal of Clinical Psychopharmacology*, **10**, 122–124.

Jenike, M.A., Buttolph, L., Baer, L., Ricciardi, J. and Holland, A., 1989. Open trial of fluoxetine in obsessive–compulsive disorder. *American Journal of Psychiatry*, **146**, 909–911.

Jenike, M.A., Hyman, S., Baer, L., Holland, A., Minichiello, W.E., Buttolph, L., Summergrad, P., Seymour, R. and Ricciardi, J., 1990b. A controlled trial of fluvoxamine in obsessive–compulsive disorder: implications for a serotonergic theory. *American Journal of Psychiatry*, **147**, 1209–1215.

Jenike, A., 1998. Neurosurgical treatment for obsessive compulsive disorder. *Br. J. Psychiatry*, **35**, 79–90.

Judd, L.L., 1994. Social phobia: a clinical overview. *Journal of Clinical Psychiatry*, **55**, 5–9.

Judge, R. and Steiner, M., 1996. The long-term efficacy and safety of paroxetine in panic disorder. Presented at the 28th CINP Congress, Melbourne.

Kent, J.M., 2000. SNaRIs, NaSSAs, and NaRIs: new agents for the treatment of depression. *Lancet*, **355**, 911–918.

Kessler, R.C., 2000. The epidemiology of pure and comorbid generalized anxiety disorder: a review and evaluation of recent research. *Acta Psychiatrica Scandinavica Supplement*, **102**, 7–13.

Kessler, R.C., Sonnega, A., Bromet, E., Hughes, M. and Nelson, C.B., 1995. Posttraumatic stress disorder in the National Comorbidity Survey. *Archives of General Psychiatry*, **52**, 1048–1060.

Kinzie, J.D. and Leung, P., 1989. Clonidine in Cambodian patients with posttraumatic stress disorder. *Journal of Nervous and Mental Disease*, **177**, 546–550.

Klein, E., Colin, V., Stolk, J. and Lenox, R.H., 1994. Alprazolam withdrawal in patients with panic disorder and generalized anxiety disorder: vulnerability and effect of carbamazepine. *American Journal of Psychiatry*, **151**, 1760–1766.

Koponen, H., Lepola, U., Leinonen, E., Jokinen, R., Penttinen, J. and Turtonen, J., 1997. Citalopram in the treatment of obsessive–compulsive disorder: an open pilot study. *Acta Psychiatrica Scandinavica*, **96**, 343–346.

Koran, L.M., Mueller, K. and Maloney, A., 1996. Will pindolol augment the response to a serotonin reuptake inhibitor in obsessive–compulsive disorder? *Journal of Clinical Psychopharmacology*, **16**, 253–254.

Kosten, T.R., Frank, J.B., Dan, E., McDougle, C.J. and Giller, E.L., 1991. Pharmacotherapy for posttraumatic stress disorder using phenelzine or imipramine. *Journal of Nervous and Mental Disease*, **179**, 366–370.

Krakow, B., Hollifield, M. and Warner, T.D., 2000. Placebo effect in posttraumatic stress disorders. *Journal of the American Medical Association*, **284**, 563–564.

Krashin, D. and Oates, E.W., 1999. Risperidone as an adjunct therapy for post-traumatic stress disorder. *Military Medicine*, **164**, 605–606.

Kronig, M.H., Apter, J., Asnis, G., Bystritsky, A., Curtis, G., Ferguson, J., Landbloom, R., Munjack, D., Riesenberg, R., Robinson, D., Roy-Byrne, P., Phillips, K. and Du, P.I., 1999. Placebo-controlled, multicenter study of sertraline treatment for obsessive–compulsive disorder. *Journal of Clinical Psychopharmacology*, **19**, 172–176.

Laverdure, B. and Boulenger, J.P., 1991. Beta-blocking drugs and anxiety. A proven therapeutic value. *Encephale*, **17**, 481–492.

Lecrubier, Y. and Judge, R., 1997. Long-term evaluation of paroxetine, clomipramine and placebo in panic disorder. Collaborative Paroxetine Panic Study Investigators. *Acta Psychiatrica Scandinavica*, **95**, 153–160.

Lecrubier, Y., Bakker, A., Dunbar, G. and Judge, R., 1997. A comparison of paroxetine, clomipramine and placebo in the treatment of panic disorder. Collaborative Paroxetine Panic Study Investigators. *Acta Psychiatrica Scandinavica*, **95**, 145–152.

Leinonen, E., Lepola, U., Koponen, H., Turtonen, J., Wade, A. and Lehto, H., 2000. Citalopram controls phobic symptoms in patients with panic disorder: randomized controlled trial. *Journal of Psychiatry & Neuroscience*, **25**, 24–32.

Leonard, H.L., Swedo, S.E., Lenane, M.C., Rettew, D.C., Cheslow, D.L., Hamburger, S.D. and Rapoport, J.L., 1991. A double-blind desipramine substitution during long-term clomipramine treatment in children and adolescents with obsessive-compulsive disorder. *Archives of General Psychiatry*, **48**, 922–927.

Leonard, H.L., Swedo, S.E., Rapoport, J.L., Koby, E.V., Lenane, M.C., Cheslow, D.L. and Hamburger, S.D., 1989. Treatment of obsessive-compulsive disorder with clomipramine and desipramine in children and adolescents. A double-blind crossover comparison. *Archives of General Psychiatry*, **46**, 1088–1092.

Lépine, J.P. and Lellouch, J., 1995. Classification and epidemiology of social phobia. *European Archives of Psychiatry and Clinical Neuroscience*, **244**, 290–296.

Lepola, U.M., Wade, A.G., Leinonen, E.V., Koponen, H.J., Frazer, J., Sjodin, I., Penttinen, J.T., Pedersen, T. and Lehto, H.J., 1998. A controlled, prospective, 1-year trial of citalopram in the treatment of panic disorder. *Journal of Clinical Psychiatry*, **59**, 528–534.

Leyba, C.M. and Wampler, T.P., 1998. Risperidone in PTSD. *Psychiatric Services*, **49**, 245–246.

Liebowitz, M.R., Schneier, F., Campeas, R., Hollander, E., Hatterer, J., Fyer, A., Gorman, J., Papp, L., Davies, S. and Gully, R., 1992. Phenelzine vs atenolol in social phobia. A placebo-controlled comparison. *Archives of General Psychiatry*, **49**, 290–300.

Lipper, S., 1988. PTSD and carbamazepine. *American Journal of Psychiatry*, **145**, 1322–1323.

Londborg, P.D., Wolkow, R., Smith, W.T., DuBoff, E., England, D., Ferguson, J., Rosenthal, M. and Weise, C., 1998. Sertraline in the treatment of panic disorder. A multi-site, double- blind, placebo-controlled, fixed-dose investigation. *British Journal of Psychiatry*, **173**, 54–60.

Looff, D., Grimley, P., Kuller, F., Martin, A. and Shonfield, L., 1995. Carbamazepine for PTSD. *Journal of the American Academic Child and Adolescent Psychiatry*, **34**, 703–704.

Lopez-Ibor, J.J., Jr, Saiz, J., Cottraux, J., Note, I., Vinas, R., Bourgeois, M., Hernandez, M. and Gomez-Perez, J.C., 1996. Double-blind comparison of fluoxetine versus clomipramine in the treatment of obsessive compulsive disorder. *European Neuropsychopharmacology*, **6**, 111–118.

Lott, M., Greist, J.H., Jefferson, J.W., Kobak, K.A., Katzelnick, D.J., Katz, R.J. and Schaettle, S.C., 1997. Brofaromine for social phobia: a multicenter, placebo-controlled, double-blind study. *Journal of Clinical Psychopharmacology*, **17**, 255–260.

Lydiard, R.B., 2000. An overview of generalized anxiety disorder: disease state — appropriate therapy. *Clinical Therapeutics*, **22**, A3–19.

Magee, W.J., Eaton, W.W., Wittchen, H.U., McGonagle, K.A. and Kessler, R.C., 1996. Agoraphobia, simple phobia, and social phobia in the National Comorbidity Survey. *Archives of General Psychiatry*, **53**, 159–168.

Malik, M.L., Connor, K.M., Sutherland, S.M., Smith, R.D., Davison, R.M. and Davidson, J.R., 1999. Quality of life and posttraumatic stress disorder: a pilot study assessing changes in SF-36 scores before and after treatment in a placebo-controlled trial of fluoxetine. *Journal of Traumatic Stress*, **12**, 387–393.

Mallya, G.K., White, K. and Waternaux, C., 1992. Short- and long-term treatment of obsessive–compulsive disorder with fluvoxamine. *Annals of Clinical Psychiatry*, **4**, 77–80.

Marks, I.M. and Gelder, M.G., 1966. Different ages of onset in varieties of phobia. *American Journal of Psychiatry*, **123**, 218–221.

Marks, I.M., Stern, R.S., Mawson, D., Cobb, J. and McDonald, R., 1980. Clomipramine and exposure for obsessive-compulsive rituals: i. *British Journal of Psychiatry*, **136**, 1–25.

Marks, I.M., Swinson, R.P., Basoglu, M., Kuch, K., Noshirvani, H., O'Sullivan, G., Lelliott, P.T., Kirby, M., McNamee, G. and Sengun, S., 1993. Alprazolam and exposure alone and combined in panic disorder with agoraphobia. A controlled study in London and Toronto. *British Journal of Psychiatry*, **162**, 776–787.

Marmar, C.R., Schoenfeld, F., Weiss, D.S., Metzler, T., Zatzick, D., Wu, R., Smiga, S., Tecott, L. and Neylan, T., 1996. Open trial of fluvoxamine treatment for combat-related posttraumatic stress disorder. *Journal of Clinical Psychiatry*, **57**, 66–70.

Marshall, J.R., 1992. The psychopharmacology of social phobia. *Bulletin of the Menninger Clinic*, **56**, A42–A49.

Marshall, J.R., 1994. The diagnosis and treatment of social phobia and alcohol abuse. *Bulletin of the Menninger Clinic*, **58**, A58–A66.

Marshall, R.D., Schneier, F.R., Fallon, B.A., Knight, C.B., Abbate, L.A., Goetz, D., Campeas, R. and Liebowitz, M.R., 1998. An open trial of paroxetine in patients with noncombat-related, chronic posttraumatic stress disorder. *Journal of Clinical Psychopharmacology*, **18**, 10–18.

Mavissakalian, M.R. and Perel, J.M., 2000. The side effects burden of extended imipramine treatment of panic disorder. *Journal of Clinical Psychopharmacology*, **20**, 547–555.

McCafferty, J.P., Bellew, K., Zaninelli, R., Iyengar, M. and Hewett, K., 2000. Paroxetine is effective in the treatment of generalized anxiety disorder, results from a randomized placebo controlled flexible dose study. Presented as an abstract at the APA, Chicago.

McDougle, C.J., Epperson, C.N., Pelton, G.H., Wasylink, S. and Price, L.H., 2000. A double-blind, placebo-controlled study of risperidone addition in serotonin reuptake inhibitor-refractory obsessive–compulsive disorder. *Archives of General Psychiatry*, **57**, 794–801.

McLeod, D.R., Hoehn-Saric, R., Porges, S.W., Kowalski, P.A. and Clark, C.M., 2000. Therapeutic effects of imipramine are counteracted by its metabolite, desipramine, in patients with generalized anxiety disorder. *Journal of Clinical Psychopharmacology*, **20**, 615–621.

McNally, R.J., 1992. Anxiety sensitivity distinguishes panic disorder from generalized anxiety disorder. *Journal of Nervous and Mental Disease*, **180**, 737–738.

McNally, R.J., 1994. *Panic Disorder: A Critical Analysis*. Guilford Press, New York.

Meltzer-Brody, S., Connor, K.M., Churchill, E. and Davidson, J.R., 2000. Symptom-specific effects of fluoxetine in post-traumatic stress disorder. *International Clinical Psychopharmacology*, **15**, 227–231.

Michelson, D., Lydiard, R.B., Pollack, M.H., Tamura, R.N., Hoog, S.L., Tepner, R., Demitrack, M.A. and Tollefson, G.D., 1998. Outcome assessment and clinical improvement in panic disorder: evidence from a randomized controlled trial of fluoxetine and placebo. The Fluoxetine Panic Disorder Study Group. *American Journal of Psychiatry*, **155**, 1570–1577.

Montgomery, S.A., McIntyre, A., Osterheider, M., Sarteschi, P., Zitterl, W., Zohar, J., Birkett, M. and Wood, A.J., 1993. A double-blind, placebo-controlled study of fluoxetine in patients with DSM-III-R obsessive–compulsive disorder. The Lilly European OCD Study Group. *European Neuropsychopharmacology*, **3**, 143–152.

Moroz, G. and Rosenbaum, J.F., 1999. Efficacy, safety, and gradual discontinuation of clonazepam in panic disorder: a placebo-controlled, multicenter study using optimized dosages. *Journal of Clinical Psychiatry*, **60**, 604–612.

Mundo, E., Bianchi, L. and Bellodi, L., 1997. Efficacy of fluvoxamine, paroxetine, and citalopram in the treatment of obsessive–compulsive disorder: a single-blind study. *Journal of Clinical Psychopharmacology*, **17**, 267–271.

Mundo, E., Maina, G. and Uslenghi, C., 2000. Multicentre, double-blind, comparison of fluvoxamine and clomipramine in the treatment of obsessive–compulsive disorder. *International Clinical Psychopharmacology*, **15**, 69–76.

Murphy, D.L. and Pigott, T.A., 1990. A comparative examination of a role for serotonin in obsessive compulsive disorder, panic disorder, and anxiety. *Journal of Clinical Psychiatry*, **51**, 53–58.

Neal, L.A., Shapland, W. and Fox, C., 1997. An open trial of moclobemide in the treatment of post-traumatic stress disorder. *International Clinical Psychopharmacology*, **12**, 231–237.

Noyes, R., Burrows, G.D., Reich, J.H., Judd, F.K., Garvey, M.J., Norman, T.R., Cook, B.L. and Marriott, P., 1996. Diazepam versus alprazolam for the treatment of panic disorder. *Journal of Clinical Psychiatry*, **57**, 349–355.

Noyes, R., DuPont, R.L., Pecknold, J.C., Rifkin, A., Rubin, R.T., Swinson, R.P., Ballenger, J.C. and Burrows, G.D., 1988. Alprazolam in panic disorder and agoraphobia: results from a multicenter trial. II. Patient acceptance, side effects, and safety. *Archives of General Psychiatry*, **45**, 423–428.

Noyes, R., Moroz, G., Davidson, J.R., Liebowitz, M.R., Davidson, A., Siegel, J., Bell, J., Cain, J.W., Curlik, S.M., Kent, T.A., Lydiard, R.B., Mallinger, A.G., Pollack, M.H., Rapaport, M., Rasmussen, S.A., Hedges, D., Schweizer, E. and Uhlenhuth, E.H., 1997. Moclobemide in social phobia: a controlled dose-response trial. *Journal of Clinical Psychopharmacology*, **17**, 247–254.

Nutt, D.J., 1998. Antidepressants in panic disorder: clinical and preclinical mechanisms. *Journal of Clinical Psychiatry*, **59**(Supp. 8), 24–28.

Oehrberg, S., Christiansen, P.E., Behnke, K., Borup, A.L., Severin, B., Soegaard, J., Calberg, H., Judge, R., Ohrstrom, J.K. and Manniche, P.M., 1995. Paroxetine in the treatment of panic disorder. A randomized, double-blind, placebo-controlled study. *British Journal of Psychiatry*, **167**, 374–379.

Otto, M.W., Pollack, M.H., Sachs, G.S., Reiter, S.R., Meltzer-Brody, S. and Rosenbaum, J.F., 1993. Discontinuation of benzodiazepine treatment: efficacy of cognitive- behavioral therapy for patients with panic disorder. *American Journal of Psychiatry*, **150**, 1485–1490.

Pallanti, S., Quercioli, L., Paiva, R.S. and Koran, L.M., 1999. Citalopram for treatment-resistant obsessive–compulsive disorder. *European Psychiatry*, **14**, 101–106.

Palatnik, A., Frolov, K., Fux, M. and Benjamin, J., 2001. Double-blind controlled cross-over trial of inositol versus fluvoxamine for the treatment of panic disorder. *Journal of Clinical Psychopharmacology*, **21**(3), 335–339.

Pande, A.C., Davidson, J.R., Jefferson, J.W., Janney, C.A., Katzelnick, D.J., Weisler, R.H., Greist, J.H. and Sutherland, S.M., 1999. Treatment of social phobia with gabapentin: a placebo-controlled study. *Journal of Clinical Psychopharmacology*, **19**, 341–348.

Papp, L.A., Sinha, S.S., Martinez, J.M., Coplan, J.D., Amchin, J. and Gorman, J.M., 1998. Low-dose venlafaxine treatment in panic disorder. *Psychopharmacology Bulletin*, **34**, 207–209.

Pato, M.T., Pigott, T.A., Hill, J.L., Grover, G.N., Bernstein, S. and Murphy, D.L., 1991. Controlled comparison of buspirone and clomipramine in obsessive–compulsive disorder. *American Journal of Psychiatry*, **148**, 127–129.

Pecknold, J.C., Luthe, L., Scott-Fleury, M.H. and Jenkins, S., 1993. Gepirone and the treatment of panic disorder: an open study. *Journal of Clinical Psychopharmacology*, **13**, 145–149.

Pecknold, J.C., Swinson, R.P., Kuch, K. and Lewis, C.P., 1988. Alprazolam in panic disorder and agoraphobia: results from a multicenter trial. III. Discontinuation effects. *Archives of General Psychiatry*, **45**, 429–436.

Perse, T.L., Greist, J.H., Jefferson, J.W., Rosenfeld, R. and Dar, R., 1987. Fluvoxamine treatment of obsessive–compulsive disorder. *American Journal of Psychiatry*, **144**, 1543–1548.

Pfanner, C., Marazziti, D., Dell'Osso, L., Presta, S., Gemignani, A., Milanfranchi, A. and Cassano, G.B., 2000. Risperidone augmentation in refractory obsessive–compulsive disorder: an open-label study. *International Clinical Psychopharmacology*, **15**, 297–301.

Phillips, M.A., Bitsios, P., Szabadi, E. and Bradshaw, C.M., 2000. Comparison of the antidepressants reboxetine, fluvoxamine and amitriptyline upon spontaneous pupillary fluctuations in healthy human volunteers. *Psychopharmacology (Berlin)*, **149**, 72–76.

Piccinelli, M., Pini, S., Bellantuono, C. and Wilkinson, G., 1995. Efficacy of drug treatment in obsessive–compulsive disorder. A meta-analytic review. *British Journal of Psychiatry*, **166**, 424–443.

Pigott, T.A. and Seay, S.M., 1999. A review of the efficacy of selective serotonin reuptake inhibitors in obsessive–compulsive disorder. *Journal of Clinical Psychiatry*, **60**, 101–106.

Pigott, T.A., Pato, M.T., Bernstein, S.E., Grover, G.N., Hill, J.L., Tolliver, T.J. and Murphy, D.L., 1990. Controlled comparisons of clomipramine and fluoxetine in the treatment of obsessive–compulsive disorder. Behavioral and biological results. *Archives of General Psychiatry*, **47**, 926–932.

Pohl, R.B., Wolkow, R.M. and Clary, C.M., 1998. Sertraline in the treatment of panic disorder: a double-blind multicenter trial. *American Journal of Psychiatry*, **155**, 1189–1195.

Pollack, M.H., Otto, M.W., Worthington, J.J., Manfro, G.G. and Wolkow, R., 1998. Sertraline in the treatment of panic disorder: a flexible-dose multicenter trial. *Archives of General Psychiatry*, **55**, 1010–1016.

Pollack, M.H., Worthington, J.J., Otto, M.W., Maki, K.M., Smoller, J.W., Manfro, G.G., Rudolph, R. and Rosenbaum, J.F., 1996. Venlafaxine for panic disorder: results from a double-blind, placebo-controlled study. *Psychopharmacology Bulletin*, **32**, 667–670.

Pomara, N., Tun, H., DaSilva, D., Hernando, R., Deptula, D. and Greenblatt, D.J., 1998. The acute and chronic performance effects of alprazolam and lorazepam in the elderly: relationship to duration of treatment and self-rated sedation. *Psychopharmacology Bulletin*, **34**, 139–153.

Price, L.H., Goodman, W.K., Charney, D.S., Rasmussen, S.A. and Heninger, G.R., 1987. Treatment of severe obsessive–compulsive disorder with fluvoxamine. *American Journal of Psychiatry*, **144**, 1059–1061.

Rasmussen, S., Eisen, J. and Pato, M., 1993. Current issues in the pharmacologic management of OCD. *Journal of Clinical Psychiatry*, **54**, 4–9.

Ravizza, L., Barzega, G., Bellino, S., Bogetto, F. and Maina, G., 1996. Drug treatment of obsessive–compulsive disorder (OCD): long-term trial with clomipramine and selective serotonin reuptake inhibitors (SSRIs). *Psychopharmacology Bulletin*, **32**, 167–173.

Reist, C., Kauffmann, C.D., Haier, R.J., Sangdahl, C., DeMet, E.M., Chicz-DeMet, A. and Nelson, J.N., 1989. A controlled trial of desipramine in 18 men with posttraumatic stress disorder. *American Journal of Psychiatry*, **146**, 513–516.

Rickels, K., DeMartinis, N., Garcia-Espana, F., Greenblatt, D.J., Mandos, L.A. and Rynn, M., 2000a. Imipramine and buspirone in treatment of patients with generalized anxiety disorder who are discontinuing long-term benzodiazepine therapy. *American Journal of Psychiatry*, **157**, 1973–1979.

Rickels, K., Pollack, M.H., Sheehan, D.V. and Haskins, J.T., 2000b. Efficacy of extended-release venlafaxine in nondepressed outpatients with generalized anxiety disorder. *American Journal of Psychiatry*, **157**, 968–974.

Rickels, K., Schweizer, E., DeMartinis, N., Mandos, L. and Mercer, C., 1997. Gepirone and diazepam in generalized anxiety disorder: a placebo-controlled trial. *Journal of Clinical Psychopharmacology*, **17**, 272–277.

Rickels, K., Schweizer, E., Garcia, E.F., Case, G., DeMartinis, N. and Greenblatt, D., 1999. Trazodone and valproate in patients discontinuing long-term benzodiazepine therapy: effects on withdrawal symptoms and taper outcome. *Psychopharmacology (Berlin)*, **141**, 1–5.

Rickels, K., Schweizer, E., Weiss, S. and Zavodnick, S., 1993. Maintenance drug treatment for panic disorder. II. S. *Archives of General Psychiatry*, **50**, 61–68.

Robinson, D.S., Alms, D.R., Shrotriya, R.C., Messina, M. and Wickramaratne, P., 1989. Serotonergic anxiolytics and treatment of depression. *Psychopathology*, **22**, 27–36.

Robinson, D.S., Rickels, K., Feighner, J., Fabre, L.F., Gammans, R.E., Shrotriya, R.C., Alms, D.R., Andary, J.J. and Messina, M.E., 1990. Clinical effects of the 5-HT1A partial agonists in depression: a composite analysis of buspirone in the treatment of depression. *Journal of Clinical Psychopharmacology*, **10**, 67S–76S.

Rocca, P., Fonzo, V., Scotta, M., Zanalda, E. and Ravizza, L., 1997. Paroxetine efficacy in the treatment of generalized anxiety disorder. *Acta Psychiatrica Scandinavica*, **95**, 444–450.

Rosenbaum, J.F. and Pollock, R.A., 1994. The psychopharmacology of social phobia and comorbid disorders. *Bulletin of the Menninger Clinic*, **58**, A67–A83.

Rosenbaum, J.F., Biederman, J., Pollock, R.A. and Hirshfeld, D.R., 1994. The etiology of social phobia. *Journal of Clinical Psychiatry*, **55**, 10–16.

Rosenbaum, J.F., Moroz, G. and Bowden, C.L., 1997. Clonazepam in the treatment of panic disorder with or without agoraphobia: a dose-response study of efficacy, safety, and discontinuance. Clonazepam Panic Disorder Dose-Response Study Group. *Journal of Clinical Psychopharmacology*, **17**, 390–400.

Rosenfeld, J.V.L., 1999. Contemporary psychosurgery. *Journal of Clinical Neuroscience*, **6**(2), 106–112.

Rothbaum, B.O., Ninan, P.T. and Thomas, L., 1996. Sertraline in the treatment of rape victims with posttraumatic stress disorder. *Journal of Traumatic Stress*, **9**, 865–871.

Roy-Byrne, P.P., 1996. Generalized anxiety and mixed anxiety–depression: association with disability and health care utilization. *Journal of Clinical Psychiatry*, **57**, 86–91.

Ruggiero, L., Pitts, C.D. and Dillingham, K., 2001. A flexible dose study of paroxetine in the treatment of PTSD. Abstract presented at the APA, New Orleans, May, 2001.

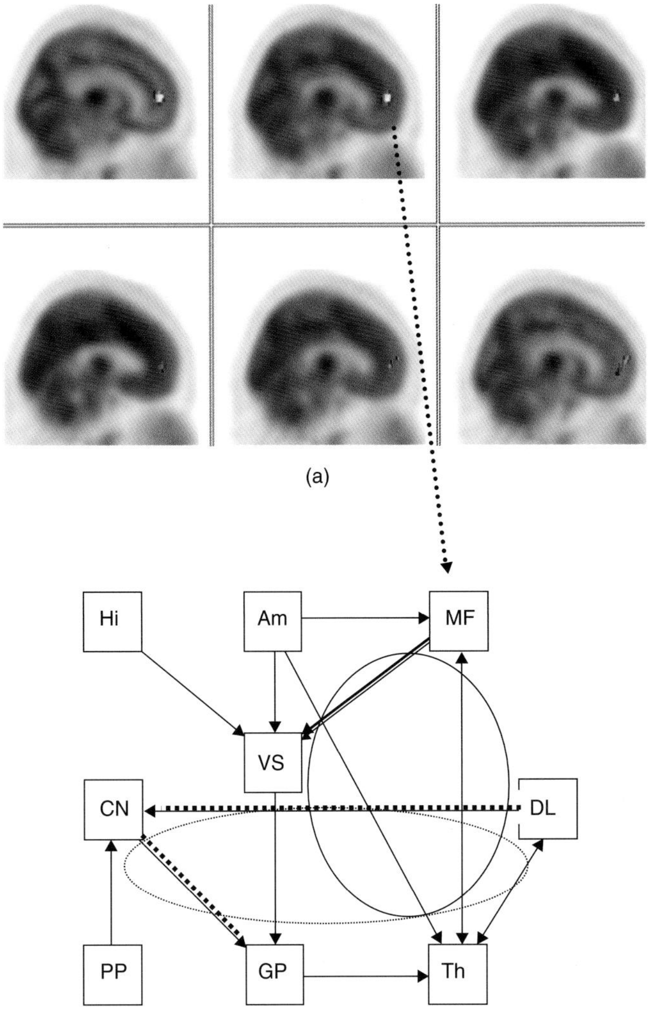

Figure XVIII-9.1 Effect of one session of TMS (5–20 Hz at 80% motor threshold over the left dorsolateral prefrontal cortex) on rCBF during a word-generation task. (a) Statistical parametric map of areas with $P < 0.01$ for effect size (z) and contiguous area (k), using Statistical Parametric Mapping, version 1996. (b) Neuroanatomical projections. Am, amygdala; CN, caudate nucleus; DL, dorsolateral prefrontal cortex; GP, globus pallidus; Hi, hippocampus; MF, medial orbitofrontal cortex; PP, posterior parietal cortex; Th, thalamus; VS, ventral striatum; Dotted ellipse, dorsolateral prefrontal loop; continuous ellipse, limbic loop; dotted arrow DL to CN, increase in regression coefficient c with significance levels in left dorsolateral loop ($c = 2.45$, $P < 0.05$); dotted arrow CN to GP, increase in regression coefficient c with significance levels in left dorsolateral loop ($c = 2.15$, $P = 0.05$); continuous arrow MF to VS, bilateral limbic loop (left: $c = 2.51$, $P < 0.05$; right: $c = 2.89$, $P < 0.05$)

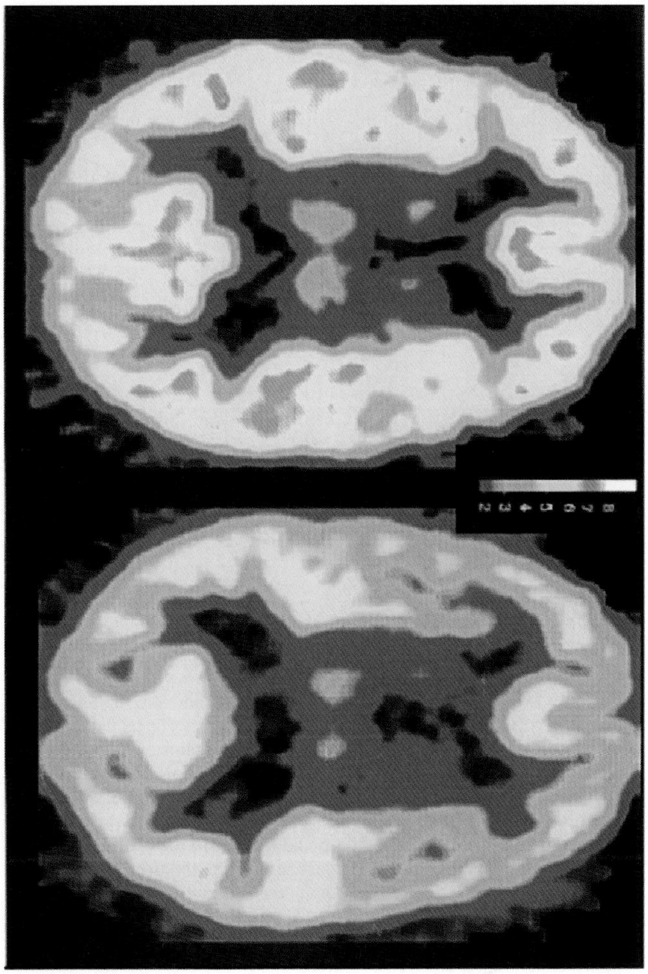

Figure XIX-10.2 A comparison of flumazenil binding between controls and panic disorder patients. The image shows a coloured scale of volume of distribution of flumazenil. The horizontal brain slice is through the middle of the brain showing occipital cortex (left) thalami amd basal ganglia (centre) temporal cortex (middle rim) and frontal cortex (right). A decrease in flumazenil binding is seen throughout the cortex and subcortical structures on the bottom which is the median map for panic disorder patients. The median map for controls is on the top

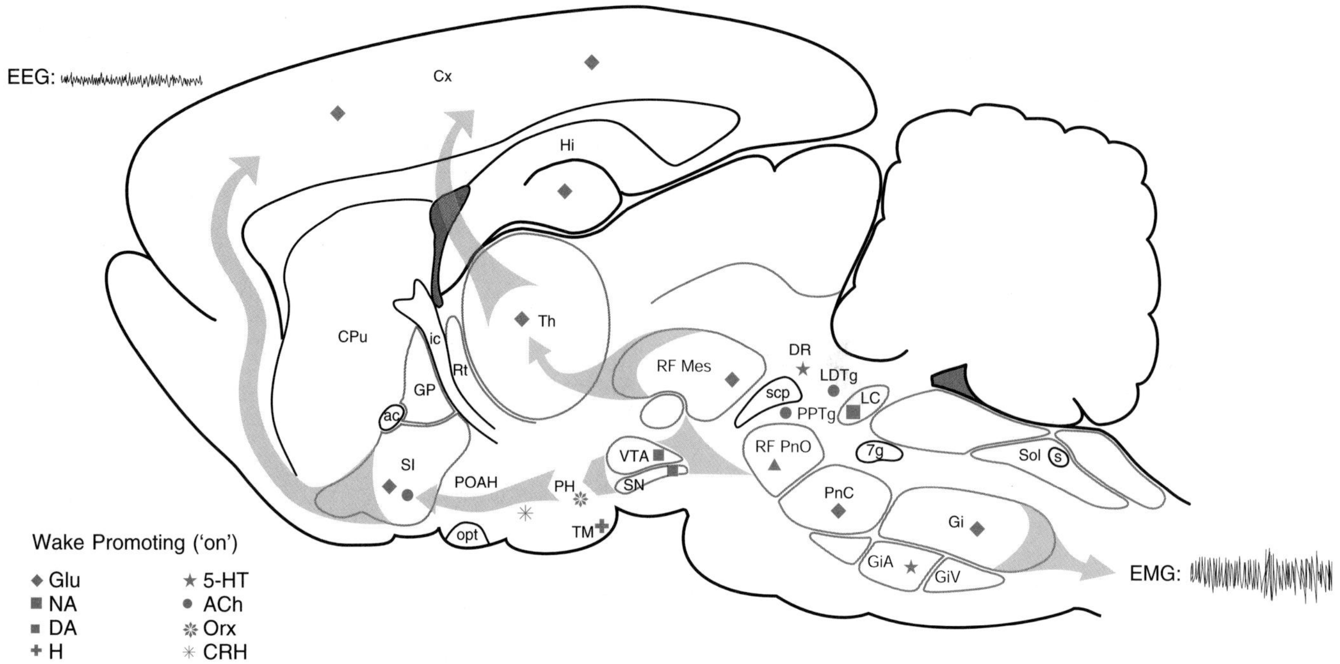

Figure XXIV-2.1 Wake-Promoting Systems. Schematic sagittal view of rat brain showing the major neuronal systems and their major excitatory pathways (arrows) involved in promoting the EEG fast activity (upper left) and EMG high muscle tone and activity (lower right) characteristic of the waking state. The major ascending pathways emerge from the brainstem reticular formation (RF, most densely from the mesencephalic, RF Mes, and oral pontine RF PnO, fields) to ascend along a) a dorsal trajectory into the thalamus (Th) where they terminate upon (midline, medial, and intralaminar) nuclei of the non-specific thalamo-cortical projection system, which projects in turn in a widespread manner to the cerebral cortex (Cx), and b) a ventral trajectory through the lateral hypothalamus up to the basal forebrain where they terminate upon neurons in the substantia innominata (SI) (and septum, not shown), which also project in turn in a widespread manner to the cerebral cortex (and hippocampus, Hi) (Jones, 1995). Descending projections collect from multiple levels of the reticular formation (though most densely from the caudal pontine, PnC, and medullary gigantocellular, Gi, fields) to form the reticulo-spinal pathways. The major transmitter systems that promote waking and discharge maximally ('on') during waking contribute to these ascending and descending systems and are represented by symbols where their cell bodies are located. Glutamatergic (Glu) neurons comprise the vast population of neurons of the reticular formation, the diffuse thalamo-cortical projection system and a contingent of the basalo-cortical projection system. Noradrenergic (NA) neurons of the locus coeruleus (LC) send axons along the major ascending and descending pathways to project in a diffuse manner to the cortex, the subcortical relay stations, brainstem and spinal cord. Dopaminergic (DA) neurons of the substantia nigra (SN) and ventral tegmental area (VTA) project along the ventral pathway in the nigro-striatal system and meso-limbo-cortical system, respectively. Histaminergic (H) neurons of the tuberomammillary nucleus (TM) project in a diffuse manner to the forebrain and cortex. Serotonergic neurons containing 5-hydroxytryptamine (5-HT) of the midbrain (including the dorsal raphe, DR) project to the forebrain, including the cerebral cortex (and hippocampus), as well as the subcortical relay stations, and those of the medulla (in raphe pallidus and obscurus, not shown, as well as pars alpha of the gigantocellular field [GiA]) project to the spinal cord. Cholinergic neurons, containing acetylcholine (ACh), are located in the laterodorsal and pedunculopontine tegmental (LDTg and PPTg) nuclei in the brainstem, from where they project along with other reticular neurons dorsally to the thalamus and ventrally to the posterior hypothalamus and basal forebrain, as well as to the brainstem reticular formation. They are also located in the substantia innominata (SI, and septum, not shown), from where they project to the cortex (and hippocampus). Orexinergic (Orx) neurons in the (perifornical and lateral) mid- and posterior hypothalamus (PH) project diffusely through the forebrain, brainstem and spinal cord to exert an excitatory influence at multiple levels. Corticotropin-releasing hormone (CRH) is contained in neurons within the paraventricular nucleus of the hypothalamus which project to the pituitary, as well as in other scattered neurons (not shown) projecting to other forebrain and brainstem areas that collectively stimulate the hypothalamo-pituitary-adrenal axis and central arousal systems. Some state-specific GABAergic neurons (triangle) may be on during waking to prevent activity of REM-promoting neurons in the oral pontine reticular formation (PnO) (Figure XXIV-2.3)

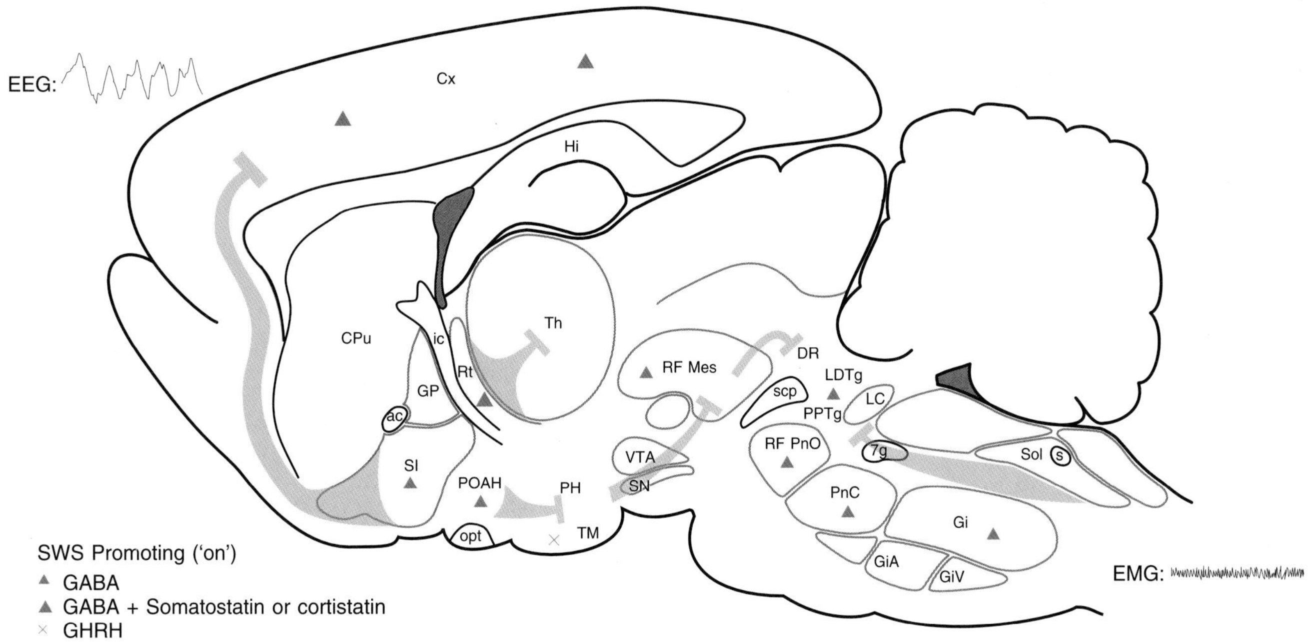

Figure XXIV-2.2 SWS-promoting systems. Schematic sagittal view of rat brain showing the major neuronal systems and their major inhibitory pathways (ending as blocks) involved in promoting the EEG slow-wave activity (upper left) and EMG reduced muscle tone (lower right) characteristic of the slow-wave sleep (SWS) state. Neurons in the region of the solitary tract nucleus (Sol) may exert an inhibitory influence on neurons in the ponto-mesencephalic tegmentum. A dampening influence on the brainstem activating system and the posterior hypothalamus (PH) also emerges from the basal forebrain and preoptic-anterior hypothalamic areas (POAH). From the basal forebrain (substantia innominata [SI]), an inhibitory influence is also exerted upon the cortex (Cx). The major transmitter systems that promote SWS and discharge maximally ('on') during SWS are represented by symbols where their cell bodies are located. These comprise largely GABAergic neurons that, by unit recording and/or c-Fos studies, have been shown to be active during SWS. Particular cortically projecting GABAergic neurons in the SI may have the capacity to dampen cortical activation directly during SWS. Locally projecting GABAergic neurons in the SI may inhibit the cholinergic and glutamatergic cortically projecting neurons. Other GABAergic neurons in the SI and POAH project caudally to the posterior hypothalamus (including the tuberomammillary nucleus [TM]) and brainstem (including RF Mes, DR, LDTg and LC), where they may inhibit multiple wake-active neurons of the activating systems. GABAergic neurons in the reticularis (Rt) nucleus, which surround and innervate the thalamic (Th) nuclei, discharge in bursts to generate spindles while inhibiting the thalamo-cortical projection neurons during SWS. These and local GABAergic neurons in the cortex (Cx) also contain somatostatin or the related peptide corticostatin, which may serve to prolong the inhibition in promoting the slow-wave activity of this state. GABAergic neurons in the brainstem may inhibit local neurons of the ascending reticular activating system as well as those of the descending reticulo-spinal system. Neurons containing growth hormone-releasing hormone (GHRH), primarily located in the arcuate nucleus and projecting to the median eminence, are actively involved in stimulating growth hormone and also promoting slow-wave activity during SWS

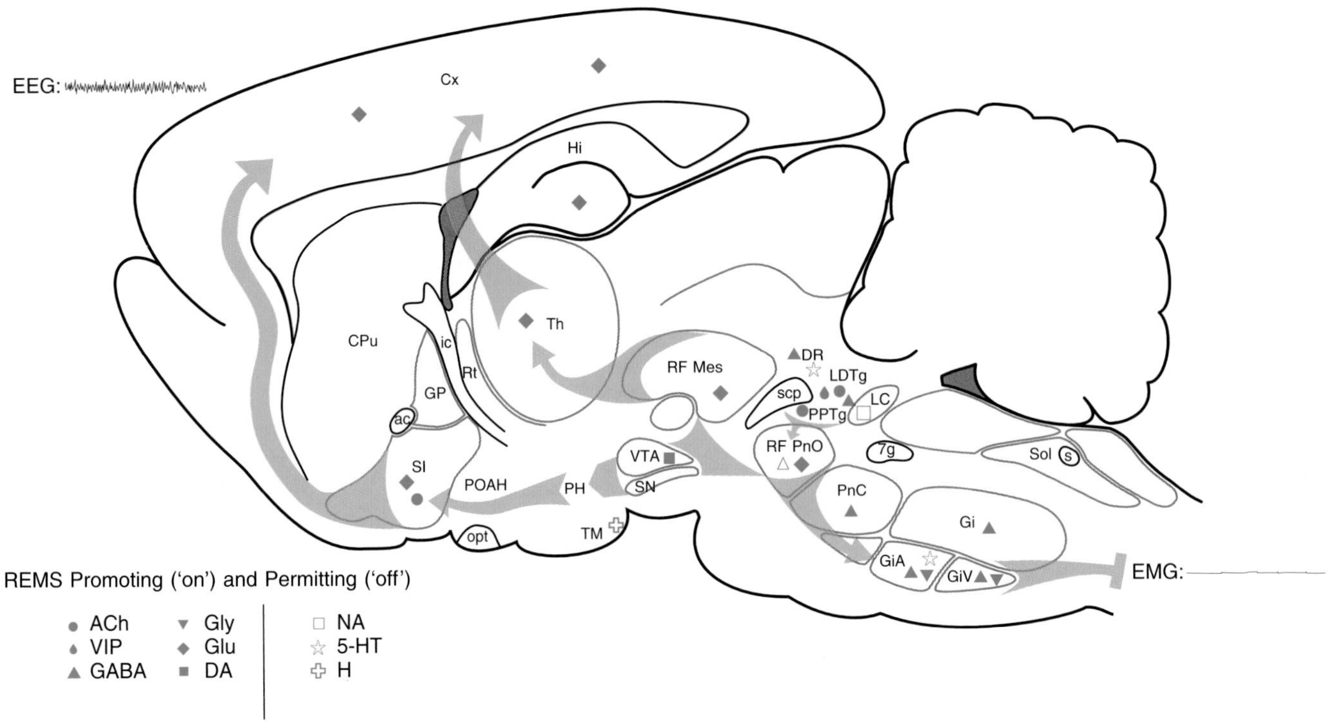

Figure XXIV-2.3 REMS-promoting and REMS-permitting systems. Schematic sagittal view of rat brain showing the major neuronal systems and their (excitatory, ending as arrows, and inhibitory, ending as blocks) pathways involved in promoting the EEG fast activity (upper left) and EMG muscle atonia (lower right) characteristic of rapid eye movement or paradoxical sleep (REMS or PS). Neurons essential for REM sleep are located in the pontine reticular formation, particularly the oral part (RF PnO). The major ascending pathways (indicated by arrows for excitation) promoting cortical activation are similar to those of the waking state; however, the extra-thalamic relay into the limbic system may be more important in REMS. The descending motor inhibition (indicated by a block) is triggered by neurons in the oral pontine reticular formation (RF PnO) and partly relayed through neurons in the alpha and ventral gigantocellular fields (GiA and GiV) of the medullary reticular formation en route to the spinal cord. The major transmitter systems that promote REMS and discharge ('on') during REMS are represented by filled symbols, whereas those that are permissive to REMS by stopping their discharge ('off') during the state are represented by empty symbols. Cholinergic neurons that release acetylcholine (ACh) and are located in the laterodorsal and pedunculopontine tegmental nuclei (LDTg and PPTg) are critically involved in promoting REMS through their projections locally into the brainstem reticular formation, and importantly to neurons in the PnO (where they excite glutamatergic neurons and could also inhibit local GABAergic neurons), as well as rostrally into the forebrain. These may be joined in promoting REMS by neurons with similar projections in the region containing vasoactive intestinal peptide (VIP). Noradrenergic (NA) locus coeruleus (LC) and serotonergic (5-HT) dorsal raphe (DR) neurons (as well as histaminergic, H, tuberomammillary neurons, TM) that directly inhibit the cholinergic neurons permit REMS to occur by ceasing their discharge. The arrest of their discharge is effected by local GABAergic neurons, which may be excited by ACh. GABAergic neurons through the caudal pontine (PnC) medullary reticular formation (Gi, GiA, and GiV) may also inhibit local reticulo-spinal and serotonergic raphe-spinal neurons to effect a disfacilitation of motor neurons. In addition, GABAergic and glycinergic neurons in the ventral medullary reticular formation (GiA and GiV) that project to the spinal cord may both directly inhibit motor neurons. One unique group of GABAergic neurons in the PnO ceases discharge during REMS to disinhibit PnO glutamatergic neurons that propagate the ascending and descending correlates of the state. In the ascending pathways, dopaminergic (DA) neurons of the ventral tegmental area (VTA), which are excited by the cholinergic neurons, may be important in activation of the limbic system. The cholinergic basal forebrain neurons (SI and septum) are particularly important in activation of the limbic cortex (hippocampus [Hi]) and neo-cortex (Cx) during REMS

Sanderson, W.C. and Barlow, D.H., 1990. A description of patients diagnosed with DSM-III-R generalized anxiety disorder. *Journal of Nervous and Mental Disease*, **178**, 588–591.

Saxena, S., Wang, D., Bystritsky, A. and Baxter, L.R., 1996. Risperidone augmentation of SRI treatment for refractory obsessive–compulsive disorder. *Journal of Clinical Psychiatry*, **57**, 303–306.

Schneier, F.R., Garfinkel, R., Kennedy, B., Campeas, R., Fallon, B., Marshall, R., O'Donnell, L., Hogan, T. and Liebowitz, M.R., 1996. Ondansetron in the treatment of panic disorder. *Anxiety*, **2**, 199–202.

Schneier, F.R., Johnson, J., Hornig, C.D., Liebowitz, M.R. and Weissman, M.M., 1992. Social phobia. Comorbidity and morbidity in an epidemiologic sample. *Archives of General Psychiatry*, **49**, 282–288.

Schneier, F.R., Spitzer, R.L., Gibbon, M., Fyer, A.J. and Liebowitz, M.R., 1991. The relationship of social phobia subtypes and avoidant personality disorder. *Comprehensive Psychiatry*, **32**, 496–502.

Schweizer, E., Rickels, K., Case, W.G. and Greenblatt, D.J., 1991. Carbamazepine treatment in patients discontinuing long-term benzodiazepine therapy. Effects on withdrawal severity and outcome. *Archives of General Psychiatry*, **48**, 448–452.

Schweizer, E., Rickels, K., Weiss, S. and Zavodnick, S., 1993. Maintenance drug treatment of panic disorder. I. Results of a prospective, placebo-controlled comparison of alprazolam and imipramine. *Archives of General Psychiatry*, **50**, 51–60.

Seedat, S. and Stein, D.J., 1999. Inositol augmentation of serotonin reuptake inhibitors in treatment-refractory obsessive–compulsive disorder: an open trial. *International Clinical Psychopharmacology*, **14**, 353–356.

Sharp, D.M., Power, K.G. and Simpson, R.J., 1996. Fluvoxamine, placebo, and cognitive behaviour therapy used alone and in combination in the treatment of panic disorder and agoraphobia. *Journal of Anxiety Disorders*, **10**, 219–242.

Shear, M.K. and Maser, J.D., 1994. Standardized assessment for panic disorder research. A conference report. *Archives of General Psychiatry*, **51**, 346–354.

Sheehan, D.V., Raj, A.B., Sheehan, K.H. and Soto, S., 1990. Is buspirone effective for panic disorder? *Journal of Clinical Psychopharmacology*, **10**, 3–11.

Sheehan, D.V., Raj, B.A., Trehan, R.R. and Knapp, E.L., 1993. Serotonin in panic disorder and social phobia. *International Clinical Psychopharmacology*, **8**, 63–77.

Sheikh, J.I., Londborg, P., Clary, C.M. and Fayyad, R., 2000. The efficacy of sertraline in panic disorder: combined results from two fixed-dose studies. *International Clinical Psychopharmacology*, **15**, 335–342.

Simpson, H.B., Schneier, F.R., Campeas, R.B., Marshall, R.D., Fallon, B.A., Davies, S., Klein, D.F. and Liebowitz, M.R., 1998. Imipramine in the treatment of social phobia. *Journal of Clinical Psychopharmacology*, **18**, 132–135.

Spiegel, D.A., 1998. Efficacy studies of alprazolam in panic disorder. *Psychopharmacology Bulletin*, **34**, 191–195.

Sramek, J.J., Fresquet, A., Marion-Landais, G., Hourani, J., Jhee, S.S., Martinez, L., Jensen, C.M., Bolles, K., Carrington, A.T. and Cutler, N.R., 1996. Establishing the maximum tolerated dose of lesopitron in patients with generalized anxiety disorder: a bridging study. *Journal of Clinical Psychopharmacology*, **16**, 454–458.

Stein, D.J., Berk, M., Els, C., Emsley, R.A., Gittelson, L., Wilson, D., Oakes, R. and Hunter, B., 1999. A double-blind placebo-controlled trial of paroxetine in the management of social phobia (social anxiety disorder) in South Africa. *South African Medical Journal*, **89**, 402–406.

Stein, D.J., Hewett, K., Oldham, M., Adams, A. and Bryson, H., 2001. PTSD, comorbid depression and paroxetine efficacy. Abstract presented at the APA, New Orleans, May 2001.

Stein, D.J., Versiani, M., Hair, T. and Kumar, R., 2001. Effectiveness and tolerability of paroxetine in the long-term treatment of social anxiety disorder: results of a placebo-controlled study. Submitted.

Stein, M.B., Fyer, A.J., Davidson, J.R., Pollack, M.H. and Wiita, B., 1999. Fluvoxamine treatment of social phobia (social anxiety disorder): a double-blind, placebo-controlled study. *American Journal of Psychiatry*, **156**, 756–760.

Stern, L., Zohar, J., Cohen, R. and Sasson, Y., 1998. Treatment of severe, drug resistant obsessive compulsive disorder with the 5HT1D agonist sumatriptan. *European Neuropsychopharmacology*, **8**, 325–328.

Stocchi, F., Nordera, G., Jokinen, R. and Lepola, U., 2001. Efficacy and tolerability of paroxetine for the long-term treatment of generalized anxiety disorder (GAD). Presented as an abstract at the APA, New Orleans.

The Expert Consensus Panels for PTSD, 1999. The expert consensus guideline series. Treatment of posttraumatic stress disorder. *Journal of Clinical Psychiatry*, **60**, 3–76.

The International Multicenter Clinical Trial Group on Moclobemide in Social Phobia, 1997. Moclobemide in social phobia. A double-blind, placebo-controlled clinical study. *European Archives of Psychiatry and Clinical Neuroscience*, **247**, 71–80.

Thompson, C., 1999. Mirtazapine versus selective serotonin reuptake inhibitors. *Journal of Clinical Psychiatry*, **60**, 18–22.

Tollefson, G.D., Birkett, M., Koran, L. and Genduso, L., 1994b. Continuation treatment of OCD: double-blind and open-label experience with fluoxetine. *Journal of Clinical Psychiatry*, **55**, 69–76.

Tollefson, G.D., Rampey, A.H., Potvin, J.H., Jenike, M.A., Rush, A.J., kominguez, R.A., Koran, L.M., Shear, M.K., Goodman, W. and Genduso, L.A., 1994a. A multicenter investigation of fixed-dose fluoxetine in the treatment of obsessive–compulsive disorder. *Archives of General Psychiatry*, **51**, 559–567.

Toni, C., Perugi, G., Frare, F., Mata, B., Vitale, B., Mengali, F., Recchia, M., Serra, G. and Akiskal, H.S., 2000. A prospective naturalistic study of 326 panic–agoraphobic patients treated with antidepressants. *Pharmacopsychiatry*, **33**, 121–131.

Tucker, P., Smith, K., Beebe, K.L., Jones, D.E., Trautman, R., Wyatt, D., Cooper-Mckenzie, J., Groff, J. and Potter-Kimball, R., 2000. Effects of paroxetine treatment on autonomic functioning in PTSD: a pilot study. Abstract presented at the 16th International Society for Traumatic Stress Studies, San Antonio, TX.

Valenca, A.M., Nardi, A.E., Nascimento, I., Mezzasalma, M.A., Lopes, F.L. and Zin, W., 2000. Double-blind clonazepam vs placebo in panic disorder treatment. *Arquivos de Neuro Psiquiatria*, **58**, 1025–1029.

van Ameringen, M., Mancini, C. and Oakman, J.M., 1999a. Selective serotonin reuptake inhibitors in the treatment of social phobia: the emerging gold standard. *CNS Drugs*, **11**, 307–315.

van Ameringen, M., Mancini, C. and Oakman, J.M., 1999b. Nefazodone in social phobia. *Journal of Clinical Psychiatry*, **60**, 96–100.

van Ameringen, M.A., Lane, R.M., Walker, J.R., Bowen, R.C., Chokka, P.R., Goldner, E.M., Johnston, D.G., Lavallee, Y.J., Nandy, S., Pecknold, J.C., Hadrava, V. and Swinson, R.P., 2001. Sertraline treatment of generalized social phobia: a 20-week, double-blind, placebo-controlled study. *American Journal of Psychiatry*, **158**, 275–281.

van Balkom, A.J., Bakker, A., Spinhoven, Ph., Blaauw, B.M.J.W., Smeenk, S. and Ruesink, B., 1997. A meta-analysis of the treatment of panic disorder with or without agoraphobia: a comparison of psychopharmacological, cognitive-behavioral, and combination treatments. *Journal of Nervous and Mental Disease*, **185**, 510–516.

van der Kolk, B.A., Dreyfuss, D., Michaels, M., Shera, D., Berkowitz, R., Fisler, R. and Saxe, G., 1994. Fluoxetine in posttraumatic stress disorder. *Journal of Clinical Psychiatry*, **55**, 517–522.

van der Linden, G.J., Stein, D.J. and van Balkom, A.J., 2000. The efficacy of the selective serotonin reuptake inhibitors for social anxiety disorder (social phobia): a meta-analysis of randomized controlled trials. *International Clinical Psychopharmacology*, **15**, S15–S23.

van Vliet, I.M., den Boer, J.A. and Westenberg, H.G.M., 1992. Psychopharmacological treatment of social phobia: clinical and biochemical effects of brofaromine, a selective MAO-A inhibitor. *European Neuropsychopharmacology*, **2**, 21–29.

van Vliet, I.M., van Veen, J.F. and Westenberg, H.G.M., 2000. Mirtazapine in social anxiety disorder. *International Journal of Neuropsychopharmacology*, S283.

van Vliet, I.M., Westenberg, H.G.M. and den Boer, J.A., 1996. Effects of the 5-HT1A receptor agonist flesinoxan in panic disorder. *Psychopharmacology (Berlin)*, **127**, 174–180.

Van Vliet, I.M., Westenberg, H.G.M., den Boer, J.A., 2001. Pindolol augmentation in panic disorder. submitted for publication.

Versiani, M., Nardi, A.E., Figueira, I., Mendlowicz, M. and Marques, C., 1997. Double-blind placebo controlled trial with bromazepam in social phobia. *J. bras. Psiq*, **46**, 167–171.

Versiani, M., Nardi, A.E., Mundim, F.D., Alves, A.B., Liebowitz, M.R. and Amrein, R., 1992. Pharmacotherapy of social phobia. A controlled study with moclobemide and phenelzine. *British Journal of Psychiatry*, **161**, 353–360.

Vythilingum, B., Cartwright, C. and Hollander, E., 2000. Pharmacotherapy of obsessive–compulsive disorder: experience with the selective serotonin reuptake inhibitors. *International Clinical Psychopharmacology*, **15**, S7–13.

Wade, A.G., Lepola, U., Koponen, H.J., Pedersen, V. and Pedersen, T., 1997. The effect of citalopram in panic disorder. *British Journal of Psychiatry*, **170**, 549–553.

Wenzel, T., Griengl, H., Stompe, T., Mirzaei, S. and Kieffer, W., 2000. Psychological disorders in survivors of torture: exhaustion, impairment and depression. *Psychopathology*, **33**, 292–296.

Wheadon, D.E., Bushnell, W.D. and Steiner, M., 1993. A fixed dose comparison of 20, 40 or 60 mg paroxetine to placebo in the treatment of obsessive compulsive disorder. Presented at the 32nd Annual Meeting of the American College of Neuropsychopharmacology, 1993.

Wingerson, D., Nguyen, C. and Roy-Byrne, P.P., 1992. Clomipramine treatment for generalized anxiety disorder. *Journal of Clinical Psychopharmacology*, **12**, 214–215.

Wittchen, H.U., Kessler, R.C., Pfister, H. and Lieb, M., 2000. Why do people with anxiety disorders become depressed? A prospective-longitudinal community study. *Acta Psychiatrica Scandinavica Supplement*, 14–23.

Wittchen, H.U., Zhao, S., Kessler, R.C. and Eaton, W.W., 1994. DSM-III-R generalized anxiety disorder in the National Comorbidity Survey. *Archives of General Psychiatry*, **51**, 355–364.

Wolf, M.E., Alavi, A. and Mosnaim, A.D., 1988. Posttraumatic stress disorder in Vietnam veterans clinical and EEG findings; possible therapeutic effects of carbamazepine. *Biological Psychiatry*, **23**, 642–644.

Wolfe, R.M., 1997. Antidepressant withdrawal reactions. *American Family Physician*, **56**, 455–462.

Worthington, J.J., Pollack, M.H., Otto, M.W., McLean, R.Y., Moroz, G. and Rosenbaum, J.F., 1998. Long-term experience with clonazepam in patients with a primary diagnosis of panic disorder. *Psychopharmacology Bulletin*, **34**, 199–205.

Yonkers, K.A., Warshaw, M.G., Massion, A.O. and Keller, M.B., 1996. Phenomenology and course of generalised anxiety disorder. *British Journal of Psychiatry*, **168**, 308–313.

Zisook, S., Chentsova-Dutton, Y.E., Smith-Vaniz, A., Kline, N.A., Ellenor, G.L., Kodsi, A.B. and Gillin, J.C., 2000. Nefazodone in patients with treatment-refractory posttraumatic stress disorder. *Journal of Clinical Psychiatry*, **61**, 203–208.

Zohar, J. and Insel, T.R., 1987. Obsessive–compulsive disorder: psychobiological approaches to diagnosis, treatment, and pathophysiology. *Biological Psychiatry*, **22**, 667–687.

Zohar, J. and Judge, R., 1996. Paroxetine versus clomipramine in the treatment of obsessive–compulsive disorder. OCD Paroxetine Study Investigators. *British Journal of Psychiatry*, **169**, 468–474.

Zohar, J., Chopra, M., Sasson, Y., Amiaz, R. and Amital, D., 2000. Obsessive Compulsive Disorder: Serotonin and Beyond. *World Journal of Biological Psychiatry*, **1**, 92–100.

Psychobiology of Somatoform Disorders

Winfried Rief and Cornelia Exner

INTRODUCTION: UNEXPLAINED PHYSICAL SYMPTOMS AND THE HEALTH CARE SYSTEM

Unexplained physical symptoms are one of the major problems of the health care system. Depending on the medical setting under investigation, between 15% and 80% of doctor visits are due to persons with physical symptoms which cannot be accounted for by a clear organic cause. Most common symptoms are pains and aches, gastrointestinal complaints, and cardiovascular symptoms. Kroenke and Mangelsdorff (1989) demonstrated that only about 16% of the most common physical symptoms can be explained by a clear organic pathology. In their longitudinal study, patients with multiple unexplained physical symptoms and with an illness duration of more than four months had the worst prognosis. As will be shown below, unfortunately this is the most frequent combination of features in patients with somatoform disorders. Accordingly, this group of patients is one of the most expensive subgroups in the health care system. Fink (1992) analysed a subgroup of high utilizers of the health care system who had had at least ten inpatient treatments during the last eight years. He found that about 20% of these frequent hospitalizations were due to unexplained physical symptoms.

Some experts believe that illness behaviour is the most typical feature of somatization. Typical features of illness behaviour are frequent doctor visits, wandering around from doctor to doctor and from treatment unit to treatment unit, taking unnecessary medication, urging doctors to do unnecessary investigations which may lead to complications, avoidance behaviour and reduction of social activities, a high number of sick-leaves, and reduced social functioning. Health anxiety is a frequent, but not a necessary condition for the development and maintenance of unexplained physical symptoms. It is unclear whether these features are consequences of the disorder or else maintaining factors, or even the cause of additional physical problems.

Patients with somatoform disorders are also characterized by a specific cognitive–perceptual style. Barsky *et al.* (1993) emphasized that patients with hypochondriasis and somatoform symptoms have an over-exclusive concept of being healthy. They conceive health as a state of perfect physical well-being without any physical discomfort. However, physical discomfort is a common sensation even to healthy persons. Therefore persons with somatoform disorders are concerned about normal bodily perceptions; they focus their attention on bodily processes, which leads to an amplified perception of physical changes. This can encourage the interpretation of physical discomfort as illness symptoms.

While Barsky's concept of somatosensory amplification (Barsky and Wyshak, 1990) related primarily to patients with *hypochondriasis*, our own group demonstrated that patients with somatization syndromes without *hypochondriasis* also tend to catastrophize their perception of physical processes (Rief *et al.*, 1998). Patients with somatization syndromes have a bias to interpret minor physical changes (e.g., heart beat acceleration while taking a hot bath) as a possible sign of a severe illness (e.g., cardiomyopathy). This cognitive–perceptual style leads to the behavioural consequences described above. Moreover, the cognitive and behavioural features of somatization interact with biological properties of the disorder and maintain a vicious circle (see Figure XX.1). Affective consequences such as demoralization, negative affectivity, or depression might present a negative feedback loop that helps to maintain the problem.

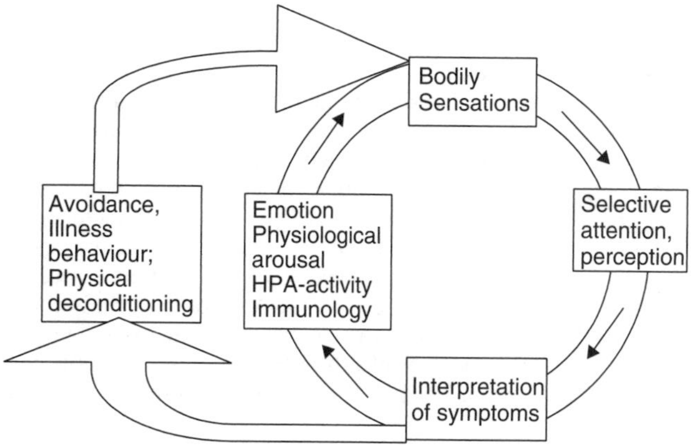

Figure XX.1 Somatization from a cognitive–psychobiological perspective (Rief and Nanke, 1999)

SYNDROMES OF SOMATIZATION AND THEIR CLASSIFICATION

The common feature of the somatoform disorders is the presence of physical symptoms which are not fully explained by a general medical condition, by the direct effect of a substance, or by another mental disorder. The symptoms must cause clinically significant distress or impairment in social functioning. Seeking medical help or para-medical consultation is very frequent. Historically, these syndromes have been labelled 'hysteria', a term which is presently less used because of stigmatizing effects.

Despite the fact that single physical complaints are very common, persons with multiple physical complaints represent the most serious subgroup for the health care system. The Diagnostic and Statistical Manual of Mental Disorders (DSM-IV) (APA, 1994) suggests the diagnosis of *somatization disorder* for polysymptomatic pictures of somatization. The disorder starts typically before age 30 years, extends over a period of years and is characterized by a

Biological Psychiatry: Edited by H. D'haenen, J.A. den Boer and P. Willner. ISBN 0-471-49198-5

combination of pain, gastrointestinal, sexual, and pseudoneurological symptoms. Eight physical symptoms out of a list of 33 suggested symptoms have to be present or had to be present in medical history. While persons with multiple somatoform symptoms are very frequent, especially in medical settings, they only rarely fulfil the complete criteria of *somatization disorder*. This is one of the most critical points concerning current classification rules of *somatization disorder*. Therefore, following DSM-IV, most patients with polysymptomatic somatoform complaints are diagnosed in the two rest categories *undifferentiated somatoform disorder* or *somatoform disorder not otherwise specified*.

Another subgroup of somatoform disorders refers to clinical pictures with a circumscribed physical symptomatology. The most frequent diagnosis of this subtype is *pain disorder*. To fulfil the criteria for this diagnosis, pain in one or more anatomical sites has to be the predominant focus of the clinical presentation; the pain causes clinically significant distress or impairment, and psychological factors are judged to have an important role in the onset, severity, exacerbation, or maintenance of pain. Especially for the diagnosis of *pain disorder*, it is nearly impossible to differentiate between the influence of psychological factors and a general medical condition. If both psychological factors and a general medical condition are judged to have important roles, the associated medical condition or anatomical site of the pain is coded on axis III. This also applies to pains where an underlying general medical condition is not yet clearly established, for example low back pain, pelvic pain, headache, joint pain, abdominal pain, and urinary pain.

Similar to pain disorder, *conversion disorder* is also characterized by circumscribed physical symptoms without sufficient organic explanation, but the typical symptoms involve voluntary motor or sensory functions. *Conversion disorder* typically suggests a neurological condition and is sometime difficult to diagnose with sufficient certainty.

The following diagnoses are not so much characterized by physical complaints, but by anxiety and cognitive preoccupations. The typical feature of *hypochondriasis* is health anxiety. The unwarranted fear or idea of having a disease persists despite medical reassurance. It can be very difficult to differentiate *hypochondriasis* from somatic delusions that may occur in psychotic disorders.

The essential feature of *body dysmorphic disorder* is the preoccupation with an imagined or exaggerated defect in physical appearance. If a slight physical anomaly is present, the person's concern is markedly excessive. While this disorder can have a dramatic course, and might have high health care relevance (e.g., cosmetic surgery), profound research relating to the condition is still rare.

Table XX.1 presents a brief guideline for the diagnostic process if a somatoform disorder is suspected. Following this guideline, three questions have to be answered.

- Does the patient describe a history of multiple somatoform complaints?
- Does the patient describe focussed, circumscribed symptoms?
- Is health anxiety or concern about the physical appearance a predominant feature?

SOMATIZATION-ASSOCIATED DISORDERS: OVERLAPPING OR DISTINCT FEATURES?

Unexplained physical symptoms are common in all disciplines of medicine. Accordingly, all disciplines have created unique terms for the description of patients with physical complaints which cannot be accounted for by a known medical condition. Examples are cephalgia, dorsalgia, recurrent abdominal pain, vulvodynia, hypomeralgia, chronic fatigue syndrome, fibromyalgia, irritable bowel syndrome, functional disorders, psychosomatic disorder, neurasthenia, multiple chemical sensitivity syndrome, somatized depression. It is

Table XX.1 The three major subgroups of somatoform disorders

Focus on multiple unexplained physical symptoms	Focus on single physical symptoms	Focus on anxiety or concerns
Somatization disorder (DSM-IV; ICD-10) Somatoform autonomic dysfunction (ICD-10)	Pain disorder (DSM-IV; ICD-10) Conversion disorder (DSM-IV; ICD-10) (Somatoform autonomic dysfunction; ICD-10)	Hypochondriasis (DSM-IV; ICD-10) Body dysmorphic disorder (DSM-IV)

Table XX.2 Case definitions for chronic fatigue syndrome

	CDC-1988	CDC-1994	Australia	UK
Minimum duration (month)	6	6	6	6
Functional impairment	50% decrease in activity	Substantial	Substantial	Disabling
Cognitive or neuropsychiatric symptoms	May be present	May be present	Required	Mental fatigue required
Other symptoms	6 or 8 required	4 required	Not specified	Not specified
New onset	Required	Required	Not required	Required
Medical exclusions	Extensive list of known physical causes	Clinically important	Known physical causes	Known physical causes
Psychiatric exclusions	Psychosis, bipolar disorder, substance abuse	Melancholic depression, substance abuse, bipolar disorders, psychosis, eating disorder	Psychosis, bipolar, substance abuse, eating disorder	Psychosis, bipolar, eating disorder, organic brain disease

obvious that there is an enormous overlap between these syndromes as well as with somatoform disorders. Despite the critique of current classification approaches to somatoform disorders, one of the major advantage of the new concept may be the provision of the one term 'somatoform' for a variety of related concepts. One common feature of all these syndromes is that although some symptoms may be the predominant focus of the clinical presentation, most of the patients also report many unspecific physical complaints. Buchwald and Garrity (1994) compared physical complaints of patients with chronic fatigue syndrome, fibromyalgia and multiple chemical sensitivity. Physical complaints that were common in chronic fatigue were also frequent symptoms of fibromyalgia and multiple chemical sensitivity. Wessely (1996) investigated the frequency of somatic symptoms in patients with chronic fatigue and reported that these patients described an enormous amount of unspecific physical complaints. The more chronic the fatigue syndrome was, the more physical complaints patients described.

To summarize, it seems that diagnoses such as fibromyalgia, chronic fatigue syndrome, multiple chemical sensitivity syndrome, etc. cannot be differentiated on the basis of somatic symptoms. The principal difference between these groups are theoretical assumptions on psychophysiological and psychobiological interactions. For some of these syndromes, well-established criteria have been defined which are useful for further research (see Table XX.2 for the example of CFS).

NEW APPROACHES TO THE CLASSIFICATION OF SOMATOFORM DISORDERS

There has been growing concern that current diagnostic concepts of *somatization disorder* fail to cover the large majority of patients presenting with unexplained somatic symptoms (Escobar *et al.*, 1989; Kroenke *et al.*, 1997). Several researchers have therefore suggested alternative diagnostic criteria for *somatization disorder* that require a smaller number of somatic symptoms and also take into consideration the higher symptom report rates of women (see below).

If the number of unexplained physical symptoms presented by the patient is the central diagnostic criterion, the first question is which symptom list should be used. Symptoms that are to be incorporated into a total score should have a sufficient base rate and a sufficient item–total correlation. In an empirical analysis Rief and Hiller (1999) demonstrated that many pseudoneurological symptoms do not fulfil these requirements. Moreover, sexual and menstruation symptoms had an insignificant item–total correlation which was due to unspecifity. These symptoms have comparable base rates in patients with somatization syndromes and in patients with other mental disorders. Our results suggest that for the diagnosis of polysymptomatic somatoform disorder one should focus on pain symptoms, gastrointestinal symptoms, cardiovascular symptoms and a reduced list of pseudoneurological symptoms.

Fink (1996) emphasized that symptom counting should not be the principal part of the diagnostic process, but that further psychological and psychobiological features should be considered, which might present additional aspects for the diagnosis of somatization disorder. In the following sections we will review the evidence concerning the possible psychobiological changes that underlie the chronic tendency to experience bodily complaints.

Abnormal Illness Behaviour

Pilowsky (1993) has outlined the concept of abnormal illness behaviour, which seems to be a predominant feature of somatization. The concept includes an abnormal behavioural reaction to physical discomfort. Doctor visits even for minor reasons, a continuous tendency to search for diagnostic evaluation and interventions, avoidance of physical demands, high number of sick-leave occasions are only some of these aspects.

Sustained Focussed Attention on Bodily Processes

Those patients with somatization syndrome show a tendency to focus attention on bodily processes. This internal attention focusing is often accompanied by a reduction of interests for external events.

Catastrophizing Interpretation of Bodily Sensations

Patients with *hypochondriasis* show a general tendency to misinterpret bodily sensations as evidence for physical illness (Barsky *et al.*, 1993; Rief *et al.*, 1998). While healthy controls can generate many normal attributions for bodily sensations, somatizing patients have a bias towards using only catastrophizing interpretations.

Self-Concept of Being Weak

Many somatizing patients (yet not all) have a self-concept of being weak which is not founded on a physical basis (Rief *et al.*, 1998). A self-concept of being weak is highly associated with disability and abnormal illness behaviour.

Following these empirical analyses, we proposed the diagnosis of *polysymptomatic somatoform disorder*. To fulfil criteria, persons should describe at least seven to eight physical symptoms affecting multiple body sites during the past two years. At least one of the psychological factors which had been mentioned above should be present as a maintaining factor. Further criteria resemble DSM-IV criteria of *somatization disorder* (symptoms not sufficiently explained by any pathological physical condition; symptoms cause clinically significant distress, etc.).

Escobar and colleagues (Escobar *et al.*, 1987, 1989) suggested using the Somatic Symptom Index (SSI) as a classification approach. The criteria for SSI-4/6 are fulfilled if men have at least four physical symptoms and women at least six physical symptoms out of the list of 35 somatoform symptoms suggested for DSM-III-*somatization disorder*. The SSI-4/6 concept of Escobar has been used in a number of studies. However, there are concerns that it may be over-inclusive and the empirical basis of this concept still needs to be improved. Kroenke *et al.* (1997) suggested a new diagnosis of *multisomatoform disorder*. The criteria for this disorder were derived from primary care studies. Patients have to present with at least three current somatoform symptoms out of a 15-symptom checklist along with at least a two-year history of somatoform symptoms. The 15 physical symptoms were chosen because they account for more than 90% of outpatient visits attributable to physical complaints. The major advantage of the Kroenke approach is its feasibility for use in primary care.

COMORBIDITY PATTERNS

Already centuries ago the high overlap between unexplained physical symptoms and depression/melancholia was described (Burton, 1621). Kielholz (1973) has postulated that depression may be the underlying disorder in many patients with bodily complaints, and that functional physical symptoms might be just epiphenomena. Empirical analyses of comorbidity patterns underline the close association of depression and somatization syndrome. In 90–100% of patients seeking help in health care settings and fulfilling the complete criteria of *somatization disorder* a comorbid affective disorder can be found. A history of major depression is reported by 65–80%

Table XX.3 Comorbidity diagnoses of distressed high users of primary care (Katon *et al.*, 1991)

Somatization syndrome	Major depression (lifetime)	Panic disorder (lifetime)
<SSI-4/6	45%	3%
SSI-4/6	75%	20%
SSI-9	71%	19%
Somatization disorder	82%	48%

of patients with *somatization disorder* (Katon *et al.*, 1991; Rief *et al.*, 1996). Despite these findings, the association between somatization and depression should be interpreted with caution. First, high prevalence of comorbid depression (especially in patients in health care settings) is not only common in somatization, but also in most other mental disorders (anxiety disorders, eating disorders and others). Second, the stricter the criteria applied for the diagnosis of *somatization disorder*, the higher is the base rate of comorbid depression (Katon *et al.*, 1991; Hiller *et al.*, 1995). Third, onset and course of depression are quite different from onset and course of somatization with somatoform symptoms having an earlier onset and very frequently a stable and chronic course (Rief *et al.*, 1992). And fourth, there seem to be significant psychobiological differences between depression and somatization, as will be shown in subsequent sections.

Somatization is not only associated with depression, but patients with somatization syndromes are at increased risk also for other disorders. There seems to be a close link to anxiety disorders (Rief *et al.*, 1996). In some studies, patients with *hypochondriasis* showed higher comorbidity rates with anxiety than with affective disorders (Barsky *et al.*, 1992). Therefore *hypochondriasis* was suggested to represent the link between somatoform disorders and anxiety disorders. Other authors emphasize the association of *hypochondriasis* and *body dysmorphic disorder* with obsessive–compulsive disorder (Starcevic, 1990; Simeon *et al.*, 1995; Bienvenu *et al.*, 2000).

Table XX.3 presents comorbidity patterns of somatoform disorders with other mental disorders. Summarizing these results, it seems that somatization, anxiety and depression (as well as other features) are risk factors one for the other.

EPIDEMIOLOGY

Patients who present with multiple physical symptoms that lack an adequate somatic explanation are commonly seen in primary care settings (Rief *et al.*, 2001). This is in contrast to the low prevalence rates of somatoform disorders according to current diagnostic systems (ICD-10 and DSM-IV). Depending on study design, diagnostic criteria (ICD-10 versus DSM-IV) and catchment area *somatization disorder* is estimated to have a lifetime prevalence between 0.03% and 3% (Escobar *et al.*, 1989; Gureje *et al.*, 1997). If less restrictive concepts are used for *somatization disorder* (SSI 4/6 or 3/5), prevalence rates are in the range of 10–20% in the general population (Escobar *et al.*, 1989; Rief *et al.*, 1996, 2001; Gureje *et al.*, 1997).

Reliable information on the prevalence rates of other diagnostic subgroups of somatoform disorders is still lacking. Hypochondrial concerns are present in at least 10–15% of the general population (Kroenke and Spitzer, 1998; Rief *et al.*, 2001). However, only 1–4% meet full diagnostic criteria for *hypochondriasis* (Faravelli *et al.*, 1997; Gureje *et al.*, 1997; Kroenke and Spitzer, 1998).

Pain is probably the most frequent complaint in medical practice. In a representative German sample, for instance, up to 30% of subjects complained about back pain in the last two years (Rief *et al.*, 2001). Pain symptoms often lack an adequate medical explanation. However, little is known about the prevalence of *somatoform pain disorder* according to current diagnostic criteria and reported rates vary from under 1% up to 5% in the general population (Gureje and Obikoya, 1992; Faravelli *et al.*, 1997).

Body dysmorphic disorder (BDD) affects approximately 1% of the general population; however, this is thought to be an underestimate because BDD is frequently underdiagnosed. In clinical populations the frequency might be much higher. Thirteen per cent of psychiatric inpatients were reported to suffer from BDD (Grant *et al.*, 2001). In dermatological patients and those seeking cosmetic surgery the rate of BDD was estimated to be between 7% and 12% (Sarwer *et al.*, 1998; Phillips *et al.*, 2000).

Reported prevalence rates of *conversion disorder* vary widely, ranging from 11/100,000 to 300/100,000 according to DSM-IV. However, in neurological patients the prevalence rates have been reported to be as high as 20% (Mace and Trimble, 1991).

GENDER EFFECTS

Unexplained physical symptoms have consistently been shown to be more frequent in women than in men (Piccinelli and Simon, 1997; Kroenke and Spitzer, 1998; Ladwig *et al.*, 2000; Rief *et al.*, 2001). Kroenke and Spitzer (1998) for instance reported the results of a mental health survey in 1000 primary care patients in the USA. Results showed that physical symptoms in general and somatoform symptoms more specifically were more common in women than in men. Odds ratios adjusted for age, race, education, medical and psychiatric comorbidity were in the range of 1.5 to 2.5. Although anxiety and depression were both strongly associated with symptom reporting the effect of gender on symptom reporting was independent of psychiatric comorbidity. While women in the general population are approximately twice as likely as men to report physical symptoms that lack an adequate somatic explanation the ratio shifts even more to the female side when only patients are considered who fully meet diagnostic criteria for a somatoform disorder. The DSM-IV reports female prevalence rates for *somatization* and *conversion disorder* to be up to 10 times higher in women than in men. However, hypercondriacal concerns in the general population as well as prevalence rates for *hypochondriasis* according to DSM-IV or ICD-10 appear to be equally frequent in women as in men (Gureje *et al.*, 1997; Kroenke and Spitzer, 1998). Men are also as likely as women to suffer from *body dysmorphic disorder*; whilst symptom localization and comorbidity patterns vary between male and female patients (Perugi *et al.*, 1997; Phillips and Diaz, 1997).

The elevated frequency of somatoform symptoms in women has been explained by several authors in terms of a biopsychosocial model of symptom perception (Pennebaker, 1982; Gijsberg van Wijk and Kolk, 1997). Accordingly, symptoms do not just result from the passive registration of bodily changes but are modulated by cognitive processes that guide attention to and the attribution of somatic information. In women there might be simply more somatic information to begin with. The female reproductive process itself produces much physical information that is absent in men. It might further exert an influence on pain perception thresholds that have been shown to be lower in women (Riley *et al.*, 1998) and to vary with the menstrual circle (Riley *et al.*, 1999). Attention towards physical symptoms, attributions applied to them and the willingness to report them to medical professionals might be further influenced by differences between women and men in socialization, sex roles and social position.

NEUROIMAGING STUDIES

Functional Neuroimaging Studies

As somatoform disorders are by their very definition thought to lack an adequate somatic explanation little research has been done to elicit possible neurophysiological abnormalities associated with this type of disorder. Tiihonen *et al.* (1995) reported the case of a 32-year-old woman with a conversive left-sided paralysis and paraesthesiae who had a single photon emission tomography (SPECT) carried out during the electric stimulation of the median nerve of her affected hand. Altered cerebral blood flow was observed with hyperfusion of the right frontal and hypofusion of the right parietal region. After recovery from her conversive symptoms cerebral blood flow measures returned to normal. Results were interpreted as reflecting a simultaneous activation of frontal inhibitory areas and inhibition of somatosensory cortex. A further case study by Marshall *et al.* (1997) reported the case of a 45-year-old woman with left-sided paralysis but without somatosensory loss in whom no organic lesion had been found. Brain activity was studied by positron emission tomography (PET) when the patient prepared to move and tried to move her paralysed (left) leg. Her good (right) leg was used as a control condition. Preparing to move or moving her good leg, and also preparing to move her paralysed leg activated motor and/or premotor areas previously described as participating in movement preparation and execution. However, the attempt to move the paralysed leg failed to activate right primary motor cortex. Instead, the right orbitofrontal and right anterior cingulate cortex were significantly activated. These areas are known from previous studies in both animals and humans as 'negative motor areas' which play a crucial role in the suppression of inappropriate motor responses (Lüders *et al.*, 1995). The interpretation was put forward by Marshall *et al.* (1997) that these two frontal areas inhibited (willed) effects on the right primary motor cortex when the patient tried to move her left leg. Interestingly, the results of their study were paralleled by those of a single case study of brain activity during hypnotic paralysis. Using an identical PET design Halligan *et al.* (2000) showed that hypnotic paralysis activated similar brain areas (orbitofrontal and anterior cingulate areas) as conversive paralysis, supporting the view that hypnosis and *conversion disorder* might share common neurophysiological mechanisms.

Both prefrontal and right parietal regions are thought to be components of a distributed neural network that integrates processes of attention and awareness (Parasuraman, 1998). Thus, the results of the studies cited above are consistent with the notion that altered inhibitory mechanisms at high levels of sensory and motor processing play a role in the formation of conversive symptoms. However, findings to date are far from forming a clear picture: Yazíci and Kostakoglu (1998) reported the results of five cases suffering from bilateral conversive symptoms (astasia-abasia) who had SPECT performed at rest. Perfusion decreases were found in left temporal and parietal areas. As symptoms were bilateral in all their cases and no activation paradigm was applied it is difficult to compare the results of Yazíci and Kostakoglu (1998) to those of Tiihonen *et al.* (1995) and Marshall *et al.* (1997). Even more care is warranted when trying to generalize neuroimaging findings in *conversion disorder* to other somatoform disorders. Studies in *somatization disorder* patients so far have yielded inconclusive results: James *et al.* (1987) reported regional cerebral blood flow changes in 14 patients with *somatization disorder* who performed a visual matching task known to activate predominantly the right hemisphere. Compared to controls they exhibited a slightly higher right posterior activation. This was interpreted as indicating a hyperactivity of the right hemisphere and the right posterior region in particular and possibly reflecting disturbed processes of selective attention. However, in a recent SPECT study of 11 cases with *somatization disorder* Garcia-Campayo *et al.* (2001) found right hemisphere or bilateral hypoperfusion in different brain areas in the majority of their patients under resting conditions. No control group was studied and no activation paradigm was applied. The seemingly contradictory results highlight the necessity for further research in this field studying larger numbers of carefully diagnosed patients under both resting and activation conditions.

To sum up, the only conclusion that can safely be drawn from functional neuroimaging findings so far is that alternations in regional cerebral blood flow accompany the expression of physical symptoms in *conversion disorder* and *somatization disorder*. These changes might be related to altered processes of attention and awareness in sensory and motor processing.

Structural Neuroimaging Studies

Again, as the definition of somatoform disorder excludes the presence of organic brain disease only few attempts have been made to discover the prevalence of (subtle) structural changes in the brains of patients with somatoform disorders. There is, however, one related condition to which structural brain imaging techniques have been applied. *Chronic fatigue syndrome* (CFS) is a debilitating multisystem condition of unknown origin. Attempts have been made to relate the clinical findings to structural changes in the brain of affected individuals but have so far yielded ambiguous results. Some researchers found an increased frequency of white matter intensities (WMI) in MRI studies of CFS patients compared to normal age-matched controls (Buchwald *et al.*, 1992; Natelson *et al.*, 1993; Schwartz *et al.*, 1994). However, others found no differences in the frequency of WMIs between CFS patients and controls (Cope *et al.*, 1995; Greco *et al.*, 1997). Reported frequencies of white matter lesions in CFS varied greatly from 8% (Cope *et al.*, 1995) to 78% (Buchwald *et al.*, 1992) depending on catchment area, age of subjects and the presence of associated disorders. Even those investigators who found increased frequencies of white matter lesions could not identify a specific pattern of radiological abnormalities and doubt their clinical usefulness (Schwartz *et al.*, 1994). The unspecific and subjective nature of the disease combined with the absence of a known causal agent and pathognomonic abnormalities makes the condition difficult to diagnose. Thus, it seems questionable whether the different investigation carried out even related to the same population of patients.

With relation to *conversion disorder* there is some evidence that lesions of the left hemisphere may present a predisposition for the development of conversive symptoms. Drake (1993) reported that patients who had sustained left hemisphere injuries or infarctions were at greater risk of developing conversion symptoms later in life.

NEUROPSYCHOLOGICAL ASPECTS

Circumstantial evidence for disturbed brain function in somatoform disorders could derive from findings of neuropsychological deficits in affected patients. Indeed, patients with unexplained physical symptoms frequently complain of cognitive deficits such as fatigue, lack of concentration and memory failure. However, little is known about how patients with somatoform disorders perform on standardized neuropsychological tests. Patients suffering from *body dysmorphic disorder* (BDD) have been reported to show performance deficits on verbal and non-verbal learning and memory tests compared to healthy controls (Deckersbach *et al.*, 2000). Learning and memory deficits in BDD patients seemed especially due to their poor organizational strategies, an aspect of memory processing that is attributed to the frontal lobes. These findings were similar to patterns previously observed in obsessive–compulsive disorder (OCD) and could thus point to the possible relationship between BDD and OCD that has repeatedly been suggested by other investigators (Bienvenu *et al.*, 2000). Further and more direct evidence for this claim comes from the study of Hanes (1998). BDD patients in this study were directly compared to OCD patients and both groups were found to show a similar pattern of neuropsychological performance. Patients with BDD showed normal performance on memory and motor tasks but were significantly impaired relative to normal controls on tests of executive functions, thus again pointing to the frontal lobes as a possible site of disturbances.

Flor-Henry *et al.* (1981) investigated cognitive functioning in 10 subjects with 'hysteria', who according to current diagnostic criteria would have been seen as suffering from *somatization disorder*. Ninety per cent of the test profiles of somatization patients were judged as 'abnormal' according to Reitan's approach (Reitan and Davison, 1974), thus suggestive of cerebral dysfunction. The somatization group was characterized by deficits on tests of sensorimotor, executive and visuospatial function. The test variables that best discriminated somatization patients from controls were Colored Progressive Matrices, Finger Localization (preferred hand) and Verbal Associative Learning. On the basis of these findings the authors concluded that dominant hemisphere dysfunction is related to the symptom of hysteria (today: *somatization disorder*). The high prevalence of cognitive impairment in somatization patients in the study of Flor-Henry *et al.* (1981) has never been replicated and might be partly due to the definition of 'abnormal' test profiles applied in this study. Further investigations of cognitive performance in patients with *somatization disorder* seem mandatory to clarify how prevalent objective cognitive deficits are in somatization patients.

Complaints about cognitive deficits mainly in the area of memory and concentration are also a core feature of *chronic fatigue syndrome* (CFS), a condition often seen as belonging to the 'somatoform spectrum' disorders. Any understanding, however, of the cognitive problems in CFS has to take account of the frequent comorbidity of CFS and depression. Affective disorders themselves are known to cause cognitive deficits (Murphy and Sahakian, 2001). In a recent review Wearden and Appleby (1996) reported that non-depressed CFS patients, although showing mild cognitive impairments, performed within normal limits on various standard neuropsychological tests. In most investigations they did not significantly differ from healthy controls. If impaired at all, CFS patients showed a tendency to perform slower especially on more complex and effortful tasks but there was no evidence for excessive fatigueability. On the basis of the current evidence Wearden and Appleby (1996) concluded that mild cognitive problems in CFS patients are unlikely to relate to grossly altered brain function; instead, psychological variables like motivation, effort, mood and arousal are likely to be involved in the explanation.

LATERALIZATION OF SYMPTOMS

The debate over whether unilateral somatization and conversion symptoms are lateralized dates back to the 1970s and has not yet led to any conclusive result. Psychogenic somatization symptoms in different psychiatric conditions (anxiety, depression, somatoform disorders) have been reported to occur more frequently on the left side of the body (Axelrod *et al.*, 1980; Min and Lee, 1997). Left-sided lateralization of conversion symptoms has been found by Stern (1977) and more recently by Pascuzzi (1994). Galin *et al.* (1977) also found a prevalence of left-sided conversion symptoms but for females only. However, others have found a predominantly right-sided lateralization of symptoms in *conversion disorders* in children (Regan and LaBabera, 1984) and adults (Fallik and Sigal, 1971) or no lateralization of symptoms (Keane, 1989; Roelofs *et al.*, 2000). Apart from the ambiguous results the integration of the existing findings on lateralization of somatoform symptoms is further complicated by differences in sample sizes, patient selection and symptom definition.

Different hypotheses have been put forward to explain the predominantly left-sided lateralization of conversion and somatization symptoms. The *evaluative hypothesis* suggests that the left side of the body is associated with negative connotations and might therefore be the preferred site for the development of somatization (bad) symptoms. This symbolic interpretation has received little empirical support. The *convenience hypothesis* claims that symptoms develop on that side of the body where they cause the least inconvenience. This would predict a left-sided predominance in right-handers and vice versa. However, this claim is contradicted by the finding that left-sided symptoms occur more frequently in both left- and right-handed patients (Galin *et al.*, 1977; Stern, 1977). By the same token, one could also propose the opposite of the convenience hypothesis, namely that symptoms are more frequently on the right side just because they are more incapacitating there and require more attention (Fallik and Sigal, 1971; Regan and LaBabera, 1984). Right-sided lateralization has also been explained as being related to *previous organic lesions* which more often occur on the dominant side of the body (Fallik and Sigal, 1971). Again, this claim is contradicted by the lack of any consistent relation between handedness and lateralization of symptoms. The predominant theory today explains symptom lateralization to the left side in terms of *hemispheric specialization* (Sierra and Berrios, 1999; Roelofs *et al.*, 2000). The right inferior parietal cortex is believed to be involved in higher-order processes of attention and awareness (Parasuraman, 1998). Disturbances of this system might thus compromise sensory and motor processing on the contralateral side of the body. This theory would also allow for the incorporation of current functional imaging findings (Tiihonen *et al.*, 1995; Marshall *et al.*, 1997; Halligan *et al.*, 2000). However, it does not seem necessary to restrict the proposed effects of a dysfunctional right-sided attention and awareness system to the contralateral body side.

To summarize, more investigations of symptom manifestation in somatoform disorder using representative samples are necessary to resolve the question of symptom lateralization. It seems important to stress that most patients suffer from symptoms that are not restricted or not attributable to only one side of the body and any explanation of a possible 'conversion' mechanism has to account for this fact (Roelofs *et al.*, 2000).

GENE–ENVIRONMENT INTERACTIONS

The aetiology and pathogenesis of somatoform disorders are still not well understood. It has been shown that adverse environmental factors such as low socioeconomic background, childhood experiences of death and illness, exposure to traumatic events or high levels of current stress increase the risk for the development of somatoform disorders (Hartvig and Sterner, 1985; Whitehead, 1994; Binzer *et al.*, 1997). There is also evidence that hereditary factors have some influence. Familial aggregation for somatization (Briquet's syndrome) has been reported for women but not for men (Cloninger *et al.*, 1986). Higher concordance rates for somatoform disorders in monozygotic than in dizygotic twins (29% vs. 10%) have been reported in a Norwegian twin study (Torgersen, 1986). However, the differences failed to reach statistical significance and shared environmental influences might have influenced the concordance rates. All the concordant pairs consisted of partners with two different somatoform disorders pointing to an aetiologic and nosologic similarity of the different subtypes of somatoform disorders.

The study further found a high frequency of anxiety disorders, especially generalized anxiety disorders, in the co-twins of somatoform disorder twins.

Familial aggregation and twin studies alone do not provide unequivocal evidence for a genetic aetiology, as shared environmental influences might be responsible for higher frequency of psychiatric disorders in the families of affected patients. More direct evidence can be drawn from adoption studies. A Swedish adoption study using the medical history data of female adoptees found an increased prevalence of alcohol abuse and antisocial behaviour in the biological fathers of somatizing women (Bohman *et al.*, 1984). The results confirmed those of earlier family studies suggesting that somatoform disorders in women and some forms of alcohol abuse and antisocial behaviour in men might share common aetiological factors.

Genetic–epidemiological approaches may also help in clarifying the relationship between somatoform disorders and other comorbid psychiatric diagnoses that are often diagnosed in the same individual. Recent studies suggest that *somatization disorder* and symptoms of anxiety and depression do not share a common genetic background (Battaglia *et al.*, 1995; Gillespie *et al.*, 2000).

The advantages of molecular biology offer new tools for studying those variations in genes and matching gene products that might be responsible for the genetic transmission of psychiatric diseases. So far, little is known about which part of the genome might hold candidate genes related to the aetiology of somatoform disorders. However, a number of the studies point to the involvement of the serotonin transmitter system in *fibromyalgia*, a syndrome of generalized muscular pain which shares clinical features with both *pain disorder* and depression. In patients with fibromyalgia the genotype distributions for both the 5-HT2A receptor gene and the serotonin transporter gene have been found to differ from healthy controls (Bondy *et al.*, 1999; Offenbacher *et al.*, 1999). These results suggest that altered serotonergic neural transmission might present a genetically transmitted vulnerability for the disorder.

NEUROTRANSMITTER SYSTEMS

The serotonergic system has repeatedly been discussed to be involved in the pathophysiology of somatoform disorders and related syndromes. Reduction of central serotonergic transmission has been linked to the pathogenesis of *pain disorder*. This notion is based first on the analgesic effects of tricyclic antidepressants and second on reports of reduced activity of the peripheral and central serotonin system (Van Kempen *et al.*, 1992). Serum levels of serotonin (5-hydroxytryptamine, 5-HT), its precursor tryptophan and its main metabolite 5-hydroxyindoleacetic acid (5-HIAA) have also been found to be decreased in patients suffering from *fibromyalgia*. Schwartz *et al.* (1999) found low levels of 5-HIAA and tryptophan to be related to higher pain scores and lower serum concentration of 5-HIAA to be associated with reduced quality of sleep in fibromyalgia patients. There was also a tendency of higher pain scores to be related to higher serum concentrations of the neuropeptide substance P, pointing to the antagonism of substance P and the serotonergic system in nociception. In a recent review Russell (1998) discussed the findings of low 5-HT and high substance P concentrations as signs of a pain amplification syndrome in fibromyalgia. The aetiology of *body dysmorphic disorder*, another somatoform disorder, has also been related to poor regulation and depletion of serotonin (Craven and Rodin, 1987; Barr *et al.*, 1992). However, altered serotonin physiology might be either a consequence or a marker of the disorder.

Current concepts of stress research point to the importance of the monoaminergic neurotransmitters for the response to and adaptation to acute and chronic stressful events. As emotional distress has been shown to be a powerful predictor of somatic complaints across gender, different age groups and different cultures (Piccinelli and Simon, 1997) one would predict that the monoaminergic neurotransmitter system should be involved in the pathophysiology of somatoform disorders. So far, there is only circumstantial evidence to support this claim. Gjerris *et al.* (1987) found CSF adrenaline but not noradrenaline levels to be reduced in 'somatizing' depressive patients. CSF adrenaline concentration was related to ratings of somatic anxiety symptoms and *hypochondriasis* on the Hamilton Depression Scale.

Taken together, most support is there for the involvement of the serotonergic neurotransmitter system in somatoform disorders especially those that are characterized by altered pain perception and obsessive–compulsive features. However, there seem to be few results specific to somatoform disorders as alternations in serotonergic transmission have been shown for other psychiatric conditions such as depression, anxiety, obsessive–compulsive disorder and eating disorders.

ENDOCRINOLOGICAL ASPECTS

Studies on endocrinological aspects of unexplained physical symptoms focus on the activity of the hypothalamic–pituitary–adrenal axis (HPA-axis). Parallels to post-traumatic stress disorder have been drawn as many patients with unexplained physical symptoms report traumatic experiences. Heim *et al.* (1998) examined women with chronic pelvic pain and analysed diurnal salivary cortisol levels and hormonal responses to a corticotropin-releasing factor (CRF) stimulation test as well as a low-dose dexamethasone suppression test. Women with chronic pelvic pain had increased prevalences of abuse experiences and post-traumatic stress disorder. Analysing endocrinological parameters, the authors found normal to low diurnal salivary cortisol levels, normal ACTH, but reduced salivary cortisol levels in the CRF stimulation test. The suppression of cortisol concentrations after dexamethasone was enhanced in patients with chronic pelvic pain.

Taking into account the tendency towards increased cortisol scores in depressive patients, the results for chronically stressed persons with syndromes other than depression are quite surprising. Pruessner *et al.* (1999) demonstrated that the associations between stress and cortisol are not as straightforward as had been thought earlier. In their study, perceived stress correlated with an increase of cortisol levels during the first hour after awakening. However, the overall cortical secretion of persons scoring high on burn-out scales showed lower cortisol concentrations on all sampling days in that study. Therefore the authors postulated differential effect of burn-out and perceived stress on HPA-access regulation.

Other studies have confirmed an association between vital exhaustion and lower basal cortisol levels (e.g., Nicolson and van Diest, 2000). These and other results stimulated Heim *et al.* (1998) to postulate a theory of hypocortisolism in the pathophysiology of stress-related bodily disorders. Chronic or very intense stress may lead to a hypoactivity of the HPA-axis. The authors assume that cortisol may have a protective function; a lack of these protective properties may be of relevance for the development of bodily disorders in chronically stressed individuals.

However, the finding of low cortisol scores in patients with unexplained physical symptoms is not as consistent as might be supposed. For chronic fatigue syndrome patients, Scott and Dinan (1998) confirmed lower urinary free cortisol excretion, while Scott *et al.* (1998) and Young *et al.* (1998) found normal cortisol scores in chronic fatigue patients. Vingerhoets *et al.* (1996) found a tendency towards lower cortisol levels in persons who described many stress-related bodily complaints, whereas Rief and Auer (2000) found normal urinary cortisol, normal salivary cortisol and normal serum cortisol after dexamethasone suppression tests for persons with somatization syndrome. In another study of Rief *et al.* (1998) we even found increased scores for salivary cortisol in somatizing patients. This effect was still evident after controlling for depression. Results contradictory to the hypocortisolism theory were also reported for persons with burn-out syndrome (Melamed *et al.*, 1999).

Therefore, the theory of hypocortisolism in the pathophysiology of stress-related bodily disorders has less empirical support than proposed by Heim *et al.* (2000). Measurement artefacts, differences in study design, or differences in comorbidity patterns of examined samples might account in part for these discrepancies. If a tendency towards reduced cortisol concentrations in somatoform disorders is confirmed in the future, it is likely to be a rather weak effect.

Neeck and Riedel (1999) presented a sophisticated outline of hormonal perturbations in fibromyalgia syndrome. According to their opinion, fibromyalgia is characterized not only by pain in defined points of the musculoskeletal system, but also by numerous additional somatoform and psychological symptoms. The authors claim that not only the HPA-axis may be deregulated in fibromyalgia, but also other hormonal axes (the thyroid system, regulation of growth hormone, and other parameters). Therefore they conclude that there must be a higher-order central rather than a peripheral origin causing perturbations of the hormonal axes. They favour a model in which hypothalamic CRH neurons play a key role not only in 'resetting' the various endocrine loops, but possibly also in regulating nociceptive and psychological mechanisms as well.

Some other studies have analysed peptides in patients with functional physical symptoms or associated disorders. Jonsson *et al.* (1998) analysed gastrin, cholecystokinin, and somatostatin in blood samples of patients with functional dyspepsia. Mean hormone values did not differ between patients with functional dyspepsia and a matched healthy control sample. Patients with a high degree of dyspeptic symptoms during the week preceding the experiment had a higher mean somatostatin level than patients with a lower degree of dyspeptic symptoms. During a stress interview, cholecystokinin levels increased in patients with functional dyspepsia, but not in controls. Somatostatin increased significantly earlier in patients than in control subjects during the stress interview. Therefore the authors postulated that cholecystokinin and somatostatin may possibly link psychological reactions to the pathophysiology of functional dyspepsia. Maes *et al.* (1998) analysed prolyl endopeptidase and dipepetidyl peptidase IV in patients with fibromyalgia. They found lower serum prolyl endopeptidase in patients with fibromyalgia than in normal volunteers. Moreover, they also described significant negative correlations between serum prolyl endopeptidase and severity of pressure hyperalgesia.

Unfortunately, for patients who were classified according to the somatoform disorders section of DSM-IV, studies on peptides are so far lacking.

IMMUNOLOGICAL ASPECTS

One of the conceptual precursors of somatoform disorders, neurasthenia, was assumed to be triggered by viral infections and other diseases. Hundreds of years later, the terminus *chronic fatigue syndrome* was created and it was postulated that viral infection and subsequent immunological processes may be underlying pathophysiological mechanisms leading to the complaints. While a uniform viral aetiology of chronic fatigue syndrome has been questioned in the following years (for an overview see Wessely *et al.*, 1999), there is convincing evidence to postulate a close link between immunological processes and the perception of physical complaints. The possible trigger function of viral infections continues to be a topic of research. For example, White *et al.* (1998) demonstrated that glandular fever is a risk factor for the development of acute and chronic fatigue syndromes, whereas ordinary upper respiratory tract infections are not (Wessely *et al.*, 1999). White (1997) summarized that specific infections can trigger chronic fatigue syndromes, but these syndromes are not maintained by the infectious agent itself, but by the patient's subsequent maladaptation. This maladaptation may be mediated by changes in sleep patterns, physical deconditioning, and endocrine and immune system changes.

One of the core features of somatization is the patient's belief and self-perception of being sick. This provides a link to the body of immunological research which focuses on 'sickness behaviour'. Sickness behaviour is characterized by reduced activity, a reduction of social interactions and sexual drive and the development of depressed mood. Interestingly, the administration of cytokines in the absence of infection produces the full syndrome of sickness behaviour. For example, all symptoms of sickness were produced by human interleukin-1b administered within rat hippocampus (Linthorst *et al.*, 1994).

Illness behaviour in somatoform disorders is phenomenologically characterized by reduced physical activity, reduced social interactions, and reduced exploration behaviour. As these features are also behavioural correlates of the acute phase-response, a close link between immunological parameters of the acute phase and the symptoms of somatoform disorders can be postulated.

Circumstantial evidence for a relationship between somatization and immunological processes is provided by the stress-dependency of immune processes. Stressors lead to increases in the levels of cytokines circulating in the blood, with IL-6 being the most frequently measured (Maier and Watkins, 1998). Moreover, several reports document the role of IL-1 in the stress response, as well as increased TNF-alpha levels following stress. Thus, both primary as well as secondary cytokines are induced *in vivo* as well as *in vitro* by stressors (Black and Berman, 1999). On the other hand, acute and chronic stressors as well as low stress tolerance are typical concomitants of somatoform syndromes.

Apart from illness behaviour and stress, there is a third line of evidence suggesting a link between somatoform disorders and immune activity. This is the interaction between immunological processes and pain sensitivity. Immune stimulation seems to activate both analgesia and hyperalgesia circuitry (Maier and Watkins, 1998). Stress-induced analgesia is a very rapid response, whereas hyperalgesia follows infectious or inflammatory processes much more slowly. The peripheral administration of LPS or IL-1 results in an increase in pain sensitivity (Watkins *et al.*, 1995). Altered pain sensitivity can lead to the perception of minor physical changes that otherwise would have gone unnoticed. These results could present a framework for research into the relationship between immune system activity and somatization.

Most of the approaches outlined above postulate increased levels of proinflammatory substances in patients with somatization. Moreover, elevated levels of proinflammatory cytokines have been found for the most frequent comorbid psychiatric disorder, major depression (Maes *et al.*, 1997). Neopterin is one of the metabolically stable markers for inflammation. In some (but not all) studies, plasma neopterin levels have been increased in major depression. Bell *et al.* (1998) found that serum neopterin is correlated with variables of somatization. However, this association was only found in a subgroup of persons with chemical intolerance, not in a subgroup of patients with depression or in normal controls.

Substance P, a neuropeptide which is involved in communication between the nervous and the immune system, seems to play a major role in the process of nociception. As outlined above, nociception and alternations of pain sensitivity can be a central process involved in the development of somatoform symptoms. Elevated levels of

Table XX.4 Immunological aspects of somatization (data from Rief *et al.* (2001) and similar studies)

Parameter	Somatization	Depression
IL-6	Reduced	Increased
IL-6R	Reduced	Reduced
IL-1	Unclear	Increased
IL-1RA	Increased	Slightly increased
CD-8 cell count	Reduced	Increased

substance P have been found in cerebrospinal fluid of patients with fibromyalgia. In some studies, there was an association between substance P serum concentrations and pain in fibromyalgia patients (Schwartz *et al.*, 1999). However, a direct investigation of substance P in patients with a DSM-IV diagnosis of somatoform disorders is still lacking.

In a study of Rief *et al.* (2001) we examined serum concentrations of immunological parameters. A total of 150 persons were divided into a subgroup of patients with major depression, patients with somatization, patients with depression and somatization, and healthy controls. Patients with multiple somatoform symptoms were characterized by reduced IL-6 concentrations, increased IL-6R concentrations, increased IL-1RA concentrations and increased concentrations of the anti-cytokine Clara cell protein CC16. Moreover, the T-lymphocyte CD-8 count was reduced for somatizing patients, while patients with major depression had increased scores in comparison to controls. This is one of the few studies comparing multiple clinical groups and providing information about the specificity of the results. To summarize, there is some evidence that immunological processes may be differentially affected in major depression and somatization. In our study we found signs of increased proinflammatory capacity in depression, while some indicators were found for anti-inflammatory capacity in somatization (see Table XX.4).

As the preceding paragraphs highlight, there are reasons for investigating the interaction of immune parameters and somatoform symptoms. To date, only a few studies have been carried out, and we are just at the beginning of understanding these associations.

PSYCHOPHYSIOLOGICAL ASPECTS

Autonomic and Peripheral Physiological Activity

Lehofer *et al.* (1998) suggested a close interrelationship between brainstem centres regulating arousal and pain sensitivity. Higher 'nervousness' has been demonstrated to be associated with increased pain sensitivity. Altered pain sensitivity, on the other hand, can be assumed to be a central feature of somatization. Following this model, somatizing patients may have a reduced threshold for perceiving physiological changes and experiencing multiple unpleasant physical sensations.

However, it is also possible that somatizing patients really have abnormal physiological reactions, and not only changed perception thresholds. There may be different ways in which physiological abnormalities may contribute to an increased risk for the perception of physical symptoms. Abnormal physiological arousal could be of importance not only for the exacerbation, but also for the maintenance of somatoform symptoms. Somatization *per se* is a state of chronic stress which is accompanied by changes of autonomic and muscular activity (Melin and Lundberg, 1997). There are different ways in which an association between arousal abnormalities and perception of symptoms may work.

(a) *Permanent over-arousal.*
Patients with somatoform symptoms can be over-aroused in challenging as well as during relaxing situations. This over-arousal can lead to the subjective feeling of exhaustion which is typical for patients with somatoform disorders.
(b) *Over-activation in response to challenging events; lack of habituation.*
Somatization may be characterized by physiological hyper-reactivity. If the body perceives challenges, physiological over presentation of energy occurs. Moreover, the process of habituation describes the tendency to reduced reactions if stimuli are repeated. If over-activation or a lack of habituation occurs, this may be associated with reduced stress tolerance.
(c) *Lack of recovery and relaxation after challenging events.*
One of the principal human adaptation processes is to relax after physical, emotional, or cognitive challenges. If people are not able to use breaks for relaxation, the activity level which is typical for challenging events remains stable even in periods without demands. Again this may lead to states of exhaustion.
(d) *Increased dishabituation.*
If people are repeating sequences of comparable demands interrupted by shorter breaks, there is a typical increase of activation after the break when people restart activity. However, another process of human adaptation is that the re-increase of arousal after breaks is reduced as the person habituates more and more to the following demands. A process of amplified dishabituation would also lead to insufficient recovery of energy, and feelings of exhaustion and stress.

Some of these pathophysiological hypotheses have been tested in patients with somatization syndrome. In the study of Rief *et al.* (1998) we demonstrated that somatized patients feel more and more tense during and after periods of mental challenges, while healthy controls habituate to the situation. A physiological correlate could be found by assessing heart rate reactions. After breaks, the heart rate of somatizing patients re-accelerated even if the task was well-known and patients were familiar with it. Healthy controls did not show signs of dishabituation in heart rate reactions in this study; obviously, the adaptation process of 'habituation to challenges' is compromised in somatizing patients.

In a subsequent study, this effect was further analysed (Rief and Auer, 2001). As in the first study, a number of muscular and autonomic parameters were assessed (e.g., electrodermal activity, peripheral temperature, muscular activity, peripheral pulse amplitude and others). Again abnormal adaptation processes in heart rate activity were demonstrated in patients with somatoform symptoms. In this study, the most pronounced effects were found for the difference between task period and subsequent breaks: heart rate activity reduced significantly in healthy controls when breaks occurred, demonstrating an adaptation of physiological activity. This process was significantly less pronounced in patients with somatization indicating a reduced ability to benefit from breaks.

Further studies have pointed to the link between cardiovascular activity and somatic complaints, while relationships with other physiological systems seem to be of less importance. Kristal-Boneh *et al.* (1998) reported an association between somatic symptoms and 24-hour ambulatory blood pressure levels. There was a direct association between systolic blood pressure and somatic complaints, while the association with diastolic blood pressure was non-significant. In their study, they also replicated the association between heart rate reactivity and somatic complaints (see Table XX.5).

Yardley *et al.* (1998) confirmed that patients with somatization-associated symptoms react to the provocation of these symptoms with physiological processes which might maintain the problems. They examined persons with vestibular dysfunction with a dizziness provocation technique. After the provocation of dizziness, a

Table XX.5 Heart rate and somatic complaints (data from Kristal-Boneh *et al.*, 1998)

	Low somatic complaints	High somatic complaints	Significance
Diurnal heart rate	76 b.p.m.	81 b.p.m.	$p < 0.001$
Nocturnal heart rate	64 b.p.m.	65 b.p.m.	NS
Work time	76 b.p.m.	83 b.p.m.	$p < 0.01$
Casual	71 b.p.m.	75 b.p.m.	NS

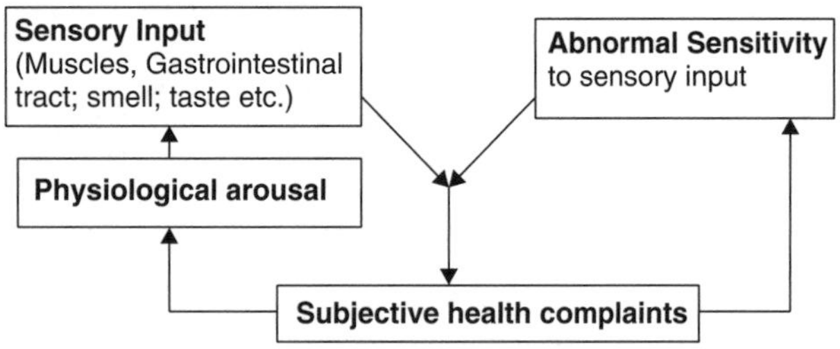

Figure XX.2 Ursin's model of a sensitization feedback loop (Ursin, 1997)

significant greater increase in respiration rate following head movements was found in those patients who complained of more somatic symptoms. These symptom-unspecific physiological effects could be associated with specific physiological changes, such as increased muscle tension or changes of blood circulation in symptom regions. Despite the face validity of the importance of these changes, they need to be better founded with empirical research.

Ursin (1997) presented a model of a psychobiological feedback loop to explain the process of somatization. Psychophysiological over-activation and the experience of complaints may lead to a sensitization of neurons. This might result in an abnormal sensitivity to sensory input from muscles or from the gastrointestinal tract, but also from smell and taste. This positive feedback loop is symbolized in Figure XX.2.

Somatoform Symptoms and the Electrophysiological Activity of the Brain (EEG, Evoked Potentials)

The perception of physical changes is a process of the central nervous system. Therefore it is possible that abnormalities of information processing in the central nervous system might be crucial for the development of somatization symptoms.

Some components of the evoked potentials are direct correlates of perceptual processes. The N1 amplitude, for example, seems to reflect processes of stimulus filtering and selective attention. Only few studies have investigated evoked potentials in somatoform disorders. However, they have yielded promising results: Gordon *et al.* (1986) used the classical 'oddball' paradigm to investigate a tone-discrimination task in *somatization disorders*. Eighty-five per cent of the tones were 1000 Hz in frequency and the remaining 15% were 2000 Hz (target tones). Participants were instructed to ignore the background tones and to count the number of target tones. The results demonstrated a trend for N1 amplitudes to be larger in the somatization group, and this was tentatively interpreted in terms of an impairment in stimulus filtering. For the other components (P1, P2, N2, P3) no significant group differences were found. The authors suggest that a more demanding task of selective attention may reveal more pronounced effects as a result of impaired stimulus processing in *somatization disorder*.

In a second study of the same group abnormalities of event-related potentials were confirmed which are thought to reflect disturbed attention processes in *somatization disorder* (James *et al.*, 1987). In this study the so-called mismatch negativity was assessed. Mismatch negativity is the difference between the potentials seen when subjects have to attend to one specific stimulus (e.g., 1000 Hz tone presented to the left ear) in comparison to potentials raised by the same stimulus when it should not be attended. Mismatch negativity starts prior to the N1 component and lasts for approximately 200 msec. This negative shift represents the difference in attention which is paid to relevant and irrelevant stimuli. In the study of James *et al.* (1987) there was less mismatch negativity in somatizers compared to normal controls at central and parietal midline sites. Somatizing patients seemed to process relevant and irrelevant stimuli more similarly than did normals; they were less capable of dividing their attention efficiently between relevant and irrelevant sensory input. This would help to explain why somatizing patients are more aware of and report more somatic symptoms.

A third study of the same group used auditory stimuli which varied in intensity (James *et al.*, 1990). The slope of P1-N1 amplitude changes as a function of stimulus intensity. This P1-N1 dependency of stimulus intensity was more pronounced in patients with *somatization disorder*, compared with controls, suggesting an enhanced central nervous system response to sensory input.

The results of these three studies are difficult to integrate. While all of them point to alternations in attention processing, the results seem not to be consistent and should be replicated and extended.

An interesting different approach was used by Wittling and colleagues (see Wittley (1997) for review). They did not investigate patients with manifest *somatization disorder*, but persons with high levels of unspecific physical complaints. Participants viewed either emotional stimuli or neutral stimuli, while topographic brain mapping procedures were used. The emotional stimuli evoked a significantly higher negativity in the period between 800 and 1200 msec over the whole posterior region. Group differences were found only for emotional stimuli, but not for the neutral stimulus conditions. Individuals with a low susceptibility to psychosomatic disorders responded to emotional stimuli with a higher negative potential than subjects with a high susceptibility to such disorders. These differences were most pronounced for the right hemisphere. Thus, these results point to abnormalities of information processing not only in simple attention tasks but also in the processing of emotional stimuli. As with other brain imaging techniques, topographic EEG can be one tool to highlight the specificities of the disturbed information processing in somatization. It would be helpful to continue this line of research.

THERAPEUTIC ARMAMENTARIUM

Management of Somatoform Disorders

In most doctor's offices, the time for diagnosis and treatment is quite limited. However, there is evidence that these few minutes can be crucial for whether the patient will be enabled to manage his complaints or whether the complaints might become chronic. Smith *et al.* (1986) and Smith *et al.* (1995) demonstrated that providing information to general practitioners on how to manage patients with somatization complaints was helpful in the avoidance of long-lasting, expensive and useless treatments. Table XX.6 contains the recommendations of Smith *et al.* (1986) as well as some extensions of our group.

Many patients with somatization symptoms are quite suspicious during the first contacts with experts. This means that the experts have to do many empathetic interventions during the first contact to install a constructive therapeutic relationship. One of these

Table XX.6 Guidelines for the management of somatization in primary care

- Confirm the credibility of the complaints
- Anticipate and inform the patient as early as possible that the most probable cause for the complaints is not a severe organic disorder, but a problem in the perception of bodily signals
- Explore the complete history and diversity of physical complaints
- Inform the patient about the next steps of investigations and about possible consequences; anticipate the time point when the procedure of organic investigations will be finished
- Avoid unnecessary investigations and alibi diagnoses
- Arrange regular dates for doctor visits of the patient; avoid spontaneous doctor visits
- Motivate for a healthy way of living and avoid physical deconditioning
- To avoid dysfunctional information processing due to the bias of the patients, use questions and ask the patient for conclusions.

steps should include the confirmation that the symptoms are 'real' for the patient and not 'just in mind'. The introduction of psychophysiological models (such as muscle over-activation, dysfunctional breathing, etc.) can be helpful at an early point in the therapeutic process. Introducing psychophysiological models only after all severe organic causes have been excluded might reduce their credibility.

Physicians may sometimes find it annoying to explore the complete history of complaints all over again. However, patients will not believe in the doctor's treatment recommendations if the doctor does not know all about the complaints. Moreover, some patients describe just those symptoms which fit in the speciality of the doctor, but do not report that they have been in gynaecological, orthopaedic or neurological treatment some weeks earlier. Therefore the diagnostician has to explore actively and ask for complaints in all parts of the body.

Some patients find it difficult to accept the doctor's opinion that no more medical investigations are necessary despite the fact that no organic reason has been found. It is easier for the patients to accept the decision to stop the diagnostic process if they have been informed in advance when this step will be taken. Unnecessary investigations increase the risk of iatrogenic harm, and unnecessary 'alibi diagnoses' reduce the probability of using successful self-help strategies.

If patients are in need of frequent doctor visits, it may be helpful to install a regular scheme for visits to avoid spontaneous, symptom-contingent procedures. The installation of regular doctor visits may be one of the first and most important steps to encourage self-help strategies for the patient: the patient knows that the doctor is still involved in the treatment process, but the patient tries to use self-help strategies in between appointments.

Some patients think that the avoidance of physical activity may be helpful to overcome the complaints. However, these patients should be informed that the avoidance of physical activity may be a helpful short-term strategy (e.g., in acute pain), but considering a long-term perspective it might increase disability. Therefore the patients should be encouraged to continue and even to expand regular physical activities.

Most patients with somatoform complaints have an information processing bias. The information provided by the doctor is transformed until it fits into the patient's reasoning. A doctor's statement of "Cancer is really improbable in your case" could be transformed into "It is probable that you have cancer" by the patient. To prevent this information transformation, the doctor can use questions and ask the patient for summaries.

As mentioned above, these simple behaviour strategies can be done even during very short-term contacts, and have a proven efficacy in the management of patients with unexplained physical symptoms. Most patients with somatoform symptoms are treated by general practitioners. Therefore it is important to transform the knowledge of experts into intervention strategies for GPs. If patients need more sophisticated psychological treatment, there are also some treatment studies demonstrating the efficacy of psychotherapeutic approaches. Kroenke and Swindle (2000) presented a critical review of controlled clinical trials for cognitive–behavioural therapy (CBT) in somatization. They summarized that CBT can be an effective treatment for patients with somatization or somatoform syndromes. Benefits can occur whether or not psychological distress is ameliorated. However, compared to some outstanding studies proving the efficacy of CBT in *hypochondriasis* (Clark *et al.*, 1998), the number of studies reporting psychotherapeutic approaches in other somatoform disorders is still small (see Figure XX.3).

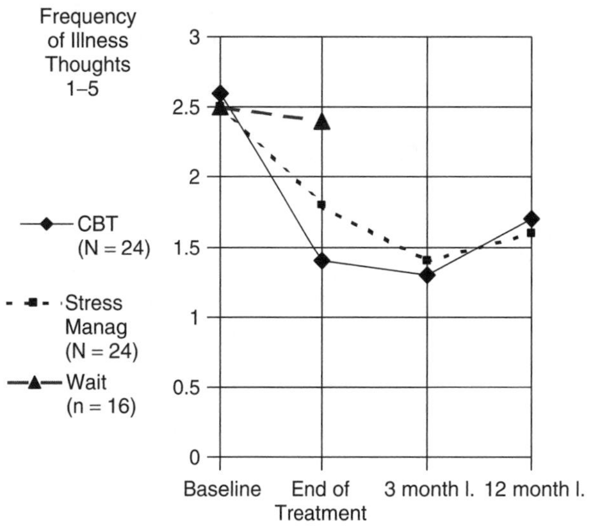

Figure XX.3 Treatment of hypochondriasis (Clark *et al.*, 1998)

Pharmacological Treatment

Although somatoform disorders are highly prevalent and present a rising problem to the health services there is still no standard pharmacological treatment. Only few placebo-controlled clinical trials have been performed. This might be partly due to the very concept of somatoform disorders that excludes somatic causes and therefore seems to call for other than pharmacological treatment. Further difficulties for the establishment of a standard pharmacological management of somatoform disorders arise from the heterogeneous characteristics of sub-syndromes summarized under the heading of somatoform disorders, inconsistencies in diagnostic concepts and outcome measures and generally elevated placebo response rates in somatoform disorder patients (Volz *et al.*, 1994). From the limited data base to date there is reason to believe that antidepressants are beneficial in the treatment of somatoform disorders (Volz *et al.*,

1994; Escobar, 1996). Open clinical trials suggest that selective serotonin reuptake inhibitors (SSRIs) like fluvoxamine might lead to improvement in about 60% of patients (Noyes *et al.*, 1998). In one of the few placebo-controlled clinical trials Volz *et al.* (2000) reported that the tricyclic antidepressant opipramol proved to be more effective than placebo in reducing somatic symptoms in patients with certain somatoform disorders (*somatization disorder, undifferentiated somatoform disorder, somatoform autonomic dysfunctions*). Additional improvement on other psychopathological outcome measures and the good tolerability profile further recommended the compound, especially for use in a patient group characterized by high psychiatric comorbidity and a focus on even minor body sensations.

Body dysmorphic disorder (BDD) has been considered an obsessive–compulsive spectrum disorder, owning to the features it shares with obsessive–compulsive disorder (OCD). As in OCD open trials suggest a good therapeutic response to serotonin reuptake inhibitors, such as clomipramine, fluoxetine and fluvoxamine; other pharmacological agents, such as neuroleptics, trazodone, lithium, benzodiazepines, tricyclics and anticonvulsants, have been less beneficial or ineffective in BDD (Hollander *et al.*, 1989; Phillips *et al.*, 2001; Phillips *et al.*, 2001). In a randomized, double-blind, crossover-design study of 29 BDD patients clomipramine, a potent serotonin reuptake inhibitor, was superior to the active control desipramine, a potent norepinephrine reuptake inhibitor in the treatment of BDD symptoms according to all outcome measures (Hollander *et al.*, 1999). As was later confirmed by other researchers delusional patients (which required the diagnosis of delusional disorder, somatic type) responded as well as non-delusional patients to SRI treatment (Hollander *et al.*, 1999; Phillips *et al.*, 2001). Thus, delusional patients may not require neuroleptic treatment and might be spared possible adverse side effects.

Another subtype of somatoform disorder, *hypochondriasis*, has also been related to obsessive–compulsive disorder. Although the comorbidity profile, clinical course and family history data do not support this hypothesis there is evidence that hypochondriac concerns respond to the same class of drugs that is effective in OCD: serotonin reuptake inhibitors. Open trial data suggest that SSRIs such as fluvoxamine might be useful therapy for hypochondriac patients (Fallon *et al.*, 1993; Perkins, 1999). A preliminary report of placebo-controlled trial in a small group of patients partly confirmed these results. However, due to high placebo response rates differences between fluvoxamine (66% responders) and placebo (50% responders) felt short of statistical significance (Fallon *et al.*, 1996). Tricyclic antidepressants seem not to be effective in *hypochondriasis* (Fallon *et al.*, 2000). As is the case in BDD there seems to be a spectrum of insight in *hypochondriasis* ranging from good to absent. Patients at the latter end of this continuum would require the diagnosis of delusional disorder, somatic type, formerly called monosymptomatic hypochondriacal psychosis. For those patients single case studies and small clinical series suggest that low doses of neuroleptics such as pimozide or olanzapine might be the treatment of choice (Opler and Feinberg, 1991; Weintraub and Robinson, 2000). However, as SSRIs have proved to be effective in treating delusionality in delusional BDD patients there might be reason to expect beneficial effects also on delusional *hypochondriasis* (Perkins, 1999).

The possible analgesic effects of antidepressants for the treatment of chronic pain have been evaluated in a number of double-blind studies. In a recent meta-analysis Fishbain *et al.* (1998) reviewed 11 randomized, placebo-controlled treatment studies on *pain disorder*. The results showed that antidepressants decreased pain intensity more than placebo in patients with psychogenic pain or *somatoform pain disorder* (mean overall effect size = 0.48). The authors argued that low dosage and short duration of treatment in most studies made it unlikely that the medication could have exerted an appreciable antidepressant effect. Thus, the analgesic effect of the treatment was considered not to be just a function of the antidepressant properties of the drugs.

The analgesic properties of both tricyclic antidepressants and new antidepressant compounds have also proved to be therapeutically useful in related syndromes such as the somatoform spectrum disorder *fibromyalgia* (Goldenberg *et al.*, 1986; Dwight *et al.*, 1998).

Taken together, there is evidence that antidepressant drugs have a beneficial effect in somatoform disorders, with traditional tricyclic antidepressants being especially useful in those conditions that are characterized by pain and multiple somatic complaints (*pain disorder, somatization disorder*) and modern SSRI antidepressants being especially effective in conditions being related to anxiety disorders and obsessive–compulsive disorder (*body dysmorphic disorder, hypochondriasis*). However, there is still a need for more controlled studies using larger patient samples. Issues of differential indication and long-term maintenance of treatment effects need considerably greater attention.

REFERENCES

American Psychiatric Association, 1994. *Diagnostic and Statistical Manual of Mental Disorders: DSM-IV*. APA, Washington, DC.

Axelrod, S., Noonan, M. and Atanacio, B., 1980. On the laterality of psychogenic somatic symptoms. *Journal of Nervous and Mental Disease*, **168**, 517–525.

Barr, L.C., Goodman, W.K. and Price, L.H., 1992. Acute exacerbation of body dysmorphic disorder during tryptophan depletion. *American Journal of Psychiatry*, **149**, 1406–1407.

Barsky, A.J., Coeytaux, R.R., Sarnie, M.K. and Cleary, P.D., 1993. Hypochondriacal patient's beliefs about good health. *American Journal of Psychiatry*, **150**, 1085–1089.

Barsky, A.J., Wyshak, G. and Klerman, G.L., 1992. Psychiatric comorbidity in DSM-III-R hypochondriasis. *Archives of General Psychiatry*, **49**, 101–108.

Barsky, A.J. and Wyshak, G.L., 1990. Hypochondriasis and somatosensory amplification. *British Journal of Psychiatry*, **157**, 404–409.

Battaglia, M., Bernardeschi, L., Politi, E., Bertella, S. and Bellodi, L., 1995. Comorbidity of panic and somatization disorder: a genetic–epidemiological approach. *Comprehensive Psychiatry*, **36**, 411–420.

Bell, I.R., Patarca, R., Baldwin, C.M., Klimas, N.G., Schwartz, G.E.R. and Hardin, E.E., 1998. Serum neopterin and somatization in women with chemical intolerance, depressives, and normals. *Neuropsychobiology*, **38**, 13–18.

Bienvenu, O.J., Samuels, J.F., Riddle, M.A., Hoehn-Saric, R., Liang, K.Y., Cullen, B.A., Grados, M.A. and Nestadt, G., 2000. The relationship of obsessive–compulsive disorder to possible spectrum disorders: results from a family study. *British Journal of Psychiatry*, **48**, 287–293.

Binzer, M., Andersen, P.M. and Kullgren, G., 1997. Clinical characteristics of patients with motor disability due to conversion disorder: a prospective control group study. *Journal of Neurology, Neurosurgery, and Psychiatry*, **63**, 83–88.

Black, P.H. and Berman, A.S., 1999. Stress and inflammation. In: Plotnikoff, N.P., Faith, R.E., Murgo, A.J. and Good, R.A. (eds), *Cytokines. Stress and Immunity*. CRC Press, Boca Raton, 115–132.

Bohman, M., Cloninger, R., von Knorring, A.-L. and Sigvardsson, S., 1984. An adoption study of somatoform disorders III. Cross-fostering analysis and genetic relationship to alcoholism and criminality. *Archives of General Psychiatry*, **41**, 872–878.

Bondy, B., Spaeth, M., Offenbacher, M., Glatzeder, K., Stratz, T., Schwarz, M., de Jonge, S., Krüger, M., Engel, R.R., Färber, L., Pongratz, D. and Ackenheil, M., 1999. The T102C polymorphism of the 5-HT2A-receptor gene in fibromyalgia. *Neurobiology of Disease*, **6**, 433–439.

Buchwald, D., Cheney, P.R., Peterson, D.L., Henry, B., Wormsley, S.B., Geiger, A., Ablashi, D.V., Salahuddin, S.Z., Saxinger, C., Biddle, R., Kikines, R., Jolesz, F.A., Folks, T., Balachandran, N., Peter, J., Gallo, R.C. and Komaroff, A.L., 1992. A chronic illness characterized by fatigue, neurologic and immunologic disorders, and active human herpesvirus type 6 infection. *Annals of Internal Medicine*, **116**, 103–113.

Buchwald, D. and Garrity, D., 1994. Comparison of patients with chronic fatigue syndrome, fibromyalgia, and multiple chemical sensitivities. *Archives of Internal Medicine*, **154**, 2049–2053.

Burton, R., 1621. *The Anatomy of Melancholia*. Oxford University Press, London (reprint 1883).

Clark, D.M., Salkovskis, P.M., Hackman, A., Wells, A., Fennell, M., Ludgate, J., Ahmad, S., Richards, H.C. and Gelder, M., 1998. Two psychological treatments for hypochondriasis. *British Journal of Psychiatry*, **173**, 218–225.

Cloninger, C.R., Martin, R.L., Guze, S.B. and Clayton, P.J., 1986. A prospective follow-up and family study of somatization in men and women. *American Journal of Psychiatry*, **143**, 873–878.

Cope, H., Pernet, A., Kendall, B. and David, A., 1995. Cognitive functioning and magnetic resonance imaging in chronic fatigue. *British Journal of Psychiatry*, **167**, 86–94.

Craven, J.L. and Rodin, G.M., 1987. Cyproheptatine dependence associated with an atypical somatoform disorder. *Canadian Journal of Psychiatry*, **32**, 143–145.

Deckersbach, T., Savage, C.R., Philipps, K.A., Wilhelm, S., Buhlmann, U., Rauch, S.L., Baer, L. and Jenike, M.A., 2000. Characteristics of memory dysfunction in body dysmorphic disorder. *Journal of the International Neuropsychological Society*, **6**, 673–681.

Drake, M.E., 1993. Conversion hysteria and dominant hemisphere lesions. *Psychosomatics*, **34**, 524–530.

Dwight, M.M., Arnold, L.M., O'Brien, H., Metzger, R., Morris-Park, E. and Keck, P.E., 1998. An open clinical trial of venlafaxine treatment of fibromyalgia. *Psychosomatics*, **39**, 14–17.

Escobar, J.I., 1996. Overview of somatization: diagnosis, epidemiology, and management. *Psychopharmacology Bulletin*, **32**, 589–596.

Escobar, J.I., Burnam, M.A., Karno, M., Forsythe, A. and Golding, J.M., 1987. Somatization in the community. *Archives of General Psychiatry*, **44**, 713–718.

Escobar, J.I., Rubio-Stipec, M., Canino, G. and Karno, M., 1989. Somatic symptom index (SSI): a new and abridged somatization construct. Prevalence and epidemiological correlates in two large community samples. *Journal of Nervous and Mental Disease*, **177**, 140–146.

Fallik, A. and Sigal, M., 1971. Hysteria, the choice of symptom site. A review of 40 cases of conversion hysteria. *Psychotherapy and Psychosomatics*, **19**, 310–318.

Fallon, B.A., Liebowitz, M.R., Salman, E., Schneider, F.R., Jusino, C., Hollander, E. and Klein, D.F., 1993. Fluoxetine for hypochondriacal patients without major depression. *Journal of Clinical Psychopharmacology*, **13**, 438–441.

Fallon, B.A., Qureshi, A.I., Laje, G. and Klein, D.F., 2000. Hypochondriasis and its relationship to obsessive–compulsive disorder. *Psychiatric Clinics of North America*, **23**, 605–616.

Fallon, B.A., Schneider, F.R., Marshall, R., Campeas, R., Vermes, D., Goetz, D. and Liebowitz, M.R., 1996. The pharmacotherapy of hypochondriasis. *Psychopharmacology Bulletin*, **32**, 607–611.

Faravelli, C., Salvatori, S., Galassi, F., Aiazzi, L., Drei, C. and Cabras, P., 1997. Epidemiology of somatoform disorders: a community survey in Florence. *Social Psychiatry and Psychiatric Epidemiology.*,

Fink, P., 1992. The use of hospitalizations by persistent somatizing patients. *Psychological Medicine*, **22**, 173–180.

Fink, P., 1996. Somatization — beyond symptom count. *Journal of Psychosomatic Research*, **40**, 7–10.

Fishbain, D.A., Cutler, R.B., Rosomoff, H.L. and Rosomoff, R.S., 1998. Do antidepressants have an analgesic effect in psychogenic pain and somatoform pain disorder? A meta-analysis. *Psychosomatic Medicine*, **60**, 503–509.

Flor-Henry, P., Fromm-Auch, D., Tapper, M. and Schopflocher, D., 1981. A neuropsychological study of the stable syndrome of hysteria. *Biological Psychiatry*, **16**, 601–626.

Galin, D., Diamond, R. and Braff, D., 1977. Lateralization of conversion symptoms. More frequent on the left. *American Journal of Psychiatry*, **134**, 578–580.

Garcia-Campayo, J., Sanz-Carrillo, C., Baringo, T. and Ceballos, C., 2001. SPECT scan in somatization disorder patients: an exploratory study of eleven cases. *Australian and New Zealand Journal of Psychiatry*, **35**, 359–363.

Gijsberg van Wijk, C.M.T. and Kolk, A.M., 1997. Sex differences in physical symptoms: the contribution of symptom perception theory. *Social Science and Medicine*, **45**, 231–246.

Gillespie, N.A., Zhu, G., Heath, A.C., Hickie, I.B. and Martin, N.G., 2000. The genetic aetiology of somatic distress. *Psychological Medicine*, **30**, 1051–1061.

Gjerris, A., Rafaelsen, O.J. and Christensen, N.J., 1987. CSF-adrenaline — low in 'somatizing depression'. *Acta Psychiatrica Scandinavica*, **75**, 516–520.

Goldenberg, D.L., Felson, D.T. and Dinerman, H., 1986. A randomized, controlled trial of amitriptyline and naproxen in the treatment of patients with fibromyalgia. *Arthritis and Rheumatism*, **29**, 1371–1377.

Gordon, E., Kraiuhin, C., Kelly, P., Meares, R. and Howson, A., 1986. A neurophysiological study of somatization disorder. *Comprehensive Psychiatry*, **27**, 295–301.

Grant, J.E., Kim, S.W. and Crow, S.J., 2001. Prevalence and clinical features of body dysmorphic disorder in adolescent and adult psychiatric inpatients. *Journal of Clinical Psychiatry*, **62**, 517–522.

Greco, A., Tannock, C., Brostoff, J. and Costa, D.C., 1997. Brain MR in chronic fatigue syndrome. *American Journal of Neuroradiology*, **18**, 1265–1269.

Gureje, O. and Obikoya, B., 1992. Somatization in primary care: pattern and correlates in a clinic in Nigeria. *Acta Psychiatrica Scandinavica*, **86**, 223–227.

Gureje, O., Simon, G.E., Ustun, T.B. and Goldberg, D.P., 1997. Somatization in cross-cultural perspective: a World Health Organization study in primary care. *American Journal of Psychiatry*, **154**, 989–995.

Gureje, O., Ustun, T.B. and Simon, G.E., 1997. The syndrome of hypochondriasis: a cross-national study in primary care. *Psychological Medicine*, **27**, 1001–1010.

Halligan, P.W., Athwal, B.S., Oakley, D.A. and Frackowiak, R.S.J., 2000. Imaging hypnotic paralysis: implications for conversion hysteria. *Lancet*, **355**, 986–987.

Hanes, K.R., 1998. Neuropsychological performance in body dysmorphic disorder. *Journal of the International Neuropsychological Society*, **4**, 167–171.

Hartvig, P. and Sterner, G., 1985. Childhood psychologic environmental exposure in women with diagnosed somatoform disorders. *Scandinavian Journal of Social Medicine*, **13**, 153–157.

Heim, C., Ehlert, U., Hanker, J.P. and Hellhammer, D., 1998. Abuse-related posttraumatic stress disorder and alterations of the hypothalamic–pituitary–adrenal axis in women with chronic pelvic pain. *Psychosomatic Medicine*, **60**, 309–318.

Heim, C., Ehlert, U. and Hellhammer, D.H., 2000. The potential role of hypocorticolism in the pathophysiology of stress-related bodily disorders. *Psychoneuroendocrinology*, **25**, 1–35.

Hiller, W., Rief, W. and Fichter, M.M., 1995. Further evidence for a broader concept of somatization disorder using the Somatic Symptom Index (SSI). *Psychosomatics*, **36**, 285–294.

Hollander, E., Allen, A., Kwon, J., Aronowitz, B., Schmeidler, J., Wong, C. and Simeon, D., 1999. Clomipramine vs desipramine crossover trial in body-dysmorphic disorder. *Archives of General Psychiatry*, **56**, 1033–1039.

Hollander, E., Liebowitz, M., Winchel, R., Klumker, A. and Klein, D., 1989. Treatment of body-dysmorphic disorder with serotonin reuptake blockers. *American Journal of Psychiatry*, **146**, 768–770.

James, L., Gordon, E., Kraiuhin, C., Howson, A. and Meares, R., 1990. Augmentation of auditory evoked potentials in somatization disorder. *Journal of Psychiatric Research*, **24**, 155–163.

James, L., Singer, A., Zurynski, Y., Gordon, E., Kraiuhin, C., Harris, A., Howson, A. and Meares, R., 1987. Evoked response potentials and regional cerebral blood flow in somatization disorder. *Psychotherapy and Psychosomatics*, **47**, 190–196.

Jonsson, B.H., Uvnäs-Moberg, K., Theorell, T. and Gotthard, R., 1998. Gastrin, cholecystokinin, and somatostatin in a laboratory experiment of patients with functional dyspepsia. *Psychosomatic Medicine*, **60**, 331–337.

Katon, W., Lin, E., von Korff, M., Russo, J., Lipscomb, P. and Bush, T., 1991. Somatization: a spectrum of severity. *American Journal of Psychiatry*, **148**, 34–40.

Keane, J.R., 1989. Hysterical gait disorder: 60 cases. *Neurology*, **39**, 586–589.

Kielholz, P., 1973. *Masked Depression*. Huber, Bern.

Kristal-Boneh, E., Melamed, S., Kushnir, T., Froom, P., Harari, G. and Ribak, J., 1998. Association between somatic symptoms and 24-h ambulatory blood pressure levels. *Psychosomatic Medicine*, **60**, 616–619.

Kroenke, K. and Mangelsdorff, D., 1989. Common symptoms in ambulatory care: incidence, evaluation, therapy and outcome. *American Journal of Medicine*, **86**, 262–266.

Kroenke, K. and Spitzer, R.L., 1998. Gender differences in the reporting of physical and somatoform symptoms. *Psychosomatic Medicine*, **60**, 150–155.

Kroenke, K., Spitzer, R.L., deGruy, F.V., Hahn, S.R., Linzer, M., Williams, J.B., Brody, D. and Davies, M., 1997. Multisomatoform disorder. An alternative to undifferentiated somatoform disorder for the somatizing patient in primary care. *Archives of General Psychiatry*, **54**, 352–358.

Kroenke, K. and Swindle, R., 2000. Cognitive–behavioral therapy for somatization and symptom syndromes: a critical review of controlled clinical trials. *Psychotherapy and Psychosomatics*, **69**, 205–215.

Ladwig, K.-H., Marten-Mittag, B., Formanek, B. and Dammann, G., 2000. Gender differences of symptom reporting and medical health care utilization in the German population. *European Journal of Epidemiology*, **16**, 511–518.

Lehofer, M., Liebmann, P.M., Moser, M. and Schauenstein, K., 1998. Nervousness and pain sensitivity: I. A positive correlation. *Psychiatry Research*, **79**, 51–53.

Linthorst, A.C., Flachskamm, C., Holsboer, F. and Reul, J.M., 1994. Local administration of recombinant human interleukin 1 beta in the rat hippocampus increases serotonergic neurotransmission, hypothalamic–pituitary–adrenocortical axis activity, and body temperature. *Endocrinology*, **135**, 520–532.

Lüders, H.O., Dinners, D.S., Morris, H.H., Wyllie, E. and Comair, Y.G., 1995. Cortical electrical stimulation in humans: the negative motor areas. In: Fahn, S., Hallet, M., Lüders, H.O. and Marsden, C.D. (eds), *Advances in Neurology, Vol. 57, Negative Motor Phenomena.* Lippencott-Raven, New York, 115–129.

Mace, C.J. and Trimble, M.R., 1991. 'Hysteria', 'functional' or 'psychogenic'? A survey of British neurologists' preferences. *Journal of the Royal Society of Medicine*, **84**, 471–475.

Maes, M., Bosmans, E., De Jongh, R., Kenis, G., Vandoolaeghe, E. and Neels, H., 1997. Increased serum IL-6 and IL-1 receptor antagonist concentrations in major depression and treatment resistant depression. *Cytokine*, **9**, 853–858.

Maes, M., Libbrecht, I., van Hunsel, F., Lin, A.H., Bonaccorso, S., Goossens, F., deMeester, I., deClerck, L., Biondi, M., Scharpe, S. and Janca, A., 1998. Lower serum activity of prolyl endopeptidase in fibromyalgia is related to severity of depressive symptoms and pressure hyperalgesia. *Psychological Medicine*, **28**, 957–965.

Maier, S.F. and Watkins, L.R., 1998. Cytokines for psychologists: implications of bidirectional immune-to-brain communication for understanding behavior, mood, and cognition. *Psychological Review*, **105**, 83–107.

Marshall, J.C., Halligan, P.W., Fink, G.R., Wade, D.T. and Frackowiak, R.S.J., 1997. The functional anatomy of a hysterical paralysis. *Cognition*, **64**, B1–B8.

Melamed, S., Ugarten, U., Shirom, A., Kahana, L., Lerman, Y. and Froom, P., 1999. Chronic burnout, somatic arousal and elevated salivary cortisol levels. *Journal of Psychosomatic Research*, **46**, 591–598.

Melin, B. and Lundberg, U., 1997. A biopsychosocial approach to work-stress and musculoskeletal disorders. *Journal of Psychophysiology*, **11**, 238–247.

Min, K.S. and Lee, B.O., 1997. Laterality in somatization. *Psychosomatic Medicine*, **59**, 236–240.

Murphy, F.C. and Sahakian, B.J., 2001. Neuropsychology of bipolar disorder. *British Journal of Psychiatry*, **178**(suppl. 41), S120–S127.

Natelson, B.H., Cohen, J.M., Brassloff, I. and Lee, H.J., 1993. A controlled study of brain magnetic resonance imaging in patients with the chronic fatigue syndrome. *Journal of the Neurological Sciences*, **120**, 213–217.

Neeck, G. and Riedel, W., 1999. Hormonal perturbations in fibromyalgia syndrome. *Annals of the New York Academy of Sciences*, **876**, 325–338.

Nicolson, N.A. and van Diest, R., 2000. Salivary cortisol patterns in vital exhaustion. *Journal of Psychosomatic Research*, **49**, 335–342.

Noyes, R.J., Happel, R.L., Muller, B.A., Holt, C.S., Kathol, R.G., Sieren, L.R. and Amos, J.J., 1998. Fluvoxamine for somatoform disorders: an open trial. *General Hospital Psychiatry*, **20**, 339–344.

Offenbacher, M., Bondy, B., de Jonge, S., Glatzeder, K., Krüger, M., Schoeps, P. and Ackenheil, M., 1999. Possible association of fibromyalgia with a polymorphism in the serotonin transporter gene regulatory region. *Arthritis and Rheumatism*, **42**, 2482–2488.

Opler, L.A. and Feinberg, S.S., 1991. The role of pimozide in clinical psychiatry: a review. *Journal of Clinical Psychiatry*, **52**, 221–233.

Parasuraman, R., 1998. *The Attentive Brain*. MIT Press, Cambridge, MA.

Pascuzzi, R.M., 1994. Nonphysiological (functional) unilateral motor and sensory syndromes involve the left more often than the right body. *Journal of Nervous and Mental Disease*, **182**, 118–120.

Pennebaker, J.W., 1982. *The Psychology of Physical Symptoms*. Springer, New York.

Perkins, R.J., 1999. SSRI antidepressants are effective for treating delusional hypochondriasis. *Medical Journal of Australia*, **170**, 140–141.

Perugi, G., Akiskal, H.S., Gianotti, D., Frafe, F., di Vaio, S. and Cassano, G.B., 1997. Gender-related differences in body dysmorphic disorder (dysmorphophobia). *Journal of Nervous and Mental Disease*, **185**, 578–582.

Phillips, K.A. and Diaz, S.F., 1997. Gender differences in body dysmorphic disorder. *Journal of Nervous and Mental Disease*, **185**, 570–577.

Phillips, K.A., Dufresne, R.G., Wilkel, C.S. and Vittorio, C.C., 2000. Rate of body dysmorphic disorder in dermatology patients. *Journal of the American Academy of Dermatology*, **185**, 570–577.

Phillips, K.A., Dwight, M.M. and McElroy, S.L., 2001. Efficacy and safety of fluvoxamine in body dysmorphic disorder. *Journal of Clinical Psychiatry*, **59**, 165–171.

Phillips, K.A., McElroy, S.L., Dwight, M.M., Eisen, J.L. and Rasmussen, S.A., 2001. Delusionality and response to open-label fluvoxamine in body dysmorphic disorder. *Journal of Clinical Psychiatry*, **62**, 87–91.

Piccinelli, M. and Simon, G., 1997. Gender and cross-cultural differences in somatic symptoms associated with emotional distress. An international study in primary care. *Psychological Medicine*, **27**, 433–444.

Pilowsky, I., 1993. Aspects of abnormal illness behaviour. *Psychotherapy and Psychosomatic*, **60**, 62–74.

Pruessner, J.C., Hellhammer, D. and Kirschbaum, C., 1999. Burnout, perceived stress, and cortisol responses to awakening. *Psychosomatic Medicine*, **61**, 197–204.

Regan, J. and LaBabera, J.D., 1984. Lateralization of conversion symptoms in children and adolescents. *American Journal of Psychiatry*, **141**, 1279–1280.

Reitan, R.M. and Davison, L.A., 1974. *Clinical Neuropsychiatry*. John Wiley & Sons, New York.

Rief, W. and Auer, C., 2000. Cortisol and somatization. *Biological Psychology*, **53**, 13–23.

Rief, W. and Auer, C., 2001. Is somatization a habituation disorder? Physiological reactivity in somatization syndrome. *Psychiatry Research*, **101**, 63–74.

Rief, W. and Hiller, W., 1999. Toward empirically based criteria for somatoform disorders. *Journal of Psychosomatic Research*, **46**, 507–518.

Rief, W. and Nanke, A., 1999. Somatization disorder from a cognitive–psychobiological perspective. *Current Opinion in Psychiatry*, **12**, 733–738.

Rief, W., Hessel, A. and Braehler, E., 2001. Somatization symptoms and hypochondrical features in the general population. *Psychosomatic Medicine*, **63**, 595–602.

Rief, W., Heuser, J., Mayrhuber, E., Stelzer, I., Hiller, W. and Fichter, M.M., 1996. The classification of multiple somatoform symptoms. *Journal of Nervous and Mental Disease*, **184**, 680–687.

Rief, W., Hiller, W. and Margraf, J., 1998. Cognitive aspects in hypochondriasis and the somatization syndrome. *Journal of Abnormal Psychology*, **107**, 587–595.

Rief, W., Pilger, F., Ihle, D., Bosmans, E., Egyed, B. and Maes, M., 2001. Immunological differences between patients with major depression and somatization syndrome. *Psychiatry Research*, in press.

Rief, W., Schaefer, S., Hiller, W. and Fichter, M.M., 1992. Lifetime diagnoses in patients with somatoform disorders: which came first? *European Archives of Psychiatry and Clinical Neuroscience*, **241**, 236–240.

Rief, W., Shaw, R. and Fichter, M.M., 1998. Elevated levels of psychophysiological arousal and cortisol in patients with somatization syndrome. *Psychosomatic Medicine*, **60**, 198–203.

Riley, J.L., Robinson, M.E., Wise, E.A., Myers, C.D. and Fillingim, R.B., 1998. Sex differences in the perception of noxious experimental stimuli: a meta-analysis. *Pain*, **74**, 181–187.

Riley, J.L., Robinson, M.E., Wise, E.A. and Price, D.D., 1999. A meta-analytic review of pain perception across the menstrual cycle. *Pain*, **81**, 225–235.

Roelofs, K., Näring, G.W.B., Moene, F.C. and Hoogduin, C.A.L., 2000. The question of symptom lateralization in conversion disorder. *Journal of Psychosomatic Research*, **49**, 21–25.

Russell, I.J., 1998. Advances in fibromyalgia: possible role for central neurochemicals. *American Journal of the Medical Sciences*, **315**, 377–384.

Sarwer, D.B., Wadden, T.A., Pertschuk, M.J. and Whitaker, L.A., 1998. Body image dissatisfaction and body dysmorphic disorder in 100 cosmetic surgery patients. *Plastic and Reconstructive Surgery*, **101**, 1644–1649.

Schwartz, M.J., Späth, M., Müller-Bardorff, H., Pongratz, D.E., Bondy, B. and Ackenheil, M., 1999. Relationship of substance P, 5-hydroxyindole acetic acid and tryptophan in serum of fibromyalgia patients. *Neuroscience Letters*, **259**, 196–198.

Schwartz, R.B., Garada, B.M., Komaroff, A.L., Tice, H.M., Gleit, M., Jolesz, F.A. and Holman, B.L., 1994. Detection of intracranial abnormalities in patients with chronic fatigue syndrome. *American Journal of Roentgenology*, **162**, 935–941.

Scott, L.V., Burnett, F., Medbak, S. and Dinan, T.G., 1998. Naloxone-mediated activation of the hypothalamic–pituitary–adrenal axis in chronic fatigue syndrome. *Psychological Medicine*, **28**, 285–293.

Scott, L.V. and Dinan, T.G., 1998. Urinary free cortisol excretion in chronic fatigue syndrome, major depression and in healthy volunteers. *Journal of Affective Disorders*, **47**, 49–54.

Sierra, M. and Berrios, G.E., 1999. Towards a neuropsychiatry of conversive hysteria. *Cognitive Neuropsychiatry*, **4**, 267–287.

Simeon, D., Hollander, E., Stein, D.J., Cohen, L. and Aronowitz, B., 1995. Body dysmorphic disorder in the DSM-IV field trial for obsessive–compulsive disorder. *American Journal of Psychiatry*, **152**, 1207–1209.

Smith, G.R., Monson, R.A. and Ray, D.C., 1986. Psychiatric consultation in somatization disorder. A randomized controlled study. *The New England Journal of Medicine*, **314**, 1407–1413.

Smith, G.R., Rost, K. and Kashner, M., 1995. A trial of the effect of a standardized psychiatric consultation on health outcomes and costs in somatizing patients. *Archives of General Psychiatry*, **52**, 238–243.

Starcevic, V., 1990. Relationship between hypochondriasis and obsessive–compulsive personality disorder: close relatives, separated by nosological schemes? *American Journal of Psychotherapy*, **19**, 340–347.

Stern, D., 1977. Handedness and the lateral distribution of conversion reaction. *Journal of Nervous and Mental Disease*, **164**, 122–128.

Tiihonen, J., Kuikka, J., Viinamäki, H., Lehtonen, J. and Partanen, J., 1995. Altered cerebral blood flow during hysterical paresthesia. *Biological Psychiatry*, **37**, 134–137.

Torgersen, S., 1986. Genetics of somatoform disorders. *Archives of General Psychiatry*, **43**, 502–505.

Ursin, H., 1997. Sensitization, somatization, and subjective health complaints. *International Journal of Behavioral Medicine*, **4**, 105–116.

Van Kempen, G.M.J., Zitman, F.G., Linssen, A.C.G. and Edelbroek, P.M., 1992. Biochemical measures in patients with a somatoform pain disorder, before, during, and after treatment with amitriptyline with or without flupentixol. *Biological Psychiatry*, **31**, 670–680.

Vingerhoets, A.J.J.M., Ratcliff-Crain, J., Jabaaij, L., Tilders, F.J.H., Moleman, P. and Menges, L.J., 1996. Self-reported stressors, symptom complaints and psychobiological functioning II: psychoneuroendocrine variables. *Journal of Psychosomatic Research*, **40**, 191–203.

Volz, H.-P., Möller, H.-J., Reimann, I. and Stoll, K.-D., 2000. Opipramol for the treatment of somatoform disorders: results from a placebo-controlled trial. *European Neuropsychopharmacology*, **10**, 211–217.

Volz, H.-P., Stieglitz, R.-D., Menges, K. and Möller, H.-J., 1994. Somatoform disorders — diagnostic concepts, controlled clinical trials, and methodological issues. *Pharmacopsychiatry*, **27**, 231–237.

Watkins, L.R., Maier, S.F. and Goehler, L.E., 1995. Immune activation: the role of pro-inflammatory cytokines in inflammation, illness responses and pathological pain states. *Pain*, **63**, 289–302.

Wearden, A.J. and Appleby, L., 1996. Research on cognitive complaints and cognitive functioning in patients with chronic fatigue syndrome (CFS): what conclusions can we draw? *Journal of Psychosomatic Research*, **41**, 197–211.

Weintraub, E. and Robinson, C., 2000. A case of monosymptomatic hypochondriacal psychosis treated with olanzapine. *Annals of Clinical Psychiatry*, **12**, 247–249.

Wessely, S., Chalder, T., Hirsch, S., Wallace, P. and Wright, D., 1996. Psychological symptoms, somatic symptoms, and psychiatric disorder in chronic fatigue and chronic fatigue syndrome: a prospective study in primary care. *American Journal of Psychiatry*, **153**, 1050–1059.

Wessely, S., Hotopf, M. and Sharpe, M., 1999. *Chronic Fatigue and its Syndromes*. Oxford University Press, Oxford.

White, P.D., 1997. The relationship between infection and fatigue. *Journal of Psychosomatic Research*, **43**, 345–350.

White, P.D., Thomas, J.M., Amess, J., Crawford, D.H., Grover, S.A., Kangro, H.O. and Clare, A.W., 1998. Incidence, risk and prognosis of acute and chronic fatigue syndromes and psychiatric disorders after glandular fever. *British Journal of Psychiatry*, **173**, 475–481.

Whitehead, W.E., 1994. Assessing the effects of stress on physical symptoms. *Health Psychology*, **13**, 99–102.

Wittley, W., 1997. The right hemisphere and the human stress response. *Acta Physiologica Scandinavica Supplementum*, **640**, 55–59.

Yardley, L., Gresty, M., Bronstein, A. and Beyts, J., 1998. Changes in heart rate and respiration rate in patients with vestibular dysfunction following head movements which provoke dizziness. *Biological Psychology*, **49**, 95–108.

Yazící, K.M. and Kostakoglu, L., 1998. Cerebral blood flow changes in patients with conversion disorder. *Psychiatry Research: Neuroimaging Section*, **83**, 163–168.

Young, A.H., Sharpe, M., Clements, A., Dowling, B., Hawton, K.E. and Cowen, P.J., 1998. Basal activity of the hypothalamus–pituitary–adrenal axis in patients with the chronic fatigue syndrome (neurasthenia). *Biological Psychiatry*, **43**, 236–237.

XXI

The Emerging Psychobiology of Trauma-Related Dissociation and Dissociative Disorders

Ellert R.S. Nijenhuis, Onno van der Hart, and Kathy Steele

INTRODUCTION

Mental dissociation is an intriguing and complex phenomenon that has been studied clinically and theoretically for more than 150 years. Major empirical studies have been conducted during the last two decades. For example, these studies have established that the prevalence rates of the DSM-IV dissociative disorders (APA, 1994) are considerable among psychiatric inpatients, with an overall prevalence among nine studies of 18.9% for dissociative disorders in general, and 4.4% for dissociative identity disorder (DID; Friedl *et al.*, 2000). Only in recent years has dissociation begun to receive attention from a combined psychological and biological perspective.

The study of dissociation has been impeded by several factors. First, conceptual confusion and controversy exist regarding the nature of this phenomenon. For example, dissociation is described as a process, as various symptoms, as mental structure, as psychological defense, and as a deficit in integrative capacity. In addition, it is confused with retraction of the field of consciousness (that which is within awareness at a given time) such as absorption, daydreaming, and states of inattention. Although negative dissociative symptoms such as amnesia are acknowledged, positive ones, such as intrusive re-experiences of trauma, are often not understood as dissociative in nature.

Second, diagnostic and aetiological issues are far from resolved in psychiatric disorders in which dissociation is an essential feature. For example, it is debatable that the DSM-IV category of dissociative disorders encompasses the actual range of dissociative disorders. As discussed below, although post-traumatic stress disorder (PTSD) is classified as an anxiety disorder, there are arguments to regard it as a dissociative disorder (e.g., Nijenhuis *et al.*, 2002b). And the ICD-10, for instance, includes dissociative disorders of movement and sensations that are defined in the DSM-IV as conversion disorders. It has been theoretically argued (Kihlstrom, 1994; Nemiah, 1991; Nijenhuis and Van der Hart, 1999a) and empirically documented (Nijenhuis, 1999) that conversion symptoms are dissociative in nature. Conversion is better conceptualized as somatoform dissociation in that the symptoms of concern are at least equally characteristic of DSM-IV dissociative disorders as dissociative symptoms that manifest in psychological variables, i.e., so-called psychoform dissociation (Van der Hart *et al.*, 2000). Moreover, somatoform dissociation correlates very strongly with psychoform dissociation (Nijenhuis, 1999; Nijenhuis *et al.*, 1996, 1997, 1999b; Sar *et al.*, 2000; Waller *et al.*, 2000), and evidence for the hypothesis that psychological conflicts can be converted into physical symptoms, and thus reduce mental strain, is lacking.

Although the DSM-IV dissociative disorders have received wide acceptance, there exists a vocal minority of clinicians and researchers who express their scepticism about the validity of the most complex dissociative disorder, DID (Spanos and Burgess, 1994). As we will discuss in more detail below, patients with DID have severe somatoform and psychoform dissociative symptoms that relate to the existence of two or more self-aware dissociative systems, i.e., dissociative systems of ideas and functions that involve a sense of self. However, sceptics doubt that dissociative personalities are genuine phenomena. Simulated or factitious cases of DID certainly exist (Draijer and Boon, 1999) along with genuine cases, and the psychobiological differences between genuine and false positive cases of DID are a fruitful area of research. Some authors have also questioned whether chronic childhood traumatization is an aetiological base for DID and other dissociative disorders, but research has converged to indicate traumatic events are a key element in the psychopathology of dissociation and dissociative disorders. Retrospective (e.g., Boon and Draijer, 1993; Coons, 1994; Kluft, 1995; Lewis *et al.*, 1997; Nijenhuis *et al.*, 1998b) and prospective studies (Ogawa *et al.*, 1997) — some of which have provided external corroboration for reported trauma — have confirmed the clinical observation that dissociative symptoms and disorders are associated with reported and factual traumatization. Studies have also demonstrated discrete and long-lasting alterations in neurobiological systems in relation to trauma and dissociation, which will be discussed below.

The current chapter focuses on dissociation related to traumatization. The first aim of the chapter is to reduce confusion about the concept of dissociation. Next, possible neuroendocrine parameters of dissociation and key brain structures that seem to be involved in the phenomenon are discussed. Several neurobiological models of dissociation will be reviewed, including Putnam's discrete behavioural states model (Putnam, 1997). Finally, the theory of structural dissociation will be presented (Nijenhuis and Van der Hart, 1999b; Van der Hart *et al.*, 1998; Nijenhuis *et al.*, 2002b; Steele *et al.*, 2001), along with supporting evidence. The theory attempts to explain trauma-related dissociation as it manifests in disorders ranging from simple PTSD to DID, and serves an important heuristic function with regard to the emerging psychobiological study of trauma-related dissociation.

THE CONCEPT OF DISSOCIATION

Dissociative symptoms are often misunderstood as indicators of other disorders or problems. Thus, it is quite common for dissociative disorder patients to hear internal voices (easily confused with psychosis); to experience disorientation to time, place and person during intrusive re-experiences (confused with intoxication, delirium, delusions, hallucinations, and psychosis); to have

Biological Psychiatry: Edited by H. D'haenen, J.A. den Boer and P. Willner. ISBN 0-471-49198-5

rapidly alternating shifts in mood (confused with bipolar disorders); to experience cognitive and attentional difficulties (confused with attention deficit disorder and cognitive processing deficits); to have intractable dissociative pain and somatoform disturbances (confused with malingering, factitious disorder; hypochondriasis, drug-seeking behaviour, and somatization disorder); to have unusual sleep disturbances due to night-time dissociation (confused with disorders of sleep); and to experience lapses in awareness (confused with malingering, manipulation, organic memory dysfunction, and iatrogenic suggestibility). Therefore, efforts to define dissociation (e.g., Braude, 1995; Cardeña, 1994; Janet, 1907; Nijenhuis *et al.*, 2002b; Putnam, 1997; Van der Hart, 2000) are important, both for clinical and research purposes.

Janet (1907, p. 332) postulated that dissociation involves a lack of integration of 'systems of ideas and functions that constitute personality' due to 'a form of mental depression'. In the context of traumatic experience, dissociation ensues when the integrative capacity of the individual is not sufficient to integrate experiences and functions. As a result, (components of) experiences can be encoded and stored as discrete systems involving sensations, body movements, affects, perceptions of the environment, and factual knowledge. Because conscious experience implies a subject, dissociative systems also involve their own sense of self, however rudimentary. While integrative failure that results in fragmentation of the personality denotes the essence of dissociation, Janet did not specify the underlying psychobiological nature of the different dissociative 'systems of ideas and functions' that traumatic experience tends to evoke.

Psychoform and Somatoform, and Negative and Positive, Dissociative Symptoms

Dissociation manifests in psychoform and somatoform symptoms (Janet, 1889; Kihlstrom, 1994; Nijenhuis and Van der Hart, 1999a; Nijenhuis *et al.*, 2002b; Van der Hart *et al.*, 2000). Both categories include negative and positive symptoms. Negative symptoms manifest when the individual fails to integrate dissociative systems of ideas and functions that, at least in principle, are available. Positive symptoms occur when these systems are retrieved (e.g., flashbacks), but without integration. Negative psychoform symptoms include losses such as amnesia, depersonalization, and derealization. Positive psychoform symptoms include re-experiencing the mental contents of traumatic memories such as thoughts, images, and feelings, as well as hearing voices that are emitted by dissociative systems (e.g., as in dissociative fugue; APA, 1994). Negative somatoform dissociative symptoms involve anaesthesia of one or more sensory modalities and motor inhibitions, such as paralysis, visual disturbances like tunnelling and haziness, deafness, or inability to feel parts of the body. Examples of positive ones are pain, sexual sensations, and freeze, flight, fight and submissive states pertaining to traumatic re-experiences.

Retraction of the Field of Consciousness and Low Levels of Conscious Awareness

Phenomena such as absorption, imaginative involvement and trance-like behaviour are often referred to as normal or non-pathological dissociation (e.g., Putnam, 1997) or as dissociative detachment (Allen *et al.*, 1999). However, these experiences result from automatic and unconscious reduction of the number of phenomena in current conscious awareness, called retraction of the field of consciousness. They do not involve encoding and storage of experience, knowledge, and skills. For example, selective attention for threat cues does not necessarily imply encoding and storage of 'peripheral' cues. While retraction of the field of consciousness may accompany dissociation (Janet, 1907; Nijenhuis *et al.*, 1996), the concepts are different.

Retraction of the field of consciousness can involve different levels of conscious awareness. The level of awareness can be high when dissociative patients focus on threat cues, but low when they enter trance states during which they are only minimally aware of themselves and their surroundings, and thus fail to encode their experience at the time. Extremely high and low levels of awareness may set the stage for dissociative processes, but are not dissociative in themselves.

The conceptual confusion with regard to dissociation continues to plague the field. For example, many instruments that evaluate the severity of dissociation suffer from under-inclusion of negative somatoform dissociative symptoms, as well as positive psychoform and somatoform dissociative symptoms, and from over-inclusion of symptoms that evaluate retraction of the field of consciousness and lowering of the level of consciousness.

PTSD, DISSOCIATION, AND STRESS RESPONSES

Defining dissociation as a lack of integration among self-aware 'systems of ideas and functions' implies that dissociation also characterizes PTSD in that this psychobiological disorder (Kardiner, 1941; Van der Kolk, 1994; cf. Vermetten and Bremner, 2001a, 2001b) involves two dissociative parts of the personality that can take control over consciousness and behaviour (Nijenhuis and Van der Hart, 1999b). One is numb and avoidant of traumatic memories and trauma-related reminders, but more or less functional in daily life, and another is enmeshed in traumatic memories. The enmeshed dissociative system intermittently intrudes or replaces the numb dissociative system. As we will discuss below, this split represents a form of structural dissociation of the personality that also constitutes the basis of more complex dissociative conditions.

To the extent that this conceptualization is correct, pre-clinical and clinical studies of severe aversive stress and PTSD are also relevant for the psychobiology of trauma-related dissociation more generally. Although a review of these studies is beyond the scope of the present chapter (for reviews, see Coupland, 2000; Van der Kolk, 1994; Vermetten and Bremner, 2001a, 2001b), the main findings are briefly noted. Animal studies have contributed to the understanding of human reactions to overwhelming events. For example, they have allowed for insights into delay conditioning of fear and defensive reactions patterns in which the conditioned stimulus immediately follows the unconditioned stimulus, as well as trace conditioning, in which the conditioned stimulus and unconditioned stimulus are separated by an interval. Delay conditioning depends on long-term potentiation within the basolateral amygdala, whereas trace conditioning requires involvement of the hippocampus. These forms of classical conditioning are relevant for dissociation, since dissociation as a process (i.e., the presumed psychobiological process that yields splits among self-aware dissociative systems) can become a conditioned response to previously neutral cues. Yet, the issue is complex: clinical observations and experimental research (Nijenhuis *et al.*, 1999a; Reinders *et al.*, in preparation; Van Honk *et al.*, 1999, 2001), to be discussed below, suggest that different dissociative systems can display different psychobiological responses to identical stimuli. Somehow the associations between unconditioned aversive stimuli (UCS) and conditioned stimuli (CS), or the responses to these associations, may depend on the particular dissociative system that dominates consciousness and behaviour.

Pre-clinical studies have also been valuable in delineating other learning processes that are relevant for trauma-related dissociative disorders. These processes include contextual conditioning (i.e., learning to respond to contextual cues such as the place where a foot shock was received), sensitization (i.e., response increment with repeated exposure to aversive cues), kindling, and extinction. It was once thought that the disappearance of conditioned responses indicated loss of the conditioned association between the CS and the UCS. However, the evidence suggests that once encoded, CS-UCS associations cannot be extinguished (Bouton, 1994), but rather become inhibited. The hippocampus and medial prefrontal and orbitofrontal cortex seem to have major roles in this process.

Animal studies provide a model for understanding a range of neurobiological alterations in PTSD, and probably are relevant for (other) dissociative disorders as well. The pathophysiology of stress reflects enduring changes in biological stress response systems with implications for learning and memory. The affected biological systems include systems mediating corticotropin-releasing factor (CRF), adrenocorticotropin hormone (ACTH), glucocorticoids (HPA-axis), neuropeptide Y (NPY), and norepinephrine (locus coeruleus/autonomic nervous system). Stressors also tend to affect serotonergic, dopaminergic, neuropeptide and central amino acid systems. Combat-related PTSD was marked by decreased benzodiazepine receptor binding in the prefrontal cortex (Bremner *et al.*, 2000b). These systems interact with brain structures involved in learning and memory, including the hippocampus, amygdala, and prefrontal cortex. Pre-clinical studies have demonstrated that the intensity and duration of the stressor, as well as the timing of the stressor in life, amplify the neurobiological effects of stressors. For example, maternal separation, lack of handling, and repetitive pain affect the developing brain of animals.

There is evidence for a number of parallels between animal responses to aversive stress and similar mechanisms in PTSD (Coupland, 2000), as well as other trauma-related disorders in humans. Thus, clinical studies of PTSD have found that brain areas such as the hippocampus, amygdala, insula, cingulate and prefrontal cortex are critically involved in responding to severe stressors, as well as in the learning from and memorization of these events (e.g., Rauch *et al.*, 1996; Van der Kolk, 1994; Vermetten and Bremner, 2001b). Some findings (to be discussed below) suggest that these brain structures are also of major importance in other dissociative conditions. Neural circuits affected in PTSD include the HPA-axis, catecholaminergic and serotonergic systems, neuropeptide systems, the hypothalamic-pituitary-thyroid axis, and neuro-immunological alterations. In both animals and humans, the HPA-axis and the autonomic nervous system are important stress response systems that, within limits, serve to maintain homeostasis during exposure to stress. Consistent with the animal studies, converging evidence has emphasized the role of early life trauma and attachment in the development of PTSD and other trauma-related disorders (Schore, 2001). Yet, there are also differences between neurobiological correlates of animal and human traumatization. An example is the finding of low cortisol levels in several studies of PTSD that contrasts with stress-induced increases of cortisol in animals (for a review see Yehuda, 2000).

POSSIBLE INVOLVEMENT OF NEUROCHEMICALS IN DISSOCIATION

Dissociation involves a failure to integrate systems of encoded and stored experiences and functions. From a biological point of view, integrative functions can be hampered by the release of neurochemicals provoked by severe threat (Ludwig, 1972; Krystal *et al.*, 1991; see also Siegel, 1999) and that are concentrated in brain regions implicated in integrative mental acts, such as the hippocampus and the prefrontal cortex.

Enhancement and Impairment of the Memory Function

The extent to which substances such as glutamate (Krystal *et al.*, 1998), norepinephrine, epinephrine, glucocorticoids, endogenous opiates, and several others (McGaugh, 1990, McGaugh *et al.*, 2000) interfere with integration is dose-dependent. For example, retention of recently learned material is enhanced when moderate doses of epinephrine are administered after training, but impaired at high doses. Memory impairment also depends on experimental conditions such as degree of arousal produced by the learning situation and the strength of the memory involved. For example, when the β-adrenergic antagonist propanolol was administered after training, memory was strongly impaired in rats that exhibited good learning during the acquisition session, but not in rats that exhibited poor learning (Cahill *et al.*, 2001, discussed in Cahill, 2000). While long-lasting exposure to threat cues such as predators may produce failure to execute previously memorized tasks (Diamond and Park, 2000; Woodson *et al.*, 2001), memories of emotional events can also be excellent, requiring little or no cognitive rehearsal (Guy and Cahill, 1999). This apparent paradox may be resolved by considering that patients with PTSD and several other dissociative conditions may alternate between hyperamnesia and memory loss. Hence, memory retrieval may depend on the dissociative part of the personality that is dominant.

Substance-Induced Dissociative-Like Symptoms in Healthy Individuals

Several substances may induce phenomena in healthy individuals that mimic dissociative symptoms, i.e., antagonists of the *N*-methyl-D-aspartate (NMDA) subtype of glutamate receptors, cannabinoids, and serotonergic hallucinogens (Krystal *et al.*, 1994a, 1994b, 1998). Because glutamate has a central role in corticocortical, thalamocortical, amygdalacortical, and hippocampocortical connectivity, higher cognitive functions could basically involve glutamatergic systems. Pre-clinical data have indeed suggested that (traumatic) stress stimulates the corticolimbic release of glutamate, and clinical studies have documented that antagonists of the NMDA receptor may transiently stimulate glutamate release, inducing symptoms that resemble dissociative symptoms in humans (Chambers *et al.*, 1999).

Ketamine blocks the NMDA receptor-mediated component of glutamatergic connections. This substance produces dose-dependent impairment of perceptual, sensory, and proprioceptive experiences that could reflect retraction of the field of consciousness, lowering of the level of consciousness, and negative dissociative symptoms. Ketamine does not seem to evoke positive dissociative symptoms, such as manifestations of dissociative parts of the personality or intrusive recollection of experiences involving negative emotions. Ketamine-induced learning and memory impairments have also been observed, as were psychotic-like symptoms such as delusions, thought disorder and negative symptoms of schizophrenia (e.g., Breier *et al.*, 1997). Hence, it seems doubtful that glutamatergic dysregulation is a *specific* inductor of dissociation, i.e., an inductor of dissociative fragmentation of the personality.

The hippocampus is implicated in the synthesis of experiences and memory encoding, and the NMDA receptor is highly concentrated in this brain structure. Since blocking of the Schaffer collateral-CA1 NMDA receptors in the hippocampus can inhibit long-term potentiation (Tsien *et al.*, 1996), ketamine could affect memory. Substances that enhance NMDA receptor function may perhaps reduce trauma-related dissociation (see Krystal *et al.*, 1998). Consistent with this hypothesis, a drug that reduces glutamate release attenuated the effects of ketamine (Chambers *et al.*, 1999). Modulatory GABAergic neurons regulate pyramidal neurons that use glutamate as their primary neurotransmitter (Krystal *et al.*, 1998). Thus, future research should assess whether substances that reduce trauma-related glutamate release or enhance gamma-aminobutyric acid (GABA) functions promote the integration of traumatic experience. Benzodiazepines are prototypical

GABA enhancers, and were useful in the treatment of some PTSD symptoms of patients with dissociative disorders (Loewenstein *et al.*, 1988). Yet, benzodiazepines can evoke positive dissociative symptoms, discussed below, and at high doses they may promote amnesia. Krystal *et al.* (1998) have proposed to evaluate whether drugs that facilitate NMDA receptor function have antidissociative effects in PTSD patients.

Depersonalization, derealization, perceptual alterations, and time distortions have also been provoked by high doses of cannabinoids (Dittrich *et al.*, 1973; Melges *et al.*, 1970), and were correlated with increased cerebral blood flow (Mathew *et al.*, 1993). Moreover, cannabinoids also produce amnestic effects due to interference with hippocampal memory functions (Hampson and Deadwyler, 1999). Some cannabinoid effects may be mediated by stimulation of glucocorticoid receptors (Eldrigde and Landfield, 1990) and blockade of NMDA receptors (Feigenbaum *et al.*, 1989). Serotonergic hallucinogens produce visual hallucinations, illusions, depersonalization, derealization, as well as body image distortion and, occasionally, emotional detachment (e.g., Freeman, 1986; Strassmann *et al.*, 1994). However, ketamine, its cousin phencyclidine, cannabinoids, and serotonergic hallucinogens do not produce dissociative disorders or positive dissociative symptoms such as hyperamnesia and flashbacks with respect to stressful and aversive experiences. As applies to ketamine, there is no evidence that the symptoms that cannabinoids and serotonergic hallucinogens produce relate to structural splits among dissociative parts of the personality.

Substance-Induced Dissociative Symptoms and States in PTSD Patients

A range of substances, including barbiturates and benzodiazepines, can reactivate traumatic memories and flashbacks in PTSD (for a review, see Krystal *et al.*, 1998). The effects of these drugs seem to be indirect, as they may reduce anxiety, and thus suppress mechanisms that inhibit access to traumatic memories (e.g., Kopelman *et al.*, 1994).

Autonomic activation, flashbacks and recall of traumatic memories can be provoked in a subset of patients with chronic PTSD using intravenous administration of sodium lactate (Rainey *et al.*, 1987), yohimbine (Southwick *et al.*, 1993), and metachlorophenylpiperazine (m-CPP; Southwick *et al.*, 1991). In some cases, yohimbine-induced flashbacks and traumatic memories were accompanied by depersonalization and derealization. Yohimbine blocks $\alpha 2$ receptors located on noradrenergic neurons that have a role in the regulation of fear and arousal. The $\alpha 2$ receptors partly mediate feedback inhibition of noradrenergic neurons (Starke *et al.*, 1975). Hence, yohimbine activates central noradrenergic neurons, producing increased release of norepinephrine in the brain. Clinical observations have suggested that autonomic arousal can reactivate traumatic memories, possibly because the autonomic arousal that was part of the traumatic experience has become a conditioned stimulus. (Thus, some PTSD patients and traumatized patients with other dissociative disorders tend to avoid aroused states, such as physical exertion, as well as negative and positive emotions.) However, Southwick (see Krystal *et al.*, 1998) reported that in some cases autonomic arousal followed yohimbine-provoked traumatic memories. This observation led Krystal and colleagues to conclude that 'noradrenergic systems might be involved in the elicitation of dissociative symptoms [i.e., traumatic memories, and accompanying features] as a direct consequence of central pharmacological actions of yohimbine on neural circuitry contributing to dissociation and memory retrieval' (p. 326). On the other hand, even small increments of arousal may perhaps trigger traumatic memories when the individual has developed a phobia for bodily arousal that originally accompanied trauma.

Norepinephrine/Locus Coeruleus

The autonomous nervous system is regulated by the locus coeruleus and its projection areas. The activity of the HPA-axis is partly mediated by the release of CRF by the paraventricular nucleus of the hypothalamus. Both systems are key players in stress responsivity and are functionally interrelated. They both have differentiated anatomical and functional responses to different kinds of stressors. For example, the hypothalamic paraventricular nucleus neuron appears to be affected by multiple sources, including brainstem aminergic and peptidergic afferents; blood-borne information; indirect input from limbic system and associated regions, including the prefrontal cortex, hippocampus, and amygdala; and local-circuit interactions (Herman *et al.*, 1996).

The locus coeruleus houses the majority of noradrenergic neurons. Exposure to chronic stress may yield long-term alterations in locus coeruleus firing and in norepinephrine release in target brain regions of the locus coeruleus (Bremner *et al.*, 1996). Norepinephrine also has a role in fear conditioning and sensitization, and there is strong evidence that noradrenergic activation of the amygdala is critical for neuromodulatory influences on memory storage (McGaugh *et al.*, 2000).

Both animal and human studies have shown that high levels of norepinephrine release are associated with a decrease in metabolism in the cerebral cortex. Following administration of yohimbine, PTSD patients had a tendency towards decreased brain metabolism in hippocampal, orbitofrontal, temporal, parietal, and prefrontal cortex areas; healthy controls had a tendency toward increased metabolism in these regions (Bremner *et al.*, 1997a).

Endorphins

Alcohol and opiate withdrawal activate central noradrenergic systems and can increase flashbacks and other PTSD symptoms (e.g., Kosten and Krystal, 1988). Many dissociative patients report that self-mutilation and substance abuse may be instrumental in temporarily reducing autonomic arousal, intrusions of traumatic memories, and internal imperative voices. These effects could be mediated by the release of β-endorphins that dampen norepinephrine firing in the locus coeruleus. Endogenous opiates contribute to stress-induced analgesia, dissociative symptoms, and possibly the high rate of opiate abuse in patients with PTSD: this disorder is associated with decreased baseline levels, but increased post-stimulation effects of β-endorphins (Newport and Nemeroff, 2000). The opioid antagonist naltrexone decreased the frequency of flashbacks and other dissociative phenomena in borderline personality disorder (Bohus *et al.*, 1999).

HPA-Axis

Several studies have suggested that PTSD involves low baseline levels of cortisol (Yehuda, 2000), and lower cortisol responses to CRF and ACTH challenge (Vermetten and Bremner, 2001b). While there is evidence for excessive CRF release from the hypothalamus in PTSD, and excessive ACTH from the pituitary, baseline cortisol is low. According to Yehuda (2000), low cortisol in PTSD is due to negative feedback inhibition in the HPA-axis. Yet, since the number of glucocorticoid receptors are high in PTSD, the HPA-axis would be very sensitive to stressors. In some studies, however, PTSD was associated with increased cortisol levels (e.g., De Bellis *et al.*, 1999; Lemieux and Coe, 1995). Bremner (1999) suggested that perhaps low cortisol characterizes chronic PTSD, and high cortisol levels the acute stages of the disorder. For example, women with a history of prior rape or assault had relatively lower cortisol levels immediately after rape than raped women without such a history (Resnick *et al.*, 1995). On the other hand, in individuals who had developed PTSD in response to motor vehicle accidents, the cortisol response in the immediate aftermath of the accident was significantly lower than in individuals who had developed major depression. This group effect remained after controlling for covariates such as minutes post accident, time of day, severity of trauma, and past PTSD (Yehuda *et al.*, 1998).

The neuropeptide CRF and ACTH are involved in the modulation of memory functions and the stress response. Bremner *et al.* (1997b) found an increase of CRF in PTSD patients, which is consistent with the impaired memory function in PTSD (Bremner *et al.*, 1998b) and the DSM-IV dissociative disorders. Heim *et al.* (2000) documented strongly increased ACTH levels and heart rate increases in response to mild stressors, but normal cortisol levels in women who had been sexually and physically abused early in life. This increase is presumably due to CRF hypersecretion.

Interactions Among Neuropeptide Y (NPY), Corticotropin-Releasing Factor (CRF), Cortisol, and Norepinephrine

Anxiety and stress vulnerability may relate to dysregulation of interrelated neurotransmitter systems that augment and attenuate threat responses. Whereas CRF promotes anxiety, pre-clinical studies suggest that NPY has anxiolytic properties (Helig *et al.*, 1989, 1993). Chronic stress exposure may result in the development of low baseline levels of NPY, as well as a blunted NPY response to subsequent stress (Corder *et al.*, 1992). It thus seems that deficits in NPY may promote anxiety and distress, whereas augmentations in NPY can buffer these effects.

The interactions between CRF and NPY are relevant to human stress responses in that abnormalities of both CRF and NPY have been noted in individuals suffering from post-traumatic stress, anxiety, and symptoms of dissociation (Bremner *et al.*, 1997b; Rasmusson *et al.*, 2000). Compared with healthy subjects, PTSD patients reported more anxiety, had low baseline levels of NPY, and had a blunted NPY response to yohimbine (Rasmusson *et al.*, 2000). Rasmusson and colleagues also found a negative correlation between the degree of combat exposure and plasma NPY and a negative correlation between baseline NPY levels and yohimbine-induced increases in plasma 3-methoxy-4-hydroxyphenylglycol and in systolic blood pressure. Thus sympathetic dysregulation in PTSD may be related to deficits in the NPY response to stress.

Twenty-four hours after cessation of uncontrollable stress during military survival school training, NPY had returned to baseline in special forces soldiers (Morgan *et al.*, 2000). However, other soldiers exhibited a significant depletion of NPY. The stress-induced release of NPY was negatively correlated to negative dissociative symptoms. Studying healthy subjects enrolled in US Army survival school, Morgan *et al.* (2001) found that release of salivary cortisol, NPY, and norepinephrine induced by stressful military interrogation during training were positively correlated. Release of cortisol, but not of NPY, was also correlated with dissociation and military performance during stress in this study. The dissociation measure (Clinician Administered Dissociative States Scale, CADSS, Bremner *et al.*, 1998a) administered in this study is problematic, however. The CADSS includes items that evaluate retraction of the field of consciousness, and lowering of the level of consciousness, disregards positive psychoform dissociative symptoms, and includes only a few items that assess somatoform dissociation. These flaws are found in many dissociation scales.

Urinary Catecholamines and CSF Norepinephrine

De Bellis *et al.* (1999) examined the relationship between trauma, psychiatric symptoms and urinary-free cortisol and epinephrine, norepinephrine, and dopamine excretion in abused pre-pubertal children with PTSD. These subjects were compared to a group of non-traumatized children with overanxious disorder, and with healthy controls. The children with PTSD excreted significantly greater concentrations of urinary dopamine and norepinephrine over 24 hours than the other subjects, had greater concentrations of 24 hour urinary-free cortisol than control subjects, and excreted greater concentrations of urinary epinephrine than subjects with overanxious disorder. They also had more dissociative symptoms and other psychiatric symptoms than control groups. Urinary catecholamine and urinary-free cortisol concentrations showed positive correlations with the duration and severity of PTSD symptoms. However, urinary catecholamine levels bear little relation to brain activity. A recent study found presence of greater central nervous system noradrenergic activity under baseline conditions in patients with chronic PTSD than in healthy individuals (Geracioti *et al.*, 2001). While plasma norepinephrine concentrations showed no significant relationship with the severity of PTSD symptoms, CSF norepinephrine levels strongly and positively correlated with PTSD symptoms.

In conclusion, progress in the study psychobiology of dissociation depends on more sophisticated conceptualization and measurement of dissociation. Excessive glutamate could be associated with negative dissociative symptoms, whereas excessive norepinephrine may provoke positive dissociative symptoms in individuals who have been traumatized. Traumatized individuals also display ACTH hypersecretion in response to even mild stressors—probably induced by hypersecretions of CRF. Assuming that the subjects studied by Heim *et al.* (2000) had increased numbers of glucocorticoid receptors, the hippocampus would be exposed to levels of cortisol that exceed normal values. The role of cortisol in dissociation requires further study. Some studies have found low-to-normal cortisol levels in PTSD, perhaps indicating negative feedback inhibition. However, abused children with PTSD and dissociative symptoms may have increased levels of cortisol. The inconsistent findings with respect to cortisol perhaps indicate that the functioning of patients with dissociative conditions depends on the dissociative system that dominates at a given time. Consistent with this hypothesis, Mason *et al.* (2001) found an inverse relationship between urinary cortisol levels and a symptom complex composed of two closely related clinical subgroupings, i.e., 'disengagement' (emotional numbing; relatively lower cortisol levels) and 'engagement' in trauma memories (relatively higher cortisol levels). Anisman *et al.* (2001) found that one month after an ice storm, salivary cortisol levels were elevated among moderately affected victims. However, they were diminished among those with the highest Impact of Event Scale scores. It seems possible that the more seriously affected victims remained in a numbed state when tested. The hypothesis that the psychobiological functioning of patients with dissociative conditions depends on dissociative systems will be discussed in detail below.

KEY BRAIN STRUCTURES IN INTEGRATIVE FUNCTIONS

The integrative failure that is characteristic of traumatized individuals may relate to structural and functional brain changes. For example, some data suggest temporal lobe abnormalities in dissociation. EEG recordings of dissociative patients usually involved temporal and frontal slow wave activity (Putnam, 1997). Studies of psychiatric patients reporting childhood abuse (Teicher *et al.*, 1993), as well as traumatized children (Ito *et al.*, 1993) have also documented EEG abnormalities. Using SPECT tomography, Yazici and Kostakoglu (1998) found regional cerebral blood flow changes in patients with somatoform dissociative disorder involving astasia–abasia, i.e., bizarre gait and the inability to stand unaided. Four of the five patients had left temporal, and one patient had left parietal perfusion decreases.

A range of temporal lobe structures have been implicated in dissociation, including the amygdala, hippocampus, and thalamus. Cortical regions involve the orbitofrontal and medial prefrontal cortex, and the sensory association areas.

Amygdala

The amygdala plays a critical role in responding to unconditioned threat stimuli, in the acquisition and expression of classical conditioning effects (Davies, 2000; Dolan, 2000), and in encoding and retrieval of the evaluative tone of episodic memories (Dolan, 2000). For example, LeDoux (2000) stressed that inactivation of the amygdala during learning prevents classical fear conditioning from taking place, and inactivation immediately after training precludes effects on memory. These data suggest that the amygdala is essential for fear learning.

There is evidence for involvement of the amygdala in PTSD. Electrical stimulation of the amygdala and hippocampus — as components of distributed neural memory networks — may automatically retrieve memories in a rather inflexible way, including sensorimotor re-experiencing of frightening experiences (Halgren *et al.*, 1978; Penfield and Perot, 1963). Relative inflexibility and involuntary retrieval are prominent features of traumatic memories (Van der Kolk and Van der Hart, 1991). The responsiveness of the amygdala to threat cues does not depend on conscious awareness of threat: Morris *et al.* (1999) found that the amygdala is responsive to masked angry faces, and Rauch *et al.* (2000) reported functional MRI-evidence for exaggerated amygdala response to masked facial stimuli in PTSD.

Hippocampus

The hippocampus supports the integration and modulation of modality-specific information (e.g., of the sensory, motor, and visual cortices). This processing is required for the development of coherent experiences and memories (Squire and Knowlton, 1995). The hippocampus also serves to evaluate context, which is important in the context-dependent modulation of acquired associations between unconditioned and conditioned (threat) stimuli. Thus, the amygdala stores (LeDoux, 1996) and modulates (Cahill, 2000; McGaugh *et al.*, 2000) the mostly permanent CS-UCS associations, but information processing involving the hippocampus is required to evaluate whether the CS-UCS association applies in the current context. If the CS does not signal the probable occurrence of the UCS in the present circumstances, the hippocampus should inhibit (with the medial prefrontal and orbitofrontal cortex) amygdala-based responses to CS.

Stress hormones interfere with functioning of the hippocampus, and may even damage it: animal studies have shown that direct glucocorticoid exposure results in a loss of pyramidal neurons and dendritic branching in the hippocampus (Woolley *et al.*, 1990). This suggests that the organic structure of the hippocampus is affected by cortisol, probably resulting in a decrease of neuronal synapses that would facilitate integration. Glucocorticoids might have similar effects on the human hippocampus. Compared with healthy controls, patients with combat-related PTSD (Bremner *et al.*, 1995), adults reporting childhood physical and sexual abuse with PTSD (Bremner *et al.*, 1997c), as well as a patient with DID (Tsai *et al.*, 1999) exhibited smaller hippocampal volume.

Whereas trauma-reporting female patients with borderline personality disorder had smaller hippocampal volumes than control groups, levels of neuropsychological functioning were associated with severity of depression but not with hippocampal volume (Driessen *et al.*, 2000). Stein *et al.* (1997) found smaller left-sided hippocampal volume for women reporting childhood sexual abuse compared to controls, with volume correlating strongly ($r = -0.73$) with dissociative symptom severity, but not with indices of explicit memory functioning. It thus seems that the relationship between hippocampal volume and memory functioning may be mediated by dissociation. Whether smaller hippocampi constitute a premorbid risk factor for PTSD and possibly for DSM-IV and ICD-10 dissociative disorders, or whether they are caused by chronic stress exposure, is a question for further study. Recently, Bonne *et al.* (2001) reported that smaller hippocampal volume was not a necessary risk factor for developing PTSD and did not occur within 6 months of expressing the disorder. A controlled study of hippocampal volume in patients with DID is underway (Ehling *et al.*, 2001).

Medial Prefrontal Cortex

Stress hormones also interfere with the activation of the medial prefrontal cortex. For example, elevated levels of norepinephrine were associated with dysfunction of the prefrontal cortex (Arnsten, 1999). This interference presents a major problem of affect regulation in that hippocampal (McCormick and Thompson, 1982) and medial prefrontal (Armony and LeDoux, 1997) information processing are crucially involved in inhibiting the amygdala. As discussed above, yohimbine-provoked traumatic memories and reduced hippocampal and medial prefrontal blood flow in PTSD.

Bremner *et al.* (2000b) found decreased benzodiazepine receptor binding in the medial prefrontal cortex and Bremner *et al.* (1999) documented medial prefrontal and anterior cingulate dysfunction in women with and without PTSD who reported childhood sexual abuse (CSA). The participants were exposed to neutral personal memories and to descriptions of personalized CSA events. CSA scripts were associated with greater increases in regional cerebral blood flow in portions of the prefrontal cortex, posterior cingulate, and motor cortex in women with PTSD than in those women without PTSD. These scripts also induced alterations in brain metabolism in the medial prefrontal cortex, i.e., decreased blood flow in subcallosal gyrus and the anterior cingulate. Compared with women who had not developed PTSD, those with PTSD also had decreased blood flow in the right hippocampus, fusiform/inferior temporal gyrus, supramarginal gyrus, and visual association cortex.

Using SPECT, Sar *et al.* (2001) assessed regional cerebral blood flow in 15 patients with DID without structural lesions and epilepsy, and in eight healthy controls. The blood flow ratio was decreased in orbitofrontal region bilaterally and increased in the left lateral temporal region among patients with DID when compared to the control group. Comorbid diagnoses or ongoing drug treatment did not have any significant effect on perfusion in these regions, and there was no statistically meaningful difference in regional cerebral blood flow ratios among dissociative parts of the personality, also described as dissociative personalities. Sar *et al.* (2001) concluded that the persistency of the findings over different dissociative personalities suggests a trait measure for DID. As we will discuss below, until specific *types* of dissociative personalities are compared, this conclusion might be premature.

In conclusion, dysfunction in the hippocampus and the prefrontal cortex may be related to memory deficits, affect dysregulation, impaired inhibition of conditioned responses, and dissociative symptoms in PTSD and possibly in more complex dissociative disorders as well.

Thalamus

Krystal *et al.* (1998) argued that dissociative-like phenomena in healthy individuals tend to ensue when they are exposed to extremely low or high levels of sensory stimulation. This led them to propose that the thalamus might contribute to dissociation-like alterations in consciousness in that it serves as a sensory gate or filter that directly and indirectly modulates the access of sensory information to the cortex, amygdala and hippocampus. In relay mode, the thalamus facilitates accurate transmission of sensory information to the cortex, amygdala, and hippocampus. When slow oscillatory firing patterns predominate, the flow of sensory information to amygdala, cingulate and frontal cortex is impeded, leaving the individual focused on internally generated thought processes and affective and sensory experiences. While Krystal *et al.* (1998) hold that this mode might be associated with dissociation, they have not detailed in what modes the thalamus would operate during detachment from and overengagement in trauma memories.

Cingulate Gyrus

The cingulate gyrus is responsive to shifts in thalamic sensory processing functions and is an important point of convergence for a network involving amygdala, prefrontal cortex, and mediodorsal thalamic nucleus (cf., Krystal *et al.*, 1998). The cingulate may be involved in dissociation. For example, Shin *et al.* (2000) reported that Vietnam veterans with PTSD failed to activate the affective division of the anterior cingulate during the Emotional Counting Stroop, while non-PTSD veterans did not (Whalen *et al.*, 1998). Maltreated children with PTSD also manifested metabolic abnormalities in the anterior cingulate (De Bellis *et al.*, 2000). Women with histories of childhood sexual abuse had increased anterior cingulate activity in response to trauma scripts, but those with PTSD had less regional cerebral blood flow increases in this region than those without PTSD (Shin *et al.*, 1999).

Motor Cortex

Marshall *et al.* (1997) reported that attempts of a patient with dissociative paralysis (somatoform dissociation) to move her affected leg failed to activate right primary motor cortex. Instead, the right orbitofrontal and the right anterior cingulate cortex were significantly activated. The authors suggested that these areas may inhibit willed effects on the right primary motor cortex. Preparing to move the paralysed leg produced normal brain activation. Findings by Spence *et al.* (2000) also suggest that somatoform dissociative motor symptoms involve intact ability to generate motor plans, but inhibition of actual motor action. All patients had deactivation of the left dorsolateral prefrontal cortex, regardless of the side of the symptoms. This frontal region is specifically activated by willed action. Feigning controls did not exhibit this deactivation but had hypofunction of the right anterior prefrontal cortex compared with controls. However, studying stress-related dissociative unilateral sensorimotor loss in seven patients using SPECT, Vuilleumier *et al.* (2001) found that these symptoms may represent lack of motor readiness. Compared with a resting condition, passive vibration of both hands-known to activate sensory and motor brain regions — generated bilateral and symmetrical regional cerebral blood flow increases in parietosomatosensory, frontal premotor, and anterior prefrontal cortical areas. Blood flow was reduced in the thalamus, putamen, and caudate contralateral to the side of the symptoms These hemispheric asymmetries disappeared in the four scanned patients who recovered. Vuilleumier *et al.* (2001) suggested that the decreased blood flow in circuits involving the basal ganglia and thalamus may reflect impaired motor readiness through inhibitory input from the amygdala and orbitofrontal cortex in response to emotional stressors.

Somatosensory Association Areas:

Depersonalization is related to several negative somatoform dissociative symptoms, e.g., experiencing the body as a foreign object. Comparing eight patients with depersonalization disorder and 24 healthy controls, Simeon *et al.* (2000) reported that the disorder was associated with functional abnormalities along sequential hierarchical areas, secondary and cross-modal areas of the sensory cortex (visual, auditory, and somatosensory), as well as areas responsible for an integrated body schema. More specifically, they found less metabolism in right temporal cortex (auditory association area), and more metabolism in parietal somatosensory association area and multimodal association area. Dissociation and depersonalization scores among the patients with depersonalization disorder were strongly correlated with metabolic activity in the posterior parietal association area. It thus seems that integrative failure with respect to bodily cues — which may be at the heart of basic forms of consciousness (Damasio, 1999) — is related to dysfunctioning of the temporal, parietal, and occipital association areas. Indeed, '[t]here is a hierarchy of sensory processing in the brain, from primary sensory areas to unimodal and then polymodal association areas and finally to the prefrontal cortex' (Simeon *et al.*, 2000, p. 1786). Depersonalization and negative somatoform dissociative symptoms may thus relate to dysfunction of the posterior association areas, that affects the input into the prefrontal cortex.

Insula:

Reiman *et al.* (2000, p. 399) observed that 'a region in the vicinity of anterior insular cortex [. . .] appears to be preferentially involved in the emotional response to potentially distressing cognitive stimuli, interoceptive sensory stimuli, and body sensations'. For example, regional cerebral blood flow increases have been observed in the anterior insular region during recall-generated sadness (Lane *et al.*, 1997), normal anticipatory anxiety, (Reiman, 1996), lactate-induced panic (Reiman *et al.*, 1998), and the perception of temperature and pain (Bushnell *et al.*, 1995). Based on these and other studies, Reiman *et al.* (2000) suggested that the insula participates in the evaluation of potentially distressing thoughts and body sensations with negative emotional significance, and may serve as an internal alarm centre, 'alerting the individual about potential dangers inside the body' (p. 399). The hypothesized alarm function could perhaps be executed in conjunction with the amygdala in that the insular cortex has afferent and efferent connections with the amygdala (Aggleton and Saunders, 2000).

Because traumatic memories essentially involve unintegrated emotional and somatosensory reactivity, re-experiences of trauma could be associated with altered metabolism in the insula. Indeed, exposing PTSD patients to recorded trauma memory scripts was associated with increased metabolism in the right insula (Rauch *et al.*, 1996). Other areas involved in processing these trauma scripts included a range of other right-sided limbic and paralimbic structures.

NEUROBIOLOGICAL MODELS OF DISSOCIATIVE DISORDERS

DID and Epilepsy

It has been suggested that DID actually represents epilepsy (e.g., Mesulam, 1981; Schenk and Bear, 1981). However, video EEG monitoring of DID patients previously diagnosed as cases of epilepsy documented EEG abnormalities, but not epileptiform EEG activity (Devinsky *et al.*, 1989). In addition, compared to patients with epilepsy, DID patients and patients with pseudo-epileptic seizures had more symptoms of psychoform and somatoform dissociation (Bowman and Coons, 2000; Devinsky *et al.*, 1989; Kuyk *et al.*, 1999; Loewenstein and Putnam, 1988). In some cases, epilepsy and DID may be concurrent disorders. In other cases, apparent epilepsy may represent dissociative convulsions

(WHO, 1992) reflecting a more complex dissociative disorder (e.g., Bowman, 1993; Kuyk *et al.*, 1996, 1999). Moreover, DID responds to psychotherapy, but not to the pharmacological treatment for epilepsy. The evidence thus reveals that DID does not represent epilepsy.

Dissociative Disorders and Cerebral Hemispheric Laterality

The hypothesis that dissociative personalities involve left- or right-sided hemispheric dominance (Tiihonen *et al.*, 1995) is difficult to reconcile with the fact that most DID patients encompass more than two dissociative personalities, and that these personalities display bilateral perfusion defects (Sar *et al.*, 2001). It has been suggested that dissociative disorders of movement and sensation involve symptom lateralization, and perhaps hemispheric lateralization (e.g., Marshall *et al.*, 1997; Tiihonen *et al.*, 1995). However, the results from different studies were contradictory, and a recent study of 114 cases found no evidence for lateralization (Roelofs *et al.*, 2000).

Dissociative Personalities as Discrete Behavioural States

While particular neuroendocrine substances and brain structures may be involved in trauma-related integrative failure, they do not explain why dissociation of the personality is not a random phenomenon, but tends to be orderly within limits. To account for this, Putnam (1997) has proposed that complex dissociative disorders involve discrete behavioural states. He argued that the first years of life are important in laying the groundwork of personality organization that is rather cohesive across contexts, such as place, time, and state. Infants tend to automatically move from one discrete state to another, initially lacking much integration. These states are referred to as discrete behavioural states because emotional states in young children are closely tied to behaviour, producing a highly state-dependent sense of self (Wolf, 1990; Wolff, 1987).

The relatively low integrative capacity of young children can be related to the immaturity of the brain regions that have major integrative functions, notably the prefrontal cortices and the hippocampus. Hippocampal maturity may not occur for up to three years (Seress, 1998), and full maturation of the orbitofrontal and prefrontal cortex requires many years (Benes, 1998). Furthermore, myelination in the hippocampus increases from childhood until adolescence, after which the pattern remains unchanged (Arnold and Trojanowski, 1996). As a result, emotional states involving the amygdala operate in relatively uncoordinated and unintegrated ways in early childhood, even under normal conditions.

The integrative capacity of children is also limited because of a relative absence of experience-derived templates that are helpful as 'attractors' (Siegel, 1999) to integrate new and/or emotionally charged experiences. Thus (young) children seem to be dependent on their social environment for regulation of instinctual emotional systems. In support of this hypothesis, Ogawa *et al.* (1997) found that dissociation in early childhood was a common response to disruption and stress, whereas persistent dissociation in adolescence and young adulthood was indicative of psychopathology.

Although little is known about the development of integration among emotional states, it is in interaction with caretakers that young children begin to acquire skills to sustain, modulate, and integrate states (Schore, 2001; Siegel, 1999). Social sharing of parallel or complementary states between the child and caretaker is associated with synchronizations of physiological processes between the child and the adult that assist the child in regulating states, and lack of synchronization has disruptive effects (Field, 1985). While adequate caretaking activities critically enhance integration of behavioural states in the child, inadequate or inconsistent caretaking will result in the child having difficulty integrating emotional states and constructing a stable sense of self.

Trauma may interfere with this developmental integrative process (Putnam, 1997) by compromising the integrative functions of the developing brain (Gurvits *et al.*, 2000; Teicher *et al.*, 1997; for reviews, see Bremner, 1999; Glaser, 2000; Schore, 2001; Siegel, 1999). Thus, repeated activation of trauma-related states can promote state-dependent functioning and concomitant neurobiological 'hard-wiring' of the brain (Perry, 1999; Perry *et al.*, 1995), depending on the child's life experiences, particularly before age six. While prospective studies should assess to what extent particular brain features are a risk factor for, or sequelae of traumatization and dissociation, the evidence to date suggests that maltreatment in childhood is associated with adverse influences on brain development (De Bellis *et al.*, 1999), and increased sensitivity to the effects of stress in later life (Graham *et al.*, 1999). Thus, adverse social experiences during early critical periods result in permanent alterations in CRF, opiate, corticosteroid, dopamine, noradrenaline, and serotonin receptors (cf. Schore, 2001).

Several studies suggest a potential causal relationship between severe traumatization in early childhood and compromised integrative functions. For example, younger children had more PTSD symptoms than adolescents (Anthony *et al.*, 1999), and the severity of psychoform and somatoform dissociation among DID patients and psychiatric controls were best predicted by reported trauma during the first six years of life (Draijer and Boon, 1993; Nijenhuis *et al.*, 1998b). Also, the age of onset, chronicity, and severity of childhood trauma were associated with psychoform dissociative symptoms up to 19 years later (Ogawa *et al.*, 1997). Recently, Nijenhuis *et al.* (2001a) found that adult psychiatric patients who reported more than five different types of traumatization during their lives had higher levels of PTSD symptoms, and more psychoform and somatoform dissociation than did psychiatric patients who reported fewer than five different types of trauma, only emotional abuse and neglect, or no traumatization at all. In most cases, the reported severe traumatization had commenced in (early) childhood, and severity of somatoform dissociation was associated with composite bodily threat scores, including age at onset, duration, and subjectively rated impact of the traumatization (Nijenhuis *et al.*, 2001a).

Dissociative Personalities in DID

Consistent with Putnam's theory (Putnam, 1997), dissociative systems in DID tend to display psychophysiological differences that are not reproduced by DID-simulating controls. Differences have been reported in electrodermal activity (skin conductance; Ludwig *et al.*, 1972; Larmore *et al.*, 1977), EEG — in particular in the beta 2 band (Coons *et al.*, 1982; Hughes *et al.*, 1990; Ludwig *et al.*, 1972; Putnam *et al.*, 1993), visual evoked potentials (Putnam *et al.*, 1992), regional cerebral blood flow (Mathew *et al.*, 1985; Saxe *et al.*, 1992), autonomic nervous system variables (Putnam *et al.*, 1990), optical variables (Birnbaum and Thomann, 1996; Miller, 1989; Miller and Triggiano, 1991; Miller *et al.*, 1991), and arousal (Putnam *et al.*, 1990).

While these studies are valuable, it is difficult to say what the data actually tell beyond suggesting that these physiological data sets 'are most parsimoniously explained by regarding the alter personalities as discrete states of consciousness' (Putnam, 1997, p. 138). Advances in the field critically depend on theoretical predictions with respect to the *kind* of differences that exist among different *types* of dissociative personalities. The theory of structural dissociation (Nijenhuis *et al.*, 2002) offers such predictions.

THE THEORY OF STRUCTURAL DISSOCIATION

Many individuals with PTSD or more complex dissociative disorders alternate between being fixated on the trauma and being detached from the experience (Nijenhuis and Van der Hart, 1999a, 1999b). Using metaphors that Myers (1940) proposed, the 'emotional' personality (EP) has encoded and stored trauma, and is dedicated to defense from major threat, in particular, threat to the integrity of the body. The 'apparently normal' personality (ANP), on the other hand, is detached from trauma, experiences some degree of amnesia or is depersonalized from some or many components of the experience, and is dedicated to fulfilling functions in daily life, some of which serve the survival of the species. According to the theory of structural dissociation (Nijenhuis *et al.*, 2002b), this alternating pattern reflects failed integration between the ANP and EP.

Structural dissociation of the personality may involve constellations of one ANP and one EP, as in PTSD; one ANP and more than one EP, as in complex PTSD (Herman, 1992), also known as disorders of extreme stress (Pelcovitz *et al.*, 1997), and more than one ANP and more than one EP, as seen only in DID. According to the theory, the extent to which the personality becomes fragmented depends on the severity of the traumatization in terms of developmental age at trauma onset, chronicity and intensity of the traumatization, and factors such as the relationship to the perpetrator and lack of support and social recognition of the trauma. A limitation of the theory of structural dissociation is that it does not address structural dissociation of the personality unrelated to trauma (for a remarkable case of latent abilities, see Braude, 2000).

ANP and EP are two different psychobiological systems, each endowed with its own sense of self. According to Damasio (1999, p. 26), consciousness and sense of self are essentially grounded in 'a feeling that accompanies the making of any kind of image — visual, auditory, tactile, visceral — within our living systems' and may involve several integrative levels: (1) the *proto-self* that emerges from the activity of brain devices that continuously and nonconsciously maintain the body state within the narrow range and relative stability required for survival; (2) the *core self* that relates to core consciousness defined as conscious awareness of the here and now based on the mental representation of how the organism's own state is affected by the organism's processing of an object; and (3) the *autobiographical self* that involves extended consciousness, i.e., conscious awareness of one's personal existence across subjective time.

The existence of the EP can be limited to re-experiencing traumatic memories, i.e., sensorimotor experiences that hardly involve narrative components, if at all (Nijenhuis *et al.*, 2001b; Van der Kolk and Fisler, 1995; Van der Kolk and Van der Hart, 1991). In this case, the EP may involve little more than core consciousness and core self. Yet clinical observations suggest that with recurrent reactivations of traumatic memories and chronic traumatization (and treatment), the EP may develop a degree of extended consciousness and autobiographical self. Even in these cases, however, extended consciousness and the sense of autobiographical self tend to remain quite limited. EPs are typically fixed in past trauma with absent or only partial awareness of the present or the passage of time. ANPs typically have developed a more substantial degree of extended consciousness, yet lack personification of the traumatic past and the associated EPs. EPs and ANPs have a narrowed field of consciousness focused on issues relevant to the functions they exert. Although Nijenhuis *et al.* (2002b) use the metaphor of dissociative personalities, it should be noted that such systems range from quite simple to highly complex: some dissociative personalities encompass just one psychobiological state, others are complex assemblies of such states. Dissociative personalities involve senses of self that are different from the pretraumatic self. However, because young children encompass psychobiological systems that are still relatively unintegrated, their pretraumatic sense of self is rather inconsistent and changeable, thus sense of self may not be stable even prior to early traumatization.

A major question is what psychobiological systems drive the EP and ANP, including their sense of self? These systems should meet a range of shared criteria: (1) they must be self-organizing and self-stabilizing within windows of homeostasis, time and context to control and integrate all the rather coherent complexes of psychobiological phenomena exhibited by ANP and EP; (2) they should be functional systems that have been developed in the course of evolution, and should be rather analogous to animal biological systems. Clinical observations suggest that the ANP typically engages in tasks of daily life such as reproduction, attachment, care taking, and socialization, and avoidance of traumatic memories that supports focus on daily life issues. In contrast, the EP primarily displays evolutionary defensive and emotional reactions to the (perceived) threat on which they seem to be fixated; (3) they should be very susceptible to classical conditioning, because, as we discuss below, the EP and ANP strongly respond to unconditioned and conditioned threat cues; (4) they should involve stable characteristics, but also allow for case-dependent variation as well, as ANP and EP exhibit both invariant and idiosyncratic variations; and (5) they should be available early in life, since dissociative disorders can manifest from a very early age.

Emotional Operating Systems

The theory of structural dissociation holds that the psychobiological systems that drive EP and ANP are *emotional operating systems*, or briefly, emotional systems, described by Panksepp (1998). Defense, attachment of offspring to parents, parental attachment to and care for offspring, procreation, sociability, energy management, exploration, and play constitute the major emotional systems, and may encompass a range of subsystems. Panksepp argued that basic emotional processes arise from distinct psychobiological systems that reflect coherent integrative processes of the nervous system (cf. Ciompi, 1991). In his view, the affective essence of emotionality is organized on subcortical and precognitive levels, and each of the emotional systems involves specific patterns of activation of neural networks and associated neurochemical activity in the brain.

Emotional systems are psychobiological in nature and closely meet the five criteria of dissociative personalities described above: they are organizational, evolutionary derived, functional, flexible within limits, and inborn but epigenetic. Emotional systems are functional in that they activate various types of affective feelings which help identify events in the world that are either biologically useful or harmful, and generate adaptive responses to many life-challenging circumstances. The basic behavioural patterns involved in emotional systems are approach and avoidance. Although the resulting behaviour is unconditionally summoned by the appropriate cues, approach and avoidance are adaptable to prevailing environmental conditions within limits, rather than being mere inflexible responses. For example, flight involves not just running away from threat, but running that is adapted to the current situation in form, direction, and duration. Thus, threat as an unconditional stimulus does not evoke a single 'unconditional' response, but integrated series of psychobiological responses.

Emotional systems are epigenetic, i.e., the result of influences by nature and nurture. Experiences, especially early ones, can change the fine details of the brain forever. These experiences include learning associations between events. Emotional systems are susceptible to classical conditioning: i.e., learning that some previously neutral events predict or refer to unconditioned stimuli. These conditioned stimuli tend to reactivate a representation of the unconditioned stimuli, and thus the once unconditionally summoned emotional system. Subsystems of defense are of particular interest in dissociation because of exposure to threat. Each defensive subsystem controls a pattern of psychobiological reactions that is adapted to meet a particular degree of threat imminence (Fanselow and Lester, 1988). This degree of imminence can be expressed in terms of the time and space that separate the subject from the threat (i.e., the distance between predator and prey), as well as in terms of an evaluation of the defensive abilities of the subject (e.g., the subject's psychosocial influence and physical force).

Pre-encounter defense involves an apprehensive state with increased arousal, potentiated startle response, interruption of 'normal life' behaviours, and nearly exclusive attentional focus on the potential threat. *Post-encounter defense* includes several subsystems: flight, freeze, with associated analgesia, and fight. *Post-strike defense* involves total submission and bodily as well as emotional anaesthesia. Upon survival, a recuperative subsystem is activated that allows for a return of affective awareness and body sensations (e.g., pain, fatigue), and that drives wound care and rest through social isolation, as well as sleep. Upon recovery, there will be a reactivation of (sub)systems that control daily life interests such as consumption of food, reproduction and taking care of offspring.

The EP is Dedicated to Survival Under Threat

According to the theory of structural dissociation, EPs are primarily manifestations of the emotional system that controls defense in the face of threat—particularly threat to the integrity of the body by a person—and potentially also of the emotional system that controls separation panic in relation to caretakers. Both systems serve survival interests and strongly influence the mental and physical experiences and actions of the EP. While EPs essentially rely on evolutionary derived mechanisms, their manifest form will be shaped by environmental conditions, especially traumatic experiences that evoke threat, in particular those that occurred in early childhood, and subsequent external and internal conditions. These conditions include the degree and quality of social support in the aftermath of trauma, repetition of trauma, and the degree of dissociation between EP and ANP.

In cases of *primary structural dissociation*, which would characterize acute stress disorder, simple PTSD, and simple cases of somatoform dissociative disorders (i.e., the ICD-10 dissociative disorders of sensation and movement), a single EP can include all defensive subsystems. *Secondary structural dissociation* is a manifestation of a range of defensive subsystems that have not, or not sufficiently, been integrated among each other. Thus the EP may become fragmented into several EPs that serve different defensive functions. In secondary structural dissociation, some EPs typically display freezing and are analgesic, others are inclined to physically resist threat and experience anger, or totally submit to threat while being severely anaesthetic. This threat often consists of re-experiencing (traumatic) memories of severe and chronic childhood abuse and neglect, or in responding to cues that are salient reminders of these events. Insecure attachment to caretakers can also become associated with one or more EPs in secondary structural dissociation. This level of integrative failure is mediated by traumatization that is more severe than that associated with simple PTSD. Secondary dissociation is characteristic of complex acute stress disorder, complex PTSD, complex cases of somatoform dissociative disorders, many cases of dissociative disorder not otherwise specified (APA, 1994), and perhaps borderline personality disorder (APA, 1994) as well.

We repeat that the literature generally refers only to states of freezing and submission as dissociative (and often these states are not regarded as different from each other), whereas sympathetic hyperarousal states are not (Perry *et al.*, 1995). However, defining dissociation as a lack of integration among emotional systems that may include single or clusters of states implies that hyperarousal states can also be dissociative. But these, as well as states involving analgesia and motor inhibition (freezing), bodily and emotional anaesthesia, disengagement from environmental cues, and submission (total submission, regulated by the parasympathetic nervous system (Porgess *et al.*, 1994; Schore, 1994)) may all be manifestations of unintegrated dissociative subsystems of defense.

The ANP Involves Systems that Manage Daily Life and Promote Survival of the Species

Clinical observations suggest that emotional systems of the ANP primarily function to direct performance of daily tasks necessary to living (work, social interaction, energy control), and of tasks related to survival of the species (reproduction; caretaking of children). Some ANPs may execute daily life emotional systems with passion, while others do so in more or less depersonalized and automatic ways (e.g., caretaking). Depersonalized functioning in caretaking and attachment may interfere with synchronizations of physiological processes between adult and child that assist the child in regulating states (Field, 1985), potentially leading to dissociation in the offspring of dissociative parents (Schore, 2001).

When trauma by caretakers begins early in the life of the child, a particular style of attachment often develops in the child, termed *disorganized/disoriented* (Liotti, 1999; Main and Morgan, 1996). In normal, middle class families about 15% of the infants develop this attachment style, but in cases of maltreatment its prevalence may be up to three times higher (Van IJzendoorn *et al.*, 1999). Thus frightened or frightening parental behaviour predicted infant disorganized attachment (Schuengel *et al.*, 1999). Prospective longitudinal research has demonstrated that disorganized and avoidant attachment in early childhood, along with age of onset, chronicity, and severity of abuse, predicted dissociation in various developmental stages, up to late adolescence (Ogawa *et al.*, 1997). Both ANP and EP may be insecurely attached to original abusive caretakers or to (positive or negative) substitute caretakers.

Disorganized attachment may neither be disorganized nor disoriented. Instead, it involves concurrent or rapid successive activation of the attachment system and the defense system when primary attachment figures are both the source of protection from threat and the threat itself for the traumatized child. Separation from attachment figures activates the innate attachment system, which evokes mental and behavioural approach to the caregiver. However, approach yields an increasing degree of imminence of threat, and therefore evokes a succession of defensive subsystems (flight, freeze, fight, submission). This approach and avoidance conflict cannot be resolved by the child and promotes a structural dissociation of the attachment and the defensive system.

In addition to secondary structural dissociation (fragmentation of the defensive system, thus of the EP), fragmentation of the ANP may also occur. Thus, this *tertiary structural dissociation* (Nijenhuis and Van der Hart, 1999b; Nijenhuis *et al.*, 2002; Van der Hart *et al.*, 1998), characteristic only of DID, involves fragmentation among two or more emotional operating systems that serve functions in daily life and in survival of the species. For example, one ANP regarded herself as the mother of her children, and another ANP engaged in a job. Remaining as the mother, the patient did not appreciate or understand the interests that she had as a worker, and vice versa. Tertiary structural dissociation does not occur during trauma, but rather emerges when certain inescapable aspects of daily life become associated with past trauma, such that systems of daily life become dissociated. Apart from extreme generalization of stimuli that reactivate traumatic memories, tertiary dissociation can also result from traumatization that started before the individual had been able to create a cohesive personality. Early and chronic traumatization may lead to some unclear mix of ANP/EP, where neither can be clearly distinguished. Such complexes are clinically observed in more dysfunctional DID patients.

SIMILARITIES BETWEEN THE HUMAN AND ANIMAL DEFENSIVE SYSTEM

At a general level, Nijenhuis *et al.* (1998c) drew a parallel between animal defensive systems/recuperative systems and characteristic somatoform dissociative responses of trauma-reporting patients with dissociative disorders. Their review suggested that there are similarities between animal and human disturbances of normal eating patterns and other normal behavioural patterns in the face of diffuse threat; freezing and stilling when serious threat materializes; analgesia and anaesthesia when strike is about to occur; and acute pain when threat has subsided and recuperation is at stake.

Nijenhuis *et al.* (1998a) performed a first empirical test of the hypothesized similarity between animal defensive reactions and certain somatoform dissociative symptoms of dissociative disorder patients who reported trauma. All 12 somatoform dissociative symptom clusters tested were found to discriminate between patients with dissociative disorders and patients with other psychiatric diagnoses. Those clusters expressive of the hypothesized similarity between animal and human models — freezing, anaesthesia–analgesia, and disturbed eating — belonged to the five most characteristic symptom clusters of dissociative disorder patients. Anaesthesia–analgesia, urogenital pain and freezing symptom clusters independently contributed to predicted caseness of dissociative disorder. Using an independent sample, it appeared that anaesthesia–analgesia best predicted caseness after controlling for symptom severity. The indicated symptom clusters correctly classified 94% of cases that constituted the original sample, and 96% of an independent second sample. These results were largely consistent with the hypothesized similarity to animal defense systems.

Among Dutch and Flemish dissociative disorders patients, the severity of somatoform dissociation — as measured by the Somatoform Dissociation Questionnaire (SDQ-20; Nijenhuis *et al.*, 1996, 1999b) — was best predicted by threat to the integrity of the body in the form of childhood physical abuse and childhood sexual trauma (Nijenhuis *et al.*, 1998b). The particularly strong association between the SDQ-20 — which includes many items that assess anaesthesia, analgesia, and motor inhibitions — and physical abuse has also been found in a range of other populations: nonclinical subjects (Waller *et al.*, 2000), gynaecology patients with chronic pelvic pain (Nijenhuis *et al.*, 1999c), women reporting childhood sexual abuse (Nijenhuis *et al.*, 2001b), psychiatric outpatients (Nijenhuis *et al.*, 2001a), as well as North American (Dell, 1997) and Ugandan patients with dissociative disorders (Van Duyl and Nijenhuis, in preparation).

According to the theory of structural dissociation, EPs involve defensive (sub)systems. We will discuss below recent experimental research suggesting that (1) animal defense-like reactions particularly characterize the EP, and that (2) EPs and ANPs have different psychophysiological stress responses to threat-related stimuli, even if these stimuli are presented preconsciously. Future research will need to decipher whether various EP-subtypes have the hypothesized features of animal defensive subsystems.

PSYCHOBIOLOGICAL INTERFERENCE WITH INTEGRATION OF ANP AND EP

Peritraumatic Integrative Failure

Evocation of the defense system or any other psychobiological system is not dissociative in itself, rather the lack of integration between various systems and subsystems is what constitutes dissociation. As discussed above, extremely high levels of arousal may interfere with the execution of normal integrative processes (Ludwig, 1972; Krystal *et al.*, 1991; see also Siegel, 1999), and integrative functions may be compromised by long-lasting neuroendocrine instability induced by severe stress in early childhood. It is likely that some emotional systems can be integrated more readily than others. As Panksepp (1998) argued, multiple feedbacks within and across emotional systems promote synthesis of components of a system (e.g., perceptions, behaviours, sense of self) and integration across emotional systems. However, integration across emotional systems that involve quite different and sometimes conflicting functions may be far more demanding than synthesizing components of a particular emotional system or integrating functionally related systems. If this is correct, the integration of systems dedicated to daily life and survival of the species (ANP), and systems dedicated to survival of the individual in the face of that threat (EP) will fail more readily than integration across subsystems of these two complex systems. Structural dissociation between the ANP and the EP will thus be the basic type of integrative failure, i.e., primary structural dissociation, when overwhelming trauma occurs. When stress levels rise, integration of subsystems of defense may be compromised as well, yielding secondary dissociation, i.e., fragmentation of the EP.

Post-traumatic Integrative Failure

Since living organisms have a natural tendency toward integration (Siegel, 1999), what maintains dissociation when trauma has ceased and stress-induced monoaminergic reactivity has returned to baseline? According to the theory of structural dissociation, apart from integrative deficiency that relates to enduring neuroendocrine changes induced by stress in early life, integrative failure in the aftermath of trauma also involves fear conditioning.

Trauma and Classical Conditioning

Trauma-related classical conditioning involves association of stimuli that saliently signalled or accompanied the overwhelming event. As a result, these previously neutral cues will thereafter reactivate a representation of the traumatic experience. Thus the essence of classical conditioning is the development of an anticipatory (CS signals UCS) or referential response (CS refers to UCS). For example, the specific mood (e.g., anger) of the caretaker when abusive, as well as the stimuli that apparently tended to elicit this mood, will tend to become conditioned stimuli.

Phobias of Traumatic Memories and Dissociative Personalities

Classical trauma conditioning can also generate effects that support continued structural dissociation (Nijenhuis *et al.*, 2002). First of all, structural dissociation is less than perfect. When the EP's traumatic memories are reactivated by potent external (e.g., certain smells, sounds, sights) or internal (e.g., feelings or body sensations) CS, they can intrude into the experiential domain of the ANP. Since traumatic memories represent the trauma, they are formally CS. But the sensorimotor and highly affectively charged properties of these unintegrated experiences are inherently aversive for the ANP and *will therefore act as UCS*. Indeed, when traumatized patients re-experience their traumas, it is as if the trauma happens ‘here and now’. When the integrative capacity of the ANP does not suffice for integration of the intruding traumatic memory, the ANP will respond to intrusions (UCS) with typical behavioural and mental defensive reactions (UCR; Nijenhuis and Van der Hart, 1999b). The ANP cannot escape from the highly stressful intrusions by behavioural means, but mental escape can be effective, as applies to factual (inescapable) trauma. Thus, typical reactions of the ANP include retracting the field of consciousness, lowering the level of consciousness (with pseudo-epileptic loss of consciousness as an extreme), and (re)dissociating the EP and the traumatic memories. At the same time, the ANP learns to fear and avoid internal and external CS that signal or refer to the EP. As time progresses and the dissociative condition continues, there is an ever widening range of CS that the ANP will avoid due to stimulus generalization.

Evaluative Conditioning

In addition to classical fear conditioning, evaluative conditioning (Baeyens *et al.*, 1993) of external and internal stimuli may occur. This type of associative learning produces robust effects and involves the presentation of two conjointly stimuli: a neutral stimulus and a stimulus that the individual evaluates in a negative (or positive) manner. As a result of this simple procedure, the previously neutral stimulus adopts a similar negative (or positive) tone. The ANP and EP evaluate traumatic memories differently (Nijenhuis *et al.*, 1999a), and clinical observations strongly suggest that evaluative conditioning applies to trauma-related dissociation. For example, when the trauma involved a shameful event, the ANP may learn to be ashamed of the EP, and to despise it.

In cases of secondary and tertiary dissociation, EPs and ANPs may learn to fear, reject, and avoid each other along similar pathways of evaluative and classical conditioning. In tertiary structural dissociation, avoidance of different ANPs may be based on similar trauma-related issues and conflicts. In summary, many dissociative personalities become phobic of each other. These conditioned effects interfere with normal integrative tendencies. Hence, *structural dissociation involves a strong tendency toward chronicity*.

In some individuals, alternations between the ANP and EP manifests from the acute phase onward, but other individuals function apparently well for extended periods of time before displaying post-traumatic stress symptoms. However, upon close scrutiny it often appears that the latency period was marked by avoidance of the trauma and associated internal and external cues, yielding a condition of chronic depersonalization. In cases of trauma-related dissociative amnesia as a disorder (APA, 1994), access to the memory of the trauma and to other parts of one's previous non-traumatic life seem to be inhibited (Markowitsch *et al.*, 2000; Van der Hart and Brom, 2000; Van der Hart and Nijenhuis, 2001; Van der Hart *et al.*, 1999).

Relational Factors that Maintain Structural Dissociation

When significant others deny trauma instead of assisting in the integration of the painful experience, or prohibit talking about it, dissociative tendencies are enhanced. These adverse social influences prevail in intrafamilial childhood sexual abuse (Freyd, 1996), and seem to promote dissociative amnesia (Vanderlinden *et al.*, 1993). PTSD has been associated with lack of support in the aftermath of trauma (King *et al.*, 1998), and in another study, patients with complex dissociative disorders reported total absence of support and consolation when abused (Nijenhuis *et al.*, 1998b). As the structural dissociation theory predicts, social support can buffer negative effects of trauma exposure (Elklit, 1997; Runtz and Schallow, 1997). It might be that social support provides safety cues, assists the individual in modulating the affective state and biological stress levels, and thus promotes the integration of the EP and ANP.

PSYCHOBIOLOGICAL RESEARCH OF ANP AND EP

To summarize the essence of the structural dissociation theory, it proposes that (1) traumatic experiences — especially trauma that occurs early in life and involves severe threat to the integrity to bodily integrity — activate evolutionary derived defensive systems, (2) these emotional operating systems may remain unintegrated to varying degrees due to extreme stress levels, classical and evaluative conditioning to traumatic memories, approach–avoidance conflicts with regard to defense and attachment, and lack of social support. ANPs involve emotional operating systems dedicated to survival of the species and normal life, and EPs systems dedicated to survival of the threatened individual. From this theory, a range of hypotheses can be derived, some of which have been tested in pioneering studies.

Differences Between ANP and EP on Subliminal Threat Exposure

Preconscious information processing plays a key role in responding to unconditioned and conditioned threat cues and in fear-related learning (Davies, 2000; Dolan, 2000; LeDoux, 1996; Morris *et al.*, 1998). The theory of structural dissociation considers that ANPs aim to avoid this threat, and that EPs will selectively attend to these cues. Thus in an original study, Van Honk *et al.* (1999, 2001) hypothesized that dissociative personality-dependent reactivity to (un)conditioned threat will be evident following exposure to cues that are presented very briefly in order to preclude consciously aware perception. More specifically, the effects of exposing the ANP and EP in DID patients to masked neutral, fearful, and angry facial expressions were tested.

Whereas ANPs named the colour of the mask that immediately followed the experimental stimuli more quickly when this stimulus involved angry facial expressions compared to exposure to neutral facial expressions, EPs did not show differential responses to these cues. DID-simulating controls showed the reverse pattern: a tendency toward longer response latencies after exposure to angry faces when enacting ANPs, and a tendency toward shorter reaction times after exposure to angry faces when enacting EPs. The interaction 'group (genuine DID vs DID-simulators) × condition (angry vs neutral faces)' was statistically significant. Because this effect was absent when comparing fearful and neutral faces, it was specific for cues that signal an increased possibility of attack. The reaction time effects were associated with a decrease of the pre-ejection period (PEP; the interval between ventricular depolarization and ventricular ejection onset) for the EP when exposed to angry faces, indicating increased sympathetic nervous system activity in this condition.

The results are consistent with the hypothesis that ANPs avoid subliminal threat cues by means of gaze aversion, and that EPs particularly attend to bodily threat from a person, with increased sympathetic tone. The response of the EP is pathological in that angry faces represent social threat that can be reduced by gaze aversion: a social cue that signals submission to a dominant individual. On the other hand, the results of the study are at odds with the theory that DID involves effects of suggestion and role-playing.

If ANPs can preconsciously avoid externally presented (un)conditioned threat cues, it is reasonable to assume that they can also preconsciously avoid *internal* (un)conditioned threatening stimuli. Hence, it seems possible that the ANP preconsciously avoids the EP and its memories, as the theory of structural dissociation holds. Some neurobiological data are consistent with the interpretation that dissociative amnesia involves inhibited access to episodic memory. Markowitsch and his colleagues have demonstrated that trauma-related dissociative amnesia as a disorder (APA, 1994) can be associated with reduced blood flow in parts of the brain that are normally activated during retrieval of autobiographical memories (Markowitsch, 1999; Markowitsch *et al.*, 1997a, 1997b, 1998, 2000). Moreover, partial regaining of these memories was correlated with a return to normal brain metabolism in these areas (Markowitsch *et al.*, 2000). The mechanisms of this presumed inhibitory process could be studied using functional MRI analysis.

Symptom Provocation by Exposure to Neutral and Trauma Memory Scripts in DID

In several studies, imagery of personal trauma, audiotaped descriptions of traumatic experiences, and videotaped traumatic scenes have been used to provoke post-traumatic stress reactions in PTSD patients. Compared to controls, many PTSD patients have increased psychophysiological responses (heart rate, blood pressure, skin conductance, EMG) to these types of trauma-related cues (Keane *et al.*, 1998; Orr *et al.*, 1993, 1998; Pitman *et al.*, 1999), and more severe pathology was associated with a higher magnitude of psychophysiological reactions to trauma cues (Orr *et al.*, 1998). However, using psychophysiological responses to trauma-related cues as a classificatory criterium of PTSD yielded a substantial number of false positives and false negatives (Keane *et al.*, 1998), i.e., the positive and negative predictive values of these factors were limited. It seems possible that the 'physiological nonresponders' to trauma cues remained as ANP, whereas 'physiological responders' failed to avoid cued intrusion by the EP, or switched into the EP. In this regard, it is interesting that physiological nonresponders with PTSD manifested less re-experiencing symptoms (Keane *et al.*, 1998), perhaps indicating ANP dominance.

In the first study of its kind, Nijenhuis *et al.* (1999a) assessed several sensorimotor, affective, and psychophysiological reactions in 11 women with DID, assessed by the SCID-D (Steinberg, 1994). Regional cerebral blood flow was evaluated with PET (Reinders *et al.*, in preparation). ANPs and EPs were subjected to audiotaped descriptions of neutral personal memories and traumatic personal memories. In support of the hypotheses, it was found that in response to the trauma scripts, EPs, but not ANPs displayed decreases of heart rate variability as measured by time domain variability. Stress induces reductions in heart rate variability. In response to the trauma scripts, EPs but not ANPs, also showed statistically significant increases of heart rate frequency and systolic blood pressure. Neither personality types had differential psychophysiological responses to the neutral memories. Whereas EPs experienced a wide range of affective and sensorimotor reactions to the trauma scripts, ANPs did not have these reactions, or only to a minor degree. The ANP's lack of psychophysiological reactivity to supraliminal threat (trauma scripts) could reveal inhibition of responding to threat cues by means of mental avoidance.

As hypothesized, there were statistically significant differences in regional cerebral blood flow between EPs and ANPs when they were exposed to trauma memory scripts, but not when they were exposed to neutral memory scripts (Reinders *et al.*, in preparation). There were also differences in brain metabolism for exposure of EPs to trauma memory scripts and neutral memory scripts. The observed neurobiological differences could not be explained as a result of the variability in subjective and psychophysiological reactivity, and thus reflected effects of the experimental conditions, i.e., types of memory scripts and types of dissociative personality. The PET scan results — described in more detail in Reinders *et al.* (in preparation) — converged with the subjective and psychophysiological data. Jointly, the findings were supportive of the hypothesis that EPs and ANPs have different patterns of psychobiological reactivity to traumatic memories, and that the psychobiological reactions of EPs to trauma memory scripts differ from their reactions to neutral memory scripts: EPs responded to trauma memory scripts in somatosensory and emotionally charged ways, whereas ANPs responded to these cues with a psychobiological pattern that reflects depersonalization and numbing.

POSITIVE FEEDFORWARD EXCITATION (EP) AND NEGATIVE FEEDFORWARD INHIBITION (ANP)?

As detailed above, the ANP tended to avoid masked angry faces, whereas the subliminal perception of angry faces interfered with performance for the EP (Van Honk *et al.*, 1999, 2001). This may imply that the ANP and EP involve different degrees or kinds of amygdala activity when exposed to external threat cues. One EP inadvertently recognized the angry faces, became very anxious, fixed her gaze on the screen, froze, and could not name the colour of the mask for several minutes. She finally mentioned the wrong colour. Remaining as ANP, the patient did not recognize the angry faces, however. (Note: the scores of this patient were excluded from the calculations.) The EP's fixation on threat cues is also suggested by the increased heart rate frequency and blood pressure, as well as the reduced heart rate variability of EPs in response to trauma memory scripts (Nijenhuis *et al.*, 1999a). Moreover, EPs but not ANPs, reported analgesia and strong negative evaluative reactions in response to the trauma scripts. A major riddle to solve regarding dissociation is how DID patients can display the EP-dependent and ANP-dependent psychobiological activity in response to identical threat stimuli (i.e., angry faces and trauma scripts).

Before presenting some thoughts on the issue, we remark that our experimental DID research was limited to women, which may have affected the results. Pre-clinical trials have suggested large gender differences with respect to responsivity to identical stressors, e.g., c-fos expression in the prefrontal cortex and other brain regions (Trentani *et al.*, 2002). Hence, the degree of activation of various brain structures may be dependent on gender. Next, there is evidence for differential responding of the left and right amygdala to stressors (Cahill *et al.*, 2001). For the time being, we disregarded this complexity, but remark that future research should control for gender.

EP-Dependent Responsivity to Threat

Exposure to major external threat causes rapid activation of the defensive system by the amygdala and related structures. This is mandatory for survival, as is learning and memorizing by means of classical conditioning that which signals or refers to threat. The range of threat-related responses orchestrated by the amygdala includes activation of the sympathetic nervous system and the HPA-axis, defensive behaviour (through the central grey), startle response, and stress-induced hypoalgesia (Aggleton, 2000). The lateral amygdala receives sensory inputs directly from the sensory thalamus and indirectly from the sensory cortex. The lateral amygdala projects to the central nucleus of the amygdala, which projects to structures controlling defensive behaviour (flight, freeze, fight, submission), autonomic arousal, hypoalgesia, stress hormones, and potentiated startle. Thus, the amygdala will be hyperactivated in the face of threat (UCS), will encode and store CS-UCS propositions (e.g., CS signals UCS), and will modulate trauma memories more generally. When CS (re)appear, the amygdala and other aspects of the emotional brain and the defensive systems tend to become reactivated.

Hyperactivation of the defensive system during traumatic stress may produce hyperamnesia through mediation of the basolateral nucleus of the amygdala. The basolateral amygdala has a major role in stress-mediated neuromodulatory influences on memory storage (Cahill, 2000; McGaugh *et al.*, 2000). Post-event memory consolidation for emotional experiences involves not only the basolateral amygdala, but the stria terminalis as well. This is a major afferent/efferent amygdala pathway, which interacts with peripheral stress hormone feedback locally in the amygdala, and with emotional memory storage elsewhere in the brain (Cahill, 2000).

Reactivated traumatic memories represent internal threat in that these memories are not narratives but somatosensory and emotionally charged experiences. Findings of Reiman and his colleagues, discussed above, suggest that internal threat cues (including body signals) are associated with activity of the insula. Because the insula have afferent/efferent connections with the amygdala, internal threat cues may activate the amygdala through this path.

Hyperactivation of the amygdala in the EPs exposed to external and internal threat cues (angry faces) may be related to failed inhibition of the amygdala and insula by the hippocampus and the medial prefrontal cortex due to excessive release of stress hormones: uninhibited positive feedforward loops would seem to stabilize the defensive system, and impede the integration of EP and ANP. In this context, reactivation of traumatic memories and the defensive system (the EP) by CS implies sensitization rather than modulation of CS-UCS propositions. Finally, hyperactivation of the defensive system/limbic structures and potent somatosensory activity combined with relatively low levels of prefrontal cortical activity could perhaps explain why in most cases EPs have only developed a quite limited degree of extended consciousness.

Thus it seems that exposure of the EP to (perceived) threat cues (re)activates defensive responses with concomitant lack of contextual information processing, uninhibited conditioned emotional responding within limits of homeostasis, and hampered integration of traumatic memories. Hyperamnesia, sensitization, and maintenance of structural dissociation between ANP and EP can co-occur.

ANP-Dependent Responsivity to Threat

Now consider the ANP. Because ANPs displayed reactivity to masked angry faces (Van Honk *et al.*, 1999, 2001), it seems unlikely that the amygdala and related brain structures were not activated at all when ANPs were exposed to these threat cues. However, in the EP, the emotional brain was strongly activated (Nijenhuis *et al.*, 1999a; Reinders *et al.*, in preparation; Van Honk *et al.*, 1999, 2001). While the EP selectively attends to threat cues, the ANP averts its gaze from threat and selectively attends to cues that matter to daily life functioning. It seems possible that the lateral amygdala is activated for a short time by means of input from the sensory thalamus when the ANP is exposed to threat. However, due to ANP's mental avoidance of threat cues and retraction of the field of consciousness to matters of daily life, the lateral amygdala could become readily subject to a form of negative feedback inhibition. When emotional systems that regulate daily life are in executive control, the amygdala — which has a role in selective attention (Gallagher, 2000) — and related structures may operate in a mode that is different from the mode associated with the defensive system.

Because ANPs are often depersonalized, studies of DID could help understand ANP reactivity to threat in various trauma-related disorders. Depersonalization is related to several negative somatoform dissociative symptoms, e.g., experiencing the body as a foreign object, and involves functional abnormalities along sequential hierarchical areas, secondary and cross-modal areas of the sensory cortex (visual, auditory, and somatosensory), as well as areas responsible for an integrated body schema (Simeon *et al.*, 2000). Perhaps the ANP's lack of sensory perception, including bodily and peripheral stress hormone feedback, could be instrumental in inhibiting the defensive system, hence, the insula and amygdala, and the responsivity it orchestrates. One way to study the presumed negative feedback and positive feedforward loops would be to apply functional MRI while ANPs and EPs are exposed to external and internal threat cues.

PSYCHOBIOLOGICAL DIFFERENCES AMONG DISSOCIATIVE PARTS OF THE PERSONALITY IN PTSD

Recent studies of PTSD have begun to appreciate that the condition in which the patient remains may affect psychobiological functioning. For example, in a recent functional MRI study using script driven imagery of traumatic situations, Lanius *et al.* (2000) found that a subgroup of PTSD patients developed a depersonalization response, while other PTSD patients relived their trauma. Both groups showed less activation of the thalami and the dorsolateral prefrontal cortices compared with healthy controls, but the depersonalization group also displayed activation of the right anterior cingulate. The depersonalization group may perhaps have represented the ANP, and the group that relived trauma, the EP. In any case, the Lanius study confirms that the activity in different brain regions depends on the dissociative part of the personality that is activated during testing. The same interpretation may apply to the finding that some PTSD patients produced (contrary to the expectation of the investigators) slower vocal responses to trauma cues in the emotional Stroop task, whereas others exhibited faster vocal responses to trauma-related than to neutral cues (Stewart *et al.*, 2000). Furthermore, Liberzon and Taylor (2000) reported that a PTSD patient who experienced a flashback in a symptom provocation study had very different regional cerebral blood flow from other PTSD patients and controls with greater uptake in subcortical regions than in cortical regions, in particular the thalamus. We conclude that future psychobiological studies of PTSD should control for the dissociative part of the personality that dominates during testing. However, controlled activation of ANPs and EPs of PTSD patients may be difficult. As a prototype that can be more readily self-controlled in ANP–EP switches, DID deserves far more study from a psychobiological angle than has been performed to date.

CONCLUSION

The integrative functions of the human mind can be hampered by overwhelming events, especially when these events begin early in life, are recurrent, involve threat to the body and to life itself, and are accompanied by compromized attachment, and lack of social recognition and support. While substances such as glutamate, norepinephrine, and CRF may have a role in dissociative processes, these substances in themselves do not define what dissociative structures ensue. Trauma-related dissociation does not split the personality in accidental ways. Clinical, empirical, and experimental evidence rather suggests that structural dissociation of the personality reflects a lack of integration among specific psychobiological systems, described in this chapter as emotional operating systems. The primary form of this structural dissociation involves failed integration between systems dedicated to daily life and survival of the species, and systems dedicated to the survival of the individual in the face of severe threat.

Key brain structures involved in responding to (perceived) threat include the amygdala, insula, locus coeruleus, HPA-axis, hippocampus, cingulate, medial prefrontal cortex, and orbitofrontal cortex, as well as the somatosensory association areas situated in the temporal, parietal and occipital cortex. The evidence to date suggests that in PTSD and the dissociative disorders, (re)activation of the defensive system — metaphorically addressed as the 'emotional' personality — by trauma-related cues implies increased activation of the amygdala, insula, and related structures, and decreased activation of the hippocampus, cingulate gyrus, medial prefrontal cortex, and perhaps other prefrontal areas as well. The amygdala orchestrates a range of unconditioned and conditioned reactions to threat, including sympathetic and parasympathetic nervous system activity, analgesia, defensive motor reaction patterns, subjective emotional feelings such as fear, and retraction of the field of consciousness to threat cues in the immediate, subjective present. These reactions seem to lack modulation by the hippocampus and prefrontal cortex. However, when the psychobiological systems that involve daily life functioning — i.e., the 'apparently normal' personality — are dominant, threat cues are avoided (gaze aversion, mental inhibition), and attention is directed to cues that have a bearing on daily life. The depersonalization and negative somatoform dissociative symptoms that characterize the ANP may be related to disturbed metabolism in the somatosensory association areas. While structural dissociation may be adaptive when the integrative level is not sufficient to integrate both systems, continued structural dissociation is maladaptive when integration of traumatic experiences would be feasible.

To date, research of PTSD and most research of dissociative disorders has largely overlooked that findings may depend on the type of dissociative psychobiological system that dominates the functioning of the patient at the time of measurement. (It must be noted that in parallel dissociation, two or more dissociative personalities may be activated simultaneously, and conflicts among them may occur.) In this regard, at a minimum, the theory of structural dissociation can serve as a heuristic for future research of trauma-related dissociation. To date, we have studied global differences between ANP and EP, but future studies should also address emotional operating subsystems. As the theory predicts, EPs engaged in flight, freeze, fight, or total submission would have different psychobiological reactivity to threat cues and, for example, ANPs engaged in work or reproduction and caretaking would have different responses to attachment cues.

ACKNOWLEDGEMENT

We kindly thank E. Vermetten and J.A. Den Boer for their assistance in preparing this chapter.

REFERENCES

Aggleton, J.P., 2000. *The Amygdala: A Functional Analysis*. Oxford University Press, New York.

Aggleton, J.P. and Saunders, R.C., 2000. The amygdala — what's happened in the last decade? In: Aggleton, J.P. (ed.), *The Amygdala: A Functional Analysis*, pp. 1–30. Oxford University Press, New York.

Allen, J.G., Console, D.A. and Lewis, L., 1999. Dissociative detachment and memory impairment: Reversible amnesia or encoding failure? *Comprehensive Psychiatry*, **40**, 160–171.

American Psychiatric Association, 1994. *Diagnostic and Statistical Manual of Mental Disorders*, (4th edn.) Author, Washington, DC.

Anisman, H., Griffiths, J., Matheson, K., Ravindran, A.V. and Merali, Z., 2001. Posttraumatic stress symptoms and salivary cortisol levels. *American Journal of Psychiatry*, **158**, 1509–1511.

Anthony, J.L., Lonigan, C.J. and Hecht, S.A., 1999. Dimensionality of posttraumatic stress disorder symptoms in children exposed to disaster: Results from confirmatory factor analyses. *Journal of Abnormal Psychology*, **108**, 326–336.

Armony, J.G. and LeDoux, J.E., 1997. How the brain processes emotional information. *Annals of the New York Academy of Sciences*, **821**, 259–270.

Arnold, S.E. and Trojanowski, J.Q., 1996. Human fetal hippocampal development: I. Cytoarchitecture, myeloarchitecture, and neuronal morphologic features. *Journal of Comprehensive Neurology*, **367**, 274–292.

Arnsten, A., 1999. Development of the prefrontal cortex: XIV. Stress impairs prefrontal cortical function. *Journal of the American Academy of Child and Adolescent Psychiatry*, **38**, 220–222.

Baeyens, F., Hermans, D. and Eelen, P., 1993. The role of CS-UCS contingency in human evaluative conditioning. *Behavior Research and Therapy*, **31**, 731–737.

Benes, F.M., 1998. Human brain growth spans decades. *American Journal of Psychiatry*, **155**, 1489.

Birnbaum, M.H. and Thomann, K., 1996. Visual function in multiple personality disorder. *Journal of American Optom Assoc.*, **67**, 327–334.

Bohus, M., Landwehrmeyer, G., Stiglmayr, C., Limberger, M., Bohme, R. and Schmal, C., 1999. Naltrexone in the treatment of dissociative symptoms in patients with borderline personality disorder. *Journal of Clinical Psychiatry*, **60**, 598–603.

Bonne, O., Brandes, D., Gilboa, A., Gomori, J.M., Shenton, M.E., Pitman, R.K. and Shalev, A.Y., 2001. Longitudinal MRI study of hippocampal volume in trauma survivors with PTSD. *American Journal of Psychiatry*, **158**, 1248–1251.

Boon, S. and Draijer, N., 1993. *Multiple Personality Disorder in The Netherlands*. Swets and Zeitlinger, Lisse.

Bouton, M.E., 1994. Context, ambiguity, and classical conditioning. *Current Directions in Psychological Science*, **3**, 49–53.

Bowman, E., 1993. Etiology and clinical course of pseudoseizures: Relationship to trauma, depression, and dissociation. *Psychosomatics*, **34**, 333–341.

Bowman, E. and Coons, P.M., 2000. The differential diagnosis of epilepsy, pseudoseizures, dissociative identity disorder and dissociative disorder not otherwise specified. *Bulletin of the Menninger Clinic*, **64**, 164–180.

Braude, S.E., 1995. *First Person Plural: Multiple Personality and the Philosophy of Mind*. Revised edition. Rowman & Littlefield, Lanham.

Braude, S.E., 2000. Dissociation and latent abilities: The strange case of Patience Worth. *Journal of Trauma and Dissociation*, **1**, 13–48.

Breier, A., Malhotra, A.K., Pinals, D.A., Weisenfeld, N.I. and Pickar, D., 1997. Association of ketamine-induced psychosis with focal activation of the prefrontal cortex in healthy volunteers. *American Journal of Psychiatry*, **154**, 805–811.

Bremner, J.D., 1999. Does stress damage the brain? *Biological Psychiatry*, **45**, 797–805.

Bremner, J.D., Innis, R.B., Ng, C.K., Staib, L.H., Salomon, R.M., Bronen, R.A., Duncan, J., Southwick, S.M., Krystal, J.H., Rich, D., Zubel, G., Dey, H., Soufer, R. and Charney, D.S., 1997a. PET measurement of central metabolic correlates of yohimbine administration in posttraumatic stress disorder. *Archives of General Psychiatry*, **54**, 246–256.

Bremner, J.D., Innis, R.B., Southwick, S.M., Staib, L., Zoghbi, S. and Charney, D.S., 2000. Decreased benzodiazepine receptor binding in prefrontal cortex in combat-related posttraumatic stress disorder. *American Journal of Psychiatry*, **157**, 1120–1126.

Bremner, J.D., Krystal, J.H., Putnam, F.W., Southwick, S.M., Marmar, C., Charney, D.S. and Mazure, C.M., 1998a. Measurement of dissociative states with the Clinician-Administered Dissociative States Scale (CADSS). *Journal of Traumatic Stress*, **11**, 125–136.

Bremner, J.D., Krystal, J.H., Southwick, S.M. and Charney, D.S., 1996. Noradrenergic mechanisms in stress and anxiety: II. Clinical studies. *Synapse*, **23**, 39–51.

Bremner, J.D., Lichio, J., Darnell, A., Krystal, J.H., Owens, M.J., Southwick, S.M., Nemeroff, C.B. and Charney, D.S., 1997b. Elevated CSF corticotropin-releasing factor concentrations in posttraumatic stress disorder. *American Journal of Psychiatry*, **154**, 624–629.

Bremner, J.D., Narayan, M., Staib, L.H., Southwick, S.M., McGlashan, T. and Charney, D.S., 1999. Neural correlates of memories of childhood sexual abuse in women with and without posttraumatic stress disorder. *American Journal of Psychiatry*, **156**, 1787–1795.

Bremner, J.D., Randall, P., Scott, T.M., Bronen, R.A., Seibyl, J.P., Southwick, S.M., Delaney, R.C., McCarthy, G., Charney, D.S. and Innis, R.B., 1995. MRI-based measures of hippocampal volume in patients with PTSD. *American Journal of Psychiatry*, **152**, 973–981.

Bremner, J.D., Randall, P., Vermetten, E., Staib, L., Bronen, R.A., Mazure, C., Capelli, S., McCarthy, G., Innis, R.B. and Charney, D.S., 1997c. Magnetic resonance imaging-based measurement of hippocampal volume in posttraumatic stress disorder related to childhood physical and sexual abuse — a preliminary report. *Biological Psychiatry*, **41**, 23–32.

Bremner, J.D., Vermetten, E., Southwick, S.M., Krystal, J.H. and Charney, D.S., 1998b. Trauma, memory, and dissociation: An integrative formulation. In: Bremner, J.D. and Marmar, C.R. (eds), *Trauma, Memory, and Dissociation*, pp. 365–402. American Psychiatric Press, Washington DC.

Bushnell, M.C., Craig, A.D., Reiman, E.M., Yun, L.S. and Evans, A., 1995. Cerebral activation in the human brain by pain, temperature and the illusion of pain. *Presented at the Annual Meeting of the Society of Neuroscience*, San Diego, CA.

Cahill, L., 2000. Modulation of long-term memory in humans by emotional arousal: Adrenergic activation and the amygdala. In: Aggleton, J.P. (ed.), *The Amygdala*, pp. 425–446. Oxford University Press, New York.

Cahill, L., Pham, C. and Setlow, B., 2001. Impaired memory consolidation in rats produced with β-adrenergic blockade. *Neurobiology of Learning and Memory* (in press).

Cardeña, E., 1994. The domain of dissociation. In: Lynn, S.J. and Rhue, J.W. (eds), *Dissociation: Clinical, Theoretical, and Research Perspectives*, pp. 15–31. Guilford, New York.

Chambers, R.A., Bremner, J.D., Moghaddam, B., Southwick, S.M., Charney, D.S. and Krystal, J.H., 1999. Glutamate and post-traumatic stress disorder: Toward a psychobiology of dissociation. *Semin Clin Neuropsychiatry*, **4**, 274–281.

Ciompi, L., 1991. Affects as central organizing and integrating factors: A new psychosocial/biological model of the psyche. *British Journal of Psychiatry*, **159**, 97–105.

Coons, P.M., Milstein, V. and Marley, C., 1982. EEG studies of two multiple personalities and a control. *Archives of General Psychiatry*, **39**, 823–825.

Coons, P.M., 1994. Confirmation of childhood abuse in child and adolescent cases of multiple personality disorder and dissociation not otherwise specified. *Journal of Nervous and Mental Disease*, **182**, 461–464.

Corder, R., Castagne, V., Rivet, J.-M., Mormede, P. and Gaillard, R.C., 1992. Central and peripheral effects of repeated stress and high NaCl diet on neuropeptide Y. *Physiol. Behav.*, **52**, 205–210.

Coupland, N.J., 2000. Brain mechanisms and neurotransmitters. In: Nutt, D., Davidson, J.R.T. and Zohar, J. (eds), *Posttraumatic Stress Disorder: Diagnosis, Management, and Treatment*, pp. 69–100. Dunitz, London.

Damasio, 1999. *The Feeling of What Happens: Body and Emotion in the Making of Consciousness*. Harcourt Brace, Orlando.

Davies, M., 2000. The role of the amygdala in conditioned and unconditioned fear and anxiety. In: Aggleton, J.P. (ed.), *The Amygdala*, pp. 213–288. Oxford University Press, New York.

De Bellis, M.D., Baum, A.S., Birmaher, B., Keshavan, M.S., Eccard, C.H., Boring, A.M., Jenkins, F.J. and Ryan, N.D., 1999. Developmental traumatology part I: Biological stress systems. *Biological Psychiatry*, **10**, 1259–1270.

De Bellis, M.D., Keshavan, M.S., Spencer, S. and Hall, J., 2000. N-acetylaspartate concentration in the anterior cingulate of maltreated children and adolescents with PTSD. *American Journal of Psychiatry*, **157**, 1175–1177.

Dell, P.F., 1997. Somatoform dissociation and reported trauma in DID and DDNOS, Paper presented at the 14th International Conference of the International Society for the Study of Dissociation, Seattle, WA, November 8–11.

Diamond, D.M. and Park, C.R., 2000. Predator exposure produces retrograde amnesia and blocks synaptic plasticity: Progress toward understanding how the hippocampus is affected by stress. *Ann. NY Acad. Sci.*, **911**, 453–455.

Dittrich, A., Bättig, K. and Von Zeppelin, I., 1973. Effects of (-)Δ^9-transtetrahydrocannabinol (Δ^9-THC) on memory, attention and subjective state: A double blind study. *Psychopharmacologica (Berl.)*, **33**, 369–376.

Dolan, R.J., 2000. Functional neuroimaging of the amygdala during emotional processing and learning. In: Aggleton, J.P. (ed.), *The Amygdala*, pp. 631–655. Oxford University Press, New York.

Draijer, N. and Boon, S., 1993. Trauma, dissociation, and dissociative disorders. In: Boon, S. and Draijer, N. (eds), *Multiple Personality Disorder in The Netherlands: A study on Reliability and Validity of the Diagnosis*, pp. 177–193. Swets and Zeitlinger, Amsterdam/Lisse.

Draijer, N. and Boon, S., 1999. The imitation of dissociative identity disorder. *Journal of Psychiatry and Law*, **27**, 423–458.

Driessen, M., Herrmann, J., Stahl, K., Zwaan, M., Meier, S., Hill, A., Osterheider, M. and Peterson, D., 2000. Magnetic resonance imaging volumes of the hippocampus and amygdala in women with borderline personality disorder and early childhood traumatization. *Archives of General Psychiatry*, **57**, 1115–1122.

Ehling, T., Nijenhuis, E.R.S. and Krikke, A., 2001. Hippocampal volume in patients with dissociative identity disorder. *Presentation at the 18th Annual Conference of the International Society for the Study of Dissociation*, New Orleans, December 1–4.

Eldridge, J.C. and Landfield, P.W., 1990. Cannabinoid interactions with glucocorticoid receptors in rat hippocampus. *Brain Research*, **534**, 135–141.

Elklit, A., 1997. The aftermath of an industrial disaster. *Acta Psychiatrica Scandinavica*, **96**, 1–25.

Fanselow, M.S. and Lester, L.S., 1988. A functional behavioristic approach to aversively motivated behavior: Predatory imminence as a determinant of the topography of defensive behavior. In: Bolles, R.C. and Beecher, M.D. (eds), *Evolution and Learning*, pp. 185–212. Erlbaum, Hillsdale, New York.

Feigenbaum, J.J., Bergmann, F., Richmond, S.A. *et al.*, 1989. Nonpsychotic cannabinoid acts as a functional *N*-methyl-D-aspartate receptor blocker. *Proc. Natl. Acad. Sci. USA*, **86**, 9584–9587.

Freyd, J.J., 1996. *Betrayal Trauma: The Logic of Forgetting Childhood Trauma*. Harvard University Press, Cambridge, MA.

Friedl, M.C., Draijer, N. and De Jonge, P., 2000. Prevalence of dissociative disorders in psychiatric in-patients: The impact of study characteristics. *Acta Psychiatrica Scandinavica*, **102**, 423–428.

Gallagher, M., 2000. The amygdala and associative learning. In: Aggleton, J.P. (ed.), *The Amygdala: A Functional Analysis*, pp. 311–329. Oxford University Press, New York.

Geracioti, T., Baker, D.G., Ekhator, N.N., West, S.A., Hill, K.K., Bruce, A.B., Schmidt, D., Rounds-Kugler, B., Yehuda, R., Keck, P.E. and Kasckow, J.W., 2001. CSF norepinephrine concentrations in posttraumatic stress disorder. *American Journal of Psychiatry*, **158**, 1227–1230.

Glaser, D., 2000. Child abuse and neglect and the brain: A review. *Journal of Child Psychology and Psychiatry*, **41**, 97–116.

Graham, Y.P., Heim, C., Goodman, S.H., Miller, A.H. and Nemeroff, C.B., 1999. The effects of neonatal stress on brain development: Implications for psychopathology. *Development and Psychopathology*, **11**, 545–565.

Gurvits, T.V., Gilbertson, M.W., Lasko, N.B., Tarhan, A.S., Simeon, D., Macklin, M.L., Orr, S.P. and Pitman, R.K., 2000. Neurologic soft signs in chronic posttraumatic stress disorder. *Archives of General Psychiatry*, **57**, 181–186.

Guy, S. and Cahill, L., 1999. Role of overt rehearsal in enhanced conscious memory for emotional events. *Consciousness and Cognition*, **8**, 114–122.

Halgren, E., Walter, R.D., Cherlow, D.G. and Crandall, P.H., 1978. Mental phenomena evoked by electrical stimulation of the human hippocampal formation and amygdala. *Brain*, **101**, 83–117.

Hampson, R.E. and Deadwyler, S.A., 1999. Cannabinoids, hippocampal function, and memory. *Life Sci.*, **65**, 715–723.

Heim, C., Newport, D.J., Heit, S., Graham, Y.P., Wilcox, M., Bonsall, R., Miller, A.H. and Nemeroff, C.B., 2000. Pituitary-adrenal and autonomic responses to stress in women after sexual and physical abuse in childhood. *JAMA*, **284**, 592–597.

Helig, M., Soderpalm, B., Engel, J. and Widerlov, E., 1989. Centrally administered neuropeptide Y (NPY) produces anxiolytic-like effects in animal anxiety models. *Psychopharmacology*, **98**, 524–529.

Helig, M., McLeod, S., Brot, M., Heinrichs, S., Menzaghi, F., Koob, G. and Britton, K., 1993. Anxiolytic-like action of neuropeptide Y: Mediation by Y1 receptors in amygdala and dissociation from food intake effects. *Neuropsychopharmacology*, **8**, 357–363.

Herman, J.P., Prewitt, C.M. and Cullinan, W.E., 1996. Neuronal circuit regulation of the hypothalamo-pituitary-adrenocortical stress axis. *Crit. Rev. Neurobiology*, **10**, 371–394.

Hughes, J.R., Kuhlman, D.T., Fichtner, C.G. and Gruenfeld, M.J., 1990. Brain mapping in a case of multiple personality. *Clinical Electroencephalography*, **21**, 200–209.

Janet, P., 1889. *L'Automatisme Psychologique*. Félix Alcan, Paris. Reprint Société Pierre Janet, Paris, 1973.

Janet, P., 1907. *The Major Symptoms of Hysteria*. Macmillan, London and New York.

Ito, Y., Teicher, M.H., Glod, C.A., Harper, D., Magnus, B.S. and Gelbard, H.A., 1993. Increased prevalence of electrophysiological abnormalities in children with psychological, physical, and sexual abuse. *Journal of Neuropsychiatry and Clinical Neurosciences*, **5**, 401–408.

Kardiner, A., 1941. *The Traumatic Neurosis of War*. Paul Hoeber: New York.

Keane, T., Kolb, L., Kaloupek, D., Orr, S., Blanchard, E., Thomas, R., Hsieh, F. and Lavori, P., 1998. Utility of psychophysiological measurement in the diagnosis of posttraumatic stress disorder: Results from a Department of Veterans Affairs cooperative study. *Journal of Consulting and Clinical Psychology*, **66**, 914–923.

Kihlstrom, J.F., 1994. One hundred years of hysteria. In: Lynn, S.J. and Rhue, J.W. (eds), *Dissociation: Clinical and Theoretical Perspectives*, pp. 365–395. Guilford, New York.

King, L.A., King, D.W., Fairbank, J.A., Keane, T.M. and Adams, G.A., 1998. Resilience–recovery factors in post-traumatic stress disorder among female and male Vietnam veterans: Hardiness, postwar social support study of reactivation of posttraumatic stress disorder symptoms: American and Cambodian psychophysiological response to viewing traumatic video scenes. *Journal of Nervous and Mental Disease*, **186**, 670–676.

Kluft, R.P., 1995. The confirmation and disconfirmation of memories of abuse in dissociative identity disorder patients. *Dissociation*, **8**, 253–258.

Kopelman, M.D., Christensen, H., Puffett, A. and Stanhope, N., 1994. The great escape: A neuropsychological study of psychogenic amnesia. *Neuropsychologia*, **32**, 675–691.

Kosten, T.R. and Krystal, J.H., 1988. Biological mechanisms in post traumatic stress disorder: Relevance for substance abuse. *Recent Dev. Alcohol*, **6**, 49–68.

Krystal, J.H., Woods, S.W., Hill, C.L., *et al.*, 1991. Characteristics of panic attack subtypes: Assessment of spontaneous panic, situational panic, sleep panic, and limited symptom attacks. *Comprehensive Psychiatry*, **32**, 474–478.

Krystal, J.H., Karper, L.P., Bennett, A. *et al.*, 1994a. Modulation of frontal cortical function by glutamate and dopamine antagonists in healthy subjects and schizophrenic patients: A neuropsychological perspective. *Neuropsychopharmacology*, **10**(suppl 3), 230S.

Krystal, J.H., Karper, L.P., Seibyl, J.P., Freeman, G.K., Delaney, R., Bremner, J.D., Heninger, G.R., Bowers, M.B. and Charney, D.S., 1994b. Subanesthetic effects of the noncompetitive NMDA antagonist, ketamine, in humans. Psychotomimetic, perceptual, cognitive, and neuroendocrine responses. *Archives of General Psychiatry*, **51**, 199–214.

Krystal, J.H., Bremner, J.D., Southwick, S.M. and Charney, D.S., 1998. The emerging neurobiology of dissociation: Implications for the treatment of posttraumatic stress disorder. In: Bremner, J.D. and Marmar, C.R. (eds), *Trauma, Memory, and Dissociation*, pp. 321–363. American Psychiatric Press, Washington DC.

Kuyk, J., Spinhoven, P., Van Emde Boas, M.D. and Van Dyck, R., 1999. Dissociation in temporal lobe epilepsy and pseudo-epileptic seizure patients. *The Journal of Nervous and Mental Disease*, **187**, 713–720.

Kuyk, J., Van Dyck, R. and Spinhoven, P., 1996. The case for a dissociative interpretation of pseudo-epileptic seizures: A review. *The Journal of Nervous and Mental Disease*, **184**, 468–474.

Lane, R.D., Reiman, E.M., Ahern, G.L., Schwartz, G.E., Davidson, R.J., Axelrod, B., Yun, L., Blocher, N. and Friston, K., 1997. Neuroanatomical correlates of happiness, sadness, and disgust. *American Journal of Psychiatry*, **154**, 926–933.

Lanius, R., Menon, R., Densmore, M., Boksman, K. and Williamson, P., 2000. Brain activation during script-driven imagery in PTSD: An fMRI investigation. *Proceedings of the 16th Annual Meeting of the International Society for the Study of Traumatic Stress Studies*, San Antonio, Texas, November 16–19: p. 96.

Larmore, K., Ludwig, A.M. and Cain, R.L., 1977. Multiple personality: An objective case study. *British Journal of Psychiatry*, **131**, 35–40.

LeDoux, J.E., 1996. *The Emotional Brain: The Mysterious Underpinning of Emotional Life*. Simon and Schuster, New York.

LeDoux, J., 2000. The amygdala and emotion: A view through fear. In: Aggleton, J.P. (ed.), *The Amygdala*, pp. 289–310. Oxford University Press, New York.

Lemieux, C.M. and Coe, C.L., 1995. Abuse-related posttraumatic stress disorder: Evidence for chronic neuroendocrine activation in women. *Psychosomatic Medicine*, **57**, 105–115.

Lewis, D.O., Yeager, C.A., Swica, Y., Pincus, J.H. and Lewis, M., 1997. Objective documentation of child abuse and dissociation in 12 murderers with dissociative identity disorder. *American Journal of Psychiatry*, **154**, 1703–1710.

Liberzon, I. and Taylor, S.F., 2000. Brain imaging studies of PTSD. In: Shalev, A.Y., Yehuda, R. and McFarlane, A.C. (eds), *International Handbook of Human Response to Trauma*, pp. 285–320. Kluwer Academic/Plenum Publishers, New York.

Liotti, G., 1999. Disorganization of attachment as a model for understanding dissociative psychopathology. In: Solomon, J. and George, C. (eds), *Attachment Disorganization*, pp. 297–317 Guilford, New York.

Loewenstein, R.J., Hornstein, N. and Farber, B., 1988. Open trial of clonazepam in the treatment of post-traumatic stress symptoms in multiple personality disorder. *Dissociation*, **1**, 3–12.

Ludwig, A.M., Brandsma, J.M., Wilbur, C.B., Bendtfeldt, F. and Jameson, D.H., 1972. The objective study of a multiple personality. *Archives of General Psychiatry*, **26**, 298–310.

Main, M. and Morgan, H., 1996. Disorganization and disorientation in infant Strange Situation behavior: Phenotypic resemblance to dissociative states? In: Michelson, L. and Ray, W. (eds), *Handbook of Dissociation*, pp. 107–137. Plenum, New York.

Markowitsch, H.J., 1999. Functional neuroimaging correlates of functional amnesia. *Memory*, **7**, 561–583.

Markowitsch, H.J., Calabrese, P., Fink, G.R., Durwen, H.F., Kessler, J., Harting, C., Konig, M., Mirzaian, E.B., Heiss, W.-D., Heuser, L. and Gehlen, W., 1997. Impaired episodic memory retrieval in a case of probably psychogenic amnesia. *Psychiatry Research: Neuroimaging Section*, **74**, 119–126.

Markowitsch, H.J., Fink, G.R., Thone, A., Kessler, J. and Heiss, W.-D., 1997. A PET study of persistent psychogenic amnesia covering the whole life span. *Cognitive Neuropsychiatry*, **2**, 135–158.

Markowitsch, H.J., Kessler, J., Van der Ven, C., Weber-Luxenburger, G., Albers, M. and Heiss, W.-D., 1998. Psychic trauma causing grossly reduced brain metabolism and cognitive deterioration. *Neuropsychologica*, **36**, 77–82.

Markowitsch, H.J., Kessler, J., Weber-Luxenburger, G., Van der Ven, C., Albers, M. and Heiss, W.-D., 2000. Neuroimaging and behavioral correlates of recovery from amnestic block syndrome and other cognitive deteriorations. *Neuropsychiatry, Neuropsychology, and Behavioral Neurology*, **13**, 60–66.

Marshall, J.C., Halligan, P.W., Fink, G.R., Wade, D.T. and Frackowiak, R.S.J., 1997. The functional anatomy of a hysterical paralysis. *Cognition*, **64**, B1–B8.

Mason, J.W., Wang, S., Yehuda, R., Riney, S., Charney, D.S. and Southwick, S.M., 2001. Psychogenic lowering of urinary cortisol levels linked to increased emotional numbing and a shame-depressive syndrome in combat-related posttraumatic stress disorder. *Psychosomatic Medicine*, **63**, 387–401.

Mathew, R.J., Jack, R.A. and West, W.S., 1985. Regional cerebral blood flow in a patient with multiple personality. *American Journal of Psychiatry*, **142**, 504–505.

Mathew, R.J., Wilson, W.H., Humphreys, D. *et al.*, 1993. Depersonalization after marijuana smoking. *Biological Psychiatry*, **33**, 431–441.

McCormick, D.D. and Thompson, R.F., 1982. Locus coeruleus lesions and resistance to extinction of a classically conditioned response: Involvement of the neocortex and hippocampus. *Brain Research*, **245**, 239–249.

McGaugh, J.L., 1990. Significance and remembrance: The role of neuromodulatory systems. *Psychological Science*, **1**, 15–25.

McGaugh, J., Ferry, B., Vazdarjanova, A. and Roozendaal, B., 2000. Amygdala: Role in modulation of memory storage. In Aggleton, J.P. (ed.), *The Amygdala*, pp. 391–424. Oxford University Press, New York.

Melges, F.T., Tinklenberg, J.R., Hollister, L.E. *et al.*, 1970. Temporal disintegration and depersonalization during marihuana intoxication. *Archives of General Psychiatry*, **23**, 204–210.

Mesulam, M.M., 1981. Dissociative states with abnormal temporal lobe EEG: Multiple personality and the illusion of possession. *Archives of Neurology*, **38**, 176–181.

Miller, S.D., 1989. Optical differences in cases of multiple personality disorder. *Journal of Nervous and Mental Disease*, **177**, 480–486.

Miller, S.D., Blackburn, T., Scholes, G., White, G.L. and Mammalis, N., 1991. Optical differences in multiple personality disorder: A second look. *Journal of Nervous and Mental Disease*, **179**, 132–135.

Miller, S.D. and Triggiano, P.J., 1992. The psychophysiological investigation of multiple personality disorder: Review and update. *American Journal of Clinical Hypnosis*, **35**, 47–61.

Morgan, C.A. III, Wang, S., Southwick, S.M., Rasmusson, A., Hauger, R. and Charney, D.S., 2000. Plasma neuropeptide-Y in humans exposed to acute uncontrollable stress. *Biol. Psychiatry* **47**, 902–909.

Morgan, C.A. III, Wang, S., Rasmusson, A., Hazlett, G., Anderson, G. and Charney, D.S., 2001. Relationship among plasma cortisol, catecholamines, neuropeptide Y, and human performance during exposure to uncontrollable stress. *Psychosomatic Medicine*, **63**, 412–422.

Morris, J.S., Ohman, A. and Dolan, R.J., 1998. Conscious and unconscious emotional learning in the human amygdala. *Nature*, **393**, 467–470.

Morris, J.S., Ohman, A. and Dolan, R.J., 1999. A subcortical pathway to the right amygdala mediating "unseen" fear. *Proceedings of the National Academy of Sciences—USA*, **96**, 1680–1685.

Myers, C.S., 1940. *Shell Shock in France 1914–1918*. Cambridge University Press, Cambridge.

Nemiah, J.C., 1991. Dissociation, conversion, and somatization. In: Tasman, A. and Goldfinger, S.M. (eds), *American Psychiatric Press Annual Review of Psychiatry, Vol. 10*, pp. 248–260. American Psychiatric Press, Washington, DC.

Newoort, D.J. and Nemeroff, C.B., 2000. Neurobiology of posttraumatic stress disorder. *Current Opinion in Neurobiology*, **10**, 211–218.

Nijenhuis, E.R.S., 1999. *Somatoform Dissociation: Phenomena, Measurement, and Theoretical Issues*. Van Gorcum, Assen, The Netherlands.

Nijenhuis, E.R.S., Quak, J., Reinders, S., Korf, J., Vos, H. and Marinkelle, A.B., 1999a. Identity-dependent processing of traumatic memories in dissociative identity disorder: Converging regional cerebral blood flow, physiological and psychological evidence. *Proceedings of the 6th European Conference on Traumatic Stress: Psychotraumatology, Clinical Practice, and Human Rights*, Istanbul, Turkey, June 5–8, p. 23.

Nijenhuis, E.R.S., Spinhoven, P., Vanderlinden, J., Van Dyck, R. and Van der Hart, O., 1998a. Somatoform dissociative symptoms as related to animal defense reactions to predatory imminence and injury. *Journal of Abnormal Psychology*, **107**, 63–73.

Nijenhuis, E.R.S., Spinhoven, P., Van Dyck, R., Van der Hart, O. and Vanderlinden, J., 1996. The development and psychometric characteristics of the Somatoform Dissociation Questionnaire (SDQ-20). *Journal of Nervous and Mental Disease*, **184**, 688–694.

Nijenhuis, E.R.S., Spinhoven, P., Van Dyck, R., Van der Hart, O. and Vanderlinden, J., 1997. The development of the Somatoform Dissociation Questionnaire (SDQ-5) as a screening instrument for dissociative disorders. *Acta Psychiatrica Scandinavica*, **96**, 311–318.

Nijenhuis, E.R.S., Spinhoven, P., Van Dyck, R., Van der Hart, O. and Vanderlinden, J., 1998b. Degree of somatoform and psychological dissociation in dissociative disorders is correlated with reported trauma. *Journal of Traumatic Stress*, **11**, 711–730.

Nijenhuis, E.R.S. and Van der Hart, O., 1999a. Somatoform dissociative phenomena: A Janetian perspective. In: Goodwin, J. and Attias, R. (eds), *Splintered Reflections: Images of the Body in Trauma*, pp. 89–127. Basic Books, New York.

Nijenhuis, E.R.S. and Van der Hart, O., 1999b. Forgetting and reexperiencing trauma. In Goodwin, J. and Attias, R. (eds), *Splintered Reflections: Images of the Body in Trauma*, pp. 39–65. Basic Books, New York.

Nijenhuis, E.R.S., Van der Hart, O. and Kruger, K., 2002a. The psychometric characteristics of the Traumatic Experiences Clinical Psychology and Psychotherapy (in press).

Nijenhuis, E.R.S., Van der Hart, O., Kruger, K. and Steele, K., 2001a. Somatoform dissociation, reported abuse, and animal defenselike reactions (submitted).

Nijenhuis, E.R.S., Van der Hart, O. and Steele, K., 2002b. Strukturale Dissoziation der Persönlichkeit: Über ihre traumatischen Wurzeln und die phobischen Mechanismen die sie in Gang halten [Structural dissociation of the personality: Traumatic origins, phobic maintenance]. In: Hofmann, A., Reddemann, L. and Gast, U. (eds), *Behandlung Dissoziativer Störungen [Treatment of Dissociative Disorders]*, Thieme Verlag, Stuttgart (in press).

Nijenhuis, E.R.S., Vanderlinden, J. and Spinhoven, P., 1998c. Animal defensive reactions as a model for dissociative reactions. *Journal of Traumatic Stress*, **11**, 243–260.

Nijenhuis, E.R.S., Van Dyck, R., Spinhoven, P., Van der Hart, O., Chatrou, M., Vanderlinden, J. and Moene, F., 1999b. Somatoform dissociation discriminates among diagnostic categories over and above general psychopathology. *Australian and New Zealand Journal of Psychiatry*, **33**, 511–520.

Nijenhuis, E.R.S., Van Dyck, R., Ter Kuile, M., Mourits, M., Spinhoven, P. and Van der Hart, O., 1999c. Evidence for associations among somatoform dissociation, psychological dissociation, and reported trauma in chronic pelvic pain patients. In: *Somatoform Dissociation: Phenomena, Measurement, and Theoretical Issues*, pp. 146–160. Nijenhuis ERS, Van Gorcum, Assen, The Netherlands.

Nijenhuis, E.R.S., Van Engen, A., Kusters, I. and Van der Hart, O., 2001b. The relationship of peritraumatic dissociation in childhood sexual abuse and subsequent recall: An exploratory study. *Journal of Trauma and Dissociation*, **2**(3), 49–68.

Ogawa, J.R., Sroufe, L.A., Weinfield, N.S., Carlson, E.A. and Egeland, B., 1997. Development and the fragmented self: Longitudinal study of dissociative symptomatology in a nonclinical sample. *Development and Psychopathology*, **9**, 855–879.

Orr, S.P., Pitman, R.K., Lasko, N.B. and Herz, L.R., 1993. Psychophysiological assessment of posttraumatic stress disorder imagery in World War II and Korean combat veterans. *Journal of Abnormal Psychology*, **102**, 152–159.

Orr, S.P., Lasko, N.B., Metzger, L.J., Berry, N.J., Ahern, C.E. and Pitman, R.K., 1998. Psychophysiologic assessment of women with posttraumatic stress disorder resulting from childhood sexual abuse. *Journal of Consulting and Clinical Psychology*, **66**, 906–913.

Panksepp, J., 1998. *Affective Neuroscience: The Foundations of Human and Animal Emotions*. Oxford University Press, New York.

Pelcovitz, D., Van der Kolk, B.A., Roth, S., Mandel, F., Kaplan, S. and Resick, P., 1997. Development of a criteria set and a structured interview for the disorders of extreme stress (SIDES). *Journal of Traumatic Stress*, **10**, 3–16.

Penfield, W. and Perot, P., 1963. The brain's record of auditory and visual experience: A final summary and discussion. *Brain*, **86**, 595–696.

Perry, B.D., 1999. The memory of states: How the brain stores and retrieves traumatic experience. In: Goodwin, J. and Attias, R. (eds), *Splintered Reflections: Images of the Body in Trauma*, pp. 9–38. Basic Books, New York.

Perry, B.D., Pollard, R.A., Blakely, T.L., Baker, W.L. and Vigilante, D., 1995. Childhood trauma, the neurobiology of adaptation, and "use dependent" development of the brain: How "states" become "traits". *Infant Mental Health Journal*, **16**, 271–291.

Pitman, R.K., Orr, S.P., Shalev, A.Y., Metzger, L.J. and Mellman, T.A., 1999. Psychophysiological alterations in post-traumatic stress disorder. *Semin. Clin. Neuropsychiatry*, **4**, 234–241.

Porgess, S.W., Doussard-Roosevelt, J.A. and Maiti, A.K., 1994. Vagal tone and the physiological regulation of emotion. *Monographs of the Society for Research in Child Development*, **59**, 167–186.

Putnam, F.W., 1997. *Dissociation in Children and Adolescents: A Developmental Perspective*. Guilford, New York.

Putnam, F.W., Buchsbaum, M.S. and Post, R.M., 1993. Differential brain electrical activity in multiple personality disorder. Unpublished manuscript.

Putnam, F.W., Buchsbaum, M.S., Howland, F. and Post, R.M., 1992. Evoked potentials in multiple personality disorder: New Research Abstract #137. *Presented at the Annual Meeting of the American Psychiatric Association*, New Orleans, May.

Putnam, F.W., Zahn, T.P. and Post, R.M., 1990. Differential autonomic nervous system activity in multiple personality disorder. *Psychiatry Research*, **31**, 251–260.

Rainey, J.M., Aleem, A., Ortiz, A. *et al.*, 1987. A laboratory procedure for the induction of flashbacks. *American Journal of Psychiatry*, **144**, 1317–1319.

Rasmusson, A., Hauger, R.L., Morgan, C.A., Bremner, J.D., Charney, D.S. and Southwick, S.M., 2000. Low baseline and yohimbine-stimulated plasma neuropeptide Y (NPY) levels in combat-related posttraumatic stress disorder. *Biological Psychiatry*, **47**, 526–539.

Rauch, S.L., Van der Kolk, B.A., Fisler, R.E., Alpert, N.M., Orr, S.P., Savage, C.R., Fischman, A.J., Jenicke, M.A. and Pitman, R.K., 1996. A symptom provocation study of posttraumatic stress disorder using positron emission tomography and script-driven imagery. *Archives of General Psychiatry*, **53**, 380–387.

Rauch, S.L., Whalen, P.J., Shin, L.M., McInerney, S.C., Macklin, M.L., Lasko, N.B., Orr, S.P. and Pitman, R.K., 2000. Exaggerated amygdala response to masked facial stimuli in posttraumatic stress disorder: A functional MRI study. *Biological Psychiatry*, **47**, 769–776.

Reiman, E.M., 1996. PET studies of anxiety, emotion, and their disorders. *Presented at the Annual Meeting of the World Congress of Psychiatry*, Madrid, Spain.

Reiman, E.M., Mintun, M.A., Raichle, M.E., Robins, E., Price, J.L., Fusselman, M., Fox, P.T. and Hackman, K., 1998. Neuroanatomical correlates of a lactate-induced anxiety attack. *Archives of General Psychiatry*, **46**, 493–500.

Reiman, E.M., Lane, R.D., Ahern, G.L., Schwartz, G.E. and Davidson, R.J., 2000. Positron emission tomography in the study of emotion, anxiety, and anxiety disorders. In: Lane, R.D. and Nadel, L. (eds), *Cognitive Neuroscience of Emotion*, pp. 389–406. Oxford University Press, New York.

Reinders, A.A.T.S., Nijenhuis, E.R.S., Quak, J. *et al.*, 2002. *Psychobiological reactivity to trauma memory scripts in dissociative identity disorder is dependent on dissociative personality types* (in preparation).

Resnick, H.S., Yehuda, R., Foy, D.W. *et al.*, 1995. Effect of prior trauma on acute hormonal response to rape. *American Journal of Psychiatry*, **152**, 1675–1677.

Roelofs, K., Näring, G.W.B., Moene, F.C. and Hoogduin, C.A.L., 2000. The question of symptom lateralization in conversion disorder. *Journal of Psychosomatic Research*, **49**, 21–25.

Runtz, M.G. and Schallow, J.R., 1997. Social support and coping strategies as mediators of adult adjustment following childhood maltreatment. *Child Abuse and Neglect*, **21**, 211–226.

Sar, V., Unal, S.N., Kiziltan, E., Kundakci, T. and Ozturk, E., 2001. HMPAO SPECT study of regional cerebral blood flow in dissociative identity disorder. *Journal of Trauma and Dissociation*, **2**(2), 5–20.

Sar, V., Kundakci, T., Kiziltan, E., Bakim, B. and Bozkurt, O., 2000. Differentiating dissociative disorders from other diagnostic groups through somatoform dissociation. *Journal of Trauma and Dissociation*, **1**, 67–80.

Saxe, G.N., Vasile, R.G., Hill, T.C., Bloomingdale, K. and Van der Kolk, B.A., 1992. SPECT imaging and multiple personality disorder. *Journal of Nervous and Mental Disease*, **180**, 662–663.

Schenk, L. and Baer, D., 1981. Multiple personality and related dissociative phenomena in patients with temporal lobe epilepsy. *American Journal of Psychiatry*, **138**, 1311–1316.

Schore, A.N., 1994. *Affect Regulation and the Origin of the Self: The Neurobiology of Emotional Development*. Erlbaum, Mahwah, NJ.

Schore, A.N., 2001. The effects of early relational trauma on right brain development, affect regulation, and infant mental health. *Infant Mental Health Journal*, **22**, 201–269.

Schuengel, C., Bakermans-Kranenburg, M.J. and Van IJzendoorn, M.H., 1999. Frightening maternal behavior linking unresolved loss and disorganized infant attachment. *Journal of Consulting and Clinical Psychology*, **67**, 54–63.

Seress, L., 1998. Neuronal connections, cell formation and cell migration in the perinatal human hippocampal dentate gyrus. *Cesk Fysiol*, **47**, 42–50.

Shin, L.M., McNally, R.J., Kosslyn, S.M., Thompson, W.L., Rauch, S.L., Alpert, N.M., Metzger, L.J., Lasko, N.B., Orr, S.P. and Pitman, R.K., 1999. Regional cerebral blood flow during script-driven imagery in childhood sexual abuse-related PTSD: A PET investigation. *American Journal of Psychiatry*, **156**, 575–584.

Shin, L.M., Whalen, P., Rauch, S.L., Orr, S.P., McInerney, S., Lasko, N.B., Macklin, M. and Pitman, R.K., 2000. fMRI study of anterior cingulate function in combat-related PTSD. *Proceedings of the 16th Annual Meeting of the International Society for the Study of Traumatic Stress*, San Antonio, USA, p. 26.

Siegel, D.J., 1999. *The Developing Mind: Toward a Neurobiology of Interpersonal Experience*. Guilford, New York.

Simeon, D., Guralnik, O., Hazlett, E.A., Spiegel-Cohen, J., Hollander, E. and Buchsbaum, M.S., 2000. Feeling unreal: A PET study of depersonalization disorder. *American Journal of Psychiatry*, **157**, 1782–1788.

Southwick, S.M., Krystal, J.H., Morgan, A. *et al.*, 1991. Yohimbine and m-chlorophenylpiperazine in PTSD. In: *1991 New Research Programs and Abstracts*, (#348). American Psychiatric Association, Washington DC.

Southwick, S.M., Krystal, J.H., Morgan, C.A., Johnson, D., Nagy, L.M., Nicolaou, A., Heninger, G.R. and Charney, D.S., 1993. Abnormal noradrenergic function in posttraumatic stress disorder. *Archives of General Psychiatry*, **50**, 266–274.

Spanos, N.P. and Burgess, C., 1994. Hypnosis and multiple personality disorder: A sociocognitive perspective. In: Lynn, S.J. and Rhue, J.W. (eds), *Dissociation: Clinical and Theoretical Perspectives*, pp. 136–155. Guilford Press, New York.

Spence, S.A., Crimlisk, H.L., Cope, H., Ron, M.A. and Grasby, P.M., 2000. Discrete neurophysiological correlates in prefrontal cortex during hysterical and feigned disorder of movement. *Lancet*, **355**, 1243–1244.

Squire, L.R. and Knowlton, B.J., 1995. Memory, hippocampus, and brain systems. In: Michael, S.G. (ed.), *The Cognitive Neurosciences*, pp. 825–837. MIT Press, Cambridge MA, USA.

Starke, K., Borowski, E. and Endo, T., 1975. Preferential blockade of presynaptic α-adrenoceptors by yohimbine. *European Journal of Pharmacology*, **34**, 385–388.

Steele, K., Van der Hart, O. and Nijenhuis, E.R.S., 2001. Allgemeine Behandlungsstrategien komplexer dissoziativer Störungen [Phase-oriented treatment of complex dissociative disorders: Overcoming trauma-related phobias.] In: Eckhart-Henn, A. and Hoffman, S.O. (eds), *Dissoziative Störungen des Bewußtseins [Dissociative Disorders of Consciousness]*. Schattauer-Verlag, Stuttgart.

Stein, M.B., Koverola, C., Hanna, C., Torchia, M.G. and McClarty, B., 1997. Hippocampal volume in women victimized by childhood sexual abuse. *Psychol. Med.*, **27**, 951–959.

Steinberg, M., 1994. *Structured Clinical Interview for DSM-IV Dissociative Disorders, Revised*. American Psychiatric Press, Washington DC.

Stewart, L., Stegman, W., Arsenaut, N. and Woodward, S., 2000. The auditory emotional Stroop in combat-related PTSD. *Proceedings of the 16th Annual Meeting of the International Society for the Study of Traumatic Stress Studies*, San Antonio, Texas, p. 100.

Teicher, M.H., Glod, C.A., Surrey, J. and Swett, C., 1993. Early childhood abuse and limbic system ratings in adult psychiatric outpatients. *Journal of Neuropsychiatry and Clinical Neuroscience*, **5**, 301–306.

Teicher, M.H., Ito, Y., Glod, C.A., Andersen, S.L., Dumont, N. and Ackerman, E., 1997. Preliminary evidence for abnormal cortical development in physically and sexually abused children using EEG coherence and MRI. *Annals of the New York Academy of Science*, **821**, 160–175.

Tiihonen, J., Kuikka, J., Viinamäki, H., Lehtonen, J. and Partanen, J., 1995. Altered cerebral blood flow during hysterical paraesthesia. *Biological Psychiatry*, **37**, 134–135.

Trentani, A., Kuipers, S., Ter Horst, G.J. and Den Boer, J.A., 2002. Intracellular signaling transduction dysregulation in depression and possible future targets for antidepressant therapy. In: Kasper, S., Den Boer, J.A. and Sitsen, J.M.A. (eds), *Handbook of Depression and Anxiety*, Marcel Dekker, New York (in press).

Tsai, G.E., Condie, D., Wu, M.T. and Chang, I.W., 1999. Functional magnetic resonance imaging of personality switches in a woman with dissociative identity disorder. *Harvard Review of Psychiatry*, **7**, 119–122.

Tsien, J.Z., Huerta, P.T. and Tonegawa, S., 1996. The essential role of hippocampal CA1 NMDA receptor dependent synaptic plasticity in spatial memory. *Cell*, **87**, 1327–1338.

Van der Hart, O., 2000. *Psychic Trauma: The Disintegrating Effects of Overwhelming Experience on Mind and Body*. 66th Beattie Smith Lecture presented at The University of Melbourne, Faculty of Medicine, Dentistry and Health Sciences, Melbourne.

Van der Hart, O. and Brom, D., 2000. When the victim forgets: Trauma-induced amnesia and its assessment in Holocaust survivors. In: Shalev, A.Y., Yehuda, R. and McFarlane, A.C. (eds), *International Handbook of Human Response to Trauma*, pp. 223–248. Kluwer Academic/Plenum Publishers, New York.

Van der Hart, O., Brown, P. and Graafland, M., 1999. Trauma-induced dissociative amnesia in World War I combat soldiers. *Australian and New Zealand Journal of Psychiatry*, **33**, 37–46.

Van der Hart, O. and Nijenhuis, E.R.S., 2001. Loss and recovery of different memory types in generalized dissociative amnesia. *Australian and New Zealand Journal of Psychiatry*, **35**(5), 589–600.

Van der Hart, O., Van der Kolk, B.A. and Boon, S., 1998. Treatment of dissociative disorders. In: Bremner, J.D. and Marmar, C.R. (eds), *Trauma, Memory, and Dissociation*, pp. 253–283. American Psychiatric Press, Washington DC.

Van der Hart, O., Van Dijke, A., Van Son, M. and Steele, K., 2000. Somatoform dissociation in traumatized World War I combat soldiers: A neglected clinical heritage. *Journal of Trauma and Dissociation*, **1**(4), 33–66.

Van Duyl, M. and Nijenhuis, E.R.S., in preparation. Dissociative possession disorder and reported trauma in Uganda.

Van IJzendoorn, M.H., Schuengel, C. and Bakersman-Kranenberg, M., 1999. Disorganized attachment in early childhood: Meta-analysis of precursors, concomitants, and sequelae. *Development and Psychopathology*, **11**, 225–249.

Van der Kolk, B.A., 1994. The body keeps the score: Memory and the evolving psychobiology of posttraumatic stress. *Harvard Review of Psychiatry*, **1**, 253–265.

Van der Kolk, B.A. and Fisler, R., 1995. Dissociation and the fragmentary nature of traumatic memories: Overview and exploratory study. *Journal of Traumatic Stress*, **8**, 505–525.

Van der Kolk, B.A., Pelcovitz, D., Roth, S., Mandel, F., McFarlane, A. and Herman, J.L., 1996. Dissociation, affect dysregulation, and somatization: The complexity of adaptation to trauma. *American Journal of Psychiatry*, **153**, Festschrift Supplement, 83–93.

Van der Kolk, B.A. and Van der Hart, O., 1991. The intrusive past: The flexibility of memory and the engraving of trauma. *American Imago*, **48**, 425–454.

Vanderlinden, J., Van Dyck, R., Vandereycken, W. and Vertommen, H., 1993. Dissociation and traumatic experiences in the general population of The Netherlands. *Hospital and Community Psychiatry*, **44**, 786–788.

Van Honk, J., Nijenhuis, E.R.S., Hermans, E., Jongen, A. and Van der Hart, O., 1999. State-dependent emotional responses to masked threatening stimuli in dissociative identity disorder. *Proceedings of the 16th International Fall Conference of the International Society for the Study of Dissociation*, Miami, November 11–13.

Van Honk, J., Nijenhuis, E.R.S., Hermans, E., Van der Hart, O. and Huntjens, R.J.C., 2001. "Ogenschijnlijk normale" en "emotionele" dissociatieve persoonlijkheden bij DIS: Reactiepatronen op gemaskeerde gezichtsuitdrukkingen. ["Apparently normal" and "emotional" dissociative personalities in DID: Response-patterns to masked facial expressions]. Proceedings Voorjaarscongres Nederlands Vereniging voor Psychiatrie, Rotterdam, April 4–6.

Vermetten, E. and Bremner, J.D., 2001a. Circuits and systems in stress: I. Preclinical studies (in press).

Vermetten, E. and Bremner, J.D., 2001b. Circuits and systems in stress: II. Application to neurobiology and treatment in PTSD (in press).

Vuilleumier, P., Chicerio, C., Assal, F., Schwartz, S., Slosmen, D. and Landis, T., 2001. Functional neuroanatomical correlates of hysterical sensorimotor loss. *Brain*, **124**, 1077–1090.

Waller, G., Hamilton, K., Elliott, P., Lewendon, J., Stopa, L., Waters, A., Kennedy, F., Lee, G., Pearson, D., Kennerley, H., Hargreaves, I., Bashford, V. and Chalkey, J., 2000. Somatoform dissociation, psychological dissociation and specific forms of trauma. *Journal of Trauma and Dissociation*, **1**, 81–98.

Whalen, P.J., Bush, G., McNally, R.J., Wilhelm, S., McInerney, S.C., Jenike, M.A. and Rauch, S.L., 1998. The emotional counting Stroop paradigm: A fMRI probe of the anterior cingulate affective division. *Biological Psychiatry*, **44**, 1219–1228.

Woodson, J.C., Park, C.R. and Diamond, D.M., 2001. Exposure to a cat produces complete retrograde amnesia in rats. *Presented at the Annual Meeting of the Society for Behavioral Neuroendocrinology*, Arizona State University, June 27–30.

Wolf, D.P., 1990. Being of several minds: Voices and versions of the self in early childhood. In: Cicchetti, D. and Beeghly, M. (eds.), *The Self in Transition: Infancy to Childhood*, pp. 183–212. The Chicago University Press, Chicago, IL.

Wolff, P.H., 1987. *The Development of Behavioral States and the Expression of Emotions in Early Childhood*. University of Chicago Press, Chicago.

Woolley, C.S., Gould, E. and McEwen, B.S., 1990. Exposure to excess glucocorticoids alters dendritic morphology of adult hippocampal pyramidal neurons. *Brain Research*, **531**, 225–231.

Yazici, K.M. and Kostakoglu, L., 1998. Cerebral blood flow changes in patients with conversion disorder. *Psychiatry Research: Neuroimaging Section*, **83**, 163–168.

Yehuda, R., 2000. Biology of posttraumatic stress disorder. *Journal of Clinical Psychiatry*, **61**, 14–21.

Yehuda, R., McFarlane, A.C. and Shalev, A.Y., 1998. Predicting the development of posttraumatic stress disorder from the acute response to a traumatic event. *Biological Psychiatry*, **44**, 1305–1313.

XXII

The Psychobiology of Sexual and Gender Identity Disorders

Cindy M. Meston and Penny F. Frohlich

INTRODUCTION

Interest in human sexual function has increased in the past decade, in large part as a result of increased recognition of the sexual side effects of various medications, the high incidence of sexual dysfunction among men and women, and the highly publicized success of some treatments for sexual dysfunction (e.g., Viagra for erectile dysfunction). This paper will describe the present knowledge of the endocrine, neurotransmitter, and central and peripheral nervous system mechanisms governing sexual function and dysfunction. The primary focus will be the underlying physiological processes although it should be noted at the outset that it would be misleading to assume that sexual dysfunction is best conceptualized in this manner.

Psychological problems, such as depression or anxiety, and relationship issues, such as marital discord or stress, can have a profound effect on sexual functioning. Although such cognitive and emotional factors are often integral to a sexual problem, these aspects will be reviewed only briefly here.

SEXUAL DESIRE DISORDERS

Hypoactive Sexual Desire Disorder

Sexual desire is commonly defined as the broad interest in sexual objects or experiences. One of the difficulties in diagnosing inhibited desire is determining exactly what constitutes low desire. Sexual desire cannot be measured exclusively by frequency of sexual activity — a person may desire sexual activity a great deal more or less often than their actual level of activity. It is problematic to measure sexual desire based on a discrepancy between partners; a man who desires sexual activity once a day may be frustrated by a partner who desires sexual activity twice a week, yet both partners have a level of sexual desire that falls within the normal range. Because there is no objective physiological criterion for desire, it is generally inferred by self-reported frequency of sexual thoughts, fantasies, dreams, wishes, and interest in initiating and/or engaging in sexual experiences. However, it is also problematic to diagnose hypoactive sexual desire based on a simple comparison with typical levels of desire. A couple who both prefer sexual activity only once a month would be exhibiting levels of desire below normal, yet it is unlikely that they would be unsatisfied with their degree of activity (LoPiccolo and Friedman, 1988). In order to meet the Diagnostic and Statistical Manual of Mental Disorders, 4th edition (DSM-IV), criteria for hypoactive sexual desire disorder, the person must not only experience a persistent or recurrent deficiency or absence of sexual fantasies and desire for sexual activity, but the situation must create marked distress or interpersonal difficulty — indeed, it should be noted at the outset that in order to be diagnosed with any of the sexual disorders a person must be experiencing significant distress or interpersonal difficulty (American Psychiatric Association, 1994).

Hypoactive sexual desire disorder is much more common in women than in men. Thirty-two percent of women between the ages of 18 and 29 years old reported a lack of sexual interest compared to 14% of men in the same age group. Women did not demonstrate a change in rates of inhibited desire according to age while men were significantly more likely to report lack of sexual interest as they aged, particularly after age 50 years old. Women did not differ in rates of inhibited desire based on marital status whereas married men were significantly less likely to report inhibited desire compared to divorced or never married men. Women who had less than a high school level of education reported significantly higher rates of inhibited desire compared to women with more education. Perhaps more educated women are more open to improving sexual communication and sexual knowledge. Exploring what is sexually pleasurable, and communicating sexual needs are techniques used for enhancing sexual desire. Unlike women, men showed no significant differences in desire according to education. African-American women reported significantly higher rates of inhibited desire compared to Caucasian or Hispanic women whereas men demonstrated no ethnic differences in sexual desire (Laumann *et al.*, 1999).

Physiological Factors

Cases of low desire in men are often related to medical conditions or treatments that affect hormone levels. Hypogonadal men (i.e., men with deficient secretion of gonadal hormones) receiving testosterone replacement therapy demonstrated a significant drop in sexual interest following removal of the hormone treatment, and a return in sexual interest when the hormone treatment was resumed. This indicates that very low testosterone levels may impair sexual desire in men. Once testosterone levels reach a certain threshold, additional testosterone does not affect sexual desire — thus, testosterone administration to a male with normal testosterone levels will not increase sexual desire. In adolescent males, higher testosterone levels are associated with increased frequency of sexual fantasies and sexual activity but this relationship does not hold true in adult men. Perhaps during and around puberty internal factors (e.g., hormones) trigger sexual appetite while in adulthood external cues (e.g., relationship factors) play more of a central role. Some evidence suggests that oestrogen and progesterone administration reduces sexual desire in men with excessive or inappropriate desire,

Biological Psychiatry: Edited by H. D'haenen, J.A. den Boer and P. Willner. ISBN 0-471-49198-5

although few studies have been published on this topic (Meston and Frohlich, 2000).

Unusually low testosterone levels that result from removal of the adrenal glands (adrenalectomy), removal of the ovaries (oophorectomy), or as a consequence of menopause, may impair sexual desire in women. Testosterone is effective in restoring sexual desire in these women with abnormally low testosterone levels. It should be noted that most women with hypoactive sexual desire disorder do not have abnormally low testosterone levels and administering exogenous testosterone to women with normal testosterone levels does not enhance sexual desire and can lead to a number of adverse side effects (e.g., acne, facial hair). Oestrogen levels do not significantly affect sexual desire in women and evidence is mixed regarding the affects of progesterone administration on sexual desire in women. Some evidence suggests that increases in prolactin levels that occur with breast-feeding may diminish sexual desire in women but myriad other psychological factors (e.g., post-partum depression) could account for these changes (Meston and Frohlich, 2000).

A variety of psychoactive medications affect sexual drive. Selective serotonin reuptake inhibitors (SSRIs, used most commonly for treating depression), which acutely increase the amount of serotonin in the synapse, produce a variety of sexual side effects including diminished libido in both men and women. Sexual dysfunction secondary to SSRI use is believed to result from the activation of the serotonin$_2$ receptor, although it is unclear whether activation of this specific receptor type is responsible for SSRI-induced loss of sexual drive *per se*.

Drugs that facilitate dopamine activity, such as the antiparkinsonian medication levodopa, tend to increase sexual desire in men. Dopamine activity also increases sexual drive in animals; selective dopamine agonists and apomorphine increased mounting behaviour in male rats (for review, see Meston and Frohlich, 2000). The role of dopamine activity in female sexual desire is not known although one report described a case of a middle-aged woman who exhibited increased sexual behaviour while receiving antiparkinsonian medication, and a return to normal sexual behaviour when the dosage was decreased (Uitti *et al.*, 1989). Long-term opioid (e.g., heroin) use diminishes libido in men and women, perhaps due to the testosterone and luteinizing hormone reducing properties of these drugs (Meston and Frohlich, 2000).

Although it is generally believed that sexual drive is controlled by the central nervous system, the specific brain regions and mechanisms controlling drive are not well understood. In male rats, lesion to the medial preoptic area impairs copulatory behaviour by disrupting the animal's ability to identify potential partners. Some evidence suggests that the medial amygdala plays an important role in sexual motivation in males. Large temporal lobe lesions have been reported to produce hypersexuality, although it is believed that damage to inhibitory neurons in the pyriform cortex may be responsible for these results (McKenna, 1999). It is feasible that activity in one or more of these regions may be abnormal in cases of hypoactive sexual desire.

Psychological Factors

Daily hassles (e.g., worrying about childcare, bills, etc.) and high stress jobs are probably the worst offenders for suppressing sexual desire, as are a multitude of relationship or partner-related issues. If the couple is experiencing conflict, one or both partners may experience a drop in desire. One member of a couple may experience a drop in desire because he or she no longer feels attracted to his or her partner. This typically occurs when the partner undergoes a dramatic change in appearance (e.g., significant weight gain). A person may experience a drop in sexual desire if their partner is unwilling to experiment sexually or lacks sexual skill, making the sexual experience frustrating, unpleasant, or in other ways unappealing. Differences in the desired amount of emotional intimacy or time spent together can impair sexual desire; one person may feel frustrated by the lack of closeness while the other may feel suffocated. Some people fear intimacy, perhaps as a result of being hurt in the past, and thus may have little desire for intimacy in the form of sexual activity. If one partner has more power in the relationship, the other partner may feel bullied or harassed, and may experience a drop in desire (LoPiccolo and Friedman, 1988). Religious concerns and certain psychological difficulties, such as depression or obsessive–compulsive disorder, may also be associated with inhibited desire.

Treatment

Treatment for inhibited sexual desire may be difficult because the person with low desire may be seeking treatment at the urging of their partner, and thus they may not be internally motivated for therapy. Provided physiological causes have been ruled out (e.g., low testosterone levels) it is essential that treatment begin by structuring the impaired desire as a couple problem, rather than as an individual problem (Pridal and LoPiccolo, 2000). Cognitive therapy is often used to restructure thoughts and beliefs about sexuality that may be inhibiting desire (e.g., good women should not desire sex) to reflect ideas more conducive to sexual enjoyment, and to address negative underlying relationship issues. Behavioural interventions are often used to treat physical expressions of affection and intimacy and to increase sexual communication. In some cases, couples have ceased not only sexual activity, but all physical affection — the partner with low desire may have stopped showing any affection for fear that it be interpreted as interest in sexual activity. In such cases, the couple is encouraged to begin expressing affection through non-sexual means such as holding hands, cuddling, hugging, and brief kissing, and then to gradually reintegrate sexual intercourse into their relationship.

Sexual Aversion Disorder

In the DSM-IV, sexual aversion disorder is defined as the recurrent or persistent extreme avoidance of or aversion to all, or nearly all, genital sexual contact with a sexual partner. The association between sexual aversion disorder and anxiety has led some to argue that sexual aversion disorder may be best conceptualized as a type of anxiety disorder, like a snake phobia or a fear of heights. Sexual aversions in some people may be related to a history of sexual trauma or unwanted sexual activity. Men may also develop sexual aversion as a result of fear of erectile failure and/or a desire to avoid unpleasant sensations associated with anxiety (Gold and Gold, 1993).

Sexual aversion disorders may be treated by addressing the underlying anxiety. Anxiolytic medications may be used to reduce the anxiety, sometimes in conjunction with sex therapy. If the sexual aversion appears to result from a history of sexual abuse, counselling directed at coming to terms with this history may be most effective. For men, treatment may involve sex education regarding realistic expectations about performance and female response (Gold and Gold, 1993).

SEXUAL AROUSAL DISORDERS

Closely connected with sexual desire, sexual arousal is defined in both psychological (e.g., 'feeling sexually excited') and physiological terms (e.g., genital blood flow). Physiological sexual arousal in males involves signals from central (brain and spinal cord) and peripheral nervous systems, and on a complex interplay between neurotransmitters, vasoactive agents and endocrine factors. Within the penis is a central artery and veins that exit and drain the erectile bodies. The muscles that line the sinusoidal spaces and the central artery are contracted during the non-aroused state. Erection begins with muscle relaxation that is controlled by autonomic nerves and by the release of nitric oxide (described below). Smooth muscle relaxation reduces vascular resistance and the erectile bodies fill with blood. Once the erectile bodies become engorged with blood, the veins are compressed under the penis's tough fibroelastic covering and blood is trapped in the penis. Normally, detumescence (i.e., loss of erection) occurs with the release of catecholamines during orgasm and ejaculation.

Physiological sexual arousal in women begins with vasocongestion of the vagina, vulva, clitoris, uterus, and possibly the urethra, and can occur within only a few seconds of sexual stimulation. Vaginal lubrication occurs when the blood vessels of the vaginal epithelium (vaginal wall) become engorged with blood, causing fluid to pass between the cells of the vaginal epithelium and emerge on the vaginal wall as sweat-like droplets. These droplets can quickly build up to form a lubricating film that facilitates penetration of the penis. Nitric oxide has also been implicated in female sexual arousal (see below).

Female Sexual Arousal Disorder

According to the DSM-IV, a woman may have female sexual arousal disorder if she experiences repeated and persistent difficulty attaining or maintaining, until sexual activity is completed, a sufficient lubrication-swelling response of sexual excitement. As with many sexual disorders, female sexual arousal disorder can be subdivided into lifelong versus acquired types, generalized versus situational types, and due to psychological versus organic, or combined factors (American Psychiatric Association, 1994). Women of all ages may experience difficulty lubricating, although it tends to be more of a problem in later life, typically after menopause. Approximately 20% of women aged 18–49 years old reported problems lubricating compared to 27% of women aged 50–59 years old. Difficulty lubricating is not associated with marital status or level of education (Laumann *et al.*, 1999).

Physiological Factors

Oestrogen levels can have a profound effect on sexual arousal. This is most apparent through the menopause transition. Oestrogen levels decline during menopause, which results in atrophy of the vaginal epithelium (vaginal walls), and a decline in blood flow into the capillaries of the vaginal wall. A loss of oestrogen following menopause can also indirectly impair sexual arousal by impairing mood. Oestrogen replacement therapy can help remedy some of the vasomotor symptoms and vaginal atrophy in postmenopausal women (Sherwin, 1991). Several researchers have examined whether hormonal fluctuations across the menstrual cycle affect sexual arousal but failed to find any consistent relationship (Meuwissen and Over, 1992).

As noted earlier, some studies have shown that activation of the sympathetic nervous system can facilitate female sexual arousal. When sexually functional women and women with low sexual desire engaged in vigorous exercise (stationary cycling, which stimulates the sympathetic nervous system), they demonstrated significantly higher levels of physiological sexual arousal to an erotic film than without exercise (Meston and Gorzalka, 1995a, 1996). Physiological sexual arousal was measured using a vaginal photoplethysmograph, a tampon-like device that the woman inserts into her vagina, which measures blood flow in the vaginal capillaries. It is important to note that in these studies exercise alone did not facilitate sexual arousal — it was only when the women viewed an erotic film that vaginal blood flow was increased. This suggests that exercise somehow prepares the women's body for sexual arousal so that when she enters a situation she views as sexually appealing, her level of physiological sexual responding is intensified. Meston and Gorzalka (1995b) found a facilitatory effect of exercise at 15 and 30 minutes following exercise. Whether the effect remains past 30 minutes has not been examined. When the sympathetic nervous system is activated using a medication to increase sympathetic nervous system activity, such as ephedrine, physiological sexual arousal to an erotic film is also facilitated (Meston and Heiman, 1998). The reverse has also been shown; medications such as clonidine that block sympathetic nervous system activity impair sexual arousal (Meston *et al.*, 1997).

Animal studies and studies examining the physiology and side effects of medications suggest that neurotransmitters in the central nervous system and neuropeptides in the periphery of the body impact sexual arousal. Nitric oxide activity in the penile tissue triggers a cascade of events leading to increased blood flow into the penile capillaries. The medication Viagra, which is an orally administered treatment for erectile dysfunction, acts by initiating these events (the mechanism of action of Viagra will be described in more detail below under the erectile dysfunction section). Recent studies show that nitric oxide is also produced in clitoral tissue.

Convergent evidence suggests that serotonin activity in the periphery of the body may be involved in female sexual function and dysfunction. Serotonin is a powerful vasoactive substance that, depending on the site and tissue type, may produce vasodilation or vasoconstriction. Normal vaginal lubrication is dependent upon adequate vasocongestion of the genital tissue and it is feasible that serotonin may be involved in this process. If so, abnormalities in serotonin mechanisms may impair vaginal vasocongestion (e.g., with SSRI use). Serotonin is also active in several other peripheral mechanisms that are likely to affect sexual functioning such as nonvascular smooth muscle contraction, endocrine functions, and the spinal cord and peripheral nerves (Frohlich and Meston, 2000).

Mild abnormalities in cutaneous sensation, the sense of touch, have been associated with difficulty becoming lubricated. Cutaneous sensation was measured using Von Frey monofilaments, hair-like fibres that when pressed against the skin reliably apply a specific amount of force — the amount of force applied depends upon the diameter and length of the hair. College aged women with sexual arousal disorder required a higher degree of stimulation (more force) to their skin before they perceived the stimulation as compared to women with normal sexual functioning. This suggests that women with sexual arousal disorder may have mild abnormalities in peripheral nervous system functioning (Frohlich and Meston, 1999).

Very little research has been published regarding brain areas involved in female sexual arousal although several studies have implicated the paraventricular nucleus of the hypothalamus. Transneural viral labelling indicates that the clitoris and uterus are connected to the paraventricular nucleus and the findings from one study in rats suggests that the paraventricular nucleus is active during copulation. During sexual arousal, oxytocin produced in the paraventricular nucleus is secreted into the blood stream by the posterior pituitary (McKenna, 1999). It is feasible that paraventricular nucleus activity is abnormal in women with sexual arousal disorder.

Psychological Factors

In addition to affecting sexual desire, factors such as performance demand, anxiety, and expectancies can also affect physiological sexual arousal (i.e., vaginal vasocongestion and lubrication). Laan *et al.* (1993) found that sexually functional women became more sexually aroused after being asked to become as sexually aroused as possible, versus being told their level of sexual arousal was not important to the study. This suggests that for women without sexual difficulties, performance demand can facilitate sexual arousal. Expectancies may interact with autonomic arousal to influence sexual arousal as well. Palace (1995) found that sexually dysfunctional women who were falsely informed that they displayed strong physiological sexual arousal to an erotic film, displayed greater physiological and self-reported sexual arousal to a subsequent erotic film. Moreover, this response was greater if the erotic stimulus was preceded by an anxiety/fear provoking film versus a neutral film. This suggests that sympathetic nervous system arousal paired with the expectation of sexual arousal may be effective in increasing physiological sexual arousal in women.

Because of the close link between sexual desire and sexual arousal in women, many of the same psychological factors that impair sexual desire also inhibit vaginal lubrication. Briefly, these include individual, relationship, and cultural factors. An estimated 49% of women who were sexually abused as children report impaired sexual arousal. Inadequate or inappropriate sexual stimulation may interfere with sexual arousal, as would negative emotions such as fear of rejection, anger, or relationship conflict (Morokoff, 1993).

Male Erectile Disorder

According to the DSM-IV, male erectile disorder is characterized by a persistent or recurrent inability to attain or maintain an adequate erection until completion of the sexual act. Erectile dysfunction may result when a medical problem or condition, such as diabetes mellitus, surgical injury, aging, or pharmaceutical intervention, affects vascular blood flow to the penis or neural innervations to and from the penis. Patients are diagnosed with erectile dysfunction when their erectile difficulties are exclusively psychogenic in nature, or are caused by a combination of psychological and medical factors (American Psychiatric Association, 1994).

Men of all ages occasionally have difficulty obtaining or maintaining an erection, but true erectile disorder is more common after age 50 years. Approximately 7% of men aged 18–29 years have erectile troubles compared to 18% of men aged 50–59 years. Level of education and ethnicity are not associated with erectile difficulties, but married men are less likely to report erectile problems compared to never married or divorced men (Laumann *et al.*, 1999).

Physiological Factors

Testosterone does not affect erectile functioning unless it falls below a critical level. Hypogonadal men, or men with unusually low testosterone levels, often experience erectile problems that are successfully treated with testosterone replacement therapy. Testosterone administration does not improve erectile response in men with normal testosterone levels. Prolactin levels also affect erectile functioning although the process is complex; men with abnormally high prolactin levels and men with abnormally low prolactin levels may experience erectile dysfunction (Besser and Thorner, 1975; Deutsch and Sherman, 1979). In normally functioning men, prolactin and oxytocin levels increase significantly during sexual arousal (Meston and Frohlich, 2000).

Acetylcholine, vasoactive intestinal peptide, and nitric oxide have also been implicated in penile tumescence (i.e., erection). Activation of cholinergic receptors produces relaxation of the penile smooth muscles, allowing blood flow into the penis, thus producing an erection (Saenz de Tejada *et al.*, 1988). Sexual stimulation leads to the production of nitric oxide in penile tissue. Nitric oxide stimulates guanylate cyclase release, which triggers the conversion of guanosine triphosphate to cGMP. cGMP activity relaxes the smooth muscles of the penile tissue allowing vasocongestion and erection (Burnett, 1995). The pharmaceutical company, Pfizer, capitalized on this process by developing the medication Viagra, which is designed to treat erectile dysfunction. Viagra potentiates the activity of cGMP by inhibiting phosphodiesterase type 5, the endogenous substance responsible for cGMP deactivation. This increases and prolongs cGMP activity, which increases and prolongs vasocongestion, and enables erection. Interestingly, Viagra was discovered by accident when researchers for Pfizer noticed that men taking an experimental drug for heart disease, which worked on nitric oxide systems, had erections as a side effect.

A variety of psychoactive medications produce erectile dysfunction. Antiparkinsonian medications are dopamine agonists and are reported to facilitate erection (Bowers *et al.*, 1971) while antipsychotic medications are dopamine antagonists and facilitate erection at low doses and impair erection at high doses (Aizenberg *et al.*, 1995; Marder and Meibach, 1994). Cocaine is a dopamine agonist and high doses can disrupt erectile capacity (Miller and Gold, 1988), perhaps due to its vasoconstrictive properties. Opioid abuse (e.g., heroin) can lead to erectile dysfunction.

Erection is dependent upon spinal reflexes and is controlled by descending inhibitory and excitatory input from the brainstem. This is most apparent when studying the effects of spinal cord injury. Transection of the spinal cord often facilitates erectile response (depending upon the region of the spinal cord injured) — animal and human studies suggest that following spinal cord injury, less stimulation is required to obtain erection and erection occurs more frequently (McKenna, 1999).

Several brain regions have been implicated in male erection. Animal studies indicate that oxytocin released from the paraventricular nucleus of the hypothalamus can produce erection as can electrical stimulation of the paraventricular nucleus of the hypothalamus and hippocampus. Electroencephalographic studies indicate that the right temporal lobe is activated when right-handed men are presented with visual sexual stimulation. Perhaps the most definitive study to date used positron emission tomography (PET scan) to examine brain activity in healthy men presented with visual sexual stimulation. The areas of the brain activated included visual, sensory, and neuroendocrine and autonomic areas. Specifically, visually presented information produced bilateral activation of the inferior temporal cortex, a visual association area, activation of the right inferior frontal cortex and right insula, paralimbic areas that relate motivational states with highly processed sensory information, and activation of the left anterior cingulated cortex, a paralimbic area that controls neuroendocrine and autonomic functions (McKenna, 1999).

Psychological Factors

It is common for men to have occasional episodes of erectile failure without it developing into a full blown erectile disorder. Barlow (1986) argued that men with erectile dysfunction respond differently in sexual situations compared to normally functioning males. When placed in a sexual situation, men with erectile dysfunction focus on non-sexual cues such as fears about inadequate performance, and worries about inability to control performance. These thoughts lead to increased anxiety, increased focus on non-erotic cues and fears of erectile failure. This process inhibits erection and thereby confirms the men's fears. Since the men's fears were confirmed, they are likely to repeat the process in subsequent sexual situations and a negative feedback loop develops. In contrast, when placed in a sexual situation, men with normal erectile responding focus on erotic cues and subsequently become aroused and are able to obtain and sustain an erection. They experience the sexual situation as pleasurable and look forward to future sexual situations creating a positive feedback loop.

Treatment

A variety of tools can be used to assess whether the erectile dysfunction is of psychological or physiological origin. If the male exhibits nocturnal erections, or obtains an erection when a vasoactive substance is injected into the corpora, the erectile problem is likely to be psychological in nature. Treatments for erectile dysfunction include vacuum devices and constriction rings, intracavernosal injections, intraurethral pharmacotherapy, topical pharmacotherapy, oral pharmacotherapy, and penile implants. The vacuum device consists of a tube that is placed over the penis, and a vacuum pump that draws blood into the penile arteries. A constriction ring is placed at the base of the penis to prevent venous outflow so that the erection is maintained until completion of the sexual act. Several medications are available that can be injected into the corpus cavernosum of the penis to induce erection including papaverine, phentolamine, and prostaglandin E_1. These all act to dilate penile capillaries, allowing blood to flow into the penis. Although intracavernosal injections are fairly effective (between 70–90%), between 50% and 80% of patients discontinue treatment, citing problems such as inconvenience, cost, and invasiveness of treatment. An intraurethral-administered medication, MUSE (Medicated Urethral System for Erection — active ingredient prostaglandin E_1), has recently been introduced. This medication is administered in suppository form and is absorbed through the urethral mucosa. It is most effective when used in conjunction with a constriction ring. Side effects of the medication include urogenital pain and urethral bleeding. Topical medications, such as Minoxidil, are also available, although these types of treatments are not commonly used, in part because their effects on vaginal mucosa are not well understood. Viagra, an orally administered treatment, was introduced to the market in 1998, and since then, many of these rather cumbersome and involved treatments have become less popular. Viagra is well tolerated by a variety of patients and is an effective treatment for both organic and psychogenic impotence (Montorsi *et al.*, 1999). Because sildenafil produces vasodilation and a minor drop in blood pressure, it may be contraindicated for patients diagnosed with or receiving treatment for cardiovascular disease. Data are not presently available regarding sildenafil-use in patients with certain cardiac conditions such as unstable angina, stroke, or recent myocardial infarction (heart attack) and/or arrhythmias. Nonetheless, sexual activity increases the likelihood of ischaemia or infarction and thus patients with cardiac risk factors are often referred for an exercise stress test prior to receiving sildenafil. Sildenafil can safely be administered in conjunction with some cardiovascular medications, such as most antihypertensives, but if it is taken in conjunction with organic nitrates, it can produce a major and life-threatening drop in blood pressure (Klonger, 2000).

Penile implants are considered a last resort and are used when tissue damage or deterioration is severe, and when other treatments have failed. Penile implants typically consist of a cylinder (implanted in the penis) that can be mechanically inflated and deflated (Rowland and Burnett, 2000).

Studies are currently underway to determine whether Viagra and other drugs that act as vasodilators on genital tissue will be effective for treating Female Sexual Arousal Disorder. The first Federal Drug Administration (FDA) approved treatment for female sexual arousal disorder was recently introduced to the market. The treatment is a hand-held battery-operated device, called the EROS-CTD, which contains a soft plastic cup and a suction device. When the cup is placed over the clitoral tissue and the device is activated it draws blood into the genital tissue.

ORGASM DISORDERS

The normal ejaculatory response typically occurs following sensory stimulation to the penis. The stimulation initiates a nerve signal that travels along the pudendal nerve (i.e., genital sensory nerve) and synapses at the sacral level of the spinal cord. The spinal cord input stimulates an autonomic and a somatic response. The autonomic response involves adrenergic neurons (within the sympathetic nervous system), which stimulate contraction of the smooth muscles of the vas deferens, seminal vesicles, and prostate. This leads to closure of the bladder neck and movement of seminal fluid into the urethral duct. In both men and women, orgasm is characterized by a peak in sexual pleasure that is accompanied by rhythmic contractions of the genital and reproductive organs, cardiovascular and respiratory changes, and a release of sexual tension. In men, during the emission stage of orgasm, seminal fluid is propelled into the bulbar urethra via the release of norepinephrine that acts on alpha-adrenergic receptors, the smooth muscles of the vas deferens, prostate, and seminal vessels. During the ejaculatory phase, which is mediated by a sacral spinal reflex, semen is released through the urethra via contractions of muscles that surround the bulbar urethra. The extent to which central neurophysiologic events are related to the intensity or experience of orgasm is not known. While orgasm is generally the result of both genital and psychological stimulation, evidence suggests central stimulation alone may trigger orgasm.

Female Orgasmic Disorder

Female orgasmic disorder is diagnosed when the woman experiences persistent or recurrent delay in, or absence of, orgasm following a normal sexual excitement phase. In order to meet DSM-IV diagnostic criteria, the woman's orgasmic capacity is less than would be reasonable for her age, sexual experience, and adequacy of sexual stimulation she receives (American Psychiatric Association, 1994). Between 22–28% of women ages 18 to 59 years report that they are unable to attain orgasm. Married women and women who have some college education are significantly less likely to report being unable to attain orgasm as compared to never married and divorced women, and women who have not attended college (Laumann *et al.*, 1999).

Physiological Factors

Among normally orgasmic women oxytocin levels were positively correlated with subjective intensity of orgasm, and prolactin levels were elevated for up to 60 minutes following orgasm (Meston and Frohlich, 2000). It is feasible that oxytocin and prolactin regulation is abnormal in women with orgasmic disorders, although a study examining oxytocin and prolactin levels in orgasmic disordered women has not yet been published.

The SSRIs frequently affect orgasmic functioning, leading to delayed orgasm or anorgasmia. The antidepressant, nefazodone, produces fewer sexual side effects in women (Feiger *et al.*, 1996), possibly because it increases serotonin activity in general while simultaneously inhibiting serotonin activity at the serotonin$_2$ receptor — the receptor implicated in SSRI-induced sexual dysfunction (Eison *et al.*, 1990). Cyproheptadine is also a serotonin$_2$ receptor antagonist and has been an effective antidote to SSRI-induced orgasmic dysfunction (although it is not an ideal antidote as it can disrupt the effectiveness of the antidepressant medication). Drugs that affect dopamine mechanisms, such as antipsychotics (which inhibit dopamine) or cocaine (which facilitate dopamine), delay or inhibit orgasm in women. Female heroin addicts also report delayed or inhibited orgasm. Taken together, these findings suggest that serotonin, dopamine, and opioid mechanisms may be functioning abnormally in orgasmic disordered women.

Studies examining blood plasma levels of neuromodulators before, during, and after orgasm suggest that epinephrine and norepinephrine levels peak during orgasm in normally functioning women (Exton *et al.*, 1999; Wiedeking *et al.*, 1979). This process may be impaired in anorgasmic women. One study showed that when vigorous exercise (which stimulates the sympathetic nervous system) is followed by an erotic stimulus, sexual arousal is facilitated in normally functioning women, but inhibited in anorgasmic women (Meston and Gorzalka, 1996).

Brain and spinal cord mechanisms are integral to the orgasm response. The neuronal pathway connecting the genitals to the brain was identified via transneuronal labelling. Virus injected into the clitoris revealed that sexual afferent neurons synapse on neurons in the lumbosacral spinal cord and connect to the nucleus paragigantocellularis in the brainstem. Lesions to the nucleus paragigantocellularis and spinal cord transection can suppress tonic inhibition of the orgasm-like response, suggesting that this pathway exerts inhibitory control over orgasm. Neurons in this region stain positively for serotonin suggesting that it may be implicated in SSRI-induced anorgasmia in women. Studies in humans suggest that the paraventricular nucleus of the hypothalamus is also involved in the orgasmic response. The paraventricular nucleus produces oxytocin that is released from the posterior pituitary during arousal and orgasm (McKenna, 1999).

The neurological disease, multiple sclerosis, often results in orgasmic disorders. In multiple sclerosis patients, orgasmic problems are related to neurological problems such as changes in genital sensation, muscle weakness in the pelvis (Lundberg and Hulter, 1996), and brain abnormalities (in the pyramidal and brain-stem regions) (Barak *et al.*, 1996). It is feasible that similar anatomical structures are involved in orgasmic disorders, albeit non-disease related.

Psychological Factors

The degree to which a woman is distracted during sexual situations may affect orgasm ability. Orgasmic women tend to focus on their own arousal and their partners' arousal throughout the sexual situation, while anorgasmic women tend to focus on trying to attain orgasm, focus on non-sexual thoughts, and are more easily distracted by non-sexual thoughts. Anorgasmic women are also more likely to report discomfort with sex compared to orgasmic women; they are more likely to be uncomfortable discussing direct clitoral stimulation, and are more likely to have guilt about sex, to endorse sex myths, and to report negative attitudes about masturbation. Anorgasmic women are less likely to be aware of their physiological sexual arousal as compared to consistently orgasmic women (Stock, 1993).

Treatment

Treatment for anorgasmia involves education about female anatomy and physiology, self-exploration, and directed masturbation. The woman is encouraged to explore her body and identify regions and types of stimulation that produce sexual arousal, to experiment with different fantasies, and to use various tools (such as a vibrator) that may enhance arousal. Once she has successfully learned to attain orgasm during masturbation, she is encouraged to teach her partner which parts of her body and which types of stimulation are likely to bring her to orgasm. Directed masturbation is a highly effective treatment for anorgasmia, with outcome studies showing up to a 90% success rate (Heiman and Meston, 1998).

Male Orgasmic Disorder

DSM-IV criteria for male orgasmic disorder include recurrent or persistent difficulty obtaining orgasm, or inability to obtain orgasm, even after sufficient sexual stimulation. The clinician takes a variety of factors into account before making the diagnosis, such as age and amount of stimulation. In most cases of inhibited male orgasm the patient is able to attain orgasm but only through manual or oral stimulation, and when orgasm occurs through intercourse it is only possible after prolonged manual or oral stimulation (American Psychiatric Association, 1994).

For the patient and his partner (male or female), sexual activity is experienced as 'hard work' (Dekker, 1993). Very few studies of male orgasmic disorder have been published, likely due to the fact that it is a rare disorder. The prevalence in the general population is estimated at 1.5 in 1000, and among those presenting for sex therapy, 0–13 in 100 (Dekker, 1993).

What is presently known about the mechanisms underlying orgasm is drawn from animal studies and from studies examining side effects of recreational and pharmaceutical drugs. One of the more common side effects of SSRI medications is delayed or inhibited orgasm, suggesting that serotonin activity may play a role in normal orgasm functioning. Animal studies indicate that serotonin$_{1A}$ receptor activation facilitates orgasm (Bitran and Hull, 1987) — it is feasible that men with inhibited orgasm have abnormal serotonin$_{1A}$ receptor activity. Dopamine may also be implicated in orgasm functioning. Dopamine agonists, such as apomorphine and cocaine, have been reported to inhibit orgasm, although apomorphine has also been reported to facilitate orgasm. The fact that dopamine can both inhibit and facilitate orgasm may be a function of dose; in rats, a low dose of a dopamine agonist increased ejaculation latency while a high dose decreased ejaculation latency (Clark *et al.*, 1983). In normally functioning men, blood plasma levels of norepinephrine significantly increased at orgasm (Kruger *et al.*, 1998) and oxytocin levels were significantly positively correlated with subjective orgasm intensity (Carmichael *et al.*, 1994). Some evidence suggests that inhibited orgasm may result from spinal reflex abnormalities. Studies examining men with spinal cord injuries and normally functioning men suggest that the dorsal penile nerve and the perineal nerve are involved in the ejaculatory response. Stimulation to these nerves in normally functioning men resulted in contraction of the bulbocavernosus muscle, the muscle involved in ejaculation (Yang and Bradley, 1999).

The brain and spinal cord are regions implicated in orgasm. The neuronal pathway from the genitals to the brain was transneuronally labelled by injecting a virus into the penile tissue. Sexual afferents enter the lumbosacral region of the spinal cord and via interneurons and neurons connect to the nucleus paragigantocellularis in the brainstem. Lesions to the nucleus paragigantocellularis impair normal tonic inhibition of the orgasmic response. Neurons in this region stain positively for serotonin suggesting this region may be implicated in SSRI-induced anorgasmia in men. During arousal and orgasm in men, oxytocin produced in paraventricular nucleus of the hypothalamus is released from the posterior pituitary (McKenna, 1999). Single photon emission computed tomography was used to examine brain physiology during orgasm in eight healthy right-handed men. During orgasm, blood flow significantly increased in the right prefrontal cortex and decreased in all other cortical regions (Tiihonen *et al.*, 1994). Although these processes have been implicated in normal orgasmic functioning in men, no evidence is currently available on men with orgasmic disorders. Nonetheless, it is feasible that these regions and mechanisms function abnormally in men with orgasmic disorders.

Premature Ejaculation

When seminal fluid enters the urethral duct, it triggers a somatic response — known as ejaculatory inevitability. The bulbocavernosus and ischiocavernosus muscles contract and semen is ejaculated through the urethral opening. This event is typically associated with the subjective pleasure of orgasm (Rowland and Burnett, 2000). When ejaculation occurs with minimal sexual stimulation before, on, or shortly after penetration, it is referred to as premature ejaculation. The clinician determines whether a diagnosis should be made after taking a variety of factors likely to affect ejaculation latency into account, such as age and novelty of partner. A diagnosis is only made if it is a recurrent or persistent problem (American Psychiatric Association, 1994).

Premature ejaculation is a fairly common problem. Approximately 30% of men ages 18 to 59 report that they orgasm too early. Marital status and ethnicity are not significantly associated with premature ejaculation, but men who have attended college or graduated from college have lower rates of premature ejaculation than men with less education (Laumann *et al.*, 1999).

Physiological Factors

As described above, several medications inhibit or delay orgasm suggesting that neurotransmitter activity affected by these medications may be involved in normal ejaculation and, possibly, premature ejaculation. Dopamine agonists such as apomorphine and cocaine have been reported to affect orgasm and SSRIs often delay ejaculation suggesting that abnormalities in serotonin and/or dopamine regulation may underlie premature ejaculation. Animal studies suggest that stimulation of the serotonin$_{1A}$ receptor decreases ejaculation latency (Ahlenius and Larsson, 1997). Usually ejaculations occur after several intromissions but in some animals the effects of serotonin$_{1A}$ stimulation are so pronounced that ejaculation occurs at the first intromission (Ahlenius *et al.*, 1981). It is feasible that the serotonin$_{1A}$ receptor is hypersensitive in men with premature ejaculation.

Kaplan (1974) proposed that men with premature ejaculation are more sensitive to erotic stimuli and thus become aroused and orgasm more quickly. They may also be less adept at perceiving the sensations leading to ejaculatory inevitability (i.e., the point when semen is in the base of the urethra and ejaculation cannot be stopped). Several studies have tested this hypothesis with mixed results. Spiess *et al.* (1984) found that men with and without premature ejaculation did not differ in how quickly they became aroused, the length of time it took for them to obtain their maximum erection, or their erectile response to an erotic film. Colpi *et al.* (1986) found that men with premature ejaculation had a more sensitive ejaculation reflex and Fanciullacci *et al.* (1988) found that men with premature ejaculation had larger areas of the somatosensory cortex devoted to the genital region compared to normal controls. Taken together, these studies suggest that some cases of premature ejaculation may be organic in nature.

Psychological Factors

Traditionally, anxiety has been implicated in the aetiology of premature ejaculation yet empirical studies have found conflicting evidence regarding its role. Strassberg *et al.* (1990) compared self-reported thoughts during sexual stimulation in men with and without premature ejaculation and found no differences in self-reported anxiety. Cooper and Magnus (1984) conducted a double-blind, placebo controlled, crossover study where men with premature ejaculation were randomly assigned to receive an anxiolytic medication versus placebo. Although the anxiolytic medication had the expected impact on anxiety (it reduced it), it did not affect ejaculation latency. Cooper *et al.* (1993) compared men with primary premature ejaculation (i.e., life-long premature ejaculation problem) to men with secondary premature ejaculation (i.e., developed the problem after a period of normal ejaculation latencies) and found that men with secondary premature ejaculation were significantly more likely to report anxiety during intercourse and scored significantly higher on a general measure of anxiety. This suggests that anxiety may play a role in secondary premature ejaculation but not primary premature ejaculation.

Treatment

Treatments for premature ejaculation include psychological as well as pharmacological interventions. The most common psychological treatment, the pause-and-squeeze technique, was introduced by Semens (1956) and popularized by Masters and Johnson (1970). This technique is fairly straightforward; the man is stimulated to a point close to orgasm, the stimulation is interrupted (pause) and firm pressure is placed under the glans of the penis (squeeze). The procedure is repeated several types (typically twice) before ejaculation is permitted. These behavioural strategies are often combined with other strategies aimed at increasing control over ejaculation such as increasing the range of sexual activities (i.e., other than intercourse) and increasing the awareness of physical sensations associated with approaching ejaculation (so that stimulation can be ceased prior to ejaculatory inevitability). Patients may also be encouraged to use sexual imagery and thoughts to slightly decrease arousal levels and thus help control ejaculation (e.g., mentally listing the players in a favourite sports team).

More recently, pharmaceutical agents that have the side-effect of delaying ejaculation have been used to treat premature ejaculation. These include antidepressants such as the SSRIs and tricyclic antidepressants, and anti-anxiety medications such as the benzodiazepines. These types of medications are often effective in delaying ejaculation, although the effectiveness can wear off after several weeks and some men do not experience any delay in ejaculation (often the men least likely to respond are also those who ejaculate the most quickly). In some people these medications can have unpleasant side effects such as gastrointestinal disturbance and headache. Topical creams that dull sensation, such as lidocaine, may also effectively delay ejaculation, although they are not appropriate for men who ejaculate prior to insertion, and the creams can be irritating to vaginal tissue (Metz and Pryor, 2000).

PAIN DISORDERS

Dyspareunia

The DSM-IV defines dyspareunia as recurrent or persistent genital pain associated with sexual intercourse. The diagnosis of dyspareunia is not given if the pain decreases or is eliminated by adequate vaginal lubrication.

Although dyspareunia is currently classified as a psychiatric disorder, experts contend that it may be better classified as a pain syndrome that results in sexual dysfunction rather than a sexual dysfunction (that involves pain). In a recent review, Binik *et al.* (2000) suggested that describing genital pain along several dimensions including location, quality, elicitors, course, intensity, and meaning could be useful in identifying the cause of the pain and directing the type and course of treatment. Some women report that the pain is localized, generalized, or wandering while some women are not able to identify the location of the pain. The pain may have a 'sharp', 'burning', 'dull', or 'shooting' quality that may reflect the type of pathology. The pain may be specific to intercourse, or may follow other types of stimulation (e.g., oral sex). It may begin before, during, or after stimulation, and may be mild, moderate, severe, or excruciating. Women may attribute meaning to the pain — they may believe it is related to a medical condition or a psychological source. Meana *et al.* (1999) found that women who attributed their pain to a psychological source rated the pain as more severe in intensity.

Dyspareunia may be caused by anatomical, pathological, iatrogenic, or psychological factors. A rigid hymen would be an anatomical factor that could result in genital pain during intercourse. Infections in the genitals could produce genital pain during intercourse, as could endometriosis and non-malignant and malignant tumours. Surgical procedures (e.g., episiotomy) could also result in dyspareunia. Following menopause, atrophy of the vulva and vaginal tissue can increase the likelihood of dyspareunia. No one disease is associated with dyspareunia and a disease or disorder can be quite extensive without causing sexual pain. A variety of psychological factors may also lead to dyspareunia. For example, it may develop as a result of attitudes and values passed down from parents that lead to fear and anxiety in sexual situations, traumatic events where sexual or non-sexual contact with the genitals was experienced as painful, or emotional or relational factors, such as depression or discord between partners (Meana and Binik, 1994).

Recent evidence suggests that some forms of dyspareunia may be associated with abnormalities in pain sensation. The sense of touch and pain was measured in women with vulvar vestibulitis and control women (vulvar vestibulitis is a condition characterized by severe pain upon attempted intercourse or vestibular touch — the vestibule refers to the area of tissue below the clitoris, between the labia minora, and the vaginal opening). Touch and pain thresholds were obtained by applying small amounts of force to the skin; touch threshold was defined as the minimum amount of force needed for the women to consciously detect the stimulation, and pain thresholds were defined as the minimum amount of force that was experienced as painful. The women with vulvar vestibulitis were more sensitive to light touch and pain than the control women suggesting greater tactile and pain acuity (Pukall *et al.*, 2000). Women with vulvar vestibulitis also had more densely packed sensory nerves in the vestibule, which may account for their increased sensitivity (Westrom and Willen, 1998).

Treatment

Regardless of the cause of dyspareunia, the symptoms are most effectively treated with cognitive-behavioural therapy. Even when the pain is a direct result of a medical condition, the pain often continues after medical intervention (Schover *et al.*, 1982). Psychological treatment typically involves one or more of the following techniques: vaginal exercises, vaginal dilation, systematic desensitization, and couples therapy (education regarding communication and sexuality). The goal is for the woman and her partner to learn, through education and direct experience, that sexual contact and intercourse do not necessarily produce pain. Vaginal exercises involve the voluntary contraction of the vaginal muscles, allowing the women to gain familiarity and greater control over her muscle contractions. Vaginal dilation involves inserting increasingly larger dilators into the vagina until the woman is able to insert one that is a similar size to her partner's penis, without experiencing pain or anxiety. Vaginal dilation is one form of systematic desensitization but systematic desensitization can also be performed by fantasizing about pain producing activities. The woman is first asked to list activities in order from least painful or anxiety provoking to most painful and anxiety provoking. She is then instructed to fantasize about the least painful activity until she is able to picture it without discomfort. Once she is able to do this, she moves to the next item on the list, until she is able to fantasize about the most painful and anxiety provoking item on the list without feeling discomfort.

Vaginismus

The DSM-IV defines vaginismus as repeated and persistent involuntary spasm of the vaginal muscles that interferes with intercourse. For many women, this difficulty is not specific to intercourse; they are often unable to insert even tampons into their vaginas and fear and avoid gynaecological exams. The condition is not necessarily a generalized sexual problem; many women with vaginismus are able to enjoy sexual stimulation and orgasm that does not involve penetration of the vagina. The prevalence of vaginismus is not known. Laumann *et al.* (1994) interviewed a random sample of 1749 women and found that 10–15% of women reported sexual pain, either dyspareunia or vaginismus. Approximately 12–17% of women seeking sexual therapy present with symptoms of vaginismus (Spector and Carey, 1990).

Although the DSM-IV indicates that vaginismus involves spasm of the musculature of the outer third of the vagina, this description is based almost exclusively on self-report rather than physical examination. One study found no difference in vaginal muscular activity (measured via EMG) between women with vaginismus and control women (van der Velde and Everaerd, 1996). No empirical studies have explored what specifically occurs to prevent penetration. It is not clear whether muscle contraction prevents penetration or makes penetration difficult or painful, or whether penetration is not attempted due to anticipatory pain. The DSM-IV does not include pain as a characteristic of vaginismus, yet some experts in the field argue that the pain, or the anticipation of pain, may be central to the disorder (Reissing *et al.*, 1999).

Vaginismus has traditionally been thought to result primarily from psychological factors. A review of the family histories of women with vaginismus reveals similar backgrounds. Often women with vaginismus were raised by parents with oppressive or authoritarian attitudes (Tugrul and Kabakci, 1997) and had parents who were engaged in frequent conflict (Silverstein, 1989).

Many women with vaginismus report having fathers who were domineering or threatening, alcoholic, seductive, or overprotective, and mothers who disliked sex or viewed sex as an obligation. Approximately 40% of women with vaginismus report a history of sexual trauma (Silverstein, 1989).

Medical conditions that could lead to vaginismus include: vaginal surgery, prolapse of the uterus, endometriosis, vaginal tumours, vaginal lesions, vaginal atrophy, congenital abnormalities, sexually transmitted diseases, abnormalities of the hymen, and pelvic congestion. In such cases, the condition may produce genital pain that develops over time into vaginismus. Medical conditions are associated with vaginismus in 23–32% of cases (Reissing *et al.*, 1999).

Treatment

Vaginismus is treated with cognitive-behavioural therapy targetted at eliminating the erroneous beliefs and the vaginal spasms. Therapy involves identifying faulty beliefs (e.g., 'my vagina is too small to accommodate his penis') and educating the woman and her partner regarding normal sexual anatomy and physiology (e.g., in the aroused and non-aroused state, the vagina is capable of accommodating even a large penis). Vaginal spasms are treated with vaginal muscle exercises and progressive vaginal dilation. The woman and her partner insert dilators into her vagina, starting with very small sized dilators, progressively increasing the size until she is able to insert a dilator that is as large as an erect penis, and finally, attempting intercourse. Few well-controlled treatment outcome studies have been conducted making it difficult to evaluate the effectiveness of therapy, but estimates suggest that 60–100% of vaginismus cases are successfully treated with this type of intervention (Reissling *et al.*, 1999).

PARAPHILIAS

According to the DSM-IV, in order to be diagnosed with a paraphilia, one must demonstrate the following features.

- "Recurrent, intense sexually arousing fantasies, sexual urges, or behaviours generally involving 1) nonhuman objects, 2) the suffering or humiliation of oneself or one's partner, or 3) children or other non-consenting persons, that occur over a period of at least 6 months."

- The behaviour, sexual urges, or fantasies cause clinically significant distress or impairment in social, occupational, or other important areas of functioning.

The DSM-IV lists eight types of paraphilic disorders but in practice, individuals displaying one paraphilia very often also exhibit other paraphilic behaviours. Incarcerated paedophiles often report, for example, that they have also engaged in other paraphilic behaviours (e.g., exhibitionism, voyeurism) and that deviant sexual behaviours other than pedophilia are their primary interest. The presence of paraphilic behaviour may represent an underlying sexual impulsivity disorder that is characterized by sexual compulsivity and hypersexuality, and in some cases, aggression (Kafka, 1997).

Fetishism

According to the DSM-IV, fetishism involves "recurrent, intense sexually arousing fantasies, sexual urges, or behaviours involving the use of nonliving objects" as sexual stimuli (American Psychiatric Association, 1994). Most fetishists are male and nearly one in four are homosexual. Common fetish items include shoes and lingerie and common materials include rubber and leather. Fetishists become aroused by stealing the object, viewing the object, or masturbating with the object. Most fetishists are aroused by a number of different objects. The aetiology of fetishism is not known. Two reported cases of fetishism have been associated with abnormalities in the temporal lobe. In one case the patient had temporal lobe epilepsy and in the other the fetish behaviour was linked to the development of a temporal lobe tumour (Wise, 1985). Some evidence suggests that fetishism may be a learned behaviour that results when a normal sexual stimulus is paired with the fetish item. Seven heterosexual males free from any prior fetish were repeatedly shown erotic stimuli paired with a slide of a black knee-length women's boot. When the slide of the boot was later shown alone, five of the seven men demonstrated penile erection, indicating that a boot fetish had been conditioned. The conditioned fetish was shown to generalize to other types of shoes in three of the men. That is, the men also became aroused when shown a slide of a high-heeled black boot and a low-heeled black shoe. They did not become aroused to a slide of a short brown boot, a brown string sandal, or a golden sandal, suggesting that the fetish only generalized to similar types of shoes (Rachman and Hodgson, 1968). A similar study was conducted in women to determine whether women could also be conditioned to become sexually aroused to a stimulus. Subjects were randomly assigned to repeatedly view an erotic film paired with a light stimulus versus an erotic film alone. No significant differences were found in physiological sexual arousal between the experimental and control groups when a light stimulus was later presented alone (Letourneau and O'Donohue, 1997). Meston and Rachman (1994) tried to condition sexual arousal to the sound of a male's voice. Even after repeated pairings of erotic video clips and the male's voice, later presentation of the male's voice alone did not produce sexual arousal. This suggests that sexual arousal is not readily classically conditioned in women and may explain why, like other paraphilias, fetishism occurs almost exclusively in men.

Transvestic Fetishism

Transvestic fetishism is diagnosed in heterosexual males who experience "recurrent, intense sexually arousing fantasies, sexual urges, or behaviours involving cross-dressing" (American Psychiatric Association, 1994). A distinction is drawn between transvestism (cross-dressing) and transvestic fetishism. A variety of people cross-dress but the behaviour is not considered a fetish unless the cross-dressing is associated with sexual feelings. For example, transsexuals, or people who feel that their external sex does not match their internal gender identity, may cross-dress in order to feel more congruent with their gender identity but do not find the cross-dressing sexually arousing. Similarly, homosexual males may cross-dress (e.g., drag-queens), but the cross-dressing is not considered to be a fetish unless it is sexually arousing.

Very few studies have been published regarding transvestic fetishism and those that have often grouped transvestic fetishists with transvestites who experienced little to no sexual arousal from cross-dressing. Doctor and Prince (1997) surveyed 1032 male transvestites between 1990 and 1992. They found that 40% of respondents found cross-dressing 'often' or 'nearly always' sexually exciting but only 9% described themselves as a "fetishist [who] favoured women's clothing". While keeping in mind that it is unclear what percentage of subjects would meet DSM-IV criteria for transvestic fetishism, the following characteristics were reported. Respondents ranged in age from 20 to 80 years of age, lived throughout the United States, and reported a range of religious affiliations (24% were Catholic, 38% were Protestant, 3% were Jewish, 10% were agnostic, and 25% were with other religious affiliations). The majority of respondents were well educated (65% had at least a BA), in committed relationships, and had children. Of those currently married, 83% reported that their wives were aware of their transvestic tendencies at present, but only 28% accepted the behaviour. The vast majority reported a heterosexual orientation (87%) although 29% reported having had homosexual experiences. The majority of respondents began cross-dressing before age 10 (66%) or between age 10 and 20 (29%), had been raised by both parents (76%), and reported that their father "provided a good masculine image" (76%).

A few cases have been reported of men with transvestic fetishism who had fathers or brothers who also cross-dressed. Since so few cases of familial co-occurrence have been reported in the literature, and because the occurrence of transvestic fetishism in the general population is not known, it is not clear whether family environment and/or genetics contributes to the likelihood of developing a cross-dressing fetish. Transvestic fetishism is associated with learning disabilities, and a few cases of transvestic fetishism have been associated with temporal lobe abnormalities (Zucker and Blanchard, 1997).

A number of studies have been published examining psychosocial causes of transvestic fetishism but most have serious methodological flaws that limit drawing confident conclusions. Some such studies suggest that adolescents with transvestic fetishism tendencies may have a history of separation from and hostility towards their mothers. The cross-dressing may serve as a means to make a connection with females, even if that connection often involves some expressions of anger and hostility (Zucker and Blanchard, 1997).

Pedophilia

Pedophilia is defined as intense and repeated sexually arousing fantasies, urges, or behaviours involving sexual activity with children, typically less than 14 years old (American Psychiatric Association, 1994). Since few paedophiles are likely to openly admit their preference, it is difficult to estimate the prevalence of pedophilia in the general population. Furthermore, individuals who feel sexual attraction to children may resist the temptation due to societal pressures, yet may nonetheless experience sexual fantasies involving children. Recent evidence suggests that pedophilia may be associated with homosexuality, mental retardation, and high maternal age. Homosexuality in the general population is estimated at 2% while homosexuality in paedophiles is estimated at up to 40%. When sexual orientation, intellectual functioning, and maternal age were measured in 991 male sex offenders, high maternal age and low intellectual functioning were significantly associated with homosexual pedophilia. The association between low intelligence and pedophilia suggests that pedophilia may reflect a developmental disorder. The association between high maternal age and pedophilia is unclear, although it may reflect differences in birth order as homosexuality is associated with being later born (discussed below under gender identity disorder) (Blanchard *et al.*, 1999).

Some researchers have speculated that a childhood history of sexual abuse contributes to an adult preference for sexual activity with children. In a large sample of men who were child sex offenders, Freund *et al.* (1990) found that heterosexual and homosexual paedophiles were significantly more likely to report childhood sexual abuse by a male abuser (versus female abuser) as compared to controls. Freund and Kuban (1994) classified child sex offenders according to whether they demonstrated phallometric (increased penile volume) preference to photographs of nude children versus adults. They found that child sex offenders who demonstrated preference for children were significantly more likely to have a childhood history of sexual abuse. It should be noted that although reports indicate approximately 49% of paedophiles have a history of childhood sexual abuse, very few people with a history of childhood sexual abuse become paedophiles (Freund and Kuban, 1994).

Paedophiles may have difficulty with gender differentiation. Freund *et al.* (1991) showed slides of nude male and female children and adults to paedophiles and controls, and measured penile volume changes. The paedophiles demonstrated less differentiation between stimuli containing males versus females as compared to non-paedophiles. Although this pattern of undifferentiated arousal has also been noted in a case study of a 20-year-old woman with multiple paraphilias (Cooper *et al.*, 1990), few cases of female pedophilia have been reported in the literature.

Paedophiles may differ from non-paedophiles on several physiological dimensions as well. Baseline plasma cortisol, prolactin, and body temperature were significantly higher in paedophiles than controls. When both groups were administered a serotonin agonist, mCPP, versus placebo, plasma cortisol levels were more elevated and remained elevated longer for paedophiles compared to controls. The paedophiles reported experiencing side effects (e.g., dizzy, restless) of mCPP administration while the controls did not. Consistent with these findings, some researchers have speculated that pedophilia may be associated with disturbances in serotonin-related aggression and impulsivity (Maes *et al.*, 2001). It has also been suggested that pedophilia may be a subtype of obsessive–compulsive disorder; a problem that is marked by repetitive, irrepressible behaviour associated with serotonin dysregulation (Balyk, 1997).

Sexual Masochism and Sexual Sadism

The DSM-IV defines sexual masochism as "recurrent, intense sexually arousing fantasies, sexual urges, or behaviours involving the act (real, not simulated) of being humiliated, beaten, bound, or otherwise made to suffer" (American Psychiatric Association, 1994). In 1886, Krafft-Ebing coined the term, masochist, after Leopold von Sacher-Masoch, who wrote novels depicting men being humiliated and bound by females. Sexual sadism is characterized by "recurrent, intense sexually arousing fantasies, sexual urges, or behaviours involving acts (real, not simulated) in which the psychological or physical suffering (including humiliation) of the victim is sexually exciting to the person" (American Psychiatric Association, 1994). The term, sadism, was derived from writings of the Marquis de Sade, an 18th century author who wrote stories depicting sexual torture and brutality. A distinction is drawn between minor versus major sexually sadistic acts. Minor sexually sadistic acts would include, for example, humiliation and bondage of a willing sexual masochist while major sexually sadistic acts would involve acts such as sexual torture and rape of an unwilling participant. The key distinction here is whether the victim was consenting or not.

The practice of sadomasochism (referred to as S&M), or the consensual participation between sexual sadist and sexual masochist, involves carrying out predetermined sexual scenarios. These scenarios commonly involve several themes: flagellation (usually on the buttocks), bondage, 'water sports' (urophilia — attraction to urine, coprophilia — attraction to feces, and mysophilia — attraction to filth), and penis and nipple torture (Arndt, 1991). Sadomasochists interviewed in New York and San Francisco between 1976 and 1983 reported S&M activities that included elements of dominance and submission, role-playing (e.g., master and slave), consensuality (i.e., both participants were willing), and were of sexual context (i.e., the role-playing was sexual) (Weinberg *et al.*, 1984). Commonly reported S&M role-play themes include: "severe boss and the naughty secretary", "the queen and many slaves", "the male barber and his customer", and "arrest scenes and military training" (Sandnabba *et al.*, 1999). Although the sexual sadist appears to be in control, often the degree of domination and humiliation is agreed upon earlier, and it is the sexual masochist who indicates with a predetermined cue when he/she has reached his/her limit (Arndt, 1991).

Female sexual masochists and sadists are outnumbered by male sexual masochists and sadists and in many cases, the females are prostitutes who specialize in sadomasochism. One study found that approximately a quarter of female sexual sadists are prostitutes (Breslow *et al.*, 1985). Approximately 80% of sadomasochists reported that they were regularly engaging in sadomasochistic activities by age 30 years (Sandnabba *et al.*, 1999). Spengler (1977) obtained questionnaire data from 245 male sadomasochists recruited through S&M magazine advertisements and via S&M clubs. The majority of respondents reported that they met partners through sadomasochism advertisements, clubs, or bars. The sample contained 30% heterosexual sadomasochists, 31% bisexual sadomasochists, and 38% homosexual sadomasochists. The respondents came from all ages, socioeconomic backgrounds and levels of education. In most cases, the families knew little if anything about the respondents' S&M activities; 41% of married respondents ($n = 109$) reported that their wives knew nothing about the sadomasochistic activity.

When queried whether they thought the sadomasochistic behaviour was acceptable, 70% indicated acceptance of the behaviour, 85% reported that they "want to do it again", "it was fun" (84%), and "sexually satisfying" (79%). Although many of the respondents reported that they enjoyed non-sadomasochistic sexual activity, they reported being more likely to orgasm with sadomasochistic activity (79%) than without (45%). About a third of respondents reported fetishisms (e.g., boots and leather).

Very few studies have been conducted examining sexual sadists who target unwilling victims. Seto and Kuban (1996) examined penile volume changes in seven sadistic rapists compared to 14 non-sadistic rapists and 20 controls. The subjects were presented audiotapes depicting five different scenarios: (1) nonviolent, non-sexual interaction with a female; (2) consensual sexual activity with a female; (3) non-sexual violence against a female; (4) rape; and (5) violent rape. Compared to controls, the sadistic rapists and non-sadistic rapists were equally aroused by the different types of sexual contact — they were less likely to differentiate between consensual sexual activity, rape, and violent rape.

A subset of sexual sadists may have abnormal endocrine activity although hormone levels typically do not differ between sexual sadists and controls. In a review of individual cases, one sexual sadist had unusually high levels of luteinizing hormone (stimulates progesterone secretion) and follicle-stimulating hormone (stimulates estradiol in women and sperm development in men), another had low testosterone levels and another Klinefelter's syndrome (XXY chromosomes rather than the typical XY male pattern). Gross examination of brain functioning revealed no differences between sexual sadists and controls, but more careful examination revealed a subtle but significant difference in the right temporal lobe. Forty-one percent of the sexual sadists had a slightly dilated right temporal horn, compared to 13% of controls. One sexual sadist had a slow growing tumour in the left frontal-temporal lobe, likely present since childhood. Another had enlargement of the ventricles, a condition typically associated with schizophrenia and suggestive of overall brain atrophy. In short, temporal lobe abnormalities may be implicated in sexual sadism, but more information is needed before any strong conclusions can be made (Langevin *et al.*, 1988).

Serial killing, which is often reported in the media and dramatized in movies, may reflect comorbid sexual sadism and antisocial personality disorder. Geberth and Turco (1997) examined records of 387 serial murderers within the United States and found that 248 had sexually assaulted their victims. These included famous cases of serial killing, such as Theodore (Ted) Bundy and the Green River Killer. Of these, they determined that 68 met DSM-IV criteria for both sexual sadism and antisocial personality disorder (in other cases, sufficient data were not available to make a determination). These 68 individuals displayed a pattern of behaviour characterized by childhood aggressiveness and antisocial behaviour, and a pattern of killing involving sexual violence, humiliation, domination and control. Examination of their records suggests that these 68 individuals engaged in sexual violence and killing because they derived pleasure from it.

Courtship Disorders: Voyeurism, Exhibitionism, and Frotteurism

Voyeurism, exhibitionism, and frotteurism may be different behavioural expressions of a single underlying courtship disorder. The overt behaviours differ, but can also be conceptualized as different stages on a continuum — different degrees of proximity to the victim. Voyeurism involves viewing the victim from a distance, exhibitionism involves approaching the victim, and frotteurism involves physically touching the victim. The preference for rape over consensual sexual activity (termed the preferential rape pattern) may represent the fourth phase in the courtship disorders (Freund *et al.*, 1983). A common aetiological factor has not been identified although evidence indicates that the courtship disorders are associated with a preference for eliciting an alarmed reaction from an unfamiliar target rather than any lack of interest in intercourse (Freund and Watson, 1990). A high degree of comorbidity exists between these disorders and even when no overt comorbid behaviour is present, some evidence suggests that presence of one disorder predisposes to another such disorder (Freund *et al.*, 1983).

Voyeurism

The DSM-IV defines voyeurism as "recurrent, intense sexually arousing fantasies, sexual urges, or behaviours involving the act of observing an unsuspecting person who is naked, in the process of disrobing or engaging in sexual activity" (American Psychiatric Association, 1994). Most men, if given the opportunity to view a woman disrobing, would not avert their eyes. A man who engages in an opportunistic 'peep' is not a voyeur, the peeping must be recurrent and the urges to do so intense. Voyeurs tend to be the youngest child in the family. Compared to other sex offenders and controls, voyeurs have fewer sisters, have a good relationship with both parents, but have parents who do not have a good marital relationship. Voyeurs are often underdeveloped socially and sexually. They tend to engage in sexual activity later than other groups, and are less likely to marry than controls and other sex offenders (Smith, 1976). The more sexually experienced a voyeur, the more frequently he is likely to engage in peeping behaviour (Langevin *et al.*, 1985). Some evidence suggests that voyeurs may be predisposed to other paraphilias as well (e.g., sadomasochism, zoophilia) (Langevin *et al.*, 1985).

Although voyeurism is rare in women, some evidence suggests that women have similar 'peeping' urges as men. Friday (1975) interviewed women from all ages (teen to retirement) and walks of life and found that women expressed fantasies about peeping and, in some cases, engaged in actual peeping behaviour.

Learning theorists have suggested that voyeurism develops when the subject is provided a voyeuristic opportunity, and then subsequently masturbates while fantasizing about the experience. Some evidence supports this hypothesis; 50% of voyeurs reported that prior to the onset of their peeping behaviour they believed that normal sexual relations were not likely to be an option for them, and so they fantasized about scenarios they believed to be more obtainable, such as peeping. In addition, 75% of voyeurs reported that the sexual scenario they envision while masturbating reflected their first peeping experience (Smith, 1976).

Exhibitionism

Exhibitionism is defined as "the exposure of one's genitals to an unsuspecting stranger" (American Psychiatric Association, 1994) and involves some form of sexual gratification. Exhibitionism occurs almost exclusively in men. Very few cases of female exhibitionists have been reported in the literature, but the characteristics of these women differed from typical male exhibitionists. Male exhibitionists tend to be timid and unassertive men who have underdeveloped social skills and who are uncomfortable with angry or hostile feelings. Some studies suggest that exhibitionists were more likely to have been raised in a sexually puritanical background. The few female exhibitionists described in the literature, and studies examining female strippers, would suggest that the majority of female exhibitionists gain no pleasure from exposing their genitals but do so either to gain money or attention (Blair and Lanyon, 1981).

Behavioural theory proposes that exhibitionism develops as a result of a learned behaviour that is subsequently reinforced. This theory has been applied successfully to the treatment of exhibitionism (i.e., a learned behaviour can be replaced with a more socially acceptable behaviour) but it is not clear whether this reflects the actually aetiology of exhibitionism. Attempts to identify a physiological cause of exhibitionism have thus far been unsuccessful.

Frotteurism

Frotteurism involves "intense sexually arousing fantasies, sexual urges, or behaviours involving touching and rubbing against a non-consenting person" (American Psychiatric Association, 1994). The majority of published articles on this disorder group frotteurism with other paraphilic disorders or report cases of men with multiple paraphilias, including frotteurism. Abel *et al.* (1987) examined 62 males diagnosed with frotteurism, as well as other paraphilic disorders, and found that, at the time of the interview, they had committed an average of 849 frottage acts. Rooth (1973) interviewed 561 nonincarcerated men with paraphilias and found that of those exhibiting frotteurism, 79% had other paraphilias, with an average of 4.8 paraphilias each.

It is unclear whether true frotteurism in women exists, perhaps in part because of the decreased likelihood that male victims would view the behaviour as unwelcome or threatening. A handful of case reports of sexual molestation of men by women have been reported in the literature. The molestation typically occurred subsequent to erectile failure or inhibited desire (Sarrel and Masters, 1982). Although these cases do not represent female frotteurism, they suggest that it is feasible that rare cases of female frotteurism may exist, but are rarely reported.

Treatment of Paraphilias

In the mid 1900s, some European countries used castration as a means of treating exhibitionism, pedophilia, and other forms of sexual crimes. In West Germany, psychosurgery, which involved removing the nucleus ventromedialis of the hypothalamus, was used as a treatment for male sex offenders. Published reports of these practices rarely provided sufficient information to determine whether this intervention was successful in eliminating the inappropriate sexual behaviour. Of course there are serious consequences to performing such extreme and permanent techniques.

Cognitive–behavioural therapies, such as aversion therapy, are often used to treat paraphilias. The arousing stimulus is paired with an aversive stimulus such as a shock or noxious odour until the paraphilic behaviour no longer produces sexual arousal. A review of the handful of studies and case reports published suggests that aversion therapy alone is effective in reducing arousal, but that relapse rates are high (Kilmann *et al.*, 1982). More recently, other forms of cognitive–behavioural therapy such as covert sensitization or orgasmic reconditioning, are being used. Orgasmic reconditioning involves fantasizing about the paraphilic behaviour while masturbating, and at the moment just before orgasm, switching the fantasy to a more acceptable stimulus, such as one's partner. The belief is that orgasm, being an intensely pleasurable sensation, will serve to reinforce the more accepted sexual fantasy. Few well-controlled treatment outcome studies have been published, however, making it difficult to determine whether these types of interventions are effective. Covert sensitization involves fantasizing about the paraphilic behaviour followed by imagining a noxious scenario, such as vomiting, or an undesirable consequence such as being discovered by one's family. It is not yet clear how successful these techniques are in eliminating the behaviour although a few reports indicate that they can be highly successful for some patients.

Pharmacological interventions include hormonal supplements or psychotropic medications. Hormonal treatments are designed to inhibit deviant sexual behaviour by reducing sexual drive and sexual arousal. They include the following: (1) oestrogen; (2) medroxyprogesterone acetate (MPA), which lowers plasma testosterone and reduces gonadotropin secretion; (3) luteinizing hormone-releasing hormone agonists (LHRH agonists), which produce the pharmacological equivalent of castration by significantly inhibiting gonadotropin secretion; and (4) antiandrogens such as cyproterone acetate (CPA), which blocks testosterone uptake and metabolism. Treatment outcome studies suggest that these treatments are effective in reducing deviant sexual behaviour provided that the treatment regimen is maintained, although more well-controlled treatment outcome studies are needed before the true effectiveness of these treatments can be determined. Psychotropic medications that affect the serotonin systems have recently been used to treat paraphilias. Clinical studies suggest that SSRIs such as Prozac are effective in reducing paraphilic arousal and may be effective in reorienting arousal to more socially acceptable scenarios. The effectiveness of SSRIs in reducing paraphilic fantasies and behaviours suggests that these disorders may have an obsessive–compulsive component, as SSRIs are often used to treat obsessive–compulsive disorders. As with hormone treatments, however, more well-controlled treatment outcome studies must be conducted before the true effectiveness of these treatments can be determined (Bradford, 2000).

GENDER IDENTITY DISORDER

The DSM-IV describes gender identity disorder as a persistent and strong cross-gender identification and a persistent unease with one's sex. Gender identity disorder is not diagnosed if these symptoms co-occur with a physical intersex condition. As with the sexual disorders, a diagnosis is only made if the symptoms produce marked distress or impairment. According to the DSM-IV, gender identity disorder can occur in childhood, adolescence, and adulthood. Sexually mature individuals may be heterosexual, homosexual, bisexual, or may feel little sexual attraction to either men or women (American Psychiatric Association, 1994). Gender identity disorder is often confused with transvestism (cross-dressing) although the two are distinct.

When biological males and females feel a cross-gender identification, it is termed male-to-female transsexualism (MF) and female-to-male transsexualism (FM), respectively. Prevalence estimates suggest that MF transsexualism is more common than FM transsexualism although a few studies have found a 1 : 1 ratio. Prevalence estimates range from 1 : 10,000 to 1 : 100,000 for MF and 1 : 30,000 to 1 : 400,000 for FM (Cohen-Kettenis and Gooren, 1999; Zucker and Green, 1992).

Studies examining the biological causes of gender identity disorder have typically examined the effects of prenatal hormones on prenatal brain development. During normal prenatal development, the presence of testosterone leads to the development of external male genitalia and to a male differentiated brain. It is hypothesized that for individuals with gender identity disorder, a discrepancy may exist between prenatal genital differentiation and brain differentiation such that the external genitals develop, for example, as male while the brain develops as female. The evidence to support this hypothesis is mixed. Genetic females exposed to high levels of testosterone *in utero* (e.g., congenital adrenal hyperplasia), rarely develop gender identity disorder. Similar prenatal exposure to antiandrogenic, androgenic, and oestrogenic drugs rarely leads to gender identity disorder in either genetic females or males although some of these individuals display abnormal gender role behaviour (Cohen-Kettenis and Gooren, 1999). The strongest evidence to suggest that abnormal prenatal brain differentiation may lead to gender identity disorder comes from a recent study examining hypothalamic brain nuclei in men with gender identity disorder. Zhou *et al.* (1995) found that the central subdivision of the bed nucleus of the stria terminalis (a region of the hypothalamus) was smaller in MF transsexuals compared to normal males but similar in size to normal females, a difference that was not accounted for by hormone therapy. Sadeghi and Fakhrai (2000) recently reported a case of 18-year-old monozygotic female twins requesting gender reassignment surgery. The twins had a childhood history of cross-dressing. Unfortunately they were lost to follow up after the initial evaluation but this case suggests that gender identity disorder may have a genetic component.

Recent studies indicate that, compared to controls, MF transsexuals have more older brothers (but not more older sisters) and a later birth order (Blanchard *et al.*, 1995; Zucker *et al.*, 1997). Conversely, FM transsexuals are more likely to have several younger sisters but not brothers compared to controls (Zucker *et al.*, 1998). The histocompatibility-Y antigen (H-Y antigen), which is responsible for the development of the male testes and brain differentiation, may be implicated in this process for males. With progressive male births, mothers may become immunized to the H-Y antigen, leading to increased production of H-Y antibodies, and a disruption in normal brain differentiation (Blanchard *et al.*, 1998).

Social, parental, or familial factors have been associated with mild gender disturbance. MF transsexuals often report over controlling, rejecting fathers. FM transsexuals often report mothers and fathers who were rejecting and mothers who were over protective. It is feasible, however, that these differences may have been the result of abnormal gender development, rather than the cause (Cohen-Kettenis and Gooren, 1999).

Childhood gender identity disorder may, in some cases, predict adult gender identity disorder. Fifty-five feminine boys with gender identity disorder were followed into early adulthood. Five of the feminine boys were diagnosed with gender identity disorder, one as a transvestite, 21 as homosexual, 14 as heterosexual, and 14 that were not rated. This suggests that childhood gender identity disorder reflects a high likelihood of either adult gender identity disorder or homosexuality (Green, 1987).

In cases where gender identity disorder is present, if the individual displays only a mild tendency, displays serious psychopathology, or is not functioning well socially, psychotherapy rather than sex reassignment surgery may be advised. For those with extreme symptoms of gender identity disorder, who are free of from psychopathology, and who are functioning well in society, sex reassignment surgery is still not permitted until the person has lived full time as the preferred gender, often for a period of 2 years. During this period, candidates may be required to change their name, inform their family, boss, and co-workers, cross-dress full time, and receive hormone treatment. This period is considered to be essential for determining whether surgery is appropriate. The candidates have the opportunity to experience what it is like to live as the other gender and to determine whether they are fully prepared for and fully comprehend the impact of living the remainder of their lives as the other sex (Cohen-Kettenis and Gooren, 1999).

A review of sex reassignment surgery outcome studies suggests that in most cases, surgery resolves the gender identity disorder. Depending on the study, between 71% and 97% of subjects were successfully treated with surgery and less than 1% later took steps to reverse the sex reassignment. Factors that predict a poor outcome include: misdiagnosed transvestism, poor surgery outcome, poor social or work functioning, suicidal tendencies, and sex reassignment surgery late in life. This suggests that the current procedure for determining appropriateness of sex reassignment surgery is effective, when applied strictly (Cohen-Kettenis and Gooren, 1999). Male to female transsexuals who are attracted to men (MF homosexuals) seem to have a better post-surgery outcome compared to MF transsexuals who are attracted to women (MF heterosexuals). MF heterosexuals may have a poorer post-surgery outcome because of the added stigma of becoming homosexual after surgery, and because they typically present for surgery much later in life than MF homosexuals and thus are likely to have more male-role investments (e.g., husband, father). FM transsexuals in general have better post-surgery outcome than MF transsexuals (Cohen-Kettenis and Gooren, 1999).

REFERENCES

Abel, G.G., Becker, J.B., Mittelman, M., Cunningham-Rathner, J., Rouleau, J.L. and Murphy, W.D., 1987. Self-reported sex crimes of nonincarcerated paraphilias. *Journal of Interpersonal Violence*, **2**(1), 3–25.

Ahlenius, S. and Larsson, K., 1997. Specific involvement of central 5-HT_{1A} receptors in the mediation of male rat ejaculatory behaviour. *Neurochemical Research*, **22**(8), 1065–1070.

Ahlenius, S., Larsson, K., Svensson, L., Hjorth, S., Carlsson, A., Lindberg, P., Wikstrom, H., Sanchez, D., Arvidsson, L.E., Hacksell, U. and Nilsson, J.L., 1981. Effects of a new type of 5-HT receptor agonist on male rat sexual behaviour. *Pharmacology, Biochemistry & Behaviour*, **15**(5), 785–792.

Aizenberg, D., Zemishlany, Z., Dorfman-Etrog, P. and Weizman, A., 1995. Sexual dysfunction in male schizophrenic patients. *Journal of Clinical Psychiatry*, **56**, 137–141.

American Psychiatric Association, 1994. *Diagnostic and Statistical Manual of Mental Disorders*, 4th edn. Author, Washington DC.

Arndt, W.B., 1991. *Gender Disorders and the Paraphilias*. International University Press, Madison, Connecticut.

Balyk, E.D., 1997. Paraphilias as a sub type of obsessive–compulsive disorder: a hypothetical bio-social model. *Journal of Orthomolecular Medicine*, **12**(1), 29–42.

Barak, Y., Achiron, A., Elizur, A. and Gavvay, U., 1996. Sexual dysfunction in relapsing–remitting multiple sclerosis: magnetic resonance imaging, clinical, and psychological correlates. *Journal of Psychiatry & Neuroscience*, **21**(4), 255–258.

Barlow, D.H., 1986. Causes of sexual dysfunction: the role of anxiety and cognitive interference. *Journal of Consulting and Clinical Psychology*, **54**(2), 140–148.

Besser, G.M. and Thorner, M.O., 1975. Prolactin and gonadal function. *Pathol Biol (Paris)*, **23**, 779–794.

Binik, Y.M., Bergeron, S. and Khalife, S., 2000. Dyspareunia. In: Leiblum, S.R. and Rosen, R.C. (eds), *Principles and Practice of Sex Therapy*, 3rd edn. The Guilford Press, New York, pp. 154–180.

Bitran, D. and Hull, E.M., 1987. Pharmacological analysis of male rat sexual behaviour. *Neuroscience and Biobehavioral Reviews*, **11**, 365–389.

Blair, C.D. and Lanyon, R.I., 1981. Exhibitionism: aetiology and treatment. *Psychological Bulletin*, **89**(3), 439–463.

Blanchard, R., Watson, M.S., Choy, A., Dickey, R., Klassen, P., Kuban, M. and Ferren, D.J., 1999. Pedophiles: mental retardation, maternal age, and sexual orientation. *Archives of Sexual Behaviour*, **28**(2), 111–127.

Blanchard, R., Zucker, K.J., Bradley, S.J. and Hume, C.S., 1995. Birth order and sibling sex ratio in homosexual male adolescents and probably prehomosexual feminine boys. *Developmental Psychology*, **31**, 22–30.

Blanchard, R., Zucker, K.J., Siegelman, M., Dickey, R. and Klassen, P., 1998. The relation of birth order to sexual orientation in men and women. *Journal of Biosocial Science*, **30**(4), 511–519.

Bowers, M.B., Woert, M.V. and Davis, L., 1971. Sexual behaviour during L-dopa treatment for parkinsonism. *American Journal of Psychiatry*, **127**, 1691–1693.

Bradford, J.M.W., 2000. The treatment of sexual deviation using a pharmacological approach. *The Journal of Sex Research*, **37**(3), 248–257.

Breslow, N., Evans, L. and Langley, J., 1985. On the prevalence and roles of females in the sadomasochistic subculture: report of an empirical study. *Archives of Sexual Behaviour*, **14**(4), 303–317.

Burnett, A.L., 1995. Role of nitric oxide in the physiology of erection. *Biological Reproduction*, **52**, 485–489.

Carmichael, M.S., Warburton, V.L., Dixen, J. and Davidson, J.M., 1994. Relationships among cardiovascular, muscular, and oxytocin responses during human sexual activity. *Archives of Sexual Behaviour*, **23**, 59–77.

Clark, J.T., Stefanick, M.L., Smith, E.R. and Davidson, J.M., 1983. Further studies on alterations in male rat copulatory behaviour induced by the dopamine-receptor agonists RDS-127. *Pharmacology, Biochemistry, & Behaviour*, **19**, 781–786.

Cohen-Kettenis, P.T. and Gooren, L.J.G., 1999. Transsexualism: a review of aetiology, diagnosis, and treatment. *Journal of Psychosomatic Research*, **46**(4), 315–333.

Colpi, G.M., Fanciullacci, F., Beretta, G., Negri, L. and Zanollo, A., 1986. Evoked sacral potentials in subjects with true premature ejaculation. *Andrologia*, **18**(6), 583–586.

Cooper, A.J., Cernovsky, Z.Z. and Colussi, K., 1993. Some clinical and psychometric characteristics of primary and secondary premature ejaculators. *Journal of Sex & Marital Therapy*, **19**(4), 276–288.

Cooper, A.J. and Magnus, R.V., 1984. A clinical trial of the beta blocker Propranolol in premature ejaculation. *Psychosomatic Research*, **28**, 331–336.

Cooper, A.J., Swaminath, S., Baxter, D. and Poulin, C., 1990. A female sex offender with multiple paraphilias: a psychologic, physiologic (laboratory sexual arousal) and endocrine case study. *Canadian Journal of Psychiatry*, **35**, 334–337.

Dekker, J., 1993. Inhibited male orgasm. In: O'Donohue, W. and Geer, J.H. (eds), *Handbook of Sexual Dysfunctions: Assessment and Treatment*. Allyn and Bacon, Boston, pp. 279–302.

Deutsch, S. and Sherman, L., 1979. Hypoprolactaemia in men with secondary sexual impotence and men with premature ejaculation [abstract]. In: *Endocrinology Society Meeting Abstracts*, Endocrinology Society, New York.

Doctor, R.F. and Prince, V., 1997. Transvestism: a survey of 1032 cross-dressers. *Archives of Sexual Behaviour*, **26**(6), 589–605.

Eison, A.S., Eison, M.S., Torrente, J.R., Wright, R.N. and Yocca, F.D., 1990. Nefazodone: preclinical pharmacology of a new antidepressant. *Psychopharmacology Bulletin*, **26**, 311–315.

Exton, M.S., Bindert, A., Kruger, T., Scheller, F., Hartmann, U. and Schedlowski, M., 1999. Cardiovascular and endocrine alterations after masturbation-induced orgasm in women. *Psychosomatic Medicine*, **61**, 280–289.

Fanciullacci, F., Colpi, G.M., Beretta, G. and Zanollo, A., 1988. Cortical evoked potentials in subjects with true premature ejaculation. *Andrologia*, **20**(4), 326–330.

Feiger, A., Kiev, A., Shrivastava, R.K., Wisselink, P.G. and Wilcox, C.S., 1996. Nefazodone versus sertraline in outpatients with major depression: focus on efficacy, tolerability, and effects on sexual function and satisfaction. *Journal of Clinical Psychology*, **57**(suppl 2), 53–62.

Freund, K. and Kuban, M., 1994. The basis of the abused abuser theory of pedophilia: a further elaboration on an earlier study. *Archives of Sexual Behaviour*, **23**(5), 553–563.

Freund, K., Scher, H. and Hucker, S., 1983. The courtship disorders. *Archives of Sexual Behaviour*, **12**(5), 369–379.

Freund, K., Watson, R. and Dickey, D., 1990. Does sexual abuse in childhood cause pedophilia: an exploratory study. *Archives of Sexual Behaviour*, **19**(6), 557–568.

Freund, K., Watson, R., Dickey, R. and Douglas, R., 1991. Erotic gender differentiation in pedophilia. *Archives of Sexual Behaviour*, **20**(6), 555–566.

Freund, K. and Watson, R., 1990. Mapping the boundaries of courtship disorder. *Journal of Sex Research*, **27**(4), 589–606.

Friday, N., 1975. *Forbidden Flowers: More Women's Sexual Fantasies*. Simon and Schuster, New York.

Frohlich, P.F. and Meston, C.M., 2000. Evidence that serotonin affects female sexual functioning via peripheral mechanisms. *Physiology & Behaviour*, **71**, 383–393.

Frohlich, P.F. and Meston, C.M., 1999. Tactile sensitivity in women with arousal difficulties. Paper presented at the Boston University School of Medicine and the Department of Urology Conference: New Perspectives in the Management of Female Sexual Dysfunction, Boston, MA.

Geberth, V.J. and Turco, R.N., 1997. Antisocial personality disorder, sexual sadism, malignant narcissism, and serial murder. *Journal of Forensic Science*, **42**(1), 49–60.

Gold, S.R. and Gold, R.G., 1993. Sexual aversions: a hidden disorder. In: O'Donohue, W. and Geer, J.H. (eds), *Handbook of Sexual Dysfunctions: Assessment and Treatment*. Allyn and Bacon, Boston, 83–102.

Green, R., 1987. *The 'Sissy Boy Syndrome' and the Development of Homosexuality*. Yale University Press, New Haven.

Heiman, J.R. and Meston, C.M., 1998. Empirically validated treatments for sexual dysfunction. In: Dobson, K.S. and Craig, K.D. (eds), *Empirically Supported Therapies: Best Practice in Professional Psychology*. Sage Publications, New York, 259–303.

Kafka, M.P., 1997. A monoamine hypothesis for the pathophysiology of paraphilic disorders. *Archives of Sexual Behaviour*, **26**(4), 343–358.

Kaplan, H., 1974. *The New Sex Therapy*. Bailliere Tindall, London.

Kilman, P.R., Sabalis, R.F., Gearing, M.L., Bukstel, L.H. and Scovern, A.W., 1982. The treatment of sexual paraphilias: a review of the outcome research. *The Journal of Sex Research*, **18**(3), 193–252.

Kloner, R.A., 2000. Sex and patients with cardiovascular risk factors: focus on sildenafil. *American Journal of Medicine*, **18**(109), 13s–21s.

Kruger, T., Exton, M.S., Pawlak, C., von zur Muhlen, A., Hartman, U. and Schedlowski, M., 1998. Neuroendocrine and cardiovascular response to sexual arousal and orgasm in men. *Psychoneuroendocrinology*, **23**, 401–411.

Laan, E., Everaerd, W., Van Aanhold, M.T. and Rebel, M., 1993. Performance demand and sexual arousal in women. *Behaviour Research & Therapy*, **31**(1), 25–35.

Langevin, R., Bain, J., Wortzman, G., Hucker, S., Dickey, R. and Wright, P., 1988. Sexual sadism: brain, blood, and behaviour. *Annals of the New York Academy of Sciences*, **528**, 163–182.

Langevin, R., Paitich, D. and Russon, A.E., 1985. Voyeurism: does it predict sexual aggression or violence in general? In: Langevin, R. (ed), *Erotic Preference, Gender Identity and Aggression in Men*. Lawrence Erlbaum Associates, Hillsdale, NJ.

Laumann, E.O., Gagnon, J.H., Michael, R.T. and Michaels, S., 1994. *The Social Organization of Sexuality: Sexual Practices in the United States*. University of Chicago Press, Chicago.

Laumann, E.O., Paik, A. and Rosen, R.C., 1999. Sexual dysfunction in the United States: prevalence and predictors. *Journal of the American Medical Association*, **281**, 537–544.

Letourneau, E.J. and O'Donohue, W., 1997. Classical conditioning of female sexual arousal. *Archives of Sexual Behaviour*, **26**(1), 63–78.

LoPiccolo, J. and Friedman, J.M., 1988. Broad-spectrum treatment of low sexual desire: integration of cognitive, behavioural, and systemic therapy. In: Leiblum, S.R. and Rosen, R.C. (eds), *Sexual Desire Disorders*. Guilford Press, New York, 107–144.

Lundberg, P.O. and Hulter, B., 1996. Female sexual dysfunction in multiple sclerosis: a review. *Sexuality & Disability*, **14**(1), 65–72.

Maes, M., West, D.van, De Vos, N., Westenberg, H., Van Hunsel, F., Hendriks, D., Cosyns, P. and Scharpe, S., 2001. Lower baseline plasma cortisol and prolactin together with increased body temperature and higher mCPP-induced cortisol responses in men with pedophilia. *Neuropsychopharmacology*, **24**(1), 37–46.

Masters, W. and Johnson, V., 1970. *Human Sexual Inadequacy*. Little, Brown, Boston.

McKenna, K., 1999. The brain is the master organ in sexual function: central nervous system control of male and female sexual function. *International Journal of Impotence Research*, **11**(1), s48–s55.

Meana, M. and Binik, Y.M., 1994. Painful coitus: a review of female dyspareunia. *The Journal of Nervous and Mental Disease*, **182**(5), 264–272.

Meana, M., Binik, Y.M., Khalife, S. and Cohen, D., 1999. Psychosocial correlates of pain attributions in women with dyspareunia. *Psychosomatics*, **40**, 497–502.

Meston, C.M. and Frohlich, P.F., 2000. The neurobiology of sexual function. *Archives of General Psychiatry*, **57**, 1012–1030.

Meston, C.M. and Gorzalka, B.B., 1995a. The effects of sympathetic activation on physiological and subjective sexual arousal in women. *Behaviour Research and Therapy*, **33**(6), 651–664.

Meston, C.M. and Gorzalka, B.B., 1995b. The effects of immediate, delayed, and residual sympathetic activation on sexual arousal in women. *Behaviour Research and Therapy*, **34**(2), 143–148.

Meston, C.M. and Gorzalka, B.B., 1996. Differential effects of sympathetic activation on sexual arousal in sexually dysfunctional and functional women. *Journal of Abnormal Psychology*, **105**(4), 582–591.

Meston, C.M., Gorzalka, B.B. and Wright, J.M., 1997. Inhibition of subjective and physiological sexual arousal in women by clonidine. *Psychosomatic Medicine*, **59**, 399–407.

Meston, C.M. and Heiman, J.R., 1998. Ephedrine-activated physiological sexual arousal in women. *Archives of General Psychiatry*, **55**(7), 652–656.

Meston, C.M. and Rachman, J.S., 1994. Conditioning sexual arousal in women. *Unpublished data*.

Metz, M.E. and Pryor, M.L., 2000. Premature ejaculation: a psychophysiological approach for assessment and management. *Journal of Sex & Marital Therapy*, **26**, 293–320.

Meuwissen, I. and Over, R., 1992. Sexual arousal across phases of the human menstrual cycle. *Archives of Sexual Behaviour*, **21**(2), 101–119.

Miller, N.S. and Gold, M.S., 1988. The human sexual response and alcohol and drugs. *Journal of Substance Abuse*, **5**, 171–177.

Montorsi, F., McDermott, T.E., Morgan, R., Olsson, A., Schultz, A., Kirkeby, H.J. and Osterloh, I.H., 1999. Efficacy in safety of fixed-dose oral Sildenafil in the treatment of erectile dysfunction of various aetiologies. *Urology*, **53**, 1011–1018.

Morokoff, P., 1993. Female sexual arousal disorder. In: O'Donohue, W. and Geer, J.H. (eds), *Handbook of Sexual Dysfunctions: Assessment and Treatment*. Allyn and Bacon, Boston, 157–200.

Palace, E.M., 1995. Modification of dysfunctional patterns of sexual response through autonomic arousal and false physiological feedback. *Journal of Consulting & Clinical Psychology*, **63**(4), 604–615.

Pridal, C.G. and LoPiccolo, J., 2000. Multielement treatment of desire disorders. In: Leiblum, S.R. and Rosen, R.C. (eds), *Principles and Practice of Sex Therapy*, 3rd edition, The Guildford Press, New York, 57–81.

Pukall, C.F., Reissing, E.D., Binik, Y.M., Khalife, S. and Abbott, F.V., 2000. New clinical and research perspectives on the sexual pain disorders. *Journal of Sex Education and Therapy*, **25**(1), 36–44.

Rachman, S. and Hodgson, R.J., 1968. Experimentally-induced 'sexual fetishism' replication and development. *Psychological Record*, **18**, 25–27.

Reissing, E.D., Binik, Y.M. and Khalife, S., 1999. Does vaginismus exist? A critical review of the literature. *The Journal of Nervous and Mental Disease*, **187**(5), 261–274.

Rooth, G., 1973. Exhibitionism, sexual violence and paedophilia. *British Journal of Psychiatry*, **122**, 705–710.

Rowland, D.L. and Burnett, A.L., 2000. Pharmacotherapy in the treatment of male sexual dysfunction. *The Journal of Sex Research*, **37**(3), 226–243.

Sadeghi, M. and Fakhrai, A., 2000. Transsexualism in female monozygotic twins: a case report. *Australian & New Zealand Journal of Psychiatry*, **34**(5), 862–864.

Saenz de Tejada, I., Blanco, R., Goldstein, I., Azadzoi, K., de las Morenas, A., Krane, R.J. and Cohen, R.A., 1988. Cholinergic neurotransmission in human corpus cavernosum, I: responses of isolated tissue. *American Journal of Physiology*, **254**, H459–H467.

Sandnabba, N.K., Santtila, P. and Nordling, N., 1999. Sexual behaviour and social adaptation among sadomasochistically-oriented males. *The Journal of Sex Research*, **36**(3), 273–282.

Sarrel, P.M. and Masters, W.H., 1982. Sexual molestation of men by women. *Archives of Sexual Behaviour*, **11**(2), 117–131.

Schover, L.R., Friedman, J.M., Weiler, S.J., Heiman, J.R. and LoPiccolo, J., 1982. Multiaxial problem-oriented system for sexual dysfunction. *Archives of General Psychiatry*, **39**, 614–619.

Semens, J., 1956. Premature ejaculation. *Southern Medical Journal*, **49**, 352–358.

Seto, M.C. and Kuban, M., 1996. Criterion-related validity of a phallometric test for paraphilic rape and sadism. *Behaviour Research and Therapy*, **34**(2), 175–183.

Sherwin, B.B., 1991. The psychoendocrinology of aging and female sexuality. *Annual Review of Sex Research*, **2**, 181–198.

Silverstein, J.L., 1989. Origins of psychogenic vaginismus. *Psychotherapy & Psychosomatics*, **52**(4), 197–204.

Smith, R.S., 1976. Voyeurism: a review of the literature. *Archives of Sexual Behaviour*, **5**(6), 585–608.

Spector, I. and Carey, M.P., 1990. Incidence and prevalence of the sexual dysfunctions: a critical review of the empirical literature. *Archives of Sexual Behaviour*, **19**(4), 389–408.

Spengler, A., 1977. Manifest sadomasochism of males: results of an empirical study. *Archives of Sexual Behaviour*, **6**(6), 441–456.

Spiess, W.F.J., Geer, J.H. and O'Donohue, W.T., 1984. Premature ejaculation: investigation of factors in ejaculatory latency. *Journal of Abnormal Psychology*, **93**, 242–245.

Stock, W., 1993. Inhibited female orgasm. In: O'Donohue, W. and Geer, J.H. (eds), *Handbook of Sexual Dysfunction: Assessment and Treatment*, Allyn and Bacon, Boston, 253–277.

Strassberg, D.S., Mohoney, J.M., Schaugaard, M. and Hale, V.E., 1990. The role of anxiety in premature ejaculation: a psychophysiological model. *Archives of Sexual Behaviour*, **19**(3), 251–257.

Tiihonen, J., Kuikka, J., Kupila, J., Partanen, K., Vainio, P., Airaksinen, J., Eronen, M., Hallikainen, T., Paanila, J. and Kinnunen, I., 1994. Increase in cerebral blood flow of right prefrontal cortex in man during orgasm. *Neuroscience Letters*, **170**(2), 241–243.

Tugrul, C. and Kabakci, E., 1997. Vaginismus and its correlates. *Sexual and Marital Therapy*, **12**(1), 23–34.

Uitti, R.J., Tanner, C.M., Rajput, A.H., Goetz, C.G., Klawans, H.L. and Thiessen, B., 1989. Hypersexuality with antiparkinsonian therapy. *Clinical Neuropharmacology*, **12**, 375–383.

van der Velde, J. and Everaerd, W., 1996. Voluntary control over pelvic floor muscles in women with and without vaginismus. Paper presented at the Annual Meeting of the International Academy of Sex Research, Rotterdam, Netherlands, June.

Weinberg, M.S., Williams, C.J. and Moser, C., 1984. The social constituents of sadomasochism. *Social Problems*, **31**(4), 379–389.

Westrom, L.V. and Willen, R., 1998. Vestibular nerve fibre proliferation in vulvar vestibulitis syndrome. *Obstetrics and Gynaecology*, **91**, 572–576.

Wiedeking, C., Ziegler, M.G. and Lake, C.R., 1979. Plasma noradrenaline and dopamine-beta-hydroxylase during human sexual activity. *Journal of Psychiatric Research*, **15**, 139–145.

Wise, T.N., 1985. Fetishism — aetiology and treatment: a review from multiple perspectives. *Comprehensive Psychiatry*, **26**(3), 249–257.

Yang, C.C. and Bradley, W.E., 1999. Somatic innervation of the human bulbocavernosus muscle. *Clinical Neurophysiology*, **110**(3), 412–418.

Zhou, J., Horman, M.A., Gooren, L.J. and Swaab, D.F., 1995. A sex difference in the human brain and its relation to transsexuality. *Nature*, **378**, 68–70.

Zucker, K.J. and Blanchard, R., 1997. Transvestic fetishism: psychopathology and theory. In: Laws, D.R. and O'Donohue, W. (eds), *Sexual Deviance: Theory, Assessment, and Treatment*. The Guildford Press, New York, 131–151.

Zucker, K.J. and Green, R., 1992. Psychosexual disorders in children and adolescents. *Journal of Child Psychology & Psychiatry & Allied Disciplines*, **33**(1), 107–151.

Zucker, K.J., Green, R., Coates, S., Zuger, B., Cohen-Kettenis, P.T., Zecca, G.M., Lertora, V., Money, J., Hahn-Burke, S., Bradley, S.J. and Blanchard, R., 1997. Sibling sex ratio of boys with gender identity disorder. *Journal of Child Psychology and Psychiatry*, **38**, 543–551.

Zucker, K.J., Lightbody, S., Pecore, K., Bradley, S.J. and Blanchard, R., 1998. Birth order in girls with gender identity disorder. *European Child & Adolescent Psychiatry*, **7**, 30–35.

XXIII

Eating Disorders

XXIII-1

Animal Models of Eating Disorders

Jeanette E. Johansen and Martin Schalling

INTRODUCTION

Eating disorders such as obesity, anorexia and bulimia are complex disorders displaying a variety of symptoms apart from an abnormal eating behaviour. Like many other motivated behaviours, feeding requires the integration of internal and external signals and it is not clear if the physiological correlates observed in these disorders are causes or effects of the altered eating behaviour. A good understanding of the physiology underlying feeding behaviour is therefore essential. This chapter deals with some of the many animal models that are being used to study feeding behaviour.

Early animal models of eating disorders include experimental studies of the effect of anorectic drugs on the amount of food consumed by rats. However, while successful in rats, pharmacological treatment of obesity is generally unimpressive in terms of weight loss in humans for a number of reasons.

That tumours in the region of the hypothalamus can cause obesity has been known for a long time. In 1940, Hetherington and Ranson confirmed the importance of the hypothalamus in the control of feeding and body weight. By performing electrolytic lesions in the hypothalamus of rats, they observed: 'A condition of marked adiposity characterized by as much as a doubling of body weight and a tremendous increase of extractable body lipids...' (Hetherington and Ranson, 1940). The damaged regions included the dorsomedial and ventromedial hypothalamic nuclei (DMH and VMH), the arcuate nucleus (Arc), the fornix, the lateral hypothalamic area (LHA) ventral to the fornix and possibly also the ventral premammillary nucleus. They also noted that lesions in the adjacent lateral hypothalamus could lead to decreased food intake. Anand and Brobeck pursued this observation and showed that bilateral electrolytic lesions of the LHA caused loss of feeding and even death by starvation (Anand and Brobeck, 1951). Thus, the concept arose of the LHA serving as a 'feeding centre' and the VMH as a 'satiety centre'—the dual centre model. This hypothesis has been widely questioned, and among the observations speaking against the dual centre model are findings that damage outside the hypothalamus can produce syndromes similar to those seen after lesions of the LHA or VMH. As cell-specific lesion methods emerged the focus was once again put on the VMH and LHA, and several studies showed that the LHA indeed could have a phagic function (Saper, 1985; Saper *et al.*, 1986; Bittencourt, 1992). Today we know that hypothalamic cell populations and nuclei play important and specific roles in the regulation of food intake and other motivated behaviours.

Most of the population practices weight control, but in spite of that, weight seems to be stable in both lean and obese individuals. Dieting is usually not successful in the long run and most obese individuals eventually regain the lost weight (Wadden, 1993). The relative stability of weight in individuals indicates that there is a feedback loop controlling energy balance and maintaining constancy of total body energy stores. In 1953, Kennedy introduced his theory on a lipostatic mechanism that maintained energy homeostasis (Kennedy, 1953). He suggested that the size of the fat depots were sensed by a lipostat, which would regulate and adjust food intake and energy metabolism accordingly, to maintain body weight at a set point. He also proposed that an impaired lipostatic mechanism could lead to obesity. Further support for this hypothesis came from a study by Hervey (1958). He performed a series of parabiosis experiments, where the circulations of two animals are surgically joined, and showed that lesions in the VMH in one of the members in a parabiotic rat pair caused the lesioned rat to become obese as the unlesioned rat starved to death (Hervey, 1958). He suggested that the obese lesioned rat produced excessive amounts of a satiety factor that was transferred to the unlesioned rat, causing it to starve itself.

Over the past five years there has been a tremendous increase in the understanding of the genetic regulation of food intake and energy expenditure, using monogenic rodent models of obesity. Several genes have been cloned that, when mutated, cause obesity in the mouse and rat (Schalling *et al.*, 1999; Barsh *et al.*, 2000). These genes and their products have unravelled biochemical pathways involved in obesity. Some of these genes have been shown to be important for the regulation of food intake and/or metabolism also in humans. Crosses of mouse, rat, pig or chicken strains that are informative with regard to body mass or body fat have produced a number of quantitative trait loci (QTL) (Chagnon *et al.*, 2000) that have opened the door to polygenic approaches in the study of obesity in animals. As with the monogenic rodent models, these QTLs can be applied to a human genetic obesity map by identifying the syntenic chromosomal regions in the human.

There has been less of a focus on genetic models of anorexia. One reason might be that there are more genetic animal models that shift the regulation of food intake, satiety or metabolic turnover towards obesity than anorexia. A possible explanation for this could be that even a relatively mild anorectic phenotype could lead to malnutrition and/or death by starvation early enough in life to affect the number and viability of the offspring (see the anorexia mouse, the dopamine-deficient mouse and the HNF-3α deficient mouse below). A number of starvation, dehydration and chemically induced models have been developed and an example of each is discussed below. There are also numerous models of anorexia induced by either infection or cancer. Anorexia, or cachexia, is a frequent complication of malignant tumours and infectious and inflammatory diseases and is contributing significantly to the mortality of these disorders (Kotler *et al.*, 1985; Tisdale, 1997; Larkin, 1998). This type of anorexia will not be dealt with in this chapter.

There are very few animal models of bulimia or binge eating. The models that exist are all based on cycles of food restriction

Biological Psychiatry: Edited by H. D'haenen, J.A. den Boer and P. Willner. ISBN 0-471-49198-5

and refeeding. The lack of animal models for bulimia and binge eating may be related to the opinion of many investigators that an animal model should mimic all the important aspects of human syndromes.

Because of the enormous toll on human health taken by eating disorders and their related disorders, there is a need for a better understanding of the underlying mechanisms for regulation of body weight and food intake. This chapter attempts to review some of the available animal models for studying eating disorders and the mechanisms behind the control of food intake. Because of the considerable uncertainty regarding the biological basis of eating disorders in humans, and the possibility that they are symptoms of personality traits, the development of animal models is complicated. Furthermore, for the same reasons validation of existing animal models of eating disorders is compromised. For face validity animal models of eating disorders should involve a change in body weight. However, there are many possible reasons why an animal lose or gain weight without having an altered eating behaviour. Therefore, measures of food intake are also required. One should also keep in mind that reduced or increased food intake is not necessarily the result of a change in appetite. Moreover, eating disorders in humans often occur under conditions where food is freely available and therefore it may be inappropriate to use models with restricted access to food as is often the case in pharmacological studies of rat feeding behaviour. Lack of potent pharmacological agents for treatment of human eating disorders make it difficult to assess predictive validity for animal models. Despite substantial research efforts, the nature of the underlying behavioural mechanisms for eating disorders remains unclear. Construct validity is therefore extremely hard to determine. A better description of the molecular mechanisms involved in human eating disorders would be invaluable to the animal modeller and paradoxically this valuable information may be gained from the study of animal models. Even though the animal models described in this chapter may not mimic all of the aspects of human eating disorders they may provide useful information on underlying causes and how to treat at least some of the symptoms. In fact, several animal models have been used as hypothesis generators and in some cases they have been most helpful in revealing the nature of specific human eating disorders.

A brief description of three genetic and three physiological models of anorexia, and one model of bulimia will be followed by a more comprehensive review of genetic models of obesity.

MODELS OF ANOREXIA

Genetic Models of Anorexia

The Anorexia Mouse

The autosomal recessive *anx* mutation arose at the Jackson laboratory (Bar Harbor, ME, USA) in 1976. Mutant mice (*anx/anx*) are characterized by poor appetite. Stomach contents are reduced compared to normal littermates at about post-natal day 5 and continue so until death (Maltais *et al.*, 1984). Interestingly, although the amount of food ingested is reduced, the daily pattern of food intake of *anx/anx* mice is very similar to that observed in normal littermates from birth to 20 days of age (Maltais *et al.*, 1984). These data indicate that *anx/anx* mice fail to properly regulate the amount of food consumed rather than failing to eat for other reasons. Other characteristics are reduced body weight, emaciated appearance and abnormal behaviour including body tremors, headweaving, hyperactivity and uncoordinated gait. The animals die at the age of 3 to 5 weeks depending on the genetic background. No organ abnormalities have been found using routine stained sections. Total RBC, hematocrits, haemoglobin and mean cell volume are within normal range (Maltais *et al.*, 1984). However, there are several dramatic alterations of peptide distributions in the hypothalamus of *anx/anx* mice, relevant to the regulation of feeding (Broberger *et al.*, 1997, 1998, 1999; Johansen *et al.*, 2000).

Abnormalities of feeding-related peptides have been described in the *anx/anx* mouse, particularly in the arcuate nucleus of the hypothalamus, which contains neuronal populations producing orexigenic as well as anorexigenic substances. The feeding stimulatory peptides neuropeptide Y (NPY) and agouti gene-related protein (AGRP) are distributed in a pattern suggestive of accumulation in the cell bodies in the arcuate nucleus of *anx/anx* mice instead of axonal transportation to their respective targets (Broberger *et al.*, 1997, 1998). Conversely, the pro-opiomelanocortin (POMC) derived peptides and cocaine- and amphetamine-regulated transcript (CART) peptides, which decrease food intake (Fan *et al.*, 1997; Kristensen *et al.*, 1998), are both decreased in the arcuate nucleus of the *anx/anx* mouse (Broberger *et al.*, 1999; Johansen *et al.*, 2000). In addition, morphological characteristics of POMC neurons are altered, as seen with immunohistochemical markers (Broberger *et al.*, 1999). Taken together these studies suggest that the reduced food intake and weight loss seen in the *anx/anx* mouse may be related to neurochemical alterations in the hypothalamus and particularly in the arcuate nucleus.

The abnormal behaviour of head weaving, body tremors, uncoordinated gait and hyperactivity of *anx/anx* mice is affected by serotonin (Maltais *et al.*, 1984). When treated with the serotonin precursor 5-hydroxy-DL-tryptophan (5-HTP) 15-day-old normal mice display the same type of abnormal behaviour as *anx/anx* mice. Similarly, 15-day-old anorexic mice show body tremors and head weaving typical for anorexic mice 18 days of age or older, when treated with 5-HTP. Conversely, treating a 20-day-old anorexic mouse with the serotonin neurotoxin 5,7-dihydroxytryptamine, diminishes the severity of the neurological symptoms (Maltais *et al.*, 1984). *anx/anx* mice have also been shown to have an increased number and density of serotonergic fibres in the forebrain and the arcuate nucleus (Son *et al.*, 1994; Jahng *et al.*, 1998), which would be consistent with the experimental data on eating and motor behaviour.

Taken together these results suggest that the abnormal feeding behaviour observed in *anx/anx* mice is caused by a CNS defect.

The Dopamine Deficient Mouse

Dopamine (DA) is a classical neurotransmitter in the central nervous system (CNS) that has been implicated in the regulation of food intake, but the neural pathways are not yet established. Some pharmacological reports suggest a stimulatory role for DA agonists, and an inhibiting role for DA antagonists in the control of food intake (Phillips and Nikaido, 1978; Dourish, 1983; Salamone *et al.*, 1990). However, opposite results have been obtained in other studies (Sanghvi *et al.*, 1975; Cooper and Al-Nasar, 1993).

Dopamine (DA) deficient mice (*DA-/-*) were created by disruption of the dopamine synthesizing enzyme tyrosine hydroxylase (TH) gene specifically in dopaminergic neurons (Zhou and Palmiter, 1995). *DA-/-* mice are born normal but gradually become hypoactive and aphagic and die prematurely at about three weeks of age (Zhou and Palmiter, 1995; Szczypka *et al.*, 1999). When *DA-/-* mice are born, they initiate suckling behaviours and nurse, however, after approximately 2 weeks, when normal mice begin to explore other sources of food, the *DA-/-* mice become lethargic and fail to eat and drink. Daily treatment with L-DOPA normalizes feeding behaviour and restores locomotor activity in *DA-/-* mice (Szczypka *et al.*, 1999). It is unlikely that the aphagia is secondary to motor deficits as *DA-/-* mice can grasp and swallow food when put in their mouth (Zhou and Palmiter, 1995). Also, *DA-/-* mice can execute behaviours necessary to seek and ingest food (Szczypka *et al.*, 1999). The *DA-/-* mice provide further evidence for the importance of dopamine for normal feeding behaviour.

That dopamine plays an important role in the regulation of food intake is a conclusion that was reached many years ago by several investigators. Studies by Anand and Brobeck (1951) showed that bilateral electrolytic lesions of the LHA in rats produced aphagia and akinesia. Evidence that DA could be a critical player in the LHA-lesion syndrome came from the demonstration that most of the symptoms of LHA ablation could be reproduced by introducing bilateral lesion of midbrain dopaminergic pathways in rats by the use of 6-hydroxydopamine (6-OHDA) (Ungerstedt, 1971; Zigmond and Stricker, 1972; Fibiger *et al.*, 1973). Furthermore, multiple connections between LHA and midbrain DA neurons have been identified (Bunney and Aghajanian, 1976; Phillipson, 1979; Wright *et al.*, 1980). It is remarkable that the phenotypes resulting from 6-OHDA and LHA lesions are so similar to the genetic model described here, given that the damage produced by a lesion greatly exceeds that resulting from the removal of one enzyme.

The Hepatocyte Nuclear Factor 3α-Deficient Mouse

The hepatocyte nuclear factor 3 (HNF-3) family of transcription factors include three different genes designated HNF-3α, HNF-3β and HNF-3γ, which have been suggested to play a critical role in pancreatic islet function (Duncan *et al.*, 1998). HNF-3α has been shown to be of importance for pancreatic alpha-cell function, including glucagon gene expression (Kaestner *et al.*, 1999). Mice lacking HNF-3α expression, due to targetted disruption of this gene, develop a complex metabolic syndrome characterized by abnormal feeding behaviour, progressive starvation, hypoglycaemia, wasting and neonatal mortality between days 2 and 14 (Shih *et al.*, 1999). The molecular and physiological mechanisms by which HNF-3α regulates food intake are currently not understood. However, HNF-3α is highly expressed in the hypothalamus (Shih *et al.*, 1999). Thus, it cannot be ruled out that the abnormal feeding behaviour observed in HNF-3α deficient mice is caused by a CNS defect.

Conclusion

There is increasing evidence suggesting that anorexia nervosa is genetic in nature (see Chapter XXIII-9: 'The evolving genetic foundations of eating disorders' by Klump *et al.*). The genetic mouse models described here probably have their strength in being hypothesis generators more than being models mimicking the human situation. The diagnostic criteria for anorexia nervosa are body weight <85% of expected weight, amenorrhea, intense fear of weight gain and inaccurate perception of own body size, weight or shape (DSM-IV, 1994). The latter two criteria are impossible to measure in animals, resulting in a low face validity for any model of anorexia. In the three models described above the face validity will be even lower as they all die prematurely before reaching puberty and amenorrhea can thus not be detected. Furthermore, the low food intake observed in the described models, is most likely caused by a reduced appetite for food. This is not the case in the human situation where the reduced food intake seems to be driven by an intense fear of weight gaining. Thus, construct validity also scores low in these models. Nevertheless, these models have their strength in allowing the identification of novel pathways involved in regulation of food intake. Genes in these pathways could certainly serve as targets for future therapeutic interventions.

Physiological Models of Anorexia

Starvation Induced Hyperactivity in Rat

If young rats are restricted to 90 minutes access to food every day, they will adapt and eat sufficient amounts to survive in good health. However, if a running wheel is available and food is restricted, the rats will start to run (Epling *et al.*, 1983). The running distance increases rapidly day by day and at the same time food consumption decreases and the rats begin to lose weight. Running may exceed 15 000 m per day, while food consumption decreases to 1 g per day or less (Epling *et al.*, 1983). In this model starvation and hyperactivity mutually reinforce each other resulting in a vicious circle where the rats starve and run themselves to death. There are major differences between male and female rats. Female rats develop running activity much faster and their activity is modulated by the menstrual cycle (Pirke *et al.*, 1993). Eventually, the menstrual cycle disappears in female rats. The reproductive function is impaired in both male and female rats, as a consequence of the starvation-induced hyperactivity (Pirke *et al.*, 1993).

It has been suggested that endogenous opioids play a role in this excessive activity (Boer *et al.*, 1990). However, data on central endorphin turnover and more detailed studies of endorphin agonists and antagonists are needed to clarify the role of opioids in this animal model. Leptin (an adipocyte derived satiety factor) has also been implicated to play a role in starvation-induced hyperactivity. Interestingly, it has been shown that leptin suppresses starvation induced hyperactivity in rats (Exner *et al.*, 2000). Also, patients with anorexia nervosa rank their motor restlessness higher when hypoleptinaemic, in the emaciated state, than after reaching maximal leptin levels, after treatment (Exner *et al.*, 2000). Thus, it is possible that hypoleptinaemia may contribute to the hyperactivity associated with anorexia nervosa. It should, however, be noted that it is not known whether the patients are restless because of the emaciation or the hypoleptinaemia.

This experimental protocol provides an animal model for the human activity anorexia syndrome (Epling *et al.*, 1983; Epling and Pierce, 1985). One should, however, keep in mind that the interpretation of the hyperactive behaviour seen in patients with anorexia nervosa has been discussed. Some argue that anorectics increase their activity for the purpose of burning more energy although this cannot explain their total weight loss, other investigators believe that the increased activity could be biological and involuntary. In 1994, Davis *et al.* showed that anorectic patients have an increased urge to be active during accelerated weight loss. This animal model, where starvation and hyperactivity mutually reinforce each other, supports the view that the increased activity is involuntary. However, there is no clear evidence for the applicability of this model in human anorexia nervosa.

Dehydration-Associated Anorexia

Dehydration is a homeostatic challenge resulting in a series of well-characterized endocrine, autonomic and behavioural motor responses. These are directed towards minimizing the impact of dehydration as rapidly as possible. Such responses are for example modifications of the ingestive behaviours so that water seeking behaviours increase and food seeking behaviours decrease (Hsaio, 1967). Thirst is the most obvious effect of dehydration, but when prolonged, dehydration also generates anorexia (Watts *et al.*, 1999). Dehydration can be induced by replacing the drinking water with 2.5% saline. By pair-feeding non-dehydrated rats with the same

Table XXIII-1.1 Animal models of anorexia

Model	Phenotype	Cause	Face validity	Construct validity
anx/anx mouse	Reduced food intake, gait disturbance, hyperactivity, premature death.	Recessive mutation in the *anx* gene.	++	++
DA-/- mouse	Aphagic, hypoactive, motor deficits, premature death.	Knockout of the TH-gene in dopaminergic neurons.	+	+
HNF3α-/- mouse	Progressive starvation, hypoglycaemia, neonatal mortality.	Knockout of the hepatocyte nuclear factor 3α.	++	−
Hyperactivity anorexia in rats	Increased activity and reduced food intake.	Starvation-induced hyperactivity.	+++	++
Dehydration-associated anorexia	Decreased food seeking behaviour.	Dehydration induced.	++	−
TCDD anorexia	Reduced food intake, wasting, permanent inhibition of weight gain.	Induced by TCDD.	++(+)	+

Lack of potent pharmacological agents makes it difficult to assess predictive validity for the models described. The genetic models of anorexia have their strength in allowing the identification of novel pathways involved in regulation of food intake serving as targets for future therapeutic interventions. Perhaps the most useful approach would be to combine the results from studies of genetic, physiological and biochemical models of anorexia, despite the weaknesses of each individual model. The 'Hyperactivity anorexia in rats' model has gained popularity as it mimics many aspects of human anorexia.

amount of food eaten by dehydrated rats and compare the neuronal and endocrine effects, one can distinguish between mechanisms causing anorectic behaviour from those occurring as a consequence of anorexia (Watts, 2000; Watts *et al.*, 1999).

This model is not applicable to human anorexia but may very well serve as a hypothesis generator and provide new insights in the complex regulation of food intake.

TCDD Induced Anorexia and Wasting Syndrome

The common environmental trace contaminant 2,3,7,8-tetrachlorodibenzo-*p*-dioxin (TCDD) is one of the most potent anorexigens known (Pohjanvirta *et al.*, 1994). TCDD causes a starvation-like or wasting syndrome with food intake refusal and consequent body weight loss (Pohjanvirta and Tuomisto, 1994; Unkila *et al.*, 1993). A sublethal dose can cause permanent inhibition of body weight gain and the new body weight gain is defended against external manipulations (Seefeld *et al.*, 1984; Pohjanvirta and Tuomisto, 1990). This is suggestive of a specific effect of TCCD on body weight regulatory systems. Despite extensive studies, the physiological mechanisms behind this wasting syndrome are unknown.

Humans suffering from anorexia will gain weight once they start eating again. Thus, this model has little validity as a model for anorexia. However, the regulation of a 'body weight set point' is unknown and this model may provide valuable information on the mechanisms behind this complex system.

Conclusions on Models of Anorexia

As mentioned several times already all the models above have their strength as hypothesis generators. Taken together these models may be very informative despite the weaknesses of each model individually. Perhaps the most useful approach at this point in time would be to combine the results from studies of genetic, physiological and biochemical models of anorexia. With such a comprehensive approach it may be possible to gain insight into many, but not all, aspects of reduced food intake as a disease. We have attempted to evaluate these models comparatively in Table XXIII-1.1.

MODELS OF BULIMIA AND BINGE EATING

Not many animal models of binge eating and/or bulimia have been described; the few existing models are all based on cycles of food restriction and refeeding. In the model described by Hagan and Moss (1997) rats were subjected to 12 restriction-refeeding cycles of 6–8 days during an 84-day period. One group of animals was cycled in a bulimic-like pattern with restriction followed by palatable refeeding and one group was cycled through a non-bulimic-like pattern. Postcycling eating behaviour was tested under conditions of hunger, satiety and availability of palatable food in both groups. Rats with a history of cycles of restriction followed by hyperphagia (bulimic-like feeding) continued to exhibit persistent binge-eating behaviour even after a 30-day period of normalization (full feeding, no restriction). This effect was shown particularly with access to palatable food in sated conditions. This model implicates restriction and overeating as biological determinants of binge-eating behaviours.

Restriction alone cannot account for bulimia. Not everyone who restricts becomes bulimic. However, restriction does seem to be a major factor in the development of binge eating, an important feature of bulimia. This model may provide clues to possible mechanisms involved in the genesis of a bulimic episode.

MODELS OF OBESITY

The Leptin System

Obese (*ob*) and diabetes (*db*) are two recessive mutations in mouse that lead to hyperphagia, decreased energy expenditure and morbid obesity (Coleman, 1978). Parabiosis experiments with lean (wild-type) mice and obese (*ob/ob*) mice suppressed weight gain in the *ob/ob* mice, while parabiosis of lean (wild-type) mice and obese (*db/db*) mice caused hypophagia and weight loss in the former (Hausberger, 1959; Coleman and Hummel, 1969; Coleman, 1973, 1978). These results were interpreted as meaning that the *ob* mutation disrupted a circulating satiety factor. In the parabiosis experiment the normal lean mouse would deliver the satiety factor to the *ob/ob* mouse with subsequent weightloss. Similarly, the *db* mutation was believed to disrupt a component required for the response to a satiety factor. Through lack of feedback inhibition the *db/db* mouse was thought to over-express the satiety factor that it could not respond to. Consequently, excess satiety factor would be delivered to the normal mouse (with a fully functioning response) leading to profound weightloss in the normal mouse in the parabiosis experiment between *db/db* and normal mouse.

The *ob* gene was positionally cloned and named leptin (*Lep*) (Zhang *et al.*, 1994). There are two mutations of the *Lep* gene in mouse, Lep^{ob} and Lep^{ob2J}. The Lep^{ob} mutation results in a premature stop codon and synthesis of a truncated protein incapable of being secreted (Zhang *et al.*, 1994; Rau *et al.*, 1999). In the Lep^{ob2J} homozygous mouse mutant, a transposon inserted into the first intron of the *Lep* gene prevents the synthesis of mature *Lep* mRNA (Zhang *et al.*, 1994). In addition to obesity, the *ob* mutations in mouse also cause hyperinsulinemia, hypoglycaemia, hypercorticism, hypothalamic hypogonadism and hypothermia (Charlton, 1984). Mutations in the human *Lep* gene are rare but there are a few cases reported (Montague *et al.*, 1997; Strobel *et al.*, 1998; Rau *et al.*, 1999). The human *ob* mutations cause hyperphagia, obesity and hypothalamic hypogonadism, but unlike the *ob/ob* mice, hyperinsulinemia, hypoglycaemia, hypercorticism and hypothermia have not been reported in leptin deficient humans. This implies that although there are many similarities in the regulatory pathways, there are also distinct differences no doubt relating to the development of regulatory systems during the evolution of the respective species. This selection process will have to be taken into account when validating leptin mutations and their role as models for obesity.

The *db* mutation phenotypically mimics the *ob* mutation and was proposed to be a mutation in an *ob* receptor gene (Coleman, 1978). The cloning of the *db* gene confirmed that *db* indeed was a mutation in the leptin receptor gene (*Lepr*) (Tartaglia *et al.*, 1995; Lee *et al.*, 1996). Similar mutations in the *Lepr* gene have been shown to underlie the obese phenotypes of the *fatty* Zucker rat and the *corpulent* Koletsky rat (Chua *et al.*, 1996; Takaya *et al.*, 1996). There are five alternatively spliced forms of the receptor, Ob–Ra, Ob–Rb, Ob–Rc, Ob–Rd and Ob–Re (Lee *et al.*, 1996). Ob–Rb (or Ob–RL) is the longest form and has a long cytoplasmic region containing several motifs required for signal transduction (Chen *et al.*, 1996; Lee *et al.*, 1996). The other forms lack some or all of these motifs and may function as transport proteins (Lee *et al.*, 1996) or act in a buffering system for free, circulating leptin. Ob–R mutations are extremely rare in humans. There is, however, one report on a family with three obese sisters with a mutation in the *Lepr* gene (Clement *et al.*, 1998).

The Melanocortin System

Pro-opiomelanocortin (POMC) is a neuropeptide precursor molecule that is cleaved post-translationally in the hypothalamus to yield multiple peptides including α-melanocyte-stimulating hormone (α-MSH) (Smith and Funder, 1988). Melanocortin peptides have been demonstrated to inhibit food intake and recent data suggest that they may play a role in energy expenditure as well (Fan *et al.*, 1997; Haynes *et al.*, 1999).

α-MSH is the principle agonist of the neuronal melanocortin receptor isoforms, MC-3R and MC-4R (Gantz *et al.*, 1993a, 1993b). Both isoforms influence body weight, but they act through distinct and complementary mechanisms. MC-4R knockout mice ($Mc4r^{-/-}$) eat excessively resulting in maturity onset obesity syndrome associated with hyperphagia, hyperinsulinemia and hypoglycaemia (Huszar *et al.*, 1997). MC-3R knockout mice ($Mc3r^{-/-}$) show an increased body fat mass at the expense of a decreased lean muscle mass (Chen *et al.*, 2000). This is not caused by increased food intake, instead $Mc3r^{-/-}$ mice gain more fat per calorie of food consumed (Chen *et al.*, 2000). Mice lacking both receptor isoforms are more obese than mice lacking just MC-3R or MC-4R, probably because the double mutants not only eat more but also store ingested calories more efficiently (Chen *et al.*, 2000). Mutations in the MC-4R have also been reported to be associated with dominantly inherited pediatric obesity and hyperphagia in humans (Vaisse *et al.*, 1998; Yeo *et al.*, 1998).

The agouti gene was the first obesity gene cloned (Bultman *et al.*, 1992; Miller *et al.*, 1993). There are five known dominant mutations in the agouti gene that result in obesity and yellow pigmentation in mice. Normally agouti mRNA is expressed exclusively in the skin of neonatal mice, but mice carrying a dominant yellow allele have a ubiquitous expression pattern (Michaud *et al.*, 1994). The agouti protein is an antagonist of MC-4R in the brain and blocking of the receptor leads to increased food intake (Lu *et al.*, 1994; Fan *et al.*, 1997). This discovery led to the cloning of an agouti homologous protein normally expressed in the brain, the agouti-related protein (AGRP) (Shutter *et al.*, 1997). AGRP was shown to be an endogenous antagonist of MC-3R and MC-4R and over-expression causes obesity in mice (Fong *et al.*, 1997; Graham *et al.*, 1997; Ollmann *et al.*, 1997). No mutations in the AGRP gene have been found in humans.

The Fat Mouse

The fat phenotype includes obesity that develops between 6 and 8 weeks of age, hypoglycaemia and hyperinsulinemia (Coleman and Eicher, 1990). The hypoglycaemia only occurs in males and is transient whereas the hyperinsulinemia is consistent throughout life and associated with hypertrophy and hyperplasia of the islets of Langerhans in the pancreas (Coleman and Eicher, 1990). The syndrome does not progress to diabetes. This phenotype is the result of a missense mutation in the carboxypeptidase E (*Cpe*) gene (Naggert *et al.*, 1995). CPE is a secretory granule enzyme involved in dibasic cleaving of proproteins and prohormones including intermediates derived from proinsulin and pro-opiomelanocortin (Naggert *et al.*, 1995). The fat mutation (Cpe^{fat})results in a loss of CPE activity and proinsulin processing is aberrant in fat mutants (Naggert *et al.*, 1995). No mutations in the human *Cpe* gene have been reported. However, a mutation in the endopeptidase, prohormone convertase 1 (*PC1*) have been found in a patient with extreme childhood obesity (Jackson *et al.*, 1997). *PC1* acts proximally to *Cpe* in the pathway of post-translational processing of prohormones and neuropeptides. Thus, it has been suggested that defects in prohormone conversion may represent a generic mechanism for obesity both in humans and rodents.

The Tubby Mouse

The recessive tubby mutation (*tub*) causes maturity-onset obesity, including insulin resistance, accompanied by retinal and cochlear degeneration (Coleman and Eicher, 1990; Ohlemiller *et al.*, 1995; Ohlemiller *et al.*, 1997). The obesity of *tub/tub* mice is relatively mild and late in onset, resembling the weight gain in human populations more closely than that observed in the *ob/ob* and *db/db* mice. Weight gain occurs slowly and *tub/tub* mice reach about twice the weight of unaffected siblings. Tubby mice are not sterile but as they develop obesity they become infertile.

The tubby gene was identified by positional cloning (Kleyn *et al.*, 1996; Noben-Trauth *et al.*, 1996). The tubby phenotype is caused by a point mutation in a donor splice site resulting in a substitution of 44 amino acids in the carboxyterminal part of the Tub protein with 24 different amino acids encoded by the unspliced intron (Kleyn *et al.*, 1996). The aberrant transcript is expressed at elevated levels in tubby mice but expression at the protein level has not been investigated. The expression pattern of *tub* mRNA appears to be specific for the nervous system (Kapeller *et al.*, 1999) but the biochemical function remains unclear. However, structure-based functional analysis suggests that Tub is a bipartite transcription factor (Boggon *et al.*, 1999). It has not been established whether all tubby phenotypes (obesity, insulin resistance and retinal and cochlear degeneration) are attributable to the *tub* gene. It has not been ruled out that some features of the phenotype could be caused by a tightly linked, but yet unidentified gene. No human examples of this mutation have been identified yet.

The Adult Mouse

The adult mutation (*Ad*) causes adult obesity and diabetes in a semidominant fashion (Wallace and MacSwiney, 1979). The obesity can be recognized at the age of 4 to 6 months and it is greater in homozygotes than in heterozygotes and it is more penetrant in heterozygote males than females (Wallace and MacSwiney, 1979). The mice are hyperinsulinemic but have normal blood glucose levels. The gene has not been identified and hence there are no known human examples of this mutation.

The 5-HT2CR Deficient Mouse

Serotonergic drugs are known to modulate appetite and serotonergic agonists with affinity for the serotonin (5-hydroxytryptamine, 5-HT) 2C receptor (5-HT2CR) such as mCPP, act as appetite suppressants (Kennett and Curzon, 1991; Kitchener and Dourish, 1994). Mice lacking 5-HT2CR, generated by the introduction of a nonsense mutation in the 5-HT2CR gene, are overweight as a result of overeating (Tecott *et al.*, 1995). 5-HT2CR transcripts have been detected in the paraventricular nucleus of the hypothalamus (Hoffman and Mezey, 1989), supporting the hypothesis of a central role for serotonin in the control of food intake. 5-HT2CR deficient mice provide a tool for elucidating some of the neurochemical pathways that underlie the regulation of food intake.

Psammomys Obesus

The sand rat *Psammomys obesus* (*P. obesus*) is a polygenic model of obesity and type II diabetes. In their native environment these animals remain lean and free from diabetes but when put on normal laboratory rodent diets a proportion of the animals develop metabolic abnormalities. These abnormalities include obesity, hyperinsulinemia, glucose intolerance, hyperleptinemia and diabetes (Barnett *et al.*, 1994a, 1994b; Collier *et al.*, 1997; Walder *et al.*, 1997). The spectrum of metabolic responses to obesity and the variability in the susceptibility to develop obesity in *P. obesus* makes this model more analogous to human obesity than the single gene obesity models.

The New Zealand Obese Mouse: A Model of the Metabolic Syndrome

New Zealand obese (NZO) mice exhibit a polygenic syndrome of hyperphagia and obesity associated with a type II diabetes-like syndrome of hyperinsulinemia and hypoglycaemia (Bielschowsky and Bielschowsky, 1953; Crofford and Davis, 1965; Veroni *et al.*, 1991). It has been shown that the NZO mouse has elevated levels of leptin in both adipose tissue and serum. Furthermore NZO mice fail to respond to peripheral recombinant leptin infusions with reduced food intake, indicating that they are leptin insensitive (Igel *et al.*, 1997). However, NZO mice respond to intracerebroventricular infusions of leptin with sensitivity similar to wild-type mice (Halaas *et al.*, 1997). It has therefore been suggested that the leptin resistance seen in NZO mice is the result of a diminished transport of leptin into the Cerebrospinal fluid (CSF) (Halaas *et al.*, 1997). Decreased levels of CSF leptin have been observed in some obese patients and the NZO mouse could thus have important implications for understanding the pathogenesis of human obesity (Schwartz *et al.*, 1996).

NZO mice also show symptoms of hypertension and hypercholesterolaemia (Ortlepp *et al.*, 2000). In humans, obesity associated with insulin resistance, dyslipidemia and hypertension is called the metabolic syndrome. The pathophysiological links between the different components of this syndrome is not fully understood and the NZO mouse presents a model for the study of these interactions.

Quantitative Trait Loci for Obesity

Quantitative trait loci (QTL) are produced by statistical analysis of genetic information derived from the offspring of crosses between informative strains with regard to, for example, body mass or fat content. It is believed that this will be a way of identifying susceptibility genes for complex disorders such as obesity. QTL

Table XXIII-1.2 Animal models of obesity

Model	Phenotype	Cause	Face validity	Predictive validity	Construct validity
ob/ob mouse	Obesity, hypoglycaemia, hypothermia, hyperinsulinemia, hypercorticism.	Recessive mutation in the *Lep* gene.	+++	+++*	+(+++)*
db/db mouse	Obesity, hypoglycaemia, hypothermia, hyperinsulinemia, hypercorticism.	Recessive mutation in the *Lepr* gene.	+++	n.d.	+(+++)*
fatty Zucker rat	Obesity, hyperphagia.	Recessive mutation in the *Lepr* gene.	+++	n.d.	+(+++)*
corpulent Koletsky rat	Obesity, hyperphagia.	Recessive mutation in the *Lepr* gene.	+++	n.d.	+(+++)*
Mc3r-/- mouse	Increased body fat mass.	Knockout of the *Mc3r* gene.	++	n.d.	+
Mc4r-/- mouse	Maturity-onset obesity, hyperphagia.	Knockout of the *Mc4r* gene.	++	n.d.	+(+++)*
Agouti yellow mouse	Obesity, yellow pigmentation.	Dominant mutations in the agouti gene.	++	n.d.	+
fat/fat mouse	Obesity, hyperinsulinemia.	Mutation in the *Cpe* gene.	+++	n.d.	+(+++)*
tub/tub mouse	Maturity-onset obesity, insulin resistance.	Recessive mutation in the *tub* gene.	+++	n.d.	+
Adult mouse	Adult obesity, diabetes.	Dominant mutation in the *Ad* gene.	+++	n.d.	+
5-HT2C-/- mouse	Obesity, hyperphagia.	Introduced nonsense mutation in the *5-HT2C-/-* gene.	++	n.d.	+
P. obesus sand rat	Obesity, type II diabetes.	Polygenic.	+++	n.d.	n.d.
NZO mouse	Obesity, type II diabetes.	Polygenic.	+++	n.d.	n.d.

*Excellent predictive and/or construct validity as models for subgroups of human obesity cases with related mutations. n.d.: not determined. Although there are several cases described where single gene mutation models have counterparts that cause obesity in the human, polygenic animal models will most likely best mimic the human situation. The monogenic models will probably have their strength as hypothesis generators and in the cases of the *ob, db, Mc4r* and *fat* mutations they have been most helpful in revealing the nature of specific human eating disorders.

analysis has become a method of choice for mimicking more closely the complex obesity in human. A total of 98 animal QTLs, from mouse, rat, pig and chicken, linked to body weight or body fat were reported in the 1999 update of 'The human obesity gene map' (Chagnon *et al.*, 2000). This number is constantly increasing as more QTL crosses are analysed. The main task of identifying and cloning the QTLs remains. Some of these QTLs will turn out to be more important than others and several will, in all likelihood, be proven to be false positives.

Conclusions on Obesity Models

Human obesity is a complex disorder influenced by both environmental as well as physiological and genetic factors. Although there are several cases described where single gene mutations cause obesity in the human the polygenic animal models will most likely mimic the human situation best. Table XXIII-1.2 contains a summary and a comparative evaluation of the models described.

CONCLUDING REMARKS

When producing valid animal models of eating disorders one is faced with two major obstacles, first the lack of accurate descriptions of the disorders and second the lack of effective treatments for these disorders. The central mechanisms of hunger and satiety are under complex physiological control. A good understanding of these mechanisms is necessary in order to understand the underlying causes for eating disorders. In this chapter we have reviewed some of the available animal models of eating behaviour that may provide clues to possible mechanisms involved in the regulation of food intake.

Given that eating disorders have become a major health concern, the combination of gene variants, mutations and environmental factors that contribute to these disorders need to be defined. Irrespective of the value of animal models for the understanding of the causes of human eating disorders, it is very probable that most of the molecules identified, using animal models, will be involved in biochemical processes regulating food intake and/or metabolism also in human. As such, these molecules constitute targets for the development of new classes of small drug pharmaceuticals that may be used to treat human eating disorders. There are thus great expectations that studies of animal models will result in new tools for the treatment and/or prevention of a major health hazard in the western world.

REFERENCES

Anand, B.K. and Brobeck, J.R., 1951. Localization of a "feeding center" in the hypothalamus of the rat. *Proc. Soc. Exp. Biol. Med.*, **77**, 323–324.

Barnett, M., Collier, G.R., Collier, F.M., Zimmet, P. and O'Dea, K., 1994a. A cross-sectional and short-term longitudinal characterization of NIDDM in *Psammomys Obesus. Diabetologica*, **37**, 671–676.

Barnett, M., Collier, G.R., Zimmet, P. and O'Dea, K., 1994b. The effect of restricting energy intake on diabetes in *Psammomys Obesus. Int. J. Obesity*, **18**, 789–794.

Barsh, G.S., Farooqi, S.F. and O'Rahilly, S., 2000. Genetics of body-weight regulation. *Nature*, **404**, 644–651.

Bielschowsky, M. and Bielschowsky, F., 1953. A new strain of mice with hereditary obesity. *Proc. Univ. Otago. Med. School*, **31**, 29–31.

Bittencourt, J.C., Presse, F., Arias, C., Peto, C., Vaughan, J., Nahon, J.L., Vale, W. and Sawchenko, P.E., 1992. The melanin concentrating hormone system of the rat brain: an immuno- and hybridization histochemical characterization. *J. Comp. Neurol.*, **319**, 218–245.

Boer, D.P., Epling, W.F., Pierce, W.D. and Russel, J.C., 1990. Suppression of food-induced high-rate wheel running in rats by naloxone. *Physiol. Behav.*, **48**, 339–342.

Boggon, T.J., Shan, W.S., Santagata, S., Myers, S.C. and Shapiro, L., 1999. Implication of tubby proteins as transcription factors by structure-based functional analysis. *Science*, **286**, 2119–2125.

Broberger, C., Johansen, J., Schalling, M. and Hökfelt, T., 1997. Hypothalamic neurohistochemistry of the murine anorexia (*anx/anx*) mutation: altered processing of neuropeptide Y in the arcuate nucleus. *J. Comp. Neurol.*, **387**, 124–135.

Broberger, C., Johansen, J., Johansson, C., Schalling, M. and Hökfelt, T., 1998. The neuropeptide Y/agouti gene-related protein (AGRP) brain circuitry in normal, anorectic, and monosodium glutamate-treated mice. *Proc. Natl. Acad. Sci. USA*, **95**, 15043–15048.

Broberger, C., Johansen, J., Brismar, H., Johansson, C., Schalling, M. and Hökfelt, T., 1999. Changes in neuropeptide Y receptors and pro-opiomelanocortin in the anorexia (*anx/anx*) mouse hypothalamus. *J. Neurosci.*, **19**, 7130–7139.

Bultman, S.J., Michaud, E.J. and Woychik, R.P., 1992. Molecular characterization of the mouse agouti locus. *Cell*, **71**, 1195–1204.

Bunney, B.S. and Aghajanian, G.K., 1976. The precise localization of nigral afferents in the rat as determined by a retrograde tracing technique. *Brain Res.*

Chagnon, Y.C., Pérusse, L., Weisnagel, S.J., Rankinen, T. and Bouchard, C., 2000. The human obesity gene map: The 1999 update. *Obesity Res.*, **8**, 89–117.

Charlton, H.M., 1984. Mouse mutants as models in endocrine research. *Q. J. Exp. Physiol.*, **69**, 655–676.

Chen, H., Charlat, O., Tartaglia, L.A., Woolf, E.A., Weng, X., Ellis, S.J., Lakey, N.D., Culpepper, J., Moore, K.J., Breitbart, R.E., Duyk, G.M., Tepper, R.I. and Morgenstern, J.P., 1996. Evidence that the diabetes gene encodes the leptin receptor: identification of a mutation in the leptin receptor gene in db/db mice. *Cell*, **84**, 491–495.

Chen, A.S., Marsh, D.J., Trumbauer, M.E., Frazier, E.G., Guan, X.M., Yu, H., Rosenblum, C.I., Vongs, A., Feng, Y., Cao, L., Metzger, J.M., Strack, A.M., Camacho, R.E., Mellin, T.N., Nunes, C.N., Min, W., Fisher, J., Gopal-Truter, S., MacIntyre, D.E., Chen, H.Y. and Van Der Ploeg, L.H., 2000. Inactivation of the mouse melanocortin-3 receptor results in increased fat mass and reduced lean body mass. *Nature Genet.*, **26**, 97–102.

Chua, S.C., Chung, W.K., Wu-Peng, X.S., Zhang, Y., Liu, S.M., Tartaglia, L. and Leibel, R.L., 1996. Phenotypes of mouse diabetes and rat fatty due to mutations in the OB (leptin) receptor. *Science*, **271**, 994–996.

Clement, K., Vaisse, C., Lahlou, N., Cabrol, S., Pelloux, V., Cassuto, D., Gourmelen, M., Dina, C., Chambaz, J., Lacorte, J.M., Basdevant, A., Bougneres, P., Lebouc, Y., Froguel, P. and Guy-Grand, B., 1998. A mutation in the human leptin receptor gene causes obesity and pituitary dysfunction. *Nature*, **392**, 398–401.

Coleman, D.L., 1973. Effects of parabiosis of obese with diabetes and normal mice. *Diabetologia*, **9**, 294–298.

Coleman, D.L., 1978. Obese and diabetes: two mutant genes causing diabetes-obesity syndromes in mice. *Diabetologia*, **14**, 141–148.

Coleman, D.L. and Eicher, E.M., 1990. Fat (fat) and tubby (tub): two autosomal recessive mutations causing obesity syndromes in the mouse. *J. Hered.*, **81**, 424–427.

Coleman, D.L. and Hummel, K.P., 1969. Effects of parabiosis of normal with genetically diabetic mice. *Am. J. Physiol.*, **217**, 1298–1304.

Collier, G., de Silva, A., Sanigorski, A., Walder, K. and Zimmet, P., 1997. Development of obesity and insulin resistance in the Israeli sand rat (*Psammomys obesus*): does leptin play a role? *Ann. New York Acad. Sci.*, **827**, 50–63.

Cooper, S.J. and Al-Nasar, H.A., 1993. D1 : D2 dopamine receptor interaction in relation to feeding responses and food intake. In: Waddington, J. (ed.), *D1 : D2 Dopamine Receptor Interactions*, pp. 203–233. Academic Press: San Diego.

Crofford, O.B. and Davis, C.K., 1965. Growth characteristics, glucose tolerance and insulin sensitivity of New Zealand Obese mice. *Metabolism*, **14**, 271–280.

Davis, C., Kennedy, S.H., Ravelski, E. and Dionne, M., 1994. The role of physical activity in the development and maintenance of eating disorders. *Psychol. Med.*, **24**, 957–967.

Diagnostic and statistical Manual of Mental Disorders, 4th edn, DSM-IV, 1994. American Psychiatric Association: Washington DC; 539–550, 729–731.

Dourish, C.T., 1983. Dopaminergic involvement in the control of drinking behaviour: a brief review. *Prog. Neuropsychopharmacol. Biol. Psychiatry*, **7**, 487–493.

Duncan, S.A., Navas, M.A., Dufort, D., Rossant, J. and Stoffel, M., 1998. Regulation of a transcription factor network required for differentiation and metabolism. *Science*, **281**, 692–695.

Epling, W.F. and Pierce, W.D., 1985. Activity-based anorexia in rats as a function of opportunity to run in an activity wheel. *Nutr. Behav.*, **2**, 37–49.

Epling, W.F., Pierce, W.D. and Stefan, L., 1983. A theory of activity-based anorexia. *Int. J. Eating Disord.*, **3**, 27–46.

Exner, C., Hebebrand, J., Remschmidt, H., Wewetzer, C., Ziegler, A., Herpertz, S., Schweiger, U., Blum, W.F., Preibisch, G., Heldmaier, G. and Klingenspor, M., 2000. Leptin suppresses semi-starvation induced hyperactivity in rats: implications for anorexia nervosa. *Mol. Psychiatry*, **5**, 476–481.

Fan, W., Boston, B.A., Kesterson, R.A., Hruby, V.J. and Cone, R.D., 1997. Role of melanocortinergic neurons in feeding and the agouti obesity syndrome. *Nature*, **385**, 165–168.

Fibiger, H.C., Zis, A.P. and McGeer, E.G., 1973. Feeding and drinking deficits after 6-hydroxydopamine administration in the rat: similarities to the lateral hypothalamic syndrome. *Brain Res.*, **55**, 135–148.

Fong, T.M., Mao, C., MacNeil, C., Kalyani, R., Smith, T., Weinberg, D., Tota, M.R. and Van der Ploeg, L.H., 1997. ART (protein product of agouti-related transcript) as an antagonist of MC-3 and MC-4 receptors. *Biochem. Biophys. Res. Commun.*, **237**, 629–631.

Gantz, I., Konda, Y., Tashiro, T., Shimoto, Y., Miwa, H., Munzert, G., Watson, S.J., DelValle, J. and Yamada, T., 1993a. Molecular cloning of a novel melanocortin receptor. *J. Biol. Chem.*, **268**, 8246–8250.

Gantz, I., Miwa, H., Konda, Y., Shimoto, Y., Tashiro, T., Watson, S.J., DelValle, J. and Yamada, T., 1993b. Molecular cloning, expression, and gene localization of a fourth melanocortin receptor. *J. Biol. Chem.*, **268**, 15174–15179.

Graham, M., Shuttre, J.R., Sarmiento, U., Sarosi, I. and Stark, K.L., 1997. Overexpression of Agrt leads to obesity in transgenic mice. *Nature Genet.*, **17**, 273–274.

Hagan, M.M. and Moss, D.E., 1997. Persistence of binge-eating patterns after a history of restriction with intermittent bouts of refeeding on palatable food in rats: Implications for bulimia nervosa. *Int. J. Eat. Disord.*, **22**, 411–420.

Halaas, J.L., Boozer, C., Blair-West, J., Fidahusein, N., Denton, D.A. and Friedman, J.M., 1997. Physiological response to long-term peripheral and central leptin infusion in lean and obese mice. *Proc. Natl. Acad. Sci. USA*, **94**, 8878–8883.

Hausberger, F.X., 1959. Parabiosis and transplantation experiments in hereditary obese mice. *Anat. Rec.*, **130**, 313.

Haynes, W.G., Morgan, D.A., Djalali, A., Sivitz, W.I. and Mark, A.L., 1999. Interactions between the melanocortin system and leptin in control of sympathetic nerve traffic. *Hypertension*, **33**, 542–547.

Hervey, G.R., 1958. The effects of lesions in the hypothalamus in parabiotic rats. *J. Physiol.*, **145**, 336–352.

Hetherington, A.W. and Ranson, S.W., 1940. Hypothalamic lesions and adiposity in the rat. *Anat. Rec.*, **78**, 149–172.

Hoffman, B.J. and Mezey, E., 1989. Distribution of serotonin 5-HT1C receptor mRNA in adult rat brain. *FEBS Lett.*, **247**, 453–462.

Hsaio, S., 1967. Saline drinking effects on food and water intake in rats. *Psychol. Rep.*, **21**, 1025–1028.

Huszar, D., Lynch, C.A., Fairchild-Huntress, V., Dunmore, J.H., Fang, Q., Berkemeier, L.R., Gu, W., Kesterson, R.A., Boston, B.A., Cone, R.D., Smith, F.J., Campfield, L.A., Burn, P. and Lee, F., 1997. Targeted disruption of the melanocortin-4 receptor results in obesity in mice. *Cell*, **88**, 131–141.

Igel, M., Becker, W., Herberg, L. and Joost, H.G., 1997. Hyperleptinemia, leptin resistance and polymorphic leptin receptor in the New Zealand Obese (NZO) mouse. *Endocrinology*, **138**, 4234–4239.

Jackson, R.S., Creemers, J.W.M., Ohagi, S., Raffin-Sanson, M.L., Sanders, L., Montague, C.T., Hutton, J.C. and O'Rahilly, S., 1997. Obesity and impaired prohormoneprocessing associated with mutations in the human prohormone convertase 1 gene. *Nature Genet.*, **16**, 303–306.

Jahng, J.W., Houpt, T.A., Kim, S.-J., Joh, T.H. and Son, J.H., 1998. Neuropeptide Y mRNA and serotonin innervation in the arcuate nucleus of anorexia mutant mice. *Brain Res.*, **790**, 67–73.

Johansen, J.E., Broberger, C., Lavebratt, C., Johansson, C., Kuhar, M.J., Hökfelt, T. and Schalling, M., 2000. Hypothalamic CART and serum leptin levels are reduced in the anorectic (*anx/anx*) mouse. *Mol. Brain Res.*, **84**, 97–105.

Kaestner, K.H., Katz, J., Liu, Y., Drucker, D.J. and Schutz, G., 1999. Inactivation of the winged helix transcription factor HNF3alpha affects glucose homeostasis and islet glucagon gene expression *in vivo*. *Genes Dev.*, **13**, 495–504.

Kapeller, R., Moriarty, A., Strauss, A., Stubdal, H., Theriault, K., Siebert, E., Chickering, T., Morgenstern, J.P., Tartaglia, L.A. and Lillie, J., 1999. Tyrosine phosphorylation of Tub and its association with Src homology 2 domain-containing proteins implicate Tub in intracellular signaling by insulin. *J. Biol. Chem.*, **275**, 24980–24986.

Kennedy, G.C., 1953. The role of depot fat in the hypothalamic control of food intake in the rat. *Proc. R. Soc. Series B*, **140**, 578–592.

Kennett, G.A. and Curzon, G., 1991. Potencies of antagonists indicate that 5-HT1C receptors mediate 1-3(chlorophenyl)piperazine-induced hypophagia. *Br. J. Pharmacol.*, **103**, 2016–2020.

Kitchener, S.J. and Dourish, C.T., 1994. An examination of the behavioural specificity of hypophagia induced by 5-HT1B, 5-HT1C and 5-HT2 receptor agonists using the post-prandial satiety sequence in rats. *Psychopharmacology*, **113**, 369–377.

Kleyn, P.W., Fan, W., Kovats, S.G., Lee, J.J., Pulido, J.C., Wu, Y., Berkmeier, L.R., Misumi, D.J., Holmgren, L., Charlat, O., Woolf, E.A., Tayber, O., Brody, T., Shu, P., Hawkins, F., Kennedy, B., Baldini, L., Ebeling, C., Alperin, G.D., Deeds, J., Lakey, N.D., Culpepper, J., Chen, H., Glücksmann-Kuis, M.A., Carlson, G.A., Duyk, G.M. and Moore, K.J., 1996. Identification and characterization of the mouse obesity gene tubby: A member of a novel gene family. *Cell*, **85**, 281–290.

Kotler, D.P., Wang, J. and Pierson, R., 1985. Body composition studies in patients with the acquired immunodeficiency syndrome. *Am. J. Clin. Nutr.*, **42**, 1255–1265.

Kristensen, P., Judge, M.J., Thim, L., Ribel, U., Christjansen, K.N., Wulff, B.S., Clausen, J.T., Jensen, P.B., Madsen, O.D., Vrang, N., Larsen, P.J. and Hastrup, S., 1998. Hypothalamic CART is a new anorectic peptide regulated by leptin. *Nature*, **393**, 72–76.

Larkin, M., 1998. Thwarting the dwindling progression of cachexia. *Lancet*, **351**, 1336.

Lee, G.H., Proenca, R., Montez, J.M., Carroll, K.M., Darvishzadeh, J.G., Lee, J.I. and Friedman, J.M., 1996. Abnormal splicing of the leptin receptor in diabetic mice. *Nature*, **379**, 632–635.

Lu, D., Willard, D., Patel, I.R., Kadwell, S., Overton, L., Kost, T., Luther, M., Chen, W., Woychik, R.P., Wilkinson, W.O. and Cone, R.D., 1994. Agouti protein is an antagonist of the melanocyte-stimulating hormone receptor. *Nature*, **371**, 799–802.

Maltais, L.J., Lane, P.W. and Beamer, W.G., 1984. Anorexia, a recessive mutation causing starvation in preweanling mice. *J. Hered.*, **75**, 468–472.

Michaud, E.J., Bultman, S.J., Klebig, M.L., van Vugt, M.J., Stubbs, L.J., Russell, L.B. and Woychik, R.P., 1994. A molecular model for the genetic and phenotypic characteristics of the mouse lethal yellow (A^y) mutation. *Proc. Natl. Acad. Sci. USA*, **91**, 2562–2566.

Miller, M.W., Duhl, D.M.J., Vrieling, H., Cordes, S.P., Ollmann, M.M., Winkes, B.M. and Barsh, G.S., 1993. Cloning of the mouse agouti gene predicts a secreted protein ubiquitously expressed in mice carrying the lethal yellow mutation. *Genes Dev.*, **7**, 454–467.

Montague, C.T., Farooqui, S., Whitehead, J.P., Soos, M.A., Rau, H., Wareham, N.J., Sewter, C.P., Digby, J.E., Mohammed, S.N., Hurst, J.A., Cheetham, C.H., Earley, A.R., Barnett, A.H., Prins, J.B. and O'Rahilly, S., 1997. Congenital leptin deficiency is associated with severe early-onset obesity in humans. *Nature*, **387**, 903–908.

Naggert, J.K., Fricker, L.D., Varlamov, O., Nishina, P.M., Rouille, Y., Steiner, D.F., Carrol, R.J., Paigen, B.J. and Leiter, E.H., 1995. Hyperproinsulinaemia in obese fat/fat mice associated with a carboxypeptidase E mutation which reduces enzyme activity. *Nature Genet.*, **10**, 135–142.

Noben-Trauth, K., Naggert, J.K., North, M.A. and Nishina, P.M., 1996. A candidate gene for the mouse mutation tubby. *Nature*, **380**, 534–538.

Ohlemiller, K.K., Huges, R.M., Mosinger-Ogilvie, J., Speck, J.D., Grosof, D.H. and Silverman, M.S., 1995. Cochlear and retinal degeneration in the tubby mouse. *Neuroreport*, **6**, 845–849.

Ohlemiller, K.K., Huges, R.M., Lett, J.M., Ogilvie, J.M., Speck, J.D., Wright, J.S. and Faddis, B.T., 1997. Progression of cochlear and retinal degeneration in the tubby (rd5) mouse. *Audiol. Neurootol.*, **2**, 175–185.

Ollmann, M.M., Wilson, B.D., Yang, Y.K., Kerns, J.A., Chen, Y., Gantz, I. and Barsh, G.S., 1997. Antagonism of central melanocortin receptors *in vitro* and *in vivo* by agouti-related protein. *Science*, **278**, 135–137.

Ortlepp, J.R., Kluge, R., Giesen, K., Plum, L., Radke, P., Hanrath, P. and Joost, H.G., 2000. A metabolic syndrome of hypertension, hyperinsulinaemia and hypercholesterolaemia in the New Zealand obese mouse. *Europ. J. Clin. Invest.*, **30**, 195–202.

Phillips, A.G. and Nikaido, N.S., 1978. Disruption of brain stimulation-induced feeding by dopamine receptor blockade. *Nature*, **258**, 750–751.

Phillipson, O.T., 1979. Afferent projections to the ventral tegmental area of Tsai and interfascicular nucleus: a horseradish peroxidase study in the rat. *J. Comp. Neurol.*, **187**, 117–144.

Pirke, K.M., Broocks, A., Wilckens, T., Marquard, R. and Schweiger, U., 1993. Starvation-induced hyperactivity in the rat: The role of endocrine and neurotransmitter changes. *Neurosci. Biobehav. Rev.*, **17**, 287–294.

Pohjanvirta, R. and Tuomisto, J., 1990. Remarkable residual alterations in responses to feeding regulatory challenges in Han/Wistar rats after recovery from the acute toxicity of TCCD. *Food Chem. Toxicol.*, **28**, 677–686.

Pohjanvirta, R. and Tuomisto, J., 1994. Short term toxicity of 2,3,7,8-chlorodibenzo-*p*-dioxin in laboratory animals: Effects, mechanisms and animal models. *Pharmacol. Rev.*, **46**, 483–549.

Pohjanvirta, R., Unkila, M. and Tuomisto, J., 1994. TCDD-induced hypophagia is not explained by nausea. *Pharmacol. Biochem. Behav.*, **47**, 273–282.

Rau, H., Reaves, B.J., O'Rahilly, S. and Whithead, J.P., 1999. Truncated human leptin (delta133) associated with extreme obesity undergoes proteasomal degradation after defective intracellular transport. *Endocrinology*, **140**, 1718–1723.

Salamone, J.D., Zigmond, M.J. and Stricker, E.M., 1990. Characterization of the impaired feeding behaviour in rats given haloperidol or dopamine-depleting brain lesions. *Neuroscience*, **39**, 17–24.

Sanghvi, I.S., Singer, G., Friedman, E. and Gershon, S., 1975. Anorexigenic effects of d-amphetamine and l-DOPA in the rat. *Pharmacol. Biochem. Behav.*, **3**, 81–86.

Saper, C.B., 1985. Organization of cerebral cortical afferent systems in the rat. II. Hypothalamocortical projections. *J. Comp. Neurol.*, **237**, 21–46.

Saper, C.B., Akil, H. and Watson, S.J., 1986. Lateral hypothalamic innervation of the cerebral cortex: immunoreactive staining for a peptide resembling but immunochemically distinct from pituitary/arcuate alpha-melanocyte stimulating hormone. *Brain Res. Bull.*, **16**, 107–120.

Schalling, M., Johansen, J., Nordfors, L. and Lönnqvist, F., 1999. Genes involved in animal models of obesity and anorexia. *J. Int. Med.*, **245**, 613–619.

Schwartz, M.W., Peskind, E., Raskind, M., Boyko, E.J. and Porte, D., 1996. Cerebrospinal fluid leptin levels: relationship to plasma levels and to adiposity in humans. *Nature Med.*, **2**, 589–593.

Seefeld, M.D., Corbett, S.W., Keesey, R.E. and Peterson, R.E., 1984. Characterization of the wasting syndrome in rats treated with 2,3,7,8-chlorodibenzo-*p*-dioxin. *Toxicol. Appl. Pharmacol.*, **73**, 311–322.

Shih, D.Q., Navas, M.A., Kuwajima, S., Duncan, S.A. and Stoffel, M., 1999. Impaired glucose homeostasis and neonatal mortality in hepatocyte nuclear factor 3alpha-deficient mice. *Proc. Natl. Acad. Sci. USA*, **96**, 10152–10157.

Shutter, J.R., Graham, M., Kinsey, A.C., Scully, S., Lüthy, R. and Stark, K.L., 1997. Hypothalamic expression of ART, a novel gene related to agouti, is up-regulated in obese and diabetic mutant mice. *Genes Develop.*, **11**, 593–602.

Smith, A.I. and Funder, J.W., 1988. Proopiomelanocortin processing in the pituitary, central nervous system, and peripheral tissues. *Endocr. Rev.*, **9**, 159–179.

Son, J.H., Baker, H., Park, D.H. and Joh, T.H., 1994. Drastic and selective hyperinnervation of central serotonergic neurones in a lethal neurodevelopmental mouse mutant, Anorexia (anx). *Mol. Brain Res.*, **25**, 129–134.

Strobel, A., Issad, T., Camoin, L., Ozata, M. and Strosberg, A.D., 1998. A leptin missense mutation associated with severe early onset obesity in humans. *Nature Genet.*, **18**, 213–215.

Szczypka, M.S., Rainey, M.A., Kim, D.S., Alaynick, W.A., Marck, B.T., Matsumoto, A.M. and Palmiter, R.D., 1999. Feeding behaviour in dopamine-deficient mice. *Proc. Natl. Acad. Sci. USA*, **96**, 12138–12143.

Takaya, K., Ogawa, Y., Hiroaka, J., Hosoda, K., Yamori, Y., Nakao, K. and Koletsky, R.J., 1996. Nonsense mutation of leptin receptor in the obese spontaneously hypertensive Koletsky rat. *Nature Genet.*, **14**, 130–131.

Tartaglia, L.A., Dembski, M., Weng, X., Deng, N., Culpepper, J., Devos, R., Richards, G.J., Campfield, L.A., Clark, F.T. and Deeds, J., 1995. Identification and Expression Cloning of a Leptin Receptor, OB-R. *Cell*, **83**, 1263–1271.

Tecott, L.H., Sun, L.M., Akana, S.F., Strack, A.M., Lowenstein, D.H., Dallman, M.F. and Julius, D., 1995. Eating disorder and epilepsy in mice lacking 5-HT2C serotonin receptors. *Nature*, **374**, 542–546.

Tisdale, M.J., 1997. Biology of cachexia. *J. Natl. Cancer Inst.*, **89**, 1763–1773.

Ungerstedt, U., 1971. Adipsia and aphagia after 6-hydroxydopamine induced degeneration of the nigrostriatal dopamine system. *Acta Physiol. Scand. (Suppl.)*, **367**, 95–122.

Unkila, M., Pohjanvirta, R., MacDonald, E. and Tuomisto, J., 1993. Differential effect of TCDD on brain serotonin metabolism in a TCDD-susceptible and a TCDD-resistant rat strain. *Chemosphere*, **27**, 401–406.

Wadden, T.A., 1993. Treatment of obesity by moderate and severe caloric restriction. Results of clinical research trials. *Ann. Intern. Med.*, **119**, 688–693.

Vaisse, C., Clement, K., Guy-Grand, B. and Frougel, P., 1998. A frameshift mutation in human MC4R is associated with a dominant form of obesity. *Nature Genet.*, **20**, 113–114.

Walder, K., Willet, M., Zimmet, P. and Collier, G.R., 1997. Ob (obese) gene expression and leptin levels in *Psammomys obesus*. *Biochim. Biophys. Acta*, **1354**, 272–278.

Wallace, M.E. and MacSwiney, F.M., 1979. An inherited mild middle-aged adiposity in wild mice. *J. Hyg.*, **89**, 309–317.

Watts, A.G., 2000. Understanding the neural control of ingestive behaviours: Helping to separate cause from effect with dehydration-associated anorexia. *Hormones Behav.*, **37**, 261–283.

Watts, A.G., Sanchez-Watts, G. and Kelly, A.B., 1999. Distinct patterns of neuropeptide gene expression in the lateral hypothalamic area and arcuate nucleus are associated with dehydration-induced anorexia. *J. Neurosci.*, **19**, 6111–6121.

Veroni, M.C., Proietto, J. and Larkins, R.G., 1991. Evolution of insulin resistance in New Zealand obese mice. *Diabetes*, **40**, 1480–1487.

Wright, A.K., Tulloch, I.F. and Arbuhnott, G.W., 1980. Possible links between hypothalamus and substantia nigra in the rat. *Appetite*, **1**, 43–51.

Yeo, G.S.H., Farooqi, I.S., Aminian, S., Halsall, D.J., Stanhope, R.G. and O'Rahilly, S., 1998. A frameshift mutation in MC4R associated with dominantly inherited human obesity. *Nature Genet.*, **20**, 111–112.

Zhang, Y., Proenca, R., Maffei, M., Barone, M., Leopold, L. and Friedman, J.M., 1994. Positional cloning of the mouse obese gene and its human homologue. *Nature*, **372**, 425–432.

Zhou, Q.-Y. and Palmiter, R.D., 1995. Dopamine-deficient mice are severely hypoactive, adipsic and aphagic. *Cell*, **83**, 1197–1209.

Zigmond, M.J. and Stricker, E.M., 1972. Deficits in feeding behaviour after intraventricular injection of 6-hydroxydopamine in rats. *Science*, **177**, 1211–1213.

XXIII-2

Transmitter Systems in the Eating Disorders

Timothy D. Brewerton

INTRODUCTION

Investigations into the role of neurotransmitters and other neuromodulators in the eating disorders have been quite productive in the last few years, especially during the last decade. The eating disorders occur in a relatively small cohort of people, primarily young women and girls, across many cultures, and they are known to be associated with significant mortality and morbidity, both medical and psychiatric (Walsh and Devlin, 1998; Becker *et al.*, 1999). Despite popular beliefs, there is no convincing evidence that cultural factors alone cause eating disorders. Recent data clearly identify strong genetic factors in the aetiology of both anorexia nervosa (AN) and bulimia nervosa (BN), which appear to share common genetic vulnerabilities (Lilenfeld *et al.*, 1998; Strober *et al.*, 2000) possibly linked to obsessionality, perfectionism, anxiety and/or behavioural inhibition (Halmi *et al.*, 2000; Kaye *et al.*, 1999a, 1999b). Such information implicates primary neurotransmitter disturbances in both disorders. One powerful piece of evidence to support monoamine involvement in the eating disorders is the observation that antidepressant medications can be beneficial in controlled studies, not only in BN patients, but also in recovered AN patients (Kaye *et al.*, 1998b).

However, it is also clear that a number of secondary disturbances come about as a result of the profound eating disturbances characteristic of these disorders (Brewerton, 1995), which then in turn only worsen or perpetuate signs and symptoms (Pollice *et al.*, 1997). This perspective, taken together with the disorders' consequences, challenges and costs, compels us towards a better understanding of the biological mechanisms underlying all stages and types of eating disorders. The identification of the psychobiological underpinnings of these conditions may be useful in many ways, including the development of improved medical and psychopharmacologic interventions, improved education and psychotherapy for patients and their families, and improved prevention efforts at a primary level.

It must be emphasized that most measurements of neurotransmitter function provide only a glimpse into the state of the organism at that moment in time. Sorting out what is trait- and what is state-related has been a challenging focus of neurotransmitter research in the eating disorders.

MONOAMINES

The classical monoaminergic neurotransmitter systems, including serotonin (5-HT), norepinephrine (NE), and dopamine (DA), have been fairly extensively studied in the eating disorders using available techniques in biological psychiatry. Most of these studies have been conducted during the disease state, which has the disadvantage of being confounded by severe nutritional compromise. Dieting and/or semi-starvation clearly deplete central monoamines and lead to altered neurotransmitter levels and receptor sensitivity in animals and humans (Cowen *et al.*, 1996; Cowen and Smith, 1999; Goodwin *et al.*, 1987a, 1987b, 1990). To avoid this problem a more recent strategy has been to study 'recovered' eating disorder patients, i.e., AN and BN patients who have attained normalization of eating and weight, resumption of menses and/or normalization of gonadal hormone levels, and abatement of typical cognitive features to sub-clinical levels. This strategy attempts to minimize starvation-state-related effects and to reveal potential trait-related disturbances or vulnerabilities. However, the long-term effects of chronic malnutrition and disordered eating behaviours on the brain (similar to substance use disorders) should not be underestimated. Studies of transmitter function in at-risk pre-morbid individuals as well as non-affected identical and fraternal twins, siblings, and other first-degree relatives of ED patients, could begin to confirm trait-related disturbances.

Neurotransmitter function in patients with EDs have been investigated using a variety of existing techniques and methodologies, each of which has its own advantages and disadvantages. Studies of cerebrospinal fluid (CSF) concentrations of the major metabolites have been a popular strategy and include measures of 5-hydroxyindoleacetic acid (5-HIAA) for serotonin (5-HT), 3-methoxy-4-hydroxyphenylglycol (MHPG) for NE, and homovanillic acid (HVA) for DA. Some studies have also examined actual concentrations of 5-HT and NE, but not DA. Such studies measure transmitter metabolism of the whole brain and spinal cord and lack any anatomical specificity.

Neuroendocrine and other psychobiological response measures have been studied following acute challenges with various agents, including amino acid precursors, e.g., L-tryptophan (L-TRP) and 5-hydroxytryptophan (5-HTP) for 5-HT, pre-synaptic receptor agonists, e.g., dl-fenfluramine (dl-FEN) or d-fenfluramine (d-FEN) for 5-HT, post-synaptic receptor agonists, e.g., m-chlorophenylpiperazine (m-CPP) for 5-HT and isoproterenol (ISOP) for NE. Longer term challenges with receptor antagonists, e.g., antipsychotics for DA and 5-HT, and antidepressants, especially the serotonin-specific reuptake inhibitors (SSRIs), also illuminate the role of neurotransmitters in the eating disorders. Acute amino acid precursor depletion, most notably of L-TRP (Delgado *et al.*, 1990; Weltzin *et al.*, 1995; Smith, Fairburn and Cowen, 1999; Kaye *et al.*, 2000), has been another important source of information about the role of central 5-HT function in eating and related disorders.

Platelet (PLT) or leukocyte studies are possibly reflective of central neurotransmitter function but are always at least step removed from the nervous system, e.g., platelet 5-HT reuptake, ^{3}H-imipramine binding, ^{3}H-paroxetine binding, platelet MAO, platelet 5-HT content, as well as platelet receptor mediated aggregation (5-HT$_2$ and alpha-adrenergic).

Plasma concentrations of neurotransmitter precursors, e.g., L-TRP, L-tyrosine (L-TYR), and their competing large neutral amino acids (LNAA), neurotransmitters themselves, e.g., NE, DA,

Biological Psychiatry: Edited by H. D'haenen, J.A. den Boer and P. Willner. ISBN 0-471-49198-5

and whole blood serotonin (WBS), as well as the usual metabolites, MHPG, HVA, and 5-HIAA.

Brain imaging-receptor-binding studies are a promising avenue but remain relatively unexplored in the eating disorders.

For each neurotransmitter, the results from controlled studies in humans will be reviewed and summarized for both AN and BN. Where applicable, comparisons between restricting AN patients, bingeing/purging AN patients, and normal-weight BN patients will be made.

NOREPINEPHRINE

There are a number of reasons to suspect NE involvement in the eating disorders. Most notably, NE pathways at the level of the hypothalamus are known to be involved in the initiation of feeding (Rowland, Morien and Li, 1996). Disturbances in these pathways may therefore be involved in the pathophysiology of the profoundly altered feeding behaviours classically associated with the eating disorders. In addition, NE's role in the modulation of mood, anxiety, neuroendocrine control, metabolic rate, sympathetic tone, and temperature make it a likely candidate of study (Jimerson *et al.*, 1987; Kaye *et al.*, 1988b, 1990a, 1990c; Lesem *et al.*, 1989; Pirke, 1996). It has been well recognized for quite some time that low-weight anorexic patients, and to some degree bulimic patients, have reduced body temperature, blood pressure, pulse and metabolic rate (Gross *et al.*, 1979; Lesem *et al.*, 1989; Obarzanek *et al.*, 1991). Investigations in this area have shown that low-weight AN patients have reduced measures of plasma, urinary and CSF MHPG (Gross *et al.*, 1979; Halmi *et al.*, 1978; Johnston *et al.*, 1984; Kaye *et al.*, 1984a, 1984b). In contrast, reports of plasma NE levels in the eating disorders has been more variable (Luck *et al.*, 1983; Kaye *et al.*, 1988a, 1988b), and this appears to be linked not only to weight but to the stresses associated with the illness (Lesem *et al.*, 1989). AN patients tend to have higher plasma NE levels at admission, which then decrease as treatment and weight gain progresses (Pahl *et al.*, 1985; Lesem *et al.*, 1989).

When ill, BN patients demonstrate lower values of plasma NE at baseline (Jimerson *et al.*, 1987; Obarzanek *et al.*, 1991) and in response to abstinence (Kaye *et al.*, 1990b), standing (Pirke *et al.*, 1985), testmeal challenge (Pirke *et al.*, 1992), and mental challenge (Pirke *et al.*, 1992). They also have other evidence of blunted sympathetic activation in response to mental stress (Koo-Loeb, Pedersen and Girdler, 1998). However, despite low baseline plasma NE levels, BN patients show normal responses to exercise (Pirke *et al.*, 1989) but reduced responses to orthostasis (Lonati-Galligani and Pirke, 1986).

In AN patients, depression has been found to be significantly worse in those patients with the lowest delta change in plasma NE concentrations to orthostasis (Pirke *et al.*, 1988). Reduced urinary MHPG levels have also been related to the presence of comorbid major depression (Biederman *et al.*, 1984a, 1984b; Halmi *et al.*, 1978). It is therefore important in such studies to control for psychiatric comorbidity.

Like the plasma NE studies, CSF NE levels have been reported to be no different in AN patients compared to controls at low weight and after short-term weight gain, but then significantly lower after weight recovery of at least 6 months (Kaye *et al.*, 1984a, 1984b, 1985; Pirke, 1996). In BN patients, reduced CSF NE levels have been reported during the active state of the illness (Kaye *et al.*, 1990a, 1990b). However, upon long-term recovery, concentrations of CSF MHPG have been reported to normalize in both AN and BN (Kaye *et al.*, 1999a, 1999b) despite earlier reports of lower levels (Kaye *et al.*, 1985). Given that CSF NE concentrations have not yet been reported in long-term (>1 year) recovered AN or BN patients, the extent to which adrenergic alterations seen in the eating disorders are trait-related is unclear. Nevertheless, available evidence suggests exquisite sensitivity of this system to malnutrition or stress.

Challenge studies using the beta-adrenergic agonist isoproterenol in underweight anorexic patients revealed erratic secretion of plasma NE in response to increasing doses (Kaye *et al.*, 1990a, 1990b). Bulimic patients demonstrated significantly increased chronotropic responses to isoproterenol (George *et al.*, 1990). Challenge studies with adrenergic agents in recovered patients have not been reported.

The number of platelet alpha-2-receptors has been reported to be reduced in both AN and BN compared to controls (Luck *et al.*, 1983; Heufelder, Warnhoff and Pirke, 1985), thereby suggesting increased post-synaptic receptor sensitivity which is probably secondary to dieting or semi-starvation. In summary, peripheral and central sympathetic nervous activity is reduced in both AN and BN, although it tends to normalize with recovery. Taken together, the preponderance of the evidence so far leads to the conclusion that these changes are a result of chronic starvation or intermittent dieting (Pirke, 1996). However, a trait-related disturbance of the adrenergic system cannot be ruled out at this time (Kaye *et al.*, 1990a, 1990b).

Studies of adrenergic receptors on human leukocytes have been another strategy to investigate adrenergic function in the eating disorders. Buckholtz *et al.* (1988) reported altered beta-adrenergic receptor affinity on circulating lymphocytes of BN patients compared to those of controls. However, in a similar study of a mixed group of eating disorder patients, Lonati-Galligani and Pirke (1986) reported lower receptor number (B_{max}) but normal affinity (K_d) in low-weight AN patients, while both measures were no different from controls in the BN patients and the weight-recovered AN patients. Gill and colleagues (1992) reported differential changes in alpha- and beta-adrenoceptor linked [$^{45}Ca^{2+}$] uptake in platelets from patients with anorexia nervosa, further documenting an adrenergic disturbance in eating disorder patients. However, the issue of cause vs. effect remains unanswered in platelet and leukocyte studies.

DOPAMINE

Dopamine (DA) is also suspect in the neuropathophysiology of the eating disorders given its reported involvement in the regulation of feeding, mood, activity, perception, sexual/social behaviour, hormone and peptide release and to some extent aggression (Hoebel, 1985; Jimerson *et al.*, 1992; Engstrom *et al.*, 1999; Kaye *et al.*, 1999a). Notably, DA is involved in the hedonic reward responses to eating and its maintenance as well as to other pleasurable activities (Hoebel, 1985; Hoebel *et al.*, 1989; Jimerson *et al.*, 1992).

The majority of studies of DA metabolism in the eating disorders have consistently shown that low-weight AN patients have reduced measures of peripheral and central DA activity, including decreased plasma (Gross *et al.*, 1979) and CSF HVA (Kaye *et al.*, 1984a, 1984b). In BN patients, reduced CSF HVA levels also have been reported in BN patients with frequent binge–purge episodes (Kaye *et al.*, 1990a; Jimerson *et al.*, 1992) but not in those less severely ill. Furthermore, binge frequency was inversely correlated with CSF HVA levels in one study (Jimerson *et al.*, 1992). Upon long-term recovery, normal concentrations of CSF HVA have been reported to normalize in BN (Kaye *et al.*, 1998a, 1998b), while a trend for decreased CSF HVA levels persisted in six restricting AN patients compared to controls and to bingeing and/or purging AN patients (Kaye *et al.*, 1999a). This suggests a possible trait-related disturbance specific to restricting AN, although this finding needs replication given the small sample size. These results could also still be due to nutritional factors given that the patients in this study weighed significantly less than the BN group and may still have been at the low end of the normal weight range.

Anecdotal reports of the successful use of dopaminergic antagonists (typical anti-psychotic agents) in the treatment of AN patients (Dally and Sargant, 1960) have been generally followed by equivocal results in controlled studies (Vandereyken and Pierloot, 1982; Vandereyken, 1984). Atypical anti-psychotic agents may show more promise in the adjunctive treatment of AN given their combined anti-dopaminergic and anti-serotonergic effects (Hansen, 1999; Jensen and Mejlhede, 2000; LaVia, Gray and Kaye, 2000), but the results of placebo-controlled studies remain to be seen.

Genetic investigations into the role of DA have been limited to the Bal I DRD3 receptor polymorphisms in which no differences were found between AN patients and controls (Bruins-Slot *et al.*, 1998). However, the polymorphisms of other genes coding for DA receptors could be tested. Interestingly, Corcos and colleagues (1999) reported significantly lower IgG and IgM autoantibodies to DA in BN patients compared to controls. There was also a trend for lower levels of IgM autoantibodies to DA in the eating disordered group. The relevance of these findings to the pathophysiology of the eating disorders remains uncertain, but invokes possible autoimmune mechanisms.

SEROTONIN

There are several lines of reasoning that point to disturbances of serotonin (5-HT) function in the pathophysiology and neuropsychopharmacology of the EDs (Kaye and Weltzin, 1991b; Brewerton, 1995; Kaye *et al.*, 1999a, 1999b), including its role in feeding (Dourish *et al.*, 1988; Leibowitz, 1999), satiety (Brewerton *et al.*, 1994a, 1994b; Leibowitz and Alexander, 1998), dieting/fasting (Cowen *et al.*, 1996; Cowen and Smith, 1999), mood regulation (Delgado *et al.*, 1990), anxiety (Anderson and Mortimore, 1999), obsessive–compulsiveness/perfectionism/behavioural inhibition (Kaye *et al.*, 1984a), harm avoidance (Brewerton, Hand and Bishop, 1993; Waller *et al.*, 1993) impulsivity/aggression (Linnoila *et al.*, 1983; Coccaro *et al.*, 1989), motor activity (Brewerton *et al.*, 1995a; Epling and Pierci, 1988), gender (Carlsson *et al.*, 1985; Goodwin, Fairburn and Cowen, 1987a), seasonality (Brewerton, 1989; Brewerton *et al.*, 1988a, 1994a, 1994b), body image/perception (Goldbloom and Olmsted, 1993), and social status (Raleigh *et al.*, 1984, 1985; McGuire and Raleigh, 1985) (see Table XXIII-2.1).

Decreases in a variety of 5-HT parameters have been consistently reported in low-weight AN patients. Although no significant differences have been found in absolute plasma L-TRP levels (Russell *et al.*, 1967; Coppen *et al.*, 1976; Hassanyeh and Marshall, 1991), the plasma L-TRP/LNAA ratio is reduced in the low-weight state (Askernazy *et al.*, 1998; Kaye *et al.*, 1984a; Johnston *et al.*, 1984) but normalizes upon short-term weight recovery (Johnston *et al.*, 1984; Kaye *et al.*, 1988b). In BN, Gendall and Joyce (2000) reported that the L-TRP/LNAA ratio inversely correlated with the desire to binge eat. In addition, symptomatic bulimic relapse or worsening of symptoms has been reported following acute L-TRP depletion in BN (Weltzin *et al.*, 1995; Smith, Fairburn and Cowen, 1999; Kaye *et al.*, 2000).

Other significant findings include decreased CSF L-TRP levels (Gerner *et al.*, 1984) and decreased CSF 5-HIAA levels (Kaye *et al.*, 1988b, 1984a; Gillberg, 1983) during low-weight status with normalization of these levels with short-term weight recovery (STWR, goal weight maintenance ≥3 weeks). Following long-term weight recovery (LTWR, goal weight maintenance ≥6–12 months), Kaye and colleagues (1991a, 1999b) have reported increased CSF 5-HIAA levels, which is associated with obsessionality and behavioural inhibition.

In BN, reduced levels of CSF 5-HIAA are consistently reported only in the subgroup of patients with more frequent binge–purge frequencies (Kaye *et al.*, 1990a, Jimerson *et al.*, 1992). In addition, binge frequency was inversely correlated with CSF 5-HIAA concentrations (Jimerson *et al.*, 1992). In a small pilot study, Brewerton and colleagues (1995a, 1995b) have reported no difference in CSF 5-HT levels between BN patients and controls. However,

Table XXIII-2.1 Monoamine involvement in the phenomenology of the eating disorders

	Norepinephrine	Dopamine	Serotonin
Feeding Initiation/Hunger	X		
Feeding Maintenance/Hedonic Reward		X	
Feeding Termination/Satiety			X
Fasting Effects	X	X	X
Activity/Exercise	X	X	X
Impulsivity/Aggression		X	X
Novelty/Sensation Seeking		X	
Mood Regulation	X	X	X
Anxiety	X		X
Harm Avoidance			X
Obsessive–Compulsiveness/Perfectionism			X
Behavioural Inhibition			X
Body Image/Perception		X	X
Social Hierarchy/Rank			X
Metabolic Rate	X		
Temperature	X		X
Blood Pressure/Pulse	X		X
Gender Differences			X
Seasonality/Light Effects			X
Circadian Rhythmicity			X
Age/Developmental Effects			X
Trauma Effects	X		X
Sexual Behaviour		X	X
Hormone Regulation	X	X	X
Neuropeptide Regulation	X	X	X

upon recovery for at least one year, BN patients have been reported to have elevated CSF 5-HIAA levels compared to healthy controls (Kaye *et al.*, 1998b). As in AN, this finding has been linked to obsessive–compulsive personality traits, perfectionism and behavioural inhibition.

Decreased prolactin (PRL) responses following m-CPP (Brewerton *et al.*, 1990; Brewerton and Jimerson, 1996; Hadagan *et al.*, 1996), L-TRP (Brewerton *et al.*, 1990; Brewerton and Jimerson, 1996), and fenfluramine (FEN) (Halmi *et al.*, 1993; Monteleone *et al.*, 1998b) have been reported in AN and indicate an anatomically specific alteration in 5-HT receptor sensitivity at the level of the hypothalamus, which could conceivably also occur in other brain pathways (Brewerton, 1995). Blunting of PRL following m-CPP persist into short-term weight recovery, although there are trends toward normalization with refeeding and weight gain (Brewerton and Jimerson, 1996). With at least a year of recovery, neurohormonal responses to m-CPP normalize in restricting AN patients (Kaye *et al.*, 1999b). Apparently, full normalization of PLR responsivity to serotonergic agents does occur after full weight restoration, normalization of hypothalamic-pituitary-gonadal function, and abatement of overt eating disorder symptoms (Kaye *et al.*, 1999b). However, the appetite-suppressing effect of FEN is significantly diminished in recovered AN patients despite normalization of hormonal release (Ward *et al.*, 1998).

In BN, there is a consistent pattern of PRL blunting following m-CPP (Brewerton *et al.*, 1992b, 1992c; Brewerton, 1995; Levitan *et al.*, 1997), fenfluramine (Halmi *et al.*, 1993; Jimerson *et al.*, 1997; McBride *et al.*, 1991; Monteleone *et al.*, 1998a), and 5-hydroxytryptophan (5-HPT) (Goldbloom *et al.*, 1996), but not L-TRP (Brewerton *et al.*, 1992b, 1992c; Brewerton, 1995). PRL responses following L-TRP are low only in the BN patients with concurrent major depression, again emphasizing the need to control for comorbidity. PRL responses following m-CPP are inversely correlated to baseline cortisol (CORT) (Brewerton, 1995). Self-reported binge frequency also has been reported to be inversely correlated to PRL responses following m-CPP (Brewerton, 1995) and fenfluramine (Jimerson *et al.*, 1997; Monteleone *et al.*, 1998a) in BN patients. Given that this presumed alteration in hypothalamic post-synaptic 5-HT functioning normalizes with recovery from BN (Kaye *et al.*, 1998a, 1998b; Wolfe *et al.*, 2000), these serotonergic abnormalities are likely a *result* of bingeing, purging, and/or dieting rather than a *cause* of these behaviours, although other vulnerabilities of the 5-HT system may also exist and interact with these psychosomatic behaviours. Dieting, bingeing and vomiting all may affect central 5-HT synthesis (Fernstrom, 1985; Goodwin *et al.*, 1987a, 1987b; Kaye *et al.*, 1988a, 1989) and could conceivably result in downregulation of post-synaptic 5-HT receptors and blunted PRL responses. In addition, these behaviours may involve activation of the HPA axis, which in turn appears to dampen 5-HT receptor sensitivity (Brewerton *et al.*, 1992b, 1992c; Brewerton, 1995).

Taken together, research findings from plasma, CSF, and pharmacologic challenge studies suggest reduced 5-HT synthesis, uptake, and turnover, as well as altered post-synaptic 5-HT receptor sensitivity during the active phases of both AN and BN. Consequently, most reported alterations in 5-HT function appear to be state-dependent, although they may play important biological roles in the perpetuation of symptoms, particularly the mood dysregulation, increased anxiety, obsessionality, impulsivity, self-aggression, and perhaps the resistance to and difficulty in learning healthier coping strategies (Riedel *et al.*, 1999).

Interestingly, other findings suggest heightened 5-HT receptor sensitivity in non-recovered eating disorder patients. Brewerton (1995) has reported enhanced temperature and migraine headache responses to m-CPP, but not L-TRP in BN patients (regardless of the comorbid presence of AN or MD) (Brewerton, 1995; Brewerton *et al.*, 1988b, 1992c). As discussed in detail elsewhere (Brewerton *et al.*, 1992c), the enhanced migraine-like HA responses in the BN patients may indicate enhanced 5-HT_2 receptor sensitivity in CNS vascular tissues. Enhanced 5-HT mediated platelet aggregation, a 5-HT_2 receptor mediated phenomenon, has also been reported in BN (Spigset *et al.*, 1999) and AN (Halmi *et al.*, 1993; McBride *et al.*, 1991; Spigset *et al.*, 1999) and lends further support to this hypothesis. The normal cortisol responses following m-CPP and L-TRP in AN and BN are compatible with this view given the involvement of both 5-HT_1 (facilitative) and 5-HT_2 receptors (inhibitive) in cortisol secretion. These presumed alterations in 5-HT receptor sensitivity, whether primary or secondary, demonstrate that 5-HT receptor sensitivity can be both decreased and increased in the same subjects depending on anatomical location of the receptor as well as receptor subtype. Brewerton (1995) has argued in favour of a dysregulation hypothesis of monoamine dysfunction in the eating and related disorders in which there is a failure in transmitter regulation in the face of a variety of psychobiological perturbations potentially affecting monoamine function, including dieting, fasting, purging, substance abuse, excessive exercising, medical illnesses, family stresses or losses, sociocultural pressures, traumatic events, puberty, other developmental tasks/challenges, and changes in the seasons.

A number of other platelet (PLT) studies contribute to the demonstration of serotonergic dysfunction in the eating disorders. Significant increases/reductions in PLT imipramine (IMI) binding (Weizman *et al.*, 1986b), but not PLT 5-HT uptake (Weizman *et al.*, 1986a; Zemishlany *et al.*, 1987) or PLT MAO content (Biederman *et al.*, 1984a, 1984b), have been reported in low-weight AN patients. However, a more recent study reported decreased PLT MAO in AN (Diaz-Marsa *et al.*, 2000), which was inversely correlated with impulsivity and positively correlated with persistence. In BN, platelet studies indicate reduced PLT IMI binding (Marazziti *et al.*, 1988) and PLT MAO (Hallman, Sakurai and Oreland, 1989). PLT 5-HT uptake has been reported to be increased in one study (Goldbloom, Hicks and Garfinkel, 1988) but not another (Hallman, Sakurai and Oreland, 1989). Steiger *et al.* (2000) reported reduced PLT paroxetine binding in a group of BN patients compared to healthy controls regardless of the presence of borderline personality disorder. Whether these changes reflect a central trait-related dysfunction remains unclear and awaits further studies in recovered patients.

In a novel study of indole metabolism, Finocchiaro and colleagues (1995) reported altered phytohaemagglutinin stimulated, light-induced [3H]thymidine incorporation into the DNA of peripheral blood mononuclear leukocytes in AN patients compared to controls. The authors concluded that the white cells of AN patients show a failure in the regulation of 5-HT and melatonin metabolism in response to light.

Genetic investigations into the role of 5-HT in the eating disorders have been more numerous and more promising than other monoamines. Collier *et al.* (1997) reported a statistically significant 5-HT2A-1438G/A receptor gene polymorphism in a group of restricting AN patients compared to healthy controls. This finding has been replicated in at least two other studies in AN (Nacmias *et al.*, 1999; Enoch *et al.*, 1998) as well as in OCD (Enoch *et al.*, 1998), but not in BN (Enoch *et al.*, 1998). Nacmias *et al.* (1999) reported that other serotonergic polymorphisms of the 5-HT2A as well as those of the 5-HT2C receptors showed no differences in AN patients compared to controls. Likewise, no differences between AN patients and controls have been reported for serotonin transporter gene linked polymorphisms (5-HTTLPR) (Hinney *et al.*, 1997; Sundaramurthy *et al.*, 2000), tryptophan hydroxylase polymorphisms (Han *et al.*, 1999), and 5-HT1Dbeta and 5-HT7 gene polymorphisms (Hinney *et al.*, 1999). 5-HT2C receptor polymorphisms showed no differences in allelic variations in a group of patients with BN or binge-eating disorder (BED) (Burnet *et al.*, 1999).

It is well known that serotonin-specific antidepressant medications can be beneficial in controlled studies of BN patients (Fluoxetine Bulimia Nervosa Collaborative Group, 1992), but not in low-weight AN patients (Attia *et al.*, 1998; Strober *et al.*, 1999). More recent data indicate a prophylactic effect of fluoxetine following weight gain in recovered AN patients (Kaye *et al.*, 1998). SSRIs don't work during the low-weight state, presumably because of central depletion of 5-HT and other monoamines with starvation. There is significantly less 5-HT centrally to inhibit the reuptake of.

Finally, recent evidence indicates significant anti-bulimic responses to 5-HT3 antagonists, such as ondansetron (Faris *et al.*, 1998, 2000). Although the authors attribute this therapeutic response to the drug's ability to reduce vagal tone, the role of the 5-HT3 receptor remains intriguing given its anti-anxiety effects (Roychoudhury and Kulkarni, 1997). These findings opens important new arenas for future research involving possible serotonergic–cholinergic mechanisms, which has been a relatively unexplored area in the eating disorders.

MAO/ISATIN

Isatin, or tribulin, is an endogenous indole associated with stress, which inhibits monoamine oxidase (MAO) (Glover *et al.*, 1988). Brewerton *et al.* (1995b) reported significantly higher CSF concentrations of isatin in BN patients compared to healthy controls. There was also a trend for CSF isatin concentrations to be inversely correlated with CSF concentrations of the serotonin metabolite, 5-hydroxyindoleacetic acid (5-HIAA) ($n = 14$, $\rho = -0.51$, $p = 0.06$), although CSF isatin levels were not significantly correlated with CSF MHPG or HVA. The increase in isatin levels has been hypothesized to be in response to the resultant monoamine depletion secondary to the effects of the illness on monoaminergic function. As noted previously, PLT MAO has been reported to be decreased in BN (Hallman, Sakurai and Oreland, 1989) and in AN (Diaz-Marsa *et al.*, 2000). This decrease may represent a compensatory change in response to monoamine depletion during the active state of the disorders.

RELATIONSHIP TO OTHER SYSTEMS

Neurotransmitter systems do not exist in a vacuum but are exquisitely interdependent with other brain and body systems and the environment as well. It is important to think about systems (e.g., 5-HT) and their subsystems (pre-synaptic, post-synaptic, receptor subtypes) in the context of larger systems (brain, environment) and interacting systems/subsystems (e.g., NE, DA, neurohormones, neuropeptides) with complex feedback and counter-feedback mechanisms at multiple anatomical levels. An extensive discussion of this rather far-reaching topic is beyond the scope of this chapter but is discussed in more detail elsewhere (Brewerton, 1995).

CONCLUSIONS

Taken together, available findings implicate abnormalities of all monoamine neurotransmitter systems during the active phases of both AN and BN. Upon normalization of weight and neurohormonal function, most transmitter abnormalities normalize, or at least improve. The strongest data show that dysregulation of 5-HT systems appears to persist and may be related to trait-related psychological characteristics found in both AN and BN that extend beyond classical eating disorder signs and symptoms, such as obsessionality, perfectionism, high harm avoidance and behavioural inhibition. Some evidence suggests prolonged alterations in NE metabolism, but this is most likely due to persistent low-grade dietary restraint following recovery. Preliminary data indicate a DA deficit in restricting AN patients, but this result remains to be replicated in larger samples. Recent findings also emphasize the importance of neurotransmitter precursor substrate availability to normal brain function and especially to the process of recovery from an eating disorder. Future research directions will include further exploration of neurotransmitter-related gene candidates, *in vivo* receptor imaging studies, and improved psychopharmacological interventions based on biological alterations characteristic of the different stages and features of these dangerous disorders.

REFERENCES

Anderson, I.M. and Mortimore, C., 1999. 5-HT and human anxiety: Evidence from studies using acute tryptophan depletion. *Advances in Experimental Medicine & Biology*, **467**, 43–55.

Attia, E., Haiman, C., Walsh, B.T. and Flater, S.R., 1998. Does fluoxetine augment the inpatient treatment of anorexia nervosa? *American Journal of Psychiatry*, **155**, 548–551.

Askenazy, F., Candito, M., Caci, H., Myquel, M., Chambon, P., Darcourt, G. and Puech, A.J., 1998. Whole blood serotonin content, tryptophan concentrations, and impulsivity in anorexia nervosa. *Biological Psychiatry*, **43**, 188–195.

Becker, A.E., Grinspoon, S.K., Klibanski, A. and Herzog, D.B., 1999. Eating disorders. *New England Journal of Medicine*, **340**, 1092–1098.

Biederman, J., Herzog, D.B., Rivinus, T.M., Ferber, R.A., Harper, G.P., Onsulak, P.J. and Schildkrautt, J.J., 1984a. Urinary MHPG in anorexia nervosa patients with and without a concomitant major depressive disorder. *Journal of Psychiatric Research*, **18**, 149–160.

Biederman, J., Rivinus, T.M., Herzog, D.B., Ferber, R.A., Harper, G.P., Onsulak, P.J., Harmatz, J.S. and Schildkrautt, J.J., 1984b. Platelet MAO activity in anorexia nervosa patients with and without a major depressive disorder. *American Journal of Psychiatry*, **141**, 1244–1247.

Blouin, A., Blouin, J., Aubin, P., Carter, J., Goldstein, C., Boyer, H. and Perez, E., 1992. Seasonal patterns of bulimia nervosa. *American Journal of Psychiatry*, **149**, 73–81.

Brewerton, T.D., 1989. Seasonal variation of serotonin function in humans: research and clinical implications. *Annals of Clinical Psychiatry*, **1**, 153–164.

Brewerton, T.D., 1995. Toward a unified theory of serotonin dysregulation in eating and related disorders. *Psychoneuroendocrinology*, **20**, 561–590.

Brewerton, T.D., Berrettini, W., Nurnburger, J. and Linnoila, M., 1988a. An analysis of seasonal fluctuations of CSF monoamines and neuropeptides in normal controls: Findings with 5-HIAA and HVA. *Psychiatry Research*, **23**, 257–265.

Brewerton, T.D., Brandt, H.A., Lesem, D.T., Murphy, D.L. and Jimerson, D.C., 1990. Serotonin in eating disorders. In: Coccaro, E. and Murphy, D. (eds), *Serotonin in Major Psychiatric Disorders*, pp. 153–184. American Psychiatric Press, Washington.

Brewerton, T.D., Hand, L.D. and Bishop, E.R., 1993. The Tridimensional Personality Questionnaire in eating disorder patients. *International Journal of Eating Disorders*, **14**, 213–218.

Brewerton, T.D. and Jimerson, D.C., 1996. Studies of serotonin function in anorexia nervosa. *Psychiatry Research*, **62**, 31–42.

Brewerton, T.D., Krahn, D., Hardin, T.A., Wehr, T.A. and Rosenthal, N.E., 1994a. Findings from the Seasonal Pattern Assessment Questionnaire (SPAQ) in patients with eating disorders and control subjects: effects of diagnosis and location. *Psychiatry Research*, **52**, 71–84.

Brewerton, T.D., Lydiard, R.B., Johnson, M., Ballenger, J.C., Fossey, M., Zealberg, J. and Roberts, J.E., 1995. CSF serotonin: Effects of diagnosis and season. *Biological Psychiatry*, **37**, 655A (Abstract #220).

Brewerton, T.D., Mueller, E.A., Lesem, M.D., Brandt, H.A., Quearry, B., George, D.T., Murphy, D.L. and Jimerson, D.C., 1992b. Neuroendocrine responses to m-chlorophenylpiperazine and L-tryptophan in bulimia. *Archives of General Psychiatry*, **49**, 852–861.

Brewerton, T.D., Murphy, D.L. and Jimerson, D.C., 1994b. Testmeal Responses Following m-chlorophenylpiperazine and L-tryptophan in bulimics and controls. *Neuropsychopharmacology*, **11**, 63–71.

Brewerton, T.D., Murphy, D.L., Lesem, M.D., Brandt, H.A. and Jimerson, D.C., 1992c. Headache responses to m-chlorophenylpiperazine and L-tryptophan in bulimia nervosa. *Headache*, **32**, 217–222.

Brewerton, T.D., Murphy, D.L., Mueller, E.A. and Jimerson, D.C., 1988b. The induction of migraine-like headaches by the serotonin agonist, m-chlorophenylpiperazine. *Clinical Pharmacology and Therapeutics*, **43**, 605–609.

Brewerton, T.D., Stellefson, E.J., Hibbs, N., Hodges, E.J. and Cochrane, C.E., 1995a. A comparison of eating disorder patients with and without compulsive exercising. *International Journal of Eating Disorders*, **17**, 413–416.

Brewerton, T.D., Zealberg, J.L., Lydiard, R.B., Glover, V., Sandler, M. and Ballenger, J.C., 1995b. CSF isatin is elevated in bulimia nervosa. *Biological Psychiatry*, **37**, 481–483.

Brown, G.L., Ebert, M.H., Goyer, P.F., Jimerson, D.C., Klein, W.J., Bunney, W.E. and Goodwin, F.K., 1982. Aggression, suicide, and serotonin: relationships to CSF amine metabolites. *American Journal of Psychiatry*, **139**, 741–746.

Bruins-Slot, L., Gorwood, P., Bouvard, M., Blot, P., Ades, J., Feingold, J., Schwartz, J.C. and Mouren-Simeoni, M.C., 1998. Lack of association between anorexia nervosa and D3 dopamine receptor gene. *Biological Psychiatry*, **43**, 76–78.

Buckholtz, N.S., George, D.T., Davies, A.O., Jimerson, D.C. and Potter, W.Z., 1988. Lymphocyte beta-adrenergic receptor modification in bulimia. *Archives of General Psychiatry*, **45**, 479–482.

Burnet, P.W., Smith, K.A., Cowen, P.J., Fairburn, C.G. and Harrison, P.J., 1999. Allelic variation of the 5-HT2C receptor (HTR2C) in bulimia nervosa and binge eating disorder. *Psychiatric Genetics*, **9**, 101–104.

Carlsson, M., Svensson, K., Eriksson, E. and Carlsson, A., 1985. Rat brain serotonin: biochemical and functional evidence for a sex difference. *Journal of Neural Transmission*, **63**, 297–313.

Casper, R.C., Eckert, E.D., Halmi, D.A., Goldberg, S.C. and Davis, J.M., 1980. Bulimia. Its incidence and clinical importance in patients with anorexia nervosa. *Archives of General Psychiatry*, **37**, 1030–1035.

Coccaro, E.F., Siever, L.J., Klar, H., Maurer, G., Cochrane, K., Cooper, T.B., Mohr, R.C. and Davis, K.L., 1989. Serotonergic studies in affective and personality disorder patients: Correlates with suicidal and impulsive aggressive behavior. *Archives of General Psychiatry*, **46**, 587–599.

Collier, D.A., Arranz, M.J., Mupita, D., Brown, N. and Treasure, J., 1997. Association between the 5-HT2A receptor gene polymorphism and anorexia nervosa. *Lancet*, **350**, 412.

Coppen, A.J., Gupta, R.K., Eccleston, E.G., Wood, K.M., Wakeling, A. and de Sousa, V.F., 1976. Plasma tryptophan in anorexia nervosa. *Lancet*, **1**, 961.

Corcos, M., Atger, F., Levy-Soussan, P., Avrameas, S., Guilbert, B., Cayol, V. and Jeammet, P., 1999. Bulimia Nervosa and autoimmunity. *Psychiatry Research*, **87**, 77–82.

Cowen, P.J., Clifford, E.M., Walsh, A.E., Williams, C. and Fairburn, C.G., 1996. Moderate dieting causes 5-HT2C receptor supersensitivity. *Psychological Medicine*, **26**, 1155–1159.

Cowen, P.J. and Smith, K.A., 1999. Serotonin, dieting, and bulimia nervosa. *Advances in Experimental Medicine & Biology*, **467**, 101–104.

Deldago, P.L., Charney, D.S., Price, L.H., Aghajanian, G.K., Landis, H. and Henninger, G.R., 1990. Serotonin function and the mechanism of antidepressant action: reversal of antidepressant-induced remission by rapid depletion of plasma tryptophan. *Archives of General Psychiatry*, **47**, 411–418.

Diaz-Marsa, M., Carrasco, J.L., Hollander, E., Cesar, J. and Saiz-Ruiz, J., 2000. Decreased platelet monoamine oxidase activity in female anorexia nervosa. *Acta Psychiatrica Scandinavica*, **101**, 226–230.

Dourish, C.T., Cooper, S.J., Gilbert, F., Coughlan, J. and Iversen, S.D., 1988. The 5-HT_{1A} agonist 8-OH-DPAT increases consumption of palatable wet mash and liquid diets in the rat. *Psychopharmacology*, **94**, 58–63.

Engstrom, G., Alling, C., Blennow, K., Regnell, G. and Traskman-Bendz, L., 1999. Reduced cerebrospinal HVA concentrations and HVA/5-HIAA ratios in suicide attempters: Monoamine metabolites in 120 suicide attempters and 47 controls. *European Neuropsychopharmacology*, **9**, 399–405.

Enoch, M.A., Kaye, W.H., Rotondo, A., Greenberg, B.D., Murphy, D.L. and Goldman, D., 1998. 5-HT2A promoter polymorphism −1438G/A, anorexia nervosa, and obsessive–compulsive disorder. *Lancet*, **351**, 1785.

Epling, F. and Pierci, D., 1988. Activity-based anorexia: a biological perspective. *International Journal of Eating Disorders*, **7**, 475–485.

Faris, P.L., Kim, S.W., Meller, W.H., Goodale, R.L., Hofbauer, R.D., Oakman, S.A., Howard, L.A., Stevens, E.R., Eckert, E.D. and Hartman, B.K., 1998. Effect of ondansetron, a 5-HT3 receptor antagonist, on the dynamic association between bulimic behaviors and pain thresholds. *Pain*, **77**, 297–303.

Faris, P.L., Kim, S.W., Meller, W.H., Goodale, R.L., Oakman, S.A., Hofbauer, R.D., Marshall, A.M., Daughters, R.S., Banerjee-Stevens, D., Eckert, E.D. and Hartman, B.K., 2000. Effect of decreasing afferent vagal activity with ondansetron on symptoms of bulimia nervosa: a randomised, double-blind trial. *Lancet*, **355**, 792–797.

Fernstrom, J.D., 1985. Dietary effects on brain serotonin synthesis: relationship to appetite regulation. *American Journal of Clinical Nutrition*, **42**, 1072–1082.

Ferrari, E., Fraschini, F. and Brambilla, F., 1990. Hormonal circadian rhythms in eating disorders. *Biological Psychiatry*, **27**, 1007–1020.

Finocchiaro, L.M., Polack, E., Nahmod, V.E. and Glikin, G.C., 1995. Cultured peripheral blood mononuclear leukocytes from anorexia nervosa patients are refractory to visible light. *Life Sciences*, **57**, 559–569.

Fluoxetine Bulimia Nervosa Collaborative Group, 1992. Fluoxetine in the treatment of bulimia nervosa: A multicenter, placebo-controlled, double-blind trial. *Archives of General Psychiatry*, **49**, 139–147.

Garfinkel, P.E., Moldofsky, H. and Garner, D.M., 1980. The heterogeneity of anorexia nervosa: Bulimia as a distinct subgroup. *Archives of General Psychiatry*, **37**, 1036–1040.

Gendall, K.A. and Joyce, P.R., 2000. Meal-induced changes in tryptophan : LNAA ratio: Effects on craving and binge eating. *Eating Behaviors*, **1**, 53–62.

George, D.T., Kaye, W.H., Goldstein, D.S., Brewerton, T.D. and Jimerson, D.C., 1990. Altered norepinephrine regulation in bulimia: effects of pharmacological challenge with isoproterenol. *Psychiatry Research*, **33**, 1–10.

Gerner, R.H., Cohen, D.J., Fairbanks, L., Anderson, G.M., Young, J.G., Scheinin, M., Linnoila, M., Shaywitz, B.A. and Hare, T.A., 1984. CSF neurochemistry of women with anorexia nervosa and normal women. *American Journal of Psychiatry*, **141**, 948–949.

Gill, J., DeSouza, V., Wakeling, A., Dandona, P. and Jeremy, J.Y., 1992. Differential changes in alpha- and beta-adrenoceptor linked [$^{45}Ca^{2+}$] uptake in platelets from patients with anorexia nervosa. *Journal of Clinical Endocrinology & Metabolism*, **74**, 441–446.

Gillberg, C., 1983. Low dopamine and serotonin levels in anorexia nervosa. *American Journal of Psychiatry*, **140**, 948–949.

Goldbloom, D.S., Garfinkel, P.E., Katz, R. and Brown, G.M., 1996. The hormonal response to intravenous 5-hydroxytryptophan in bulimia nervosa. *Journal of Psychosomatic Research*, **40**, 289–297.

Goldbloom, D.S., Hicks, L.K. and Garfinkel, P.E., 1988. Platelet serotonin uptake in bulimia nervosa. *Biological Psychiatry*, **28**, 644–647.

Goldbloom, D.S. and Olmsted, M.P., 1993. Pharmacotherapy of bulimia nervosa with fluoxetine: assessment of clinically significant attitudinal change. *American Journal of Psychiatry*, **50**, 770–774.

Goodwin, G.M., Cowen, P.J., Fairburn, C.G., Parry-Billings, M., Calder, P.C. and Newsholme, E.A., 1990. Plasma concentrations of tryptophan and dieting. *British Medical Journal*, **300**, 1499–1500.

Goodwin, G.M., Fairburn, C.G. and Cowen, P.J., 1987a. Dieting changes serotonergic function in women, not men: implications for the etiology of anorexia nervosa. *Psychological Medicine*, **17**, 839–842.

Goodwin, G.M., Fairburn, C.G. and Cowen, P.J., 1987b. The effects of dieting and weight loss upon neuroendocrine responses to tryptophan, clonidine and apomorphine in volunteers: important implications for neuroendocrine investigations in depression. *Archives of General Psychiatry*, **44**, 952–957.

Goodwin, G.M., Fraser, S., Stump, K., Fairburn, C.G., Elliott, J.M. and Cowen, P.J., 1987c. Dieting and weight loss in volunteers increases the number of $alpha_2$-adrenoceptors and 5-HT receptors on blood platelets without effect on [^{3}H]imipramine binding. *Journal of Affective Disorders*, **12**, 267–274.

Gross, H.A., Lake, C.R., Ebert, M.H., Ziegler, M.G. and Kopin, I.J., 1979. Catecholamine metabolism in primary anorexia nervosa. *Journal of Clinical Endocrinology & Metabolism*, **49**, 805–809.

Gwirtsman, H.E., Guze, B.H., Yager, J. *et al.*, 1990. Fluoxetine treatment of anorexia nervosa: an open clinical trial. *Journal of Clinical Psychiatry*, **51**, 378–382.

Hadigan, C.M., Walsh, B.T., Buttinger, C. and Hollander, E., 1995. Behavioral and neuroendocrine responses to metaCPP in anorexia nervosa. *Biological Psychiatry*, **37**, 504–511.

Hallman, J., Sakurai, E. and Oreland, L., 1989. Blood platelet monoamine oxidase activity, serotonin uptake and release rates in anorexia and bulimia patients and in healthy controls. *Acta Psychiatrica Scandanavica*, **81**, 73–77.

Halmi, K.A., 1981. Catecholamine metabolism in anorexia nervosa. *International Journal of Psychiatry in Medicine*, **11**, 251–254.

Halmi, K.A., Dekirmenjian, H., Dav, J.M., Casper, R. and Goldberg, S., 1978. Catecholamine metabolism in anorexia nervosa. *Archives of General Psychiatry*, **35**, 458–460.

Halmi, K.A., Sunday, S.R., Strober, M., Kaplan, A., Woodside, D.B., Fichter, M., Treasure, J., Berrettini, W.H. and Kaye, W.H., 2000. Perfectionism in anorexia nervosa: Variation by clinical subtype, obsessionality, and pathological eating behavior. *American Journal of Psychiatry*, **157**, 1799–1805.

Han, L., Nielsen, D.A., Rosenthal, N.E., Jefferson, K., Kaye, W., Murphy, D., Altemus, M., Humphries, J., Cassano, G., Rotondo, A., Virkkunen, M., Linnoila, M. and Goldman, D., 1999. No coding variant of the tryptophan hydroxylase gene detected in seasonal affective disorder, obsessive–compulsive disorder, anorexia nervosa, and alcoholism. *Biological Psychiatry*, **45**, 615–619.

Hansen, L., 1999. Olanzapine in the treatment of anorexia nervosa. *British Journal of Psychiatry*, **175**, 592.

Hardin, T.A., Wehr, T.A., Brewerton, T.D., Kasper, S., Berrettini, W., Rabkin, J. and Rosenthal, N.E., 1991. Evaluation of seasonality in six clinical populations and two normal populations. *Journal of Psychiatric Research*, **25**, 75–87.

Hassanyeh, F. and Marshall, E.F., 1991. Measures of serotonin metabolism in anorexia nervosa. *Acta Psychiatrica Scandinavica*, **84**, 561–563.

Heufelder, A., Warnhoff, M. and Pirke, K.M., 1985. Platelet alpha 2-adrenoceptor and adenylate cyclase in patients with anorexia nervosa and bulimia. *Journal of Clinical Endocrinology & Metabolism*, **61**, 1053–1060.

Hinney, A., Barth, N., Ziegler, A., von Prittwitz, S., Hamann, A., Hennighausen, K., Pirke, K.M., Heils, A., Rosenkranz, K., Roth, H., Coners, H., Mayer, H., Herzog, W., Siegfried, A., Lehmkuhl, G., Poustka, F., Schmidt, M.H., Schafer, H., Grzeschik, K.H., Lesch, K.P., Lentes, K.U., Remschmidt, H. and Hebebrand, J., 1997. Serotonin transporter gene-linked polymorphic region, allele distributions in relationship to body weight and in anorexia nervosa. *Life Sciences*, **61**, 295–303.

Hinney, A., Herrmann, H., Lohr, T., Rosenkranz, K., Ziegler, A., Lehmkuhl, G., Poustka, F., Schmidt, M.H., Mayer, H., Siegfried, W., Remschmidt, H. and Hebebrand, J., 1999. No evidence for an involvement of alleles of polymorphisms in the serotonin1Dbeta and 7 genes in obesity, underweight or anorexia nervosa. *International Journal of Obesity and Related Metabolic Disorders*, **23**, 760–763.

Hoebel, B.G., 1985. Brain neurotransmitters in food and drug reward. *American Journal of Clinical Nutrition*, **42**, 1133–1150.

Hoebel, B.G., Hernandez, L., Schwartz, D.H., Mark, P. and Hunter, G.A., 1989. Microdialysis studies of brain norepinephrine, serotonin, and dopamine release during ingestive behavior. *The Psychobiology of Human Eating Disorders. Annals of the New York Academy of Sciences*, Vol. 575, pp. 171–193.

Jensen, V.S. and Mejlhede, A., 2000. Anorexia nervosa: treatment with olanzapine. *British Journal of Psychiatry*, **177**, 87.

Jimerson, D.C., George, D.T., Kaye, W., Brewerton, T.D. and Goldstein, D.S., 1987. Norepinephrine regulation in bulimia. In: Hudson, J.I. and Pope, H.G. (eds), *Psychobiology of Bulimia*, pp. 145–146. American Psychiatric Press, Washington.

Jimerson, D.C., Lesem, M.D., Kaye, W.H. and Brewerton, T.D., 1992. Low serotonin and dopamine metabolite concentrations in CSF from bulimic patients with frequent binge episodes. *Archives of General Psychiatry*, **49**, 132–138.

Jimerson, D.C., Wolfe, B.E., Metzger, E.D., Finkelstein, D.M., Cooper, T.B. and Levine, J.M., 1997. Decreased serotonin function in bulimia nervosa. *Archives of General Psychiatry*, **54**, 529–534.

Johnston, J.L., Leiter, L.A., Burrow, G.N., Garfinkel, P.E. and Anderson, G.H., 1984. Excretion of urinary catecholamine metabolites in anorexia nervosa: effect of body composition and energy intake. *American Journal of Clinical Nutrition*, **40**, 1001–1006.

Kassett, J.A., Gershon, E.S., Maxwell, M.E., Guroff, J.J., Kazuba, D.M., Smith, A.L., Brandt, H.A. and Jimerson, D.C., 1989. Psychiatric disorders in the first-degree relatives of probands with bulimia nervosa. *American Journal of Psychiatry*, **146**, 1468–1471.

Kaye, W.H., Ballenger, J.C., Lydiard, R.B., Stuart, G.W., Laraia, M.T., O'Neil, P., Fossey, M.D., Stevens, V., Lesser, S. and Hsu, G., 1990a. CSF monoamine levels in normal-weight bulimia: evidence for abnormal noradrenergic activity. *American Journal of Psychiatry*, **147**, 225–229.

Kaye, W.H., Ebert, M.H., Gwirtsman, H.E. and Weiss, S.R., 1984a. Differences in brain serotonergic metabolism between nonbulimic and bulimic patients with anorexia nervosa. *American Journal of Psychiatry*, **141**, 1598–1601.

Kaye, W.H., Ebert, M.H., Raleigh, M. and Lake, C.R., 1984b. Abnormalities in CNS monoamine metabolism in anorexia nervosa. *Archives of General Psychiatry*, **41**, 350–355.

Kaye, W.H., Gendall, K.A., Fernstrom, M.H., Fernstrom, J.D., McConaha, C.W. and Weltzin, T.E., 2000. Effects of acute tryptophan depletion on mood in bulimia nervosa. *Biological Psychiatry*, **47**, 151–157.

Kaye, W.H., Gendall, K.A. and Strober, M., 1998a. Serotonin neuronal function and selective reuptake inhibitor treatment in anorexia nervosa and bulimia nervosa. *Biological Psychiatry*, **44**, 825–838.

Kaye, W.H., George, D.T., Gwirtsman, H.E., Jimerson, D.C., Goldstein, D.S., Ebert, M.H. and Lake, C.R., 1990b. Isoproterenol infusion test in anorexia nervosa: assessment of pre- and post-beta-noradrenergic receptor activity. *Psychopharmacology Bulletin*, **26**, 355–359.

Kaye, W.H., Greeno, C.G., Moss, H., Fernstrom, J., Fernstrom, M., Lilenfeld, L.R., Weltzin, T.E. and Mann, J.J., 1998b. Alterations in serotonin activity and psychiatric symptoms after recovery from bulimia nervosa. *Archives of General Psychiatry*, **55**, 927–935.

Kaye, W.H., Guido, K.W.F., Frank, G.K. and McConaha, C., 1999a. Altered dopamine activity after recovery from restricting anorexia nervosa. *Neuropsychopharmacology*, **21**, 503–506.

Kaye, W.H., Gwirtsman, H.E., Brewerton, T.D., George, D.T., Jimerson, D.C. and Wurtman, R.J., 1988a. Bingeing behavior and plasma amino acids: a possible involvement of brain serotonin in bulimia. *Psychiatry Research*, **23**, 31–43.

Kaye, W.H., Gwirtsman, H.E., George, D.T., Jimerson, D.C. and Ebert, M.H., 1988b. CSF 5-HIAA concentrations in anorexia nervosa: reduced values in underweight subjects normalize after weight gain. *Biological Psychiatry*, **23**, 102–105.

Kaye, W.H., Gwirtsman, H.E. and George, D.T., 1989. The effects of bingeing and vomiting on hormonal secretion. *Biological Psychiatry*, **25**, 768–780.

Kaye, W.H., Gwirtsman, H.E., George, D.T. and Ebert, M.H., 1991a. Altered serotonin activity in anorexia nervosa after long-term weight restoration. *Archives of General Psychiatry*, **48**, 556–562.

Kaye, W.H., Gwirtsman, H.E., George, D.T., Jimerson, D.C., Ebert, M.H. and Lake, C.R., 1990c. Disturbances of noradrenergic systems in normal weight bulimia: relationship to diet and menses. *Biological Psychiatry*, **27**, 4–21.

Kaye, W.H., Jimerson, D.C., Lake, C.R. and Ebert, M.H., 1988b. Altered norepinephrine metabolism following long-term weight recovery in patients with anorexia nervosa. *Psychiatry Research*, **14**, 333–342.

Kaye, W., Strober, M., Stein, D. and Gendall, K., 1999b. New directions in treatment research of anorexia and bulimia nervosa. *Biological Psychiatry*, **45**, 1285–1292.

Kaye, W.H. and Weltzin, T.E., 1991b. Serotonin activity in anorexia and bulimia nervosa: relationship to the modulation of feeding and mood. *Journal of Clinical Psychiatry*, **52**(suppl), 41–48.

Kaye, W.H., Weltzin, T.E., Hsu, L.K.G. and Bulik, C.M., 1991c. An open trial of fluoxetine in patients with anorexia nervosa. *Journal of Clinical Psychiatry*, **52**, 464–471.

Koo-Loeb, J.H., Pedersen, C. and Girdler, S.S., 1998. Blunted cardiovascular and catecholamine stress reactivity in women with bulimia nervosa. *Psychiatry Research*, **80**, 13–27.

Laessle, R.G., Schweiger, U. and Pirke, K.M., 1988. Mood and orthostatic norepinephrine response in anorexia nervosa. *Psychiatry Research*, **24**, 87–94.

Lam, R., Goldner, E.M., Solyom, L. and Resnick, R.A., 1994. A controlled study of light therapy for bulimia nervosa. *American Journal of Psychiatry*, **151**, 744–750.

LaVia, M., Gray, N. and Kaye, W.H., 2000. Case reports of olanzapine treatment of anorexia nervosa. *International Journal of Eating Disorders*, **27**, 363–366.

Leibowitz, S.F. and Alexander, J.T., 1998. Hypothalamic serotonin in control of eating behavior, meal size, and body weight. *Biological Psychiatry*, **44**, 851–864.

Lesem, M.D., George, D.T., Kaye, W.H., Goldstein, D.S. and Jimerson, D.C., 1989. State-related changes in norepinephrine regulation in anorexia nervosa. *Biological Psychiatry*, **25**, 509–512.

Levitan, R.D., Kaplan, A.S., Joffe, R.T. and Levitt, A.J., 1997. Hormonal and subjective responses to intravenous meta-chlorophenylpiperazine in bulimia nervosa. *Archives of General Psychiatry*, **54**, 521–527.

Lilenfeld, L.R., Kaye, W.H., Greeno, C.G., Merikangas, K.R., Plotnicov, K., Pollice, C., Radhika, R., Strober, M., Bulik, C. and Nagy, L., 1998. A controlled family study of anorexia nervosa and bulimia nervosa. *Archives of General Psychiatry*, **55**, 603–610.

Linnoila, M., Virkhunen, M., Scheinin, M., Nuutila, A., Rimon, R. and Goodwin, F.K., 1983. Low cerebrospinal fluid 5-hydroxyindoleacetic acid concentration differentiates impulsive from nonimpulsive violent behavior. *Life Sciences*, **33**, 2609–2614.

Lonati-Galligani, M. and Pirke, K.M., 1986. Beta 2-adrenergic receptor regulation in circulating mononuclear leukocytes in anorexia nervosa and bulimia. *Psychiatry Research*, **19**, 189–198.

Luck, P., Mikhailid, D.P., Dashwood, M.R., Barradas, M.A., Sever, P.S., Dandona, P. and Wakeling, A., 1983. Platelet hyperaggregability and increased alpha-adrenoceptor density in anorexia nervosa. *Journal of Clinical Endocrinology & Metabolism*, **57**, 911–914.

Marazziti, D., Macchi, E., Rotondo, A., Placidi, G.F. and Cassano, G.B., 1988. Involvement of serotonin system in bulimia. *Life Sciences*, **43**, 2123–2126.

McBride, P.A., Anderson, G.M., Khait, V.D., Sunday, S.R. and Halmi, K.A., 1991. Serotonergic responsivity in eating disorders. *Psychopharmacology Bulletin*, **27**, 365–372.

McGuire, M.T. and Raleigh, M.J., 1985. Serotonin-behavior interactions in vervet monkeys. *Psychopharmacology Bulletin*, **21**, 458–463.

Monteleone, P., Brambilla, F., Bortolot, F., Ferraro, C. and Maj, M., 1998a. Plasma prolactin response to D-fenfluramine blunted in bulimic patients with frequent binge episodes. *Psychological Medicine*, **28**, 975–983.

Monteleone, P., Brambilla, F., Bortolot, F., La Rocca, A. and Maj, M., 1998b. Prolactin response to d-fenfluramine blunted in people with anorexia nervosa. *British Journal of Psychiatry*, **172**, 439–442.

Nacmias, B., Ricca, V., Tedde, A., Mezzani, B., Rotella, C.M. and Sorbi, S., 1999. 5-HT2A receptor gene polymorphisms in anorexia nervosa and bulimia nervosa. *Neuroscience Letters*, **277**, 134–136.

Nielsen, S., 1992. Seasonal variation in anorexia nervosa? Some preliminary findings from a neglected area of research. *International Journal of Eating Disorders*, **11**, 25–35.

Obarzanek, E., Lesem, M.D., Goldstein, D.S. and Jimerson, D.C., 1991. Reduced resting metabolic rate in patients with bulimia nervosa. *Archives of General Psychiatry*, **48**, 456–462.

O'Dwyer, A.M., Lucey, J.V. and Russell, G.F., 1996. Serotonin activity in anorexia nervosa after long-term weight restoration: response to D-fenfluramine challenge. *Psychological Medicine*, **26**, 353–359.

Pahl, J., Pirke, K.M., Schweiger, U., Warnhoff, M., Gerlinghoff, M., Brinkmann, W., Berger, M. and Krieg, C., 1985. Anorectic behavior, mood, and metabolic and endocrine adaptation to starvation in anorexia nervosa during inpatient treatment. *Biological Psychiatry*, **20**, 874–887.

Pirke, K.M., 1996. Central and peripheral noradrenalin regulation in eating disorders. *Psychiatry Research*, **62**, 43–49.

Pirke, K.M., Eckert, M., Ofers, B., Goebl, G., Spyra, B., Schweiger, U., Tuschl, R.J. and Fichter, M.M., 1989. Plasma norepinephrine response to exercise in bulimia, anorexia nervosa, and controls. *Biological Psychiatry*, **25**, 799–802.

Pirke, K.M., Kellner, M., Philipp, E., Laessle, R., Krieg, J.C. and Fichter, M.M., 1992. Plasma norepinephrine after a standardized test meal in acute and remitted patients with anorexia nervosa and in healthy controls. *Biological Psychiatry*, **31**, 1074–1077.

Pirke, K.M., Platte, P., Laessle, R., Seidl, M. and Fichter, M.M., 1992. The effect of a mental challenge test of plasma norepinephrine and cortisol in bulimia nervosa and in controls. *Biological Psychiatry*, **32**, 202–206.

Pirke, K.M., Jorg, P., Schweiger, U. and Warnhoff, M., 1985. Metabolic and endocrine indices of starvation in bulimia: a comparison with anorexia nervosa. *Psychiatry Research*, **15**, 33–39.

Pollice, C., Kaye, W.H., Greeno, C.G. and Weltzin, T.E., 1997. Relationship of depression, anxiety, and obsessionality to state of illness in anorexia nervosa. *International Journal of Eating Disorders*, **21**, 367–376.

Raleigh, M.J., Brammer, G.L., McGuire, M.T. and Yuwiler, A., 1985. Dominant social status facilitates the behavioral effects of serotonergic agonists. *Brain Research*, **348**, 274–282.

Raleigh, M.J., McGuire, M.T., Brammer, G.L. and Yuwiler, A., 1984. Social and environmental influences on blood serotonin concentrations in monkeys. *Archives of General Psychiatry*, **41**, 405–410.

Riedel, W.J., Klaassen, T., Deutz, N.E., van Someren, A. and van Praag, H.M., 1999. Tryptophan depletion in normal volunteers produces selective impairment in memory consolidation. *Psychopharmacology*, **141**, 362–369.

Rowland, N.E., Morien, A. and Li, B.H., 1996. The physiology and brain mechanisms of feeding. *Nutrition*, **12**, 626–639.

Roychoudhury, M. and Kulkarni, S.K., 1997. Anti-anxiety profile of ondansetron, a selective 5-HT3 antagonist, in a novel animal model. *Methods & Findings in Experimental & Clinical Pharmacology*, **19**, 107–111.

Smith, K.A., Fairburn, C.G. and Cowen, P.J., 1999. Symptomatic relapse in bulimia nervosa following acute tryptophan depletion. *Archives of General Psychiatry*, **56**, 171–176.

Sorbi, S., Nacmias, B., Tedde, A., Ricca, V., Mezzani, B. and Rotella, C.M., 1998. 5-HT2A promoter polymorphism in anorexia nervosa. *Lancet*, **351**, 1785.

Spigset, O., Andersen, T., Hagg, S. and Mjondal, T., 1999. Enhanced platelet serotonin 5-HT2A receptor binding in anorexia nervosa and bulimia nervosa. *European Neuropsychopharmacology*, **9**, 469–473.

Steiger, H., Leonard, S., Kin, N.Y., Ladouceur, C., Ramdoyal, D. and Young, S.N., 2000. Childhood abuse and platelet tritiated-paroxetine binding in bulimia nervosa: implications of borderline personality disorder. *Journal of Clinical Psychiatry*, **61**, 428–435,

Strober, M., 1981. The significance of bulimia in juvenile anorexia nervosa: an exploration of possible etiologic factors. *International Journal of Eating Disorders*, **1**, 28–43.

Strober, M., Freeman, R., Lampert, C., Diamond, J. and Kaye, W.H., 2000. Controlled family study of anorexia nervosa and bulimia nervosa: Evidence of shared liability and transmission of partial syndromes. *American Journal of Psychiatry*, **157**, 393–401.

Strober, M., Pataki, C., Freeman, R. and DeAntonio, M., 1999. No effect of adjunctive fluoxetine on eating behavior or weight phobia during the inpatient treatment of anorexia nervosa: an historical case-control study. *Journal of Child & Adolescent Psychopharmacology*, **9**, 195–201.

Sundaramurthy, D., Pieri, L.F., Gape, H., Markham, A.F. and Campbell, D.A., 2000. Analysis of serotonin transporter gene linked polymorphism (5-HTTLPR) in anorexia nervosa. *American Journal of Medical Genetics*, **96**, 53–55.

Vandereycken, W. and Pierloot, R., 1982. Pimozide combined with behavior therapy in the short-term treatment of anorexia nervosa. A double-blind placebo-controlled cross-over study. *Acta Psychiatrica Scandinavica*, **66**, 445–450.

Vandereycken, W., 1984. Neuroleptics in the short-term treatment of anorexia nervosa: A double-blind placebo-controlled, cross-over trial with sulpride. *British Journal of Psychiatry*, **144**, 288–292.

von Ranson, K.M., Kaye, W.H., Weltzin, T.E., Rao, R. and Matsunaga, H., 1999. Obsessive–Compulsive Disorder symptoms before and after recovery from bulimia nervosa. *American Journal of Psychiatry*, **156**, 1703–1708.

Waller, D.A., Gullion, C.M., Petty, F., Hardy, B.W., Murdock, M.V. and Rush, A.J., 1993. Tridimensional Personality Questionnaire and serotonin in bulimia nervosa. *Psychiatry Research*, **48**, 9–15.

Walsh, B.T. and Devlin, M.J., 1998. Eating disorders: progress and problems. *Science*, **280**, 1387–1390.

Ward, A., Brown, N., Lightman, S., Campbell, I.C. and Treasure, J., 1998. Neuroendocrine, appetitive and behavioural responses to d-fenfluramine in women recovered from anorexia nervosa. *British Journal of Psychiatry*, **172**, 351–358.

Weizman, R., Carmi, M., Tyano, S., Apter, A. and Rehavi, M., 1986b. High affinity [^{3}H]imipramine binding and serotonin uptake to platelets of adolescent females suffering from anorexia nervosa. *Life Sciences*, **38**, 1235–1242.

Weltzin, T.E., Fernstrom, M.H., Fernstrom, J.D., Neuberger, S.K. and Kaye, W.H., 1995. Acute tryptophan depletion and increased food intake and irritability in bulimia nervosa. *American Journal of Psychiatry*, **152**, 1668–1671.

Wolfe, B.E., Metzger, E.D., Levine, J.M., Finkelstein, D.M., Cooper, T.B. and Jimerson, D.C., 2000. Serotonin function following remission from bulimia nervosa. *Neuropsychopharmacology*, **22**, 257–263.

Zemishlany, Z., Modai, I., Apter, A., Jerushalmy, Z., Samuel, E. and Tyano, S., 1987. Serotonin (5-HT) uptake by blood platelets in anorexia nervosa. *Acta Psychiatrica Scandanavica*, **75**, 127–130.

XXIII-3

Neuroendocrinology

Frances Connan

INTRODUCTION

Although over a single day food intake is poorly matched to energy expenditure, longer term food intake and energy expenditure can be extremely well balanced such that weight may remain remarkably stable over time (Edholm, 1977). However, the systems governing energy homeostasis appear to function more effectively to defend against starvation than they do in defence of overweight. Indeed, it has been argued that the capacity of the system to maintain healthy weight in the face of high availability of energy dense food and low physical activity levels is poor: there is a marked tendency to over consume, resulting in a high prevalence of obesity (Pinel *et al.*, 2000). In addition to the significant morbidity associated with obesity in its own right, a tendency toward overweight may be a vulnerability factor for the most common of the eating disorders, bulimia nervosa (BN) and binge-eating disorder (BED). These disorders are associated with elevated subjective reward value of food (Karhunen *et al.*, 1997a; Wisniewski *et al.*, 1997), reduced subjective sense of satiety (Kissileff *et al.*, 1996) and premorbid or family history of obesity (Fairburn *et al.*, 1997, 1998).

At the other end of the weight spectrum, anorexia nervosa (AN) is characterized by reduced food intake, but the question of whether appetite is impaired remains controversial and poorly researched. Studies employing subjective assessment have consistently reported reduced hunger and desire to eat and enhanced satiety and sensation of fullness in people with AN (e.g., Halmi and Sunday, 1991; Robinson, 1989). Furthermore, the subjective reward value of food is reduced (Drewnowski *et al.*, 1987; Sunday and Halmi, 1990), and the rate of eating is slow (Halmi and Sunday, 1991). Some authors argue that these findings reflect tight cognitive control of normal appetite (Palmer, 2000). However, relative to healthy comparison women, those with AN show reduced salivation (LeGoff *et al.*, 1988) and a heightened autonomic response to food (Leonard *et al.*, 1998). Images of food elicit fear and disgust (Ellison *et al.*, 1998). These objective data suggest that appetite may indeed be impaired in AN (Pinel *et al.*, 2000), although some capacity to respond to hunger and satiety cues clearly remains (Cugini *et al.*, 1998; Rolls *et al.*, 1992). A predisposition to leanness may be a risk factor for AN (Hebebrand and Remschmidt, 1995), supporting the notion that heritable risk for the disorder may be exerted through the biological systems regulating appetite and weight.

If we are to understand the neuroendocrinology of appetite and weight regulation in eating disorders, we must first understand the normal function of these systems and their responses to changes in body weight. It is well recognized that starvation causes profound changes in neuroendocrine systems and thus many of the findings associated particularly with AN, are liable to be consequence rather than cause of the disorder. Accordingly, the first section provides an overview of current models for understanding the neuroendocrine regulation of appetite and weight. Subsequent sections examine neuroendocrine data relating to each of the eating disorders in turn before presenting a synthesis and considering the implications for treatment and future research.

SECTION 1: REGULATION OF APPETITE AND WEIGHT

Leptin — A Peripheral Energy Sensor

The discovery of leptin in 1995 led to dramatic advances in the understanding of central pathways regulating appetite and weight. Leptin is a 146 amino acid protein that is synthesized and secreted by fat cells. When energy balance is stable, leptin concentration is proportional to fat mass (Considine *et al.*, 1996). However, acute changes in energy balance modulate leptin expression, such that fasting is associated with a greater fall in leptin than might be expected for the change in fat mass and conversely, overeating results in an enhanced postprandial rise in circulating leptin (Ahima *et al.*, 1996; Kolaczynski *et al.*, 1996a). The leptin system therefore responds to potential weight change before fat mass actually changes.

The importance of leptin as a signal of energy balance is demonstrated by genetic strains of mice lacking functional leptin (*ob/ob* mice) or its receptor (*db/db* mice). These animals are hyperphagic, hypothermic, hyperinsulinaemic and obese (Chua-SC *et al.*, 1996; Lee *et al.*, 1996; Zhang *et al.*, 1994). Although rare, genetic deficits of leptin signalling in humans are associated with a similar phenotype (Clement *et al.*, 1998; Montague *et al.*, 1997). Exogenous leptin administration reduces food intake and weight in normal and leptin deficient individuals (Farooqi *et al.*, 1999; Halaas *et al.*, 1997; Pelleymounter *et al.*, 1995). Thus, despite the obese phenotype, genetic leptin deficiency is actually a model of starvation: reduced leptin levels signal reduced fat mass and appetite is appropriately elevated.

Leptin enters the brain via an active transport mechanism and its functional long-arm receptors are located in areas of the hypothalamus, such as the arcuate, ventromedial, paraventricular and dorsomedial nuclei (Elmquist *et al.*, 1998): areas important for the function of neuroendocrine systems, including those regulating appetite and weight. The leptin system is therefore an excellent candidate for a peripheral signal of energy homeostasis and adequacy of fat stores to central systems coordinating the adaptive response to starvation.

Other Peripheral Signals of Energy Homeostasis

Several other peripheral hormones play a significant role in the central regulation of appetite. Insulin was one of the first hormonal signals known to be secreted in proportion to adipose mass. Insulin is actively transported across the blood–brain barrier and both insulin receptor mRNA and specific insulin binding sites

Biological Psychiatry: Edited by H. D'haenen, J.A. den Boer and P. Willner. ISBN 0-471-49198-5

have been demonstrated in regions of the brain important in the control of appetite such as the arcuate nucleus of the hypothalamus (Werther *et al.*, 1987). Chronic central infusion of insulin dose-dependently reduces daily food intake (Chavez *et al.*, 1995; Foster *et al.*, 1991). This effect is not immediate and is maximal only after 24 hours. Central administration of insulin not only reduces appetite but also activates brown fat thermogenesis and increases energy expenditure (Muller *et al.*, 1997). Animals that are insulin deficient show marked hyperphagia and this effect can be reversed by central administration of insulin (Sipols *et al.*, 1995). Central administration of anti-insulin antibodies enhances appetite and weight gain in normal animals (Strubbe and Mein, 1977).

Reciprocal regulatory effects have been demonstrated between leptin and insulin. Insulin has a delayed stimulatory effect on adipocyte leptin production (Kolaczynski *et al.*, 1996b; Utriainen *et al.*, 1996). Conversely, the hyperglycaemia, hyperinsulinaemia and insulin resistance of leptin deficient mice (*ob/ob* mice) is reversed by leptin replacement (Pelleymounter *et al.*, 1995), suggesting that leptin may modulate insulin expression and sensitivity. Recent evidence from the study of diabetic hyperphagia suggests that the role of leptin is more critical to energy homeostasis than that of insulin (Sindelar *et al.*, 1999).

Whilst leptin and insulin inhibit appetite, the recently identified peptide ghrelin stimulates appetite (Tschop *et al.*, 2000). This 28 amino acid peptide was identified in 1999 having been purified from rat stomach and subsequently cloned in man. Ghrelin is the endogenous agonist of the growth hormone secretagogue receptor (GHS-R), which is present in the hypothalamus. Recent work has demonstrated that serum ghrelin concentrations increase with fasting and fall with refeeding whilst intraperitoneal and intracerebroventricular injection of ghrelin increases food intake and body weight in rats and mice (Asakawa *et al.*, 2001; Tschop *et al.*, 2000). In obese humans, ghrelin levels are low and inversely correlated with serum leptin and insulin concentrations (Tschop *et al.*, 2001).

Hypothalamic Regulation of Appetite

First Order Neurones of the Arcuate Nucleus

The hypothalamus has long been recognized as a key component of the pathways regulating food intake. For example, destruction of the arcuate nucleus (ARC) causes hyperphagia and obesity (Olney, 1969). The ARC lies outside the blood–brain barrier and expresses receptors for leptin, insulin and ghrelin (Elmquist *et al.*, 1998; Tschop *et al.*, 2000; Werther *et al.*, 1987). It is therefore ideally placed to communicate peripheral signals to central pathways for energy regulation. Indeed, microinjection of leptin into the ARC reduces food intake (Satoh *et al.*, 1997) and if the arcuate nucleus is destroyed, there is no response to leptin (Dawson *et al.*, 1997).

A variety of orexigenic and anorexigenic peptides are expressed in the ARC. Neuropeptide Y (NPY) is perhaps the most powerful of the orexigenic peptides. Centrally administered NPY is a potent stimulant of feeding and reduces energy expenditure, but repeated administration is needed to elicit significant weight gain (Billington *et al.*, 1991; Stanley *et al.*, 1986). Agouti gene related peptide (Agrp) has a less potent, but more prolonged orexigenic activity, increasing feeding for up to a week after single central administration (Hagan *et al.*, 2000). NPY and Agrp are co-localized to a sub-population of neurones located in the medial ARC that up-regulate expression of both peptides in response to fasting (Broberger *et al.*, 1998; Hahn *et al.*, 1998).

The melanocortin system is perhaps the most important anorexigenic system of the hypothalamus. Mutations of the melanocortin (MC4) receptor gene in both mice (Huszar *et al.*, 1997) and humans (Vaisse *et al.*, 1998; Yeo *et al.*, 1998) are associated with a hyperphagic, obese phenotype, suggesting that activity of this receptor tonically inhibits appetite. Alpha melanocyte stimulating hormone (αMSH), cleaved from pro-opiomelanocortin (POMC), is an endogenous agonist at MC4 receptors (Mezey *et al.*, 1985), whilst Agrp exerts its orexigenic effect by antagonizing the effect of αMSH at this receptor (Ollmann *et al.*, 1997).

Cocaine- and amphetamine-regulated transcript (CART) is thought to be a second contributor to the anorexigenic system of the ARC. Intraventricular administration inhibits both normal and starvation induced feeding (Kristensen *et al.*, 1998). CART is co-expressed with αMSH in a sub-population of neurones in the lateral ARC (Elias *et al.*, 1998) and, as might be predicted, activity of these POMC/CART neurones is inhibited by fasting (Vrang *et al.*, 1999). More recently however, microinjection studies have demonstrated that whilst CART inhibits feeding when injected into the third ventricle, it has the opposite effect when administered directly into the ARC or other hypothalamic nuclei involved in the regulation of appetite (Abbott *et al.*, 2001). It appears therefore that POMC/CART neurones may have mixed anorexigenic and orexigenic activity.

Leptin receptors are expressed on both NPY/Agrp and POMC/CART neurones (Baskin *et al.*, 1999; Cheung *et al.*, 1997). Leptin inhibits the expression of NPY and Agrp (Mizuno and Mobbs, 1999; Stephens *et al.*, 1995) whilst stimulating activity in POMC/CART neurones (Elias *et al.*, 1998). Furthermore, if the fasting induced fall in leptin is prevented by administration of exogenous leptin, the rise in NPY expression is also prevented and the rate of weight gain during refeeding is blunted (Ahima *et al.*, 1996). Insulin also inhibits the expression of NPY mRNA (Schwartz *et al.*, 1992) whilst fasting induced ghrelin elevates NPY and Agrp expression (Asakawa *et al.*, 2001; Kamegai *et al.*, 2000). Thus the fasting induced fall in the peripheral signals leptin and insulin and rise in ghrelin stimulates NPY/Agrp neurones and inhibits POMC/CART neuronal pathways of the arcuate, generating an appropriate appetitive response.

Second Order Hypothalamic Pathways

NPY/Agrp and POMC/CART neurones of the ARC project to other areas of the hypothalamus thought to play a role in the regulation of appetite and weight, including the lateral hypothalamus (LH) and paraventricular nucleus (PVN) (Broberger *et al.*, 1998; Dall *et al.*, 2000; Elias *et al.*, 1999). Lesion studies indicate that bilateral ablation of the LH causes anorexia and weight loss (Stellar, 1954) whilst destruction of the PVN results in hyperphagic obesity (Weingarten *et al.*, 1985). Furthermore, almost all known orexigenic and anorexigenic peptides modulate appetite when injected into the PVN. Schwartz *et al.* (2000) have therefore proposed a two stage model of hypothalamic pathways regulating appetite: second order PVN and LH neurones function as down-stream effectors for the first order ARC neurones terminating in these regions.

Melanin concentrating hormone (MCH) is an orexigenic peptide (Herve and Fellmann, 1997) for which the LH is a major site of expression in the human brain (Viale *et al.*, 1997). The recently identified MCH receptor (MCH-R/SLC-1) (Shimomura *et al.*, 1999) is widely distributed in the CNS, including hypothalamic sites such as the ventromedial, dorsomedial and arcuate nuclei (Chambers *et al.*, 1999; Saito *et al.*, 2001). Expression of MCH and MCH-R is up-regulated by fasting, an effect that is blocked by central administration of leptin (Kokkotou *et al.*, 2001; Tritos *et al.*, 2001). If these are second order neurones, co-expression of NPY, MC4 and CART receptors should be demonstrable but this remains to be proven.

The orexins, first identified in 1998 (de Lecea *et al.*, 1998; Sakurai *et al.*, 1998), also stimulate feeding, albeit less potently than NPY and MCH (Edwards *et al.*, 1999). These peptides are expressed in a distinct population of LH neurones that lie in close proximity to MCH neurones and NPY/Agrp nerve terminals (Broberger *et al.*, 1998). As with other orexigenic peptides, a fasting induced rise in the expression of orexin and its receptor can be prevented by the administration of leptin (Lopez *et al.*, 2000). Although orexin has been hypothesized to contribute to second order appetitive signalling, recent evidence suggests a role upstream of NPY: NPY-Y1 receptor antagonists block the feeding effect of exogenous orexin (Jain *et al.*, 2000). In addition to a role in appetite regulation, orexin increases arousal, locomotor activity and metabolic rate (Hagan *et al.*, 1999; Lubkin and Stricker-Krongrad, 1998). Orexin deficient mice exhibit narcolepsy, hypophagia and late onset obesity (Hara *et al.*, 2001). Orexin's primary role may therefore be regulation of the sleep–wake cycle and the modulation of appetite and energy expenditure in accordance with state of arousal (Willie *et al.*, 2001).

One last orexigenic peptide for consideration here is galanin (Smith *et al.*, 1994). Although preprogalanin mRNA is present in both ARC and PVN (Gundlach *et al.*, 1990), microinjection studies suggest that the orexigenic action of galanin may be restricted to the PVN (Kyrkouli *et al.*, 1990). Once more, expression is decreased by central administration of leptin (Sahu, 1998), as predicted for an orexigenic peptide.

The PVN is also rich in anorexigenic peptides, including thyrotrophin releasing hormone (TRH) and corticotrophin-releasing hormone (CRH). TRH expression is reduced by fasting, an effect that is mediated by low leptin levels and dependent upon an intact ARC (Legradi *et al.*, 1997; Legradi and Lechan, 1999; Seoane *et al.*, 2000). Leptin inhibits TRH expression directly via leptin receptors co-expressed on TRH neurones, and indirectly via regulation of αMSH and NPY which respectively stimulate and inhibit TRH expression (Fekete *et al.*, 2001; Nillni *et al.*, 2000).

The anorectic effect of leptin is at least partially mediated by CRH (Gardner *et al.*, 1998; Okamoto *et al.*, 2001; Uehara *et al.*, 1998) and several studies demonstrate enhanced expression of CRH in response to leptin (Costa *et al.*, 1997; Morimoto *et al.*, 2000; Schwartz *et al.*, 1996). However, leptin may also inhibit the expression of CRH (Arvaniti *et al.*, 2001; Heiman *et al.*, 1997) suggesting an indirect mechanism for leptin regulation of CRH. This hypothesis is supported by the finding that the fasting induced fall in CRH expression is mediated at least in part by reduced αMSH activity (Fekete *et al.*, 2001). These data are consistent with a putative role for TRH and CRH as second order anorectic effectors (Schwartz *et al.*, 2000). In addition to the anorectic effect of these neuropeptides, each also plays a role in peripheral energy regulation, via the thyroid and adrenal axis respectively (see below).

Integration of Anorexigenic and Orexigenic Signals within the PVN

GABA interneurones in the PVN are thought to be the substrate for functional integration of anorexigenic and orexigenic pathways of the hypothalamus (Cowley *et al.*, 1999). Since GABA is an inhibitory neurotransmitter, this model is consistent with studies demonstrating an inability to adequately restrain eating following bilateral PVN ablation. Electrophysiological and immunohistochemical studies indicate that NPY/Agrp and POMC/CART neurones converge on GABA interneurones expressing both MC4 and NPY receptors. NPY receptor activation inhibits adenylate cyclase activity via the Gi subunit of the plasma membrane G protein. Reduced availability of intracellular cyclic AMP results in decreased GABA release, which in turn reduces inhibition of feeding. Conversely, MC4 receptors are coupled to the Gs subunit. αMSH therefore stimulates adenylate cyclase, activating GABA neurones. Agrp inhibits GABA activity via prolonged antagonism of MC4 mediated activation of adenylate cyclase. Thus when food intake is restricted, reduced leptin signalling gives rise to increased NPY/Agrp activity and reduced POMC activity which in turn inhibits the activity of GABA interneurones to enhance appetite (see Figure XXIII-3.1). It is not yet known whether CART inhibits or stimulates GABA interneurone activity, but if CART is an orexigenic peptide an inhibitory effect would be predicted.

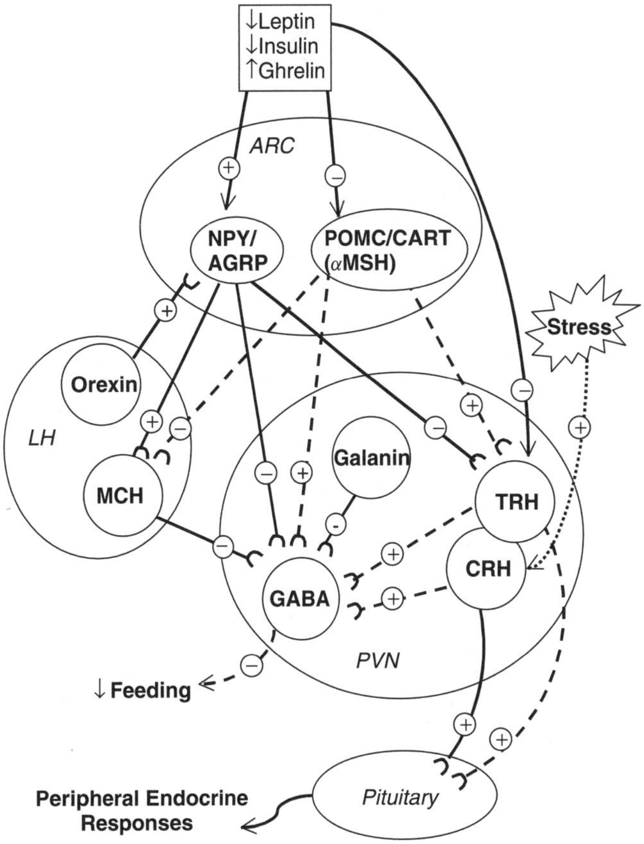

Figure XXIII-3.1 Proposed Model for the Neuroendocrine Response to Starvation. In response to acute food restriction, leptin levels fall below that expected for body fat mass, facilitating an early response to reduced energy availability. If food intake does not increase, falling body mass maintains this low leptin response. Reduced leptin signal to the ARC enhances activity of orexigenic NPY/Agrp neurones, whilst inhibiting anorexigenic αMSH activity. The appetitive effects of CART remain to be clarified. NPY/Agrp and POMC/CART neurones in the ARC project to the PVN and LH where putative second order orexigenic peptides MCH and galanin are up-regulated and anorexigenic peptides such as CRH and TRH are inhibited. Stress-induced CRH release may enhance anorexigenic activity in the PVN. Orexin appears to function upstream of NPY, perhaps providing a link between sleep–wake cycles and feeding behaviour. Orexigenic and anorexigenic signals may be functionally integrated via G protein coupled receptors on GABAergic interneurones in the PVN. When the leptin signal is low, inhibition of GABA activity reduces inhibition on feeding. Additionally, low leptin levels modulate the function of hypothalamic–pituitary endocrine axes such that energy is mobilized from peripheral stores and energy expenditure for growth and reproduction is minimized. In the case of the HPA axis, although fasting may inhibit CRH release in the PVN, a fasting induced increase of NPY expression stimulates CRH release in the median eminence, giving rise to enhanced HPA axis activity. (ARC = arcuate nucleus; LH = lateral hypothalamus; PVN = paraventricular nucleus; NPY = neuropeptide Y; Agrp = agouti related peptide; POMC = pro – opiomelanocortin; αMSH = alpha melanocyte stimulating hormone; CART = cocaine amphetamine related peptide; MCH = melanin concentrating hormone; TRH = thyrotrophin releasing hormone; CRH = corticotrophin releasing hormone. ——— = enhanced pathways; - - - - = suppressed pathways)

The effector neurones upon which GABA interneurones act have yet to be elucidated, but it is likely that at least some of the hypothesized second order neurones function in this way (Schwartz *et al.*, 2000). However, MCH receptors are also coupled to the inhibitory G protein subunit and CRH receptors are coupled to the Gs subunit. It is therefore possible that activity within the proposed second order anorexigenic and orexigenic pathways can also be functionally integrated at the GABA interneurone (Cowley *et al.*, 1999). Further studies are clearly needed to test these hypotheses.

Multiple orexigenic and anorexigenic peptides therefore contribute to the appetitive pathways of the hypothalamus, giving rise to a degree of redundancy within the system. NPY knockout mice, for example, are of normal weight (Erickson *et al.*, 1996), indicating that other neuropeptides, such as Agrp, compensate for this genetic deficit. However, it seems likely that our current model for understanding is an over-simplification of a highly complex network in which the different neuroendocrine systems contribute unique links with important higher functions. For example, the orexin system appears to provide a link between energy regulation and arousal, whilst the CRH system provides a link with stress responsivity. CRH inhibits the expression of NPY (Van Huijsduijnen *et al.*, 1993) and mediates stress-induced anorexia (Krahn *et al.*, 1986; Shibasaki, 1988). Thus even if undernourished, appetite may be impaired in the context of CRH hyperactivity (Schwartz *et al.*, 1995). This hypothesis may be particularly relevant to eating disorders, given their association with premorbid stressful life events and difficulties (Schmidt *et al.*, 1997) and impaired coping (Troop and Treasure, 1997).

Effector Systems

Second order PVN neurones provide a link between leptin and peripheral effectors that mediate adaptations to altered energy availability. One such mechanism involves the hypothalamic–pituitary hormonal axes. In humans, genetic deficits of leptin signalling are associated with widespread neuroendocrine abnormality of the type seen in starvation, including failure of puberty and reduced secretion of thyrotrophin and growth hormone (Clement *et al.*, 1998). Furthermore, if the fall in leptin associated with fasting is prevented by exogenous replacement, changes within the gonadal (HPG), adrenal (HPA) and thyroid hormone (HPT) axes are blunted (Ahima *et al.*, 1996).

Leptin suppresses HPA axis activity at both the central and adrenal level of the axis (Ahima *et al.*, 1996; Bornstein *et al.*, 1997; Heiman *et al.*, 1997), such that cortisol levels are elevated during fasting. Whilst the action of cortisol at high concentrations is catabolic in the periphery, generating glucose and ketone bodies from stored energy, at the central level, cortisol stimulates expression of NPY and is thus anabolic (Strack *et al.*, 1995). In turn, NPY further stimulates HPA axis activity via increased CRH expression in the median eminence, but not other hypothalamic regions (Haas and George, 1987). Thus a feed-forward system is generated in which cortisol and NPY are reciprocally positively regulated in order to maintain a robust central appetite response coupled with mobilization of peripheral energy stores. Schwartz *et al.* (1995) have suggested that persistently dysregulated CRH release in the PVN could impair this feed-forward system via inhibition of NPY expression.

During fasting, low leptin levels suppress prothyrotropin-releasing hormone expression, reducing peripheral thyroid hormone activity (Legradi *et al.*, 1997) and thus reducing energy expenditure. Low leptin levels also suppress growth hormone (GH) secretion during fasting (Carro *et al.*, 1997; LaPaglia *et al.*, 1998) and in genetic leptin deficiency (Clement *et al.*, 1998). This effect appears to be mediated by enhanced expression of NPY (Vuagnat *et al.*, 1998). Interestingly, the fasting induced fall in insulin-like growth factor (IGF-1) levels is not reversed by leptin (Carro *et al.*, 1997; LaPaglia *et al.*, 1998). In contrast to an acute fast, severe starvation is associated with elevated GH secretion, GH resistance and low IGF-1 and insulin levels (Soliman *et al.*, 2000). This pattern of GH-IGF-1 axis activity is thought to promote muscle catabolism, rather than growth, and is therefore adaptive to the starving state.

Leptin regulates gonadal axis activity via stimulation of both hypothalamic and pituitary components of the axis (Yu *et al.*, 1997) and plays a pivotal role in the onset of ovulation at puberty and cessation during starvation (Ahima *et al.*, 1997; Chehab *et al.*, 1996; Miller *et al.*, 1998). The effects of leptin upon gonadal and other anabolic hormone axes may be mediated by NPY (Catzeflis *et al.*, 1993). Since oestrogen enhances leptin production (Mannucci *et al.*, 1998), oestrogen deficiency arising from HPG axis suppression during starvation may amplify orexigenic signalling.

The adaptive response to leptin deficiency may therefore be as important as its role in the regulation of appetite. It is characterized by reduced energy expenditure, via suppression of reproductive and thyroid axis activity, and mobilization of stored energy via the actions of cortisol and altered GH-IGF-1 axis function. Leptin deficiency therefore defends against starvation by both increasing appetite and reducing energy expenditure (see Figure XXIII-3.1).

Similarly, excessive leptin production in the context of obesity may also elicit adaptive changes. POMC/CART neurones project to sympathetic preganglionic neurones in thoracic spinal cord (Elias *et al.*, 1998) suggesting these pathways may contribute to enhanced thermogenesis and energy expenditure when anorexigenic pathways are activated by elevated leptin. Pituitary endocrine axis changes in obesity include reduced GH and elevated cortisol release, which in this context may serve to promote growth and central adiposity. Excess leptin therefore appears to be somewhat less effective in defending healthy body weight than leptin deficiency. Central leptin resistance, perhaps arising from saturation of active leptin transport mechanisms, may contribute (Caro *et al.*, 1996). Indeed, the ratio of CSF to plasma leptin is reduced in obese subjects (Caro *et al.*, 1996; Schwartz *et al.*, 1996). These findings support the hypothesis that the primary role of leptin is to defend against starvation rather than obesity.

SECTION 2: NEUROENDOCRINOLOGY OF APPETITE AND WEIGHT IN EATING DISORDERS

Anorexia Nervosa

Leptin

The wealth of studies examining a putative role for leptin in the aetiology of AN have produced little evidence to support a functional abnormality. In acute AN, leptin levels are low and proportional to BMI and fat mass (Ferron *et al.*, 1997; Grinspoon *et al.*, 1996; Lear *et al.*, 1999; Mathiak *et al.*, 1999) except at extremely low BMI (Balligand *et al.*, 1998; Casanueva *et al.*, 1997; Eckert *et al.*, 1998; Pauly *et al.*, 2000). Even in the severely emaciated state, leptin diurnal rhythm and temporal relationship with insulin and IGF-1 are preserved (Casanueva *et al.*, 1997; Eckert *et al.*, 1998; Herpertz *et al.*, 2000), although the temporal relationship with cortisol is disrupted until weight is restored (Herpertz *et al.*, 2000). During weight gain, plasma leptin levels are relatively elevated for BMI (Hebebrand *et al.*, 1997; Mantzoros *et al.*, 1997) and this could at least partially explain the difficulty achieving full weight restoration during rapid refeeding. Similarly, leptin levels are greater than expected for BMI in those with the purging subtype of AN (Mehler *et al.*, 1999). An elevated CSF : plasma leptin ratio in acute AN (Mantzoros *et al.*, 1997) suggests that enhanced central leptin signalling could contribute to impairment of appetite. However, normalization of both plasma leptin levels (Gendall *et al.*, 1999; Hebebrand *et al.*, 1997; Polito *et al.*, 2000) and the CSF : plasma ratio (Mantzoros *et al.*, 1997) following full recovery indicates that altered leptin dynamics are a state related phenomena.

Insulin and Ghrelin

Although studies of insulin and glucose dynamics in acute AN have not been entirely consistent, on balance, the evidence suggests that basal and fasting insulin levels are reduced in acute AN (Alderdice *et al.*, 1985; de Rosa *et al.*, 1983; Uhe *et al.*, 1992), consistent with the need to promote gluconeogenesis in the starving state. Delayed absorption and, in chronic cases, impaired pancreatic beta cell function (Nozaki *et al.*, 1994) may contribute to reduced insulin response to nutrients in AN (Alderdice *et al.*, 1985; Blickle *et al.*, 1984). Insulin sensitivity varies greatly between subjects (Kiriike *et al.*, 1990) and there may be a tendency toward increased glucose utilization rather than storage (Franssila-Kallunki *et al.*, 1991). These altered dynamics appear to resolve with full recovery from AN (Casper, 1996). The role of insulin as a central signal of peripheral energy balance has not been investigated in AN. Similarly, ghrelin has yet to be examined in AN.

Hypothalamic Regulation of Appetite and Weight

Several authors have postulated an imbalance between anorexigenic and orexigenic pathways of the hypothalamus in the aetiology of AN (Kaye *et al.*, 1989; Menzaghi *et al.*, 1993). Despite obvious methodological problems limiting the scope of available data, there is some indirect evidence to support this hypothesis. An association between an Agrp gene polymorphism and AN raises the possibility that this variant could be a less effective MC4-R antagonist, conferring susceptibility to AN via reduced ability to inhibit anorexigenic pathways (Vink *et al.*, 2001). NPY levels are elevated in CSF during the acute illness (Kaye *et al.*, 1990), consistent with a reduced leptin signal from the periphery. Levels normalize with full recovery, at which time CSF polypeptide Y (PPY) levels are also reported normal (Gendall *et al.*, 1999; Kaye *et al.*, 1990; Sapolsky, 1992). The NPY Y5 receptor mediates the orexigenic effects of NPY (Schaffhauser *et al.*, 1997) and there is no evidence for an association between receptor gene polymorphisms and AN (Rosenkranz *et al.*, 1998). However, low CSF galanin in women fully recovered from AN (Frank *et al.*, 2001) could reflect a functional impairment of orexigenic pathways of the hypothalamus in those vulnerable to AN.

One recent study found elevated plasma CART concentrations in those with the acute disorder, and normal concentrations in women who had fully recovered (Sarah Stanley, personal communication). This finding perhaps adds weight to the hypothesized orexigenic role of CART in the ARC, LH and PVN (Abbott *et al.*, 2001).

In terms of anorexigenic pathways in AN, there is no evidence of an MC4 receptor mutation or polymorphism associated with AN (Hinney *et al.*, 1999) and no other studies of the melanocortin system have yet been reported. CSF TRH levels are reduced at low weight and are not fully normalized at attainment of target weight (Lesem *et al.*, 1994). This is not inconsistent with an adaptive response to starvation. CSF CRH levels are elevated during the acute illness (Kaye *et al.*, 1987) and this appears to be in contrast to animal models of food restriction in which CRH activity in the PVN is reduced (Brady *et al.*, 1990).

Studies of HPA axis activity in AN suggest that an impairment of feedback inhibition at the level of the hypothalamus gives rise to elevated CRH activity. This is turn is thought to override intact feedback inhibition at the level of the pituitary (Kling *et al.*, 1993), giving rise to the HPA axis hyperactivity associated with AN (Kaye *et al.*, 1987; Licinio *et al.*, 1996). Elevated concentrations of CRH in the CSF (Kaye *et al.*, 1987) and blunting of the ACTH and β-endorphin responses to exogenous CRH (Brambilla *et al.*, 1996; Hotta *et al.*, 1986) are consistent. with this hypothesis. Although HPA axis arginine vasopressin (AVP) activity is up-regulated in the context of chronic stress in animals and depression in humans, there is no evidence of elevated AVP activity in acute AN (Connan *et al.*, 2001a, 2001b). This is significant because AVP modulates CRH release and sensitivity of the axis to feedback inhibition via altered glucocorticoid receptor activity (Felt *et al.*, 1984; Plotsky *et al.*, 1984). An abnormal HPA axis response to chronic stress may therefore contribute to persistently elevated CRH activity in AN. In addition to the inhibitory effect on appetite and feeding, the widespread behavioural and physiological effects of CRH include many of the features of AN including increased locomotor activity, cardiovascular changes, reduced social and sexual behaviour, impaired sleep and increased anxiety behaviours (Dunn and Berridge, 1990).

There is some evidence to suggest that a heightened cortisol response to stress and a blunted cortisol response to a meal may persist even after full recovery (Connan *et al.*, 2001c; Ward *et al.*, 1998). Subtle abnormalities of HPA axis regulation could therefore contribute to susceptibility to AN. Whilst genetic factors are likely to be important, the elevated prevalence of perinatal stress (Cnattingius *et al.*, 1999; Foley *et al.*, 2001) and insecure attachment (Ward *et al.*, 2000) in those vulnerable to AN suggest that early environmental modulation of HPA axis responsivity (Heim and Nemeroff, 1999) may also contribute.

Effector Systems

In acute AN, basal and fasting IGF-1 concentrations are reduced (Argente *et al.*, 1997; Fukuda *et al.*, 1999; Stoving *et al.*, 1999a) whilst GH (de Rosa *et al.*, 1983; Stoving *et al.*, 1999b) and cortisol concentrations are elevated. These findings are consistent with the need to promote gluconeogenesis in the starving state and resolve with weight gain (Casper *et al.*, 1988a; Casper, 1996; Golden *et al.*, 1994), suggesting that they arise as an adaptive response to prolonged negative energy balance.

GH hypersecretion in AN is associated with a disorganized pattern of both basal and pulsatile release (Stoving *et al.*, 1999b). Neuroendocrine challenge studies suggest that hypersecretion is attributable to impaired somatostatinergic inhibition rather than elevated GHRH activity (Ghigo *et al.*, 1994). Low T3 concentrations may also contribute (Valcavi *et al.*, 1990). Peripheral GH resistance, reflected in reduced availability of GH binding protein (GHBP), is characteristic of both AN and other forms of malnutrition (Stoving *et al.*, 1999a, for review). Since IGF-1 mediates many of the anabolic effects of GH, reduced levels in the starving state likely contribute to GH resistance. Reduced central IGF-1 feedback inhibition may also contribute to GH axis hyperactivity (Melmed *et al.*, 1996). It therefore appears that reciprocal interactions between IGF-1 and GH function effectively in AN, generating a feed-forward system of low IGF-1 and elevated GH. A paradoxical increase in the GH response to intravenous glucose in AN could reflect abnormality of hypothalamic appetite and satiety responses (Tamai *et al.*, 1991).

Altered thyroid function in acute AN does not differ from that associated with malnutrition (de Rosa *et al.*, 1983) and normalizes with maintenance of healthy weight and eating (e.g., Kiyohara *et al.*, 1987; Komaki *et al.*, 1992). Specifically, serum total and free thyroxine (T4) are low or normal, tri-iodothyronine (T3) is reduced and reverse T3 (rT3) is elevated (e.g., Boyar *et al.*, 1977; de Rosa *et al.*, 1983; Komaki *et al.*, 1992). Altered peripheral conversion of T4 to T3 contributes to these abnormalities. However, whilst TSH levels are normal, the TSH response to TRH is delayed and prolonged and T3 response to TRH is reduced, suggesting that central HPT axis dysregulation may also play a role (Casper and Frohman, 1982; Kiyohara *et al.*, 1989).

In terms of the HPG axis, gonadotrophin releasing hormone (GnRH) release is reduced and gonadotrophin secretion exhibits a pre-pubertal pattern (e.g., van Binsbergen *et al.*, 1990), as would be expected in a low leptin state. Leptin levels are predictive of amenorrhoea in eating disordered patients (Kopp *et al.*, 1997) and restoration of normal levels is necessary, although not sufficient, for restoration of menses (Audi *et al.*, 1998). Similarly, leptin levels are positively correlated with HPG function in males recovering from AN (Wabitsch *et al.*, 2001). Although there is a critical BMI threshold for menstruation to return, the presence of anorexic attitudes and behaviours during recovery from AN appears to be more predictive of persistent amenorrhoea than BMI (Falk and Halmi, 1982). Interestingly, CSF NPY levels following weight gain were normal only in those women with return of menses (Kaye *et al.*, 1990), consistent with the hypothesized role of NPY in mediating the effects of leptin deficiency on HPG axis function.

Bulimia Nervosa

Leptin

The fall in leptin levels associated with fasting is blunted in those with BN (Monteleone *et al.*, 2000a). Additionally, although plasma leptin levels are positively correlated with BMI (Monteleone *et al.*, 2000b), leptin levels are lower than those of healthy comparison women, even after adjusting for low BMI (Brewerton *et al.*, 2000; Monteleone *et al.*, 2000b), a finding that persists even after recovery (Jimerson *et al.*, 2000). Duration of illness and severity of disorder are related to the reduced leptin levels in BN (Monteleone *et al.*, 2000a). Amongst obese binge eaters, lower leptin levels are associated with greater dietary restraint (d'Amore *et al.*, 2001) and restraint might similarly contribute to low leptin levels in those vulnerable to BN. These data suggest that whilst the body fat sensing function of leptin is intact, there is a tendency for a lower leptin secretion per fat mass and thus a higher settling point for weight in BN. A degree of restrained eating may therefore be necessary to maintain a healthy low weight in these individuals. The impaired capacity for the leptin system to respond to acute changes in energy intake could contribute to maintenance of disordered eating in BN.

Hypothalamic Regulation of Appetite and Weight

Following short-term abstinence from binge–purge behaviour, CSF levels of PYY and somatostatin are elevated relative to both acute BN and healthy controls (Kaye *et al.*, 1988, 1990). A relative excess activity in the orexigenic pathways of the hypothalamus might therefore be stimulating overeating in BN. However, levels of both PYY and NPY in CSF are normal after full recovery suggesting that this is unlikely to be a trait phenomenon (Gendall *et al.*, 1999). There are currently no published data regarding other orexigenic and anorexigenic neuropeptides in BN.

Effectors

Milder variants of HPG, HPT, HPA and GH axis changes associated with AN also occur in BN (Coiro *et al.*, 1992; Kennedy *et al.*, 1989; Levy, 1989; Pirke *et al.*, 1988). It is likely that these changes reflect undernutrition despite healthy weight, consistent with the hypothesis that women with BN are maintaining weight at a lower level than is necessary to switch off anabolic systems. The finding that a current weight of less than 85% of previous highest weight is predictive of impaired HPG function in BN (Weltzin *et al.*, 1994) further supports this. There is some suggestion of an association between polycystic ovary syndrome (PCO) and BN, but the nature and extent of such an association have been little studied (Michelmore *et al.*, 2001; Morgan, 1999). Raphael and colleagues (Raphael *et al.*, 1995) found a high prevalence of polycystic ovaries on ultrasound scan, but this was not associated with elevated levels of luteinizing hormone or the metabolic features of PCO. The ultrasound findings may therefore reflect multifollicular ovaries rather than true PCO (Treasure, 1988).

Women with BN exhibit reduced cortisol and sympathetic nervous system (SNS) responses to mental stress, relative to healthy comparison women (Laessle *et al.*, 1992), suggesting that in contrast to AN, BN may be associated with stress hyporesponsivity.

Binge-Eating Disorder

At the opposite end of the eating and weight spectrum from AN, binge-eating disorder (BED) is associated with obesity and overeating, in the absence of behaviours to compensate. The biology of BED is therefore likely to overlap with that of BN, but in the absence of the biological consequences of food restriction. When presented with food, those with BED experience a greater subjective desire to eat than women with simple obesity, although the salivary response to food exposure is reduced (Karhunen *et al.*, 1997a). Binge eating may therefore be driven more by emotional cues than hunger in BED.

The few available data examining biological contributions to dysregulated appetite and weight in obese binge eaters can be summarized as follows. This group do not differ from obese non-binge eaters in terms of resting energy expenditure, body composition, serum lipids, insulin and thyroid hormones (Adami *et al.*, 1995; Wadden *et al.*, 1993). Cephalic phase plasma insulin, free fatty acid and glucose levels also do not differ between binge- and non-binge-eating obese people (Karhunen *et al.*, 1997b). Leptin levels are elevated and proportional to BMI in women with BED (Monteleone *et al.*, 2000b), but it remains to be seen whether leptin levels differ between obese binge and non-binge eaters after adjustment for BMI. It is likely that obese binge eaters have a degree of leptin resistance, as occurs in simple obesity, but again, this remains to be demonstrated. Simple peripheral obesity is associated with elevated morning cortisol and high diurnal variability, whilst visceral obesity is associated with low morning cortisol and blunting of the diurnal rhythm, as well as reduced GH and HPG axis activity (Rosmond *et al.*, 1998). These endocrine changes are thought to be responsible for the metabolic and haemodynamic features of visceral obesity as well as reduced fertility in women (Bjorntorp and Rosmond, 2000a). Termed the Metabolic Syndrome by Bjorntorp and colleagues, an interaction between genetic factors, such as an associated glucocorticoid receptor polymorphism, and environmental stress in early and adult life is thought to contribute to aetiology (Bjorntorp and Rosmond, 2000b). Given the association between early adversity and BED (Fairburn *et al.*, 1998), one might predict that those with BED are more likely to exhibit visceral obesity and the associated metabolic syndrome than simple peripheral obesity.

Synthesis and Implications

Eating disorders can be conceptualized as stress related disorders. A severe life event or difficulty can be identified prior to onset in the majority of cases (Schmidt *et al.*, 1997) and there is evidence of abnormal coping (Troop and Treasure, 1997). Additionally, early adversity is a risk factor for each of the disorders, as it is for psychiatric disorders in general (Fairburn *et al.*, 1997, 1998, 1999). The capacity for adverse early life experience to modulate HPA axis development is now well recognized (Heim and Nemeroff, 1999) and such experience may also affect appetite and weight regulation in adulthood (McIntosh *et al.*, 1999). Interestingly, feeding ameliorates the adverse effect of maternal deprivation upon HPA axis function (van Oers, de Kloet, and Levine, 1999), providing a potential precursor to emotion driven eating in later life. It seems likely that genetic and early environmental factors interact to generate specific vulnerabilities in the systems regulating appetite, weight and stress responsivity. For AN, the phenotype is characterized by impaired appetite and heightened stress responsivity. In contrast, the BN phenotype may be a tendency toward obesity, eating as a strategy to manage emotional experience and reduced stress responsivity.

In terms of the neuroendocrine data, leptin appears to signal low peripheral energy availability to hypothalamic networks effectively in AN, giving rise to elevated NPY expression and appropriate adaptations to the starving state. These include amenorrhoea, and enhanced metabolic efficiency arising from altered thyroid and IGF-1/GH axis function. Relatively elevated central leptin concentrations could play a role in maintenance of the disorder, whilst elevated leptin for BMI during rapid refeeding may contribute to difficulty restoring weight. There is some evidence to support a hypothesized imbalance between anorexigenic and orexigenic pathways of the hypothalamus. Specifically, impaired Agrp function and reduced galanin expression may impair orexigenic pathways, whilst hyper-reactivity of CRH expression may enhance activity in anorexigenic networks. These abnormalities could underlie the association between AN and premorbid tendency toward leanness. An aberrant HPA axis response to chronic stress, characterized by persistently elevated CRH activity, may be one factor that contributes to the onset and pathophysiology of AN. However, it is likely that other neuropeptide and neurotransmitter systems also play an important role. Indeed, the serotonin system may be particularly relevant in this regard because of the well recognized effects on appetite (Blundell, 1986; Dourish *et al.*, 1986) and reciprocal regulatory interactions with the HPA axis (Dinan, 1996; Grignaschi *et al.*, 1996; Lowry *et al.*, 2000). This may underpin some of the response to treatment. Preliminary evidence suggests that olanzepine, which acts on the serotonin system at multiple sites, may improve weight gain during refeeding in AN (Hanson, 1999; La Via *et al.*, 2000; Mehler *et al.*, 2000). There is also weak evidence to support the use of fluoxetine in preventing relapse after weight restoration (Kaye *et al.*, 2001). As in the treatment of depressive disorder, antidepressant modulation of GR levels, and thus HPA axis function, could be as important as serotonergic modulation for efficacy in AN.

In BN, a tendency toward overweight may arise from a variety of constitutional factors, including reduced leptin signalling from stored body fat. Overweight in the context of low self-esteem and emotional dysregulation increases the risk of engaging in weight reduction behaviours. Once initiated, food restriction gives rise to both hunger and dysphoric mood, which are key triggers for binge eating. At the central level, overactivity of orexigenic pathways in acute BN is in keeping with leptin levels that are relatively low for body mass. However, other factors are likely to contribute because orexigenic peptide levels in CSF return to normal after recovery, despite persistence of low leptin levels. The high reward value of food for those with BN may also be secondary to chronic food restriction and low leptin levels, and could serve to both establish and reinforce binge eating as a strategy for emotional regulation. Reduced satiety signalling from peripheral factors such as CCK (Devlin *et al.*, 1997) and the vagus nerve (Faris *et al.*, 2000) may impair the capacity to terminate binges, whilst the rapid fall in serum insulin and glucose associated with purging may play an important role in perpetuating binge–purge behaviour (Johnson *et al.*, 1994). However, there is no evidence currently to suggest that these are primary problems.

Understanding the biological components of appetite and weight regulation is vital if we are to develop better aetiological and treatment models for eating disorders. Functional neuroimaging, neuroendocrine and molecular genetic studies will help to further elucidate the central mechanisms maintaining low appetite and weight in AN, and the drive to overeat in BN and BED. However, emerging differences in the biology of restricting and binge–purge subtypes of AN, as well as between peripherally and centrally distributed obesity, highlight the need for good phenotypic description of study participants. A consensus definition of diagnostic subtypes, stage of illness and recovery is urgently needed.

Peptides that increase appetite and ultimately body weight have potential for the treatment of AN. Agrp analogues may be particularly interesting because of their long-lasting effect in promoting food intake and fat storage in animals. CRH antagonists may also prove fruitful therapeutic options for the treatment of AN. Safe and effective anti-obesity drugs that target central orexigenic pathways are likely to proliferate in the future, providing potentially useful treatments for BN and BED.

REFERENCES

Abbott, C.R., Rossi, M., Wren, A.M., Murphy, K.G., Kennedy, A.R., Stanley, S.A., Zollner, A.N., Morgan, D.G., Morgan, I., Ghatei, M.A., Small, C.J. and Bloom, S.R., 2001. Evidence of an orexigenic role for cocaine and amphetamine-regulated transcript (CART) following administration into discrete hypothalamic nuclei. *Endocrinol.*, **142**(8), 3457–3463.

Adami, G.F., Gandolfo, P., Campostano, A., Cocchi, F., Bauer, B. and Scopinaro, N., 1995. Obese binge eaters: metabolic characteristics, energy expenditure and dieting. *Psychol. Med.*, **25**(1), 195–198.

Ahima, R.S., Dushay, J., Flier, S.N., Prabakaran, D. and Flier, J.S., 1997. Leptin accelerates the onset of puberty in normal female mice. *J. Clin. Invest.*, **99**(3), 391–395.

Ahima, R.S., Prabakaran, D., Mantzoros, C., Qu, D., Lowell, B., Maratos, F.E. and Flier, J.S., 1996. Role of leptin in the neuroendocrine response to fasting. *Nature*, **382**(6588), 250–252.

Alderdice, J.T., Dinsmore, W.W., Buchanan, K.D. and Adams, C., 1985. Gastrointestinal hormones in anorexia nervosa. *J. Psychiatr. Res.*, **19**(2–3), 207–213.

Argente, J., Caballo, N., Barrios, V., Munoz, M.T., Pozo, J., Chowen, J.A., Morande, G. and Hernandez, M., 1997. Multiple endocrine abnormalities of the growth hormone and insulin-like growth factor axis in patients with anorexia nervosa: effect of short- and long-term weight recuperation. *J. Clin. Endocrinol. Metab*. **82**(7), 2084–2092.

Arvaniti, K., Huang, Q. and Richard, D., 2001. Effects of leptin and corticosterone on the expression of corticotropin-releasing hormone, agouti-related protein, and proopiomelanocortin in the brain of ob/ob mouse. *Neuroendocrinology*, **73**(4), 227–236.

Asakawa, A., Inui, A., Kaga, T., Yuzuriha, H., Nagata, T., Ueno, N., Makino, S., Fujimiya, M., Niijima, A., Fujino, M.A. and Kasuga, M., 2001. Ghrelin is an appetite-stimulatory signal from stomach with structural resemblance to motilin. *Gastroenterology*, **120**(2), 337–345.

Audi, L., Mantzoros, C.S., Vidal-Puig, A., Vargas, D., Gussinye, M. and Carrascosa, A., 1998. Leptin in relation to resumption of menses in women with anorexia nervosa [see comments]. *Mol. Psychiatry*, **3**(6), 544–547.

Balligand, J.L., Brichard, S.M., Brichard, V., Desager, J.P. and Lambert, M., 1998. Hypoleptinemia in patients with anorexia nervosa: loss of circadian rhythm and unresponsiveness to short-term refeeding. *Eur. J. Endocrinol.*, **138**(4), 415–420.

Baskin, D.G., Hahn, T.M. and Schwartz, M.W., 1999. Leptin sensitive neurons in the hypothalamus. *Horm. Metab. Res.*, **31**(5), 345–350.

Billington, C.J., Briggs, J.E., Grace, M. and Levine, A.S., 1991. Effects of intracerebroventricular injection of neuropeptide Y on energy metabolism. *Am. J. Physiol.*, **260**(2), R321–R327.

Bjorntorp, P. and Rosmond, R., 2000b. Neuroendocrine abnormalities in visceral obesity. *Int. J. Obes. Relat. Metab. Disord.*, **24**(2), S80–S85.

Bjorntorp, P. and Rosmond, R., 2000a. Obesity and cortisol. *Nutrition*, **16**(10), 924–936.

Blickle, J.F., Reville, P., Stephan, F., Meyer, P., Demangeat, C. and Sapin, R., 1984. The role of insulin, glucagon and growth hormone in the regulation of plasma glucose and free fatty acid levels in anorexia nervosa. *Horm. Metab. Res.*, **16**(7), 336–340.

Blundell, J.E., 1986. Serotonin manipulations and the structure of feeding behaviour. *Appetite*, **7**(suppl), 39–56.

Bornstein, S.R., Uhlmann, K., Haidan, A., Ehrhart-Bornstein, M. and Scherbaum, W.A., 1997. Evidence for a novel peripheral action of leptin as a metabolic signal to the adrenal gland: leptin inhibits cortisol release directly. *Diabetes*, **46**(7), 1235–1238.

Boyar, R.M., Hellman, L.D., Roffwarg, H., Katz, J., Zumoff, B., O'Connor, J., Bradlow, H.L. and Fukushima, D.K., 1977. Cortisol secretion and metabolism in anorexia nervosa. *N. Engl. J. Med.*, **296**(4), 190–193.

Brady, L.S., Smith, M.A., Gold, P.W. and Herkenham, M., 1990. Altered expression of hypothalamic neuropeptide mRNAs in food-restricted and food-deprived rats. *Neuroendocrinology*, **52**(5), 441–447.

Brambilla, F., Ferrari, E., Brunetta, M., Peirone, A., Draisci, A., Sacerdote, P. and Panerai, A., 1996. Immunoendocrine aspects of anorexia nervosa. *Psychiatry Res.*, **62**(1), 97–104.

Brewerton, T.D., Lesem, M.D., Kennedy, A. and Garvey, W.T., 2000. Reduced plasma leptin concentrations in bulimia nervosa. *Psychoneuroendocrinology*, **25**(7), 649–658.

Broberger, C., Johansen, J., Johansson, C., Schalling, M. and Hokfelt, T., 1998. The neuropeptide Y/agouti gene-related protein (AGRP) brain circuitry in normal, anorectic, and monosodium glutamate-treated mice. *Proc. Natl. Acad. Sci. USA*, **95**(25), 15043–15048.

Caro, J.F., Kolaczynski, J.W., Nyce, M.R., Ohannesian, J.P., Opentanova, I., Goldman, W.H., Lynn, R.B., Zhang, P.L., Sinha, M.K. and Considine, R.V., 1996. Decreased cerebrospinal-fluid/serum leptin ratio in obesity: a possible mechanism for leptin resistance. *Lancet*, **348**(9021), 159–161.

Carro, E., Senaris, R., Considine, R.V., Casanueva, F.F. and Dieguez, C., 1997. Regulation of *in vivo* growth hormone secretion by leptin. *Endocrinology*, **138**(5), 2203–2206.

Casanueva, F.F., Dieguez, C., Popovic, V., Peino, R., Considine, R.V. and Caro, J.F., 1997. Serum immunoreactive leptin concentrations in patients with anorexia nervosa before and after partial weight recovery. *Biochem. Mol. Med.*, **60**(2), 116–120.

Casper, R.C., 1996. Carbohydrate metabolism and its regulatory hormones in anorexia nervosa. *Psychiatry Res.*, **62**(1), 85–96.

Casper, R.C. and Frohman, L.A., 1982. Delayed TSH release in anorexia nervosa following injection of thyrotropin-releasing hormone (TRH). *Psychoneuroendocrinology*, **7**(1), 59–68.

Casper, R.C., Pandey, G., Jaspan, J.B. and Rubenstein, A.H., 1988b. Eating attitudes and glucose tolerance in anorexia nervosa patients at 8-year followup compared to control subjects. *Psychiatry Res.*, **25**(3), 283–299.

Casper, R.C., Pandy, G.N., Jaspan, J.B. and Rubenstein, A.H., 1988a. Hormone and metabolite plasma levels after oral glucose in bulimia and healthy controls. *Biol. Psychiatry*, **24**(6), 663–674.

Catzeflis, C., Pierroz, D.D., Rohner-Jeanrenaud, F., Rivier, J.E., Sizonenko, P.C. and Aubert, M.L., 1993. Neuropeptide Y administered chronically into the lateral ventricle profoundly inhibits both the gonadotropic and the somatotropic axis in intact adult female rats. *Endocrinology*, **132**(1), 224–234.

Chambers, J., Ames, R.S., Bergsma, D., Muir, A., Fitzgerald, L.R., Hervieu, G., Dytko, G.M., Foley, J.J., Martin, J., Liu, W.S., Park, J., Ellis, C., Ganguly, S., Konchar, S., Cluderay, J., Leslie, R., Wilson, S. and Sarau, H.M., 1999. Melanin-concentrating hormone is the cognate ligand for the orphan G-protein-coupled receptor SLC-1. *Nature*, **400**(6741), 261–265.

Chavez, M., Kaiyala, K., Madden, L.J., Schwartz, M.W. and Woods, S.C., 1995. Intraventricular insulin and the level of maintained body weight in rats. *Behav. Neurosci.*, **109**(3), 528–531.

Chehab, F.F., Lim, M.E. and Lu, R., 1996. Correction of the sterility defect in homozygous obese female mice by treatment with the human recombinant leptin. *Nat. Genet.*, **12**(3), 318–320.

Cheung, C.C., Clifton, D.K. and Steiner, R.A., 1997. Proopiomelanocortin neurons are direct targets for leptin in the hypothalamus. *Endocrinology*, **138**(10), 4489–4492.

Chua-SC, J., Chung, W.K., Wu, P.X., Zhang, Y., Liu, S.M., Tartaglia, L. and Leibel, R.L., 1996. Phenotypes of mouse diabetes and rat fatty due to mutations in the OB (leptin) receptor [see comments]. *Science*, **271**(5251), 994–996.

Clement, K., Vaisse, C., Lahlou, N., Cabrol, S., Pelloux, V., Cassuto, D., Gourmelen, M., Dina, C., Chambaz, J., Lacorte, J.M., Basdevant, A., Bougneres, P., Lebouc, Y., Froguel, P. and Guy-Grand, B., 1998. A mutation in the human leptin receptor gene causes obesity and pituitary dysfunction. *Nature*, **392**(6674), 398–401.

Cnattingius, S., Hultman, C.M., Dahl, M. and Sparen, P., 1999. Very preterm birth, birth trauma, and the risk of anorexia nervosa among girls. *Arch. Gen. Psychiatry*, **56**(7), 634–638.

Coiro, V., Volpi, R., Marchesi, C., Capretti, L., Speroni, G., Rossi, G., Caffarri, G., De Ferri, A., Marcato, A. and Chiodera, P., 1992. Abnormal growth hormone and cortisol, but not thyroid-stimulating hormone, responses to an intravenous glucose tolerance test in normal-weight, bulimic women. *Psychoneuroendocrinology*, **17**(6), 639–645.

Connan, F., Campbell, I.C., Lightman, S.L., Landau, S., Wheeler, M. and Treasure, J., 2001. An arginine vasopressin challenge test in anorexia nervosa. In press.

Connan, F., Campbell, I.C., Lightman, S.L., Landau, S., Wheeler, M. and Treasure, J., 2001. Hypercortisolaemia in anorexia nervosa. In press.

Connan, F., Campbell, I.C., Lightman, S.L., Landau, S., Wheeler, M. and Treasure, J., 2001. The combined dexamethasone/corticotrophin releasing hormone challenge test in anorexia nervosa. In press.

Considine, R.V., Sinha, M.K., Heiman, M.L., Kriauciunas, A., Stephens, T.W., Nyce, M.R., Ohannesian, J.P., Marco, C.C., McKee, L.J. and Bauer, T.L., 1996. Serum immunoreactive-leptin concentrations in normal-weight and obese humans [see comments]. *N. Engl. J. Med.*, **334**(5), 292–295.

Copeland, P.M., Herzog, D.B., Carr, D.B., Klibanski, A., MacLaughlin, R.A. and Martin, J.B., 1988. Effect of dexamethasone on cortisol and prolactin responses to meals in bulimic and normal women. *Psychoneuroendocrinology*, **13**(3), 273–278.

Costa, A., Poma, A., Martignoni, E., Nappi, G., Ur, E. and Grossman, A., 1997. Stimulation of corticotrophin-releasing hormone release by the obese (ob) gene product, leptin, from hypothalamic explants. *Neuroreport*, **8**(5), 1131–1134.

Cotrufo, P., Monteleone, P., d'Istria, M., Fuschino, A., Serino, I. and Maj, M., 2000. Aggressive behavioural characteristics and endogenous hormones in women with bulimia nervosa. *Neuropsychobiology*, **42**(2), 58–61.

Cowley, M.A., Pronchuk, N., Fan, W., Dinulescu, D.M., Colmers, W.F. and Cone, R.D., 1999. Integration of NPY, AGRP, and melanocortin signals in the hypothalamic paraventricular nucleus: evidence of a cellular basis for the adipostat. *Neuron*, **24**(1), 155–163.

Cugini, P., Ventura, M., Ceccotti, P., Cilli, M., Marciano, F., Salandri, A., Di Marzo, A., Fontana, S., Pellegrino, A.M., Vacca, K. and Di Siena, G., 1998. Hunger sensation: a chronobiometric approach to its within-day and intra-day recursivity in anorexia nervosa restricting type. *Eat. Weight. Disord.*, **3**(3), 115–123.

d'Amore, A., Massignan, C., Montera, P., Moles, A., De Lorenzo, A. and Scucchi, S., 2001. Relationship between dietary restraint, binge eating, and leptin in obese women. *Int. J. Obes. Relat. Metab. Disord.*, **25**(3), 373–377.

Dall, V.S., Lambert, P.D., Couceyro, P.C., Kuhar, M.J. and Smith, Y., 2000. CART peptide immunoreactivity in the hypothalamus and pituitary in monkeys: analysis of ultrastructural features and synaptic connections in the paraventricular nucleus. *J. Comp. Neurol.*, **416**(3), 291–308.

Dawson, R., Pelleymounter, M.A., Millard, W.J., Liu, S. and Eppler, B., 1997. Attenuation of leptin-mediated effects by monosodium glutamate-induced arcuate nucleus damage. *Am. J. Physiol.*, **273**(1), E202–E206.

de Lecea, L., Kilduff, T.S., Peyron, C., Gao, X., Foye, P.E., Danielson, P.E., Fukuhara, C., Battenberg, E.L., Gautvik, V.T., Bartlett, F.S., Frankel, W.N., van den Pol, A.N., Bloom, F.E., Gautvik, K.M. and Sutcliffe, J.G., 1998. The hypocretins: hypothalamus-specific peptides with neuroexcitatory activity. *Proc. Natl. Acad. Sci. USA*, **95**(1), 322–327.

de Rosa, G., Corsello, S.M., de Rosa, E., Della, C.S., Ruffilli, M.P., Grasso, P. and Pasargiklian, E., 1983. Endocrine study of anorexia nervosa. *Exp. Clin. Endocrinol.*, **82**(2), 160–172.

Devlin, M.J., Walsh, B.T., Guss, J.L., Kissileff, H.R., Liddle, R.A. and Petkova, E., 1997. Postprandial cholecystokinin release and gastric emptying in patients with bulimia nervosa. *Am. J. Clin. Nutr.*, **65**(1), 114–120.

Dinan, T.G., 1996. Serotonin and the regulation of hypothalamic–pituitary–adrenal axis function. *Life Sci.*, **58**(20), 1683–1694.

Dourish, C.T., Hutson, P.H., Kennett, G.A. and Curzon, G., 1986. 8-OH-DPAT-induced hyperphagia: its neural basis and possible therapeutic relevance. *Appetite*, **7**(suppl), 127–140.

Drewnowski, A., Halmi, K.A., Pierce, B., Gibbs, J. and Smith, G.P., 1987. Taste and eating disorders. *Am. J. Clin. Nutr.*, **46**(3), 442–450.

Dunn, A.J. and Berridge, C.W., 1990. Physiological and behavioural responses to corticotropin-releasing factor administration: is CRF a mediator of anxiety or stress responses? *Brain Res. Brain Res. Rev.*, **15**(2), 71–100.

Eckert, E.D., Pomeroy, C., Raymond, N., Kohler, P.F., Thuras, P. and Bowers, C.Y., 1998. Leptin in anorexia nervosa [see comments]. *J. Clin. Endocrinol. Metab.*, **83**(3), 791–795.

Edholm, O.G., 1977. Energy balance in man studies carried out by the Division of Human Physiology, National Institute for Medical Research. *J. Hum. Nutr.*, **31**(6), 413–431.

Edwards, C.M., Abusnana, S., Sunter, D., Murphy, K.G., Ghatei, M.A. and Bloom, S.R., 1999. The effect of the orexins on food intake: comparison with neuropeptide Y, melanin-concentrating hormone and galanin. *J. Endocrinol.*, **160**(3), R7–R12.

Elias, C.F., Aschkenasi, C., Lee, C., Kelly, J., Ahima, R.S., Bjorbaek, C., Flier, J.S., Saper, C.B. and Elmquist, J.K., 1999. Leptin differentially regulates NPY and POMC neurons projecting to the lateral hypothalamic area. *Neuron*, **23**(4), 775–786.

Elias, C.F., Lee, C., Kelly, J., Aschkenasi, C., Ahima, R.S., Couceyro, P.R., Kuhar, M.J., Saper, C.B. and Elmquist, J.K., 1998. Leptin activates hypothalamic CART neurons projecting to the spinal cord. *Neuron*, **21**(6), 1375–1385.

Ellison, Z., Foong, J., Howard, R., Bullmore, E., Williams, S. and Treasure, J., 1998. Functional anatomy of calorie fear in anorexia nervosa [letter]. *Lancet*, **352**(9135), 1192.

Elmquist, J.K., Ahima, R.S., Elias, C.F., Flier, J.S. and Saper, C.B., 1998. Leptin activates distinct projections from the dorsomedial and ventromedial hypothalamic nuclei. *Proc. Natl. Acad. Sci. USA*, **95**(2), 741–746.

Erickson, J.C., Clegg, K.E. and Palmiter, R.D., 1996. Sensitivity to leptin and susceptibility to seizures of mice lacking neuropeptide Y. *Nature*, **381**(6581), 415–421.

Fairburn, C.G., Cooper, Z., Doll, H.A. and Welch, S.L., 1999. Risk factors for anorexia nervosa: three integrated case-control comparisons. *Arch. Gen. Psychiatry*, **56**(5), 468–476.

Fairburn, C.G., Doll, H.A., Welch, S.L., Hay, P.J., Davies, B.A. and O'Connor, M.E., 1998. Risk factors for binge eating disorder: a community-based, case-control study [see comments]. *Arch. Gen. Psychiatry*, **55**(5), 425–432.

Fairburn, C.G., Welch, S.L., Doll, H.A., Davies, B.A. and O'Connor, M.E., 1997. Risk factors for bulimia nervosa. A community-based case-control study. *Arch. Gen. Psychiatry*, **54**(6), 509–517.

Falk, J.R. and Halmi, K.A., 1982. Amenorrhea in anorexia nervosa: examination of the critical body weight hypothesis. *Biol. Psychiatry*, **17**(7), 799–806.

Faris, P.L., Kim, S.W., Meller, W.H., Goodale, R.L., Oakman, S.A., Hofbauer, R.D., Marshall, A.M., Daughters, R.S., Banerjee-Stevens, D., Eckert, E.D. and Hartman, B.K., 2000. Effect of decreasing afferent vagal activity with ondansetron on symptoms of bulimia nervosa: a randomised, double-blind trial. *Lancet*, **355**(9206), 792–797.

Farooqi, I.S., Jebb, S.A., Langmack, G., Lawrence, E., Cheetham, C.H., Prentice, A.M., Hughes, I.A., McCamish, M.A. and O'Rahilly, S., 1999. Effects of recombinant leptin therapy in a child with congenital leptin deficiency [see comments]. *N. Engl. J. Med.*, **341**(12), 879–884.

Fekete, C., Kelly, J., Mihaly, E., Sarkar, S., Rand, W.M., Legradi, G., Emerson, C.H. and Lechan, R.M., 2001. Neuropeptide Y has a central inhibitory action on the hypothalamic–pituitary–thyroid axis. *Endocrinology*, **142**(6), 2606–2613.

Felt, B.T., Sapolsky, R.M. and McEwen, B.S., 1984. Regulation of hippocampal corticosterone receptors by a vasopressin analogue. *Peptides*, **5**(6), 1225–1227.

Ferron, F., Considine, R.V., Peino, R., Lado, I.G., Dieguez, C. and Casanueva, F.F., 1997. Serum leptin concentrations in patients with anorexia nervosa, bulimia nervosa and non-specific eating disorders correlate with the body mass index but are independent of the respective disease. *Clin. Endocrinol. (Oxf.)*, **46**(3), 289–293.

Foley, D.L., Thacker, L.R., Aggen, S.H., Neale, M.C. and Kendler, K.S., 2001. Pregnancy and perinatal complications associated with risks for common psychiatric disorders in a population-based sample of female twins. *Am. J. Med. Genet.*, **105**(5), 426–431.

Foster, L.A., Ames, N.K. and Emery, R.S., 1991. Food intake and serum insulin responses to intraventricular infusions of insulin and IGF-I. *Physiol. Behav.*, **50**(4), 745–749.

Frank, G.K., Kaye, W.H., Sahu, A., Fernstrom, J. and McConaha, C., 2001. Could reduced cerebrospinal fluid (csf) galanin contribute to restricted eating in anorexia nervosa? *Neuropsychopharmacology*, **24**(6), 706–709.

Franssila-Kallunki, A., Rissanen, A., Ekstrand, A., Eriksson, J., Saloranta, C., Widen, E., Schalin-Jantti, C. and Groop, L., 1991. Fuel metabolism in anorexia nervosa and simple obesity. *Metabolism*, **40**(7), 689–694.

Fukuda, I., Hotta, M., Hizuka, N., Takano, K., Ishikawa, Y., Asakawa-Yasumoto, K., Tagami, E. and Demura, H., 1999. Decreased serum levels of acid-labile subunit in patients with anorexia nervosa. *J. Clin. Endocrinol. Metab.*, **84**(6), 2034–2036.

Gardner, J.D., Rothwell, N.J. and Luheshi, G.N., 1998. Leptin affects food intake via CRF-receptor-mediated pathways. *Nat. Neurosci.*, **1**(2), 103.

Gendall, K.A., Kaye, W.H., Altemus, M., McConaha, C.W. and La Via, M.C., 1999. Leptin, neuropeptide Y, and peptide YY in long-term recovered eating disorder patients. *Biol. Psychiatry*, **46**(2), 292–299.

Ghigo, E., Arvat, E., Gianotti, L., Nicolosi, M., Valetto, M.R., Avagnina, S., Bellitti, D., Rolla, M., Muller, E.E. and Camanni, F., 1994. Arginine but not pyridostigmine, a cholinesterase inhibitor, enhances the GHRH-induced GH rise in patients with anorexia nervosa. *Biol. Psychiatry*, **36**(10), 689–695.

Golden, N.H., Kreitzer, P., Jacobson, M.S., Chasalow, F.I., Schebendach, J., Freedman, S.M. and Shenker, I.R., 1994. Disturbances in growth hormone secretion and action in adolescents with anorexia nervosa. *J. Pediatr.*, **125**(4), 655–660.

Grignaschi, G., Sironi, F. and Samanin, R., 1996. Stimulation of 5-HT2A receptors in the paraventricular hypothalamus attenuates neuropeptide Y-induced hyperphagia through activation of corticotropin releasing factor. *Brain Res.*, **708**(1–2), 173–176.

Grinspoon, S., Gulick, T., Askari, H., Landt, M., Lee, K., Anderson, E., Ma, Z., Vignati, L., Bowsher, R., Herzog, D. and Klibanski, A., 1996. Serum leptin levels in women with anorexia nervosa. *J. Clin. Endocrinol. Metab.*, **81**(11), 3861–3863.

Gundlach, A.L., Wisden, W., Morris, B.J. and Hunt, S.P., 1990. Localization of preprogalanin mRNA in rat brain: *in situ* hybridization study with a synthetic oligonucleotide probe. *Neurosci. Lett.*, **114**(3), 241–247.

Gwirtsman, H.E., Kaye, W.H., George, D.T., Jimerson, D.C., Ebert, M.H. and Gold, P.W., 1989. Central and peripheral ACTH and cortisol levels in anorexia nervosa and bulimia. *Arch. Gen. Psychiatry*, **46**(1), 61–69.

Haas, D.A. and George, S.R., 1987. Neuropeptide Y administration acutely increases hypothalamic corticotropin-releasing factor immunoreactivity: lack of effect in other rat brain regions. *Life Sci.*, **41**(25), 2725–2731.

Hagan, J.J., Leslie, R.A., Patel, S., Evans, M.L., Wattam, T.A., Holmes, S., Benham, C.D., Taylor, S.G., Routledge, C., Hemmati, P., Munton, R.P., Ashmeade, T.E., Shah, A.S., Hatcher, J.P., Hatcher, P.D., Jones, D.N., Smith, M.I., Piper, D.C., Hunter, A.J., Porter, R.A. and Upton, N., 1999. Orexin A activates locus coeruleus cell firing and increases arousal in the rat. *Proc. Natl. Acad. Sci. USA*, **96**(19), 10911–10916.

Hagan, M.M., Rushing, P.A., Pritchard, L.M., Schwartz, M.W., Strack, A.M., Van Der Ploeg, L.H., Woods, S.C. and Seeley, R.J., 2000. Long-term orexigenic effects of AgRP-(83–132) involve mechanisms other than melanocortin receptor blockade. *Am. J. Physiol. Regul. Integr. Comp. Physiol.*, **279**(1), R47–R52.

Hahn, T.M., Breininger, J.F., Baskin, D.G. and Schwartz, M.W., 1998. Coexpression of Agrp and NPY in fasting-activated hypothalamic neurons. *Nat. Neurosci.*, **1**(4), 271–272.

Halaas, J.L., Boozer, C., Blair-West, J., Fidahusein, N., Denton, D.A. and Friedman, J.M., 1997. Physiological response to long-term peripheral and central leptin infusion in lean and obese mice. *Proc. Natl. Acad. Sci. USA*, **94**(16), 8878–8883.

Halmi, K.A., Struss, A. and Goldberg, S.C., 1978. An investigation of weights in the parents of anorexia nervosa patients. *J. Nerv. Ment. Dis.*, **166**(5), 358–361.

Halmi, K.A. and Sunday, S.R., 1991. Temporal patterns of hunger and fullness ratings and related cognitions in anorexia and bulimia. *Appetite*, **16**(3), 219–237.

Hanson, L., 1999. Olanzepine in the treatment of anorexia nervosa [letter]. *British Journal of Psychiatry*, **175**(592).

Hara, J., Beuckmann, C.T., Nambu, T., Willie, J.T., Chemelli, R.M., Sinton, C.M., Sugiyama, F., Yagami, K., Goto, K., Yanagisawa, M. and Sakurai, T., 2001. Genetic ablation of orexin neurons in mice results in narcolepsy, hypophagia, and obesity. *Neuron*, **30**(2), 345–354.

Hebebrand, J., Blum, W.F., Barth, N., Coners, H., Englaro, P., Juul, A., Ziegler, A., Warnke, A., Rascher, W. and Remschmidt, H., 1997. Leptin levels in patients with anorexia nervosa are reduced in the acute stage and elevated upon short-term weight restoration [see comments]. *Mol. Psychiatry*, **2**(4), 330–334.

Hebebrand, J. and Remschmidt, H., 1995. Anorexia nervosa viewed as an extreme weight condition: genetic implications. *Hum. Genet.*, **95**(1), 1–11.

Heim, C. and Nemeroff, C.B., 1999. The impact of early adverse experiences on brain systems involved in the pathophysiology of anxiety and affective disorders. *Biol. Psychiatry*, **46**(11), 1509–1522.

Heiman, M.L., Ahima, R.S., Craft, L.S., Schoner, B., Stephens, T.W. and Flier, J.S., 1997. Leptin inhibition of the hypothalamic–pituitary–adrenal axis in response to stress. *Endocrinology*, **138**(9), 3859–3863.

Herpertz, S., Albers, N., Wagner, R., Pelz, B., Kopp, W., Mann, K., Blum, W.F., Senf, W. and Hebebrand, J., 2000. Longitudinal changes of circadian leptin, insulin and cortisol plasma levels and their correlation during refeeding in patients with anorexia nervosa. *Eur. J. Endocrinol.*, **142**(4), 373–379.

Herve, C. and Fellmann, D., 1997. Changes in rat melanin-concentrating hormone and dynorphin messenger ribonucleic acids induced by food deprivation. *Neuropeptides*, **31**(3), 237–242.

Hinney, A., Schmidt, A., Nottebom, K., Heibult, O., Becker, I., Ziegler, A., Gerber, G., Sina, M., Gorg, T., Mayer, H., Siegfried, W., Fichter, M., Remschmidt, H. and Hebebrand, J., 1999. Several mutations in the melanocortin-4 receptor gene including a nonsense and a frameshift mutation associated with dominantly inherited obesity in humans. *J. Clin. Endocrinol. Metab.*, **84**(4), 1483–1486.

Hotta, M., Shibasaki, T., Masuda, A., Imaki, T., Demura, H., Ling, N. and Shizume, K., 1986. The responses of plasma adrenocorticotropin and cortisol to corticotropin-releasing hormone (CRH) and cerebrospinal fluid immunoreactive CRH in anorexia nervosa patients. *J. Clin. Endocrinol. Metab.*, **62**(2), 319–324.

Huszar, D., Lynch, C.A., Fairchild-Huntress, V., Dunmore, J.H., Fang, Q., Berkemeier, L.R., Gu, W., Kesterson, R.A., Boston, B.A., Cone, R.D., Smith, F.J., Campfield, L.A., Burn, P. and Lee, F., 1997. Targeted disruption of the melanocortin-4 receptor results in obesity in mice. *Cell*, **88**(1), 131–141.

Jain, M.R., Horvath, T.L., Kalra, P.S. and Kalra, S.P., 2000. Evidence that NPY Y1 receptors are involved in stimulation of feeding by orexins (hypocretins) in sated rats. *Regul. Pept.*, **87**(1–3), 19–24.

Jimerson, D.C., Mantzoros, C., Wolfe, B.E. and Metzger, E.D., 2000. Decreased serum leptin in bulimia nervosa. *J. Clin. Endocrinol. Metab.*, **85**(12), 4511–4514.

Johnson, W.G., Jarrell, M.P., Chupurdia, K.M. and Williamson, D.A., 1994. Repeated binge/purge cycles in bulimia nervosa: role of glucose and insulin. *Int. J. Eat. Disord.*, **15**(4), 331–341.

Kamegai, J., Tamura, H., Shimizu, T., Ishii, S., Sugihara, H. and Wakabayashi, I., 2000. Central effect of ghrelin, an endogenous growth hormone secretagogue, on hypothalamic peptide gene expression. *Endocrinology*, **141**(12), 4797–4800.

Karhunen, L., Haffner, S., Lappalainen, R., Turpeinen, A., Miettinen, H. and Uusitupa, M., 1997b. Serum leptin and short-term regulation of eating in obese women. *Clin. Sci. (Colch.)*, **92**(6), 573–578.

Karhunen, L.J., Lappalainen, R.I., Tammela, L., Turpeinen, A.K. and Uusitupa, M.I., 1997a. Subjective and physiological cephalic phase responses to food in obese binge-eating women. *Int. J. Eat. Disord.*, **21**(4), 321–328.

Kaye, W.H., Berrettini, W., Gwirtsman, H. and George, D.T., 1990. Altered cerebrospinal fluid neuropeptide Y and peptide YY immunoreactivity in anorexia and bulimia nervosa. *Arch. Gen. Psychiatry*, **47**(6), 548–556.

Kaye, W.H., Berrettini, W.H., Gwirtsman, H.E., Gold, P.W., George, D.T., Jimerson, D.C. and Ebert, M.H., 1989. Contribution of CNS neuropeptide (NPY, CRH, and beta-endorphin) alterations to psychophysiological abnormalities in anorexia nervosa. *Psychopharmacol. Bull.*, **25**(3), 433–438.

Kaye, W.H., Gwirtsman, H.E., George, D.T., Ebert, M., Jimerson, D.C., Tomai, T.P., Chrousos, G.P. and Gold, P.W., 1987. Elevated cerebrospinal fluid levels of immunoreactive corticotrophin-releasing hormone in anorexia nervosa: relation to state of nutrition, adrenal function and intensity of depression. *Journal of Clinical Endocrinology and Metabolism.*, **64**, 203–208.

Kaye, W.H., Nagata, T., Weltzin, T.E., Hsu, L.K., Sokol, M.S., McConaha, C., Plotnicov, K.H., Weise, J. and Deep, D., 2001. Double-blind placebo-controlled administration of fluoxetine in restricting-type anorexia nervosa. *Biol. Psychiatry*, **49**(7), 644–652.

Kaye, W.H., Rubinow, D., Gwirtsman, H.E., George, D.T., Jimerson, D.C. and Gold, P.W., 1988. CSF somatostatin in anorexia nervosa and bulimia: relationship to the hypothalamic–pituitary–adrenal cortical axis. *Psychoneuroendocrinology*, **13**(3), 265–272.

Kennedy, S.H., Garfinkel, P.E., Parienti, V., Costa, D. and Brown, G.M., 1989. Changes in melatonin levels but not cortisol levels are associated with depression in patients with eating disorders. *Arch. Gen. Psychiatry*, **46**(1), 73–78.

Kiriike, N., Nishiwaki, S., Nagata, T., Okuno, Y., Yamada, J., Tanaka, S., Fujii, A. and Kawakita, Y., 1990. Insulin sensitivity in patients with anorexia nervosa and bulimia. *Acta Psychiatr. Scand.*, **81**(3), 236–239.

Kissileff, H.R., Wentzlaff, T.H., Guss, J.L., Walsh, B.T., Devlin, M.J. and Thornton, J.C., 1996. A direct measure of satiety disturbance in patients with bulimia nervosa. *Physiol. Behav.*, **60**(4), 1077–1085.

Kiyohara, K., Tamai, H., Karibe, C., Kobayashi, N., Fujii, S., Fukino, O., Nakagawa, T., Kumagai, L.F. and Nagataki, S., 1987. Serum thyrotropin (TSH) responses to thyrotropin-releasing hormone (TRH) in patients with anorexia nervosa and bulimia: influence of changes in body weight and eating disorders. *Psychoneuroendocrinology*, **12**(1), 21–28.

Kiyohara, K., Tamai, H., Takaichi, Y., Nakagawa, T. and Kumagai, L.F., 1989. Decreased thyroidal triiodothyronine secretion in patients with anorexia nervosa: influence of weight recovery. *Am. J. Clin. Nutr.*, **50**(4), 767–772.

Kling, M.A., Demitrack, M.A., Whitfield, H.J., Jr, Kalogeras, K.T., Listwak, S.J., DeBellis, M.D., Chrousos, G.P., Gold, P.W. and Brandt, H.A., 1993. Effects of the glucocorticoid antagonist RU 486 on pituitary–adrenal function in patients with anorexia nervosa and healthy volunteers: enhancement of plasma ACTH and cortisol secretion in underweight patients. *Neuroendocrinology*, **57**(6), 1082–1091.

Kokkotou, E.G., Tritos, N.A., Mastaitis, J.W., Slieker, L. and Maratos-Flier, E., 2001. Melanin-concentrating hormone receptor is a target of leptin action in the mouse brain. *Endocrinology*, **142**(2), 680–686.

Kolaczynski, J.W., Considine, R.V., Ohannesian, J., Marco, C., Opentanova, I., Nyce, M.R., Myint, M. and Caro, J.F., 1996a. Responses of leptin to short-term fasting and refeeding in humans: a link with ketogenesis but not ketones themselves. *Diabetes*, **45**(11), 1511–1515.

Kolaczynski, J.W., Nyce, M.R., Considine, R.V., Boden, G., Nolan, J.J., Henry, R., Mudaliar, S.R., Olefsky, J. and Caro, J.F., 1996b. Acute and chronic effects of insulin on leptin production in humans: studies *in vivo* and *in vitro*. *Diabetes*, **45**(5), 699–701.

Komaki, G., Tamai, H., Mukuta, T., Kobayashi, N., Mori, K., Nakagawa, T. and Kumagai, L.F., 1992. Alterations in endothelium-associated proteins and serum thyroid hormone concentrations in anorexia nervosa. *Br. J. Nutr.*, **68**(1), 67–75.

Koo-Loeb, J.H., Pedersen, C. and Girdler, S.S., 1998. Blunted cardiovascular and catecholamine stress reactivity in women with bulimia nervosa. *Psychiatry Res.*, **80**(1), 13–27.

Kopp, W., Blum, W.F., von Prittwitz, S., Ziegler, A., Lubbert, H., Emons, G., Herzog, W., Herpertz, S., Deter, H.C., Remschmidt, H. and Hebebrand, J., 1997. Low leptin levels predict amenorrhea in underweight and eating disordered females [see comments]. *Mol. Psychiatry*, **2**(4), 335–340.

Krahn, D.D., Gosnell, B.A., Grace, M. and Levine, A.S., 1986. CRF antagonist partially reverses CRF- and stress-induced effects on feeding. *Brain Res. Bull.*, **17**(3), 285–289.

Kristensen, P., Judge, M.E., Thim, L., Ribel, U., Christjansen, K.N., Wulff, B.S., Clausen, J.T., Jensen, P.B., Madsen, O.D., Vrang, N., Larsen, P.J. and Hastrup, S., 1998. Hypothalamic CART is a new anorectic peptide regulated by leptin. *Nature*, **393**(6680), 72–76.

Kyrkouli, S.E., Stanley, B.G., Seirafi, R.D. and Leibowitz, S.F., 1990. Stimulation of feeding by galanin: anatomical localization and behavioural specificity of this peptide's effects in the brain. *Peptides*, **11**(5), 995–1001.

La Via, M.C., Gray, N. and Kaye, W.H., 2000. Case reports of olanzapine treatment of anorexia nervosa. *Int. J. Eat. Disord.*, **27**(3), 363–366.

Laessle, R.G., Fischer, M., Fichter, M.M., Pirke, K.M. and Krieg, J.C., 1992. Cortisol levels and vigilance in eating disorder patients. *Psychoneuroendocrinology*, **17**(5), 475–484.

LaPaglia, N., Steiner, J., Kirsteins, L., Emanuele, M. and Emanuele, N., 1998. Leptin alters the response of the growth hormone releasing factor — growth hormone — insulin-like growth factor-I axis to fasting. *J. Endocrinol.*, **159**(1), 79–83.

Lear, S.A., Pauly, R.P. and Birmingham, C.L., 1999. Body fat, caloric intake, and plasma leptin levels in women with anorexia nervosa. *Int. J. Eat. Disord.*, **26**(3), 283–288.

Lee, G.H., Proenca, R., Montez, J.M., Carroll, K.M., Darvishzadeh, J.G., Lee, J.I. and Friedman, J.M., 1996. Abnormal splicing of the leptin receptor in diabetic mice. *Nature*, **379**(6566), 632–635.

LeGoff, D.B., Leichner, P. and Spigelman, M.N., 1988. Salivary response to olfactory food stimuli in anorexics and bulimics. *Appetite*, **11**(1), 15–25.

Legradi, G., Emerson, C.H., Ahima, R.S., Flier, J.S. and Lechan, R.M., 1997. Leptin prevents fasting-induced suppression of prothyrotropin-releasing hormone messenger ribonucleic acid in neurons of the hypothalamic paraventricular nucleus. *Endocrinology*, **138**(6), 2569–2576.

Legradi, G. and Lechan, R.M., 1999. Agouti-related protein containing nerve terminals innervate thyrotropin-releasing hormone neurons in the hypothalamic paraventricular nucleus. *Endocrinology*, **140**(8), 3643–3652.

Leonard, T., Perpina, C., Bond, A. and Tresaure, J., 1998. Assessment of test meal induced autonomic arousal in anorexic, bulimic and control females. *European Eating Disorders Review*, **6**, 188–200.

Lesem, M.D., Kaye, W.H., Bissette, G., Jimerson, D.C. and Nemeroff, C.B., 1994. Cerebrospinal fluid TRH immunoreactivity in anorexia nervosa. *Biol. Psychiatry*, **35**(1), 48–53.

Levy, A.B., 1989. Neuroendocrine profile in bulimia nervosa. *Biol. Psychiatry*, **25**(1), 98–109.

Licinio, J., Wong, M.-L. and Gold, P.W., 1996. The hypothalamic–pituitary–adrenal axis in anorexia nervosa. *Psychiatry Res.*, **62**, 75–83.

Lopez, M., Seoane, L., Garcia, M.C., Lago, F., Casanueva, F.F., Senaris, R. and Dieguez, C., 2000. Leptin regulation of prepro-orexin and orexin receptor mRNA levels in the hypothalamus. *Biochem. Biophys. Res. Commun.*, **269**(1), 41–45.

Lowry, A.C., Plant, A., Ingram, C.D. and Lightman, S.L., 2000. Corticotrophin-releasing factor (CRF) alters serotonin metabolism in neuroanatomical loci associated with anxiety and conditioned fear: an integrative analysis of evidence for a functionally distinct mesolimbocortical serotonergic system. In press.

Lubkin, M. and Stricker-Krongrad, A., 1998. Independent feeding and metabolic actions of orexins in mice. *Biochem. Biophys. Res. Commun.*, **253**(2), 241–245.

Mannucci, E., Ognibene, A., Becorpi, A., Cremasco, F., Pellegrini, S., Ottanelli, S., Rizzello, S.M., Massi, G., Messeri, G. and Rotella, C.M., 1998. Relationship between leptin and oestrogens in healthy women. *Eur. J. Endocrinol.*, **139**(2), 198–201.

Mantzoros, C., Flier, J.S., Lesem, M.D., Brewerton, T.D. and Jimerson, D.C., 1997. Cerebrospinal fluid leptin in anorexia nervosa: correlation with nutritional status and potential role in resistance to weight gain. *J. Clin. Endocrinol. Metab*, **82**(6), 1845–1851.

Mathiak, K., Gowin, W., Hebebrand, J., Ziegler, A., Blum, W.F., Felsenberg, D., Lubbert, H. and Kopp, W., 1999. Serum leptin levels, body fat deposition, and weight in females with anorexia or bulimia nervosa. *Horm. Metab. Res.*, **31**(4), 274–277.

McIntosh, J., Anisman, H. and Merali, Z., 1999. The Neuroendocrinology of Eating Disorders. *Brain Res. Dev. Brain Res.*, **113**(1–2), 97–106.

Mehler, C., Wewetzer, C., Schulze, U., Theisen, F., Dittman, W. and Warnke, A., 2000. Olanzepine in children and adolescents with chronic anorexia nervosa. A study of five cases. *European Journal of Child and Adolescent Psychiatry*. In press.

Mehler, P.S., Eckel, R.H. and Donahoo, W.T., 1999. Leptin levels in restricting and purging anorectics. *Int. J. Eat. Disord.*, **26**(2), 189–194.

Melmed, S., Yamashita, S., Yamasaki, H., Fagin, J., Namba, H., Yamamoto, H., Weber, M., Morita, S., Webster, J. and Prager, D., 1996. IGF-I receptor signalling: lessons from the somatotroph. *Recent Prog. Horm. Res.*, **51**, 189–215.

Menzaghi, F., Heinrichs, S.C., Pich, E.M., Tilders, F.J. and Koob, G.F., 1993. Functional impairment of hypothalamic corticotropin-releasing factor neurons with immunotargeted toxins enhances food intake induced by neuropeptide Y. *Brain Res.*, **618**(1), 76–82.

Mezey, E., Kiss, J.Z., Mueller, G.P., Eskay, R., O'Donohue, T.L. and Palkovits, M., 1985. Distribution of the pro-opiomelanocortin derived peptides, adrenocorticotrope hormone, alpha-melanocyte-stimulating hormone and beta-endorphin (ACTH, alpha-MSH, beta-END) in the rat hypothalamus. *Brain Res.*, **328**(2), 341–347.

Michelmore, K.F., Balen, A.H. and Dunger, D.B., 2001. Polycystic ovaries and eating disorders: are they related? *Hum. Reprod.*, **16**(4), 765–769.

Miller, K.K., Parulekar, M.S., Schoenfeld, E., Anderson, E., Hubbard, J., Klibanski, A. and Grinspoon, S.K., 1998. Decreased leptin levels in normal weight women with hypothalamic amenorrhea: the effects of body composition and nutritional intake. *J. Clin. Endocrinol. Metab.*, **83**(7), 2309–2312.

Mizuno, T.M. and Mobbs, C.V., 1999. Hypothalamic agouti-related protein messenger ribonucleic acid is inhibited by leptin and stimulated by fasting. *Endocrinology*, **140**(2), 814–817.

Montague, C.T., Farooqi, I.S., Whitehead, J.P., Soos, M.A., Rau, H., Wareham, N.J., Sewter, C.P., Digby, J.E., Mohammed, S.N., Hurst, J.A., Cheetham, C.H., Earley, A.R., Barnett, A.H., Prins, J.B. and O'Rahilly, S., 1997. Congenital leptin deficiency is associated with severe early-onset obesity in humans. *Nature*, **387**(6636), 903–908.

Monteleone, P., Bortolotti, F., Fabrazzo, M., La Rocca, A., Fuschino, A. and Maj, M., 2000a. Plasma leptin response to acute fasting and refeeding in untreated women with bulimia nervosa. *J. Clin. Endocrinol. Metab.*, **85**(7), 2499–2503.

Monteleone, P., Brambilla, F., Bortolotti, F., La Rocca, A. and Maj, M., 1998. Prolactin response to d-fenfluramine is blunted in people with anorexia nervosa. *Br. J. Psychiatry*, **172**, 439–442.

Monteleone, P., Di Lieto, A., Tortorella, A., Longobardi, N. and Maj, M., 2000b. Circulating leptin in patients with anorexia nervosa, bulimia nervosa or binge-eating disorder: relationship to body weight, eating patterns, psychopathology and endocrine changes [in process citation]. *Psychiatry Res.*, **94**(2), 121–129.

Monteleone, P., Maes, M., Fabrazzo, M., Tortorella, A., Lin, A., Bosmans, E., Kenis, G. and Maj, M., 1999. Immunoendocrine findings in patients with eating disorders. *Neuropsychobiology*, **40**(3), 115–120.

Morgan, J.F., 1999. Polycystic ovary syndrome, gestational diabetes, and bulimia nervosa. *J. Clin. Endocrinol. Metab.*, **84**(12), 4746.

Morimoto, I., Yamamoto, S., Kai, K., Fujihira, T., Morita, E. and Eto, S., 2000. Centrally administered murine-leptin stimulates the hypothalamus-pitui. *Neuroendocrinology*, **71**(6), 366–374.

Muller, C., Voirol, M.J., Stefanoni, N., Surmely, J.F., Jequier, E., Gaillard, R.C. and Tappy, L., 1997. Effect of chronic intracerebroventricular infusion of insulin on brown adipose tissue activity in fed and fasted rats. *Int. J. Obes. Relat. Metab. Disord.*, **21**(7), 562–566.

Nillni, E.A., Vaslet, C., Harris, M., Hollenberg, A., Bjorbak, C. and Flier, J.S., 2000. Leptin regulates prothyrotropin-releasing hormone biosynthesis. Evidence for direct and indirect pathways. *J. Biol. Chem.*, **275**(46), 36124–36133.

Nozaki, T., Tamai, H., Matsubayashi, S., Komaki, G., Kobayashi, N. and Nakagawa, T., 1994. Insulin response to intravenous glucose in patients with anorexia nervosa showing low insulin response to oral glucose. *J. Clin. Endocrinol. Metab.*, **79**(1), 217–222.

Okamoto, S., Kimura, K. and Saito, M., 2001. Anorectic effect of leptin is mediated by hypothalamic corticotropin-releasing hormone, but not by urocortin, in rats. *Neurosci. Lett.*, **307**(3), 179–182.

Ollmann, M.M., Wilson, B.D., Yang, Y.K., Kerns, J.A., Chen, Y., Gantz, I. and Barsh, G.S., 1997. Antagonism of central melanocortin receptors *in vitro* and *in vivo* by agouti-related protein. *Science*, **278**(5335), 135–138.

Olney, J.W., 1969. Brain lesions, obesity, and other disturbances in mice treated with monosodium glutamate. *Science*, **164**(880), 719–721.

Palmer, R.L., 2000. *Management of Eating Disorders*. Wiley, Chichester.

Pauly, R.P., Lear, S.A., Hastings, F.C. and Birmingham, C.L., 2000. Resting energy expenditure and plasma leptin levels in anorexia nervosa during acute refeeding [in process citation]. *Int. J. Eat. Disord.*, **28**(2), 231–234.

Pelleymounter, M.A., Cullen, M.J., Baker, M.B., Hecht, R., Winters, D., Boone, T. and Collins, F., 1995. Effects of the obese gene product on body weight regulation in ob/ob mice. *Science*, **269**(5223), 540–543.

Pinel, J.P.J., Assanand, S. and Lehman, D.R., 2000. Hunger, eating, and ill health. *American Psychologist*, **55**(10), 1105–1116.

Pirke, K.M., Dogs, M., Fichter, M.M. and Tuschl, R.J., 1988. Gonadotrophins, oestradiol and progesterone during the menstrual cycle in bulimia nervosa. *Clin. Endocrinol. (Oxf.)*, **29**(3), 265–270.

Plotsky, P.M., Bruhn, T.O. and Vale, W., 1984. Central modulation of immunoreactive corticotrophin-releasing factor secretion by arginine vasopressin. *Endocrinology*, **115**, 1639–1641.

Polito, A., Fabbri, A., Ferro-Luzzi, A., Cuzzolaro, M., Censi, L., Ciarapica, D., Fabbrini, E. and Giannini, D., 2000. Basal metabolic rate in anorexia nervosa: relation to body composition and leptin concentrations. *Am. J. Clin. Nutr.*, **71**(6), 1495–1502.

Raphael, F.J., Rodin, D.A., Peattie, A., Bano, G., Kent, A., Nussey, S.S. and Lacey, J.H., 1995. Ovarian morphology and insulin sensitivity in women with bulimia nervosa. *Clin. Endocrinol. (Oxf.)*, **43**(4), 451–455.

Robinson, P.H., 1989. Perceptivity and paraceptivity during measurement of gastric emptying in anorexia and bulimia nervosa. *Br. J. Psychiatry*, **154**, 400–405.

Rolls, B.J., Andersen, A.E., Moran, T.H., McNelis, A.L., Baier, H.C. and Fedoroff, I.C., 1992. Food intake, hunger, and satiety after preloads in women with eating disorders. *Am. J. Clin. Nutr.*, **55**(6), 1093–1103.

Rosenkranz, K., Hinney, A., Ziegler, A., von Prittwitz, S., Barth, N., Roth, H., Mayer, H., Siegfried, W., Lehmkuhl, G., Poustka, F., Schmidt, M.,

Schafer, H., Remschmidt, H. and Hebebrand, J., 1998. Screening for mutations in the neuropeptide Y Y5 receptor gene in cohorts belonging to different weight extremes. *Int. J. Obes. Relat. Metab. Disord.*, **22**(2), 157–163.

Rosmond, R., Dallman, M.F. and Bjorntorp, P., 1998. Stress-related cortisol secretion in men: relationships with abdominal obesity and endocrine, metabolic and hemodynamic abnormalities. *J. Clin. Endocrinol. Metab.*, **83**(6), 1853–1859.

Sahu, A., 1998. Evidence suggesting that galanin (GAL), melanin-concentrating hormone (MCH), neurotensin (NT), proopiomelanocortin (POMC) and neuropeptide Y (NPY) are targets of leptin signaling in the hypothalamus. *Endocrinology*, **139**(2), 795–798.

Saito, Y., Cheng, M., Leslie, F.M. and Civelli, O., 2001. Expression of the melanin-concentrating hormone (MCH) receptor mRNA in the rat brain. *J. Comp. Neurol.*, **435**(1), 26–40.

Sakurai, T., Amemiya, A., Ishii, M., Matsuzaki, I., Chemelli, R.M., Tanaka, H., Williams, S.C., Richardson, J.A., Kozlowski, G.P., Wilson, S., Arch, J.R., Buckingham, R.E., Haynes, A.C., Carr, S.A., Annan, R.S., McNulty, D.E., Liu, W.S., Terrett, J.A., Elshourbagy, N.A., Bergsma, D.J. and Yanagisawa, M., 1998. Orexins and orexin receptors: a family of hypothalamic neuropeptides and G protein-coupled receptors that regulate feeding behaviour. *Cell*, **92**(4), 573–585.

Sapolsky, R.M., 1992. Do glucocorticoid concentrations rise with age in the rat? *Neurobiol. Aging*, **13**(1), 171–174.

Satoh, N., Ogawa, Y., Katsuura, G., Hayase, M., Tsuji, T., Imagawa, K., Yoshimasa, Y., Nishi, S., Hosoda, K. and Nakao, K., 1997. The arcuate nucleus as a primary site of satiety effect of leptin in rats. *Neurosci. Lett.*, **224**(3), 149–152.

Schaffhauser, A.O., Stricker-Krongrad, A., Brunner, L., Cumin, F., Gerald, C., Whitebread, S., Criscione, L. and Hofbauer, K.G., 1997. Inhibition of food intake by neuropeptide Y Y5 receptor antisense oligodeoxynucleotides. *Diabetes*, **46**(11), 1792–1798.

Schmidt, U., Tiller, J., Blanchard, M., Andrews, B. and Treasure, J., 1997. Is there a specific trauma precipitating anorexia nervosa? *Psychol. Med.*, **27**(3), 523–530.

Schwartz, M.W., Dallman, M.F. and Woods, S.C., 1995. Hypothalamic response to starvation: implications for the study of wasting disorders. *Am. J. Physiol.*, **269**(5), R949–R957.

Schwartz, M.W., Seeley, R.J., Campfield, L.A., Burn, P. and Baskin, D.G., 1996. Identification of targets of leptin action in rat hypothalamus. *J. Clin. Invest.*, **98**(5), 1101–1106.

Schwartz, M.W., Sipols, A.J., Marks, J.L., Sanacora, G., White, J.D., Scheurink, A., Kahn, S.E., Baskin, D.G., Woods, S.C. and Figlewicz, D.P., 1992. Inhibition of hypothalamic neuropeptide Y gene expression by insulin. *Endocrinology*, **130**(6), 3608–3616.

Schwartz, M.W., Woods, S.C., Porte, D., Seeley, R.J. and Baskin, D.G., 2000. Central nervous system control of food intake. *Nature*, **404**(6778), 661–671.

Seoane, L.M., Carro, E., Tovar, S., Casanueva, F.F. and Dieguez, C., 2000. Regulation of *in vivo* TSH secretion by leptin. *Regul. Pept.*, **92**(1–3), 25–29.

Shibasaki, T.Y.N.K.Y. *et al.*, 1988. Involvement of corticotrophin-releasing factor in restraint stress-induced anorexia and reversion of the anorexia by somatostatin in the rat. *Life Sciences*, **43**, 1103–1110.

Shimomura, Y., Mori, M., Sugo, T., Ishibashi, Y., Abe, M., Kurokawa, T., Onda, H., Nishimura, O., Sumino, Y. and Fujino, M., 1999. Isolation and identification of melanin-concentrating hormone as the endogenous ligand of the SLC-1 receptor. *Biochem. Biophys. Res. Commun.*, **261**(3), 622–626.

Sindelar, D.K., Havel, P.J., Seeley, R.J., Wilkinson, C.W., Woods, S.C. and Schwartz, M.W., 1999. Low plasma leptin levels contribute to diabetic hyperphagia in rats. *Diabetes*, **48**(6), 1275–1280.

Sipols, A.J., Baskin, D.G. and Schwartz, M.W., 1995. Effect of intracerebroventricular insulin infusion on diabetic hyperphagia and hypothalamic neuropeptide gene expression. *Diabetes*, **44**(2), 147–151.

Smith, B.K., York, D.A. and Bray, G.A., 1994. Chronic cerebroventricular galanin does not induce sustained hyperphagia or obesity. *Peptides*, **15**(7), 1267–1272.

Soliman, A.T., ElZalabany, M.M., Salama, M. and Ansari, B.M., 2000. Serum leptin concentrations during severe protein-energy malnutrition: correlation with growth parameters and endocrine function. *Metabolism*, **49**(7), 819–825.

Stanley, B.G., Kyrkouli, S.E., Lampert, S. and Leibowitz, S.F., 1986. Neuropeptide Y chronically injected into the hypothalamus: a powerful neurochemical inducer of hyperphagia and obesity. *Peptides*, **7**(6), 1189–1192.

Stellar, E., 1954. The physiology of motivation. *Psychological Reviews*, **61**, 5–22.

Stephens, T.W., Basinski, M., Bristow, P.K., Bue-Valleskey, J.M., Burgett, S.G., Craft, L., Hale, J., Hoffmann, J., Hsiung, H.M. and Kriauciunas, A., 1995. The role of neuropeptide Y in the antiobesity action of the obese gene product. *Nature*, **377**(6549), 530–532.

Stoving, R.K., Flyvbjerg, A., Frystyk, J., Fisker, S., Hangaard, J., Hansen-Nord, M. and Hagen, C., 1999a. Low serum levels of free and total insulin-like growth factor I (IGF-I) in patients with anorexia nervosa are not associated with increased IGF-binding protein-3 proteolysis. *J. Clin. Endocrinol. Metab.*, **84**(4), 1346–1350.

Stoving, R.K., Veldhuis, J.D., Flyvbjerg, A., Vinten, J., Hangaard, J., Koldkjaer, O.G., Kristiansen, J. and Hagen, C., 1999b. Jointly amplified basal and pulsatile growth hormone (GH) secretion and increased process irregularity in women with anorexia nervosa: indirect evidence for disruption of feedback regulation within the GH-insulin-like growth factor I axis. *J. Clin. Endocrinol. Metab.*, **84**(6), 2056–2063.

Strack, A.M., Sebastian, R.J., Schwartz, M.W. and Dallman, M.F., 1995. Glucocorticoids and insulin: reciprocal signals for energy balance. *Am. J. Physiol.*, **268**(1), R142–R149.

Strubbe, J.H. and Mein, C.G., 1977. Increased feeding in response to bilateral injection of insulin antibodies in the VMH. *Physiol. Behav.*, **19**(2), 309–313.

Sunday, S.R. and Halmi, K.A., 1990. Taste perceptions and hedonics in eating disorders. *Physiol. Behav.*, **48**(5), 587–594.

Tamai, H., Kiyohara, K., Mukuta, T., Kobayashi, N., Komaki, G., Nakagawa, T., Kumagai, L.F. and Aoki, T.T., 1991. Responses of growth hormone and cortisol to intravenous glucose loading test in patients with anorexia nervosa. *Metabolism*, **40**(1), 31–34.

Treasure, J.L., 1988. The ultrasonographic features in anorexia nervosa and bulimia nervosa: a simplified method of monitoring hormonal states during weight gain. *J. Psychosom. Res.*, **32**(6), 623–634.

Tritos, N.A., Mastaitis, J.W., Kokkotou, E. and Maratos-Flier, E., 2001. Characterization of melanin concentrating hormone and preproorexin expression in the murine hypothalamus. *Brain Res.*, **895**(1–2), 160–166.

Troop, N.A. and Treasure, J.L., 1997. Psychosocial factors in the onset of eating disorders: responses to life-events and difficulties. *Br. J. Med. Psychol.*, **70**(4), 373–385.

Tschop, M., Smiley, D.L. and Heiman, M.L., 2000. Ghrelin induces adiposity in rodents. *Nature*, **407**, 908–913.

Tschop, M., Weyer, C., Tataranni, P.A., Devanarayan, V., Ravussin, E. and Heiman, M.L., 2001. Circulating ghrelin levels are decreased in human obesity. *Diabetes*, **50**(4), 707–709.

Uehara, Y., Shimizu, H., Ohtani, K., Sato, N. and Mori, M., 1998. Hypothalamic corticotropin-releasing hormone is a mediator of the anorexigenic effect of leptin. *Diabetes*, **47**(6), 890–893.

Uhe, A.M., Szmukler, G.I., Collier, G.R., Hansky, J., O'Dea, K. and Young, G.P., 1992. Potential regulators of feeding behaviour in anorexia nervosa. *Am. J. Clin. Nutr.*, **55**(1), 28–32.

Utriainen, T., Malmstrom, R., Makimattila, S. and Yki-Jarvinen, H., 1996. Supraphysiological hyperinsulinemia increases plasma leptin concentrations after 4 h in normal subjects. *Diabetes*, **45**(10), 1364–1366.

Vaisse, C., Clement, K., Guy-Grand, B. and Froguel, P., 1998. A frameshift mutation in human MC4R is associated with a dominant form of obesity. *Nat. Genet.*, **20**(2), 113–114.

Valcavi, R., Zini, M. and Portioli, I., 1990. Triiodothyronine administration reduces serum growth hormone levels and growth hormone responses to thyrotropin-releasing hormone in patients with anorexia nervosa. *Psychoneuroendocrinology*, **15**(4), 287–295.

van Binsbergen, C.J., Coelingh Bennink, H.J., Odink, J., Haspels, A.A. and Koppeschaar, H.P., 1990. A comparative and longitudinal study on endocrine changes related to ovarian function in patients with anorexia nervosa. *J. Clin. Endocrinol. Metab.*, **71**(3), 705–711.

Van Huijsduijnen, O.B., Rohner-Jeanrenaud, F. and Jeanrenaud, B., 1993. Hypothalamic neuropeptide Y messenger ribonucleic acid levels in pre-obese and genetically obese (fa/fa) rats: potential regulation thereof by corticotrophin releasing factor. *Journal of Neuroendocrinology*, **5**, 381–386.

van Oers, H.J., de Kloet, E.R. and Levine, S., 1999. Persistent effects of maternal deprivation on HPA regulation can be reversed by feeding and stroking, but not by dexamethasone. *J. Neuroendocrinol.*, **11**(8), 581–588.

Viale, A., Zhixing, Y., Breton, C., Pedeutour, F., Coquerel, A., Jordan, D. and Nahon, J.L., 1997. The melanin-concentrating hormone gene in human: flanking region analysis, fine chromosome mapping, and tissue-specific expression. *Brain Res. Mol. Brain Res.*, **46**(1–2), 243–255.

Vink, T., Hinney, A., van Elburg, A.A., van Goozen, S.H., Sandkuijl, L.A., Sinke, R.J., Herpertz-Dahlmann, B.M., Hebebrand, J., Remschmidt, H., van Engeland, H. and Adan, R.A., 2001. Association between an agouti-related protein gene polymorphism and anorexia nervosa. *Mol. Psychiatry*, **6**(3), 325–328.

Vrang, N., Tang, C.M., Larsen, P.J. and Kristensen, P., 1999. Recombinant CART peptide induces c-Fos expression in central areas involved in control of feeding behaviour. *Brain Res.*, **818**(2), 499–509.

Vuagnat, B.A., Pierroz, D.D., Lalaoui, M., Englaro, P., Pralong, F.P., Blum, W.F. and Aubert, M.L., 1998. Evidence for a leptin–neuropeptide Y axis for the regulation of growth hormone secretion in the rat. *Neuroendocrinology*, **67**(5), 291–300.

Wabitsch, M., Ballauff, A., Holl, R., Blum, W.F., Heinze, E., Remschmidt, H. and Hebebrand, J., 2001. Serum leptin, gonadotropin, and testosterone concentrations in male patients with anorexia nervosa during weight gain. *J. Clin. Endocrinol. Metab.*, **86**(7), 2982–2988.

Wadden, T.A., Foster, G.D., Letizia, K.A. and Wilk, J.E., 1993. Metabolic, anthropometric, and psychological characteristics of obese binge eaters. *Int. J. Eat. Disord.*, **14**(1), 17–25.

Ward, A., Brown, N., Lightman, S., Campbell, I.C. and Treasure, J., 1998. Neuroendocrine, appetitive and behavioural responses to d-fenfluramine in women recovered from anorexia nervosa. *Br. J. Psychiatry*, **172**, 351–358.

Ward, A., Ramsay, R. and Treasure, J., 2000. Attachment research in eating disorders. *Br. J. Med. Psychol.*, **73**(1), 35–51.

Weingarten, H.P., Chang, P.K. and McDonald, T.J., 1985. Comparison of the metabolic and behavioural disturbances following paraventricular- and ventromedial-hypothalamic lesions. *Brain Res. Bull.*, **14**(6), 551–559.

Weltzin, T.E., Cameron, J., Berga, S. and Kaye, W.H., 1994. Prediction of reproductive status in women with bulimia nervosa by past high weight. *Am. J. Psychiatry*, **151**(1), 136–138.

Werther, G.A., Hogg, A., Oldfield, B.J., McKinley, M.J., Figdor, R., Allen, A.M. and Mendelsohn, F.A., 1987. Localization and characterization of insulin receptors in rat brain and pituitary gland using *in vitro* autoradiography and computerized densitometry. *Endocrinology*, **121**(4), 1562–1570.

Willie, J.T., Chemelli, R.M., Sinton, C.M. and Yanagisawa, M., 2001. To eat or to sleep? Orexin in the regulation of feeding and wakefulness. *Annu. Rev. Neurosci.*, **24**, 429–458.

Wisniewski, L., Epstein, L.H., Marcus, M.D. and Kaye, W., 1997. Differences in salivary habituation to palatable foods in bulimia nervosa patients and controls. *Psychosom. Med.*, **59**(4), 427–433.

Yeo, G.S., Farooqi, I.S., Aminian, S., Halsall, D.J., Stanhope, R.G. and O'Rahilly, S., 1998. A frameshift mutation in MC4R associated with dominantly inherited human obesity. *Nat. Genet.*, **20**(2), 111–112.

Yu, W.H., Kimura, M., Walczewska, A., Karanth, S. and McCann, S.M., 1997. Role of leptin in hypothalamic–pituitary function [published erratum appears in *Proc Natl Acad Sci USA* 1997 Sep 30;**94**(20):11108]. *Proc. Natl. Acad. Sci. USA*, **94**(3), 1023–1028.

Zhang, Y., Proenca, R., Maffei, M., Barone, M., Leopold, L. and Friedman, J.M., 1994. Positional cloning of the mouse obese gene and its human homologue [published erratum appears in *Nature* 1995 Mar 30;**374**(6521):479] [see comments]. *Nature*, **372**(6505), 425–432.

XXIII-4

Neuroimmunology of Eating Disorders

Jan Pieter Konsman and Robert Dantzer

INTRODUCTION

Eating is a behaviour familiar to all of us. Despite this familiarity, regulation of eating in humans is complex and involves biological, psychological, social as well as cultural factors (Fischler, 2001). Most of our current knowledge concerning the biological factors involved in the regulation of food intake has been gained from investigations of eating behaviour in animals. The results obtained have recently been incorporated into a neurobiological model of the regulation of food intake (see for review Schwartz *et al.*, 2000) that most probably bears important implications for a better understanding of eating behaviour and disorders in humans.

In this paper, we will, therefore, first review the neurobiological basis of the regulation of food intake before addressing two of the most common causes of anorexia in the absence of lesions or dysfunction of the gastro-intestinal tract, namely anorexia associated with infectious diseases and anorexia nervosa. Factors inhibiting food intake will be discussed in more depth than signals promoting eating since the focus of this paper is on anorexia. Besides, our present day understanding of how feeding is initiated is limited and the prevailing model of the regulation of food intake is based on the assumption that ingestion of food generates signals that subsequently inhibit eating.

NEUROBIOLOGY OF EATING

Food intake needs to be regulated to assure the supply of amino acids and energy to cells throughout the body. All macronutrients, carbohydrates, lipids and proteins, can provide usable cellular energy, albeit with different efficiencies. Most cells are, however, capable of using carbohydrates in the form of glucose or lipids in the form of free fatty acids as energy substrates.

The early so-called depletion–repletion model of food intake postulated that organisms start eating when energy substrates, for example glucose levels, are low (depleted) and stop ingesting food as soon as energy substrate levels are replenished. According to this model a relationship should exist between the size of a meal and the time passed since the preceding meal. However, no such relationship is found when measuring meal size and the interval between meals in rats with free access to food (Le Magnen and Tallon, 1966). Instead, a relationship exists between the size of a meal and the time lag before the rat eats its next meal (Le Magnen and Tallon, 1966). These findings indicate that the ingestion of a meal generates satiety signals that suppress food intake.

Cholecystokinin Acts as a Satiety Signal Reducing Meal Size

During the 1970s and 1980s it became clear that the gut peptide cholecystokinin (CCK) constitutes a meal-generated satiety signal. CCK is synthesized in endocrine cells within the mucosa of the proximal small intestine (Buchan *et al.*, 1978) and secreted upon ingestion of food (Liddle *et al.*, 1985). Intraperitoneal administration of a synthetic peptide corresponding to the eight amino acids at the C-terminal portion of CCK (CCK-8) in rats just prior to food presentation causes a dose-dependent decrease in meal size, but not in water intake (Gibbs *et al.*, 1973). CCK-8 administered intravenously to humans also induces earlier satiation without reports or signs of sickness (Geary *et al.*, 1992).

Low concentrations of CCK-8 act on afferent fibres of the vagus nerves to reduce food intake in rats (Smith *et al.*, 1981). Vagal afferent fibres express CCK receptors (Lin and Miller, 1992) and terminate in the brain stem at the level of the nucleus of the solitary tract. Lesioning this brain structure attenuates the satiety effects of CCK-8 (Edwards *et al.*, 1986) indicating that it plays a role in the CCK-induced reduction of meal size. Although forebrain structures most probably influence brain stem circuits activated by CCK-8, it is important to note that brain stem circuits are sufficient to mediate the inhibitory effects of peripheral CCK-8 administration on sucrose intake (Grill and Smith, 1988).

More recently, with the development of CCK receptor antagonists, it has become possible to test the hypothesis that abdominal release of endogenous CCK constitutes a satiety signal. The expected effect of a CCK receptor antagonist would be to increase meal size. Indeed, administration of a CCK_A (CCK type A) receptor antagonist increases meal size by about 25% in rats (Brenner and Ritter, 1995). It is important to note here that these results were obtained with an antagonist that did not enter the brain, since CCK receptors are also present in the CNS. Altogether, these findings indicate that the peripheral release of CCK after ingestion of food constitutes a satiety signal suppressing eating by acting on the vagus nerve and activating hind brain circuits.

Leptin Constitutes an Adiposity Signal Inhibiting Long-Term Meal Size

Although CCK clearly inhibits the ingestion of food during a meal, systematic administration of CCK-8 to rats at the start of each spontaneous meal turns out to have no effect on body weight, since animals eat meals more frequently (West *et al.*, 1984). This indicates that other factors regulate eating over a longer time span to maintain energy stores. The hypothesis that the regulation of food intake is linked to the amount of energy stocked, for example in the form of fat, was first formulated in the 1950s by Kennedy (1953). This so-called lipostatic model of food intake and energy balance postulates that the organism eats to maintain a set point level of body adiposity. This stock of energy in the form of fat is used to meet the energetic demands of the organism. In this model the existence of adiposity signals reflecting the amount of energy stocked in the form of fat was postulated and proposed to act on

Biological Psychiatry: Edited by H. D'haenen, J.A. den Boer and P. Willner. ISBN 0-471-49198-5

the brain to inhibit feeding and body adiposity (Kennedy, 1953). These adiposity signals are integrated with other factors regulating food intake, such as satiety signals (see above), energy needs as well as the physiological state of the animal and food properties.

It was not until the mid 1990s that a factor proportional to body fat mass was identified in the form of leptin, also known as ob protein (Frederich *et al.*, 1995; Zhang *et al.*, 1994). Leptin is released mainly by subcutaneous and visceral adipose tissue. Leptin levels increase with feeding and quickly fall after starvation (Ahima *et al.*, 1996; Maffei *et al.*, 1995). Mice carrying mutations in the leptin gene or its receptor are obese (Chen *et al.*, 1996; Zhang *et al.*, 1994) indicating that leptin inhibits feeding and adiposity. Indeed, repeated Intraperitoneal administration of leptin reduces food intake and, in contrast to CCK (see above), induces weight loss in leptin deficient mice, but not in mice lacking the leptin receptor (Halaas *et al.*, 1995). Moreover, repeated subcutaneous administration of a stabilized form of leptin in rats reduces meal size through several days after the last injection and does not induce the compensatory overeating (Kahler *et al.*, 1998) that develops after repeated CCK administration (see above). Interestingly, injection of regular leptin into the lateral brain ventricle of the rat reduces meal size for at least 12 hours and at much lower doses than needed after peripheral injection (Flynn *et al.*, 1998). Moreover, neutralization of leptin in the CNS augments food intake in rats without any subsequent compensatory changes in eating patterns (Brunner *et al.*, 1997). These findings clearly show that leptin acts in the CNS to inhibit meal size in both the short and long term.

The Adiposity Signal Leptin Interacts with the Satiety Signal CCK, but Inhibits Long-Term Food Intake by its Action on the Hypothalamus

One of the predictions of the lipostatic model for the regulation of food intake is that adiposity signals, such as leptin, are integrated with satiety signals, such as CCK (see above). Leptin acts in the CNS to inhibit food intake (Brunner *et al.*, 1997) and its receptors are found at the level of the nucleus of the solitary tract (Elmquist *et al.*, 1998). Given that this brain structure is involved in the satiety effects of CCK (Edwards *et al.*, 1986), leptin might interact with the brain circuits mediating the effects of CCK to inhibit food intake. Indeed, intracerebroventricular administration of leptin at a dose that by itself does not affect food intake, increases the suppression of intake induced by Intraperitoneal injection of CCK-8 (Emond *et al.*, 1999). Moreover, combined leptin and CCK-8 treatment augments the number of activated neurons in the nucleus of the solitary tract compared with either leptin or CCK-8 treatment alone (Emond *et al.*, 1999) indicating that leptin and CCK signals interact at the level of the brainstem (see Figure XXIII-4.1).

However, intracerebroventricular injection of leptin still inhibits food intake in rats lacking the CCK_A receptor (Niimi *et al.*, 1999), the receptor responsible for the satiety effects of CCK (see above). In addition, intracerebroventricular leptin induces activation of hypothalamic structures in these rats (Niimi *et al.*, 1999) indicating that leptin inhibits food intake by acting on the hypothalamus independently from CCK. Strong expression of leptin receptors in the CNS is found in the arcuate nucleus at the basis of the hypothalamus in both humans and rodents (Couce *et al.*, 1997; Elmquist *et al.*, 1998). This hypothalamic structure that regulates long-term food intake and energy balance (Dawson and Lorden, 1981; Morris *et al.*, 1998) is pivotal in mediating the anorectic effects of leptin, since lesions of the arcuate nucleus prevent the inhibitory effects of leptin administered into the lateral brain ventricle (Tang-Christensen *et al.*, 1999). Moreover, intravenously injected leptin is taken up by the arcuate nucleus (Banks *et al.*, 1996) possibly by diffusion from the nearby median eminence which lacks a blood-brain barrier. Taken together, these results indicate that leptin acts as a hormone at the level of the arcuate hypothalamus to reduce food intake (see Figure XXIII-4.1).

The Arcuate Hypothalamus Contains Two Neuronal Populations Exerting Opposite Effects on Food Intake and Fat Tissue and Senses Adiposity Signals as well as Energy Needs

Leptin receptors in the arcuate nucleus of the hypothalamus are found on two populations of neuropeptide-expressing neurons (Hakansson *et al.*, 1998; Mercer *et al.*, 1996). The first population expresses neuropeptide Y and projects to the paraventricular nucleus of the hypothalamus (Baker and Herkenham, 1995). Local injection of neuropeptide Y into the paraventricular nucleus promotes food intake (Stanley and Leibowitz, 1985) and inhibits sympathetic output to fat tissue (Egawa *et al.*, 1991), thus inhibiting catabolic pathways (Schwartz *et al.*, 2000). Conversely, food intake is decreased by damaging arcuate NPY neurons immunologically (Burlet *et al.*, 1995) or by local administration of NPY antigens oligonucleotides (Akabayashi *et al.*, 1994).

The effects of NPY are countered by a second population of arcuate neurons that also project to the paraventricular hypothalamus, but express the neuropeptide alpha-melanocyte-stimulating hormone (α-MSH) (Cowley *et al.*, 1999), a product of the pro-opiomelanocortin gene. α-MSH acts on so-called melanocortin receptors and intracerebroventricular injection of a melanocortin-4 receptor agonist, that mimics α-MSH action, inhibits food intake (Murphy *et al.*, 1998) and increases sympathetic nervous system outflow to adipose tissue (Haynes *et al.*, 1999). Conversely, administration of a melanocortin-4 receptor antagonist into the paraventricular nucleus stimulates feeding (Giraudo *et al.*, 1998).

Feeding increases metabolic rate by 25–40% (Shibata and Bukowiecki, 1987; Sims and Danforth, 1987), and decreases NPY contents in the paraventricular hypothalamus while increasing POMC expression in the arcuate nucleus (Hagan *et al.*, 1999; Kalra *et al.*, 1991). Food restriction, on the other hand, increases NPY, but decreases POMC expression in the arcuate nucleus (Brady *et al.*, 1990; Mizuno *et al.*, 1998; Schwartz *et al.*, 1993) and leads to a reduction in energy expenditure (Leibel *et al.*, 1995).

As might be predicted from its inhibitory effects on food intake, leptin decreases arcuate levels of neuropeptide Y (Stephens *et al.*, 1995; Wang *et al.*, 1997) (see insert Figure XXIII-4.1). Leptin receptors are also found on neurons expressing the pro-opiomelanocortin gene that gives rise to α-MSH in the arcuate nucleus (Cheung *et al.*, 1997) and leptin increases expression of pro-opiomelanocortin (Schwartz *et al.*, 1997). Furthermore, the anorectic effect of leptin directly injected into the brain ventricle is attenuated by administration of a melanocortin receptor antagonist (Seeley *et al.*, 1997) indicating that leptin inhibits food intake by stimulating α-MSH release from arcuate neurons (see insert Figure XXIII-4.1).

In summary, leptin inhibits food intake and promotes fat breakdown by stimulation of an α-MSH containing projection and inhibition of a neuropeptide Y-expressing projection from the arcuate to the paraventricular nucleus of the hypothalamus. In addition to sensing energy supplies via leptin receptors, the arcuate nucleus also contains receptors for growth hormone (Minami *et al.*, 1993), corticosterone (Fuxe *et al.*, 1987) and the pro-inflammator cytokine interleukin-1 (Ericsson *et al.*, 1995). These factors signal energy needs in conditions of growth, stress and disease. The presence of their receptors at the level of the arcuate nucleus indicates that the integration of adiposity signals and factors signalling energy needs, as postulated in the lipostatic model of the regulation of food intake (see above), occurs at the level of the arcuate hypothalamus.

Rewarding and Motivational Aspects of Feeding

In addition to its energetic value, food has rewarding properties. In fact, it has been suggested that the energetic value and rewarding

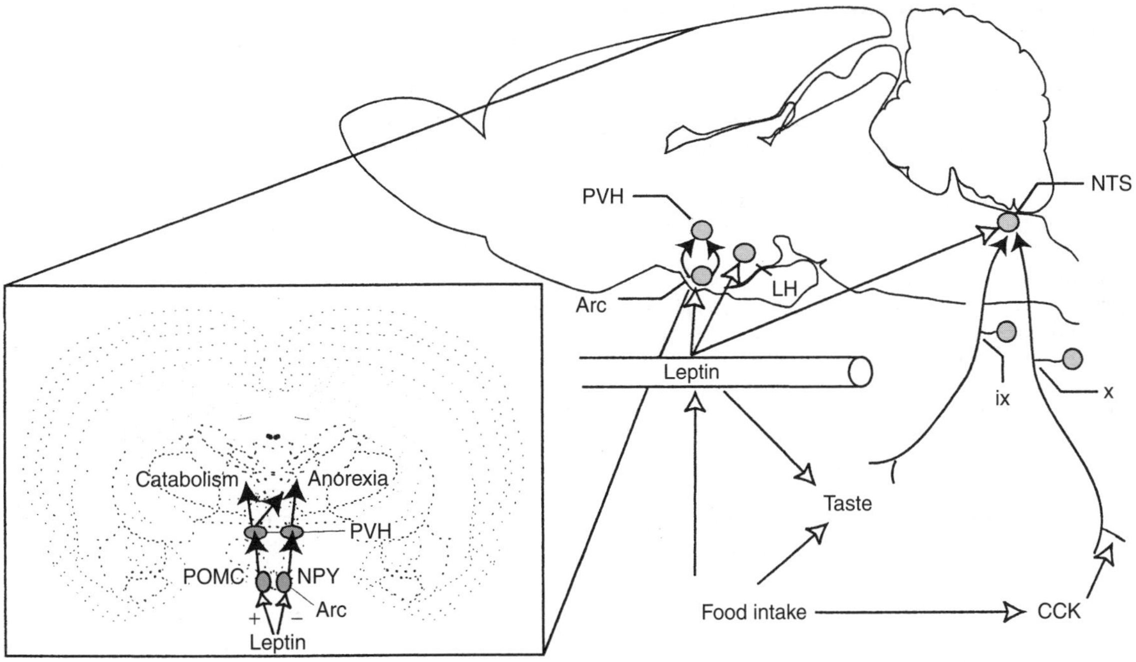

Figure XXIII-4.1 Saggital view of the rat brain to illustrate mechanisms by which leptin reduces food intake. Ingestion of food intake leads to an increase in intestinal cholecystokinin and circulating leptin. At the level of the nucleus of the solitary tract in the brainstem, leptin augments the anorectic signal induced by action of cholecystokinin on the vagus nerve. Leptin also acts at the level of the arcuate hypothalamic nucleus to inhibit the neuropeptide Y containing neuronal projection to the paraventricular hypothalamus which promotes food intake (see insert showing a coronal section at the level of the arcuate and paraventricular hypothalamus). At the same time, leptin increases the synthesis of α-melanocyte-stimulating hormone, a product of the pro-opiomelanocortin gene in neurons of the arcuate hypothalamus. These latter neurons project to the paraventricular hypothalamus to activates anorectic and catabolic pathways. Other mechanisms underlying the anorectic effects of leptin may include modulation of lateral hypothalamic (LH) circuits mediating the rewarding properties of food intake and inhibition of sweet taste sensitivity (see text). Open arrowheads indicate humoral or paracrine action, closed arrowheads neuronal projections. Abbreviations: ix: glossopharyngeal nerve, x: vagus nerve, Arc: arcuate hypothalamic nucleus, CCK: cholecystokinin, LH: lateral hypothalamus, NPY: neuropeptide Y, NTS: nucleus of the solitary tract, POMC: pro-opiomelanocortin, PVH: paraventricular hypothalamus. Drawings of rat brain sections were modified from Swanson (1998)

properties of a food are correlated in that highly palatable foods, such as chocolate, are more energy dense (Drewnowski, 1998). Palatability increases appetite and thus food intake and can be measured as the perceived pleasantness of a food or the intent to eat in humans (Drewnowski, 1998).

The term reward, which connotes pleasure, infers a subjective state and is therefore strictly spoken problematic when referring to animal experiments. Obviously, an animal cannot report the perceived pleasantness of a food or its intent to eat. However, since this term is widely used in the scientific literature, it will also be employed here. Despite this fundamental difficulty, there are ways to measure the rewarding properties of food in laboratory animals. One approach is to electrically activate the brain regions that mediate reward by a micro-electrode when the animal presses an operant lever and to study how natural stimuli like food affect the rate of lever pressing. It is well known that animals work vigorously in the form of lever pressing in order to trigger electrical stimulation of certain brain regions, for example the lateral hypothalamus, as if the stimulation had rewarding properties (Shizgal, 1997). When rats are forced to choose between brain-stimulation reward and a natural reward in the form of a sucrose solution, they choose sucrose when the electrical stimulation is weak. However, at higher stimulation frequencies, rats prefer brain stimulation over sucrose ingestion (Shizgal, 1997).

The rewarding properties of a stimulus also depend on the physiological state of the organism. A hungry animal will choose a more concentrated sucrose solution rather than a less concentrated solution, whereas a sated animal is likely to ingest both solutions with indifference, and an overfed animal chooses not to ingest at all. A hungry animal is also more sensitive to stimulation of the lateral hypothalamus (Abrahamsen *et al.*, 1995; Carr and Papadouka, 1994). Furthermore, mildly food-deprived rats choose to ingest sucrose and stimulate their lateral hypothalamus rather than apply brain stimulation alone (Shizgal, 1997). Since brain stimulation and natural stimuli compete with and add to each other, both signals are likely to activate the same brain circuits that mediate reward.

Interestingly, both food reward and self-stimulation of the lateral hypothalamus increase dopamine release in the nucleus accumbens (Hernandez and Hoebel, 1988). Dopamine containing terminals at the level of the nucleus accumbens are part of the so-called mesolimbic dopamine system that plays an important role in mediating reward (Berridge and Robinson, 1998). Finally, the findings described above are not restricted to the ingestion of sucrose, but also occur when a saline solution is provided to salt-deprived animals (Shizgal, 1997). Altogether, these data are in accordance with the hypothesis that self-stimulation of the lateral hypothalamus is an appropriate model to study reward mechanisms in animals.

From the experiments described above it is also clear that both the properties of a stimulus, such as sweetness, and the physiological state of the organism determine the rewarding properties of that stimulus and the motivational state of the animal. The animal's degree of motivation can be assessed by its capacity to work for a goal, for example by studying the number of times the animal is willing to press a lever in order to obtain a food pellet.

Leptin Modulates Brain Circuits Involved in the Rewarding Aspects of Feeding

According to the lipostatic model of the regulation of food intake, adiposity signals, such as leptin, should interact with the physiological state of the animal and food properties. Intracerebroventricular administration of leptin reduces intake of a sucrose solution from a bottle in rats (Ammar *et al.*, 2000) indicating that leptin is likely to act on those brain circuits that mediate the rewarding properties of food.

However, leptin also inhibits the sensitivity for sweet taste in peripheral taste cells of rodents (Kawai *et al.*, 2000). An alternative explanation would therefore be that leptin does not modulate brain circuits mediating reward, but merely alters the taste of a sucrose solution (see Figure XXIII-4.1). Although the modulation of taste by leptin most probably contributes to the reduction of sucrose intake, evidence exists to indicate that this is not the only factor. As discussed above, food deprivation enhances hypothalamic self-stimulation, an operant model to study reward in animals. Interestingly, intracerebroventricular injection of leptin inhibits the deprivation-induced enhancement of self-stimulation (Fulton *et al.*, 2000) indicating that leptin does indeed modulate brain circuits mediating reward (see Figure XXIII-4.1).

So, in addition to its interaction with brain circuits controlling energy balance at the level of the arcuate nucleus of the hypothalamus, leptin also interacts with CNS circuits mediating the rewarding properties of food. Although the brain circuits that mediate reward are not yet fully unravelled, leptin might act directly on the lateral hypothalamus as its receptors are expressed present in this structure (Elmquist *et al.*, 1998). In contrast to what occurs in the arcuate nucleus which is located close to the median eminence where the blood-brain barrier is absent, circulating leptin does not appear to reach the lateral hypothalamus by diffusion from the blood. Instead, an active transport system involving a shorter form of the leptin receptor might be responsible for leptin action on the lateral hypothalamus (Banks *et al.*, 1996).

ANOREXIA ASSOCIATED WITH INFECTIOUS DISEASES

Suppression of food intake is seen in humans and animals with a variety of systemic diseases as well as with more localized infections (Hart, 1988). By decreasing their food intake the organism reduces the chance of raising plasma concentrations of free iron, which is an essential element that many bacteria need to replicate (Weinberg, 1984). Low iron levels alone do not impair bacterial growth, but proliferation of bacteria is inhibited when iron levels are low and body temperature is elevated (Kluger and Rothenburg, 1979). This is probably due to decreased bacterial synthesis of iron-chelating compounds at temperatures above 37°C (Garibaldi, 1972). So, anorexia together with fever limits bacterial proliferation.

The low incidence of infections in iron-deficient humans is in accordance with this hypothesis. In the late 1970s Murray *et al.*, described a five-fold increase in the incidence of infectious episodes after treatment of iron-deficient nomads with iron (Murray *et al.*, 1978). Based on this finding and their experience with famines in Africa these authors proposed that therapeutic refeeding during infection can be harmful (Murray *et al.*, 1978). When this hypothesis was tested experimentally, it was indeed found that forced feeding of mice during acute bacterial infection reduces survival time and increases mortality (Murray and Murray, 1979), while food deprivation increases survival (Wing and Young, 1980). These findings indicate that anorexia upon acute infection is an adaptive response.

Anorexia during disease has long been thought to be either the consequence of fever or to result from a general weakness of the sick individual. However, hyperthermia alone does not suppress food intake (McCarthy *et al.*, 1984), indicating that anorexia during disease is not a necessary consequence of fever. Since muscle weakness and pain are common symptoms of infectious diseases (Hart, 1988), anorexia during disease might be due to difficulty or pain interfering with hoarding of food. Hoarding of food requires a high locomotor activity, but allows rodents to consume food safely and to anticipate food scarceness. When rats that are dependent for their food intake on the amount of food they hoard are injected with bacterial fragments, food hoarding decreases only by 22%, whereas food consumption drops by 70–75% (Aubert *et al.*, 1997). These findings indicate that the difficulty to move does not play a major factor in anorexia during infectious disease.

During infectious disease anorexia is accompanied by fever as a result of increased heat production in adipose tissue. However, normally when food intake diminishes, adipose tissue metabolism is decreased, a response mediated by the effects of low circulating leptin on the central nervous system (see above). The concomitant occurrence of fever and anorexia suggests, therefore, that the central nervous circuits controlling food intake and energy metabolism are altered during infectious disease.

Interleukin-1β Acts on the Vagus Nerve to Induce Anorexia

Soluble factors secreted by immune cells are proposed to act on the nervous system to induce anorexia during infectious disease (Hart, 1988). One of the soluble factors secreted by tissue macrophages upon detection of bacterial fragments is the pro-inflammatory cytokine interleukin-1β (IL-1β). Intraperitoneal administration of IL-1β induces a reduction in total caloric intake thus mimicking the effect of injection of bacterial fragments (Aubert *et al.*, 1995). To explain its anorectic effects, IL-1β was proposed to act on vagus nerve (Dantzer, 1994). The first evidence indicating that IL-1β affects functioning of the vagus nerve was obtained by Niijima, who showed an increase in firing frequency of the hepatic vagus nerve after injection of IL-1β into the hepatoportal system (Niijima, 1996).

Based on Niijima's initial findings, experiments were performed in our laboratory to study the role of subdiaphragmatic vagal branches in anorexia associated with infectious diseases. A modified Skinner box was used to study the effects of bacterial fragments or IL-1β on food-motivated behaviour in mice of which the vagus nerve was sectioned under the diaphragm. The depressing effects of Intraperitoneal administration of bacterial fragments or IL-1β on a food-motivated lever-pressing response were found to be abolished by subdiaphragmatic vagotomy (Bret-Dibat *et al.*, 1995) and were independent from the well-known anorectic effect of cholecystokinin on the vagus nerve (Bret-Dibat and Dantzer, 2000). These findings indicate that IL-1β acts directly on the vagus nerve to induce anorexia during infectious disease. The discovery of IL-1 receptors on cell bodies of the vagus nerve (Ek *et al.*, 1998) is in accordance with the idea of direct IL-1β action on the vagus nerve (see Figure XXIII-4.2).

The vagus nerve projects to the nucleus of the solitary tract in the brainstem which plays an important role in meal termination (Treece *et al.*, 1998, 2000). Peripheral administration of bacterial fragments (Gaykema *et al.*, 1995) or IL-1β (Ericsson *et al.*, 1994) activates in part the same neurons as the ingestion of a meal (Rinaman *et al.*, 1998) or a physiological dose of cholecystokinin (Rinaman *et al.*, 1993) (see above). However, an additional neuronal population is activated at the level of the nucleus of the solitary tract in response to immunological stimuli. This neuronal population contains the neuropeptide glucagon-like peptide 1 (GLP-1) and seems to mediate nausea during illness (Rinaman, 1999). Moreover, intracerebroventricular administration of an antagonist of GLP receptors attenuates anorexia induced by an Intraperitoneal injection of bacterial fragments as well as activation of the paraventricular nucleus of the hypothalamus (Rinaman, 2000). This latter structure is important in the control of food intake and energy metabolism (see above), since neuropeptide containing neurons in the paraventricular nucleus of the hypothalamus have been proposed to give rise to pathways that stimulate breakdown of body fat and promote anorexia (Schwartz *et al.*, 2000). In addition to abolishing the anorectic effects of Intraperitoneal administration of bacterial fragments, subdiaphragmatic vagotomy prevents activation of neurons in the nucleus of the solitary tract as well as in the paraventricular nucleus of the hypothalamus (Konsman *et al.*, 2000). Altogether, these findings indicate that during infectious disease IL-1β acts on the vagus nerve to activate GLP-1 neurons in the nucleus of the solitary tract that signal nausea and by consequence induce anorexia.

Although subdiaphragmatic vagotomy prevents the decrease in food-motivated behaviour in response to Intraperitoneal injection of a low dose of IL-1β, it only attenuates the effect of a higher dose (Bret-Dibat *et al.*, 1995). Moreover, vagotomy does not affect activation of neurons in nucleus of the solitary tract and the paraventricular hypothalamus after intravenous injection of LPS or IL-1β (Ericsson *et al.*, 1997; Wan *et al.*, 1994). These observations suggest that still other pathways exist by which IL-1 can act on the central nervous system to induce anorexia during disease.

Interleukin-1β Acts in the Central Nervous System to Induce Anorexia

Observations by several authors show that IL-1 receptors are expressed in the central nervous system (Cunningham *et al.*, 1992; Ericsson *et al.*, 1995; Konsman *et al.*, 2000; Parnet *et al.*, 1994; Yabuuchi *et al.*, 1994), thus raising the possibility that IL-1β acts in the central nervous system to induce anorexia. An experiment was designed in our laboratory to study the role of brain IL-1 receptors in anorexia during infectious disease by infusing an IL-1 receptor antagonist into the lateral brain ventricle of mice after Intraperitoneal injection of bacterial fragments. Intracerebroventricular infusion of the IL-1 receptor antagonist was indeed found to attenuate the reduction in food intake induced by bacterial fragments (Layé *et al.*, 2000).

Although these findings clearly indicate that IL-1 acts in the central nervous system to mediate anorexia during infectious disease, they also give rise to the question as to how IL-1β enters the central nervous system. Blood-borne IL-1β, with its relatively high molecular weight and hydrophilic profile, cannot cross the blood-brain barrier passively. Therefore, circulating IL-1β can only enter the brain by active transport (Banks *et al.*, 1991) or by leakage at the level of circumventricular organs where the blood-brain barrier is non-functional. Circumventricular organs contain fenestrated capillaries that by consequence do not form a functional blood-brain barrier (Gross, 1992). Circulating IL-1β can thus leak from the blood stream into circumventricular organs and possibly into adjacent central nervous tissue. Circumventricular organs also contain phagocytic cells (Murabe *et al.*, 1981) and express receptors for bacterial fragments (Laflamme and Rivest, 2000) raising the possibility that these organs synthesize IL-1β during infectious disease. IL-1β immunoreactivity is, indeed, found in phagocytic cells of circumventricular organs after Intraperitoneal injection of bacterial fragments (Konsman *et al.*, 1999).

One of the circumventricular organs, the median eminence is juxtaposed to the arcuate nucleus of the hypothalamus, a structure involved in the integration of factors signalling energy stocks and needs (see above). The part of the arcuate nucleus of the hypothalamus just adjacent to the median eminence contains capillaries rich in vesicles suggesting transport of molecules through these cells (Gross, 1992). Furthermore, these capillaries are surrounded by perivascular spaces that are thought to be confluent with those around fenestrated capillaries in the median eminence (Gross, 1992), suggesting that circulating molecules reach at least this part of the arcuate hypothalamus. Physiological experiments using intravenous tracer injections in the rat revealed that the capillary and perivascular space available for blood-tissue exchange is four times larger and tissue penetration 34 times greater in the arcuate nucleus proximal to the median eminence compared to the distal arcuate nucleus (Shaver *et al.*, 1992). Since IL-1 receptor mRNA is expressed in the arcuate nucleus of the hypothalamus (Ericsson *et al.*, 1995; Konsman *et al.*, 2000), it is tempting to speculate that IL-1β acts on arcuate neurons to induce anorexia associated with infectious disease. Further research is necessary to establish which neuronal population expresses IL-1 receptors and to what extent IL-1β reaches its receptors in arcuate nucleus of the hypothalamus (see Figure XXIII-4.2).

In summary, IL-1β seems to induce anorexia during infectious disease by provoking nausea via its action on the vagus nerve and possibly by altering central nervous circuits regulating food intake and energy metabolism at the level of the arcuate nucleus of the hypothalamus. In contrast to leptin (see above), IL-1β does not modulate brain circuits mediating reward directly (Anisman *et al.*, 1998). However, both the administration of bacterial fragments and IL-1β do induce a rise in plasma levels of leptin at later time points (Faggioni *et al.*, 1998; Sarraf *et al.*, 1997). The role of leptin in anorexia associated with infectious diseases needs therefore to be addressed in future studies (see Figure XXIII-4.2).

ANOREXIA NERVOSA

Anorexia nervosa is an eating disorder common among teenage girls and characterized by self-starvation and weight loss. This disorder has a very poor prognosis with less than 50% chance of recovery and a mortality rate of 9% (Woodside, 1995). Despite intensive research and numerous hypotheses, the causes of this disorder remain at present unknown.

In view of the anorectic effects of pro-inflammatory cytokines during infectious and probably neoplasic diseases (see above), it was tempting to hypothesize that pro-inflammatory cytokines play a role in the aetiology of anorexia nervosa (Holden and Pakula, 1996; Vaisman and Hahn, 1991). Despite numerous studies aimed at measuring circulating cytokines or *in vitro* cytokine secretion by white blood cells, no clear-cut conclusion can be drawn from these studies (Marcos, 1997). Among the difficulties in interpreting these findings are the fact that cytokines may have paracrine or autocrine effects that do not result in elevated plasma levels and the fact that starvation alters cytokine production (Grimble, 1994). Besides, virtually all reported alternations of immune responses in anorexia nervosa patients improve with refeeding (Marcos, 1997) suggesting that they are a consequence rather than a cause of anorexia nervosa.

A closer look at the symptoms of anorexia nervosa and the non-specific symptoms of infectious disease indicates, however, that it is rather unlikely that pro-inflammatory cytokines play an important role in the aetiology of anorexia nervosa. Anorexia induced by bacterial fragments or interleukin-1 concerns mostly protein intake and not carbohydrates (Aubert *et al.*, 1995). On the contrary, the diet of a typical anorexia nervosa patient is deficient in carbohydrates, while relatively sufficient in protein and fat (Crisp and Stonehill, 1971; Russell, 1967). Another striking difference between anorexia nervosa and infectious diseases is that both infection and pro-inflammatory cytokines provoke depression of behavioural activity (Bluthe *et al.*, 1992), whereas anorexia nervosa is characterized by increased physical activity (Davis *et al.*, 1994). Taken together, these findings indicate that it is unlikely that pro-inflammatory cytokines play a causative role in anorexia nervosa.

Although it seems at first sight counter intuitive that starvation is accompanied by enhanced physical activity, the combination

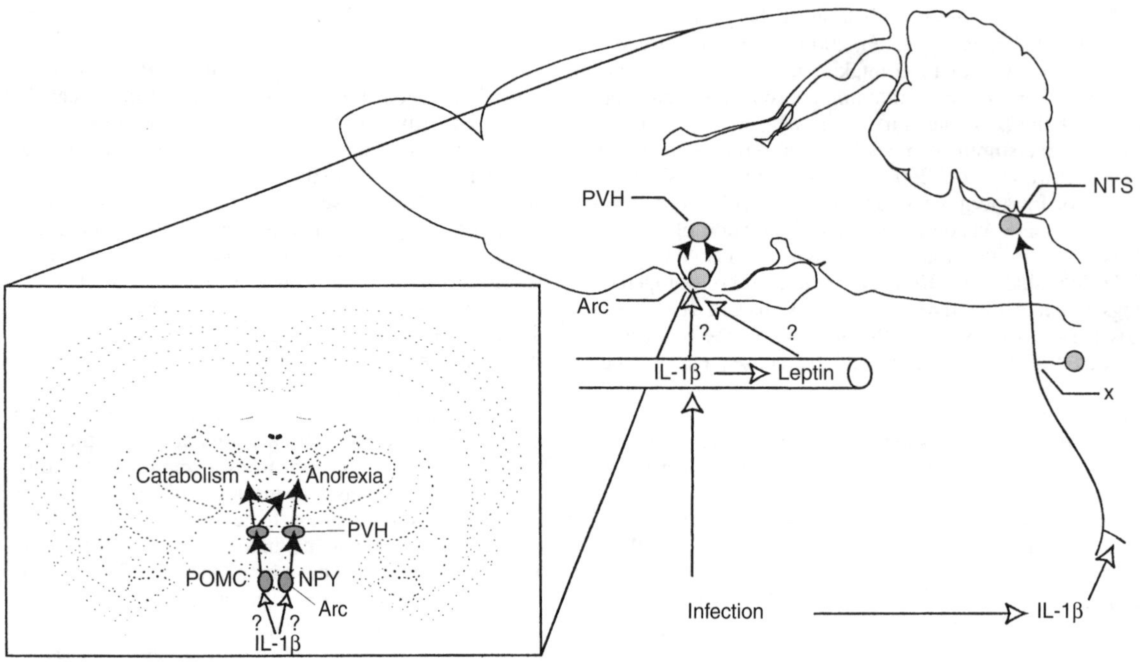

Figure XXIII-4.2 Saggital view of the rat brain to illustrate mechanisms by which interleukin-1β reduces food intake after infection. After detection of bacterial fragments by tissue macrophages, these cells produce interleukin-1β. Interleukin-1β produced by macrophages in the abdominal cavity then acts on the vagus nerve to induce anorexia. Interleukin-1β also acts directly in the brain to induce anorexia after infection. The mechanisms by which interleukin-1β acts in the brain are at present unknown. Circulating interleukin-1β or interleukin-1 produced by phagocytic cells in brain circumventricular organs may act at the level of the arcuate hypothalamus to inhibit the production of neuropeptide Y and to increase that of pro-opiomelanocortin. Interestingly, interleukin-1β induces a rise in circulating levels of leptin, raising the possibility that leptin also plays a role in mediating infection-induced anorexia. Abbreviations and arrowheads see Figure XXIII-4.1

of these two symptoms was considered to be most striking and distinctive in the eyes of Sir William Gull, who coined the disorder anorexia nervosa at the end of the 19th century (Bergh and Sodersten, 1996, 1998). Recent studies in both humans and animals suggest that enhanced physical activity may indeed play an important role in the development and maintenance of anorexia. Analysis of interviews with 32 anorexia nervosa patients revealed that 78% engaged in excessive exercise, 60% were competitive athletes prior to the onset of anorexia nervosa, 60% engaged in sports or exercise before dieting and 75% reported that their physical activity steadily increased during the period when food intake and weight loss decreased the most (Davis *et al.*, 1994). Moreover, earlier studies pointed out that both reducing food intake and exercise are rewarding and agreeable to the patient (reviewed in Bergh and Sodersten, 1996). Interestingly, when rats that have restricted access to food are given access to a running wheel, they also engage in excessive exercise, lose control over body weight and eventually even die (Morrow *et al.*, 1997). The findings both in humans and animals indicate that increased physical activity plays an important role in maintaining and perhaps even in the development of reduced food intake in anorexia nervosa.

The inverse relationship between food intake and energy expenditure indicates that, just like during infectious diseases, the inverse relationship between energy stocks reflected by leptin levels and food intake that normally regulates food intake is overridden in anorexia nervosa. In the case of anorexia nervosa this may be due to an increased release of endogenous opioids or of the neuropeptide corticotropin-releasing hormone. Interestingly, plasma endogenous morphine activities are increased in anorexia nervosa patients (Marrazzi *et al.*, 1997). Furthermore, injections of morphine can reduce food intake when animals are food deprived or have been engaged in intense physical activity (Gulati *et al.*, 1991; Sanger and McCarthy, 1980; White *et al.*, 1977). So, starvation and overactivity might potentate one another through the release of endogenous opioids. In view of the fact that morphine injection increases dopamine release in the nucleus accumbens (Rada *et al.*, 1991) which plays an important role in mediating reward (see above), it can be hypothesized that the rewarding properties of food restriction and exercise in anorexia nervosa are due to activation of brain circuits associated with reward (Bergh and Sodersten, 1996).

Another neuropeptide that may play a role in the association of reduced food intake and increased activity typical of anorexia nervosa is corticotropin-releasing hormone. This peptide controls the activity of the hypothalamus-pituitary adrenal axis, but is also involved in other manifestations of responses to stress (Dunn and Berridge, 1990). Interestingly, corticotropin-releasing hormone is involved in the reduction of food intake after exercise in rats (Rivest and Richard, 1990). In view of the elevated concentrations of corticotropin-releasing hormone in cerebrospinal fluid of anorexia nervosa patients (Kaye *et al.*, 1987), this neuropeptide may indeed play a role in maintaining reduced food intake in anorexia nervosa.

CONCLUSION

There is now ample evidence to suggest that pro-inflammatory cytokines are important mediators of the profound alterations in food intake and energy metabolism that develop during infection and probably during wasting syndromes associated with cancer and AIDS (Argilés and López-Soriano, 1999; Chang *et al.*, 1998). A role for cytokines in other pathological conditions such as geriatric cachexia is also likely especially in view of the increased production of pro-inflammatory cytokines that occurs with ageing (Yeh and

Schuster, 1999). In all these cases, however, the mechanisms of effects of cytokines have not yet been fully elucidated, and their exact targets within the central nervous system remain to be determined. Despite their potent anorectic and metabolic effects, cytokines do not appear to play a major role in anorexia nervosa.

REFERENCES

Abrahamsen, G.C., Berman, Y. and Carr, K.D., 1995. Curve-shift analysis of self-stimulation in food-restricted rats: relationship between daily meal, plasma corticosterone and reward sensitization. *Brain Research*, **695**, 186–194.

Ahima, R.S., Prabakaran, D., Mantzoros, C., Qu, D., Lowell, B., Maratos-Flier, E. and Flier, J.S., 1996. Role of leptin in the neuroendocrine response to fasting. *Nature*, **382**, 250–252.

Akabayashi, A., Wahlestedt, C., Alexander, J.T. and Leibowitz, S.F., 1994. Specific inhibition of endogenous neuropeptide Y synthesis in arcuate nucleus by antigens oligonucleotides suppresses feeding behavior and insulin secretion. *Brain Research. Molecular Brain Research*, **21**, 55–61.

Ammar, A.A., Sederholm, F., Saito, T.R., Scheurink, A.J., Johnson, A.E. and Sodersten, P., 2000. NPY-leptin: opposing effects on appetitive and consummatory ingestive behavior and sexual behavior. *Am. J. Physiol. Regul. Integr. Comp. Physiol.*, **278**, R1627–1633.

Anisman, H., Kokkinidis, L., Borowski, T. and Merali, Z., 1998. Differential effects of interleukin (IL)-1beta, IL-2 and IL-6 on responding for rewarding lateral hypothalamic stimulation. *Brain Research*, **779**, 177–187.

Argilés, J.M. and López-Soriano, F.J., 1999. The role of cytokines in cancer cachexia. *Medicinal Research Reviews*, **19**, 223–248.

Aubert, A., Goodall, G. and Dantzer, R., 1995. Compared effects of cold ambient temperature and cytokines on macronutrient intake in rats. *Physiology and Behavior*, **57**, 869–873.

Aubert, A., Kelley, K.W. and Dantzer, R., 1997. Differential effect of lipopolysaccharide on food hoarding behavior and food consumption in rats. *Brain, Behavior, and Immunity*, **11**, 229–238.

Baker, R.A. and Herkenham, M., 1995. Arcuate nucleus neurons that project to the hypothalamic paraventricular nucleus: neuropeptidergic identity and consequences of adrenalectomy on mRNA levels in the rat. *Journal of Comparative Neurology*, **358**, 518–530.

Banks, W.A., Kastin, A.J., Huang, W., Jaspan, J.B. and Maness, L.M., 1996. Leptin enters the brain by a saturable system independent of insulin. *Peptides*, **17**, 305–311.

Banks, W.A., Ortiz, L., Plotkin, S.R. and Kastin, A.J., 1991. Human interleukin (IL) 1 alpha, murine IL-1 alpha and murine IL-1 beta are transported from blood to brain in the mouse by a shared saturable mechanism. *Journal of Pharmacology and Experimental Therapeutics*, **259**, 988–996.

Bergh, C. and Sodersten, P., 1996. Anorexia nervosa, self-starvation and the reward of stress. *Nature Medicine*, **2**, 21–22.

Bergh, C. and Sodersten, P., 1998. Anorexia nervosa: rediscovery of a disorder. *Lancet*, **351**, 1427–1429.

Berridge, K.C. and Robinson, T.E., 1998. What is the role of dopamine in reward: hedonic impact, reward learning, or incentive salience? *Brain Research. Brain Research Reviews*, **28**, 309–369.

Bluthe, R.M., Dantzer, R. and Kelley, K.W., 1992. Effects of interleukin-1 receptor antagonist on the behavioral effects of lipopolysaccharide in rat. *Brain Research*, **573**, 318–320.

Brady, L.S., Smith, M.A., Gold, P.W. and Herkenham, M., 1990. Altered expression of hypothalamic neuropeptide mRNAs in food-restricted and food-deprived rats. *Neuroendocrinology*, **52**, 441–447.

Brenner, L. and Ritter, R.C., 1995. Peptide cholecystokinin receptor antagonist increases food intake in rats. *Appetite*, **24**, 1–9.

Bret-Dibat, J.L., Bluthé, R.M., Kent, S., Kelley, K.W. and Dantzer, R., 1995. Lipopolysaccharide and interleukin-1 depress food-motivated behavior in mice by a vagal-mediated mechanism. *Brain, Behavior, and Immunity*, **9**, 242–246.

Bret-Dibat, J.L. and Dantzer, R., 2000. Cholecystokinin receptors do not mediate the suppression of food-motivated behavior by lipopolysaccharide and interleukin-1 beta in mice. *Physiology and Behavior*, **69**, 325–331.

Brunner, L., Nick, H.P., Cumin, F., Chiesi, M., Baum, H.P., Whitebread, S., Stricker-Krongrad, A. and Levens, N., 1997. Leptin is a physiologically important regulator of food intake. *International Journal of Obesity and Related Metabolic Disorders*, **21**, 1152–1160.

Buchan, A.M., Polak, J.M., Solcia, E., Capella, C., Hudson, D. and Pearse, A.G., 1978. Electron immunohistochemical evidence for the human intestinal I cell as the source of CCK. *Gut*, **19**, 403–407.

Burlet, A., Grouzmann, E., Musse, N., Fernette, B., Nicolas, J.P. and Burlet, C., 1995. The immunological impairment of arcuate neuropeptide Y neurons by ricin A chain produces persistent decrease of food intake and body weight. *Neuroscience*, **66**, 151–159.

Carr, K.D. and Papadouka, V., 1994. The role of multiple opioid receptors in the potentiation of reward by food restriction. *Brain Research*, **639**, 253–260.

Chang, H.R., Dulloo, A.G. and Bistrian, B.R., 1998. Role of cytokines in AIDS wasting. *Nutrition*, **14**, 853–863.

Chen, H., Charlat, O., Tartaglia, L.A., Woolf, E.A., Weng, X., Ellis, S.J., Lakey, N.D., Culpepper, J., Moore, K.J., Breitbart, R.E., Duyk, G.M., Tepper, R.I. and Morgenstern, J.P., 1996. Evidence that the diabetes gene encodes the leptin receptor: identification of a mutation in the leptin receptor gene in db/db mice. *Cell*, **84**, 491–495.

Cheung, C.C., Clifton, D.K. and Steiner, R.A., 1997. Proopiomelanocortin neurons are direct targets for leptin in the hypothalamus. *Endocrinology*, **138**, 4489–4492.

Couce, M.E., Burguera, B., Parisi, J.E., Jensen, M.D. and Lloyd, R.V., 1997. Localization of leptin receptor in the human brain. *Neuroendocrinology*, **66**, 145–150.

Cowley, M.A., Pronchuk, N., Fan, W., Dinulescu, D.M., Colmers, W.F. and Cone, R.D., 1999. Integration of NPY, AGRP and melanocortin signals in the hypothalamic paraventricular nucleus: evidence of a cellular basis for a cellular basis for the adipostat. *Neuron*, **24**, 155–163.

Crisp, A.H. and Stonehill, E., 1971. Relation between aspects of nutritional disturbance and menstrual activity in primary anorexia nervosa. *British Medical Journal*, **3**, 149–151.

Cunningham, E.T.J., Wada, E., Carter, D.B., Tracey, D.E., Battey, J.F. and De Souza, E.B., 1992. *In situ* histochemical localization of type I interleukin-1 receptor messenger RNA in the central nervous system, pituitary, and adrenal gland of the mouse. *Journal of Neuroscience*, **12**, 1101–1114.

Dantzer, R., 1994. How do cytokines say hello to the brain? Neural versus humoral mediation. *European Cytokine Network*, **5**, 271–273.

Davis, C., Kennedy, S.H., Ravelski, E. and Dionne, M., 1994. The role of physical activity in the development and maintenance of eating disorders. *Psychological Medicine*, **24**, 957–967.

Dawson, R.J. and Lorden, J.F., 1981. Behavioral and neurochemical effects of neonatal administration of monosodium L-glutamate in mice. *Journal of Comparative and Physiological Psychology*, **95**, 71–84.

Drewnowski, A., 1998. Energy density, palatability, and satiety: implications for weight control. *Nutrition Reviews*, **56**, 347–353.

Dunn, A.J. and Berridge, C.W., 1990. Physiological and behavioral responses to corticotropin-releasing factor administration: is CRF a mediator of anxiety or stress responses? *Brain Research. Brain Research Reviews*, **15**, 71–100.

Edwards, G.L., Ladenheim, E.E. and Ritter, R.C., 1986. Dorsomedial hindbrain participation in cholecystokinin-induced satiety. *American Journal of Physiology*, **251**, R971–977.

Egawa, M., Yoshimatsu, H. and Bray, G.A., 1991. Neuropeptide Y suppresses sympathetic activity to interscapular brown adipose tissue in rats. *American Journal of Physiology*, **260**, R328–334.

Ek, M., Kurosawa, M., Lundeberg, T. and Ericsson, A., 1998. Activation of vagal afferents after intravenous injection of interleukin-1beta: role of endogenous prostaglandins. *Journal of Neuroscience*, **18**, 9471–9479.

Elmquist, J.K., Bjørbaek, C., Ahima, R.S., Flier, J.S. and Saper, C.B., 1998. Distributions of leptin receptor mRNA isoforms in the rat brain. *Journal of Comparative Neurology*, **395**, 535–547.

Emond, M., Schwartz, G.J., Ladenheim, E.E. and Moran, T.H., 1999. Central leptin modulates behavioral and neural responsivity to CCK. *American Journal of Physiology*, **276**, R1545–1549.

Ericsson, A., Arias, C. and Sawchenko, P.E., 1997. Evidence for an intramedullary prostaglandin-dependent mechanism in the activation of stress-related neuroendocrine circuitry by intravenous interleukin-1. *Journal of Neuroscience*, **17**, 7166–7179.

Ericsson, A., Kovács, K.J. and Sawchenko, P.E., 1994. A functional anatomical analysis of central pathways subserving the effects of interleukin-1 on stress-related neuroendocrine neurons. *Journal of Neuroscience*, **14**, 897–913.

Ericsson, A., Liu, C., Hart, R.P. and Sawchenko, P.E., 1995. Type 1 interleukin-1 receptor in the rat brain: distribution, regulation, and relationship to sites of IL-1-induced cellular activation. *Journal of Comparative Neurology*, **361**, 681–698.

Faggioni, R., Fantuzzi, G., Fuller, J., Dinarello, C.A., Feingold, K.R. and Grunfeld, C., 1998. IL-1 beta mediates leptin induction during inflammation. *American Journal of Physiology*, **274**, R204–208.

Fischler, C., 2001. *L'hommivore*. Editions Odile Jacob, Paris.

Flynn, M.C., Scott, T.R., Pritchard, T.C. and Plata-Salaman, C.R., 1998. Mode of action of OB protein (leptin) on feeding. *American Journal of Physiology*, **275**, R174–179.

Frederich, R.C., Hamann, A., Anderson, S., Lollmann, B., Lowell, B.B. and Flier, J.S., 1995. Leptin levels reflect body content in mice: evidence for diet-induced resistance to leptin action. *Nature Medicine*, **1**, 1311–1314.

Fulton, S., Woodside, B. and Shizgal, P., 2000. Modulation of brain reward circuitry by leptin. *Science*, **287**, 125–128.

Fuxe, K., Cintra, A., Agnati, L.F., Harfstrand, A., Wikstrom, A.C., Okret, S., Zoli, M., Miller, L.S., Greene, J.L. and Gustafsson, J.A., 1987. Studies on the cellular localization and distribution of glucocorticoid receptor and oestrogen receptor immunoreactivity in the central nervous system of the rat and their relationship to the monoaminergic and peptidergic neurons of the brain. *Journal of Steroid Biochemistry*, **27**, 159–170.

Garibaldi, J.A., 1972. Influence of temperature on the biosynthesis of iron transport compounds by Salmonella typhimurium. *Journal of Bacteriology*, **110**, 262–265.

Gaykema, R.P., Dijkstra, I. and Tilders, F.J., 1995. Subdiaphragmatic vagotomy suppresses endotoxin-induced activation of hypothalamic corticotropin-releasing hormone neurons and ACTH secretion. *Endocrinology*, **136**, 4717–4720.

Geary, N., Kissileff, H.R., Pi-Sunyer, F.X. and Hinton, V., 1992. Individual, but not simultaneous, glucagon and cholecystokinin infusions inhibit feeding in men. *American Journal of Physiology*, **262**, R975–980.

Gibbs, J., Young, R.C. and Smith, G.P., 1973. Cholecystokinin elicits satiety in rats with open gastric fistulas. *Nature*, **245**, 323–325.

Giraudo, S.Q., Billington, C.J. and Levine, A.S., 1998. Feeding effects of hypothalamic injection of melanocortin 4 receptor ligands. *Brain Research*, **809**, 302–306.

Grill, H.J. and Smith, G.P., 1988. Cholecystokinin decreases sucrose intake in chronic decerebrate rats. *American Journal of Physiology*, **254**, R853–856.

Grimble, R.F., 1994. Malnutrition and the immune response. 2. Impact of nutrients on cytokine biology in infection. *Transactions of the Royal Society of Tropical Medicine and Hygiene*, **88**, 615–619.

Gross, P.M., 1992. Circumventricular organ capillaries. *Progress in Brain Research*, **91**, 219–233.

Gulati, K., Ray, A. and Sharma, K.K., 1991. Role of diurnal variation and receptor specificity in the opioidergic regulation of food intake in free-fed and food-deprived rats [published erratum appears in *Physiol. Behav.* (1993) **54**(3): 613]. *Physiology and Behavior*, **49**, 1065–1071.

Hagan, M.M., Rushing, P.A., Schwartz, M.W., Yagaloff, K.A., Burn, P., Woods, S.C. and Seeley, R.J., 1999. Role of the CNS melanocortin system in the response to overfeeding. *Journal of Neuroscience*, **19**, 2362–2367.

Hakansson, M.L., Brown, H., Ghilardi, N., Skoda, R.C. and Meister, B., 1998. Leptin receptor immunoreactivity in chemically defined target neurons of the hypothalamus. *Journal of Neuroscience*, **18**, 559–572.

Halaas, J.L., Gajiwala, K.S., Maffei, M., Cohen, S.L., Chait, B.T., Rabinowitz, D., Lallone, R.L., Burley, S.K. and Friedman, J.M., 1995. Weight-reducing effects of the plasma protein encoded by the obese gene. *Science*, **269**, 543–546.

Hart, B.L., 1988. Biological basis of the behavior of sick animals. *Neuroscience and Biobehavioral Reviews*, **12**, 123–137.

Haynes, W.G., Morgan, D.A., Djalali, A., Sivitz, W.I. and Mark, A.L., 1999. Interactions between the melanocortin system and leptin in control of sympathetic nerve traffic. *Hypertension*, **33**, 542–547.

Hernandez, L. and Hoebel, B.G., 1988. Food reward and cocaine increase extracellular dopamine in the nucleus accumbens as measured by microdialysis. *Life Sciences*, **42**, 1705–1712.

Holden, R.J. and Pakula, I.S., 1996. The role of tumor necrosis factor-alpha in the pathogenesis of anorexia and bulimia nervosa, cancer cachexia and obesity. *Medical Hypotheses*, **47**, 423–438.

Kahler, A., Geary, N., Eckel, L.A., Campfield, L.A., Smith, F.J. and Langhans, W., 1998. Chronic administration of OB protein decreases food intake by selectively reducing meal size in male rats. *American Journal of Physiology*, **275**, R180–185.

Kalra, S.P., Dube, M.G., Sahu, A., Phelps, C.P. and Kalra, P.S., 1991. Neuropeptide Y secretion increases in the paraventricular nucleus in association with increased appetite for food. *Proceedings of the National Academy of Sciences of the United States of America*, **88**, 10931–10935.

Kawai, K., Sugimoto, K., Nakashima, K., Miura, H. and Ninomiya, Y., 2000. Leptin as a modulator of sweet taste sensitivities in mice. *Proceedings of the National Academy of Sciences of the United States of America*, **97**, 11044–11049.

Kaye, W.H., Gwirtsman, H.E., George, D.T., Ebert, M.H., Jimerson, D.C., Tomai, T.P., Chrousos, G.P. and Gold, P.W., 1987. Elevated cerebrospinal fluid levels of immunoreactive corticotropin-releasing hormone in anorexia nervosa: relation to state of nutrition, adrenal function, and intensity of depression. *Journal of Clinical Endocrinology and Metabolism*, **64**, 203–208.

Kennedy, G.C., 1953. The role of depot fat in the hypothalamic control of food intake in the rat. *Proceedings of the Royal Society of London B*, **140**, 479–592.

Kluger, M.J. and Rothenburg, B.A., 1979. Fever and reduced iron: their interaction as a host defense response to bacterial infection. *Science*, **203**, 374–376.

Konsman, J.P., Kelley, K. and Dantzer, R., 1999. Temporal and spatial relationships between lipopolysaccharide-induced expression of Fos, interleukin-1beta and inducible nitric oxide synthase in rat brain. *Neuroscience*, **89**, 535–548.

Konsman, J.P., Luheshi, G.N., Bluthé, R.M. and Dantzer, R., 2000. The vagus nerve mediates behavioral depression, but not fever, in response to peripheral immune signals; a functional anatomical analysis. *European Journal of Neuroscience*, **12**, 4434–4446.

Konsman, J.P., Rees, G., Ek, M., Dantzer, R., Ericsson-Dahlstrand, A. and Blomqvist, A., 2000. Distribution of interleukin-1 receptor type 1 mRNA and protein in rat brain. *Society for Neuroscience Abstracts*, **26**, 242–241.

Laflamme, N. and Rivest, S., 2000. Toll-like receptor 4: the missing link of the cerebral innate immune response triggered by circulating gram-negative bacterial cell wall components. *Society for Neuroscience Abstracts*, **26**, 242–217.

Layé, S., Gheusi, G., Cremona, S., Combe, C., Kelley, K., Dantzer, R. and Parnet, P., 2000. Endogenous brain IL-1 mediates LPS-induced anorexia and hypothalamic cytokine expression. *American Journal of Physiology*, **179**, R93–98.

Le Magnen, J. and Tallon, S., 1966. The spontaneous periodicity of ad libitum food intake in white rats. *Journal de Physiologie*, **58**, 323–349.

Leibel, R.L., Rosenbaum, M. and Hirsch, J., 1995. Changes in energy expenditure resulting from altered body weight. *New England Journal of Medicine*, **332**, 621–628.

Liddle, R.A., Goldfine, I.D., Rosen, M.S., Taplitz, R.A. and Williams, J.A., 1985. Cholecystokinin bioactivity in human plasma. Molecular forms, responses to feeding, and relationship to gallbladder contraction. *Journal of Clinical Investigation*, **75**, 1144–1152.

Lin, C.W. and Miller, T.R., 1992. Both CCK-A and CCK-B/gastrin receptors are present on rabbit vagus nerve. *American Journal of Physiology*, **263**, R591–595.

Maffei, M., Halaas, J., Ravussin, E., Pratley, R.E., Lee, G.H., Zhang, Y., Fei, H., Kim, S., Lallone, R., Ranganathan, S. *et al.*, 1995. Leptin levels in human and rodent: measurement of plasma leptin and ob RNA in obese and weight-reduced subjects. *Nature Medicine*, **1**, 1155–1161.

Marcos, A., 1997. The immune system in eating disorders: an overview. *Nutrition*, **13**, 853–862.

Marrazzi, M.A., Luby, E.D., Kinzie, J., Munjal, I.D. and Spector, S., 1997. Endogenous codeine and morphine in anorexia and bulimia nervosa. *Life Sciences*, **60**, 1741–1747.

McCarthy, D.O., Kluger, M.J. and Vander, A.J., 1984. The role of fever in appetite suppression after endotoxin administration. *American Journal of Clinical Nutrition*, **40**, 310–316.

Mercer, J.G., Hoggard, N., Williams, L.M., Lawrence, C.B., Hannah, L.T., Morgan, P.J. and Trayhurn, P., 1996. Coexpression of leptin receptor and preproneuropeptide Y mRNA in arcuate nucleus of mouse hypothalamus. *Journal of Neuroendocrinology*, **8**, 733–735.

Minami, S., Kamegai, J., Hasegawa, O., Sugihara, H., Okada, K. and Wakabayashi, I., 1993. Expression of growth hormone receptor gene in rat hypothalamus. *Journal of Neuroendocrinology*, **5**, 691–696.

Mizuno, T.M., Kleopoulos, S.P., Bergen, H.T., Roberts, J.L., Priest, C.A. and Mobbs, C.V., 1998. Hypothalamic pro-opiomelanocortin mRNA is reduced by fasting and corrected in ob/ob and db/db mice, but is stimulated by leptin. *Diabetes*, **47**, 294–297.

Morris, M.J., Tortelli, C.F., Filippis, A. and Proietto, J., 1998. Reduced BAT function as a mechanism for obesity in the hypophagic, neuropeptide Y deficient monosodium glutamate-treated rat. *Regulatory Peptides*, **75–76**, 441–447.

Morrow, N.S., Schall, M., Grijalva, C.V., Geiselman, P.J., Garrick, T., Nuccion, S. and Novin, D., 1997. Body temperature and wheel running predict survival times in rats exposed to activity-stress. *Physiology and Behavior*, **62**, 815–825.

Murabe, Y., Nishida, K. and Sano, Y., 1981. Cells capable of uptake of horseradish peroxidase in some circumventricular organs of the cat and rat. *Cell and Tissue Research*, **219**, 85–92.

Murphy, B., Nunes, C.N., Ronan, J.J., Harper, C.M., Beall, M.J., Hanaway, M., Fairhurst, A.M., Van der Ploeg, L.H., MacIntyre, D.E. and Mellin, T.N., 1998. Melanocortin mediated inhibition of feeding behavior in rats. *Neuropeptides*, **32**, 491–497.

Murray, J., Murray, A. and Murray, N., 1978. Anorexia: sentinel of host defense? *Perspectives in Biology and Medicine*, **22**, 134–142.

Murray, M.J. and Murray, A.B., 1979. Anorexia of infection as a mechanism of host defense. *American Journal of Clinical Nutrition*, **32**, 593–596.

Murray, M.J., Murray, A.B., Murray, M.B. and Murray, C.J., 1978. The adverse effect of iron repletion on the course of certain infections. *British Medical Journal*, **2**, 1113–1115.

Niijima, A., 1996. The afferent discharges from sensors for interleukin 1 beta in the hepatoportal system in the anesthetized rat. *Journal of the Autonomic Nervous System*, **61**, 287–291.

Niimi, M., Sato, M., Yokote, R., Tada, S. and Takahara, J., 1999. Effects of central and peripheral injection of leptin on food intake and on brain Fos expression in the Otsuka Long-Evans Tokushima Fatty rat with hyperleptinaemia. *Journal of Neuroendocrinology*, **11**, 605–611.

Parnet, P., Amindari, S., Wu, C., Brunke-Reese, D., Goujon, E., Weyhenmeyer, J.A., Dantzer, R. and Kelley, K.W., 1994. Expression of type I and type II interleukin-1 receptors in mouse brain. *Brain Research. Molecular Brain Research*, **27**, 63–70.

Rada, P., Mark, G.P., Pothos, E. and Hoebel, B.G., 1991. Systemic morphine simultaneously decreases extracellular acetylcholine and increases dopamine in the nucleus accumbens of freely moving rats. *Neuropharmacology*, **30**, 1133–1136.

Rinaman, L., 1999. Interoceptive stress activates glucagon-like peptide-1 neurons that project to the hypothalamus. *American Journal of Physiology*, **277**, R582–590.

Rinaman, L., 2000. Central glucagon-like peptide-1 signaling pathways contribute to anorexia in diverse models of nausea and disease. In: *Anorexia During Disease Workshop*.

Rinaman, L., Baker, E.A., Hoffman, G.E., Stricker, E.M. and Verbalis, J.G., 1998. Medullary c-Fos activation in rats after ingestion of a satiating meal. *American Journal of Physiology*, **275**, R262–268.

Rinaman, L., Verbalis, J.G., Stricker, E.M. and Hoffman, G.E., 1993. Distribution and neurochemical phenotypes of caudal medullary neurons activated to express cFos following peripheral administration of cholecystokinin. *Journal of Comparative Neurology*, **338**, 475–490.

Rivest, S. and Richard, D., 1990. Involvement of corticotropin-releasing factor in the anorexia induced by exercise. *Brain Research Bulletin*, **25**, 169–172.

Russell, G.F., 1967. The nutritional disorder in anorexia nervosa. *Journal of Psychosomatic Research*, **11**, 141–149.

Sanger, D.J. and McCarthy, P.S., 1980. Differential effects of morphine on food and water intake in food deprived and freely-feeding rats. *Psychopharmacology*, **72**, 103–106.

Sarraf, P., Frederich, R.C., Turner, E.M., Ma, G., Jaskowiak, N.T., Rivet, D., Jr, Flier, J.S., Lowell, B.B., Fraker, D.L. and Alexander, H.R., 1997. Multiple cytokines and acute inflammation raise mouse leptin levels: potential role in inflammatory anorexia. *Journal of Experimental Medicine*, **185**, 171–175.

Schwartz, M.W., Seeley, R.J., Woods, S.C., Weigle, D.S., Campfield, L.A., Burn, P. and Baskin, D.G., 1997. Leptin increases hypothalamic pro-opiomelanocortin mRNA expression in the rostral arcuate nucleus. *Diabetes*, **46**, 2119–2123.

Schwartz, M.W., Sipols, A.J., Grubin, C.E. and Baskin, D.G., 1993. Differential effect of fasting on hypothalamic expression of genes encoding neuropeptide Y, galanin, and glutamic acid decarboxylase. *Brain Research Bulletin*, **31**, 361–367.

Schwartz, M.W., Woods, S.C., Porte, D., Jr, Seeley, R.J. and Baskin, D.G., 2000. Central nervous system control of food intake. *Nature*, **404**, 661–671.

Seeley, R.J., Yagaloff, K.A., Fisher, S.L., Burn, P., Thiele, T.E., van Dijk, G., Baskin, D.G. and Schwartz, M.W., 1997. Melanocortin receptors in leptin effects. *Nature*, **390**, 349.

Shaver, S.W., Pang, J.J., Wainman, D.S., Wall, K.M. and Gross, P.M., 1992. Morphology and function of capillary networks in subregions of the rat tuber cinereum. *Cell and Tissue Research*, **267**, 437–448.

Shibata, H. and Bukowiecki, L.J., 1987. Regulatory alterations of daily energy expenditure induced by fasting or overfeeding in unrestrained rats. *Journal of Applied Physiology*, **63**, 465–470.

Shizgal, P., 1997. Neural basis of utility estimation. *Current Opinion in Neurobiology*, **7**, 198–208.

Sims, E.A. and Danforth, E.J., 1987. Expenditure and storage of energy in man. *Journal of Clinical Investigation*, **79**, 1019–1025.

Smith, G.P., Jerome, C., Cushin, B.J., Eterno, R. and Simansky, K.J., 1981. Abdominal vagotomy blocks the satiety effect of cholecystokinin in the rat. *Science*, **213**, 1036–1037.

Stanley, B.G. and Leibowitz, S.F., 1985. Neuropeptide Y injected in the paraventricular hypothalamus: a powerful stimulant of feeding behavior. *Proceedings of the National Academy of Sciences of the United States of America*, **82**, 3940–3943.

Stephens, T.W., Basinski, M., Bristow, P.K., Bue-Valleskey, J.M., Burgett, S., Craft, L., Hale, J., Hoffmann, J., Hsiung, H.M. and Kriauciunas, A., 1995. The role of neuropeptide in anti-obesity action of the ob gene product. *Nature*, **377**, 530–532.

Swanson, L.W., 1998. *Brain Maps: Structure of the Rat Brain*. Elsevier, Amsterdam.

Tang-Christensen, M., Holst, J.J., Hartmann, B. and Vrang, N., 1999. The arcuate nucleus is pivotal in mediating the anorectic effects of centrally administered leptin. *Neuroreport*, **10**, 1183–1187.

Treece, B.R., Covasa, M., Ritter, R.C. and Burns, G.A., 1998. Delay in meal termination follows blockade of N-methyl-D-aspartate receptors in the dorsal hindbrain. *Brain Research*, **810**, 34–40.

Treece, B.R., Ritter, R.C. and Burns, G.A., 2000. Lesions of the dorsal vagal complex abolish increases in meal size induced by NMDA receptor blockade. *Brain Research*, **872**, 37–43.

Vaisman, N. and Hahn, T., 1991. Tumor necrosis factor-alpha and anorexia–cause or effect? *Metabolism: Clinical and Experimental*, **40**, 720–723.

Wan, W., Wetmore, L., Sorensen, C.M., Greenberg, A.H. and Nance, D.M., 1994. Neural and biochemical mediators of endotoxin and stress-induced c-fos expression in the rat brain. *Brain Research Bulletin*, **34**, 7–14.

Wang, Q., Bing, C., Al-Barazanji, K., Mossakowaska, D.E., Wang, X.M., McBay, D.L., Neville, W.A., Taddayon, M., Pickavance, L., Dryden, S., Thomas, M.E., McHale, M.T., Gloyer, I.S., Wilson, S., Buckingham, R., Arch, J.R., Trayhurn, P. and Williams, G., 1997. Interactions between leptin and hypothalamic neuropeptide Y neurons in the control of food intake and energy homeostasis in the rat. *Diabetes*, **46**, 335–341.

Weinberg, E.D., 1984. Iron withholding: a defense against infection and neoplasia. *Physiological Reviews*, **64**, 65–102.

West, D.B., Fey, D. and Woods, S.C., 1984. Cholecystokinin persistently suppresses meal size but not food intake in free-feeding rats. *American Journal of Physiology*, **246**, R776–787.

White, N., Sklar, L. and Amit, Z., 1977. The reinforcing action of morphine and its paradoxical side effect. *Psychopharmacology*, **52**, 63–66.

Wing, E.J. and Young, J.B., 1980. Acute starvation protects mice against Listeria monocytogenes. *Infection and Immunity*, **28**, 771–776.

Woodside, D.B., 1995. A review of anorexia nervosa and bulimia nervosa. *Current Problems in Pediatrics*, **25**, 67–89.

Yabuuchi, K., Minami, M., Katsumata, S. and Satoh, M., 1994. Localization of type I interleukin-1 receptor mRNA in the rat brain. *Brain Research. Molecular Brain Research*, **27**, 27–36.

Yeh, S.S. and Schuster, M.W., 1999. Geriatric cachexia: the role of cytokines. *American Journal of Clinical Nutrition*, **70**, 183–197.

Zhang, Y., Proenca, R., Maffei, M., Barone, M., Leopold, L. and Friedman, J.M., 1994. Positional cloning of the mouse obese gene and its human homologue. *Nature*, **372**, 425–432.

XXIII-5

Psychophysiology and Eating Disorders

Patricia P. Sanchez Gomez, Nicholas A. Troop and Janet L. Treasure

INTRODUCTION

For psychiatric disorders such as eating disorders in which psychological conflicts seem to be essentially played out on the body, psychophysiology is an important avenue of exploration. Apparently abnormal behaviours in relation to food and weight may be associated with an abnormal psychophysiological response to such stimuli.

One advantage of taking psychophysiological measures, is that this approach is relatively objective and may therefore overcome some of the characteristic biases of other techniques (Lattimore, Gowers and Wagner, 2000) such as the confounding in self-report measures caused by patients' motivational states (e.g. trying to make sense of the illness or even to punish/reward a therapist) and co-morbidity with mood or personality disorders. For example, several studies have shown elevated rates of alexithymia in individuals with eating disorders (Bourke *et al.*, 1992; Schmidt, Jiwany and Treasure, 1993). Alexithymia is a personality construct denoting difficulties in identifying and expressing feelings, an impoverished imaginative life, and an externally oriented cognitive style with thoughts characterized by pragmatic contents (Taylor *et al.*, 1996; Corcos *et al.*, 2000). Individuals displaying these characteristics may systematically misreport their inner states. Thus an objective assessment of emotional responses to food stimuli by monitoring of indices of autonomic arousal can be informative. Among these indices heart rate, blood pressure, skin conductance, finger temperature, respiration and eye movement variability are the most widely used (Léonard *et al.*, 1998; Parrott and Hertel, 1999).

There has been a relative lack of psychophysiological research in patients with either anorexia or bulimia nervosa. However, eating disorders can be set within a dimensional framework in which the clinical conditions merge on the continuum of eating behaviour from dietary restraint to overeating and on the continuum of body weight from emaciation to obesity. Therefore, in addition to studies using clinical groups of patients, we include in this review those studies that report on the psychophysiological responses of dieters and overeaters and in people of different weight groups.

Studies have generally used two types of provocative stimuli to elicit a physiological response. The first relates directly to the symptoms and includes food and body shapes (either real, pictorial or imagined). The second involves exposing participants to some kind of stressor such as a difficult cognitive task (such as unsolvable anagrams) or speech threat (where participants prepare a talk that they believe they will have to present to a group of judges). Below we review studies that measure psychophysiological responses to both of these kinds of stimuli. These studies are summarized in Table XXIII-5.1.

LIMITATIONS OF PSYCHOPHYSIOLOGICAL ASSESSMENT IN EATING DISORDERS

There are some limitations in using psychophysiological methods to assess the autonomic arousal in patients with eating disorders. In the first place, basal autonomic tone may differ from that of non-eating disordered women, particularly, for example, in those who are emaciated. Leptin levels are lower in those who are in a state of starvation and leptin is known to affect activity in the autonomic nervous system. Research has shown that patients with anorexia nervosa and bulimia report high levels of anxiety and depression (de Zwaan *et al.*, 1996; Phillips, Tiggeman and Wade, 1997; Godart *et al.*, 2000) and these variables should also be taken into account. Any differences in arousal between patients with eating disorders and controls could be partially due to their higher baseline levels of anxiety and depression (Léonard *et al.*, 1998; Staiger, Dawe and McCarthy, 2000).

In addition, it is often difficult to get patients with eating disorders to eat foods that they consider 'forbidden', let alone get them to consume as much as non-eating disordered groups (Williamson, 1988). Simple differences in the amount eaten may directly influence psychophysiological measures independently of any pathology. One way round this may be to ask participants to imagine or to look at pictures of food, rather than consume it. However, even here it is possible that patients with anorexia may use cognitive strategies such as avoidance.

Another variable to take into account is the individualization of food cues. As Staiger and co-workers (2000) suggest, an individual's favourite binge food may elicit a greater activation than a standard food. Although some studies have used individualized favourite foods (e.g. Bulik *et al.*, 1996; Staiger, Dawe and McCarthy, 2000) others have used standardized foods or meals (e.g. Léonard *et al.*, 1998). In studies on psychophysiological responses to stress it can also be questioned whether the stressors used approximate to the type and severity of problems that are associated with eating disorders outside of the laboratory. For example, it is severe events and difficulties (such as the ending of a relationship) that typically provoke the onset of an eating disorder rather than being taxed by mental arithmetic or preparing a brief speech. On the other hand, laboratory studies using tasks such as these have been shown successfully to disinhibit dietary restraint (e.g. Heatherton, Herman and Polivy, 1991).

Any or all of these reasons may account for why there is very little psychophysiological research in patients with anorexia nervosa or bulimia nervosa.

Furthermore, psychophysiological measurement is very complex, involving influences due to both situational and person factors. This creates variability in the data and one of the consequences is that only very salient effects can be established using psychophysiological methods. It is also difficult to control other variables that may influence results, such as the amount of food eaten prior to the

Biological Psychiatry: Edited by H. D'haenen, J.A. den Boer and P. Willner. ISBN 0-471-49198-5

Table XXIII-5.1 Psychophysiological responses to two types of stimuli

Authors	Stimuli	Participants	Psychophysiological measures	Results
Test meal				
Williamson *et al.* (1988)	Test meal	12 BN 12 obese 24 comparison women (12 ate test meal, 12 did not) Mean ages for all the groups ranged from 21.5 to 22.0 yrs. Weight ranges: obese subjects (mean percent overweight = 28%); the two normal groups had weights from −10% to +20% under/overweight of population norms.	Heart rate Vasomotor response Skin temperature Skin resistance Forearm electromyogram	After test meal, increase in heart rate and EMG in BN women. No other significant differences.
Léonard *et al.* (1998)	Standardized test-meal	14 AN women (Age: X = 23.9; BMI: X = 16.2) 10 BN women (Age: X = 27.8; BMI: X = 21.1) 18 comparison women (Age: X = 29.3; BMI: X = 21.1)	Skin conductance Heart rate ECG	Increase in skin conductance during meal in ANs only. No other significant differences between groups.
Food cues exposure and food consumption				
Bulik *et al.* (1996)	Exposure to individualized high-risk binge food	31 BN women (Age: X = 26; BMI<30 $kg\,m^{-2}$)	Salivation Blood pressure Heart rate	Pre-treatment, no change in salivation after presentation of foods. Post-treatment, increased salivary reactivity. Salivation negatively related to blood pressure, not heart rate.
Vögele and Florin (1996)	Exposure and consumption of individualized binge food	30 female binge eaters (Age: X = 27.5; BMI: X = 23.4) 30 female non-binge eaters (Age: X = 24.3; BMI: X = 22.0)	Heart rate Blood pressure Electrodermal activity Respiration rate	Binge eaters show higher reactivity than comparison women. Heart rate during food exposure predicted amount subsequently consumed.
Overduin *et al.* (1997)	Slides of favourite binge food and subject's own body	11 restrained eaters (non-clinical but disinhibitive) (Age: X = 21.5; BMI: X = 21.8) 13 unrestrained eaters (controls) (Age: X = 20.3; BMI: X = 19.9)	Skin conductance Heart rate Startle eyeblink EMG	No significant differences between groups for any stimuli on any measure.
Nederkoorn *et al.* (2000)	Exposure and consumption of favourite foods	24 healthy students (Age: X = 20.1; BMI: X = 21.5)	Heart rate Blood pressure Peripheral pulse amplitude Electrogastrography Salivation Skin conductance level Temperature	Increases in salivation, temperature, heart rate, skin conductance, diastolic and systolic blood pressure during the exposure. Same changes for saliva, temperature, blood pressure, heart rate and gastric activity during food intake. Blood pressure related to restraint during exposure to food.
Staiger *et al.* (2000)	Sight and smell or sight, smell and taste of individualized binge/favourite and neutral food	17 BN women (Age: X = 21.8; BMI: X = 22.3) 17 comparison women (Age: X = 23.5; BMI: X = 21.1)	Salivation	No significant difference between groups.
Drobes *et al.* (2001) — Study 1	Emotional and food related pictures	105 male and female students	Heart rate Skin conductance Facial EMG	Food deprivation led to greater reactivity (an enhanced startle reflex and increased heart rate) in response to food stimuli but not emotion stimuli.
Drobes *et al.* (2001) — Study 2	Emotional and food-related pictures	76 female students: Binge eaters (Age: X = 19.1; BMI: X = 22.04)	Heart rate Skin conductance	Binge eater and food-deprived groups showed startle potentiation to food cues but not emotional stimuli.

Table XXIII-5.1 (*continued*)

Authors	Stimuli	Participants	Psychophysiological measures	Results
		Restrained eaters (Age: X = 18.5; BMI: X = 21.75) Food deprived (Age: X = 18.3; BMI: X = 21.00) Food non-deprived (Age: X = 18.7; BMI: X = 22.18)		
Stress stimuli				
Cattanach *et al.* (1988)	Interpersonal conflict vignette Audiovisual conflict task Speech delivery Social interaction vignette	15 BN students 15 non-BN students Mean age for both groups: ranging from 17 to 21 yrs.	Blood pressure Pulse	No significant group differences in psychophysiological responses.
Koo-Loeb *et al.* (1998)	Paced auditory task Serial addition task Interpersonal speech task	15 BN (Age: X = 25.3; Weight: X = 130.9 pounds; Height: X = 65.3 inches) 15 comparison women (Age: X = 24.4; Weight: X = 131.5 pounds; Height: X = 64.9 inches)	Blood pressure Heart rate Epinephrine Norepinephrine Systolic time interval Peripheral resistance	Blunted sympathetic activation in BN in response to mental stressors.
Tuschen-Caffier and Vögele (1999)	Achievement challenge Interpersonal conflict	27 BN women (Age: X = 24.5; BMI: X = 20.9) 27 women restrained eaters (Age: X = 26.5; BMI: X = 22.6) 27 women unrestrained eaters (Age: X = 24.6; BMI: X = 21.4)	Heart rate Blood pressure Skin conductance Respiration rate	No significant group differences in psychophysiological reactivity.
Lattimore *et al.* (2000)	Low and high conflict discussion tasks	20 AN (Age: X = 15.7; BMI: X = 17.1) and their mothers 14 psychiatric controls (Age: X = 15.2; BMI: X = 21.8) and their mothers	Heart rate Skin conductance	Higher arousal in AN patients than their mothers and psychiatric controls.

experimental session or the anticipatory anxiety due to participation in the study itself (Williamson *et al.*, 1988).

Another problematic aspect of these studies is that the appropriateness of some parameters to measure autonomic responses (e.g. heart rate, heart rate variability, blood pressure) is still uncertain and we do not exactly know what changes in these parameters mean (Nederkoorn, Smulders and Jansen, 2000). Most of the studies on cue reactivity have used non-specific autonomic responses (e.g. heart rate, blood pressure) that are multidetermined. Changes in these parameters may reflect a range of biological, affective and cognitive events that may or may not be related to the cue exposure (Bulik *et al.*, 1996).

Therefore, and although psychophysiological measures potentially offer an objective measure of emotional arousal, it is in fact likely that, due to the limitations noted above, other types of assessment in addition to psychophysiological measures should be included in the experimental procedure. Direct behavioural observation of participants throughout the experimental session, subjective ratings, and data from self-report inventories may be necessary to support psychophysiological data (Williamson *et al.*, 1988) in order that an overall picture of responses emerges. This is in line with current componential definitions of emotions which emphasize that an emotion includes a cognitive appraisal of the situation, a subjective feeling, an action tendency (or actual behaviour) as well as a psychophysiological response.

CUE REACTIVITY

Notable animal and human research has proved the role of conditioning in the mediation of the appetitive reflex modulation and motivation to eat (Drobes *et al.*, 2001). Classical conditioning models, derived from addiction research have been recently applied to binge eating (Overduin, Jansen and Eilkes, 1997; Overduin and Jansen, 1997).

'Cue reactivity' is defined as a range of physiological, cognitive and emotional responses elicited by cues (conditioned stimuli) that have been repeatedly paired with a specific behaviour such as alcohol, drug administration or binge eating (Staiger, Dawe and McCarthy, 2000). Over a hundred studies have found autonomic responding, such as increased heart rate, skin conductance and salivation, in addicts who were confronted with drug-related cues (Jansen, 1998). However, in contrast to addiction research, relatively few laboratory cue reactivity studies have been carried out in individuals with eating disorders (Overduin, Jansen and Eilkes, 1997; Staiger, Dawe and McCarthy, 2000) and the results are rather contradictory.

Conditioning models of binge eating assume that, through a learning process, cues predictive of binge eating (e.g. feelings of depression, anxiety, loneliness or boredom, or the sight and smell of food) acquire the power to elicit a variety of anticipatory physiological, behavioural, affective and cognitive responses (Bulik *et al.*, 1996; Vögele and Florin, 1996; Overduin, Jansen and Eilkes, 1997). These responses are subjectively experienced as craving, leading to increased food consumption, and play a significant role in dysfunctional eating behaviour (Jansen, 1998; Nederkoorn, Smulders and Jansen, 2000). The reduction of cue reactivity may be an essential part of treatment and continued elevated cue reactivity after treatment could predict relapse (Bulik *et al.*, 1996).

REACTIVITY TO FOOD CUES IN STATES OF NORMAL AND ABNORMAL PHYSIOLOGY OR PSYCHOPATHOLOGY

Now we will review some of the studies that have been carried out to examine the arousal elicited by food cues in individuals with eating disorders and sub-clinical samples of restrained and binge eaters.

Restrained Eating

Homeostatic drives are thought to lead to periodic phases of disinhibited eating in people who chronically restrain their eating. Both bulimic and restrained subjects are characterized by failed attempts to restrict eating, overconcern with body shape and weight and an elevated frequency of binge eating (Overduin *et al.*, 1997). The conditioning model of binge eating predicts that cue reactivity should be larger in restrained eaters than in normal individuals. However, and contrary to these predictions, psychophysiological studies carried out in restrained and unrestrained eaters (Overduin, Jansen and Eilkes, 1997; Drobes *et al.*, 2001) have not found significant differences in the responses of both groups to food cues.

Binge Eating

Food cue reactivity has been investigated in sub-clinical samples of binge eaters and in individuals with a clear diagnosis of bulimia nervosa. For example, Vögele and Florin (1996) examined reactivity to exposure to favourite foods in non-binge eaters and to binge foods in binge eaters. All subjects responded with increased physiological arousal and feelings of hunger and desire to binge but significant differences between groups were also found. Binge eaters showed higher psychophysiological reactivity (increased blood pressure and electrodermal activity) throughout food exposure relative to controls. Interestingly, heart rate during food exposure predicted the later amount of food consumed in all subjects. This relationship was more marked in binge eaters than in the comparison group. In a later study, Drobes *et al.* (2001) also studied the emotional responding to food cues in binge eaters. Since binge eaters typically report high levels of dietary restraint, these authors predicted that they would show similar responses to food-deprived subjects given that these two groups might have an enhanced approach-oriented bias to food. Their hypothesis was confirmed as both groups showed enhanced startle reflexes while viewing food pictures. The same result was previously reported by Mauler *et al.* (1997) (cited in Drobes *et al.*, 2001) who found augmented probe startle responses to the presentation of food pictures in a bulimic group and in food-deprived normal eaters. Thus it appears that people with bulimia nervosa have arousal of the sympathetic nervous system in response to food cues.

Results from this research therefore suggest that binge eaters show an enhanced overall psychophysiological arousal to the presentation of food cues than do controls. However, the physiological response in terms of parasympathetic reactivity such as salivation to food cues in bulimia nervosa is less clear cut. Staiger and co-workers (2000) examined psychophysiological reactivity to individualized binge/favourite food exposure in bulimic subjects. They hypothesized that increasing cue salience would correlate with augmented reactivity and examined salivation and subjective responses to sensory properties of food (the sight and smell and the sight, smell, and taste of a binge/favourite food) and compared this to the responses elicited by a neutral food. Results confirmed the hypothesis that bulimic subjects would show greater urge to binge, stress and loss of control than the control group and this relationship would be more pronounced when exposed to the sight, smell and taste condition. However, there were no significant differences between groups in salivary reactivity.

In a longitudinal study, Bulik *et al.* (1996) examined salivary reactivity to individualized binge foods in a group of bulimic subjects. Before treatment (eight sessions of cognitive behavioural therapy), there was no evidence of an increase in salivation with the presentation of food. After treatment, however, food cues did lead to greater salivary reactivity. Thus it is possible that, before treatment, arousal of the sympathetic nervous system may have inhibited the parasympathetic response to food cues, namely salivation.

This result contrasts with those of other studies (LeGoff, Leichner and Spigelman, 1988) however, in which a greater increase in salivation was found in individuals with bulimia nervosa compared to controls. It is not easy to suggest a single conclusion for the contradictory results obtained in salivary reactivity in bulimic subjects. It has been hypothesized that variables such as body mass index, anxiety, depression, food restriction, dehydration, volume depletion or parotid gland hypertrophy could influence salivary reactivity and confound the results (Bulik *et al.*, 1996). In order to test this, Bulik *et al.* (1996) correlated all these variables with salivary reactivity but they failed to find any connection between them. Clearly, further research is needed to elucidate the possible variables affecting salivary reactivity in individuals with bulimia nervosa.

Another interesting topic of research in the addiction area has been to experimentally induce negative mood states and observe changes in the response to specific cues. In line with this, Laberg *et al.* (1991) assessed the physiological and subjective response of restrained eaters and patients with bulimia nervosa to slides before and after an experimental induction of negative mood. The slides consisted of pictures of the subject's actual body, food previously identified by the individual as typical binge food and control images of landscapes and houses. Heart rate was recorded continuously and self-reports of mood, craving and self-efficacy were obtained before and after the presentations of the slides. Patients with bulimia nervosa and restrained eaters did not differ in their responses prior to the negative mood induction. All participants had an initial deceleration in heart rate to food slides. After the induction of negative mood, patients with bulimia nervosa showed a greater deceleration in heart rate in response to food and body shape pictures than comparison women. Furthermore, bulimic patients reported an increased craving for food in the negative mood state. These findings suggest that negative affect focuses attention on food and increases craving in patients with bulimia nervosa and are congruent with clinical data suggesting that binge episodes are more likely in negative mood states.

Anorexia Nervosa

Very few studies of cue reactivity have included a group of individuals with anorexia nervosa. As noted above, one difficulty in interpreting the results of such studies is that starvation is associated with changes in autonomic nervous activity, and this may confound the response. One of the first reported studies of cue reactivity in anorexia nervosa was that by Salkind, Fincham and Silverstone (1980). These authors were interested in testing the conceptualization of anorexia nervosa as a fear-based disorder (i.e. fear of weight gain, weight phobia, morbid dread of fatness) and so also included as a control group patients with a specific phobia. The skin conductance changes in patients with anorexia and related feeding disturbances following exposure to food- and weight-related stimuli were either absent or small. This contrasted with the marked responses to the feared stimuli in subjects with specific phobias. Therefore, the hypothesis that anorexia might be considered a phobic disorder was not supported. However, 'fear of weight gain' remains one of the criteria for a diagnosis of anorexia nervosa in DSM-IV (APA, 1994).

Conclusion

Overall we can conclude that abnormal eating behaviours alter physiological and subjective reactivity to food cues. However, responses on some parameters are still uncertain. It is unclear whether the difference in these results arises from differences in food cues or technology used from the studies or whether the negative results can be attributed to low power or to inappropriateness of some response parameters. Finally, it is not clear whether this reactivity to food cues confirms the conditioning model of binge eating or not. Future research should be aimed to clarify the veracity of this model and its accuracy to explain abnormal eating patterns.

REACTIVITY TO FOOD INTAKE IN STATES OF NORMAL AND ABNORMAL PHYSIOLOGY OR PSYCHOPATHOLOGY

Weight and appetite are regulated homeostatically. Food is more attractive and the drive to eat is increased in states of starvation (Keys *et al.*, 1950). Food intake is governed not only by states of depletion but also by the hedonic properties of food (Pinel, Assanand and Lehman, 2000). The sensory properties of foods influence food choice and intake (Shepherd and Farleigh, 1989). Therefore the physiological and psychological state of the individual as well as salience of the cue will impact on the psychophysiological response.

The anticipation of food or the exposure to the sensory properties of food (visual, olfactory and taste) as well as cognitive processes (such as the thought of food or eating) elicit cephalic phase responses which prepare the body to optimize the digestion, absorption and use of nutrients, and play a role in the amount of food that an individual can tolerate (Jansen, 1998; Nederkoorn, Smulders and Jansen, 2000). Therefore, it is hypothesized that they are also important in eating disorders in which the intake of a large amount of food is a characteristic feature (Nederkoorn, Smulders and Jansen, 2000). Specifically, the cue reactivity model predicts that the frequent large food intake of binge eaters and their chaotic eating pattern (alternating between dieting and binge eating) will induce stronger conditioned responses in binge eaters than in normal subjects, and that these anticipatory responses will be subjectively experienced as craving, making it more difficult for the subject to abstain from eating (Nederkoorn, Smulders and Jansen, 2000; Jansen, 1998). Although this relationship is particularly marked in individuals with eating disorders, food cues also increase feelings of hunger and craving in healthy individuals (Overduin, Jansen and Eilkes, 1997; Vögele and Florin, 1996; Nederkoorn, Smulders and Jansen, 2000).

Animal and human research has found that food exposure increases salivation, gastric activity, and insulin release. Woods and Strubbe (1994) found that the temperature of rats increased prior to a meal. Nederkoorn and co-workers (2000) found a similar increase in temperature of humans during food exposure. The response to eating differs from that of exposure alone. Skin conductance increased during food exposure and decreased during and after the meal. A parallel pattern of change was seen in the low frequency component of heart rate variability.

Léonard *et al.* (1998) also assessed the emotional response to food intake in patients with anorexia nervosa, bulimia nervosa and in a comparison group using three measures of psychophysiological response (skin conductance, heart rate and electroencephalogram). The results showed that meal intake did not lead to significant changes in skin conductance in controls or in people with bulimia nervosa. However, in people with anorexia nervosa there was a significant increase in skin conductance during eating. No changes were found on other physiological variables in any of the groups. It is possible that the negative finding in bulimia nervosa may be because the study was underpowered (there were only 10 women with bulimia) and also the cue may have been less salient for women with bulimia than for women with anorexia.

In an early study, Williamson *et al.* (1988) assessed sympathetic arousal following eating. Four groups were included in this study: bulimia nervosa, obese and a normal control group who all ate a test meal and another normal control group who did not eat the test meal. Results showed that both the bulimic and obese groups responded with increased heart rate after eating the test meal, differing from the normal control group who showed a deceleration in heart rate after eating. All groups had vasoconstriction immediately after eating but this rapidly reversed within 20 minutes in the bulimia nervosa group. All groups responded with decreased skin temperature. The bulimic group also differed from all other groups because subjects with bulimia nervosa responded to eating with an immediate augment in skin resistance followed by a subsequent decline. Contrasting to both normal groups, the obese group responded to food intake with decreased skin resistance. Finally, results for forearm EMG suggested that bulimic and obese groups responded to eating with enhanced EMG, whereas both normal groups showed a decrease in this response. Therefore, some of these physiological responses were congruent with a higher level of sympathetic arousal, whereas others showed opposite results, especially in bulimia nervosa. A possible explanation for these mixed results is that vomiting may produce reduced autonomic arousability and therefore it may be particularly hard to find a global sympathetic arousal response in individuals with bulimia nervosa.

Overall it is difficult to draw a general conclusion from these studies due to the different methodologies used in them. For example, the type of food and caloric content of the test meals, the amount of food the subjects were allowed to eat, sample characteristics and previous exposure of food cues were different for each study. Further research characterized by the use of a single methodology and similar groups of subjects is needed to clarify differences in psychophysiological responses to eating in individuals with and without an eating disorder.

STRESS AND BULIMIA NERVOSA

Stress, in particular interpersonal stress (Cattanach, Malley and Rodin, 1988; Polivy and Herman, 1993; Leal, Weise and Dodd, 1995; Koo-Loeb *et al.*, 2000), plays an important role in the aetiology and maintenance of eating disorders. Eating disorder patients subjectively report high levels of perceived stress as well as the presence of objectively determined severe life events and difficulties both concurrently (Soukup, Beiler and Terrell, 1990; Troop, Holbrey and Treasure, 1998) and at onset (Schmidt *et al.*, 1997; Welch, Doll and Fairburn, 1997). In addition, patients with eating disorders show poorer coping in terms of individual coping strategies (such as cognitive and behavioural avoidance of problems), lower confidence in coping and increased helplessness (e.g. Soukup, Beiler and Terrell, 1990; Neckowitz and Morrison, 1991; Troop *et al.*, 1994, 1998; Yager, Rorty and Rossotto, 1995). It is thought that the abnormal eating behaviours arise from a maladaptive response to stress and that individuals with eating disorders, therefore, will respond to stress with a greater psychophysiological reactivity relative to non-eating disordered controls.

In an early study that tested this hypothesis, Cattanach and co-workers (1988) assessed cardiovascular and affective responses to achievement challenge and interpersonal stress in women with bulimia nervosa. Strong cardiovascular responses and negative mood states were seen in both groups but, relative to the comparison group, bulimic individuals did not show significant differences in blood pressure, pulse rate or affective responses to the stressors. Subjective responses were significantly different between both groups. Individuals with bulimia reported a higher desire to binge than controls (particularly during interpersonal stress) and more global stress, lower self-esteem, and lower mastery than the normal control group. Consistent with these results, Tuschen-Caffier and Vögele (1999) did not find significant differences in heart rate, blood pressure, respiration rate, and electrodermal activity between patients with bulimia nervosa, restrained eaters and controls during achievement challenge and interpersonal stress. However, subjective ratings did show substantial differences between groups since bulimic patients responded to the stressful tasks with enhanced desire to binge and hunger.

In contrast, however, Tuschen *et al.* (1995) found lower cardiovascular reactivity during achievement challenge in the bulimic group relative to the normal comparison group. Koo-Loeb, Pedersen and Girdler (1998) also found elongated PEP intervals, blunted blood pressure and heart rate in response to mental stressors in individuals with bulimia nervosa relative to a normal comparison group. Psychosocial responses of bulimic individuals also suggested that the bulimic group perceived more stress and were more anxious and depressed than the comparison group.

Overall, subjective ratings from these studies suggest that individuals with bulimia nervosa show higher levels of distress to mental stressors than control subjects and this is accompanied by an increased desire to binge. However, psychophysiological data are confusing. This dissociation between emotional responses and physiological reactivity could be due to a variety of factors. For example, the low power of the studies or the type and range of the stressors used through the different studies (see Table XXIII-5.1). Therefore, and as we suggested above, more studies using a similar methodology should be carried out to clarify physiological reactivity in response to stressors. It is also important to discern what kind of stressors may be important for stress-induced eating.

SUMMARY AND CONCLUSION

Research on psychophysiological factors and eating disorders has provided limited and confusing results (Laberg *et al.*, 1991). The psychophysiological reactivity to food cues remains unclear (Nederkoorn, Smulders and Jansen, 2000). As Nederkoon and coworkers (2000) suggest, deriving a global conclusion from these studies is problematic due to the diversity of groups (restrained eaters, bulimic patients, obese), cues (standardized food, individualized favourite food, pictures of food, real food) and psychophysiological measures (salivation, heart rate, skin conductance) used in these studies. Besides this, most of the studies present methodological problems, such as inadequate test stimuli, small sample size, inappropriate control groups and limited analysis of psychophysiological reactivity (Laberg *et al.*, 1991). Results from studies on psychophysiological responses to stress are similarly inconsistent. While some studies report no difference in psychophysiological responses between patients with bulimia nervosa and non-eating disordered women, others do find differences. More consistently, however, self-reports of urge to binge are greater in patients than in comparison women.

So what are we to make of the results reviewed? What are the implications for the theory and therapy of eating disorders? For the cue reactivity to food- and body-related stimuli, if not for responses to stress, the weight of evidence suggests there are differences in physiological arousal to food when people are in a state of deprivation. This is seen in normals who have missed a meal, in restrained eaters and in women with bulimia and anorexia nervosa.

It is uncertain as to whether the psychophysiological abnormalities that have been found represent aetiological risk factors for eating disorders or whether they are consequences of the illness or even factors that may maintain the illness. The psychophysiological differences found in the normal controls as a result of food deprivation suggest that it may be a maintaining factor.

Regardless of any possible role in the development of eating disorders, the use of psychophysiological measures in response to food-related stimuli may provide a useful marker of improvement and recovery. Measures of outcome tend to rely on objective behavioural indicators as these are relatively unequivocal in terms of making diagnoses (notwithstanding debates about the validity of particular criteria or diagnostic categories). However, there is considerable debate as to what constitutes 'recovery' rather than simply 'abstinence' from eating disordered behaviours. Perhaps it is here, potentially, that psychophysiological measures may be of greatest value in identifying differences between asymptomatic rather than recovered patients. One study has explored changes across treatment (Bulik *et al.*, 1996) but not specifically addressed whether 'normal' psychophysiological reactivity to food and food cues can be used as a marker of recovery. Future research on this possibility might be a useful line of enquiry.

REFERENCES

American Psychiatric Association, 1994. *Diagnostic and Statistical Manual of Mental Disorders 4th Edition*. APA, Washington DC.

Bourke, M.P., Taylor, G.J., Parker, J.D.A. and Bagby, R.M., 1992. Alexithymia in women with anorexia nervosa. *British Journal of Psychiatry*, **161**, 240–243.

Bulik, C.M., Sullivan, P.F., Lawson, R.H. and Carter, F.A., 1996. Salivary reactivity in women with bulimia nervosa across treatment. *Biological Psychiatry*, **39**, 1009–1012.

Cattanach, L., Malley, R. and Rodin, J., 1988. Psychologic and physiologic reactivity to stressors in eating disordered individuals. *Psychosomatic Medicine*, **50**, 591–599.

Corcos, M., Guilbaud, O., Speranza, M., Paterniti, S., Loas, G., Stephan, P. and Jeammet, P., 2000. Alexithymia and depression in eating disorders. *Psychiatry Research*, **93**, 263–266.

De Zwaan, M., Biener, D., Bach, M., Wiesnagrotzki, S. and Stacher, G., 1996. Pain sensitivity, alexithymia, and depression in patients with eating disorders: Are they related? *Journal of Psychosomatic Research*, **41**, 65–70.

Drobes, D.J., Miller, E.J., Hillman, C.H., Bradley, M.M., Cuthbert, B.N. and Lang, P.J., 2001. Food deprivation and emotional reactions to food cues: implications for eating disorders. *Biological Psychology*, **57**, 153–177.

Godart, N.T., Flament, M.F., Lecrubier, Y. and Jeammet, P., 2000. Anxiety disorders in anorexia nervosa and bulimia nervosa: co-morbidity and chronology of appearance. *European Psychiatry*, **15**, 38–45.

Heatherton, T.F., Herman, C.P. and Polivy, J., 1991. Effects of physical threat and ego threat on eating behavior. *Journal of Personality and Social Psychology*, **60**, 138–143.

Jansen, A., 1998. A learning model of binge eating: cue reactivity and cue exposure. *Behaviour Research and Therapy*, **36**, 257–272.

Keys, A., Brozek, J., Henschel, A., Mickelson, O. and Taylor, H.L., 1950. *The Biology of Human Starvation*. University of Minnesota Press, Minneapolis.

Koo-Loeb, J.H., Costello, N., Light, K. and Girdler, S., 2000. Women with eating disorder tendencies display altered cardiovascular, neuroendocrine, and psychosocial profiles. *Psychosomatic Medicine*, **62**, 539–548.

Koo-Loeb, J.H., Pedersen, C. and Girdler, S.S., 1998. Blunted cardiovascular and catecholamine stress reactivity in women with bulimia nervosa. *Psychiatry Research*, **80**, 13–27.

Laberg, J.C., Wilson, G.T., Eldredge, K. and Nordby, H., 1991. Effects of mood on heart rate reactivity in bulimia nervosa. *International Journal of Eating Disorders*, **10**, 169–178.

Lattimore, P., Gowers, S. and Wagner, H.L., 2000. Autonomic arousal and conflict avoidance in anorexia nervosa: A pilot study. *European Eating Disorders Review*, **8**, 31–39.

Leal, L., Weise, S.M. and Dodd, D.K., 1995. The relationship between gender, symptoms of bulimia, and tolerance for stress. *Addictive Behaviors*, **20**, 105–109.

LeGoff, D., Leichner, P. and Spigelman, M., 1988. Salivary responses to olfactory food stimuli in anorexics and bulimics. *Appetite*, **11**, 15–25.

Léonard, T., Pepinà, C., Bond, A. and Treasure, J., 1998. Assessment of test-meal induced autonomic arousal in anorexic, bulimic and control females. *European Eating Disorders Review*, **6**, 188–200.

Neckowitz, P. and Morrison, T.L., 1991. Interactional coping strategies of normal-weight bulimic women in intimate and nonintimate stressful interactions. *Psychological Reports*, **69**, 1167–1175.

Nederkoorn, C., Smulders, F.T.Y. and Jansen, A., 2000. Cephalic phase responses, craving and food intake in normal subjects. *Appetite*, **35**, 45–55.

Overduin, J. and Jansen, A., 1997. Conditioned insulin and blood sugar responses in humans in relation to binge eating. *Physiology and Behavior*, **61**, 569–575.

Overduin, J., Jansen, A. and Eilkes, H., 1997. Cue reactivity to food- and body-related stimuli in restrained and unrestrained eaters. *Addictive Behaviors*, **22**, 395–404.

Parrott, W.G. and Hertel, P., 1999. Research methods in cognition and emotion. In: Dalgleish, T. and Power, M. (eds), *Handbook of Cognition and Emotion*. John Wiley & Sons Ltd, London.

Phillips, L., Tiggemann, M. and Wade, T., 1997. Comparison of cognitive style in bulimia nervosa and depression. *Behaviour Research and Therapy*, **35**, 939–948.

Pinel, J.P., Assanand, S. and Lehman, D.R., 2000. Hunger, eating, and ill health. *The American Psychologist*, **55**(10), 105–1116.

Polivy, J. and Herman, C.P., 1993. Etiology of binge eating: Psychological mechanisms. In: Fairburn, C.G. and Wilson, G.T. (eds), *Binge Eating: Nature, Assessment, and Treatment*, pp. 173–205. Guilford, New York.

Salkind, M.R., Fincham, J. and Silverstone, T., 1980. Is anorexia nervosa a phobic disorder? A psychophysiological enquiry. *Biological Psychiatry*, **15**, 803–808.

Schmidt, U., Jiwany, A. and Treasure, J., 1993. A controlled study of alexithymia in eating disorders. *Comprehensive Psychiatry*, **34**, 54–58.

Schmidt, U.H., Tiller, J.M., Andrews, B., Blanchard, M. and Treasure, J.L., 1997. Is there a specific trauma precipitating onset of anorexia nervosa? *Psychological Medicine*, **27**, 523–530.

Sheperd, R. and Farleigh, C.A., 1989. Sensory assessment of foods and the role of sensory attributes in determining food choice. In: Sheperd, R. (ed.), *Handbook of the Psychophysiology of Human Eating*, pp. 25–56. John Wiley & Sons Ltd, New York.

Soukup, V.M., Beiler, M.E. and Terrell, F., 1990. Stress, coping style and problem solving ability among eating disordered inpatients. *Journal of Clinical Psychology*, **46**, 592–599.

Staiger, P., Dawe, S. and McCarthy, R., 2000. Responsivity to food cues in bulimic women and controls. *Appetite*, **35**, 27–33.

Taylor, G.J., Parker, J.D.A., Bagby, R.M. and Bourke, M.P., 1996. Relationships between alexithymia and psychological characteristics associated with eating disorders. *Journal of Psychosomatic Research*, **41**, 561–568.

Troop, N.A., Holbrey, A. and Treasure, J.L., 1998. Stress, coping and crisis support in eating disorders. *International Journal of Eating Disorders*, **24**, 157–166.

Troop, N.A., Holbrey, A., Trowler, R. and Treasure, J.L., 1994. Ways of coping in women with eating disorders. *The Journal of Nervous and Mental Disease*, **182**, 535–540.

Tuschen-Caffier, B. and Vögele, C., 1999. Psychological and physiological reactivity to stress: An experimental study on bulimic patients, restrained eaters and controls. *Psychotherapy and Psychosomatics*, **68**, 333–340.

Vögele, C. and Florin, I., 1996. Psychophysiological responses to food exposure: An experimental study in binge eaters. *International Journal of Eating Disorders*, **21**, 147–157.

Welch, S.L., Doll, H.A. and Fairburn, C.G., 1997. Life events and the onset of bulimia nervosa: A controlled study. *Psychological Medicine*, **27**, 515–522.

Williamson, D.A., Goreczny, A.J., Davis, C.J., Ruggiero, L. and McKenzie, S.J., 1988. Psychophysiological analysis of the anxiety model of bulimia nervosa. *Behavior Therapy*, **19**, 1–9.

Woods, S.C. and Strubbe, J.H., 1994. The psychobiology of meals. *Psychonomic Bulletin and Review*, **1**, 141–155.

Yager, J., Rorty, M. and Rossotto, E., 1995. Coping styles differ between recovered and nonrecovered women with bulimia nervosa but not between recovered women and non-eating disordered control subjects. *Journal of Nervous and Mental Disease*, **183**, 86–94.

XXIII-6

Neuropsychological Findings in Eating Disorders

Christoph J. Lauer

INTRODUCTION

Neuropsychological research in eating disorders initially was driven by the observation that anorexic patients with evidence for perinatal brain injury showed a poor treatment outcome; particularly, a smaller weight gain was found to be associated with more frequent complications in pregnancy and delivery. Such complications were suggested to increase the susceptibility to subtle cerebral damage, which then may lead to a poor clinical prognosis. Hereby, neuropsychological testing was thought to comprise the advantage of favouring identification of cortical dysfunctions caused by these subtle brain damages below anatomically or physiologically detectable levels. The general hypothesis formulated proposed that the pattern of neurocognitive deficits might be suggestive of dysfunction of relative specific brain systems (Braun and Chouinard, 1992). In following these assumptions, most of the early neuropsychological investigations applied formal test batteries such as the 'Luria-Nebraska Neuropsychological Battery' or the 'Wechsler Intelligence Scales' (WAIS). However, while such test batteries are useful in making general conclusions about the presence of impairments in individuals with a given brain injury, they are not flexible enough to allow the investigator to assess the variety of functions that may underlie a performance deficit on a complex cognitive task in patients with, for example, an eating disorder. Poor performance may be the result of a broad range of possibilities, including damage to one of several areas, the accumulative effect of mild deficits in multiple areas, or factors unrelated to specific brain dysfunctions (see: Keefe, 1995). Therefore, neuropsychology should provide more than a window into the everyday mental processes of psychiatric patients; it should provide an objective description of what areas of behaviour and cognition are likely to be a problem for the patient and — more important — what areas are not.

This paper is divided into five sections. First, a short overview of neurocognitive observations in non-eating disordered subjects (e.g. dieters) will be provided; thereafter, the findings obtained during the acute state of an eating disorders will be summarized, followed by the presentation of neurocognitive changes after treatment, the attempt to identify neuropsychological predictors of the treatment outcome and a short section aiming at the neurocognitive-based identification of patients dropping out of therapy. Finally, the significance of various factors mediating the neurocognitive deficits in eating disorder patients will be discussed.

Because little scientific effort has so far been undertaken to evaluate the neurocognitive function in overweight and obese subjects not suffering from an additional disease known to affect neuropsychological task performance (such as the Prader–Willy syndrome, the sleep apnoea syndrome, the Down syndrome), these types of eating disorders will not be considered in this paper.

NEUROPSYCHOLOGICAL FINDINGS IN FORMER PRISONERS OF WAR AND IN NON-EATING DISORDERED, NORMAL WEIGHT DIETERS

In the following the suggestion that severe starvation and weight loss may cause sustained impairments in brain morphology and cognitive functioning, Sutker and co-workers (1987, 1990) evaluated the neuropsychological task performances in former prisoners of war (POW) who had experienced severe weight loss during captivity due to biological and psychological stress. Compared to combat veterans not captured and interned, the high weight-loss POW (loss of more than 35% of preconfinement weight) were deficient on the 'Attention-Concentration' Factor of the WAIS-R and on measures of immediate and delayed memory as assessed by the Wechsler-Memory-Scale (WMS); on the other hand, no significant impairment was obvious on the WAIS-R subtests 'digit symbol' (sustained attention), 'block design' (visuospatial construction) and 'digit span' (span of attention, working memory). The authors concluded that their findings of deficits on measures of immediate recall combined with lowered 'Attention-Concentration' factor performances raises the possibility that memory problems cited frequently in POW self-reports may be more attributable to deficiencies in attention, concentration and perhaps organizing functions than to memory storage or retrieval processes.

In healthy normal weight non-dieting females, various degrees of 'acute' food deprivation (miss one meal, miss two meals and miss all food for 24 hours) did not result in obvious effects on neurocognitive functions such as sustained attention, attentional focus, simple reaction time or immediate memory, except for a significant slower psychomotor speed performance (finger tapping) after 24-hour of food deprivation (Green, Elliman and Rogers, 1995). However, the same group reported that normal weight female *dieters* displayed poorer vigilance performance, slower reaction times and poorer immediate recall of words when they were dieting compared to a period of normal food intake. Performance on psychomotor speed was not impaired (Green and Rogers, 1995). Because self-reported dietary restraint, but not anxiety and depression, was increased during dieting, the authors related their findings to an association between dieting behaviour and high levels of distractibility; they proposed that impaired cognitive performance is closely related to dieting or the perceived need to diet *per se*. An increased distractibility (reduced capacity to inhibit responding to task irrelevant information and to facilitate responses that are goal-directed; assessed by the Stroop Colour Naming Task) was also reported in restrained eaters after a 'high-caloric' preload (single Twix bar) compared to a 'low-caloric' preload (cream cracker) and to unrestrained eaters (Odgen and Greville, 1993); the restrained females took longer to colour name active state words, food words and body size words after the high-caloric preload than unrestrained eating females. Interestingly, not only do acute food deprivation and prolonged periods of dieting affect some facets of neurocognitive

Biological Psychiatry: Edited by H. D'haenen, J.A. den Boer and P. Willner. ISBN 0-471-49198-5

performance but also the micro-composition of the nourishment *per se*. Investigating the acute effects of isocaloric lunches differing in fat and carbohydrate content Lloyd and colleagues (1994) observed a slower reaction time following the fat- as well as the carbohydrate-rich lunches compared to the fat- and carbohydrate-balanced meals. However, because the subjects reported themselves as more drowsy and muddled after the fat- and carbohydrate-rich lunches, the reported limited attentional capacity might simply reflect the well-known phenomenon of a 'post lunch dip'.

Thus, the findings reported so far in non-eating disordered *dieters* demonstrate that various manipulations of individual eating habits result in a mild impairment of attention and concentration, as indicated by a slower reaction time, an increased distractibility and a slightly reduced capacity of the working memory. However, in non-eating disordered and non-dieting subjects such manipulations failed to provoke any changes in their neurocognitive task profile.

NEUROPSYCHOLOGICAL FINDINGS IN THE ACUTE STATE OF THE EATING DISORDER

One of the initial studies that investigated a broad range of neurocognitive test performances in patients with anorexia nervosa was conducted by Hamsher and colleagues about 20 years ago (1981). The authors followed the concept that at least some forms of anorexia nervosa may occur in the context of subtle brain dysfunction. Applying the cut-off scores that were known to differentiate well between patients with brain lesions and patients with other clinical disorders, the authors reported 45% of their anorexic patients to show impaired performances on two or more of the applied tasks; most frequently a retarded reaction time on a forced-choice task (35% of the patients) was observed, followed by an impairment on mental arithmetic tasks (15%; sustained attention), short-term visual memory (30%) and long-term information retrieval (20%; long-term memory). Other neurocognitive abilities assessed were more or less well preserved (percentage of affected patients <15%; e.g. psychomotor speed, perceptual-analytic ability, spatial orientation and verbal fluency). The rather non-specific and sporadic nature of the test failures was described by the authors as being most characteristic of an attention-concentration deficit or cognitive inefficiency. The assumption of a reduced attentional capacity in eating disorder patients, along with other but sporadic reported difficulties, was underlined in most of the subsequent studies in anorexic and in bulimic patients (*vigilance and sustained attention*: Laessle *et al.*, 1989, 1990; Green *et al.*, 1996; Kingston *et al.*, 1996; *divided attention*: Lauer *et al.*, 1999; attentional capacity necessary for *response execution/inhibition*: Fairburn *et al.*, 1991; Cooper and Fairburn, 1992; Kingston *et al.*, 1996; *attentional flexibility*: Pendleton Jones *et al.*, 1991; Szmukler *et al.*, 1992; *speed of information processing*: Pendleton Jones *et al.*, 1991; Kingston *et al.*, 1996). Because psychomotor speed and reaction time are among the critical variables on almost all tasks assessing the various aspects of attention, one might simply attribute these findings to the general slowing of motor responses associated with starvation (Maxwell, Tucker and Townes, 1984; Green *et al.*, 1996). Alternatively, the poor performances on these tasks may be related to an increased susceptibility to interference and an increased distractibility (Ben-Tovim *et al.*, 1989; Fairburn *et al.*, 1991; Perpina *et al.*, 1993; Long, Hinton and Gillespie, 1994). In other words, most of the attentional deficits in patients with eating disorders seem to depend on an insufficient functioning of selective and flexible processing of more than one piece of relevant information.

In a number of studies, working (immediate) memory capacity, learning abilities, as well as short-term and long-term memory, were found to be impaired to a similar extent in both anorexia and bulimia nervosa (Touyz, Beumont and Johnstone, 1986; Pendleton Jones *et al.*, 1991; Green *et al.*, 1996; Kingston *et al.*, 1996; Mathias and Kent, 1998). In contrast to the rather 'unspecific' impairments of attention, these findings of mnemonic disabilities are suggestive of a 'specific' deficit and have been primarily discussed in terms of an impaired working memory that, according to Baddeley (1992), is formed by the phonological loop and the visuospatial sketch-pad in conjunction with a central executive component. However, other studies failed to demonstrate a significantly reduced capacity of either the phonological loop (e.g. Digit Span) or the visuospatial sketch pad (e.g. Block/Corsi Span) (see Hamsher, Halmi and Benton, 1981; Szmukler *et al.*, 1992; Lauer *et al.*, 1999), implying that the central executive component was dysfunctional; however, this component is particularly dependent on preserved attentional processes. Of interest here are also the findings of Beatty and colleagues (1990). These authors reported the process of learning to be deficient in their patients; however, the delayed recall (short- and long-termed) of that previously learned material was not. Thus, whereas the acquisition period of the new material was affected probably due to impaired attentional demands and information processing, the final encoding and the memory retrieval processes were undisturbed. Interestingly, Strupp and colleagues (1986) reported the effortful information processing (conscious learning) to be quite normal in their patient sample; however, the automatic information processing (learning without conscious intent) was found to be impaired. The authors discussed their finding in terms of heightened arousal (for example, anxiety and preoccupations concerning food and body weight) and attentional focusing. According to Bacon (1974), they suggested that arousal both narrows attentional focus and reduces overall cognitive capacity; therefore, an aroused subject might be expected to have sufficient cognitive capacity to perform well on the designated (effortful) aspect of the task, but to have insufficient capacity to automatically process additional information. Again, the suggestion of an insufficient attentional capacity allowed a satisfactory explanation without dealing with more complex neurocognitive functioning such as working memory or the ability to appropriately encode, store and retrieve information from the memory.

In only a few studies were higher order cognitive skills such as problem solving capacity, categorization and abstraction evaluated (Palazidou, Robinson and Lishman, 1990; Szmukler *et al.*, 1992; Lauer *et al.*, 1999). The performances of tasks measuring such skills depend on complex neurocognitive functioning (for example, to solve the Wisconsin Card Sorting Test, at least auditory attention, visual attention, motor skills, learning, abstraction, categorization, working memory, short-term memory and executive control are needed). No obvious impairments could be ascertained in two investigations applying the WCST (Palazidou, Robinson and Lishman, 1990; Lauer *et al.*, 1999), while Szmukler and co-workers (1992) reported a poor performance in the Austin Maze, which assesses complex serial learning, error utilization, flexibility, planning and adaptive behaviour abilities.

According to the cited findings, no definite conclusion can be drawn as to which neurocognitive functions are impaired in the acute state of the eating disorder. However, as already proposed by Hamsher and colleagues (1981) there is fairly good evidence that the most characteristic failure is a cognitive inefficiency in the form of attentional deficits irrespective of the type of eating disorder (restricting anorexics, bulimic anorexics, and bulimics). Although this conclusion sounds rather non-specific, most of the investigations revealed that especially the selective processing of information is affected in eating disorder patients. This results in a general slowing not limited to specific types of mental decision-making processes. However, this deficiency apparently seems not to diminish the final encoding, storage and retrieval of the information—as long as the information was subjected to conscious learning. In more popular terms, patients with an eating disorder need a bit more time than healthy subjects for sufficient information encoding, because their overall attentional capacity is limited by additionally processing a certain amount of task irrelevant (disease related?) information. However, this conclusion does not refer to all eating disorder patients; as far as explicitly indicated in the respective reports, only about 38% of the patients presented with more or less obvious neurocognitive impairments (see: Lauer *et al.*, 1999).

RECTIFICATION OF THE NEUROPSYCHOLOGICAL MEASURES AFTER TREATMENT

A number of investigations followed the hypothesis that the neurocognitive deficits assessed at hospital admission might ameliorate in parallel with improvement of the primary and secondary eating disorder symptomatology (weight gain, decreased frequency of bingeing and purging episodes, rectification of the abnormalities in brain morphology and neuroendocrinology). A second, and probably more important point was to identify cognitive deficits predictive for a good but also for a poor clinical prognosis. Such identification would allow the development of additional and specific treatment strategies to increase the likelihood of a favourable outcome.

In addressing this question, two investigations applied a cross-sectional design. In the first study (Strupp *et al.*, 1986), which mainly focused on effortful versus automatic information processing, there were no obvious differences between acute underweight and weight-recovered anorexic patients. Pendleton Jones and colleagues (1991) found a poorer performance on tasks corresponding to attentional focusing, verbal memory and visuospatial reasoning in their underweight anorexics compared to weight-restored anorexics; however, these differences were subtle and nonsignificant.

In contrast, all the prospective studies (Hamsher, Halmi and Benton, 1981; Small *et al.*, 1983; Szmukler *et al.*, 1992; Kingston *et al.*, 1996; Lauer *et al.*, 1999) reported a rectification of the impaired neurocognitive skills, in particular of the attentional capacity, when the patients had successfully completed the respective therapeutic schedules (weight gain, reduction in the frequency of bingeing and purging). In one study, however, the mnemonic disabilities observed in the acute state of anorexia nervosa, continued to persist after a weight gain of at least 10% of the body mass index (Kingston *et al.*, 1996); the authors related their finding to an insufficient weight gain (incomplete nutritional rehabilitation) at the time of re-testing; but they also speculated that the mnemonic disability might have antedated the onset of the illness, although a relationship with the history of perinatal injury could be excluded.

Because one methodological problem is inherent to all neuropsychological prospective study designs — that is the repeated application of the same tasks at different time points — one might argue that the neurocognitive rectifications observed after clinical remission of the eating disorder simply are due to practice effects. However, in most of the studies, methodological attention had been paid to choose measures for which acceptable alternative forms were available, in order to minimize this effect. In addition, the time interval between pre- and post-treatment sessions lasted between 70 days (Szmukler *et al.*, 1992) and seven months (Lauer *et al.*, 1999), a timely length that further lowers the probability of significant practice effects. Therefore, it is certainly possible that the improved attentional abilities are, in part, related to a decrease in susceptibility to interferences and an increase of the flexibility/inhibition functions, as was reported by Kingston *et al.* (1996). This is further supported by the finding of Lauer and colleagues (1999) that the percentage of eating disorder patients who were able to resolve a Daily-Living Problem Task without any cues had increased from 73% at pretreatment to about 90% at post-treatment.

Thus, the neurocognitive deficits that had been present in eating disorder patients before the onset of a specific treatment schedule appear to vanish in parallel with the amelioration of the eating disorder symptomatology, irrespective of whether the patients suffered from an anorexic or a bulimic disorder. However, as will be outlined in more detail in the following section, this conclusion sounds too optimistic, because it refers to only 11% of the eating disorder patients (see below).

DO NEUROPSYCHOLOGICAL MEASURES PREDICT THE CLINICAL OUTCOME?

In four investigations, the authors attempted to identify neurocognitive predictors of the clinical outcome. However, the results reported were conflicting. Hamsher and colleagues (1981) found their anorexic patients who showed impaired performance on two or more neuropsychological tasks at *post*-treatment examination to be more likely to exhibit an unfavourable outcome (weight loss) after one year of follow-up than patients with very mild or no cognitive deficits at hospital discharge. Regarding the task performances at pretreatment examination, however, no such predictions could be confirmed. Small and colleagues (1983) reported the performance in the digit span task, which measures immediate (working) memory capacity, to be a powerful predictor of weight gain in their anorexic patients. In contrast, Szmukler and co-workers (1992) as well as Lauer and colleagues (1999) failed to identify any valuable predictors for the clinical outcome (either just prior to or eight weeks after hospital discharge), although they had applied a broad range of neuropsychological tasks.

NEUROPSYCHOLOGICAL FINDINGS IN PATIENTS DROPPING THE TREATMENT

In one study, the authors aimed at the neuropsychological identification of those patients who dropped out of the therapeutical schedule (Lauer *et al.*, 1999). However, the neurocognitive task performances as well as the personal and clinical characteristics of these patients were fairly good comparable to those patients who completed the programme. Again, the type of the eating disorder appeared not to be of importance.

Percentage of Patients with Neuropsychological Deficits

At present, one would suggest that certain cognitive deficits are evident in anorexic and bulimic patients, but disappear when the eating disorder patients recover. However, when looking at an *individual* level, this suggestion is not reasonable. Considering two or more impaired task performances as a cut-off, only 38% of patients are reported to be cognitively affected in the acute episode of the eating disorder (38 patients out of a total of 101 patients; Hamsher, Halmi and Benton, 1981; Szmukler *et al.*, 1992; Kingston *et al.*, 1996; Lauer *et al.*, 1999) and this figure drops to 27% at post-treatment. In other words, 62% of the patients with an acute eating disorder have well-preserved cognitive skills, while in the remaining patients displaying cognitive deficits (38%) a rectification can be observed in only 11%. Therefore, it appears not surprising that the reports on the cognitive abilities in eating disorders published so far do not provide a very consistent picture, especially as 'positive' findings depend not only on the severity of cognitive deficits but, more importantly, on the number of patients displaying such deficits. It is important to note also that the attempt to distinguish 'poor' and 'good' performing eating disorder patients on a personal (e.g. age, years of education) and a clinical level (e.g. Beck Depression Inventory, BDI; Eating Disorder Inventory, EDI) yielded completely negative results (Hamsher, Halmi and Benton, 1981; Lauer *et al.*, 1999).

FACTORS MODULATING NEUROCOGNITIVE PERFORMANCE IN EATING DISORDER PATIENTS

Eating Disorder Symptomatology

Interestingly, in only a few studies was the performance on neurocognitive tasks directly related to the degree of underweight, the frequency of bingeing and purging, and the severity of the psychopathology in the eating disordered patients (e.g. as measured by the EDI) and their ameliorations during treatment, respectively. The results reported, however, are somewhat disappointing. Correlations calculated between task performances and eating disorder symptomatology were all far from reaching statistical significance. In addition, group comparisons of 'good' performing and 'poor' performing patients revealed no obvious differences in the severity of the eating disorder. And finally, although in all prospective studies the rectification of the cognitive deficits had run in parallel with that of the eating disorder symptomatology, little evidence was found that the two processes are closely interrelated (Strupp *et al.*, 1986; Laessle *et al.*, 1990; Green *et al.*, 1996; Lauer *et al.*, 1999).

'Secondary' Psychopathology

It can also be speculated that the impaired cognitive functions in eating disorder patients are due to secondary psychopathological symptoms, in particular of depression. However, in almost all of the studies performed so far no evidence was found that the severity of depressive symptomatology had influenced the respective cognitive findings in these patients (Hamsher, Halmi and Benton, 1981; Beatty *et al.*, 1990; Pendleton Jones *et al.*, 1991; Szmukler *et al.*, 1992; Cooper and Fairburn, 1993; Green *et al.*, 1996; Kingston *et al.*, 1996; Lauer *et al.*, 1999). Occasionally, however, an association was reported between level of vigilance and severity of depression (Green *et al.*, 1996), a finding that closely matches that generally observed in patients with affective disorders (see further papers in this chapter). In addition, the actual level ('state') of anxiety at neuropsychological examination appeared not to affect task performances (Szmukler *et al.*, 1992; Kingston *et al.*, 1996; Green *et al.*, 1996; Mathias and Kent, 1998). However, the more enduring level of anxiety ('trait'; as measured by the MMPI) was closely associated with the neuropsychological task performances at pretreatment (Hamsher, Halmi and Benton, 1981) and accounted for nearly all of the neuropsychological deficits, though rather subtle ones, reported in the study by Pendleton Jones and colleagues (1991). Therefore, it could be argued that the neurocognitive deficits observed in eating disorder patients reflect simply the effect of more enduring anxiety (this chapter).

Unspecific Stress due to Hospital Admission

In 1981, Hamsher and colleagues had speculated that stress due to hospital admission might obscure task performance in eating disorder patients. A comparable effect also could be expected in those investigations evaluating the neurocognitive status of their patients two to three weeks after admission, that is, during the re-feeding/treatment period. To control for such a bias, Lauer *et al.* (1999) had investigated their patients four weeks *before* admission. However, the profile of cognitive deficits they observed was surprisingly similar to that usually found at or shortly *after* hospital admission. Therefore, it is rather unlikely that the level of performance in patients with eating disorders is affected by unspecific stress due to hospital admission.

Sleep Disorders

Recent observations in sleep research provide fairly good evidence for a relationship between learning and sleep states, particularly rapid eye movement (REM) sleep or dream sleep (Smith, 1996). Furthermore, patients suffering from severe insomnia were found to perform poorly on tasks measuring the capacity of attention and working memory (Pedrosi *et al.*, 1995; Hauri, 1997), observations that are comparable to the neurocognitive task profile in eating disorder patients. The initial electroencephalographic (EEG) sleep studies in patients with anorexia nervosa reported a decreased sleep maintenance caused by frequent awakenings associated with a prolonged wake time during the night, while the amount of REM sleep was unaffected (Crisp, Stonehill and Fenton, 1970); thus, the attentional deficits present in anorexia nervosa might be attributed to a disturbed nocturnal sleep profile. However, the sleep of bulimic patients, who display similarly impaired task performances, was quite undisturbed (Walsh *et al.*, 1985). Moreover, subsequent EEG sleep studies failed to replicate a definite disturbance of the sleep profile (increased numbers of arousals and wake time, decreased amounts of slow wave sleep or REM sleep) in both anorexic and bulimic patients (see: Lauer and Krieg, 2002). Therefore, it appears unlikely that disturbances in the regulation and the maintenance of nocturnal sleep account for the impaired neuropsychological performance in eating disorder patients.

Morphological and Functional Brain Alterations

As already mentioned, neuropsychological research in eating disorder patients initially was driven by the assumption that neurocognitive impairments might be due to subtle cerebral damage acquired by complications in pregnancy and delivery. However, Hamsher and co-workers (1981) were not able to confirm this initial hypothesis by using their patients' case records. One might also speculate that the cognitive deficits depend on morphological and functional brain alterations that are present in the acute episode of an eating disorder, but tend to normalize with clinical recovery (Krieg *et al.*, 1988, 1989; Herholz, 1996; Delvenne *et al.*, 1996; Kingston *et al.*, 1996). Palazidou and co-workers (1990) reported on a significant association between *morphological* brain alterations (size of the cortical sulci) and the performance on the digit symbol test; however, Laessle *et al.* (1989) and Kingston *et al.* (1996) failed to replicate such associations indicating that crude morphological measurements are too insensitive for matching with cognitive deficits. A more conclusive picture can be expected from studies in which neuropsychological assessments are combined with *functional* brain imaging. Several investigations have revealed a relative hypermetabolism in the caudate nuclei and the inferior frontal cortex associated with a relative hypometabolism in the parietal and superior frontal cortex in both anorexics and bulimics (Herholz *et al.*, 1987; Delvenne *et al.*, 1996, 1997; Naruo *et al.*, 2000; see also this chapter). After weight restoration, the parietal hypometabolism and the inferior frontal hypermetabolism tended to persist, whereas the remaining changes had normalized (Delvenne *et al.*, 1996). These findings appear to coincide with the assumption that the capacity of the working memory, which is functionally 'localized' in the frontal and parietal lobes (Shallice, 1982), is particularly affected in eating disorder patients (Green *et al.*, 1996), but also agree with the assumption that primarily the attentional capacity is deficient in these patients (Hamsher, Halmi and Benton, 1981; Pendleton Jones *et al.*, 1991; Lauer *et al.*, 1999).

Neurochemical Changes

Finally, one has to consider several neurochemical substances as the factors mediating the neurocognitive impairments. For example, steroid hormones are known to be specifically altered in the acute eating disorder but normalize with clinical remission (Pirke, Vandereycken and Ploog, 1988; Schweiger, 1991). In addition, these steroid hormones obviously influence human cognitive functions

(Wolkowitz *et al.*, 1990, 1993; Squire, 1992; Sapolsky, 1992). To date, two studies have demonstrated that patients with elevated cortisol concentrations performed poorer on tasks assessing vigilance, attentional demands and memory (Laessle *et al.*, 1992; Seed *et al.*, 2000). However, a direct correlation between the neurocognitive deficits and the cortisol measures could not be established. In a further investigation, Laessle and colleagues (1990) determined the association between β-hydroxybutyric acid (BHBA; elevated levels indicate metabolic adaptation to starvation) and vigilance performance in patients with bulimia nervosa. Interestingly, only the patients with pathologically high BHBA values performed worse on that vigilance task. The authors concluded that biological adaptation to (acute) starvation might be associated with alterations in CNS transmitter systems that regulate and allocate information processing capacity. Thus, although direct evidence is scarce at present, several neurochemical substances appear to be potential candidates that may serve as factors mediating between eating disorder symptomatology and neuropsychological deficits.

SUMMARY

The most robust neurocognitive finding in patients suffering from an eating disorder — and also but to a lesser extent in non-eating disordered dieters — can be characterized by a non-specific attention-concentration deficit. In particular, the selective information processing (enhanced distractibility) and the flexibility/inhibition functions (response selection) appear to be affected. These neurocognitive failures tend to vanish in parallel with the amelioration of the eating disorder. However, there is little evidence that any neuropsychological deficit assessed before the onset of a therapeutical regime might predict the clinical outcome. In addition, eating disorder patients with impaired task performances do not differ in their personal and clinical characteristics from patients presented with well-preserved neurocognitive functioning. Nevertheless, there is some evidence that elevated and enduring anxiety, neurochemical disturbances and, probably, metabolic brain alterations might mediate neuropsychological task performance. Finally, the fact that only fewer than 40% of eating disorder patients show obvious neurocognitive impairments should not limit our efforts to improve therapy by adding specific neuropsychological training programs that aim to ameliorate the attentional deficits. With this, a better clinical prognosis for *all* eating disorder patients might be achieved.

REFERENCES

Bacon, S.J., 1974. Arousal and the range of cue utilization. *Journal of Experimental Psychology*, **102**, 81–93.

Baddeley, A.D., 1992. Working memory. *Science*, **255**, 556–559.

Beatty, W.W., Wonderlich, S.A., Staton, R.D. and Ternes, L.A., 1990. Cognitive functioning in bulimia: Comparison with depression. *Bulletin of the Psychonomic Society*, **28**, 289–292.

Ben-Tovim, D.I., Walker, M.K., Fok, D. and Yap, E., 1989. An adaptation of the Stroop Test for measuring shape and food concerns in eating disorders: A quantitative measure of psychopathology? *International Journal of Eating Disorders*, **8**, 681–687.

Braun, C.M.J. and Chouinard, M.J., 1992. Is anorexia nervosa a neuropsychological disease? *Neuropsychology Review*, **3**, 171–212.

Cooper, M.J. and Faiburn, C.G., 1992. Selective processing of eating, weight and shape related words in patients with eating disorders and dieters. *British Journal of Clinical Psychology*, **31**, 363–365.

Cooper, M.J. and Fairburn, C.G., 1993. Demographic and clinical correlates of selective information processing in patients with bulimia nervosa. *International Journal of Eating Disorders*, **13**, 109–116.

Crisp, A.H., Stonehill, E. and Fenton, G.W., 1970. An aspect of the biological basis of the mind–body apparatus: the relationship between sleep, nutritional state and mood in disordered weight. *Psychotherapy and Psychosomatic*, **18**, 16–175.

Delvenne, V., Goldman, S., De Maertelaer, V., Simon, Y., Luxen, A. and Lotstra, F., 1996. Brain hypometabolism of glucose in anorexia nervosa: normalization after weight gain. *Biological Psychiatry*, **40**, 761–768.

Delvenne, V., Goldman, S., Simon, Y., De Maertelaer, V. and Lotstra, F., 1997. Brain hypometabolism of glucose in bulimia nervosa. *International Journal of Eating Disorders*, **21**, 313–320.

Fairburn, C.G., Cooper, P.J., Cooper, M.J., McKenna, F.P. and Anastasiades, P., 1991. Selective information processing in bulimia nervosa. *International Journal of Eating Disorders*, **10**, 415–422.

Green, M.W. and Rogers, P.J., 1995. Impaired cognitive functioning during spontaneous dieting. *Psychological Medicine*, **25**, 1003–1010.

Green, M.W., Elliman, N.A. and Rogers, P.J., 1995. Lack of effect of short-term fasting on cognitive function. *Journal of Psychiatric Research*, **29**, 245–253.

Green, M.W., Elliman, N.A., Wakeling, A. and Rogers, P.J., 1996. Cognitive functioning, weight change and therapy in anorexia nervosa. *Journal of Psychiatric Research*, **30**, 401–410.

Hamsher, K.S., Halmi, K.A. and Benton, A.L., 1981. Prediction of outcome in anorexia nervosa from neuropsychological status. *Psychiatry Research*, **4**, 79–88.

Hauri, P.J., 1997. Cognitive deficits in insomnia patients. *Acta Neurologica Belgium*, **97**, 113–117.

Herholz, K., 1996. Neuroimaging in anorexia nervosa. *Psychiatry Research*, **62**, 105–110.

Herholz, K., Krieg, J.C., Emrich, H.M., Pawlik, G., Beil, C., Pirke, K.M., Wagner, R., Wienhard, K., Ploog, D. and Heiss, W.D., 1987. Regional cerebral glucose metabolism in anorexia nervosa measured by positron emission tomography. *Biological Psychiatry*, **22**, 43–51.

Keefe, R.S.E., 1995. The contribution of neuropsychology to psychiatry. *American Journal of Psychiatry*, **152**, 6–15.

Kingston, K., Szmukler, G., Andrewes, D., Tress, B. and Desmond, P., 1996. Neuropsychological and structural brain changes in anorexia nervosa before and after refeeding. *Psychological Medicine*, **26**, 15–28.

Krieg, J.C., Pirke, K.M., Lauer, C.J. and Backmund, H., 1988. Endocrine, metabolic, and cranial computed tomographic findings in anorexia nervosa. *Biological Psychiatry*, **23**, 377–387.

Krieg, J.C., Lauer, C.J. and Pirke, K.M., 1989. Structural brain abnormalities in patients with bulimia nervosa. *Psychiatry Research*, **27**, 39–48.

Laessle, R.G., Krieg, J.C., Fichter, M.M. and Pirke, K.M., 1989. Cerebral atrophy and vigilance performance in patients with anorexia nervosa and bulimia nervosa. *Neuropsychobiology*, **21**, 187–191.

Laessle, R.G., Bossert, S., Hank, G., Hahlweg, K. and Pirke, K.M., 1990. Cognitive performance in patients with bulimia nervosa: Relationship to intermittent starvation. *Biological Psychiatry*, **27**, 549–551.

Laessle, R.G., Fischer, M., Fichter, M.M., Pirke, K.M. and Krieg, J.C., 1992. Cortisol levels and vigilance in eating disorder patients. *Psychoneuroendocrinology*, **17**, 475–484.

Lauer, C.J., Gorzewski, B., Gerlinghoff, M., Backmund, H. and Zihl, J., 1999. Neuropsychological assessments before and after treatment in patients with anorexia nervosa and bulimia nervosa. *Journal of Psychiatric Research*, **33**, 129–138.

Lauer, C.J. and Krieg, J.C., 2002. Electroencephalographic sleep in patients with eating disorder. *Sleep Medicine Review*, in press.

Lloyd, H.M., Green, M.W. and Rogers, P.J., 1994. Mood and cognitive performance effects of isocaloric lunches differing in fat and carbohydrate content. *Physiology & Behavior*, **56**, 51–57.

Long, C.G., Hinton, C. and Gillespie, N.K., 1994. Selective processing of food and body size words: Application of the Stroop Test with obese restrained eaters, anorexics, and normals. *International Journal of Eating Disorders*, **15**, 279–283.

Matias, J.L. and Kent, P.S., 1998. Neuropsychological consequences of extreme weight loss and dietary restriction in patients with anorexia nervosa. *Journal of Clinical & Experimental Neuropsychology*, **20**, 548–564.

Maxwell, J.K., Tucker, D.M. and Townes, B.D., 1984. Asymmetric cognitive function in anorexia nervosa. *International Journal of Neuroscience*, **24**, 37–44.

Naruo, T., Nakabeppu, Y., Sagiyama, K., Munemoto, T., Homan, N., Deguchi, D., Nakajo, M. and Nozoe, S., 2000. Characteristic regional cerebral blood flow patterns in anorexia nervosa patients with binge/purge behavior. *American Journal of Psychiatry*, **157**, 1520–1522.

Ogden, J. and Greville, L., 1993. Cognitive changes to preloading in restrained and unrestrained eaters as measured by the Stroop task. *International Journal of Eating Disorders*, **14**, 185–195.

Palazidou, E., Robinson, P. and Lishman, W.A., 1990. Neuroradiological and neuropsychological assessment in anorexia nervosa. *Psychological Medicine*, **20**, 521–527.

Pedrosi, B., Roehrs, T.A., Rosenthal, L., Forter, J. and Roth, T., 1995. Daytime functioning and benzodiazepine effects in insomniacs compared to normals. In: Chase, M., Rosenthal, L. and O'Connor, C. (eds), *Sleep Research*, Vol. 24, p. 48. Brain Information Service, Los Angeles.

Pendleton Jones, B., Duncan, C.C., Brouwers, P. and Mirsky, A.F., 1991. Cognition in eating disorders. *Journal of Clinical and Experimental Neuropsychology*, **13**, 711–728.

Perpina, C., Hemsley, D., Treasure, J. and de Silva, P., 1993. Is the selective information processing of food and body words specific to patients with eating disorders? *International Journal of Eating Disorders*, **14**, 359–366.

Pirke, K.M., Vandereycken, W. and Ploog, D., 1988. *The Psychobiology of Bulimia Nervosa*. Berlin, Springer Verlag.

Sapolsky, R.M., 1992. Stress, glucocorticoids, and damage to the nervous system: The current state of confusion. *Stress*, **1**, 1–19.

Schweiger, U., 1991. Menstrual function and luteal-phase deficiency in relation to weight changes and dieting. *Clinical Obstetrics and Gynecology*, **34**, 191–197.

Seed, J.A., Dixon, R.A., McCluskey, S.E. and Young, A.H., 2000. Basal activity of the hypothalamic-pituitary-adrenal axis and cognitive function in anorexia nervosa. *European Archives of Psychiatry & Clinical Neuroscience*, **250**, 11–15.

Shallice, T., 1982. Specific impairments of planning. *Philosophical Transactions of the Royal Society London B*, **298**, 199–209.

Small, A., Madero, J., Teagno, L. and Ebert, M., 1983. Intellect, perceptual characteristics and weight gain in anorexia nervosa. *Journal of Clinical Psychology*, **39**, 780–782.

Smith, C., 1996. Sleep stages, memory processes and synaptic plasticity. *Behavioural Brain Research*, **78**, 49–56.

Squire, L.R., 1992. Memory and the hippocampus: A synthesis from findings with rats, monkeys, and humans. *Psychological Reviews*, **2**, 195–231.

Strupp, B.J., Weingartner, H., Kaye, W. and Gwirtsman, H., 1986. Cognitive processing in anorexia nervosa: A disturbance in automatic information processing. *Neuropsychobiology*, **15**, 89–94.

Sutker, P.B., Allain, A.N. and Winstead, D.K., 1987. Cognitive performances in former WWII and Korean-Conflict POWs. *VA Practitioner*, **4**, 77–85.

Sutker, P.B., Galina, Z.H., West, J.A. and Allain, A.N., 1990. Trauma-induced weight loss and cognitive deficits among former prisoners of war. *Journal of Consulting and Clinical Psychology*, **58**, 323–328.

Szmukler, G.I., Andrewes, D., Kingston, K., Chen, L., Stargatt, R. and Stanley, R., 1992. Neuropsychological impairment in anorexia nervosa: Before and after refeeding. *Journal of Clinical and Experimental Neuropsychology*, **14**, 247–352.

Touyz, S.W., Beumont, P.J.V. and Johnstone, L.C., 1986. Neuropsychological correlates of dieting disorders. *International Journal of Eating Disorders*, **5**, 1025–1034.

Walsh, B.T., Goetz, R., Roose, S.P., Fingeroth, S. and Glassman, A.H., 1985. EEG-monitored sleep in anorexia nervosa and bulimia. *Biological Psychiatry*, **20**, 947–956.

Wolkowitz, O.M., Reus, V.I., Weingartner, H., Thompson, K., Breier, A., Doran, A., Rubinow, D. and Pickar, D., 1990. Cognitive effects of corticosteroids. *American Journal of Psychiatry*, **147**, 1297–1303.

Wolkowitz, O.M., Weingartner, H., Rubinow, D.R., Jimerson, D., Kling, M., Berretini, W., Thompson, K., Breier, A., Doran, A., Reus, V.I. and Pickar, D., 1993. Steroid modulation of human memory: Biochemical correlates. *Biological Psychiatry*, **33**, 744–746.

XXIII-7

Neuroanatomical Bases of Eating Disorders

Rudolf Uher, Janet Treasure and Iain C. Campbell

INTRODUCTION

There are several lines of evidence that may eventually converge to provide an integrated model of brain dysfunction in eating disorders (ED). In this section we have combined current knowledge and have constructed a neuroanatomically based explanation of ED. The picture is far from clear; and consequently, much of what is written contains suggestions and hypotheses rather than established explanations.

Diagnostic categories of ED span a spectrum of heterogeneous conditions, ranging from anorexia to obesity, in which maladaptive eating habits constitute a major symptom and which are thought to arise from primarily psychological disturbance. The inclusion of simple obesity in ED is controversial (Bruch, 1973; Treasure and Collier, 2001). Restrictive anorexia nervosa (RAN), one of the extreme conditions at the end of the ED spectrum, constitutes probably the most clear-cut syndrome, and is therefore a useful model for research. Much more knowledge has been collected for anorexia nervosa (AN) than for other ED. Therefore, this chapter will be substantially based on AN research and bulimia nervosa (BN) will be discussed to a lesser extent.

In the second part of this paper (Symptoms and Physiology) four groups of ED symptoms and their neural correlates are examined (eating and hunger/satiety perception, body image, pain perception and cognitive functions). A third part (Direct evidence of neural disturbance in ED) summarizes evidence from lesions, electrophysiological and neuroimaging studies. Finally, the fourth part provides a conclusion.

SYMPTOMS AND PHYSIOLOGY

Given the heterogeneity of symptoms and syndromes within the spectrum of ED (Treasure and Collier, 2001), it is unlikely that a particular neuroanatomically defined disturbance will match on to DSM IV or ICD10 diagnostic categories, rather it may be helpful at this stage to examine brain function in relation to individual symptoms. However, a question may be raised: can these diverse symptoms be considered as separate disturbances or do they (all or some of them) represent several facets of a common psychopathological mechanism? For example, the apparent insensitivity of AN patients to hunger, pain and physical fatigue could be attributed to a general impairment or inhibition of signalling coming from the body. Moreover, as body image representation is dependent on interoceptive and exteroceptive sensory information, its distortion in ED may also be caused by primary or secondary sensory insensitivity (Smeets and Kosslyn, 2001). The concept of a 'proto-self' (Damasio, 1999) as a representation of bodily awareness that constitutes a basic level of consciousness can be considered as a model which links these various symptoms. The proposed neuroanatomical substrate for this representation of body physical status is comprised of brainstem nuclei, hypothalamus, basal forebrain, insular, secondary sensory and medial parietal cortices.

Four groups of ED symptoms and their neural correlates are examined in this section: eating and hunger/satiety, body image, pain perception and cognitive functions. Although not clinically apparent, the insensitivity to pain is dealt with in detail, because considerable research has been carried out on this topic and it may provide a useful link in the pathophysiology of ED. Other constituents of ED symptomatology: affective and emotional disturbance, impulsivity and obsessive–compulsive symptoms are shared with other psychiatric disorders (affective disorders, personality disorders, obsessive–compulsive disorder) and their description and neural mechanisms can be found in other sections of this book.

Eating, Hunger and Satiety

Deleterious eating behaviour, the most obvious manifestation of ED, is associated with an abnormal perception of hunger and satiety. People with AN seem to lack the feeling of hunger, whereas those with BN have diminished feelings of satiety and still feel hungry after having eaten a large meal (Owen *et al.*, 1985; Halmi, 1988; Halmi and Sunday, 1991; Hetherington and Rolls, 1991, 2001). The complementarity between hunger and satiety states seems to disappear in ED and people with AN of the bingeing–purging subtype (BPAN) may report feeling both full and hungry at the same time (Halmi and Sunday, 1991). In response to provocation by insulin or 2-deoxy-D-glucose the subjective rating of hunger by AN patients paradoxically decreases (Nakai and Koh, 2001). Despite this subjective absence of hunger, when AN patients were shown palatable food, they responded by increasing insulin secretion to an even greater extent than did healthy controls, but then chose not to eat the food (Broberg and Bernstein, 1989). This suggests that although their body is preparing for meal ingestion, people with AN do not follow this with appropriate behaviour (eating the food). In summary, hunger/satiety sensing is apparently disrupted in people with eating disorders and the subjective experience and behaviour are disconnected from the body's needs and autonomic functions. Several important questions remain unresolved: Do patients with AN not feel hunger or do they just not admit feeling it? Is this disturbance in hunger/satiety sensing primary (and possibly causative) or is it acquired during the course of the illness? Hetherington and Rolls (2001) in a recent review have argued in favour of a secondary, learned disturbance in ED.

Neural mechanisms involved in the response to food and its modulation by hunger and satiation have been extensively investigated with single neuron activity mapping in primates (Rolls, 1999). It has been established that taste, olfactory and visual pathways which process food-related stimuli converge to the amygdala and the caudal orbitofrontal cortex, where their

Biological Psychiatry: Edited by H. D'haenen, J.A. den Boer and P. Willner. ISBN 0-471-49198-5

reward value is appraised and a choice is made whether to engage in action aimed at ingesting the potential food. Whereas the amygdala provides a relatively slow and rigid mechanism of learned stimulus-reinforcement associations, the hierarchically superior orbitofrontal cortex adds the flexibility necessary to rapidly adapt the behaviour to a changing environment. Information on the organism's energy needs is conveyed from the hypothalamus and in both the caudal orbitofrontal cortex and in the lateral hypothalamus, the representation of food-related stimuli depends on whether the organism is hungry or satiated. The ventral striatum is implicated in the representation of reward value of food-related stimuli and also constitutes a link to the motor system. In the head of the caudate nucleus, which receives a direct input from the orbitofrontal cortex, an appropriate behavioural (motor) response is selected, once the decision is made. (For a detailed review of findings in primates, see Rolls, 1999.)

Human neuroimaging studies suggest that the neural circuitry involved in eating might be more widespread than suggested by primate studies. In the human amygdala, parahippocampal gyrus and anterior fusiform gyrus, neural activity in response to visual food-related cues was found to be hunger-dependent (LaBar *et al.*, 2001). Several loci in the orbitofrontal and medial prefrontal cortex are activated by food stimuli in a sensory specific manner — i.e. they are activated only to food that has not been eaten to satiety (O'Doherty *et al.*, 2000). A positron emission tomography (PET) study in healthy men identified hypothalamus, posterior orbitofrontal cortex, anterior cingulate cortex and insular cortex, but also hippocampus, precuneus, caudate nucleus, putamen and cerebellum as being activated in a hungry state (36 hours fasting) compared to the state of satiety (Tataranni *et al.*, 1999). Satiation on the other hand was associated with increased neural activity in the dorsolateral and anterior ventromedial prefrontal cortices and left inferior parietal lobule, whereas the activity in the hypothalamus, orbitofrontal cortex and insula decreased (Tataranni *et al.*, 1999). The influence of satiety on eating-related brain processing has been further investigated in a study, where chocolate was eaten to satiety and beyond, so that its reward value gradually diminished and even became negative. The activity (measured as regional cerebral blood flow — rCBF — with $H_2{}^{15}O$-PET) in response to eating another piece of chocolate gradually decreased in subcallosal and medial orbitofrontal cortex, insula, striatum and midbrain, whereas lateral orbitofrontal, prefrontal and parahippocampal regions became activated with increasing satiety (Small *et al.*, 2001). The human central appetite control system apparently is comprised of an orexigenic network and an inhibitory control (or anorexigenic) circuit and the balance between these two subsystems determines eating behaviour (Tataranni *et al.*, 1999). The orexigenic network (consisting of orbitofrontal and insular cortices, hypothalamus, parts of striatum and hippocampal formation) activates with fasting and it promotes feeding behaviour. The inhibitory anorexigenic circuit consists of anterior ventromedial and dorsolateral prefrontal cortices and acts to terminate eating, probably by direct inhibition of the orexigenic system (Karhunen *et al.*, 1997; Tataranni *et al.*, 1999; Gautier *et al.*, 2000; Small *et al.*, 2001), see Figure XXIII-7.1.

Little is known about neural correlates of the feeling of hunger. This subjective feeling is not separable from the biological state of acute negative energy balance (fasting) in the available studies on healthy volunteers but in AN the sensation of hunger and the energy balance status are dissociated. Furthermore, most but not all (Karhunen *et al.*, 1997; Gordon *et al.*, 2000), human studies have been performed on male volunteers, whereas the majority of ED patients are females. A PET study of food stimuli perception in females yielded results that were rather inconsistent with other studies; no increase of brain activity was recorded in the fasted state in this study and only parietal deactivation was seen (Gordon *et al.*, 2000). The question of gender differences in the neurophysiology of eating has however not yet been addressed.

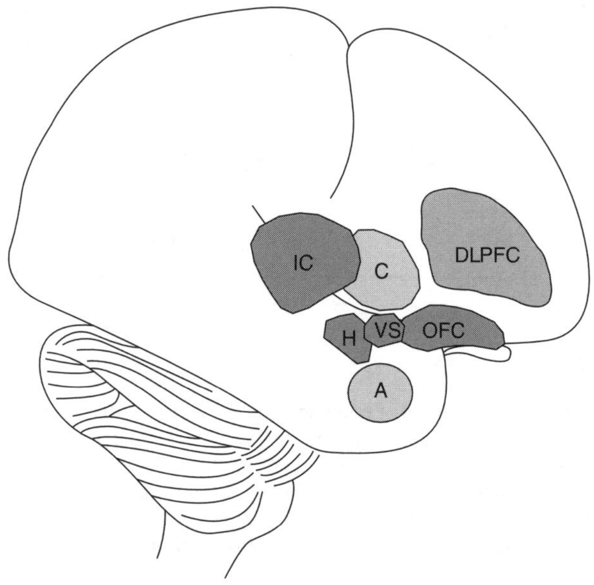

Figure XXIII-7.1 Brain circuits controlling eating behaviour: components of the **orexigenic circuit** are shown in dark shading (OFC — orbitofrontal cortex; VS — ventral striatum; H — hypothalamus; IC — insular cortex); other structures important for eating behaviour in light shading (A-amygdala, C — head of the caudate nucleus); and dorsolateral prefrontal cortex (DLPFC) is shown in medium shading as a structure inhibiting feeding and thus constituting the anorexigenic circuit

Body Image and Anosognosia

Patients with both AN and BN commonly believe their objectively thin bodies or body parts to be fat and large even though their perception of the bodies of other people is usually not distorted (Bruch, 1962; Slade, 1988). Furthermore, any subjective concern about emaciation and its consequences is conspicuously absent (Bruch, 1962), contrasting with their general concern for health and healthy eating in particular. The degree of abnormal body perception and/or conception in ED is akin to neurological disorders such as asomatognosia, microsomatognosia or neglect syndromes or indeed frank delusions or hallucinations. AN is not usually mentioned in writings on anosognosia, but the striking denial of being ill and the body image disturbance are in many ways reminiscent of neurological descriptions of anosognosic patients. As the disturbance in body image is an important constituent of ED psychopathology, we will review the concepts of body representation and its possible contribution to a neuroanatomically based theory of ED.

The body scheme (representing spatial aspects of size, shape and posture) and body image (including also the emotional and cognitive attitudes towards it) depend on multimodal sensory input including proprioception, visual, and haptic tactile sensations (Cumming, 1988; Damasio, 1999; Smeets and Kosslyn, 2001). Unlike early concepts localizing body representation to brain structures in a form of a homunculus, body image is currently viewed as a complex function of a widely distributed network spanning structures from the brainstem to associative cortices (Damasio, 1999). The importance of some of these structures has been highlighted by lesion studies. Considerable evidence implicates the associative parietal cortices, especially in the right hemisphere, and their connections to the thalamus, as lesions in these areas often produce gross alteration of body perception such as asomatognosia and anosognosia (Cumming, 1988; McGlynn and Schacter, 1989). Anosognosia — unawareness of an obvious deficit is a common phenomenon in many neurological conditions: hemiplegia, cortical blindness (Anton's syndrome), hemianopia, visual agnosia, dementia, amnesia and aphasia, poriomania but also in personality disorder and personality change due to a head injury. In most cases, these disturbances are associated with extensive right parietal lesions (especially in somatic conditions like hemiplegia) or with prefrontal lesions (personality changes) (McGlynn and Schacter, 1989). It has been suggested that the right parietal cortex is the dominant locus for body scheme representation and the proximal prefrontal cortex is important for self-monitoring of the cognitive processes (McGlynn and Schacter, 1989). Thus, damage to these structures would prevent the somatic or cognitive deficits respectively from entering the consciousness. Furthermore, an association of temporal epilepsy with such experiences as micro- or macro-somatognosia (perceiving one's body as smaller or larger) (Trimble, 1988) provides evidence for the participation of temporal lobes in body image representation.

The laterality aspect of body image representation in AN has been examined in a recent study, where body images were morphed to various proportions (thicker and thinner than the real person) and projected separately to the left or right hemisphere in a divided visual field experiment. The left hemisphere tended to identify the subject's own (but not other's) body image with the falsely fatter morphed pictures more often and more quickly than the right hemisphere. The authors suggest that the memory of the subject's own proto-image in the left hemisphere is distorted, whereas the concrete examples represented in the right hemisphere are more accurate (Smeets and Kosslyn, 2001).

In summary, body image representation appears to be a widely distributed and complex function of the CNS with associative cortices of parietal, and possibly frontal and temporal lobes playing important roles; their functioning is nevertheless dependent on multimodal sensory information processing. A pathological disturbance of these structures may be suspected in ED but no particular evidence has been given.

Pain Perception

BN and AN patients have been reported to be less sensitive to pain but the mechanism of this insensitivity is not known (Lautenbacher *et al.*, 1990, 1991). In AN patients, the pain threshold correlates significantly negatively with the local skin temperature, which is suggestive of a primary thermoregulation deficit in AN. In BN patients, the pain threshold tends to correlate positively with body weight (Lautenbacher *et al.*, 1991). The decreased pain sensitivity in ED is not influenced by administration of naloxone and therefore an opiate mechanism seems unlikely to be an important factor. As the pain threshold correlated with the height of patients, it has been hypothesized that a subclinical neuropathy could be the cause (Lautenbacher *et al.*, 1990). The clinical observation that a large proportion of AN patients frequently complain of neuropathic symptoms such as paraesthesias and diminished position sense, also supports the notion of a peripheral neuropathy in AN. Nevertheless, a study aimed at identifying features of a peripheral neuropathy in AN found a selective deficit in pain perception with preserved warmth, cold and vibration recognition in both AN and BN. There was no difference between pain perception from proximal and distal loci, which is considered as an argument against a peripheral neuropathic cause, and therefore the authors concluded that a neuropathy is unlikely to account for elevated pain threshold in ED (Pauls *et al.*, 1991). An autonomic nervous system imbalance has also been suggested as a possible mechanism (Yamamotova and Papezova, 2000).

Decreased pain sensitivity appears to be state dependent in anorexia, because people recovered from AN have normal thresholds (Krieg *et al.*, 1993). Normal pain sensitivity was also found in healthy females after severe food restriction for three weeks (Lautenbacher *et al.*, 1991).

As both BN and AN patients often indulge in self-injurious behaviours, it is interesting that an elevated pain threshold (measured by the cold-pressor test) has also been found in people with borderline personality disorder who reported that they do not experience pain during self-harm (Russ *et al.*, 1992).

Neural mechanisms underlying decreased pain sensitivity in ED are unknown and no relay on the pain pathway can be pinpointed or excluded: receptors, afferent nerve fibres, spinal, medullar, thalamic or cortical mechanisms may be involved. Contrary to earlier views, cortical representation is also essential for pain perception. Neocortical areas surrounding the lateral sulcus (Sylvian fissure), notably the parietal operculum and anterior insula, have been identified as playing a crucial role (Treede *et al.*, 2000). Lesions of the anterior insular cortex produce asymbolia for pain (pain is recognized but not accompanied by negative emotions), which implicates this region in the affective underpinning of pain (Berthier, Starkstein and Leiguarda, 1988; Greenspan, Lee and Lenz, 1999). The anterior cingulate cortex performs the integration of a painful affect and behavioural response selection (Devinsky, Morrell and Vogt, 1995).

In summary, people with eating disorders have an elevated pain threshold, which may be a consequence of starvation as it is not present after weight recovery. Most authors consider primarily peripheral causes of this pain insensitivity, but a central mechanism cannot be excluded. While a peripheral mechanism would probably be restricted to pain perception, a central mechanism may be shared with other disturbances found in ED, such as cognitive impairment, hunger insensitivity and emotional dysregulation.

Cognitive Deficit

Neuropsychological examination of cognitive functioning is a valuable tool for detecting and localizing brain dysfunction and Lauer provides a comprehensive review of ED neuropsychology in Chapter XXIII-6 of this book. In this section, these findings will be summarized according to the neuroanatomical correlates of the cognitive functions impaired in ED.

Both deficits in attention and in visuospatial and tactile spatial processing have been consistently found across studies in AN patients (Fox, 1981; Hamsher, Halmi and Benton, 1981; Kingston *et al.*, 1996; Lauer *et al.*, 1999; Maxwell, Tucker and Townes, 1984; Rovet *et al.*, 1988; Szmukler *et al.*, 1992). Patients with anorexia nervosa are particularly impaired in tasks of spatial abilities which require them to copy a complex figure, complete missing parts of a picture or analyse spatial constructions. The right parietal associative cortex is considered to be central in visuospatial processing and spatial attention and several authors raised the suggestion of right parietal dysfunction in AN (Kinsbourne and Bemporad, 1984; Maxwell, Tucker and Townes, 1984; Braun and Chouinard, 1992; Neumarker *et al.*, 2000; Grunwald *et al.*, 2001). As further evidence for right-rather than left-hemispheric neural disturbance in AN, non-verbal and numeric processing have been reported to be more impaired in AN compared to relatively preserved verbal functions and often excellent language-based academic performance (Fox, 1981; Maxwell, Tucker and Townes, 1984; Strupp *et al.*, 1986; Neumarker *et al.*, 2000). Other studies do not however support this distinction (Jones *et al.*, 1991; Kingston *et al.*, 1996).

Deficits in executive functions, which are mainly attributable to the prefrontal cortices, have also been reported in AN. Problem solving (Szmukler *et al.*, 1992; Lauer *et al.*, 1999), working memory (Green *et al.*, 1996; Kingston *et al.*, 1996), and cognitive and perceptual set shifting (Kingston *et al.*, 1996; Tchanturia *et al.*, 2001, 2002) have all been reported to be impaired in AN.

As cerebral atrophy is a common finding in AN, several studies combined neuropsychological tests and MRI (magnetic resonance imaging) structural measurements to address the question of whether there is a relationship between structural atrophy and cognitive deficits, but the correlations were generally insignificant (Kingston *et al.*, 1996; Neumarker *et al.*, 2000).

Neuropsychological studies in BN are scarce, but the available evidence indicates cognitive impairments similar to those in AN, with the addition of increased impulsivity (Ferraro, Wonderlich and Jocic, 1997; Lauer *et al.*, 1999, Tchanturia *et al.*, 2001).

In conclusion, there appears to be widespread cognitive impairment in AN. Deficits in attention, visuospatial and numeric processing, problem solving and set shifting are established (see Table XXIII-7.1). This pattern of cognitive impairment is suggestive of a predominantly parietal and prefrontal cortical dysfunction but this association has not been demonstrated in the available morphological neuroimaging studies. As the degree of cognitive disturbance is relatively mild, a rather subtle deficit can be expected, perhaps detectable by functional neuroimaging.

Table XXIII-7.1 Cognitive deficits in AN and their possible neuroanatomical correlates

Function	Evidence	Anatomical correlate
Attention, concentration	Hamsher, 1981 Szmukler, 1992 Laessle, 1989 Jones, 1991 Kingston, 1996 Lauer, 1999	Right frontal, Right parietal, Thalamus
Visuospatial	Fox, 1981; Hamsher, 1981 Szmukler, 1992 Jones, 1991 Kingston, 1996	Right parietal
(Haptic perception)	Grunwald, 2001	
Numeral processing	Fox, 1981 Witt, 1985 Small, 1983 Szmukler, 1992 Palazidou, 1990 Neumarker, 2000	Parietal
Automatic processing	Strupp, 1986 Kingston, 1996	Prefrontal/basal ganglia
Set shifting, flexibility	Tchanturia, 2001 Kingston, 1996	DLPF
Working memory	Green, 1996	DLPF, parietal
Problem solving	Szmukler, 1992 Lauer, 1999	Prefrontal
Psychomotor speed	Kingston, 1996 Lauer, 1999 Maxwell, 1984 Green, 1996	Brainstem + neocortex
Memory (immediate)	Jones, 1991 Kingston, 1996	Prefrontal, temporal, hippocampus
Verbal	Jones, 1991	LH
Non-verbal processing	Maxwell, 1984	RH

DLPF, dorsolateral prefrontal cortex; LH, left hemisphere; RH, right hemisphere.

DIRECT EVIDENCE OF NEURAL DISTURBANCE IN ED

In this section we provide an overview of the evidence from brain lesions and from electrophysiological and neuroimaging studies in ED patients.

Due to the ethical limitations of human studies, most of the knowledge on ED neuroanatomy *in vivo* derives from functional neuroimaging and surface electrophysiology studies. The fact that both these methods appear to be relatively more sensitive to the changes in cortical activity than to those occurring in deep subcortical structures, may have contributed to focus the attention on neocortical functions. The relative importance of some subcortical structures implicated in eating behaviour by the primate single neuron recording studies, e.g. hypothalamus and ventral striatum, cannot be adequately assessed by these methods. There is a relative dearth of the electrophysiological studies compared to the rapidly expanding neuroimaging research.

While functional neuroimaging simply implicates a region as active under certain conditions, the lesion studies provide valuable information on the indispensability of a structure for physiological eating behaviour. In human lesion studies it is however not possible to differentiate between cellular and fibre damage and between acute effects and subsequent adaptation.

Given these methodological differences and limitations, a careful comparison between results of various studies is necessary and only findings replicated by different methods should be taken into account, when constructing an integrated model of brain dysfunction in ED.

Disorders of Eating Associated with Brain Lesions

Although primarily genetic and psychological explanations for ED are prevalent in the recent literature, there is also evidence that relates disordered eating to specific brain lesions and neurological disease. Cases with an obvious somatic cause constitute a small minority of ED, but they are helpful in understanding neural mechanisms underlying eating and its disorders.

Lesions of prefrontal and temporal cortices, mesiotemporal structures and the hypothalamus have all been reported to produce the clinical manifestations of ED, notably AN (Chipkevitch, 1994; Griffith and Hochberg, 1988; Regard and Landis, 1997; Signer and Benson, 1990; Ward *et al.*, 2000). Lesion studies also provide evidence for a right-hemispheric dominance for eating physiology and pathology. Tumours causing anorexia were found to be predominantly located in the right anterior quadrant (Griffith and Hochberg, 1988) as were lesions causing the so-called 'gourmand syndrome', a benign preoccupation with fine eating (Regard and Landis, 1997). Both right temporal and right frontal lesions are associated with eating-related symptoms. Fisher (1994) reported a case where a sudden feeling of hunger was a first symptom of right anterior temporal haemorrhage and hunger is prominent among the symptoms of temporal lobe epilepsy (Gastaut, 1955). An association of AN with temporal lobe epilepsy has also been reported (Signer and Benson, 1990). Bilateral damage to the temporal lobes leads to the Klüver–Bucy syndrome which includes, among other symptoms, hyperphagia and hyperorality (Klüver and Bucy, 1939; Terzian and Ore, 1955). There are several case studies of anorexia associated with tumours affecting the hypothalamus (Heron and Johnston, 1976; Lewin, Mattingly and Millis, 1972; Weller and Weller, 1982) but only one of these tumours was limited to the hypothalamus alone (Lewin, Mattingly and Millis, 1972). An association of AN syndrome with right prefrontal lesions has been reported in several cases (Ward *et al.*, 2000).

In conclusion, lesion studies indicate the hypothalamus and frontal and temporal lobes as physiologically indispensable for eating. Predominance of the right-hemispheric cortical regions is supported by considerable evidence. Especially the right frontal lesions seem to be causally associated with clear-cut AN syndrome in its whole complexity.

Electrophysiology

Sixty percent of adolescent AN patients have some disturbance of spontaneous electrical activity in their resting electroencephalogram (EEG) which, in most cases, does not improve with weight gain (Rothenberger, Blanz and Lehmkuhl, 1991). Poor modulation of brain responses to auditory stimuli of various intensity and uncoupling of cortical and subcortical systems has been suggested, based on an augmenting/reducing paradigm auditory evoked potential study; this partially normalizes with weight gain (Rothenberger, Blanz and Lehmkuhl, 1991). A study of event-related potentials (ERP) in eating disorders found a prolonged P300 latency (but normal P300 amplitude) in all three ED groups (BN, BPAN, RAN); this may reflect slowness of cognitive processing (Otagaki *et al.*, 1998). Finally, an extensive ERP study by Bradley and coworkers (1997) provides further support for a right hemisphere dysfunction in AN, demonstrating that AN patients fail to show the normal $R > L$ asymmetry for non-verbal tasks seen in control subjects. They also found that the ERP's latency and amplitude abnormalities in AN were most pronounced in the central-parietal region.

Neuroimaging

Neuroimaging research provides direct information on brain dysfunction in eating disorders and Naruo gives a detailed review of both structural and functional neuroimaging studies in Chapter XXIII-8. Only findings most relevant to the neuroanatomy of eating disorders are summarized here.

Whereas most structural imaging findings point to an overall decrease in brain white and grey matter, functional imaging studies, performed either at rest or under a specific challenge, have reported dysfunction of specific brain regions. When AN patients are examined at rest, both global and regional changes in brain function have been reported in terms of increased or decreased brain perfusion or metabolism (Delvenne *et al.*, 1995, 1999; Takano *et al.*, 2001; Naruo *et al.*, 2001). The most frequently reported functional brain abnormalities include global cerebral hypofunction (Delvenne *et al.*, 1995, 1999), anterior cingulate and frontal hypofunction (Delvenne *et al.*, 1995; Nozoe *et al.*, 1995; Takano *et al.*, 2001; Naruo *et al.*, 2001), parietal hypofunction (Delvenne *et al.*, 1995, 1999), and basal ganglia hyperfunction (Delvenne *et al.*, 1999; Herholz *et al.*, 1987). Takano *et al.* (2001) also reported increased perfusion in thalamus and in the hippocampo–amygdalar complex, but these findings have not yet been replicated. Global brain hypometabolism most pronounced in the temporoparietal and frontal regions persists after recovery from AN (Rastam *et al.*, 2001).

In BN patients parietal hypometabolism (Delvenne *et al.*, 1999) and a loss of the normal right > left asymmetry of brain glucose metabolism (Wu *et al.*, 1990) (Andreason *et al.*, 1992) were demonstrated.

To further explore the neural basis of ED symptomatology, specific behavioural challenges (e.g. eating or viewing caloric food) have been used. In AN patients perfusion of the frontal lobes increased in reaction to eating a cake (Nozoe *et al.*, 1993), viewing colour photographs of food and drink activated the right orbitofrontal cortex (Uher *et al.*, 2001) and labelled high-caloric drinks elicited a response in amygdala, insula, anterior cingulate and prefrontal cortex (Ellison *et al.*, 1998). Interestingly, patients with anorexia and bulimia displayed inverse patterns of cerebral perfusion before and after eating a cake: in BN high frontotemporal perfusion at rest abated after eating a cake; in the AN group low frontotemporal perfusion at rest contrasted with an increase while eating (Nozoe *et al.*, 1995). Patients with binge-purging AN (but not restrictive AN) showed increases in glucose metabolism in the right frontal and parietal regions while visualizing a custard cake (Naruo *et al.*, 2000).

In summary, neuroimaging research provides most convincing evidence for a frontal lobe dysfunction in anorexia nervosa; this comprises a decreased resting activity as well as an overreaction of some frontal regions to specific stimuli. Some abnormalities (e.g. parietal hypometabolism) are common to AN and BN, whereas other findings differ between these diagnoses (e.g. frontal lobe reaction to eating).

CONCLUSION

As eating disorders are primarily psychiatric diseases, their genesis and symptomatology are presumed to result from alterations in brain neural networks. In this paper, evidence from physiology, neuropathology, neuropsychology and neuroimaging has been brought together to identify the underlying neural abnormalities. Data obtained with various research methods are summarized in Table XXIII-7.2 according to the brain structures they implicate.

Table XXIII-7.2 Brain structures possibly dysfunctional in ED

Structure	Indirect evidence	Direct evidence
Prefrontal cortex (including orbitofrontal cortex and anterior cingulate)	Eating behaviour Executive cognitive functions deficit (set shifting, problem solving) Personality characteristics	Brain lesions: Ward, 2000; Griffith and Hochberg, 1988; Regard and Landis, 1997 Neuroimaging: Nozoe, 1993, 1995; Delvenne, 1993, 1999; Takano, 2001; Naruo, 2000, 2001; Ellison, 1998; Uher, 2001
Parietal cortex	Visuospatial abilities Number processing Haptic perception Body image Awareness of bodily status Anosognosia Pain perception	Neuroimaging: Delvenne, 1995, 1999 Electrophysiology: Bradley *et al.*, 1997; Grunwald, 2001
Right hemisphere	Cognitive deficit predominantly in non-verbal and spatial skills Right-hemispheric dominance for eating behaviour	Brain lesions: Griffith and Hochberg, 1988; Regard and Landis, 1997; Ward, 2000 Neuroimaging: Nozoe, 1993, 1995; Naruo, 2000; Uher, 2001 Electrophysiology: Bradley *et al.*, 1997
Temporal cortex	Contributes to hunger (Fisher, 1994) and taste recognition (Small, 1997) Klüver–Bucy syndrome	Neuroimaging: Nozoe, 1993, 1995
Insular cortex	Taste, visceral sensing, pain, disgust, body scheme representation	Neuroimaging: Ellison, 1998
Striatum (basal ganglia)	Eating behaviour	Neuroimaging: Herholtz, 1987; Delvenne, 1999
Hypothalamus	Neurohumoral disturbances Eating behaviour	Tumours associated with anorexia: Lewin, 1972

This table reflects an apparent shift in emphasis from hypothalamic and endocrine mechanisms to the neocortical circuits based theories, which is characteristic of much of the current research. The structures in Table XXIII-7.2 are listed roughly in the order of their importance with the reservation that there is functional interdependency within cerebral networks. The available data consistently implicates the association cortices of frontal and parietal lobes as probable loci of dysfunction. Primary involvement of these high-order associative cortices with a multiplicity of functions may reflect the complexity of these diseases. In the face of this complexity and relative lack of consistency in some research results, substantial changes in our concept of ED are still likely to occur and a consensus on the aetiology and neural basis of eating disorders will remain a challenge for future research.

REFERENCES

Andreason, P.J., Altemus, M., Zametkin, A.J., King, A.C., Lucinio, J. and Cohen, R.M., 1992. Regional cerebral glucose metabolism in bulimia nervosa. *American Journal of Psychiatry*, **149**, 1506–1513.

Berthier, M., Starkstein, S. and Leiguarda, R., 1988. Asymbolia for pain: a sensory-limbic disconnection syndrome. *Annals of Neurology*, **24**, 41–49.

Bradley, S.J., Taylor, M.J., Rovet, J.F., Goldberg, E., Hood, J., Wachsmuth, R., Azcue, M.P. and Pencharz, P.B., 1997. Assessment of brain function in adolescent anorexia nervosa before and after weight gain. *Journal of Clinical and Experimental Neuropsychology*, **19**, 20–33.

Braun, C.M. and Chouinard, M.J., 1992. Is anorexia nervosa a neuropsychological disease? *Neuropsychological Review*, **3**, 171–212.

Broberg, D.J. and Bernstein, I.L., 1989. Cephalic insulin release in anorexic women. *Physiology and Behaviour*, **45**, 871–874.

Bruch, H., 1962. Perceptual and conceptual disturbances in anorexia nervosa. *Psychosomatic Medicine*, **24**, 187–195.

Bruch, H., 1973. *Eating Disorders*. Basic Books, New York.

Chipkevitch, E., 1994. Brain tumors and anorexia nervosa syndrome. *Brain Development*, **16**, 175–179.

Cumming, W.J., 1988. The neurobiology of the body schema. *British Journal of Psychiatry*, **153**(Suppl 2), 7–11.

Damasio, A., 1999. *The Feeling of What Happens*. Harcourt Brace, New York.

Delvenne, V., Goldman, S., De, M.V. and Lotstra, F., 1999. Brain glucose metabolism in eating disorders assessed by positron emission tomography. *International Journal of Eating Disorders*, **25**, 29–37.

Delvenne, V., Lotstra, F., Goldman, S., Biver, F., De, M.V., Appelboom-Fondu, J., Schoutens, A., Bidaut, L.M., Luxen, A. and Mendelwicz, J., 1995. Brain hypometabolism of glucose in anorexia nervosa: a PET scan study. *Biological Psychiatry*, **37**, 161–169.

Devinsky, O., Morrell, M.J. and Vogt, B.A., 1995. Contributions of anterior cingulate cortex to behaviour. *Brain*, **118 (Pt 1)**, 279–306.

Ellison, Z., Foong, J., Howard, R., Bullmore, E., Williams, S. and Treasure, J., 1998. Functional anatomy of calorie fear in anorexia nervosa. *Lancet*, **352**, 1192.

Ferraro, F.R., Wonderlich, S. and Jocic, Z., 1997. Performance variability as a new theoretical mechanism regarding eating disorders and cognitive processing. *Journal of Clinical Psychology*, **53**, 117–121.

Fisher, C.M., 1994. Hunger and the temporal lobe. *Neurology*, **44**, 1577–1579.

Fox, C.F., 1981. Neuropsychological correlations of anorexia nervosa. *International Journal of Psychiatry in Medicine*, **11**, 285–290.

Gastaut, H., 1955. Les troubles du comportement alimentaire chez les epileptiques psychomoteurs. *Revue Neurologique (Paris)*, **92**, 55–62.

Gautier, J.F., Chen, K., Salbe, A.D., Bandy, D., Pratley, R.E., Heiman, M., Ravussin, E., Reiman, E.M. and Tataranni, P.A., 2000. Differential brain responses to satiation in obese and lean men. *Diabetes*, **49**, 838–846.

Gordon, C.M., Dougherty, D.D., Rauch, S.L., Emans, S.J., Grace, E., Lamm, R., Alpert, N.M., Majzoub, J.A. and Fischman, A.J., 2000. Neuroanatomy of human appetitive function: A positron emission tomography investigation. *International Journal of Eating Disorders*, **27**, 163–171.

Green, M.W., Elliman, N.A., Wakeling, A. and Rogers, P.J., 1996. Cognitive functioning, weight change and therapy in anorexia nervosa. *Journal of Psychiatric Research*, **30**, 401–410.

Greenspan, J.D., Lee, R.R. and Lenz, F.A., 1999. Pain sensitivity alterations as a function of lesion location in the parasylvian cortex. *Pain*, **81**, 273–282.

Griffith, J.L. and Hochberg, F.H., 1988. Anorexia and weight loss in glioma patients. *Psychosomatics*, **29**, 335–337.

Grunwald, M., Ettrich, C., Assmann, B., Dahne, A., Krause, W., Busse, F. and Gertz, H.J., 2001. Deficits in haptic perception and right parietal theta power changes in patients with anorexia nervosa before and after weight gain. *International Journal of Eating Disorders*, **29**, 417–428.

Halmi, K.A., 1988. Appetite regulation in anorexia nervosa. *Current Concepts in Nutrition*, **16**, 125–135.

Halmi, K.A. and Sunday, S.R., 1991. Temporal patterns of hunger and fullness ratings and related cognitions in anorexia and bulimia. *Appetite*, **16** 219–237.

Hamsher, K.S., Halmi, K.A. and Benton, A.L., 1981. Prediction of outcome in anorexia nervosa from neuropsychological status. *Psychiatry Research*, **4**, 79–88.

Herholz, K., Krieg, J.C., Emrich, H.M., Pawlik, G., Beil, C., Pirke, K.M., Wagner, R., Wienhard, K., Ploog, D. and Heiss, W.D., 1987. Regional cerebral glucose metabolism in anorexia nervosa measured by positron emission tomography. *Biological Psychiatry*, **22**, 43–51.

Heron, G.B. and Johnston, D.A., 1976. Hypothalamic tumor presenting as anorexia nervosa. *American Journal of Psychiatry*, **133**, 580–582.

Hetherington, M.M. and Rolls, B.J., 1991. Eating behavior in eating disorders: response to preloads. *Physiology and Behaviour*, **50**, 101–108.

Hetherington, M.M. and Rolls, B.J., 2001. Dysfunctional eating in the eating disorders. *Psychiatric Clinics of North America*, **24**, 235–248.

Jones, B.P., Duncan, C.C., Brouwers, P. and Mirsky, A.F., 1991. Cognition in eating disorders. *Journal of Clinical and Experimental Neuropsychology*, **13**, 711–728.

Karhunen, L.J., Lappalainen, R.I., Vanninen, E.J., Kuikka, J.T. and Uusitupa, M.I., 1997. Regional cerebral blood flow during food exposure in obese and normal-weight women. *Brain*, **120 (Pt 9)** 1675–1684.

Kingston, K., Szmukler, G., Andrewes, D., Tress, B. and Desmond, P., 1996. Neuropsychological and structural brain changes in anorexia nervosa before and after refeeding. *Psychological Medicine*, **26**, 15–28.

Kinsbourne, M. and Bemporad, B., 1984. Lateralization of emotions. In: Fox, N.A. and Davidson, R.J. (eds), *The Psychobiology of Affective Development*. Lawrence Erlbaum Associates, Hillsdale, NJ.

Klüver, H. and Bucy, P.C., 1939. Preliminary analysis of functions of the temporal lobes in monkeys. *Archives of Neurology and Psychiatry*, **42**, 979–1000.

Krieg, J.C., Roscher, S., Strian, F., Pirke, K.M. and Lautenbacher, S., 1993. Pain sensitivity in recovered anorexics, restrained and unrestrained eaters. *Journal of Psychosomatic Research*, **37**, 595–601.

LaBar, K.S., Gitelman, D.R., Parrish, T.B., Kim, Y.H., Nobre, A.C. and Mesulam, M.M., 2001. Hunger selectively modulates corticolimbic activation to food stimuli in humans. *Behavioral Neuroscience*, **115**, 493–500.

Lauer, C.J., Gorzewski, B., Gerlinghoff, M., Backmund, H. and Zihl, J., 1999. Neuropsychological assessments before and after treatment in patients with anorexia nervosa and bulimia nervosa. *Journal of Psychiatric Research*, **33**, 129–138.

Lautenbacher, S., Pauls, A.M., Strian, F., Pirke, K.M. and Krieg, J.C., 1990. Pain perception in patients with eating disorders. *Psychosomatic Medicine*, **52**, 673–682.

Lautenbacher, S., Pauls, A.M., Strian, F., Pirke, K.M. and Krieg, J.C., 1991. Pain sensitivity in anorexia nervosa and bulimia nervosa. *Biological Psychiatry*, **29**, 1073–1078.

Lewin, K., Mattingly, D. and Millis, R.R., 1972. Anorexia nervosa associated with hypothalamic tumor. *British Medical Journal*, **2**, 629–630.

Maxwell, J.K., Tucker, D.M. and Townes, B.D., 1984. Asymmetric cognitive function in anorexia nervosa. *International Journal of Neuroscience*, **24**, 37–44.

McGlynn, S.M. and Schacter, D.L., 1989. Unawareness of deficits in neuropsychological syndromes. *Journal of Clinical and Experimental Neuropsychology*, **11**, 143–205.

Nakai, Y. and Koh, T., 2001. Perception of hunger to insulin-induced hypoglycemia in anorexia nervosa. *International Journal of Eating Disorders*, **29**, 354–357.

Naruo, T., Nakabeppu, Y., Deguchi, D., Nagai, N., Tsutsui, J., Nakajo, M. and Nozoe, S., 2001. Decreases in blood perfusion of the anterior cingulate gyri in anorexia Nervosa restricters assessed by SPECT image analysis. *BMC Psychiatry*, **1**, 2.

Naruo, T., Nakabeppu, Y., Sagiyama, K., Munemoto, T., Homan, N., Deguchi, D., Nakajo, M. and Nozoe, S., 2000. Characteristic regional cerebral blood flow patterns in anorexia nervosa patients with binge/purge behavior. *American Journal of Psychiatry*, **57**, 1520–1522.

Neumarker, K.J., Bzufka, W.M., Dudeck, U., Hein, J. and Neumarker, U., 2000. Are there specific disabilities of number processing in adolescent patients with Anorexia nervosa? Evidence from clinical and neuropsychological data when compared to morphometric measures from magnetic resonance imaging. *European Child and Adolescent Psychiatry*, **9**(Suppl 2), II111–II121.

Nozoe, S., Naruo, T., Nakabeppu, Y., Soejima, Y., Nakajo, M. and Tanaka, H., 1993. Changes in regional cerebral blood flow in patients with anorexia nervosa detected through single photon emission tomography imaging. *Biological Psychiatry*, **34**, 578–580.

Nozoe, S., Naruo, T., Yonekura, R., Nakabeppu, Y., Soejima, Y., Nagai, N., Nakajo, M. and Tanaka, H., 1995. Comparison of regional cerebral blood flow in patients with eating disorders. *Brain Research Bulletin*, **36**, 251–255.

O'Doherty, J., Rolls, E.T., Francis, S., Bowtell, R., McGlone, F., Kobal, G., Renner, B. and Ahne, G., 2000. Sensory-specific satiety-related olfactory activation of the human orbitofrontal cortex. *Neuroreport*, **11**, 399–403.

Otagaki, Y., Tohoda, Y., Osada, M., Horiguchi, J. and Yamawaki, S., 1998. Prolonged P300 latency in eating disorders. *Neuropsychobiology*, **37**, 5–9.

Owen, W.P., Halmi, K.A., Gibbs, J. and Smith, G.P., 1985. Satiety responses in eating disorders. *Journal of Psychiatric Research*, **19**, 279–284.

Pauls, A.M., Lautenbacher, S., Strian, F., Pirke, K.M. and Krieg, J.C., 1991. Assessment of somatosensory indicators of polyneuropathy in patients with eating disorders. *European Archives of Psychiatry and Clinical Neuroscience*, **241**, 8–12.

Rastam, M., Bjure, J., Vestergren, E., Uvebrant, P., Gillberg, I.C., Wentz, E. and Gillberg, C., 2001. Regional cerebral blood flow in weight-restored anorexia nervosa: a preliminary study. *Developmental Medicine and Child Neurology*, **43**, 239–242.

Regard, M. and Landis, T., 1997. "Gourmand syndrome": eating passion associated with right anterior lesions. *Neurology*, **48**, 1185–1190.

Rolls, E.T., 1999. *Brain and Emotions*. Oxford University Press, Oxford.

Rothenberger, A., Blanz, B. and Lehmkuhl, G., 1991. What happens to electrical brain activity when anorectic adolescents gain weight? *European Archives of Psychiatry and Clinical Neuroscience*, **240**, 144–147.

Rovet, J., Bradley, E., Goldberg, E. and Wachsmuth, R., 1988. Hemispheric lateralisation in anorexia nervosa. *Journal of Clinical and Experimental Neuropsychology*, **10**, 24.

Russ, M.J., Roth, S.D., Lerman, A., Kakuma, T., Harrison, K., Shindledecker, R.D., Hull, J. and Mattis, S., 1992. Pain perception in self-injurious patients with borderline personality disorder. *Biological Psychiatry*, **32**, 501–511.

Signer, S.F. and Benson, D.F., 1990. Three cases of anorexia nervosa associated with temporal lobe epilepsy. *American Journal of Psychiatry*, **147**, 235–238.

Slade, P.D., 1988. Body image in anorexia nervosa. *British Journal of Psychiatry*, **153**(Suppl 2), 20–22.

Small, D.M., Zatorre, R.J., Dagher, A., Evans, A.C. and Jones-Gotman, M., 2001. Changes in brain activity related to eating chocolate: From pleasure to aversion. *Brain*, **124**, 1720–1733.

Smeets, M.A. and Kosslyn, S.M., 2001. Hemispheric differences in body image in anorexia nervosa. *International Journal of Eating Disorders*, **29**, 409–416.

Strupp, B.J., Weingartner, H., Kaye, W. and Gwirtsman, H., 1986. Cognitive processing in anorexia nervosa: A disturbance in automatic information processing. *Neuropsychobiology*, **15**, 89–94.

Szmukler, G.I., Andrewes, D., Kingston, K., Chen, L., Stargatt, R. and Stanley, R., 1992. Neuropsychological impairment in anorexia nervosa: Before and after refeeding. *Journal of Clinical and Experimental Neuropsychology*, **14**, 247–352.

Takano, A., Shiga, T., Kitagawa, N., Koyama, T., Katoh, C. and Tsukamoto, E., 2001. Abnormal neuronal network in anorexia nervosa studied with I-123-IMP SPECT. *Psychiatry Research*, **107**, 45–50.

Tataranni, P.A., Gautier, J.F., Chen, K., Uecker, A., Bandy, D., Salbe, A.D., Pratley, R.E., Lawson, M., Reiman, E.M. and Ravussin, E., 1999. Neuroanatomical correlates of hunger and satiation in humans using positron emission tomography. *Proceedings of the National Academy of Sciences of the United States of America*, **96**, 4569–4574.

Tchanturia, K., Morris, R.G., Surguladze, S. and Treasure, J., 2002. Evidence of mental rigidity in anorexia nervosa: set shifting paradigms. *Eating and Weight Disorders* (in press).

Tchanturia, K., Serpell, L., Troop, N. and Treasure, J., 2001. Perceptual illusions in eating disorders: rigid and fluctuating styles. *Journal of Behavioral Therapy and Experimental Psychiatry*, **32**, 1007–1115.

Terzian, H. and Ore, C.D., 1955. Syndrome of Klüver and Bucy. *Neurology*, **5**, 373–380.

Treasure, J. and Collier, D., 2001. Spectrum of eating disorders. In: Owen, J.B., Treasure, J. and Collier, D. (eds), *Animal Models of Eating Behaviour and Body Composition Disorders*. Kluwer Academic Publishers B.V., Amsterdam.

Treede, R.D., Apkarian, A.V., Bromm, B., Greenspan, J.D. and Lenz, F.A., 2000. Cortical representation of pain: functional characterization of nociceptive areas near the lateral sulcus. *Pain*, **87**, 113–119.

Trimble, M.R., 1988. Body image and the temporal lobes. *British Journal of Psychiatry*, **153**(Suppl 2), 12–14.

Uher, R., Murphy, T., Ng, V., Phillips, M. and Dalgleish, T.T.J., 2001. Perception of food and emotional stimuli in anorexia nervosa. *Neuroimage*, **13**, S1022–S1022.

Ward, A., Tiller, J., Treasure, J. and Russell, G., 2000. Eating disorders: psyche or soma? *International Journal of Eating Disorders*, **27**, 279–287.

Weller, R.A. and Weller, E.B., 1982. Anorexia nervosa in a patient with an infiltrating tumor of the hypothalamus. *American Journal of Psychiatry*, **139**, 824–825.

Wu, J.C., Hagman, J., Buchsbaum, M.S., Blinder, B., Derrfler, M., Tai, W.Y., Hazlett, E. and Sicotte, N., 1990. Greater left cerebral hemispheric metabolism in bulimia assessed by positron emission tomography. *American Journal of Psychiatry*, **147**, 309–312.

Yamamotova, A. and Papezova, H., 2000. Does the pain perception depend on the type of vegetative reactivity? Comparison of healthy women with eating disorders patients. *Homeostasis*, **40**, 134–136.

XXIII-8

Brain Imaging

Tetsuro Naruo

INTRODUCTION

There is a general consensus that the aetiology of eating disorders is multidetermined, affected by biological, psychological and social factors that interact in a complex fashion (Garfinkel, Kennedy and Kaplan, 1995). And while it is clear that no one cause for eating disorders will be discovered, the role of the central nervous system (CNS) deserves special attention as the CNS must play a central role in mediating and maintaining eating behaviours. A fuller understanding of CNS control of eating may lead to improvements in the medical treatment of various disorders of eating. For these reasons, direct and non-invasive analytic methods of brain imaging are now widely applied in the study of eating disorders (Ellison and Foog, 1998; Krishnan and Gadde, 1998; Grady, 1999; Demaerel, 2000; Hendren, De Backer and Pandina, 2000).

This chapter will review the research findings from brain imaging techniques focusing on anorexia nervosa and bulimia nervosa, and categorizing the studies as either structural or functional. The literature on obesity will also be reviewed, as a substantial proportion of the obese in weight control programs have binge-eating behaviour (De Zwaan *et al.*, 1994) and are reported to have many characteristics in common with patients suffering from eating disorders (Stunkard, 1996).

Tables XXIII-8.1 and XXIII-8.2 present a brief summary of the studies reviewed in this chapter according to the brain imaging techniques used.

STRUCTURAL IMAGING FINDINGS

Computed Tomography

Anorexia Nervosa

Numerous important findings in patients with anorexia nervosa were detected by computed tomography (CT) in studies performed in the 1980s. These structural changes are characterized by an enlargement of the cortical and cerebellar sulci, the interhemispheric fissure and the cisterns, and a widening of internal cerebrospinal fluid (CSF) spaces (Datlof *et al.*, 1986; Lankenau *et al.*, 1985). According to these studies, as body weight increased, these changes, labelled 'pseudoatrophy' returned to normal (Kohkmeyer, Lemkuhl and Poutska, 1983; Artmann *et al.*, 1985).

However, there may be different patterns of recovery for the cortical sulci and ventricles over the course of weight restoration. In one of these studies, 15 anorexic patients out of 25 displayed enlarged ventricles and cortical sulci. After 3 month's treatment, the cortical sulci returned to normal while the ventricles remained enlarged (Dolan, Mitchell and Wakeling, 1988). The authors suggested that ventricular enlargement might require longer than 3 months to recover, or that with sufficient chronicity the observed changes in ventricular size might be irreversible. The observed reversal of sulcal widening following refeeding was interpreted as upholding a hypothesis that the observed changes are secondary to malnourishment.

Table XXIII-8.1 Brain imaging studies of eating disorders: structural brain imaging studies

Instruments	Reference	Subjects	Main findings
CT	Dolan *et al.* (1988)	25 AN	Decreased sulcal widening and persisting ventricular enlargement in recovered AN
CT	Krieg *et al.* (1989)	50 BN vs 50 AN vs 50 C	Enlarged CSF spaces in both AN and BN patients
MRI	Hoffman *et al.* (1989)	8 BN vs 8 C	Greater cortical atrophy in BN patients indicated by SCCR
MRI	Golden *et al.* (1996)	12 AN	Inverse correlation between BMI and total ventricular enlargement
MRI	Kingston *et al.* (1996)	46 AN vs 41 C	Association between lower BW and disturbed flexibility/inhibition and memory
MRI	Lamabe *et al.* (1997)	12 AN vs 18 C	Persisting cerebral grey-matter volume deficits after weight recovery

Table XXIII-8.2 Brain imaging studies of eating disorders: functional brain imaging studies

Instruments	Reference	Subjects	Main findings
SPECT	Gordon *et al.* (1997)	15 AN	Unilateral temporal lobe hypoperfusion
SPECT	Karhunen *et al.* (2000)	19 Obese vs 12 C	Correlation between hunger and the rCBF of the lt. frontal and temporal regions
SPECT	Naruo *et al.* (2000)	7 AN-R vs 7 AN-BPvs 7 C	Activation on the rCBF in rt. frontal cortical regions in AN-BP during imagining food
PET	Andreason *et al.* (1992)	11 BN vs 18 HC	Functional links between depressive symptoms and lt. prefrontal hypometabolism
PET	Delvenne *et al.* (1999)	10 AN vs 10 BN vs 10 C	Global hypometabolism in AN and a common parietal cortex dysfunction in ED
PET	Gautier *et al.* (2000)	11 Obese vs 11 C	Greater increases in rCBF in the prefrontal cortex in obese men to satiation
fMRI	Ellison *et al.* (1998)	6 AN vs 6 C	Activation in a limbic and paralimbic network in AN under food stimuli

Biological Psychiatry: Edited by H. D'haenen, J.A. den Boer and P. Willner. ISBN 0-471-49198-5

In another study, enlarged external CSF spaces were found in 43 (86%) of 50 anorectic patients (Krieg, Lauer and Pirke, 1989a). In a subgroup of 25 subjects examined both at admission and discharge the authors showed that while external CSF was still greater than normal controls, significant decreased had occurred compared to pre-treatment. Among several possible pathogenetic mechanisms thought to be responsible for these morphological brain alterations in patients with anorexia nervosa, hypercortisolemia was suggested as a possible mechanism as reversible changes on CT scan are found not to be unique to anorexia nervosa and have been reported in Cushing's disease, following therapeutic administration of corticosteroids, and in alcohol abuse and dependence.

Bulimia Nervosa

Morphological brain alterations have also been found in patients with bulimia nervosa via CT examinations. A study revealed that patients suffering from bulimia displayed enlarged external CSF spaces. The larger number of patients (13 of 28) than control subjects (2 of 18) displaying signs of cortical atrophy was statistically significant (Krieg, Backmund and Pirke, 1987). It is interesting to note that nine patients who had no history of anorexia nervosa also displayed cortical atrophy. The authors discussed various possible pathogenetic mechanisms, such as changes in the permeability of the blood vessels, diminished blood volume, protein loss with a subsequent movement of intracellular fluid into extracellular spaces or inhibition of brain protein biosynthesis, that have been thought to be responsible for the enlargement of the CSF spaces.

A comparison of 50 bulimia nervosa patients to 50 anorexia nervosa patients and 50 age-matched control subjects, showed increased rates and severity of sulcal widening and ventricular enlargement in both anorexia nervosa and bulimia nervosa subjects compared to controls though the degree and frequency of atrophic changes in bulimics were not so pronounced as in anorexics (Krieg *et al.*, 1989a, 1989b). In this study, the authors assumed that the morphological brain alterations might reflect the endocrine and metabolic reactions to starvation or abnormal eating behaviours as a low concentration of the plasma level of triiodothyronine was inversely correlated with ventricular size in the patients.

Magnetic Resonance Imaging

Anorexia Nervosa

Studies performed using magnetic resonance imaging (MRI) began to appear in the late 1980s, reporting similar findings to those using CT (Palazidou, Robinson and Lishman, 1990; Swayze *et al.*, 1996). MRI studies have expanded on the work done in earlier CT studies. For example, in a study of 12 subjects with anorexia nervosa after 11 months treatment, there was an inverse relationship between body mass index and total ventricular volume (Golden *et al.*, 1996).

Another study compared 12 weight recovered anorexic patients with 13 low-weight anorexic patients and 18 normal controls (Lambe *et al.*, 1997). The weight recovered patient's average BMI was 20.5 and time since weight recovery was more than 1 year. The low-weight patients' average BMI was 15.6. While weight recovered anorexia nervosa patients showed significantly larger grey-matter volume compared to ill subjects, it was still smaller than in the normal controls. The weight recovered group showed no significant difference from the control group on total white-matter volumes though remaining higher than the ill group.

Another study comparing anorexic patients before and after weight gain demonstrated correlations between structural brain abnormalities and neuropsychological function (Kingston *et al.*, 1996). Forty-six patients with anorexia nervosa were compared to 41 normal controls and found to be poor in performance on the attention, visuospatial and memory tasks. On tasks assessing flexibility and learning, no group differences were evident although an examination of deficits in individuals revealed that more anorexics were impaired on both types of tasks. Attention tasks improved, after the patients had gained 10% (BMI = 17.9) of their body weight. The enlarged ventricles and dilatated sulci were both reduced, but showed no correlation with the observed cognitive impairments. The authors also reported that lower weight, but not duration of illness, was associated with poorer performance on tasks assessing flexibility/inhibition and memory, and greater MRI ventricular size. The findings here should be interpreted with caution, but the study is important since it speculates on the relationship between cognitive function and structural findings.

A prospective cohort study using MRI was performed to examine the brains of female adolescents after weight recovery from AN (Katzman *et al.*, 1997). Of 13 patients who underwent an MRI study at low weight, six patients were re-scanned after weight recovery. Quantitative analysis showed that white matter and CSF volumes changed significantly on weight recovery but that there were significant grey-matter volume deficits and enlarged CSF spaces compared to aged-matched female controls. Both of these findings suggest that anorexia nervosa may exert different effects on grey-matter and white-matter volumes, with the former appearing to be more closely related to the degree of weight loss. These results suggest that the abnormalities found in grey matter, white matter, and CSF volumes may resolve to varying degrees and over time with weight restoration.

Since it is well established that glucocorticoids inhibit the proliferation of progenitor cells that occurs in the hippocampal dentate gyrus of adult mammals (Kuhn, Dickinson-Anson and Gage, 1996), hypercortisolemia and other abnormal factors induced by malnutrition may have a specific role in producing the distorted recovery processes of remyelination of grey- and white-matter volumes in patients with anorexia nervosa.

Bulimia Nervosa

Patients with bulimia nervosa have also been investigated with MRI scans. In one study, eight consecutive unmedicated bulimics without a history of anorexia nervosa or alcohol abuse were compared with eight sex and age-matched controls (Hoffman *et al.*, 1989). Using the sagittal cerebral/cranial ratio (SCCR): an easily obtainable and replicable method of quantifying relative cerebral size, the authors found cortical atrophy to be significantly greater in the bulimic group compared to controls. But they failed to find significant differences in ventricle/brain ration (VBR) between bulimics and controls. Methodologic differences in measuring or different metabolic patterns in various brain areas were thought to be responsible for the atrophy found in the two different areas because the correlation between VBR and SCCR was quite low. In discussion the authors described that hypercortisolisms, elevated beta-hydroxy-butyric acid and a loss of brain tissue water due to changes in vascular permeability might be possible causes of brain atrophy.

Anorexia Nervosa and Bulimia Nervosa

Another small study, comparing 18 eating disorder patients (eight anorexia nervosa, 10 bulimia nervosa patients) to 13 normal controls, examined the size and morphology of the pituitary gland using MRI (Doraiswamy *et al.*, 1990). Both anorexics and bulimics showed smaller pituitary gland areas compared with controls. Though the mean values were longer, none of the pituitary measurements in the bulimics differed significantly from those of the anorexics. The authors mentioned that the smaller pituitary sizes

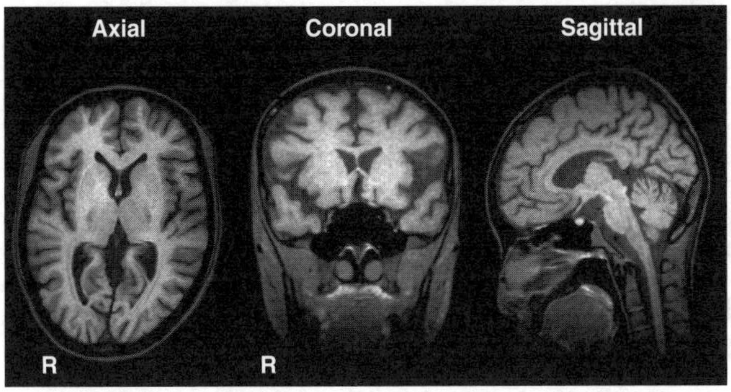

Figure XXIII-8.1 MRI displaying typical brain atrophy of a young female patient with severe anorexia nervosa. Three T1-weighted images show an enlargement of the cortical and cerebellar sulci, cisterns and ventricular dilatation

in the group of patients compared to controls may reflect pituitary atrophy secondary to nutritional or endocrine alterations.

Summary

In summary, early studies using CT and MRI indicated that the morphological alterations in patients with anorexia nervosa were due to weight loss. However, the occurrence of cortical atrophy in normal weight bulimics, as well as relative absence of ventricular enlargement in these patients, suggest more complicated possible mechanisms inducing cerebral atrophy in eating disorders.

Figure XXIII-8.1 shows an example of pseudo cerebral atrophy in anorexia nervosa revealed with MRI. There are obvious structural abnormalities such as an enlargement of the cortical and cerebellar sulci and cisterns, and ventricular dilatation.

FUNCTIONAL IMAGE FINDINGS

Single Photon Emission Computed Tomography

Anorexia Nervosa

Anorexia nervosa has been studied by single photon emission computed tomography (SPECT) since 1989. These studies have used radioactive tracers, allowing the measurement of brain blood flow. In the earlier studies regional cerebral blood flow (rCBF) was measured by the xenon-133 inhalation method.

One early study compared 12 anorexic patients to 12 normal controls at rest using CT and SPECT with xenon-133. This study revealed that the anorexic patients showed no significant reduction in rCBF compared to controls. However, there was a significant inverse relationship between VBR measured by CT and rCBF (Krieg *et al.*, 1989b).

Since the early 1990s ^{99m}Tc-hexamethylpropylene amineoxime (HM-PAO) has become available for the investigation of rCBF. HM-PAO behaves like a chemical microsphere quasipermanently trapped in the brain and allows imagings of regional cerebral perfusion (Inugami, 1988).

SPECT study using HM-PAO observed changes in rCBF before and after weight gain. Subjects were 15 patients with anorexia nervosa, three of whom were re-examined after weight gain. Eight of 15 subjects showed unilateral left-sided temporal lobe hypoperfusion and five of 15 right temporal lobe hypoperfusion. The three subjects re-scanned after weight gain showed a further 10% reduction in perfusion (Gordon *et al.*, 1997). Another study comparing rCBF of anorexic patients before and after 3 months of treatment, reported that the low blood flow in frontal, parietal and frontotemporal areas normalized after weight gain (Kuruoglu *et al.*, 1998).

HM-PAO also allows for activation studies. One preliminary study using a food intake stimulus in five normal controls and seven anorexic patients analysed ratios of the radioactive counts in a region of interest to the cerebellum in various cortical regions before and after eating, and before and after weight gain (Nozoe *et al.*, 1993). Patients showed a significant increase of the percentage of rCBF in the left inferior frontal region but had no significant difference of the ratios before treatment. After weight gain, the patients failed to show significant differences in the percentage of rCBF though they significantly increased the ratios in both sides of the temporal cortex in the rest period.

Another study using a food sight stimulus revealed different response patterns of the percentage of rCBF in anorexic patients with binge/purge behaviour compared to restricting anorexics (Naruo *et al.*, 2000). The results of this study indicate that anorexic patients with habitual binge/purge behaviour display increases in regional cerebral blood flow in the right cerebral hemisphere, especially in the inferior frontal and parietal region with a food-related visual stimulus.

There has recently been progress in converting the techniques of PET imaging into SPECT. Two recent studies using statistical parametric mapping (SPM) 96 analysis reported hypoperfusion in the anterior frontal areas in untreated restricting anorexia nervosa at baseline. The first study using HM-PAO found hypoperfusion in the frontal area, mainly bilaterally in the anterior cingulate cortex (ACC) in restricting anorexia nervosa patients compared to anorexia nervosa patients with binge/purge behaviour and healthy volunteers (Naruo *et al.*, 2001). The other SPECT study using Iodin-123-iodoamphetamine (IMP) and SPM analysis also found hypoperfusion in the ACC and medial prefrontal area. Furthermore, a significant hyperperfusion was found in the thalamus and the amygdala–hippocampus complex when compared to the normal subjects (Takano *et al.*, 2001). Since the frontal regions including the ACC have often been reported to be very important in controlling a wide range of higher brain functions, the identical finding concerning the ACC in these two studies suggested that dysfunction of the ACC may possibly be associated with the causing or maintaining of abnormal eating behaviour in anorexia nervosa patients.

Anorexia Nervosa and Bulimia Nervosa

A study using the same experimental design and radioactive tracer examined eight untreated patients with anorexia nervosa, five patients with bulimia nervosa, and nine normal controls (Nozoe *et al.*, 1995). Comparisons across the three groups using a food intake stimulus showed an increase in ratios of the radioactive counts in a region of interest to the cerebellum in the bilateral inferior frontal and left temporal regions in the bulimic patients at baseline. In the anorexic patients, an overall decrease of the normalized radioactivity before stimulus and a significant decrease in the left temporal region were observed at baseline. After exposure to food the intake stimulus only the anorexic patients showed an increased blood flow in a wide region of the cortex, more specifically bilaterally in the inferior frontal, parietal and occipital regions. The authors hypothesized that the increases in rCBF after a food intake stimulus in both studies could reflect changes necessary for patients with anorexia nervosa to control their eating behaviour. On the other hand, the small or negative changes in rCBF in the superior and inferior frontal regions in the bulimia nervosa patients could be correlated with their eating behaviour.

Bulimia Nervosa

Using iodine-labelled [^{123}I]-2β-carbomethoxy-3β-(4-iodophenyl) tropane ([^{123}I] β-CIT) and SPECT, the first exploratory investigation of brain serotonin and dopamine transporter availability in bulimia nervosa has recently been reported (Tauscher *et al.*, 2001). These authors found that 10 bulimic patients showed a 17% reduction in brain serotonin transporter availability in the hypothalamus and thalamus and a 15% reduction in striatal dopamine transporter availability as compared to controls. In particular, the reduction of [^{123}I] β-CIT binding in the hypothalamus and thalamus was reported to be in line with a previous study demonstrating decreased serotonergic transmission in bulimia nervosa. The authors note that it remains unclear whether the reduced serotonin transporter availability is an aetiologic defect, an adaptive mechanism, or an unrelated epiphenomenona of some other process.

Positron Emission Tomography

Anorexia Nervosa

The first preliminary study on anorexia nervosa using (18-F)-fluordeoxyglucose (FDG) and positron emission tomography (PET) was reported in 1987. It was a comparison study of five female patients with anorexia nervosa, before and after treatment, and 15 young male controls (median 29 years) (Herholz *et al.*, 1987). The results were that the anorexic patients before treatment displayed significant bilateral hypermetabolism in the caudate nuclei and temporal cortex compared to post-treatment. Whole brain metabolism was also reported to be higher in the anorexic patients before treatment compared to post-treatment and controls. The authors mentioned that since cortical pseudoatrophy would be associated with hypometabolism in the atrophic structures the observed hypermetabolism cannot be explained by partial volume effects.

Another study examined cerebral glucose metabolism using FDG in 20 patients with anorexia nervosa and 10 healthy controls. Compared to controls, the anorexic group showed global hypometabolism and an absolute as well as relative hypometabolism of glucose in cortical regions, with the most significant differences found in the frontal and the parietal cortices (Delvenne *et al.*, 1995). Within the anorexic and the normal volunteer groups, no correlations were found between absolute or relative cerebral glucose metabolism (rCMRglu) and BMI, anxiety, or Hamilton Depression Rating Scale scores. Different factors may explain the reduced glucose metabolism in anorexia nervosa. It might be the consequence of neurophysiological or morphological aspects of anorexia nervosa and/or the result of some associated symptoms such as anxiety or depression. Supported by cognitive studies, the authors also hypothesized a primary corticocerebral dysfunctioning in anorexia nervosa.

Bulimia Nervosa

Several studies in bulimia nervosa using PET and FDG or [^{15}O]water have been reported as follows.

A preliminary study of eight female bulimia nervosa patients, eight depressed women and eight normal controls revealed that the normal controls and the depressed patients had high metabolic rates in the right cortical regions, whereas the bulimic group instead had high rCMRglu in the basal ganglia (Hagman *et al.*, 1990). From these findings the authors concluded that although women with bulimia nervosa frequently present with symptoms of depression, the pathophysiologic changes associated with bulima differ from depression.

A study of 11 bulimia nervosa patients and 18 normal controls investigated the relationship between rCMRglu and the symptoms of depression, obsessive–compulsive disorder, and bulimia nervosa (Andreason *et al.*, 1992). It was demonstrated that in the patients with bulimia nervosa a lower left anterolateral prefrontal rCMRglu correlated with a greater amount of depressive symptoms, while left temporal lobe hypermetabolism and asymmetries observed in the bulimic patients appeared to be independent of the mood state. The authors also reported that they failed to observe a pattern characteristic of obsessive–compulsive disorder in the patients with bulimia nervosa.

In a study comparing 10 patients with bulimia nervosa of normal body weight, 10 patients with anorexia nervosa and 10 normal controls, the absolute rCMRglu was reduced only in the anorexic patients (Delvenne *et al.*, 1999). This was hypothesized to be related to the low body weight. On the other hand, both anorexic and bulimic patients displayed a decreased in rCMRglu in the parietal cortex. The authors hypothesized that this region might be particularly sensitive to nutritional factors, leading to characteristic changes in this region.

Recently a PET study using [^{15}O]water investigated rCBF in recovered bulimia nervosa patients (Frank *et al.*, 2000). Comparing nine recovered patients to 13 normal controls, a significant inverse relationship between rCFB in several cortical regions and the thalamus and length of recovery was found. The authors suggest that previously reported alterations in rCBF in bulimia nervosa patients during the ill state is a state-related phenomenon that remits with recovery.

Functional Magnetic Resonance Imaging

Anorexia Nervosa

Functional magnetic resonance imaging (fMRI) is a good tool for investigating regional brain abnormalities associated with specific cognitive processes. Because it can map fine changes in cerebral blood flow without using radioactivity, it is expected to be a useful way to investigate brain function in eating disorders.

Up to now, only one fMRI study has been published. The study compared with six patients with anorexia nervosa and six normal controls using videotaped pictures of drinks labelled high (e.g. chocolate milkshake) and low (e.g. still mineral water) calories, respectively (Ellison *et al.*, 1998). The anorexic group showed a higher level of anxiety along with an increased blood flow in response to the contrasting stimuli, especially in the left insula, anterior, cingulate gyrus and left amygdala-hippocampal region.

The authors suggested that the findings provided evidence that the fear associated with high caloric food in people who have anorexia nervosa is associated with activation in a limbic and paralimbic network. The abnormal activity in this area of the brain was suggested to be a linked with an abnormal preoccupation with food-related items.

Magnetic Resonance Spectroscopy

Anorexia Nervosa

Analysis of the chemical composition of the brain in anorexia nervosa using magnetic resonance spectroscopy (MRS) has been the subject of a few reports.

One study of four anorexic patients suggested that the main cause of the brain structure changes such as brain atrophy, was an abnormality in membrane phospholipid metabolism due to the starving state of anorexia nervosa patients (Kato *et al.*, 1997). Another study, comparing 12 anorexic patients with seven normal controls revealed that the ratio of choline containing compounds relative to total creatine in the grey matter was significantly higher in anorexia nervosa subjects compared to controls, but that anorexia nervosa subjects showed significantly lower ratios of N-acetyl-aspartate relative to choline containing compounds compared to controls (Schlemmer *et al.*, 1998).

Anorexia Nervosa and Bulimia Nervosa

A study comparing a group of anorexia nervosa patients, bulimia nervosa patients, and normal controls using MRI and MRS in three regions of the brain, found that reductions in the myo-inositol and lipid compounds (containing lipids, proteins and lactate) within the frontal white matter correlated with reductions in body weight (Roser *et al.*, 1999). Furthermore, reduced lipid signals were found in the occipital grey matter, but on the other hand, in the cerebellum, the concentration of all metabolites except lipid was increased. The authors suggested that decrease in myo-inositol was related to hyponatoremia or hypercortisolemia in patients with eating disorders. They also suggested that both altered glucose oxidation and fatty acid metabolism in anorexic patients could explain the reduced spectral intensity of these compounds probably caused by a reduced concentration of free lipoproteins in brain parenchyma.

Summary

Progress in functional imaging techniques have made it possible to identify specific areas of abnormal brain functions regardless of structural changes. Interestingly, the recent studies have reported that untreated anorexia nervosa patients showed decreases in regional blood perfusion and metabolism of the anterior frontal areas. However, we should be careful in understanding the localized abnormal areas of brain functions because it is still very difficult to specify the neuronal projections that account for the observed changes in regional activity.

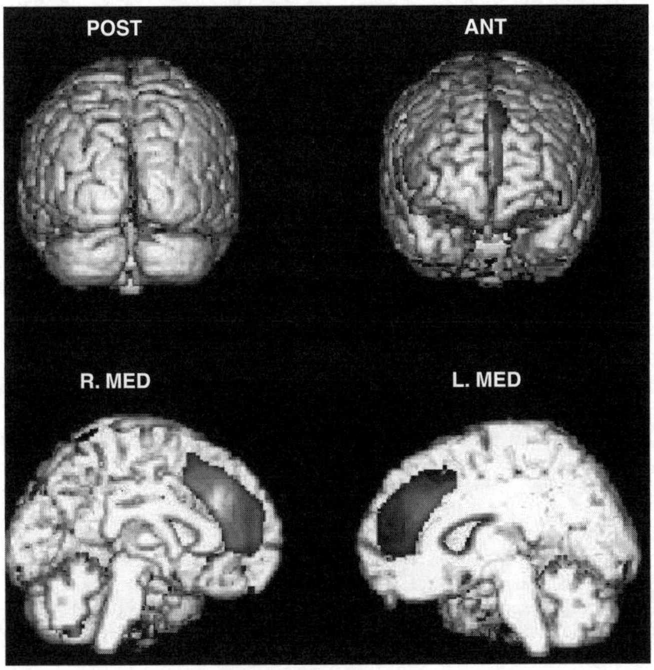

Figure XXIII-8.2 The 3D rendering image displaying area of hypoperfusion. The SPM 96 analysis of SPECT data shows significantly decreased of rCBF in the anorexia nervosa restricters in the bilateral ACC and parts of frontal regions when compared to controls. Height threshold = 3.09, $p = 0.001$, extent threshold = 550

Figure XXIII-8.2 shows the rendering images of an SPM analysis of SPECT data with HM-PAO displaying hypoperfusion both bilaterally in the medial prefrontal regions and in the ACC in restricting anorexia nervosa patients.

RESEARCH ON OBESITY

Although the aetiology of obesity is still unclear, genetic, metabolic, and social factors are all believed to play a role in its development and progression (Stunkard, 1996). Recently, behaviourally distinct subsets of obese persons have been considered to display particular patterns of disordered eating and elevated rates of psychopathology (Devlin, Yanovski and Wilson, 2000). Brain imaging investigations in obese patients may shed light on the mechanisms of the onset and maintenance of obesity. A literature review of this area revealed no studies of structure using CT or MRI, but did locate some functional brain imaging studies.

One study using ^{99m}Tc–ethyl-cysteine-dimer (ECD) and SPECT compared 11 obese women without binge-eating behaviour to 12 normal control females using a food-exposure stimulus. The obese women show higher rCB in right parietal and temporal cortices compared to controls (Karhunen *et al.*, 1997). In addition, higher activity in the right parietal cortex was found to be associated with an enhanced feeling of hunger when looking at food. The authors concluded that the increase in the rCBF of the right cortex after exposure to food could be associated with difficulties in the control of eating since the right hemisphere plays a role in the recognition and control of emotional expressions and related behaviours.

In another study using the same radiotracer in eight obese binge-eating patients and 12 normal controls, regional cerebral blood flow was mapped by SPECT, while the subjects were looking at a picture of a landscape or at a portion of food (Karhunen *et al.*, 2000). When exposed to food the obese patients showed different changes in the cerebral blood flow of the right and left hemisphere, especially in the frontal and prefrontal lobe compared to controls. The increase in blood flow in obese patients was positively correlate with the intensity of hunger. The authors concluded that the left frontal and prefrontal regions could play a role in binge-eating behaviour in humans.

Another study used PET to investigate the functional anatomy of satiation, comparing 11 obese and 11 lean men. It was demonstrated that refeeding after 36 hours of fasting resulted in increases in rCBF in the ventromedial and dorsolateral prefrontal cortex, and decreases in limbic/paralimbic areas and striatum in both groups (Gautier *et al.*, 2000). However, the obese group displayed a significant increase in blood flow in the prefrontal cortex, but a significant decrease in blood flow in the limbic/paralimbic areas, temporal and occipital cortex and cerebellum. The authors suggested that obese individuals have a greater activation of the prefrontal cortex and a greater deactivation of the limbic/paralimbic areas in response to satiation. They also speculated that differences in postprandial amino acid metabolism between lean and obese men might underlie the observed differences in neural activity.

CONCLUSION

The majority of structural studies have examined subjects with anorexia nervosa; few studies have reported on structural changes in bulimia nervosa or obesity. It is now generally agreed upon that alterations in structures such as cerebral atrophy and enlargement of the ventricles are secondary to low body weight (Addolorato *et al.*, 1998). The more recent use of volumetric methods assessing grey- and white-matter volumes has made it possible to assess these changes. While these structural abnormalities typically revert to normal with weight restoration, the process of this recovery is poorly understood. The precise aetiology of these changes is controversial, hypercortisolemia being an attractive explanation, as associations have been demonstrated between hypercortisolemia and the magnitude of structural brain abnormalities (Katzman *et al.*, 2001).

The use of functional brain imaging techniques has led to significant improvements in our understanding of the characteristic brain functional changes in eating disorders and obesity. However, the limitations of these techniques must be acknowledged because of the following reasons. Changes in regional brain activity are considered to reflect the activity of terminal neuronal fields which include those from local interneurons and afferent projections arising in other sites (Tataranni *et al.*, 1999). Comparisons of studies across countries are complicated by varying diagnostic criteria and differences in establishing appropriate comparison groups. Spatial resolution, contrast resolution of individual subtraction images, and accuracy of the image deformation algorithm make it difficult to specify in greater detail the structures that are responsible for the observed increases in regional brain activity (Woods, 1996).

Furthermore, significant challenges remain for functional imaging. These include the effects of prolonged starvation, the administration of medication, and the effect of comorbidity such as depression and obsessive–compulsive disorders. It is also not clear as to what constitutes optimal experimental designs to compare scans at rest or after specific stimuli or tasks. Technical problems in accounting for individual variations in the shape and volume of the brain have yet to be overcome. It is not yet clear whether the findings to date are only state effects, secondary to starvation, or whether any might be pre-existing trait phenomena. Future studies should try to address these various problems.

Finally, brain imaging techniques are believed to serve as the bridge between the molecular clinical domains of this field (Mazzoitta, 2000). Therefore, using the rapidly developing brain imaging techniques in the study of eating disorders is likely to provide us with important information regarding the understanding of the disease and its possible treatment.

ACKNOWLEDGEMENTS

I would like to thank Dr S. Nozoe and Dr D.B. Woodside for comments and corrections to this manuscript, and Dr Y. Nakabeppu and Ms J. Tsutsui for their assistance in preparing this manuscript.

REFERENCES

Addolorato, G., Taranto, C., Capristo, E. and Gasbarrini, G., 1998. A case of marked cerebellar atrophy in a woman with anorexia nervosa and cerebral atrophy and a review of the literature. *International Journal of Eating Disorders*, **24**, 443–447.

Andreason, P.J., Altemus, M., Zametkin, A.J., King, A.C., Lucinio, J. and Cohen, R.M., 1992. Regional cerebral glucose metabolism in bulimia nervosa. *American Journal of Psychiatry*, **149**, 1506–1513.

Artmann, H., Grau, H., Adelmann, M. and Schleiffer, R., 1985. Reversible and non-reversible enlargement of cerebrospinal fluid spaces in anorexia nervosa. *Neuroradiology*, **27**, 304–312.

Datlof, S., Coleman, P.D., Forbes, G.B. and Kreipe, R.E., 1986. Ventricular dilation on CAT scans of patients with anorexia nervosa. *American Journal of Psychiatry*, **143**, 96–98.

Delvenne, V., Goldman, S., DeMaertelaer, V. and Lotstra, F., 1999. Brain glucose metabolism in eating disorders assessed by positron emission tomography. *International Journal of Eating Disorders*, **25**, 29–37.

Delvenne, V., Lotstra, F., Goldman, S., Biver, F., DeMaertelaer, F., Appelboom, F.J., Schoutens, A., Bidaut, L.M., Luxen, A. and Mendelwicz, J., 1995. Brain hypometabolism of glucose in anorexia nervosa: a PET scan study. *Biological Psychiatry*, **37**, 161–169.

Demaerel, P., 2000. Magnetic resonance imaging in psychiatry. *Acta Neurologica Belgium*, **100**, 18–23.

Devlin, M., Yanovski, S. and Wilson, G., 2000. Obesity: What mental health professionals need to know. *American Journal of Psychiatry*, **157**, 854–866.

De Zwaan, M., Mitchell, J.E., Raymond, N.C. and Spitzer, R.L., 1994. Binge eating disorder: Clinical features and treatment of a new diagnosis. *Harvard Review of Psychiatry*, **1**, 310–325.

Dolan, R.J., Mitchell, J. and Wakeling, A., 1988. Structural brain changes in patients with anorexia nervosa. *Psychological Medicine*, **18**, 349–353.

Doraiswamy, P.M., Krishnan, K., Figiel, G., Husain, M.M., Boyko, O.B., Rockwell, W.J. and Ellinwood, E.H. Jr, 1990. A brain magnetic resonance imaging study of pituitary gland morphology in anorexia nervosa and bulimia. *Biological Psychiatry*, **28**, 110–116.

Ellison, Z.R. and Foong, J., 1998. *Neurobiology in the Treatment of Eating Disorders*, pp. 255–270. John Wiley & Sons, Chichester.

Ellison, Z., Foong, J., Howard, R., Bullmore, E., Williams, S. and Treasure, J., 1998. Functional anatomy of calorie fear in anorexia nervosa. *Lancet*, **352**, 1192.

Frank, G.K., Kaye, W.H., Greer, P., Meltzer, C.C. and Price, J.C., 2000. Regional cerebral blood flow after recovery from bulimia nervosa. *Psychiatry Research*, **100**, 1–9.

Garfinkel, P.E., Kennedy, S.H. and Kaplan, A.S., 1995. View on classification and diagnosis of eating disorders. *Canadian Journal of Psychiatry*, **40**, 445–456.

Gautier, J.F., Chen, K., Salbe, A.D., Bandy, D., Pratley, R.E., Heiman, M., Ravussin, E., Reiman, E.M. and Tataranni, P.A., 2000. Differential brain responses to satiation in obese and lean men. *Diabetes*, **49**, 838–846.

Golden, N.H., Ashtari, M., Kohn, M.R., Patel, M., Jacobson, M.S., Fletcher, A. and Shenker, I.R., 1996. Reversibility of cerebral ventricular enlargement in anorexia nervosa, demonstrated by quantitative magnetic resonance imaging. *Journal of Pediatrics*, **128**, 296–301.

Gordon, I., Lask, B., Bryant-Waugh, R., Christie, D. and Timini, S., 1997. Childhood-onset anorexia nervosa: Towards identifying a biological substrate. *International Journal of Eating Disorders*, **22**, 159–165.

Grady, C.L., 1999. *The Human Frontal Lobes*, pp. 196–230. The Guilford Press, New York.

Hagman, J.O., Buchsbaum, M.S., Wu, J.C., Rao, S.J., Reynolds, C.A. and Blinder, B.J., 1990. Comparison of regional brain metabolism in bulimia nervosa and affective disorder assessed with positron emission tomography. *Journal of Affective Disorders*, **19**, 153–162.

Hendren, R.L., De Backer, I. and Pandina, G.L., 2000. Review of neuroimaging studies of child and adolescent psychiatric disorders from the past 10 years. *Journal of the American Academy of Child and Adolescent Psychiatry*, **39**, 815–828.

Herholz, K., Krieg, J.C., Emrich, H.M., Pawlik, G., Beil, C., Pirke, K.M., Pahl, J.J., Wagner, R., Wienhard, K., Ploog, D. and Heiss, W.D., 1987. Regional cerebral glucose metabolism in anorexia nervosa measured by positron emission tomography. *Biological Psychiatry*, **22**, 43–51.

Hoffman, G.W. Jr, Ellinwood, E.H. Jr, Rockwell, W.J.K., Herfkens, R.J., Nishita, J.K. and Guthrie, L.F., 1989. Cerebral atrophy in anorexia nervosa; a pilot study. *Biological Psychiatry*, **25**, 894–902.

Inugami, A., Kanno, I., Uemura, K., Shishido, F., Murakami, M., Tomura, N., Fujita, H. and Higano, S., 1988. Linearization correction of 99mTc-labeled hexamethyl-prophylene amine oxime (HM-PAO) image in terms of regional CBF distribution: comparison to C15O2 inhalation steady-state method measured by positron emission tomography. *Journal of Cerebral Blood Flow and Metabolism*, **8**, s52–s60.

Karhunen, L.J., Lappalainen, R.I., Vanninen, E.J., Kuikka, J.T. and Uusitupa, M.I.J., 1997. Regional cerebral blood flow during food-exposure in obese women. *Brain*, **120**, 1675–1684.

Karhunen, L.J., Vanninen, E.J., Kuikka, J.T., Lappalaien, R.I., Tiihonen, J. and Uusitupa, M.I., 2000. Regional cerebral blood flow during exposure to food obese binge eating women. *Psychiatry Research*, **10**, 29–42.

Kato, T., Shioiri, T., Murashita, J. and Inubushi, T., 1997. Phosphorus-31 magnetic resonance spectroscopic observations in 4 cases with anorexia nervosa. *Progress in Neuropsychopharmacology and Biological Psychiatry*, **21**, 719–724.

Katzman, D.K., Zipursky, R.B., Lambe, E.K. and Mikulis, D.J., 1997. A longitudinal magnetic resonance imaging study of brain change in adolescents with anorexia nervosa. *Archives of Pediatrics and Adolescent Medicine*, **151**, 793–797.

Katzman, D.K., Christensen, B., Young, A.R. and Zipursky, R.B., 2001. Starving the brain; Structural abnormalities and cognitive impairment in adolescents with anorexia nervosa. *Seminars in Clinical Neuropsychiatry*, **6**, 146–152.
Kingston, K., Szmukler, G., Andrewes, D., Tress, B. and Desmond, P., 1996. Neuropsychological and structural brain changes in anorexia nervosa before and after refeeding. *Psychological Medicine*, **26**, 15–28.
Kohkmeyer, K., Lemkuhl, G. and Poutska, F., 1983. Computed tomography of anorexia nervosa. *AJNR American Journal Neuroradiology*, **4**, 437–438.
Krieg, J.C., Backmund, H. and Pirke, K.M., 1987. Cranial computed tomography findings in bulimia. *Acta Psychiatrica Scanavica*, **75**, 144–149.
Krieg, J.C., Pirke, K.M., Lauer, C. and Backmund, H., 1988. Endocrine, metabolic and cranial computed tomographic findings in anorexia nervosa. *Biological Psychiatry*, **23**, 377–387.
Krieg, J.C., Lauer, C. and Pirke, K.M., 1989a. Structural brain abnormalities in patients with bulimia nervosa. *Psychiatry Research*, **27**, 39–48.
Krieg, J.C., Lauer, C., Leinsinger, G., Pahl, J., Schreiber, W., Pirke, K.M. and Moser, E.A., 1989b. Brain morphology and regional cerebral blood flow in anorexia nervosa. *Biological Psychiatry*, **25**, 1041–1048.
Krishnan, K.R. and Gadde, K.M., 1998. Psychoneuroendocrinology and brain imaging in depression. *Psychiatric Clinics of North America*, **21**, 465–472.
Kuhn, H.G., Dickinson-Anson, H. and Gage, F.H., 1996. Neurogenesis in the dentate gyrus of the adult rat: age-related decrease of neuronal progenitor proliferation. *Journal of Neuroscience*, **16**, 2027–2033.
Kuruoglu, A.C., Kapucu, O., Atasever, T., Arikan, Z., Isik, E. and Unlu, M., 1998. Technetium-99m-HMPAO brain SPECT in anorexia nervosa. *Journal of Nuclear Medicine*, **39**, 304–306.
Lambe, E.K., Katzman, D.K., Mikulis, D.J., Kennedy, S.H. and Zipursky, R.B., 1997. Cerebral gray matter volume deficits after weight recovery from anorexia nervosa. *Archives of General Psychiatry*, **54**, 537–542.
Lankenau, H., Swigar, M.E., Bhimani, S., Luchins, D. and Quinlan, D.M., 1985. Cranial CT scans in eating disorder patient and controls. *Comprehensive Psychiatry*, **26**, 136–147.
Mazzoitta, J.C., 2000. Imaging: window on the brain. *Archives of Neurology*, **57**, 1413–1421.
Naruo, T., Nakabeppu, Y., Deguchi, D., Nagai, N., Tsutsui, J., Nakajo, M. and Nozoe, S., 2001. Decreases in blood perfusion of the anterior cingulate gyri in anorexia nervosa restricters assessed by SPECT image analysis. *BMC Psychiatry*, **1**, 2.
Naruo, T., Nakabeppu, Y., Sagiyama, K., Munemoto, T., Homan, N., Deguchi, D., Nakajo, M. and Nozoe, S., 2000. Characteristic regional cerebral blood flow patterns in anorexia nervosa patients with binge/purge behavior. *American Journal of Psychiatry*, **57**, 1520–1522.
Nozoe, S., Naruo, T., Nakabeppu, Y., Soejima, Y., Nakajo, M. and Tanaka, H., 1993. Change in regional cerebral blood flow in patients with anorexia nervosa detected through single photon emission tomography imaging. *Biological Psychiatry*, **34**, 578–580.
Nozoe, S., Naruo, T., Yonekura, R., Nakabeppu, Y., Soejima, Y., Nagai, N., Nakajo, M. and Tanaka, H., 1995. Comparison of regional cerebral blood flow in patients with eating disorders. *Brain Research Bulletin*, **36**, 251–255.
Palazidou, E., Robinson, P. and Lishman, W.A., 1990. Neuroradiological and neuropsychological assessment in anorexia nervosa. *Psychological Medicine*, **20**, 521–527.
Rolls, E.T., 1994. Appetite, Neural and Behavioral Bases, pp. 11–53. Oxford University Press, Oxford.
Roser, W., Bubl, R., Buergin, D., Seelig, J., Radue, E.W. and Rost, B., 1999. Metabolic changes in the brain of patients with anorexia and bulimia nervosa as detected by proton magnetic resonance spectroscopy. *International Journal of Eating Disorders*, **26**, 119–126.
Schlemmer, H.P., Moeckel, R., Marcus, A., Hentschel, F., Goepel, C., Becker, G., Koepke, J., Guckel, F., Schmidt, M.H. and Georgi, M., 1998. Proton magnetic resonance spectroscopy in acute, juvenile anorexia nervosa. *Psychiatry Research*, **82**, 171–179.
Stunkard, A.J., 1996. Current views on obesity. *American Journal of Medicine*, **100**, 230–236.
Swayze, V.W. IInd, Andersen, A., Arndt, S., Rajarethinam, R., Fleming, F., Sato, Y. and Andreasen, N.C., 1996. Reversibility of brain tissue loss in anorexia nervosa assessed with a computerized Talairach 3-D proportional grid. *Psychological Medicine*, **26**, 381–390.
Takano, A., Shiga, T., Kitagawa, N., Koyama, T., Katoh, C. and Tsukamoto, E., 2001. Abnormal neuronal network in anorexia nervosa studied with I-123-IMP SPECT. *Psychiatry Research*, **107**, 45–50.
Tataranni, P.A., Gautier, J.F., Chen, K., Uecker, A., Bandy, D., Salbe, A.D., Pratley, R.E., Lawson, M., Reiman, E.M. and Ravussin, E., 1999. Neuroanatomical correlates of hunger and satiation in humans using positron emission tomography. *Proceedings of the National Academy of Sciences of the United States of America*, **96**, 4569–4574.
Tauscher, J., Pirker, W., Willeit, M., Zwaan, M., Bailer, U., Neumeister, A., Asenbaum, S., Lennkh, C., Praschak-Rieder, N., Brucke, T. and Kasper, S., 2001. [^{123}I] β-CIT and single photon emission computed tomography reveal reduced brain serotonin transporter availability in bulimia nervosa. *Biological Psychiatry*, **49**, 326–332.
Woods, R.P., 1996. Modeling for intergroup comparisons of imaging data. *Neuroimage*, **4**, s84–94.

XXIII-9

The Genetics of Eating Disorders

Kelly L. Klump, Cynthia M. Bulik, Walter H. Kaye and Michael Strober

INTRODUCTION

Anorexia nervosa (AN) and bulimia nervosa (BN) are disorders characterized by abnormal patterns of eating behaviour and disturbances in attitudes and perceptions toward weight and shape. In AN, there is an extreme fear of weight gain despite increasing emaciation. BN usually emerges after a period of dieting (Bulik *et al.*, 1997; Mussell *et al.*, 1997) and is characterized by alternating patterns of binge eating and compensatory behaviour. Binge eating, which is the consumption of a large amount of food in an uncontrollable manner, is typically followed by either self-induced vomiting, excessive exercise, fasting, and/or the misuse of laxatives, diuretics or enemas. Although abnormally low body weight excludes a BN diagnosis, 25% to 30% of patients with BN have a prior history of AN (Eckert *et al.*, 1995; Bulik *et al.*, 1997; Strober, Freeman and Morrell, 1997; Garfinkel, Moldofsky and Garner, 1980). Common to individuals with AN and BN are pathological concern with weight and shape, depression, and anxiety (Mitchell *et al.*, 1986; Keck *et al.*, 1990; Fornari *et al.*, 1992; Bulik *et al.*, in press).

The aetiology of these disorders is presumed to be multiply influenced by developmental, social, and biological processes (Garner, 1993; Treasure and Campbell, 1994). However, the exact nature of these interactive processes remains incompletely understood. Cultural attitudes towards thinness have relevance to the psychopathology of eating disorders, but they are unlikely to be sufficient to account for the pathogenesis of these disorders. Notably, dieting behaviour is quite common in industrialized countries throughout the world, yet AN and BN affect only an estimated 0.3% to 0.7%, and 1.7% to 2.5%, respectively, of females in the general population (APA, 1994). Moreover, numerous descriptions of AN date from the middle of the 19th century suggesting that factors other than modern culture play an aetiologic role. In addition, both syndromes have a relatively homogeneous clinical presentation, sex distribution, and age-of-onset, supporting the possibility of some biological susceptibility. This is not to discount the role of culture, as the introduction of Western ideals of thinness may serve to release a biological propensity toward eating disorders (Becker, 1999) possibly by increasing behaviours such as dieting that may trigger the spiral of disordered eating.

Recent findings from behaviour genetic studies suggest that this biological vulnerability might be genetic in nature. In this paper, we will highlight these emerging findings and suggest areas for future research.

HERITABILITY

Family Studies

Family studies provide initial data regarding genetic influence on a disorder by establishing whether it clusters amongst biologically-related individuals. Controlled family studies have generally found increased rates of eating disorders in relatives of women with AN and BN compared to relatives of controls (Biederman *et al.*, 1985; Lilenfeld *et al.*, 1998; Strober *et al.*, 1990, 2000). Findings from the largest and most systematic studies (Lilenfeld *et al.*, 1998; Strober *et al.*, 2000) suggest a 7–12-fold increase in the prevalence of AN and BN in relatives of eating disordered probands. This clustering of eating disorders in families of AN and BN individuals provides strong support for familial transmission of both disorders. However, given that first-degree relatives share both genes and environments, these studies cannot differentiate genetic versus environmental causes for the observed familiality. Systematic studies of twins are the means by which to disentangle the relative aetiological influence of genes and environment.

Twin Studies

Twin studies differentiate genetic from environmental effects by comparing similarity for a trait/disorder between identical (monozygotic (MZ)) and fraternal twins (dizygotic (DZ)). This comparison is based on the fact that MZ twins share all of their genes identical by descent, whereas DZ twins share, on average, half of their genes identical by descent. Consequently, MZ twin correlations that are $\simeq$ two times greater than DZ twin correlations suggest genetic effects. In general, greater MZ relative to DZ twin similarity for AN and BN has generally been found (Holland *et al.*, 1984, 1988; Fichter and Noegel, 1990; Treasure and Holland, 1990). Estimates indicate that roughly 58–76% of the variance in the liability to AN (Klump *et al.*, 2001; Wade *et al.*, 2000), and 54–83% of the variance in the liability to BN (Bulik, Sullivan and Kendler, 1998; Kendler *et al.*, 1991) can be accounted for by genetic factors. Although the confidence intervals on these estimates are wide, consistent findings across studies support moderate heritability of these traits (Bulik *et al.*, 2000). For both AN and BN, the remaining variance in liability appears to be due to unique environmental factors (i.e., factors that are unique to siblings in the same family) rather than shared or common environmental factors (i.e., factors that are shared by siblings in the same family).

Eating disorder symptoms themselves also appear to be moderately heritable. Twin studies of binge eating, self-induced vomiting, and dietary restraint suggest that these behaviours are roughly 46–72% heritable (Sullivan, Bulik and Kendler, 1998; Klump *et al.*, 2000). Likewise, pathological attitudes such as body dissatisfaction, eating and weight concerns, and weight preoccupation show heritabilities of roughly 32–72% (Klump *et al.*, 2000; Rutherford *et al.*, 1993; Wade *et al.*, 1998, 1999). Taken together, findings suggest a significant genetic component to AN and BN as well as the attitudes and behaviours that contribute to, and correlate with, clinical eating pathology.

Biological Psychiatry: Edited by H. D'haenen, J.A. den Boer and P. Willner. ISBN 0-471-49198-5

Developmental Differences

A caveat to the above conclusions is that there appears to be developmental differences in genetic effects across adolescence. Two recent twin studies (Klump *et al.*, 2000, in press) from the Minnesota Twin Family Study (MTFS) have examined this issue by comparing genetic influences on eating attitudes and behaviours in population-based samples of 680 11-year-old twins and 602 17-year-old twins. In the first of these studies, essentially no genetic influence was found for weight preoccupation scores and overall eating pathology in 11 year-old twins, whereas 52–57% of the variance in these attitudes and behaviours could be accounted for by genetic factors in the older cohort (Klump *et al.*, 2000). Increased genetic influence across age was also found for body dissatisfaction scores, although effects were much less dramatic. The authors speculated that these findings may reflect an activation of aetiologic genes during puberty.

In a follow-up study (Klump, McGue and Iacono, in press), the 11-year-old cohort was divided into a pre- and post-pubertal group in order to directly examine the effect of puberty on the heritability of these traits and behaviours. Findings revealed a pattern of results similar to those reported in the initial study (Klump *et al.*, 2000). Genetic factors accounted for 0% of the variance in overall eating pathology scores in pre-pubertal twins, but accounted for 53% of the variance in post-pubertal twins. Although sample sizes were small in the post-pubertal group ($n = 39$ pairs), the similar pattern of twin correlations in the two studies suggested that puberty may account for the dramatic age differences observed earlier. Increased heritability in post-pubertal relative to pre-pubertal twins *who were the same age* provided strong evidence of potential pubertal activation of the heritability of eating pathology that may be mediated by ovarian hormones. These findings are important for highlighting not only developmental differences in genetic effects, but also the potential role of ovarian steroids in the heritability of these disorders.

COMORBIDITY

Individuals with AN and BN commonly present with comorbid psychopathology — most notably affective and anxiety disorders (Bulik *et al.*, 2000). Family and twin studies have been effective in illuminating the causes of comorbidity (Neale and Kendler, 1995) and addressing to what extent comorbidity among these disorders might arise as a function of a shared genetic effect.

Psychopathology

Substance Use Disorders

Family studies investigating substance use disorders suggest relatively low prevalence among relatives of restricting AN probands (Holderness, Brooks-Gunn and Warren, 1994; Lilenfeld *et al.*, 1998). In contrast, rates are elevated in relatives of probands with BN. However, results from three studies (Kaye *et al.*, 1996; Schuckit *et al.*, 1996; Miller *et al.*, 1998) indicate that there is no evidence of a cross-transmission of BN and substance use disorder in families, and twin data (Kendler *et al.*, 1995) have shown that the genes influencing susceptibility to alcoholism were independent of those underlying risk to BN.

Major Depression

Several family and twin studies have examined the covariation between eating disorders and major depression. Studies of AN probands have yielded relative risk estimates for depression in the range of 2.1 to 3.4 (Strober *et al.*, 1990; Lilenfeld *et al.*, 1998). Likewise, studies of BN probands indicate that their first-degree relatives are significantly more likely to develop major depression than relatives of controls (Lilenfeld *et al.*, 1998). However, most studies considering the effects of proband comorbidity on familial risk have shown that affective illness is more likely to be transmitted by probands with this same diagnostic comorbidity (Strober *et al.*, 1990; Lilenfeld *et al.*, 1998). These later studies suggest that although eating disorders and depression may share some aetiologic factors, there are also unique factors specific to each. Two recent twin studies support this conclusion, as both found evidence for shared as well as unique genetic influences on major depression and both AN and BN (Walters *et al.*, 1992; Wade *et al.*, 2000).

Anxiety Disorders

Several different anxiety disorders have been examined for their genetic relationships with eating pathology. In general, evidence supports shared genetic transmission between these disorders and both AN and BN. For example, although obsessive–compulsive disorder (OCD) appears to segregate independently from AN and BN in families (Lilenfeld *et al.*, 1998), shared familial transmission has been found between obsessive-personality disorder (OCPD) and AN and BN (Lilenfeld *et al.*, 1998). In addition, shared familial transmission has been found between broadly defined AN and BN and separation anxiety and overanxious disorder (Keel *et al.*, submitted), and between BN and both simple phobia and panic disorder (Kendler *et al.*, 1995). Taken together, these findings suggest the existence of a broad, genetically influenced obsessive phenotype with core features of rigid perfectionism, anxiety, and a propensity towards behavioural constraint.

Personality and Physical Characteristics

Personality Traits

Individuals with AN and BN exhibit characteristic personality traits including high levels of stress reactivity, negative emotionality, and harm avoidance (Brewerton, Hand and Bishop, 1983; Casper, 1990; Kleifield *et al.*, 1994a, 1994b; Bulik *et al.*, 1995, 2000; O'Dwyer, Lucey and Russell, 1996; Klump *et al.*, 1999, 2000). These characteristics persist after recovery (Casper, 1990; O'Dwyer, Lucey and Russell, 1996; Klump *et al.*, 1999) from the disorder and are independent of body weight (Klump *et al.*, 2000), suggesting that they may be trait disturbances contributing to the disorders' development. The moderately heritable nature of these traits (Tellegen *et al.*, 1988) suggests that relationships may be genetic in nature.

Four studies have examined familial relationships between personality traits and eating disorders, with many suggesting familial co-transmission. Klump *et al.* (1999) found increased levels of negative emotionality and stress reactivity, and decreased levels of well-being, in family members of restricting AN probands compared to control relatives. Likewise, Lilenfeld *et al.* (2000) found increased perfectionism and stress reactivity scores in non-eating disordered relatives of bulimic probands compared to control relatives. Carney, Yates and Cizadlo (1990) failed to find shared transmission between DSM-III-R personality disorder characteristics and BN, although their use of lower prevalence personality disorder symptoms rather than more normative personality characteristics may have prohibited detection of significant effects.

Recent twin study results suggest that familial relationships between personality and eating pathology may be genetic in nature (Klump, McGue and Iacono, in press), as genetic rather than environmental influences have been found to underlie phenotypic and familial relationships between these characteristics. However, genetic influences that are independent of those operating in personality also appear to contribute to eating pathology (Klump, McGue and Iacono, in press).

Body Mass Index

Vulnerability to obesity has been found to be a risk factor for bulimia nervosa (Fairburn *et al.*, 1997). Body weight is highly heritable (Stunkard *et al.*, 1990) leading to questions of shared genetic transmission between body weight and eating pathology. One study directly examined this question by investigating shared genetic transmission of body mass index (BMI) and disordered eating including body dissatisfaction, weight preoccupation, overall eating pathology, and the use of compensatory behaviours such as self-induced vomiting and laxative abuse (Klump *et al.*, 2000). Findings suggested some shared genetic transmission, although again, the majority of genetic influence on these disordered eating variables was independent of the genes influencing BMI.

Shared Transmission between AN and BN

Cumulating evidence suggests that AN and BN likely share some aetiologic features. Clinically, approximately 50% of women with AN develop BN during the course of their illness and ~30% of women with BN report a history of AN (Bulik *et al.*, 1997; Eckert *et al.*, 1995; Garfinkel, Moldofsky and Garner, 1980; Strober, Freeman and Morrell, 1997).

Family and twin studies indicate an increased risk of both AN and BN in relatives of AN and BN probands (Walters and Kendler, 1995; Lilenfeld *et al.*, 1998; Strober *et al.*, 2000), suggesting a shared familial component between the two disorders. In addition, subthreshold forms of eating disorders appear to lie on a continuum of liability with full eating disorders (Kendler *et al.*, 1991). These findings suggest the existence of a broad eating disorder phenotype with possible shared genetic predispositions.

Summary

Research reviewed above suggests that AN and BN may share genetic transmission with each other and with body weight, personality, anxiety, and possibly major depression. However, findings also suggest that there are genetic influences on eating pathology that are independent of those influencing the traits/disorders mentioned above. This complexity is the norm rather than the exception in psychiatric genetics and highlights the need for additional research to further characterize the genetic variance of these disorders.

MOLECULAR GENETIC STUDIES

A detailed comparison of the molecular genetic designs that can be brought to bear upon complex traits is beyond the scope of this chapter (Lander and Schork, 1994; Risch and Merikangas, 1996; Martin, Boomsma and Machin, 1997). Briefly, there are two general strategies in humans: linkage and association studies (Sham, 1998).

Linkage studies can be used in gene discovery: with a sufficiently large number of multiplex pedigrees or extreme sibling pairs (Allison *et al.*, 1998), anonymous genetic markers scattered across the genome can be used to identify the chromosomal regions that may contain genes that contribute to a disorder such as AN or BN. This appealing strength is tempered by the low power (Risch and Zhang, 1996) and resolution (Roberts *et al.*, 1999) likely for linkage studies of complex traits.

Association studies are conceptually equivalent to the familiar case-control design. This design is particularly useful and powerful when prior knowledge of the pathophysiology of a trait suggests a number of candidate genes. However, the use of this design is controversial because of the risk of false positive findings when studying a sample that contains individuals of evolutionary diverse ancestry (Kidd, 1993). Obtaining genotypes on other family members can reduce this risk but at the cost of reduced statistical power.

Association Studies

Evidence linking AN and BN to monoamine functioning (Gorwood *et al.*, 1998) have led researchers to target serotonin and dopamine-related genes in association studies. Several groups have reported an increase in the −1438/A allele of the 5-HT$_{2A}$ receptor gene in AN women compared to controls (Collier *et al.*, 1997; Enoch *et al.*, 1998; Sorbi *et al.*, 1998; Nacmias *et al.*, 1999). However, additional studies of this and other serotonin-related genes (5-HT$_{1D\beta}$, 5-HTT, 5-HT7, tryptophan hydroxylase receptor (TPH)) have failed to find significant associations in AN (Hinney *et al.*, 1997a, 1997b, 1999a; Campbell *et al.*, 1998, Han *et al.*, 1999; Ziegler *et al.*, 1999) or BN (Burnet *et al.*, 1999; Nacmias *et al.*, 1999) individuals. Studies have also failed to find increased allele frequencies of the dopamine D_3 (Bruins-Slot *et al.*, 1998) and D_4 (Hinney *et al.*, 1999b) receptor genes in AN relative to controls. These genes have not yet been examined in individuals with BN.

The primary role of weight control, feeding, and energy expenditure in the pathology of AN and BN has lead researchers to examine genes related to these processes. Results thus far have been mixed, as tests for association between AN and neuropeptide Y5 and Y1 (Rosenkranz *et al.*, 1998), the β_3 adrenergic receptor gene (Hinney *et al.*, 1997c), the melanocortin-4 receptor gene (Hinney *et al.*, 1999c), and the leptin gene (Hinney *et al.*, 1998) were all negative. However, studies have found an increase in the D11S911 allele located near the UCP-2/UCP-3 gene in AN subjects relative to controls (Campbell *et al.*, 1999), as well as an increase in the oestrogen receptor β 1082/G allele in AN relative to obese and overweight subjects (Rosenkranz *et al.*, 1998). Once again, associations between most of these genes and BN have not been investigated.

Findings suggest possible associations between the 5-HT$_{2A}$ receptor gene, the UCP-2/UCP-3 gene, and the oestrogen receptor β gene with AN. However, additional research is necessary to clarify conflicting findings and replicate initial results. Moreover, association studies of BN are needed, as this disorder has been much less studied than AN and findings thus far have been generally negative.

Linkage Studies

We and a number of collaborators (Kaye *et al.*, 2000) have recently completed the first study to date (Grice *et al.*, submitted) using genome-wide linkage analyses in AN or BN. This multicentre study is funded by the Price Foundation of Switzerland and uses allele-sharing linkage analyses to identify genes contributing to eating disorders in 196 families with two or more family members with AN, BN, or eating disorder not otherwise specified (EDNOS). Initial analyses of this dataset show only modest evidence for linkage, with peaks observed on chromosomes 4, 11, 13, and 15 with NPL scores >1. The highest peak was a NPL score on chromosome 4 (Grice *et al.*, in preparation). These modest results are likely due to decreased power to detect linkage as a result of large number of loci influencing the phenotype as well as considerable sample heterogeneity (i.e., inclusion of AN, BN, and EDNOS). These possibilities suggest that additional studies using more homogeneous phenotypes and larger numbers of subjects would increase power to identify genetic effects.

We have recently completed a larger, genome-wide linkage study of approximately 400 families with two or more family members with AN, BN, or EDNOS. This larger study will provide the necessary power to detect linkage and may prove to be the first to identify susceptibility loci for these disorders. In addition, we are currently in the process of collecting genetic data on approximately 700 AN individuals and their parents. This homogeneous sample will be used to conduct association analyses such as those described above and will provide additional power to detect genes of modest to large effect.

CONCLUSIONS

Data described above are clear in establishing a role for genes in the development of eating pathology. Estimates from the most rigorous studies suggest that >50% of the variance in liability to eating disorders and disordered eating behaviours can be accounted for by additive genetic effects. The remaining variance appears to be due to unique rather than common environmental effects. These high estimates indicate a need for studies identifying the specific genes contributing to this large proportion of variance. Twin and family studies suggest that a number of heritable characteristics that are frequently comorbid with AN and BN may share genetic transmission with these disorders, including anxiety disorders/traits, body weight, and possibly major depression. Developmental twin research is beginning to shed light on why eating disorders tend to develop within a relatively narrow developmental window. Additional work is required to enhance our understanding of how puberty (and which aspects of puberty) influences the apparent activation of genetic effects on disordered eating.

Molecular genetic research of these disorders is in its infancy. However, promising areas for future research have already been identified (e.g., 5-HT2A receptor gene, UCP-2/UCP-3 gene, oestrogen receptor β gene), and several large-scale linkage and association studies are currently underway. These studies are likely to provide invaluable information regarding both the appropriate phenotypes to be included in genetic studies as well as the genes with the most influence on the development of these disorders.

REFERENCES

Allison, D.B., Heo, M., Schork, N.J., Wong, S.L. and Elston, R.C., 1998. Extreme selection strategies in gene mapping studies of oligogenic quantitative traits do not always increase power. *Human Heredity*, **48**(2), 97–107.

American Psychiatric Association, 1994. *Diagnostic and Statistical Manual of Mental Disorders (DSM-IV)*. American Psychiatric Association, Washington, DC.

Becker, A., 1999. *Eating Disorders in Fiji*. Paper presented at the American Psychiatric Association, Washington, DC.

Biederman, J., Rivinus, T., Kemper, K., Hamilton, D., MacFadyen, J. and Harmatz, J., 1985. Depressive disorders in relatives of anorexia nervosa patients with and without a current episode of nonbipolar major depression. *Am. J. Psychiatry*, **142**, 1495–1496.

Brewerton, T.D., Hand, L.D. and Bishop, E.R., 1993. The Tridimensional Personality Questionnaire in eating disorder patients. *International Journal of Eating Disorders*, **14**(2), 213–218.

Bruins-Slot, L., Gorwood, P., Bouvard, M., Blot, P., Ades, J., Feingold, J., Schwartz, J.C., Mouren, S. and Marie, C., 1998. Lack of association between anorexia nervosa and D3 dopamine receptor gene. *Biol. Psychiatry*, **43**(1), 76–78.

Bulik, C., Sullivan, P., Carter, F. and Joyce, P., 1997. Initial manifestation of disordered eating behavior: dieting versus binging. *International Journal of Eating Disorders*, **22**, 195–201.

Bulik, C.M., Sullivan, P.F., Fear, J.L. and Pickering, A., 2000. The outcome of anorexia nervosa: Eating attitudes, personality, and parental bonding. *International Journal of Eating Disorders*, **28**, 139–147.

Bulik, C., Sullivan, P.F., Fear, J. and Pickering, A., 1997. Predictors of the development of bulimia nervosa in women with anorexia nervosa. *Journal of Nervous and Mental Disease*, **185**, 704–707.

Bulik, C., Sullivan, P., Wade, T. and Kendler, K., 2000. Twin studies of eating disorders: a review. *International Journal of Eating Disorders*, **27**, 1–20.

Bulik, C.M., Sullivan, P.F., Weltzin, T.E. and Kaye, W.H., 1995. Temperament in eating disorders. *International Journal of Eating Disorders*, **17**(3), 251–261.

Bulik, C.M., Sullivan, P.F. and Kendler, K.S., 1998. Heritability of binge-eating and broadly-defined bulimia nervosa. *Biological Psychiatry*, **44**, 1210–1218.

Burnet, P.W., Smith, K.A., Cowen, P.J., Fairburn, C.G. and Harrison, P.J., 1999. Allelic variation of the 5-HT2C receptor (HTR2C) in bulimia nervosa and binge eating disorder. *Psychiatric Genetics*, **9**(2), 101–104.

Campbell, D.A., Sundaramurthy, D., Gordon, D., Markham, A.F. and Pieri, L.F., 1998. Lack of association between 5-HT2A gene promoter polymorphism and susceptibility to anorexia nervosa. *Lancet*, **351**, 499.

Campbell, D.A., Sundaramurthy, D., Gordon, D., Markham, A.F. and Pieri, L.F., 1999. Association between a marker in the UCP-2/UCP-3 gene cluster and genetic susceptibility to anorexia nervosa. *Molecular Psychiatry*, **4**(1), 68–70.

Carney, C.P., Yates, W.R. and Cizadlo, B., 1990. A controlled family study of personality in normal-weight bulimia nervosa. *International Journal of Eating Disorders*, **9**(6), 659–665.

Casper, R.C., 1990. Personality features of women with good outcome from restricting anorexia nervosa. *Psychosomatic Medicine*, **52**, 156–170.

Collier, D.A., Arranz, M.J., Li, T., Mupita, D., Brown, N. and Treasure, J., 1997. Association between 5-HT2A gene promoter polymorphism and anorexia nervosa. *Lancet*, **350**, 412.

Eckert, E.D., Halmi, K.A., Marchi, P., Grove, W. and Crosby, R., 1995. Ten-year follow-up of anorexia nervosa: Clinical course and outcome. *Psychological Medicine*, **25**(1), 143–156.

Enoch, M.A., Kaye, W.H., Rotondo, A., Greenberg, B.D., Murphy, D.L. and Goldman, D., 1998. 5-HT2A promoter polymorphism — 1438G/A, anorexia nervosa, an obsessive–compulsive disorder. *Lancet*, **351**, 1785–1786.

Fairburn, C.G., Welch, S.L., Doll, H.A., Davies, B.A. and O'Connor, M.E., 1997. Risk factors for bulimia nervosa: A community-based case-control study. *Archives of General Psychiatry*, **54**, 509–517.

Fichter, M.M. and Noegel, R., 1990. Concordance for bulimia nervosa in twins. *Int. J. Eating Disorders*, **9**, 255–263.

Fornari, V., Kaplan, M., Sandberg, D.E., Matthews, M., Skolnick, N. and Katz, J.L.L., 1992. Depressive and anxiety disorders in anorexia nervosa and bulimia nervosa. *International Journal of Eating Disorders*, **12**, 21–29.

Garfinkel, P.E., Moldofsky, H. and Garner, D.M., 1980. The heterogeneity of anorexia nervosa. *Archives of General Psychiatry*, **37**, 1036–1040.

Garner, D.M., 1993. Pathogenesis of anorexia nervosa. *Lancet*, **341**, 1631–1635.

Gorwood, P., Bouvard, M., Mouren-Simeoni, M.C., Kipman, A. and Ades, J., 1998. Genetics and anorexia nervosa: a review of candidate genes. *Psychiatric Genetics*, **8**, 1–12.

Grice, D.E., Berrettini, W.H., Halmi, K.A., Fichter, M., Strober, M., Woodside, D.B., Treasure, J., Kaplan, A.S., Magistretti, P.J., Goldman, D. and Kaye, W.H., submitted. Genome-wide affected relative pair analysis of anorexia nervosa.

Han, L., Nielson, D.A., Rosenthal, N.E., Jefferson, K., Kaye, W., Murphy, D., Altemus, M., Humphries, J., Casssano, G., Rotondo, A., Virkkhunen, M., Linnoila, M. and Goldman, D., 1999. No coding variant of the tryptophan hydroxylase gene detected in seasonal affective disorder, obsessive–compulsive disorder, anorexia nervosa, and alcoholism. *Biological Psychiatry*, **45**(5), 615–619.

Hinney, A., Barth, N., Ziegler, A., von-Prittwitz, S., Hamann, A., Hennighausen, K., Pirke, K.M., Heils, A., Rosenkranze, K., Roth, H., Coners, H., Mayer, H., Herzog, W., Siegfried, A., Lehmkuhl, G., Poustka, F., Schmidt, M.H., Schafer, H., Grzeschik, K.H., Lesch, K.P., Lentes, K.U., Remschmidt, H. and Hebebrand, J., 1997a. Serotonin transporter gene-linked polymorphic region: allele distributions in relationship to body weight and in anorexia nervosa. *Life Sciences*, **61**(21), 295–303.

Hinney, A., Bornscheuer, A., Depenbusch, M., Mierke, B., Tolle, A., Middeke, K., Ziegler, A., Roth, H., Schmidt, M.H., Hermann, H., Herpetz-Dahlmann, B.M., Fichter, M., Remschmidt, H. and Hebebrand, J., 1998. No evidence for involvement of the leptin gene in anorexia nervosa, bulimia nervosa, underweight or early onset extreme obesity: identification of two novel mutations in the coding sequence and a novel polymorphism in the leptin gene linked upstream region. *Molecular Psychiatry*, **3**(6), 539–543.

Hinney, A., Herrmann, H., Lohr, T., Rosenkranz, K., Ziegler, A., Lehmkuhl, G., Poustka, R., Schmidt, M.H., Mayer, H., Siegfried, W., Remschmidt, H. and Hebebrand, J., 1999a. No evidence for involvement of alleles of polymorphisms in the serotonin 1Dbeta and 7 receptor genes in obesity, underweight or anorexia nervosa. *International Journal of Obesity and Related Metabolic Disorders*, **23**(7), 760–763.

Hinney, A., Lentes, K.U., Rosenkranz, K., Barth, N., Roth, H., Ziegler, A., Hennighausen, K., Coners, H., Wurmers, H., Jacob, K., Romer, G., Winnikes, U., Mayer, H., Herzog, W., Lehmkuhl, G., Poustka, F., Schmidt, M.H., Blum, W.F., Pirke, K.M., Schafer, H., Grzeschik, K.H., Remschmidt, H. and Hebebrand, J., 1997c. Beta 3-adrenergic-receptor allele distributions in children, adolescents and young adults with obesity, underweight or anorexia nervosa. *International Journal of Obesity and Related Metabolic Disorders*, **21**(3), 224–230.

Hinney, A., Schmidt, A., Nottebom, K., Heibult, O., Becker, I., Ziegler, A., Gerber, G., Sina, M., Gorg, T., Mayer, H., Siegfried, W., Fichter, M., Remschmidt, H. and Hebebrand, J., 1999c. Several mutations in the melanocorton-4 receptor gene including a nonsense and a frameshift mutation associated with dominantly inherited obesity in humans. *Journal of Clinical Endocrinology and Metabolism*, **84**(4), 1483–1486.

Hinney, A., Schneider, J., Ziegler, A., Lehmkuhl, G., Poustka, F., Schmidt, M.H., Mayer, H., Siegfried, W., Remschmidt, H. and Hebebrand, J., 1999b. No evidence for involvement of polymorphisms of the dopamine D4 receptor gene in anorexia nervosa, underweight, and obesity. *American Journal of Medical Genetics*, **88**(6), 594–597.

Hinney, A., Ziegler, A., Nothen, M.M., Remschmidt, H. and Hebebrand, J., 1997b. 5-HT2A receptor gene polymorphisms, anorexia nervosa, and obesity. *Lancet*, **350**, 1324–1325.

Holderness, C.C., Brooks-Gunn, J. and Warren, W.P., 1994. Co-morbidity of eating disorders and substance abuse: Review of the literature. *International Journal of Eating Disorders*, **16**, 1–34.

Holland, A.J., Hall, A., Murray, R., Russell, G.F.M. and Crisp, A.H., 1984. Anorexia nervosa: a study of 34 twin pairs. *British Journal of Psychiatry*, **145**, 414–419.

Holland, A.J., Sicotte, N. and Treasure, J., 1988. Anorexia nervosa: evidence for a genetic basis. *Journal of Psychosomatic Research*, **32**, 561–571.

Hsu, L.K.G., Chesler, B.E. and Santhouse, R., 1990. Bulimia nervosa in eleven sets of twins: A clinical report. *International Journal of Eating Disorders*, **9**, 275–282.

Kaye, W.H., Lilenfeld, L.R.R., Berrettini, W.H., Strober, M., Devlin, B., Klump, K.L., Goldman, D., Bulik, C.M., Halmi, K.A., Fichter, M.M., Kaplan, A., Woodside, D.B., Treasure, J., Plotnicov, K.H., Pollice, C., Rao, R. and McConaha, C., 2000. A search for susceptibility loci for anorexia nervosa: methods and sample description. *Biological Psychiatry*, **47**, 794–803.

Kaye, W.H., Lilenfeld, L.R., Plotnikov, K., Merikangas, K.R., Nagy, L., Strober, M., Bulik, C.M., Moss, H. and Greeno, C.G., 1996. Bulimia nervosa and substance dependence: association and family transmission. *Alcoholism, Clinical & Experimental Research*, **20**, 878–881.

Keck, P.E., Pope, H.G., Hudson, J.L., McElroy, S.L., Yurgelun-Todd, D. and Hundert, E.M., 1990. A controlled study of phenomenology and family history in outpatients with bulimia nervosa. *Comprehensive Psychiatry*, **31**, 275–283.

Keel, P.K., Klump, K.L., Miller, K.B., McGue, M. and Iacono, W.G. (submitted). Shared transmission of eating disorders and comorbid disorders.

Kendler, K.S., MacLean, C., Neale, M.C., Kessler, R.C., Heath, A.C. and Eaves, L.J., 1991. The genetic epidemiology of bulimia nervosa. *American Journal of Psychiatry*, **148**, 1627–1635.

Kendler, K.S., Walters, E.E., Neale, M.C., Kessler, R., Heath, A. and Eaves, L., 1995. The structure of genetic and environmental risk factors for six major psychiatric disorders in women. *Archives of General Psychiatry*, **52**, 374–383.

Kidd, K.K., 1993. Associations of disease with genetic markers: deja vu all over again. *American Journal of Medical Genetics*, **48**(2), 71–73.

Kleifield, E.I., Sunday, S., Hurt, S. and Halmi, K.A., 1994a. The Tridimensional Personality Questionnaire: An exploration of personality traits in eating disorders. *Journal of Psychiatric Research*, **28**(5), 413–423.

Kleifield, E.I., Sunday, S., Hurt, S. and Halmi, K.A., 1994b. The effects of depression and treatment on the Tridimensional Personality Questionnaire. *Biological Psychiatry*, **36**, 68–70.

Klump, K.L., Bulik, C.M., Pollice, C., Halmi, K.H., Fichter, M.M., Berrettini, W.H., Devlin, B., Strober, M., Kaplan, A., Woodside, D.B., Treasure, J., Shabbout, M., Lilenfeld, L.R.R., Plotnicov, K.H. and Kaye, W.H., 2000. Temperament and character in women with anorexia nervosa. *Journal of Nervous and Mental Disease*, **188**(9), 559–567.

Klump, K.L., Kaye, W.H., Plotnicov, K., Pollice, C. and Rao, R., 1999. Familial transmission of personality traits in women with anorexia nervosa and their first-degree relatives. Poster presented at the Academy for Eating Disorders Annual Meeting, San Diego, California.

Klump, K.L., McGue, M. and Iacono, W.G., in press. Genetic relationships between personality and disordered eating. *Journal of Abnormal Psychology*.

Klump, K.L., McGue, M. and Iacono, W.G., 2000. Age differences in genetic and environmental influences on eating attitudes and behaviors in preadolescent and adolescent Twins. *Journal of Abnormal Psychology*, **109**(2), 239–251.

Klump, K.L., McGue, M. and Iacono, W.G., in press. Differential heritability of eating pathology in pre-pubertal versus pubertal twins. *International Journal of Eating Disorders*.

Klump, K.L., Miller, K.B., Keel, P.K., Iacono, W.G and McGue, M., in press. Genetic and environmental influences on anorexia nervosa syndromes in a population-based twin sample. *Psychological Medicine*.

Lander, E.S. and Schork, N.J., 1994. Genetic dissection of complex traits. *Science*, **265**(5181), 2037–2048.

Lilenfeld, L.R., Kaye, W.H., Greeno, C.G., Merikangas, K.R., Plotnicov, K., Pollice, K., Rao, R., Strober, M., Bulik, C.M. and Nagy, L., 1998. A controlled family study of anorexia nervosa and bulimia nervosa: Psychiatric disorders in first-degree relatives and effects of proband comorbidity. *Archives of General Psychiatry*, **55**, 603–610.

Lilenfeld, L.R.R., Stein, D., Bulik, C.M., Strober, M., Plotnicov, K., Pollice, C., Rao, R., Merikangas, K.R., Nagy, L. and Kaye, W.H., 2000. Personality traits among currently eating disordered, recovered and never ill first-degree female of bulimic and control women. *Psychological Medicine*, **30**, 1399–1410.

Martin, N., Boomsma, D. and Machin, G., 1997. A twin-pronged attack on complex traits. *Nature Genetics*, **17**, 387–392.

Miller, K.B., Klump, K.L., Keel, P.K., McGue, M. and Iacono, W.G., 1998. A population-based twin study of anorexia and bulimia nervosa: Heritability and shared transmission with anxiety disorders. Paper presented at the Eating Disorder Research Society Meeting, Boston, MA.

Mitchell, J.E., Hatsukami, D., Pyle, R.L. and Eckert, E.D., 1986. The bulimia syndrome: course of illness and associated problems. *Comprehensive Psychiatry*, **27**, 165–170.

Mussell, M., Mitchell, J., Fenna, C., Crosby, R., Miller, J. and Hoberman, H.M., 1997. A comparison of onset of binge eating versus dieting in the development of bulimia nervosa. *International Journal of Eating Disorders*, **21**, 353–360.

Nacmias, B., Ricca, V., Tedde, A., Mezzani, B., Rotella, C.M. and Sorbi, S., 1999. 5-HT2A receptor gene polymorphisms in anorexia and bulimia nervosa. *Neuroscience Letters*, **277**(2), 134–136.

Neale, M. and Kendler, K., 1995. Models of comorbidity for multifactorial disorders. *American Journal of Human Genetics*, **57**, 935–953.

O'Dwyer, A.M., Lucey, J.V. and Russell, G.F.M., 1996. Serotonin activity in anorexia nervosa after long-term weight restoration: Response to d-fenfluramine challenge. *Psychological Medicine*, **26**(2), 353–360.

Risch, N. and Merikangas, K., 1996. The future of genetic studies of complex human diseases. *Science*, **273**, 1516–1517; Erratum, 1997, 1275, 1329–1330.

Risch, N. and Zhang, H., 1996. Mapping quantitative trait loci with extreme discordant sib pairs: sampling considerations. *American Journal of Human Genetics*, **58**, 836–843.

Roberts, S.B., MacLean, C.J., Neale, M.C., Eaves, L.J. and Kendler, K.S., 1999. Replication of linkage studies of complex traits: an examination of variation in location estimates. *American Journal of Human Genetics*, **65**(3), 876–884.

Rosenkranz, K., Hinney, A., Ziegler, A., Hermann, H., Fichter, M., Mayer, H., Siegfried, W., Young, J.K., Remschmidt, H. and Hebebrand, J., 1998. Systematic mutation screening of the estrogen receptor beta gene in probands of different weight extremes: identification of several genetic variants. *Journal of Clinical Endocrinology and Metabolism*, **83**(12), 4524–4527.

Rosenkranz, K., Hinney, A., Ziegler, A., von-Prittwitz, S., Barth, N., Roth, H., Mayer, H. and Siegfried, W., 1998. Screening for mutations in the neuropeptide Y Y5 receptor gene in cohorts belonging to different weight extremes. *International Journal of Obesity and Related Metabolic Disorders*, **22**(2), 157–163.

Rutherford, J., McGuffin, P., Katz, R.J. and Murray, R.M., 1993. Genetic influences on eating attitudes in a normal female twin pair population. *Psychological Medicine*, **23**, 425–436.

Schuckit, M.A., Tipp, J.E., Anthenall, R.M., Bucholz, K.K., Hesselbrock, V.M. and Nurnberger, J.I., 1996. Anorexia nervosa and bulimia nervosa in alcohol-dependent men and women and their relatives. *American Journal of Psychiatry*, **153**, 74–82.

Sham, P., 1998. *Statistics in Human Genetics*. Arnold, London.

Sorbi, S., Nacmias, B., Tedde, A., Ricca, V., Mezzani, B. and Rotella, C.M., 1998. 5-HT2A promoter polymorphis in anorexia nervosa. *Lancet*, **351**, 1785.

Strober, M. and Bulik, C.M., in press. The genetic epidemiology of eating disorders. In: Fairburn, C. and Brownell, K. (eds), *Eating Disorders and Obesity: A Comprehensive Handbook (2nd Edition)*. Guilford Press, New York.

Strober, M., Freeman, R., Lampert, C., Diamond, J. and Kaye, W.H., 2000. Controlled family study of anorexia and bulimia nervosa: Evidence of shared liability and transmission of partial syndromes. *American Journal of Psychiatry*, **157**(3), 393–400.

Strober, M., Freeman, R. and Morrell, W., 1997. The long-term course of severe anorexia nervosa in adolescents: Survival analysis of recovery, relapse, and outcome predictors over 10–15 years in a prospective study. *International Journal of Eating Disorders*, **22**(4), 339–360.

Strober, M., Lampert, C., Morrell, W., Burroughs, J. and Jacobs, C., 1990. A controlled family study of anorexia nervosa: evidence of familial aggregation and lack of shared transmission with affective disorders. *International Journal of Eating Disorders*, **9**, 239–253.

Stunkard, A.J., Harris, J.R., Pedersen, N.L. and McClearn, G.E., 1990. The body-mass index of twins who have been reared apart. *New England Journal of Medicine*, **322**, 1483–1487.

Sullivan, P.F., Bulik, C.M. and Kendler, K.S., 1998. Genetic epidemiology of binging and vomiting. *British Journal of Psychiatry*, **173**, 75–79.

Tellegen, A., Lykken, D.T., Bouchard, T.J., Wilcox, K.J., Segal, N.L. and Rich, S., 1988. Personality similarity in twins reared apart and together. *Journal of Social and Personality Psychology*, **54**, 1031–1039.

Treasure, J. and Campbell, I., 1994. The case for biology in the aetiology of anorexia nervosa. *Psychological Medicine*, **24**, 3–8.

Treasure, J. and Holland, A., 1990. Genetic vulnerability to eating disorders: Evidence from twin and family studies. In: Remschmidt, H. and Schmidt, M.H. (eds), *Child and Youth Psychiatry: European Perspectives*. Hogrefe & Huber, Lewiston, NY.

Wade, T.D., Bulik, C.M., Neale, M. and Kendler, K.S., 2000. Anorexia nervosa and major depression: An examination of shared genetic and environmental risk factors. *American Journal of Psychiatry*, **157**, 469–471.

Wade, T., Martin, N.G. and Tiggeman, M., 1998. Genetic and environmental risk factors for the weight and shape concerns characteristic of bulimia nervosa. *Psychological Medicine*, **28**, 761–771.

Wade, T., Martin, N.G., Neale, M.C., Tiggemann, M., Treloar, S.A., Bucholz, K.K., Madden, P.A. and Heath, A.C., 1999. The structure of genetic and environmental risk factors for three measures of disordered eating. *Psychological Medicine*, **29**(4), 925–934.

Walters, E.E. and Kendler, K.S., 1995. Anorexia nervosa and anorexic-like syndromes in a population-based female twin sample. *American Journal of Psychiatry*, **152**, 64–71.

Walters, E.E., Neale, M.C., Eaves, L.J., Heath, A.C., Kessler, R.C. and Kendler, K.S., 1992. Bulimia nervosa and major depression: a study of common genetic and environmental factors. *Psychological Medicine*, **22**, 617–622.

Ward, A., Brown, N., Lightman, S., Campbell, I.C. and Treasure, J., 1998. Neuroendocrine, appetitive, and behavioural responses to d-fenfluramine in women recovered from anorexia nervosa. *British Journal of Psychiatry*, **172**, 351–358.

Ziegler, A. and Gorg, T., 1999. 5-HT2A gene promotor polymorphism and anorexia nervosa. *Lancet*, **353**, 929.

Ziegler, A., Hebebrand, J., Gorg, T., Rosenkranz, K., Fichter, M.M., Herpertz-Dahlmann, B., Remschmidt, H. and Hinney, A., 1999. Further lack of association between the 5-HT2A gene promoter polymorphism and susceptibility to eating disorders and a meta-analysis pertaining to anorexia nervosa. *Molecular Psychiatry*, **4**(5), 410–412.

XXIII-10

The Therapeutic Armamentarium in Eating Disorders

James E. Mitchell, Scott Crow, Tricia Cook Myers and Steve Wonderlich

INTRODUCTION

In this paper we will briefly summarize the available literature on the empirically tested treatments for patients suffering from eating disorders. We will address the traditional eating disorders of anorexia nervosa and bulimia nervosa, and will also include binge-eating disorder, a condition included as an example of 'eating disorders — not otherwise specified' in the DSM-IV as a disorder for further study. We focus on treatments that have been shown to be effective in randomized trials, but include other clinical information when it appears relevant and necessary to the reader's understanding of that particular area.

In perusing this text, many readers will notice several trends that typify this literature. First and of greatest clinical concern, the reader will notice the relative paucity of literature on the treatment of patients with anorexia nervosa, despite the fact that anorexia nervosa was the first identified eating disorder and clearly is the most severe, with a significant well-documented risk for morbidity and mortality. There are a number of factors that have contributed to the relative lack of research in this area, including the following: (1) anorexia nervosa is a relatively rare condition and it is difficult for individual treatment centres to acquire the necessary number of subjects to complete randomized trials; (2) patients with anorexia nervosa, by virtue of their illness, many times are not particularly motivated to be cooperative with treatment and therefore it is difficult for them to be compliant with research treatment protocols; (3) when initially seen many patients with anorexia nervosa are critically ill, and require a multiplicity of interventions (e.g., medical stabilization, occasionally hospitalization, family involvement, individual counselling, medication management) which markedly complicates the ability of researchers to design clinical trials which adequately control for all of these variables; (4) anorexia nervosa patients are often quite difficult to treat, again given the nature of their illness, and this undoubtedly dissuades many potential investigators from pursuing work in this area. All of these factors have contributed to what currently is an apparent and quite worrisome lack of knowledge regarding the best treatments for patients with this disorder.

Second, readers of this text will probably also notice that although the treatment literature on bulimia nervosa is better developed, this entire literature has been published in the last 20 years. This is attributable to the fact that bulimia nervosa was only first identified as a discrete diagnostic entity in 1979 (Russell, 1979) and randomized clinical trials were first implemented several years after that.

Third, readers may notice that the literature on binge-eating disorder is also quite limited. This again is attributable to the fact that binge-eating disorder was only described in its current form in the DSM-IV, which was published in 1994. At that time there were little data regarding this group of patients, and our current understanding of this disorder has developed since then.

Fourth, an observation that may strike some readers as surprising is the finding that psychotherapy plays a clearly important and, in some cases, central role in the treatment of patients with eating disorders. The reader is therefore reminded that psychological interventions that result in psychological changes often result in corollary changes in the underlying biology, and therefore discussions of such therapies in a text on biological psychiatry is quite appropriate.

We turn now to the treatment literature on these three conditions.

Pharmacotherapy of Bulimia Nervosa

The pharmacotherapy of bulimia nervosa can be conveniently divided into three areas: (1) antidepressant trials, which have employed a variety of types of agents using various experimental designs ranging from acute treatment studies to relapse prevention studies; (2) studies examining the utility of non-antidepressant pharmacological approaches — none of which have been definitive, but several of which are interesting and show promise; and (3) a handful of studies regarding the relative efficacy of pharmacotherapy and psychotherapy for patients with bulimia nervosa.

Antidepressant Therapy of Bulimia Nervosa

Early in the course of our understanding of bulimia nervosa, research groups studying this condition noted that many of the patients were depressed (Russell, 1979). Based on this observation, it was hypothesized that patients might be better able to control their bulimic symptoms if their depression were treated. Some researchers even went so far as to hypothesize that bulimia nervosa might be a variant of affective disorders, although few would endorse such a model currently (Pope *et al.*, 1983).

Given this background, a number of antidepressants were tried. Following the initial observation that tricyclic and MAO inhibitors both seemed beneficial for these patients, a series of randomized treatment trials were undertaken. These studies are summarized in Table XXIII-10.1, and as can be seen the list has grown rather lengthy. In examining these studies, several issues emerge. First, the number of compounds studied and the classes of compounds studied (e.g., MAOIs, tricyclics, SSRIs) is large but not exhaustive. Second, the sample size in most of the studies has been modest, the exceptions being the large multicentre studies involving fluoxetine that were funded by Eli Lilly, who subsequently sought and received FDA approval to market fluoxetine for bulimia nervosa in the US. Third, although not illustrated, there is a great deal of variability in response rates to placebo. This probably speaks to a number of issues, one of which is the lack of standardization of the protocols for administering agents in this population, a problem we have discussed previously in the literature (Mitchell *et al.*, 2000). Fourth, the reductions in the frequencies of target eating behaviours

Biological Psychiatry: Edited by H. D'haenen, J.A. den Boer and P. Willner. ISBN 0-471-49198-5

Table XXIII-10.1 Placebo-controlled antidepressant trials for bulimia nervosa

Reference	N	Duration (weeks)	Treatment	Outcome ↓ BE (%)	Outcome AB (%)
Pope *et al.*, 1983	36	8	Imipramine		0
Sabine *et al.*, 1983	19	8	Mianserin		
Mitchell and Groat, 1984	32	8	Amitriptyline	72	19
Hughes *et al.*, 1986	22	6	Desipramine	91	68
Agras *et al.*, 1987	22	16	Imipramine	72	30
Horne *et al.*, 1988	81	8	Bupropion	67	30
Barlow *et al.*, 1988	24	6	Desipramine	4	
Blouin *et al.*, 1988	10	6	Desipramine	45*	
Kennedy *et al.*, 1988	18	13	Isocarboxazid		33
Walsh *et al.*, 1988	50	12	Phelelzine	64	35
Pope *et al.*, 1989	42	4	Trazadone	31	10
Fichter *et al.*, 1991	40	35 (days)	Fluoxetine	**	
Kennedy *et al.*, 1993	36	8	Brofaromine	62	
FBNC, 1992	387	12	Fluoxetine	67	
Goldstein *et al.*, 1995	398	16	Fluoxetine	50	
Romano, 1999	150	52	Fluoxetine	**	

*Vomiting frequency;
**Relapse prevention trials.

are generally large and consistently superior to those seen with placebo. Fifth, despite this finding, the majority of subjects treated with these agents are not free of symptoms at the end of treatment, a particularly worrisome finding given the fact that research suggests that subjects who are not abstinent at the end of treatment may subsequently relapse to a more severe syndrome.

A few other studies have addressed relapse prevention (Walsh *et al.*, 1991; Fichter *et al.*, 1996; Romano, 1999), and indeed the data suggest that there is clearly an effect for drug therapy, although findings in these studies are also discouraging in that some patients relapse on medication, and a high dropout rate occurs at long-term follow-up, suggesting that the maintenance of patients on drug therapy, even if their initial response is favourable, may be difficult to accomplish.

Given these limitations, the agent that has been studied in the largest number of clinical trials is fluoxetine hydrochloride, and of particular importance clinically, the first multicentre trial demonstrated superiority for 60 mg over 20 mg in the treatment of bulimia nervosa (FBNC, 1992). The second multicentre treatment study (Goldstein *et al.*, 1995) and the relapse prevention trial (Romano, 1999) both employed 60 mg as an initial dosage. This suggests that subjects can either be started at this dosage or should have the dosage fairly rapidly escalated to this dosage to achieve optimal results.

Although such data cannot be easily summarized, studies using antidepressants have also demonstrated significant improvement on other variables such as mood, anxiety, and measures of core psychopathology as measured by various instruments. Therefore, the drugs do not appear just to suppress the core symptoms of binge eating and vomiting, but appear to have more global effects on the syndrome.

Accompanying this growing literature has been a growing acceptance of pharmacotherapy on the part of non-medical mental health practitioners and on the part of patients. While there was initial resistance on the part of health care professionals in the early 1980s to refer patients for pharmacotherapy, and while many patients were very resistant to the idea of drug treatment, most therapists now appreciate the worth of this approach, and not uncommonly patients seek treatment with pharmacotherapy.

Other Pharmacotherapies for Bulimia Nervosa

A variety of other agents have been tried, some for intriguing theoretical reasons. Phenytoin was tried for bulimia nervosa following the observation that a group of patients with binge-eating behaviour had abnormal electroencephalograms (Green and Rau, 1974), although subsequent studies have failed to find an exaggerated rate of EEG abnormalities in patients with bulimia nervosa (Mitchell, Hosfield and Pyle, 1983). The results of this study were ambiguous, yet surprisingly no attempt has been made to further examine the utility of this agent (Wermuth *et al.*, 1977).

Narcotic antagonists were used following the observation that the endogenous opioid system is involved in the modulation of feeding, particularly stress-induced and hedonically driven feeding in various animal models (de Zwaan and Mitchell, 1992). While some early work using short acting narcotic antagonists suggested positive effects (Jonas and Gold, 1986, 1987), randomized treatment trials at usually applied dosages have failed to find evidence of efficacy (Ingoin-Apfelbaum and Apfelbaum, 1987; Mitchell *et al.*, 1989), while open-label trials employing higher doses, which can only be used if one is willing to accept the risk of possible hepatotoxicity, suggested positive effects (Jonas and Gold, 1988). Given the current state of knowledge, until non-hepatotoxic agents are available, narcotic antagonists cannot be recommended as treatment, although their utility as adjunctive agents in other situations at usual doses could reasonably be explored.

d-Fenfluramine was not found to be particularly useful (Russell *et al.*, 1988; Fahy, Eisler and Russell, 1993). However, this compound has been shown subsequently to cause valvular heart disease (Cannistra and Gaasch, 1999). This is a moot point now, given the removal of both fenfluramine and d-fenfluramine from the market secondary to drug-induced valvular dysfunction.

A report demonstrating the efficacy of ondansetron, marketed as an anti-nauseant, over placebo in a randomized clinical trial recently appeared (Hartman *et al.*, 1997). The results are interesting theoretically but the magnitude of the improvement was not in excess of those achieved in trials finding modest benefits with antidepressants.

Psychotherapy of Bulimia Nervosa

Since the early 1980s numerous studies have investigated the efficacy of psychotherapy for bulimia nervosa. Cognitive-behavioural therapy (CBT) has been shown to be more beneficial than placebo antidepressant medication (Whittal, Agras and Gould, 1999) in the treatment of bulimia nervosa. Randomized trials indicate that CBT is superior to both support groups and wait-list controls (Lacey, 1983; Lee and Rush, 1986; Leitenberg *et al.*, 1988; Agras *et al.*, 1989). CBT has also been shown to be as effective or more effective than non-directive (Kirkley *et al.*, 1985), short-term focal (Fairburn *et al.*, 1986), supportive–expressive (Garner *et al.*, 1993), and supportive non-directive therapies (Walsh *et al.*, 1997). In fact most controlled treatment research to date has supported CBT as the psychotherapy of choice in the treatment of bulimia nervosa.

Recently, however, there has been some evidence that a therapy that does not specifically address the bulimic behaviours may be as effective as CBT in decreasing bulimic symptoms. Specifically, interpersonal therapy (IPT), originally developed as a treatment for depression (Klerman *et al.*, 1984), may also be efficacious for the treatment of bulimia nervosa. Fairburn and colleagues (1991) compared CBT, behavioural therapy and a therapy that contained many elements of IPT and concluded that although CBT was most helpful in reducing bulimic symptoms at the end of treatment, at one- and six-year follow-up IPT and CBT were found to be equally effective. More recently, a multicentre study replicated this finding using IPT in its originally developed form (Agras *et al.*, 2000).

CBT and IPT differ in some significant ways. CBT addresses eating-related thoughts and behaviours and can be divided into three stages. The first stage focuses on education about the cognitive model of bulimia nervosa, which proposes that bulimic behaviours are maintained by weight and shape-related thoughts and attitudes, and specific behavioural techniques such as self-monitoring, regular eating, alternative behaviours and weekly weighings. The second stage continues to address these behavioural techniques; however, the main emphasis is on restructuring faulty cognitions and increasing problem solving skills. Additionally, this stage of treatment may also address low self-esteem, if applicable. Relapse prevention is the focus of the final stage of treatment.

CBT appears to be effectively delivered in both individual and group formats with a typical treatment length of 20 sessions. There appears to be considerable benefit to asking the patient to attend sessions twice per week during the first month of treatment, after which sessions are held on a weekly basis. CBT can also include, or be augmented with some form of dietary counseling. Lastly, there is evidence that CBT can be effectively delivered in the form of self-help manuals when guided by a non-specialist (Cooper, 1994; Waller *et al.*, 1996).

IPT, on the other hand, concentrates on current interpersonal functioning and tends to eschew issues related to eating problems and weight. During the initial phase of IPT treatment, interpersonal problems associated with the eating disorder are identified with the remainder of the therapy sessions geared toward resolving these interpersonal deficits.

One drawback of all treatments for bulimia nervosa, including antidepressant medication, is the low rate of abstinence from bulimic behaviour at the end of treatment. Another problem is the unavailability of empirically supported psychotherapies for those with bulimia nervosa due to lack of psychotherapist training (Mussell *et al.*, 2000). In addition, there is evidence that if a patient hasn't responded to CBT by the sixth session, she is unlikely to improve with additional sessions of CBT (Agras *et al.*, 2000).

These concerns have prompted researchers to begin to examine alternative approaches, such as stepped care models of treatment. Although controlled trials have supported the use of CBT and, in two studies, IPT, in the treatment of bulimia nervosa, the majority of psychotherapists are not trained to deliver such treatments. Stepped care models have arisen due to this growing disparity between research and practice. Given that supervised CBT self-help manuals and antidepressant medication are more readily available than full CBT, they seem to be appropriate first line interventions. Full CBT could then be offered to those individuals who fail to respond to these initial interventions. A study examining this approach is currently underway.

Pharmacotherapy vs Psychotherapy in the Treatment of Bulimia Nervosa

Given the growing literature on the efficacy of antidepressant treatments for bulimia nervosa, as well as the growing literature on the efficacy of various forms of psychotherapy, one logical step was to compare the relative efficacy of each approach versus the efficacy of the combination of these approaches. Five such studies have been published. In an initial trial comparing imipramine to intensive outpatient cognitive-behavioural group psychotherapy to the combination, clear superiority was found for CBT, with evidence of greater improvement on some variables (e.g., depression and anxiety) when active medication was added (Mitchell *et al.*, 1990). A second trial utilizing desipramine and individual CBT found similar results with added benefit on some variables (e.g., dietary restraint) with the combination (Agras *et al.*, 1992). Two studies are difficult to interpret because of a high dropout rate during treatment and a high dropout rate to follow-up (Leitenberg *et al.*, 1994; Goldbloom, Olmsted and Davis, 1996). The fifth study employed the most sophisticated design. Published by Walsh *et al.* (1997), the study involved randomization of outpatient bulimia nervosa subjects to one of five treatment cells: (a) medication management, which involved treatment with desipramine followed by treatment with fluoxetine if abstinence was not achieved; (b) and (c) treatment with individual cognitive-behavioural therapy with medication management or placebo; and (d) and (e) treatment with a control psychotherapy condition — supportive psychotherapy — with medication management or placebo.

The results showed that CBT was superior to supportive psychotherapy, and medication management was superior to placebo. In a *post-hoc* analysis, the best results overall were achieved using both medication management and CBT.

In summary, the literature on psychotherapy versus drug therapy versus combined treatment suggests that CBT is clearly superior to drug therapy alone, and arguments can be made for using the combination, particularly among patients who are depressed at baseline.

Pharmacotherapy of Binge-Eating Disorder

There are both similarities and differences in the state of our knowledge concerning the pharmacologic treatment of bulimia nervosa and binge-eating disorder. On the one hand, many of the trials conducted using subjects with binge-eating disorder thus far have been informed by previous work in bulimia nervosa. Often the same agents have been employed (for example, SSRIs and desipramine). Similarly, the major focus of treatment has been on the diminishment of binge-eating frequency as the major outcome variable. Much as with bulimia nervosa, the attendant symptoms have received less focus. One point of departure from the treatment of bulimia nervosa involves the issue of weight. The majority of individuals with binge-eating disorder have body mass indices that would currently be classified as overweight or obese, and presumably are at increased risk for the medical morbidity and mortality typically associated with obesity. Previous work suggests that binge eating may or may not be a predictor of poor outcome in weight loss therapy and of weight regain after treatment (Ho *et al.*, 1995; Hsu, Betancourt and Sullivan, 1996; McGuire *et al.*, 1999; Sherwood, Jeffery and Wing, 1999). However, most overweight or obese individuals seeking treatment for binge-eating disorder are very interested in losing weight, so treatments which result in control of binge eating but not weight loss are relatively disappointing to them. Therefore, it appears that successful treatment of those with binge-eating disorder would include the successful treatment of their weight problem as well.

Most of the drug trials completed to date have involved antidepressants, with the SSRIs being used most commonly (Marcus *et al.*, 1990; McCann and Agras, 1990; Alger *et al.*, 1991; de Zwaan, Nutinger and Schonbeck, 1992; Stunkard *et al.*, 1996; Hudson *et al.*, 1998; McElroy *et al.*, 2000). These studies have reported outcomes in terms of both binge-eating frequency and weight loss, but have targeted the issue of weight loss to varying degrees. Trials involving desipramine, fenfluramine, fluvoxamine, and sertraline have all found greater decreases in binge eating and greater rates of abstinence at the end of treatment in drug-treated patients compared to those receiving placebo. On the other hand, trials of fluoxetine and imipramine have been negative in terms of binge-eating outcome.

Only three studies, Marcus *et al.* (1990), using fluoxetine, Hudson *et al.* (1998), using fluvoxamine, and McElroy *et al.* (2000), using sertraline, have shown active drug to produce more weight loss than placebo. In the Marcus *et al.* fluoxetine trial, which was lengthy (approximately one year), there was substantially more weight loss in the active drug group (13.9 kg vs 0.6 kg). Most of the weight loss occurred early in the trial, and subjects appeared to reach a plateau. Additionally, after the end of treatment, fluoxetine patients experienced fairly prompt regain of lost weight. In the fluvoxamine trial, although there was more weight loss in individuals receiving active drug, the difference between drug and placebo-treated patients was quite small (1.3 kg). In the sertraline trial, a weight loss of 5.6 kg occurred with active drug vs 2.4 kg with placebo.

Of historical note, there is one report of a trial of d-Fenfluramine in the treatment of binge-eating disorder (Stunkard *et al.*, 1996). Interestingly, d-Fenfluramine was superior to placebo in terms of binge-eating outcome, but there was no evidence for difference in weight loss over only eight weeks. However, d-Fenfluramine has been taken off the market in the United States.

Psychotherapy of Binge-Eating Disorder

A number of treatment studies targeting weight loss have examined the outcome for binge eating versus non-binge-eating obese subjects. The available studies are ambiguous as to whether or not obese binge eaters lose comparable amounts of weight as non-binge eaters in obesity treatment (Marcus *et al.*, 1988, 1990; Wadden, Foster and Letizia, 1992; de Zwaan, Mitchell and Mussell, 1992) but do suggest that abstinence from binge eating can be promoted by instituting a regimented diet (Yanovski, Gormally and Lese, 1994). In fact, these studies suggest that behavioural therapy in conjunction with dietary interventions for weight loss may be adequate to treat binge-eating disorder, at least in the short term. Because the presence of binge eating does not seem to increase dropout rates, it seems reasonable to include individuals with binge-eating disorder in weight management programs (Ho *et al.*, 1995).

Comorbid psychopathology is also common in individuals with binge-eating disorder. Therefore, another subset of studies has targeted binge eating as well as comorbid depression and anxiety. Initially, treatment manuals for bulimia nervosa were modified to address binge-eating disorder (e.g., Fairburn, 1995). Similar to treatment for bulimia nervosa, CBT for binge-eating disorder includes self-monitoring, stimulus control, alternative behaviours, and a pattern of regular eating, as well as cognitive restructuring, problem solving, and relapse prevention. These treatments successfully reduce the frequency of binge eating; however, weight reduction, a primary goal for many of these patients, has been modest at best with the cognitive-behavioural interventions (Wilfley *et al.*, 1993). As a result, many BED treatment approaches have been expanded to include a weight loss component. This subset of studies has incorporated sequential or concurrent treatment for obesity, binge eating and comorbid psychopathology.

In a series of studies (Agras *et al.*, 1995, 1997; Eldredge *et al.*, 1997), overweight participants were initially treated with 12 weeks of CBT. Participants who stopped binge eating then received weight loss therapy while those who continued to binge eat received IPT or additional sessions of CBT. The results showed that participants lost weight when treated with subsequent weight loss therapy and were still able to maintain abstinence from binge eating. Although there was no added benefit for treatment with subsequent IPT, a substantial number of participants who initially failed to reduce binge-eating frequency were successful with an extended course of CBT. At one-year follow-up those treated with CBT and weight loss therapy showed a 64% reduction in binge eating and a 33% abstinence rate. Those who were abstinent from binge eating were able to maintain a 4 kg weight loss while participants who were still binge eating gained an average of 3.6 kg.

Another study investigated the addition of CBT to the refeeding phase of a combined treatment of behavioural weight loss and VLCD for binge-eating obese (de Zwaan, Mitchell and Mussell, 1996). These authors found that although the acute treatment package was effective in reducing binge eating and in inducing weight loss, the addition of CBT did not prevent weight regain compared to the rate of regain in those not receiving CBT.

Cognitive-behavioural self-help manuals can also be beneficial for individuals with binge-eating disorder. When guided by a non-specialist, this type of therapy is cost-effective, timely, and may be less stigmatizing than traditional CBT. This method of treatment seems to be effective when guidance is provided via videotape and written instructions (Peterson *et al.*, 1998), or by telephone (Wells *et al.*, 1997), and in a face-to-face format (Carter and Fairburn, 1998).

In conclusion, the available evidence seems to support an integrated treatment of CBT and dietary intervention for optimum treatment of binge-eating disorder. Binge eating, weight loss and comorbid psychopathology should all be addressed. In addition, it may be appropriate to recommend guided self-help prior to implementing more formalized treatments, although this question needs further study.

Pharmacotherapy of Anorexia Nervosa

As noted above, relatively little information exists about effective pharmacologic strategies for the treatment of anorexia nervosa. We will review the limited number of controlled trials that have been conducted. In looking at this literature a few generalizations should be considered. First, a wide variety of different classes of agents have been tried. This undoubtedly reflects the difficult challenge of treating individuals with this illness, and the fact that most trials to date have been negative. Second, the outcome measures used to decide whether treatments are beneficial usually have been either weight gain or the maintenance of a relatively healthy body weight. As described elsewhere in this volume, fear of becoming fat, body image disturbance and perfectionism and obsessionality are critical core features of anorexia nervosa; addressing these problems in pharmacologic treatment seems a desirable and probably a necessary goal. Unfortunately, to date, these symptoms have received little attention in the controlled treatment literature. Third, anorexia nervosa is uniformly viewed as an illness needing long-term treatment, yet most of our knowledge to date is limited to short-term trials.

The placebo-controlled drug trials for anorexia nervosa that have been conducted are listed in Table XXIII-10.2. In contrast to bulimia nervosa, for which antidepressants are the most commonly tried agents, only a minority of trials have employed antidepressants. Typically, these trials have been conducted in individuals in intensive outpatient or inpatient treatment setting, with a goal of increasing body weight. To date, one study has shown support for the use of medication to aid short-term weight gain in subjects at low weight. That study (Halmi *et al.*, 1986) compared cyproheptadine in a dose of 32 mg per day, amitriptyline in a dose of 175 mg per day, and placebo over a short period. In that trial, the rates of weight gain with both active drugs exceeded that seen with placebo. Unfortunately, other trials of cyproheptadine (Vigersky and Loriaux, 1977; Goldberg *et al.*, 1979) and amitriptyline (Biederman *et al.*, 1985) have been negative. Similarly, in a small trial the antidepressant clomipramine was not more effective than placebo (Lacey and Crisp, 1980). Given the high rate of comorbidity between anorexia nervosa and obsessive–compulsive

Table XXIII-10.2 Placebo-controlled drug trials for anorexia nervosa

Reference	*N*	Duration (weeks)	Treatment	Outcome (weight gain vs placebo)
Virgersky and Loriaux, 1977	24	8	Cyproheptadine	No difference
Goldberg *et al.*, 1979	81	Variable	Cyproheptadine	No difference
Halmi *et al.*, 1986	72	4	Cyproheptadine	Cyproheptadine > placebo in rate of weight regain
Lacey and Crisp, 1980	16	Variable	Clomipramine	No difference
Gross *et al.*, 1981	16	4	Lithium	No difference
Biederman *et al.*, 1985	25	5	Amitriptyline	No difference
Halmi *et al.*, 1986	72	4	Amitriptyline	Amitriptyline > placebo in rate of weight regain
Vandereycken and Pierloot, 1982	18	6	Pimozide	No difference
Vandereycken, 1984	18	6	Sulpiride	No difference
Gross *et al.*, 1983	11	4	Tetrahydrocannabinol	No difference
Casper *et al.*, 1987	4	8	Clonidine	No difference
Stacher *et al.*, 1993	12	12	Cisapride	No difference

disorder, clomipramine would seem a logical choice; however, the dose (50 mg) was relatively low and might well have been subtherapeutic.

A wide range of other agents have been tried. These include lithium (Gross *et al.*, 1981), the antipsychotics pimozide (Vandereycken, and Pierloot, 1982) and sulpiride (Vandereycken, 1984), and drugs noted to increase appetite, tetrahydrocannabinol (Gross *et al.*, 1983) and clonidine (Casper, Schlemner and Javaid, 1987). In each case, active drug and placebo did not differ in efficacy. Finally, of historical note, cisapride was used in one trial (Stacher *et al.*, 1993). This agent was theoretically appealing given the symptoms of impaired intestinal motility among anorectic individuals, but this drug, too, was no more effective than placebo, and it has been taken off the market in the United States due to concerns about cardiovascular toxicity.

Another area of interest in the pharmacotherapy of anorexia nervosa involves the use of medications in individuals restored to a normal or near normal body weight, in an attempt to prevent relapse. One controlled trial has been reported thus far (Kaye, 1996). In this relapse prevention trial, subjects receiving active drug were less likely to relapse than those receiving placebo. The results of this trial are interesting in light of other work using fluoxetine in acutely ill, low weight anorectic individuals. In one double-blind, placebo-controlled protocol, fluoxetine in a dose of up to 60 mg per day did not differ from placebo in terms of weight gain or other measures in a series of inpatients (Attia *et al.*, 1998). Similarly, in a separate study, neither the short-term in-hospital course nor the long-term follow-up course of the group of anorectic patients was improved by the use of fluoxetine (Strober *et al.*, 1999). One potential explanation for these seemingly contradictory results could be that the efficacy of fluoxetine in anorexia nervosa may be highly dependent on the phase of the illness in which it is being used. The results of these trials seem to concur with the prevailing clinical opinion that when individuals are at very low weight, pharmacotherapy is unlikely to be effective. On the other hand, pharmacotherapy both for anorexia nervosa and perhaps for comorbid problems as well, appears to be more effective once weight has been restored.

Based on the results of these studies, pharmacotherapy for anorexia nervosa at this time is typically confined to one of two situations. The first is the use of medications, typically fluoxetine, in an attempt to maintain weight in weight-recovered individuals. Second, a variety of psychopharmacologic agents are used to provide the appropriate treatment for comorbid psychopathology.

Psychotherapy of Anorexia Nervosa

Despite the fact that anorexia nervosa has been studied for a long period of time, the number of empirical trials in patients in this population has been quite limited. Part of this reflects the difficulty in conducting trials in this area, as detailed in the introduction to this chapter. However, this situation is beginning to be remedied, in that the number of randomized trials which have recently appeared or which are now underway has increased dramatically, and one can only hope that the result of these studies will better inform our treatment of this group of patients, many of whom remain chronically ill, and some of whom die of the disorder.

One group of investigators that has been quite interested in examining various treatment methodologies for patients with anorexia nervosa includes Arthur Crisp and his colleagues at St. George's Hospital in London. In a series of publications, treatment techniques for anorexia nervosa have been examined (Hall and Crisp, 1987; Deeble *et al.*, 1990; Crisp *et al.*, 1999; Gowers *et al.*, 1994). This series of studies has documented that 'dietary advice' can be useful in inducing weight gain, compared to psychotherapy alone. Perhaps in the most controversial of these studies, 90 subjects with anorexia nervosa were randomly allocated to one of four treatment cells: inpatient treatment, assessment interview only, and one of two outpatient treatment cells. All three of the active treatment regimens resulted in improvement, and there appeared to be no significant advantage for the inpatient treatment program, despite the fact that the outpatient treatment programs offered were of relatively brief duration.

In another series of studies, Russell, Dare, Isler, and colleagues (for summaries please see Russell *et al.*, 1987; Eisler *et al.*, 1997) have sequentially examined different models of outpatient treatment for weight restored anorectic patients. In an initial study, these investigators found that family therapy was more effective for younger patients who had been ill for a briefer period of time, while the older more chronic patients did better with individual therapy. The second study, which included adult patients with anorexia nervosa who had been weight restored, found that family therapy was superior to individual psychoanalytic or individual supportive therapy. A third study found that a conjoint therapy approach, wherein patients were seen with their families, was less effective in inducing weight gain, but more effective in changing various psychological parameters, than family therapy where the patients and the family were each seen alone.

Another group of investigators has examined family therapy versus individual therapy with adolescents, employing either a behavioural family systems therapy approach or an ego-oriented individual therapy approach (Robin *et al.*, 1994, 1995, 1999). The results of these studies suggest that the behavioural family systems therapy produced greater overall weight gain and was more likely to be associated with resumption of menses; however, both treatments were effective in producing improvement in eating attitudes, depression and eating-related family conflict.

Also of note, a pilot study by Treasure *et al.* (1995) found that a group of adult anorexia nervosa patients reported subjectively greater improvement when treated with cognitive analytical treatment as opposed to educational behavioural treatment, but there were no differences in other outcome parameters. Most recently Geist *et al.* (2000) contrasted family therapy versus family psychoeducational treatment in 25 adolescents requiring hospitalization for eating disorders, and found no significant group differences, suggesting that both interventions appeared to be effective, in a study with a relatively small sample size.

Taken together, these studies indicate quite clearly that structured forms of psychotherapy appear to benefit patients with anorexia nervosa. The findings regarding inpatient versus outpatient treatment in the protocol by Crisp and colleagues are of concern, and seems to be in conflict with the clinical impression of many researchers in the field, and clearly needs to be replicated. Other work suggests that many patients, particularly younger patients, may benefit from family involvement.

DISCUSSION

Both pharmacotherapy and psychotherapy play a role in the treatment of all three eating disorders. Bulimia nervosa appears to respond optimally to treatment with CBT, with the possible addition of fluoxetine in those comorbidly depressed. Pharmacotherapy plays a more limited role in the treatment of anorexia nervosa, but is probably useful in preventing relapse is limited among those also receiving counselling. Our knowledge of the treatment of binge-eating disorder, although results to date suggest that interventions that target both weight loss and binge eating are most useful.

ACKNOWLEDGEMENTS

This work was supported in part by Grants R01-MH59100, R01-MH59674, and R01-MH/DK-58820 from the National Institute of Health and a Center Grant from the McKnight Foundation.

REFERENCES

Agras, W.S., Crow, S.J., Halmi, K.A., Mitchell, J.E., Wilson, G.T. and Kraemer, H.C., 2000. Outcome predictors for the cognitive behavior treatment of bulimia nervosa: Data from a multisite study. *Am. J. Psychiatry*, **157**, 1302–1308.

Agras, W.S., Dorian, B., Kirkley, B.G., Arnow, B. and Bachman, J., 1987. Imipramine in the study of bulimia: A double-blind, controlled study. *Int. J. Eat. Dis.*, **6**, 29–38.

Agras, W.S., Rossiter, E.M., Arnow, B., Schneider, J.A., Telch, C.F., Raeburn, S.D., Bruce, B., Perl, M. and Koran, L.M., 1992. Pharmacologic and cognitive-behavioral treatment for bulimia nervosa: A controlled comparison. *Am. J. Psychiatry*, **149**, 82–87.

Agras, W.S., Schneider, J.A., Arnow, B., Raeburn, S.D. and Telch, C.F., 1989. Cognitive-behavioral and response prevention treatments for bulimia nervosa. *J. Consult. Clin. Psychol.*, **57**, 215–221.

Agras, W.S., Telch, C.F., Arnow, B., Eldredge, K. and Marnell, M., 1997. One-year follow-up of cognitive-behavioral therapy for obese individuals with binge eating disorder. *J. Consult. Clin. Psychol.*, **65**, 343–347.

Agras, W.S., Telch, C.F., Arnow, B., Eldredge, K., Detzer, M.J., Henderson, J. and Marnel, M., 1995. Does interpersonal therapy help patients with binge eating disorder who fail to respond to cognitive-behavioral therapy? *J. Consult. Clin. Psychol.*, **63**, 356–360.

Agras, W.S., Telch, C.F., Arnow, B., Rossiter, E.M., Raeburn, S.D. and Koran, L.M., 1994. Weight loss, cognitive-behavioral, and desipramine treatments in binge eating disorder. An additive design. *Behavior Therapy*, **25**, 225–238.

Agras, W.S., Walsh, B.T., Fairburn, C.G., Wilson, G.T. and Kraemer, H.C., 2000. A multicenter comparison of cognitive behavioral therapy and interpersonal psychotherapy for bulimia nervosa. *Arch. Gen. Psychiatry*, **57**, 459–466.

Alger, A., Schwalberg, M.D., Bigouette, J.M., Michalek, A.V. and Howard, L.J., 1991. Effect of a tricyclic antidepressant and opiate antagonist on binge-eating behavior in normoweight bulimic and obese, binge-eating subjects. *Am. J. Clin. Nutr.*, **53**, 865–871.

Attia, E., Haiman, C., Walsh, B.T. and Flater, S.R., 1998. Does fluoxetine augment the inpatient treatment of anorexia nervosa? *American Journal of Psychiatry*, **155**, 548–551.

Barlow, J., Blouin, J., Blouin, A. and Perez, A., 1988. Treatment of bulimia with desipramine: A double-blind, crossover study. *Can. J. Psychiatry*, **33**, 129–133.

Biederman, J., Herzog, D.B., Rivinus, T.M., Harper, G.P., Ferber, R.A., Rosenbaum, J.F., Harmatz, J.S., Tondorf, R., Orsulak, P.J. and Schildkraut, J.J., 1985. Amitriptyline in the treatment of anorexia nervosa: A double-blind, placebo-controlled study. *J. Clin. Psychopharmacology*, **5**, 10–16.

Blouin, A.G., Blouin, J.H., Perez, E.L., Bushnik, T., Zuro, C. and Mulder, E., 1988. Treatment of bulimia with fenfluramine and desipramine. *J. Clin. Psychopharmacol.*, **8**, 261–269.

Cannistra, L.B. and Gaasch, W.H., 1999. Appetite-suppressant drugs and valvular heart disease. *Cardiol. Rev.*, **7**, 356–361.

Carter, J.C. and Fairburn, C.G., 1998. Cognitive-behavioral self-help for binge eating disorder: A controlled effectiveness study. *J. Consult. Clin. Psychol.*, **66**, 616–623.

Casper, R.C., Schlemner, R.F. Jr and Javaid, J.I., 1987. A placebo-controlled crossover study of oral clonidine in acute anorexia nervosa. *Psychiatry Research*, **20**, 249–260.

Cooper, P.J., 1994. *Bulimia Nervosa and Binge-eating: A Guide to Recovery*. New York University Press, New York.

Crisp, A.H., Norton, K., Gowers, S., Halek, C., Bowyer, C., Yeldham, D., Levett, G. and Bhat, A., 1991. A controlled study of the effect of therapies aimed at adolescent and family psychopathology in anorexia nervosa. *British Journal of Psychiatry*, **159**, 325–333.

Deeble, E.A., Crisp, A.H., Lacey, J.H. and Bhat, A.V., 1990. A comparison between women seeking self-help and psychiatric treatment in anorexia nervosa and bulimia. *British Journal of Medical Psychology*, **63**, 65–72.

de Zwaan, M. and Mitchell, J.E., 1992. Opioid antagonists and feeding in humans: A review of the literature. *J. Clin. Pharmacol.*, **32**, 1060–1072.

de Zwaan, M., Mitchell, J.E. and Mussell, M.P., 1996. Does CBT improve treatment outcome in obese binge eaters participating in a very-low-calorie-diet treatment? Presented at the Second Meeting of the Eating Disorders Research Society, Pittsburgh, PA, November.

de Zwaan, N., Nutinger, D.O. and Schonbeck, G., 1992. Binge eating in overweight females. *Compr. Psychiatry*, **33**, 256–261.

Eisler, I., Dare, C., Hodes, M., Russell, G., Dodge, E. and Le Grange, D., 2000. Family therapy for adolescent anorexia nervosa: The results of a controlled comparison of two family interventions. *J. Child Psychol. Psychiatry*, **41**, 727–736.

Eisler, I., Dare, C., Russell, G.F., Szmukler, G., Le Grange, D. and Dodge, E., 1997. Family and individual therapy in anorexia nervosa. A 5-year follow-up. *Archives of General Psychiatry*, **54**, 1025–1030.

Eldredge, K.L., Agras, W.S., Arnow, B., Telch, C.F., Bell, S., Castonguay, L. and Marnell, M., 1997. The effects of extending cognitive-behavioral therapy for binge eating disorder among initial treatment non-responders. *Int. J. Eat. Disord.*, **21**, 347–352.

Fahy, T.A., Eisler, I. and Russell, F.M., 1993. A placebo-controlled trial of d-Fenfluramine in Bulimia Nervosa. *Br. J. Psychiatry*, **162**, 597–603.

Fairburn, C.G., Jones, R., Peveler, R.C., Hope, R.A. and O'Connor, M., 1986. Psychotherapy and bulimia nervosa: Longer-term effects of interpersonal psychotherapy, behavior therapy, and cognitive behavior therapy. *Arch. Gen. Psychiatry*, **50**, 419–428.

Fairburn, C.G., Jones, R.T., Peveler, R.C., Carr, S.J., Solomon, R.A., O'Connor, M.E., Burton, J. and Hope, R.A., 1991. Three psychological treatments for bulimia nervosa. *Arch. Gen. Psychiatry*, **48**, 463–469.

Fairburn, C.G., 1995. *Overcoming Binge Eating*. Guilford Press, New York.

FBNC (Fluoxetine Bulimia Nervosa Collaborative Study Group), 1992. Fluoxetine in the treatment of bulimia nervosa. *Arch. Gen. Psychiatry*, **49**, 139–147.

Fichter, M.M., Kruger, R., Rief, W., Holland, R. and Dohne, J., 1996. Fluvoxamine in prevention of relapse in bulimia nervosa: Effects on eating-specific psychopathology.

Fichter, M.M., Leibl, K., Rief, W., Brunner, E., Schmidt-Auberger, S. and Engel, R.R., 1991. Fluoxetine versus placebo: A double-blind study with bulimic inpatients undergoing intensive psychotherapy. *Pharmacopsychiatry*, **24**, 1–7.

Garner, D.M., Rockert, W., Davis, R., Garner, M.V., Olmsted, M.P. and Eagle, M., 1993. Comparison of cognitive-behavioral and supportive-expressive therapy for bulimia nervosa. *Am. J. Psychiatry*, **150**, 37–46.

Geist, R., Heinmaa, M., Stephens, D., Davis, R. and Katzman, D.K., 2000. Comparison of family therapy and family group psychoeducation in adolescents with anorexia nervosa. *Canadian Journal of Psychiatry*, **45**, 173–178.

Goldberg, S.C., Halmi, K.A., Eckert, E.D., Casper, R.C. and Davis, J.M., 1979. Cyproheptadine in anorexia nervosa. *British Journal of Psychiatry*, **134**, 67–70.

Goldbloom, D., Olmsted, M. and Davis, R., 1996. A randomized controlled trial of fluoxetine and individual cognitive behavioral therapy for women with bulimia nervosa: Short-term outcome. Presented at the American Psychiatric Association meeting, New York, NY, May.

Goldstein, D.J., Wilson, M.G., Thompson, V.L., Potvin, J.H. and Rampey, A.H. Jr, 1995. Long-term fluoxetine treatment of bulimia nervosa: Fluoxetine Bulimia Nervosa Research Group. *Br. J. Psychiatry*, **166**, 660–666.

Gowers, S., Norton, K., Halek, C. and Crisp, A.H., 1994. Outcome of outpatient psychotherapy in a random allocation treatment study of anorexia nervosa. *International Journal of Eating Disorders*, **15**, 165–177.

Green, R.S. and Rau, J.H., 1974. Treatment of compulsive eating disturbances with anticonvulsant medication. *Am. J. Psychiatry*, **131**, 428–432.

Gross, H.A., Ebert, M.H., Faden, V.B., Goldberg, S.C., Nee, L.E. and Kaye, W.H., 1983. A double-blind trial of D^9-tetrahydrocannabinol in primary anorexia nervosa. *Journal of Clinical Psychopharmacology*, **3**, 165–171.

Gross, H.A., Ebert, M.H., Faden, V.B., Goldberg, S.C., Nee, L.E. and Kaye, K.H., 1981. A double-blind trial of lithium carbonate in primary anorexia nervosa. *Journal of Clinical Psychopharmacology*, **51**, 378–381.

Hall, A. and Crisp, A.H., 1987. Brief psychotherapy in the treatment of anorexia nervosa. Outcome at one year. *British Journal of Psychiatry*, **151**, 185–191.

Halmi, K.A., Eckert, E.D., LaDu, T.J. and Cohen, J., 1986. Anorexia nervosa: Treatment efficacy of cyproheptadine and amitriptyline. *Archives of General Psychiatry*, **43**, 177–181.

Hartman, B.K., Faris, P.L., Kim, S.W., Raymond, N.C., Goodale, R.L., Meller, W.H. and Eckert, E.D., 1997. Treatment of bulimia nervosa with ondansetron (letter). *Arch. Gen. Psychiatry*, **54**, 969–970.

Ho, K.S., Nichaman, M.Z., Taylor, W.C., Lee, E.S. and Foreyt, J.P., 1995. Binge eating disorder, retention, and dropout in an adult obesity program. *Int. J. Eat. Disord.*, **18**, 291–294.

Horne, R.L., Ferguson, J.M., Pope, H.G. Jr, Hudson, J.I., Lineberry, C.G., Ascher, J. and Cato, A., 1988. Treatment of bulimia with bupropion: A multicenter controlled trial. *J. Clin. Psychiatry*, **49**, 262–266.

Hsu, L.K., Betancourt, S. and Sullivan, S.P., 1996. Eating disturbances before and after vertical banded gastroplasty: A pilot study. *International Journal of Eating Disorders*, **19**, 23–34.

Hudson, J.I., McElroy, S.L., Raymond, N.C., Crow, S., Keck, P.E., Carter, W.P., Mitchell, J.E., Strakowski, S.M., Pope, H.G., Coleman, B. and Jonas, J.M., 1998. Fluvoxamine in the treatment of binge eating disorder: A multicenter placebo-controlled double blind trial. *Am. J. Psychiatry*, **155**, 1756–1762.

Hughes, P.L., Wells, L.A., Cunningham, C.J. and Ilstrup, D.M., 1986. Treating bulimia with desipramine. A double-blind, placebo-controlled study. *Arch. Gen. Psychiatry*, **43**, 182–186.

Ingoin-Apfelbaum, L. and Apfelbaum, M., 1987. Naltrexone and bulimic symptoms. *Lancet*, 1087–1088.

Jonas, J.M. and Gold, M.S., 1986. Naltrexone reverses bulimic symptoms. *Lancet*, **1**, 807.

Jonas, J.M. and Gold, M.S., 1988. The use of opiate antagonists in treating bulimia: A study of low-dose versus high-dose naltrexone. *Psychiatry Res.*, **24**, 195–199.

Jonas, J.M. and Gold, M.S., 1987. Treatment of antidepressant-resistant bulimia with naltrexone. *Int. J. Psychiatry in Med.*, **16**, 305–309.

Kaye, W.H., 1996. The use of fluoxetine to prevent relapse in anorexia nervosa. Paper presented at the Annual Meeting of the Eating Disorder research Society, Pittsburgh, PA, November.

Kennedy, S.H., Goldbloom, D.S., Ralevski, E., Davis, C., D'Souza, J.D. and Lofchy, J., 1993. Is there a role for selective monoamine oxidase inhibitor therapy in bulimia nervosa? A placebo-controlled trial of brofaromine. *J. Clin. Psychopharmacol.*, **13**, 415–422.

Kennedy, S.H., Piran, N. and Garfinkel, P.E., 1985. Monoamine oxidase inhibitor therapy for anorexia nervosa and bulimia: A preliminary trial of isocarboxazide. *J. Clin. Psychopharmacol.*, **5**, 279–286.

Kirkley, G.B., Schneider, J.A., Agras, W.S. and Bachman, J.A., 1985. Comparison of two group treatments for bulimia. *J. Consul. Clin. Psychol.*, **53**, 43–48.

Klerman, G.L., Weissman, M.M., Rounsaville, B.J. and Chevron, E.S., 1984. *Interpersonal Psychotherapy of Depression*. Basic Books, New York, NY.

Lacey, H., 1983. Bulimia nervosa, binge-eating, and psychogenic vomiting: A controlled treatment study and long-term outcome. *Br. Med. J.*, **2**, 1609–1613.

Lacey, J.H. and Crisp, A.H., 1980. Hunger, food intake and weight: The impact of clomipramine on a refeeding anorexia nervosa population. *Postgraduate Medical Journal*, **56**, S70–S85.

LaPorte, D.J., 1992. Treatment response in obese binge eaters: Preliminary results using a very low calorie diet (VLCD) and behavior therapy. *Addict. Behav.*, **17**, 247–257.

Lee, N.I. and Rush, A.J., 1986. Cognitive-behavioral group therapy for bulimia. *Int. J. Eat. Disord.*, 599–615.

Leitenberg, H., Rosen, J., Gross, J., Nudelman, S. and Vara, L.S., 1988. Exposure plus response-prevention treatment of bulimia nervosa. *J. Consult. Clin. Psychol.*, **56**, 535–541.

Leitenberg, H., Rosen, J.C., Wolf, J., Vara, L.S., Detzer, M.J. and Srebnik, D., 1994. Comparison of cognitive-behavioral therapy and desipramine in the treatment of bulimia nervosa. *Behav. Res. Ther.*, **32**, 37–45.

Marcus, M.D., Wing, R.R. and Hopkins, J., 1988. Obese binge eaters: Affect, cognitions, and response to behavioral weight control. *J. Consult. Clin. Psychol.*, **56**, 433–439.

Marcus, M.D., Wing, R.R., Ewing, L., Kern, E., McDermott, M. and Gooding, W., 1990. A double-blind, placebo-controlled trial of fluoxetine plus behavior modification in the treatment of obese binge-eaters and non-binge-eaters. *Am. J. Psychiatry*, **147**, 876–881.

McCann, U.D. and Agras, W.S., 1990. Successful treatment of non-purging bulimia nervosa with desipramine: A double-blind, placebo-controlled study. *American Journal of Psychiatry*, **147**, 1509–1513.

McElroy, S.L., Casuto, L.S., Nelson, E.R., Lake, K.A., Soutullo, C.A., Keck, P.E., Jr and Hudson, J.I., 2000. Placebo-controlled trial of sertraline in the treatment of binge eating disorder. *American Journal of Psychiatry*, **157**, 1004–1006.

McGuire, M.T., Wing, R.R., Klem, M.L., Lang, W. and Hill, J.O., 1999. What predicts weight regain in a group of weight losers? *Journal of Consulting and Clinical Psychology*, **67**, 177–185.

Mitchell, J.E. and Groat, R., 1984. A placebo-controlled, double-blind trial of amitriptyline in bulimia. *J. Clin. Psychopharmacol.*, **4**, 186–193.

Mitchell, J.E., Christenson, G., Jennings, J., Huber, M., Thomas, B., Pomeroy, C. and Morley, J., 1989. A placebo-controlled, double-blind crossover study of naltrexone hydrochloride in outpatients with normal weight bulimia. *J. Clin. Psychopharmacol.*, **9**, 94–97.

Mitchell, J.E., Hosfield, W. and Pyle, R.L., 1983. EEG findings in patients with bulimia syndrome. *Int. J. Eat. Disord.*, **2**, 17–23.

Mitchell, J.E., Pyle, R.L., Eckert, E.D., Hatsukami, D., Pomeroy, C. and Zimmerman, R., 1990. A comparison study of antidepressants and structured intensive group psychotherapy in the treatment of bulimia nervosa. *Arch. Gen. Psychiatry*, **47**, 149–157.

Mitchell, J.E., Tareen, B., Sheehan, W., Agras, S., Brewerton, T.D., Crow, S., Devlin, M., Eckert, E., Halmi, K., Herzog, D., Marcus, M., Powers, P., Stunkard, A. and Walsh, B.T., 2000. Establishing guidelines for pharmacotherapy trials in bulimia nervosa and anorexia nervosa. *Int. J. Eat. Disord.*, **28**, 1–7.

Mussell, M.P., Crosby, R.D., Crow, S.J., Knopke, A.J., Peterson, C.B., Wonderlich, S.A. and Mitchell, J.E., 2000. Utilization of empirically supported psychotherapy treatments for individuals with eating disorders: A survey of psychologists. *Int. J. Eat. Disord.*, **27**, 230–327.

Peterson, C.A., Mitchell, J.E., Engbloom, S., Nugent, S., Mussell, M.P. and Miller, J.P., 1998. Group cognitive-behavioral treatment of binge eating disorder: A comparison of therapist led versus self-help formats. *Int. J. Eat. Disord.*, **24**, 125–136.

Pope, H.G. Jr, Hudson, J.I., Jonas, J.M. and Yurgelun-Todd, D., 1983. Bulimia treated with imipramine: A placebo-controlled, double-blind study. *Am. J. Psychiatry*, **140**, 544–558.

Pope, H.G. Jr, Keck, P.E. Jr, McElroy, S.L. and Hudson, J.I., 1989. A placebo-controlled study of trazodone in bulimia nervosa. *J. Clin. Psychopharmacol.*, **9**, 254–259.

Robin, A.L., Siegel, P.T. and Moye, A., 1995. Family versus individual therapy for anorexia: Impact on family conflict. *International Journal of Eating Disorders*, **17**, 313–322.

Robin, A.L., Siegel, P.T., Koepke, T., Moye, A.W. and Tice, S., 1994. Family therapy versus individual therapy for adolescent females with anorexia nervosa. *Journal of Developmental and Behavioural Pediatrics*, **15**, 111–116.

Robin, A.L., Siegel, P.T., Moye, A.W., Gilroy, M., Dennis, A.B. and Sikand, A., 1999. A controlled comparison of family versus individual therapy for adolescents with anorexia nervosa. *Journal of the American Academy of Child and Adolescent Psychiatry*, **38**, 1482–1489.

Romano, S., 1999. Fluoxetine maintenance therapy for bulimia nervosa. Paper presented at the Eating Disorders Research Society Annual Meeting, San Diego, CA, November.

Russell, G., 1979. Bulimia nervosa: An ominous variant of anorexia nervosa. *Psychol. Med.*, **9**, 429–488.

Russell, G.F., Checkley, S.A., Feldman, J. and Eisler, I., 1988. A controlled trial of d-fenfluramine in bulimia nervosa. *Clin. Neuropharmacol.*, **11**, S146–S59.

Russell, G.F., Szmukler, G.I., Dare, C. and Eisler, I., 1987. An evaluation of family therapy in anorexia nervosa and bulimia nervosa. *Archives of General Psychiatry*, **44**, 1047–1056.

Sabine, E.J., Yonace, A., Farrington, A.J., Barra, H.K.H. and Wakeling, A., 1983. Bulimia nervosa: A placebo-controlled, double-blind therapeutic trial of mianserin. *Br. J. Clin. Pharmacol.*, **15**, S195–S202.

Sherwood, N.E., Jeffery, R.W. and Wing, R.R., 1999. Binge status as a predictor of weight loss treatment outcome. *International Journal of Obesity Related Metabolic Disorders*, **23**, 485–493.

Stacher, G., Abutzi-Wentzel, T.A., Wiesnagrotzki, S., Bergmann, H., Schneider, C. and Gaupmann, G., 1993. Gastric emptying, body weight and symptoms in primary anorexia nervosa: Long-term effects of cisapride. *British Journal of Psychiatry*, **162**, 398–402.

Strober, M., Pataki, C., Freeman, R. and DeAntonio, M., 1999. No effect of adjunctive fluoxetine on eating behavior or weight phobia during the inpatient treatment of anorexia nervosa: An historical case-control study. *Journal of Child and Adolescent Psychopharmacology*, **9**, 195–201.

Stunkard, A., Berkowitz, R., Tanrikut, C., Reiss, E. and Young, L., 1996. d-Fenfluramine treatment of binge eating disorder. *Am. J. Psychiatry*, **153**, 1455–1459.

Treasure, J., Todd, G., Brolly, M., Tiller, J., Nehmed, A. and Denman, F., 1995. A pilot study of randomized trial of cognitive behavioral analytical therapy versus educational behavioral therapy for adult anorexia nervosa. *Behaviour Research and Therapy*, **33**, 363–367.

Vandereycken, W. and Pierloot, R., 1982. Pimozide combined with behavior therapy in the short-term treatment of anorexia nervosa. *Acta Psychiatrica Scandinavica*, **66**, 445–450.

Vandereycken, W., 1984. Neuroleptics in the short-term treatment of anorexia nervosa: A double-blind placebo-controlled study with sulpride. *British Journal of Psychiatry*, **144**, 288–292.

Vigersky, R.A. and Loriaux, D.L., 1997. The effect of cyproheptadine in anorexia nervosa: A double-blind trial. In: Vigersky, R.A. (ed.), *Anorexia Nervosa*. Raven Press, New York.

Wadden, T.A., Foster, G.D. and Letizia, K.A., 1992. Response of obese binge eaters to treatment by behavioral therapy combined with very low calorie diet. *J. Consult. Clin. Psychol.*, **60**, 808–811.

Waller, D., Fairburn, C.G., McPherson, A., Kay, R., Lee, A. and Nowell, T., 1996. Treating bulimia nervosa in primary care: A pilot study. *Int. J. Eat. Disord.*, **19**, 99–103.

Walsh, B.T., Gladis, M., Roose, S.P., Stewart, J.W., Stetner, F. and Glassman, A.H., 1988. Phenelzine vs placebo in 50 patients with bulimia. *Arch. Gen. Psychiatry*, **45**, 471–475.

Walsh, B.T., Hadigan, C.M., Devlin, M.J., Gladis, M. and Roose, S.P., 1991. Long-term outcome of antidepressant treatment for bulimia nervosa. *Am. J. Psychiatry*, **148**, 1206–1212.

Walsh, B.T., Wilson, G.T., Loeb, K.L., Devlin, M.J., Pike, K.M., Roose, S.P., Fleiss, J. and Waternaux, C., 1997. Medication and psychotherapy in the treatment of bulimia. *Am. J. Psychiatry*, **154**, 523–531.

Wells, A.M., Garvin, V., Dohm, F.A. and Striegel-Moore, R.H., 1997. Telephone-based guided self-help for binge eating disorder: A feasibility study. *Int. J. Eat. Disord.*, **21**, 341–346.

Wermuth, B.M., Davis, K.L., Hollister, L.E. and Stunkard, A.J., 1977. Phenytoin treatment of the binge-eating syndrome. *Am. J. Psychiatry*, **134**, 1249–1253.

Whittal, M.L., Agras, W.S. and Gould, R.A., 1999. Bulimia nervosa: A meta-analysis of psychosocial and pharmacological treatments. *Behav. Ther.*, **30**, 117–135.

Wilfley, D.E., Agras, W.S., Telch, C.F., Rossiter, E.M., Schneider, J.A., Cole, A.G., Sifford, L.A. and Raeburn, S.D., 1993. Group cognitive-behavioral therapy and group interpersonal psychotherapy for the non-purging bulimic: A controlled comparison. *J. Consult. Clin. Psychol.*, **61**, 296–305.

Yanovski, S.Z., Gormally, J.F. and Lese, M.S., 1994. Binge eating disorder affects outcome of comprehensive very low calorie diet treatment. *Obes. Res.*, **2**, 205–212.

XXIV

Sleep Disorders

XXIV-1

Animal Models of Sleep Disturbances: Intrinsic and Environmental Determinants

Peter Meerlo, Bernard M. Bergmann and Fred W. Turek

INTRODUCTION

Although each mammalian species has its own sleep characteristics in terms of the total amount and distribution of sleep over the day (Campbell and Tobler, 1984; Zepelin, 2000), most of them share the fundamental regulatory principles with human beings (Borbely, 1982, Mistlberger *et al.*, 1983; Tobler, 2000). First, most species display a daily rhythm in sleep and wakefulness that is under the control of an endogenous biological clock in the brain. Second, within sleep, there is a cyclic alternation of two different states, non-rapid-eye-movement sleep (NREM) and rapid-eye-movement sleep (REM). And third, there is a homeostatic drive for each of the two sleep states that accumulates when the sleep state is absent. The longer an organism is awake, the higher its need for sleep. Remarkably, the exact functions of NREM and REM sleep are still unknown, but both states apparently serve vital functions. Studies in rats have shown that prolonged deprivation of either or both sleep states ultimately results in death (Rechtschaffen *et al.*, 1983; 1989). Studies of biological rhythms and sleep states in animals have greatly extended our knowledge of the regulatory mechanisms of sleep and provided clues to its functions. In addition, because of the similarities in sleep between human beings and other mammalian species, laboratory animals also provide a useful tool to gain insight into human sleep disorders.

Sleep disturbances can have a variety of underlying causes and contributing factors, and often are the outcome of a complex interplay between intrinsic factors and environmental influences. This chapter will summarize how sleep in animals can be affected by intrinsic factors (e.g., the physiological profile of an individual as determined by its genes, development, and age) as well as external factors (such as stressors and other environmental influences). Animal research allows detailed studies of each of these possible components and, as such, animal models can be a relevant source of information on the aetiology and mechanisms of sleep disorders.

We have chosen to categorize and present the animal literature on sleep disturbances roughly according to their intrinsic or extrinsic cause since that is what many studies use as a starting point. Although there are a number of animal models that mimic a specific sleep disorder (e.g., narcolepsy), a more common approach is to examine the influence of a certain intrinsic factor or environmental condition on sleep rather than modelling a sleep disorder *per se* (e.g., the influence of ageing or stress). The results of studies using the latter approach do not always allow a symptom-based classification as generally is used for human sleep disorders. For example, since insomnia in humans is often ascribed to stress, studying the influence of stressors on sleep in animals and its possible physiological pathways is highly relevant to the understanding of human sleep disorders. However, studies in mice and rats show that various stressors induce dynamic and complex changes in sleep that cannot simply be listed as insomnia. Therefore, we choose to present these models under the heading of stress, rather than insomnia.

The first sections hereafter describe how sleep disorders may be related to genes and development. The genetic models include successful models of narcolepsy as well as selected lines of rats with changes in particularly REM sleep. The developmental models show how influences during early stages of life can affect adult sleep and potential sensitivity to sleep disorders. These models also are characterized in particular by changes in adult REM sleep regulation. The following section discusses animal models of sleep in ageing, and the paragraphs thereafter deal with alterations in sleep due to disturbances of the circadian clock. Finally, a number of sections summarize the changes and disturbances in sleep that may occur in response to environmental factors, such as light and temperature, and, probably the most commonly cited cause of disturbed sleep, stress.

GENETIC MODELS

A variety of genetic tools and approaches are used to study gene effects on sleep in animals, including comparisons of different strains of rats or mice, knockout mice, or mice strains with other mutations. Whereas many of these studies are undertaken to unravel basic physiological mechanisms underlying sleep regulation, some of the models provide relevant information on genetic factors in sleep disturbances or genetic influences on the sensitivity to sleep disorders.

Narcoleptic Dogs and Mice

Probably the first true animal model of a sleep disorder was the finding of narcoleptic behaviour in dogs (Mitler *et al.*, 1974). Narcolepsy is a seriously disabling neurological disease that is characterized by disturbed night-time sleep and excessive daytime sleepiness, as well as pathological manifestations of REM sleep and cataplexy, often triggered by emotional expressions (Bassetti and Aldrich, 1996; Guilleminault and Anagnos, 2000). Early studies identified a narcoleptic phenotype in several breeds of dogs, including Doberman pinchers, which have played an important role in unravelling the genetic basis of the disease and also contributed to the development of treatment strategies (Baker *et al.*, 1982; Nishino and Mignot, 1997). More recently, mice were discovered with narcoleptic phenomena similar to those seen in dogs

Biological Psychiatry: Edited by H. D'haenen, J.A. den Boer and P. Willner. ISBN 0-471-49198-5

(Chemelli *et al.*, 1999). Taken together, the different animal models point to a link between narcolepsy and a dysfunction of the hypocretin/orexin neuropeptide system in the brain (for review, see Siegel, 1999). Hypocretin/orexin neurons are located in the hypothalamus and have widespread projections to various brain areas, including the brainstem, the limbic system, and the cerebral cortex (Peyron *et al.*, 1998). Originally, the hypocretin and orexin peptides were discovered independently by different research groups, and the function of these peptides appeared to be related to the regulation of food intake (De Lecea *et al.*, 1998; Sakurai *et al.*, 1998). In subsequent studies the orexins and hypocretins not only turned out to be identical, but also were found to have a major effect on sleep. The narcoleptic dogs, which are now known to have a mutation in one of the hypocretin receptors, have disturbed sleep and cataplexy attacks much like those in human patients (Lin *et al.*, 1999). Moreover, mice whose gene coding for the hypocretin/orexin peptide has been inactivated exhibit clear, narcolepsy-like symptoms, including an increase in sleep time during their normal activity phase, sleep-onset REM sleep episodes, and sudden behavioural arrests (Chemelli *et al.*, 1999). Pharmacological studies in rats have confirmed a role for hypocretins/orexin in sleep-wake regulation, and administration of the peptide increases wakefulness and suppresses REM sleep (Hagan *et al.*, 1999; Piper *et al.*, 2000).

Taken together, the results suggest that hypocretins/orexins serve as an arousal factor and suppress REM sleep, and a lack of hypocretin/orexin signalling might be the cause for much of the narcoleptic symptomatology (Siegel, 1999). Based on these results from animal research, subsequent studies found that human narcolepsy is indeed associated with a specific loss of hypocretin/orexin neurons and undetectable levels of the peptide in the brain and cerebrospinal fluid, supporting a role for hypocretin peptides in sleep disorders such as narcolepsy, and opening new avenues for drug development and treatment procedures (Nishino *et al.*, 2000; Peyron *et al.*, 2000; Thannickal *et al.*, 2000).

Rat Strains with REM Sleep Disorders

A number of studies on selected lines of rats have explored alterations in REM sleep regulation and its possible relevance to human disorders such as depression. Human depression is characterized by changes in REM sleep regulation, especially an increase in REM sleep early in the night, and it has been suggested that a dysregulation of REM sleep may be linked to the development of the mood disturbance (Berger and Riemann, 1993; Vogel *et al.*, 1980). Two rat lines in particular have been studied in this context, the Flinders Sensitive Line rats (Shiromani *et al.*, 1988) and the Wistar Kyoto rats (Dugovic *et al.*, 2000). The Flinders Sensitive Line was selectively bred for hypersensitivity of the cholinergic system (Overstreet, 1993) whereas the Wistar Kyoto rat was originally bred as a normotensive control for spontaneously hypertensive rats (Louis and Howes, 1990). Both of these rat strains show behavioural abnormalities that have been suggested as a model of human depression (Overstreet, 1993; Pare and Redei, 1993). Subsequent analysis of sleep in the Flinders Sensitive rats indeed revealed an increase in the amount of REM sleep, without major changes in NREM sleep (Shiromani *et al.*, 1988; Benca *et al.*, 1996). The Wistar Kyoto rats were found to have more fragmented sleep and an overall increase in the total amount of REM sleep (Dugovic *et al.*, 2000). These models thus support the hypothesis of a link between alterations of REM sleep regulation and mood disturbances such as depression. Although originally these selection lines of rats were not developed as models of sleep disorders, they hold great potential to study whether altered REM sleep regulation has detrimental effects and perhaps is a causal factor in the development of depression-like behavioural disturbances.

DEVELOPMENTAL FACTORS

In addition to genetic models of sleep disturbances, there is evidence from animal research that adult sleep characteristics and perhaps sensitivity to sleep disorders may depend on developmental factors as well. Manipulations and environmental stimuli around the time of birth can lead to profound changes in physiological function and behaviour later in life. Maternal stress, malnutrition, and alcohol ingestion are among several factors that induce developmental changes in the fetus and cause alterations in the offspring's sleep regulation that last into adulthood.

Maternal Stress

One example of developmental influences on sleep regulation is the effect of so-called maternal or prenatal stress. In this model, pregnant female rats are repeatedly subjected to stress, which often comprises immobilization several times a day during the last 1–2 weeks of gestation (Barbazanges *et al.*, 1996). Some of the effects of prenatal stress on the development of the young appear to be mediated by an increase in maternal corticosterone (Barbazanges *et al.*, 1996). After birth, the young are raised in a standard way until adulthood, when physiological function and behaviour are studied. In adulthood, the offspring of mothers subjected to such stress have increased sleep fragmentation and increased amount of REM sleep (Dugovic *et al.*, 1999). Maternal immobilization stress also induces certain alterations in HPA axis function and behaviour that are reminiscent of human depression (Weinstock, 1997). It has therefore been proposed that prenatal stress, similar to the genetic models with increased REM sleep, may be a valuable model to study the relationship between altered sleep and mood disorders (Dugovic *et al.*, 1999). Important in this context is the finding that experimentally depriving adult rats of REM sleep results in hyperactivity, fearlessness, and aggression (Hicks and Moore, 1979; Hicks *et al.*, 1979). Thus, whereas too much REM sleep may be associated with passive and depression-like behaviour, too little REM sleep may result in hyperemotionality and mania.

Maternal Food and Alcohol Intake

There is considerable evidence from studies in female rodents that the caloric content and composition of food, as well as alcohol and drugs during pregnancy, strongly affect the development of the foetuses. Especially maternal malnutrition and alcohol ingestion can result in serious morphological, physiological, and behavioural abnormalities in the offspring, including alterations in sleep regulation. A study on maternal protein malnutrition in rats showed that during adulthood the offspring had more NREM sleep but their REM sleep was less than half that of control animals (Datta *et al.*, 2000). In rat pups that were exposed to alcohol in utero, quiet sleep was reduced and more frequently interrupted by waking episodes (Hilakivi, 1986). In adulthood, the offspring showed a strong reduction in the amount of REM sleep (Stone *et al.*, 1996), an effect that, for unknown reasons, may be particularly severe in the female offspring (Sylvester *et al.*, 2000). Although the changes in sleep after maternal malnutrition and alcohol intake were not hypothesized to reflect a specific sleep disorder, it has been suggested that such sleep changes, particularly the decrease in REM sleep, may have detrimental effects on cognitive functions. Importantly, in rats that are exposed to alcohol in utero, the deficits in REM sleep during adulthood seem to predict certain cognitive deficits during ageing (Stone *et al.*, 1996).

It is noteworthy that the reduction in REM sleep in offspring after maternal malnutrition and alcohol intake is opposite to the increase in REM sleep seen after maternal stress. Apparently, developmental influences on adult sleep-wake patterns strongly depend on the nature of the stimulus. Moreover, these studies on maternal malnutrition and alcohol intake support the hypothesis that not only too much, but also too little REM sleep may be associated with specific malfunctions and disease-like manifestations. As already mentioned above, REM sleep deprivation appears to result in hyperemotionality. In addition, although the evidence is contradictory, other studies have linked REM sleep loss to a decrease in cognitive performance and disturbances in learning and memory (for review, see Graves *et al.*, 2001; Siegel, 2001; Smith, 1996).

AGEING

Many reports suggest that the prevalence of certain sleep disorders and insomnia increase during human ageing (for review, see Bliwise, 2000). However, the study of sleep and human ageing is severely complicated by factors such as disease and medication, and several reports suggest that poor sleep in the elderly is in many cases secondary to medical illness rather than chronological age (Foley *et al.*, 1995; Gislason and Almqvist, 1987). Controlled studies in animals can shed light on such issues, and measurements in a variety of mammalian species have explored the changes in sleep that occur with ageing. The most commonly used animal model for studies on ageing and sleep is the rat. In old rats of about 20–24 months, ageing-related changes in sleep include a dampening of the sleep-wake rhythm amplitude, more fragmentation of sleep, a decrease in deep NREM sleep, and, sometimes, slight overall decreases in the amount of sleep, especially REM sleep (Mendelson and Bergmann, 1999; Rosenberg *et al.*, 1979; Van Gool and Mirmiran, 1983). However, the changes can be fairly subtle, and not all studies have found clear changes in basal sleep patterns in old rats (see Mendelson and Bergmann, 1999; Zepelin *et al.*, 1972). The age-related changes in sleep may vary considerably between individual animals as well as between strains of rats (Li and Satinoff, 1995; Shiromani *et al.*, 2000), suggesting that the consequences of ageing may strongly depend on genetically determined individual characteristics.

Importantly, although age-related changes in *baseline* sleep may not always be consistent, there seems to be a more robust change in the compensatory sleep *rebound* after a period of sleep deprivation (Mendelson and Bergmann, 2000; Shiromani *et al.*, 2000). Young rats respond to extended wakefulness with an increase in the time spent in NREM sleep and an increase in NREM sleep intensity, as reflected in an increase in EEG slow waves, as well as an increase in REM sleep (Borbely and Neuhaus, 1979; Tobler and Borbely, 1986). In old animals, however, the compensatory NREM sleep rebound is diminished (Mendelson and Bergman, 2000; Shiromani *et al.*, 2000). The REM sleep rebound after sleep deprivation was also found to be attenuated, but only after a very long period of sleep deprivation of 48 h (Mendelson and Bergmann, 2000), and not after milder 12-h sleep deprivation (Shiromani *et al.*, 2000). Moreover, whereas in young animals extended wakefulness is generally followed by an immediate recovery rebound, in aged rats the rebound is not only attenuated but also sometimes delayed (Mendelson and Bergmann, 2000). Taken together, the results seem to point to a decline in the homeostatic response to sleep loss in ageing rats.

Age-related changes in sleep have been reported for several other mammalian species, including mice (Welsh *et al.*, 1986), hamsters (Naylor *et al.*, 1998), and cats (Bowersox *et al.*, 1984). Many of the sleep changes that occur during ageing in these species are comparable with those seen in the rat. A notable difference is that, in both hamsters and cats, ageing is associated with a slight increase in the total daily amount of NREM sleep. The reason for this difference is not fully understood, but it has been explained as an attempt to compensate for lower sleep efficiency as reflected in a decrease in electroencephalographic (EEG) slow waves (Naylor *et al.*, 1998).

Some of the ageing-related changes in sleep in the various animal models, such as a higher fragmentation of sleep and a decrease in sleep-wake rhythm amplitude, are thought to be due to alterations in the biological clock that is driving the sleep-wake rhythm (see next section). In addition, the decline in the compensatory response to sleep deprivation in the rat suggests that also the homeostatic mechanisms underlying NREM sleep regulation are affected by age. Interestingly, part of the age-related sleep changes in rats can be prevented by housing them in an enriched environment (Van Gool and Mirmiran, 1986), an observation which suggests that an increase in behavioural activity and sensory input may alleviate the consequences of ageing. A recent study in humans indeed confirmed that structured physical and social activity can improve night-time sleep in the elderly (Naylor *et al.*, 2000). These latter findings illustrate the potential value of animal models in finding treatment strategies and therapies for sleep disturbances in ageing.

CLOCK DISTURBANCES

In most mammalian species, the alternation of sleep and wakefulness occurs in a rhythmic fashion, and sleep is preferentially consolidated to certain periods of the day. The regulation of such daily rhythmicity, which is not restricted to sleep but is manifest in most biological functions, is under the control of an endogenous oscillator, or 'clock', located in the suprachiasmatic nuclei (SCN) of the hypothalamus (Moore and Eichler, 1972; Stephan and Zucker, 1972; for review, see Klein *et al.*, 1991). Since the periodicity of endogenous circadian rhythms often slightly deviates from 24 h, synchronization to the environment occurs through daily adjustment of the clock by light (Pittendrigh, 1981). For this purpose, the clock in the SCN receives photic information from the environment via a direct neuronal input from the retina (Moore and Lenn, 1972).

Several studies have shown that destruction of the clock by lesioning the SCN results in a fragmented sleep pattern without a clear daily rhythm in mice (Ibuka *et al.*, 1980), rats (Eastman *et al.*, 1984; Mistlberger *et al.*, 1983; Mouret *et al.*, 1978; Tobler *et al.*, 1983), and squirrel monkeys (Edgar *et al.*, 1993). In the mice and rat studies, destruction of the SCN abolished the normal expression of the circadian sleep-wake cycle, but it did not change the total amount of sleep. In the squirrel monkeys, however, lesioning the central oscillator resulted not only in an arrhythmic sleep-wake pattern but also in a pronounced increase in total sleep time. This finding may imply that, at least in some species, alterations in clock function may affect not only the timing and consolidation of sleep but also the homeostatic regulation of sleep duration.

The *Clock* Mutation

An alternative approach to study the effects of changes in clock function on sleep is to examine animals that have a genetically altered clock system. One such model is the *Clock* mouse, which has a mutation in one of the genes that is involved in the regulation of circadian rhythmicity (Vitaterna *et al.*, 1994). Under a normal light-dark cycle, homozygote *Clock* mice still maintain fairly normal activity patterns. However, under conditions of constant darkness, when the endogenous clock is no longer synchronized to the environment, the *Clock* mice have unstable activity rhythms with an abnormally long, 28-h period. Eventually, the animals even become arrhythmic (Vitaterna *et al.*, 1994). Under both conditions of synchronization to a light-dark cycle and constant darkness, the *Clock* mice have a dampened amplitude of the sleep-wake rhythm and spend less time in NREM sleep than their wild-type counterparts (Naylor *et al.*, 2000). This study confirms that changes in circadian clock function are a potential pathway to disturbance of sleep.

The Ageing Clock

As discussed in a previous section, ageing is often associated with increased sleep fragmentation and reduced sleep-wake rhythm amplitude, part of which may be due to an age-related decline in the functional activity of the endogenous pacemaker in the SCN (for review, see Turek *et al.*, 2001; Weinert, 2000). In line with this, aged rodents sometimes exhibit decreased numbers of SCN cells with vasopressin, one of the primary neurotransmitters in the clock (Van der Zee *et al.*, 1999). Moreover, peak neuronal discharge in the SCN is reduced and more irregular in old animals (Satinoff *et al.*, 1993). In addition, advanced age has been associated with a decrease in responsiveness of the circadian clock to the phase-shifting effects of light and other synchronizers (Penev *et al.*, 1995; Van Reeth *et al.*, 1993; Zee *et al.*, 1992). Taken together, the data from animal studies indicate that in the aged the endogenous oscillator in the SCN is less sensitive to input stimuli that are normally involved in synchronizing the clock to the environment, and that the SCN has an altered output to the rest of the brain and body. However, although a great deal is known about the molecular machinery of the biological clock in the SCN and studies in rodents have revealed several pathways by which the SCN might affect the sleep-wake rhythm (Aston-Jones *et al.*, 2001), it is still unclear which of these pathways might deteriorate during ageing (Shiromani *et al.*, 2000).

Dissociations Between Clock and Environment

In addition to alterations in the central circadian clock itself, disturbed sleep may also arise from a misalignment between the endogenous clock and environmental determinants of the sleep-wake rhythm. In humans, this can occur, for instance, after a long-distance flight when the internal clock is temporarily out of synchrony with the environmental light-dark cycle at the place of arrival, a condition that is referred to as jet lag. In animals, the effects of long-distance flights can easily be mimicked by shifting the light-dark cycle of the housing facility. In one study, rats were subjected to an 8-h advance of the light-dark cycle, comparable to a transatlantic flight from the USA to Europe (Sei *et al.*, 1992). Sleep patterns were studied for 3 days preceding, and 5–7 days following the shift. Especially the rhythm of NREM sleep was severely disturbed and had a strongly dampened amplitude. The daily REM sleep rhythm, however, was less affected. Perhaps the REM sleep rhythm was strongly determined by the clock whereas the dampening of the NREM sleep rhythm may have been the result of interactive effects of the endogenous clock and direct effects of light (see next section). Overall, the amount of both NREM and REM sleep was somewhat increased during the simulated jet lag. Eventually, light input to the clock will lead to resynchronization of the endogenous clock to the new light-dark cycle, but in this particular study recordings did not extend beyond 5–7 days, when alterations in the sleep-wake rhythm were far from normalized. This in itself suggests that long-distance flight may have quite persistent effects. Animal models for jet lag hold great potential for studying concomitant sleep disturbances and treatment strategies.

Taken together, studies on the circadian regulation of sleep and wakefulness imply that alterations in the biological clock or in the light input to the clock can be a major cause of disrupted sleep. The progress that has been made in identifying the molecular and neurobiological substrates of circadian rhythms in animals has broadened our understanding of clock function and the way rhythm disturbances may contribute to disrupted sleep in our society.

ENVIRONMENTAL INFLUENCES

There are a variety of environmental factors, such as light and ambient temperature, that can directly or indirectly affect sleep quality. In human beings, the possibility of self-regulating light exposure and temperature conditions has turned these environmental influences into lifestyle factors that can have positive effects on sleep but may also contribute to the occurrence of disrupted sleep. Although most of the animal studies on light and ambient temperature were undertaken from a fundamental interest and were not presented as models of sleep disorders, some of them provide information that is relevant in the context of disrupted sleep due to inadequate sleep hygiene.

Light Effects

Light is a factor that may have both positive and negative effects on sleep. As mentioned in a previous section, light is important for the regulation of normal circadian rhythmicity, and well-timed exposure to light keeps the sleep-wake rhythm in synchrony with the outside world. However, light at the wrong time of day for prolonged periods of time may shift the clock and lead to disrupted sleep. In addition to direct input to the SCN, there is light input to various other brain regions, including the serotonergic raphe nuclei in the brainstem (Shen and Sembra, 1994), via which route light may modulate sleep and arousal as well (Jouvet, 1999; Portas *et al.*, 2000).

Rodents such as rats are primarily nocturnal animals. Maintained under a 12-h light:12-h dark schedule in the laboratory, both NREM and REM sleep in the rat predominantly occur during the light phase. However, under natural conditions, rats would probably avoid light and spend most of the daytime hours in the darkness of their burrows (Terman *et al.*, 1991). Thus, as in human beings, sleep would most likely occur mainly in darkness. Several studies in rats have shown that light can have potent effects on sleep architecture and sleep intensity. A number of studies that compared sleep under a light-dark cycle with sleep under constant darkness showed that *removal* of the light influence significantly enhances sleep continuity and increases NREM sleep EEG amplitude, a measure of sleep intensity (Tobler *et al.*, 1994; Trachsel *et al.*, 1986). Under these conditions, the overall amount of NREM sleep is not strongly affected by light, but the amount of REM sleep is sometimes suppressed (Trachsel *et al.*, 1986). Another approach that has been used to investigate the effects of light on sleep involves exposing rats to ultra-short light-dark cycles — for instance, cycles with consecutive periods of 1-h light and 1-h darkness (for review, see Borbely, 1978). Also under these conditions, the amount of REM sleep is lower in the light than in the dark. The amount of NREM sleep, however, is higher in the short light phases than in the short dark phases (Alfoldi *et al.*, 1991; Borbely, 1976; Lelkes *et al.*, 1990). Clearly, the effects of light on the amount of NREM sleep are complex, but the data suggest that exposure to light during the normal sleeping phase may disrupt sleep by at least suppressing NREM sleep intensity and REM sleep duration. Animal studies on the effects of light on sleep and the mechanism by which it acts become increasingly important in our rapidly developing 24-h society where we are frequently exposed to artificial light at unusual times, as in shift work.

Ambient Temperature

Another environmental variable that can have both positive and disruptive effects on sleep is the ambient temperature. The effects of ambient temperature on sleep have been studied in various mammalian species, including mice (Roussel *et al.*, 1984), rats (Schmidek *et al.*, 1972), hamsters (Sichieri and Schmidek, 1984), and cats (Parmeggiani and Rabini, 1970). A number of studies suggest that moderate and short-lasting thermal loads may promote NREM sleep (Moriarty *et al.*, 1993; Obal *et al.*, 1995), a finding that is in agreement with increases in NREM sleep in human beings after heating in a warm bath or a sauna (Horne and Reid, 1985; Putkonen *et al.*, 1973). However, exposure to more extreme ambient temperatures for prolonged periods of time may seriously disrupt sleep and reduce NREM sleep time. The amount of REM sleep is generally maximal around thermoneutrality, that is, the ambient temperature at which the metabolic rate is minimal. Both higher and lower ambient temperatures cause a decrease in REM sleep time (Parmeggiani and Rabini, 1970; Rosenthal and Vogel, 1993; Schmidek *et al.*, 1972; Szymusiak and Satinoff, 1981). Studies of rats under very low ambient temperatures around or below 0 °C have shown severe reductions and even complete loss of REM sleep (Amici *et al.*, 1994; 1998). During recovery from cold exposure, REM sleep levels are markedly increased above baseline levels, indicating that during cold exposure the animals are deprived of REM sleep. Clearly, these data indicate that extreme ambient temperatures should be avoided in order to prevent sleep from being disturbed. However, the sleep-stimulating effect of a mild temperature load preceding sleep could perhaps be used as a basis for developing treatments to alleviate sleep complaints.

STRESS

Probably the most frequently cited cause of disrupted sleep and insomnia in humans is 'stress' (Roehrs *et al.*, 2000). Accordingly, there is a great interest in using stress as a starting point for animal models of sleep disturbances. However, animal research shows that the relationship between stress and sleep is rather complex. Stress-induced changes in sleep show a dynamic temporal pattern that depends on the nature and duration of the stressor.

Acute Stress

Stress is usually defined as a non-specific physiological response to any kind of demand that an organism is facing (Selye, 1936). Traditionally, the autonomic sympatho-adrenal axis and the hypothalamic-pituitary-adrenal (HPA) axis are considered to be the main neuroendocrine systems involved in the integrated stress response (Axelrod and Reisine, 1984; Johnson *et al.*, 1992). The increased catecholaminergic activity and HPA axis activity, in a complex interplay with various other neuroendocrine systems, orchestrate an adequate response to the challenge an animal or human being is dealing with. Obviously, coping with environmental challenges requires alertness, and since stress is a state of physiological activation and arousal, by definition, it inhibits sleep. Indeed, exposing animals to stressors is invariably associated with at least a short-lasting increase in wakefulness. Moreover, many of the classical neuropeptides and hormones involved in the stress response are known to promote wakefulness, including catecholamines (Jones *et al.*, 1977; Cespuglio *et al.*, 1982; Lin *et al.*, 1992), corticotropin-releasing factor (CRF) (Ehlers *et al.*, 1986; Opp, 1995), and adrenocorticotropic hormone (ACTH) (Chastrette *et al.*, 1990; Gillin *et al.*, 1974). These data support the notion that acute stress and the concomitant physiological arousal may be an important cause of sleep disruption. The acute stress-induced arousal in animals can be used as a model to study and test the effects of potential hypnotic compounds (James and Piper, 1978).

Interestingly, studies in rats and mice have shown that upon removal of a stressor the arousing effect is rapidly overcome, and that stress may actually promote and increase sleep during the subsequent recovery period (Meerlo *et al.*, 1997; Meerlo and Turek, 2001; Meerlo *et al.*, 2001; Rampin *et al.*, 1991). In addition to this biphasic effect of stress on sleep, the picture is further complicated by the finding that different stressors may have different effects on NREM sleep and REM sleep. For example, whereas *immobilization* of rats and mice in a small tube results in an increase of REM sleep during subsequent recovery (Meerlo *et al.*, 2001; Rampin *et al.*, 1991), a *social conflict* with an aggressive conspecific was found to promote NREM sleep (Meerlo *et al.*, 1997; Meerlo and Turek, 2001). Importantly, although both social conflict and immobilization cause strong sympathetic and HPA axis activation, the respective increases in NREM sleep or REM sleep are apparently due to certain specific aspects of the stimuli. In this respect, one should perhaps not speak in general terms about the effects of stressors on sleep but, rather, refer to the effects of specific stimuli.

What are the specific elements of the different stressors that affect sleep? Clearly, the effects of a stressor may very well consist of multiple, interacting components, some non-specific, and some specific to a particular stimulus. The mechanism underlying an increase in NREM sleep as it is seen after a social conflict is still unknown, but for stressful stimuli that increase REM sleep, various factors have been proposed, including CRF (Gonzalez and Valatx, 1997), corticotropin-like intermediate lobe peptide (CLIP) (Bonnet *et al.*, 1997; Bonnet *et al.*, 2000), and prolactin (Bodosi *et al.*, 2000; Meerlo *et al.*, 2001). In particular, differences in prolactin release may explain some of the differential effects of stress on REM sleep. Prolactin is commonly referred to as a stress hormone, but the change in prolactin levels strongly depends on the nature of the stressor. In line with its effects on sleep, immobilization stress in rodents indeed appears to be characterized by an increase in prolactin that is much larger than what is observed after other stressors such as social conflict or cold stress (Lenox *et al.*, 1980; Meerlo *et al.*, 2001). Moreover, in a comparison between two different strains of mice, immobilization stress induced an increase in REM sleep during recovery only in one strain of mice, which had a large prolactin response (Meerlo *et al.*, 2001). The latter finding also illustrates how modulation of sleep by environmental factors depends not only on the nature of the stimulus but also on the genetic make-up of the individual.

Taken together, studies in rodents show that the final effect of an acute and short-lasting stress on sleep depends not only on the non-specific arousal common to all stressors but also on the specific aspects of a given stimulus. Whereas many of the classical *non-specific* stress response factors initially increase arousal and inhibit sleep, factors *specific* to a particular situation or stimulus may increase either NREM sleep or REM sleep during recovery sleep. Importantly, an increase in NREM sleep or REM sleep after exposure to a particular stressful stimulus is not necessarily a manifestation of dysregulation. Rather, it may be interpreted as a necessary homeostatic recovery process, although the exact nature of this recovery process is still unknown, in the case of both stress-induced sleep and sleep in general (Meerlo *et al.*, 1997).

Although exposure to an acute stressor in animals is generally associated with an increase in wakefulness for as long as the stimulus persists, it seems puzzling that this arousing and sleep-inhibiting effect of the stressor is so rapidly overcome. Moreover, especially the finding of an increase in sleep following certain stressful stimuli may seem to contrast with the general notion that stress is a major cause of sleep disturbances in human beings. However, there is very little information about the effects of acute stressors on human sleep, at least not in response to traumatic experiences comparable to, for instance, social defeat in rodents. Thus, on the basis of the animal studies, one could hypothesize that, also in our own species, specific stressors may have a stimulatory effect on sleep systems shortly after the initial arousing effects. In fact, anecdotal information suggests that this may indeed be true (Oswald, 1962).

Studying the influence of acute and severe stressors may be a valid approach that mimics what could happen in real life, but, given the minimal and short-lasting wakefulness that occurs afterwards, these acute stress models do not appear to be extremely useful as models for the persistent insomnia so common in our society. For that purpose, one should perhaps use other or chronic stress models.

Repeated or Chronic Stress

In contrast to the acute and severe stress models discussed above, the 'stress' causing sleep disturbances in humans often seems to relate to a subtle cognitive phenomenon, that is, feelings of discomfort, not necessarily associated with an acute challenge (Roehrs *et al.*, 2000). Often, such feelings of discomfort may be based on memories of past events as well as worries and expectations about the future. In that respect, the human brain may be capable of turning a single acute stressor or life event that occurred in the past into a more persistent and chronic stress state. Although certain human cognitive processes may be difficult to model in animals, there are a number of studies that have examined the effects of chronic stress on sleep-wakefulness patterns in the rat.

In one model of chronic stress, sleep was measured in rats that were subjected to a paradigm of around-the-clock intermittent electrical shocks (Kant *et al.*, 1995). In this model of sustained stress, the animals display a wide variety of stress symptoms including elevated plasma levels of stress hormones such as corticosterone, a decrease in food intake and body weight, and disturbed temperature rhythm and activity pattern. The amount of sleep was remarkably reduced the first day of the treatment but normalized in the course of the days thereafter. However, the distribution of sleep over the 24-h cycle remained somewhat disturbed throughout the stress period. The amount of sleep was reduced in the light phase, the normal resting phase of rats, but this was compensated for by an increase in sleep during the dark phase. However, whereas rats under laboratory conditions have the possibility of such compensatory responses, human beings often do not have that possibility. These data show that, although a rat may rapidly overcome the arousal of a single stressful event, repetition of the stressor may add up and culminate in disrupted sleep.

In another study that applied a model of 'chronic mild stress', male rats were subjected to a mixture of noxious stimuli, once or twice a day, for various durations. The stimuli included cage tilt, soiled cage, deprivation of food and water, and housing in a mouse cage, which rats apparently dislike, but also exposure to continuous lighting and stroboscopic lighting (Cheeta *et al.*, 1997). The most significant finding from this study was a reduction in REM sleep latency during the protocol. The day after 3 weeks of a chronic mild stress treatment, the overall amount of sleep as well as the amount of REM sleep was somewhat increased, a finding which may in part reflect a rebound due to sleep that was lost during the actual stress exposure. Unfortunately, stimuli such as the lighting that was applied, although relevant in the context of environmental influences on sleep discussed earlier, may have effects on sleep that have little to do with stress *per se*.

Moreover, both models of chronic stress discussed here partly rely on direct stimulation of the animals, a fact which may explain some of the changes in sleep, whereas stress-related sleep disturbances in humans often appear to be of a more psychological nature. It may very well be that the physiological and neurobiological mechanisms resulting in disrupted sleep due to repeated electrical shocks and stroboscopic light are quite different from those involved in psychological stress in humans. These models are important first steps toward developing relevant models for stress-related sleep disturbances and insomnia, but, perhaps, research on the relationship between stress and sleep would gain by models that are based on, for instance, conditioned fear and arousal in which animals anticipate the occurrence of adverse events. Such an approach may have more resemblance to the psychological stress in humans, and with such a model one may be able to study the central mechanisms by which sleep is disrupted and how such disturbances could best be treated.

CONCLUDING REMARKS

Although the function of sleep is still an unresolved mystery, sleep is clearly necessary for optimal performance and well-being. The results from studies in a wide variety of animal models show that alterations and disruptions of sleep are often associated with changes in cognitive performance, emotionality, and disease. Sleep disturbances are a widespread and serious problem in our society, but animal research continues to push advances in the understanding of the causes and mechanisms of human sleep disorders, and to aid the improvement of treatment procedures and medicines.

ACKNOWLEDGEMENTS

The preparation of this chapter was supported in part by the National Alliance for Research on Schizophrenia and Depression (NASAD), NIH grants R01-AG-18200 and PO1-AG-11412, and a grant from the National Aeronautics and Space Administration through NASA Cooperative Agreement NCC 9–58 with the National Space Biomedical Research Institute.

REFERENCES

Alfoldi, P., Franken, P., Tobler, I. and Borbely, A.A., 1991. Short light-dark cycles influence sleep stages and EEG power spectra in the rat. *Behavioral Brain Research*, **43**, 125–131.

Amici, R., Zamboni, G., Perez, E., Jones, C.A., Toni, I.I., Culin, F. and Parmeggiani, P.L., 1994. Pattern of desynchronised sleep during deprivation and recovery induced in the rat by changes in ambient temperature. *Journal of Sleep Research*, **3**, 250–256.

Amici, R., Zamboni, G., Perez, E., Jones, C.A. and Parmeggiani, P.L., 1998. The influence of a heavy thermal load on REM sleep in the rat. *Brain Research*, **781**, 252–258.

Aston-Jones, G., Chen, S., Zhu, Y. and Oshinsky, M.L., 2001. A neural circuit for circadian regulation of arousal. *Nature Neuroscience*, **4**, 732–738.

Axelrod, J. and Reisine, T.D., 1984. Stress hormones: their interaction and regulation. *Science*, **224**, 452–459.

Baker, T.L., Foutz, A.S., McNerney, V., Mitler, M.M. and Dement, W.C., 1982. Canine model of narcolepsy: genetic and developmental determinants. *Experimental Neurology*, **75**, 729–742.

Barbazanges, A., Piazza, P.V., Le Moal, M. and Maccari, S., 1996. Maternal glucocorticoid secretion mediates long-term effects of prenatal stress. *Journal of Neuroscience*, **16**, 3943–3949.

Bassetti, C. and Aldrich, M.S., 1996. Narcolepsy. *Neurologic Clinics*, **14**, 545–571.

Benca, R.M., Overstreet, D.E., Gilliland, M.A., Russell, D., Bergmann, B.M. and Obermeyer, W.H., 1996. Increased basal REM sleep but no differences in dark induction or light suppression of REM sleep in Flinders rats with cholinergic supersensitivity. *Neuropsychopharmacology*, **15**, 45–51.

Berger, M. and Riemann, D., 1993. REM sleep in depression: an overview. *Journal of Sleep Research*, **2**, 211–223.

Bliwise, D.L., 2000. Normal aging. In: Kryger, M.H., Roth, T. and Dement, W.C. (eds), *Principles and Practices of Sleep Medicine* (3rd edn), pp. 26–42. WB Saunders, Philadelphia.

Bodosi, B., Obal, F., Gardi, J., Komlodi, J., Fang, J. and Krueger, J.M., 2000. An ether stressor increases REM sleep in rats: possible role of prolactin. *American Journal of Physiology*, **279**, R1590–R1598.

Bonnet, C., Leger, L., Baubet, V., Debilly, G. and Cespuglio, R., 1997. Influence of a 1-h immobilization stress on sleep states and corticotropin-like intermediate lobe peptide (CLIP or $ACTH_{18-39}$, Ph-$ACTH_{18-39}$) brain contents in the rat. *Brain Research*, **751**, 54–63.

Bonnet, C., Marinesco, S., Debilly, G., Kovalzon, V. and Cespuglio, R., 2000. Influence of a 1-h immobilization stress on sleep and CLIP ($ACTH_{18-39}$) brain contents in adrenalectomized rats. *Brain Research*, **853**, 323–329.

Borbely, A.A., 1976. Sleep and motor activity of the rat under ultra-short light-dark cycles. *Brain Research*, **114**, 305–317.

Borbely, A.A., 1978. Effects of light on sleep and activity rhythms. *Progress in Neurobiology*, **10**, 1–31.

Borbely, A.A. and Neuhaus, H.U., 1979. Sleep deprivation: effects on sleep and EEG in the rat. *Journal of Comparative Physiology A*, **133**, 71–87.

Borbely, A.A., 1982. Sleep regulation: circadian rhythms and homeostasis. *Current Topics in Neuroendocrinology*, **1**, 83–103.

Bowersox, S.S., Baker, T.L. and Dement, W.C., 1984. Sleep-wakefulness patterns in the aged cat. *Electroencephalography and Clinical Neurophysiology*, **58**, 240–252.

Campbell, S.S. and Tobler, I., 1984. animal sleep: a review of sleep duration across phylogeny. *Neuroscience and Biobehavioral Reviews*, **8**, 269–300.

Cespuglio, R., Gomez, M.E., Faradji, H. and Jouvet, M., 1982. Alterations in the sleep-waking cycle induced by cooling of the locus coeruleus area. *Electroencephalography and Clinical Neurophysiology*, **54**, 570–578.

Chastrette, N., Cespuglio, R. and Jouvet, M., 1990. Proopiomelanocortin (POMC)-derived peptides and sleep in the rat. I. Hypnogenic properties of ACTH derivates. *Neuropeptides*, **15**, 61–74.

Cheeta, S., Ruigt, G., Van Proosdij, J. and Willner, P., 1997. Changes in sleep architecture following chronic mild stress. *Biological Psychiatry*, **41**, 419–427.

Chemelli, R.M., Willie, J.T., Sinton, C.M., Elmquist, J.K., Scammell, T., Lee, C., Richardson, J.A., Williams, S.C., Xiong, Y., Kisanuki, Y., Fitch, T.E., Nakazato, M., Hammer, R.E., Saper, C.B. and Yanagisawa, M., 1999. Narcolepsy in orexin knockout mice: molecular genetics of sleep regulation. *Cell*, **98**, 437–451.

Datta, S., Patterson, E.H., Vincitore, M., Tonkiss, J., Morgane, P.J. and Galler, J.R., 2000. Prenatal protein malnourished rats show changes in sleep/wake behavior as adults. *Journal of Sleep Research*, **9**, 71–79.

De Lecea, L., Kilduff, T.S., Peyron, C., Gao, X.B., Foye, P.E., Danielson, P.E., Fukuhura, C., Battenburg, E.L.F., Gautvik, V.T., Bartlett, F.S., Frankel, W.N., Van den Poll, A.N., Bloom, F.E., Gautvik, K.M. and Sutcliffe, J.G., 1998. The hypocretins: hypothalamus specific peptides with neuroexcitatory activity. *Proceedings of the National Academy of Sciences of the United States of America*, **95**, 322–327.

Dugovic, C., Maccari, S., Weibel, L., Turek, F.W. and Van Reeth, O., 1999. High corticosterone levels in prenatally stressed rats predict persistent paradoxical sleep alterations. *Journal of Neuroscience*, **19**, 8656–8664.

Dugovic, C., Solberg, L.C., Redei, E., Van Reeth, O. and Turek, F.W., 2000. Sleep in the Wistar-Kyoto rat, a putative genetic animal model for depression. *Neuroreport*, **11**, 627–631.

Eastman, C.I., Mistlberger, R.E. and Rechtschaffen, A., 1984. Suprachiasmatic nuclei lesions eliminate circadian temperature and sleep rhythms in the rat. *Physiology and Behavior*, **32**, 357–368.

Edgar, D.M., Dement, W.C. and Fuller, C.A., 1993. Effect of SCN lesions on sleep in squirrel monkeys: evidence for opponent processes in sleep-wake regulation. *Journal of Neuroscience*, **13**, 1065–1079.

Ehlers, C.L., Reed, T.K. and Henriksen, S.J., 1986. Effects of corticotropin-releasing factor and growth hormone-releasing factor on sleep and activity in rats. *Neuroendocrinology*, **42**, 467–474.

Foley, D.J., Monjan, A.A. and Brown, S.L., 1995. Sleep complaints among elderly persons: an epidemiological study of three communities. *Sleep*, **18**, 425–432.

Gillin, J.C., Jacobs, L.S., Snyder, S. and Henken, R.I., 1974. Effects of ACTH on the sleep of normal subjects and patients with Addison's disease. *Neuroendocrinology*, **15**, 21–31.

Gislason, T. and Almqvist, M., 1987. Somatic diseases and sleep complaints. *Acta Medica Scandinavica*, **221**, 475–481.

Gonzalez, M. and Valatx, J.L., 1997. Effect of intracerebroventricular administration of α-helical CRH (9–41) on the sleep/waking cycle in rats under normal conditions or after subjection to an acute stressful stimulus. *Journal of Sleep Research*, **6**, 164–170.

Graves, L., Pack, A. and Abel, T., 2001. Sleep and memory: a molecular perspective. *Trends in Neuroscience*, **24**, 237–243.

Guilleminault, C. and Anagnos, A., 2000. Narcolepsy. In *Principles and Practices of Sleep Medicine* (3rd edn), Kryger, M.H., Roth, T. and Dement, W.C. (eds), WB Saunders, Philadelphia, 676–686.

Hagan, J.J., Leslie, R.A., Patel, S., Evans, M.L., Wattam, T.A., Holmes, S., Benham, C.D., Taylor, S.G., Routledge, C., Hemmati, P., Munton, R.P., Ashmeade, T.E., Shah, A.S., Hatcher, C.P., Hatcher, P.D., Jones, D.N., Smith, M.I., Piper, D.C., Hunter, A.J., Porter, R.A. and Upton, N., 1999. Orexin A activates locus coeruleus cell firing and increases arousal in the rat. *Proceedings of the National Academy of Sciences of the United States of America*, **96**, 10911–10916.

Hicks, R.A. and Moore, J.D., 1979. REM sleep deprivation diminishes fear in rats. *Physiology and Behavior*, **22**, 689–692.

Hicks, R.A., Moore, J.D., Hayes, C., Phillips, N. and Hawkins, J., 1979. REM sleep deprivation increases aggressiveness in male rats. *Physiology and Behavior*, **22**, 1097–1100.

Hilakivi, L., 1986. Effects of prenatal alcohol exposure on neonatal sleep-wake behaviour and adult alcohol consumption in rats. *Acta Pharmacologica et Toxicologica*, **59**, 36–42.

Horne, J.A. and Reid, J.A., 1985. Night-time sleep EEG changes following body heating in a warm bath. *Electroencephalography and Clinical Neurophysiology*, **60**, 154–157.

Ibuka, N., Nihonmatsu, I. and Sekiguchi, S., 1980. Sleep-wakefulness rhythms in mice after suprachiasmatic nucleus lesions. *Waking Sleeping*, **4**, 167–173.

James, G.W.L. and Piper, D.C.A., 1978. A method for evaluating potential hypnotic compounds in rats. *Journal of Pharmacological Methods*, **1**, 145–154.

Johnson, E.O., Kamilaris, T.C., Chrousos, G.P. and Gold, P.W., 1992. Mechanisms of stress: a dynamic overview of hormonal and behavioral homeostasis. *Neuroscience and Biobehavioral Reviews*, **16**, 115–130.

Jones, B.E., Harper, S.T. and Halaris, A.E., 1977. Effects of locus coeruleus lesions upon cerebral monoamine content, sleep-wakefulness states and the response to amphetamine. *Brain Research*, **124**, 473–496.

Jouvet, M., 1999. Sleep and serotonin: an unfinished story. *Neuropsychopharmacology*, **21**(Suppl 2), 24S–27S.

Kant, G.J., Pastel, R.H., Bauman, R.A., Meininger, G.R., Maughan, K.R., Robinson, T.N., Wright, W.L. and Covington, P.S., 1995. Effects of chronic stress on sleep in rats. *Physiology and Behavior*, **57**, 359–365.

Klein, D.C., Moore, R.Y. and Reppert, S.M., 1991. *Suprachiasmatic Nucleus: The Mind's Clock*. Oxford University Press, New York.

Lelkes, Z., Benedek, G., Alfoldi, P. and Hideg, J., 1990. Effects of alternating 45-min light dark cycles on sleep in the rat. *Acta Physiologica Hungarica*, **76**, 229–236.

Lenox, R.H., Kant, G.J., Sessions, G.R., Pennington, L.L., Mougey, E.H. and Meye, J.L., 1980. Specific hormonal and neurochemical responses to different stressors. *Neuroendocrinology*, **30**, 300–308.

Li, H. and Satinoff, E., 1995. Changes in circadian rhythms of body temperature and sleep in old rats. *American Journal of Physiology*, **269**, R208–214.

Lin, J.S., Roussel, B., Akaoka, H., Fort, P., Debilly, G. and Jouvet, M., 1992. Role of catecholamines in the modafinil and amphetamine induced wakefulness, a comparative pharmacological study in the cat. *Brain Research*, **591**, 319–326.

Lin, L., Faraco, J., Li, R., Kadotani, H., Rogers, W., Lin, X., Qiu, X., De Jong, P.J., Nishino, S. and Mignot, E., 1999. The sleep disorder canine narcolepsy is caused by a mutation in the hypocretin (orexin) receptor 2 gene. *Cell*, **98**, 365–376.

Louis, W.J. and Howes, L.G., 1990. Genealogy of the spontaneously hypertensive rat and Wistar-Kyoto strains: implications for studies of inherited hypertension. *Journal of Cardiovascular Pharmacology*, **16**(Suppl 7), S1–5.

Meerlo, P., Pragt, B. and Daan, S., 1997. Social stress induces high intensity sleep in rats. *Neuroscience Letters*, **225**, 41–44.

Meerlo, P. and Turek, F.W., 2001. Effects of social stimuli on sleep in mice: non-rapid-eye movement (NREM) sleep is promoted by aggressive interaction but not by sexual interaction. *Brain Research*, **907**, 84–92.

Meerlo, P., Easton, A., Bergmann, B.M. and Turek, F.W., 2001. Restraint increases prolactin and rapid eye movement (REM) sleep in C57BL/6J mice but not in BALB/cJ mice. *American Journal of Physiology*, **281**, R846–R854.

Mendelson, W.B. and Bergmann, B.M., 1999. Age-related changes in sleep in the rat. *Sleep*, **22**, 145–150.

Mendelson, W.B. and Bergmann, B.M., 2000. Age-dependent changes in recovery sleep after 48 h of sleep deprivation in rats. *Neurobiology of Aging*, **21**, 689–693.

Mistlberger, R.E., Bergmann, B.M., Waldenar, W. and Rechtschaffen, A., 1983. Recovery sleep following sleep deprivation in intact and suprachiasmatic nuclei-lesioned rats. *Sleep*, **6**, 217–233.

Mitler, M.M., Boyse, B.G., Campbell, L. and Dement, W.C., 1974. Narcolepsy-cataplexy in a female dog. *Experimental Neurology*, **45**, 322–340.

Moore, R.Y. and Eichler, V.B., 1972. Loss of circadian adrenal corticosterone rhythm following suprachiasmatic lesions in the rat. *Brain Research*, **42**, 201–206.

Moore, R.Y. and Lenn, N.J., 1972. A retinohypothalamic projection in the rat. *Journal of Comparative Neurology*, **146**, 1–14.

Moreau, J.L., Scherschlicht, R.R., Jenck, F.F. and Martin, J.R., 1995. Chronic mild stress-induced anhedonia model of depression; sleep abnormalities and curative effects of electroshock treatment. *Behavioral Pharmacology*, **6**, 682–687.

Moriarty, S.R., Szymusiak, R., Thomson, D. and McGinty, D.J., 1993. Selective increases in non-rapid eye movement sleep following whole body heating in rats. *Brain Research*, **617**, 10–16.

Mouret, J., Coindet, J., Debilly, G. and Chouvet, G., 1978. Suprachiasmatic nuclei lesions in the rat: alterations in sleep circadian rhythms. *Electroencephalography and Clinical Neurophysiology*, **45**, 402–408.

Naylor, E., Buxton, O.M., Bergmann, B.M., Easton, A., Zee, P.C. and Turek, F.W., 1998. Effects of aging on sleep in the golden hamster. *Sleep*, **21**, 687–693.

Naylor, E., Penev, P.D., Orbeta, L., Janssen, I., Ortiz, R., Colecchia, E.F., Keng, M., Finkel, S. and Zee, P.C., 2000. Daily social and physical activity increases slow-wave sleep and daytime neuropsychological performance in the elderly. *Sleep*, **23**, 87–95.

Naylor, E., Bergmann, B.M., Krauski, K., Zee, P.C., Takahashi, J.S., Vitaterna, M.H. and Turek, F.W., 2000. The circadian clock mutation alters sleep homeostasis in the mouse. *Journal of Neuroscience*, **20**, 8138–8143.

Nishino, S. and Mignot, E., 1997. Pharmacological aspects of human and canine narcolepsy. *Progress in Neurobiology*, **52**, 27–78.

Nishino, S., Ripley, B., Overeem, S., Lammers, G.J. and Mignot, E., 2000. Hypocretin (orexin) deficiency in human narcolepsy. *Lancet*, **355**, 39–40.

Obal, F., Alfoldi, P. and Rubicsek, G., 1995. Promotion of sleep by heat in young rats. *Pflugers Archiv*, **430**, 729–738.

Opp, M.R., 1995. Corticotropin-releasing hormone involvement in stressor-induced alterations in sleep and in the regulation of wakefulness. *Advances in Neuroimmunology*, **5**, 127–143.

Oswald, I., 1962. *Sleeping and Waking: Physiology and Psychology*. Elsevier, Amsterdam.

Overstreet, D.H., 1993. The Flinders sensitive line rats: a genetic model of depression. *Neuroscience and Biobehavioral Reviews*, **17**, 51–68.

Palma, B.D., Suchecki, D. and Tufik, S., 2000. Differential effects of acute cold and foot shock on the sleep of rats. *Brain Research*, **861**, 97–104.

Pare, W.P. and Redei, E., 1993. Depressive behavior and stress ulcer in Wistar Kyoto rats. *Journal of Physiology, Paris*, **87**, 229–238.

Parmeggiani, P.L. and Rabini, C., 1970. Sleep and environmental temperature. *Archives Italiennes de Biologie (Pisa)*, **108**, 369–387.

Penev, P.D., Zee, P.C., Wallen, E.P. and Turek, F.W., 1995. Aging alters the phase-resetting properties of a serotonin agonist on hamster circadian rhythmicity. *American Journal of Physiology*, **268**, R293–298.

Peyron, C., Tighe, D.K., Van den Pol, A.N., De Lecea, L., Heller, H.C., Sutcliffe, J.G. and Kilduff, T.S., 1998. Neurons containing hypocretin (orexin) project to multiple neuronal systems. *Journal of Neuroscience*, **18**, 9996–10015.

Peyron, C., Faraco, J., Rogers, W., Ripley, B., Overeem, S., Charnay, Y., Nevsimalova, S., Aldrich, M., Reynolds, D., Albin, R., Li, R., Hungs, M., Pedrazzoli, M., Padigaru, M., Kucherlapati, M., Fan, J., Maki, R., Lammers, G.J., Bouras, C., Kucherlapati, R., Nishino, S. and Mignot, E., 2000. A mutation in a case of early onset narcolepsy and a generalized absence of hypocretin peptides in human narcoleptic brains. *Nature Medicine*, **6**, 991–997.

Piper, D.C., Upton, N., Smith, M.I. and Hunter, A.J., 2000. The novel brain neuropeptide, orexin-A, modulates the sleep-wake cycle of rats. *European Journal of Neuroscience*, **12**, 726–730.

Pittendrigh, C.S., 1981. Circadian systems: entrainment. In: Aschoff, J. (ed.), *Handbook of Behavioural Biology, Volume 4: Biological Rhythms*, pp. 95–124. Plenum Press, New York.

Portas, C.M., Bjorvatn, B. and Ursin, R., 2000. Serotonin and the sleep/wake cycle: special emphasis on microdialysis studies. *Progress in Neurobiology*, **60**, 13–35.

Putkonen, P.T.S., Eloman, E. and Kotilnen, P.V., 1973. Increase in delta (3–4) sleep after heat stress in sauna. *Journal of Clinical Laboratory Investigation*, **32**(Suppl 130), 19.

Rampin, C., Cespuglio, R., Chastrette, N. and Jouvet, M., 1991. Immobilization stress induces a paradoxical sleep rebound in the rat. *Neuroscience Letters*, **126**, 113–118.

Rechtschaffen, A., Gilliland, M.A., Bergmann, B.M. and Winter, J.B., 1983. Physiological correlates of prolonged sleep deprivation in rats. *Science*, **221**, 182–184.

Rechtschaffen, A., Bergmann, B.M., Everson, C.A., Kushida, C.A. and Gilliland, M.A., 1989. Sleep deprivation in the rat. X. Integration and discussion of the findings. *Sleep*, **12**, 68–87.

Roehrs, T., Zorick, F.J. and Roth, T., 2000. Transient and short-term insomnias. In: Kryger, M.H., Roth, T. and Dement, W.C. (eds), pp. 624–632. *Principles and Practices of Sleep Medicine* (3rd edn), WB Saunders, Philadelphia.

Rosenberg, R.S., Zepelin, H. and Rechtschaffen, A., 1979. Sleep in young and old rats. *Journal of Gerontology*, **34**, 525–532.

Rosenthal, M.S. and Vogel, G.W., 1993. The effect of a 3-day increase of ambient temperature toward the thermoneutral zone on rapid eye movement sleep in the rat. *Sleep*, **16**, 702–705.

Roussel, B., Turrillot, P. and Kitahama, K., 1984. Effect of ambient temperature on the sleep-waking cycle in two strains of mice. *Brain Research*, **294**, 67–73.

Sakurai, T., Amemiya, A., Ishii, M., Matsuzaki, I., Chemelli, R.M., Tanaka, H., Williams, S.C., Richardson, J.A., Kozlowski, G.P., Wilson, S., Arch, J.R., Buckingham, R.E., Haynes, A.C., Carr, S.A., Annan, R.S., McNulty, D.E., Liu, W.S., Terrett, J.A., Elshourbagy, N.A., Bergsma, D.J. and Yanagisawa, M., 1998. Orexins and orexin receptors: a family of hypothalamic neuropeptides and G protein-coupled receptors that regulate feeding behavior. *Cell*, **92**, 573–585.

Satinoff, E., Li, H., Tcheng, T.K., Liu, C., McArthur, A.J., Medanic, M. and Gillette, M.U., 1993. Do the suprachiasmatic nuclei oscillate in old rats as they do in young ones? *American Journal of Physiology*, **265**, R1216–1222.

Schmidek, W.R., Hoshino, K., Schmidek, M. and Timo-Iaria, C., 1972. Influence of environmental temperature on the sleep-wakefulness cycle in the rat. *Physiology and Behavior*, **8**, 363–371.

Sei, H., Kiuchi, T., Chang, H.Y. and Morita, Y., 1992. Effects of an eight-hour advance of the light-dark cycle on sleep-wake rhythm in the rat. *Neuroscience Letters*, **137**, 161–164.

Selye, H., 1936. A syndrome produced by diverse nocuous agents. *Nature*, **138**, 32.

Shen, H. and Semba, K., 1994. A direct retinal projection to the dorsal raphe nucleus in the rat. *Brain Research*, **635**, 159–168.

Shiromani, P.J., Overstreet, D., Levy, D., Goodrich, C.A., Campbell, S.S. and Gillin, S.S., 1988. Increased REM sleep in rats selectively bred for cholinergic hyperactivity. *Neuropsychopharmacology*, **1**, 127–133.

Shiromani, P.J., Lu, J., Wagner, D., Thakker, J., Greco, M.A., Basheer, R. and Thakkar, M., 2000. Compensatory sleep response to 12-h wakefulness in young and old rats. *American Journal of Physiology*, **278**, R125–R133.

Sichieri, R. and Schmidek, W.R., 1984. Influence of ambient temperature on the sleep-wakefulness cycle in the golden hamster. *Physiology and Behavior*, **33**, 871–877.

Siegel, J.M., 1999. Narcolepsy: a key role for hypocretins (orexins). *Cell*, **98**, 409–412.

Siegel, J.M., 2001. The REM sleep-memory consolidation hypothesis. *Science*, **294**, 1058–1063.

Smith, C., 1996. Sleep states, memory processes and synaptic plasticity. *Behavioral Brain Research*, **78**, 49–56.

Stephan, F.K. and Zucker, I., 1972. Circadian rhythms in drinking behavior and locomotor activity of rats are eliminated by hypothalamic lesions. *Proceedings of the National Academy of Sciences of the United States of America*, **69**, 1583–1586.

Stone, W.S., Altman, H.J., Hall, J., Arankowsky-Sandoval, G., Parekh, P. and Gold, P.E., 1996. Prenatal exposure to alcohol in adult rats: relationships between sleep and memory deficits, and effects of glucose administration on memory. *Brain Research*, **742**, 98–106.

Sutcliffe, J.G. and De Lecea, L., 2000. The hypocretins: excitatory neuromodulatory peptides for multiple homeostatic systems, including sleep and feeding. *Journal of Neuroscience Research*, **62**, 161–168.

Sylvester, L., Kapron, C.M. and Smith, C., 2000. In utero ethanol exposure decreases rapid eye movement sleep in female Sprague-Dawley rat offspring. *Neuroscience Letters*, **289**, 13–16.

Szymusiak, R. and Satinoff, E., 1981. Maximal REM sleep time defines a narrower thermoneutral zone than does minimal metabolic rate. *Physiology and Behavior*, **26**, 687–690.

Terman, M., Reme, C.E. and Wirz-Justice, A., 1991. The visual input stage of the mammalian circadian pacemaker system: the effect of light and drugs on retinal function. *Journal of Biological Rhythms*, **6**, 31–48.

Thannickal, T., Moore, R.Y., Nienhuis, R., Ramanathan, L., Gulyani, S., Aldrich, M., Cornford, M. and Siegel, J.M., 2000. Reduced number of hypocretin neurons in human narcolepsy. *Neuron*, **27**, 460–474.

Tobler, I., Borbely, A.A. and Groos, G., 1983. The effects of sleep deprivation on sleep in rats with suprachiasmatic lesions. *Neuroscience Letters*, **42**, 49–54.

Tobler, I. and Borbely, A.A., 1986. Sleep EEG in the rat as a function of prior waking. *Electroencephalography and Clinical Neurophysiology*, **64**, 74–76.

Tobler, I., Franken, P., Alfoldi, P. and Borbely, A.A., 1994. Room light impairs sleep in the albino rat. *Behavioral Brain Research*, **63**, 205–211.

Tobler, I., 2000. The phylogeny of sleep regulation. In: Kryger, M.H., Roth, T. and Dement, W.C. (eds), *Principles and Practices of Sleep Medicine* (3rd edn), pp. 72–81. WB Saunders, Philadelphia.

Trachsel, L., Tobler, I. and Borbely, A.A., 1986. Sleep regulation in rats: effects of sleep deprivation, light, and circadian phase. *American Journal of Physiology*, **251**, R1037–1044.

Turek, F.W., Scarbrough, K., Penev, P., Labyak, S., Valentinuzzi, V.S. and Van Reeth, O., 2001. Aging of the mammalian circadian system. In: Takahashi, J.S., Turek, F.W. and Moore, R.Y. (eds), *Handbook of Behavioral Neurobiology, Volume 12: Circadian Clocks*, pp. 292–317. Kluwer Academic/Plenum, New York.

Van der Zee, E.A., Jansen, K. and Gerkema, M., 1999. Severe loss of vasopressin-immunoreactive cells in the suprachiasmatic nucleus of aging voles coincides with reduced circadian organization of running wheel activity. *Brain Research*, **816**, 572–579.

Van Gool, W.A. and Mirmiran, M., 1983. Age-related changes in the sleep pattern of male adult rats. *Brain Research*, **279**, 394–398.

Van Gool, W.A. and Mirmiran, M., 1986. Effects of aging and housing in an enriched environment on sleep-wake patterns in rats. *Sleep*, **9**, 335–347.

Van Reeth, O., Zhang, Y., Zee, P.C. and Turek, F., 1993. The effects of aging on the entraining properties of activity-inducing stimuli on the circadian clock. *Brain Research*, **607**, 286–292.

Vitaterna, M.H., King, D.P., Chang, A.M., Kornhauser, J.M., Lowrey, P.L., McDonald, J.D., Dove, W.F., Pinto, L.H., Turek, F.W. and Takahashi, J.S., 1994. Mutagenesis and mapping of a mouse gene, *Clock*, essential for circadian behavior. *Science*, **264**, 719–725.

Vogel, G.W., Vogel, F., McAbee, R.S. and Thurmond, A.J., 1980. Improvement of depression by REM sleep deprivation. *Archives of General Psychiatry*, **37**, 247–253.

Weinert, D., 2000. Age-dependent changes of the circadian system. *Chronobiology International*, **17**, 261–183.

Weinstock, M., 1997. Does prenatal stress impair coping and regulation of hypothalamic-pituitary-adrenal axis? *Neuroscience and Biobehavioral Reviews*, **21**, 1–10.

Welsh, D.K., Richardson, G.S. and Dement, W.C., 1986. Effect of age on the circadian pattern of sleep and wakefulness in the mouse. *Journal of Gerontology*, **41**, 579–586.

Zee, P., Rosenberg, R. and Turek, F., 1992. Effects of aging on entrainment and rate of resynchronization of circadian locomotor activity. *American Journal of Physiology*, **263**, R1099–1103.

Zepelin, H., Whitehead, W.E. and Rechtschaffen, A., 1972. Aging and sleep in the albino rat. *Behavioral Biology*, **7**, 65–74.

Zepelin, H., 2000. Mammalian sleep. In: Kryger, M.H., Roth, T. and Dement, W.C. (eds), *Principles and Practices of Sleep Medicine* (3rd edn), pp. 82–92. WB Saunders, Philadelphia.

XXIV-2

Neurotransmitter Systems Regulating Sleep-Wake States

Barbara E. Jones

Three distinct physiological and cognitive states exist in mammals: waking, slow-wave sleep (SWS) and rapid-eye-movement sleep (REMS). Waking is a multifarious state but is generally characterized by fast waves on the electroencephalographic (EEG) record in association with behavioural activity and responsiveness; SWS is characterized by slow waves on the EEG record in association with behavioural quiescence and decreased responsiveness; however, REMS, or 'paradoxical sleep' (PS), is characterized by a unique dissociation of EEG, characterized by fast waves indicative of cortical arousal, and behaviour, characterized by quiescence and diminished responsiveness, indicative of sleep. Viewed in terms of metabolism and energy expenditure, waking requires variable yet relatively high levels of energy expenditure by the brain and body; SWS requires low levels and thus allows conservation and restoration of energy stores in both brain and body; however, REMS requires high levels of energy expenditure by the brain while maintaining minimal energy use by the body. These states occur within a circadian cycle and an ultradian cycle. Depending upon the species, the active, waking phase of the circadian cycle occurs either during the day and light, as in humans, or during the night and darkness, as in cats and rats. Sleep is concentrated to differing degrees in the opposite phase, when it occurs, according to an ultradian rhythm. Across the phylogenetic scale, the period of the ultradian sleep-wake rhythm is correlated with basal metabolic rate and body weight, and thus is apparently determined in part by energy expenditure, storage, conservation and restoration. In addition to their regulation by underlying rhythms, the sleep-wake states are also regulated by homeostatic processes, such that the deprivation of sleep results in an increased drive for sleep and increased occurrence of sleep upon recovery. The rhythmic and homeostatic nature of sleep-wake states indicates the existence of underlying, alternating and accumulating processes that may depend upon changes in chemical transmitters and their receptors in the brain.

Neurotransmitters include small molecules such as glutamate and GABA, acetylcholine and the monoamines, which may act directly upon ion channels or indirectly upon them through second messengers to modify membrane potentials and activity of neurons. They may also include peptides, which function as transmitters, modulators or hormones. Although, to date, no single transmitter/modulator molecule has been found that serves a specific or exclusive function in promoting or generating waking, SWS or REMS, specific neuronal systems containing particular neurotransmitters have been shown to be integral to the promotion of each of these states.

From early physiological studies, it has been known that no specific centres are present in the brain for the generation of any one state, but that redundant neuronal systems are distributed through the brainstem and forebrain, systems which are collectively important for the promotion and maintenance of individual states (Jones, 2000). For **waking** (Figure XXIV-2.1), neurons distributed through the brainstem reticular formation (RF) and concentrated within the oral pontine and mesencephalic fields comprise the ascending reticular activating system, which, by lesions in humans and animals, is known to be critical for the generation and maintenance of the EEG and behavioural components of waking (Moruzzi and Magoun, 1949). This system of neurons gives rise to ascending pathways projecting dorsally into the non-specific thalamo-cortical projection system, which in turn stimulates widespread activation of the cerebral cortex (Dempsey *et al.*, 1941). Other fibres ascend ventrally into and through the hypothalamus up to the level of the basal forebrain (substantia innominata [SI]), from where cortical activation is also relayed in a widespread manner (Starzl *et al.*, 1951). These systems collectively stimulate cortical activation, characterized by high-frequency (beta and gamma) EEG activity. Fibres also terminate in the posterior hypothalamus, where lesions are known in humans and animals to produce a comatose state (Ranson, 1939). As evident as well from electrical stimulation (Hess, 1957), the posterior hypothalamus is an important higher control centre for the sympathetic nervous system, thus coordinating peripheral autonomic responses (increased temperature, respiration, heart rate, blood pressure) with cortical activation. In addition, the descending projections from the brainstem reticular formation, including the caudal pontine and medullary reticular formation, serve to stimulate somatic motor activity, reactivity and postural muscle tonus (as evident in electromyographic [EMG] activity) through facilitatory reticulo-spinal influences (Magoun and Rhines, 1946).

For **SWS** (Figure XXIV-2.2), the medulla appears, to play a role in promoting sleep, particularly neurons in the region of the solitary and vagal, parasympathetic nuclei, which may inhibit the activating neurons located in the ponto-mesencephalic tegmentum (Batini *et al.*, 1959; Favale *et al.*, 1961). Within the forebrain, sleep marked by EEG slow waves may be elicited by low-frequency stimulation of the thalamo-cortical projection neurons (Akert *et al.*, 1952). Most potent there is the influence shown to emanate from the preoptic and anterior hypothalamic (POAH) region, where lesions have produced insomnia and electrical stimulation has promoted sleep, probably in part due to inhibition of the posterior hypothalamus and ponto-mesencephalic reticular formation (von Economo, 1931; Nauta, 1946; Hess, 1954). This region serves in an antagonistic manner to the posterior hypothalamus, inhibiting sympathetic activity and facilitating parasympathetic responses (decreased temperature, respiration, heart rate, blood pressure). SWS appears to emerge from the dampening of cortical activation, somatic motor activity (as evident by decreased EMG) and sympathetic nervous activity along with a shift to a predominance of parasympathetic activity.

For **REMS** (or PS, as it is often also called in animals) (Figure XXIV-2.3), the brainstem appears to contain the essential structures for the generation of the state (Jouvet, 1962). The oral pontine reticular formation (PnO) is necessary for the triggering of ascending and descending parameters of the state, including

Biological Psychiatry: Edited by H. D'haenen, J.A. den Boer and P. Willner. ISBN 0-471-49198-5

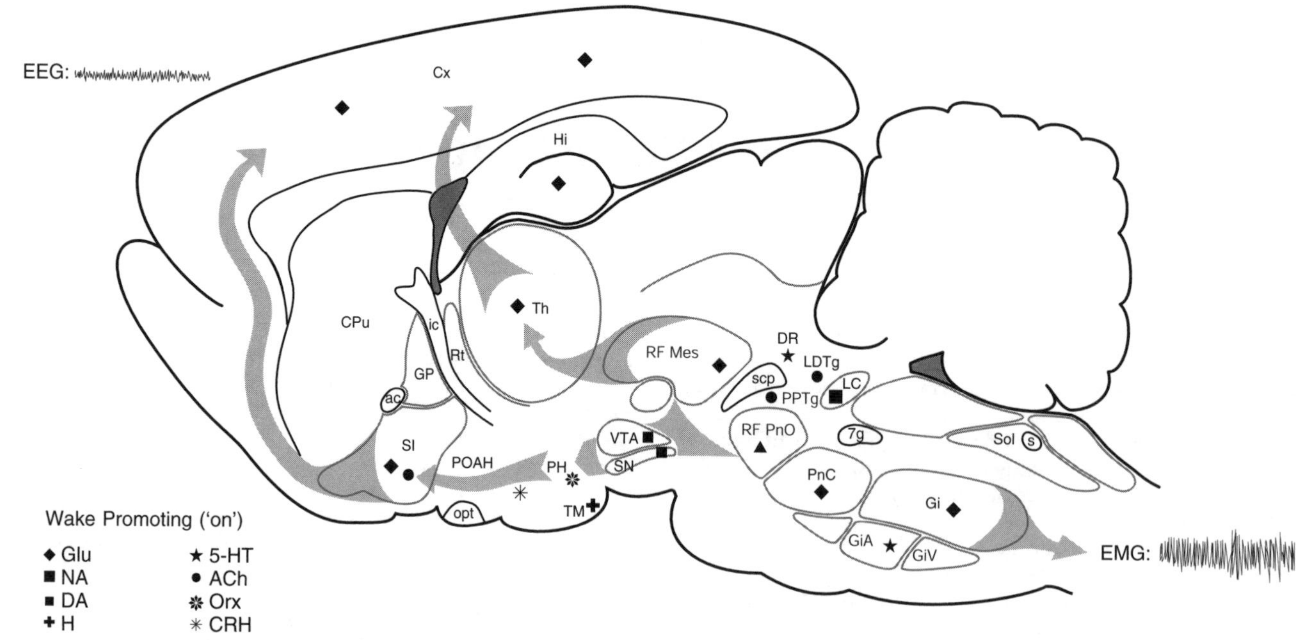

Figure XXIV-2.1 Wake-Promoting Systems. Schematic sagittal view of rat brain showing the major neuronal systems and their major excitatory pathways (arrows) involved in promoting the EEG fast activity (upper left) and EMG high muscle tone and activity (lower right) characteristic of the waking state. The major ascending pathways emerge from the brainstem reticular formation (RF, most densely from the mesencephalic, RF Mes, and oral pontine RF PnO, fields) to ascend along a) a dorsal trajectory into the thalamus (Th) where they terminate upon (midline, medial, and intralaminar) nuclei of the non-specific thalamo-cortical projection system, which projects in turn in a widespread manner to the cerebral cortex (Cx), and b) a ventral trajectory through the lateral hypothalamus up to the basal forebrain where they terminate upon neurons in the substantia innominata (SI) (and septum, not shown), which also project in turn in a widespread manner to the cerebral cortex (and hippocampus, Hi) (Jones, 1995). Descending projections collect from multiple levels of the reticular formation (though most densely from the caudal pontine, PnC, and medullary gigantocellular, Gi, fields) to form the reticulo-spinal pathways. The major transmitter systems that promote waking and discharge maximally ('on') during waking contribute to these ascending and descending systems and are represented by symbols where their cell bodies are located. Glutamatergic (Glu) neurons comprise the vast population of neurons of the reticular formation, the diffuse thalamo-cortical projection system and a contingent of the basalo-cortical projection system. Noradrenergic (NA) neurons of the locus coeruleus (LC) send axons along the major ascending and descending pathways to project in a diffuse manner to the cortex, the subcortical relay stations, brainstem and spinal cord. Dopaminergic (DA) neurons of the substantia nigra (SN) and ventral tegmental area (VTA) project along the ventral pathway in the nigro-striatal system and meso-limbo-cortical system, respectively. Histaminergic (H) neurons of the tuberomammillary nucleus (TM) project in a diffuse manner to the forebrain and cortex. Serotonergic neurons containing 5-hydroxytryptamine (5-HT) of the midbrain (including the dorsal raphe, DR) project to the forebrain, including the cerebral cortex (and hippocampus), as well as the subcortical relay stations, and those of the medulla (in raphe pallidus and obscurus, not shown, as well as pars alpha of the gigantocellular field [GiA]) project to the spinal cord. Cholinergic neurons, containing acetylcholine (ACh), are located in the laterodorsal and pedunculopontine tegmental (LDTg and PPTg) nuclei in the brainstem, from where they project along with other reticular neurons dorsally to the thalamus and ventrally to the posterior hypothalamus and basal forebrain, as well as to the brainstem reticular formation. They are also located in the substantia innominata (SI, and septum, not shown), from where they project to the cortex (and hippocampus). Orexinergic (Orx) neurons in the (perifornical and lateral) mid- and posterior hypothalamus (PH) project diffusely through the forebrain, brainstem and spinal cord to exert an excitatory influence at multiple levels. Corticotropin-releasing hormone (CRH) is contained in neurons within the paraventricular nucleus of the hypothalamus which project to the pituitary, as well as in other scattered neurons (not shown) projecting to other forebrain and brainstem areas that collectively stimulate the hypothalamo-pituitary-adrenal axis and central arousal systems. Some state-specific GABAergic neurons (triangle) may be on during waking to prevent activity of REM-promoting neurons in the oral pontine reticular formation (PnO) (Figure XXIV-2.3) (See Colour Plate XXIV-2.1)

cortical activation, phasic REM along with motor twitches, and tonic postural muscle atonia (Carli and Zanchetti, 1965). The ascending pathways stimulating cortical activation travel along the same routes as those utilized in waking, although the ventral extrathalamic pathway through the basal forebrain and into the limbic cortex appears to be most important (Jouvet, 1962). The descending motor inhibition (as evident from the flat EMG) appears to emerge from the oral pontine reticular formation and to relay through the ventral medullary reticular formation (Magoun and Rhines, 1946). Both visceral and somatic sensory-motor circuits and reflexes are inhibited by this system.

The representation from the classical physiological studies of the distribution of neuronal systems most critically involved in generating waking, SWS and REMS remains valid today. Within those regions and neuronal systems, particular transmitters/modulators have been localized and shown through specific lesions, unit recording, and pharmacological or more recently genetic modulation to play, if not specific, nonetheless differentiated, important roles in promoting waking, SWS or REMS.

WAKE-PROMOTING TRANSMITTER SYSTEMS

Glutamate (Glu) is the most common excitatory neurotransmitter in the brain and is critical for the waking state (Figure XXIV-2.1). It is utilized as the primary transmitter of the neurons within the brainstem reticular formation (RF) and thus is the transmitter of the ascending reticular activating system (Jones, 1995). It is also the transmitter of the non-specific thalamo-cortical projection system (Ottersen *et al.*, 1983) and of a contingent of the basalo-cortical

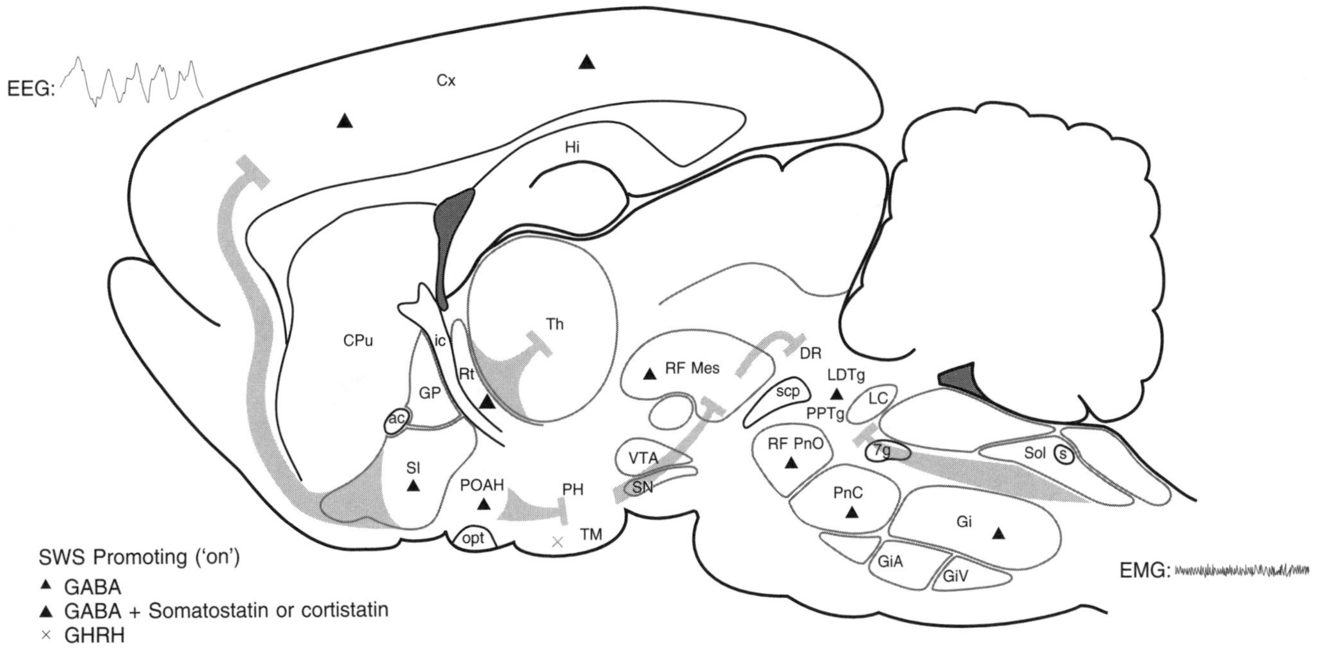

Figure XXIV-2.2 SWS-promoting systems. Schematic sagittal view of rat brain showing the major neuronal systems and their major inhibitory pathways (ending as blocks) involved in promoting the EEG slow-wave activity (upper left) and EMG reduced muscle tone (lower right) characteristic of the slow-wave sleep (SWS) state. Neurons in the region of the solitary tract nucleus (Sol) may exert an inhibitory influence on neurons in the ponto-mesencephalic tegmentum. A dampening influence on the brainstem activating system and the posterior hypothalamus (PH) also emerges from the basal forebrain and preoptic-anterior hypothalamic areas (POAH). From the basal forebrain (substantia innominata [SI]), an inhibitory influence is also exerted upon the cortex (Cx). The major transmitter systems that promote SWS and discharge maximally ('on') during SWS are represented by symbols where their cell bodies are located. These comprise largely GABAergic neurons that, by unit recording and/or c-Fos studies, have been shown to be active during SWS. Particular cortically projecting GABAergic neurons in the SI may have the capacity to dampen cortical activation directly during SWS. Locally projecting GABAergic neurons in the SI may inhibit the cholinergic and glutamatergic cortically projecting neurons. Other GABAergic neurons in the SI and POAH project caudally to the posterior hypothalamus (including the tuberomammillary nucleus [TM]) and brainstem (including RF Mes, DR, LDTg and LC), where they may inhibit multiple wake-active neurons of the activating systems. GABAergic neurons in the reticularis (Rt) nucleus, which surround and innervate the thalamic (Th) nuclei, discharge in bursts to generate spindles while inhibiting the thalamo-cortical projection neurons during SWS. These and local GABAergic neurons in the cortex (Cx) also contain somatostatin or the related peptide corticostatin, which may serve to prolong the inhibition in promoting the slow-wave activity of this state. GABAergic neurons in the brainstem may inhibit local neurons of the ascending reticular activating system as well as those of the descending reticulo-spinal system. Neurons containing growth hormone-releasing hormone (GHRH), primarily located in the arcuate nucleus and projecting to the median eminence, are actively involved in stimulating growth hormone and also promoting slow-wave activity during SWS (See Colour Plate XXIV-2.2)

projection system (Manns *et al.*, 2001). Cortical activation thus depends upon glutamatergic transmission. Glutamate release from the cerebral cortex is highest in association with cortical activation (Jasper *et al.*, 1965). The reticulo-spinal neurons important for increasing muscle tonus, enhancing behavioural responsiveness and stimulating locomotion are also glutamatergic (Grillner *et al.*, 1995).

Drugs that block glutamate transmission by pre- and/or postsynaptic mechanisms (especially the NMDA receptor) comprise some of the anaesthetics, including ketamine (Yamamura *et al.*, 1990) and halothane (MacIver *et al.*, 1996), that produce a loss of consciousness and sensory-motor responsiveness.

Noradrenaline (NA) is a wake- and arousal-promoting transmitter/modulator that is contained in the diffuse projecting locus coeruleus (LC)/subcoeruleus neurons of the pons (Figure XXIV-2.1) and in other hypothalamically projecting and spinally projecting pontine and medullary cell groups. Although lesions of the locus coeruleus nucleus do not result in long-term deficits in cortical activation or waking (Jones *et al.*, 1977), stimulation of the locus coeruleus by electrical or chemical means elicits cortical activation and a vigilant, waking state (Berridge and Foote, 1991). Locus coeruleus neurons discharge at their highest rates during waking, decrease their rate during SWS and cease firing during REMS (Hobson *et al.*, 1975; Aston-Jones and Bloom, 1981b). During waking, they discharge maximally in association with arousal, including attentive and active behaviours, orientation to sensory stimuli, response to painful stimuli and reaction to stressful conditions (Foote *et al.*, 1980; Aston-Jones and Bloom, 1981a; Rasmussen *et al.*, 1986; Abercrombie and Jacobs, 1987a, b). Release of noradrenaline is greatest in association with cortical activation and behavioural arousal, including stress (Nisenbaum *et al.*, 1991; Shouse *et al.*, 2000). In situations of stress, the increased activity of these neurons occurs in parallel with activation of the sympathetic nervous system and the hypothalamo-pituitary-adrenal axis. Through their diffuse projection system that includes the entire forebrain and spinal cord, the locus coeruleus neurons have the capacity to stimulate cortical activation, to activate sympathetic and hypothalamo-pituitary-adrenal systems in the hypothalamus and to excite sympathetic and somatic motor neurons in the spinal cord. Therefore, even though it may not be necessary for maintaining a waking state, the noradrenergic system is important for stimulating a coordinated response to significant sensory stimuli or conditions and thus promoting a maximally attentive and active waking state.

Drugs that diminish noradrenaline, such as alpha-methyl tyrosine (AMT), through inhibition of its synthetic enzyme decrease arousal and enhance both SWS and REMS (King and Jewett, 1971). Drugs that act as agonists at postsynaptic alpha1 receptors

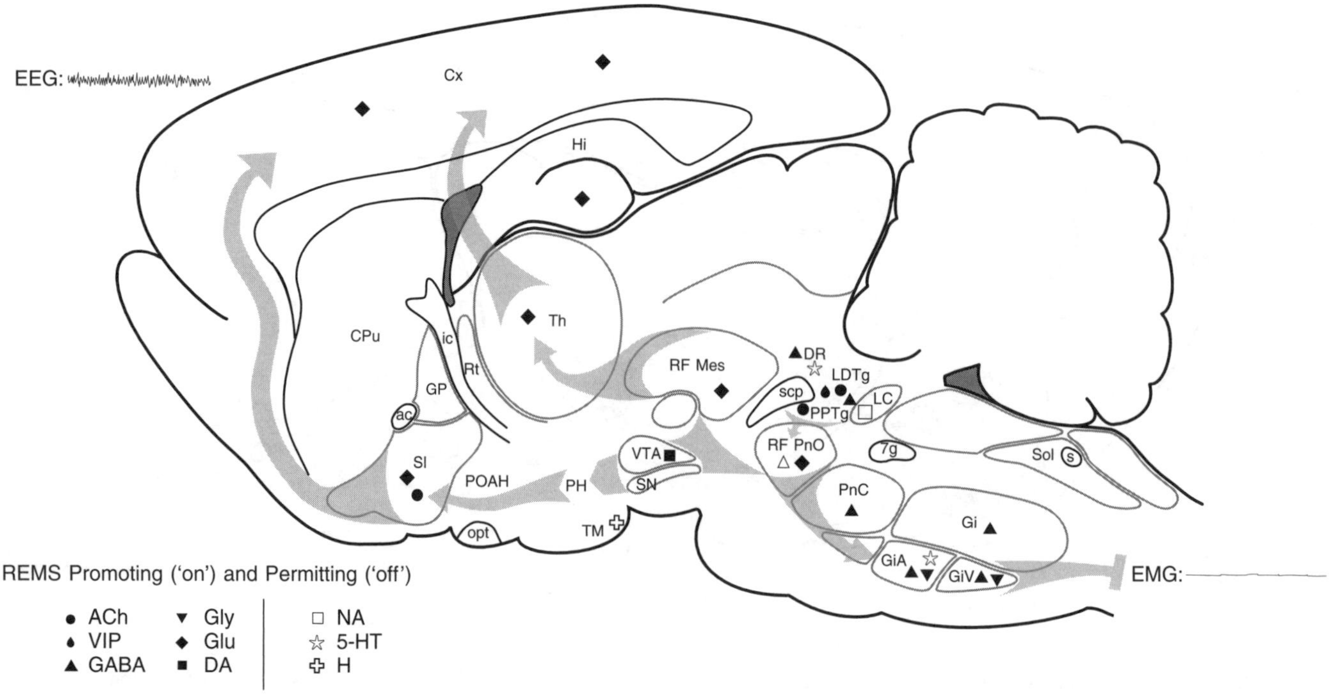

Figure XXIV-2.3 REMS-promoting and REMS-permitting systems. Schematic sagittal view of rat brain showing the major neuronal systems and their (excitatory, ending as arrows, and inhibitory, ending as blocks) pathways involved in promoting the EEG fast activity (upper left) and EMG muscle atonia (lower right) characteristic of rapid eye movement or paradoxical sleep (REMS or PS). Neurons essential for REM sleep are located in the pontine reticular formation, particularly the oral part (RF PnO). The major ascending pathways (indicated by arrows for excitation) promoting cortical activation are similar to those of the waking state; however, the extrathalamic relay into the limbic system may be more important in REMS. The descending motor inhibition (indicated by a block) is triggered by neurons in the oral pontine reticular formation (RF PnO) and partly relayed through neurons in the alpha and ventral gigantocellular fields (GiA and GiV) of the medullary reticular formation en route to the spinal cord. The major transmitter systems that promote REMS and discharge ('on') during REMS are represented by filled symbols, whereas those that are permissive to REMS by stopping their discharge ('off') during the state are represented by empty symbols. Cholinergic neurons that release acetylcholine (ACh) and are located in the laterodorsal and pedunculopontine tegmental nuclei (LDTg and PPTg) are critically involved in promoting REMS through their projections locally into the brainstem reticular formation, and importantly to neurons in the PnO (where they excite glutamatergic neurons and could also inhibit local GABAergic neurons), as well as rostrally into the forebrain. These may be joined in promoting REMS by neurons with similar projections in the region containing vasoactive intestinal peptide (VIP). Noradrenergic (NA) locus coeruleus (LC) and serotonergic (5-HT) dorsal raphe (DR) neurons (as well as histaminergic, H, tuberomammillary neurons, TM) that directly inhibit the cholinergic neurons permit REMS to occur by ceasing their discharge. The arrest of their discharge is effected by local GABAergic neurons, which may be excited by ACh. GABAergic neurons through the caudal pontine (PnC) medullary reticular formation (Gi, GiA, and GiV) may also inhibit local reticulo-spinal and serotonergic raphe-spinal neurons to effect a disfacilitation of motor neurons. In addition, GABAergic and glycinergic neurons in the ventral medullary reticular formation (GiA and GiV) that project to the spinal cord may both directly inhibit motor neurons. One unique group of GABAergic neurons in the PnO ceases discharge during REMS to disinhibit PnO glutamatergic neurons that propagate the ascending and descending correlates of the state. In the ascending pathways, dopaminergic (DA) neurons of the ventral tegmental area (VTA), which are excited by the cholinergic neurons, may be important in activation of the limbic system. The cholinergic basal forebrain neurons (SI and septum) are particularly important in activation of the limbic cortex (hippocampus [Hi]) and neo-cortex (Cx) during REMS (See Colour Plate XXIV-2.3)

stimulate wakefulness. These drugs appear to include modafinil, which stimulates prolonged cortical activation and behavioural arousal, since its effects are blocked by alpha1-receptor antagonists (Duteil *et al.*, 1990; Lin *et al.*, 1992). Through second messengers, alpha1-adrenergic receptors close potassium channels on thalamic and cortical neurons, resulting in their tonic depolarization and the increased excitation that underlies cortical activation (McCormick, 1992). Noradrenaline also acts on alpha2-adrenergic receptors, which commonly open potassium channels through second messengers to hyperpolarize neurons. These receptors are located presynaptically on noradrenergic neurons, as well as postsynaptically on other target neurons. For this reason, drugs that act upon alpha2 receptors are associated with complex, dose-dependent effects upon the sleep-waking cycle. However, the postsynaptic inhibition associated with alpha2 receptors may be important in inhibiting sleep-promoting neurons during waking (see below). Drugs that enhance synaptic levels of noradrenaline through stimulating release and/or blocking reuptake, such as desipramine or amphetamine and possibly also modafinil, enhance arousal, including both cortical activation and muscle tone, and thereby enforce wakefulness, while preventing the onset of both SWS and REMS (Mignot *et al.*, 1993).

Dopamine (DA), like noradrenaline, is principally a wake-promoting transmitter/modulator; however, unlike noradrenaline, it is particularly associated with the pleasurable and rewarding emotional states that may also occur during sleep. Dopaminergic neurons are located in the ventral mesencephalic tegmentum, within the substantia nigra (SN) and ventral tegmental area (VTA) (Figure XXIV-2.1). Dopaminergic neurons of the substantia nigra project predominantly to the striatum, whereas those of the ventral tegmental area project to limbic and medial cortical areas forming the respective nigro-striatal and meso-limbo-cortical projection systems. Lesions of the dopaminergic neurons in the ventral mesencephalic tegmentum result in reduced behavioural arousal; major lesions result in akinesia, along with anorexia and adipsia (Ungerstedt, 1971; Jones *et al.*, 1973). Whereas lesions of the dopaminergic nigro-striatal neurons decrease locomotion, lesions of the meso-limbo-cortical neurons diminish attentive immobility and simultaneously decrease the high-frequency EEG activity associated with that behavioural state (Galey *et al.*, 1977; Montaron *et al.*, 1982). Lesions have also produced a decrease in REMS (Lai *et al.*, 1999). Surprisingly, however, dopaminergic unit activity has not been found to vary significantly across sleep-wake states when measured as average rate of discharge (Miller *et al.*, 1983; Trulson and Preussler, 1984). Similarly, the average release of dopamine has not been found to vary across the sleep-waking cycle (Trulson, 1985; de Saint Hilaire *et al.*, 2000; Shouse *et al.*, 2000). However, dopaminergic neurons discharge in different patterns such that although continuing at the same average firing rate, they may fire in either a tonic or a bursting pattern. Dopaminergic neurons discharge in bursts during arousing situations and particularly when presented with positively rewarding stimuli or conditions (Mirenowicz and Schultz, 1996). Moreover, dopamine release is greatest during waking when animals are aroused and in positively rewarding situations, including those associated with food and drug reward (Di Chiara and Imperato, 1988; Richardson and Gratton, 1996). Accordingly, dopaminergic neurons would be maximally active by bursting in highly aroused, motivated or rewarding situations during waking. They may also be differentially active during sleep, according to the evidence of a change in pattern of discharge during REMS relative to SWS (Miller *et al.*, 1983). Thus, unlike the other monoamine neurons, they do not cease firing during REMS and may discharge in a manner to contribute to the cognitive correlate of that state, as they do in waking (see below).

Drugs that diminish dopamine through inhibition of its synthesis also diminish noradrenaline, and their soporific effects must accordingly be attributed to the simultaneous depletion of both transmitters. Interpreting the effects of drugs acting upon different dopamine receptors is also difficult because of the presynaptic (D2) and multiple postsynaptic (D1/D2) sites of the receptors. More than EEG activity, dopamine-receptor antagonists most markedly alter behaviour and cognitive state. Neuroleptic drugs that block postsynaptic dopamine receptors, such as pimozide, induce a state of anhedonia (Wise *et al.*, 1978). Drugs that act to enhance synaptic levels of dopamine by blocking reuptake or stimulating release, particularly amphetamine and cocaine, have positively rewarding, pleasurable effects associated with their addictive properties (Di Chiara and Imperato, 1988). These drugs also enhance cortical activation and behavioural arousal (Wisor *et al.*, 2001). Drugs that are used in the treatment of hypersomnolence and narcolepsy, and that accordingly prevent both SWS and REMS, include the amphetamines and modafinil. Although to differing degrees, both these drugs most likely act simultaneously upon dopaminergic and noradrenergic transmission to enforce wakefulness (see above) (Wisor *et al.*, 2001).

Histamine (H) is a wake-promoting transmitter/modulator. The neurons containing histamine are located in the tuberomammillary nucleus (TM) of the posterior hypothalamus (Figure XXIV-2.1) and give rise to diffuse projections through the forebrain. Lesions or pharmacological inactivation of these neurons leads to an acute decrease in waking (Lin *et al.*, 1989; Sakai *et al.*, 1990) and increase in REMS as well as SWS (Sallanon *et al.*, 1988). Like noradrenergic neurons, presumed histaminergic neurons discharge at their maximal rate during waking, decrease their rate during SWS and cease firing during REMS (Sakai *et al.*, 1990).

Drugs that antagonize postsynaptic histamine receptors (particularly H1), the common antihistaminergic drugs used for antiallergy medication, as well as those that occupy the presynaptic autoreceptor (H3), which decrease histamine release, produce somnolence and a decrease in waking and vigilance (Monti *et al.*, 1986; Lin *et al.*, 1988, 1990). Conversely, drugs that act as agonists upon the postsynaptic receptors have the capacity to enforce attentive waking and prevent the onset of SWS (Lin *et al.*, 1988). Through these receptors, histamine blocks potassium channels on target thalamic and cortical neurons and thus stimulates a depolarization of those cells underlying cortical activation (McCormick, 1992; Reiner and Kamondi, 1994).

Serotonin (5-hydroxytryptamine [5-HT]) may promote waking, yet it appears to promote a quiet, satiated waking state that can also facilitate the passage into sleep. It is contained in neurons located in the raphe nuclei within the mesencephalon and pons (including the dorsal raphe [DR]), from which diffuse ascending projections into the forebrain arise, and the medulla, from which descending projections to the spinal cord arise (Figure XXIV-2.1). Lesions of the raphe nuclei have produced complete insomnia in association with a behaviourally agitated state (Jouvet, 1972), leading to the postulate that serotonergic neurons generate SWS. However, electrical stimulation of the midbrain raphe arrested waking behaviours, including eating, although it did not produce sleep (Jacobs, 1973). Moreover, most presumed serotonergic raphe neurons discharge during waking and decrease their discharge during SWS, becoming virtually silent during REMS (McGinty and Harper, 1976; Trulson and Jacobs, 1979). During waking, some presumed serotonergic neurons discharge in association with rhythmic motor activities, such as grooming in cats (Jacobs and Fornal, 1991). Accordingly, they may not generate SWS, although they can promote a quiet waking state that is more conducive to sleep onset. Release of serotonin is also, on average, lower during SWS than during waking (Wilkinson *et al.*, 1991; Portas *et al.*, 1998), but appears to increase during prolonged waking and prior to SWS onset (Python *et al.*, 2001).

Drugs that diminish serotonin levels through inhibition of its synthesis (by *p*-chlorophenylalanine [PCPA]) produce complete insomnia with acute administration (Jouvet, 1972) and a recovery of sleep with chronic administration (Dement *et al.*, 1973). Under both conditions, certain behaviours are increased, including eating, and sexual and aggressive activities, and appear along with a release of the phasic activity (ponto-geniculo-occipital [PGO] spikes) of REMS. The insomnia elicited by PCPA can be reversed with very low quantities of the 5-HT precursor, 5-hydroxytryptophan (5-HTP) (Jouvet, 1972). This effect is also present with local injections of the precursor into the preoptic region (Denoyer *et al.*, 1989). The effects of drugs that act upon individual serotonin receptors are difficult to interpret since they act at multiple presynaptic (5-HT1) and postsynaptic (5-HT1/2/3) sites. Increased synaptic levels of serotonin elicited by the serotonin reuptake inhibitors generally produce relatively quiet waking states, characterized by satiety and thus reduced appetite for food and sex, as well as the psychologically reported reduction in anxiety common in humans (Ursin, 1976, 1980; Sommerfelt and Ursin, 1991; Foreman *et al.*, 1992; Leibowitz and Alexander, 1998; Halford and Blundell, 2000; Kennedy *et al.*, 2000). Like the effects of the precursor, tryptophan, those of the reuptake blockers are best characterized as dampening cortical activation (Ursin, 1980). This effect may be mediated in part by serotonin's inhibitory effect upon cholinergic basal forebrain neurons (see below) through 5-HT1 receptors, which indirectly open potassium channels to hyperpolarize these cells (Khateb *et al.*, 1993). Local microinjections of serotonin into the region of the cholinergic neurons results in the decrease of high-frequency (gamma) cortical activity and the appearance of slow-wave activity with SWS (Cape and Jones, 1998). Through input to the septum, serotonin also dampens theta activity in the limbic system (Vertes *et al.*, 1994). It similarly inhibits cholinergic ponto-mesencephalic neurons that also serve to stimulate cortical activation through their thalamic and other subcortical relay stations (Luebke *et al.*, 1992). In the hypothalamus, serotonin appears to act as a satiety factor in the feeding system (Leibowitz and Alexander, 1998). In the brainstem and spinal cord, serotonin has the capacity to stimulate muscle tone in skeletal muscles (Kubin *et al.*, 1992). Accordingly, serotonin may promote a waking state during which cortical activation is minimal, and feeding, sexual and aggressive behaviours are dampened, yet rhythmic motor activities and postural muscle tonus are maintained. Serotonergic systems may thus produce a sated, quiet waking state that precedes and facilitates SWS, but prevents REMS (see below).

Acetylcholine (ACh) promotes cortical activation that can be associated with either the state of waking or REMS (see below), as it also stimulates, through brainstem mechanisms, motor inhibition and muscle atonia. Cholinergic neurons are located in the ponto-mesencephalic tegmentum (laterodorsal and pedunculopontine tegmental nuclei [LDTg and PPTg]), as well as the medullary reticular formation, and, like neurons of the ascending reticular activating system, give rise to ascending projections to the thalamus, posterior hypothalamus and basal forebrain (Figure XXIV-2.1). Lesions of the cholinergic ponto-mesencephalic neurons have minimal effects upon waking but eliminate the state of REMS (Webster and Jones, 1988). Another major cholinergic cell group is located in the basal forebrain (substantia innominata [SI] corresponding to the nucleus basalis of Meynert, as well as the septum and diagonal band nuclei) and gives rise to widespread projections to the cerebral cortex (and hippocampus). Lesions of the cholinergic basal forebrain neurons lead to deficits in cortical activation and attention during waking (Stewart *et al.*, 1984; Dunnett *et al.*, 1991). Unit recording of presumed cholinergic neurons in the ponto-mesencephalic tegmentum has indicated that these cells discharge at higher rates during waking than during SWS; most also discharge during REMS and some at higher rates than during waking (El Mansari *et al.*, 1989; Kayama *et al.*, 1992). In the basal forebrain, unidentified but possibly cholinergic neurons discharge at higher rates during waking and REMS than during SWS (Detari *et al.*, 1984; Szymusiak and McGinty, 1986). Release of acetylcholine from both the thalamus and cortex is highest in association with cortical activation and high in both waking and REMS relative to slow-wave sleep (Celesia and Jasper, 1966; Jasper and Tessier, 1971; Williams *et al.*, 1994; Marrosu *et al.*, 1995). During waking, acetylcholine release is high in association with appetitive behaviours, such as eating (Inglis *et al.*, 1994). Acetylcholine release in the hippocampus is highest during REMS (Marrosu *et al.*, 1995); in the brainstem, it is also highest during REMS and the muscle atonia that accompanies that state (see below) (Kodama *et al.*, 1990; 1992).

Drugs that block the muscarinic postsynaptic action of acetylcholine, such as atropine, lead to the loss of fast cortical activity and its replacement by slow waves, despite the persistence of waking behaviours (Longo, 1966; Stewart *et al.*, 1984). This effect is marked behaviourally, nonetheless, by deficits in attention and memory. In addition to affecting glutamate receptors (see above), some anaesthetics, such as ketamine and halothane, appear to block nicotinic receptors (Flood and Krasowski, 2000; Mori *et al.*, 2001). Drugs such as eserine that enhance acetylcholine by blocking its catabolism through the acetylcholinesterase enzyme enhance and prolong cortical activation and diminish cortical slow waves and SWS (Jouvet, 1975; Vanderwolf, 1975). Direct administration of muscarinic agonists into the brain (done of necessity, since most do not cross the blood–brain barrier) also enhances cortical activation. Through second messengers, multiple muscarinic receptors (M1/M3) block potassium channels and lead to prolonged depolarization and increased excitation of their target neurons in the thalamus and cortex (McCormick, 1992). Nicotine also stimulates cortical activation and enhances vigilance (Domino, 1967; Koelega, 1993). Directly linked to sodium ion channels, the nicotinic receptor is associated with rapid depolarization and excitation of target neurons. The muscarinic-nicotinic mixed agonist, carbachol, when injected directly into subcortical sites, stimulates cortical, including limbic, activation accompanied by theta activation, and reduces locomotor activity (Brudzynski and Mogenson, 1986). Such injections can also induce REMS with muscle atonia, particularly when administered into the ponto-mesencephalic tegmentum (see below) (Hernandez-Peon and Chavez Ibarra, 1963; Baxter, 1969; Mitler and Dement, 1974; Amatruda *et al.*, 1975). Acetylcholine thus plays an important role in cortical and limbic activation associated with aroused, attentive, yet also immobile behavioural states, including REMS (see below).

Orexin (Orx), also known as hypocretin, is a wake-promoting neuromodulator that also stimulates eating, for which it was named. It is contained within neurons of the mid- and posterior hypothalamus (PH) that give rise to very diffuse projections through the brain, including the forebrain, brainstem and spinal cord (Figure XXIV-2.1). It appears to have the capacity to enforce waking with muscle tonus since in its absence or that of its postsynaptic receptor, as produced by genetic knockout, narcolepsy results in mice and dogs (Chemelli *et al.*, 1999; Lin *et al.*, 1999). As recently established in human cases, the Orx-containing cells in the hypothalamus are reduced in number with narcolepsy (Thannickal *et al.*, 2000). Orexin acts upon other activating systems including, importantly, the noradrenergic locus coeruleus (Bourgin *et al.*, 2000), histaminergic tuberomammillary (Huang *et al.*, 2001; Bayer *et al.*, 2002) and cholinergic basal forebrain neurons (Eggermann *et al.*, 2001), all of which it excites.

The drug which stimulates waking and vigilance and is used in the treatment of narcolepsy, modafinil, was recently shown by c-Fos immunostaining to activate Orx-containing cells (in addition to other neurons of the activating system) (Estabrooke *et al.*, 2001).

Corticotrophin-releasing hormone (CRH) is a wake-promoting neuromodulator and hormone. It is contained within neurons of the paraventricular nucleus of the hypothalamus (Figure XXIV-2.1) that stimulate release of adrenocorticotrophic hormone (ACTH) from the pituitary. A circadian rhythm of the activity of these neurons is presumably responsible for the circadian rise in human cortisol secretion that occurs in the morning, reaching a maximum upon waking, and more so in the presence of bright light (Leproult *et al.*, 2001). Also contained within other neurons in the hypothalamus and brainstem (not shown) with more widespread projections, corticotropin-releasing hormone may act upon many systems in the brain. Injected into the ventricles of animals, it promotes cortical activation and waking while diminishing slow-wave activity and SWS (Ehlers *et al.*, 1986). It also acts through other transmitter systems, including the locus coeruleus, to promote waking, cortical activation and arousal (Valentino *et al.*, 1993). Such circuits would be highly active during conditions of stress when an attentive waking state is maintained. In addition, however, CRH and ACTH may stimulate REM sleep in association with stress, as evident during REM sleep rebound following deprivation (Marrosu *et al.*, 1990; Gonzalez and Valatx, 1998).

In summary, multiple transmitter/modulator systems play partially redundant yet differentiated roles in promoting and maintaining the cortical activation and behavioural arousal of waking. Glutamatergic neurons, through the reticular activating system, diffuse thalamo-cortical projection system and basalo-cortical system, as well as the cortex, maintain fast excitatory activity through the brain during waking. In the most attentive and aroused conditions, including stress, noradrenergic locus coeruleus neurons, through diffuse projections, promote, maintain and enhance cortical activation and sympathetic and hypothalamo-pituitary-adrenal activation, as well as sensory-motor readiness. Histaminergic hypothalamic neurons, also through diffuse projections, maintain cortical activation and vigilance. These systems work mutually with corticotropin-releasing hormone and orexinergic hypothalamic neurons that serve to enforce a state of waking and prevent the onset of sleep. Serotonergic raphe neurons through diffuse projections also prevent the onset of REMS and loss of muscle tonus associated with that state, but they promote a quiet waking state that precedes and can expedite the onset of SWS. Cholinergic brainstem and basal forebrain neurons that project to the thalamus and cortex stimulate activation of the limbic cortex and the neo-cortex during waking, but do not oppose and may actually stimulate the loss of muscle tonus that occurs during REMS, when they also promote cortical activation. Dopaminergic mesencephalic neurons may join cholinergic neurons during waking and REMS to stimulate limbic and cortical activation associated particularly with pleasurable states.

SLOW-WAVE SLEEP-PROMOTING TRANSMITTER SYSTEMS

GABA (gamma-hydroxy-butyric acid) is the most common inhibitory amino-acid transmitter in the central nervous system and, as such, is involved in almost all inhibitory processes that occur during different states. It is contained in interneurons through the cortex, hippocampus, thalamus, brainstem and spinal cord. It is also contained in certain long-projection neurons. In addition to suppressing discharge of neurons, GABAergic neurons can pace the activity of neurons in fast or slow rhythms. It should thus be mentioned that GABAergic interneurons and projection neurons are important in contributing to activating gamma and theta activities in the limbic cortex and the neo-cortex (Soltesz and Deschenes, 1993; Whittington *et al.*, 2000). The activity of particular GABAergic neurons is similarly important for pacing slower sleep rhythms while inhibiting activating systems (Figure XXIV-2.2). Through a bursting discharge, GABAergic neurons of the thalamic reticular nuclei play a critical role in the generation of thalamo-cortical spindle activity, by both inhibiting and pacing the thalamic relay neurons in association with the spindles and then slower delta activity through SWS (Steriade and Llinas, 1988). These GABAergic neurons appear to be responsible for closing the afferent gateway through the thalamus to the cerebral cortex during SWS (Hofle *et al.*, 1997). GABA is also contained within long-projection neurons, including those ascending to the cortex from the basal forebrain (Gritti *et al.*, 1997). Such long-projecting GABAergic neurons may be involved in dampening cortical activity in association with cortical slow-wave activity and SWS (Szymusiak and McGinty, 1989; Manns *et al.*, 2000). In addition, GABA is contained in locally projecting neurons within the basal forebrain that may inhibit the cholinergic neurons during SWS (Manns *et al.*, 2000; Szymusiak *et al.*, 2000). It is also contained in neurons projecting to the posterior hypothalamus and brainstem from the basal forebrain and the preoptic-anterior hypothalamic regions (Gritti *et al.*, 1994). It appears from c-Fos expression, in addition to neural firing profiles, that such GABAergic cells are most active with EEG slow-wave activity and SWS (Sherin *et al.*, 1996; Szymusiak *et al.*, 1998; Gong *et al.*, 2000; Manns *et al.*, 2000). Such cells have been identified in the substantia innominata and preoptic region, concentrated particularly in the ventro-lateral preoptic area (VLPO), as well as in the more medial and median preoptic nuclei. These GABAergic neuronal systems serve as gating mechanisms for state changes, since when they are on (closing the gate), neurons in the posterior hypothalamus and brainstem are inhibited, thus allowing sleep; when they are off (opening the gate), neurons in the posterior hypothalamus and brainstem are disinhibited, preventing sleep and promoting waking. Consistent with this view, GABA release is greatest in the posterior hypothalamus during SWS (Nitz and Siegel, 1996), and it is higher in brainstem dorsal raphe and locus coeruleus regions during SWS than waking (Nitz and Siegel, 1997a, b). Collectively, the preoptic GABAergic neurons form an integral part of the regulatory system for autonomic and hypothalamo-pituitary function, inhibiting sympathetic and hypothalamo-pituitary adrenal activity, while dampening the cortical activating system.

GABAergic neurons in the VLPO have been shown to be inhibited by noradrenaline (presumably through an alpha2-adrenergic receptor that opens potassium channels) (Gallopin *et al.*, 2000). Thus, in the absence of noradrenergic input, GABAergic preoptic area neurons may serve to decrease temperature, lower metabolism and decrease blood pressure while dampening activating systems and bringing on sleep. GABAergic neurons are also distributed within the reticular formation among the more numerous glutamatergic neurons (Jones, 1995) and among or around the cholinergic and noradrenergic neurons of the brainstem, from where they may exert a local inhibitory action to dampen the activity of these neurons at sleep onset and during SWS, as well as more markedly during REMS (see below). Local GABAergic neurons may inhibit neurons in the lower brainstem reticular formation to dampen the excitatory reticulo-spinal influence, resulting in the decrease in muscle tonus evident in the EMG during that state. Whereas many GABAergic neurons in the brainstem may be active during both SWS and REMS, others (such as those in the pontine reticular formation) may become inactive during REMS (see below).

Drugs that enhance GABAergic transmission include the major anaesthetic agents, such as pentobarbital (Schulz and Macdonald, 1981), and hypnotic drugs, including the benzodiazepines and benzodiazepine-like drugs (Mendelson, 1985; Smith, 2001). Most of these drugs act via $GABA_A$ receptors, which hyperpolarize and inhibit neurons through opening chloride channels. Whereas barbiturates and other anaesthetic agents directly stimulate this receptor, the benzodiazepines amplify the action of GABA upon the receptor, thus enhancing and prolonging its natural effect in the circuits within which it is released. Accordingly, benzodiazepines may serve to facilitate SWS by facilitating GABA's action within particular circuits that dampen cortical activation. Although the hypnotic drugs in this class increase SWS, they do not increase delta activity but instead increase spindling (Feinberg *et al.*, 2000).

Interestingly, in a case of idiopathic recurring stupor, the blocking of $GABA_A$ receptors could reverse the stupor and normalize the EEG, which was characterized by 14-Hz activity (Tinuper *et al.*, 1992). Gamma hydroxybutyrate (GHB) is another drug that facilitates delta SWS along with REMS within the natural sleep cycle (Broughton and Mamelak, 1980; Lapierre *et al.*, 1990). It restored sleep in a case of fatal familial insomnia (Reder *et al.*, 1995). It appears to act upon $GABA_B$ receptors that hyperpolarize neurons through second messengers that open potassium channels (Williams *et al.*, 1995). Transmitters or their agonists that open potassium channels allow a deeper hyperpolarization (to $\sim -90\,\text{mV}$) than those that open chloride channels (to $\sim -70\,\text{mV}$), perhaps explaining the enhancement of slow, delta activity with GHB. GHB, as well as other drugs acting upon $GABA_A$ receptors, such as clonazepam, also serve to diminish muscle tone during sleep (see below).

Somatostatin and cortistatin are related peptides that are colocalized with GABA in many neurons within the brain, including those of the reticular thalamic nucleus and the cerebral cortex (Figure XXIV-2.2) (Schmechel *et al.*, 1984; de Lecea *et al.*, 1997), and may be important in inhibiting through those neurons other thalamo-cortical systems, and promoting slow-wave activity during SWS (de Lecea *et al.*, 1996). Since somatostatin inhibits release of most hormones/transmitters, it could act to dampen the release of other transmitters with activating influences in multiple areas. Nonetheless, it should be kept in mind that somatostatin release in the hypothalamo-pituitary-somatic axis is specifically turned off during sleep to allow the SWS-dependent release of growth hormone.

Growth hormone-releasing hormone (GHRH) facilitates SWS (Ehlers *et al.*, 1986; Obal *et al.*, 1996; Zhang *et al.*, 1999). The neurons containing growth hormone-releasing hormone are located principally in the arcuate nucleus, from where they project to the median eminence (Figure XXIV-2.2). Together with the decrease in somatostatin release, growth hormone-releasing hormone is responsible for the increase in human growth hormone release from the pituitary that occurs in association with cortical slow-wave activity at night during SWS (Van Cauter *et al.*, 1998). Growth hormone-releasing hormone is also contained in other neurons within the hypothalamus (not shown) to provide an innervation to other hypothalamic and preoptic nuclei. Intraventricular administration of the releasing hormone enhances slow-wave activity and SWS in animals (Ehlers *et al.*, 1986). Peripheral administration of a long-lasting analogue of somatostatin, which centrally blocks growth hormone release, decreases SWS, indicating that the releasing factor and the hormone itself may normally promote slow-wave activity and SWS through central mechanisms (Beranek *et al.*, 1997).

Adenosine may facilitate SWS (Benington *et al.*, 1995). It is the by-product of ATP catabolism as well as formation, and it is not associated with any particular group of neurons. Released with most synaptic vesicles, it is potentially released from most active nerve terminals. Acting through second messengers upon receptors (A1) that open potassium channels, adenosine has the capacity to hyperpolarize and inhibit neurons and nerve terminals. Like GABA, it could accordingly function within specific circuits to promote sleep. Its release is increased with prolonged waking episodes (Porkka-Heiskanen *et al.*, 1997).

The drug that is very well known to promote wakefulness and enhance vigilance (Koelega, 1993), caffeine, acts as an antagonist upon adenosine receptors, supporting the notion that adenosine normally acts to promote somnolence and sleep (Yanik *et al.*, 1987).

Insulin, cholecystokinin (CCK) and bombesin can facilitate SWS. These modulators/hormones are released peripherally in association with food intake and digestion. They may act upon the brain to promote SWS through transmission of impulses by the vagal nerve to the solitary tract nucleus or through access to the brain by circulation within regions of the brainstem and hypothalamus that are outside the blood–brain barrier (Danguir and Nicolaidis, 1984; DeMesquita and Hershel Haney, 1986; de Saint Hilaire-Kafi *et al.*, 1989). Cholecystokinin and bombesin are also contained in multiple central neurons in the brain (not shown), where they may also act in association with feeding. Their intraventricular administration facilitates sleep. Collectively, they mediate the postprandial satiety that facilitates sleep onset.

In summary, multiple transmitter/modulator/hormonal systems play differential roles in facilitating the onset of SWS or in generating and maintaining it. Whereas sleep onset is prevented by those systems stimulating the sympathetic and hypothalamo-pituitary-adrenal axis, as during conditions of strong motivational states or stress (see above), it is facilitated by those systems activating the parasympathetic and hypothalamo-pituitary-somatic axis, as during conditions of satiety. Insulin, cholecystokinin and bombesin released with food intake and digestion all facilitate sleep onset. In this manner, serotonin associated with low motivational states, satiety and quiescence may also facilitate sleep onset (see above). Adenosine, which may accumulate in the region of the most active neurons during waking, may selectively inhibit those neurons after prolonged waking to induce sleep. Ultimately, specific GABAergic neurons through the brainstem reticular formation, thalamus and hypothalamus/preoptic area, and basal forebrain are responsible for inhibiting activating and sympathetic systems, as well as enabling the slow rhythms within thalamo-cortical systems that characterize mammalian SWS. Colocalized with GABA in certain thalamic and cortical neurons, somatostatin/corticostatin may enhance this process.

REMS-PROMOTING AND REMS-PERMITTING TRANSMITTER SYSTEMS

Acetylcholine (ACh) is a REMS-promoting transmitter. The neurons containing acetylcholine within the ponto-mesencephalic tegmentum (Figure XXIV-2.3) are critically involved in the generation of REMS, as is evident by its loss following their destruction (Webster and Jones, 1988). In addition to projecting to the forebrain, they provide a dense innervation to the brainstem reticular formation, and particularly to the adjacent oral pontine reticular formation (RF PnO) (Jones, 1991). Electrophysiological studies have established that putative cholinergic neurons in this region discharge in both waking and REMS, and many discharge at their highest rates during REMS (El Mansari *et al.*, 1989). By the use of c-Fos expression as an indicator of neuronal activity, immunohistochemically identified cholinergic neurons were revealed to be maximally active as a population during REMS (Maloney *et al.*, 1999). Acetylcholine release is also maximal during REMS within the brainstem reticular formation (Kodama *et al.*, 1990; Kodama *et al.*, 1992). The cholinergic neurons of the basal forebrain can also promote REMS (Reid *et al.*, 1998; Cape *et al.*, 2000). Moreover, acetylcholine release from the hippocampus is maximal during REMS (Marrosu *et al.*, 1995).

Drugs that enhance acetylcholine levels by blocking its catabolism, such as eserine, promote waking under normal circumstances (see above). However, following depletion of the monoamines by reserpine (see below), eserine stimulates the appearance of REMS (Karczmar *et al.*, 1970). It can also stimulate REMS in depressed patients, who are believed to have increased pressure for REMS, perhaps due to enhanced cholinergic and/or deficient monoaminergic transmission (Sitaram *et al.*, 1976; Gillin and Sitaram, 1984). Carbachol, the muscarinic-nicotinic agonist, when injected into the oral pontine reticular formation (RF PnO), can trigger the state of REMS, including limbic theta activity, phasic oculomotor activity and tonic muscle atonia (Baghdoyan *et al.*, 1987; Vanni-Mercier *et al.*, 1989; Vertes *et al.*, 1993). It presumably mimics acetylcholine there, which is normally released by a rich fibre plexus therein emanating from the ponto-mesencephalic cholinergic neurons. Carbachol's effect, presumably like acetylcholine's, appears to depend upon nicotinic receptors and probably multiple muscarinic receptors, of which the M1/M3, which commonly indirectly close potassium channels, are thought to be important in REMS induction through direct excitation of particular reticular neurons (Velazquez-Moctezuma *et al.*, 1990; Sakai and Onoe, 1997). However, M2 receptors, which may indirectly open potassium channels to hyperpolarize neurons, could be important in selectively inhibiting certain neurons that would otherwise prevent the occurrence of the state and associated muscle atonia (see below).

Noradrenaline, serotonin and histamine (NA, 5-HT and H) play permissive roles in the occurrence of REMS (Figure XXIV-2.3). The importance of this role was first documented in the pharmacological studies (see above) showing that eserine could stimulate REMS, but only under conditions when the monoamines were depleted by reserpine (Karczmar *et al.*, 1970). It was subsequently discovered that the serotonergic neurons (McGinty and Harper, 1976), then found that the noradrenergic neurons (McCarley and Hobson, 1975), and more recently also found that the histaminergic (Vanni-Mercier *et al.*, 1984) neurons cease firing prior to and during REMS. It was proposed that the monoaminergic and cholinergic neurons discharge in a reciprocal manner across the sleep-waking cycle (McCarley and Hobson, 1975). Such a reciprocal relationship is apparent in c-Fos patterns of activation occurring in identified serotonergic and noradrenergic as opposed to cholinergic neurons in association with REMS deprivation as opposed to recovery (Maloney *et al.*, 1999). Since the cessation of firing by the noradrenergic, serotonergic and histaminergic neurons appears to be important for the occurrence of REMS, it is considered that they serve a permissive role in this state. The more recent evidence that serotonin and noradrenaline both hyperpolarize and inhibit the cholinergic ponto-mesencephalic neurons (through 5-HT1 and alpha2 receptors) lends further support to this thesis, indicating that these systems would normally exert an inhibitory influence upon REMS-promoting cholinergic neurons (Luebke *et al.*, 1992; Williams and Reiner, 1993; Thanker *et al.*, 1998). Both noradrenaline and serotonin are also important for the maintenance of muscle tone characteristic of waking and thus prevention of the loss of muscle tone that occurs with REMS.

Drugs that enhance synaptic noradrenaline or 5-HT, such as amphetamines and tricycles, prevent the occurrence of REMS and associated loss of muscle tonus, as applied in their use in the treatment of narcolepsy (Noising and Mignot, 1997).

Dopamine (DA) is neither clearly REMS-permissive nor REMS-promoting as a transmitter. That dopaminergic neurons continue to discharge (Miller *et al.*, 1983) and dopamine to be released during REMS (see above) suggests that dopamine, in contrast to noradrenaline, does not prevent the occurrence of REMS. Since the dopaminergic neurons in the ventral mesencephalic tegmentum receive an excitatory input from the cholinergic ponto-mesencephalic neurons, which are active during REMS, it is not surprising that dopaminergic neurons are also active during REMS. Recent results from c-Fos studies indicate that immunohistochemically identified dopaminergic neurons of the ventral tegmental area are indeed highly active during REMS, such that they could be discharging in a manner during this state similar to that during highly motivated or rewarding waking states (see above) (Maloney *et al.*, 2002). Accordingly, the dopaminergic neurons could be responsible for some of the ascending components of REMS, including limbic and cognitive changes that could accompany dreaming (Maloney *et al.*, 2002) (Figure XXIV-2.3). The role of dopamine in hallucinations, to which dreams have often been likened, might reflect similar processes underlying these cognitive states (Yeoman, 1995).

Most drugs, like the amphetamines, that enhance dopamine release, as well as noradrenaline and serotonin release, stimulate waking and arousal (see above), and not REMS. However, reports of increased vivid dreams and nightmares, along with increased incidences of hallucinations and psychosis, have been reported with amphetamine and also in the treatment of Parkinsonism with l-DOPA (Moskovitz *et al.*, 1978; Thompson and Pierce, 1999).

GABA serves as a critical transmitter in gating the state of REMS in the brainstem and probably contributing to the muscle atonia of REMS there and in the spinal cord (Figure XXIV-2.3) (Maloney *et al.*, 2000). Many GABAergic neurons appear from c-Fos to be active during REMS, including those surrounding the monoaminergic cells, which they probably are responsible for inhibiting during REMS (Gervasoni *et al.*, 1998; Maloney *et al.*, 1999). Consonant with this action, GABA release is maximal during REMS in the locus coeruleus and dorsal raphe (Nitz and Siegel, 1997a, b). Active GABAergic neurons through the brainstem reticular formation may contribute to muscle atonia indirectly by inhibiting excitatory inputs from pontine and medullary reticulo-spinal and serotonergic raphe-spinal neurons to motor neurons, and thus effecting a disfacilitation of the motor neurons (Maloney *et al.*, 2000). Furthermore, spinally projecting GABAergic neurons in the ventral medullary reticular formation (alpha and ventral gigantocellular fields [GiA and GiV]) may contribute directly to the inhibition of spinal motor neurons. A unique group of GABAergic neurons located in the oral pontine reticular formation (PnO) appear to be less active (or 'off') during REMS relative to SWS (Maloney *et al.*, 2000). Injections of bicuculline into this region were shown to trigger a state of REMS (Xi *et al.*, 1999). In this area, GABAergic neurons may thus act as a gate that, when open (GABA neurons off), allows REMS to occur, but, when closed (GABA neurons on), prevents the occurrence of REMS by inhibiting local reticular neurons that drive REMS. These GABAergic cells could in turn be inhibited by cholinergic neurons or other ponto-mesencephalic GABAergic neurons during REMS.

Drugs that enhance GABA transmission through $GABA_A$ receptors (see above), such as clonazepam, are used in the treatment of REMS behaviour disorder to improve the deficient motor inhibition underlying that condition (Mahowald and Schenck, 1989). Gamma hydroxybutyrate (GHB), which serves as an agonist on the $GABA_B$ receptor (see above), has been used to enhance REMS with muscle atonia, in addition to SWS, during the night in narcoleptic patients in order to diminish narcoleptic attacks during the following day (Broughton and Mamelak, 1980).

Glycine (Gly) is responsible (probably together with GABA) for the postsynaptic inhibition of cranial and spinal motor neurons during REM sleep (Figure XXIV-2.3) (Chase *et al.*, 1989). Together with GABA, it is the other major inhibitory neurotransmitter within the spinal cord. It is also contained in neurons within the medullary reticular formation (alpha and ventral gigantocellular fields [GiA and GiV]) that project to the spinal cord. The drug that blocks glycine, strychnine, can reverse the motor inhibition during REM sleep when applied locally in the region of the motor neurons (Chase *et al.*, 1989).

Glutamate (Glu) plays an important role in the excitation and excitatory action of neuronal systems involved in REMS (Figure XXIV-2.3). It is contained in the majority of neurons within the brainstem reticular formation (above) and in those neurons within the oral pontine reticular formation (PnO) that appear to be critically involved in the generation of REMS and muscle atonia. Glutamate agonists can stimulate REMS when injected into the ponto-mesencephalic tegmentum (Onoe and Sakai, 1995).

Vasoactive intestinal peptide (VIP) is a peptide with REMS-promoting activity, as, when injected into the pontine reticular formation in regions where carbachol stimulates REMS, it can also do so (Riou *et al.*, 1982; Bourgin *et al.*, 1997). Often a cotransmitter with acetylcholine, and located in the region of the cholinergic neurons in the ponto-mesencephalic tegmentum (Figure XXIV-2.3), VIP may act upon similar systems in a more prolonged manner.

In summary, multiple transmitter/modulator systems participate by a particular progression and constellation of events in the generation of REMS. First, the activity of multiple wake-promoting systems is progressively dampened during the SWS that normally precedes REMS. This dampening is effected by particular inhibitory GABAergic neurons that must increase their activity to effect a complete inhibition of noradrenergic, serotonergic and histaminergic cell groups in order to permit the onset of REMS. Lifted from the inhibitory influence of noradrenergic and serotonergic neurons, cholinergic ponto-mesencephalic neurons (and vasoactive intestinal peptide neurons) increase their discharge. Perhaps by a direct inhibitory influence of acetylcholine or by an indirect one through an excitatory influence of acetylcholine on other inhibitory interneurons, specific GABAergic neurons in the oral pontine reticular formation are turned off, opening a gate for the occurrence of REMS through the activity of the oral pontine reticular neurons that release glutamate. These neurons are also directly excited by acetylcholine. Through selective inhibition and excitation of particular reticular neurons, ascending pathways for cortical activation and descending pathways, including glycinergic as well as GABAergic neurons, for motor inhibition are activated. One important ascending pathway may involve dopaminergic neurons that would contribute to the limbic activation and special cognitive components underlying dreaming.

In conclusion, multiple neurotransmitter systems are involved in redundant and interactive ways in promoting waking, SWS and REMS. Glutamate, as the basic excitatory transmitter of the activating system, as well as its forebrain and spinal targets, is critical to the waking state, while noradrenaline, dopamine, histamine, serotonin, acetylcholine and orexin modulate the activating system and its targets in ways that enhance and prolong but also shape particular waking behaviours and motivational states. GABA, as the basic inhibitory transmitter through the forebrain and brainstem, is critical for SWS and acts through particular neurons in the pacing as well as inhibiting of projection neurons of the activating system and its targets. GABA is also critically involved in REMS, effecting the inhibition of noradrenergic, serotonergic, and histaminergic neurons, which by their cessation permit the occurrence of the state. Released from monoaminergic inhibition, cholinergic neurons by their activity promote REMS, and in this process they excite glutamatergic oral pontine reticular neurons, which are also released from GABAergic inhibition, to propagate the unique ascending forebrain activation and descending motor inhibition of that state.

ACKNOWLEDGEMENTS

The author would like to thank Elida Arriza for her help with the illustrations, Ian Manns for consultation on the manuscript, Lynda Mainville for technical assistance and Naomi Takeda for secretarial assistance.

REFERENCES

Abercrombie, E.D. and Jacobs, B.L., 1987a. Single-unit response of noradrenergic neurons in the locus coeruleus of freely moving cats. I. Acutely presented stressful and nonstressful stimuli. *J Neurosci*, **7**, 2837–2843.

Abercrombie, E.D. and Jacobs, B.L., 1987b. Single-unit response of noradrenergic neurons in the locus coeruleus of freely moving cats. II. Adaptation to chronically presented stressful stimuli. *J Neurosci*, **7**, 2844–2848.

Akert, K., Koella, W.P. and Hess, R.J., 1952. Sleep produced by electrical stimulation of the thalamus. *Am J Physiol*, **168**, 260–267.

Amatruda, T.T., Black, D.A., McKenna, T.M., McCarley, R.W. and Hobson, J.A., 1975. Sleep cycle control and cholinergic mechanisms: differential effects of carbachol injections at pontine brain stem sites. *Brain Res*, **98**, 501–515.

Aston-Jones, G. and Bloom, F.E., 1981a. Norepinephrine-containing locus coeruleus neurons in behaving rats exhibit pronounced responses to non-noxious environmental stimuli. *J Neurosci*, **1**, 887–900.

Aston-Jones, G. and Bloom, F.E., 1981b. Activity of norepinephrine-containing locus coeruleus neurons in behaving rats anticipates fluctuations in the sleep-waking cycle. *J Neurosci*, **1**, 876–886.

Baghdoyan, H.A., Rodrigo-Angulo, M.L., McCarley, R.W. and Hobson, J.A., 1987. A neuroanatomical gradient in the pontine tegmentum for the cholinoceptive induction of desynchronized sleep signs. *Brain Res*, **414**, 245–261.

Batini, C., Moruzzi, G., Palestini, M., Rossi, G.F. and Zanchetti, A., 1959. Effects of complete pontine transections of the sleep-wakefulness rhythm: the midpontine pretrigeminal preparation. *Arch Ital Biol*, **97**, 1–12.

Baxter, B.L., 1969. Induction of both emotional behavior and a novel form of REM sleep by chemical stimulation applied to cat mesencephalon. *Exp Neurol*, **23**, 220–230.

Bayer, L., Eggermann, E., Serafin, M., Saint-Mleux, B., Machard, D., Jones, B. and Muhlethaler, M., 2002. Orexins (hypocretins) directly excite tuberomammillary neurones. *Eur J Neurosci*, **14**, 1571–1575.

Benington, J.H., Kodali, S.K. and Heller, H.C., 1995. Stimulation of A_1 adenosine receptors mimics the electroencephalographic effects of sleep deprivation. *Brain Res*, **692**, 79–85.

Beranek, L., Obal, F., Jr., Taishi, P., Bodosi, B., Laczi, F. and Krueger, J.M., 1997. Changes in rat sleep after single and repeated injections of the long-acting somatostatin analog octreotide. *Am J Physiol*, **273**, R1484–1491.

Berridge, C.W. and Foote, S.L., 1991. Effects of locus coeruleus activation on electroencephalographic activity in neocortex and hippocampus. *J Neurosci*, **11**, 3135–3145.

Bourgin, P., Lebrand, C., Escourrou, P., Gaultier, C., Franc, B., Hamon, M. and Adrien, J., 1997. Vasoactive intestinal polypeptide microinjections into the oral pontine tegmentum enhance rapid eye movement sleep in the rat. *Neuroscience*, **77**, 351–360.

Bourgin, P., Huitron-Resendiz, S., Spier, A.D., Fabre, V., Morte, B., Criado, J.R., Sutcliffe, J.G., Henriksen, S.J. and de Lecea, L., 2000. Hypocretin-1 modulates rapid eye movement sleep through activation of locus coeruleus neurons. *J Neurosci*, **20**, 7760–7765.

Broughton, R. and Mamelak, M., 1980. Effects of nocturnal gamma-hydroxybutyrate on sleep/waking patterns in narcolepsy-cataplexy. *Can J Neurol Sci*, **7**, 23–31.

Brudzynski, S.M. and Mogenson, G.J., 1986. Decrease of locomotor activity by injections of carbachol into the anterior hypothalamic/preoptic area of the rat. *Brain Res*, **376**, 38–46.

Cape, E.G. and Jones, B.E., 1998. Differential modulation of high frequency gamma electroencephalogram activity and sleep-wake state by noradrenaline and serotonin microinjections into the region of cholinergic basalis neurons. *J Neurosci*, **18**, 2653–2666.

Cape, E.G., Manns, I.D., Alonso, A., Beaudet, A. and Jones, B.E., 2000. Neurotensin-induced bursting of cholinergic basal forebrain neurons promotes gamma and theta cortical activity together with waking and paradoxical sleep. *J Neurosci*, **20**, 8452–8461.

Carli, G. and Zanchetti, A., 1965. A study of pontine lesions suppressing deep sleep in the cat. *Arch Ital Biol*, **103**, 751–788.

Celesia, G.G. and Jasper, H.H., 1966. Acetylcholine released from cerebral cortex in relation to state of activation. *Neurology*, **16**, 1053–1064.

Chase, M.H., Soja, P.J. and Morales, F.R., 1989. Evidence that glycine mediates the postsynaptic potentials that inhibit lumbar motoneurons during the atonia of active sleep. *J Neurosci*, **9**, 743–751.

Chemelli, R.M., Willie, J.T., Sinton, C.M., Elmquist, J.K., Scammell, T., Lee, C., Richardson, J.A., Williams, S.C., Xiong, Y., Kisanuki, Y., Fitch, T.E., Nakazato, M., Hammer, R.E., Saper, C.B. and Yanagisawa, M., 1999. Narcolepsy in orexin knockout mice: molecular genetics of sleep regulation. *Cell*, **98**, 437–451.

Danguir, J. and Nicolaidis, S., 1984. Chronic intracerebroventricular infusion of insulin causes selective increase of slow wave sleep in rats. *Brain Res*, **306**, 97–103.

de Lecea, L., del Rio, J.A., Criado, J.R., Alcantara, S., Morales, M., Danielson, P.E., Henriksen, S.J., Soriano, E. and Sutcliffe, J.G., 1997. Cortistatin is expressed in a distinct subset of cortical interneurons. *J Neurosci*, **17**, 5868–5880.

de Lecea, L., Criado, J.R., Prospero-Garcia, O., Guatvik, K.M., Schweitzer, P., Danielson, P.E., Dunlop, C.L.M., Siggins, G.R., Henriksen, S.J. and Sutcliffe, J.G., 1996. A cortical neuropeptide with neuronal depressant and sleep-modulating properties. *Nature*, **381**, 242–248.

de Saint Hilaire, Z., Orosco, M., Rouch, C., Python, A. and Nicolaidis, S., 2000. Neuromodulation of the prefrontal cortex during sleep: a microdialysis study in rats. *Neuroreport*, **11**, 1619–1624.

de Saint Hilaire-Kafi, A., Gibbs, J. and Nicolaidis, S., 1989. Satiety and sleep: the effects of bombesin. *Brain Res*, **478**, 152–155.

Dement, W., Henriksen, S., Jacobs, B. and Mitler, M., 1973. Biogenic amines, phasic events, and behavior. In: Bloom, F.E. and Acheson, G.H. (eds), *Pharmacology and the Future of Man*, pp. 74–89. Karger, New York.

DeMesquita, S. and Hershel Haney, W., 1986. Effect of chronic intracerebroventricular infusion of cholecystokinin on respiration and sleep. *Brain Res*, **378**, 127–132.

Dempsey, E.W., Morison, R.S. and Morison, B.R., 1941. Some afferent diencephalic pathways related to cortical potentials in the cat. *Am J Physiol*, **131**, 718–731.

Denoyer, M., Sallanon, M., Kitahama, K., Aubert, C. and Jouvet, M., 1989. Reversibility of para-chlorophenylalanine-induced insomnia by intrahypothalamic microinjection of L-5-hydroxytryptophan. *Neuroscience*, **28**, 83–94.

Detari, L., Juhasz, G. and Kukorelli, T., 1984. Firing properties of cat basal forebrain neurones during sleep-wakefulness cycle. *Electroencephalogr Clin Neurophysiol*, **58**, 362–368.

Di Chiara, G. and Imperato, A., 1988. Drugs abused by humans preferentially increase synaptic dopamine concentrations in the mesolimbic system of freely moving rats. *Proc Natl Acad Sci USA*, **85**, 5274–5278.

Domino, E.F., 1967. Electroencephalographic and behavioral arousal effects of small doses of nicotine: a neuropsychopharmacological study. *Ann N Y Acad Sci*, **142**, 216–244.

Dunnett, S.B., Everitt, B.J. and Robbins, T.W., 1991. The basal forebrain-cortical cholinergic system: interpreting the functional consequences of excitotoxic lesions. *Trends Neurosci*, **14**, 494–501.

Duteil, J., Rambert, F.A., Pessonnier, J., Hermant, J.F., Gombert, R. and Assous, E., 1990. Central alpha 1-adrenergic stimulation in relation to the behaviour stimulating effect of modafinil; studies with experimental animals. *Eur J Pharmacol*, **180**, 49–58.

Eggermann, E., Serafin, M., Bayer, L., Machard, D., Sanit-Mleux, B., Jones, B.E. and Muhlethaler, M., 2001. Orexins/hypocretins excite basal forebrain cholinergic neurones. *Neuroscience*, **108**, 177–188.

Ehlers, C., Reed, T.K. and Henriksen, S.J., 1986. Effects of corticotropin-releasing factor and growth hormone-releasing factor on sleep and activity in rats. *Neuroendocrinology*, **42**, 467–474.

El Mansari, M., Sakai, M. and Jouvet, M., 1989. Unitary characteristics of presumptive cholinergic tegmental neurons during the sleep-waking cycle in freely moving cats. *Exp Brain Res*, **76**, 519–529.

Estabrooke, I.V., McCarthy, M.T., Ko, E., Chou, T.C., Chemelli, R.M., Yanagisawa, M., Saper, C.B. and Scammell, T.E., 2001. Fos expression in orexin neurons varies with behavioral state. *J Neurosci*, **21**, 1656–1662.

Favale, E., Loeb, C., Rossi, G.F. and Sacco, G., 1961. EEG synchronization and behavioral signs of sleep following low frequency stimulation of the brain stem reticular formation. *Arch Ital Biol*, **99**, 1–22.

Feinberg, I., Maloney, T. and Campbell, I.G., 2000. Effects of hypnotics on the sleep EEG of healthy young adults: new data and psychopharmacologic implications. *J Psychiatr Res*, **34**, 423–438.

Flood, P. and Krasowski, M.D., 2000. Intravenous anesthetics differentially modulate ligand-gated ion channels. *Anesthesiology*, **92**, 1418–1425.

Foote, S.L., Aston-Jones, G. and Bloom, F.E., 1980. Impulse activity of locus coeruleus neurons in awake rats and monkeys is a function of sensory stimulation and arousal. *Proc Natl Acad Sci USA*, **77**, 3033–3037.

Foreman, M.M., Hall, J.L. and Love, R.L., 1992. Effects of fenfluramine and para-chloroamphetamine on sexual behavior of male rats. *Psychopharmacology*, **107**, 327–330.

Galey, D., Simon, H. and Le Moal, M., 1977. Behavioral effects of lesions in the A10 dopaminergic area of the rat. *Brain Res*, **124**, 83–97.

Gallopin, T., Fort, P., Eggermann, E., Cauli, B., Luppi, P.H., Rossier, J., Audinat, E., Muhlethaler, M. and Serafin, M., 2000. Identification of sleep-promoting neurons *in vitro*. *Nature*, **404**, 992–995.

Gervasoni, D., Darracq, L., Fort, P., Souliere, F., Chouvet, G. and Luppi, P.-H., 1998. Electrophysiological evidence that noradrenergic neurons of the rat locus coeruleus are tonically inhibited by GABA during sleep. *Eur J Neurosci*, **10**, 964–970.

Gillin, J.C. and Sitaram, N., 1984. Rapid eye movement (REM) sleep: cholinergic mechanisms. *Psychol Med*, **14**, 501–506.

Gong, H., Szymusiak, R., King, J., Steininger, T. and McGinty, D., 2000. Sleep-related c-Fos protein expression in the preoptic hypothalamus: effects of ambient warming. *Am J Physiol Regul Integr Comp Physiol*, **279**, R2079–2088.

Gonzalez, M.M. and Valatx, J.L., 1998. Involvement of stress in the sleep rebound mechanism induced by sleep deprivation in the rat: use of alpha-helical CRH (9-41). *Behav Pharmacol*, **9**, 655–662.

Grillner, S., Deliagina, T., Ekeberg, O., el Manira, A., Hill, R.H., Lansner, A., Orlovsky, G.N. and Wallen, P., 1995. Neural networks that co-ordinate locomotion and body orientation in lamprey. *Trends Neurosci*, **18**, 270–279.

Gritti, I., Mainville, L. and Jones, B.E., 1994. Projections of GABAergic and cholinergic basal forebrain and GABAergic preoptic-anterior hypothalamic neurons to the posterior lateral hypothalamus of the rat. *J Comp Neurol*, **339**, 251–268.

Gritti, I., Mainville, L., Mancia, M. and Jones, B.E., 1997. GABAergic and other non-cholinergic basal forebrain neurons project together with cholinergic neurons to meso- and iso-cortex in the rat. *J Comp Neurol*, **383**, 163–177.

Halford, J.C. and Blundell, J.E., 2000. Pharmacology of appetite suppression. *Prog Drug Res*, **54**, 25–58.

Hernandez-Peon, R. and Chavez Ibarra, G., 1963. Sleep induced by electrical or chemical stimulation of the forebrain. *Electroencephalogr Clin Neurophysiol*, **24**, 188–198.

Hess, W.R., 1954. *Diencephalon. Autonomic and Extrapyramidal Functions*. Grune & Stratton, New York.

Hess, W.R., 1957. *The Functional Organization of the Diencephalon*. Grune & Stratton, New York.

Hobson, J.A., McCarley, R.W. and Wyzinski, P.W., 1975. Sleep cycle oscillation: reciprocal discharge by two brainstem neuronal groups. *Science*, **189**, 55–58.

Hofle, N., Paus, T., Reutens, D., Fiset, P., Gotman, J., Evans, A.C. and Jones, B.E., 1997. Regional cerebral blood flow changes as a function of delta and spindle activity during slow wave sleep in humans. *J Neurosci*, **17**, 4800–4808.

Huang, Z.L., Qu, W.M., Li, W.D., Mochizuki, T., Eguchi, N., Watanabe, T., Urade, Y. and Hayaishi, O., 2001. Arousal effect of orexin A depends on activation of the histaminergic system. *Proc Natl Acad Sci USA*, **98**, 9965–9970.

Inglis, F.M., Day, J.C. and Fibiger, H.C., 1994. Enhanced acetylcholine release in hippocampus and cortex during the anticipation and consumption of a palatable meal. *Neuroscience*, **62**, 1049–1056.

Jacobs, B.L., 1973. Electrophysiological and behavioral effects of electrical stimulation of the raphe nuclei in cats. *Physiol Behav*, **11**, 489–495.

Jacobs, B.L. and Fornal, C.A., 1991. Activity of brain serotonergic neurons in the behaving animal. *Pharmacol Rev*, **43**, 563–578.

Jasper, H.H. and Tessier, J., 1971. Acetylcholine liberation from cerebral cortex during paradoxical (REM) sleep. *Science*, **172**, 601–602.

Jasper, H.H., Khan, R.T. and Elliott, K.A.C., 1965. Amino acids released from the cerebral cortex in relation to its state of activation. *Science*, **147**, 1448–1449.

Jones, B.E., 1991. Paradoxical sleep and its chemical/structural substrates in the brain. *Neuroscience*, **40**, 637–656.

Jones, B.E., 1995. Reticular formation. Cytoarchitecture, transmitters and projections. In: Paxinos, G. (ed.), *The Rat Nervous System* (2nd edn), pp. 155–171. Academic Press Australia, New South Wales.

Jones, B.E., 2000. Basic mechanisms of sleep-wake states. In: Kryger, M.H., Roth, T. and Dement, W.C. (eds), *Principles and Practice of Sleep Medicine* (3rd edn), pp. 134–154. Saunders, Philadelphia.

Jones, B.E., Harper, S.T. and Halaris, A.E., 1977. Effects of locus coeruleus lesions upon cerebral monoamine content, sleep-wakefulness states and the response to amphetamine. *Brain Res*, **124**, 473–496.

Jones, B.E., Bobillier, P., Pin, C. and Jouvet, M., 1973. The effect of lesions of catecholamine-containing neurons upon monoamine content of the brain and EEG and behavioral waking in the cat. *Brain Res*, **58**, 157–177.

Jouvet, M., 1962. Recherches sur les structures nerveuses et les mécanismes responsables des différentes phases du sommeil physiologique. *Arch Ital Biol*, **100**, 125–206.

Jouvet, M., 1972. The role of monoamines and acetylcholine-containing neurons in the regulation of the sleep-waking cycle. *Ergeb Physiol*, **64**, 165–307.

Jouvet, M., 1975. Cholinergic mechanisms and sleep. In: Waser, P.G. (ed.), *Cholinergic Mechanisms*, pp. 455–476. Raven Press, New York.

Karczmar, A.G., Longo, V.G. and Scotti de Carolis, A., 1970. A pharmacological model of paradoxical sleep: the role of cholinergic and monoamine systems. *Physiol Behav*, **5**, 175–182.

Kayama, Y., Ohta, M. and Jodo, E., 1992. Firing of 'possibly' cholinergic neurons in the rat laterodorsal tegmental nucleus during sleep and wakefulness. *Brain Res*, **569**, 210–220.

Kennedy, S.H., Eisfeld, B.S., Dickens, S.E., Bacchiochi, J.R. and Bagby, R.M., 2000. Antidepressant-induced sexual dysfunction during treatment with moclobemide, paroxetine, sertraline, and venlafaxine. *J Clin Psychiatry*, **61**, 276–281.

Khateb, A., Fort, P., Alonso, A., Jones, B.E. and Muhlethaler, M., 1993. Pharmacological and immunohistochemical evidence for a serotonergic input to cholinergic nucleus basalis neurons. *Eur J Neurosci*, **5**, 541–547.

King, C.D. and Jewett, R.E., 1971. The effects of α-methyltyrosine on sleep and brain norepinephrine in cats. *J Pharmacol Exp Ther*, **177**, 188–195.

Kodama, T., Takahashi, Y. and Honda, Y., 1990. Enhancement of acetylcholine release during paradoxical sleep in the dorsal tegmental field of the cat brain stem. *Neurosci Lett*, **114**, 277–282.

Kodama, T., Lai, Y.Y. and Siegel, J.M., 1992. Enhancement of acetylcholine release during REM sleep in the caudomedial medulla as measured by *in vivo* microdialysis. *Brain Res*, **580**, 348–350.

Koelega, H.S., 1993. Stimulant drugs and vigilance performance: a review. *Psychopharmacology*, **111**, 1–16.

Kubin, L., Tojima, H., Davies, R.O. and Pack, A.I., 1992. Serotonergic excitatory drive to hypoglossal motoneurons in the decerebrate cat. *Neurosci Lett*, **139**, 243–248.

Lai, Y.Y., Shalita, T., Hajnik, T., Wu, J.P., Kuo, J.S., Chia, L.G. and Siegel, J.M., 1999. Neurotoxic *N*-methyl-D-aspartate lesion of the ventral midbrain and mesopontine junction alters sleep-wake organization. *Neuroscience*, **90**, 469–483.

Lapierre, O., Montplaisir, J., Lamarre, M. and Bedard, M.A., 1990. The effect of gamma-hydroxybutyrate on nocturnal and diurnal sleep of normal subjects: further considerations on REM sleep-triggering mechanisms. *Sleep*, **13**, 24–30.

Leibowitz, S.F. and Alexander, J.T., 1998. Hypothalamic serotonin in control of eating behavior, meal size, and body weight. *Biol Psychiatry*, **44**, 851–864.

Leproult, R., Colecchia, E.F., L'Hermite-Baleriaux, M. and Van Cauter, E., 2001. Transition from dim to bright light in the morning induces an immediate elevation of cortisol levels. *J Clin Endocrinol Metab*, **86**, 151–157.

Lin, J.S., Roussel, B., Akaoka, H., Fort, P., Debilly, G. and Jouvet, M., 1992. Role of catecholamines in the modafinil and amphetamine induced wakefulness, a comparative pharmacological study in the cat. *Brain Res*, **591**, 319–326.

Lin, J.-S., Sakai, K. and Jouvet, M., 1988. Evidence for histaminergic arousal mechanisms in the hypothalamus of cats. *Neuropharmacol*, **27**, 111–122.

Lin, J.-S., Sakai, K., Vanni-Mercier, G. and Jouvet, M., 1989. A critical role of the posterior hypothalamus in the mechanisms of wakefulness determined by microinjection of muscimol in freely moving cats. *Brain Res*, **479**, 225–240.

Lin, J.-S., Sakai, K., Vanni-Mercier, G., Arrang, J.-M., Garbarg, M., Schwartz, J.-C. and Jouvet, M., 1990. Involvement of histaminergic neurons in arousal mechanisms demonstrated with H3-receptor ligands in the cat. *Brain Res*, **523**, 325–330.

Lin, L., Faraco, J., Li, R., Kadotani, H., Rogers, W., Lin, X., Qiu, X., de Jong, P.J., Noising, S. and Mignot, E., 1999. The sleep disorder canine narcolepsy is caused by a mutation in the hypocretin (orexin) receptor 2 gene. *Cell*, **98**, 365–376.

Longo, V.G., 1966. Behavioral and electroencephalographic effects of atropine and related compounds. *Pharamacol Rev*, **18**, 965–996.

Luebke, J.I., Greene, R.W., Semba, K., Kamondi, A., McCarley, R.W. and Reiner, P.B., 1992. Serotonin hyperpolarizes cholinergic low-threshold burst neurons in the rat laterodorsal tegmental nucleus *in vitro*. *Proc Natl Acad Sci USA*, **89**, 743–747.

MacIver, M.B., Mikulec, A.A., Amagasu, S.M. and Monroe, F.A., 1996. Volatile anesthetics depress glutamate transmission via presynaptic actions. *Anesthesiology*, **85**, 823–834.

Magoun, H.W. and Rhines, R., 1946. An inhibitory mechanism in the bulbar reticular formation. *J Neurophysiol*, **9**, 165–171.

Mahowald, M.W. and Schenck, C.H., 1989. REM sleep behavior disorder. In: Kryger, M.H., Roth, T. and Dement, W.C. (eds), *Principles and Practice of Sleep Medicine*, pp. 389–401. Saunders, Philadelphia.

Maloney, K.J., Mainville, L. and Jones, B.E., 1999. Differential c-Fos expression in cholinergic, monoaminergic and GABAergic cell groups of the pontomesencephalic tegmentum after paradoxical sleep deprivation and recovery. *J Neurosci*, **19**, 3057–3072.

Maloney, K.J., Mainville, L. and Jones, B.E., 2000. c-Fos expression in GABAergic, serotonergic and other neurons of the pontomedullary reticular formation and raphe after paradoxical sleep deprivation and recovery. *J Neurosci*, **20**, 4669–4679.

Maloney, K., Mainville, L. and Jones, B.E., 2002. c-Fos expression in dopaminergic and GABAergic neurons of the ventral mesencephalic tegmentum after paradoxical sleep deprivation and recovery. *Eur J Neurosci*, **15**, 1–6.

Manns, I.D., Alonso, A. and Jones, B.E., 2000. Discharge profiles of juxtacellularly labeled and immunohistochemically identified GABAergic basal forebrain neurons recorded in association with the electroencephalogram in anesthetized rats. *J Neurosci*, **20**, 9252–9263.

Manns, I.D., Mainville, L. and Jones, B.E., 2001. Evidence for glutamate, in addition to acetylcholine and GABA, neurotransmitter synthesis in basal forebrain neurons projecting to the entorhinal cortex. *Neuroscience*, **107**, 249–263.

Marrosu, F., Gessa, G.L., Giagheddu, M. and Fratta, W., 1990. Corticotropin-releasing factor (CRF) increases paradoxical sleep (PS) rebound in PS-deprived rats. *Brain Res*, **515**, 315–318.

Marrosu, F., Portas, C., Mascia, S., Casu, M.A., Fa, M., Giagheddu, M., Imperato, A. and Gessa, G.L., 1995. Microdialysis measurement of cortical and hippocampal acetylcholine release during sleep-wake cycle in freely moving cats. *Brain Res*, **671**, 329–332.

McCarley, R.W. and Hobson, J.A., 1975. Neuronal excitability modulation over the sleep cycle: a structural and mathematical model. *Science*, **189**, 58–60.

McCormick, D.A., 1992. Neurotransmitter actions in the thalamus and cerebral cortex and their role in neuromodulation of thalamocortical activity. *Progr Neurobiol*, **39**, 337–388.

McGinty, D. and Harper, R.M., 1976. Dorsal raphe neurons: depression of firing during sleep in cats. *Brain Res*, **101**, 569–575.

Mendelson, W.B., 1985. GABA-benzodiazepine receptor-chloride ionophore complex: implications for the pharmacology of sleep. In: Wauquier, A., Monti, J.M., Gaillard, J.M. and Radulovacki, M. (eds), *Sleep. Neurotransmitters and Neuromodulators*, pp. 229–236. Raven Press, New York.

Mignot, E., Renaud, A., Noising, S., Arrigoni, J., Guilleminault, C. and Dement, W.C., 1993. Canine cataplexy is preferentially controlled by adrenergic mechanisms: evidence using monoamine selective uptake inhibitors and release enhancers. *Psychopharmacology*, **113**, 76–82.

Miller, J.D., Farber, J., Gatz, P., Roffwarg, H. and German, D.C., 1983. Activity of mesencephalic dopamine and non-dopamine neurons across stages of sleep and waking in the rat. *Brain Res*, **273**, 133–141.

Mirenowicz, J. and Schultz, W., 1996. Preferential activation of midbrain dopamine neurons by appetitive rather than aversive stimuli. *Nature*, **379**, 449–451.

Mitler, M.M. and Dement, W.C., 1974. Cataplectic-like behavior in cats after microinjections of carbachol in pontine reticular formation. *Brain Res*, **68**, 335–343.

Montaron, M.-F., Bouyer, J.-J., Rougeul, A. and Buser, P., 1982. Ventral mesencephalic tegmentum (VMT) controls electrocortical beta rhythms and associated attentive behaviour in the cat. *Behav Brain Res*, **6**, 129–145.

Monti, J.M., Pellejero, T. and Jantos, H., 1986. Effects of H1- and H2-histamine receptor agonists and antagonists on sleep and wakefulness in the rat. *J Neural Transm*, **66**, 1–11.

Mori, T., Zhao, X., Zuo, Y., Aistrup, G.L., Nishikawa, K., Marszalec, W., Yeh, J.Z. and Narahashi, T., 2001. Modulation of neuronal nicotinic acetylcholine receptors by halothane in rat cortical neurons. *Mol Pharmacol*, **59**, 732–743.

Moruzzi, G. and Magoun, H.W., 1949. Brain stem reticular formation and activation of the EEG. *Electroencephalogr Clin Neurophysiol*, **1**, 455–473.

Moskovitz, C., Moses, H., 3rd and Klawans, H.L., 1978. Levodopa-induced psychosis: a kindling phenomenon. *Am J Psychiatry*, **135**, 669–675.

Nauta, W.J.H., 1946. Hypothalamic regulation of sleep in rats. An experimental study. *J Neurophysiol*, **9**, 285–316.

Nisenbaum, L.K., Zigmond, M.J., Sved, A.F. and Abercrombie, E.D., 1991. Prior exposure to chronic stress results in enhanced synthesis and release of hippocampal norepinephrine in response to a novel stressor. *J Neurosci*, **11**, 1478–1484.

Noising, S. and Mignot, E., 1997. Pharmacological aspects of human and canine narcolepsy. *Prog Neurobiol*, **52**, 27–78.

Nitz, D. and Siegel, J.M., 1996. GABA release in posterior hypothalamus across sleep-wake cycle. *Am J Physiol*, **271**, R1707–R1712.

Nitz, D. and Siegel, J., 1997a. GABA release in the dorsal raphe nucleus: role in the control of REM sleep. *Am J Physiol*, **273**, R451–R455.

Nitz, D. and Siegel, J.M., 1997b. GABA release in the locus coeruleus as a function of sleep/wake state. *Neuroscience*, **78**, 795–801.

Obál, F., Jr., Floyd, R., Kapas, L., Bodosi, B. and Krueger, J.M., 1996. Effects of systemic GHRH on sleep in intact and hypophysectomized rats. *Am J Physiol*, **270**, E230–237.

Onoe, H. and Sakai, K., 1995. Kainate receptors: a novel mechanism in paradoxical (REM) sleep generation. *Neuroreport*, **6**, 353–356.

Ottersen, O.P., Fischer, B.O. and Storm-Mathisen, J., 1983. Retrograde transport of D-[3H]aspartate in thalamocortical neurones. *Neurosci Lett*, **42**, 19–24.

Porkka-Heiskanen, T., Strecker, R.E., Thanker, M., Bjorkum, A.A., Greene, R.W. and McCarley, R.W., 1997. Adenosine: a mediator of the sleep-inducing effects of prolonged wakefulness. *Science*, **276**, 1265–1268.

Portas, C.M., Bjorvatn, B., Fagerland, S., Gronli, J., Mundal, V., Sorensen, E. and Ursin, R., 1998. On-line detection of extracellular levels of serotonin in dorsal raphe nucleus and frontal cortex over the sleep/wake cycle in the freely moving rat. *Neuroscience*, **83**, 807–814.

Python, A., Steimer, T., de Saint Hilaire, Z., Mikolajewski, R. and Nicolaidis, S., 2001. Extracellular serotonin variations during vigilance states in the preoptic area of rats: a microdialysis study. *Brain Res*, **910**, 49–54.

Ranson, S.W., 1939. Somnolence caused by hypothalamic lesions in the monkey. *Arch Neurol Psychiatry*, **41**, 1–23.

Rasmussen, K., Morilak, D.A. and Jacobs, B.L., 1986. Single unit activity of locus coeruleus neurons in the freely moving cat. I. During naturalistic behaviors and in response to simple and complex stimuli. *Brain Res*, **371**, 324–334.

Reder, A.T., Mednick, A.S., Brown, P., Spire, J.P., Van Cauter, E., Wollmann, R.L., Cervenakova, L., Goldfarb, L.G., Garay, A., Ovsiew, F., Gajdusek, C.D. and Roos, R.P., 1995. Clinical and genetic studies of fatal familial insomnia. *Neurology*, **45**, 1068–1075.

Reid, M.S., Noising, S., Tafti, M., Siegel, J.M., Dement, W.C. and Mignot, E., 1998. Neuropharmacological characterization of basal forebrain cholinergic stimulated cataplexy in narcoleptic canines. *Exp Neurol*, **151**, 89–104.

Reiner, P.B. and Kamondi, A., 1994. Mechanisms of antihistamine-induced sedation in the human brain: H1 receptor activation reduces a background leakage potassium current. *Neuroscience*, **59**, 579–588.

Richardson, N.R. and Gratton, A., 1996. Behavior-relevant changes in nucleus accumbens dopamine transmission elicited by food reinforcement: an electrochemical study in rat. *J Neurosci*, **16**, 8160–8169.

Riou, F., Cespuglio, R. and Jouvet, M., 1982. Endogenous peptides and sleep in the rat. III. The hypnogenic properties of vasoactive intestinal polypeptide. *Neuropeptides*, **2**, 265–277.

Sakai, K. and Onoe, H., 1997. Critical role for M3 muscarinic receptors in paradoxical sleep generation in the cat. *Eur J Neurosci*, **9**, 415–423.

Sakai, K., El Mansari, M., Lin, J.-S., Zhang, G. and Vanni-Mercier, G., 1990. The posterior hypothalamus in the regulation of wakefulness and paradoxical sleep. In: Mancia, M. and Marini, G. (eds), *The Diencephalon and Sleep*, pp. 171–198. Raven Press, New York.

Sallanon, M., Sakai, K., Buda, C., Puymartin, M. and Jouvet, M., 1988. Increase of paradoxical sleep induced by microinjections of ibotenic acid into the ventrolateral part of the posterior hypothalamus in the cat. *Arch Ital Biol*, **126**, 87–97.

Schmechel, D., Vickrey, B., Fitzpatrick, D. and Elde, R., 1984. GABAergic neurons of mammalian cerebral cortex: widespread subclass defined by somatostatin content. *Neurosci Lett*, **47**, 227–232.

Schulz, D.W. and Macdonald, R.L., 1981. Barbiturate enhancement of GABA-mediated inhibition and activation of chloride ion conductance: correlation with anticonvulsant and anesthetic actions. *Brain Res*, **209**, 177–188.

Sherin, J.E., Shiromani, P.J., McCarley, R.W. and Saper, C.B., 1996. Activation of ventrolateral preoptic neurons during sleep. *Science*, **271**, 216–219.

Shouse, M.N., Staba, R.J., Saquib, S.F. and Farber, P.R., 2000. Monoamines and sleep: microdialysis findings in pons and amygdala. *Brain Res*, **860**, 181–189.

Sitaram, N., Wyatt, R.J., Dawson, S. and Gillin, J.C., 1976. REM sleep induction by physostigmine infusion during sleep. *Science*, **191**, 1281–1283.

Smith, T.A., 2001. Type A gamma-aminobutyric acid (GABAA) receptor subunits and benzodiazepine binding: significance to clinical syndromes and their treatment. *Br J Biomed Sci*, **58**, 111–121.

Soltesz, I. and Deschenes, M., 1993. Low- and high-frequency membrane potential oscillations during theta activity in CA1 and CA3 pyramidal neurons of the rat hippocampus under ketamine-xylazine anesthesia. *J Neurophysiol*, **70**, 97–116.

Sommerfelt, L. and Ursin, R., 1991. Behavioral, sleep-waking and EEG power spectral effects following the two specific 5-HT uptake inhibitors zimeldine and alaproclate in cats. *Behav Brain Res*, **45**, 105–115.

Starzl, T.E., Taylor, C.W. and Magoun, H.W., 1951. Ascending conduction in reticular activating system, with special reference to the diencephalon. *J Neurophysiol*, **14**, 461–477.

Steriade, M. and Llinas, R.R., 1988. The functional states of the thalamus and the associated neuronal interplay. *Physiol Rev*, **68**, 649–742.

Stewart, D.J., Macfabe, D.F. and Vanderwolf, C.H., 1984. Cholinergic activation of the electrocorticogram: role of the substantia innominata and effects of atropine and quinuclidinyl benzilate. *Brain Res*, **322**, 219–232.

Szymusiak, R. and McGinty, D., 1986. Sleep-related neuronal discharge in the basal forebrain of cats. *Brain Res*, **370**, 82–92.

Szymusiak, R. and McGinty, D., 1989. Sleep-waking discharge of basal forebrain projection neurons in cats. *Brain Res Bull*, **22**, 423–430.

Szymusiak, R., Alam, N. and McGinty, D., 2000. Discharge patterns of neurons in cholinergic regions of the basal forebrain during waking and sleep. *Behav Brain Res*, **115**, 171–182.

Szymusiak, R., Alam, N., Steininger, T.L. and McGinty, D., 1998. Sleep-waking discharge patterns of ventrolateral preoptic/anterior hypothalamic neurons in rats. *Brain Res*, **803**, 178–188.

Thanker, M.M., Strecker, R.E. and McCarley, R.W., 1998. Behavioral state control through differential serotonergic inhibition in the mesopontine cholinergic nuclei: a simultaneous unit recording and microdialysis study. *J Neurosci*, **18**, 5490–5497.

Thannickal, T.C., Moore, R.Y., Nienhuis, R., Ramanathan, L., Gulyani, S., Aldrich, M., Cornford, M. and Siegel, J.M., 2000. Reduced number of hypocretin neurons in human narcolepsy. *Neuron*, **27**, 469–474.

Thompson, D.F. and Pierce, D.R., 1999. Drug-induced nightmares. *Ann Pharmacother*, **33**, 93–98.

Tinuper, P., Montagna, P., Cortelli, P., Avoni, P., Lugaresi, A., Schoch, P., Bonetti, E.P., Gallassi, R., Sforza, E. and Lugaresi, E., 1992. Idiopathic recurring stupor: a case with possible involvement of the gamma-aminobutyric acid (GABA)ergic system. *Ann Neurol*, **31**, 503–506.

Trulson, M.E., 1985. Simultaneous recording of substantia nigra neurons and voltammetric release of dopamine in the caudate of behaving cats. *Brain Res Bull*, **15**, 221–223.

Trulson, M.E. and Jacobs, B.L., 1979. Raphe unit activity in freely moving cats: correlation with level of behavioral arousal. *Brain Res*, **163**, 135–150.

Trulson, M.E. and Preussler, D.W., 1984. Dopamine-containing ventral tegmental area neurons in freely moving cats: activity during the sleep-waking cycle and effects of stress. *Exp Neurol*, **83**, 367–377.

Ungerstedt, U., 1971. Adipsia and aphagia after 6-hydroxydopamine induced degeneration of the nigro-striatal dopamine system. *Acta Physiol Scand Suppl*, **367**, 95–122.

Ursin, R., 1976. The effects of 5-hydroxytryptophan and L-tryptophan on wakefulness and sleep patterns in the cat. *Brain Res*, **106**, 105–115.

Ursin, R., 1980. Deactivation, sleep and serotonergic functions. In: Koukkou, M., Lehmann, D. and Angst, J. (eds), *Functional States of the Brain: Their Determinants*, pp. 163–171. Elsevier, Amsterdam.

Valentino, R.J., Foote, S.L. and Page, M.E., 1993. The locus coeruleus as a site for integrating corticotropin-releasing factor and noradrenergic mediation of stress responses. *Ann NY Acad Sci*, **697**, 173–188.

Van Cauter, E., Plat, L. and Copinschi, G., 1998. Interrelations between sleep and the somatotropic axis. *Sleep*, **21**, 553–566.

Vanderwolf, C.H., 1975. Neocortical and hippocampal activation in relation to behavior: effects of atropine, eserine, phenothiazines and amphetamine. *J Comp Physiol Psychol*, **88**, 300–323.

Vanni-Mercier, G., Sakai, K. and Jouvet, M., 1984. Neurones spécifiques de l'éveil dans l'hypothalamus postérieur. *CR Acad Sci Paris*, **298 (III)**, 195–200.

Vanni-Mercier, G., Sakai, K., Lin, J.-S. and Jouvet, M., 1989. Mapping of cholinoceptive brainstem structures responsible for the generation of paradoxical sleep in the cat. *Arch Ital Biol*, **127**, 133–164.

Velazquez-Moctezuma, J., Shalauta, M.D., Gillin, J.C. and Shiromani, P.J., 1990. Differential effects of cholinergic antagonists on REM sleep components. *Psychopharmacol Bull*, **26**, 349–353.

Vertes, R.P., Colom, L.V., Fortin, W.J. and Bland, B.H., 1993. Brainstem sites for the carbachol elicitation of the hippocampal theta rhythm in the rat. *Exp Brain Res*, **96**, 419–429.

Vertes, R.P., Kinney, G.G., Kocsis, B. and Fortin, W.J., 1994. Pharmacological suppression of the median raphe nucleus with sertonin$_{1A}$ agonists, 8-OH-DPAT and buspirone, produces hippocampal theta rhythm in the rat. *Neuroscience*, **60**, 441–451.

von Economo, C., 1931. *Encephalitis Lethargica. Its Sequelae and Treatment*. Oxford University Press, London.

Webster, H.H. and Jones, B.E., 1988. Neurotoxic lesions of the dorsolateral pontomesencephalic tegmentum-cholinergic cell area in the cat. II. Effects upon sleep-waking states. *Brain Res*, **458**, 285–302.

Whittington, M.A., Traub, R.D., Kopell, N., Ermentrout, B. and Buhl, E.H., 2000. Inhibition-based rhythms: experimental and mathematical observations on network dynamics. *Int J Psychophysiol*, **38**, 315–336.

Wilkinson, L.O., Auerbach, S.B. and Jacobs, B.L., 1991. Extracellular serotonin levels change with behavioral state but not with pyrogen-induced hyperthermia. *J Neurosci*, **11**, 2732–2741.

Williams, J.A., Comisarow, J., Day, J., Fibiger, H.C. and Reiner, P.B., 1994. State-dependent release of acetylcholine in rat thalamus measured by *in vivo* microdialysis. *J Neurosci*, **14**, 5236–5242.

Williams, J.A. and Reiner, P.B., 1993. Noradrenaline hyperpolarizes identified rat mesopontine cholinergic neurons *in vitro*. *J Neurosci*, **13**, 3878–3883.

Williams, S.R., Turner, J.P. and Crunelli, V., 1995. Gamma-hydroxybutyrate promotes oscillatory activity of rat and cat thalamocortical neurons by a tonic GABA$_B$ receptor-mediated hyperpolarization. *Neuroscience*, **66**, 135–141.

Wise, R.A., Spindler, J., deWit, H. and Gerberg, G.J., 1978. Neuroleptic-induced 'anhedonia' in rats: pimozide blocks reward quality of food. *Science*, **201**, 262–264.

Wisor, J.P., Noising, S., Sora, I., Uhl, G.H., Mignot, E. and Edgar, D.M., 2001. Dopaminergic role in stimulant-induced wakefulness. *J Neurosci*, **21**, 1787–1794.

Xi, M.-C., Morales, F.R. and Chase, M.H., 1999. Evidence that wakefulness and REM sleep are controlled by a GABAergic pontine mechanism. *J Neurophysiol*, **82**, 2015–2019.

Yamamura, T., Harada, K., Okamura, A. and Kemmotsu, O., 1990. Is the site of action of ketamine anesthesia the *N*-methyl-D-aspartate receptor? *Anesthesiology*, **72**, 704–710.

Yanik, G., Glaum, S. and Radulovacki, M., 1987. The dose-response effects of caffeine on sleep in rats. *Brain Res*, **403**, 177–180.

Yeoman, J.S., 1995. Role of tegmental cholinergic neurons in dopaminergic activation, antimuscarinic psychosis and schizophrenia. *Neuropsychopharmacol*, **12**, 3–16.

Zhang, J., Obal, F., Jr., Zheng, T., Fang, J., Taishi, P. and Krueger, J.M., 1999. Intrapreoptic microinjection of GHRH or its antagonist alters sleep in rats. *J Neurosci*, **19**, 2187–2194.

XXIV-3

Neuroendocrinology of Sleep Disorders

Axel Steiger

INTRODUCTION

The two major methods for the investigation of human sleep are the sleep electroencephalogram (EEG) and the collection of nocturnal hormone profiles. The combination of these electrophysiological and neuroendocrinological methods in young and elderly, female and male normal control subjects; in patients with psychiatric, endocrine and sleep disorders, under baseline conditions and after administration of synthetic and endogenous central nervous system (CNS) active compounds, particularly neuropeptides and neuroactive steroids; and in related animals models has shown that, firstly, during sleep a considerable activity of various endocrine systems occurs, and, secondly, a bidirectional interaction exists between the electrophysiological and neuroendocrine components of sleep. The aim of this chapter is to summarize the current knowledge in this field, which is thought to be the prerequisite for major achievements in the therapy of sleep disorders and of psychiatric disorders as well.

SLEEP EEG AND SLEEP-ASSOCIATED HORMONE SECRETION IN YOUNG NORMAL HUMAN ADULTS

When subjects spend a night in the sleep laboratory, their sleep EEG is analysed either visually by coding each 30-s interval of the night as a sleep stage according to standard guidelines (Rechtschaffen and Kales, 1968), resulting in a hypnogram (Figure XXIV-3.1), or by EEG spectral analysis (Steiger *et al.*, 1993a; Trachsel *et al.*, 1992). The hypnogram shows the cyclic occurrence of periods of non-REM sleep (NREMS) and rapid-eye-movement sleep (REMS). In young normal subjects during the first period of NREMS, the major portion of slow-wave sleep (SWS) occurs. Correspondingly, in EEG spectral analysis, the major portion of slow-wave activity (SWA) is detected. The amounts of SWS and SWA are relatively low during the second half of the night. During this interval, stage 2 sleep preponderates during NREMS. The mean value for the occurrence of the first period of REMS is about 90 min. This first REMS period is relatively short. During 8 h of night sleep, 3–6 sleep cycles are found. The duration of the REMS periods increases throughout the night. Correspondingly, the amount of REMS is higher in the second half of the night than in the first half.

Near to sleep onset in a rather strict, although not absolute, association with the first period of SWS, the major peak of growth hormone (GH) secretion in 24 h is found (Quabbe *et al.*, 1966; Steiger *et al.*, 1987; Takahashi *et al.*, 1968). This GH surge appears to be widely sleep dependent and is suppressed during sleep deprivation (Beck *et al.*, 1975; Sassin *et al.*, 1969). However, in sleep-deprived, but relaxed young men in a supine position, an unchanged nocturnal GH peak was observed (Mullington *et al.*, 1996). During the second half of the night, GH concentrations are low. The pattern of cortisol secretion is inverse to that of GH. After sleep onset, cortisol reaches its nadir. Between 0200 and 0300, the first pulse of cortisol release occurs, and it is followed by further pulses until awakening (Weitzman, 1976). Adrenocorticotrophic hormone (ACTH) is the prime stimulus of nocturnal cortisol secretion in man. Nevertheless, the secretion of ACTH and cortisol may dissociate (Fehm *et al.*, 1984). In summary, during the first half of the night, SWS, SWA and GH preponderate while ACTH and cortisol levels are low. In contrast, during the second half of the night, the amounts of REMS, ACTH and cortisol are high while SWS and GH secretion are low. This pattern suggests

(1) a reciprocal interaction of the hypothalamo-pituitary-somatotrophic (HPS) and the hypothalamo-pituitary-adrenocortical (HPA) systems (the corresponding peripheral end points are GH and cortisol, respectively)
(2) the existence of common regulators of sleep EEG and sleep-associated hormone secretion.

Indeed, there is now a good evidence that a reciprocal interaction of the key hormones of the HPS and HPA systems, GH-releasing hormone (GHRH) and corticotrophin-releasing hormone (CRH), plays a major role in sleep regulation, as indicated in more detail below.

Prolactin rises after sleep onset and reaches its peak during the second or the last third of the night. In males, testosterone rises constantly throughout the night (Weitzman, 1976). Melatonin secretion is related to the light-dark cycle and has its peak during the early morning (Zhdanova *et al.*, 1997).

The secretion of thyroidea-stimulating hormone (TSH) and of the thyroid hormone thyroxin is related to circadian rhythm (Brabant *et al.*, 1987; Chan *et al.*, 1978). The minimum TSH level is found during daytime. TSH rises during the night and reaches its maximum by midnight. Then the levels decline during the early morning hours. The course of thyroxin release is inverse to that of TSH. Thyroxin levels are low during the night and increase during daytime. One study reported declining TSH levels during REMS periods (Follenius *et al.*, 1988).

The hormone most clearly linked to the NREMS-REMS cycle is renin. Plasma renin activity oscillates throughout the night and reaches its peak during NREMS and its acrophase during REMS (Brandenberger *et al.*, 1988) (Figure XXIV-3.6).

Most sleep-endocrine studies have been done on males. A sexual dimorphism is reported in young normal humans. Cortisol secretion is higher in females than in males. A lower amount of SWS during the second half of the night and a greater decrease in SWS and SWA from the first to the second half of the night were found in young normal women (Antonijevic *et al.*, 1999).

Leptin, the protein product of the obese *(ob)* gene, is released from adipocytes in the periphery. It acts within in the hypothalamus (Elmquist *et al.*, 1997) and reduces food intake, probably by

Biological Psychiatry: Edited by H. D'haenen, J.A. den Boer and P. Willner. ISBN 0-471-49198-5

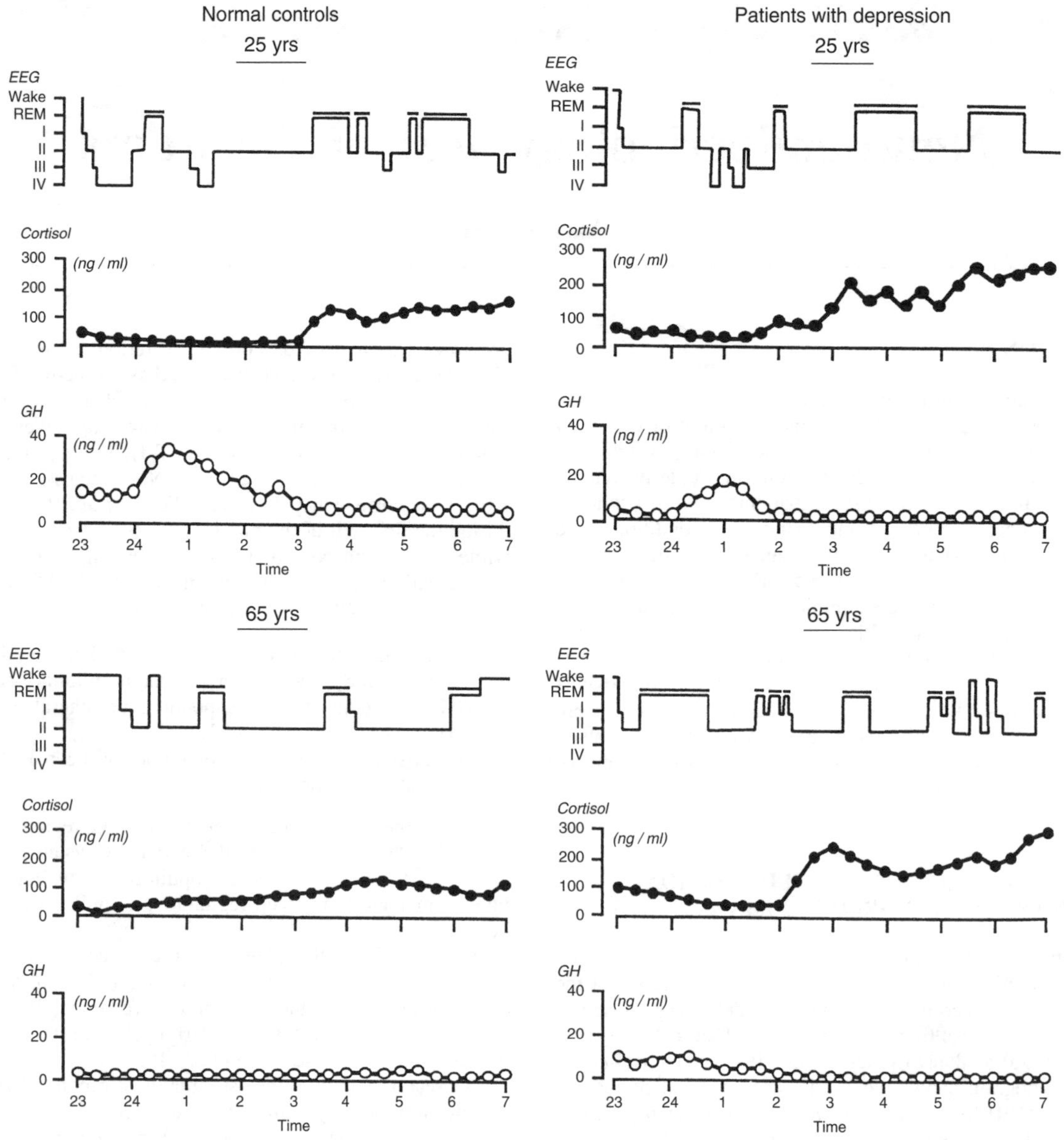

Figure XXIV-3.1 Individual hypnograms and patterns of cortisol and growth hormone (GH) secretion in four male subjects (young and old patients with depression and normal controls)

inhibition of neuropeptide Y (NPY) release (Hanson *et al.*, 1997; Tomaszuk *et al.*, 1996). A circadian rhythm of serum leptin with a maximum between 0000 and 0400, an inverse relationship between leptin and cortisol (Licinio *et al.*, 1997), and a sexual dimorphism with higher leptin levels in women than in men were reported (Deuschle *et al.*, 1996; Saad *et al.*, 1997). Higher nocturnal leptin levels in normal female control subjects than in males were confirmed in a recent study, whereas an inverse correlation between leptin and cortisol was observed in women rather than men (see Figure XXIV-3.2) (Antonijevic *et al.*, 1998).

CHANGES OF SLEEP DURING AGEING

Sleep EEG and nocturnal hormone secretion change throughout the lifespan. There is a controversy whether deterioration of sleep due to ageing starts during puberty or during early adolescence (Bliwise, 1993). It is well established, however, that as early as the third decade of the lifespan, distinct parallel decreases of SWS, SWA and GH secretion start. Near to the onset of the fifth decade, the GH pause occurs. In women, the menopause is a major turning point towards impaired sleep in older age (Ehlers *et al.*, 1993), whereas in men the sleep quality declines continuously during ageing. Correspondingly, in the elderly the amounts of SWS and SWA are low, or SWS may even be totally absent (Figure XXIV-3.1). Furthermore, sleep continuity is disturbed, as is evident from, prolonged sleep-onset latency, increases in the number and duration of nocturnal awakenings, and decreases in sleep efficiency and sleep period time. Finally, REMS time and REMS latency decrease in older age. Controversial reports exist on the effects of age on HPA hormones. Elevated and unchanged cortisol levels have been reported in the elderly. Most studies agree that the amplitude of the cortisol rhythm is blunted. Accordingly, cortisol concentrations during the first half of the night and at the

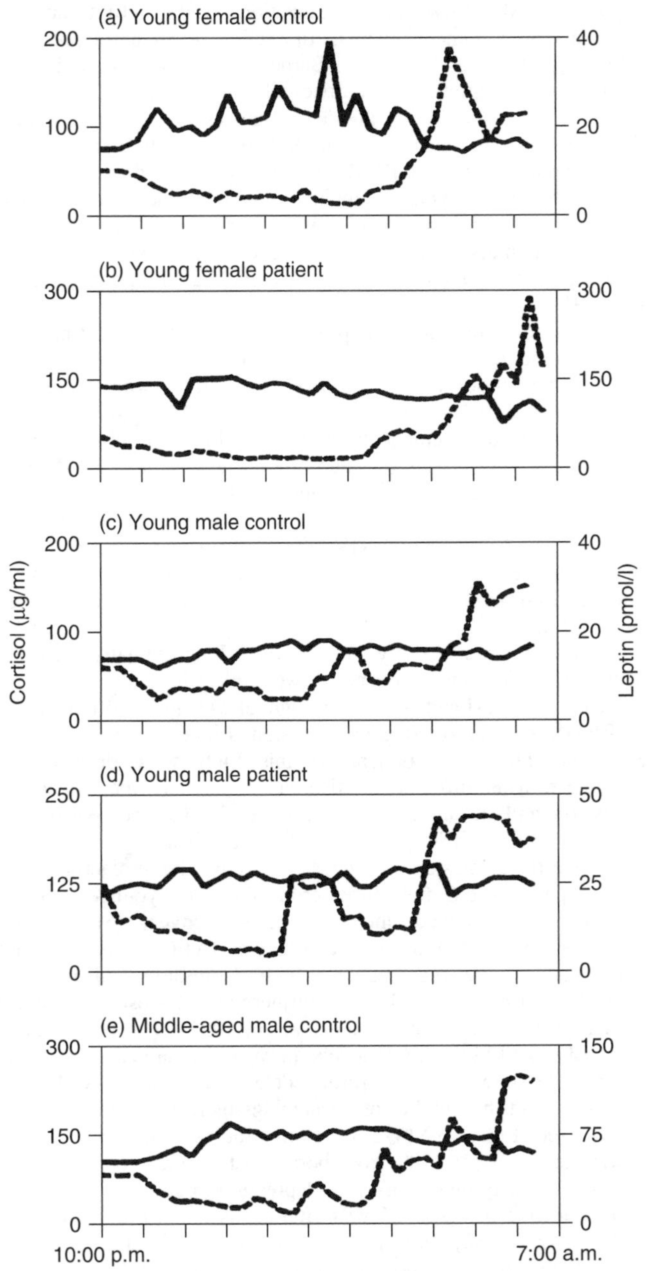

Figure XXIV-3.2 (A–E) Nocturnal profiles of leptin and cortisol. Representative profiles of nocturnal serum levels of leptin and cortisol are shown and correlation analysis between the two hormones was performed: A) young female control ($r = -0.61$, $P < 0.001$); B) young female patient ($r = -0.64$, $P < 0.001$); C) young male control ($r = -0.08$, n.s.); D) young male patient ($r = -0.22$, n.s.); E) middle-aged (42 years old) male control (-0.44, $P < 0.01$). Left y-axis represents plasma cortisol concentrations (dotted line); right y-axis represents serum leptin concentrations (black line) (Reproduced from Antonijevic *et al.*, 1998 with permission of Elsevier Science)

nadir are elevated. Similar results derive from the analysis of the largest sample ($n = 149$) of normal male control subjects (aged 16–83 years) investigated so far (Van Cauter *et al.*, 2000). These authors reported a modest effect of ageing on the 24-h mean cortisol level. Ageing was associated with an elevation of the evening cortisol nadir, but morning maximum cortisol values remained stable across all age ranges. Increases in evening cortisol levels became apparent after the age of 50 years, when sleep became more fragmented and REMS declined. Furthermore, a trend to an association between lower amounts of REMS and higher evening cortisol levels independent of age was found.

Melatonin and, in males, testosterone levels also decrease during ageing. The melatonin levels of older people who reported sleep maintenance problems in a questionnaire did not differ from those of older people reporting normal sleep (Baskett *et al.*, 2001). In contrast to most other hormones, prolactin levels remain widely unaffected by ageing (Van Coevorden *et al.*, 1991).

This complex pattern of age-related changes of sleep-endocrine activity mirrors a central process of ageing with major consequences to mental and physical health. The changes of sleep EEG correspond to a high incidence of insomnia and a high prescription rate of hypnotics in the elderly. A lack of GH is linked to risk of frailty. Elevated HPA activity impairs the capacity to cope with stress and elevates the risk of depression and cardiovascular diseases in higher age.

CHANGES OF SLEEP-ENDOCRINE ACTIVITY RELATED TO DISEASES

Psychiatric Disorders

Depression in Adult Patients

Disturbed sleep is a frequent symptom in most psychiatric disorders. Interestingly, sleep-endocrine changes in patients with depression are similar to those during normal ageing. Characteristically, sleep-EEG findings in depressed patients include disturbed sleep continuity, a decrease of SWS (in younger patients, a shift of the major portion of SWS from the first to the second sleep cycle) and REMS disinhibition (shortened REMS latency, prolonged first REMS period and elevated REMS density, a measure of the amount of rapid-eye movements during REMS) (reviewed by Benca *et al.*, 1992; Reynolds and Kupfer, 1987). Several endocrine aberrations are well documented in affective disorders, particularly HPA overactivity (reviewed in Holsboer, 1999) and HPS dysfunction (reviewed in Steiger *et al.*, 1989). Elevated cortisol and ACTH levels were reported in most sleep-endocrine studies in patients with depression throughout the night or during 24 h, respectively, in comparison to normal control subjects (Antonijevic *et al.*, 2000c; Linkowski *et al.*, 1987) (Figure XXIV-3.1). The circadian pattern of cortisol secretion is preserved during depression. Particularly in females, a positive correlation between age and cortisol levels was found (Antonijevic *et al.*, 2000c). Recently, enhanced cortisol plasma and norepinephrine levels but normal ACTH plasma and CRH cerebrospinal fluid (CSF) levels throughout 30 h were reported (Wong *et al.*, 2000). GH secretion was blunted in most (Jarrett *et al.*, 1990; Sakkas *et al.*, 1998; Steiger *et al.*, 1989; Voderholzer *et al.*, 1993), but not in all (Linkowski *et al.*, 1987) studies. These findings suggest a crucial relationship between shallow sleep, blunted GH and HPA overdrive in depression. In adult patients, ageing and depression exert synergistic effects on sleep-endocrine activity (Antonijevic *et al.*, 2000c). As a result of this synergism, sleep-endocrine changes are most distinct in elderly patients with depression (Figure XXIV-3.1).

As depression is frequently associated with loss of appetite, reduced food intake and weight loss, the secretion of leptin in patients with depression is of interest since leptin is involved in the regulation of food intake. In drug-free patients with major depression, nocturnal serum leptin was significantly higher than in age- and sex-matched controls (Antonijevic *et al.*, 1998). The sexual dimorphism with higher leptin levels in females than in males as described before was confirmed in patients and in controls.

Serum leptin was correlated with body mass index in controls, but not in patients, supporting an altered regulation of leptin secretion in depression. Neither in patients with depression nor male controls was a clear increase in leptin between 0000 and 0400 (as reported by Licinio *et al.*, 1997) or at any other time during the night observed. However, in the group of young female controls (younger than 35 years), an increase in leptin levels between 0000 and 0400 was found, showing the trend to be greater than in young female patients (see Figure XXIV-3.2). This finding suggests that in young female patients with depression the nocturnal leptin surge is blunted. As expected, cortisol levels were enhanced in the patients. As glucocorticoids can prevent the fasting-induced decline of serum leptin, we suggest that hypercortisolism in depression might counteract the reduction in leptin release due to decreased food intake and weight loss. Elevated leptin levels in depression might, in turn, further promote the release of CRH, as shown in animals (Raber *et al.*, 1997; Schwartz *et al.*, 1996), and contribute to HPA system overactivity in depression.

Simultaneous investigation of nocturnal TSH and ACTH levels in drug-free male patients with depression and matched controls showed a blunted TSH and elevated ACTH secretion in the patients. ACTH was negatively correlated to TSH in the first half of the night. These data support the hypothesis that both hypophyseal hormones reflect a common dysregulation of the HPA and the hypothalamo-pituitary thyroid systems in depression, probably as a result of impaired action of the corticotropin-release inhibiting factor (Peteranderl *et al.*, in press).

During antidepressant therapy with tricyclics (amitriptyline, imipramine), a decrease of nocturnal cortisol levels and of REMS and an increase of SWS were found in comparison to baseline values. At this examination, the Hamilton Depression Rating Scale (HAMD) score was improved by about 50% in comparison to the examination before treatment (Steiger *et al.*, 1993b). The effect of subchronic treatment with several antidepressants on sleep EEG and sleep-related hormone secretion was examined in normal male control subjects. The volunteers received first placebo for 3 days, then increasing dosages of antidepressants (the tricyclics amitriptyline, clomipramine and trimipramine, and the selective, reversible, short-acting inhibitors of monoamine oxidase type A, moclobemide and brofaromine for 7–10 days), and finally again placebo after drug withdrawal for 4–8 days (Steiger *et al.*, 1993b). Furthermore, the effects of acute oral administration of the selective serotonin-uptake inhibitor, fluoxetine, and placebo were compared (von Bardeleben *et al.*, 1989). As shown in Table XXIV-3.1, active antidepressant treatment decreased REMS after all substances except trimipramine. Whereas cortisol levels increased after some of the drugs, a distinct blunting of cortisol was observed after trimipramine. After cessation of trimipramine, cortisol levels distinctly exceeded baseline values. It was suggested previously that REMS suppression is the way of action of antidepressants (Vogel *et al.*, 1975). But this hypothesis is challenged by the fact that some antidepressants, including trimipramine, do not suppress REMS. However, normalization of HPA activity appears to be a common mechanism in the action of all antidepressants (Holsboer, 2000; Holsboer and Barden, 1996). This view is supported by the blunting of cortisol after trimipramine, which is known to be an effective antidepressant, although the substance does not share the classical neurobiological effects of most other antidepressants such as REMS suppression, beta-downregulation and inhibition of synaptic uptake of monoamines. In a similar vein, corticosteroid receptor density increased in the rat brain when the animals were treated during several weeks with various antidepressants from several classes, including trimipramine (Reul *et al.*, 1993).

Finally, in a double-blind protocol, the effect of treatment by trimipramine or imipramine on sleep EEG, hormone secretion and psychopathology was compared in patients with depression (Sonntag *et al.*, 1996). Both treatments produced rapid and significant clinical improvement. Imipramine and trimipramine differed, however, in their effects on neurobiological variables. REMS was suppressed and sleep continuity impaired after imipramine, whereas REMS and SWS increased and the sleep quality improved under trimipramine (see Figure XXIV-3.3). Cortisol levels were blunted throughout the night and prolactin was increased after trimipramine, whereas imipramine showed no effect on hormone secretion (see Figure XXIV-3.4).

Sleep-endocrine activity was studied longitudinally between acute depression and recovery in two studies in adult patients. A decrease of ACTH and cortisol throughout 24 h and a normalization of REMS were reported after remission (Linkowski *et al.*, 1987). Since not all of the patients in this study were drug-free at the retest, it is difficult to distinguish between the effects of remission and of antidepressants. Intraindividual comparison of drug-free patients (Steiger *et al.*, 1989) confirmed a decrease of cortisol after remission. In the same study, the prolactin levels of the patients did not differ from those of younger normal controls and remained unchanged after recovery (Steiger and Holsboer, 1997a). Similarly, nocturnal prolactin levels were not distinguishable between patients with depression and matched controls (Jarrett *et al.*, 1987). Furthermore, testosterone levels increased after remission (Steiger *et al.*, 1991). The pathological sleep EEG and blunted GH levels, however, remained unchanged. Sleep EEG showed even a further deterioration, as stage 4 sleep decreased and the number of awakenings increased (Steiger *et al.*, 1989) (see Figure XXIV-3.5). Both studies (Linkowski *et al.*, 1987; Steiger *et al.*, 1989) corroborate that hypersecretion of HPA hormones is a symptom of acute depression in adults.

The decline of cortisol levels after remission (Linkowski *et al.*, 1987; Steiger *et al.*, 1989) is similar to the normalization of results of challenge tests of the HPA system and of CRH CSF levels after recovery (reviewed by Holsboer, 1999). The persistence of most sleep-EEG changes (Kupfer *et al.*, 1993) and of blunted GH levels (Jarrett *et al.*, 1990) in remitted depressed patients has been confirmed over a period of 3 years. Obviously, HPA activity

Table XXIV-3.1 Changes of sleep EEG and nocturnal hormone secretion in normal control subjects after subchronic treatment with antidepressants

				Hormone secretion			
	REMS	NRREMS stages 1 and 2	SWS	Under medication		After withdrawal	
Brofaromine	↓	↑	↓	GH ↓		GH↓	
Moclobemide	↓	ø	ø	Cortisol ↑		Cortisol ↑	
Clomipramine	↓	↑	↓	Cortisol ↑		Cortisol ø	
Amitriptyline	↓	ø	↑	Cortisol ↑	GH ↓	Cortisol ø	GH ↓
Trimipramine	ø	ø	ø	Cortisol ↓	PRL ↑	Cortisol ↑	PRL ↓
Fluoxetine	↓	ø	ø	Cortisol ↑			

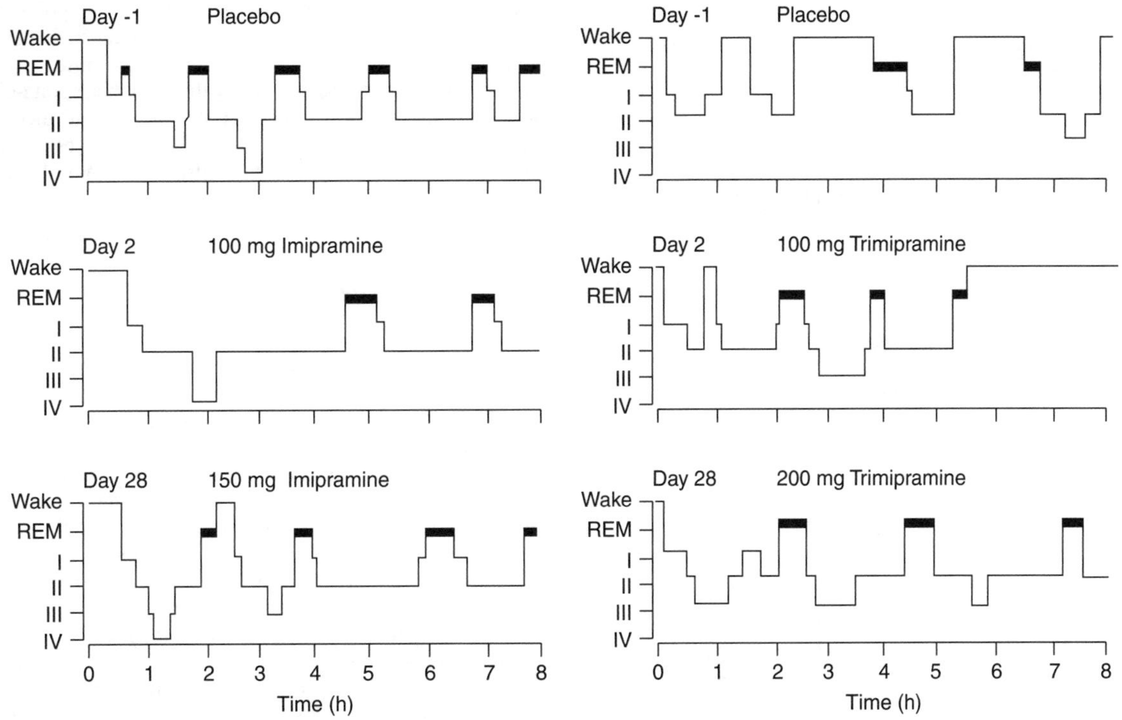

Figure XXIV-3.3 Changes in plasma cortisol concentration during treatment with trimipramine or imipramine (Reproduced from Sonntag *et al.*, 1996. Reprinted by permission of Wiley-Liss, Inc., a subsidiary of John Wiley & Sons, Inc.)

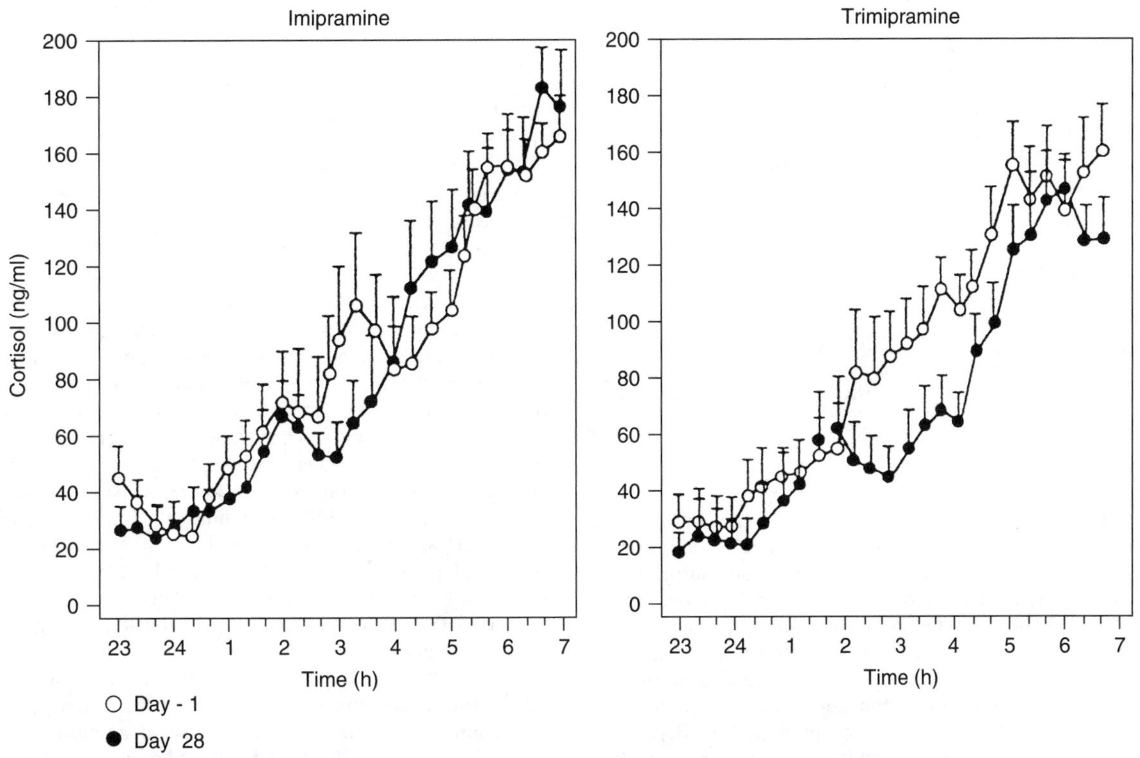

Figure XXIV-3.4 Changes in sleep-EEG variables during treatment with trimipramine or imipramine (Reproduced from Sonntag *et al.*, 1996. Reprinted by permission of Wiley-Liss, Inc., a subsidiary of John Wiley & Sons, Inc.)

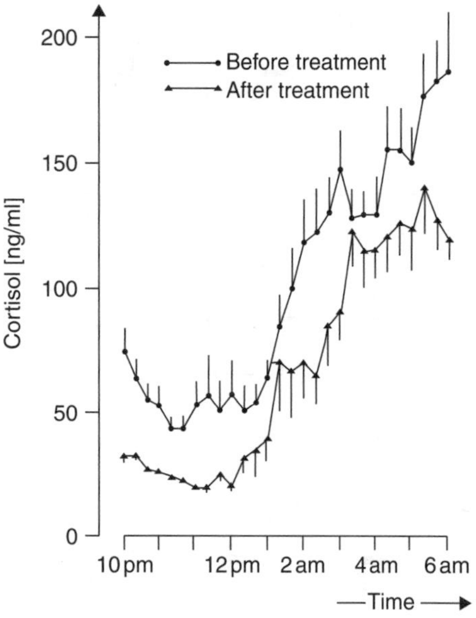

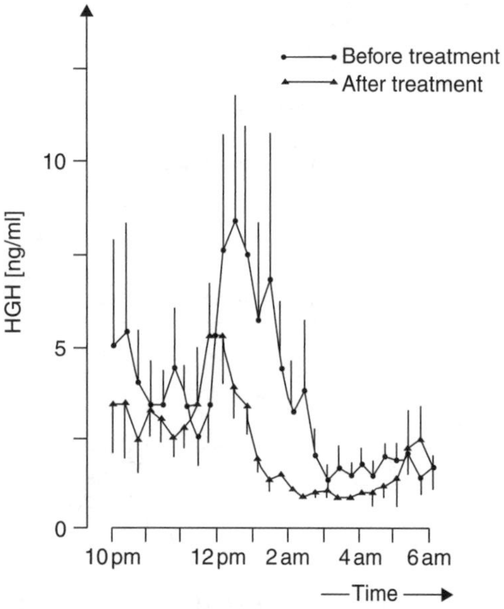

Figure XXIV-3.5 Courses of the mean nocturnal concentrations ± SEM of cortisol and GH in 10 depressed patients before treatment and after remission (Reproduced from Steiger *et al.*, 1989 with permission of Elsevier Science)

normalizes independently of sleep architecture. This observation clarifies that hypercortisolism in depression is not a consequence of shallow sleep. Blunted testosterone levels in males during acute depression, however, appear to be secondary to HPA overdrive. Finally, prolactin is not affected by either depression or ageing. The persistence of aberrations of sleep EEG and GH secretion in remitted patients may be explained as a biological scar due to the metabolic aberrations during acute depression. An alternative explanation is that these changes represent a trait in depressed patients. This issue will remain unclear as long as no data are available for comparing intraindividually the premorbid and depressed state in patients. Interestingly, in healthy relatives of patients with depression, some depression-like neurobiological changes were observed. In the Munich Vulnerability Study, healthy subjects with high familial risk of affective disorders were investigated by assessing the neuroendocrine, polysomnographic and psychometric status. Like patients with an acute episode of major depression, the healthy relatives exhibited signs of HPA system overactivity, as shown by the dexamethasone-CRH test, as well as reduced SWS in the first sleep cycle and increased REMS density. On a single case level, 32% of these high-risk probands exhibited depression-like features in at least two of the three areas assessed (Krieg *et al.*, 2001).

Depression in Children and Adolescents

Most but not all sleep-EEG studies in depressed children and adolescents did not find differences between patients and age-matched controls (reviewed by Lauer *et al.*, 1991). Similarly, changes of sleep-related hormone secretion are more subtle in depressed children and adolescents than in adults. In one study in prepubertal children with depression, sleep EEG and cortisol profiles throughout 24 h did not differ from those of children with other psychiatric disorders and controls. Only four of the 45 depressed children showed hypercortisolism. In a retest after recovery, cortisol hypersecretion persisted in only one of the four young patients (Puig-Antich *et al.*, 1989). In another study, prepubertal depressed children had lower cortisol levels during the first 4 h after sleep onset than controls. ACTH, prolactin and GH concentrations did not differ between patients and controls. Examination of clinical characteristics in patient groups revealed lower nocturnal ACTH in depressed inpatients than depressed outpatients and in depressed, sexually abused than depressed, non-abused children (De Bellis *et al.*, 1996). Depressed children who had experienced at least one clearly adverse, stressful life event during the prior year hypersecreted GH at night compared to depressed children without the experience of such an event and normal controls with and without stressful life events (Williamson *et al.*, 1996). This finding is in line with an elevated responsiveness of GH to CRH in adult patients with depression during daytime (Lesch *et al.*, 1988).

In a set of studies, the relationship between the longitudinal clinical course and sleep-endocrine findings in adolescent patients with depression was studied. In one study on sleep and cortisol, the patients and matched controls were retested about 7 years after the initial study. Although initial group comparisons failed to detect significant differences in sleep-endocrine variables, analyses incorporating clinical follow-up showed that changes in sleep EEG and cortisol are associated with differential longitudinal course. Normal controls who would develop depression had shown initially higher REM density and, by trend, shortened REM latency compared to controls without psychiatric disorder. Depressed patients with a recurrent unipolar course showed elevated cortisol levels around sleep onset compared to depressed patients with no further episodes during the follow-up interval (Rao *et al.*, 1996). Nocturnal GH secretion was studied in a large sample of adolescent depressed patients and matched controls. Clinical follow-up was performed approximately one decade later. The original adolescent nocturnal GH data were analysed in the light of the information obtained regarding clinical course into adulthood. Normal controls who developed at least one episode of major depression or dysthymia during the follow-up period differed from depression-free controls by a more rapid increase of nocturnal GH secretion after sleep onset. Of the subjects who had at least one major depressive episode during the follow-up, those who would go on to make suicide attempts released greater amounts of GH during the first 4 h of sleep. Adults with lifetime depression showed blunted GH in the 100 min preceding sleep onset (Coplan *et al.*, 2000).

Mania and Schizophrenia

Only two studies deal with sleep-endocrine activity in psychiatric disorders other than depression. Elevated cortisol levels were also found in acute mania (Linkowski *et al.*, 1994). Cortisol levels were enhanced in the first 3 h of the night, and prolactin was elevated distinctly around sleep onset in patients with schizophrenia. The sleep latency was prolonged, and the sleep efficiency and the time spent in REMS were reduced (Van Cauter *et al.*, 1991).

Sexual Dysfunction

Blunted sleep-related testosterone levels were reported in males with reduced sexual interest in comparison to normal controls (Schiavi *et al.*, 1986).

Dyssomnias

Experts have generated a host of diagnoses of sleep disorders. So far sleep-endocrine data are available only on some of these disorders. 'Dyssomnia' is defined as a disturbance of initiating or maintaining sleep or as excessive sleepiness (American Sleep Disorders Association, 1997). It should be kept in mind that hypersomnia during the daytime in the same patient can be the consequence of disturbed sleep during the night.

Insomnia

In patients with primary insomnia, elevated nocturnal cortisol levels and a shorter quiescent period of cortisol secretion were found in comparison to controls (Rodenbeck *et al.*, 1999). In a sample of younger adult patients with insomnia, a positive correlation between total wake time and 24-h urinary free cortisol was found (Vgontzas *et al.*, 1998). Furthermore, in a group of 10 patients with insomnia, wakefulness was increased and ACTH and cortisol levels were enhanced throughout 24 h in comparison to controls. The most distinct elevations were observed between 1400 and 1730 and between 2100 and 0300 (Vgontzas *et al.*, 2000). These observations point to an elevated activity of the HPA system in primary insomnia. There appear to be similarities in the pathophysiology of primary insomnia and of depression. This is of particular interest, since several epidemiological studies reported a highly increased risk of the development of a depressive episode in patients with persistent insomnia (Vollrath *et al.*, 1989). Unfortunately, so far, the literature offers no studies that integrate sleep-endocrine data in patients with primary insomnia and with depression.

Sleep Apnoea

Sleep apnoea is a disorder characterized by repetitive upper airway occlusion resulting in progressive hypoxaemia that induces arousals and termination of the obstruction. Consequently, marked sleep fragmentation and decrease of SWS are associated with this disease (Bradley and Phillipson, 1985). Nasal continuous positive airway pressure (CPAP) therapy has been shown to eliminate sleep apnoea and related hypoxaemia (Sullivan *et al.*, 1981). In one study, the effect of nasal CPAP therapy on sleep EEG and hormone secretion was investigated in obese patients with obstructive sleep apnoea syndrome. Under baseline conditions, the time spent in SWS and REMS was low, the number of apnoeas was elevated and the arterial oxygen saturation was reduced. With nasal CPAP therapy, all these variables turned significantly to normalization over one night. Furthermore, GH secretion, which was blunted at baseline, significantly increased on the CPAP night. Cortisol secretion did not differ significantly between both conditions (Cooper *et al.*, 1995). Similarly, cessation of nasal CPAP in eight patients regularly using this device led to an immediate recurrence of sleep apnoea, whereas ACTH and cortisol levels remained unchanged (Grunstein *et al.*, 1996). Krieger *et al.* (1991) compared sleep EEG, plasma renin activity and aldosterone levels in male patients with obstructive sleep apnoea at baseline and during one night with CPAP therapy. In untreated patients, frequent awakenings, absence of SWS, and few and short REMS periods were reported. CPAP therapy led to improvements in sleep depth and REMS. In some treated patients, regular NREMS-REMS cycles occurred; in others, the sleep structure remained irregular. Plasma renin activity profiles reflected the pattern of NREMS-REMS distribution as known from normal controls. Increasing plasma renin activity levels coincided with NREMS phases, and declining levels with REMS. When sleep cycles were regular in some of the treated patients, the oscillating plasma renin activity levels also became regular. Irregularities in sleep EEG, such as short sleep cycles and varying length of sleep-phase duration, led to fluctuations of smaller amplitude and to a general non-oscillatory pattern of plasma renin activity. The mean levels of plasma renin activity and aldosterone were significantly enhanced by nasal CPAP treatment.

Narcolepsy

Narcolepsy is thought to be a disorder of REMS regulation. Accordingly, patients with narcolepsy show several abnormalities of their sleep-wake organization throughout 24 h and of the internal sleep structure. Prominent symptoms are cataplexy and excessive daytime sleepiness, which often results in sleep attacks. The sleep EEG of these patients frequently shows sleep-onset REMS episodes, e.g., the occurrence of REMS directly at or during the first 10 min after sleep onset, frequent awakenings and REMS fragmentation. Normal cortisol and melatonin secretion was reported in narcoleptic patients. Blunted prolactin levels were found, and studies on GH release are contradictory, reporting either high or blunted secretion (reviewed by Schulz *et al.*, 1992). Schulz *et al.* (1992) investigated 24-h plasma renin activity and sleep EEG in patients with narcolepsy and in normal control subjects. The mean concentrations of plasma renin activity was similar in patients and controls. The individual hormone profiles reveal that the already mentioned association between renin oscillations and the NREMS-REMS cycle was preserved. Plasma renin activity profiles exactly reflected the irregularities and disturbances in the sleep structure of the patients with narcolepsy (see Figure XXIV-3.6). In contrast to controls, in these patients no upward trend of plasma renin activity was found. The authors argued that this phenomenon is probably induced in the control subjects by the repetitive occurrence of longer episodes of NREMS. Due to marked sleep fragmentations in the narcoleptic patients, the duration of NREMS was often insufficient to stimulate plasma renin activity. This hypothesis is supported by the more recent finding that SWA stimulates plasma renin activity (Luthringer *et al.*, 1995). In accordance with this observation, sleep-onset REMS episodes that are not preceded by NREMS are not accompanied by relative decline of plasma renin activity.

In patients with narcolepsy, leptin levels were examined in CSF and serum from a blood sample collected in the morning. When these were compared to two control groups of patients with depression and patients with a non-inflammatory neurological disorder, respectively, leptin serum levels were blunted, whereas CSF levels did not differ significantly between groups (Schuld *et al.*, 2000). The authors suggested that reduced leptin production in narcolepsy may be caused by deficiency of hypocretin. It is thought that hypocretins are involved in the pathophysiology of narcolepsy, because mice whose hypocretin gene has been inactivated exhibit a narcolepsy-like phenotype. Furthermore, CSF levels of hypocretins are blunted in patients with narcolepsy (Sutcliffe and de Lecea, 2000).

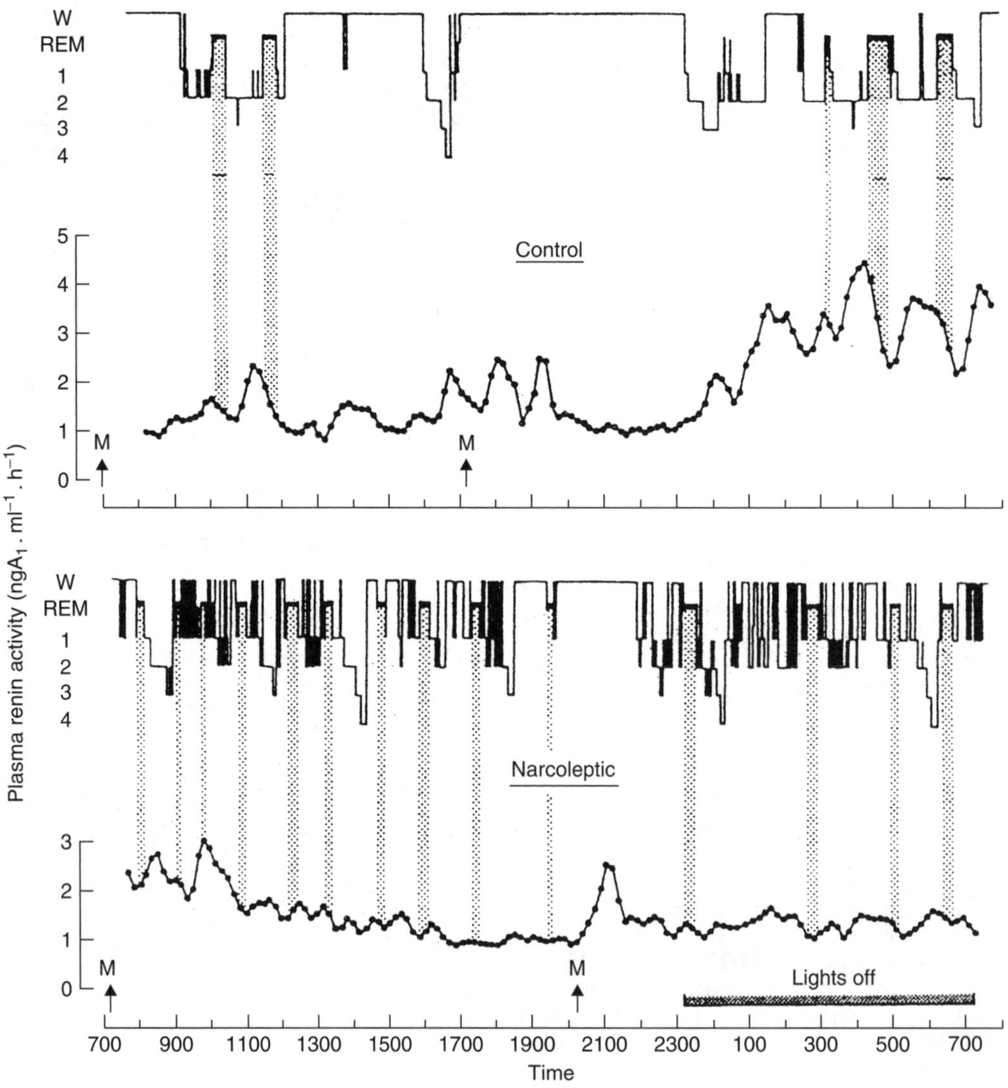

Figure XXIV-3.6 Individual 24-h profiles of plasma renin activity and the corresponding sleep-stage pattern for one control subjects and one patient with narcolepsy (Reproduced from Schulz *et al.*, 1992 by permission of SLEEP)

Restless Legs Syndrome

Restless legs syndrome is a clinical entity characterized by uncomfortable dysaesthesia or paraesthesia in the legs and less frequently in the arms, occurring primarily at rest in the evening hours. Ten male, never-medicated patients with chronically mild to moderate symptoms of this disorder did not show aberration of sleep EEG and of 24-h hormone profiles of cortisol, GH and prolactin, in comparison to age-matched male controls (Wetter *et al.*, in press).

Sleep-Wake Rhythm Disorders

The circadian rhythm of circulating melatonin and the sleep-wake rhythm were investigated in five patients with chronic sleep-wake rhythm disorder and matched controls (Rodenbeck *et al.*, 1998). All the patients showed altered circadian melatonin rhythm variables. The melatonin onset to sleep onset interval varied between the patients, and the melatonin acrophase of sleep- onset interval was prolonged in four patients. The authors concluded that individual phase relations exist between the circadian melatonin rhythm and the sleep-wake cycle in patients with chronic sleep-wake rhythm disorders. Since a prolonged melatonin acrophase to sleep-onset interval was the most consistent finding regardless of aetiology, this abnormality is thought to be a maintaining factor in this disorder as a result of the reduced phase-resetting properties of the circadian pacemarker. Furthermore, rather low circadian melatonin amplitudes and a subsensitivity to daylight are thought to maintain the disorder, at least in some patients.

Familial Advanced Sleep-Phase Syndrome

Familial sleep-phase syndrome is a rare disorder with disabling early evening sleepiness and early morning awakening. Three kindreds with a profound phase advance were identified. In the patients, polysomnographic measures of sleep phase were advanced by almost 4 h compared with those of control subjects. The melatonin and temperature rhythms were also both phase advanced by 3–5 h. The patients tended to fall asleep during solar clock times corresponding to the 'maintenance of wakefulness zone' in healthy subjects. They also tended to wake up during solar clock times corresponding to the circadian peak of sleepiness in controls. These findings define a hereditary circadian rhythm variant associated with a short endogenous period (Jones *et al.*, 1999).

Disturbed Sleep Associated to Medical Disorders

Fatal Familial Insomnia

Fatal familial insomnia is a rare disease with selective thalamic degeneration that results in chronic sleep loss (Lugaresi *et al.*, 1986). Cortisol levels have been reported to be elevated from the early stages of the disease, further increasing with disease progression. ACTH concentrations, however, remained normal even in later stages (Montagna *et al.*, 1995). In two patients, 24-h profiles of GH and prolactin were studied longitudinally (Portaluppi *et al.*, 1995). The nocturnal GH peak disappeared simultaneously with sleep loss whereas the physiological rhythm of prolactin secretion with normally placed nocturnal acrophases was still present for months after total disruption of the sleep-wake cycle. Complete obliteration of the prolactin rhythm was found only in the advanced stages of the disease as the result of a progressive decrease in the circadian amplitude of variation.

Blindness

A high prevalence of sleep disorders is known in blind people. Subjects with no conscious light perception (NPL) have a higher occurrence and more severe sleep disorders than those with some degree of light perception. It was shown that patients with NPL are likely to have free running circadian rhythms of melatonin, cortisol and sleep (Skene *et al.*, 1999).

Brain Injury

As mentioned before, the persistent changes of sleep EEG and GH in depressed patients after recovery (Steiger *et al.*, 1989) may represent a biological scar due to the metabolic aberrations during acute depression. A recent study on young male patients who survived severe brain injury supports this view (Frieboes *et al.*, 1999). Several months after the injury, the cortisol concentrations of these patients did not differ from normal controls. The GH levels and sleep-stage 2 time of the patients, however, were lower than in the controls. These findings point to similarities between the sleep-endocrine activity of patients who survived brain injury and of those who recovered from depression. In the survivors of brain injury, it appears likely that either HPA overactivity due to stress under the intensive care situation or treatment with glucocorticoids in a subgroup contributed to the changes of NREMS and GH.

Obesity

Several studies report blunted nocturnal GH secretion in obese patients (Ferini-Strambi *et al.*, 1991). Ferini-Strambi *et al.* (1991) examined sleep EEG and sleep-related GH secretion in obese patients without obstructive sleep apnoea before and after weight loss due to a hypocaloric diet. They were compared with lean control subjects. Sleep-EEG parameters did not differ significantly between groups. Before weight loss, there was nearly a total lack of GH secretion in the obese subjects. After weight loss, the mean body mass index in these patients decreased from 37.1 to 31.4 (controls 22.3). Although the sleep architecture in obese patients was unchanged after weight loss, GH concentrations increased, suggesting a partial restoration of GH secretion.

Whipple's Disease

In a patient with long-lasting nearly complete sleep loss due to cerebral Whipple's disease (Lieb *et al.*, 1999), GH secretion was nearly flattened over 24 h. The methodological limitation of this case report is the fact that GH concentrations were determined every 30 min. Therefore, it appears possible that some minor peaks were not detected. Nevertheless, these data suggest that severe chronic sleep loss is accompanied by marked blunting of GH release (Lieb *et al.*, 2000).

Sleeping Sickness

The sleep-wake cycle is distinctly changed in human African trypanosomiasis (sleeping sickness). Sleep EEG and 24-h hormone profiles were compared in patients with sleeping sickness and controls (Brandenberger *et al.*, 1994). A marked sleep fragmentation was found in the patients. The circadian rhythm of cortisol was attenuated in all but one of the six patients. In patients and normal subjects, SWS was associated with the declining phases of cortisol secretion. In the patients, profiles of prolactin and plasma renin activity did not show the increase normally associated with long sleep periods but reflected the disturbances of sleep and wakefulness throughout 24 h. In both patients and controls, REMS began during the descending phases of prolactin pulses. In both groups, plasma renin activity reflected the sleep-stage distribution, with NREMS occurring during the ascending phases and REMS during the descending phases of the oscillations. However, in the patients, sleep fragmentation often did not allow sufficient time for plasma renin activity to increase, as known in regular sleep cycles.

Disturbed Rhythms due to Environmental Influences

Modern civilization influences the physiological sleep-wake schedule of millions of people throughout the world. Intercontinental air travel, shift work and prolonged awake time due to artificial light exert distinct effects on sleep-endocrine activity.

Jet Lag

In an experiment, sleep, EEG and hormone secretion were studied in normal subjects before and after a flight from Europe to the USA. The GH secretion adapted quickly to the new sleep schedule, but it took 2 weeks for the cortisol pattern to be totally adjusted (Desir *et al.*, 1981). Dissociation of sleep and cortisol rhythm during the first few days after long-distance travel may contribute to the symptoms of jet lag.

Light

The major environmental factor influencing the timing of neuroendocrine rhythms via the suprachiasmatic nucleus is light. This view is further supported by studies in which 24-h hormone profiles were sampled in normal control subjects on two separate occasions, once after they were chronically exposed to simulated short (8-h) 'summer nights' and once after they were chronically exposed to simulated long (14-h) 'winter nights'. The duration of the period of rising cortisol levels, active melatonin secretion and high prolactin secretion was longer during the 'winter nights' than during the 'summer nights' (Wehr, 1998).

Shift Work

In shift workers, a long-lasting resistance of the cortisol rhythm to total adaptation to an inverted sleep schedule was detected. Young male night workers who had been permanently on night shift for at least 2 years were compared to day-active control subjects. Sleep EEG and hormone secretion were examined in each group during the usual sleep time (0700–1500 in the night workers, and 2300–0700 in the control subjects, respectively). Furthermore, hormone secretion was investigated during the usual work time. Sleep-EEG variables did not show major differences between the groups. In contrast, cortisol levels were enhanced and TSH levels were blunted in the night workers during the usual sleep time. However, cortisol levels were blunted in the night workers during their work hours. During this interval, a transient increase of prolactin occurred (Weibel and Brandenberger, 1998). Another study from the same laboratory (Weibel *et al.*, 1997) found a more random distribution of GH pulses during sleep in the daytime sleep of night workers than controls.

Sleep in Endocrine Disorders

Hypo- and hypersecretion of various hormones is regularly linked to disturbed sleep. Insomnia is the most frequent sleep-related symptom in these disorders. Only in patients with prolactinoma has enhanced sleep depth been reported so far.

Disorders of HPS System

Given the strong association between SWS and GH secretion, it was interesting to investigate patients with inborn or acquired lack of GH secretion and those with excessive GH levels in acromegaly.

In eight patients, isolated GH deficiency was initially diagnosed by slow growth velocity, an abnormal insulin hypoglycaemia test and retarded bone age. In comparison to normal controls, SWS in these patients was reduced, whereas total sleep time and time spent in stages 1 and 2 were increased (Åström and Lindholm, 1990). The same laboratory reported a decrease in SWA in these patients (Åström and Jochumsen, 1989). Guilhaume *et al.* (1982) examined a small sample of children with psychosocial dwarfism. At the initial examination, the amount of SWS was low. After several weeks in a new environment, an improvement of sleep quality was observed during recovery of growth, particularly an increase of SWS.

In patients with acromegaly, obstructive sleep apnoea syndrome is frequent due to hyperplasia of the upper airway soft tissue (Hart *et al.*, 1985). But also patients with acromegaly but without sleep apnoea have daytime sleepiness and an abnormal sleep structure. One year after adenectomy, REMS time and SWS time increased in patients with acromegaly (Åström and Trojaborg, 1992).

HPA System Aberrations

The capacity of the adrenal glands to produce corticosteroids is severely reduced in Addison's disease (Gillin *et al.*, 1974). There exist only a few case reports on these patients, and these reports do not suggest major changes of their sleep EEG. Garcia-Borreguero *et al.* (2000) compared patients with Addison's disease under two conditions, either continuous hydrocortisone replacement therapy or shorter hydrocortisone withdrawal. Under hydrocortisone replacement, REMS latency was shortened, and REMS time and intermittent wakefulness were increased in comparison to hydrocortisone withdrawal. The authors suggest that cortisol may be needed to facilitate the initiation and maintenance of REMS.

Excessive cortisol levels are produced in patients with Cushing's disease, of either central or peripheral origin. SWS is decreased in these patients (Krieger and Glick, 1974; Shipley *et al.*, 1992). In one study, increases of sleep latency and intermittent wake time and disinhibition of REMS (shortened REM latency, elevated REMS density) were also reported (Shipley *et al.*, 1992). Particularly the latter report suggests that sleep-EEG changes in Cushing's disease and in depression are similar.

Hypothyroidism and Hyperthyroidism

Changes of sleep-wake behaviour are characteristic symptoms of diseases of the thyroid gland. From clinical practice, it is well known that hyperthyroidism is linked with insomnia, whereas fatigue is frequently observed in patients with hypothyroidism. Astonishingly, there are only a few data on sleep EEG in these diseases. One study reported that SWS was reduced in patients with hypothyroidism in comparison to normal controls. The sleep EEG normalized after therapy (Kales *et al.*, 1967).

Prolactinoma

Comparison of patients with hyperprolactinoma and normal controls showed a separate increase of SWS in the patients (Frieboes *et al.*, 1998).

EXPERIMENTAL MODELS OF CHANGES OF SLEEP-ENDOCRINE ACTIVITY

A host of preclinical, human and clinical studies have investigated the interaction of sleep EEG and endocrine activity. The applied methods include transgenic animals; manipulation of endocrine activity in animals by surgery; manipulation of sleep-wake behaviour in normal human control subjects, as by partial or total sleep deprivation; and exogenous administration of hormones, particularly peptides and steroids, to animals and humans. The knowledge accumulated from these studies helps us to understand the pathophysiology of the aberrations reported before in this chapter. Ehlers and Kupfer (1987) were the first to advance the hypothesis that the key peptides of the HPS and the HPA systems, GHRH and CRH, play a major role in sleep regulation. Today this view is corroborated by many data. Besides stimulating GH release, GHRH has been shown to promote NREMS, particularly SWS, in various species including the human (male subjects) (reviewed in Krueger and Obál, 1993), and to blunt HPA hormones in human males (Steiger *et al.*, 1992; Antonijevic *et al.*, 2000b; Antonijevic *et al.*, 2000c). In contrast to GHRH, CRH stimulates the HPA hormones ACTH and cortisol, blunts GH release, impairs sleep and enhances vigilance. Furthermore, a REMS-promoting effect of CRH has been discussed (Steiger, in press). It is thought that changes of the GHRH/CRH ratio result in changes in sleep-endocrine activity. Besides GHRH and CRH, there are other endocrine factors which appear to participate in sleep regulation (see Figure XXIV-3.7).

HPA Hormones

The synthesis and release of CRH is reduced by a hypothalamic gene defect in the Lewis rat. Lewis rats spend less time awake and show more SWS than intact control rats. After intracerebroventricular (ICV) administration of CRH, waking increased

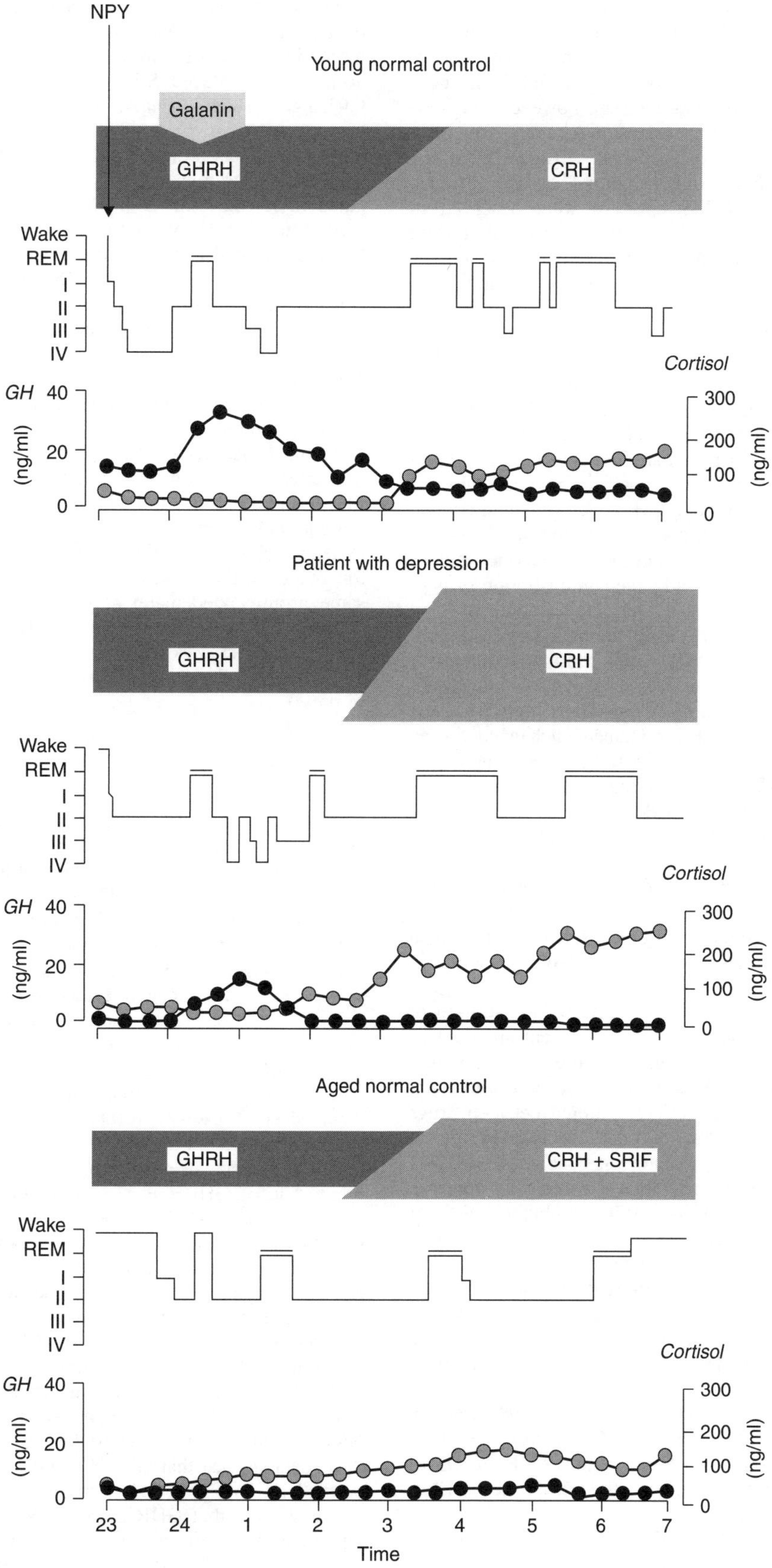

Figure XXIV-3.7 Model of peptidergic sleep regulation

similarly in Lewis and control rats. The sleep-disturbing effects of CRH are suggested by this study (Opp, 1997). In rats, after adrenalectomy and corticosterone replacement, the concentration of this hormone remained about $100\,\mathrm{ng\,ml^{-1}}$ throughout 24 h. In the sham-operated control group, however, corticosterone levels ranged between peak levels of about $240\,\mathrm{ng\,ml^{-1}}$ in the evening and the minimum of about $20\,\mathrm{ng\,ml^{-1}}$ in the morning. Sleep EEG differed only slightly between groups. Slightly more, but shorter, REMS episodes were observed in the adrenalectomized group than the control rats. Obviously, the tonic levels of corticosterone exerted only minor effects on spontaneous sleep-wake behaviour (Langebartels and Lancel, 2000).

ICV administration of CRH diminished SWS in rats (Ehlers *et al.*, 1986) and rabbits (Opp *et al.*, 1989). Moreover, after 72 h of sleep deprivation, SWS was reduced in rats. Furthermore, sleep latency and REMS time increased (Marrosu *et al.*, 1990). Similarly, in young, normal, male control subjects after pulsatile intravenous (IV) administration of $4 \times 50\,\mu\mathrm{g}$ human CRH between 2200 and 0100, SWS decreased during the second half of the night, whereas REMS decreased. Furthermore, the GH peak was blunted and during the first hours of the night, cortisol concentration was elevated (Holsboer *et al.*, 1988). In human sleep-endocrine studies, the time, the dosage and the protocol of the administration of peptides are crucial methodological issues. Repetitive administration around sleep onset (Holsboer *et al.*, 1988) mimics the physiological partial release of CRH. In contrast, after continuous nocturnal infusion of CRH, no effect on the sleep EEG was found (Fehm *et al.*, 1993). Moreover, after hourly IV injections of $10\,\mu\mathrm{g}$ CRH between 0800 and 1800, sleep EEG remained unchanged during the following night (Kellner *et al.*, 1997). In this study, melatonin levels were blunted after CRH. This finding suggests that the low melatonin syndrome in patients with depression is secondary to CRH overdrive. The responsiveness of sleep to CRH appears to increase during ageing. This theory is suggested by a study comparing the influence of a single dose of ovine CRH given 10 min after sleep onset between young and middle-aged normal control subjects (Vgontzas *et al.*, 2001). In young men, sleep EEG remained unchanged, whereas wakefulness increased and SWS decreased in the middle-aged subjects.

Two studies reported conflicting results after administration of CRH antagonists to rats. In one study, two different antagonists, alpha-helical CRH and astressin, were given before the dark period. These substances reduced wakefulness in a dose-dependent manner, whereas the time courses of these effects differed between drugs (Chang and Opp, 1998). Administration of the substances before the light period had no effect on sleep. The authors concluded that CRH contributes to the regulation of physiological waking. In contrast, in another study (Gonzalez and Valatx, 1997), alpha-helical CRH was effective only in stressed animals. In these rats, REMS was elevated and declined to values of the nonstressed condition after the drug. In sleep-deprived rats, REMS rebound, but not SWS rebound, was diminished by alpha-helical CRH during recovery sleep. The authors suggested that stress acting via CRH may be the major factor inducing the REMS rebound after sleep deprivation (Gonzalez and Valatx, 1998). Some of the cited preclinical work (Gonzalez and Valatx, 1997; Gonzalez and Valatx, 1998; Marrosu *et al.*, 1990) suggests that CRH promotes REMS. From the study in young human controls, the role of endogenous CRH in REMS regulation is uncertain, however, since CRH diminished REMS (Holsboer *et al.*, 1988).

Studies on the effects of ACTH and cortisol on sleep may help to differentiate the central and peripherally mediated sleep-EEG changes after CRH in human subjects. As reviewed elsewhere (Steiger, in press), suppression of REMS is a common effect of the acute administration of CRH, ACTH and cortisol in humans, whereas a synthetic ACTH (4-9) analogue affected neither cortisol release nor REMS (Steiger and Holsboer, 1997b). Furthermore, inhibition of cortisol synthesis by metyrapone in young normal men reduced SWS and cortisol while REMS remained unchanged (Steiger *et al.*, 1998). It is likely that endogenous CRH was enhanced in this study since ACTH was elevated. Interestingly, the effects of subchronic treatment with steroids differ from acute administration in normal controls. Sleep EEG was investigated in female patients with multiple sclerosis at baseline and after 2 and 9 days of administration of the glucocorticoid receptor agonist methylprednisolone. After 2 days, no major effects were found. After 9 days, REMS latency was shortened, REMS density increased and a major portion of SWS shifted from the first to the second NREMS period. These effects are similar to sleep-EEG aberrations in patients with depression (Steiger and Antonijevic, 2001).

Furthermore, the administration of the mixed glucocorticoid and progesterone receptor antagonist, mifepriston, is a method to modulate the HPA system. In a single case study in a normal control after oral mifepriston, ACTH and cortisol were enhanced. Sleep quality was disturbed markedly as sleep latency and intermittent wakefulness increased and SWS and REMS decreased (Wiedemann *et al.*, 1992). The sleep-disturbing effects of mifepriston were further corroborated by a set of studies from the same group (Wiedemann *et al.*, 1994; Wiedemann *et al.*, 1998). Whereas HPA hormones are widely dependent on a circadian rhythm, most studies report increases of ACTH and cortisol after awakenings and during sleep deprivation (reviewed by Steiger, in press).

HPS System

Hormones of the HPA system can modulate sleep. GHRH is the endogenous substance with the best-documented sleep-promoting activity. ICV administration of GHRH to rats and rabbits increases SWS (Ehlers *et al.*, 1986; Obál *et al.*, 1988). The same effect is seen when GHRH is injected into the medial preoptic area in rats (Zhang *et al.*, 1999) or IV in rats (Obál *et al.*, 1996). NREMS increases when GHRH is inhibited by receptor antagonists (Obál *et al.*, 1991) or by negative feedback inhibition of GHRH after administration of GH (Mendelson *et al.*, 1980; Stern *et al.*, 1975) or insulin-like growth factor-1 (Obál *et al.*, 1999). Hypothalamic GHRH mRNA is dependent on a circadian rhythm. In the rat, the highest concentration is found at the beginning of the light period when sleep propensity reaches its maximum in these nocturnal animals (Bredow *et al.*, 1996). Furthermore, hypothalamic GHRH contents display sleep-related variations (Gardi *et al.*, 1999). A major role of GHRH in sleep promotion by sleep deprivation is indicated since GHRH antibodies antagonize this effect in the rat (Obál *et al.*, 1992). Furthermore, hypothalamic GHRH mRNA has been found to be increased after sleep deprivation in rats (Toppila *et al.*, 1997; Zhang *et al.*, 1999). The sleep rebound following sleep deprivation was inhibited by microinjections of a GHRH antagonist into the area preoptica of the rat (Zhang *et al.*, 1999). Very big 'supermice' slept more than normal mice (Lachmansingh and Rollo, 1994). However, dwarf rats with deficits in the central GHRHergic transmission and reduced hypothalamic GHRH content had less NREMS than control rats (Obál *et al.*, 2001). Taken together, these data suggest that GHRH is a common stimulus for NREMS, particularly SWS and GH secretion.

We showed that GHRH promotes sleep also in humans. After repetitive IV administration of GHRH during the first few hours of the night, SWS and GH secretion increased in young normal male controls and cortisol secretion decreased (Steiger *et al.*, 1992). Sleep promotion in young men by GHRH was confirmed after IV(Kerkhofs *et al.*, 1993; Marshall *et al.*, 1999) and intranasal

(Perras *et al.*, 1999a) administration. We investigated the effects of GHRH on sleep-endocrine activity in three states with a change of the GHRH/CRH ratio in favour of CRH: first, the second half of the night in young normal men; second, in elderly normal men and women; and, third, in patients with depression.

In the first case, in young normal men, administration of GHRH during the early morning hours (0400–0700) prompted no major effects on sleep EEG, particularly no change of SWS. GH increased whereas HPA hormones remained unchanged (Schier *et al.*, 1997). In the second case, in the normal elderly, during the daytime, the response of GH to GHRH was blunted (Iovino *et al.*, 1989). Similarly, we found only a weak sleep-promoting effect of GHRH in the elderly. The first NREMS period was prolonged and the time of awakenings decreased, whereas SWS remained unchanged (Guldner *et al.*, 1997). In the third case, the influence of pulsatile IV administration of GHRH during the first few hours of the night was tested in 42 drug-free patients of both sexes with major depression (age range 19–76 years) and matched controls. Interestingly, a sexual dimorphism in the response to GHRH was found. In male patients and controls, GHRH inhibited ACTH levels during the first half of the night and cortisol levels during the second half of the night. In contrast, these hormones were enhanced in females, regardless whether they were healthy or depressed. Similarly, NREMS and stage 2 sleep increased in male patients and controls, whereas opposite sleep-impairing effects occurred in women. These data confirm a reciprocal antagonism of GHRH and CRH in males, whereas a synergism of GHRH and CRH is suggested in females. The latter issue may be an explanation for the increased prevalence of mood disorders in women (Antonijevic *et al.*, 2000b; Antonijevic *et al.*, 2000c).

The major antagonist of GHRH in the regulation of GH is somatostatin. In rats, systemic administration of the somatostatin analogue octreotide decreased NREMS (Beranek *et al.*, 1999). Similarly, SWS was reduced in young normal men after subcutaneous administration of octreotide (Ziegenbein *et al.*, 2000). Octreotide is known to be more potent than exogenous somatostatin. This is shown by the fact that repetitive IV administration of somatostatin impaired sleep in normal elderly controls (Frieboes *et al.*, 1997), whereas it had no effect in young normal men (Steiger *et al.*, 1992).

Galanin

Under repetitive IV administration of galanin to young normal men, SWS and the duration of REMS periods increased, whereas the secretion of GH and cortisol remained unchanged (Murck *et al.*, 1999).

Neuropeptide Y (NPY)

Besides GHRH, NPY appears to be a physiological antagonist of CRH. Originally, this theory was based on the opposite effects of CRH and NPY in animal models of anxiety (reviewed in Steiger and Holsboer, 1997b). This view is supported by recent studies on the sleep-EEG effects of NPY. After ICV administration of NPY to rats, EEG spectral activity changed in a way similar to the effects of benzodiazepines (Ehlers *et al.*, 1997a). Furthermore, the prolongation of sleep-onset latency by CRH was antagonized dose-dependently by NPY in rats (Ehlers *et al.*, 1997b). Similar effects were observed in young normal men. Repetitive IV administration of NPY prompted decreases of sleep latency and the first REMS period, and increases of stage 2 sleep and sleep period time, and blunted cortisol and ACTH secretion (Antonijevic *et al.*, 2000a). Moreover, in patients with depression of both sexes with a wide age range and age-matched controls, the sleep latency was shortened after NPY, whereas cortisol and ACTH levels and the first REM period remained unchanged (Held *et al.*, 1999). These data suggest that NPY participates in sleep regulation, particularly in the timing of sleep onset as an antagonist of CRH acting via the $GABA_A$ receptor.

Vasoactive Intestinal Polypeptide (VIP)

Pulsatile IV administration of vasoactive intestinal polypeptide (VIP) in young normal male control subjects decelerated the NREMS-REMS cycles. Each cycle was prolonged, the cortisol nadir appeared to be advanced and the GH surge was blunted (Murck *et al.*, 1996). These findings suggest that VIP exerts a specific effect on the temporal organization of sleep-endocrine activity, including the timing of the cortisol nadir. It appears likely that VIP affects the circadian clock, resulting in prolonged sleep cycles and earlier occurrence of the cortisol nadir. Blunted GH surge may be explained as a result of the advanced elevated HPA activity.

HORMONES AS THERAPY IN SLEEP DISORDERS

Several approaches were applied to use hormones or synthetic analogues in the treatment of sleep disorders. In most cases, the rational was the substitution of declining hormone levels.

Oestrogen Replacement Therapy

In postmenopausal women oestrogen replacement therapy by skin patch (50 µg of estradiol per day) enhanced REMS and reduced intermittent wakefulness during the first two sleep cycles. The normal decrease in SWS and SWA from the first to the second sleep cycle was restored by oestrogen (Figure XXIV-3.8) (Antonijevic *et al.*, 2000d). These data suggest that oestrogen treatment after the menopause can help to restore the normal sleep-EEG pattern in women.

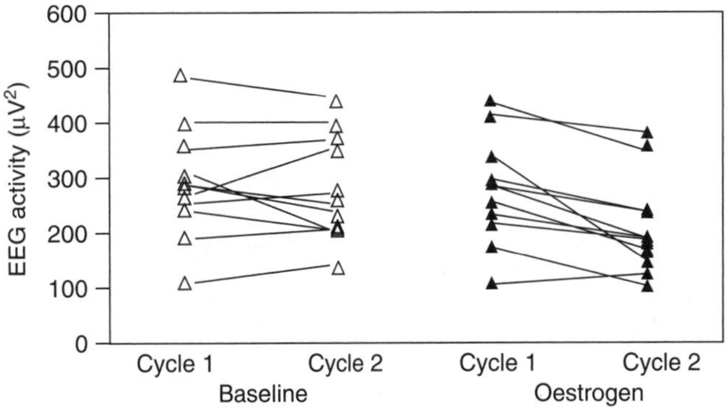

Figure XXIV-3.8 Changes in delta electroencephalographic activity from first to second cycle during baseline and oestrogen replacement therapy (ERT). A change in delta electroencephalographic (EEG) activity from first to second non-rapid-eye movement during baseline (open circles) was not consistently observed, whereas during ERT (filled circles) a normal decrease in delta activity from first to second non-rapid-eye movement period was observed in most subjects (expressed as percentage change of the respective value from first to second non-rapid-eye movement period: −2.4% ± 5.4% during baseline versus −20.4% ± 5.7% during ERT; univariate F test after one-factorial (treatment) analysis of variance, including covariate short-term versus long-term ERT; $n = 11$; F1, 9 = 8.8; $P < 0.05$)

GHRH and GH Secretagogues

Acute repetitive IV (Guldner *et al.*, 1997) and intranasal (Perras *et al.*, 1999b) administration of GHRH in elderly subjects had only a relatively weak sleep-promoting effect compared to the increase of SWS in young men after this peptide. A pilot study tested the hypothesis that after priming (e.g., daily IV administration of GHRH every 2 days for 12 days) the sleep-promoting effect of GHRH would be restored in the elderly. The study results in two subjects do not support this hypothesis (Murck *et al.*, 1997). GH secretagogues are synthetic peptides. These substances share the capacity of GHRH to stimulate GH release, although they act via a specific GH secretagogue receptor, and not at the GHRH receptor. As in the observations after GHRH, oral administration of one GH secretagogue, MK-677, for 1 week, had a distinct sleep-promoting effect in young men and only a weak effect in elderly controls (Copinschi *et al.*, 1997). Obviously, the capacity of GHRH and GH secretagogues to promote sleep in the elderly is reduced. It might be necessary to start with the substitution of GHRH or related analogues earlier during the lifespan in order to counteract the sequelae of their declining endogenous activity.

Vasopressin

After 3 months' daily intranasal administration of vasopressin to elderly subjects, SWS was enhanced markedly, whereas intermittent wakefulness and self-rated sleep quality remained unchanged (Perras *et al.*, 1999b).

Melatonin

Study results on a beneficial effect of melatonin in young and elderly subjects are ambiguous (Baskett *et al.*, 2001). A possible side effect of long-term treatment with melatonin is a blunting of sexual steroids in men and women. So far, there is a lack of sufficient data from clinical studies to recommend melatonin as an effective alternative sleeping pill. Some studies suggest that, as a result of its phase-shifting properties, melatonin may be helpful in the treatment of rhythm disturbances, such as jet lag and disturbed rhythms in blind patients (Sack *et al.*, 2000; Zhdanova *et al.*, 1997).

CONCLUSIONS

The data reported in this chapter corroborate the bidirectional action of sleep EEG and endocrine activity. Shallow sleep and sleep loss due to various causes are frequently linked to elevated secretion of cortisol and ACTH and blunted GH levels. Another clear link has been shown between changes of the sleep-wake rhythm and the pattern of melatonin activity. The link between the NREMS-REMS cycle and the oscillations of plasma renin activity known from normal controls appears to be preserved in disrupted sleep patterns. Although it is so far unknown what factors are the common regulators of sleep and plasma renin activity, the role of GHRH and CRH as links between sleep EEG and peripheral hormone secretion is well established. At least in male subjects, GHRH appears to stimulate GH and SWS and to inhibit HPA hormones. CRH exerts opposite effects. Changes of the GHRH/CRH ratio occur during normal ageing (reduced GHRH activity) and in depression (CRH overactivity). Common features of these states are shallow sleep, blunted GH and elevated cortisol levels. Sleep-EEG changes in dwarfs (low GHRH) and subjects with acromegaly (feedback inhibition of GHRH due to excessive GH levels) can be similarly explained. Gender differences in sleep regulation are suggested by the opposite effects of GHRH in normal and depressed women in comparison to men. This issue needs further clarification.

Besides GHRH and CRH, other peptides and steroids are thought to participate in sleep regulation. Like CRH, somatostatin is sleep-impairing factor, and, like GHRH, NPY and galanin promote sleep. VIP appears to be involved in the temporal organization of sleep. The similarities between sleep-EEG in patients with depression and with Cushing's disease and in patients with multiple sclerosis after subchronic administration of a glucocorticoid agonist suggest, that besides CRH, elevated glucocorticoid levels also contribute to the sleep-EEG changes in depression. So far, the use of hormones in the therapy of sleep disorders is rare. Since the hypnotics of today do not induce physiological sleep (Steiger and Lancel, 2000), novel substances are needed that correspond better to human physiology. The progress in sleep-endocrine research should help to develop such therapeutic strategies. In the related field of antidepressants, the recent development of CRH antagonists (Holsboer, 1999; Zobel *et al.*, 2000) is an encouraging example.

REFERENCES

Åström, C. and Jochumsen, P.L., 1989. Decrease in delta sleep in growth hormone deficiency assessed by a new power spectrum analysis. *Sleep*, **12**, 508–515.

Åström, C. and Lindholm, J., 1990. Growth hormone-deficient young adults have decreased deep sleep. *Neuroendocrinology*, **51**, 82–84.

Åström, C. and Trojaborg, W., 1992. Effect of growth hormone on human sleep energy. *Clinical Endocrinology*, **36**, 241–245.

American Sleep Disorders Association, 1997. *ICSD—International Classification of Sleep Disorders, Revised: Diagnostic and Coding Manual*. American Sleep Disorders Association, Rochester, Minnesota.

Antonijevic, I.A., Murck, H., Frieboes, R.M., Horn, R., Brabant, G. and Steiger, A., 1998. Elevated nocturnal profiles of serum leptin in patients with depression. *Journal of Psychiatric Research*, **32**, 403–410.

Antonijevic, I.A., Murck, H., Frieboes, R.M., Holsboer, F. and Steiger, A., 1999. On the gender differences in sleep-endocrine regulation in young normal humans. *Neuroendocrinology*, **70**, 280–287.

Antonijevic, I.A., Murck, H., Bohlhalter, S., Frieboes, R.M., Holsboer, F. and Steiger, A., 2000a. NPY promotes sleep and inhibits ACTH and cortisol release in young men. *Neuropharmacology*, **39**, 1474–1481.

Antonijevic, I.A., Murck, H., Frieboes, R.M., Barthelmes, J. and Steiger, A., 2000b. Sexually dimorphic effects of GHRH on sleep-endocrine activity in patients with depression and normal controls. I. The sleep EEG. *Sleep Research Online*, **3**, 5–13.

Antonijevic, I.A., Murck, H., Frieboes, R.M. and Steiger, A., 2000c. Sexually dimorphic effects of GHRH on sleep-endocrine activity in patients with depression and normal controls. II. Hormone secretion. *Sleep Research Online*, **3**, 15–21.

Antonijevic, I.A., Stalla, G.K. and Steiger, A., 2000d. Modulation of the sleep electroencephalogram by estrogen replacement in postmenopausal women. *American Journal of Obstetrics and Gynecology*, **182**, 277–282.

Baskett, J.J., Wood, P.C., Broad, J.B., Duncan, J.R., English, J. and Arendt, J., 2001. Melatonin in older people with age-related sleep maintenance problems: a comparison with age-matched normal sleepers. *Sleep*, **24**, 418–424.

Beck, U., Brezinova, V., Hunter, W.M. and Oswald, I., 1975. Plasma growth hormone and slow wave sleep increase after interruption of sleep. *Journal of Clinical Endocrinology and Metabolism*, **40**, 812–815.

Benca, R.M., Obermeyer, W.H., Thisted, R.A. and Gillin, J.C., 1992. Sleep and psychiatric disorders. A meta-analysis. *Archives of General Psychiatry*, **49**, 651–668.

Beranek, L., Hajdu, I., Gardi, J., Taishi, P., Obál, F., Jr. and Krueger, J.M., 1999. Central administration of the somatostatin analog octreotide induces captopril-insensitive sleep responses. *American Journal of Physiology*, **277**, R1297–R1304.

Bliwise, D.L., 1993. Sleep in normal aging and dementia. *Sleep*, **16**, 40–81.

Brabant, G., Brabant, A., Ranft, U., Ocran, K., Köhrle, J., Hesch, R.D. and Von zur Mühlen, A., 1987. Circadian and pulsatile thyrotropin secretion in euthyroid man under the influence of thyroid hormone and glucocorticoid administration. *Journal of Clinical Endocrinology and Metabolism*, **65**, 83–88.

Bradley, T.D. and Phillipson, E.A., 1985. Pathogenesis and pathophysiology of the obstructive sleep apnoea syndrome. *Medical Clinics of North America*, **69**, 1169–1185.

Brandenberger, G., Follenius, M., Simon, C., Ehrhart, J. and Libert, J.P., 1988. Nocturnal oscillations in plasma renin activity and REM-NREM sleep cycles in humans: a common regulatory mechanism? *Sleep*, **11**, 242–250.

Brandenberger, G., Buguet, A., Spiegel, K., Stanghellini, A., Mouanga, G., Bogui, P., Montmayeur, A. and Dumas, M., 1994. Maintenance of the relation between the pulsed secretion of hormones and the internal sleep structure in human African trypanosomiasis [in French]. *Bulletin de la Société de Pathologie Exotique*, **87**, 383–389.

Bredow, S., Taishi, P., Obál, F., Jr., Guha-Thakurta, N. and Krueger, J.M., 1996. Hypothalamic growth hormone-releasing hormone mRNA varies across the day in rat. *Neuroreport*, **7**, 2501–2505.

Chan, V., Jones, A., Liendo, Ch P., McNeilly, A., Landon, J. and Besser, G.M., 1978. The relationship between circadian variations in circulating thyrotrophin, thyroid hormones and prolactin. *Clinical Endocrinology*, **9**, 337–349.

Chang, F.C. and Opp, M.R., 1998. Blockade of corticotropin-releasing hormone receptors reduces spontaneous waking in the rat. *American Journal of Physiology*, **275**, R793–R802.

Cooper, B.G., White, J.E., Ashworth, L.A., Alberti, K.G. and Gibson, G.J., 1995. Hormonal and metabolic profiles in subjects with obstructive sleep apnea syndrome and the acute effects of nasal continuous positive airway pressure (CPAP) treatment. *Sleep*, **18**, 172–179.

Copinschi, G., Leproult, R., Van Onderbergen, A., Caufriez, A., Cole, K.Y., Schilling, L.M., Mendel, C.M., De Lepeleire, I., Bolognese, J.A. and Van Cauter, E., 1997. Prolonged oral treatment with MK-677, a novel growth hormone secretagogue, improves sleep quality in man. *Neuroendocrinology*, **66**, 278–286.

Coplan, J.D., Wolk, S.I., Goetz, R.R., Ryan, N.D., Dahl, R.E. and Weissman, M.M., 2000. Nocturnal growth hormone secretion studies in adolescents with or without major depression re-examined: integration of adult clinical follow-up data. *Biological Psychiatry*, **47**, 594–604.

De Bellis, M.D., Dahl, R.E., Perel, J.M., Birmaher, B., al-Shabbout, M., Williamson, D.E., Nelson, B. and Ryan, N.D., 1996. Nocturnal ACTH, cortisol, growth hormone and prolactin secretion in prepubertal depression. *Journal of the American Academy of Child and Adolescent Psychiatry*, **35**, 1130–1138.

Desir, D., Van Cauter, E., Fang, V.S., Martino, E., Jadot, C., Spire, J.P., Noel, P., Refetoff, S., Copinschi, G. and Golstein, J., 1981. Effects of 'jet lag' on hormonal patterns. I. Procedures, variations in total plasma proteins, and disruption of adrenocorticotropin-cortisol periodicity. *Journal of Clinical Endocrinology and Metabolism*, **52**, 628–641.

Deuschle, M., Blum, W.F., Englaro, P., Schweiger, U., Weber, B., Pflaum, C.D. and Heuser, I., 1996. Plasma leptin in depressed patients and healthy controls. *Hormone and Metabolic Research*, **28**, 714–717.

Ehlers, C.L. and Kupfer, D.J., 1987. Hypothalamic peptide modulation of EEG sleep in depression: a further application of the S-process hypothesis. *Biological Psychiatry*, **22**, 513–517.

Ehlers, C.L., Reed, T.K. and Henriksen, S.J., 1986. Effects of corticotropin-releasing factor and growth hormone-releasing factor on sleep and activity in rats. *Neuroendocrinology*, **42**, 467–474.

Ehlers, C.L., Kaneko, W.M., Owens, M.J. and Nemeroff, C.B., 1993. Effects of gender and social isolation on electroencephalogram and neuroendocrine parameters in rats. *Biological Psychiatry*, **33**, 358–366.

Ehlers, C.L., Somes, C., Lopez, A., Kirby, D. and Rivier, J.E., 1997a. Electrophysiological actions of neuropeptide Y and its analogs: new measures for anxiolytic therapy? *Neuropsychopharmacology*, **17**, 34–43.

Ehlers, C.L., Somes, C., Seifritz, E. and Rivier, J.E., 1997b. CRF/NPY interactions: a potential role in sleep dysregulation in depression and anxiety. *Depression and Anxiety*, **6**, 1–9.

Elmquist, J.K., Ahima, R.S., Maratos-Flier, E., Flier, J.S. and Saper, C.B., 1997. Leptin activates neurons in ventrobasal hypothalamus and brainstem. *Endocrinology*, **138**, 839–842.

Fehm, H.L., Klein, E., Holl, R. and Voigt, K.H., 1984. Evidence for extrapituitary mechanisms mediating the morning peak of cortisol secretion in man. *Journal of Clinical Endocrinology and Metabolism*, **58**, 410–414.

Fehm, H.L., Späth-Schwalbe, E., Pietrowsky, R., Kern, W. and Born, J., 1993. Entrainment of nocturnal pituitary-adrenocortical activity to sleep processes in man — a hypothesis. *Experimental and Clinical Endocrinology*, **101**, 267–276.

Ferini-Strambi, L., Franceschi, M., Cattaneo, A.G., Smirne, S., Calori, G. and Caviezel, F., 1991. Sleep-related growth hormone secretion in human obesity: effect of dietary treatment. *Neuroendocrinology*, **54**, 412–415.

Follenius, M., Brandenberger, G., Simon, C. and Schlienger, J.L., 1988. REM sleep in humans begins during decreased secretory activity of the anterior pituitary. *Sleep*, **11**, 546–555.

Frieboes, R.M., Murck, H., Schier, T., Holsboer, F. and Steiger, A., 1997. Somatostatin impairs sleep in elderly human subjects. *Neuropsychopharmacology*, **16**, 339–345.

Frieboes, R.M., Murck, H., Stalla, G.K., Antonijevic, I.A. and Steiger, A., 1998. Enhanced slow wave sleep in patients with prolactinoma. *Journal of Clinical Endocrinology and Metabolism*, **83**, 2706–2710.

Frieboes, R.M., Müller, U., Murck, H., von Cramon, D.Y., Holsboer, F. and Steiger, A., 1999. Nocturnal hormone secretion and the sleep EEG in patients several months after traumatic brain injury. *Journal of Neuropsychiatry and Clinical Neurosciences*, **11**, 354–360.

Garcia-Borreguero, D., Wehr, T.A., Larrosa, O., Granizo, J.L., Hardwick, D., Chrousos, G.P. and Friedman, T.C., 2000. Glucocorticoid replacement is permissive for rapid eye movement sleep and sleep consolidation in patients with adrenal insufficiency. *Journal of Clinical Endocrinology and Metabolism*, **85**, 4201–4206.

Gardi, J., Obál, F., Jr., Fang, J., Zhang, J. and Krueger, J.M., 1999. Diurnal variations and sleep deprivation-induced changes in rat hypothalamic GHRH and somatostatin contents. *American Journal of Physiology*, **277**, R1339–R1344.

Gillin, J.C., Jacobs, L.S., Snyder, F. and Henkin, R.I., 1974. Effects of ACTH on the sleep of normal subjects and patients with Addison's disease. *Neuroendocrinology*, **15**, 21–31.

Gonzalez, M.M.C. and Valatx, J.L., 1997. Effect of intracerebroventricular administration of alpha-helical CRH (9-41) on the sleep/waking cycle in rats under normal conditions or after subjection to an acute stressful stimulus. *Journal of Sleep Research*, **6**, 164–170.

Gonzalez, M.M.C. and Valatx, J.L., 1998. Involvement of stress in the sleep rebound mechanism induced by sleep deprivation in the rat: use of alpha-helical CRH (9-41). *Behavioral Pharmacology*, **9**, 655–662.

Grunstein, R.R., Stewart, D.A., Lloyd, H., Akinci, M., Cheng, N. and Sullivan, C.E., 1996. Acute withdrawal of nasal CPAP in obstructive sleep apnoea does not cause a rise in stress hormones. *Sleep*, **19**, 774–782.

Guilhaume, A., Benoit, O., Gourmelen, M. and Richardet, J.M., 1982. Relationship between sleep stage IV deficit and reversible hGH deficiency in psychosocial dwarfism. *Pediatric Research*, **16**, 299–303.

Guldner, J., Schier, T., Friess, E., Colla, M., Holsboer, F. and Steiger, A., 1997. Reduced efficacy of growth hormone-releasing hormone in modulating sleep endocrine activity in the elderly. *Neurobiology of Aging*, **18**, 491–495.

Hanson, E.S., Levin, N. and Dallman, M.F., 1997. Elevated corticosterone is not required for the rapid induction of neuropeptide Y gene expression by an overnight fast. *Endocrinology*, **138**, 1041–1047.

Hart, T.B., Radow, S.K., Blackard, W.G., Tucker, H.S.G. and Cooper, K.R., 1985. Sleep apnoea in active acromegaly. *Archives of Internal Medicine*, **145**, 865–866.

Held, K., Murck, H., Antonijevic, I.A., Künzel, H., Ziegenbein, M. and Steiger, A., 1999. Neuropeptide Y (NPY) does not differentially affect sleep-endocrine regulation in depressed patients and controls. *Pharmacopsychiatry*, **32**, 184.

Holsboer, F., 1999. The rationale for corticotropin-releasing hormone receptor (CRH-R) antagonists to treat depression and anxiety. *Journal of Psychiatric Research*, **33**, 181–214.

Holsboer, F., 2000. The corticosteroid receptor hypothesis of depression. *Neuropsychopharmacology*, **23**, 477–501.

Holsboer, F. and Barden, N., 1996. Antidepressants and hypothalamic-pituitary-adrenocortical regulation. *Endocrine Reviews*, **17**, 187–205.

Holsboer, F., von Bardeleben, U. and Steiger, A., 1988. Effects of intravenous corticotropin-releasing hormone upon sleep-related growth hormone surge and sleep EEG in man. *Neuroendocrinology*, **48**, 32–38.

Iovino, M., Monteleone, P. and Steardo, L., 1989. Repetitive growth hormone-releasing hormone administration restores the attenuated growth hormone (GH) response to GH-releasing hormone testing in normal aging. *Journal of Clinical Endocrinology and Metabolism*, **69**, 910–913.

Jarrett, D.B., Miewald, J.M., Fedorka, I.B., Coble, P., Kupfer, D.J. and Greenhouse, J.B., 1987. Prolactin secretion during sleep: a comparison between depressed patients and healthy control subjects. *Biological Psychiatry*, **22**, 1216–1226.

Jarrett, D.B., Miewald, J.M. and Kupfer, D.J., 1990. Recurrent depression is associated with a persistent reduction in sleep-related growth hormone secretion. *Archives of General Psychiatry*, **47**, 113–118.

Jones, C.R., Campbell, S.S., Zone, S.E., Cooper, F., DeSano, A., Murphy, P.J., Jones, B., Czajkowski, L. and Ptacek, L.J., 1999. Familial advanced sleep-phase syndrome: a short-period circadian rhythm variant in humans. *Nature Medicine*, **5**, 1062–1065.

Kales, A., Heuser, G., Jacobson, A., Kales, J.D., Hanley, J., Zweizig, J.R. and Paulson, M.J., 1967. All night sleep studies in hypothyroid patients, before and after treatment. *Journal of Clinical Endocrinology and Metabolism*, **27**, 1593–1599.

Kellner, M., Yassouridis, A., Manz, B., Steiger, A., Holsboer, F. and Wiedemann, K., 1997. Corticotropin-releasing hormone inhibits melatonin secretion in healthy volunteers — a potential link to low-melatonin syndrome in depression? *Neuroendocrinology*, **16**, 339–345.

Kerkhofs, M., Van Cauter, E., Van Onderbergen, A., Caufriez, A., Thorner, M.O. and Copinschi, G., 1993. Sleep-promoting effects of growth hormone-releasing hormone in normal men. *American Journal of Physiology*, **264**, E594–E598.

Krieg, J.C., Lauder, C.J., Schreiber, W. and Holsboer, F., 2001. Neuroendocrine, polysomnographic and psychometric observations in healthy subjects at high familial risk for affective disorders: the current state of the 'Munich vulnerability study'. *Journal of Affective Disorders*, **62**, 33–37.

Krieger, D.T. and Glick, S.M., 1974. Sleep EEG stages and plasma growth hormone concentration in states of endogenous and exogenous hypercortisolemia or ACTH elevation. *Journal of Clinical Endocrinology and Metabolism*, **39**, 986–1000.

Krieger, J., Follenius, M., Sforza, E. and Brandenberger, G., 1991. Effects of treatment with nasal continuous positive airway pressure on atrial natriuretic peptide and arginine vasopressin release during sleep in patients with obstructive sleep apnoea. *Clinical Science*, **80**, 443–449.

Krueger, J.M. and Obál, F., Jr., 1993. Growth hormone-releasing hormone and interleukin-1 in sleep regulation. *FASEB Journal*, **7**, 645–652.

Kupfer, D.J., Ehlers, C.L., Frank, E., Grochocinski, V.J., McEachran, A.B. and Buhari, A., 1993. Electroencephalographic sleep studies in depressed patients during long-term recovery. *Psychiatry Research*, **49**, 121–138.

Lachmansingh, E. and Rollo, C.D., 1994. Evidence for a trade-off between growth and behavioural activity in giant 'supermice' genetically engineered with extra growth hormone genes. *Canadian Journal of Zoology*, **72**, 2158–2168.

Langebartels, A. and Lancel, M., 2000. Influence of constant corticosterone levels on spontaneous and lipopolysaccharide-induced sleep in the rat. *Journal of Sleep Research*, **9**(Suppl 1), 109.

Lauer, C., Riemann, D., Wiegand, M. and Berger, M., 1991. From early to late adulthood. Changes in EEG sleep of depressed patients and healthy volunteers. *Biological Psychiatry*, **29**, 979–993.

Lesch, K.P., Laux, G., Schulte, H.M., Pfuller, H. and Beckmann, H., 1988. Abnormal responsiveness of growth hormone to human corticotropin-releasing hormone in major depressive disorder. *Journal of Affective Disorders*, **14**, 245–250.

Licinio, J., Mantzoros, C., Negrao, A.B., Cizza, G., Wong, M.L., Bongiorno, P.B., Chrousos, G.P., Karp, B., Allen, C., Flier, J.S. and Gold, P.W., 1997. Human leptin levels are pulsatile and inversely related to pituitary-adrenal function. *Nature Medicine*, **3**, 575–579.

Lieb, K., Maiwald, M., Berger, M. and Voderholzer, U., 1999. Insomnia for 5 years. *Lancet*, **354**, 1966.

Lieb, K., Reincke, M., Riemann, D. and Voderholzer, U., 2000. Sleep deprivation and growth-hormone secretion. *Lancet*, **356**, 2096–2097.

Linkowski, P., Mendlewicz, J., Kerkhofs, M., Leclercq, R., Golstein, J., Brasseur, M., Copinschi, G. and Van Cauter, E., 1987. 24-hour profiles of adrenocorticotropin, cortisol, and growth hormone in major depressive illness: effect of antidepressant treatment. *Journal of Clinical Endocrinology and Metabolism*, **65**, 141–152.

Linkowski, P., Kerkhofs, M., Van Onderbergen, A., Hubain, P., Copinschi, G., L'Hermite-Balériaux, M., Leclercq, R., Brasseur, M., Mendlewicz, J. and Van Cauter, E., 1994. The 24-hour profiles of cortisol, prolactin, and growth hormone secretion in mania. *Archives of General Psychiatry*, **51**, 616–624.

Lugaresi, E., Medori, R., Montagna, P., Baruzzi, A., Cortelli, P., Lugaresi, A., Tinuper, P., Zucconi, M. and Gambetti, P., 1986. Fatal familial insomnia and dysautonomia with selective degeneration of thalamic nuclei. *New England Journal of Medicine*, **315**, 997–1003.

Luthringer, R., Brandenberger, G., Schaltenbrand, N., Muller, G., Spiegel, K., Macher, J.P., Muzet, A. and Follenius, M., 1995. Slow wave electroencephalic activity parallels renin oscillations during sleep in humans. *Electroencephalography and Clinical Neurophysiology*, **95**, 318–322.

Marrosu, F., Gessa, G.L., Giagheddu, M. and Fratta, W., 1990. Corticotropin-releasing factor (CRF) increases paradoxical sleep (PS) rebound in PS-deprived rats. *Brain Research*, **515**, 315–318.

Marshall, L., Derad, L., Starsburger, C.J., Fehm, H.L. and Born, J., 1999. A determinant factor in the efficacy of GHRH administration in the efficacy of GHRH administration in promoting sleep: high peak concentration versus recurrent increasing slopes. *Psychoneuroendocrinology*, **24**, 363–370.

Mendelson, W.B., Slater, S., Gold, P. and Gillin, J.C., 1980. The effect of growth hormone administration on human sleep: a dose-response study. *Biological Psychiatry*, **15**, 613–618.

Montagna, P., Cortelli, P., Gambetti, P. and Lugaresi, E., 1995. Fatal familial insomnia: sleep, neuroendocrine and vegetative alterations. *Advances in Neuroimmunology*, **5**, 13–21.

Mullington, J., Hermann, D., Holsboer, F. and Pollmächer, T., 1996. Age-dependent suppression of nocturnal growth hormone levels during sleep deprivation. *Neuroendocrinology*, **64**, 233–241.

Murck, H., Guldner, J., Colla-Müller, M., Frieboes, R.M., Schier, T., Wiedemann, K., Holsboer, F. and Steiger, A., 1996. VIP decelerates non-REM-REM cycles and modulates hormone secretion during sleep in men. *American Journal of Physiology*, **271**, R905–R911.

Murck, H., Frieboes, R.M., Schier, T. and Steiger, A., 1997. Long-time administration of growth hormone-releasing hormone (GHRH) does not restore the reduced efficiency of GHRH on sleep endocrine activity in 2 old-aged subjects — a preliminary study. *Pharmacopsychiatry*, **30**, 122–124.

Murck, H., Antonijevic, I.A., Frieboes, R.M., Maier, P., Schier, T. and Steiger, A., 1999. Galanin has REM-sleep deprivation-like effects on the sleep EEG in healthy young men. *Journal of Psychiatric Research*, **33**, 225–232.

Obál, F., Jr., Alföldi, P., Cady, A.B., Johannsen, L., Sary, G. and Krueger, J.M., 1988. Growth hormone-releasing factor enhances sleep in rats and rabbits. *American Journal of Physiology*, **255**, R310–R316.

Obál, F., Jr., Payne, L., Kapás, L., Opp, M. and Krueger, J.M., 1991. Inhibition of growth hormone-releasing factor suppresses both sleep and growth hormone secretion in the rat. *Brain Research*, **557**, 149–153.

Obál, F., Jr., Payne, L., Opp, M., Alföldi, P., Kapás, L. and Krueger, J.M., 1992. Growth hormone-releasing hormone antibodies suppress sleep and prevent enhancement of sleep after sleep deprivation. *American Journal of Physiology*, **263**, R1078–R1085.

Obál, F., Jr., Floyd, R., Kapás, L., Bodosi, B. and Krueger, J.M., 1996. Effects of systemic GHRH on sleep in intact and in hypophysectomized rats. *American Journal of Physiology*, **270**, E230–E237.

Obál, F., Jr., Kapás, L., Gardi, J., Taishi, P., Bodosi, B. and Krueger, J.M., 1999. Insulin-like growth factor-1 (IGF-1)-induced inhibition of growth hormone secretion is associated with sleep suppression. *Brain Research*, **818**, 267–274.

Obál, F., Jr., Fang, J., Taishi, P., Kacsóh, B., Gardi, J. and Krueger, J.M., 2001. Deficiency of growth hormone-releasing hormone signaling is associated with sleep alterations in the dwarf rat. *Journal of Neuroscience*, **21**, 2912–2918.

Opp, M.R., 1997. Rat strain differences suggest a role for corticotropin-releasing hormone in modulating sleep. *Physiology and Behavior*, **63**, 67–74.

Opp, M., Obál, F., Jr. and Krueger, J.M., 1989. Corticotropin-releasing factor attenuates interleukin 1-induced sleep and fever in rabbits. *American Journal of Physiology*, **257**, R528–R535.

Perras, B., Marshall, L., Köhler, G., Born, J. and Fehm, H.L., 1999a. Sleep and endocrine changes after intranasal administration of growth hormone-releasing hormone in young and aged humans. *Psychoneuroendocrinology*, **24**, 743–757.

Perras, B., Pannenborg, H., Marshall, L., Pietrowsky, R., Born, J. and Fehm, H.L., 1999b. Beneficial treatment of age-related sleep disturbances with prolonged intranasal vasopressin. *Journal of Clinical Psychopharmacology*, **19**, 28–36.

Peteranderl, C., Antonijevic, I.A., Steiger, A., Murck, H., Frieboes, R.M., Uhr, M. and Schaaf, L., 2002. Reduced TSH/ACTH ratio in patients with depression and healthy controls. *Journal of Psychiatric Research*, in press.

Portaluppi, F., Cortelli, P., Avoni, P., Vergnani, L., Pavani, A., Sforza, E., Manfredini, R., Montagna, P. and Roiter, I., 1995. Dissociated 24-hour patterns of somatotropin and prolactin in fatal familial insomnia. *Neuroendocrinology*, **61**, 731–737.

Puig-Antich, J., Dahl, R., Ryan, N., Novacenko, H., Goetz, D., Goetz, R., Twomey, J. and Klepper, T., 1989. Cortisol secretion in prepubertal children with major depressive disorder. *Archives of General Psychiatry*, **46**, 801–809.

Quabbe, H.J., Schilling, E. and Helge, H., 1966. Pattern of growth hormone secretion during a 24-hour fast in normal adults. *Journal of Clinical Endocrinology and Metabolism*, **26**, 1173–1177.

Raber, J., Chen, S., Mucke, L. and Feng, L., 1997. Corticotropin-releasing factor and adrenocorticotrophic hormone as potential central mediators of OB effects. *Journal of Biological Chemistry*, **272**, 15057–15060.

Rao, U., Dahl, R.E., Ryan, N.D., Birmaher, B., Williamson, D.E., Giles, D.E., Rao, R., Kaufman, J. and Nelson, B., 1996. The relationship between longitudinal clinical course and sleep and cortisol changes in adolescent depression. *Biological Psychiatry*, **40**, 474–484.

Rechtschaffen, A. and Kales, A., 1968. *A Manual of Standardized Terminology, Techniques and Scoring System for Sleep Stages of Human Subjects*. US Department of Health, Education and Welfare, Neurological Information Network, Bethesda, MD.

Reul, J.M., Stec, I., Söder, M. and Holsboer, F., 1993. Chronic treatment of rats with the antidepressant amitriptyline attenuates the activity of the hypothalamic-pituitary-adrenocortical system. *Endocrinology*, **133**, 312–320.

Reynolds, C.F., 3rd and Kupfer, D.J., 1987. Sleep research in affective illness: state of the art *circa* 1987. *Sleep*, **10**, 199–215.

Rodenbeck, A., Huether, G., Rüther, E. and Hajak, G., 1999. Enhanced evening plasma cortisol secretion may induce the vicious cycle of chronification in primary insomnia. *Sleep Research Online*, **2**(Suppl 1), 184.

Rodenbeck, A., Huether, G., Ruther, E. and Hajak, G., 1998. Altered circadian melatonin secretion patterns in relation to sleep in patients with chronic sleep-wake rhythm disorders. *Journal of Pineal Research*, **25**, 201–210.

Saad, M.F., Damani, S., Gingerich, R.L., Riad-Gabriel, M.G., Khan, A., Boyadjian, R., Jinagouda, S.D., el-Tawil, K., Rude, R.K. and Kamdar, V., 1997. Sexual dimorphism in plasma leptin concentration. *Journal of Clinical Endocrinology and Metabolism*, **82**, 579–584.

Sack, R.L., Brandes, R.W., Kendall, A.R. and Lewy, A.J., 2000. Entrainment of free-running circadian rhythms by melatonin in blind people. *New England Journal of Medicine*, **343**, 1070–1077.

Sakkas, P.N., Soldatos, C.R., Bergiannaki, J.D. and Stefanis, C.N., 1998. Growth hormone secretion during sleep in male depressed patients. *Progress in Neuro-Psychopharmacology and Biological Psychiatry*, **22**, 467–483.

Sassin, J.F., Parker, D.C., Mace, J.W., Gotlin, R.W., Johnson, L.C. and Rossman, L.G., 1969. Human growth hormone release: relation to slow-wave sleep and sleep-waking cycles. *Science*, **165**, 513–515.

Schiavi, R.C., Davis, D.M. and Fogel, M., 1986. Luteinizing hormone and testosterone during nocturnal sleep: relation to penile tumescent cycles. In: Shagass, C., Josiassen, R.C. and Bridger, W.H. (eds), *Biological Psychiatry*, pp. 153–155. Elsevier, New York.

Schier, T., Guldner, J., Colla, M., Holsboer, F. and Steiger, A., 1997. Changes in sleep-endocrine activity after growth hormone-releasing hormone depend on time of administration. *Journal of Neuroendocrinology*, **9**, 201–205.

Schuld, A., Blum, W.F., Uhr, M., Haack, M., Kraus, T., Holsboer, F. and Pollmächer, T., 2000. Reduced leptin levels in human narcolepsy. *Neuroendocrinology*, **72**, 195–198.

Schulz, H., Brandenberger, G., Gudewill, C., Hasse, D., Kiss, E., Löhr, K., Pollmächer, T. and Follenius, M., 1992. Plasma renin activity and sleep-wake structure of narcoleptic patients and control subjects under continuous bed rest. *Sleep*, **15**, 423.

Schwartz, M.W., Seeley, R.J., Campfield, L.A., Burn, P. and Baskin, D.G., 1996. Identification of targets of leptin action in rat hypothalamus. *Journal of Clinical Investigation*, **98**, 1101–1106.

Shipley, J.E., Schteingart, D.E., Tandon, R. and Starkman, M.N., 1992. Sleep architecture and sleep apnea in patients with Cushing's disease. *Sleep*, **15**, 514–518.

Skene, D.J., Lockley, S.W. and Arendt, J., 1999. Melatonin in circadian sleep disorders in the blind. *Biological Signals and Receptors*, **8**, 90–95.

Sonntag, A., Rothe, B., Guldner, J., Yassouridis, A., Holsboer, F. and Steiger, A., 1996. Trimipramine and imipramine exert different effects on the sleep EEG and on nocturnal hormone secretion during treatment of major depression. *Depression*, **4**, 1–13.

Steiger, A., 2002. Sleep and the hypothalamo-pituitary-adrenocortical system. *Sleep Medicine Reviews*, in press.

Steiger, A. and Antonijevic, I.A., 2001. Sleep-EEG changes after methylprednisolone therapy in multiple sclerosis are similar to those in depression. *Experimental and Clinical Endocrinology and Diabetes*, **109**(Suppl 1), S64.

Steiger, A. and Holsboer, F., 1997a. Nocturnal secretion of prolactin and cortisol and the sleep EEG in patients with major endogenous depression during an acute episode and after full remission. *Psychiatry Research*, **72**, 81–88.

Steiger, A. and Holsboer, F., 1997b. Neuropeptides and human sleep. *Sleep*, **20**, 1038–1052.

Steiger, A. and Lancel, M., 2000. Hypnotika der Zukunft. *Nervenheilkunde*, **19**, 134–138.

Steiger, A., Herth, T. and Holsboer, F., 1987. Sleep-electroencephalography and the secretion of cortisol and growth hormone in normal controls. *Acta Endocrinologica (Copenhagen)*, **116**, 36–42.

Steiger, A., von Bardeleben, U., Herth, T. and Holsboer, F., 1989. Sleep EEG and nocturnal secretion of cortisol and growth hormone in male patients with endogenous depression before treatment and after recovery. *Journal of Affective Disorders*, **16**, 189–195.

Steiger, A., von Bardeleben, U., Wiedemann, K. and Holsboer, F., 1991. Sleep EEG and nocturnal secretion of testosterone and cortisol in patients with major endogenous depression during acute phase and after remission. *Journal of Psychiatric Research*, **25**, 169–177.

Steiger, A., Guldner, J., Hemmeter, U., Rothe, B., Wiedemann, K. and Holsboer, F., 1992. Effects of growth hormone-releasing hormone and somatostatin on sleep EEG and nocturnal hormone secretion in male controls. *Neuroendocrinology*, **56**, 566–573.

Steiger, A., Trachsel, L., Guldner, J., Hemmeter, U., Rothe, B., Rupprecht, R., Vedder, H. and Holsboer, F., 1993a. Neurosteroid pregnenolone induces sleep-EEG changes in man compatible with inverse agonistic $GABA_A$-receptor modulation. *Brain Research*, **615**, 267–274.

Steiger, A., von Bardeleben, U., Guldner, J., Lauer, C., Rothe, B. and Holsboer, F., 1993b. The sleep EEG and nocturnal hormonal secretion. Studies on changes during the course of depression and on effects of CNS-active drugs. *Progress in Neuro-Psychopharmacology and Biological Psychiatry*, **17**, 125–137.

Steiger, A., Antonijevic, I.A., Bohlhalter, S., Frieboes, R.M., Friess, E. and Murck, H., 1998. Effects of hormones on sleep. *Hormone Research*, **49**, 125–130.

Stern, W.C., Jalowiec, J.E., Shabshelowitz, H. and Morgane, P.J., 1975. Effects of growth hormone on sleep-waking patterns in cats. *Hormones and Behavior*, **6**, 189–196.

Sullivan, C.E., Issa, F.G., Berthon-Jones, M. and Eves, L., 1981. Reversal of obstructive sleep apnoea by continuous positive airway pressure applied through the nares. *Lancet*, **1**, 862–865.

Sutcliffe, J.G. and de Lecea, L., 2000. The hypocretins: excitatory neuromodulatory peptides for multiple homeostatic systems, including sleep and feeding. *Journal of Neuroscience Research*, **62**, 161–168.

Takahashi, Y., Kipnis, D.M. and Daughaday, W.H., 1968. Growth hormone secretion during sleep. *Journal of Clinical Investigation*, **47**, 2079–2090.

Tomaszuk, A., Simpson, C. and Williams, G., 1996. Neuropeptide Y, the hypothalamus and the regulation of energy homeostasis. *Hormone Research*, **46**, 53–58.

Toppila, J., Alanko, L., Asikainen, M., Tobler, I., Stenberg, D. and Porkka-Heiskanen, T., 1997. Sleep deprivation increases somatostatin and growth hormone-releasing hormone messenger RNA in the rat hypothalamus. *Journal of Sleep Research*, **6**, 171–178.

Trachsel, L., Edgar, D.M., Seidel, W.F., Heller, H.C. and Dement, W.C., 1992. Sleep homeostasis in suprachiasmatic nuclei-lesioned rat: effects of sleep deprivation and triazolam administration. *Brain Research*, **598**, 253–261.

Van Cauter, E., Leproult, R. and Plat, L., 2000. Age-related changes in slow wave sleep and REM sleep and relationship with growth hormone and cortisol levels in healthy men. *JAMA*, **284**, 861–868.

Van Cauter, E., Linkowski, P., Kerkhofs, M., Hubain, P., L'Hermite-Balériaux, M., Leclercq, R., Brasseur, M., Copinschi, G. and Mendlewicz, J., 1991. Circadian and sleep-related endocrine rhythms in schizophrenia. *Archives of General Psychiatry*, **48**, 348–356.

Van Coevorden, A., Mockel, J., Laurent, E., Kerkhofs, M., L'Hermite-Balériaux, M., Decoster, C., Neve, P. and Van Cauter, E., 1991. Neuroendocrine rhythms and sleep in aging men. *American Journal of Physiology*, **260**, E651–E661.

Vgontzas, A.N., Bixler, E.O., Lin, H.M., Kales, A. and Chrousos, G.P., 2000. Chronic insomnia is associated with hypothalamic-pituitary-adrenal axis activation: role of sleep disturbance. *Journal of Sleep Research*, **9**(Suppl 1), 201.

Vgontzas, A.N., Bixler, E.O., Wittman, A.M., Zachman, K., Lin, H.M., Vela-Bueno, A., Kales, A. and Chrousos, G.P., 2001. Middle-aged men show higher sensitivity of sleep to the arousing effects of corticotropin-releasing hormone than young men: clinical implications. *Journal of Clinical Endocrinology and Metabolism*, **86**, 1489–1495.

Vgontzas, A.N., Tsigos, C., Bixler, E.O., Stratakis, C.A., Kales, A., Vela-Bueno, A. and Chrousos, G.P., 1998. Chronic insomnia and activity of the stress system: a preliminary study. *Journal of Psychosomatic Research*, **45**, 21–31.

Voderholzer, U., Laakmann, G., Wittmann, R., Daffner-Bujia, C., Hinz, A., Haag, C. and Baghai, T., 1993. Profiles of spontaneous 24-hour and stimulated growth hormone secretion in male patients with endogenous depression. *Psychiatry Research*, **47**, 215–227.

Vogel, G.W., Thurmond, A., Gibbons, P., Sloan, K. and Walker, M., 1975. REM sleep reduction effects on depression syndromes. *Archives of General Psychiatry*, **32**, 765–777.

Vollrath, M., Wicki, W. and Angst, J., 1989. The Zurich Study. VIII. Insomnia: association with depression, anxiety, somatic syndromes, and course of insomnia. *European Archives of Psychiatry and Neurological Sciences*, **239**, 113–124.

von Bardeleben, U., Steiger, A., Gerken, A. and Holsboer, F., 1989. Effects of fluoxetine upon pharmacoendocrine and sleep-EEG parameters in normal controls. *International Clinical Psychopharmacology*, **4**(Suppl 1), 1–5.

Wehr, T.A., 1998. Effect of seasonal changes in daylength on human neuroendocrine function. *Hormone Research*, **49**, 118–124.

Weibel, L. and Brandenberger, G., 1998. Disturbances in hormonal profiles of night workers during their usual sleep and work times. *Journal of Biological Rhythms*, **13**, 202–208.

Weibel, L., Follenius, M., Spiegel, K., Gronfier, C. and Brandenberger, G., 1997. Growth hormone secretion in night workers. *Chronobiology International*, **14**, 49–60.

Weitzman, E.D., 1976. Circadian rhythms and episodic hormone secretion in man. *Annual Review of Medicine*, **27**, 225–243.

Wetter, T.C., Collado-Seidel, V., Oertel, H., Uhr, M., Yassouridis, A. and Trenkwalder, C., 2002. Endocrine rhythms in patients with restless legs syndrome. *Journal of Neurology*, in press.

Wiedemann, K., Lauer, C., Loycke, A., Pollmächer, T., Durst, P., Macher, J.P. and Holsboer, F., 1992. Antiglucocorticoid treatment disrupts endocrine cycle and nocturnal sleep pattern. *European Archives of Psychiatry and Clinical Neuroscience*, **241**, 372–375.

Wiedemann, K., Lauer, C., Pollmächer, T. and Holsboer, F., 1994. Sleep-endocrine effects of antigluco- and antimineralocorticoids in healthy males. *American Journal of Physiology*, **267**, E109–E114.

Wiedemann, K., Lauer, C.J., Hirschmann, M., Knaudt, K. and Holsboer, F., 1998. Sleep-endocrine effects of mifepristone and megestrol acetate in healthy men. *American Journal of Physiology: Endocrinology and Metabolism*, **274**, E139–E145.

Williamson, D.E., Birmaher, B., Dahl, R.E. and al-Shabbout, M., 1996. Stressful life events influence nocturnal growth hormone secretion in depressed children. *Biological Psychiatry*, **40**, 1176–1180.

Wong, M.L., Kling, M.A., Munson, P.J., Listwak, S., Licinio, J., Prolo, P., Karp, B., McCutcheon, I.E., Geracioti, T.D. Jr., De Bellis, M.D., Rice, K.C., Goldstein, D.S., Veldhuis, J.D., Chrousos, G.P., Oldfield, E.H., McCann, S.M. and Gold, P.W., 2000. Pronounced and sustained central hypernoradrenergic function in major depression with melancholic features: relation to hypercortisolism and corticotropin-releasing hormone. *Proceedings of the National Academy of Sciences of the United States of America*, **97**, 325–330.

Zhang, J., Obál, F. Jr., Zheng, T., Fang, J., Taishi, P. and Krueger, J.M., 1999. Intrapreoptic microinjection of GHRH or its antagonist alters sleep in rats. *Journal of Neuroscience*, **19**, 2187–2194.

Zhdanova, I.V., Lynch, H.J. and Wurtman, R.J., 1997. Melatonin: a sleep-promoting hormone. *Sleep*, **20**, 899–907.

Ziegenbein, M., Künzel, H.E., Held, K., Murck, H. and Antonijevic, I.A., 2000. Effect of the long lasting somatostatin analogue octreotide on sleep EEG in young men. *European Neuropsychopharmacology*, **10**, Supplement 3, S 407.

Zobel, A.W., Künzel, H., Sonntag, A. and Holsboer, F., 2000. Effects of the high-affinity corticotropin-releasing hormone receptor 1 antagonist R121919 in major depression: the first 20 patients treated. *Journal of Psychiatric Research*, **34**, 171–181.

XXIV-4

Neuroimmunology of Sleep

Jeannine A. Majde and James M. Krueger

INTRODUCTION

Sleep consumes a third of our lives, but its functions are unknown. Excess, inhibited, or fragmented sleep often accompanies psychiatric disorders or their treatments. The fatigue and confusion associated with the abnormal sleep may constitute a major complaint of the patient. Before we can begin to understand the pathological sleep associated with psychiatric disorders, it is essential that we have a better understanding of normal sleep and its functions. Ironically, the major insights we have gained into the regulation of normal sleep come from another class of pathologies, acute infectious diseases. This chapter will summarize what we have learned about sleep regulation through analysis of the molecular changes associated with infections.

Acute infections are generally detected clinically by the manifestations of fever and malaise. Included in the concept of malaise is the subjective feeling of profound fatigue and the overwhelming need to sleep. Sleep is detected and measured primarily through analysis of electroencephalographic (EEG) patterns, as has been described elsewhere in this text. Over the last 20 years we have characterized the EEG changes that occur in response to several acute infections. These changes will be described in more detail later in this chapter, but consistent features are the manifestation of increased slow-wave or non-rapid-eye-movement sleep (NREMS), increased slow-wave amplitudes, and often the reduction of total REM sleep (Krueger and Majde, 1994). These sleep characteristics are seen regardless of whether the stimulus is a purely microbial component or an actual infection. A major breakthrough in our conceptualization of sleep regulation is the realization that the peripheral cytokines produced in response to an infectious or other inflammatory stimulus are responsible for triggering the subjective need to sleep as well as the characteristic sleep changes. Furthermore, these same cytokines are actively involved in regulating physiological sleep.

Cytokines are a large class of protein hormones produced primarily by cells of the immune system or by damaged epithelial cells. Over 100 cytokines have been identified to date. One subclass of cytokines, the chemokines, appears to act primarily in a paracrine fashion to regulate inflammation at the site of tissue damage. However, a large and loosely defined subclass of cytokines, the proinflammatory cytokines, act not only locally but also systemically to trigger all of the characteristic responses to inflammatory challenge, including fever, anorexia, and somnolence. Thus, at least one function of proinflammatory cytokines appears to be signalling the brain that the host is threatened by invading micro-organisms and that adaptive responses are required (Hart, 1988). The best-characterized proinflammatory cytokines are the interleukin-1s (IL1α and IL1β), IL6, and tumour necrosis factor-α (TNF-α). The array of physiological, behavioural, haematological, and biochemical responses initiated by these cytokines is termed the acute-phase response (APR). In addition to proinflammatory cytokines, growing evidence points to an important systemic role of anti-inflammatory cytokines such as IL10, IL4, IL13, and transforming growth factor-β (TGF-β) in the inhibition of the APR, including the excess sleep component. In the sections to follow, we will outline the evidence that proinflammatory and anti-inflammatory cytokines regulate both pathological and physiological sleep.

In addition to cytokines, several classical hormones, such as growth hormone-releasing hormone (GHRH), corticotrophin-releasing hormone (CRH), and prolactin, have been implicated in sleep regulation. Growth factors such as nerve growth factor (NGF), neurotropins, epidermal growth factor, and fibroblast growth factor are involved as well (reviewed by Krueger and Obál, 1997). The gaseous neurotransmitter nitric oxide (NO) has also been implicated (Kapás *et al.*, 1994; Kapás and Krueger, 1996). The regulation of these hormones and NO synthesis by cytokines may form the basis for the association of cytokines and sleep.

INDIGENOUS MICROBIAL FLORA AND CYTOKINE STIMULATION IN THE HEALTHY INDIVIDUAL

It is widely recognized from such conditions as rheumatic heart disease that bacteraemia can occur in response to dental work. Profound immunodeficiency disorders such as AIDS have also demonstrated that the massive microbial flora that lines our mucosal surfaces, particularly the intestine, can escape protective mucosal barriers when normal immune defences are impaired. Much less is known about our day-to-day exposure to these micro-organisms because this exposure is not perceptible. However, studies of the intraintestinal lymphoid tissue, the Peyer's patches, reveal specialized epithelial cells that can transport bacteria to adjacent macrophages for degradation (Owen *et al.*, 1986). Bacteria and their breakdown products accumulating in the Peyer's patches then can enter the portal circulation or the mesenteric lymph (Sartor *et al.*, 1988). Though not quantified, it is thought that millions of bacteria may be cleared by this mechanism daily.

The first insights into the relationship of microbial products to sleep were gained from structural studies on a sleep factor isolated from human urine (Krueger *et al.*, 1982a). This factor proved to share the unique chemical properties of the peptidoglycans found in the cell walls of bacteria (Krueger *et al.*, 1982a). Peptidoglycans comprise 90% of the cell wall of Gram-positive bacteria and 5–20% of the cell wall of Gram-negative bacteria (Krueger and Majde, 1990). Subsequent sleep studies with various natural and synthetic peptidoglycans revealed that the minimally active unit is a glycopeptide consisting of the sugar *N*-acetylmuramic acid (found only in bacteria) and the dipeptide L-alanine-D-alanine, termed muramyl dipeptide (MDP) (Krueger *et al.*, 1982b). MDP and certain derivatives have immunological

Biological Psychiatry: Edited by H. D'haenen, J.A. den Boer and P. Willner. ISBN 0-471-49198-5

adjuvant properties. Peptidoglycans also contain the bacterially unique amino acids D-glutamic acid (eukaryotes employ primarily L-amino acids) and diaminopimelic acid, as well as L-lysine. Many peptidoglycan derivatives are pyrogenic as well as somnogenic.

In addition to the peptidoglycans found in all bacterial cell walls, the lipopolysaccharide (LPS) moiety of the endotoxin component of Gram-negative bacterial cell walls also potently alters sleep through induction of proinflammatory cytokines (Krueger and Majde, 1994). A majority of studies on cytokine induction by microbial products have employed LPS as the stimulus. Other bacterial components such as lipoteichoic acid and lipoproteins also stimulate proinflammatory cytokine induction, although their effects on sleep have not been analysed. Recently, it has been recognized that structural differences in bacterial DNA are recognized by the immune system with the production of cytokines (Sweet *et al.*, 1998). It is not yet known whether bacterial DNA plays a role in bacterial illness or in sleep responses to bacteria.

It has recently been determined that bacterial and fungal cell-wall components, although structurally distinct, are detected by phagocytes through activation of Toll-like receptors (TLRs), a receptor type first demonstrated as a host-defence mechanism in fruit flies (Aderem and Ulevitch, 2000). Activated TLRs then signal the phagocyte to release proinflammatory cytokines.

A common feature of all microbial components (with the possible exception of bacterial DNA) capable of inducing cytokines is their chemical resistance to biodegradation (Krueger and Majde, 1994). While mature macrophages and neutrophils carry enzymes capable of degrading peptidoglycans (lysozyme, *N*-acetylmuramyl-L-alanine amidase, Hoijer *et al.*, 1997), these enzymes do not always achieve complete degradation and fragments may be secreted extracellularly (Pabst *et al.*, 1999). These secreted partial degradation products can then serve as steady stimulators of cytokine release by neighbouring phagocytes. Little direct evidence exists for this cytokine source from the intestine, however, because the portal blood and mesenteric lymph of healthy individuals are rarely accessed. Furthermore, it is clear that soluble receptors and other binding factors exist in body fluids that are capable of neutralizing and facilitating the clearance of cytokines (Dinarello, 2000). Low levels of cytokines, especially IL1s, routinely circulate in association with intrinsic binding factors. These binding factors are likely to play a significant role in determining the levels of cytokines free to bind to cell receptors and activate neighbouring or distant cells.

While there are substantial gaps in our knowledge of physiological cytokine regulation, indirect evidence supports a role for indigenous flora in the regulation of both body temperature and sleep, in that animals with reduced indigenous flora have lower body temperatures and sleep less (Krueger and Majde, 1994). Rats treated with antibiotics that reduce intestinal flora have reduced NREMS but normal REMS (Brown *et al.*, 1990). Furthermore, neutralization of the proinflammatory cytokines IL1β and TNFα with antibodies or endogenous binding factors also reduces spontaneous sleep (see section below on *IL1β and TNFα*).

Whereas much remains to be elucidated regarding the exact source of the cytokines regulating physiological sleep, the means by which cytokines produced in the periphery can affect the brain have been extensively investigated. Three possible routes to the brain for peripheral cytokines have been implicated: brain circumventricular organs (Blatteis and Sehic, 1997), specific transporters in the blood–brain barrier (Banks *et al.*, 1991), and sub-diaphragmatic vagal afferents (Kapás *et al.*, 1998; Hansen and Krueger, 1997). Of these three routes, stimulation of the vagal nerve has been most closely linked with sleep regulation. The liver paraganglia contain IL1 receptors (Goehler *et al.*, 1997). Systemic bacterial LPS and IL1 both induce increased IL1β mRNA production in the brain, and this effect is blocked by vagotomy (Hansen *et al.*, 1998a; Layé *et al.*, 1995). Excess NREMS in response to systemic IL1β is also blocked by vagotomy (Hansen and Krueger, 1997). Other events that promote NREMS such as excessive food intake are also dependent on vagal innervation (Hansen *et al.*, 1998b). The relative importance of these three brain access routes in regulating both physiological and pathological sleep under different conditions is unknown, although direct action on the brain via circumventricular organs and/or blood–brain barrier transporters would require elevation of unbound cytokines in the circulation.

CHANGES IN SLEEP DURING ACUTE INFECTIONS OR CHALLENGE WITH MICROBIAL COMPONENTS

Acute infections such as influenza are associated with an overwhelming need to sleep and an increase in total sleep time. Our knowledge of polysomnographic sleep changes in acute infections is derived from animal studies, as only subjective sleep reports have been acquired during acute infections in man (Smith, 1992). As mentioned previously, acutely infected animals demonstrate increased NREMS and diminished REMS as well as increased amplitudes of EEG slow waves, which are considered an index of the intensity of sleep (Krueger and Majde, 1994). These gross changes occur in bacterial, fungal, and viral infections, but with different kinetics depending on the infective organism, dose, and route (Toth, 1999).

The sleep alterations in acute bacterial, fungal, and viral infections have been recently reviewed in detail (Toth, 1999) and in summary form (Krueger *et al.*, 2001). Studies with bacteria in rabbits include both human pathogens (*Staphylococcus aureus*, *Streptococcus pyogenes*, and *Escherichia coli*) and the rabbit pathogen *Pasturella multocida* (Toth, 1999). Challenge of rats with baker's yeast or rabbits with *Candida albicans* induces sleep alterations similar to those seen in animals challenged with Gram-positive bacteria (Toth, 1999). Viral sleep alterations have been analysed in an abortive rabbit model of influenza virus and an abortive mouse model of Newcastle disease virus. NREMS and delta-wave amplitudes are increased and REMS decreased during the febrile period in all of these infections (Toth, 1999). A similar but more prolonged sleep alteration is seen in an active influenza infection in mice when virus is administered in such a manner as to cause pneumonitis, whether or not a lethal infection ensues (Fang *et al.*, 1995a; Toth, 1999). When the same amount of virus is delivered only to the upper respiratory tract, no changes in sleep or other symptoms are seen (Fang *et al.*, 1996).

The same fundamental sleep changes occur in response to challenge with bacterial cell-wall peptidoglycans or LPS, with biodegradation-resistant fungal cell-wall polysaccharides, or with synthetic or virus-associated double-stranded RNA derived from viral replication intermediates (Krueger and Majde, 1994). These fungal and viral components stimulate proinflammatory cytokine induction similarly to that induced by bacterial cell-wall components, though by different mechanisms.

It is the central thesis of this chapter that microbially upregulated cytokines initiate the sleep changes associated with acute infections, presumably because the amounts of cytokines produced exceed the levels that can be bound and cleared by the body. Unbound cytokines produced in the periphery then act upon the brain, probably via vagal afferents (Hansen *et al.*, 1998a), to induce IL1β in relevant brain regions. This thesis is supported by the observation that excess NREMS, fever, and other behavioural responses induced by systemic LPS, muramyl peptides, or IL1β are attenuated by central inhibition of IL1β (Kent *et al.*, 1992; Klir *et al.*, 1994; Takahashi *et al.*, 1996). The extensive evidence that IL1 and TNF play a role in physiological and pathological sleep regulation is discussed in the section below on humoral regulation.

It should be noted that, whereas we have focused on cytokines as triggers of the APR, other inflammatory mediators such as the eicosenoids may also play a role in the CNS response to infection. It is widely recognized that prostaglandin E_2 (PGE_2) is an important mediator of the fever response to infection (Kluger, 1991). PGD_2 and PGE_2 have also been implicated in sleep regulation (Hayaishi, 1988; Terao *et al.*, 1998). IL1 induces brain astrocytes to produce both prostaglandins (Hayaishi, 1988), and IL1 promotes sleep when injected into a PGD_2-sensitive brain region (Terao *et al.*, 1998). Thus, IL1 within the brain may regulate sleep in part through eicosenoid induction.

The proinflammatory cytokine response to microbes or their stimulatory components is grossly indistinguishable from the proinflammatory cytokine response to other inflammatory stimuli such as tissue damage, although infections are more commonly associated with sleep alterations than are other acute inflammatory states. Whether the relative potency of infections is qualitative or quantitative is unknown.

SLEEP ALTERATIONS IN CHRONIC INFECTIONS AND CHRONIC INFLAMMATORY STATES

Chronic infections with such agents as human immunodeficiency virus (HIV) or hepatitis virus are much more difficult to dissect than are acute infections because they are inevitably associated with diffuse chronic inflammation. In addition to the proinflammatory cytokine cascade characteristic of acute inflammation, chronic inflammation has the added complexity of manifesting a simultaneous anti-inflammatory cytokine cascade. Sleep responses have been examined following administration of single anti-inflammatory cytokines (Krueger and Majde, 1994), and IL10, IL4, and TGFβ all have been found to reduce sleep (Kushikata *et al.*, 1998). However, no studies have attempted to characterize the sleep effects of the complex mixture of pro- and anti-inflammatory cytokines that occurs in chronic inflammation. Studies of sleep in chronic infections suggest, however, that the proinflammatory cytokines dominate sleep regulation in clinical disease.

The chronic infections that have been most extensively investigated with respect to sleep changes are the immunodeficiency virus infections of humans and cats; trypanosome infections of rabbits, rats and humans; and prion infections of mice, rats, cats, and humans (reviewed by Toth, 1999). All of these infections directly affect the brain, and their associated sleep alterations may reflect inflammatory changes within the brain. Because patients infected with the human immunodeficiency virus HIV-1 or the prion causing Creutzfeldt-Jakob disease often manifest psychiatric disorders, what is known about their sleep changes is summarized here.

Sleep changes in HIV-1 infections have been studied during asymptomatic and symptomatic phases. Asymptomatic HIV-1-infected men express increased NREMS during the second half of the night, sleep fragmentation, and abnormal REMS architecture (reviewed by Toth, 1999). These altered sleep patterns precede neurological involvement or onset of secondary infections (Darko *et al.*, 1995). Progression to overt AIDS is marked by reduced NREMS, marked sleep fragmentation, and profound disruption of sleep architecture.

Prions, infectious agents associated with profound dementia, also cause alterations in sleep. Rats inoculated with the scrapie prion demonstrate unusual spiking patterns in the EEG during wakefulness 4 months after inoculation (Toth, 1999). Later NREMS and active wakefulness are reduced and drowsiness is increased (Toth, 1999). Cats challenged with Creutzfeldt-Jakob brain homogenate demonstrate increased NREMS, reduced wakefulness, and abnormal REMS 20 months after inoculation (Toth, 1999). The condition known as fatal familial insomnia is associated with prion-related thalamic neurodegeneration (Toth, 1999). Deletion of the prion protein gene results in altered sleep and circadian rhythms in mice (Toth, 1999).

Less is known about the specific sleep alterations associated with chronic inflammatory diseases, although sleep disorders are prominent components of such diseases as rheumatoid arthritis, fibromyalgia, and chronic fatigue syndrome. Sleep alterations in these three diseases will be briefly described here, as they may affect the psychiatric patient or cause the patient to seek psychiatric help.

Fatigue is a common symptom of all chronic inflammatory diseases. In autoimmune disorders such as rheumatoid arthritis, the fatigue is probably due to the associated sleep fragmentation with frequent movement of the extremities and frequent arousal (Mahowald *et al.*, 1989). Alpha-delta sleep patterns where EEG NREMS intrudes on delta sleep are characteristic. Increasing sleep though treatment with the hypnotic drug triazolam reduces morning stiffness and daytime sleepiness without improving sleep fragmentation (Walsh *et al.*, 1996). Rats experiencing chronic adjuvant arthritis display fragmented sleep, sleep less during the normal sleeping period, and thus lose their normal diurnal sleep rhythms (Landis *et al.*, 1988). Non-steroidal anti-inflammatory analgesics have complex effects on the sleep in these animals (Landis *et al.*, 1989). The pain associated with rheumatic diseases does not appear to cause the fragmented sleep (Hirsch *et al.*, 1994), but the disrupted sleep may contribute to the pain (Moldofsky *et al.*, 1993).

Syndromes associated with chronic fatigue, subjective cognitive impairment, and diffuse myalgia rather than focal inflammation (joint swelling) of the type seen in rheumatic diseases include fibromyalgia and chronic fatigue syndrome. Fibromyalgia is distinguished from chronic fatigue syndrome clinically by its associated marked fibrositis. Depression is also commonly associated with both these disorders. Recently, the depression in chronic fatigue syndrome was shown to be associated with a characteristic REM latency that has been associated with other depressive disorders (Morehouse *et al.*, 1998). Most patients with these syndromes complain of non-restorative sleep, and sleep fragmentation similar to that in rheumatoid arthritis is characteristic of fibromyalgia (Branco *et al.*, 1994). One study has indicated that the association of these two syndromes with sleep disorders is no greater than in patients with psychiatric disorders not associated with pain (Buchwald *et al.*, 1994). Both syndromes are frequently preceded by a febrile illness, but fibromyalgia is also commonly associated with both psychological distress and primary sleep disorders such as sleep apnoea and periodic limb movement (Moldofsky, 1993).

The sleep disorder in chronic fatigue syndrome is essentially the same as that in fibromyalgia (Moldofsky, 1993), although the association with primary sleep disorders such as sleep apnoea is not seen. Circadian rhythm disruption of melatonin secretion and core temperature is seen in chronic fatigue syndrome, which may or may not be a consequence of the sleep disorder (Williams *et al.*, 1996). It has been proposed that fibromyalgia and chronic fatigue are both clinical manifestations of the reciprocal relationship between the immune and sleep-wake systems. Interference with either the immune system (by an infection generating large amounts of cytokines) or the sleep-wake system (by sleep deprivation) affects the other system and will be accompanied by symptoms of chronic fatigue (Moldofsky, 1993). Interestingly, a study of the chronic fatigue and arthralgia syndrome that commonly follows infection with the tick-borne spirochete causing Lyme disease reveals sleep features similar to those of other chronic inflammatory diseases (Bujak *et al.*, 1996).

HUMORAL REGULATION OF SLEEP — THE INVOLVEMENT OF IMMUNE SYSTEM PRODUCTS

While our discussion above has focused on microbial products and inflammatory mediators in sleep regulation, we would be remiss if we failed to emphasize that sleep is ultimately regulated by both neural and humoral mechanisms that interact and are inseparable. Neural mechanisms of sleep regulation have been extensively reviewed elsewhere (Steriade and McCarley, 1990); here we will focus on humoral mechanisms.

The involvement of specific neurotransmitters in sleep regulation is often included within the concept of humoral regulation of sleep. Almost all well-characterized neurotransmitters have been implicated in one or more aspects of sleep-wake regulation. In this section we will focus on neuromodulator involvement in sleep regulation, specifically IL1β, TNFα, and GHRH in physiological NREMS regulation, and prolactin (PRL) and vasoactive intestinal peptide (VIP) in REMS regulation, because for these substances there is extensive evidence for their involvement in physiological sleep regulation. In the section below on central targets in the brain, we will present evidence for the concept that IL1, TNF, and other somnogenic growth factors such as NGF induce sleep via nuclear factor kappa B (NFκB)-dependent mechanisms; several events downstream from NFκB activation, such as cyclooxygenase-2 (COX-2) and inducible-nitric oxide synthase (iNOS) induction, also seem to be involved in sleep regulation.

IL1β and TNFα

IL1β or TNFα given centrally or systemically induce prolonged large increases in the amount of time spent in NREMS in every species thus far tested (rats, rabbits, mice, monkeys, sheep, and cats). For example, 3 µg of TNF given intraperitoneally to mice induces about 90 extra min of NREMS during the first 9 h after injection (Fang *et al.*, 1997). The excess NREMS induced by IL1β or TNFα is associated with high-amplitude EEG slow waves (Krueger *et al.*, 1984). Similar supranormal EEG slow waves occur during NREMS after sleep deprivation (Pappenheimer *et al.*, 1975) or during the initial sleep responses to infectious challenge (Toth and Krueger, 1988). These supranormal EEG slow waves are posited to reflect a higher intensity of NREMS (Borbély and Tobler, 1989). Low somnogenic doses of IL1β and TNFα have little effect on REMS, whereas doses that induce large increases in NREMS often reduce duration of REMS. In rats (Lancel *et al.*, 1996; Opp *et al.*, 1991) and cats (Susic and Totic, 1989), higher doses of IL1β inhibit sleep.

The excess NREMS induced by either IL1β or TNFα appears to be physiological in the sense that after low somnogenic doses, sleep architecture remains normal; animals continue to cycle through stages of sleep and wakefulness, although within each cycle there may be more NREMS. After IL1β or TNFα treatment, sleep remains readily reversible; for example, the entry of the experimenter into the room quickly awakens the cytokine-treated

Table XXIV-4.1 Putative sleep-regulatory substances

Sleep-promoting substances	Sleep-inhibitory substances
Interleukin-1$\beta^{1,4}$ (ILβ)	Hypocretin
Interleukin-1α^4 (IL1α)	Corticotropin-releasing hormone[4] (CRH)
Interleukin-2[4] (IL2)	Adrenocorticotropin hormone[4] (ACTH)
Interleukin-6[4] (IL6)	Alpha melanocyte-stimulating hormone[4] (αMSH)
Interleukin-15[4] (IL15)	Interleukin-4[4] (IL4)
Interleukin-18[4] (IL18)	Interleukin-10[4] (IL10)
Epidermal growth factor[4] (EGF)	Interleukin-13[4] (IL13)
Acidic fibroblast growth factor[4] (aFGF)	Transforming growth factor β^4 (TGFβ)
Nerve growth factor[3,4] (NGF)	Somatostatin (SRIH)
Brain-derived neurotropic factor[3] (BDNF)	Insulin-like growth factor-1[4] (IGF-1)
Neurotropin-3 (NT3)	Soluble TNF receptor[4] (STNFR)
Neurotropin-4 (NT4)	Soluble IL1 receptor[4] (sIL1R)
Interferon-α^4 (IFNα)	Interleukin-1-receptor antagonist[4] (IL1RA)
Interferon-γ^4 (IFNγ)	Glucocorticoid[4]
Tumour necrosis factor $\alpha^{1,4}$ (TNFα)	Prostaglandin E_2^4 (PGE_2)
Tumour necrosis factor β^4 (TNFβ)	
Oleamide	
Growth hormone-releasing hormone[1,3,4] (GHRH)	
Adenosine[1,3,4]	
Prostaglandin $D_2^{1,3,4}$ (PGD_2)	
Nitric oxide[1,3,4] (NO)	
Nuclear factor kappa B[4] (NFκB)	
Uridine	
Vasoactive intestinal peptide[1,2] (VIP)	
Growth hormone[2,4] (GH)	
Prolactin[1,2,4] (PRL)	
Insulin[4]	

[1]Substances for which there is extensive evidence for their involvement in physiological sleep regulation.
[2]Promotes REMS only.
[3]Promotes both NREMS and REMS.
[4]Also involved in host defence.

animals. After such a disturbance, the return to NREMS is generally more rapid after IL1β- or TNFα-treatment than in control animals. After somnogenic doses of either IL1β or TNFα, there are no gross behavioural abnormalities; sleep postures remain normal and no motor dysfunction is evident. Changes in sleep-coupled autonomic functions also remain intact; for example, changes in brain temperature associated with sleep state persist in IL1β- or TNFα-treated animals.

As mentioned earlier, inhibition of either IL1 or TNF reduces spontaneous NREMS, thereby strongly implicating these substances in physiological sleep regulation. Thus, anti-TNF or IL1 antibodies, soluble IL1 or TNF receptors, and the IL1 receptor-antagonist cytokine inhibit spontaneous NREMS and the expected NREMS rebound induced by sleep deprivation (Krueger and Majde, 1994). The latter data suggest that IL1 and TNF are also involved in sleep-deprivation-induced excess NREMS. In contrast, inhibition of IL18 (related to IL1) does not affect spontaneous NREMS, although it does attenuate bacterial cell-wall product-induced sleep (Kubota *et al.*, 2001). Other physiological inhibitors of IL1 or TNF also inhibit spontaneous sleep; the list includes IL4 (Kushikata *et al.*, 1998), IL10 (Opp *et al.*, 1995), IL13, TGFβ, PGE_2, α-melanocyte-stimulating hormone, glucocorticoids, and CRH (reviewed by Krueger & Obál, 1997) (Table XXIV-4.1) (Figure XXIV-4.1). Many of these substances form part of a feedback mechanism dampening the proinflammatory cytokine cascade (Figure XXIV-4.1).

There are diurnal variations within the brain of IL1β mRNA (Taishi *et al.*, 1997) and TNF mRNA levels (Bredow *et al.*, 1997), as well as IL1β (Nguyen *et al.*, 1998) and TNFα (Floyd & Krueger, 1997) protein levels. These diurnal variations occur in the hypothalamus (an area involved in sleep regulation) and several other brain areas including the hippocampus and the cerebral cortex. After sleep deprivation, hypothalamic IL1β mRNA levels (Taishi *et al.*, 1998; Mackiewicz *et al.*, 1996) and TNF mRNA levels (Veasey *et al.*, 1997) increase. In contrast, related molecules such as the IL1 receptor accessory protein are not affected by sleep deprivation (Taishi *et al.*, 1998). IL1β also seems to be involved in the excess NREMS associated with excess food intake; rats on a cafeteria diet express increased IL1β mRNA in the hypothalamus during peak food-induced sleep responses (Hansen *et al.*, 1998c). In humans, there is a diurnal rhythm in plasma levels of TNFα, and plasma levels of TNFα correlate with EEG-slow-wave activity (Darko *et al.*, 1995). Furthermore, in humans, plasma levels of TNFα increase after sleep deprivation (Yamusa *et al.*, 1992), and the ability of circulating white blood cells to produce TNFα increases after sleep deprivation (Uthgenannt *et al.*, 1995; Hohogen *et al.*, 1993).

Mutant mice lacking the TNF 55-kDa receptor do not exhibit sleep responses if given TNFα, although they are responsive to IL1β (Fang *et al.*, 1997). In contrast, mutant mice lacking the IL1 type I receptor are unresponsive if given IL1β, but do exhibit robust NREMS responses if given TNFα (Fang *et al.*, 1998). Both strains of mice sleep less than strain controls, although the sleep deficit in the TNF-receptor knockout mice occurs mostly during daylight hours while that in the IL1 type I receptor knockout mice occurs during the night-time. In humans, sleep deprivation induces enhanced levels of the 55-kDa soluble TNF receptor, but not the 75-kDa soluble TNF receptor (Shearer *et al.*, 2001).

Certain clinical conditions associated with excessive sleepiness also seem to involve cytokines; that is, sleep apnoea patients have elevated TNF plasma levels (Entzian *et al.*, 1996; Vgontzas *et al.*, 1997). HIV-AIDS patients have disrupted TNF rhythms (Darko *et al.*, 1995). Treatment of rheumatoid arthritis patients with the TNF 75-kDa soluble receptor alleviates the fatigue associated with the disease (Franklin, 1999). TNFα is elevated in chronic fatigue patients (Moss *et al.*, 1999). Elevated TNF also occurs in pre-eclampsia patients accompanied by excess sleep (Edwards *et al.*, 2000). Postdialysis fatigue is also associated with elevated TNF levels (Dreisbach *et al.*, 1998; Sklar *et al.*, 1998), and cancer patients receiving either TNFα or IL1β report fatigue (e.g., Eskander *et al.*, 1997). Infectious challenge induces a plethora of proinflammatory cytokines and many other substances implicated

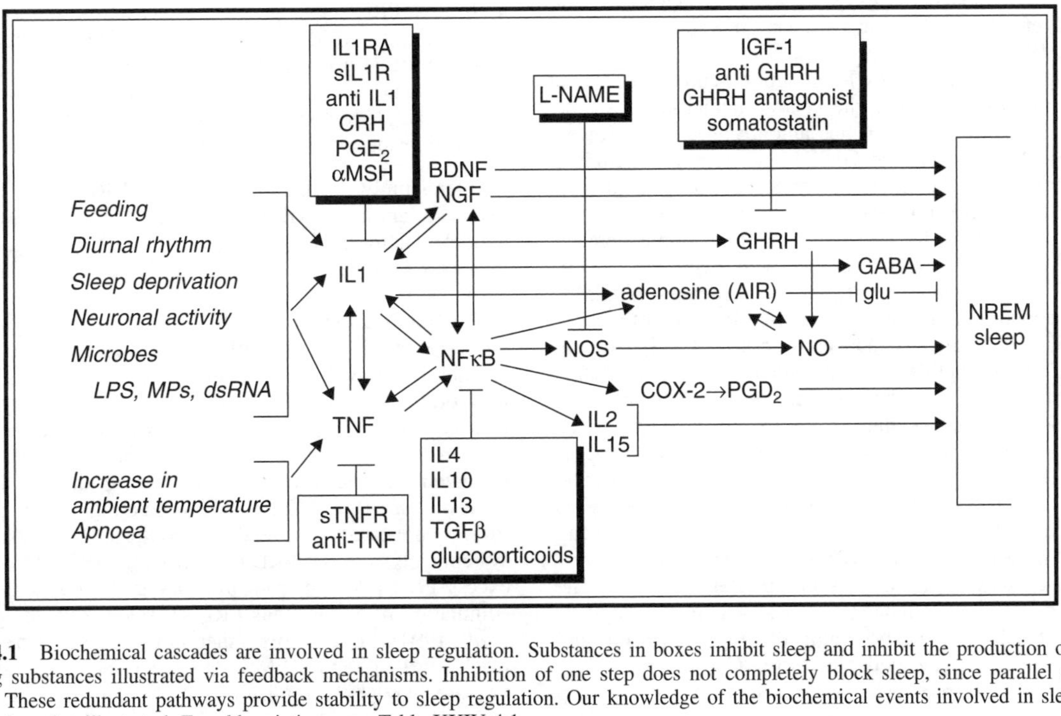

Figure XXIV-4.1 Biochemical cascades are involved in sleep regulation. Substances in boxes inhibit sleep and inhibit the production or actions of the sleep-promoting substances illustrated via feedback mechanisms. Inhibition of one step does not completely block sleep, since parallel sleep-promoting pathways exist. These redundant pathways provide stability to sleep regulation. Our knowledge of the biochemical events involved in sleep regulation is more extensive than that illustrated. For abbreviations, see Table XXIV-4.1

in sleep regulation. These same substances also play a role in host defence (Table XXIV-4.1).

The Somatotrophic Axis

In humans, a major peak in growth hormone (GH) release occurs during the first period of deep, slow-wave sleep (Takahashi *et al.*, 1968). Furthermore, abnormal GH secretory patterns are associated with sleep disorders (e.g., Aström and Linhölm, 1990). In addition, during extended wakefulness, GH release is suppressed, and when subjects are allowed to sleep, excess GH secretion occurs (e.g., Moldofsky *et al.*, 1988). Nevertheless, dissociation between GH release and sleep can occur (Carlson *et al.*, 1972), and it is thus posited that GHRH provides the link between GH release and sleep (Obál *et al.*, 1988; reviewed by Krueger *et al.*, 1999).

GHRH administration induces increases in the amount of time spent in NREMS in several species including rats, rabbits, and humans (reviewed by Krueger and Obál, 1997). For instance, in humans, systemic injection of GHRH (e.g., Steiger *et al.*, 1992) and a GHRH-containing nasal spray (Perras *et al.*, 1989) enhance NREMS. The GHRH-induced NREMS is characterized by supranormal EEG slow waves and, thus, is thought to be of greater intensity. GHRH can also induce increases in REMS (Obál *et al.*, 1988). However, in hypophysectomized animals, GHRH induces only NREMS (Obál *et al.*, 1996), and the REMS-promoting actions of GHRH are thought to be the result of pituitary GH release. The sleep induced by GHRH appears normal in the sense that it is easily reversible if animals are disturbed, and no abnormal behaviours are evident.

Inhibition of GHRH — for example, by using an anti-GHRH antibody or a GHRH peptide antagonist — inhibits spontaneous NREMS and sleep rebound after sleep loss (e.g., Zhang *et al.*, 1999). Transgenic mice that overexpress GH in the brain have less NREMS, but not REMS; these mice have less GHRH and more somatostatin (SRIH) in the brain (Zhang *et al.*, 1996). Furthermore, dwarf rats and lit/lit mice, which underexpress GHRH receptors in the hypothalamus, also have reduced NREMS and REMS (Obál *et al.*, 2001; Alt *et al.*, 2001). Inhibition of GHRH by antibodies also attenuates IL1β-induced excess NREMS, thus suggesting that IL1β elicits its effects on sleep, in part, via GHRH (reviewed by Krueger *et al.*, 1999).

Within the hypothalamus, GHRH-containing neurons are found in the arcuate nucleus and around the ventral medial nucleus. The former project to the median eminence and are probably involved in GH release. The ventromedial GHRHergic neurons, including those in the paraventricular nucleus, project to both the median eminence and to the basal forebrain. The preoptic area — basal forebrain — is involved in NREMS regulation; for example, damage of this area is associated with insomnia (von Economo, 1930), and rapid electrical stimulation of this area induces NREMS. This area also contains GHRH receptors. Microinjection of GHRH into the anterior hypothalamus induces excess NREMS, whereas injection of the GHRH peptide antagonist into the same area inhibits NREMS and attenuates sleep rebound after sleep loss (Zhang *et al.*, 1999). There is a diurnal rhythm of GHRH mRNA within the hypothalamus, but not other areas of brain; the highest levels occur during the onset of daylight hours, which is the peak sleep period in rats (Bredow *et al.*, 1996). After sleep deprivation, there also is an increase in GHRH mRNA levels in the hypothalamus (Zhang *et al.*, 1998). These changes in GHRH mRNA are found only in the extra-arcuate GHRHergic neurons (Toppila *et al.*, 1997). The GHRH content of the hypothalamus also has a diurnal rhythm, with the highest values at the beginning of the dark period, and decreased amounts associated with sleep loss (Gardi *et al.*, 1998), suggesting that GHRH release is associated with higher sleep propensity.

Other members of the somatotropic axis also influence sleep and GHRH secretion. SRIH inhibits GHRH and GH release, and it inhibits NREMS, presumably via its effects of GHRH. In contrast, SRIH stimulates REMS despite the fact that it inhibits GH release (Beranek *et al.*, 1997). GH by itself stimulates REMS (reviewed by Krueger and Obál, 1997), and the promotion of REMS by GHRH in thought to be mediated via release of pituitary GH. Furthermore, microinjection of GHRH into the basal forebrain induces NREMS, but not REMS. GH may, via its metabolic actions, have a NREMS-promoting activity; sleep is reduced in rats treated with anti-GH antibodies (Obál *et al.*, 1997a). In contrast, GH stimulates insulin-like growth factor-1 (IGF-1); IGF-1 has a brief inhibitory action on both REMS and NREMS (Obál *et al.*, 1998).

The role of the somatotrophic axis in sleep responses elicited by infectious agents remains relatively uninvestigated. However, GH release is increased during infection, and is induced by cytokines such as IL1 and TNF. GH also has many direct actions on immunocytes, and the effects of IL1 on sleep involve, in part, GHRH. Finally, preliminary data from our laboratory indicate that lit/lit mice that lack functional GHRH receptors sleep less after being challenged with influenza virus; normal mice sleep much more (Alt *et al.*, 2001). Collectively, such data suggest a role for the somatotropic axis hormones in sleep regulation in health as well as in disease.

Prolactin

REMS is enhanced in response to systemic administration of PRL in hypophysectomized pontine cats (Jouvet *et al.*, 1986). Since this initial anecdotal report, several additional lines of evidence have implicated PRL in the regulation of REMS (reviewed by Roky *et al.*, 1995). The major findings are as follows:

1. Administration of exogenous PRL stimulates REMS in cats, rabbits, and rats.
2. PRL-induced increases in REMS develop slowly, over 2–3 h, and are then maintained for several hours.
3. PRL-induced changes in sleep are restricted to REMS; that is, NREMS is not altered after bolus injection of PRL.
4. In rats, PRL enhances REMS only during the light period.
5. In contrast, REMS is suppressed during the light period and is enhanced at night in PRL-deficient rats (Valatx *et al.*, 1990).
6. Rats made chronically hyperprolactinaemic, by grafting pituitaries under the kidney capsule, have increases in REMS during the light period of the day (Obál *et al.*, 1997b).

Interestingly, small enhancements in NREMS were also observed in these animals. REMS and NREMS are also enhanced in hyperprolactinaemic pseudopregnant rats (Zhang, 1995). Slight increases in NREMS might be attributed to a GH-like effect of chronically increased PRL.

The modulation of REMS is a central action of PRL. Thus, intracerebral injection of PRL or anti-PRL antibodies stimulates or inhibits REMS, respectively (Roky *et al.*, 1995). Brain PRL may originate from two sources: it is produced by hypothalamic neurons, and PRL is also released by the anterior pituitary, and circulating PRL is transported into the brain via a specific receptor-mediated transport mechanism residing in the choroid plexus (Walsh *et al.*, 1987). The REMS-promoting activity of blood-borne PRL is suggested by several observations. REMS is enhanced after systemically injected PRL (Jouvet *et al.*, 1986; Obál *et al.*, 1989), excess PRL released from pituitary grafts (Obál *et al.*, 1989), or stimulation of endogenous PRL secretion from the pituitary (Obál *et al.*, 1994). Furthermore, ether stress induces increases in plasma levels of PRL and REMS; the latter increases do not occur if rats are hypophysectomized or if they are treated with anti-PRL antibodies before being exposed to the ether stressor (Bodosi *et al.*,

2000). Nevertheless, only small decreases in REMS occur when basal, non-stimulated blood PRL is immunoneutralized (Obál *et al.*, 1992). Increases in plasma PRL stimulate REMS, but, at normal concentrations, circulating PRL has only a slight effect on REMS regulation. The impact of increased blood PRL on REMS is, in part, attributed to a stimulation of the expression of PRL receptors in the choroid plexus because PRL enhances its own transport into the brain. It is likely that intracerebral PRL modulates REMS under physiological conditions whereas pituitary PRL provides additional stimulating influence when PRL secretion is high, as in stress. Furthermore, intracerebroventricular injections of VIP and PACAP promote REMS (Obál *et al.*, 1989; Fang *et al.*, 1995b) and elicit expression of PRL mRNA in the hypothalamus (Bredow *et al.*, 1994). Anti-PRL antibodies block VIP-induced REMS response. In conclusion, the observation that PRL is probably involved in modulating REMS and is also involved in host-defence provides another link between sleep and host-defence mechanisms.

CENTRAL TARGETS IN THE BRAIN: NFκB AND NO SYNTHASES

The biochemical regulation of NREMS is undoubtedly complex, involving many biochemical cascades operating in several cell types within the brain. Several of the sleep-regulatory substances (Figure XXIV-4.1) are either upregulated in response to NFκB activation or themselves induce NFκB activation. For instance, several sleep-promoting substances activate NFκB; the list includes IL1, TNF, NGF, interferon-α, epidermal growth factor, acidic fibroblast growth factor, insulin, and insulin-like growth factor (reviewed by Krueger and Majde, 1994; Krueger *et al.*, 1999). Furthermore, NFκB is involved in the expression of IL2, cyclooxygenase-2, inducible NOS (reviewed by Eizirik *et al.*, 1996), IL1, TNF (reviewed by Ballou *et al.*, 1996), NGF, and the adenosine A_1 receptor (Nie *et al.*, 1998), all of which are part of the biochemical network involved in sleep regulation (Figure XXIV-4.1). Other substances, such as IL4, IL10 (e.g., Clarke *et al.*, 1998), and glucocorticoids (see Barnes, 1997), directly or indirectly inhibit NFκB activation, and they inhibit sleep (Krueger *et al.*, 1999). Furthermore, sleep deprivation promotes NFκB activation in murine cerebral cortex, and cortical NFκB activation has a diurnal rhythm, with higher levels of activation occurring during daylight hours (the sleep period in mice) than during the dark period (Chen *et al.*, 1999). Thus, the activation of NFκB correlates with high sleep propensity. Furthermore, a NFκB cell-permeable inhibitor peptide, given centrally, inhibits spontaneous NREMS and REMS, and attenuates IL1β-enhanced NREMS (Kubota *et al.*, 2000). Finally, NFκB is involved in the production of several other transcription factors that could also be involved in sleep regulation, such as c-fos (Shiromani *et al.*, 1998).

NO also seems to function as an endogenous sleep-promoting substance. NO is produced by three distinct NO synthases (NOSs), all of which are found in the brain. NOS inhibitors injected systemically or intracerebroventricularly (i.c.v.) suppress REMS and NREMS in rats and rabbits (reviewed by Kápas *et al.*, 1993). Conversely, systemically or i.c.v. administered, the NO donors *S*-nitrosyl-*N*-acetylpenicillamine (SNAP) and 3-morpholinosydnonimine (SIN-1) mimic the effects of sleep deprivation, in that each induced prolonged increases in the duration and intensity of NREMS in rats after a 7–9-h delay (Kapás *et al.*, 1996). Furthermore, NREMS responses after sleep deprivation are diminished in rats given a NOS inhibitor prior to deprivation (Riberio *et al.*, 2000). Inducible NOS (iNOS or NOS-2) is stimulated by proinflammatory cytokines and is dependent on NFκB activation, making this isoform an attractive candidate for sleep regulation.

While the specific signalling mechanisms involved in sleep responses to NO stimulation remain incompletely understood, one effect probably involves modulation of cholinergic signalling within pontine nuclei linked to sleep-wake regulation. Thus, decreased acetylcholine release occurs in the pontine reticular formation (PRF) of cats injected into the PRF with NOS inhibitors (Leonard and Lydic, 1995; 1997), and is accompanied by decreased REMS. Injection of the pedunculopontine tegmental nucleus (PPT) with NOS inhibitors likewise affects sleep, with reduced REMS and NREMS observed in cats (Datta *et al.*, 1997) and rabbits (Williams *et al.*, 1997). Conversely, increases in REMS and NREMS occur after PPT injection of the NO precursor L-arginine in rats (Hars, 1999), or the NO donor SNAP (*S*-nitroso-*N*-acetylpenicillamine) in cats (Leonard and Lydic, 1997). Thus, manipulation of NO levels in this neuronal circuit appears to influence sleep and waking states through modulation of the cholinergic neurotransmission involved in ascending reticular activation.

NO may also affect sleep through interaction with other sleep-regulatory pathways. For instance, NO production is induced by a number of other sleep-regulatory substances, including IL1, GHRH, adenosine (Rosenberg *et al.*, 2000), and TNFα (reviewed by Krueger and Majde, 1994). The somnogenic effects of IL1 signalling may be exerted, in part, by its induction of NO, as enhanced sleep in rabbits after i.c.v. IL1 injection is abolished if the rabbits are given a NOS inhibitor (Kapás *et al.*, 1994).

It is hypothesized (L. Kapás, personal communication) that opposing influences of NO on circadian and homeostatic sleep-regulatory mechanisms are responsible for sleep-wake regulation. In the suprachiasmatic nucleus (SCN) of rats, NO sensitivity is highest during the dark, behaviourally active period. NO production in the SCN is enhanced by retinohypothalamic glutamate release, and functions to promote arousal, possibly via a cGMP-dependent enhancement of neurotransmission. Conversely, NO promotes sleep within the brain structures involved in homeostatic sleep regulation. Within these sites, NO sensitivity does not exhibit circadian variation. Rather, NO production progressively increases in a neuronal use-dependent manner, such that its tonic release may influence multiple potential effectors, which collectively may increase sleep propensity. NO is elevated in mouse influenza-infected lungs (Akaike *et al.*, 1996), but NOS activity in the brain has not been examined in influenza. However, mice lacking inducible NOS do not have as large a NREMS response after influenza viral challenge (Chen *et al.*, unpublished).

SLEEP DEPRIVATION AND IMMUNE CONSEQUENCES

Rats deprived of sleep for 2–3 weeks die (Rechtschaffen *et al.*, 1983). The probable cause of death is septicaemia; the bacteria cultured from the blood are primarily facultative anaerobes indigenous to the host (Everson, 1993). Whether death or septicaemia occurs in other species after sleep deprivation has not been determined. In any case, the results with rats suggest that loss of sleep leads to host-defence breakdown. Consistent with this notion are the more recent findings that after just a few days of sleep deprivation viable bacteria can be cultured from organs of filtration such as mesenteric lymph nodes (Everson & Toth, 1997; Landis *et al.*, 1997), and the number of bacteria in the intestine increases (Everson, 1993; Bergmann *et al.*, 1996b). The mechanisms responsible for these effects remain unknown, although, as described below, several immune system measures are altered by sleep deprivation. Furthermore, these sleep-linked changes in bacteria could be related to a normal endosymbiotic relationship between bacteria and the host. Rats treated with antibiotics (neomycin and metronidazole) have reduced NREMS but normal REMS (Brown *et al.*, 1990), thereby suggesting that bacterial products could affect everyday sleep (reviewed by Krueger and Majde, 1994), as discussed above in the section on indigenous microbial flora.

In contrast to long-term sleep deprivation, short-term sleep deprivation does not result in death and, under some circumstances, may even enhance host-defence mechanisms. For example, in one study, rats deprived of sleep had smaller tumours than corresponding control animals (Bergmann *et al.*, 1996a). Other studies suggest that short-term sleep deprivation has little effect on infection. In human studies of sleep deprivation, there has been a failure to demonstrate an increased incidence of infection. However, most of these studies involve healthy young volunteers in unchallenging environmental conditions. In fact, if studies were designed to increase the probability of infection, they probably would not be approved. Consistent with these human studies is a report that sleep deprivation of rabbits failed to exacerbate *E. coli*-induced clinical illness (Toth *et al.*, 1995). Nevertheless, there is a wealth of data indicating that short-term sleep deprivation is associated with changes in immune system parameters.

Several laboratories have measured natural killer cell (NK) activity in conjunction with sleep and sleep loss. In several of these studies, circulating NK activity decreased after sleep deprivation (Moldofsky *et al.*, 1989; Irwin *et al.*, 1994, 1996). In other studies, circulating NK activity increased after sleep deprivation (Born *et al.*, 1997; Dinges *et al.*, 1994). Although there is a reduction of NK activity in depressed insomniac patients (Irwin *et al.*, 1992), in normal individuals NK activity may decrease during sleep (Moldofsky *et al.*, 1989). In summary, it seems likely that sleep or sleep loss may affect NK activity, but the magnitude and direction of such effects is sensitive to specific experimental conditions and the subject population.

Sleep deprivation affects several other facets of the immune system, including antigen uptake (Casey *et al.*, 1974), lymphocyte DNA synthesis (Palmblad *et al.*, 1979), phagocytosis (Palmbald *et al.*, 1976), mitogen responses (Moldofsky *et al.*, 1989), circulating immune complexes (Isenberg *et al.*, 1981), circulating IgG levels (Renegar *et al.*, 1998), secondary antibody responses (Brown *et al.*, 1989), and a variety of lymphocyte subsets (Dinges *et al.*, 1994). Sleep deprivation is also associated with changes in cytokines. Sleep loss is associated with an enhanced ability of lymphocytes to produce interferon (Palmblad *et al.*, 1976), increased white blood cell and monocyte TNF production (Yamasu *et al.*, 1992; Uthgenannt *et al.*, 1995), increased production of IL1β and IFNα by cultures of whole blood (Hohagen *et al.*, 1993), and increased plasma IL1 activity in humans and rats (Moldofsky *et al.*, 1989; Opp & Krueger, 1994). In normal people, and in people with sleep disorders, plasma levels of cytokines are related to the sleep-wake cycle or sleep disturbance. For example, IL1 plasma levels peak at the onset of NREMS (Moldofsky *et al.*, 1986), and TNF levels vary with EEG-slow-wave amplitude (Darko *et al.*, 1995). Patients with obstructive sleep apnoea syndrome have altered plasma TNF (Entzian *et al.*, 1996; Vgontzus *et al.*, 1997). Patients with psychoses who have reduced sleep have enhanced IL1β plasma levels (Appelberg *et al.*, 1997).

Collectively, the data cited above strongly suggest that sleep and sleep loss affect immune function. Nevertheless, few studies have directly measured the effect of sleep on host outcome. Study results often leave one uninformed as to whether the effects of sleep or sleep loss is adverse or beneficial to the host. Despite such limitations, it does appear that sleep influences immune function. Furthermore, currently, it appears that short-term sleep loss may enhance host defences, whereas long-term sleep loss is devastating.

RECUPERATIVE PROPERTIES OF SLEEP

There is no direct evidence that sleep per se aids in recuperation from infectious diseases or inflammation, primarily because of the difficulty of isolating sleep as an independent variable. Thus, during manipulations of sleep, such as sleep deprivation many physiological parameters vary. For example, sleep deprivation, is associated with changes in hormonal and cytokine production, body temperature, food intake, metabolic rate, etc. However, there are some data consistent with the notion that sleep is beneficial during infectious disease. After microbial challenge, rabbits that had robust NREMS responses within the first 12 h had a higher probability of survival than animals that failed to exhibit NREMS responses (Toth *et al.*, 1993). Although this evidence is correlative in nature, it suggests that perhaps our grandmothers' folk wisdom of the curative and preventative properties of sleep may, in fact, be correct. In any event, it is likely that physicians will continue to prescribe bed rest and sleep because this is often just what the patient wants to do.

ACKNOWLEDGEMENTS

This work was supported in part by the National Institutes of Health, grant numbers HD 36520, NS25378, NS27250, and NS31453, and by the Office of Naval Research, grant N00014-98-1-0144.

REFERENCES

Aderem, A. and Ulevitch, R.J., 2000. Toll-like receptors in the induction of the innate immune response. *Nature*, **406**, 782–787.

Akaike, T., Nogushi, Y., Ijiri, Y., Setoguchi, S., Suga, M., Yong, M.-Z., Dietzschold, B. and Maeda, H., 1996. Pathogenesis of influenza virus-induced pneumonia: involvement of both nitric oxide and oxygen radicals. *Proceedings of the National Academy of Science of the United States of America*, **93**, 2448–2453.

Alt, J.A., Obál, F., Jr., Majde, J.A. and Krueger, J.M., 2001. Impairment of the sleep response to influenza infection in mice with a defective GHRH-receptor. *Sleep*, **24**, A144–A145.

Appelberg, B., Katila, H. and Rimon, R., 1997. Plasma interleukin-1 beta and sleep architecture in schizophrenia and other nonaffective psychoses. *Psychosomatic Medicine*, **59**, 529–532.

Aström, C. and Linhölm, J., 1990. Growth hormone-deficient young adults have decreased sleep. *Neuroendocrinology*, **51**, 82–84.

Ballou, L.R., Laulederkind, S.J., Rosloniec, E.F. and Raghow, R., 1996. Ceramide signaling and the immune response. *Biochimica Biophysica Acta*, **1301**, 273–287.

Banks, W.A., Ortiz, L., Plotkin, S.R. and Kastin, J.A., 1991. Human interleukin (IL)-1α, murine IL1α and murine IL1β are transported from blood to brain in the house by a shared saturable mechanism. *Journal of Pharmacology and Experimental Therapeutics*, **259**, 988–996.

Barnes, P.J., 1997. Nuclear factor κB. *International Journal of Biochemistry and Cell Biology*, **29**, 867–870.

Beranek, L., Obál, F., Jr., Taishi, P., Bodosi, B., Laczi, F. and Krueger, J.M., 1997. Changes in rat sleep after single and repeated injections of long-acting somatostatin analog, octreotide. *American Journal of Physiology*, **42**, R1484–R1491.

Bergmann, B.J., Rechtschaffen, A., Gilliland, M.A. and Quintans, J., 1996a. Effect of extended sleep deprivation on tumor growth in rats. *American Journal of Physiology*, **271**, R1460–R1464.

Bergmann, B.M., Gilliland, M.A., Feng, P.-F., Russell, D.R., Shaw, P., Wright, M., Rechtschaffen, A. and Alverdy, J.C., 1996b. Sleep deprivation and sleep extension: are physiological effects of sleep deprivation in the rat mediated by bacterial invasion? *Sleep*, **19**, 554–562.

Blatteis, C.M. and Sehic, E., 1997. Fever: how may circulating pyrogens signal the brain? *News of Physiological Science*, **12**, 1–9.

Bodosi, B., Obál, F., Jr., Gardi, J., Komlodi, J. and Krueger, J.M., 2000. Ether stress induces increases in REM sleep in the rat: possible role of prolactin. *American Journal of Physiology*, **279**, R1590–R1598.

Borbély, A. and Tobler, I., 1989. Endogenous sleep-promoting substances and sleep regulation. *Physiological Reviews*, **69**, 605–670.

Born, J., Lange, T., Hansen, K., Molle, M. and Fehm, H.L., 1997. Effects of sleep and circadian rhythm on human circulating immune cells. *Journal of Immunology*, **158**, 4454–4464.

Branco, J., Atalaia, A. and Paiva, T., 1994. Sleep cycles and alpha-delta sleep in fibromyalgia syndrome. *Journal of Rheumatology*, **21**, 1113–1117.

Bredow, S., Kacsoh, B., Obál, F., Jr., Fang, J. and Krueger, J.M., 1994. Increase of prolactin mRNA in the rat hypothalamus after intracerebroventricular injection of VIP or PACAP. *Brain Research*, **660**, 301–308.

Bredow, S., Taishi, P., Obál, F., Jr., Guha-Thakurta, N. and Krueger, J.M., 1996. Hypothalamic growth hormone-releasing hormone mRNA varies across the day in rats. *Neuroreport*, **7**, 2501–2505.

Bredow, S., Guha-Thakurta, N., Taishi, P., Obál, F., Jr. and Krueger, J.M., 1997. Diurnal variations of tumor necrosis factor-α mRNA and α-tubulin mRNA in rat brain. *Neuroimmunomodulation*, **4**, 84–90.

Brown, R., Price, R.J., King, M.G. and Husband, A.J., 1989. Interleukin-1β and muramyl dipeptide can prevent decreased antibody response associated with sleep deprivation. *Brain, Behavior and Immunity*, **3**, 320–330.

Brown, R., Price, J.R., King, M.G. and Husband, A.J., 1990. Are antibiotic effects on sleep behavior in the rat due to modulation of gut bacteria? *Physiology and Behavior*, **48**, 561–565.

Buchwald, D., Pascualy, R., Bombardier, C. and Kith, P., 1994. Sleep disorders in patients with chronic fatigue. *Clinical Infectious Disease*, **18**(Suppl 1), S68–S72.

Bujak, D.I., Weinstein, A. and Dornbush, R.L., 1996. Clinical and neurocognitive features of the post Lyme syndrome. *Journal of Rheumatology*, **23**, 1392–1397.

Carlson, H.E., Gillin, J.C., Gorden, P. and Snyder, F., 1972. Absence of sleep-related growth hormone peaks in aged normal subjects and in acromegaly. *Journal of Clinical Endocrinology and Metabolism*, **34**, 1102–1105.

Casey, F.B., Eisenberg, J., Peterson, D. and Pieper, O., 1974. Altered antigen uptake and distribution due to exposure to extreme environmental temperatures or sleep deprivation. *Journal of the Reticuloendothelial Society*, **15**, 87–90.

Chen, Z., Gardi, J., Kushikata, T., Fang, J. and Krueger, J.M., 1999. Nuclear factor-κB-like activity increases in murine cerebral cortex after sleep deprivation *American Journal of Physiology Regulatory Integrative Comparative Physiology*, **276**, R1812–R1818.

Clarke, C.J., Hales, A., Hunt, A. and Foxwell, B.M., 1998. IL10-mediated suppression of TNF-α production is independent of its ability to inhibit NF-κB activity. *European Journal of Immunology*, **28**, 1719–1726.

Darko, D.F., Miller, J.C., Gallen, C., White, W., Koziol, J., Brown, S.J., Hayduk, R., Atkinson, J., Assmus, J., Munnell, D.T., Naitoh, P., McCutchen, J.A. and Mitler, M.M., 1995. Sleep electroencephalogram delta frequency amplitude, night plasma levels of tumor necrosis factor α and human immunodeficiency virus infection. *Proceedings of the National Academy of Science of the United States of America*, **92**, 12080–12086.

Datta, S., Patterson, E.H. and Siwek, D.F., 1997. Endogenous and exogenous nitric oxide in the pedunculopontine tegmentum induces sleep. *Synapse*, **27**, 69–78.

Dinarello, C.A., 2000. Proinflammatory cytokines. *Chest*, **118**, 503–508.

Dinges, D.F., Douglas, S.D., Zaugg, L., Campbell, D.E., McMann, J.M., Whitehouse, W.G., Orene, E.C., Kapoor, S.C., Icaza, E. and Orne, M.T., 1994. Leukocytosis and natural killer cell function parallel neurobehavioural fatigue induced by 64 hours of sleep deprivation. *Journal of Clinical Investigation*, **93**, 1930–1939.

Dreisbach, A.W., Hendrickson, T., Beezhold, D., Riesenberg, L.A. and Sklar, A.H., 1998. Elevated levels of tumor necrosis factor alpha in postdialysis fatigue. *International Journal of Artificial Organs*, **21**, 83–86.

Edwards, N., Blyton, D.M., Kesby, G.J., Wilcox, I. and Sullivan, C.E., 2000. Pre-eclampsia is associated with marked alterations in sleep architecture. *Sleep*, **23**, 619–623.

Eizirik, D.L., Flodstrom, M., Karlsen, A.E. and Welsh, N., 1996. The harmony of the spheres: inducible nitric oxide synthase and related genes in pancreatic beta cells. *Diabetologia*, **39**, 875–890.

Entzian, P., Linnemann, K., Schlaak, M. and Zabel, P., 1996. Obstructive sleep apnoea syndrome and circadian rhythms of hormones and cytokines. *American Journal of Respiratory Critical Care Medicine*, **153**, 1080–1086.

Eskander, E.D., Harvey, H.A., Givant, E. and Lipton, A., 1997. Phase I study combining tumor necrosis factor with interferon-alpha and interleukin-2. *American Journal of Clinical Oncology*, **20**, 511–514.

Everson, C.A., 1993. Sustained sleep deprivation impairs host defence. *American Journal of Physiology*, **265**, R1148–R1154.

Everson, C.A. and Toth, L.A., 1997. Abnormal control of viable bacteria in body tissues during sleep deprivation in rats. *APSS Abstracts*, **254**.

Fang, J., Sanborn, C.K., Renegar, K.B., Majde, J.A. and Krueger, J.M., 1995a. Influenza viral infections enhance sleep in mice. *Proceedings of the Society for Experimental Biology and Medicine*, **210**, 242–252.

Fang, J., Payne, L. and Krueger, J.M., 1995b. Pituitary adenylate activating polypeptide enhances rapid eye movement sleep in rats. *Brain Research*, **686**, 23–28.

Fang, J., Tooley, D., Gatewood, C., Renegar, K.B., Majde, J.A. and Krueger, J.M., 1996. Differential effects of total and upper airway influenza viral infection on sleep in mice. *Sleep*, **19**, 337–342.

Fang, J., Wang, Y. and Krueger, J.M., 1997. Mice lacking the TNF 55-kD receptor fail to sleep more after TNFα treatment. *Journal of Neuroscience*, **17**, 5949–5955.

Fang, J., Wang, Y. and Krueger, J.M., 1998. The effects of interleukin-1β on sleep are mediated by the type I receptor. *American Journal of Physiology*, **274**, R655–R660.

Floyd, R.A. and Krueger, J.M., 1997. Diurnal variations of TNFα in the rat brain. *Neuroreport*, **8**, 915–918.

Franklin, C.M., 1999. Clinical experience with soluble TNF p75 receptor in rheumatoid arthritis. *Seminars on Arthritis and Rheumatism*, **29**, 172–181.

Gardi, J., Obál, F., Jr., Fang, J., Zhang, J. and Krueger, J.M., 1998. Diurnal variations and sleep-deprivation-induced changes in GHRH contents of the rat hypothalamus. *Journal of Sleep Research*, **7**, 97.

Goehler, L.E., Relton, J.K., Dripps, D., Kiechle, R., Tartaglia, N., Maier, S.F. and Watkins, L.R., 1997. Vagal paraganglia bind biotinylated interleukin-1 receptor antagonist: a possible mechanism for immune-to-brain communication. *Brain Research Bulletin*, **43**, 357–364.

Hansen, M.K. and Krueger, J.M., 1997. Subdiaphragmatic vagotomy blocks the sleep- and fever-promoting effects of interleukin-1β. *American Journal of Physiology*, **273**, 1246–1253.

Hansen, M.K., Taishi, P., Chen, Z. and Krueger, J.M., 1998a. Vagotomy blocks the induction of interleukin-1β (IL1β) mRNA in the brain of rats in response to system IL1β. *Journal of Neuroscience*, **18**, 2247–2253.

Hansen, M.K., Kapás, L., Fang, J. and Krueger, J.M., 1998b. Cafeteria diet-induced sleep is blocked by sub-diaphragmatic vagotomy in rats. *American Journal of Physiology*, **274**, R168–R174.

Hansen, M.K., Taishi, P., Chen, Z. and Krueger, J.M., 1998c. Cafeteria-feeding induces interleukin-1β mRNA expression in rat liver and brain. *American Journal of Physiology*, **43**, R1734–R1739.

Hars, B., 1999. Endogenous nitric oxide in the rat pons promotes sleep. *Brain Research*, **816**, 209–219.

Hart, B.L., 1988. Biological basis of the behavior of sick animals. *Neuroscience and Biobehavior Reviews*, **12**, 123–137.

Hayaishi, O., 1988. Sleep-wake regulation by prostaglandins D2 and E2. *Journal of Biological Chemistry*, **263**, 14593–14596.

Hirsch, M., Carlander, B., Verge, M., Tafti, M., Anaya, J.M., Billiard, M. and Sany, J., 1994. Objective and subjective sleep disturbances in patients with rheumatoid arthritis. A reappraisal. *Arthritis and Rheumatism*, **37**, 41–49.

Hohogan, F., Timmer, J., Weyerbrock, A., Firtsch-Montero, R., Ganter, U., Krieger, S., Berger, M. and Bauer, J., 1993. Cytokine production during sleep and wakefulness and its relationship to cortisol in healthy humans. *Neuropsychobiology*, **28**, 9–16.

Hoijer, M.A., Melief, M.J., Calafat, J., Roos, D., van den Beemd, R.W., van Dongen, J.J. and Hazenberg, M.P., 1997. Expression and intracellular localization of the human *N*-acetylmuramyl-L-alanine amidase, a bacterial cell wall-degrading enzyme. *Blood*, **90**, 1246–1254.

Irwin, M., Smith, T.L. and Gillin, J.C., 1992. Electroencephalographic sleep and natural killer activity in depressed patients and control subject. *Psychosomatic Medicine*, **54**, 10–21.

Irwin, M., Mascovich, A., Gillin, J.C., Willoughby, R., Pike, J. and Smith, T.L., 1994. Partial sleep deprivation reduces natural killer cell activity in humans. *Psychosomatic Medicine*, **56**, 493–498.

Irwin, M., McClintick, J., Costlow, C., Fortner, M., White, J. and Gilling, J.C., 1996. Partial night sleep deprivation reduces natural killer and cellular immune responses in humans. *FASEB Journal*, **10**, 643–653.

Isenberg, D.A., Crisp, A.J., Morrow, W.J., Newham, D. and Snaith, M.L., 1981. Variation in circulating immune complex levels with diet, exercise, and sleep: a comparison between normal controls and patients with systemic lupus erythematosus. *Annals of the Rheumatic Diseases*, **40**, 466–469.

Jouvet, M., Buda, C., Cespuglio, R., Castrette, N., Denoyer, M., Sallanon, M. and Sastre, J.P., 1986. Hypnogenic effects of some hypothalamo-pituitary peptides. *Clinical Neuropharmacology*, **9**, 465–467.

Kapás, L., Obál, F., Jr. and Krueger, J.M., 1993. Humoral regulation of sleep. *International Reviews of Neurobiology*, **35**, 131–160.

Kapás, L., Shibata, M., Kimura, M. and Krueger, J.M., 1994. Inhibition of nitric oxide synthesis suppresses sleep in rabbits. *American Journal of Physiology*, **266**, R151–R157.

Kapás, L. and Krueger, J.M., 1996. Nitric oxide donors SIN-1 and SNAP promote non-rapid eye movement sleep in rats. *Brain Research Bulletin*, **41**, 293–298.

Kapás, L., Hansen, M.K., Chang, H.-Y. and Krueger, J.M., 1998. Vagotomy attenuates but does not prevent the somnogenic and febrile effects of lipopolysaccharide in rats. *American Journal of Physiology*, **274**, R406–R411.

Kent, S., Bluthé, R.-M., Kelley, K.W. and Dantzer, R., 1992. Sickness behavior as a new target for drug development. *Trends in Pharmacological Sciences*, **13**, 24–28.

Klir, J.J., McClellan, J.L. and Kluger, M.J., 1994. Interleukin-1β causes the increase in anterior hypothalamic interleukin-6 during LPS-induced fever in rats. *American Journal of Physiology*, **266**, 1845–1848.

Kluger, M.J., 1991. Fever: role of pyrogens and cryogens. *Physiological Reviews*, **71**, 93–127.

Krueger, J.M., Pappenheimer, J.R. and Karnovsky, M.L., 1982a. The composition of sleep-promoting factor isolated from human urine. *Journal of Biological Chemistry*, **257**, 1664–1669.

Krueger, J.M., Pappenheimer, J.R. and Karnovsky, M.L., 1982b. Sleep-promoting effects of muramyl peptides. *Proceedings of the National Academy of Sciences of the United States of America*, **79**, 6102–6106.

Krueger, J.M., Walter, J., Dinarello, C.A., Wolff, S.M. and Chedid, L., 1984. Sleep-promoting effects of endogenous pyrogen (interleukin-1). *American Journal of Physiology*, **246**, R994–999.

Krueger, J.M. and Majde, J.A., 1990. Sleep as a host defence: its regulation by microbial products and cytokines. *Clinical Immunology and Immunopathology*, **57**, 188–199.

Krueger, J.M. and Majde, J.A., 1994. Microbial products and cytokines in sleep and fever regulation. *Critical Reviews of Immunology*, **14**, 355–379.

Krueger, J.M. and Obál, F., Jr., 1997. Sleep regulatory substances. In: Schwartz, W.J. (ed.), *Sleep Science: Integrating Basic Research and Clinical Practice*, pp. 175–194. *Monograph of Clinical Neuroscience*, Vol. 15. Karger, Basel.

Krueger, J.M., Obál, F., Jr. and Fang, J., 1999. Humoral regulation of physiological sleep: cytokines and GHRH. *Journal of Sleep Research*, **8**, 53–59.

Krueger, J.M., Fang, J. and Majde, J.A., 2001. Sleep in health and disease. In: Ader, B., Felton, D. and Cohen, N. (eds), *Psychoneuroimmunology*, (3rd edn), pp. 667–685. Academic Press, New York.

Kubota, T., Fang, J., Brown, R.A. and Krueger, J.M., 2001. Interleukin-18 promotes sleep in rabbits and rats. *American Journal of Physiology*, **281**, R828–R838.

Kubota, T., Kushikata, T., Fang, J. and Krueger, J.M., 2000. Nuclear factor-κB inhibitor peptide inhibits spontaneous and interleukin-1β-induced sleep. *American Journal of Physiology*, **279**, R404–R413.

Kushikata, T., Fang, J., Wang, Y. and Krueger, J.M., 1998. Interleukin-4 inhibits spontaneous sleep in rabbits. *American Journal of Physiology*, **275**, R1185–R1191.

Lancel, M., Mathias, S., Faulhaber, J. and Schiffelholz, T., 1996. Effect of interleukin-1 beta on EEG power density during sleep depends on circadian phase. *American Journal of Physiology*, **270**, R830–R835.

Landis, C.A., Robinson, C.R. and Levine, J.D., 1988. Sleep fragmentation in the arthritic rat. *Pain*, **34**, 93–99.

Landis, C.A., Robinson, C.R., Helms, C. and Levine, J.D., 1989. Differential effects of acetylsalicylic acid and acetaminophen on sleep abnormalities in a rat chronic pain model. *Brain Research*, **488**, 195–201.

Landis, C., Pollack, S. and Helton, W.S., 1997. Microbial translocation and NK cell cytotoxicity in female rats sleep deprived on small platforms. *APSS Abstracts*, **188**.

Layé, S., Bluthé, R.-M., Kent, S., Combe, C., Médina, C., Parnet, P., Kelley, D. and Dantzer, R., 1995. Subdiaphragmatic vagotomy blocks the induction of interleukin-1β mRNA in the brain of mice in response to peripherally administered lipopolysaccharide. *American Journal of Physiology*, **268**, 1327–1331.

Leonard, T.O. and Lydic, R., 1995. Nitric oxide synthase inhibition decreases pontine acetylcholine release. *Neuroreport*, **6**, 1525–1529.

Leonard, T.O. and Lydic, R., 1997. Pontine nitric oxide modulates acetylcholine release, rapid eye movement sleep generation, and respiratory rate. *Journal of Neuroscience*, **17**, 774–785.

Mackiewicz, M., Sollars, P.J., Ogilvie, M.D. and Pack, A.I., 1996. Modulation of IL1β gene expression in the rat CNS during sleep deprivation. *Neuroreport*, **7**, 529–533.

Mahowald, M.W., Mahowald, M.L., Bundlie, S.R. and Ytterberg, S.R., 1989. Sleep fragmentation in rheumatoid arthritis. *Arthritis and Rheumatism*, **32**, 974–983.

Moldofsky, H., Lue, F.A., Eisen, J., Keystone, E. and Gorczynski, R.M., 1986. The relationship of interleukin-1 and immune functions to sleep in humans. *Psychosomatic Medicine*, **48**, 309–318.

Moldofsky, H., Davidson, J.R. and Lue, F.A., 1988. Sleep-related patterns of plasma growth hormone and cortisol following 40 hours of wakefulness. *Sleep Research*, **17**, 69.

Moldofsky, H., Lue, F.A., Davidson, J.R. and Gorczynski, R., 1989. Effects of sleep deprivation on human immune functions. *FASEB Journal*, **3**, 1972–1977.

Moldofsky, H., Leu, F.A. and Smythe, H.A., 1993. Alpha EEG sleep and morning symptoms in rheumatoid arthritis. *Journal of Rheumatology*, **10**, 373–379.

Morehouse, R.L., Flanigan, M., MacDonald, D.D., Braha, D. and Shapiro, C., 1998. Depression and short REM latency in subjects with chronic fatigue syndrome. *Psychosomatic Medicine*, **60**, 347–351.

Moss, R.B., Mercandetti, A. and Vojdani, A., 1999. TNF-alpha and chronic fatigue syndrome. *Journal of Clinical Immunology*, **19**, 314–316.

Nguyen, K.T., Deak, T., Owens, S.M., Kohno, T., Fleshner, M., Watkins, L.R. and Maier, S.F., 1998. Exposure to acute stress induces brain interleukin-1β protein in the rat. *Journal of Neuroscience*, **18**, 2239–2246.

Nie, Z., Mei, Y., Ford, M., Rybak, L., Marcuzzi, A., Ren, H., Stiles, G.L. and Ramkumar, V., 1998. Oxidative stress increases A1 adenosine receptor expression by activating nuclear factor κB. *Molecular Pharmacology*, **53**, 663–669.

Obál, F., Jr., Alföldi, P., Cady, A.B., Johannsen, L., Sáry, G. and Krueger, J.M., 1988. Growth hormone releasing factor enhances sleep in rats and rabbits. *American Journal of Physiology*, **255**, R310–R316.

Obál, F., Jr., Opp, M., Cady, A.A., Johannsen, L. and Krueger, J.M., 1989. Prolactin, vasoactive intestinal peptide, and peptide histidine methionine elicit selective increases in REM sleep in rabbits. *Brain Research*, **490**, 292–300.

Obál, F., Jr., Kacsoh, B., Alföldi, P., Payne, L., Markovic, O., Grosvenor, C. and Krueger, J.M., 1992. Antiserum to prolactin decreases rapid eye movement sleep (REM sleep) in the male rat. *Physiology and Behavior*, **52**, 1063–1968.

Obál, F., Jr., Payne, L., Kacsoh, B., Opp, M., Kapás, L., Grosvenor, C.E. and Krueger, J.M., 1994. Involvement of prolactin in the REM sleep-promoting activity of systemic vasoactive intestinal peptide (VIP). *Brain Research*, **645**, 143–149.

Obál, F., Jr., Floyd, R., Kapás, L., Bodosi, B. and Krueger, J.M., 1996. Effects of systemic GHRH on sleep in intact and hypophysectomized rats. *American Journal of Physiology*, **270**, E230–E237.

Obál, F., Jr., Bodosi, B., Szilágyi, A., Kacsóh, B. and Krueger, J.M., 1997a. Antiserum to growth hormone decreases sleep in the rat. *Neuroendocrinology*, **66**, 9–16.

Obál, F., Jr., Kacsoh, B., Bredow, S., Guha-Thakurta, N. and Krueger, J.M., 1997b. Sleep in rats rendered chronically hyperprolactinemic with anterior pituitary grafts. *Brain Research*, **755**, 130–136.

Obál, F., Jr., Kapás, L., Bodosi, B. and Krueger, J.M., 1998. Changes in sleep in response to intracerebral injection of insulin-like growth factor-1 (IGF-1) in the rat. *Sleep Research Online*, **2**, 87–91.

Obál, F., Jr., Fang, J., Taishi, P., Kacsoh, B., Gardi, J. and Krueger, J.M., 2001. Deficiency of growth hormone-releasing hormone signaling is associated with sleep alterations in the dwarf rat. *Journal of Neuroscience*, **21**, 2912–2918.

Opp, M.R., Obál, F., Jr. and Krueger, J.M., 1991. Interleukin-1 alters rat sleep: temporal and dose-related effects. *American Journal of Physiology*, **260**, R52–R58.

Opp, M.R. and Krueger, J.M., 1994. Anti-interleukin-1β reduces sleep and sleep rebound after sleep deprivation in rats. *American Journal of Physiology*, **266**, R688–R695.

Opp, M.R., Smith, E.M. and Hughes, T.K., 1995. Interleukin-10 acts in the central nervous system of rats to reduce sleep. *Journal of Neuroimmunology*, **60**, 165–168.

Owen, R.L., Pierce, N.F., Apple, R.T. and Cray, W.C., Jr., 1986. M cell transport of *Vibrio cholerae* from the intestinal lumen into

Peyer's patches: a mechanism for antigen sampling and for microbial transepithelial migration. *Journal of Infectious Disease*, **153**, 1108–1118.

Pabst, M.J., Beranova, S. and Krueger, J.M., 1999. A review of the effects of muramyl peptides on macrophages, monokines and sleep. *Neuroimmunomodulation*, **6**, 261–283.

Palmblad, J., Cantell, K., Strander, H., Fröberg, J., Karlsson, C.G., Levi, L., Granström, M. and Unger, P., 1976. Stressor exposure and immunological response in man: interferon producing capacity and phagocytosis. *Psychosomatic Research*, **20**, 193–199.

Palmblad, J., Petrini, B., Wasserman, J. and Akerstedt, T., 1979. Lymphocyte and granulocyte reactions during sleep deprivation. *Psychosomatic Medicine*, **41**, 273–278.

Pappenheimer, J.R., Koski, G., Fencl, V., Karnovsky, M.L. and Krueger, J.M., 1975. Extraction of sleep-promoting factor S from cerebrospinal fluid and from brains of sleep-deprived animals. *Journal of Neurophysiology*, **38**, 1299–1311.

Perras, B., Marshall, L., Kohler, G., Born, J. and Fehm, H.L., 1999. Sleep and endocrine changes after intranasal administration of growth hormone-releasing hormone in young and aged humans. *Psychoneuroendocrinology*, **24**, 743–757.

Rechtschaffen, A., Gilliland, M.A., Bergmann, B.M. and Winter, J.B., 1983. Physiological correlation of prolonged sleep deprivation in rats. *Science*, **221**, 182–184.

Ribeiro, A.C., Gilligan, J.G. and Kapás, L., 2000. Systemic injection of a nitric oxide synthase inhibitor suppresses sleep responses to sleep deprivation in rats. *American Journal of Physiology*, **278**, R1048–R1056.

Roky, R., Obál, F., Jr., Valatx, J.L., Bredow, S., Fang, J., Pagano, L.P. and Krueger, J.M., 1995. Prolactin and rapid eye movement sleep regulation. *Sleep*, **18**, 536–542.

Rosenberg, P.A., Li, Y., Le, M. and Zhang, Y., 2000. Nitric oxide-stimulated increase in extracellular adenosine accumulation in rat forebrain neurons in culture is associated with ATP hydrolysis and inhibition of adenosine kinase activity. *Journal of Neuroscience*, **20**, 6294–6301.

Sartor, R.B., Bond, T.M. and Schwab, J.H., 1988. Systemic uptake and intestinal inflammatory effects of luminal bacterial cell wall polymers in rats with acute colonic injury. *Infection and Immunity*, **56**, 2101–2108.

Shearer, W.T., Reuben, J.M., Mullington, J.M., Price, N.J., Lee, B.N., Smith, E.O., Szuba, M.P., Van Dongen, H.P. and Dinges, D.F., 2001. Soluble TNF-alpha receptor 1 and IL6 plasma levels in humans subjected to the sleep deprivation model of spaceflight. *Journal of Allergy and Clinical Immunology*, **107**, 167–170.

Shiromani, P.J., Basheer, R., Greco, M.A., Ramanathan, L. and McCarley, R.W., 1998. Emerging evidence on the role of transcription factors in sleep. *Journal of Sleep Research*, **7**, 248.

Sklar, A.H., Beezhold, D.H., Newman, N., Hendrickson, T. and Dreisbach, A.W., 1998. Postdialysis fatigue: lack of effect of a biocompatible membrane. *American Journal of Kidney Disease*, **31**, 1007–1010.

Smith, A., 1992. Sleep, colds, and performance. In: Broughton, R.J. and Ogilvie, R.D. (eds), *Sleep, Arousal and Performance*, pp. 233–242. Birkhauser, Boston.

Steiger, A., Guldner, J., Hemmeter, U., Rothe, B., Wiedemann, K. and Holsboer, F., 1992. Effects of growth hormone-releasing hormone and somatostatin on sleep EEG and nocturnal hormone secretion in male controls. *Neuroendocrinology*, **56**, 566–573.

Steriade, M.D. and McCarley, R.N., 1990. *Brainstem Control of Wakefulness and Sleep*. Plenum Press, New York.

Susic, V. and Totic, S., 1989. 'Recovery' function of sleep: effects of purified human interleukin-1 on the sleep and febrile response of cats. *Metabolic Brain Disease*, **4**, 73–80.

Sweet, M.J., Stacey, K.J., Kakuda, D.K., Markovich, D. and Hume, D.A., 1998. IFN-γ primes macrophage responses to bacterial DNA. *Journal of Interferon and Cytokine Research*, **18**, 263–271.

Taishi, P., Bredow, S., Guha-Thakurta, N., Obál, F., Jr. and Krueger, J.M., 1997. Diurnal variations of interleukin-1β mRNA and β-actin mRNA in rat brain. *Journal of Neuroimmunology*, **75**, 69–74.

Taishi, P., Chen, Z., Obál, F., Jr. Zhang, J., Hansen, M., Fang, J. and Krueger, J.M., 1998. Sleep associated changes in interleukin-1β mRNA in the brain. *Journal of Interferon and Cytokine Research*, **18**, 793–798.

Takahashi, S., Kapás, L., Fang, J., Wang, Y., Seyer, J.M. and Krueger, J.M., 1996. An interleukin-1 receptor fragment inhibits spontaneous sleep and muramyl dipeptide-induced sleep in rabbits. *American Journal of Physiology*, **271**, R101–R108.

Takahashi, Y., Kipnis, D.M. and Daughaday, W.H., 1968. Growth hormone secretions during sleep. *Journal of Clinical Investigation*, **47**, 2079–2090.

Terao, A., Matsumura, H. and Saito, M., 1998. Interleukin-1 induces slow wave sleep at the prostaglandin D_2-sensitive sleep-promoting zone in the rat brain. *Journal of Neuroscience*, **18**, 6599–6607.

Toppila, J., Alanko, L., Asikainen, M., Tobler, I., Stenberg, D. and Porkka-Heiskanen, T., 1997. Sleep deprivation increases somatostatin and growth hormone releasing hormone messenger RNA in the rat hypothalamus. *Journal of Sleep Research*, **6**, 171–178.

Toth, C.A., Tolley, E.A. and Krueger, J.M., 1993. Sleep as a prognostic indicator during infectious disease in rabbits. *Proceedings of the Society for Experimental Biological Medicine*, **203**, 179–192.

Toth, L.A., Opp, M.R. and Mao, L., 1995. Somnogenic effects of sleep deprivation and *Escherichia coli* inoculation in rabbits. *Journal of Sleep Research*, **4**, 30–40.

Toth, L.A. and Krueger, J.M., 1988. Alterations of sleep in rabbits by *Staphylococcus aureus infection. Infection and Immunity*, **56**, 1785–1791.

Toth, L.A., 1999. Microbial modulation of sleep. In: Lydic, R. and Baghdoyan, H. (eds), *Handbook of Behavioural State Control: Cellular and Molecular Mechanisms*, pp. 641–657. CRC Press, Boca Raton, FL.

Uthgenannt, D., Schoolmann, D., Pietrowsky, R., Fehm, H.L. and Born, J., 1995. Effects of sleep on the production of cytokines in humans. *Psychosomatic Medicine*, **57**, 97–104.

Valatx, J.L., Roky, R. and Paut-Pagano, L., 1990. Prolactin and sleep regulation. In: Horne, J. (ed.), *Sleep '90*, pp. 346–348. Pontenagel Press, Bochum, Germany.

Veasey, S.C., Mackiewicz, M., Fenik, P., Ro, M., Olgilvie, M.D. and Pack, A.I., 1997. IL1β knockout mice lack the TNFα response to sleep deprivation but have normal sleep and sleep recovery. *Society for Neuroscience Abstracts B*, **23**, 792.

Vgontzas, A.N., Papanicolaou, D.A., Bixler, E.O., Kales, A., Tyson, K. and Chrousos, G.P., 1997. Elevation of plasma cytokines in disorders of excessive daytime sleepiness: role of sleep disturbance and obesity. *Journal of Clinical Endocrinology Metabolism*, **82**, 1313–1316.

Von Economo, C., 1930. Sleep as a problem of localization. *Journal of Nervous and Mental Disorders*, **71**, 249–259.

Walsh, J.K., Muehlbach, M.J., Lauter, S.A., Hilliker, N.A. and Schweitzer, P.K., 1996. Effects of triazolam on sleep, daytime sleepiness, and morning stiffness in patients with rheumatoid arthritis. *Journal of Rheumatology*, **23**, 245–252.

Walsh, R.J., Slaby, F.J. and Posner, B.I., 1987. A receptor-mediated mechanism for the transport of prolactin from blood to cerebrospinal fluid. *Endocrinology*, **120**, 1846–1850.

Williams, G., Pirmohamed, J., Minors, D., Waterhouse, J., Buchan, I., Arendt, J. and Edwards, R.H., 1996. Dissociation of body-temperature and melatonin secretion circadian rhythms in patients with chronic fatigue syndrome. *Clinical Physiology*, **16**, 327–337.

Williams, J.A., Vincent, S.R. and Reiner, P.B., 1997. Nitric oxide production in rat thalamus changes with behavioural state, local depolarization, and brainstem stimulation. *Journal of Neuroscience*, **117**, 420–427.

Yamasu, K., Shimada, Y., Sakaizumi, M., Soma, G. and Mizuno, D., 1992. Activation of the systemic production of tumor necrosis factor after exposure to acute stress. *European Cytokine Network*, **3**, 391–398.

Zhang, J., Obál, F., Jr. Fang, J., Collins, B.J. and Krueger, J.M., 1996. Sleep is suppressed in transgenic mice with a deficiency in the somatotropic system. *Neuroscience Letters*, **220**, 97–100.

Zhang, J., Chen, Z., Taishi, P., Obál, F., Jr., Fang, J. and Krueger, J.M., 1998. Sleep deprivation increases rat hypothalamic growth hormone-releasing hormone mRNA. *American Journal of Physiology*, **275**, R1755–R1761.

Zhang, J., Obál, F., Jr., Zheng, T., Fang, J., Taishi, P. and Krueger, J.M., 1999. Intrapreoptic microinjection of GHRH or its antagonist alters sleep in rats. *Journal of Neuroscience*, **19**, 2187–2194.

Zhang, S.Q., Kimura, M. and Inoue, S., 1995. Sleep patterns in cyclic and pseudopregnant rats. *Neuroscience Letters*, **193**, 125–128.

XXIV-5

Psychophysiology of Sleep Disorders

R.T. Pivik

INTRODUCTION

Understanding the disordered presupposes a fundamental knowledge of the normal reference state or behaviour. It should come as no surprise, therefore, that our understanding of the psychophysiology of sleep disorders is limited, given that our knowledge of the characteristics and processes associated with normal sleep physiology and related variations in cognition can, in many respects, be considered elementary. Until relatively recent times, the development of knowledge about sleep was restricted by conceptual limitations and behavioural barriers. The emphasis on wakefulness as the state during which the most important behavioural and cognitive accomplishments occurred diminished the importance of sleep as a behaviour worthy of or even requiring investigation. This attitude was reflected in the view of the waking state as 'the sole portion of ... existence that "counts" in any way, sleep appearing as "time out" from the game of living' (Kleitman, 1963: p. 3) — an attitude reinforced by the behavioural inertness characteristic of the sleeping organism. Still, the influence of sleep on waking behaviour is undeniable and evident both in its timing and duration. The occurrence of sleep can be considered to be subject to limited volitional control since it is possible to remain awake for long periods of time or to select convenient times and environments for sleeping. However, at times the pressure for sleep is irresistible and sleep will occur despite the known likelihood of potentially deadly consequences, as while driving an automobile. The amount of sleep obtained has also been shown to be important for normal waking activities. The adverse effects of reduced sleep on alertness and performance are well documented (Monk, 1991; Gillberg and Åkerstedt, 1994), and, in the extreme, the long-term absence of sleep may lead to death (Horne, 1988; Everson, 1995; Bentivoglio and Grassi-Zucconi, 1997). From these observations, two important inferences can be drawn: 1) sleep is not simply a passive state during which physical activities are suspended; and 2) sleep processes interact with those occurring during waking in complementary and synergistic ways to maintain and extend life. Until the mid-20th century, insight into the nature of this codependence was prevented by the inability to obtain information regarding ongoing processes from the sleeping organism. Technologic developments during the past half-century have largely removed obstacles to these efforts. Notable among these developments has been the ability to conduct recordings of central nervous system and related autonomic and peripheral nervous system activities over the extended time periods that sleep typically occurs. More recently, these measures have been supplemented with assessments of state-related variations in brain metabolism using imaging procedures.

The interest in applying these technologic tools to chart variations in sleep physiology across the night was accompanied by an equally intense curiosity regarding what these measures might reveal about the occurrence of mental activity during sleep. The long-standing belief that experiences of mental activity continue during sleep in the form of dreams suggested that sleep was not a mental void. Furthermore, since these mental experiences occur during times of sustained disengagement from the environment, the nature of psychophysiological relationships under these circumstances could be different than those present during wakefulness. The advent of the new methods brought the study of these relationships within the range of effective experimental control. Investigations using these new procedures revolutionized the study of sleep, and the findings from this research have forced a redefinition of concepts regarding physiological and psychological activities and events that can be considered normal.

Although it is apparently the natural order that the states of sleep and wakefulness remain separate, their codependence renders them inseparable and interactive. Some aspects of these state interactions are fixed, and others more variable. Since the existence of higher mammals can be considered a closed system generally dichotomized into states of sleep and wakefulness (although conditions exist which do not clearly fall into either of these categories, such as coma and anaesthetic states), interactions based on state duration are constrained and essentially hydraulic in nature — that is, increases in time spent in one state are at the expense of time spent in the other.

It can be assumed that an important determinant of state duration is the time needed to satisfy functional requirements. Consequently, an important source of sleep-wakefulness interactions derives from the manner in which within-state behaviours (or processes) affect, or are reflective of, the realization of these requirements. Broad examples of such variations would include the nature of waking activity (e.g., resting vs. vigorous physical activity) or sleep quality (e.g., quiescent vs. disturbed). Such variations have both immediate within-state effects as well as longer-term, between-state consequences.

The relative inaccessibility of sleep processes to systematic study delayed the recognition of these interactions and consequences as significant determinants of behaviour. This delayed acknowledgement was evident in the absence of sleep-related variables among factors considered contributory to mental disorders in the initial publications of the *Diagnostic and Statistical Manual of Mental Disorders* (DSM) in 1917 and 1952 (DSM-I). The publication of DSM-I occurred near the time that rapid-eye-movement (REM) sleep was discovered (Aserinsky and Kleitman, 1953) — a revelation that effectively launched the new era of sleep research. Fifteen years later (1968), DSM-II appeared, and for the first time sleep disorders were included (referenced under 'Special Symptoms'). By 1979, an understanding of sleep had developed to the point that a 'Diagnostic Classification of Sleep and Arousal Disorders' could be published. Beginning with the publication of DSM-III one year later, the involvement of sleep disorders in the determination of mental status has been consistently and more fully represented.

Biological Psychiatry: Edited by H. D'haenen, J.A. den Boer and P. Willner. ISBN 0-471-49198-5

As background for a consideration of the associations between disordered sleep and mental processes, a brief overview of fundamental observations that have been made regarding normative sleep physiology and sleep-associated cognition will be provided.

SLEEP PHYSIOLOGY: DESCRIPTIVE ASPECTS

As previously mentioned, the technology that provided the window through which investigators could view sleep processes in progress was the ability to conduct long-term recordings of electrophysiological activities. Although this technology was available and being used to describe sleep-related variations in electroencephalographic (EEG) activities in the 1930s (Loomis *et al.*, 1937, 1938), it would be another 15 years before the discoveries that brought renewed attention to the study of sleep would begin to be made. These discoveries consisted of reports of recurring episodes of physiological activation during sleep that were related to the occurrence of dreaming (Aserinsky and Kleitman, 1953, 1955; Dement, 1955; Dement and Kleitman, 1957a, 1957b; Dement and Wolpert, 1958a, 1958b). Subsequent research has provided a detailed map of the physiological and psychological dimensions of sleep.

The work begun by Loomis *et al.* (1937, 1938) in describing sequential brain potential patterns during sleep has been expanded to include the additional physiological descriptors (measures of autonomic and muscle activities), and stages of sleep have been defined and their variations charted across the night (Dement and Kleitman, 1957a; Rechtschaffen and Kales, 1968). Examples of physiological variations characteristic of sleep-wakefulness and within sleep-stage differentiations are presented in Figures XXIV-5.1 and XXIV-5.2. Sleep-stage determinations in these figures are based on the standardized criteria for the

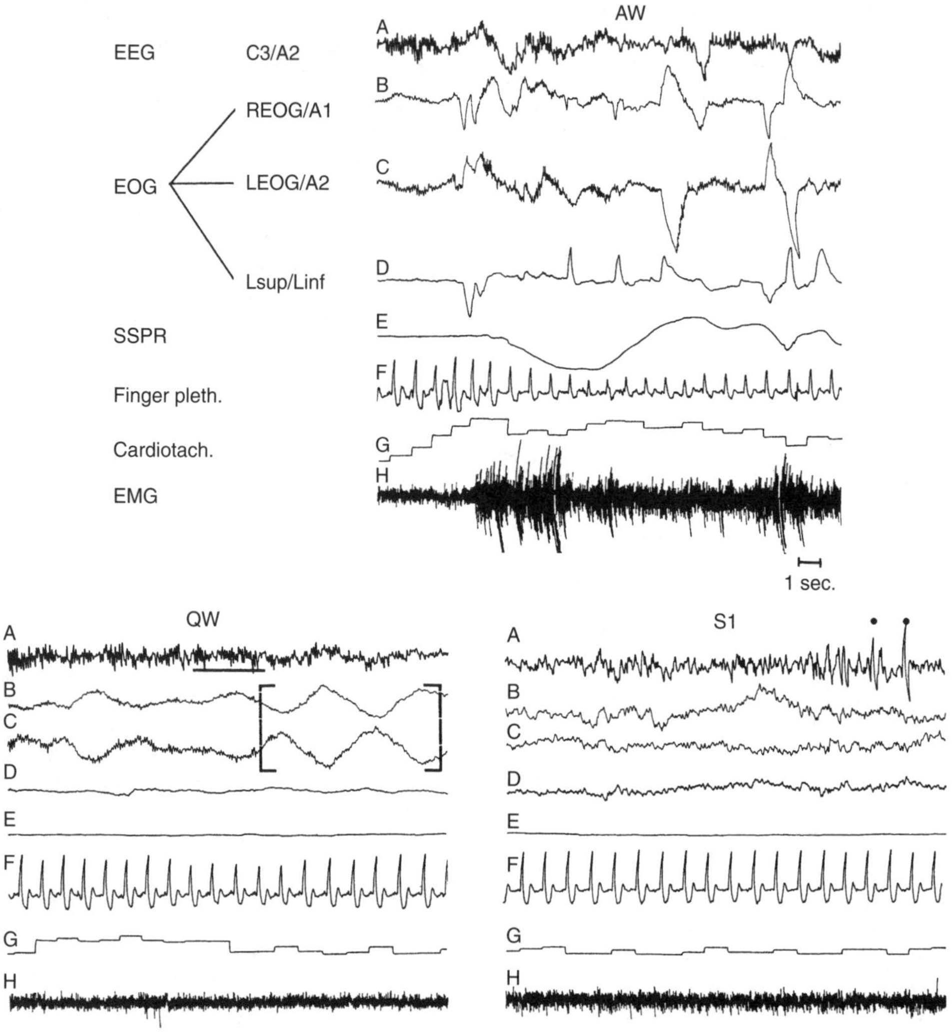

Figure XXIV-5.1 Polygraphic tracings of physiological measures associated with sleep-wakefulness state variations. Eight channels of activity (A–H) are depicted during active and quiet wakefulness (AW and QW, respectively) and the first stage of sleep (NREM stage 1, or S1). The recorded variables include the electroencephalogram (EEG; C3/A2, channel A), the electro-oculogram (EOG; horizontal [right and left outer canthi] and vertical [placements superior and inferior to right eye orbit], channels B, C, and D, respectively), autonomic activity (spontaneous skin potential response [SSPR], channel E), finger plethysmogram (channel F), cardiotachometer recordings (channel G), and the facial (orbicularis oris) electromyogram (EMG; channel H). In these examples, the passive decrease in EMG activity which commonly occurs at sleep onset (S1) does not become evident until slow-wave sleep (Figure XXIV-5.2, S3 and S4). Electrophysiological features of note are alpha activity (underscored, channel A) and slow, rolling eye movements (channels B and C) preceding sleep onset in QW, and vertex sharp waves in stage 1 (see dots, channel A). See text for discussion of sleep-stage definitions and electrophysiologic composition (Reproduced from Pivik, 2000, by permission of Cambridge University Press)

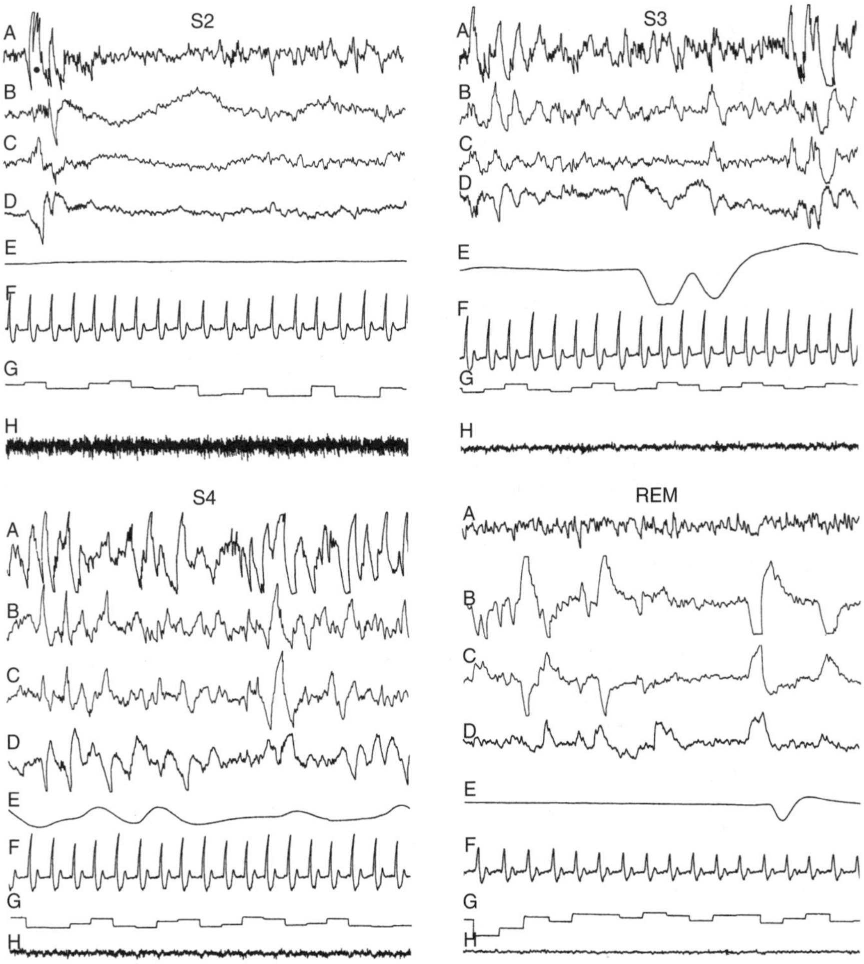

Figure XXIV-5.2 Polygraphic tracings of physiological measures associated with variations in sleep stages (NREM stages 2–4 [S2–S4] and REM). For explanation of channels A–H, see Figure XXIV-5.1. Of note is the occurrence of stage 2 K-complexes (see dot, channel A). See text for discussion of sleep stage definitions and electrophysiological composition (Reproduced from Pivik, 2000, by permission of Cambridge University Press)

sleep-stage analysis of adult human sleep published by Rechtschaffen and Kales (1968). These figures include the basic measures required for sleep evaluation (EEG, EOG, and EMG; channels A, B, C, and H), as well as optional measures, such as recordings of vertical eye movements (channel D) and autonomic activity (channels E, F, and G). In these illustrations, wakefulness (AW and W) is associated with a low-voltage, mixed-frequency EEG, blinking, rapid eye movements, and variations in the levels of tonic facial EMG activity.

As accurately described by Davis *et al.* (1938), 8–12 Hz alpha activity is diminished during the transition from wakefulness to sleep. This is accompanied by a slowing of EEG activity, an increase in 4–7 Hz theta activity, the sporadic occurrence of vertex sharp waves, and the appearance of slow horizontal eye movements, while facial muscle tonus may decrease relative to levels present during relaxed wakefulness (see Figure XXIV-5.1, S1). Stage 2 is defined by the intermittent occurrence of K-complexes and 12–14 Hz spindle activity against a background of relatively low amplitude, mixed-frequency EEG activity (Figure XXIV-5.2). Relative to stage 2, during stages 3 and 4 (slow-wave sleep) there are increasing amounts of delta activity (0.5–4 Hz) present in each scoring epoch. Stage 3 epochs must contain 20–50%, and stage 4 epochs more than 50%, of this activity (Figure XXIV-5.2). Collectively, stages 1–4 are referred to as non-REM (NREM) sleep. REM sleep is defined by a relatively low-voltage, mixed-frequency EEG, the absence of K-complexes or spindles, the sporadic occurrence of eye movements, and reduced levels of submental and facial EEG activity (Figure XXIV-5.2). Other distinctive EEG features which may be present during REM sleep are bursts of theta activity (sawtooth waves) preceding clusters of eye movements (Berger *et al.*, 1962), and alpha activity which is 1–2 Hz slower than subjects' waking alpha frequency (Johnson *et al.*, 1967).

Associated with these sleep stages are other variations in physiologic measures which, although not integral to stage determination, serve to reinforce and validate stage differentiation. Prominent among these are the presence of generalized physiologic activation during REM sleep, including increases in the rate and irregularity of respiratory (Snyder *et al.*, 1964; Aserinsky, 1965) and cardiovascular (Snyder *et al.*, 1963, 1964; Pivik *et al.*, 1996) activities, and increased density of eye movements as a function of time both within individual REM periods and within REM periods across the night (Aserinsky, 1969, 1971). Electrodermal activity in REM sleep is reduced and more similar in form to responses of this system during wakefulness (Broughton *et al.*, 1965; Hauri and Van de Castle, 1973b). These REM-associated variations occur against a background of centrally mediated inhibition of facial and submental musculature and spinal monosynaptic reflexes (Jouvet and Michel, 1959; Berger, 1961; Hodes and Dement, 1964; Jacobson *et al.*,

1964; Pompeiano, 1966, 1967). Other notable physiologic variations that occur in association with REM sleep include increases in body movements and K-complexes just prior to REM periods (Dement and Kleitman, 1957a; Pivik and Dement, 1968, Halasz *et al.*, 1977) and reduced numbers of K-complexes and increased spindle activity in the few minutes following REM periods (Pivik and Dement, 1968; Azumi *et al.*, 1975).

With the exception of unusual levels of autonomic, hormonal, and motor activation present during slow-wave sleep, physiological activation during most NREM sleep is unremarkable. During stage 4, for example, dramatic increases in electrodermal activity are common (Broughton *et al.*, 1965; Johnson and Lubin, 1966) (Figure XXIV-5.2). Electrodermal activation of this intensity would normally indicate enhanced arousal, yet the arousal threshold during stage 4 is higher than that of all other sleep stages (Goodenough *et al.*, 1965; Bonnet and Moore, 1982; Lammers and Badia, 1991; Busby *et al.*, 1994). An explanation consistent with these data attributes this overactivity to the release of subcortical control areas involved in the production of these responses from inhibition by higher centres, and not to a condition of enhanced physiological arousal (Johnson and Lubin, 1966; Johnson, 1973). During slow-wave sleep, approximately 80% of the total daily secretion of growth hormone is released (Takahashi *et al.*, 1968; Sassin *et al.*, 1969; Born *et al.*, 1988). It is also during this time that a variety of arousal disorders (termed parasomnias), characterized by varying degrees of motor and autonomic activity, occurs (Roffwarg, 1979). More detailed considerations of the nosology, description, and treatment of these and other sleep-related disorders are available (*International Classification of Sleep Disorders Diagnostic and Coding Manual* [*ICSD*, 1990] or *Principles and Practice of Sleep Medicine* [Kryger *et al.*, 2000]).

The nature and organization of the physiologic variations described above differ distinctly from those present during wakefulness, and these differences can be summarized as follows:

1. The presence of waveforms unique to sleep — for example, endogenously determined K-complexes, 12 to 14 Hz spindle activity, vertex sharp waves, and frontal sawtooth waves.
2. The prevalence and concentration of activities — for example, the enhancement of slower EEG frequencies (delta and theta), and the concentration of these and other activities, such as eye movements or galvanic skin responses (GSRs), at specific times of the night. With respect to EEG activity, computerized analyses have shown that in only rare instances is the EEG composed of a single frequency; even in the desynchronized low-voltage EEG of wakefulness in normal individuals, there is a small but nonetheless real component of delta activity present (Lubin *et al.*, 1969; Hoffman *et al.*, 1979). The shift away from the higher frequencies associated with arousal during wakefulness and the concentration on slower activities are what make sleep unique.
3. The predictable constellations of physiological patterns that occur — for example, concentrations of delta activity are associated with high GSR activation during slow-wave sleep, and indices of cortical, ocular-motor, and autonomic arousal are associated with sustained muscular inhibition during REM sleep (Pivik, 1986: p. 384).

In the course of studying the global patterns of state change during sleep another fundamental observation was made, that is, that sleep-stage pattern variations across the night were largely predictable from night to night, indicating the existence of the sleep cycle (Dement and Kleitman, 1957a) (Figure XXIV-5.3). Sleep profiles such as those illustrated in Figure XXIV-5.3 are useful for representing general sleep characteristics, such as latencies, cyclicity, stage distribution, and relative amounts of sleep disturbance. These graphs underscore the concentration of stage 4 in the first third of the night and REM sleep in the last third (Williams

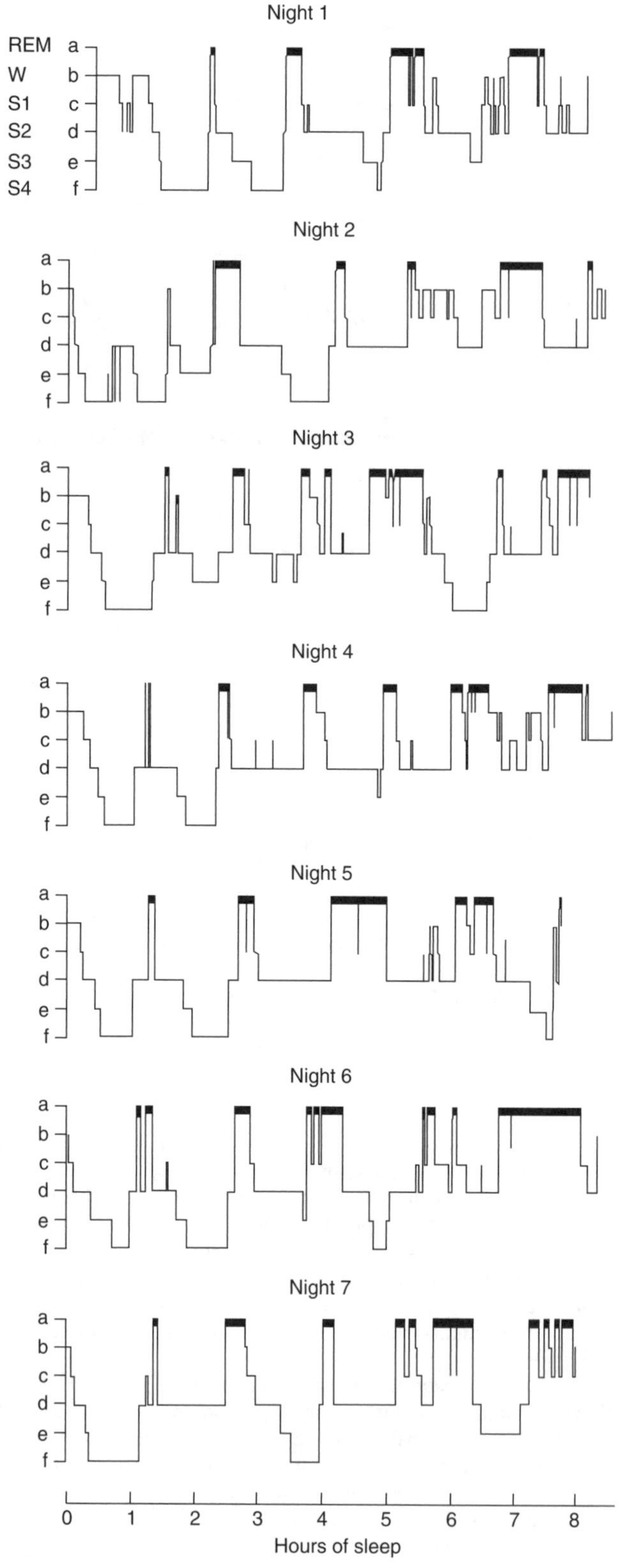

Figure XXIV-5.3 Sleep profiles depicting variations in sleep stages (ordinate) as a function of time asleep (abscissa). These profiles, based on seven consecutive nights of baseline sleep in a young adult, illustrate the stability of sleep patterns across nights, the presence of patterned oscillations between REM (darkened rectangles) and NREM sleep (i.e., sleep cycle), and the decrease in stage 4 and increase in REM sleep as a function of sleep time within a given night (Reproduced from Pivik, 2000, by permission of Cambridge University Press)

et al., 1964, 1966) — observations consistent with the exponential decrease in delta activity across the night as determined from computerized analyses of EEG sleep data (Feinberg *et al.*, 1978; 1980). Figure XXIV-5.3 also illustrates the relative difficulty in initiating REM mechanisms early in the night, as indicated by the latency to REM sleep (normally about 90 min) and the general brevity of REM periods that may occur during the first 2 h of sleep (Dement and Kleitman, 1957a; Berger and Oswald, 1962; Roffwarg *et al.*, 1966).

SLEEP COGNITION: DESCRIPTIVE ASPECTS

The discovery that dreaming is associated with a physiological state that recurs predictably across each night and which normally accounts for one quarter of each night of sleep in the adult, forced a reconsideration of beliefs that dreams occur only sporadically and under special conditions. It is not surprising, therefore, that the initial wave of psychophysiological studies of sleep following the discovery of REM sleep was significantly influenced by the belief that REM sleep provides an objective measure of dreaming, and that dreaming occurs only during these periods. These studies commonly reported high recall following arousals from REM sleep (approximately 80%) and a relative mental void in NREM sleep (less than 10% recall). There were also reports of subjects who typically failed to recall dreams even from REM sleep (Goodenough *et al.*, 1959; Goodenough, 1978). However, reports of mental activity following arousals from NREM sleep (Goodenough *et al.*, 1959) persisted. By 1967, there were nine such studies reporting NREM recall values of 23–74% (reviewed in Foulkes, 1967). The apparent discrepancy between the early and later studies regarding the presence of mental activity during NREM sleep can be attributed in part to differences in what investigators accepted as a dream report. The early studies did not provide a definition of what was required for an acceptable dream report, but relied rather on an intuitive and implicit understanding of the nature of the dream. Nevertheless, these studies provided an important insight into the nature of the dreaming process by indicating that in most individuals this process was most evident during REM sleep.

However, a systematic and effective evaluation of mental activity during sleep requires an operational definition of what would be accepted as a dream, and the suggested definitions have been wide-ranging. For example, Berger (1967: p. 16) defined the dream as a 'verbal report describing an occurrence involving multisensory images and sensations, frequently of a bizarre and unreal nature and involving the narrator himself', whereas Foulkes (1978: p. 3) extended this definition to include simply 'thinking'. The acceptance of more fragmentary and less perceptual reports as valid data revealed the presence of a much more extensive mental life during sleep; thus, reports of greater than 50% recall from NREM sleep arousals were not uncommon (Goodenough *et al.*, 1959; Foulkes, 1962; Pivik and Foulkes, 1968; Molinari and Foulkes, 1969; Zimmerman, 1970; Herman *et al.*, 1978). There were, however, qualitative distinctions between REM and NREM reports (Rechtschaffen *et al.*, 1963; Foulkes and Rechtschaffen, 1964; Pivik, 1971; Antrobus, 1983), and these may be characterized as follows:

> Reports obtained in periods of REM activity showed more organismic involvement in affective, visual and muscular dimensions and were more highly elaborated than non-REMP reports. REMP reports showed less correspondence to the waking life of the subjects than did reports from spindle and delta sleep. The relatively frequent occurrence of thinking and memory processes in spindle and delta sleep was an especially striking result (Foulkes, 1962: pp. 24–25).

Although REM reports were generally more complex, vivid, and bizarre, and NREM reports more mundane and less 'dream-like', NREM reports characterized as dreaming can be as common (Goodenough *et al.*, 1965) or more common (Foulkes, 1960, 1962; Rechtschaffen *et al.*, 1963; Bosinelli *et al.*, 1968; Pivik and Foulkes, 1968; Zimmerman, 1968; Pivik, 1971) than NREM thinking reports. However, with one exception, REM and NREM rep ts can be reliably distinguished (Monroe *et al.*, 1965; Bosinelli *et al.*, 1968). The exception relates to mentation elicited following arousals during sleep onset. Sleep onset mentation is similar to REM sleep on variables such as incidence, hallucinatory dramatic quality, and report length (Foulkes and Vogel, 1965; Foulkes *et al.*, 1966; Vogel *et al.*, 1966; Vogel, 1978), as well as perceptual and emotional qualities (Vogel *et al.*, 1972). The finding that dream-like mental activity is not restricted to REM sleep forced a rethinking of concepts such as those equating REM sleep deprivation with dream deprivation (Dement, 1960) or those suggesting that REM sleep dreams are vital to psychological normality during wakefulness (Sampson, 1965, 1966; Vogel *et al.*, 1975).

Recent research has suggested even more drastic revisions of traditional concepts regarding the occurrence and process of dreaming. For example, the presence of large amounts (40–70% of total sleep time) of REM sleep in infants presented an obvious problem for a strict identification of dreaming with this sleep stage (Roffwarg *et al.*, 1966; Pivik, 1983; Louis *et al.*, 1997). The implausibility of infants experiencing such an extensive dream life was recognized, and it forced the question of when in the course of early development the REM sleep dreaming association did become evident. When systematic studies of dreaming in early childhood were conducted (Foulkes, 1982; Foulkes *et al.*, 1990), they revealed that dreams with the formal properties present in adult dreams did not begin to appear until the age of 8 or 9 years, and required the processes used for imagery during waking. The conclusion was drawn that dreaming 'is a symbolic process with strong cognitive prerequisites and with a developmental history much like that of waking symbolic thought [and waking consciousness]' (Foulkes, 1996: p. 619). This parallelism between cognitive processes during waking and sleep is apparent in reports indicating the absence of visual imagery in the dreams of the congenitally blind or those blinded before the time when dreaming with properties similar to those in adults appears, but the presence of such imagery in the dreams of those blinded after this time (Foulkes, 1993; Kerr, 1993).

One implication of the developmental findings reviewed above is that the association between dreaming and REM sleep is not automatic and inevitable. There is a growing literature suggesting not only that dreaming is not confined to a particular sleep stage, but that it may even occur independently of sleep (Foulkes, 1985; Ellman and Antrobus, 1991; Antrobus and Bertini, 1992; Cavallero and Foulkes, 1993; Cicogna *et al.*, 2000). This more pervasive view of the occurrence of dreaming follows if the conditions and properties associated with this experience are distinguished from the larger state contexts in which they may occur. Accordingly, dreaming may be understood as 'the form assumed by consciousness whenever there is residual but somewhat dissociated cognitive/cerebral activation in the relative absence of direction either from the person's environment or from voluntary self-control' (Foulkes, 1997: p. 3). However, a better understanding of the processes defining or contributing to these experiences will require a more specific knowledge of the various brain areas and systems differentially active during dream and non-dream experiences. The use of functional imaging technology in the study of physiological and cognitive processes during sleep (Hong *et al.*, 1995; Maquet *et al.*, 1996; Braun *et al.*, 1997, 1998) promises to provide the kind of psychophysiological specificity necessary for these determinations. Of course, other processes integral to the study of dream experiences are also subject to state-determined influences and variations; for example, learning and memory are being examined in this regard (Maquet, 2001; Stickgold *et al.*, 2001; Siegel, 2001).

PSYCHOPHYSIOLOGICAL VARIATIONS ASSOCIATED WITH SLEEP DISORDERS

The preceding overview has shown that the marked behavioural and physiological differences between wakefulness and sleep are generally associated with equally marked differences in associated cognitive activity, with waking cognition being generally more organized, rational, and self-directed and sleep cognition more disorganized, irrational, and under little volitional control. Recognizing these state and condition influences on cognitive activity, and appreciating the nature and extent of differences between normal wakefulness and sleep along these dimensions, we may expect the physiological and behavioural correlates defining disorders of sleep to present with unusual and informative psychophysiological relationships. The full range of such relationships remains to be determined since the identification of sleep disorders is an ongoing process. Some appreciation of the breadth and complexity of these disorders can be gained from the number of listings presented in *The International Classification of Sleep Disorders* (1990) — the only systematic updating of sleep disorders since the first diagnostic classification appeared in 1979. This volume identifies 66 disorders, and includes a section describing another 11 disorders which are under consideration for inclusion pending further investigation. The organizational principles used to classify sleep disorders in this publication were generally adopted in the sleep disorders section of the most recent DSM edition (American Psychiatric Association, 1994). Basically, these disorders are differentiated according to whether they are considered primary sleep disorders, that is, those that are 'presumed to arise from endogenous abnormalities in sleep-wake generating or timing mechanisms' (American Psychiatric Association, 1994: p. 551), or whether they result from other conditions — specifically, mental disorders, medical conditions, or substance abuse. The following review will focus on disorders for which the nature of the psychophysiological relationships has been most thoroughly described, namely, those classified among the primary sleep disorders and those associated with mental disorders.

PRIMARY SLEEP DISORDERS

The primary sleep disorders present a wide array of behavioural conditions reflecting the consequences of disturbed sleep-wake control processes. These conditions have been divided into two general categories, namely, those associated with difficulties involving the amount, quality, or timing of sleep (the dyssomnias), and those characterized by disorders of arousal and state transition (the parasomnias).

Dyssomnias

One of the most prevalent of sleep disturbances — primary insomnia — is classified among the dyssomnias. The incidence of this problem in the general population has not been accurately determined. However, of those referred to sleep disorders clinics with complaints of chronic insomnia, 15–25% receive a diagnosis of primary insomnia, placing this second in prevalence only to diagnoses of insomnia related to mental disorders (46%) (American Psychiatric Association, 1994; Hajak, 2000). Although the term 'insomnia' implies an absence of sleep, the nature of the sleep disturbances associated with this disorder commonly involves difficulties in initiating (increased sleep latency) and maintaining sleep (frequent awakenings, and increases in stage 1 and decreases in stages 3 and 4 sleep). One type of primary insomnia, psychophysiological insomnia, is characterized by a combination of somatized tension, resulting in increased physiological arousal, and learned sleep-preventing associations, that is, a conditioning of bad sleep habits. It is therefore commonly referred to as 'learned' or 'behavioural' insomnia (Hauri, 2000). Studies have indicated a high level of dream recall in these subjects, attributed in part to the high frequency of awakenings (Schredl *et al.*, 1998). The dreams of these individuals have been reported to reflect waking life stressors (Schredl *et al.*, 1998), and reports following arousals from fragmented REM sleep have been characterized as vivid and frightening (Lee *et al.*, 1993), suggesting a complementarity of waking and sleep cognition in terms of concerns and affect.

The abutment of wakefulness and sleep states occurs nowhere as unexpectedly and suddenly as it does in patients with 'narcolepsy'. This term was first used in 1880 to describe the pathological occurrence of repetitive, brief episodes of irresistible sleep (Gélineau, 1880). Since that time, the association of these sleep attacks with a distinct set of clinical features has been recognized, and the latter now comprise the diagnostic criteria for this disorder. These features include: excessive daytime sleepiness; cataplexy — the sudden loss of muscle tone, most frequently precipitated by emotional behaviour such as laughter, surprise, or intense excitement; sleep paralysis — a condition of motor inhibition occurring while falling asleep or on awakening during which the individual is fully conscious and aware but unable to initiate any volitional motor activity; and hallucinations — either hypnogogic (occurring while falling asleep) or hypnopompic (occurring while awakening). This syndrome clearly involves a dysfunction of REM sleep mechanisms, as evidenced by the initiation of sleep by full-blown REM periods, or the presence of elements of REM sleep, that is, motor inhibitory processes and hallucinations, during waking-sleep state transitions (reviewed by Guilleminault and Anagnos, 2000). The abrupt and irresistible imposition of elements of REM sleep on the waking subject not only creates potentially hazardous physical situations for the many individuals afflicted with this disorder (prevalence estimated at ~0.05% [Dement *et al.*, 1972, 1973]), but may also introduce psychological disturbances. The latter have been related to the unusual psychophysiological circumstances brought about by the rapid transition from waking consciousness to that associated with REM sleep physiology — a state transition that is associated with striking changes in state-related brain functional relationships (Hong *et al.*, 1995; Braun *et al.*, 1998).

Normally, the transition from wakefulness to sleep is characterized by a gradual relinquishing of waking conscious control that occurs across a succession of introspective stages. Kleitman (1963) considered Vihvelin's (1948) three-stage description as representative of this process and summarized these stages as follows: '(a) a progressive narrowing of the field of consciousness, as a quantitative change in psychological processes; (b) a stage of "pure" hypnagogic hallucinations, as a qualitative change in psychological processes; and (c) a vacillation between wakefulness and sleep, when hypnagogic hallucinations are confused with dreams' (pp. 79–80). Later studies (Foulkes and Vogel, 1965; Vogel *et al.*, 1966) tied the sleep onset-associated psychological changes to EEG and EOG patterns present during this time. Vogel *et al.* (1966), in summarizing the corresponding psychophysiological changes occurring during this state transition, noted that the progression from relaxed wakefulness (characterized by alpha activity and occasional rapid eye movements), through stage 1 sleep and into stage 2 sleep was associated with a progressive loss of control over the course of mental activity, then a loss of awareness of the environment, and finally a loss of reality orientation and the onset of hallucinations. These progressive variations characteristic of normal wakefulness-sleep transitions are bypassed during narcoleptic sleep attacks. During these episodes, the sudden interruption of waking physiological processes by those of REM sleep can create an unusual and disturbing mental state in which the hallucinatory processes characteristic of REM sleep cognition are joined with the incorporation of elements from the patient's waking environment. The result is a confusing mental experience in which the boundaries between dreaming and reality are blurred to the extent that patients question their sanity (Broughton, 1982; Zarcone and Fuchs, 1976) or may sincerely believe that a hallucinatory experience, such as sexual abuse, was real (Hays, 1992). Many of the dreams of narcoleptics, whether occurring at sleep onset or during nocturnal sleep, are particularly intense, bizarre, and frightening (Ribstein, 1976; Broughton, 1982; Lee *et al.*, 1993; American Psychiatric Association, 1994; Schredl, 1998). In part, these characteristics may reflect the influence of the fragmentation of REM sleep (Montplaisir *et al.*, 1978) or the effects associated with motor inhibitory processes (that is, sleep paralysis) (Ribstein, 1976; Honda, 1988).

Parasomnias

The disorders represented among the parasomnias include behaviours disruptive of sleep that develop during sleep-wake transitions or during sleep. Many of these are behaviours that are normally confined to wakefulness (walking, talking, or urinating) and others, such as sleep terrors and nightmares, reflect intense physiological or behavioural disturbances peculiar to sleep. These disorders may be sleep-stage specific in their expression (sleepwalking and sleep terrors during slow-wave sleep and nightmares during REM sleep) or may occur throughout sleep (sleep talking and enuresis). Several develop early in life and resolve before adulthood (night terrors, sleepwalking, and enuresis), whereas others typically emerge in adults (REM sleep behaviour disorder).

The study of mental activity associated with various parasomnias has provided informative, and at times surprising, insights into brain–behaviour relationships. For example, consistent with findings indicating reduced recall of sleep mentation after awakenings from slow-wave sleep (Pivik and Foulkes, 1968; Pivik, 1971; Armitage, 1980), the recall of mental experiences associated with parasomnias occurring during slow-wave sleep (sleepwalking and sleep terrors) is limited and fragmentary (see Pivik, 2000a and Nielsen and Zadra, 2000 for reviews). This relative absence of recall seems particularly remarkable when associated with the marked physiological arousal and expressiveness that occurs during sleep terrors. During these episodes, subjects appear to be responding to frightful and horrific thoughts and images. Although an identification of these experiences with nightmares may seem warranted, sleep terrors and nightmares have been shown to be clearly differentiated along several dimensions — including time of occurrence — as well as in terms of behavioural and physiological correlates (Nielsen and Zadra, 2000).

The inability to access mental experiences more directly during sleep behaviours such as sleep terrors and nightmares while these experiences are ongoing frustrates our attempts at better understanding of these behaviours. Verbal communication with the sleeping subject could circumvent this barrier, and the spontaneous occurrence of talking during sleep would appear to provide unique access to the sleeping mind. Furthermore, this access would span both REM and NREM sleep since sleep talking — although most prevalent during slow-wave sleep — may occur in all sleep stages (Arkin, 1991). Unfortunately, it has not been possible to initiate and maintain intelligent dialogue with subjects while they are asleep, and attempts to induce subjects to relate ongoing mentation while remaining asleep via posthypnotic suggestions have not been successful (Arkin *et al.*, 1970; Arkin, 1978). Moreover, when reports have been available to assess the relationship between what was said and what was reported, the degree of concordance is quite variable, and often no discernible association is evident (Arkin, 1991).

The unique physiological and psychological attributes that set REM sleep apart from other waking and sleep states provide the basis for an unusual group of parasomnias associated with this state. These can be quite dramatic and exceptionally intense in their expression, and their consequences may include immediate and extended effects that are both mental and physical in nature. Perhaps the most readily recognized among these disorders is the nightmare. The essential characteristics and ramifications of these frightening dream experiences have been succinctly summarized as follows:

> Nightmares typically occur in a lengthy, elaborate dream sequence that is highly anxiety provoking or terrifying. Dream content most often focuses on imminent physical danger to the individual (e.g., pursuit, attack, injury). In other cases, the perceived danger may be more subtle, involving personal failure or embarrassment. Nightmares that occur after traumatic experiences may replicate the original dangerous or threatening situation, but most nightmares do not recount actual events. On awakening, individuals with this disorder can describe the dream sequence and content in detail. Nightmares usually terminate with an awakening that is associated with a rapid return to full alertness and a lingering sense of fear or anxiety. These factors often lead to difficulty returning to sleep. Nightmare Disorder causes significant subjective distress more often than it causes demonstrable social or occupational impairment. However, if nocturnal awakenings are frequent, or if the individual avoids sleeping because of fear of nightmares, the individual may experience excessive sleepiness, poor concentration, depression, anxiety, or irritability that can disrupt daytime functioning. (American Psychiatric Association, 1994: p. 580).

Nightmares are experienced by individuals of all ages, but because of a variety of factors — such as diverse study populations, varying frequency criteria, and different methods of assessment (retrospective self-report vs. daily logs) — reliable estimates of prevalence have been difficult to determine. It is agreed, however, that although this disorder is most common in children (rates of 10–90%), its presence in the adult population remains substantial (8–25%) (Neilsen and Zadra, 2000; Partinen and Hublin, 2000). Despite the prevalence of this form of dream disturbance, the causal factors for these experiences have not been extensively studied and are not well understood. Psychopathology has been implicated, but the findings have not been consistent (reviewed by Nielsen and Zadra, 2000). Possible insights into the mechanisms underlying the nightmare that might come from physiological studies of sleep have been limited because of the paucity of such investigations. Although the general nature of the findings has not been particularly surprising, that is, increased autonomic activation (Fisher *et al.*, 1970, 1973; Nielsen and Zadra, 1997) and signs of increased EEG arousal (Nielsen *et al.*, in press), the degree of autonomic activation was unexpectedly low given the intensity of the associated psychological experiences. As a possible explanation for these findings, it has been suggested that a dissociative process similar to that thought to be effected by behavioural therapies, such as systematic desensitization and flooding, may be invoked. This process is postulated to reduce the level of sympathetic activation that normally occurs in association with the processing of stressful imagery, effectively desomatizing the imagery (Fisher *et al.*, 1970; Perlis and Nielsen, 1993; Nielsen and Zadra, 2000). Although the persistence of such complex functional relationships across sleep-waking states is uncommon, the uncoupling of physiological activation and cognitive activity during sleep is not. For example, the intense levels of electrodermal activity that regularly occur during stages 3 and 4 sleep (Burch, 1965) apparently have little effect on the recall or qualitative aspects of sleep mentation (Hauri and Rechtschaffen, 1963; Pivik, 1971; Tracy and Tracy, 1974). Similarly, it might be expected that because of the common occurrence during REM sleep of penile erections (Fisher *et al.*, 1965; Karacan *et al.*, 1966) and clitoral engorgement

(Cohen and Shapiro, 1970), many REM reports would contain overt sexual content. However, with the exception of lucid dream reports (LaBerge *et al.*, 1983; Laberge, 1985), REM reports with such features are uncommon (Fisher, 1966; Hall and Van de Castle, 1966). Furthermore, even during lucid dreams containing sexual activity, there is some dissociation between content and associated autonomic activity; that is, expected variations have been observed for respiration and skin conductance measures, but not for heart rate (LaBerge, 1985; 1992).

A final example of psychophysiological relationships present during wakefulness that do not persist unchanged during sleep comes from studies examining the correspondence between the visual aspects of dream imagery and the rapid eye movements of REM sleep. The discovery that dreams are associated with a physiological sleep state during which eye movements are prominent suggested the possibility that these eye movements serve the same function during sleep as they do during wakefulness, that is, to track positional changes in visual targets. Attempts to demonstrate this relationship, which came to be known as the scanning hypothesis (Roffwarg *et al.*, 1962), have been largely unsuccessful (reviewed by Rechtschaffen, 1973; Pivik, 1991). However, more positive relationships between eye movement and dream imagery may exist in lucid dreams (LaBerge, 1992), and imaging procedures have indicated that the same cortical areas are involved in the control of eye movements during waking and REM sleep (Hong *et al.*, 1995).

Two other types of REM-associated parasomnias — sleep paralysis and REM sleep behaviour disorder — can be viewed as cases of dissociative behaviours. This perspective is understandable when it is recognized that the REM state consists of the integration of activities from different sensory and motor systems — as evidenced in the disparate physiological activities that define and characterize this state, that is, EEG activation, motor inhibition, eye movements, and autonomic variability — and that these various systems are selectively susceptible to malfunctions that compromise normal sleep-wake state boundaries and result in abnormal amalgamations of sleep and waking behaviours. Sleep paralysis — the experience of motor inhibition during the process of falling asleep or waking up — is an example of such a malfunction. In this case, inhibitory processes involved in the suppression of motor activity during REM sleep occur independently of REM sleep and in conjunction with conscious awareness (Hishikawa and Shimuzu, 1995; Hishikawa, 1976). Sleep paralysis is a cardinal symptom of narcolepsy, but occurs independently of this disorder at least once in the lifetimes of 25–50% of the general population (Spanos *et al.*, 1995; Fukuda *et al.*, 1998; Cheyne *et al.*, 1999; ICSD, 1990). As a chronic complaint, isolated sleep paralysis is reported to have only a 3–6% prevalence rate (ICSD, 1990).

The psychological experiences accompanying these sleep paralysis episodes are distinguished by elements of fear, terror, and panic, often occurring together with sensory hallucinations (Hishikawa, 1976; Hufford, 1982; Buzzi and Cirignotta, 2000). Although these episodes occur at times of state transition during which hallucinatory experiences are common, it is clear that the latter experiences can, and generally do, occur independently of this motor inhibition (Buzzi and Cirignotta, 2000; Nielsen and Zadra, 2000). Even during sleep, arousals made during times of tonic EMG suppression occurring just prior to, but still independently of, REM sleep onset are not associated with either greater recall frequency or reports that are more dream-like (Larson and Foulkes, 1969; Pivik, 1971). Clearly, however, the awareness of motor inhibitory effects during these transitory states can contribute directly to the concurrent cognitive experiences. This is apparent in the reports of the threatening and terrifying feelings that develop in association with the restrictions in movement and respiration that characterize this condition (Hishikawa, 1976; Hufford, 1982). It has been suggested, however, that mental experiences occurring in association with sleep paralysis may be intensified relative to hypnagogic and hypnopompic experiences not accompanied by this motor inhibition (Hufford, 1982; Takeuchi *et al.*, 1994), but the processes involved have not been specified.

Whereas sleep paralysis represents the displacement of REM-associated motor inhibitory processes from REM sleep to sleep-wake transitional states, REM sleep behaviour disorder (RBD) results from the failure of these inhibitory processes to be maintained during REM sleep. This disorder typically develops later in life (after the age of 50 years) and occurs predominantly in men (Mahowald and Schenck, 2000; Olson *et al.*, 2000). The overall prevalence rate for this disorder has been reported to be 0.5% (Ohayon *et al.*, 1997). Recognized as a distinct clinical disorder in 1986 (Schenck *et al.*, 1986), this disorder was included for the first time in the latest edition of the *Diagnostic and Statistical Manual of Mental Disorders* (American Psychiatric Association, 1994).

It is not uncommon for motor inhibition to vary in intensity during REM sleep. Depending on the duration of such reduced inhibition and covariations in other physiological measures, these intervals would normally be interpreted as interruptions in the continuity of REM sleep periods and would be scored as stage 1 sleep or relaxed wakefulness. Certainly, these episodes would go behaviourally unnoticed. What sets these transient reductions in inhibition apart from the loss of inhibition in RBD is the remarkable behaviours that occur at these times in RBD. These outbursts are characterized by excessive motor activity that often results in injuries to individuals or their sleeping partner (Mahowald and Schenck, 2000; Olson *et al.*, 2000). These behaviours are usually related to the associated dream content which commonly deals with themes involving acts of aggression and defence, and may be considered to represent instances where dreams are being acted out. The notion that the motor inhibition during REM sleep may function to prevent the expression of hallucinatory activities finds support in animal studies in which selective subcortical lesions are followed by hallucinatory-like behaviours at times when REM sleep periods are expected to occur (Jouvet and Delorme, 1965; Henley and Morrison, 1974; Morrison *et al.*, 1979). However, the general restriction of these outbursts in RBD to dream behaviour of a violent nature (Nielsen and Zarda, 2000; Mahowald and Schenck, 2000; Olson *et al.*, 2000) and evidence that RBD behaviours can occur despite the presence of full muscle atonia (Schenck *et al.*, 1988; Lapierre and Montplaisir, 1992) precludes the general conclusion that muscle atonia during REM sleep normally functions to prevent the acting out of dreams.

MENTAL DISORDERS

The association between disordered minds and disordered sleep has been recognized for centuries. In the fifth century AD, Caelius Aurelianus noted that 'those who are on the verge of phrenitis or are slipping into the disease show the following signs: continual sleeplessness or troubled sleep with confused dreams' (p. 21). He later advised, 'Then in all cases let the patients sleep — for timely sleep refreshes no less than food' (p. 49) (Drabkin, 1950). Hundreds of years later, in 1892, Hammond, a psychiatrist, stated: 'In my opinion no one cause is so productive of cerebral afflictions as persistent wakefulness' (Hammond, 1892: p. 174). It was to be expected, therefore, that when methods allowing a more extensive and thorough evaluation of sleep became available, they would be applied to the study of sleep in patients with psychiatric disorders. It is of historical interest that the new sleep research became focused almost immediately upon studies of psychiatric patients. To a great extent, this was determined by one of the more remarkable revelations made regarding sleep — namely, the finding that dreaming was associated with a physiological sleep state that occurred predictably each night. The opening up of this new cognitive territory to systematic study and the influence of earlier speculations linking dreams and psychoses (Wundt, 1897; Jackson, 1958) served to attract many psychiatrists and psychologists to this new discipline, thereby ensuring a cognitive emphasis for these early studies. Among mental disorders, those receiving the greatest attention from sleep researchers have been schizophrenia, and mood and anxiety disorders.

Schizophrenia

The earliest investigations applying the new technology to the study of sleep were conducted in individuals diagnosed with schizophrenia (Dement, 1955; Koresko *et al.*, 1963; Rechtschaffen *et al.*, 1964). Schizophrenia is a very debilitating illness, characterized by a wide range of cognitive and motor symptoms — including the presence of delusions and hallucinations, disorganized speech, and disturbed affect — that occurs in 0.4–2.7% of the population (Benson and Zarcone, 2000). Beliefs of an identity between the processes underlying hallucinations and dreams (Jackson, 1958; Jung, 1960) raised exciting possibilities that studies of sleep in these patients might provide significant insights into the pathophysiology of their disorder. The initial wave of studies failed to find evidence of REM sleep abnormalities (Dement, 1955; Koresko *et al.*, 1963) or indications of REM sleep physiology during waking hallucinations in these patients (Rechtschaffen *et al.*, 1964).

Although subsequent research has identified parameters which distinguish sleep in schizophrenia from that in age-matched comparison groups, such as poor sleep efficiency, shorter latency to the onset of the first REM period (REM latency), and reduced amounts of slow-wave sleep (see Benson and Zarcone, 2000), the research emphasis in this population has been on relationships between REM sleep mechanisms and hallucinations. A significant role in this research has been played by a procedure designed to determine the consequences of the elimination of dreaming upon behaviour. This procedure, originally termed ‘dream deprivation’, involved awakening subjects at the onset of each REM period and was based on the premise that if REM periods were prevented from occurring, dreaming could not take place. The initial studies applied this technique to non-schizophrenic subjects, and the results were interpreted as indicating that dreaming or REM sleep was essential to waking psychological normality (Dement, 1960; Dement and Fisher, 1963; Sampson, 1965, 1966). Not only has subsequent research failed to support this interpretation of those data (Vogel, 1975), but there are indications that for some clinical groups REM deprivation may have beneficial effects on waking symptomatology (Vogel, 1968; Vogel *et al.*, 1975).

Although the psychological sequelae of REM deprivation did not indicate the existence of a simple transfer function between hallucinatory activity during sleep and wakefulness in schizophrenia, there were other consequences of REM deprivation that offered possible explanations of how such interactions might take place. The most prominent of these were increases in the amount of time spent in REM sleep following deprivation (the REM rebound) and an apparent intensification of physiological activity within REM periods, such as increases in phasic events such as brief muscle twitches and eye movements (Dement, 1960; Dement *et al.*, 1966; Dement *et al.*, 1969). Reports indicating reductions in the amount of REM rebound in actively ill schizophrenics compared to those in remission or to normal subjects raised the possibility that REM-associated behaviours were being expressed during, or ‘leaking out’ into, wakefulness (Azumi *et al.*, 1967; Zarcone *et al.*, 1968; Gillin *et al.*, 1974; Jus *et al.*, 1977). However, these findings were not consistently observed (see Vogel, 1975), and adverse psychological effects of REM deprivation in such subjects have not been observed (Vogel, 1975; Vogel *et al.*, 1975; Hoyt and Singer, 1978; Benson and Zarcone, 2000). Similarly, extensive examination of variations in indices of REM sleep phasic activity during sleep in these patients, as well as investigations into the relationship of these events to sleep cognition in normal subjects, has not demonstrated the hoped-for identity between these events and hallucinatory activity (Pivik, 1986, 2000b; Benson and Zarcone, 2000).

Relative to the research effort that has been expended in investigating the physiology of sleep in schizophrenia, the research devoted to the study of dream content in these patients has been minimal. It would be quite amazing if the mental experiences of these patients during sleep did not reflect their waking psychopathology, and observations made by Dement (1955) in the first study of these patients after the discovery of REM sleep appeared to confirm this expectation. In that study, he noted the unusual presence of inanimate, stationary objects in over half the reports he obtained. A review of reports limited to the characteristics of dream content in schizophrenia that have been verified, that is, have been replicated at least once (Kramer and Roth, 1979), was limited to 22 studies — only 11 of which were conducted in sleep laboratories. From the entire series of studies, the authors characterized the dreams of schizophrenics as ‘more hostile, more affective, and containing more evidence of the schizophrenic thought disorder, i.e., unrealistic, bizarre, and so on, than those of non-schizophrenics’ (p. 381). A subsequent review more than two decades later could add only six more papers to this list, and concluded that these ‘few additional articles on dreaming in schizophrenia contributed little to our knowledge of the dreams of these patients. The inattention to dreams in schizophrenia may be part of the shift from the psychological to the biological study of psychiatric disorders, and more particularly to the greater interest in mood disorders than in schizophrenia’ (Kramer, 2000: p. 513).

Mood Disorders

It is true that mood disorders have been the subject of intense study. This interest appears to be proportional to the prevalence rate of these disorders in the general population and to the prevalence of sleep disturbance among those with this diagnosis. Major depression, the most common of the mood disorders, is present in 5–12% of men and 10–25% of women (Boyd and Weissman, 1981). Furthermore, as indicated in a recent review, this disorder ‘has been studied polysomnographically more than any other psychiatric disorder, and the majority of patients have shown objective sleep disturbances’ (Benca, 2000, pp. 1142–1143). Common subjective complaints regarding sleep problems in these patients emphasize difficulties in initiating and maintaining sleep and include reports of disturbing dreams (Benca 2000). The sleep disturbances are generally pervasive throughout sleep and are not limited to a specific time of night, sleep stage, or process. They are reflected in measures indicating compromised sleep continuity (increased sleep latency, sleep fragmentation by awakenings, and early morning awakening [Oswald *et al.*, 1963; Zung *et al.*, 1964; Gresham *et al.*, 1965]), decreased slow-wave sleep (Hawkins and Mendels, 1966; Gillin *et al.*, 1979; Kupfer *et al.*, 1985), and REM sleep abnormalities (reduced latency to the first REM period [Kupfer and Foster, 1972; Akiskal *et al.*, 1982; Emslie *et al.*, 1990], prolonged duration of the first REM period [Feinberg *et al.*, 1982; Borbély *et al.*, 1984], and increased eye movement density during REM sleep [Kupfer *et al.*, 1985; Waller *et al.*, 1989]).

The general reliability of these findings, together with insights provided by various treatment procedures that have proven to have antidepressant effects — such as pharmacologic and behavioural (sleep deprivation) interventions—have led to the development of several hypotheses to account for the observed interactions among depression, sleep, and treatment variables. Prominent among these have been explanations attributing various features of these interactions to the adverse effects of excessive REM sleep in these patients (the REM pressure hypothesis [Vogel, 1975; Vogel *et al.*, 1975]), irregularities in the neurochemical control of REM sleep (the cholinergic-aminergic imbalance hypothesis [Jankowski *et al.*, 1972; McCarley, 1982; Sitaram *et al.*, 1984]), variations in the circadian control of REM sleep, and autonomic and hormonal variables (the phase-advance hypothesis [Wehr and Wirz-Justice, 1981; Wehr *et al.*, 1983]), and a deficiency in homeostatic sleep-inducing processes (the process S deficiency hypothesis [Borbély and Wirz-Justice, 1982]). A recent review that summarized the rationale, strengths, and weaknesses of these hypotheses concluded that, although each offered plausible explanations for some of the recognized sleep and depression relationships, none provided a full accounting for these findings (Benca, 2000).

From his review of 31 studies examining dream characteristics in depressed individuals, Kramer (2000) concluded that 'in depression there is a decrease in the frequency and length of dream reports. The dreams are commonplace, but have content characteristics of interest. There is an increase in death themes in depressed suicidal patients and in bipolar patients before becoming manic.... It is evident that a past focus is not universal in depression, nor indeed was it unique to the depressed state. Affects such as anxiety and hostility are not prominent in their dreams' (p. 514).

Some observations that have been made in these studies are especially relevant to issues of the interactions between cognitive activity during sleep and wakefulness. For example, poorer treatment outcome or greater difficulty in problem resolution has been associated with distinct qualitative dream features, as in disorganized dreams without human characters (Greenberg *et al.*, 1990), masochism (Cartwright and, Wood, 1993), or the extent to which problems are incorporated into the dream (Cartwright, 1991). Such findings not only have prognostic implications, but are consistent with suggestions that dreams in these patients may facilitate waking coping functions (Kramer, 1993).

Anxiety Disorders

That an experience may have profound extended effects on both waking and sleep behaviour is nowhere better exemplified than in subjects with post-traumatic stress disorder. Following the traumatic experience, these subjects typically exhibit a range of anxiety and fear-related symptoms and repeatedly relive or re-experience the event in the form of intrusive images and thoughts during wakefulness, and arousal disturbances and nightmares during sleep (American Psychiatric Association, 1994). In a general population survey, Helzer *et al.* (1987) reported a 1% general prevalence among those surveyed, with an increase to 3.5% if they had been physically attacked or had served in Vietnam.

Sleep-related disturbances are a common, and often the principal, complaint among patients with this disorder (Kramer, 1979; Kramer *et al.*, 1984; Mellman and Davis, 1985). These disturbances are reflected as problems with initiating or maintaining sleep, and sleep disturbance as a result of nightmares occurs in over half of these patients (Horowitz *et al.*, 1980; van der Kolk *et al.*, 1980; Mellman and Davis, 1985). In addition to the obvious REM-related nature of many of these disturbances (Ross *et al.*, 1989), arousals may also develop from NREM sleep (Schlosberg and Benjamin, 1978; van der Kolk *et al.*, 1984; Hefez *et al.*, 1987). However, Uhde (2000) has noted that, despite the absence of a specific REM sleep parameter that was consistently deviant in this disorder, 'it is nevertheless impressive how often *some* type of REM-related abnormality is reported in patients with post-traumatic stress disorder' (p. 1135).

The nature of dreams in patients with this disorder has been a focus of extensive research. Kramer (1979) has argued that disturbing dreams are more defining as characteristics of this disorder than are the other observed sleep disturbances. In summarizing his review of 61 articles that have been published on this topic during the past 34 years, Kramer concluded: 'An adequate characterization of the phenomenology of the disturbing dream remains to be done. It can be confirmed that the dream is disturbing and that the dream events may be outside the realm of current waking experience. The literature does not support the position that the dream is affect-laden or that the dream is easy to recall. It is not known if the dream is any more or less vivid than other dreams' (p. 516).

CONCLUSIONS

This review began with a statement about how understanding what is normal is a prerequisite for understanding what is not. Often, what comes to be recognized as normal borders on the unbelievable. For example, 50 years ago it was inconceivable that hallucinations accompanied by paralysis would occur predictably 4–6 times each night (that is, REM sleep). The nature of some abnormalities also strains the imagination. For example, how could it be that individuals would not only stop breathing while asleep, but also remain unaware this had happened even though it occurred hundreds of time during the night (that is, sleep apnoea)? The cataloguing of normal and abnormal sleep behaviours in this paper, while not exhaustive, does give an indication of the wide range of forms these behaviours may assume, and does provide a glimpse of the complexity of the physiological and psychological processes that accompany these variations.

The generally negative impact of disordered processes on both sleep and waking behaviours—whether emanating primarily from sleep or wakefulness—would seem to force the conclusion that whatever individual or symbiotic functions are served by these states, they are best satisfied with as little between-state interference as possible. However, the dependence of these states on the same biological substrates—although functionally reorganized for some behaviours—makes it inevitable that the barrier separating sleep and wakefulness would be vulnerable to cross-state influences. Usually, these border violations result in minor disturbances in state continuity (sleep fragmentation or decreases in waking attention), but they may also be expressed as dramatic and debilitating full-scale invasions when inappropriate waking behaviours erupt during sleep (as in REM behaviour disorder) or wakefulness is abruptly terminated by the imposition of sleep (as in narcolepsy).

Presumably, if a condition of functional balance were to be achieved between states, it would be reflected in the absence of adverse cross-state influences. However, since achieving such a condition of détente is obviously difficult (but perhaps not impossible; see Carskadon, 1979; Dement and Carskadon, 1982), the biological permission for between-state interactions that exists—even though it may at times work to great behavioural disadvantage—must be considered normal and perhaps functional. It is the task of future research—guided rather than constrained by prevailing theories—to re-examine and revise current concepts and definitions of state and normality, and to provide a more informed understanding of the bases for ordered and disordered behaviours and their relationships to one another.

ACKNOWLEDGEMENTS

The author gratefully acknowledges the assistance of Patricia Sumner, Marcy Young and Kevin Tennal in the preparation of this paper.

REFERENCES

Akiskal, H.S., Lemmi, H., Yerevanian, B., King, D. and Belluomini, J., 1982. The utility of the REM latency test in psychiatric diagnosis: a study of 81 depressed outpatients. *Psychiatry Research*, **7**, 101–110.

American Psychiatric Association, 1917. *Diagnostic and Statistical Manual of Mental Disorders*. American Psychiatric Association Press, Washington, DC.

American Psychiatric Association, 1952. *Diagnostic and Statistical Manual of Mental Disorders*. American Psychiatric Association Press, Washington, DC.

American Psychiatric Association, 1968. *Diagnostic and Statistical Manual of Mental Disorders* (2nd edn). American Psychiatric Association Press, Washington, DC.

American Psychiatric Association, 1980. *Diagnostic and Statistical Manual of Mental Disorders* (3rd edn). American Psychiatric Association Press, Washington, DC.

American Psychiatric Association, 1994. *Diagnostic and Statistical Manual of Mental Disorders* (4th edn). American Psychiatric Association Press, Washington, DC.

Antrobus, J.S., 1983. REM and NREM sleep reports: comparison of word frequencies by cognitive classes. *Psychophysiology*, **20**, 562–568.

Antrobus, J.S. and Bertini, M. (eds), 1992. *The Neuropsychology of Sleep and Dreaming*. Erlbaum, Hillsdale, New Jersey.

Arkin, A.M., 1978. Sleep talking. In: Arkin, A.M., Antrobus, J.S. and Ellman, S.J. (eds), *The Mind in Sleep: Psychology and Psychophysiology*, pp. 513–532. Erlbaum, Hillsdale, New Jersey.

Arkin, A.M., 1991. Sleep talking. In: Arkin, A.M., Antrobus, J.S. and Ellman, S.J. (eds), *The Mind in Sleep: Psychology and Psychophysiology*, pp. 415–436. Erlbaum, Hillsdale, New Jersey.

Arkin, A.M., Toth, M., Baker, J. and Hastey, J.M., 1970. The frequency of sleep-talking in the laboratory among chronic sleep-talkers and good dream recallers. *Journal of Nervous and Mental Disorders*, **151**, 369–374.

Armitage, R., 1980. Changes in Dream Content as a Function of Time of Night, Stage of Awakening and Frequency of Recall. Master's Thesis, Carleton University, Ottawa, Ontario, Canada.

Aserinsky, E., 1965. Periodic respiratory pattern occurring in conjunction with eye movements during sleep. *Science*, **150**, 763–766.

Aserinsky, E., 1969. The maximal capacity for sleep: rapid eye movement density as an index of sleep satiety. *Biological Psychiatry*, **1**, 147–159.

Aserinsky, E., 1971. Rapid eye movement density and pattern in the sleep of normal young adults. *Psychophysiology*, **8**, 361–375.

Aserinsky, E. and Kleitman, N., 1953. Regularly occurring periods of eye motility and concomitant phenomena during sleep. *Science*, **118**, 273–275.

Aserinsky, E. and Kleitman, N., 1955. Two types of ocular motility occurring during sleep. *Journal of Applied Physiology*, **8**, 1–10.

Association of Sleep Disorder Centers, 1979. *Diagnostic Classification of Sleep and Arousal Disorders.* Sleep Disorders Classification Committee, HP Roffwarg, Chairman, *Sleep*, **2**, 1–137.

Azumi, K., Shirakawa, S. and Takahashi, S., 1975. Periodicity of sleep spindle appearance in normal adults. *Sleep Research*, **4**, 263 [Abstract].

Azumi, K., Takahashi, S., Takahashi, K., Maruyama, N. and Kikuti, S., 1967. The effects of dream deprivation on chronic schizophrenics and normal adults: a comparative study. *Folia Psychiatrica et Neurologica Japonica*, **21**, 205–225.

Benca, R.M., 2000. Mood disorders. In: Kryger, M.H., Roth, T. and Dement, W.C. (eds), *Principles and Practices of Sleep Medicine* (3rd edn), pp. 1140–1158. WB Saunders, Philadelphia.

Benson, K.L. and Zarcone, V.P., 1994. Sleep abnormalities in schizophrenia and other psychotic disorders. In: Oldham, J.M. and Riba, M.B. (eds), *Review of Psychology (Volume 13)*, pp. 677–705. American Psychiatric Press, Washington, DC.

Benson, K.L. and Zarcone, V.P., 2000. Schizophrenia. In: Kryger, M.H., Roth, T. and Dement, W.C. (eds), *Principles and Practices of Sleep Medicine* (3rd edn), pp. 1159–1167. WB Saunders, Philadelphia.

Bentivoglio, M. and Grassi-Zucconi, G., 1997. The pioneering experimental studies on sleep deprivation. *Sleep*, **20**, 570–576.

Berger, R.J., 1961. Tonus of extrinsic laryngeal muscles during sleep and dreaming. *Science*, **134**, 840.

Berger, R.J., 1967. When is a dream is a dream is a dream? *Experimental Neurology*, **19**, 15–28.

Berger, R.J., Olly, P. and Oswald, L., 1962. The EEG, eye movements, and dreams of the blind. *Quarterly Journal of Experimental Psychology*, **14**, 183–186.

Berger, R.J. and Oswald, I., 1962. Effects of sleep deprivation on behaviour, subsequent sleep, and dreaming. *Journal of Mental Science*, **108**, 457–465.

Bonnet, M.H. and Moore, S.E., 1982. The threshold of sleep: perception of sleep as a function of time asleep and auditory threshold. *Sleep*, **5**, 267–276.

Borbély, A.A., Tobler, I., Loepfe, M., Kupfer, D.J., Ulrich, R.F., Grochocinski, V., Doman, J. and Matthews, G., 1984. All-night spectral analyses of the sleep EEG in untreated depressives and controls. *Psychiatric Research*, **12**, 27–33.

Borbély, A.A. and Wirtz-Justice, A., 1982. Sleep, sleep deprivation and depression: a hypothesis derived from a model of sleep regulation. *Human Neurobiology*, **1**, 205–210.

Born, J., Muth, S. and Fehm, H.L., 1988. The significance of sleep onset and slow wave sleep for nocturnal release of growth hormone (GH) and cortisol. *Psychoneuroendocrinology*, **13**, 233–243.

Bosinelli, M., Molinari, S., Bagnaresi, G. and Salzarulo, P., 1968. Caratteristiche dell attitiva psycofisiologica durante il sonno: un contributo alle techniche di valutazion. *Rivista Sperimentale Freiatria*, **92**, 128–150.

Boyd, J.H. and Weissman, M.M., 1981. Epidemiology of affective disorders: a reexamination and future directions [Review]. *Archives of General Psychiatry*, **38**, 1039–1046.

Broughton, R.J., 1982. Neurology and dreaming. *Psychiatric Journal of the University of Ottawa*, **7**, 101–110.

Broughton, R.J., Poire, R. and Tassinari, C.A., 1965. The electrodermogram (Tarchanoff effect) during sleep. *Electroencephalography and Clinical Neurophysiology*, **18**, 691–708.

Braun, A.R., Balkin, T.J., Wesensten, N.L., Carson, R.E., Varga, M., Baldwin, P.S., Selbie, J., Belenky, G. and Herscovitch, P., 1997. Regional cerebral blood flow throughout the sleep-wake cycle: a H215O PET study. *Brain*, **120**, 1173–1197.

Braun, A.R., Balkin, T.J., Wesensten, N.L., Carson, R.E., Varga, M., Baldwin, P.S., Selbie, J., Belenky, G. and Herscovitch, P., 1998. Dissociated pattern of activity in visual cortices and their projections during human rapid eye movement sleep. *Science*, **279**, 91–95.

Burch, N., 1965. Data processing of psychophysiological recordings. In: Proctor, L.D. and Adey, W.R. (eds), *Symposium on the Analysis of Central Nervous System and Cardiovascular Data using Computer Methods*, pp. 165–180. National Aeronautics and Space Administration, Washington, DC.

Busby, K.A., Mercier, L. and Pivik, R.T., 1994. Ontogenetic variations in auditory arousal threshold during sleep. *Psychophysiology*, **31**, 182–188.

Buzzi, G. and Cirignotta, F., 2000. Isolated sleep paralysis: a web survey. *Sleep Research Online*, **3**, 61–66.

Carskadon, M.A., 1979. Determinants of Daytime Sleepiness: Adolescent Development, Extended and Restricted Nocturnal Sleep. PhD Dissertation, Stanford University, Palo Alto, California.

Cartwright, R., 1991. Dreams that work: the relation of dream incorporation to adaptation to stressful events. *Dreaming*, **1**, 3–9.

Cartwright, R. and Wood, E., 1993. The contribution of dream masochism to the sex ratio difference in major depression. *Psychiatric Research*, **46**, 165–173.

Cavallero, C. and Foulkes, D. (eds), 1993. *Dreaming as Cognition*. Harvester Wheatsheaf, New York.

Cheyne, J.A., Rueffer, S.D. and Newby-Clark, I.R., 1999. Hypnagogic and hypnopompic hallucinations during sleep paralysis: neurological and cultural construction of the nightmare. *Consciousness and Cognition*, **8**, 319–337.

Cicogna, P., Natale, V., Occhionero, M. and Bosinelli, M., 2000. Slow wave and REM sleep mentation. *Sleep Research Online*, **3**, 67–72.

Cohen, H.D. and Shapiro, A., 1970. Vaginal blood flow during sleep. *Psychophysiology*, **1**, 338 [Abstract].

Davis, H., Davis, P.A., Loomis, A.L., Harvey, E.N. and Hobart, G., 1938. Human brain potentials during the onset of sleep. *Journal of Neurophysiology*, **1**, 24–38.

Dement, W.C., 1955. Dream recall and eye movement during sleep in schizophrenics and normals. *Journal of Nervous and Mental Disorders*, **122**, 263–269.

Dement, W.C., 1960. The effect of dream deprivation. *Science*, **131**, 1705–1707.

Dement, W.C. and Carskadon, M.A., 1982. Current perspectives on daytime sleepiness: the issues. *Sleep*, **5**, S56–S66.

Dement, W.C. and Fisher, C., 1963. Experimental interference with the sleep cycle. *Canadian Psychiatric Association Journal*, **8**, 400–405.

Dement, W.C. and Kleitman, N., 1957a. Cyclic variations in EEG during sleep and their relation to eye movements, bodily motility and dreaming. *Electroencephalography and Clinical Neurophysiology*, **9**, 673–690.

Dement, W.C. and Kleitman, N., 1957b. The relation of eye movements during sleep to dream activity: an objective method for the study of dreaming. *Journal of Experimental Psychology*, **53**, 339–346.

Dement, W. and Wolpert, E., 1958a. Interrelations in the manifest content of dreams occurring on the same night. *Journal of Nervous and Mental Disorders*, **126**, 568–578.

Dement, W. and Wolpert, E., 1958b. The relation of eye movements, body motility, and external stimuli to dream content. *Journal of Experimental Psychology*, **55**, 543–554.

Dement, W.C., Carskadon, M.A. and Ley, R., 1973. The prevalence of narcolepsy. *Sleep Research*, **2**, 147 [Abstract].

Dement, W.C., Greenberg, S. and Klein, R., 1966. The effect of partial REM sleep deprivation and delayed recovery. *Journal of Psychiatric Research*, **4**, 141–152.

Dement, W., Zarcone, V., Ferguson, J., Cohen, H., Pivik, T. and Barchas, J., 1969. Some parallel findings in schizophrenic patients and serotonin-depleted cats. In: Sankar, D.V. (ed.), *Schizophrenia: Current Concepts and Research*, pp. 775–811. PJD Publications, Hicksville, NY.

Dement, W.C., Zarcone, V., Varner, V., Hoddes, E., Nassau, S., Jacobs, B., Brown, J., McDonald, A., Horan, K., Glass, R., Gonzales, P., Friedman, E. and Phillips, R., 1972. The prevalence of narcolepsy. *Sleep Research*, **1**, 148 [Abstract].

Drabkin, I.E., 1950. *Caelius Aurelianus on Acute Diseases and Chronic Diseases*, pp. 21, 49. University of Chicago Press, Chicago.

Ellman, S.J. and Antrobus, J.S. (eds), 1991. *The Mind in Sleep: Psychology and Psychophysiology* (2nd edn). Wiley, New York.

Emslie, G.J., Rush, A.J., Weinberg, W.A., Rintelmann, J.W. and Roffwarg, H.P., 1990. Children with major depression show reduced rapid eye movement latencies. *Archives of General Psychiatry*, **47**, 119–124.

Everson, C.A., 1995. Functional consequences of sustained sleep deprivation in the rat. *Behavioural Brain Research*, **69**, 43–54.

Feinberg, I., Fein, G. and Floyd, T.C., 1980. Period and amplitude analysis of NREM EEG in sleep: repeatability of results in young adults. *Electroencephalography and Clinical Neurophysiology*, **48**, 212–221.

Feinberg, I., March, J.D., Fein, G., Floyd, T.C., Walker, J.M. and Price, L., 1978. Period of amplitude analysis of 0.5–3 c/sec activity in NREM sleep of young adults. *Electroencephalography and Clinical Neurophysiology*, **44**, 202–213.

Feinberg, M., Gillin, J.C., Carroll, B.J., Greden, J.F. and Zis, A.P., 1982. EEG studies of sleep in the diagnosis of depression. *Biological Psychiatry*, **17**, 305–316.

Fisher, C., 1966. Dreaming and sexuality. In: Lowenstein, R., Newman, L., Shur, M. and Solnit, A. (eds), *Psychoanalysis: A General Psychology*, pp. 537–569. International Universities Press, New York.

Fisher, C., Byrne, J., Edwards, A. and Kahn, E., 1970. A psychophysiological study of nightmares. *Journal of the American Psychoanalytical Association*, **18**, 747–782.

Fisher, C., Kahn, E., Edwards, A. and Davis, S.M., 1973. A psychophysiological study of nightmares and night terrors. I. Physiological aspects of the stage 4 night terror. *Journal of Nervous and Mental Disorders*, **157**, 75–98.

Fisher, C., Gross, J. and Zuch, J., 1965. Cycles of penile erection synchronous with dreaming (REM) sleep. *Archives of General Psychiatry*, **12**, 29–45.

Foulkes, D., 1960. Dream Reports From Different Stages of Sleep. Doctoral Dissertation, University of Chicago.

Foulkes, D., 1962. Dream reports from different stages of sleep. *Journal of Abnormal Social Psychology*, **65**, 14–25.

Foulkes, D., 1967. Nonrapid eye movement mentation. *Experimental Neurology*, **19**, 28–38.

Foulkes, D., 1978. *A Grammar of Dreams*. Basic Books, New York.

Foulkes, D., 1982. *Children's Dreams: Longitudinal Studies*. Wiley, New York.

Foulkes, D., 1985. *Dreaming: A Cognitive-Psychological Analysis*. Erlbaum., Hillsdale, New Jersey.

Foulkes, D., 1993. Children's dreaming. In: Cavallero, C. and Foulkes, D. (eds), *Dreaming as Cognition*, pp. 114–132. Harvester Wheatsheaf, New York.

Foulkes, D., 1996. Dream research: 1953–1993. *Sleep*, **19**, 609–624.

Foulkes, D., 1997. A contemporary neurobiology of dreaming. *Sleep Research Society Bulletin*, **3**, 2–4.

Foulkes, D. and Rechtschaffen, A., 1964. Presleep determinants of dream content: effects of two films. *Perceptual Motor Skills*, **19**, 983–1005.

Foulkes, D., Spear, P.S. and Symonds, J., 1966. Individual differences in mental activity at sleep onset. *Journal of Abnormal Psychology*, **71**, 280–286.

Foulkes, D. and Vogel, G., 1965. Mental activity at sleep onset. *Journal of Abnormal Psychology*, **70**, 231–243.

Foulkes, D., Hollifield, M., Bradley, L., Terry, R. and Sullivan, B., 1991. Waking self-understanding, REM-dream self representation, and cognitive ability variables at ages 5–8. *Dreaming*, **1**, 41–51.

Foulkes, D., Hollifield, M., Sullivan, B., Bradley, L. and Terry, R., 1990. REM dreaming and cognitive skill at ages 5–8: a cross-sectional study. *International Journal of Behaviour Development*, **13**, 447–465.

Fukuda, K., Ogilvie, R.D., Chilcott, L., Vendittelli, A.M. and Takeuchi, T., 1998. The prevalence of sleep paralysis among Canadian and Japanese college students. *Dreaming*, **8**, 59–66.

Gélineau, J., 1880. De la narcolepsie. *Gazette des Hôpiteaux (Paris)*, **53**, 626–628.

Gillberg, M. and Äkerstedt, T., 1994. Sleep restriction and SWS-suppression: effects on daytime alertness and night-time recovery. *Journal of Sleep Research*, **3**, 144–151.

Gillin, J.C., Buchsbaum, M.S., Jacobs, L.S., Fram, D.H., Williams, R.B. Jr., Vaughn, T.B. Jr., Mellon, E., Snyder, F. and Wyatt, R.J., 1974. Partial REM sleep deprivation, schizophrenia and field articulation. *Archives of General Psychiatry*, **30**, 653–662.

Gillin, J.C., Duncan, W.C., Pettigrew, K.D., Frankel, B.L. and Snyder, F., 1979. Successful separation of depressed, normal, and insomniac subjects by EEG sleep data. *Archives of General Psychiatry*, **36**, 85–90.

Goodenough, D.R., 1978. Dream recall: history and current status of the field. In: Arkin, A.M., Antrobus, J.S. and Ellman, S.J. (eds), *The Mind in Sleep: Psychology and Psychophysiology*, pp. 113–140. Erlbaum, Hillsdale, New Jersey.

Goodenough, D.R., Lewis, H.B., Shapiro, A. and Sleser, I., 1965. Some correlates of dream reporting following laboratory awakenings. *Journal of Nervous Mental Disorders*, **140**, 365–373.

Goodenough, D.R., Shapiro, A., Holden, M. and Steinschriber, L., 1959. A comparison of 'dreamers' and 'nondreamers': eye movements, electroencephalograms and the recall of dreams. *Journal of Abnormal Psychology*, **59**, 295–302.

Greenberg, R., Pearlman, C., Blacher, R., Katz, H., Sashin, J. and Gottlieb, P., 1990. Depression: variability of intrapsychic and sleep parameters. *Journal of the American Academy of Psychoanalysis*, **18**, 233–246.

Gresham, S.C., Agnew, H.W. Jr. and Williams, R.L., 1965. The sleep of depressed patients: an EEG and eye movement study. *Archives of General Psychiatry*, **13**, 503–507.

Guilleminault, C. and Anagnos, A., 2000. Narcolepsy. In: Kryger, M.H., Roth, T. and Dement, W.C. (eds), *Principles and Practices of Sleep Medicine* (3rd edn), pp. 676–686. WB Saunders, Philadelphia.

Hajak, G., 2000. Insomnia in primary care. *Sleep*, **23**(Suppl 3), S54–S64.

Halasz, P., Rajna, P., Pal, I., Kundra, O., Vargha, A., Balogh, A. and Kemeny, A., 1977. K-complexes and micro-arousals as functions of the sleep process. In: Koella, W.P. and Levin, P. (eds), *Sleep 1976*, pp. 292–294. Karger, Basel.

Hall, C. and Van de Castle, R.L., 1966. *The Content Analysis of Dreams*. Appleton-Century-Crofts, New York.

Hammond, W.A., 1892. *Sleep, Sleeplessness, and Derangements of Sleep*, p. 174. Sumpkin, Marshall and Company, London.

Hauri, P., 2000. Primary insomnia. In: Kryger, M.H., Roth, T. and Dement, W.C. (eds), *Sleep Medicine* (3rd edn), pp. 633–639. WB Saunders, Philadelphia.

Hauri, P. and Rechtschaffen, A., 1963. An unsuccessful attempt to find physiological correlates of NREM recall. Paper presented at the meeting of the Association for the Psychophysiological Study of Sleep, New York.

Hauri, P. and Van de Castle, R.L., 1973a. Psychophysiological parallelism in dreams. *Psychosomatic Medicine*, **35**, 297–308.

Hauri, P. and Van de Castle, R.L., 1973b. Psychophysiological parallels in dreams. In: Jovanovic, U.J. (ed.), *The Nature of Sleep*, pp. 140–142. Fischer, Stuttgart.

Hawkins, D.R. and Mendels, J., 1966. Sleep disturbance in depressive syndromes. *American Journal of Psychiatry*, **123**, 682–690.

Hays, P., 1992. False but sincere accusations of sexual assault made by narcoleptic patients. *Medical Legal Journal*, **60**, 1–8.

Hefez, A., Metz, L. and Laire, P., 1987. Long-term effects of extreme situational stress on sleep and dreaming. *American Journal of Psychiatry*, **144**, 344–347.

Helzer, J., Robins, L. and McEvoy, M., 1987. Post traumatic stress disorder in the general population: findings of the epidemiologic catchment area survey. *New England Journal of Medicine*, **317**, 1630–1634.

Henley, K. and Morrison, A.R., 1974. A reevaluation of the effects of lesions of the pontine tegmentum and locus coeruleus on phenomena of paradoxical sleep in the cat. *Acta Neurogiologiae Experimentalis*, **34**, 215–232.

Herman, J.H., Ellman, S.J. and Roffwarg, H.P., 1978. The problem of NREM dream recall re-examined. In: Arkin, A.M., Antrobus, J.S. and Ellman, S.J. (eds), *The Mind in Sleep: Psychology and Psychophysiology*, pp. 59–92. Erlbaum, Hillsdale, New Jersey.

Hishikawa, Y., 1976. Sleep paralysis. In: Guilleminault, C., Dement, W.C. and Passouant, P. (eds), *Advances in Sleep Research, Vol. 3*, pp. 97–124. Spectrum, New York.

Hishikawa, Y. and Shimuzu, T., 1995. Physiology of REM sleep, cataplexy, and sleep paralysis. In: Fahn, S., Hallet, M., Luders, H.O. and Marsden, C.D. (eds), *Advances in Neurology, Vol. 3*, pp. 245–271. Lippincott-Raven, Philadelphia.

Hodes, R. and Dement, W.C., 1964. Depression of electrically induced reflexes ('H'-reflexes) in man during low voltage EEG 'sleep'. *Electroencephalography and Clinical Neurophysiology*, **17**, 617–629.

Hoffman, R.F., Moffitt, A.R., Shearer, J.C., Sussman, P.S. and Wells, R.B., 1979. Conceptual and methodological considerations towards the development of computer-controlled research on the electro-physiology of sleep. *Waking and Sleeping*, **3**, 1–16.

Honda, Y., 1988. Clinical features of narcolepsy: Japanese experiences. In: Honda, Y. and Juji, T. (eds), *HLA in Narcolepsy*, pp. 24–57. Springer Verlag, New York.

Hong, C.C.H., Gillin, J.C., Dow, B.M., Wu, J. and Buchsbaum, M.S., 1995. Localized and lateralized cerebral glucose metabolism associated with eye movements during REM sleep and wakefulness: a positron emission tomography (PET) study. *Sleep*, **18**, 570–580.

Horne, J., 1988. *Why We Sleep. The Functions of Sleep in Humans and Other Mammals*. Oxford University Press, London.

Horowitz, M.J., Wilner, N., Kaltreider, N. and Alvarez, W., 1980. Signs and symptoms of post-traumatic stress disorder. *Archives of General Psychiatry*, **37**, 85–92.

Hoyt, M.F. and Singer, J.L., 1978. Psychological effects of REM ('dream') deprivation upon waking mentation. In: Arkin, A.M., Antrobus, J.S. and Ellman, S.J. (eds), *The Mind in Sleep: Psychology and Psychophysiology*, pp. 487–510. Erlbaum, Hillsdale, New Jersey.

Hufford, D.J., 1982. *The Terror That Comes in the Night*. University of Pennsylvania Press, Philadelphia.

ICSD (International Classification of Sleep Disorders): Diagnostic and Coding Manual, 1990. Thorpy, M.J. (Chairman, Diagnostic Classification Steering Committee, ed.), American Sleep Disorders Association, Rochester, MN.

Jackson, J.H., 1958. *Selected Writings*, Taylor, J., Holmes, G., Walshe, F.M.R. (eds), Basic Books, New York.

Jacobson, A., Kales, A., Lehmann, D. and Hoedemaker, F.S., 1964. Muscle tonus in human subjects during sleep and dreaming. *Experimental Neurology*, **10**, 418–424.

Janowsky, D.S., el Yousef, M.K., Davis, J.M. and Sekerke, J.H., 1972. A cholinergic-adrenergic hypothesis of mania and depression. *Lancet*, **2**, 632–635.

Johnson, L.C., 1973. Are stages of sleep related to waking behaviour? *American Scientist*, **61**, 326–338.

Johnson, L.C. and Lubin, A., 1966. Spontaneous electrodermal activity during waking and sleeping. *Psychophysiology*, **3**, 8–17.

Johnson, L.C., Nute, C., Austin, M.J. and Lubin, A., 1967. Spectral analysis of the EEG during waking and sleeping. *Electroencephalography and Clinical Neurophysiology*, **23**, 80.

Jouvet, M. and Delorme, J., 1965. Locus coeruleus et sommeil paradoxal. *Comptes Rendus des Séances de la Société de Biologie et de Ses Filiales*, **159**, 895–899.

Jouvet, M. and Michel, F., 1959. Correlations électromyographiques du sommeil chez le chat décortique et mésencéphalique chronique. *Compte Rendu Sociologie et Biologie (Paris)*, **153**, 422–425.

Jung, C., 1960. *The Psychology of Dementia Praecox*. Princeton University Press, Princeton, New Jersey.

Jus, K., Gagnon-Binette, M., Desjardins, D. and Brunelle, R., 1977. Effets de la déprivation du sommeil rapide pendant la première et la seconde partie de la nuit chez les schizophrènes chroniques. *La Vie Medicine Canadien Française*, **6**, 1234–1242.

Karacan, I., Goodenough, D.R., Shapiro, A. and Starker, S., 1966. Erection cycle during sleep in relation to dream anxiety. *Archives of General Psychiatry*, **15**, 183–189.

Kerr, M.H., 1993. Mental imagery, dreams and perception. In: Cavallero, C. and Foulkes, D. (eds), *Dreaming as Cognition*, pp. 18–37. Harvester Wheatsheaf, New York.

Kleitman, N., 1963. *Sleep and Wakefulness* (2nd edn). University of Chicago Press, Chicago.

Koresko, R., Snyder, F. and Feinberg, I., 1963. 'Dream time' in hallucinating and non-hallucinating schizophrenic patients. *Nature*, **199**, 1118–1119.

Kramer, M., 1979. Dream disturbances. *Psychiatric Annals*, **9**, 50–68.

Kramer, M., 1993. The selective mood regulatory function of dreaming: an update and revision. In: Moffitt, A., Kramer, M., Hoffman, R. (eds), *The Functions of Dreaming*, pp. 139–195. State University of New York Press, Albany, New York.

Kramer, M., 2000. Dreams and psychopathology. In Kryger, M.H., Roth, T. and Dement, W.C. (eds), *Principles and Practices of Sleep Medicine* (3rd edn), pp. 511–520. WB Saunders, Philadelphia.

Kramer, M. and Roth, T., 1979. Dreams in psychopathology. In: Wolman, B. (ed.), *Handbook of Dreams: Research, Theories and Applications*, pp. 361–387. Van Nostrand Reinhold, New York.

Kramer, M., Schoen, L.W. and Kinney, L., 1984. The dream experience in dream-disturbed Vietnam veterans. In: van der Kolk, B.A. (ed.), *PTSD: Psychological and Biological Sequelae*, pp. 81–95. American Psychiatric Press, Washington, DC.

Kryger, M.H., Roth, T. and Dement, W.C. (eds), 2000. *Principles and Practice of Sleep Medicine*, (3rd edn). WB Saunders, Philadelphia.

Kupfer, D.J., Ulrich, R.F., Coble, P.A., Jarrett, D.B., Grochocinski, V.J., Doman, J., Matthews, G. and Borbély, A.A., 1985. Electroencephalographic sleep of younger depressives: comparison with normals. *Archives of General Psychiatry*, **42**, 806–810.

Kupfer, D.J. and Foster, F.G., 1972. Interval between onset of sleep and rapid-eye-movement sleep as an indicator of depression. *Lancet*, **2**, 684–686.

LaBerge, S., 1985. *Lucid Dreaming*. JP Tarcher, Los Angeles.

LaBerge, S., 1992. The postawakening testing technique in the investigation of cognitive asymmetries during sleep. In: Antrobus, J.S. and Bertini, M. (eds), *The Neuropsychology of Sleep and Dreaming*, pp. 289–303. Erlbaum, Hillsdale, New Jersey.

LaBerge, S., Greenleaf, W. and Kedzierski, B., 1983. Physiological responses to dreamed sexual activity during lucid REM sleep. *Psychophysiology*, **20**, 454–455.

Lammers, W.J. and Badia, P., 1991. Motor responsiveness to stimuli presented during sleep: the influence of time-of-testing on sleep stage analyses. *Physiology and Behaviour*, **50**, 867–868.

Lapierre, O. and Montplaisir, J., 1992. Polysomnographic features of REM sleep behaviour disorder: development of a scoring method. *Neurology*, **42**, 1371–1374.

Larson, J.D. and Foulkes, D., 1969. Electromyogram suppression during sleep, dream recall and orientation time. *Psychophysiology*, **5**, 548–555.

Lee, J.H., Bliwise, D.L., Lebret-Borles, E., Guilleminault, C. and Dement, W.C., 1993. Dream-disturbed sleep in insomnia and narcolepsy. *Journal of Nervous and Mental Disorders*, **181**, 320–324.

Loomis, A.L., Harvey, E.N. and Hobart, G.A., 1937. Cerebral states during sleep as studied by human brain potentials. *Journal of Experimental Psychology*, **21**, 127–144.

Loomis, A.L., Harvey, E.N. and Hobart, G.A., III, 1938. Distribution of disturbance-patterns in the human electroencephalogram, with special reference to sleep. *Journal of Neurophysiology*, **1**, 413–430.

Louis, J., Cannard, C., Bastuji, H. and Challamel, M.J., 1997. Sleep ontogenesis revisited: a longitudinal 24-hour home polygraphic study on 15 normal infants during the first two years of life. *Sleep*, **20**, 323–333.

Lubin, A., Johnston, L.C. and Austin, M.J., 1969. Discrimination among states of consciousness using EEG spectra. *Psychophysiology*, **6**, 122–132.

Mahowald, M.W. and Schenck, C.H., 2000. REM sleep parasomnias. In: Kryger, M.H., Roth, T. and Dement, W.C. (eds), *Principles and Practices of Sleep Medicine* (3rd edn), pp. 724–741. WB Saunders, Philadelphia.

Maquet, P., 2001. The Role of sleep in learning and memory. *Science*, **294**, 1048–1051.

Maquet, P., Péters, J.M., Aerts, J., Delfiore, G., Degueldre, C., Luxen, A. and Granck, G., 1996. Functional neuroanatomy of human rapid-eye-movement sleep and dreaming. *Nature*, **383**, 163–166.

McCarley, R.W., 1982. REM sleep and depression: common neurobiological control mechanisms. *American Journal of Psychiatry*, **139**, 565–570.

Mellman, T.A. and Davis, G.C., 1985. Combat-related flashbacks in post traumatic stress disorder: phenomenology and similarity to panic attacks. *Journal of Clinical Psychiatry*, **46**, 379–382.

Molinari, S. and Foulkes, D., 1969. Tonic and phasic events during sleep: psychological correlates and implications. *Perceptual Motor Skills*, **29**, 343–368.

Monk, T.H., 1991. *Sleep, Sleepiness and Performance*. Wiley, New York.

Monroe, L.J., Rechtschaffen, A., Foulkes, D. and Jensen, J., 1965. Discriminability of REM and NREM reports. *Journal of Personality and Social Psychology*, **2**, 456–460.

Montplaisir, J., Billiard, M., Takahashi, S., Bell, I.R., Guilleminault, C. and Dement, W.C., 1978. Twenty-four-hour recording in REM-narcoleptics with special reference to nocturnal sleep disruption. *Biological Psychiatry*, **13**, 73–89.

Morrison, A.R., Mann, G., Hendricks, J.C. and Starkenweather, C., 1979. Release of exploratory behaviour in wakelike lesions which produce paradoxical sleep without atonia. *Anatomical Record*, **193**, 628 [Abstract].

Nielsen, T.A. and Zadra, A., 1997. Laboratory studies of idiopathic nightmares. In: *Abstracts of the Journée académique du départment de psychiatrie*, Centre Fernand-Séguin, Louis H. Lafontaine Hospital, Montreal, 16 May.

Nielsen, T.A. and Zadra, A., 2000. Dreaming disorders. In: Kryger, M.H., Roth, T. and Dement, W.C. (eds), *Principles and Practices of Sleep Medicine* (2nd edn), pp. 753–772. WB Saunders, Philadelphia.

Nielsen, T.A., Zadra, A. and Germain, A., 2002. Topography of REM sleep nightmares. *American Journal of Psychiatry* (in press).

Ohayon, M.M., Caulet, M. and Priest, R.G., 1997. Violent behaviour during sleep. *Journal of Clinical Psychiatry*, **58**, 369–376.

Olson, E.J., Bradley, F.B. and Silber, M.H., 2000. Rapid eye movement sleep behaviour disorder: demographic, clinical and laboratory findings in 93 cases. *Brain*, **123**, 331–339.

Oswald, I., Berger, R.J., Jaramillo, R.A., Keddie, K.M.G., Ollcy, P.C. and Plunkett, G.B., 1963. Melancholia and barbiturates: a controlled EEG, body and eye movement study of sleep. *British Journal of Psychiatry*, **109**, 66–78.

Partinen, M. and Hublin, C., 2000. Epidemiology of sleep disorders. In: Kryger, M.H., Roth, T. and Dement, W.C. (eds), *Principles and Practices of Sleep Medicine* (3rd edn), pp. 558–579. WB Saunders, Philadelphia.

Perlis, M.L. and Nielsen, T.A., 1993. Mood regulation, dreaming and nightmares: evaluation of a desensitization function for REM sleep. *Dreaming*, **3**, 243–257.

Pivik, R.T., 1971. Mental Activity and Phasic Events During Sleep. Unpublished Doctoral Dissertation, Stanford University, Palo Alto, California.

Pivik, R.T., 1983. Order and disorder during sleep ontogeny: a selective review. In: Firestone, P., McGrath, P.J. and Feldman, W. (eds), *Advances in Behavioural Medicine for Children and Adolescents*, pp. 75–102. Erlbaum, Hillsdale, New Jersey.

Pivik, R.T., 1986. Sleep: physiology and psychophysiology. In: Coles, G.H., Donchin, E. and Porges, S.W. (eds), *Psychophysiology*, pp. 378–406. Guilford Press, New York.

Pivik, R.T., 1991. Tonic states and phasic events in relation to sleep mentation. In: Arkin, A.M., Antrobus, J.S. and Ellman, S.J. (eds), *The Mind in Sleep: Psychology and Psychophysiology* (2nd edn), pp. 214–247. Erlbaum, Hillsdale, New Jersey.

Pivik, R.T., 2000a. Psychophysiology of dreams. In: Kryger, M.H., Roth, T. and Dement, W.C. (eds), *Principles and Practices of Sleep Medicine* (3rd edn), pp. 491–501. WB Saunders, Philadelphia.

Pivik, R.T., 2000b. Sleep and dreaming. In: Cacioppo, J.T., Tassinary, L.G. and Berntson, G.G. (eds), *Handbook of Psychophysiology* (2nd edn), pp. 687–716. Cambridge University Press, Cambridge.

Pivik, T. and Foulkes, D., 1968. NREM mentation: relation to personality, orientation time, and time of night. *Journal of Consulting Clinical Psychology*, **37**, 144–151.

Pivik, R.T., Busby, K.A., Gill, E., Hunter, P. and Nevins, R., 1996. Heart rate variations during sleep in preadolescents. *Sleep*, **19**, 117–135.

Pivik, R.T. and Dement, W.C., 1968. Amphetamine, REM deprivation and K-complexes. *Psychophysiology*, **5**, 241 [Abstract].

Pompeiano, O., 1966. Muscular afferents and motor control during sleep. In: Granit, R. (ed.), *Muscular Afferents and Motor Control*, pp. 415–436. Almquist & Siksell, Stockholm.

Pompeiano, O., 1967. The neurophysiological mechanism of the postural and motor events during desynchronized sleep. In: Kety, S.S., Evarts, E.V. and Williams, H.L. (eds), *Sleep and Altered States of Consciousness*, pp. 351–423. Williams and Wilkins, Baltimore.

Rechstschaffen, A., 1973. The psychophysiology of mental activity during sleep. In: McGuigan, F.J. and Schoonover, R.A. (eds), *The Psychophysiology of Thinking*, pp. 153–205. Academic Press, New York.

Rechstschaffen, A. and Kales, A. (eds), 1968. *A Manual of Standardized Terminology, Techniques and Scoring system for Sleep Stages of Human Subjects* (NIM Publ. No. 204). US Government Printing Office, Washington, DC.

Rechstschaffen, A., Schulsinger, F. and Mednick, S., 1964. Schizophrenia and physiological indices of dreaming. *Archives of General Psychiatry*, **10**, 89–93.

Rechtschaffen, A., Vogel, G. and Shaikun, G., 1963. Interrelatedness of mental activity during sleep. *Archives of General Psychiatry*, **9**, 536–547.

Ribstein, M., 1976. Hypnagogic hallucinations. In *Narcolepsy*, Guilleminault, C., Dement, W.C. and Passouant, P. (eds), Spectrum, New York, pp. 145–160.

Roffwarg, H., Muzio, J.N. and Dement, W.C., 1966. Ontogenetic development of the human sleep-dream cycle. *Science*, **152**, 604–619.

Roffwarg, H., Dement, W., Muzio, J. and Fisher, C., 1962. Dream imagery: relationship to rapid eye movements of sleep. *Archives of General Psychiatry*, **7**, 235–258.

Ross, R.J., Ball, W.A., Sullivan, K.A. and Caroff, S.N., 1989. Sleep disturbance as the hallmark of post traumatic stress disorder. *American Journal of Psychiatry*, **146**, 697–707.

Sampson, H., 1965. Deprivation of dreaming sleep by two methods. I. Compensatory REM time. *Archives of General Psychiatry*, **13**, 79–86.

Sampson, H., 1966. Psychological effects of deprivation of dreaming sleep. *Journal of Nervous and Mental Disorders*, **143**, 305–317.

Sassin, J.F., Parker, D.C., Mace, J.W., Gotlin, R.W., Johnson, L.C. and Rossman, L.G., 1969. Human growth hormone release: relation to slow-wave sleep and sleep-waking cycles. *Science*, **165**, 513–515.

Schenck, C.H., Bundlie, S.R., Ettinger, M.G. and Mahowald, M.W., 1986. Chronic behavioural disorders of human REM sleep: a new category of parasomnia. *Sleep*, **9**, 293–308.

Schenck, C.H., Duncan, E., Hopwood, J., Garfinkel, B., Bundlie, S. and Mahowald, M.W., 1988. The human REM sleep behaviour disorder (RBD): quantitative polygraphic and behaviour analysis of 9 cases. *Sleep Research*, **17**, 14.

Schlosberg, A. and Benjamin, M., 1978. Sleep patterns in three acute combat fatigue cases. *Journal of Clinical Psychiatry*, **39**, 546–549.

Schredl, M., 1998. Dream content in narcoleptic patients: preliminary findings. *Dreaming*, **8**, 103–107.

Schredl, M., Schafer, G., Weber, B. and Heuser, I., 1998. Dreaming and insomnia: dream recall and dream content of patients with insomnia. *Journal of Sleep Research*, **7**, 191–198.

Siegel, J.M., 2001. The REM sleep-memory consolidation hypothesis. *Science*, **294**, 1058–1063.

Sitaram, N., Gillin, J.C. and Bunney, W.E.J., 1984. Cholinergic and catecholaminergic receptor sensitivity in affective illness: strategy and theory. In: Post, R.M., Ballenger, J.C. (eds), *Neurobiology of Mood Disorders*, pp. 629–651. Williams and Wilkins, Baltimore, Maryland.

Snyder, F., Hobson, J. and Goldfrank, F., 1963. Blood pressure changes during human sleep. *Science*, **142**, 1313–1314.

Snyder, F., Hobson, J., Morrison, D. and Goldfrank, F., 1964. Changes in respiration, heart rate, and systolic blood pressure in human sleep. *Journal of Applied Physiology*, **19**, 417–422.

Spanos, N.P., McNulty, S.A., DuBreuil, S.C., Pires, M. and Burgess, M.F., 1995. The frequency and correlates of sleep paralysis in a university sample. *Journal of Research in Personality*, **29**, 285–305.

Stickgold, R., Hobson, J.A., Fosse, R. and Fosse, M., 2001. Sleep, learning, and dreams: off-line memory reprocessing. *Science*, **294**, 1052–1057.

Takahashi, Y., Kipnis, D.M. and Daughaday, W.H., 1968. Growth hormone secretion during sleep. *Journal of Clinical Investigations*, **47**, 2079–2090.

Takeuchi, T., Miyasita, A., Inugami, M., Sasaki, Y. and Fukuda, K., 1994. Laboratory-documented hallucinations during sleep-onset REM period in a normal subject. *Perceptual and Motor Skills*, **78**, 979–895.

Tracy, R.L. and Tracy, L.N., 1974. Reports of mental activity from sleep stages 2 and 4. *Perceptual Motor Skills*, **38**, 647–648.

Uhde, T.W., 2000. Anxiety disorders. In: Kryger, M.H., Roth, T. and Dement, W.C. (eds), *Principles and Practices of Sleep Medicine*, (3rd edn), pp. 1123–1139. WB Saunders, Philadelphia.

van der Kolk, B.A., Hartmann, E., Burr, A. and Blitz, R., 1980. A survey of nightmare frequencies in a veterans outpatient clinic. *Sleep Research*, **9**, 229 [Abstract].

van der Kolk, B.A., Blitz, R., Burr, W., Sherry, S. and Hartmann, E., 1984. Nightmares and trauma: a comparison of nightmares after combat with lifelong nightmares in veterans. *American Journal of Psychiatry*, **141**, 187–190.

Vihvelin, H., 1948. On the differentiation of some typical forms of hypnagogic hallucinations. *Acta Psychiatry Neurology*, **23**, 359–389.

Vogel, G.W., 1968. REM deprivation. III. Dreaming and psychosis. *Archives of General Psychiatry*, **18**, 312–329.

Vogel, G.W., 1975. Review of REM sleep deprivation. *Archives of General Psychiatry*, **32**, 749–761.

Vogel, G.W., 1978. Sleep-onset mentation. In: Arkin, A.M., Antrobus, J.S. and Ellman, S.J. (eds), *The Mind in Sleep: Psychology and Psychophysiology*, pp. 97–108. Erlbaum, Hillsdale, New Jersey.

Vogel, G.W., Barrowclough, B. and Giesler, D., 1972. Limited discriminability of REM and sleep onset reports and its psychiatric implications. *Archives of General Psychiatry*, **26**, 449–455.

Vogel, G.W., Foulkes, D. and Trosman, H., 1966. Ego functions and dreaming during sleep onset. *Archives of General Psychiatry*, **14**, 238–248.

Vogel, G.W., Thurmond, A., Gibbons, P., Sloan, K., Boyd, M. and Walker, M., 1975. REM sleep reduction effects on depression syndromes. *Archives of General Psychiatry*, **32**, 765–777.

Waller, D.A., Hardy, B.W., Pole, R., Giles, D., Gullion, C.M., Rush, A.J. and Roffwarg, H.P., 1989. Sleep EEG in bulimic, depressed, and normal subjects. *Biological Psychiatry*, **25**, 661–664.

Wehr, T.A., Gillin, J.C. and Goodwin, F.K., 1983. Sleep and circadian rhythms in depression. In: Chase, M. (ed.), *Sleep Disorders: Basic and Clinical Research*, pp. 195–225. Spectrum, New York.

Wehr, T.A. and Wirz-Justice, A., 1981. Internal coincidence model for sleep deprivation and depression. In: Koella, W.P. (ed.), *Sleep 1980*, pp. 26–33. Karger, Basel, Switzerland.

Williams, R.L., Agnew, H.W. Jr. and Webb, W.B., 1964. Sleep patterns in young adults: an EEG study. *Electroencephalography and Clinical Neurophysiology*, **17**, 376–381.

Williams, R.L., Agnew, H.W. Jr. and Webb, W.B., 1966. Sleep patterns in the young adult female: an EEG study. *Electroencephalography and Clinical Neurophysiology*, **20**, 264–266.

Wundt, W., 1897. *Outlines of Psychology*. Scholar Publications, East St Clair Shores, Michigan.

Zarcone, V.P. and Fuchs, H.E., 1976. Psychiatric disorders and narcolepsy. In: Guilleminault, C., Dement, W.C. and Passouant, P. (eds), *Narcolepsy*, pp. 231–255. Spectrum, New York.

Zarcone, V., Gulevich, G., Pivik, T. and Dement, W., 1968. Partial REM phase deprivation and schizophrenia. *Archives of General Psychiatry*, **18**, 194–202.

Zimmerman, W.B., 1968. Psychological and physiological differences between 'light' and 'deep' sleepers. *Psychophysiology*, **4**, 387 [Abstract].

Zimmerman, W.B., 1970. Sleep mentation and auditory awakening thresholds. *Psychophysiology*, **6**, 540–549.

Zung, W., Wilson, W. and Dodson, W., 1964. Effect of depressive disorders on sleep EEG responses. *Archives of General Psychiatry*, **10**, 429–445.

XXIV-6

The Neuropsychology of Sleep Disorders

Raymond Cluydts and Edwin Verstraeten

INTRODUCTION

Within the vast area of the life sciences, sleep and sleep disorders have received increasing attention and interest during recent decades from governmental and health authorities, the news media, and the public in general. A big step forward in the recognition of sleep as an important aspect of our health was based on findings revealing the numerous effects of poor or inadequate sleep on daytime functioning and quality of life in general.

Epidemiological studies show (Partinen and Hublin, 2000) that a vast majority of children, adolescents, adults, and the elderly can expect to suffer for either a short or longer period in their lives, from some kind of sleep problem. In addition to primary insomnia, sleep disturbances associated with breathing problems, muscular contractions, or irritability during the night, as well as narcolepsy and circadian rhythm disorders, have been identified. These conditions have selective effects on either sleep stages, such as REM or non-REM sleep, or sleep onset, the continuity of sleep, or sleep architecture. This disturbance or lack of sleep has been associated with serious safety consequences not only for the patient, but also for the public. Daytime sleepiness has been recognized as a major intervening factor. A sleepy brain cannot function normally and attend to ongoing activities. Many disasters witnessed in recent years, such as train, coach, and car crashes, may be related to ignorance of the limits of human performance after sleep loss.

On the individual level, extensive clinical and neuropsychological investigation of the sleep-disordered patient seems necessary to understand fully the impact of sleep disorders on the patient's daily activities. But, next to the process of diagnosis, the results obtained from this neuropsychological examination can provide the clinician with clues for a comprehensive treatment plan and outcome measures of the therapy.

Neuropsychological Findings in Sleep-Wake Disorders

The fact that sleep loss and poor sleep result in daytime impairment of cognitive functioning is inferred not only from real disasters but also mainly from two types of research and clinical findings. First there are research data on the effects of total and partial sleep deprivation and sleep fragmentation; secondly, we can rely on clinical data gathered from patients suffering from sleep disorders.

Decades of research on sleep deprivation show the consistently detrimental effects of sleep shortage on next-day performance. Good reviews on this topic are numerous (Walsh and Lindblom, 1997; Bonnet, 2000; Pilcher and Hufcutt, 1996; Dinges and Kribbs, 1991). Most of these studies were performed to reveal the function(s) of sleep, providing us with key information about areas in the neurocognitive field that are susceptible to these experimental manipulations. These areas include attentional performance (impact of daytime sleepiness), mood changes, and memory function. But can these experimentally induced sleep disturbance be compared to the sleep disturbance experienced by insomniacs? Probably not. At best, this experimentally induced sleep fragmentation and partial sleep deprivation can be compared to the effects of an acute shift-work or jet-lag situation. We do not consider induced sleep deprivation a condition of 'insomnia' but one of 'sleeplessness'. Furthermore, these experiments are conducted in laboratory situations and are very much affected by selection bias (students as volunteers), experimental set-effects (motivation), and testing and instrumentation effects (learning), so that a generalization of these findings to a sleep disorder population is absolutely unwarranted. Our patients are mostly confronted with non-stimulating situations and lack of motivation in everyday life. Nevertheless, the findings in the three areas described above can give us some clues on promising areas to explore in insomniacs. However, we should certainly not restrict our studies to these areas only. Moreover, the finding that, in many studies on partial sleep deprivation in volunteers, few neurocognitive effects were evidenced cannot be simply generalized to the patient population.

From clinical practice, we know that patients suffering from sleep disorders complain not only of poor sleep, but also of significant impairment of their daytime activities. This includes cognitive impairment such as memory deficits (both encoding and retrieval) and limited attention span; some patients even report specific disorders such as visuoperceptual and spatial orientation difficulties. These clinical observations became the focus of some population-based studies in recent years. These studies confirm that patients with insomnia experience more problems with memory, concentration, thinking, and ability to accomplish tasks (Roth and Ancoli-Israel, 1999). These problems not only affect quality of life scales (Zammit *et al.*, 1999) but are also associated with poor occupational performance and increased absenteeism. Leger (1999) estimated the annual economic impact of insomnia in France to be around US$ 2 billion.

A crucial question is whether these neurocognitive phenomena are just one part of a larger 'neurotic' complex that is 'complaint'-driven, or whether a causal relationship between the sleep complaint and the reported daytime neurocognitive impairment can be demonstrated. In the next sections, we will discuss the data available on neurocognitive functioning in patients suffering from following sleep disorders: primary insomnia, sleep apnoea syndrome, and narcolepsy.

PRIMARY INSOMNIA

Insomnia is usually defined according to the *Diagnostic and Statistical Manual of Mental Disorders* (4th edition) (DSM-IV) (American Psychiatric Association, 1994) or the *International Classification of Sleep Disorders* (ICSD) (Revised) (American

Biological Psychiatry: Edited by H. D'haenen, J.A. den Boer and P. Willner. ISBN 0-471-49198-5

Sleep Disorders Association, 1997). The DSM-IV criteria for 'primary insomnia' are not exactly the same, but overlap largely with the ICSD categories psychophysiological insomnia, sleep stage misperception and idiopathic insomnia. We can assume that in many studies very heterogeneous groups of patients were tested in the morning so that results obtained need to be interpreted with care. Earlier studies performed in the 1970s and 1980s used 'poor sleepers' as research subjects without screening for sleep-related breathing disturbances, movement disorders, or other medical conditions. Therefore, we will discuss only recent studies that used appropriate screening methods. Extensive reviews on the topic can be found in Riedel and Lichstein (2000) and Fulda and Schulz (2001) [see also References]. We will focus on recent studies by Hauri (1997), Edinger *et al.* (1997), and Rosa and Bonnet (2000). Three areas of interest already identified in sleep deprivation studies will be considered: sleepiness, mood, and cognition.

Sleepiness

Three methods for assessing daytime sleepiness are well accepted: the Stanford Sleepiness Scale (SSS) (Hoddes *et al.*, 1973), a 7-point sleepiness rating scale and the Epworth Sleepiness Scale (ESS) (Johns, 1991), which asks patients about the likelihood of falling asleep in eight situations, are subjective measures. The former is a measure of 'state' sleepiness, whereas the latter measures 'trait' aspects of sleepiness.

As an objective test to be performed in a laboratory under strictly standardized conditions, the Multiple Sleep Latency Test (MSLT) (Carkadon *et al.*, 1986) is accepted worldwide as a routine procedure in all sleep disorders centres: it measures sleep onset latency in five 20-min naps with 2-h intervals during the day.

The study of Edinger *et al.*, (1997) is typical: in sharp contrast to the effects of sleep deprivation on daytime napping, insomniacs do not show shortened sleep latencies on the MSLT recorded either in the sleep laboratory or at home. The study of Bonnet and Arand (1995) even found an increased mean sleep onset latency in insomniacs. This finding suggests that insomniacs have difficulty in falling asleep, either at night or during the day; in them, a neurobiological substrate that introduces sleep (sleep drive) seems to be defective and/or the wake drive is too elevated.

Hauri (1997) found higher scores on the SSS in insomniacs, and this finding has been confirmed in other studies that also administered this state measure of sleepiness during the day after a polysomnographic (PSG) recording. Data with the ESS are conflicting and less available, as this scale is much more often used in patient groups presenting with high daytime sleepiness. A floor effect may be the reason for this negative finding in primary insomniacs.

Mood

The Profile of Mood States (POMS) (McNair *et al.*, 1981) is a self-administered rating scale comprising six well-defined dimensions of affect: tension-anxiety, depression, anger, fatigue-inertia, vigour-activity, and confusion-bewilderment. It assesses intensity of a mood state and can cover any time period, but the scale is usually administered in reference to how someone feels at the moment of completion. It is an interesting procedure to be used in insomnia for at least two reasons. Firstly, it allows one to detect an underlying anxiety and/or depressive component. Although primary insomniacs do not fit the criteria for generalized anxiety or major depressive disorder, we see in our consultation primary insomniacs who present with elevated anxiety and depression at non-clinical levels. This was also observed in the study by Bonnet and Arand (1995).

Secondly, as primary insomniacs may confuse feelings of fatigue and sleepiness, the fatigue scale of the POMS can depict this particular state in the absence of sleepiness. Indeed, primary insomniacs complain more about fatigue than sleepiness, as was found by Fichten *et al.* (1995). Maybe we should reconsider more the impact of feelings of fatigue in these patients. In contrast to sleepiness and cognition, there is a clear bidirectionality between mood and sleep. Rosa and Bonnet (2000) found that patients complaining about their sleep had higher tension, depression, anger, and confusion scores on the POMS in comparison to controls, but when the same group of subjects in the study were grouped by poor EEG sleep instead of the complaint itself, the same results were found, indicating dysphoric mood in both situations. Interestingly, the POMS fatigue scale was related only to the poor EEG criterion, and not to the complaint factor.

Cognition

The studies by Hauri (1997) and Edinger *et al.* (1997) will be discussed, as both are methodologically sound and original. Hauri compared not only insomniacs with normal controls, but also the performance of the insomniacs after their best night with that after their poorest of three nights. Edinger compared performance after a PSG recording in the sleep laboratory with performance after an ambulatory recording at the patient's home.

Hauri's study included 26 insomniacs, starting from a screening total of 75. They filled out a sleep diary and the SSS for 1 week, slept in the laboratory on 3–4 occasions, and were tested by a well-validated test battery (Roehrs *et al.*, 1995), tapping many neurocognitive functions. The insomniacs performed worse than matched controls, and, in particular, were more variable on a simple visual reaction time test (initiation time). A complex reaction time test showed less variability but again a slower initiation and total reaction time. Insomniacs also remembered fewer digits in the Wechsler Digit Span Test, but the Digit-Symbol Substitution, Auditory Verbal Learning, and Auditory Vigilance Task were performed at the same level as the healthy controls. Of most importance, no significant differences on the cognitive tasks could be found in comparing performances after the worst and the best nights in the insomniacs.

The Edinger *et al.* (1997) study found no differences in the Simple Reaction Time Test performance between insomniacs and controls, but made an interesting observation in the Continuous Performance Test. This test is a signal detection task in which target letters have to be identified from background letters. Insomniacs recorded in the sleep laboratory performed better at this task than those who were recorded at home; the reverse was found for healthy controls. Moreover, among those who slept at home, the normal sleepers performed better during daytime testing than the insomniacs, whereas after a night in the sleep laboratory the reverse was found. This indicates that after a night in the sleep laboratory, normal sleepers might have been somewhat sleep deprived and perform worse, whereas the worst performance in insomniacs was observed the day after a sleep recording in their usual sleep environment. The sleep laboratory environment may have produced some extra arousal, or there may be a 'reversed first night' effect (Hauri, 1989) in the insomniacs.

In a further study, Rosa and Bonnet (2000) reported that when patients were grouped on the basis of poor EEG nights, a poorer performance on the memory test (number of words recalled) was associated with two nights of poor EEG sleep, but the same phenomenon was observed when the subjects were grouped on the basis of their complaint: subjects with sleep complaints remembered fewer words. All other performance tests (vigilance, motor steadiness, etc.) were not significantly different whatever comparison was made.

Conclusion

It seems that neurocognitive deficits in primary insomniacs are very difficult to demonstrate at this time. Some of problems we encounter in these studies are as follows:

- types of insomnia patients included and characteristics of the insomnia (type, severity, and duration of the sleep problem)
- home versus sleep laboratory PSG recordings
- types of tests/tasks used (real world?)
- effects of age, gender, and education on test performance
- control of confounding variables such as motivation, mood
- robustness of the effect (test-retest).

These issues will be considered in turn.

A selection bias is one possible source of unreliability. The selection criteria in earlier studies were most probably not adequately defined, resulting in very heterogeneous groups of insomnia patients. We can rule out possible medical/psychiatric origins during a screening night, but then we still have different subtypes of primary insomniacs: psychophysiological, idiopathic, and possibly sleep-stage misperception as well. Another possible selection bias is the type of referral. In most studies, patients are solicited by newspaper advertisement, but sometimes they are referred from a sleep disorders centre. In some studies (Rosa and Bonnet, 2000), patients were recruited from both sources. There might have been a tendency towards morbidity in those patients seeking help via a sleep laboratory or their physician. Edinger *et al.* (1997) have posed an interesting question: when studying patients with insomnia, should we study their sleep in the sleep laboratory or at home? Regarding their daytime performance testing, Edinger *et al.* suggest that a sleep laboratory PSG put insomniacs at an advantage and healthy controls at a disadvantage, and that when insomniacs are recorded at home they show the attentional/concentration deficits of which they typically complain. Maybe the daytime performance testing should be administered at home as well to find even more of these daytime complaints, as the trip to the laboratory might induce a certain arousal in these patients.

This brings us to the next point of interest, which is the type of tests used. Some studies use a broad range of clinical psychological tests, mostly multifactorial in nature, whereas other authors prefer tasks developed by cognitive psychologists. Unfortunately, we lack a rationale for the selection of tests or tasks used or a theoretical framework of the neurocognitive functions that are assessed. Given the recent findings on the important role of sleep on memory consolidation (Maquet *et al.*, 2000; Poe *et al.*, 2000), we probably should look in more detail at this phenomenon and at test encoding at night and recall in the morning in these patients. Given the effects of age and gender on sleep, and given the skewed distribution of sleep complaints with respect to these factors (more females and more elderly with complaints), we must not forget that these same factors can also have a tremendous effect on performance testing.

Controlling for confounding factors in these highly complex matters is difficult. Factors such as motivation and mood, which are probably highly influenced by sleep quality, can interfere with daytime performance testing. Therefore, a good definition of the dependent variables and the possible confounders that can be controlled for by analysis of covariance is a necessity. Certainly, simple, univariate analyses lead to simplistic conclusions, given these highly interrelated variables. More studies investigating the robustness of the daytime neurocognitive effects in insomniacs are needed. One good example is the Pilcher *et al.* (1996) study, which shows — albeit in young adults, and not in insomniacs — that there is a stable relationship over time between sleep quality ratings and health, well-being, and daytime sleepiness. Longitudinal studies with insomniacs are rarely found, but therapeutic intervention studies might offer an opportunity here. They obviously include more assessments over time, and if daytime performance outcome measures are included, in addition to mood and other relevant measures, it would be a big step forward if the reversibility of the morbidity at baseline in these patients could be demonstrated.

Patients with primary insomnia do complain about daytime complications comprising the domains of cognition and affect. However, several studies show that it is difficult to demonstrate a clear-cut daytime neurocognitive deficit that is causally related to the sleep problem. Some factors contributing to this have been explained. A subjective sleep complaint itself does not mean a PSG-objectified sleep disturbance *per se*. Only a complaint of 'non-restorative' sleep might be related to an increased number of arousals during sleep.

Thus, there certainly exists a gap in our understanding of primary insomnia, and promising hypotheses have been formulated. Sleep-stage misperception, a disorder in which a complaint of insomnia or excessive sleepiness occurs without objective evidence of sleep disturbance, and psychophysiological insomnia have been related to fast EEG during sleep onset (Perlis *et al.*, 2001). Hyperarousal certainly explains why insomniacs who cannot fall asleep at night have the same difficulty during the daytime multiple sleep latency tests, but hyperarousal itself does not predict poor EEG sleep (Bonnet and Rosa, 2001). In addition to sleep drive, the wake-drive system needs careful consideration in our patients (Bonnet, 1997; Cluydts *et al.*, 2002).

Tension, anxiety, and mild psychopathology in primary insomniacs have repeatedly been demonstrated (Nowell *et al.*, 1997; Buysse *et al.*, 1994; Cluydts *et al.*, 1996), but these phenomena can be the result of years of non-successful searching for help in these patients. Saletu-Zyhlarz *et al.* (1997) showed that generalized anxiety disorder (GAD) patients who complain about poor sleep quality do well in some attention, concentration, and memory tasks, whereas their motor performance decreases, and they related these findings to a state of hypervigilance and hyperarousal. This agrees well with the proposed neurocognitive model of insomnia (Perlis *et al.*, 1999; 2001), which suggests that beta and gamma activity is enhanced during sleep onset in primary insomniacs.

Incorrect beliefs, expectations, and attributes concerning sleep have been identified in insomniacs, and these can be corrected successfully by cognitive-behavioural therapy (Edinger *et al.*, 2001; Morin *et al.*, 1993). Again, are these cognitions the cause or the result of years of suffering? The model of Spielman (1987) might offer some help here, as it describes predisposing, precipitating, and perpetuating factors in the development of insomnia. Within a biopsychosocial perspective, one might consider a 'fragile sleep system' or a hyperaroused nervous system as a predisposing factor that could develop into a sleep complaint in acute stress but could also develop more insidiously. The well-known conditioning processes may then contribute to the perpetuation or exacerbation of the complaint. All these hypotheses need to be further developed and evaluated.

Future research might also redirect our attention to the concept of 'sleep quality' which is so strongly related to daytime well-being and health. A better understanding of the biopsychosocial factors that contribute to the perception of the quality of our sleep might eventually result in the full recognition of the 'non-restorative sleep' syndrome.

SLEEP APNOEA

Obstructive sleep apnoea syndrome (OSAS) is a sleep-related breathing disorder characterized by repetitive episodes of complete cessation of airflow (apnoea) or decreases in airflow (hypopnoea) due to upper airway obstruction. Nocturnal apnoea and hypopnoea result in brief arousals from sleep and are frequently associated with intermittent hypoxaemia. The apnoea-hypopnoea index (AHI) is defined by the average number of episodes of apnoea plus hypopnoea per hour of sleep. 'Mild', 'moderate', and 'severe' cases of OSAS are defined as AHI of 5–15, 16–30, and >30, respectively (American Academy of Sleep Medicine, 1999). These respiratory disturbances are associated with daytime symptoms, the most important being sleepiness and neuropsychological dysfunctioning. Obstructive sleep apnoea is the most common cause of excessive daytime sleepiness among patients evaluated at sleep disorder centres. The prevalence of this syndrome is about 4% in middle-aged men meeting minimal diagnostic criteria (AHI > 5) (Young *et al.*, 1993), is higher among males than females (Partinen and Telakivi, 1992), and increases in the elderly (Ancoli-Israel *et al.*, 1987).

We begin by discussing excessive daytime sleepiness. Furthermore, the literature on neurocognitive dysfunction is reviewed. This is followed by a discussion of some relevant methodological considerations that are particularly important in hypersomnia research. We also point out pathophysiological mechanisms of the neuropsychological impairments. Next, an overview of sleep apnoea patients' driving performance is provided. Finally, we summarize reported psychosocial symptoms and the effects of treatment in sleep apnoea.

Sleepiness

Excessive daytime sleepiness is the most common complaint in apnoea patients, as evidenced by subjective ratings such as the Stanford Sleepiness Scale (Kribbs *et al.*, 1993; Sforza and Lugaresi, 1995), the POMS (Kribbs *et al.*, 1993), and the ESS (Engleman *et al.*, 1996; Hardinge *et al.*, 1995). Objective measures of sleepiness/alertness also demonstrate clinically significant impairments. The MSLT demonstrates sleep onset latencies in apnoea patients consistently below the normal threshold of 10 min, suggesting mild to moderate sleepiness (Cheshire *et al.*, 1992; Engleman *et al.*, 1994; Kribbs *et al.*, 1993; Lamphere *et al.*, 1989). In severe apnoea patients, the mean sleep onset latency is usually in the pathological range of 5 min or less (Bédard *et al.*, 1991b; Sforza and Lugaresi, 1995). In mild sleep apnoea patients, however, average ESS ratings and average sleep onset latencies on the MSLT are at the high end of the normal range (Engleman *et al.*, 1997; Redline *et al.*, 1997). The Maintenance of Wakefulness Test requires the subject to remain awake while sitting up in bed during four 40-min trials at 2-h intervals throughout the day (Mitler *et al.*, 1982). This procedure provides evidence of significant decreases in sleep onset latency in OSAS patients (Poceta *et al.*, 1992; Sforza and Krieger, 1997). The ability to stay awake may be a more important parameter of daytime performance than the propensity to fall asleep (Roth *et al.*, 1980; Johnson, 1992). The same protocol as in the Maintenance of Wakefulness Test is used in the Oxford Sleep Resistance Test, which is a procedure to evaluate sleepiness from a behavioural perspective by measuring lapses in reaction time responses to a light-emitting diode regularly illuminated for one in every three seconds. This test distinguishes healthy subjects (mean latency to lapsing 39.8 min) from sleep apnoea patients (10.5 min) (Bennett *et al.*, 1997).

In most studies, weak to moderate positive correlations ($r = 0.3$–0.5) are found between severity of sleep apnoea and severity of daytime sleepiness measured by self-report (Johns, 1993; Rosenthal *et al.*, 1997) or by objective assessment (Poceta *et al.*, 1992; Roehrs *et al.*, 1989; Roth *et al.*, 1980). Some studies, though, report no significant correlations between sleep parameters and MSLT scores, thus suggesting hypoxaemia as a major determinant of daytime sleepiness (Bédard *et al.*, 1991a; Cheshire *et al.*, 1992). Notwithstanding this, most findings indicate sleep fragmentation as the primary cause of excessive daytime sleepiness (Day *et al.*, 1999). For example, Colt *et al.* (1991) found that OSAS patients showed similar improvements in daytime sleepiness after two nights of treatment with nasal continuous positive airway pressure, whether or not the researchers induced repetitive nocturnal hypoxaemia. Therefore, they concluded that sleep disruption, rather than hypoxaemia, leads to daytime sleepiness. It should be noted, however, that, in this study, a small sample size was used (seven patients) and that hypoxaemia could be induced for only two nights. Conversely, in a study in which nocturnal oxygen was administered to improve oxygenation without having an effect on sleep fragmentation, no improvement in daytime sleepiness was found (Gold *et al.*, 1986). Moreover, multiple regression research has identified sleep fragmentation as the best predictor of daytime sleepiness in apnoea patients (Roehrs *et al.*, 1989; Verstraeten *et al.*, 1996).

Cognition

Neurocognitive performance reported in the moderate to severe sleep apnoea literature can be subdivided into the areas of attention, executive function, memory and learning, and psychomotor function.

Attention

Sleep apnoea patients typically show vigilance decrements. The so-called Steer Clear, a simulated driving programme, has been used to assess vigilance. It measures simple reaction time performance on a 30-min task that requires the subject to avoid about 780 obstacles presented at varying intervals. Significantly higher obstacle hit rates in severe or older OSAS patients have been demonstrated (Findley *et al.*, 1991; 1995), as well as time-on-task decrements (Findley *et al.*, 1999). However, Ingram *et al.* (1994) found no significant correlation between mild apnoea in community-dwelling older adults and Steer Clear performance. On another laboratory-based Divided Attention Driving Test, 21 severe apnoea patients performed worse than 21 normal controls on all measures, with the largest decrement in tracking error. The performance of half of the patients was worse than any control subject, some even performing worse than alcohol-intoxicated control subjects (George *et al.*, 1996). In addition, community-acquired subjects with mild to moderate sleep-disordered breathing (AHI 10–30) performed worse during the last 2 min on a 10-min visual vigilance test (perceptual sensitivity) than healthy controls (Redline *et al.*, 1997), while severe OSAS patients (mean AHI 65) performed worse on the Continuous Performance Test than chronic obstructive pulmonary disease patients that experience both daytime and night-time hypoxaemia (Roehrs *et al.*, 1995).

In view of the relationship of working memory to attention (see, e.g., Baddeley, 1992), we discuss working-memory function in this section as far as the 'slave systems' are concerned. The 'visuospatial sketch pad' is assumed to be a slave system capable of holding visuospatial information, while the 'phonological loop' performs a similar function for speech-based information. These systems are coordinated and linked to long-term memory by the 'central executive', being concerned with attentional control rather than storage (see *Executive function* section). It has been shown that moderate to severe apnoea patients exhibit decreased working-memory spans for both verbal (digit span) and visual (Corsi block-tapping) information (Kales *et al.*, 1985; Naëgelé *et al.*, 1995). Severe OSAS patients also performed poorly on the Wechsler Digit-Symbol Substitution (Bédard *et al.*, 1991b), which is a measure of information processing speed, or their AHI was significantly correlated with performance on this test (Cheshire *et al.*, 1992). However, information processing speed in subjects with mild to moderate sleep-disordered breathing did not differ from controls (AHI < 5) (Kim *et al.*, 1997; Redline *et al.*, 1997).

Executive Function

The concept of 'executive function' refers to a multidimensional construct of (loosely) related higher-order cognitive processes such as planning, cognitive flexibility, response initiation and inhibition, problem solving, goal-directed behaviour, and self-regulation, of which the central executive of working memory is an important subordinate operation. Relatively few controlled studies exist on executive functioning in sleep apnoea. A frequently used neuropsychological task of executive function is the Trail Making Test. In this test, the subject has to connect in proper order 25 circled numbers randomly arranged on a page (part A), and 25 circled numbers and letters by alternating between these numbers and letters (part B). Some authors have found that patients performed worse on the Trail Making Test, part B, assessing cognitive flexibility (Bédard *et al.*, 1991b; Findley *et al.*, 1986), whereas others have not found such deficits (Naëgelé *et al.*, 1995; Greenberg *et al.*, 1987; Kim *et al.*, 1997). As performance on Trail Making, part A, was not included in the former studies, appropriate interpretation may be problematic (see methodological considerations below). Moreover, hypoxaemic patients in the study of Findley *et al.* (1986) showed oxygen desaturation even during the day, thus hampering the evaluation of the specific impact of sleep apnoea. Both moderate to severe (Naëgelé *et al.*, 1995) and mild to moderate (Redline *et al.*, 1997) apnoea patients remembered fewer Wechsler digits backwards, a test which is a measure of the 'central executive' of the working memory. However, Naëgelé *et al.*'s (1995) findings showed that patients also remembered fewer forward digits, while Redline *et al.* (1997) presented no data on forward digits (see methodological considerations below). The latter authors also found no deficits in their mild to moderate OSAS sample in performance on the Trail Making Test, the Wisconsin Card Sorting Test (number of perseverative errors), and a serial digit-subtraction task (Redline *et al.*, 1997). No significant decreases in verbal fluency were found in moderate to severe (Naëgelé *et al.*, 1995) or in mild to moderate OSAS (Kim *et al.*, 1997). In contrast, Bédard *et al.* (1991b) did demonstrate such an impairment. Interestingly, no deficit and no significant association were found between verbal fluency and severity of hypoxaemia in chronic obstructive pulmonary disease patients (Stuss *et al.*, 1997). Regarding planning abilities, apnoeics made more errors on the Wechsler Mazes Test (Bédard *et al.*, 1991b). They also needed a higher number of moves in a three-disc Tower of Toronto (a simplified version of the Tower of Hanoi) experiment, whereas, surprisingly, there was no significant difference between patients and controls on the more difficult four-disc Tower of Toronto (Naëgelé *et al.*, 1995). Furthermore, Naëgelé *et al.* (1995) found that patients needed more time to complete the so-called interference condition of the Stroop Color-Word Test measuring focused attention and inhibition of interfering habitual responses. Unfortunately, no data were provided on the 'easy' test conditions (see methodological considerations below). Scores on a modified Wisconsin Card Sorting Test, another frequently used test of executive function, in 17 moderate to severe OSAS patients, were not impaired as far as the number of categories achieved and total number of errors are concerned. However, these patients made more perseverative errors than the control group matched for age, verbal IQ, and educational level (Naëgelé *et al.*, 1995). When moderate patients (either AHI 10–40 or oxygen saturation level of <85% below 10 min) were compared to severe patients (either AHI > 40 or oxygen saturation level of <85% over 10 min), no significant differences in perseverative errors emerged, a finding which is in agreement with the lack of relationship between severity of hypoxaemia and Wisconsin Card Sorting performance in chronic obstructive pulmonary disease patients (Stuss *et al.* 1997).

Memory and Learning

It has been repeatedly found that moderate to severe apnoea patients show reduced short-term memory of both verbal and visual material (Bédard *et al.*, 1991b; Borak *et al.*, 1996; Kales *et al.*, 1985; Klonoff *et al.*, 1987; Naëgelé *et al.*, 1995) (see also *Attention* section above). In addition, these patients exhibited delayed recall deficits for both verbal and visual information (Bédard *et al.*, 1991b; Naëgelé *et al.*, 1995). In mild to moderate sleep-disordered breathing, however, neither immediate nor delayed verbal recall memory deficits was found (Kim *et al.*, 1997; Redline *et al.*, 1997). Moreover, these patients showed no procedural memory dysfunction, as measured with a 'pursuit rotor' task (Redline *et al.*, 1997).

Psychomotor Function

Manual dexterity was found to be impaired in moderate to severe OSAS patients (Bédard *et al.*, 1991b; Greenberg *et al.*, 1987), but not in mild to moderate patients (Kim *et al.*, 1997). Block *et al.* (1986) also found lowered psychomotor speed in mildly sleep-disordered breathing. Interestingly, a relationship between hypoxaemia and reduced complex perceptual motor and simple motor performance has been repeatedly demonstrated in chronic obstructive pulmonary disease patients (Krop *et al.*, 1973; Grant *et al.*, 1982; Grant *et al.*, 1987). Moreover, these lung patients exhibit a lower finger-tapping speed than OSAS patients (Roehrs *et al.*, 1995).

Before concluding this overview of neurocognitive function, we now return to the available executive function data. In general, it has been claimed that OSAS patients exhibit executive control deficits (see Day *et al.*, 1999; Décary *et al.*, 2000; Engleman and Joffe, 1999, for reviews). It should be noted, however, that research on higher attentional (executive) dysfunction should be guided by sound theoretical neuropsychological models of attention. This is especially important in sleep disorders characterized by excessive daytime sleepiness, since it is well known that sleepiness, as a result of sleep deprivation and/or sleep fragmentation, has significant effects on cognitive function (Bonnet, 2000; Dinges and Kribbs, 1991; Tilley and Brown, 1992), not the least of which is general cognitive slowing. As cognitive slowing underlies the higher executive functions, the effect of this basal slowing in information processing should be controlled for. This can be illustrated using the already mentioned Trail Making Test. Part A of this test is a measure of visual search, psychomotor speed, and visuomotor tracking. Part B, in addition to the same visuomotor activity and visual search processes as in part A, also requires task switching. Because of this additional demand, part B is considered to be a measure of cognitive flexibility. This test is scored in terms of the time in seconds required for part A and part B, respectively. However, it should be kept in mind that performance on part B can never be evaluated without taking into account the performance on task A. In other words, an underlying impaired basic process, such as in part A, can be responsible for a deficit in part B. Overall, this is true for all complex attention tests. Data from other tasks or other task conditions within the same test should always be considered to interpret neuropsychological data appropriately (van Zomeren and Brouwer, 1994). Other typical examples of such tests are the Digit Span Forwards and Backwards (Lehto, 1996) and the Stroop Color-Word Task (Henik, 1996). As the pervasive effects of sleepiness on cognitive function are not fully taken into account in the sleep apnoea literature, the findings of executive deficits should be regarded as tentative.

Aetiological Factors of Cognitive Dysfunction

The pathophysiological mechanisms that cause neurocognitive deficits in sleep apnoea have been argued to be sleep fragmentation and nocturnal hypoxaemia. The relative contribution of these aetiological factors is still a contentious issue (e.g., Verstraeten *et al.*, 1996). The investigation of the specific impact of these causal factors is complicated by the fact that sleep fragmentation is highly correlated with nocturnal respiratory disturbances. In any case, most studies suggest that both sleep fragmentation and nocturnal hypoxaemia contribute to the neurocognitive impairments (see Engleman and Joffe, 1999, for a detailed review). Some researchers have suggested differential effects of alertness impairment and nocturnal hypoxaemia (Bédard *et al.*, 1991b). According to their interpretations, reductions in psychomotor and executive function seem to be related to the extent of hypoxaemia, whereas attention and memory dysfunction appear to be associated with daytime sleepiness. As there is no agreement on this, further research is needed. One strategy to assess the impact of the two hypothesized pathophysiological mechanisms is to examine to what extent treatment leads to improvement in neuropsychological function (see below).

Driving Performance

For an excellent review on the relationship between sleepiness and motor and working accidents, the reader is referred to the December 1995 Supplement of the *Journal of Sleep Research* (Åkerstedt, 1995). It has been repeatedly shown that sleepiness may account for a considerable portion of automobile accidents (e.g., Horne and Reyner, 1995). To investigate the relationship of motor vehicle accidents to sleep-disordered breathing, Young *et al.* (1997) performed a population-based study in which 913 employed adults were involved and objective governmental records of accidents were used. Men with AHI of >5, compared to those without sleep-disordered breathing, were significantly more likely to have at least one accident in 5 years (odds ratios = 3.4 for habitual snorers, 4.2 for AHI 5–15, and 3.4 for AHI of >15). Men and women combined with AHI of >15 were more likely to have multiple motor vehicle accidents in 5 years (odds ratio = 7.3). Laboratory-based driving simulators were employed to assess driving ability in OSAS. For instance, the 20-min Divided Attention Driving Test requires division of attention between tracking and visual search. Severe apnoea patients performed worse than age-matched normal controls in mean tracking error (George *et al.*, 1996). The MSLT and AHI explained less than 25% of the variance in tracking error. Self-reported accident frequency does not appear to be significantly related to the severity of sleep-disordered breathing (Stoohs *et al.*, 1994). These findings indicate the difficulty of identifying individual OSAS patients at increased risk of accidents by PSG or behavioural testing.

Psychosocial Impact

The most frequently, though not always reported, psychological problem in the sleep apnoea literature is depression, as assessed with personality inventories or psychiatric screening questionnaires. It should be noted, however, that depressive symptoms on, for instance, the Zung self-rating depression scale and symptoms of sleep apnoea may overlap (e.g., fatigue, sleep disruption, impaired task performance, indecisiveness, decreased libido, and constipation from inactivity), indicating that such scales have not been adequately validated for use in sleep-disordered patients (Lee, 1990). Therefore, it is recommended in medical disorders to use assessment instruments that exclude many somatic items. For instance, the Freiburger Personality Inventory, a questionnaire measuring 12 personality traits, has only two out of 138 items confounded with daytime sleepiness. Using this inventory, it was found that even severe OSAS patients' average values were within the normal range of all scales (Cassel, 1993). In another interesting study, severe OSAS patients waiting for surgical treatment were compared to patients awaiting coronary artery bypass surgery (Klonoff *et al.*, 1987). Both patient groups showed similar subclinical elevations on the Minnesota Multiphasic Personality Inventory scales of depression, hysteria, and hypochondriasis. Moreover, these elevated levels of emotional distress before surgery in both groups were significantly ameliorated 3 months after successful surgical intervention for the respective diseases. Overall, these findings are in line with the consensus nowadays that the psychological problems of OSAS patients are not unique to sleep apnoea, but are rather a characteristic response to any chronic medical disorder (Roth *et al.*, 1995), and that psychological well-being is normalized after treatment (Engleman *et al.*, 1994; Platon and Sierra, 1992).

Treatment Effects

Nasal continuous positive airway pressure (CPAP) has become the non-surgical treatment of choice for obstructive sleep apnoea. Overall, CPAP treatment has shown, either by self-report (Engleman *et al.*, 1996) or by randomized placebo-controlled crossover design (Engleman *et al.*, 1994), that daytime function improves significantly. CPAP therapy reduces effectively both subjective (Hardinge *et al.*, 1995; Kribbs *et al.*, 1993) and objective daytime sleepiness (Sforza and Lugaresi, 1995; Kribbs *et al.*, 1993; Poceta *et al.*, 1992). Driving performance on a realistic simulator (Haraldsson *et al.*, 1995), on Steer Clear (Engleman *et al.*, 1994), or on the Divided Attention Driving Test (George *et al.*, 1997) recovers significantly after therapy. In addition, research shows that CPAP therapy reverses most neurocognitive deficits (Bédard *et al.*, 1993; Engleman *et al.*, 1994; Naëgelé *et al.*, 1998). However, Naëgelé *et al.* (1998) found no improvements in verbal and visual short-term memory. Furthermore, Bédard *et al.* (1993) demonstrated persistent deficits in planning abilities and manual dexterity after CPAP treatment. As these functions were related to hypoxaemia in their study, these researchers have suggested irreversible anoxic frontal brain damage. However, poor treatment compliance (Berthon-Jones *et al.*, 1996; Hoy *et al.*, 1999; Reeves-Hoche *et al.*, 1994: average duration of use ranging from 3.2 to 4.7 h/night) may explain the residual deficits, all the more so because some daytime somnolence, although greatly improved, persisted compared to healthy controls. Finally, as already noted, enhancements in psychological well-being were consistently found after nasal CPAP therapy (Engleman *et al.*, 1994; Platon and Sierra, 1992).

NARCOLEPSY

The narcoleptic tetrad was well described by Gélineau (1880) in a classic paper: excessive daytime sleepiness with sleep attacks, cataplexy, sleep paralysis, and hypnagogic hallucinations. The onset of adolescence is often the beginning of this neurological condition, which is more prevalent in males than females. Regarding cognitive dysfunction, these patients often complain of memory disturbances (especially encoding). Lhermitte (1930) gave a neuropsychological description of the amnesic phenomena, and Broughton *et al.* (1981), in a series of studies, repeatedly encountered subjective memory complaints in narcoleptics.

More recent studies, such as that of Beusterien *et al.* (1999), with large patient groups ($n = 558$) also found that, in addition to other psychosocial and intrapersonal problems, narcoleptics have difficulty in maintaining concentration and attention, a problem which can be reversed by appropriate treatment. Brain-imaging studies (Bassetti *et al.*, 1997; Heyde *et al.*, 2001) did not provide evidence of structural anatomical anomalies. As the emphasis in narcolepsy research moved towards the hypocretin/orexin deficiency (Siegel, 1999; Nishino *et al.*, 2000) (hypocretinergic neurons are located in the lateral hypothalamus and are believed to control monoaminergic and cholinergic activity during sleep), interest has rekindled in possible neurocognitive deficits associated with this disorder. Initially, these deficits were thought to be related to a suspected monoaminergic and cholinergic involvement. Can the subjective attention and memory complaints of these patients be objectified by formal neuropsychological testing?

Aguirre *et al.* (1985) compared 10 untreated narcoleptics with matched controls on a battery of verbal and non-verbal memory tests and could not detect a memory deficit. They concluded that it is these patients' drowsiness that induces a subjective memory problem, as the short duration of the tests and the test session itself made it possible for the patients to counteract sleepiness. Henry *et al.* (1988) found a reduced vigilance and diminished memory encoding with longer response latencies in a classic Sternberg task in four of their eight patients when they were not treated. (The Sternberg task is a recognition memory-scanning task in which subjects need to make a reaction time response to indicate whether or not a test digit is a member of a previously memorized list of digits. The reaction time increases with the size of the set to be memorized.) Under treatment, these deficits almost fully recovered. Rogers and Rosenberg (1990) recorded on-task EEG in 30 narcoleptics and 30 healthy controls during the Wechsler Memory Scale and Digit Substitution tests, Rey's Auditory Verbal Learning and Complex Figure test, and the Profile of Mood States. No significant differences on the different measures of attention/concentration or memory tests could be detected. The continuous EEG recordings did show changes in alertness that were not accompanied by poor test performance. In a 'temporal isolation' study in which six untreated narcoleptics were allowed to follow their free-running circadian rhythm for a part of the study (Pollak *et al.*, 1992), only very minor differences in neuropsychological test performance were found. Again, the impairment of an accuracy measure in a serial search task was related to occasional lapses in attention, according to the authors. The only evidence of a very specific perceptual encoding deficit that underlies poor memory and complex reaction time performance comes from Henry *et al.* (1993), who compared 10 unmedicated narcoleptic patients with controls.

It is a common observation that most studies on cognitive processes in narcolepsy include a very small number of patients and use short duration tests that are often too engaging and stimulating. Often a theoretical rationale for the tests selected is missing and, finally, no comparison group comprising other hypersomnia, but non-narcoleptic, patients is introduced in the study design, so that it is difficult to detect narcolepsy-specific cognitive deficits.

Schulz and Wilde-Frenz (1995) used a monotonous task, the Critical Flicker Fusion Test, during a period of 10 h and found that the 10 narcoleptic patients were unable to maintain a steady performance level throughout the experiment. Finally, Hood and Bruck (1996) used an experimental protocol in which narcoleptic patients were tested in a low- and in a high-arousal condition. During the high-arousal condition, narcoleptics performed at the same level as healthy controls in the task under automatic control. On the contrary, complex tasks such as word fluency, semantic reasoning, and the paced auditory serial addition task were highly dependent on fluctuations in arousal.

From the evidence available, it seems correct to conclude that cognitive impairment in narcoleptic patients is a function of the daytime sleepiness they suffer from. These episodes of sleepiness have a temporal character, making it difficult to demonstrate cognitive deficits without an appropriate experimental protocol.

GENERAL CONCLUSION

Summarizing the currently available evidence on the existence of neuropsychological impairment as a consequence of disturbed sleep, we find few hard data on significant daytime cognitive deficits in chronic primary insomnia. Memory and attention problems often occur, but they can also be interpreted as symptoms of a more general malaise in these patients. They worry excessively about their sleep, and the possible consequences of poor sleep, and behavioural treatment seems to be their first choice. Studies on both pharmacological and behavioural interventions should include these cognitive outcome measures to find out whether the above described morbidity can be reversed.

Regarding sleep apnoea syndrome, the size and range of cognitive deficits increase with the severity of sleep-disordered breathing. Most of the community-based studies with only mild sleep-disordered breathing have documented no or only weak relationships between sleep apnoea and neuropsychological function. In contrast, studies using clinic patients have found neuropsychological impairments. These impairments may exist only in patients with more severe sleep-disordered breathing and/or in conjunction with significant daytime sleepiness. Narcoleptic patients do present with specific memory and attention problems, but these seem to be related to the attacks of daytime sleepiness they suffer from.

We have chosen to discuss possible daytime dysfunctions following some selective sleep disorders, thereby inevitably making a selection. Other sleep disorders such as idiopathic hypersomnia, and shift-work and jet-lag-related sleep disturbances are also suspected to result in cognitive deficits, as has been shown by Cho (2001). The mechanisms involved, including prolonged higher cortisol levels affecting sensible brain structures such as the hippocampus, should also be investigated and explored in chronic primary insomnia.

Further research is certainly needed to address the many methodological considerations we discussed in the previous paragraphs. Fine-grained analyses to divide cognitive abilities into their subcomponents in well-defined groups of insomnia, sleep apnoea, idiopathic hypersomnia, and narcoleptic patients are urgently needed.

REFERENCES

Aguirre, M., Broughton, R. and Stuss, D., 1985. Does memory impairment exist in narcolepsy-cataplexy? *Journal of Clinical and Experimental Neuropsychology*, **7**, 14–24.

Åkerstedt, T., 1995. Work hours, sleepiness and accidents: introduction and summary. *Journal of Sleep Research*, **4**, 1–3.

American Academy of Sleep Medicine, 1999. Sleep related breathing disorders in adults: recommendation for syndrome definition and measurement techniques in clinical research. *Sleep*, **22**, 667–689.

American Psychiatric Association, 1994. *Diagnostic and Statistical Manual of Mental Disorders* (4th edn). American Psychiatric Association, Washington, DC.

American Sleep Disorders Association, 1997. *International Classification of Sleep Disorders. Diagnostic and Coding Manual Revised*. American Sleep Disorders Association, Rochester MN.

Ancoli-Israel, S., Kripke, D.F. and Mason, W., 1987. Characteristics of obstructive and central sleep apnea in the elderly: an interim report. *Biological Psychiatry*, **22**, 741–750.

Baddeley, A.D., 1992. Working memory. *Science*, **255**, 556–559.

Bassetti, C., Aldrich, M.S. and Quint, D.J., 1997. MRI findings in narcolepsy. *Sleep*, **20**, 630–631.

Bédard, M.A., Montplaisir, J., Richer, F. and Malo, J., 1991a). Nocturnal hypoxemia as a determinant of vigilance impairment in sleep apnea syndrome. *Chest*, **100**, 367–370.

Bédard, M.A., Montplaisir, J., Richer, F., Rouleau, I. and Malo, J., 1991b. Obstructive sleep apnea syndrome: pathogenesis of neuropsychological deficits. *Journal of Clinical and Experimental Neuropsychology*, **13**, 950–964.

Bédard, M.A., Montplaisir, J., Malo, J., Richer, F. and Rouleau, I., 1993. Persistent neuropsychological deficits and vigilance impairment in sleep apnea syndrome after treatment with continuous positive airways pressure (CPAP). *Journal of Clinical and Experimental Neuropsychology*, **15**, 330–341.

Bennett, L.S., Stradling, J.R. and Davies, R.J.O., 1997. A behavioural test to assess daytime sleepiness in obstructive sleep apnoea. *Journal of Sleep Research*, **6**, 142–145.

Berry, D.T., Phillips, B.A., Cook, Y.R., Schmitt, F.A., Gilmore, R.L., Patel, R., Keener, T.M. and Tyre, E., 1987. Sleep-disordered breathing in healthy aged persons: possible daytime sequelae. *Journal of Gerontology*, **42**, 620–626.

Berry, D.T., Phillips, B.A., Cook, Y.R., Schmitt, F.A., Honeycutt, N.A., Edwards, C.L., Lamb, D.G., Magan, L.K. and Allen, R., 1989. Sleep-disordered breathing in healthy aged persons: one-year follow-up of daytime sequelae. *Sleep*, **12**, 211–215.

Berthon-Jones, M., Lawrence, S., Sullivan, C.E. and Grunstein, R., 1996. Nasal continuous positive airway pressure treatment: current realities and future. *Sleep*, **19**, S131–S135.

Beusterien, K.M., Rogers, A.E., Walsleben, J.A., Emsellem, H.A., Reblando, J.A., Wang, L., Goswami, M. and Steinwald, B., 1999. Health-related quality of life effects of modafinil for treatment of narcolepsy. *Sleep*, **22**, 757–765.

Block, A.J., Berry, D. and Webb, W., 1986. Nocturnal hypoxemia and neuropsychological deficits in men who snore. *European Journal of Respiratory Disease*, **69**, 405–408.

Bonnet, M.H., 2000. Sleep deprivation. In: Kryger, M.H., Roth, T. and Dement, W.C. (eds), *Principles and Practice of Sleep Medicine*, pp. 53–71. WB Saunders, New York.

Bonnet, M.H. and Arand, D.L., 1995. 24-Hour metabolic rate in insomniacs and matched normal sleepers. *Sleep*, **18**, 581–588.

Bonnet, M.H. and Arand, D.L., 1997. Hyperarousal and insomnia. *Sleep Medicine Reviews*, **1**, 97–108.

Bonnet, M.H. and Arand, D.L., 2000. Activity, arousal and the MSLT in patients with insomnia. *Sleep*, **23**, 205–211.

Bonnett, M.H. and Rosa, R.R., 2001. Predictors of objective sleepiness in insomniacs and normal sleepers. *Sleep*, **24**, 128.

Borak, J., Cieslicki, J.K., Koziej, M., Matuszewski, A. and Zielinski, J., 1996. Effects of CPAP treatment on psychological status in patients with severe obstructive sleep apnoea. *Journal of Sleep Research*, **5**, 123–127.

Broughton, M., Ghanem, Q., Hishikawa, Y., Sugita, Y., Nevsimalova, S. and Roth, B., 1981. Life effects of narcolepsy in 180 patients from North America, Asia and Europe compared to matched controls. *Canadian Journal of Neurological Sciences*, **8**, 299–304.

Buysse, D.J., Reynolds, C.F., Kupfer, D.J., Thorpy, M.J., Bixler, E., Manfredi, R., Kales, A., Vgontzas, A., Stepanski, E., Roth, T. and Hauri, P., 1994. Clinical diagnoses in 216 insomnia patients using the International Classification of Sleep Disorders (ICSD), DSM-IV and ICD-10 categories — a report from the APA/NIMH DSM-IV field trial. *Sleep*, **17**, 630–637.

Carscadon, M.A. and Dement, W.C., 1982. Nocturnal determinants of daytime sleepiness. *Sleep*, **5**, S73–91.

Carskadon, M.A., Dement, W.C., Mitler, M.M., Roth, T., Westbrook, P.R. and Keenan, S., 1986. Guidelines for the multiple sleep latency test (MSLT): a standard measure of sleepiness. *Sleep*, **9**, 519–524.

Cassel, W., 1993. Sleep apnea and personality. *Sleep*, **16**, S56–S58.

Chambers, M.J. and Kim, J.Y., 1993. The role of state-trait anxiety in insomnia and daytime restedness. *Behavioral Medicine*, **19**, 42–46.

Cheshire, K., Engleman, H., Deary, I., Shapiro, C. and Douglas, N.J., 1992. Factors impairing daytime performance in patients with sleep apnea/hypopnea syndrome. *Archives of Internal Medicine*, **152**, 538–541.

Cho, K., 2001. Chronic 'jet lag' produces temporal lobe atrophy and spatial cognitive deficits. *Nature Neuroscience*, **4**, 567–568.

Cluydts, R., De Valck, E., Verstraeten, E. and Theys, P., 2002. Evaluation of sleepiness. *Sleep Medicine Reviews*, in press.

Cluydts, R., Rouckhout, D. and Vandeputte, M., 1996. MMPI-2 Characteristics of chronic insomniacs. *International Journal of Psychology*, **31**, 228.

Cohen, R., 1993. *The Neuropsychology of Attention*. Plenum Press, New York.

Colt, H.G., Haas, H. and Rich, G.B., 1991. Hypoxemia vs sleep fragmentation as cause of excessive daytime sleepiness in obstructive sleep apnea. *Chest*, **100**, 1542–1548.

Day, R., Gerhardstein, R., Lumley, A., Roth, T. and Rosenthal, L., 1999. The behavioral morbidity of obstructive sleep apnea. *Progress in Cardiovascular Diseases*, **41**, 341–354.

Décary, A., Rouleau, I. and Montplaisir, J., 2000. Cognitive deficits associated with sleep apnea syndrome: a proposed neuropsychological test battery. *Sleep*, **23**, 369–381.

Dinges, D. and Kribbs, N., 1991. Performing while sleepy: effects of experimentally-induced sleepiness. In: Monk, T. (ed.), *Sleep, Sleepiness and Performance*, pp. 97–128. Wiley, West Sussex, England.

Edinger, J.D., Fins, A.I., Sullivan, R.J., Marsh, G.R., Dailey, D.S., Hope, T.V., Young, M., Shaw, E., Carlson, D. and Vasilas, D., 1997. Do our methods lead to insomniacs' madness? Daytime testing after laboratory and home-based polysomnographic studies. *Sleep*, **20**, 1127–1134.

Edinger, J.D., Wohlgemuth, W.K., Radtke, R.A., Marsh, G.R. and Quillian, R.E., 2001. Cognitive behavioral therapy for treatment of chronic primary insomnia. *Journal of the American Medical Association*, **285**, 1856–1864.

Engleman, H. and Joffe, D., 1999. Neuropsychological function in obstructive sleep apnoea. *Sleep Medicine Reviews*, **3**, 59–78.

Engleman, H.M., Martin, S.E., Deary, I.J. and Douglas, N.J., 1994. The effect of continuous positive airway pressure therapy on daytime function in the sleep apnoea/hypopnoea syndrome. *Lancet*, **343**, 572–575.

Engleman, H.M., Asgari-Jirhandeh, N., McLeod, A.L., Ramsay, C.F., Deary, I.J. and Douglas, N.J., 1996. Self-reported use of CPAP and benefits of CPAP therapy: a patient survey. *Chest*, **109**, 1470–1476.

Engleman, H.M., Martin, S.E., Deary, I.J. and Douglas, N.J., 1997. Effect of CPAP therapy on daytime function in patients with mild sleep apnoea/hypopnoea syndrome. *Thorax*, **52**, 114–119.

Fichten, C.S., Creti, L., Amsel, R., Brender, W., Weinstein, N. and Libman, E., 1995. Poor sleepers who do not complain of insomnia — myths and realities about psychological and life-style. *Journal of Behavioral Medicine*, **18**, 189–223.

Findley, L.J., Barth, J.T., Powers, M.E., Wilhoit, S.C., Boyd, D.G. and Suratt, P.M., 1986. Cognitive impairment in patients with obstructive sleep apnea and associated hypoxemia. *Chest*, **90**, 686–690.

Findley, L.J., Weiss, J.W. and Jabour, E.R., 1991. Drivers with untreated sleep apnea: a cause of death and serious injury. *Archives of Internal Medicine*, **151**, 1451–1452.

Findley, L., Unverzagt, M., Guchu, R., Fabrizio, M., Buckner, J. and Suratt, P., 1995. Vigilance and automobile accidents in patients with sleep apnea or narcolepsy. *Chest*, **108**, 619–624.

Findley, L.J., Suratt, P.M. and Dinges, D.F., 1999. Time-on-task decrements in 'Steer Clear' performance of patients with sleep apnea and narcolepsy. *Sleep*, **22**, 804–809.

Fulda, S. and Schulz, H., 2001. Cognitive dysfunction in sleep disorders. *Sleep Medicine Reviews*, **5**, 423–445.

Gélineau, J., 1880. De la narcolepsie. *Gazette des Hôpiteaux (Paris)*, **53**, 535–637.

George, C.F.P., Boudreau, A.C. and Smiley, A., 1996. Simulated driving performance in patients with obstructive sleep apnea. *American Journal of Respiratory and Critical Care Medicine*, **154**, 175–181.

George, C.F.P., Boudreau, A.C. and Smiley, A., 1997. Effects of nasal CPAP on simulated driving performance in patients with obstructive sleep apnoea. *Thorax*, **52**, 648–653.

Gold, A.R., Schwartz, A.R., Bleecker, E.R. and Smith, P.L., 1986. The effect of nocturnal oxygen administration upon sleep apnea. *American Review of Respiratory Disease*, **134**, 925–929.

Grant, I., Heaton, R.K., McSweeny, A.J., Adams, K.M. and Timms, R.M., 1982. Neuropsychologic findings in hypoxemic chronic obstructive pulmonary disease. *Archives of Internal Medicine*, **142**, 1470–1476.

Grant, I., Prigatano, G.P., Heaton, R.K., McSweeny, A.J., Wright, E.C. and Adams, K.M., 1987. Progressive neuropsychologic impairment and hypoxemia. *Archives of General Psychiatry*, **44**, 999–1006.

Greenberg, G.D., Watson, R.K. and Deptula, D., 1987. Neuropsychological dysfunction in sleep apnea. *Sleep*, **10**, 254–262.

Haraldsson, P.O., Carenfelt, C., Lysdahl, M. and Tornros, J., 1995. Long-term effect of uvulopalatopharyngoplasty on driving performance. *Archives of Otolaryngology, Head and Neck Surgery*, **121**, 90–94.

Hardinge, F.M., Pitson, D.J. and Stradling, J.R., 1995. Use of the Epworth sleepiness scale to demonstrate response to treatment with nasal continuous positive airway pressure in patients with obstructive sleep apnoea. *Respiratory Medicine*, **89**, 617–620.

Hataway, S.R. and McKinley, J.C., 1967. *The Minnesota Multiphasic Personality Inventory Manual*. Psychological Corporation, New York.

Hauri, P.J., 1997. Cognitive deficits in insomnia patients. *Acta Neurologica Belgica*, **97**, 113–117.

Hauri, P.J. and Olmstead, E.M., 1989. Reverse 1st night effect in insomnia. *Sleep*, **12**, 97–105.

Hayward, L., Mant, A., Eyland, A., Hewitt, H., Purcell, C., Turner, J., Goode, E., Le Count, A., Pond, D. and Saunders, N., 1992. Sleep disordered breathing and cognitive function in a retirement village population. *Age and Ageing*, **21**, 121–128.

Henik, A., 1996. Paying attention to the Stroop effect? *Journal of the International Neuropsychological Society*, **2**, 467–470.

Henry, G.K., Hart, R.P., Kwentus, J.A. and Sicola, M.J., 1988. Effects of protriptyline on vigilance and information processing in narcolepsy. *Psychopharmacology*, **95**, 109–112.

Henry, G.K., Satz, P. and Heibroner, R.L., 1993. Evidence of a perceptual-encoding deficit in narcolepsy? *Sleep*, **16**, 123–127.

Heyde, K., De Volder, I., Estercam, S., Van den Haude, L. and Cluydts, R., 2001. No relevant MRI findings in narcolepsy. *Sleep*, **24**, 313–314.

Hoddes, E., Zarcone, V., Smythe, H., Phillips, R. and Dement, W.C., 1973. Quantification of sleepiness: a new approach. *Psychophysiology*, **10**, 431–436.

Hood, B. and Bruck, D., 1996. Sleepiness and performance in narcolepsy. *Journal of Sleep Research*, **5**, 128–134.

Horne, J.A. and Reyner, L.A., 1995. Sleep related vehicle accidents. *British Medical Journal*, **310**, 565–567.

Hoy, C.J., Vennelle, M., Kingshott, R.N., Engleman, H.M. and Douglas, N.J., 1999. Can intensive support improve continuous positive airway pressure use in patients with the sleep apnea/hypopnea syndrome? *American Journal of Respiratory and Critical Care Medicine*, **159**, 1096–1100.

Ingram, F., Henke, K.G., Levin, H.S., Fishel Ingram, P.T. and Kuna, S.T., 1994. Sleep apnea and vigilance performance in a community-dwelling older sample. *Sleep*, **17**, 248–252.

Johns, M.W., 1991. A new method for measuring daytime sleepiness: the Epworth sleepiness scale. *Sleep*, **14**, 540–545.

Johns, M.W., 1993. Daytime sleepiness, snoring and obstructive sleep apnea: the Epworth sleepiness scale. *Chest*, **103**, 30–36.

Johnson, L.C., 1992. Daytime sleepiness in good sleepers: measurements and correlates. In: Broughton, R.J. and Ogilvie, R.D. (eds), *Sleep, Arousal and Performance*, pp. 220–229. Raven Press, Boston.

Kales, A., Caldwell, A.B., Cadieux, R.J., Vela-Bueno, A., Ruch, L.G. and Mayes, S.D., 1985. Severe obstructive sleep apnea-II: associated psychopathology and psychosocial consequences. *Journal of Chronic Diseases*, **38**, 427–434.

Kim, H.C., Young, T., Matthews, C.G., Weber, S.M., Woodward, A.R. and Palta, M., 1997. Sleep-disordered breathing and neuropsychological deficits: a population-based study. *American Journal of Respiratory and Critical Care Medicine*, **156**, 1813–1819.

Klonoff, H., Fleetham, J., Taylor, D.R. and Clark, C., 1987. Treatment outcome of obstructive sleep apnea: physiological and neuropsychological concomitants. *Journal of Nervous and Mental Disease*, **175**, 208–212.

Kribbs, N.B. and Dinges, D., 1994. Vigilance decrement and sleepiness. In: Harsh, J.R. and Ogilvie, R.D. (eds), *Sleep Onset: Normal and Abnormal Processes*, pp. 113–125. American Psychological Association, Washington, DC.

Kribbs, N.B., Pack, A.I., Kline, L.R., Getsy, J.E., Schuett, J.S., Henry, J.N., Maislin, G. and Dinges, D.F., 1993. Effects of one night without nasal CPAP treatment on sleep and sleepiness in patients with obstructive sleep apnea. *American Review of Respiratory Disease*, **147**, 1162–1168.

Krop, H.D., Block, A.J. and Cohen, E., 1973. Neuropsychologic effects of continuous oxygen therapy in chronic obstructive pulmonary disease. *Chest*, **64**, 317–322.

Lamphere, J., Roehrs, T., Wittig, R., Zorick, F., Conway, W.A. and Roth, T., 1989. Recovery of alertness after CPAP in apnea. *Chest*, **96**, 1364–1367.

Lee, S., 1990. Depression in sleep apnea: a different view. *Journal of Clinical Psychiatry*, **51**, 309–310.

Leger, D., Levy, E. and Paillard, M., 1999. The direct costs of insomnia in France. *Sleep*, **22**, S394–401.

Lehto, J., 1996. Are executive function tests dependent on working memory capacity? *Quarterly Journal of Experimental Psychology*, **49A**, 29–50.

Lhermitte, J., 1930. Les narcolepsies. *Progrès en Médecine*, 962–975.

Lichstein, K.L., Durrence, H.H., Bayen, U.J. and Riedel, B.W., 2001. Primary versus secondary insomnia in older adults: subjective sleep and daytime functioning. *Psychology of Aging*, **16**, 264–271.

Maquet, P., Laureys, S., Peigneux, P., Fuchs, S., Petiau, C., Phillips, C., Aerts, J., Del Fiore, G., Degueldre, C., Meulemans, T., Luxen, A., Franck, G., Van der Linden, M., Smith, C. and Cleeremans, A., 2000). Experience-dependent changes in cerebral activation during human REM sleep. *Nature Neuroscience*, **3**, 831–836.

McNair, D.M., Lorr, M. and Droppleman, L.F., 1981. *Manual for the Profile of Mood States*. Educational and Industrial Testing Service, San Diego.

Mitler, M.M., Gujavarty, K.S. and Browman, C.P., 1982. Maintenance of wakefulness test: a polysomnographic technique for evaluating treatment efficacy in patients with excessive somnolence. *Electroencephalography and Clinical Neurophysiology*, **53**, 658–661.

Morin, C.M., Stone, J. and Trinkle, D., 1993. Dysfunctional beliefs and attitudes about sleep among older adults with and without insomnia complaints. *Psychology of Aging*, **8**, 463–467.

Naëgelé, B., Thouvard, V., Pépin, J-L., Levy, P., Bonnet, C., Perret, J.E., Pellat, J. and Feuerstein, C., 1995. Deficits of cognitive executive functions in patients with sleep apnea syndrome. *Sleep*, **18**, 43–52.

Naëgelé, B., Pepin, J.L., Levy, P., Bonnet, C., Pellat, J. and Feuerstein, C., 1998. Cognitive executive dysfunction in patients with obstructive sleep apnea syndrome (OSAS) after CPAP treatment. *Sleep*, **21**, 392–397.

Nishino, S., Ripley, B., Overeem, S., Lammers, G.J. and Mignot, E., 2000). Hypocretin (orexin) deficiency in human narcolepsy. *Lancet*, **355**, 39–40.

Nowell, P.D., Buysse, D.J., Reynolds, C.F., Hauri, P.J., Roth, T., Stepanski, E.J., Thorpy, M.J., Bixler, E., Kales, A., Manfredi, R.L., Vgontzas, A.N., Stapf, D.M., Houck, P.R. and Kupfer, D.J., 1997. Clinical factors contributing to the differential diagnosis of primary insomnia and insomnia related to mental disorders. *American Journal of Psychiatry*, **154**, 1412–1416.

Palinkas, L.A., Houseal, M. and Miller, C., 2000. Sleep and mood during a winter in Antarctica. *Int. J. Circumpolar Health*, **59**, 63–73.

Partinen, M. and Hublin, C., 2000. Epidemiology of sleep disorders. In: Kryger, M.H., Roth, T. and Dement, W.C. (eds), *Principles and Practice of Sleep Medicine* (3rd edn), pp. 558–579. WB Saunders, New York.

Partinen, M. and Telakivi, T., 1992. Epidemiology of obstructive sleep apnea syndrome. *Sleep*, **15**, S1–S4.

Perlis, M.L., Giles, D.E., Mendelson, W.B., Bootzin, R.R. and Wyatt, J.K., 1999. Psychophysiological insomnia: the behavioral model and a neurocognitive perspective. *Journal of Sleep Research*, **8**, 161–162.

Perlis, M.L., Kehr, E., Smith, M.T., Andrews, P.J., Orff, H. and Giles, D.E., 2001. Temporal and stagewise distribution of high frequency EEG activity in patients with primary and secondary insomnia and in good sleeper controls. *Journal of Sleep Research*, **10**, 93–104.

Phillips, B.A., Berry, D.T., Schmitt, F.A., Harbison, L. and Lipke-Molby, T., 1994. Sleep-disordered breathing in healthy aged persons: two- and three-year follow-up. *Sleep*, **17**, 411–415.

Pilcher, J.J. and Hufcutt, A.I., 1996. Effects of sleep deprivation on performance: a meta-analysis. *Sleep*, **19**, 318–326.

Pilcher, J.J., Ott, E.S., Her, C. and Faulkner, E.E., 1996. The relationship between sleep and measures of health, well-being, and sleepiness: a repeated measures approach. *Sleep Research*, **25**, 173.

Platon, M.J.R. and Sierra, J.E., 1992. Changes in psychopathological symptoms in sleep apnea patients after treatment with nasal continuous positive airway pressure. *International Journal of Neuroscience*, **62**, 173–195.

Poceta, J.S., Timms, R.M., Jeong, D.U., Ho, S.L., Erman, M.K. and Mitler, M.M., 1992. Maintenance of wakefulness test in obstructive sleep apnea syndrome. *Chest*, **101**, 893–897.

Poe, G.R., Nitz, D.A., McNaughton, B.L. and Barnes, C.A., 2000. Experience-dependent phase-reversal of hippocampal neuron firing during REM sleep. *Brain Research*, **855**, 176–180.

Pollak, C.P., Wagner, D.R., Moline, M.L. and Monk, T.H., 1992. Cognitive and motor performance of narcoleptic and normal subjects living in temporal isolation. *Sleep*, **15**, 202–211.

Redline, S., Strauss, M.E., Adams, N., Winters, M., Roebuck, T., Spry, K., Resenberg, C. and Adams, K., 1997. Neuropsychological function in mild sleep-disordered breathing. *Sleep*, **20**, 160–167.

Reeves-Hoche, M.K., Meck, R. and Zwillich, C.W., 1994. Nasal CPAP: an objective evaluation of patient compliance. *American Journal of Respiratory and Critical Care Medicine*, **149**, 149–154.

Riedel, B.W. and Lichstein, K.L., 2000. Insomnia and daytime functioning. *Sleep Medicine Reviews*, **4**, 277–298.

Roehrs, T., Zorick, F., Wittig, R., Conway, W. and Roth, T., 1989. Predictors of objective level of daytime sleepiness in patients with sleep-related breathing disorders. *Chest*, **95**, 1202–1206.

Roehrs, T., Merrion, M., Pedrosi, B., Stepanski, E., Zorick, F. and Roth, T., 1995. Neuropsychological function in obstructive sleep apnea syndrome

(OSAS) compared to chronic obstructive pulmonary disease (COPD). *Sleep*, **18**, 382–388.

Rogers, A.E. and Rosenberg, R.S., 1990. Tests of memory in narcoleptics. *Sleep*, **13**, 42–52.

Rosa, R.R. and Bonnet, M.H., 2000. Reported chronic insomnia is independent of poor sleep as measured by electroencephalography. *Psychosomatic Medicine*, **62**, 474–482.

Rosenthal, L., Bishop, C., Guido, P., Syron, M.L., Helmus, T., Rice, F.M. and Roth, T., 1997. The sleep/wake habits of patients diagnosed as having obstructive sleep apnea. *Chest*, **111**, 1494–1499.

Roth, T. and Ancoli-Israel, S., 1999. Daytime consequences and correlates of insomnia in the United States: results from the 1991 National Sleep Foundation Survey. II. *Sleep*, **22**, S354–358.

Roth, T., Hartse, K.M., Zorick, F. and Conway, W., 1980. Multiple naps and the evaluation of daytime sleepiness in patients with upper airway sleep apnea. *Sleep*, **3**, 425–439.

Roth, T., Roehrs, T. and Rosenthal, L., 1995. Hypersomnolence and neurocognitive performance in sleep apnea. *Current Opinion in Pulmonary Medicine*, **1**, 488–490.

Saletu-Zyhlarz, G., Saletu, B., Anderer, P., Brandstatter, N., Frey, R., Klosch, G., Mandl, M., Grunberger, J. and Linzmayer, L., 1997. Nonorganic insomnia in generalized anxiety disorder. Controlled studies on sleep, awakening and daytime vigilance utilizing polysomnography and EEG mapping. *Neuropsychobiology*, **36**, 117–129.

Schulz, H. and Wilde-Frenz, J., 1995. Cognitive processes and sleep disturbances: the disturbance of cognitive processes in narcolepsy. *Journal of Sleep Research*, **4**, 10–14.

Sforza, E. and Krieger, J., 1997. Daytime sleepiness after long-term continuous positive airway pressure (CPAP) treatment in obstructive sleep apnea syndrome. *Journal of Neurological Science*, **110**, 21–26.

Sforza, E. and Lugaresi, E., 1995. Daytime sleepiness and nasal continuous positive airway pressure therapy in obstructive sleep apnea syndrome patients: effects of chronic treatment and 1-night withdrawal. *Sleep*, **18**, 195–201.

Siegel, J.M., 1999. Narcolepsy: a key role for hypocretins (orexins). *Cell*, **98**, 437–451.

Spielman, A.J., Caruso, L.S. and Glovinsky, P.B., 1987. A behavioral-perspective on insomnia treatment. *Psychiatric Clinics of North America*, **10**, 541–553.

Stoohs, R.A., Guilleminault, C., Itoi, A. and Dement, W.C., 1994. Traffic accidents in commercial long-haul truck drivers: the influence of sleep-disordered breathing and obesity. *Sleep*, **17**, 619–623.

Stuss, D.T., Peterkin, I., Guzman, D.A., Guzman, C. and Troyer, A.K., 1997. Chronic obstructive pulmonary disease: effects of hypoxia on neurological and neuropsychological measures. *Journal of Clinical and Experimental Neuropsychology*, **19**, 515–524.

Tilley, A. and Brown, S., 1992. Sleep deprivation. In: Smith, A. and Jones, D. (eds), *Handbook of Human Performance. Vol. 3: Trait and State*, pp. 237–259. Academic Press, London.

van Zomeren, A. and Brouwer, W., 1994. *Clinical Neuropsychology of Attention*. Oxford University Press, New York.

Verstraeten, E., Cluydts, R., Verbraecken, J. and De Roeck, J., 1996. Neuropsychological functioning and determinants of morning alertness in patients with obstructive sleep apnea syndrome. *Journal of the International Neuropsychological Society*, **2**, 306–314.

Walsh, J.K. and Lindblom, S.S., 1997. Psychophysiology of sleep deprivation and disruption. In: Pressman, M.R. and Orr, W.C. (eds), *Understanding Sleep*, pp. 73–110. American Psychological Association, Washington, DC.

Young, T., Palta, M., Dempsey, J., Skatrud, J., Weber, S. and Badr, S., 1993. The occurrence of sleep-disordered breathing among middle-aged adults. *New England Journal of Medicine*, **328**, 1230–1235.

Young, T., Blustein, J., Finn, L. and Palta, M., 1997. Sleep-disordered breathing and motor vehicle accidents in a population-based sample of employed adults. *Sleep*, **20**, 608–613.

Zammit, G.K., Weiner, J., Damato, N., Sillup, G.P. and McMillan, C.A., 1999. Quality of life in people with insomnia. *Sleep*, **22**, S379–385.

Zorick, J.F. and Wash, J.K., 2000. Evaluation and management of insomnia: an overview. In: Kryger, M.H., Roth, T. and Dement, W.C. (eds), *Principles and Practice of Sleep Medicine* (3rd edn), pp. 615–623. WB Saunders, New York.

XXIV-7

Sleep Disorders — Functional Neuroanatomy

Pierre Maquet

INTRODUCTION

Sleep is probably the last complex and integrated behaviour of which the functions remain poorly understood. Nevertheless, since the last half of the 20th century, an impressive body of knowledge has been accumulated on sleep in mammals, especially cats and rodents. Much is now known on the mechanisms that maintain wakefulness, non-rapid eye movement (non-REM) sleep and rapid eye movement (REM) sleep, down to cellular and molecular levels.

In parallel, studies on patients and normal human subjects suggest that similar mechanisms generate sleep and sustain wakefulness in humans. However, we are still far from a comprehensive understanding of human sleep and its disorders at the fine-grained level of description reached in animal studies. Therefore, at present, it remains difficult to interpret the human pathology of sleep in terms of the underlying neuronal disturbances. Some exceptions, however, are mentioned in this chapter. For instance, recent breakthrough in molecular biology shed some light on the pathophysiology of narcolepsy in animals and, hopefully, in humans.

Sleep regulation does not involve only the generation of wakefulness and sleep periods. It also includes the interaction of sleep processes with the internal circadian rhythms and the external synchronizers, especially light. These aspects of sleep regulation are also important to consider because of the related human pathology.

This chapter provides an overview on the generation of sleep and wakefulness. It is not meant to review these mechanisms in the greatest detail but to put emphasis on the mechanisms that might be disturbed in sleep disorders. It is divided into two parts: (a) the regulation of circadian cycles and (b) the generation of wakefulness, non-REM sleep and REM sleep.

GENERALITIES ABOUT SLEEP

Sleep is not a homogeneous process. It is composed of two main sleep states: non-REM sleep and REM sleep. These two types of sleep differ in many aspects, such as their circadian distribution, their pattern of cellular activity and their physiological regulation. Non-REM sleep is usually recognized by the appearance of sleep spindles and K-complexes, the hallmarks of the light non-REM sleep (stage 2 sleep). The deepest stage of non-REM sleep, called slow-wave sleep (SWS), is defined by the presence of large-amplitude, low-frequency EEG waves. The power density of these slow waves is maximal at sleep onset and decreases exponentially during the night (Borbely, 1982).

Rapid eye movement sleep, also called paradoxical sleep (PS), is characterized by low amplitude, relatively fast rhythms on EEG recordings, ocular saccades and muscular atonia interspersed by muscular twitches. REM sleep typically occurs by periods of about 20 min, recurring every 90 min. In contrast to non-REM sleep, the duration of REM sleep episodes increases as the night progresses.

REGULATION OF CIRCADIAN RHYTHMS

Sleep/waking cycles, like many other physiological and behavioural parameters, occur with circadian periodicity. In mammals, a large body of data proves that the suprachiasmatic nucleus (SCN) of the hypothalamus is the site which controls these circadian rhythms, especially sleep/wakefulness cycles.

First, in animals, lesions of the SCN abolish the rest/activity rhythmicity and alter sleep/waking patterns (Ibuka and Kawamura, 1975; Mouret *et al.*, 1978). Second, circadian rhythms are reinstated by SCN transplants, the restored rhythms being derived from the donor SCN (Ralph and Lehman, 1991). Third, individual SCN cells maintain for long periods a near 24-h periodicity in their firing rates (Welsh *et al.*, 1995). This observation suggests that the periodicity of the SCN activity does not emerge from local networks but reflects the genuine pacemaker properties of the SCN cells. This hypothesis was confirmed at the molecular level. The circadian rhythms are generated by autoregulatory feedback loops of transcription and translation of a set of clock genes and their gene products (for review, see King and Takahashi, 2000; Wager-Smith and Kay, 2000). Manipulation of these clocks genes can lead to mutant individuals with intrinsic circadian rhythms different than the wild type (King and Takahashi, 2000; Vitaterna *et al.*, 1994).

In addition, the clock of the SCN does not tick only on its own. It is entrained to the night/day cycle by light. Anatomically, SCN is in position both to receive light signal and synchronize several physiological rhythms. The SCN receives light signal from the retina, mainly through the retino-hypothalamic tract (Dai *et al.*, 1998; Morin, 1994). It projects primarily to hypothalamic nuclei and, to a smaller extent, to limbic, thalamic and mesencephalic structures (van Esseveldt *et al.*, 2000). The SCN can influence sleep/waking cycles via the secretion of melatonin, using a specific polysynaptic pathway (paraventricular nucleus, intermedio-lateral column of the spinal cord, superior cervical ganglion, and pineal gland) (see Moore, 1996).

Biological rhythms in humans seem to be generated by similar molecular and cellular mechanisms, which thus have important implications in sleep or circadian disorders. SCN is described in humans and, as in other mammals, it receives fibres from the retina and projects extensively to other hypothalamic nuclei (Dai *et al.*, 1998). The disturbances of biological rhythms in demented patients have been attributed to structural modifications of the SCN (Swaab *et al.*, 1985). As in other mammals, circadian rhythms in humans can be entrained by light (Lewy and Sack, 1996; Shanahan and Czeisler, 2000) and by melatonin (Cagnacci, 1997; Lewy and Sack, 1996). Blind people are known to suffer from sleep disorders due to free-running circadian rhythms (Nakagawa *et al.*, 1992), with a circadian period rather longer than normal subjects (Sack *et al.*, 2000). Melatonin may help these patients to entrain circadian rhythms and improve their condition (Sack *et al.*, 2000). Finally, polymorphisms have been identified in several human clock genes.

Biological Psychiatry: Edited by H. D'haenen, J.A. den Boer and P. Willner. ISBN 0-471-49198-5

A link was reported between such a polymorphism and human diurnal preferences (Katzenberg *et al.*, 1999). Likewise, probands of a familial advance sleep-phase syndrome have been shown to have an intrinsic circadian rhythm of 23 h (Jones *et al.*, 1999), 1 h less than normal (Czeisler *et al.*, 1999). This trait segregates as an autosomal dominant with high penetrance. These examples provide a clear evidence of the direct effect of genotype on the phenotype of human biological rhythms.

GENERATION OF WAKEFULNESS, NON-REM-SLEEP AND REM SLEEP

The Hypothalamic Control of Sleep and Wakefulness

Wakefulness and sleep are generated continuously, in an ordered succession, through the action of interacting structures of the brainstem and the diencephalon. In particular, the anterior hypothalamus and the posterior hypothalamus play an important role in the generation of sleep and wakefulness, respectively. Two neuronal populations seem critical in this respect, the ventrolateral preoptic nucleus (VLPO) in the anterior hypothalamus and the tuberomammillary nucleus (TMN) in the posterior hypothalamus.

Lesions of the anterior preoptic area of the anterior hypothalamus (POAH) and adjacent basal forebrain (BF) cause prolonged insomnia in mammals (for review, see Szymusiak, 1995; for the most recent study using lesions restricted to the VLPO only, see Lu *et al.*, 2000). In contrast, local stimulation of this region induces sleep (McGinty *et al.*, 1994; Sterman and Clemente, 1962). In this area, electrophysiological studies have detected neurons with firing rates two or three times higher during sleep than during wakefulness (Szymusiak *et al.*, 1998). It was also shown that the number of Fos-immunoreactive cells in VLPO increases after sleep and is proportional to the duration of sleep episode during the preceding hour (Sherin *et al.*, 1996). These data indicate that VLPO plays an instrumental role in the generation of sleep. VLPO receives a sparse projection from the SCN, thereby allowing the modulation of sleep by circadian rhythms (Novak and Nunez, 2000). VLPO neurons in turn project to the tuberomammillary nucleus of the posterior hypothalamus (Sherin *et al.*, 1998) and to other wakefulness-sustaining structures such as the locus coeruleus (LC) (Steininger *et al.*, 2001).

By contrast, the posterior hypothalamus seems to sustain arousal. Lesions of the posterior hypothalamus (Von Economo, 1926), as its inactivation (Lin *et al.*, 1988; 1989; 1990; 1994), decrease wakefulness and favour sleep. Within the posterior hypothalamus, a population of histaminergic neurons in the tuberomammillary nucleus have been particularly involved in wakefulness (Lin *et al.*, 1988; 1989; 1990; 1994). It is also a common clinical observation that antihistaminic drugs induce somnolence (Meltzer, 1990). Histaminergic neurons project to a wealth of structures (such as cortex, POAH, thalamus, and mesopontine tegmentum) thereby controlling the arousal state of the whole brain (Lin *et al.*, 1996).

It seems that feedback loops exist between the anterior and the posterior hypothalamus and regulate the succession of sleep and wakefulness periods. The GABAergic VLPO neurons probably have an inhibitory effect on TMN cells (Sherin *et al.*, 1998) but are themselves inhibited by wakefulness-sustaining neurotransmitters such as 5HT and NA (Gallopin *et al.*, 2000). Moreover, enhancement of histaminergic neurotransmission in the POAH decreases sleep and favours wakefulness periods (Lin *et al.*, 1994).

Finally, a small hypothalamic neuronal population was recently the subject of great experimental scrutiny. Located in the lateral posterior hypothalamus, they project throughout the brain and, importantly, to arousal-related structures (LC, raphe nuclei, and thalamus) (Peyron *et al.*, 1998). They secrete two newly described peptides, the hypocretins 1 and 2 (de Lecea *et al.*, 1998). Their effect is essentially neuroexcitatory and is mediated by two different receptors (hypocretin receptors 1 and 2), which are differently expressed in the cerebrum (Kilduff and Peyron, 2000). The presumptive functions of hypocretins concern eating behaviour and sleep (Sutcliffe and de Lecea, 2000). Local administration of hypocretin 1 into the LC suppresses REM sleep and increases wakefulness in a dose-dependent manner (Bourgin *et al.*, 2000) while perfusion of hypocretin 2 receptor antisense in the pontine reticular formation increases REM sleep (Thakkar *et al.*, 1999). These discoveries bear directly on one major sleep disorder, narcolepsy. In narcoleptic dogs, a mutation of the hypocretin 2 receptor gene leads to a truncated receptor protein (Lin *et al.*, 1999). Furthermore, systemic administration of hypocretin-1 reduces cataplexy and normalizes sleep/waking cycles in these dogs (John *et al.*, 2000). Likewise, knockout mice in which the hypocretin gene was inactivated suffered from cataplectic attacks, a hallmark of human narcolepsy (Chemelli *et al.*, 1999). Finally, perfusion of hypocretin 2 receptor antisense in the pontine reticular formation induces cataplectic attacks in rats (Thakkar *et al.*, 1999). It is unlikely that human narcolepsy is due, as in the dog, to a mutation of a single gene, because epidemiological studies do not point to a simple genetic transmission (Mignot, 1998). However, it was recently found that hypocretin concentration in the cerebrospinal fluid was undetectable in seven out of nine narcoleptic patients (Nishino *et al.*, 2000). Moreover, post-mortem examination of the narcoleptic hypothalamus revealed a decreased number of hypocretin cells (Thannickal *et al.*, 2000). It remains to be shown whether human narcolepsy is caused by a defect in hypocretin production, secretion or signalling. These pathological mechanisms could be due to genetic, viral or autoimmune causes (van den Pol, 2000).

HOW IS WAKEFULNESS MAINTAINED?

Besides hypothalamic sites, the generation of wakefulness depends on the mesencephalic reticular formation, and on the modulation of cerebral activity by the aminergic neurotransmission: acetylcholine (mesopontine reticular formation and basal forebrain), serotonin (raphe nuclei) and noradrenaline (locus coeruleus) (for review, see Steriade and McCarley, 1990).

The mesencephalic reticular formation, as well as the cholinergic neurons of the mesopontine tegmentum, maintain wakefulness by tonically bombarding the thalamic nuclei, thereby supporting a tonic firing in thalamocortical neurons and, consequently, a cortical arousal (Datta and Siwek, 1997; Datta *et al.*, 2001; Steriade and McCarley, 1990).

The cholinergic magnocellular neurons of the basal forebrain project directly to the whole cortex and are thought to be critical for the cortical arousal. Ibotenic acid lesions of the BF reduce acetylcholinesterase cortical staining and result in an ipsilateral increase in slow waves (Buzsaki *et al.*, 1988). In contrast, electrical and chemical BF stimulation elicits a shift of the spike discharge pattern of cortical neurons from phasic to tonic and consequently leads to EEG activation (Metherate *et al.*, 1992). By the same token, the unit activity of cortically projecting BF neurons (most of which are cholinergic) increases their discharge rate during EEG activation (Detari and Vanderwolf, 1987).

Serotonergic cells of the raphe nuclei and noradrenergic neurons of the locus coeruleus can also influence the firing pattern of thalamic cells, maintaining a tonic firing in thalamocortical neurons. They also project to widespread areas of the cortex, thereby influencing the activity of large neuronal population in the telencephalon.

THALAMOCORTICAL LOOPS AND THE GENERATION OF NON-REM SLEEP

Current theories of non-REM sleep generation put a strong emphasis on the activity patterns in the thalamocortical loops. Several rhythms and activities coalesce during non-REM sleep: spindles, delta rhythm, slow rhythm and K-complexes. All these rhythms occur through complex interactions between the reticular thalamic cells, the relay thalamic neurons and cortical networks. For didactic reasons, they are described as separate processes but, in practice, these oscillations coexist (spindles and slow rhythm, delta and slow rhythm [Steriade and Amzica, 1998]) or smoothly alternate (spindles and delta rhythm [Merica and Fortune, 1997]).

In animals, it is known that thalamic neurons become hyperpolarized because the activating brainstem structures described above decrease progressively during their firing rate at sleep onset. Due to this disfacilitation mechanism, thalamic neurons change their firing mode from tonic to phasic (Steriade and McCarley, 1990). First, due to their intrinsic membrane properties, GABAergic cells of the reticular thalamic nucleus burst in the spindle frequency range and entrain thalamocortical neurons in spindle oscillation (Steriade and McCarley, 1990; Steriade *et al.*, 1993b). As sleep deepens, thalamic neurons get more hyperpolarized and a clock-like delta rhythm appears in thalamocortical cells, due to their intrinsic membrane properties (Steriade *et al.*, 1993a). This delta rhythm arises from the interplay between a low threshold calcium current (It) and a hyperpolarization-activated K^+ current (Ih) (Steriade *et al.*, 1993a). Thalamic delta rhythm is conveyed to the cortex, which further reorganizes it and incorporates it into a cortically-induced, slow rhythm (Steriade and Amzica, 1998).

Neuroimaging data support the role of thalamic nuclei in non-REM sleep generation. A significant regression was found between thalamic blood flow and the power density within the spindle frequency band (Hofle *et al.*, 1997). Likewise, significant changes in thalamic blood flow and glucose metabolism is the most consistent feature reported in human non-REM sleep (Maquet, 2000). The observation of patients with thalamic lesions also confirms the role of thalamic nuclei in non-REM sleep. Thalamotomized Parkinson patients show significant changes in their pattern of spindles (Roth *et al.*, 2000). Likewise, fatal insomnia, a prion disease characterized by a severe loss of sleep, is related to thalamic lesions and a decrease in thalamic metabolism (Cortelli *et al.*, 1997).

The slow rhythm relies on the properties of the cortical networks and the alternate silent periods of hyperpolarization with activity periods (Steriade *et al.*, 1993a; Steriade *et al.*, 1993c). The slow rhythm was recently identified in humans (Achermann and Borbely, 1997). Moreover, K-complexes, a hallmark of human stage 2 sleep, are viewed as an expression of the slow rhythm (Amzica and Steriade, 1997; Amzica and Steriade, 1998). The long-lasting silent periods appear to be due to a cascade of disfacilitation (Contreras *et al.*, 1996). Activity periods depend on aminoacidergic neurotransmission (Steriade *et al.*, 1993a). The participation of intracortical inhibitory neurons (Steriade *et al.*, 1993a), as well as cortico-cortical connection fibres (Amzica and Steriade, 1995a; Amzica and Steriade, 1995b), has also been emphasized. Recent data suggest that the slow rhythm is actively generated in the cortex. The depolarization state is related to recurrent excitatory interactions between pyramidal cells, regulated by inhibitory networks. The hyperpolarization state is characterized by an after-hyperpolarization in pyramidal cells and the withdrawal of synaptic barrages (Sanchez-Vives and McCormick, 2000).

REM SLEEP: BRAINSTEM MECHANISMS AND LIMBIC/PARALIMBIC ACTIVATION

Two aspects of REM sleep are worth describing: its generation by brainstem nuclei and the characteristic activation of limbic and paralimbic structures.

The widely held theory on REM sleep generation relies on the balance between, on the one hand, the activity of cholinergic REM sleep-on neurons of the mesopontine tegmentum (laterodorsal tegmenti [LDT], pedunculo-pontine nucleus [PPT], and peri-locus coeruleus alpha [periLCa]) and, on the other hand, the noradrenergic cells of the LC and serotonergic neurons of the raphe nuclei (Hobson *et al.*, 1975). The reciprocal interaction model is based on the observation that, during REM sleep, raphe nuclei and LC cells remain silent while, at the same time, mesopontine cholinergic cells increase their firing rate (Steriade and McCarley, 1990). The inhibition of LC and raphe nuclei cells could be due to a direct effect of cholinergic cells, but other mechanisms are possible, such as the inhibition of LC by GABAergic or glycinergic periaqueductal grey (PAG) neurons (Gervasoni *et al.*, 2000; Rampon *et al.*, 1999). Recently, it was also shown that the midbrain structures responsible for REM sleep generation were themselves modulated by higher structures, such as the central nucleus of the amygdala (Morrison *et al.*, 1999).

The activation of cholinergic mesopontine neurons leads to the three characteristics of REM sleep: the cortical activation, the muscular atonia and rapid eye movements. Mesopontine neurons project monosynaptically to the thalamic nuclei. The thalamic activation is then conveyed to the cortex. The ensuing cortical activation would explain the small-voltage, relatively high-frequency EEG activity characteristic of REM sleep (Steriade and McCarley, 1990).

The characteristic muscular atonia observed in REM sleep also depends originally on cholinergic mesopontine neurons (Lai and Siegel, 1999). Cells in or near the periLCα project and stimulate the bulbar reticular formation, directly or via a polysynaptic pathway through the pontine reticular formation. Bulbar reticular formation in turn projects and inhibits motoneurons in the spinal cord, through glycinergic neurotransmission, leading to a tonic decrease in muscle tone. In animals, lesions in the pontine reticular formation lead to REM sleep without atonia. A similar condition, the REM sleep behaviour disorder, was recently described in humans (Schenck *et al.*, 1986). It is characterized by movements of the limbs or body associated with dream mentation and at least one of the following criteria: dreams that appear acted out or sleep behaviour that disturbs sleep continuity (American Sleep Disorder Association, 1997). This condition is related to extrapyramidal disorders (Parkinson's disease, multiple system atrophy). In some of these patients, symptoms have been related to the marked neuronal loss in brainstem nuclei, such as the locus coeruleus, that usually inhibit cholinergic mediated atonia during REM sleep (Turner *et al.*, 2000).

Finally, ocular saccades in REM sleep also depend on cholinergic mesopontine neurons, especially the peribrachial region (Datta, 1999). In animals, saccades are related to ponto-geniculo-occipital (PGO) waves, prominent transient activities that are readily (although not exclusively) recorded in the pons, the lateral geniculate nucleus and the occipital cortex (Datta, 1999). These PGO waves have not been directly recorded in humans, but many arguments suggest that they exist in humans (Peigneux *et al.*, 2000).

The other striking aspect of REM sleep is the predominant activation of limbic and paralimbic structures. Although described in animals for some time (Lydic *et al.*, 1991; Ramm and Frost, 1986), this aspect of REM sleep was recently emphasized in humans by functional neuroimaging studies (Maquet, 2000). Activation in both amygdala and hippocampal formation was reported. Moreover, amygdalo-cortical functional relationships specific to REM sleep were observed. These results suggest that brain function during REM sleep is mainly driven by an interplay between the limbic areas and posterior (temporal and occipital) cortices. The relation between this cortico-limbic interplay and the dreaming activity, although sensible, remains to be formally assessed (Maquet, 2000).

CONCLUSIONS

Sleep is not a state of complete cerebral quiescence. The patterns of brain activity certainly are different in sleep than during wakefulness but do not correspond to the absence of brain activity. The understanding of sleep mechanisms is crucial since they probably underlie some important — or even vital (Rechtschaffen *et al.*, 1989) — function.

REFERENCES

Achermann, P. and Borbely, A.A., 1997. Low-frequency (<1 Hz) oscillations in the human sleep electroencephalogram. *Neuroscience*, **81**, 213–222.

Amzica, F. and Steriade, M., 1995a. Disconnection of intracortical synaptic linkages disrupts synchronization of a slow oscillation. *J Neurosci*, **15**, 4658–4677.

Amzica, F. and Steriade, M., 1995b. Short- and long-range neuronal synchronization of the slow (<1 Hz) cortical oscillation. *J Neurophysiol*, **73**, 20–38.

Amzica, F. and Steriade, M., 1997. The K-complex: its slow (<1-Hz) rhythmicity and relation to delta waves. *Neurology*, **49**, 952–995.

Amzica, F. and Steriade, M., 1998. Cellular substrates and laminar profile of sleep K-complex. *Neuroscience*, **82**, 671–686.

Association ASD, 1997. *International Classification of Sleep Disorders and Codgin Manual*, pp. 177–180. Rochester, MN.

Borbély, A.A., 1982. A two process model of sleep regulation. *Hum Neurobiol*, **1**, 195–204.

Bourgin, P., Huitron-Resendiz, S., Spier, A.D., Fabre, V., Morte, B., Craido, J.R., Sutcliffe, J.G., Henriksen, S.J. and de Lecea, L., 2000. Hypocretin-1 modulates rapid eye movement sleep through activation of locus coeruleus neurons. *J Neurosci*, **20**, 7760–7765.

Buzsaki, G., Bickford, R.G., Ponomareff, G., Thal, L.J., Mandel, R. and Gage, F.H., 1988. Nucleus basalis and thalamic control of neocortical activity in the freely moving rat. *J Neurosci*, **8**, 4007–4026.

Cagnacci, A., 1997. Influences of melatonin on human circadian rhythms. *Chronobiol Int*, **14**, 205–220.

Chemelli, R.M., Willie, J.T., Sinton, C.M., Elmquist, J.K., Scammell, T., Lee, C., Richardson, J.A., Williams, S.C., Xiong, Y., KiChesanauki, Y., Fitch, T.E., Nakazato, M., Hammer, R.E., Saper, C.B. and Yanagisawa, M., 1999. Narcolepsy in orexin knockout mice: molecular genetics of sleep regulation. *Cell*, **98**, 437–451.

Contreras, D., Timofeev, I. and Steriade, M., 1996. Mechanisms of long lasting hyperpolarizations underlying slow sleep oscillations in cat corticothalamic networks. *J Physiol* (*London*), **494**, 251–264.

Cortelli, P., Perani, D., Parchi, P., Grassi, F., Montagna, P., De Martin, M., Castellani, R., Tinuper, P., Gambetti, P., Lugaresi, E. and Fazio, F., 1997. Cerebral metabolism in fatal familial insomnia: relation to duration, neuropathology, and distribution of protease-resistant prion protein. *Neurology*, **49**, 126–133.

Czeisler, C.A., Duffy, J.F., Shanahan, T.L., Brown, E.N., Mitchell, J.F., Rimmer, D.W., Ronda, J.M., Silva, E.J., Allan, J.S., Emens, J.S., Dijk, D.J. and Kronauer, R.E., 1999. Stability, precision, and near-24-hour period of the human circadian pacemaker. *Science*, **284**, 2177–2181.

Dai, J., Van der Vliet, J., Swaab, D.F. and Buijs, R.M., 1998. Human retinohypothalamic tract as revealed by *in vitro* post-mortem tracing. *J Comp Neurol*, **397**, 357–370.

Datta, S., 1999. PGO wave generation: mechanism and functional significance. In: Mallick, B., Inoue, S. (eds), *Rapid Eye Movement Sleep*, pp. 91–106. Narosa Publishing, New Delhi.

Datta, S. and Siwek, D.F., 1997. Excitation of the brain stem pedunculopontine tegmentum cholinergic cells induces wakefulness and REM sleep. *J Neurophysiol*, **77**, 2975–2988.

Datta, S., Spoley, E.E. and Patterson, E.H., 2001. Microinjection of glutamate into the pedunculopontine tegmentum induces REM sleep and wakefulness in the rat. *Am J Physiol Regul Integr Comp Physiol*, **280**, R752–R759.

de Lecea, L., Kilduff, T.S., Peyron, C., Gao, X., Foye, P.E., Danielson, P.E., Fukuhara, C., Battenberg, E.L., Gautvik, V.T., Barlett, F.S., Frankel, W.N., Van den Pol, A.N., Bloom, F.E., Gautvik, K.M. and Sutcliffe, J.G., 1998. The hypocretins: hypothalamus-specific peptides with neuroexcitatory activity. *Proc Natl Acad Sci USA*, **95**, 322–327.

Detari, L. and Vanderwolf, C.H., 1987. Activity of identified cortically projecting and other basal forebrain neurons during large slow waves and cortical activation in anaesthetized rats. *Brain Res*, **437**, 1–8.

Gallopin, T., Fort, P., Eggermann, E., Cauli, B., Luppi, P.H., Rossier, J., Audinat, E., Muhlethaler, M., Serafin, M. and Luppi, P.H., 2000. Identification of sleep-promoting neurons *in vitro*. *Nature*, **404**, 992–995.

Gervasoni, D., Peyron, C., Rampon, C., Barbagli, B., Chouvet, G., Urbain, N. and Fort, P., 2000. Role and origin of the GABAergic innervation of dorsal raphe serotonergic neurons. *J Neurosci*, **20**, 4217–4225.

Hobson, J.A., McCarley, R.W. and Wyzinski, P.W., 1975. Sleep cycle oscillation: reciprocal discharge by two brainstem neuronal groups. *Science*, **189**, 55–58.

Hofle, N., Paus, T., Reutens, D., Fiset, P., Gotman, J., Evans, A.C. and Jones, B.E., 1997. Regional cerebral blood flow changes as a function of delta and spindle activity during slow wave sleep in humans. *J Neurosci*, **17**, 4800–4808.

Ibuka, N. and Kawamura, H., 1975. Loss of circadian rhythm in sleep-wakefulness cycle in the rat by suprachiasmatic nucleus lesions. *Brain Res*, **96**, 76–81.

John, J., W.u., M. and Siegel, J., 2000. Systemic administration of hypocretin-1 reduces cataplexy and normalizes sleep and waking durations in narcoleptic dogs. *Sleep Res Online*, **3**, 23–28.

Jones, C.R., Campbell, S.S., Zone, S.E., Cooper, F., DeSano, A., Murphy, P.J., Jones, B., Czajkowski, L. and Ptacek, L.J., 1999. Familial advanced sleep-phase syndrome: A short-period circadian rhythm variant in humans. *Nat Med*, **5**, 1062–1065.

Katzenberg, D., Young, T., Lin, L., Finn, L. and Mignot, E., 1999. A human period gene (HPER1) polymorphism is not associated with diurnal preference in normal adults. *Psychiatr Genet*, **9**, 107–109.

Kilduff, T.S. and Peyron, C., 2000. The hypocretin/orexin ligand-receptor system: implications for sleep and sleep disorders. *Trends Neurosci*, **23**, 359–365.

King, D.P. and Takahashi, J.S., 2000. Molecular genetics of circadian rhythms in mammals. *Annu Rev Neurosci*, **23**, 713–742.

Lai, Y. and Siegel, J., 1999. Muscle atonia in REM sleep. In Mallick, B., Inoue, S. (eds), *Rapid Eye Movement Sleep*, pp. 69–90. Narosa Publishing, New Delhi.

Lewy, A.J. and Sack, R.L., 1996. The role of melatonin and light in the human circadian system. *Prog Brain Res*, **111**, 205–216.

Lin, J.S., Hou, Y., Sakai, K. and Jouvet, M., 1996. Histaminergic descending inputs to the mesopontine tegmentum and their role in the control of cortical activation and wakefulness in the cat. *J Neurosci*, **16**, 1523–1537.

Lin, J.S., Sakai, K. and Jouvet, M., 1988. Evidence for histaminergic arousal mechanisms in the hypothalamus of cat. *Neuropharmacology*, **27**, 111–122.

Lin, J.S., Sakai, K. and Jouvet, M., 1994. Hypothalamo-preoptic histaminergic projections in sleep-wake control in the cat. *Eur J Neurosci*, **6**, 618–625.

Lin, J.S., Sakai, K., Vanni-Mercier, G., Arrang, J.M., Garbarg, M., Schwartz, J.C. and Jouvet, M., 1990. Involvement of histaminergic neurons in arousal mechanisms demonstrated with H3-receptor ligands in the cat. *Brain Res*, **523**, 325–330.

Lin, J.S., Sakai, K., Vanni-Mercier, G. and Jouvet, M., 1989. A critical role of the posterior hypothalamus in the mechanisms of wakefulness determined by microinjection of muscimol in freely moving cats. *Brain Res*, **479**, 225–240.

Lin, L., Faraco, J., Li, R., Kadotani, H., Rogers, W., Lin, X., Qiu, X., de Jong, P.J., Nishino, S. and Mignot, E., 1999. The sleep disorder canine narcolepsy is caused by a mutation in the hypocretin (orexin) receptor 2 gene. *Cell*, **98**, 365–376.

Lu, J., Greco, M.A., Shiromani, P. and Saper, C.B., 2000. Effect of lesions of the ventrolateral preoptic nucleus on NREM and REM sleep. *J Neurosci*, **20**, 3830–3842.

Lydic, R., Baghdoyan, H.A., Hibbard, L., Bonyak, E.V., DeJoseph, M.R. and Hawkins, R.A., 1991. Regional brain glucose metabolism is altered

during rapid eye movement sleep in the cat: a preliminary study. *J Comp Neurol*, **304**, 517–529.
Maquet, P., 2000. Functional neuroimaging of normal human sleep by positron emission tomography. *J Sleep Res*, **9**, 207–231.
McGinty, D., Szymusiak, R. and Thomson, D., 1994. Preoptic/anterior hypothalamic warming increases EEG delta frequency activity within non-rapid eye movement sleep. *Brain Res*, **667**, 273–277.
Meltzer, E.O., 1990. Performance effects of antihistamines. *J Allergy Clin Immunol*, **86**, 613–619.
Merica, H. and Fortune, R.D., 1997. A neuronal transition probability model for the evolution of power in the sigma and delta frequency bands of sleep EEG. *Physiol Behav*, **62**, 585–589.
Metherate, R., Cox, C.L. and Ashe, J.H., 1992. Cellular bases of neocortical activation: modulation of neuronal oscillations by the nucleus basalis and endogenous acetylcholine. *J Neurosci*, **12**, 4701–4711.
Mignot, E., 1998. Genetic and familial aspects of narcolepsy. *Neurology*, **50**, S16–22.
Moore, R.Y., 1996. Neural control of the pineal gland. *Behav Brain Res*, **73**, 125–130.
Morin, L.P., 1994. The circadian visual system. *Brain Res Brain Res Rev*, **19**, 102–127.
Morrison, A., Sanford, L. and Ross, R., 1999. Initiation of rapid eye movement sleep: beyond the brainstem. In: Mallick, B., Inoue, S. (eds), *Rapid Eye Movement Sleep*, pp. 51–68. Narosa Publishing, New Delhi.
Mouret, J., Coindet, J., Debilly, G. and Chouvet, G., 1978. Suprachiasmatic nuclei lesions in the rat: alterations in sleep circadian rhythms. *Electroencephalogr Clin Neurophysiol*, **45**, 402–408.
Nakagawa, H., Sack, R.L. and Lewy, A.J., 1992. Sleep propensity free-runs with the temperature, melatonin and cortisol rhythms in a totally blind person. *Sleep*, **15**, 330–336.
Nishino, S., Ripley, B., Overeem, S., Lammers, G.J. and Mignot, E., 2000. Hypocretin (orexin) deficiency in human narcolepsy. *Lancet*, **355**, 39–40.
Novak, C.M. and Nunez, A.A., 2000. A sparse projection from the suprachiasmatic nucleus to the sleep active ventrolateral preoptic area in the rat. *Neuroreport*, **11**, 93–96.
Peigneux, P., Laureys, S., Aerts, J., Fuchs, S., Delbeuck, X., Del Fiore, G., Dequeldre, C., Franck, G., Luxen, A. and Maquet, P., 2000. Generation of rapid eye movements during paradoxical sleep in humans. *Society for Neuroscience Abstracts*, **30**, 215.
Peyron, C., Tighe, D.K., vanden Pol, AN., de Lecea, L. Heller, H.C., Sutcliffe, J.G. and Kilduff, T.S., 1998. Neurons containing hypocretin (orexin) project to multiple neuronal systems. *J Neurosci*, **18**, 9996–10015.
Ralph, M.R. and Lehman, M.N., 1991. Transplantation: a new tool in the analysis of the mammalian hypothalamic circadian pacemaker. *Trends Neurosci*, **14**, 362–366.
Ramm, P. and Frost, B.J., 1986. Cerebral and local cerebral metabolism in the cat during slow wave and REM sleep. *Brain Res*, **365**, 112–124.
Rampon, C., Peyron, C., Gervasoni, D., Pow, D.V., Luppi, P.H. and Fort, P., 1999. Origins of the glycinergic inputs to the rat locus coeruleus and dorsal raphe nuclei: a study combining retrograde tracing with glycine immunohistochemistry. *Eur J Neurosci*, **11**, 1058–1066.
Rechtschaffen, A., Bergmann, B.M., Everson, C.A., Kushida, C.A. and Gilliland, M.A., 1989. Sleep deprivation in the rat. X. Integration and discussion of the findings. *Sleep*, **12**, 68–87.
Roth, C., Jeanmonod, D., Magnin, M., Morel, A. and Achermann, P., 2000. Effects of medial thalamotomy and pallido-thalamic tractotomy on sleep and waking EEG in pain and Parkinsonian patients. *Clin Neurophysiol*, **111**, 1266–1275.
Sack, R.L., Brandes, R.W., Kendall, A.R. and Lewy, A.J., 2000. Entrainment of free-running circadian rhythms by melatonin in blind people. *N Engl J Med*, **343**, 1070–1077.
Sanchez-Vives, M.V. and McCormick, D.A., 2000. Cellular and network mechanisms of rhythmic recurrent activity in neocortex. *Nat Neurosci*, **3**, 1027–1034.
Schenck, C.H., Bundlie, S.R., Ettinger, M.G. and Mahowald, M.W., 1986. Chronic behavioral disorders of human REM sleep: a new category of parasomnia. *Sleep*, **9**, 293–308.
Shanahan, T.L. and Czeisler, C.A., 2000. Physiological effects of light on the human circadian pacemaker. *Semin Perinatol*, **24**, 299–320.
Sherin, J.E., Elmquist, J.K., Torrealba, F. and Saper, C.B., 1998. Innervation of histaminergic tuberomammillary neurons by GABAergic and galaninergic neurons in the ventrolateral preoptic nucleus of the rat. *J Neurosci*, **18**, 4705–4721.
Sherin, J.E., Shiromani, P.J., McCarley, R.W. and Saper, C.B., 1996. Activation of ventrolateral preoptic neurons during sleep. *Science*, **271**, 216–219.
Steininger, T.L., Gong, H., McGinty, D. and Szymusiak, R., 2001. Subregional organization of preoptic area/anterior hypothalamic projections to arousal-related monoaminergic cell groups. *J Comp Neurol*, **429**, 638–653.
Steriade, M. and Amzica, F., 1998. Coalescence of sleep rhythms and their chronology in corticothalamic networks. *Sleep Res Online*, **1**, 1–10.
Steriade, M., Contreras, D., Curro Dossi, R and Nunez, A., 1993a. The slow (<1 Hz) oscillation in reticular thalamic and thalamocortical neurons: scenario of sleep rhythm generation in interacting thalamic and cortical networks. *J Neurosci*, **13**, 3284–3299.
Steriade, M. and McCarley, R.W., 1990. *Brainstem Control of Wakefulness and Sleep*, New York: Plenum Press.
Steriade, M., McCormick, D.A. and Sejnowski, T.J., 1993b. Thalamocortical oscillations in the sleeping and aroused brain. *Science*, **262**, 679–685.
Steriade, M., Nunez, A. and Amzica, F., 1993c: A novel slow (<1 Hz) oscillation of neocortical neurons *in vivo*: depolarizing and hyperpolarizing components. *J Neurosci*, **13**, 3252–3265.
Sterman, M. and Clemente, C., 1962. Forebrain inhibitory mechanisms: cortical synchronisation induced by basal forebrain stimulation. *Exp Neurol*, **6**, 91–102.
Sutcliffe, J.G. and de Lecea, L., 2000. The hypocretins: excitatory neuromodulatory peptides for multiple homeostatic systems, including sleep and feeding. *J Neurosci Res*, **62**, 161–168.
Swaab, D.F, Fliers, E. and Partiman, T.S., 1985. The suprachiasmatic nucleus of the human brain in relation to sex, age and senile dementia. *Brain Res*, **342**, 37–44.
Szymusiak, R., 1995. Magnocellular nuclei of the basal forebrain: substrates of sleep and arousal regulation. *Sleep*, **18**, 478–500.
Szymusiak, R., Alam, N., Steininger, T.L. and McGinty, D., 1998. Sleep-waking discharge patterns of ventrolateral preoptic/anterior hypothalamic neurons in rats. *Brain Res*, **803**, 178–188.
Thakkar, M., Ramesh, V., Cape, E., Winston, S., Strecker, R. and McCarley, R., 1999. REM sleep enhancement and behavioral cataplexy following orexin (hypocretin)-II receptor antisense perfusion in the pontine reticular formation. *Sleep Res Online*, **2**, 113–120.
Thannickal, T.C., Moore, R.Y., Nienhuis, R., Ramanathan, L., Gulyani, S., Aldrich, M., Cornford, M. and Siegel, J.M., 2000. Reduced number of hypocretin neurons in human narcolepsy. *Neuron*, **27**, 469–474.
Turner, R.S., D'Amato, C.J., Chervin, R.D. and Blaivas, M., 2000. The pathology, of REM sleep behavior disorder with comorbid Lewy body dementia. *Neurology*, **55**, 1730–1732.
van den Pol, A.N., 2000. Narcolepsy: a neurodegenerative disease of the hypocretin system? *Neuron*, **27**, 415–418.
van Esseveldt, K.E., Lehman, M.N. and Boer, G.J., 2000. The suprachiasmatic nucleus and the circadian time-keeping system revisited. *Brain Res Brain Res Rev*, **33**, 34–77.
Vitaterna, M.H., King, D.P., Chang, A.M., Kornhauser, J.M., Lowrey, P.L., McDonald, J.D., Dove, W.F., Pinto, L.H., Turek, F.W. and Takahashi, J.S., 1994. Mutagenesis and mapping of a mouse gene, Clock, essential for circadian behavior. *Science*, **264**, 719–725.
Von Economo, C., 1926. Die Pathologie des Schlafes. In: Von Bethe, A., Von Bergmann, G., Embden, G. and Ellinger, A. (eds), *Handbuch des normalen und Pathologischen Physiologie*, Vol. 17, pp. 591–610. Springer-Verlag, Berlin.
Wager-Smith, K. and Kay, S.A., 2000. Circadian rhythm genetics: from flies to mice to humans. *Nat Genet*, **26**, 23–27.
Welsh, D.K., Logothetis, D.E., Meister, M. and Reppert, S.M., 1995. Individual neurons dissociated from rat suprachiasmatic nucleus express independently phased circadian firing rhythms. *Neuron*, **14**, 697–706.

XXIV-8

Functional Neuroimaging in Sleep and Sleep Disorders

Pierre Maquet

INTRODUCTION

Functional neuroimaging characterizes the human brain function in time and space, using various techniques such as electroencephalography (EEG), positron emission tomography (PET), single photon emission computed tomography (SPECT), functional magnetic resonance imaging (fMRI) or near infrared spectroscopy (NIRS). In this chapter, we review the studies of human sleep using PET, SPECT or fMRI, all techniques which allow us to investigate the whole cerebral volume. In the following sections, we consider successively studies performed in normal subjects and in several sleep disorders.

FUNCTIONAL NEUROIMAGING OF NORMAL HUMAN SLEEP

The regional organization of brain activity is completely different in sleep than in wakefulness and reflects cellular processes similar to the ones described in sleeping animals.

Functional neuroimaging by PET has recently yielded original data on the functional neuroanatomy of human sleep. A more comprehensive discussion of these results, which is beyond the scope of the present chapter, can be found in a recent review paper (Maquet, 2000). These recent data describe the very reproducible functional neuroanatomy in sleep. The core characteristics of this 'canonical' sleep may be summarized as follows. In slow-wave sleep (SWS), the most deactivated areas are located in the dorsal pons and mesencephalon, cerebellum, thalami, basal ganglia, basal forebrain/hypothalamus, prefrontal cortex, anterior cingulate cortex, precuneus and the mesial aspect of the temporal lobe. Briefly, these findings are in keeping with the generation of non-rapid eye movement (REM) sleep in mammals, whereby the decreased firing in brainstem structures causes hyperpolarization of the thalamic neurons and triggers a cascade of processes responsible for the generation of various non-REM sleep rhythms (spindles, theta, and slow rhythm; see Chapter XXIV-7). The human data showed for the first time that the pattern of cortical deactivation was not homogeneous but predominated in various associative cortices, particularly the dorso-lateral and orbital prefrontal cortex. There seems to be a functional link between these cortical regions and sleep processes. Indeed, these areas are known to be involved in mood regulation and in various cognitive functions (such as planning or probability matching) that help to adapt individual behaviour and are known to deteriorate after a short deprivation of sleep (Harrison and Horne, 1998, 1999; Horne, 1988, 1993; Pilcher and Huffcutt, 1996).

During REM sleep, significant activations were found in the pontine tegmentum, thalamic nuclei, limbic areas:amygdaloid complexes (Maquet *et al.*, 1996; Nofzinger *et al.*, 1997), hippocampal formation (Braun *et al.*, 1997; Nofzinger *et al.*, 1997), and anterior cingulate cortex (Braun *et al.*, 1997; Maquet *et al.*, 1996; Nofzinger *et al.*, 1997). The posterior cortices in temporo-occipital areas were also activated (Braun *et al.*, 1997) and their functional interactions are different in REM sleep than in wakefulness (Braun *et al.*, 1998). In contrast, the dorso-lateral prefrontal cortex and parietal cortex, as well as the posterior cingulate cortex and precuneus, were the least active brain regions (Braun *et al.*, 1997; Maquet *et al.*, 1996). Once again, these regional distributions of brain activity are in good accordance with the knowledge already acquired on sleep in animals (see Chapter XXIV-7). REM sleep is generated by neuronal populations of the meso-pontine reticular formation that monosynaptically activate the thalamic nuclei and in turn the cortex. Although early animals studies had mentioned the high limbic activity during REM sleep (Lydic *et al.*, 1991), functional neuroimaging in humans highlighted the contrast between this activation of limbic, paralimbic and posterior cortical areas, and the relative quiescence of associative frontal and parietal cortices. This particular pattern of activation has been thought to account for the main characteristics of human dreaming activity (Hobson *et al.*, 1998; Maquet, 2000; Maquet *et al.*, 1996). The perceptual aspects of dreams may be related to the activation of the posterior (occipital and temporal) cortices and the emotional features to the activation of the amygdalar complexes and related mesio-temporal areas. In contrast, the lack of insight, the loss of time perception, and the amnesia on awakening may be related to the relative hypoactivation of the prefrontal cortex.

Sleep as a Period Favourable to Brain Plasticity

In the adult brain, it is believed that sleep periods participate in memory trace consolidation (Hennevin *et al.*, 1995; Smith, 1995). If this were the case, the regional brain activity in sleep would not be fixed and stereotyped but would depend on previous waking experience. It was recently shown that waking experience indeed influences regional brain activity during subsequent sleep (Maquet *et al.*, 2000). During REM sleep, several brain areas, activated during the execution of a serial reaction time (SRT) task during wakefulness, are significantly more active in subjects previously trained on the task than in non-trained subjects. The functional connectivity of these brain regions was also examined (Laureys *et al.*, unpublished data). One of the reactivated areas, the left premotor cortex, was functionally more tightly correlated with the posterior parietal cortex and the supplementary motor area (SMA) during post-training REM sleep than in 'typical' REM sleep. It was hypothesized that this increase of functional connectivity during post-training REM sleep reflects some processing of the memory traces recently acquired during wakefulness and embodied in the parietal-premotor-SMA network. It remains to be shown that these processes lead to memory trace consolidation.

Biological Psychiatry: Edited by H. D'haenen, J.A. den Boer and P. Willner. ISBN 0-471-49198-5

The Brain's Reactivity to External Stimulation in Sleep

During sleep, the brain remains able to process external stimuli (see, for instance, Perrin *et al.*, 1999). During non-REM sleep, as during wakefulness, several areas continue to be activated by external auditory stimulation: the thalamic nuclei, the auditory cortices and the caudate nucleus (Portas *et al.*, 2000). However, in contrast to wakefulness, no activation is observed in the left parietal, or in the prefrontal and cingulate cortices. Furthermore, in sleeping normal subjects, the activation related to the subject's own name, as compared to beeps, involved the amygdala and the prefrontal cortex (Portas *et al.*, 2000). This demonstrated the persistence during sleep of specific responses to meaningful or emotionally loaded stimuli.

Sleep Drugs and Regional Brain Function

Functional neuroimaging can also be used to explore the effect of a therapeutic agent on brain function. For instance, during REM sleep, zolpidem administration decreased regional blood flow in the anterior cingulate cortex during REM sleep, and in the prefrontal cortex and the insula during non-REM sleep. The results indicate that some differences in regional cerebral blood flow (rCBF) from wakefulness to sleep are modulated by zolpidem (Finelli *et al.*, 2000).

SLEEP DISORDERS

Sleep is deteriorated in a wide range of conditions, ranging from environmental situations (such as jet lag, shift work, and noisy environment) to medical diseases (such as endocrine disorders, chronic pain, brain lesions, sleep apnoea) and psychiatric disorders (such as anxiety and depression). Only a handful of these situations have been explored by functional neuroimaging. Our relative ignorance of the pathophysiology of most sleep disorders and the technical difficulties related to sleep studies probably explain why neuroimaging techniques have not been widely used in the exploration of human sleep disorders and certainly less than in other neurological conditions such as epilepsy or degenerative diseases. In this chapter, we will cover only a few disorders of sleep. We exclude single-case reports, however interesting they may be in their own right (see, for instance, the report on Kleine-Levine syndrome by Lu *et al.*, 2000). Depression is extensively dealt with elsewhere in this book and will be only briefly mentioned here in the context of sleep and sleep deprivation studies.

Narcolepsy

To our knowledge, the voxelwise functional neuroanatomy of the waking state, REM sleep or SWS is not yet described in narcoleptic patients. Nor have been the brain areas related to the other cardinal symptoms of diseases — cataplectic attacks and hypnapompic/hypnagogic hallucinations or sleep paralyses — characterized.

Early observations using ^{133}Xe inhalation showed that during wakefulness, brainstem and cerebellar blood flow was lower in narcoleptic patients than in normal subjects (Meyer *et al.*, 1980). During sleep (3 out of 13 subjects in REM sleep), the cerebral blood flow increased in all regions, and particularly in the temporo-parietal regions. This pattern was putatively attributed to dreaming activity. More recently, a HMPAO-SPECT study compared the waking state to REM sleep (Asenbaum *et al.*, 1995). The global uptake was similar in both conditions. Analysis by regions of interest indicated again an activation of parietal regions. These parietal activations are not in agreement with the parietal deactivation observed by PET studies during normal REM sleep (Maquet, 2000). Further observations are required, using present technology of the acquisition and analysis of functional neuroimaging data, to characterize better the functional organization of the narcoleptic brain during wakefulness and sleep.

Some ligand studies have been reported. Because acetylcholine is an important neurotransmitter in the generation of REM sleep, it was thought that some disturbance in the cholinergic system might underlie narcolepsy. Unfortunately, no change in muscarinic cholinergic receptors could be observed in narcoleptic patients (Sudo *et al.*, 1998). Likewise, post-mortem examination of the brain of narcoleptic patients indicated an increased dopamine D2 binding (Aldrich *et al.*, 1992). This finding was not confirmed by *in vivo* measurements by PET or SPECT, three studies out of four not showing any change in dopamine receptor-binding potential in narcoleptic patients, as compared to controls (Hublin *et al.*, 1994; MacFarlane *et al.*, 1997; Rinne *et al.*, 1996; Rinne *et al.*, 1995). In one study, there was a significant increase in the uptake of ^{11}C-raclopride, a specific D2-receptor ligand, in the putamen of narcoleptic subjects older than 31 years (Khan *et al.*, 1994). Finally, although the binding of IBZM, another D2 receptor ligand, was similar in narcoleptic patients and normal controls, treatment by stimulants and antidepressants for 3 months significantly changed the ligand uptake in four out of five patients. This suggested that the post-mortem findings were more related to treatment than to the disorder itself (Staedt *et al.*, 1996).

The effects of stimulant drugs on cerebral function in narcoleptic patients was assessed in two fMRI studies. The first one tested the effect of modafinil, a sleep-preventing drug (Ellis *et al.*, 1999). First, it was observed that the activation related to visual or auditory stimulation was dependent on the time of day. Normal subjects show higher levels of activation at 10 am than at 3 pm. In a group of 12 narcoleptic patients, the reverse pattern was observed. The administration of modafinil did not modify the average level of activation in either normals or narcoleptics ($n = 8$). However, in both populations, the post-drug activation level was inversely proportional to the pre-drug activation level. This finding is not easily interpreted, but it suggests that modafinil can modulate the brain activation to external stimuli.

Finally, an fMRI study assessed the effects of amphetamines in a small sample of patients with narcoleptic syndrome ($n = 2$, Howard *et al.*, 1996). As compared to three normal control subjects, the activation related to auditory and visual stimulation was decreased in extent after amphetamine administration in normal subjects. The reverse pattern was observed in patients. Once again, these findings are difficult to interpret, and larger samples should be studied before any generalization can be made.

Following the advances made recently in the understanding of narcolepsy (see Chapter XXIV-7) and the discovery of the implication of the hypocretin system in this disorder, it is expected that new neuroimaging studies will soon appear that provide a better description of regional brain function in the various aspects of the disease, such as excessive daytime somnolence, cataplexy and hypnapompic/hypnagogic hallucinations.

Periodic Leg Movements

Periodic leg movements during sleep (PLMS) are characterized by repetitive flexion of the extremities. PLMS can occur in isolation or together with other sleep disorders (narcolepsy, sleep apnoea syndrome or REM sleep behaviour disorder [RBD]). In any case, PLMS disturbs sleep, being responsible for repeated brief arousals. A disinhibition of the descending inhibitory pathways, involving the dopaminergic, adrenergic and opiate systems, is thought to cause PLMS (Wetter and Pollmacher, 1997). Among other therapeutic possibilities, dopaminergic drugs were shown to relieve PLMS (Montplaisir *et al.*, 1991). Only one group has tested the hypothesis of a decreased dopaminergic activity in PLMS patients. In a series of reports, they mention a decreased IBZM striatal uptake, indicating a lower D2 receptor occupancy in PLMS patients (Staedt *et al.*, 1993; Staedt *et al.*, 1995a; Staedt *et al.*, 1995b). Treating patients with dopamine replacement therapy increased the IBZM binding and improved the sleep quality in these patients (Staedt *et al.*, 1995b).

REM Sleep Behaviour Disorder (RBD)

This condition, which has been described only recently (Schenck *et al.*, 1986), is characterized by movements of the limbs or body associated with dream mentation and at least one of the following criteria: dreams that appear to be acted out or sleep behaviour that disturbs sleep continuity (American Sleep Disorders Association, 1997). Patients with REM sleep behaviour disorder are likely to develop extrapyramidal disorders (Schenck *et al.*, 1996) as multiple system atrophy (Plazzi *et al.*, 1997), i.e., degenerative disorders related to alteration in the central dopaminergic system.

With SPECT and IPT (a ligand of striatal presynaptic dopamine transporter), it was recently shown that IPT binding in RBD patients ($n = 5$) is lower than in normal controls but higher than in Parkinson patients ($n = 14$; Eisensehr *et al.*, 2000). These results suggest that the number of presynaptic dopamine transporters is decreased in both Parkinson and RBD patients. It remains to be shown whether this alteration plays a causal role in the pathophysiology of RBD. Although there is evidence that some Parkinson patients do show excessive nocturnal movements (Trenkwalder, 1998), it is intriguing that not all Parkinson patients develop full-blown RBD. This suggests that modifications of other systems of neurotransmission are probably necessary for RBD to occur.

Depression: Studies of Sleep and Sleep Deprivation

There are good reasons to study brain function during sleep in depressed patients. Sleep disturbances are an integral feature of depressive disorders, ranging from hypersomnia to marked difficulty in maintaining sleep. The architecture of sleep itself is modified and characterized by a reduced SWS, an early onset of the first episode of REM sleep, and increased phasic REM sleep (Thase, 1998).

Sleep deprivation had rapid beneficial effects on about 60% of depressed patients (Wirz-Justice and Van den Hoofdakker, 1999). Responders to sleep deprivation are usually patients with high behavioural activation and low levels of tiredness (Bouhuys *et al.*, 1995; Szuba *et al.*, 1991). The hypothesis has been put forward of an increased arousal in depressed patients. Functional neuroimaging lends support to this hypothesis. Beta activity was proposed as a marker of arousal during sleep (Nofzinger *et al.*, 2000). Beta power is negatively correlated with subjective sleep quality, in both normal and depressed individuals. Depressed patients tend to have increased beta activity during the night as compared to normal controls. Finally, beta power is correlated with the glucose metabolism of ventro-medial prefrontal cortex, one of the most deactivated regions during consolidated SWS (see above).

Brain activity during sleep differs in several aspects from normal human sleep. Early studies indicated that cerebral metabolism during non-REM sleep in depressed patients is higher than in normal subjects (Ho *et al.*, 1996). The greatest increases was observed in the posterior cingulate, the amygdala, the hippocampus, and the occipital and temporal cortex (Ho *et al.*, 1996). During REM sleep, more recent data showed that the anterior paralimbic areas (anterior cingulate cortex, right insula, right parahippocampal gyrus) were less active, as compared to wakefulness, in depressed patients than in normal subjects (Nofzinger *et al.*, 1999).

Sleep deprivation has profound effects on brain metabolism, in both normals and depressed subjects. After 24 h of total sleep deprivation in normal subjects, cerebral glucose metabolism decreases by 8% (Thomas *et al.*, 2000). This decline involves the brain as a whole but is particularly prominent in the thalamic nuclei and associative cortices of the frontal and parietal lobes. No brain area increases its glucose metabolic rates after 24 h of continuous wakefulness. In depressed patients who respond to sleep deprivation, the baseline brain activity (measured in the awake patient) is higher in the anterior cingulate cortex (Wu *et al.*, 1992) or nearby mesial frontal cortex (Ebert *et al.*, 1994; Wu *et al.*, 1999) than in nonresponders. This feature normalizes after sleep deprivation. The same pattern was observed in elderly depressed patients, the normalization of anterior cingulate metabolism persisting even after recovery sleep (Smith *et al.*, 1999).

These data suggest a close link between the mood alteration and the activity in limbic and paralimbic structures. In particular, it is as if the anterior cingulate cortex were hyperactive in depressed patients during wakefulness, masking any further increase in REM sleep. Sleep deprivation would decrease both the activity in the anterior cingulate cortex and depression ratings. Further studies are needed to understand the causes and consequences of these mesial frontal metabolic disturbances.

CONCLUSIONS

Functional neuroimaging provides unprecedented possibilities to explore the brain function during sleep. In the near future, it should help to clarify the functions of sleep and the mechanisms underlying sleep disorders.

REFERENCES

Aldrich, M.S., Hollingsworth, Z., Penney, J.B., 1992. Dopamine-receptor autoradiography of human narcoleptic brain. *Neurology*, **42**, 410–415.

Asenbaum, S., Zeithofer, J., Saletu, B., Frey, R., Brucke, T., Podreka, I., Deecke, L., 1995. Technetium-99m-HMPAO SPECT imaging of cerebral blood flow during REM sleep in narcoleptics. *J Nucl Med*, **36**, 1150–1155.

American Sleep Disorder Association ASDA, 1997. International Classification of Sleep Disorders and Coding Manual. *Rochester MN*, 177–180.

Braun, A.R., Balkin, T.J., Wesensten, N.J., Carson, R.E., Varga, M., Baldwin, P., Selbie, S., Belenky, G., Herscovitch, P., 1997. Regional cerebral blood flow throughout the sleep-wake cycle — an (H2O)-O-15 PET study. *Brain*, **120**, 1173–1197.

Braun, A.R., Balkin, T.J., Wesensten, N.J., Gwadry, F., Carson, R.E., Varga, M., Baldwin, P., Belenky, G., Herscovitch, P., 1998. Dissociated pattern of activity in visual cortices and their projections during human rapid eye movement sleep. *Science*, **279**, 91–95.

Eisensehr, I., Linke, R., Noachtar, S., Schwarz, J., Gildehaus, F.J., Tatsch, K., 2000. Reduced striatal dopamine transporters in idiopathic rapid eye movement sleep behaviour disorder. Comparison with Parkinson's disease and controls. *Brain*, **123**, 1155–1160.

Ellis, C.M., Monk, C., Simmons, A., Lemmens, G., Williams, S.C., Brammer, M., Bullmore, E., Parkes, J.D., 1999. Functional magnetic resonance imaging neuroactivation studies in normal subjects and subjects with the narcoleptic syndrome. *Actions of Modafinil. J Sleep Res*, **8**, 85–93.

Finelli, L.A., Landolt, H.P., Buck, A., Roth, C., Berthold, T., Borbely, A.A., Achermann, P., 2000. Functional neuroanatomy of human sleep states after zolpidem and placebo: a H215O-PET study. *J Sleep Res*, **9**, 161–173.

Harrison, Y., Horne, J.A., 1998. Sleep loss affects risk-taking. *J Sleep Res*, **7**(Suppl. 2), 113.

Harrison, Y., Horne, J.A., 1999. One night of sleep loss impairs innovative thinking and flexible decision making. *Organ Beh and Hum Decis Processes*, **78**, 128–145.

Hennevin, E., Hars, B., Maho, C., Bloch, V., 1995. Processing of learned information in paradoxical sleep: relevance for memory. *Behav Brain Res*, **69**, 125–135.

Ho, A.P., Gillin, J.C., Buchsbaum, M.S., Wu, J.C., Abel, L., Bunney, W.E., 1996. Brain glucose metabolism during non-rapid eye movement sleep in major depression. A positron emission tomography study. *Arch Gen Psychiatry*, **53**, 645–652.

Hobson, J.A., Pace-Schott, E.F., Stickgold, R., Kahn, D., 1998. To dream or not to dream? Relevant data from new neuroimaging and electrophysiological studies. *Curr Opin Neurobiol*, **8**, 239–244.

Horne, J.A., 1988. Sleep loss and 'divergent' thinking ability. *Sleep*, **11**, 528–536.

Horne, J.A., 1993. Human sleep, sleep loss and behaviour. Implications for the prefrontal cortex and psychiatric disorder. *Br J Psychiatry*, **162**, 413–419.

Howard, R.J., Ellis, C., Bullmore, E.T., Brammer, M., Mellers, J.D., Woodruff, P.W., David, A.S., Simmons, A., Williams, S.C., Parkes, J.D., 1996. Functional echoplanar brain imaging correlates of amphetamine administration to normal subjects and subjects with the narcoleptic syndrome. *Magn Reson Imaging*, **14**, 1013–1016.

Hublin, C., Launes, J., Nikkinen, P., Partinen, M., 1994. Dopamine D2-receptors in human narcolepsy: a SPECT study with 123I-IBZM. *Acta Neurol Scand*, **90**, 186–189.

Khan, N., Antonini, A., Parkes, D., Dahlitz, M.J., Meier-Ewert, K., Weindl, A., Leenders, K.L., Firnau, G., Chen, J.J., Szechtman, H., Garnett, S., Nahmias, C., 1994. Striatal dopamine D2 receptors in patients with narcolepsy measured with PET and 11C-raclopride. *Neurology*, **44**, 2102–2104.

Laureys, S., Faymonville, M.E., Degueldre, C., *et al.*, 2000. Auditory processing in the vegetative state. *Brain*, **123**, 1589–1601.

Lu, M.L., Liu, H.C., Chen, C.H., Sung, S.M., 2000. Kleine-Levin syndrome and psychosis: observation from an unusual case. *Neuropsychiatry Neuropsychol Behav Neurol*, **13**, 140–142.

Lydic, R., Baghdoyan, H.A., Hibbard, L., Bonyak, E.V., DeJoseph, M.R., Hawkins, R.A., 1991. Regional brain glucose metabolism is altered during rapid eye movement sleep in the cat: a preliminary study. *J Comp Neurol*, **304**, 517–529.

MacFarlane, J.G., List, S.J., Moldofsky, H., Firnau, G., Chen, J.J., Szechtman, H., Garnett, S., Nahmias, C., 1997. Dopamine D2 receptors quantified *in vivo* in human narcolepsy. *Biol Psychiatry*, **41**, 305–310.

Maquet, P., 2000. Functional neuroimaging of normal human sleep by positron emission tomography. *J Sleep Res*, **9**, 207–231.

Maquet, P., Laureys, S., Peigneux, P., Fuchs, S., Petiau, C., Phillips, C., Aerts, J., Del Fiore, G., Degueldre, C., Meulemans, T., Luxen, A., Franck, G., van der Linden, M., Smith, C., Cleeremans, A., 2000. Experience-dependent changes in cerebral activation during human REM sleep. *Nat Neurosci*, **3**, 831–836.

Maquet, P., Péters, J.M., Aerts, J., Delfiore, G., Degueldre, C., Luxen, A., Franck, G., 1996. Functional neuroanatomy of human rapid eye movement sleep and dreaming. *Nature*, **383**, 163–166.

Meyer, J.S., Sakai, F., Karacan, I., Derman, S., Yamamoto, M., 1980. Sleep apnea, narcolepsy, and dreaming: regional cerebral hemodynamics. *Ann Neurol*, **7**, 479–485.

Nofzinger, E.A., Mintun, M.A., Wiseman, M., Kupfer, D.J., Moore, R.Y., 1997. Forebrain activation in REM sleep: an FDG PET study. *Brain Res*, **770**, 192–201.

Nofzinger, E.A., Price, J.C., Meltzer, C.C., Buysse, D.J., Villemagne, V.L., Miewald, J.M., Sembrat, R.C., Steppe, D.A., Kupfer, D.J., 2000. Towards a neurobiology of dysfunctional arousal in depression: the relationship between beta EEG power and regional cerebral glucose metabolism during NREM sleep. *Psychiatry Res*, **98**, 71–91.

Perrin, F., Garcia-Larrea, L., Mauguiere, F., Bastuji, H., 1999. A differential brain response to the subject's own name persists during sleep. *Clin Neurophysiol*, **110**, 2153–2164.

Pilcher, J.S., Huffcutt, A.I., 1996. Effects of sleep deprivation on performance: a meta-analysis. *Sleep*, **19**, 318–326.

Plazzi, G., Corsini, R., Provini, F., Pierangeli, G., Martinelli, P., Montagna, P., Lugaresi, E., Cortelli, P., 1997. REM sleep behavior disorders in multiple system atrophy. *Neurology*, **48**, 1094–1097.

Portas, C.M., Krakow, K., Allen, P., Josephs, O., Armony, J.L., Frith, C.D., 2000. Auditory Processing across the sleep-wake cycle. Simultaneous EEG and fMRI monitoring in humans. *Neuron*, **28**, 991–999.

Rinne, J.O., Hublin, C., Partinen, M., Rinne, J.O., Hublin, C., Partinen, M., Ruottinen, H., Nagren, K., Lehikoinen, P., Ruotsalainen, U., Laihinen, A., 1996. Striatal dopamine D1 receptors in narcolepsy: a PET study with [11C]NNC 756. *J Sleep Res*, **5**, 262–264.

Rinne, J.O., Hublin, C., Partinen, M., Ruottinen, H., Ruotsalainen, U., Nagren, K., Lehikoinen, P., Laihinen, A., 1995. Positron emission tomography study of human narcolepsy: no increase in striatal dopamine D2 receptors. *Neurology*, **45**, 1735–1738.

Schenck, C.H., Bundlie, S.R., Ettinger, M.G., Mahowald, M.W., 1986. Chronic behavioral disorders of human REM sleep: a new category of parasomnia. *Sleep*, **9**, 293–308.

Schenck, C.H., Bundlie, S.R., Mahowald, M.W., 1996. Delayed emergence of a parkinsonian disorder in 38% of 29 older men initially diagnosed with idiopathic rapid eye movement sleep behaviour disorder. *Neurology*, **46**, 388–393.

Smith, C., 1995. Sleep states and memory processes. *Behav Brain Res*, **69**, 137–145.

Smith, G.S., Reynolds, C.F., Pollock, B., Derbyshire, S., Nofzinger, E., Dew, M.A., Houch, P.R., Milko, D., Meltzer, C.C., Kupfer, D.J., 1999. Cerebral glucose metabolic response to combined total sleep deprivation and antidepressant treatment in geriatric depression. *Am J Psychiatry*, **156**, 683–689.

Staedt, J., Stoppe, G., Kogler, A., Munz, D., Riemann, H., Emrich, D., Ruther, E., 1993. Dopamine D2 receptor alteration in patients with periodic movements in sleep (nocturnal myoclonus). *J Neural Transm Gen Sect*, **93**, 71–74.

Staedt, J., Stoppe, G., Kogler, A., Riemann, H., Hajak, G., Munz, D.L., Emrich, D., Ruther, E., 1995a. Nocturnal myoclonus syndrome (periodic movements in sleep) related to central dopamine D2-receptor alteration. *Eur Arch Psychiatry Clin Neurosci*, **245**, 8–10.

Staedt, J., Stoppe, G., Kogler, A., Riemann, H., Hajak, G., Munz, D.L., Emrich, D., Ruther, E., 1995b. Single photon emission tomography (SPET) imaging of dopamine D2 receptors in the course of dopamine replacement therapy in patients with nocturnal myoclonus syndrome (NMS). *J Neural Transm Gen Sect*, **99**, 187–193.

Staedt, J., Stoppe, G., Kogler, A., Riemann, H., Hajak, G., Rodenbeck, A., Mayer, G., Steinhoff, B.J., Munz, D.L., Emrich, D., Ruther, E., 1996. [123I]IBZM SPET analysis of dopamine D2 receptor occupancy in narcoleptic patients in the course of treatment. *Biol Psychiatry*, **39**, 107–111.

Sudo, Y., Suhara, T., Honda, Y., Nakajima, T., Okubo, Y., Suzuki, K., Nakashima, Y., Yoshikawa, K., Okauchi, T., Sasaki, Y., Matsushita, M., 1998. Muscarinic cholinergic receptors in human narcolepsy: a PET study. *Neurology*, **51**, 1297–1302.

Thomas, M., Sing, H., Belenky, G., Holcomb, H., Mayberg, H., Dannals, R., Wagner, H., Thorne, D., Popp, K., Rowland, L., Welsh, A., Balwinski, S., Redmond, D., 2000. Neural basis of alertness and cognitive performance impairments during sleepiness. I. Effects of 24 h of sleep deprivation on waking human regional brain activity. *J Sleep Res*, **9**, 335–352.

Trenkwalder, C., 1998. Sleep dysfunction in Parkinson's disease. *Clin Neurosci*, **5**, 107–114.

Wu, J.C., Gillin, J.C., Buchsbaum, M.S., Hershey, T., Johnson, J.C., Bunney, W.E., 1992. Effect of sleep deprivation on brain metabolism of depressed patients. *Am J Psychiatry*, **149**, 538–543.

XXIV-9

Genetics of Sleep and Sleep Disorders

Paul Linkowski

INTRODUCTION

The relationship of genes to behaviour has always been a major topic of research and interest in the neurosciences. In the study of sleep, the traditional way to determine whether distinct phenotypes have a familial component was to study family pedigrees or to investigate sleep in monozygotic (MZ) and dizygotic (DZ) twins, a classical method in human and psychological research. In animals, the inheritance of sleep traits was previously studied by Valatx *et al.* (1972) in cross-breeding mice strains. The developments of molecular genetics and gene technology favoured a renewed interest in the behavioural neurobiology of sleep, leading to an increasing number of papers on the genetics of sleep and the molecular aspects of sleep disorders.

Current scientific investigations address various phenotypic dimensions, including the genetic components of rapid-eye-movement (REM) sleep and delta sleep, and the circadian components of human sleep.

In the present paper we will review some of the classical genetic studies of sleep and summarize important recent results.

GENETICS OF SLEEP IN NORMAL MAN: TWIN STUDIES

The importance of the investigation of the genetic aspects of sleep was demonstrated in some early studies that focused mainly on the investigation of twin pairs in man. In 1937, Geyer (quoted in Vogel, 1958) reported that concordance for a number of sleep characteristics was much better in MZ than in DZ twins. Other pioneering efforts were made by Vogel (1958), who was the first to study the sleep EEG in MZ twins, and by Zung and Wilson (1967), who performed computations of the sleep EEG of three pairs of MZ and three pairs of DZ twins. They reported that the all-night-sleep EEG and REM patterns of MZ twins were similar, whereas those of DZ twins were dissimilar and variable.

It should be noted, however, that some further studies relied mainly on questionnaire investigations of sleep habits (duration of sleep, subjective reports of sleep timing and quality) in MZ and DZ twins (Partinen *et al.*, 1983; Heath *et al.*, 1990). These studies were conducted mainly in adult twins, and, in general, correlations were higher for MZ than for DZ twins, with a significant synchronizing effect of cohabitational status on sleep length (Partinen *et al.*, 1983). Heath *et al.* (1990) found that genetic influences accounted for at least 33% of the variance in sleep quality and sleep disturbance, and 40% of the variance in sleep pattern. A substantial genetic effect was also reported for some parasomnias such as sleepwalking and nocturnal enuresis (Kales *et al.*, 1980).

The hereditary components of sleep were also suggested by some polygraphic twin studies of newborns (Gould *et al.*, 1978), of a limited number of adolescent twin pairs, and of single nights of identical and fraternal twins. In the study of Webb and Campbell (1983), measures of awakening and REM sleep amounts were found to be significantly correlated in identical twins. In a study of seven twin pairs, Hori (1986) suggested that sleep spindles were determined by a genetic trait.

The inheritance of properties of the wake EEG has also been a focus of interest in recent years, since the pioneering observations of Vogel (1958). Stassen *et al.* (1987) reviewed 22 twin studies and noted that MZ co-twins were generally more alike than DZ co-twins, indicating the presence of genetic influences on the spontaneous EEG. In a more recent study, Van Beijsterveldt *et al.* (1996) measured four frequency bands (delta, theta, alpha, and beta) and reported that the average heritability of brain functioning, as indexed by rhythmic brain electrical activity, is one of the most heritable characteristics in humans.

Finally, a large number of animal studies also indicate unequivocally that certain aspects of sleep might be genetically determined.

These studies have mainly suggested a genetic determination of sleep length in rodents (Valatx *et al.*, 1972; Friedman, 1974; Franken *et al.*, 1999) as well as a significant genetic effect on REM sleep in mice (Valatx *et al.*, 1980; Valatx, 1984).

Taken together, most studies that addressed the issue of genetic aspects of sleep in normal men have relied on the twin method, which allows the determination of heritability estimates and is frequently used to partition variance of phenotypic quantitative traits into environmental and genetic components.

The twin design has also been frequently used to evaluate the heritability of other primary sleep disorders such as sleepiness, nightmares and sleepwalking. This will be reviewed later in the chapter. We will first present the results of the Brussels twin study, which was conducted between 1986 and 1990 (see Table XXIV-9.1) (Linkowski *et al.*, 1989; 1991).

In this study of two samples of 26 pairs of male twins, we have found that stages 2, 3, 3 + 4 and 4 were significantly determined by genetic components. This was also the case for REM density. No genetic effect was found for total sleep period, period of sleep, total sleep time, sleep onset latency and REM latency. Waking was found to be significantly determined by genetic factors in one of the two samples.

Therefore, our results substantiate previous reports suggesting that some components of human sleep might be genetically determined (Partinen *et al.*, 1983; Webb and Campbell, 1983). In our study, stages 2, 4 and delta sleep (stages 3 + 4) unequivocally show a strong genetic component: the same is true, but is less pronounced for REM density measures. It is of interest that the stages with the strongest genetic component show the best relative stability from night to night (Merica and Gaillard, 1985). This is also supported by previous reports of substantial within-subject, night-to-night correlation of stage 4 (Webb and Agnew, 1968) and a greater inter- than intraindividual variation of stage 4 (Merica and Gaillard, 1985).

Biological Psychiatry: Edited by H. D'haenen, J.A. den Boer and P. Willner. ISBN 0-471-49198-5

Table XXIV-9.1 Selected heritability estimates of markers of sleep-wake homeostasis

Parameter	Authors	No. of pairs	Gender	Age range (years)	Heritability 2 ($r_{MZ}-r_{DZ}$)
Minimum of stages 2 + 4	Linkowski *et al.*, 1989	14 MZ 12 DZ	M	16–35	0.50
REM density Minimum of stages 3 + 4	Linkowski *et al.*, 1991	11 MZ 15 DZ	M	20–36	0.95 0.52
REM density Minimum of stages 3 + 4 (with catheter)	Linkowski *et al.*, 1998	9 MZ 8 DZ	M	16–35	0.64 0.90
Minimum of stages 3 + 4 (with catheter)	Linkowski *et al.*, unpublished	11 MZ 11 DZ	M	16–35	0.68

More recently, Franken *et al.* (2001) have reported that the increase of slow-wave sleep need after sleep deprivation is under strong genetic control in the mouse. Our data also show that regulation of REM stage variability shows substantial environmental determination rather than evidence of significant genetic effect, in opposition to what is observed in animals (Valatx, 1984).

GENETIC ASPECTS OF SLEEP DISORDERS

For most of the disorders of sleep, twin or family studies support a genetic component in a majority of sleep disorders such as sleepwalking nightmares, hypersomnia, restless legs syndrome (RLS), insomnia, obstructive sleep apnoea and narcolepsy. With reference to the last disease, the gene responsible for dog narcolepsy has recently been cloned (Lin *et al.*, 1999), also implicating the dysfunction of orexins (hypocretins), neuropeptides active in energy homeostasis and arousal (Thannickal *et al.*, 2000; van den Pol *et al.*, 2001).

FAMILY ASPECTS OF INSOMNIA

A family history of insomnia is a well-known symptom among patients with a complaint of chronic insomnia (Hauri and Olmstead, 1980; Bastien and Morin, 2000). In the study of Bastien and Morin (2000), 35% of the patients consulting for insomnia had a positive family history of sleep disturbances. Insomnia was the most common type of sleep disturbance identified (76%), and the mother was the most frequently afflicted family member.

The reported sleep disturbances among family members were more prevalent when the onset of insomnia was before 40 years of age than when it was later in life. These findings are supported by other reports such as that of Dashevsky and Kramer (1998), which shows that 42% of patients with psychiatric disturbances have a positive family history of insomnia.

Another major contribution to the genetic studies of insomnia came from the studies that explored the clinical and molecular genetics of a new syndrome: fatal familial insomnia (FFI) (Lugaresi *et al.*, 1986; Cortelli *et al.*, 1999). FFI is a rare autosomal dominant disease clinically characterized by sleep loss that inevitably proves fatal, disordered sleep-wake cycle, dysautonomia (increased perspiration and salivation, impotence, constipation, tachycardia, systemic hypertension and fever progressively worsening), and motor signs (ataxia, dysarthria, astasia-abasia and myoclonic jerks). At autopsy, both in the thalamus and in the cortex, the limbic structures (the orbito-frontal cortex, the cingulate gyrus and the mediodorsal and ventral thalamic nuclei) are those most consistently and severely involved.

Genetically, the disease is characterized by a missense mutation at codon 178 coupled with methionine at the polymorphic codon 129 of the prion protein gene (Goldfarb *et al.*, 1992; Medori *et al.*, 1992). The selective atrophy of the limbic thalamus that characterizes FFI might be due to the binding of toxic prion proteins to specific receptors on thalamolimbic neurons, leading to this rare but well-characterized inherited prion disease in humans.

SLEEPINESS

Carmelli *et al.* (2001) have explored the responses to the eight-item Epworth Sleepiness Scale obtained from 1560 World War II male veteran twin pairs to determine the extent to which genetic influences are involved in self-reported daytime sleepiness in the elderly. The heritability of responses to the Epworth Sleepiness Scale was estimated to be 38% while environmental influences not shared by twin brothers accounted for the remaining variance in daytime sleepiness. The authors interpreted the heritability of the responses to the Epworth Sleepiness Scale as related to a genetic susceptibility to disordered breathing during night sleep.

NIGHTMARES, SLEEPWALKING AND SLEEPTALKING

The twin design was also applied to quantify the genetic influences affecting the liability to nightmares, sleepwalking, night terrors and sleeptalking.

Nightmares are frightening dreams that usually awaken the sleeper from REM sleep. They are usually long and complicated, exhibiting a progressive content that becomes increasingly frightening toward the end (Broughton, 1994).

Sleepwalking belongs to the group of parasomnias characterized by a series of complex behaviours that are initiated during slow-wave sleep and result in walking during sleep.

Talking, screaming, striking out or walking during the nightmare rarely occurs, distinguishing the nightmare from sleep terror and REM sleep behaviour disorder (ASDA, 1990). No firm evidence for a familial basis of nightmares was available until the study of Hublin *et al.* (1999), who investigated 1298 MZ and 2419 DZ twin pairs by questionnaire. They showed a persistent genetic effect on the disposition to nightmares in both childhood and adulthood. Of the phenotypic variance, the estimated proportion of genetic effect in childhood was 44% in males and 45% in females. In adults the values were 36% in males and 38% in females. Nightmare frequency and psychiatric disorders were linearly associated.

The same authors explored the prevalence a genetic predisposition to sleepwalking in the same population of twins and reported a substantial genetic effect in both childhood and adulthood (Hublin *et al.*, 1997). The proportion of total phenotypic variance attributed to genetic influences was 80% in men and 36% in women. The same values were 60% in men and 57% in children for sleepwalking.

RESTLESS LEGS SYNDROME (RLS)

RLS is a common sleep disorder, present in about 6% of the adult population. It is characterized by motor restlessness and painful sensations during sleep in the legs. RLS has been reported to be familial: 30–64% of RLS patients have positive family history (Lazzarini *et al.*, 1999). It has been shown that familial RLS follows an autosomal dominant mode of inheritance with variable expressivity (Becker *et al.*, 1993). It is also important to note that genetic anticipation (increased severity with age and an earlier age of onset of the illness in successive generations) has been suggested for RLS indicating a possible trinucleotide repeat expansion in the molecular mechanisms of the disease (Lazzarini *et al.*, 1999).

NARCOLEPSY

Narcolepsy is a disabling sleep disorder which typically arises during adolescence and early adulthood, and affects 0.02–0.18% of the general population (Mignot, 1998). This syndrome is characterized by excessive daytime sleepiness and pathological manifestations of REM sleep. These include cataplexy (a sudden loss of muscle tone generally caused by a strong emotion), sleep paralysis (muscle atonia when falling asleep or at awakening) and hypnagogic hallucinations, a complex state that occurs between waking and sleep. The full tetrad of excessive daytime sleepiness, cataplexy, sleep paralysis and hypnagogic hallucinations is present in only 15% of the patients (Aldrich, 1998).

Familial narcolepsy is rare (sporadic cases are more frequent) and the risk to first-degree relatives is estimated at 1–2%; only 8–10% of narcoleptic patients identify another member of the family as having the narcolepsy-cataplexy syndrome. Furthermore, a risk of 2% is 10 times higher than what is observed in the general population, suggesting the existence of predisposing genetic factors (Mignot, 1998).

The importance of environmental factors is supported by the fact that up to 30% of MZ twin factors are concordant for narcolepsy. This led some authors to suggest that undefined environmental factors act on a susceptible genetic background to initiate the disease. Several studies have reported a strong association between certain HLA haplotypes on human chromosome 6 and human narcolepsy; HLA DQB1*0602 and DQA1*0102 are found in 90% of narcoleptics, but in only 30% of the general population, suggesting that autoimmunity plays a role in the disorder (Kadotani *et al.*, 1998).

The major breakthrough, however, occurred recently, shedding new light on the physiopathological and molecular basis of the disease. In 1998, two peptides were identified in the hypothalamus, and were termed hypocretin-1 (HCRT-1) and hypocretin-2 (HCRT-2), reflecting their hypothalamic origin. They project to monoaminergic and cholinergic components of the ascending reticular activating system (Kilduff and Peyron, 2000). The sleepiness in narcolepsy appears to reflect lack of hypocretin excitatory inputs on histaminergic, dopaminergic and cholinergic components of the ascending reticular activating system, which normally promote thalamo-cortical arousal (Silber and Rye, 2001).

Other recent molecular and post-mortem studies further support the role of hypocretins, indicating a mutation in a case of early-onset narcolepsy and a generalized absence of hypocretin peptides in human narcoleptic brains (Peyron *et al.*, 2001). These studies are paralleled by similar studies in mice (Hara *et al.*, 2001) and canine narcolepsy (Hungs *et al.*, 2001). HLA and hypocretin findings can be integrated into a concept of immunologically mediated destruction of hypocretin-containing cells in human narcolepsy (Mignot *et al.*, 2001). The genetic contribution of HLA to narcolepsy might also be estimated by the use of the lambda statistic (Risch, 1987), which computes the relationship between increased risk in relatives and population prevalence. The results indicate that complex HLA-DR and -DQ interactions contribute to the genetic predisposition to human narcolepsy but that additional susceptibility loci are also probably involved.

HCRT-1 was undetectable in the CSF of seven of nine patients with narcolepsy (Nishino *et al.*, 2001). In an autopsy study, hypocretin neurons were damaged in 95% of narcoleptic brains (Thannickal *et al.*, 2000). Finally, Dalal *et al.* (2001) confirmed low to absent HCRT-1 concentrations in the CSF of narcoleptic patients and demonstrated that serum HCRT-1 was normal in narcolepsy.

These results add further fascinating details to the neurochemical aspects of sleep and offer a new potential for the discovery of pharmacological tools targeting hypocretin receptors in order to cure the disorders of excessive sleep.

CONCLUSION

Current research suggests that both normal sleep and various sleep disorders either have a genetic basis or are influenced by genetically determined physiological or environmental predispositions. Identifying the genes that influence the various components of sleep may ultimately contribute to a better understanding of the processes that control normal sleep, and also to the understanding of sleep disorders, and might add new pathways to the development of interventions to alleviate these disabling conditions.

REFERENCES

Aldrich, M.S., 1998. Diagnostic aspects of narcolepsy. *Neurology*, **50** (Suppl 1), S2–S7.

American Sleep Disorders Association (ASDA), 1990. *International Classification of Sleep Disorders. Diagnostic and Coding Manual*. ASDA, Rochester, MN.

Bastien, C.H. and Morin, C.M., 2000. Familial incidence of insomnia. *Journal of Sleep Research*, **9**, 49–54.

Becker, P.M., Jamieson, A.O. and Brown, W.D., 1993. Dopaminergic agents in restless legs syndrome and periodic limb movements of sleep: response and complications of extended treatment in 49 cases. *Sleep*, **16**, 713–716.

Broughton, R.J., 1994. Parasomnias. In: Chokroverty, S (ed.), *Sleep Disorders Medicine*, pp. 381–399. Butterworths-Heinemann, Stoneham, M.A.

Carmelli, D., Bliwise, D., Swan, G. and Reed, T., 2001. A genetic analysis of the Epworth Sleepiness Scale in 1,560 World War II male veteran twins in the NAS-NRC Twin Registry. *Journal of Sleep Research*, **10**, 53–58.

Cortelli, P., Gambetti, P., Montagna, P. and Lugaresi, E., 1999. Fatal familial insomnia: clinical features and molecular genetics. *Journal of Sleep Research*, **8**(Suppl 1), 23–29.

Dalal, M.A., Schuld, A. and Haack, M., 2001. Normal plasma levels of cresein A (hypocretin-1) in narcoleptic patients. *Neurology*, **56**, 1749–1751.

Dashevsky, B.A. and Kramer, M., 1998. Behavioral treatment of chronic insomnia in psychiatric patients. *Journal of Clinical Psychiatry*, **59**, 693–699.

De Lecea, L., Kilduff, T.S. and Peyron, C., 1998. The hypocretins: hypothalamus-specific peptides with neuroexcitatory activity. *Proceedings of the National Academy of Sciences of the United States of America*, **18**, 9996–10015.

Franken, P., Chollet, D. and Tafti, M., 2001. The homeostatic regulation of sleep is under genetic control. *Journal of Neuroscience*, **21**, 2610–2621.

Franken, P., Malafosse, A. and Tafti, M., 1999. Genetic determinants of sleep regulation in inbred mice. *Sleep*, **22**, 155–169.

Friedman, J.K., 1974. A diallellic analysis of the genetic underpinnings of mouse sleep. *Physiology and Behaviour*, **12**, 169–175.

Gilber, M.H. and Ryl, D.B., 2001. Solving the mysteries of narcolepsy: the hypocretin story. *Neurology*, **56**, 1616–1618.

Goldfarf, L.G., Petersen, R.B., Tabaton, M., Brown, P., Leblanc, A.C., Montagna, P., Cortelli, P., Julien, J., Vital, C., Pendelburg, W., Hallia, M., Wills, P.R., McKeever, P.E., Monari, L., Schrank, B., Swergold, G.D., Autilio-Gambetti, L., Gajdusek, D.C., Lugaresi, E. and Gambetti, P., 1992. Fatal familial insomnia and familial Creutzfeld-Jakob disease: disease phenotype determined by a DNA polymorphism. *Science*, **258**, 806–808.

Gould, J., Austin, F. and Cook, P.A., 1978. Genetic analysis of sleep stage organization in new-born twins. *Sleep Research*, **7**, 132.

Hara, J., Beuckmann, C.T., Nambre, T., Willi, J.T., Chemelli, R.M., Sinton, C.M., Sugiyama, F., Yagami, K., Goto, K., Yanagisawa, M. and Sakurai, T., 2001. Genetic ablation of orexin neurones in mice results in narcolepsy, hyperphagia and obesity. *Neuron*, **30**, 2, 345–354.

Hauri, P.J. and Olmstead, E.M., 1980. Childhood-onset insomnia. *Sleep*, **13**, 318–355.

Heath, A.C., Kendler, K.S., Eaves, L. and Martin, N.G., 1990. Evidence for genetic influences on sleep disturbance and sleep pattern in twins. *Sleep*, **13**, 318–335.

Hori, A., 1986. Sleep characteristics in twins. *Japanese Journal of Psychiatry and Neurology*, **40**, 35–46.

Hublin, C., Kaprio, J., Partinen, M., Heikkila, K. and Koskenvuo, M., 1997. Prevalence and genetics of sleepwalking: a population-based twin study. *Neurology*, **48**, 177–181.

Hublin, C., Kaprio, J., Partinen, M. and Koskenvuo, M., 1999. Nightmares: familial aggregation and association with psychiatric disorders in a nationwide twin cohort. *American Journal of Medical Genetics*, **88**, 329–336.

Hungs, M., Fan, J., Lin, L., Lin, X., Maki, R.A. and Mignot, E., 2001. Identification and functional analysis of mutations in the hypocretin (orexin) genes of narcoleptic canines. *Genome Research*, **11**, 531–539.

Kadotani, H., Faraco, J. and Mignot, E., 1998. Genetic studies in the sleep disorder narcolepsy. *Genome Research*, **8**, 427–434.

Kales, A., Soldatos, C.R. and Bixter, E.O., 1980. Hereditary factors in sleepwalking and nightmares. *British Journal of Psychiatry*, **137**, 111–118.

Kilduff, F. and Peyron, C., 2000. The hypocretin (orexin ligand-receptor system): implications for sleep and sleep disorders. *Trends in Neurosciences*, **23**, 359–365.

Lazzarini, A., Walters, A.S., Hickey, K., Coccagua, G., Lugaresi, E., Ehrenberg, B.L., Picchietti, D.L., Brin, M.F., Stenroos, E.S., Verico, J. and Johnson, W.G., 1999. Studies of penetrance and anticipation in five autosomal-dominant restless legs syndrome pedigrees. *Movement Disorders*, **14**, 111–116.

Lazzarini, A., Walters, A.S. and Slickey, K., 1999. Studies of penetrance and anticipation in five autosomal-dominant restless legs syndrome pedigrees. *Movement Disorders*, **14**, 111–116.

Linkowski, P., Kerkhofs, M., Hauspie, R. and Mendlewicz, J., 1991. Genetic determinants of EEG sleep: a study in twins living apart. *Electroencephalography and Clinical Neurophysiology*, **79**, 114–118.

Linkowski, P., Kerkhofs, M., Hauspie, R., Susanne, C. and Mendlewicz, J., 1989. EEG sleep patterns in man: a twin study. *Electroencephalography and Clinical Neurophysiology*, **73**, 279–284.

Linkowski, P., Spiegel, K., Kerkhofs, M.L., Hermite-Baleriaux, M., Van Onderbergen, A., Leproult, R., Mendlewicz, J. and van Cauter, E., 1998. Genetic and environmental influences on prolactin secretion during wake and during sleep. *American Journal of Physiology*, **274**(5pt 1), E909–919.

Lugaresi, E., Medori, R., Montagna, P., Baruzzi, A., Cortelli, P., Longarssi, A., Tinuper, P., Zucconi, M. and Gambetti, P., 1986. Fatal familial insomnia and dysautonomia with selective degeneration of thalamic nuclei. *New England Journal of Medicine*, **315**, 997–1003.

Medori, R., Tritschler, H.J., Leblanc, A., Villare, F., Manetto, V., Chen, H.Y., Xue, R., Leal, S., Montagna, P., Cortelli, P., Tinuper, P., Avoni, P., Mochi, M., Barsurri, A., Haew, J.J., Ott, J., Lugaresi, E., Autilio-Gambetti, L. and Gambetti, P., 1992. Fatal familial insomnia: a prion disease with a mutation on codon 178 of the prion protein gene. *New England Journal of Medicine*, **326**, 444–449.

Merica, H. and Gaillard, J.M, 1985. Statistical description and evaluation of the interrelationships of standard sleep variables for normal subjects. *Sleep*, **8**, 261–273.

Mignot, E, 1998. Genetic and familial aspects of narcolepsy. *Neurology*, **50**(Suppl 1), S16–S22.

Mignot, E., Lin, L., Rogers, W., Houda, Y., Oju, X., Lin, X., Okun, M., Slohjoh, J.L., Miki, T., Itsu, S., Leffel, M., Grumet, F., Fernandez-Vina, M., Houda, M. and Risch, N., 2001. Complex HLA-DR and -DQ interactions confer risk of narcolepsy-cataplexy in three ethnic groups. *American Journal of Human Genetics*, **68**, 686–699.

Nishino, S., Ripley, B., Overeem, S., Lammers, G.J. and Mignot, E., 2000. Hypocretin deficiency in human narcolepsy. *Lancet*, **355**, 39–40.

Partinen, M., Kaprio, J., Koshenvuo, M., Putkonen, P. and Langinvanio, H., 1983. Genetic and environmental determination of human sleep. *Sleep*, **6**, 179–185.

Peyron, C., Farceo, J., Rogers, W., Ripley, B., Overeem, S., Charnay, Y., Newsimalova, S., Aldrich, M., Reynolds, D., Albin, R., Li, R., Hungs, M., Pedrazzoli, M., Padigaro, M., Kucherlapati, M., Kan, J., Maki, R., Lammers, G.J., Bouras, C., Nishino, S. and Mignot, E., 2000. A mutation in a case of early onset narcolepsy and a generalized absence of hypocretin peptides in human narcoleptic brains. *Nature Medicine*, **6**, 991–997.

Risch, N., 1987. Assessing the role of HLA-linked and unlinked determinants of disease. *American Journal of Human Genetics*, **40**, 1–14.

Stassen, H., Bomben, G. and Propping, P., 1987. Genetic aspects of the EEG: an investigation into the within-pairs similarity of monozygotic and dizygotic twins with a new method of analysis. *Electroencephalography and Clinical Neurophysiology*, **66**, 489–501.

Thannickal, T.C., Moore, R.Y., Nienhuis, R., Ramarrathan, L., Gulyani, S., Aldrich, M., Cornford, M. and Siegal, J., 2000. Reduced number of hypocretin neurons in human narcolepsy. *Neuron*, **27**, 469–474.

Valatx, J.L., 1984. Genetics as a model for studying the sleep-waking cycle. In: Borbély, A. and Valatx, J.L. (eds), *Sleep Mechanisms. Experimental Brain Research*, pp. 135–145. Springer, Berlin.

Valatx, J.L., Buget, R. and Jouvet, M., 1972. Genetic studies of sleep in mice. *Nature*, **238**, 226–227.

Valatx, J.L., Cespuglio, R. and Paut, L., 1980. Etude génétique du sommeil paradoxal chez la souris. *Waking Sleeping*, **4**, 1975–1983.

Van Beijsterveldt, C.E.M., Molenaar, P.C.M., De Geus, E.J.C. and Boomsma, D.I., 1996. Heritability of human brain functioning as assessed by electroencephalography. *American Journal of Human Genetics*, **58**, 562–573.

van den Pol, A.N., Patrylo, P.R., Ghosh, P.K. and Gao X.B., 2001. Lateral hypothalamus:early developmental expression and response to hypocretin (orexin). *Journal of Comparative Neurology*, **433**, 349–363.

Vogel, F., 1958. *Über die Erblichkeit des Normalen Electroencephalograms*. Stuttgart, Thieme.

Webb, W.B. and Campbell, S.S., 1983. Relationship in sleep characteristics of identical and fraternal twins. *Archives of General Psychiatry*, **410**, 1093–1095.

Webb, W.B. and Agnew, H.W., 1968. Measurement and characteristics of nocturnal sleep. In: Abt, L. and Riess, B. (eds), *Progress in Clinical Physiology*, pp. 2–27. Grune and Stratton, New York.

Zai, C., Wigg, K. and Barr, C.L., 2000. Genetics and sleep disorders. *Seminars in Clinical Neuropsychiatry*, **5**, 33–43.

Zung, W.I.C. and Wilson, W.P., 1967 Sleep and dream patterns in twins: Markov analysis of a genetic trait. In: Wortis, J. (ed.), *Recent Advances in Biological Psychiatry*, Vol. 9, pp. 119–130. Plenum Press, New York.

XXIV-10

Gender Issues Related to Sleep

Joyce Walsleben

Sleep is an active cyclic process that involves both physiological and behavioural changes. There are two major states of sleep: rapid-eye-movement (REM) sleep, commonly known as 'dream sleep', and non-REM (NREM) sleep. In the adult, these states cycle every 70–90 min across the night, usually beginning with NREM sleep. The state of NREM is divided into four stages: stages 1–4, which denote the 'depth' of sleep, based upon one's ability to respond to stimulation. Stage 1 is thought to be transitional and the lightest. Stage 2 fills approximately 50% of the night and is frequently felt to be the first definite stage of sleep. The deepest stages are 3 and 4, called delta sleep, or slow-wave sleep (SWS). SWS is felt to be the most restorative stage. The depiction of these states and stages of sleep in a histogram shows the structure or architecture of one's sleep at any given time point.

Originally, scoring of sleep stages was performed visually only by comparison to standard guidelines which evaluated the EEG frequency and amplitude (Rechtschaffen and Kales, 1968) of the electroencephalogram (EEG), electro-oculogram (EOG) and electromyogram (EMG). For instance, delta sleep is represented by an EEG frequency of 0.5–4 Hz and an amplitude $>75\,\mu V$, with steady EOG and decreased EMG, and it is further delineated into stages 3 or 4 by the percentage of a 30-s epoch which displays this frequency and amplitude. More recently, with the advent of computer scoring and spectral analysis, more definitive changes of EEG power can be documented, allowing subtle changes across and between stages of sleep to be noted.

Two main biological drives regulate the timing and amount of sleep. They are the circadian drive, or 24-h sleep/wake cycle, and the homeostatic drive, which may represent the accumulation of sleep factors or toxins produced during wake. These drives change as we age, altering the normal flow of sleep across our 24-h 'day'.

We begin to form the various stages of sleep around the fourth month of life. Sleep architecture continues to evolve throughout childhood and adolescence, and subtle differences of architecture between sexes may exist at times during this period. Sleep then reaches a fairly stable period until mid-life when gender differences begin to be more noticeable and suggest a female advantage. Sleep architecture continues to change subtly with ageing, sometimes affected by health and lifestyle.

Besides the biological changes that occur in sleep across age and gender, sleep disorders may develop, and certain of these have a higher prevalence or impact in one sex than the other. Furthermore, females' sleep is often affected by significant hormonal influences that may cause day-to-day alterations from menarche through menopause. Some women are more sensitive to these influences than others. Finally, psychosocial issues, particularly stressful lifestyle, affect one's ability to sleep well and cannot be ignored in a discussion of gender differences in sleep. Females, perhaps secondary to hormonal influences, appear to be more affected by stress than men. In addition, the psychosocial demands of mothering and caregiving frequently have a negative impact on woman's sleep.

SLEEP CHANGES ACROSS AGE AND SEX

A seminal work examining sleep in normal subjects was reported by Williams *et al.* (1974), who showed sleep architectural changes across ages and between genders (Table XXIV-10.1)

Table XXIV-10.1 Comparison of gender differences in sleep characteristics (Williams *et al.*, 1974)

Age (years)	Females	Males
3–5	Increased SWS, decreased stage 2	Increased TIB, SPT, TST
6–9	Increased SWS	
10–12	Increased SWS, no. of stage changes	
13–15	Same, begin to see decreased TIB, TST and TSP	
16–19	Same, decreased REM	
20–29	Increased stage 2	Increased awakenings
30–39	No differences	
40–49	Increased TST, SE	Increased WASO, decreased SE
50–59	Increased SWS, REM	
60–69	Increased SWS (50% have it)	Increased wake, only 10% have SWS
70–79	Increased stage shifts, SWS, REM	Increased TIB

SWS = slow-wave sleep, TST = total sleep time, TSP = total sleep period, TIB = time in bed, REM = rapid-eye-movement sleep, WASO = wake after sleep onset.

Biological Psychiatry: Edited by H. D'haenen, J.A. den Boer and P. Willner. ISBN 0-471-49198-5

Non-complaining sleepers, categorized by decade and gender, were studied with full laboratory-based polysomnography. While not all variables that could influence sleep were controlled for at this early time in the science, this work did attempt to control for the influence of the menstrual cycle by studying only adult women in their follicular phase. Sleep differences between males and females were seen to begin around 9–10 months of age, with female babies sleeping longer. Around the age of 3 years, males showed greater time in bed (TIB), longer total sleep time (TST), longer REM cycle length and higher percentage of stage 2 sleep. Females demonstrated a trend toward increased SWS that continued throughout most of their lives. Teenage females tended to show less TIB, and in the later teens females slept less than males. In their twenties, females demonstrated more TST than men and continued to do so throughout life. Additionally, they showed more stage 2 sleep. Males began to show increased levels of arousal and decreased SWS toward the end of the second decade. The decline of SWS continued throughout their life, but it did not begin in females until the fourth or fifth decade. Males continued to show increased levels of arousal and decline in REM sleep during their fourth decade. Women began to show less SWS in their fifties and began to exhibit patterns like those of men in their thirties. Sleep became fragmented in women during the perimenopausal years with increased arousal. During the sixth decade, larger differences were seen in the amount of SWS; only 10% of males showed SWS while 50% of females did 50. In their seventh decade, women showed more stage changes than men did, perhaps simply because they continued to show all stages of sleep. By seventy, few men showed appreciable amounts of SWS. In addition, they tended to show shorter REM cycles. The REM cycles of younger adults showed increasing length across the night such that the last REM cycle of the night was the longest. This pattern changed in the elderly, with REM cycles becoming more even in length across the night.

While numerous smaller studies have confirmed these findings using visually scored sleep staging, many have resulted in controversy, particularly regarding the sleep of infants. Some studies of infants have shown no gender-related differences (Parmalee *et al.*, 1961, Hoppenbrowers *et al.*, 1989). Others have shown increased variability in males (Moore and Ucko, 1957) or females (Cornwell, 1992). The environment is one influence that could alter findings. To examine infant sleep and the influence of environment, Bach *et al.* (2000) examined the relationship between gender-related sleep differences with a thermal challenge. Healthy preterm neonates were studied (21 males/17 females) during three consecutive morning sleep sessions while sleeping in their closed, convectively heated incubators. The first morning served as a screen at thermoneutral conditions. The second session provided baseline data at thermoneutral conditions. The experimental condition, day 3, monitored sleep at cool conditions (<1.5°C from baseline). Sleep continuity and architecture were altered in both males and females. Active sleep (AS) increased at the expense of quiet sleep (QS). Males exhibited a larger variability in their sleep than females, sleeping less, waking more frequently and showing more AS. Since QS is believed to be highly controlled by developing brain centres, the investigators suggested that stable QS might mark the more advanced development of the female infants. The investigators also proposed that the increased variability seen in male infant sleep might be similar to that seen in older males. Furthermore, they suggested the need to consider the role of environmental factors in the variability noted in infants' sleep.

Few differences have been noted among young adults by visual scoring. However, Dijk *et al.* (1989) studied gender differences in young adults aged 19–28 years (13 males/15 females), using computer-quantified spectral analysis of EEG. He noted no change between sexes in the distribution of sleep stages but saw an increase of delta power in the EEG (0.25–11 Hz) of women during NREM sleep and higher power densities in women during REM sleep that was consistent across the night. The changes were independent of those seen after sleep deprivation or increased homeostatic drive for sleep, which should have dissipated across the night. The authors suggest that these differences may reflect gender differences in skull size or thickness, which has previously been shown to be negatively correlated to EEG amplitude (Pfefferbaum and Rosenbloom, 1987) rather than physiological differences between the sexes. Unfortunately, nine of the females in this study used oral contraceptives, which may have acted to blunt the temperature changes that affected sleep.

Also using visually scored staging and period-analysis algorithms, Armitage (1995) studied young men and women (mean age 25 years, 11 men/11 women) to examine EEG frequencies during sleep. She evaluated EEG in five conventional frequency categories: delta (0.5–4 Hz), seen in SWS; theta (4–8 Hz), predominantly seen other stages of sleep; alpha (8–12 Hz), found in quiet wakefulness; sigma (12–16 Hz), seen in spindle activity of stage 2; and beta (16–32 Hz), seen in lighter stages of sleep and wake. No striking gender-related differences were noted. However, when the global delta power of NREM was examined, females again showed significantly more delta across the sleep period. Unfortunately, all the women were taking oral or injectable contraceptives, a factor that may have altered the findings. As we will see, this may have an important impact on the findings.

To examine the effects of ageing on the EEG, Ehlers and Kupfer (1997) studied young adults aged 20–40 years, using visually scored sleep staging and spectral analysis of EEG characteristics. No gender differences in SWS or delta wave activity were seen among subjects in their twenties. Both sexes had a decline in the spectral power of spindles with age. No significant change of a visually scored sleep variable was noted for women across the groups. However, significant reductions of delta activity and percent SWS were noted for men in their thirties. Additionally, males showed significant reductions of REM time, and REM density, activity and intensity, with an increase of stage 2 sleep. These authors suggested this might indicate that men and women age differently over the second and third decade.

To avoid confounds of the laboratory environment, numerous studies have evaluated sleep in the subject's home. Kobayashi *et al.* (1998) studied 18 older subjects (8 males/10 females, mean age 60.6 and 61.7 years, respectively) during two 36-h sleep/wake periods. Full polysomnography was obtained in the home. They noted that men napped more frequently, had lower sleep efficiency, more stage 1 sleep, less stage 3/4 sleep, less REM sleep, and more state changes than females. However, no mention was made of concomitant sleep disorders, such as apnoea, that could be expected to produce similar patterns.

In another small study, Fukuda *et al.* (1999) evaluated sleep in older subjects (8 males/8 females, aged 54–72), also using full polysomnography in their homes. Visually scored sleep staging and spectral analysis of two frequency bands (0.5–2 HZ and 2–4 Hz) were done. No significant gender differences were noted in the following visually scored sleep parameters (percent wake, stages 1 and 2 sleep, REM sleep and REM latency, TIB, TST, sleep efficiency (SE), and awakenings). However, females had a higher percentage of SWS (stages 3 and 4). With spectral analysis, the investigators report females had larger amounts of delta power across the night than men. Furthermore, the females maintained clearer periodicity of delta power across the night. The authors suggest that the SWS generator is better conserved in middle-aged and elderly females than in males of the same age.

In another home-monitored study, Reyner and Horne (1995) studied 400 adults (211 female/189 males) aged 20–70 years for 15 consecutive nights, using sleep logs and actigraphy. Actigraphy provides objective confirmation of sleep length and timing as well as sleep continuity. Subjects were divided into three age groups: young, 20–34 years; middle-aged, 35–49; and older, 50–70. Home environmental factors were not controlled in this field study. Overall, there appeared to be minimal effects of ageing in both the subjective and objective parameters. However, women, particularly the older ones, tended to go to bed earlier than men and stay in bed longer, but they reported worse sleep with frequent awakenings, a report which was confirmed by actigraphy. They also reported longer sleep latency (time needed to fall asleep). There was also a significant difference in rising time between middle-aged men and women, with men rising earlier. Both men and women awoke earlier with age. Young men slept longer than both their middle-aged and older counterparts and middle-aged women slept longer than middle-aged men. Women in all age groups had significantly more awakenings than men. Many of these awakenings were noted to be environmental (children's needs).

CIRCADIAN RHYTHMICITY

As previously noted, sleep is regulated in part by our circadian cycle, with input from the pacemaker located in the suprachiasmatic nuclei, as well as from exogenous factors such as food, light and ambient temperature. Body temperature also has a circadian rhythm, oscillating between a nadir at night and a maximum in the afternoon, and is thought to influence sleep onset and offset. There has been interest as to whether the circadian rhythm of temperature and sleep is disrupted in ovulatory women who have a menstrual cycle, with increased body temperatures in the luteal phase, or in women taking oral contraceptives.

To examine this question, Baker *et al.* (2001) studied eight normally cycling women, eight women taking birth-control pills, and eight men (all aged 21–22). All subjects had a screen/adaptation night in the laboratory. Women were alternately studied in their mid-follicular and mid-luteal phases over a 3-month period. Polysomnography and continuous core body temperature were measured along with levels of estradiol and progesterone in the women. Both subjective and objective sleep measures were compared. Rectal temperatures of the normally cycling women were elevated, as expected in the luteal phase of the menstrual cycle compared to that in the follicular cycle, and they had blunted nocturnal drops of temperature compared to men, but not compared to the follicular phase. Both groups of women attained temperature minima earlier than men, suggesting a gender effect. The temperatures of the women taking exogenous hormones were similar to that of the luteal phase in normally cycling women. Therefore, hormonal supplementation may render these women poor subjects for sleep evaluations since the hormones alter the temperature phase. There was no significant difference in the sleep architecture (macrostructure) of men and women except that more SWS was seen in the luteal phase of normally cycling women. Those women on exogenous hormones demonstrated less SWS than normally cycling women.

Buysee *et al.* (1993) studied 17 healthy, 20–30-year-old men ($n = 9$) and women ($n = 8$) and 18 healthy 80-year-olds (11 men/7 women) during a 36-h constant routine paradigm to evaluate temporal patterns of unintended sleep episodes. The constant routine followed a 24-h adaptation period of normal routines. During the constant routine, balanced nutrition was supplied every hour. Core body temperatures were tracked on line, and cortisol and melatonin levels were sampled over the entire period. All subjects had continuous EEG with measurement of mood and sleepiness every hour. Women showed stronger rhythmic trends for sleep than men, and the older women in this study showed higher temperature amplitudes than the younger women. All temperature measurements of the younger women were taken during their follicular menstrual phase. However, three of the younger women were taking oral contraceptives, and this could have served to blunt the temperature curves for younger women.

To examine further the relationship between age-related changes in sleep and the circadian timing system, Campbell and Murphy (1998) studied 60 subjects (32 females/28 males) aged 40–84. For some analyses, the group was divided by age: a group of 40–60 middle-aged subjects, and two older groups of 65–81. One of the older groups was a subset that had experienced sleep difficulties for at least 1 year prior to the study. Polysomnography and measures of core body temperature were performed at an adaptation and baseline night. There was no difference between the sleep quality of non-complaining older subjects and that of those middle-aged; however, there was an advance of minimum body temperature in older subjects. Complaining older subjects had decreased TST, SE, and REM with increased wake after sleep onset (WASO) compared to non-complaining older subjects. There was no difference in the rhythm of body temperature between complaining and non-complaining older subjects. With age controlled for, women showed significantly higher temperature amplitude than men. In addition, there was a significant age effect on amplitude in women, but not men. According to the authors, these findings argue that older women maintain a stronger circadian rhythmicity than older men, as measured by temperature curve amplitude, and that age-related sleep disturbances may have multiple causes.

Parry *et al.* (1997) studied the nocturnal patterns of melatonin in women with premenstrual dysphoric disorder (PMDD) and controls, and noted a delay in the secretion of melatonin and a decrease in melatonin secretion during the luteal menstrual phase, as compared to the follicular phase in women with PMDD. The authors suggest that the circadian pacemaker of women with PMDD is more responsive to the hormonal changes of the menstrual cycle. Furthermore, they postulate that this sensitivity may render these women more subject to mood, cognitive and sleep disturbances as a result of endogenous and exogenous stimuli.

HORMONAL INFLUENCES: MENSTRUATION, PREGNANCY, LACTATION, AND MENOPAUSE

Limited data suggest that secretions of gonadal hormones influence/modulate sleep physiology in animals, and both the physiology and disorders of sleep in humans. Neuroendocrine function is influenced at both the pre- and postsynaptic levels. However, most animal studies have been carried out in males of species where the direct influence of exogenous hormones may differ from that endogenously produced. Animal studies show that neurosteroids (oestrogen, progesterone and testosterone) play a pivotal role in the mediation of stress and the effect on brain functions. In humans, studies examining the role of these hormones have been small-scale, and few studies have taken even menstrual cycling into consideration in any systematic way. Nevertheless, both animal and human studies indicate neurosteroidal effects at both the genomic and nongenomic levels. Furthermore, effects have been noted in brain regions related to the control of sleep and wake (medial preoptic nuclei, medial hypothalamus) and limbic areas such as the hippocampus and amgydala.

For instance, oestrogen has been shown to increase the turnover of norepinephrine in the brainstem, hypothalamus, nucleus accumbens and locus coeruleus, as well as to alter expression of c-fos proteins in A2 adrenergic neurons. These effects act to decrease REM sleep, but the action appears to depend on the phase of the circadian cycle. Temperature phase may be altered, suggesting that oestrogen may weaken the coupling between the core body temperature and the sleep/wake cycle, or otherwise modulate circadian rhythms (Dijk, 1989).

Oestrogen acts as an excitatory stimulus by increasing the production and receptor concentrations of neurotransmitters such as serotonin, norepinephrine and dopamine, as well as the B-endorphins, and increasing the availability of glutamate, which stimulates the excitatory *N*-methyl-D-asparate system (NMDA) (Arpels, 1996). In theory, increased levels of oestrogen occurring as a consequence of oestrogen hormone replacement therapy (HRT) could increase activity and irritability and lessen sleep. However, studies evaluating HRT in post-menopausal women demonstrate increased sleep times; that is, less fragmentation and enhanced REM sleep compared to baseline and placebo controls (Leproult *et al.*, 1998).

Progesterone and its metabolites act directly on the $GABA_A$ receptor and, through a complex mechanism, this action results in either a hyperpolarization and decrease in neuronal excitability (allopregnanolone and pregnanolone) or an antagonistic reaction that limits GABA-induced chloride transport (pregnenolone sulphate) (Mellon, 1994). The sedating action of progesterone is comparable to that of the benzodiazepines and is dose-dependent (Lancel *et al.*, 1997). Progesterone has been shown to decrease sleep latency, decrease wakefulness and increase EEG spindle activity in both REM and NREM sleep, in both animal and human studies. Furthermore, the progesterone antagonist, mifepristone (RU-486), has been shown to produce an increase of wake time, longer sleep latencies and decreased REM and SWS when administered to healthy men (Wiedemann *et al.*, 1998). Progesterone also acts as an anti-oestrogen and downregulates the oestrogen receptors.

Antonijevic *et al.* (1999) note the likelihood that ovarian steroids, such as estradiol and progesterone, may modulate GABA receptors, as well as the adrenergic system, thus effecting changes in sleep between the sexes. Women secrete more cortisol early in the night and show a pulsatile pattern of release of growth hormone (gH) across the night as compared to men, who typically show a single peak at the start of sleep.

Researchers have also detected changes in cellular immune function across the menstrual cycle that appear to be associated with fluctuations of progesterone. Moldofsky *et al.* (1995) have shown that there is less natural killer (NK) cell activity during the luteal phase, when progesterone is high. During the follicular phase, the NK responses are the same as in men. This suggests that progesterone may modify immune function and may affect women's risk of lupus and rheumatoid diseases that also alter their ability to sleep.

Human sleep changes during the perimenopausal years may therefore reflect the impact of fluctuating and ultimately decreasing levels of oestrogen and progesterone. Additionally, sleep across the menstrual cycle, for those women sensitive to subtle hormonal changes, can be problematic. Numerous studies and surveys of subjective complaints of sleep disturbance demonstrate large numbers of women with occasional, menstrual-related sleep difficulty (National Sleep Foundation, 1998). However, few objective studies confirm these complaints. This may be partly because few studies have accurately measured hormonal levels, many dividing the menstrual cycle into a variety of phases that could not be matched for meta-analysis, and most studies having few subjects. Furthermore, the two well-controlled studies that follow illustrate the subtlety of sleep changes across the menstrual cycle in healthy, non-complaining women.

Ito *et al.* (1995) studied seven women aged 18–19 who spent three consecutive days in each of five successive weeks in the laboratory. The investigators studied the plasma melatonin circadian pattern under controlled conditions with measurements every hour for 24 h on the third day of each week. They divided the menstrual cycle into four phases. Plasma melatonin was raised in the late luteal phase, and the rise time was delayed on the first of the three days in the laboratory. Additionally, SWS was increased in the follicular phase as was TIB and TST, suggesting that the menstrual cycle did affect melatonin and sleep/wake rhythm.

In a study of nine menstruating women free of oral contraceptives, Driver *et al.* (1996) evaluated 138 sleep episodes spaced every other night throughout a 36-day period. Menstrual status was measured with biphasic temperature rhythms, to capture pre/postovulatory phases, urinary luteal hormone (LH), and mid-luteal plasma levels of oestrogen and progesterone. Lighting, activity, and alcohol and caffeine intake were controlled. Subjective and objective measures of sleep showed no significant change over the menstrual cycle, with the exception of an increase of spindle (14.25–15 Hz) activity that had large variations across the cycle, reaching a high in the luteal phase in parallel with body temperature.

Animal work also suggests that the androgens (testosterone) play a role in the sexual dimorphism of REM sleep during a critical period of brain development around the perinatal time (Manber and Armitage, 1998). The administration of exogenous testosterone to adult animals has been shown to have little effect on sleep. However, it is felt that in humans it is the lessening of progesterone, as well as the change in the ratio of oestrogen to testosterone, that may influence the sleep changes around the perimenopause.

Pregnancy

Significant changes in sleep occur during pregnancy, in part due to hormonal changes and changes in the woman's girth. Profound sleepiness occurs during the first trimester secondary to elevated levels of progesterone. Progesterone also affects smooth muscle and the resultant urinary frequency disturbs sleep. Restless legs and pain begin to disrupt sleep during the second trimester. In the third trimester, women are uncomfortable due to the gravid uterus.

Using quantitative EEG, Brunner *et al.* (1994) studied nine healthy pregnant women, on two consecutive nights during each trimester. WASO was elevated across the pregnancy. No other significant differences were noted by visual scoring, but the quantitative techniques revealed significant changes across trimesters. There was an increase in WASO from trimester 2 to trimester 3, a decrease in REM sleep from trimester 1 to trimester 2, and a progressive reduction in NREM power density of spindle bands of >14.25–15 Hz across the pregnancy.

A second study of this type confirmed a loss of SWS as the pregnancy progressed. Schoor *et al.* (1998) studied four pregnant women and four non-pregnant controls with polysomnography in each trimester. There were no differences between groups on comparing time until sleep onset, latency to stage 2 and latency to REM. There were no differences in cardiopulmonary indices. However, there was a decrease in SWS even during the first trimester, and alpha intrusion into SWS was noted in the pregnant women.

Not only does pregnancy affect sleep but also sleep problems continue into the post-partum phase for many women. Lee and Zaffke (1999) followed 24 primiparous and 18 multiparous women to evaluate perceived levels of fatigue and energy before, during and after pregnancy. Studies were carried out in the subjects' homes during the follicular and luteal phase of menstruation prior to conception that served as baseline. Studies were repeated during each trimester and again at months 1 and 3 of the post-partum period. The measures included polysomnography, and scales such as the Lee Fatigue Scale, the POMS and the Dupuy General Well-Being and Vitality subscale. Serum chemistries included iron (Hg, HCT, ferritin, B_{12} and folic acid); progesterone; and thyroid serum T3, serum T4, T3 resin uptake, free T4 index, and thyroid antimicrosomal antibody titre. Complaints of fatigue during the first trimester were related to younger age and lower levels of iron, haemoglobin and ferritin. Haemoglobin levels remained low normal throughout the pregnancy while ferritin levels dipped more slowly across trimesters. During the third trimester, fatigue was related to decreased TST. Post-partum, fatigue was related to decreased sleep, ferritin and haemoglobin. Even at 3 months post-partum, these women still felt less energy than their baseline levels. The perception of energy appeared to be influenced by parity, with multiparas having less energy throughout pregnancy. This suggests that pregnancy takes a significant toll on the sleep patterns and energy levels of women. Poor sleep may incline women to profound mood changes and depression during the post-partum period. Some believe the 'baby blues' may be a consequence of prolonged sleep deprivation.

Additionally, during pregnancy, changes in respiration and airway mechanics occur. Snoring and apnoea are not uncommon. To evaluate the extent of this problem, Loube *et al.* (1996) carried out a large survey of pregnant women, determining snoring status and comparing infant outcomes to examine the impact of self-reported snoring on infant health. A total of 350 pregnant women and 110 age-matched women as controls answered a survey about snoring and daytime sleepiness. Those with reported daytime sleepiness and snoring were given full sleep evaluations. Fourteen percent of pregnant women snored versus 4% of the non-pregnant. Eleven women reported anecdotal apnoea. Of these, only four were recorded. Two of them met the criteria for mild apnoea; one had positional apnoea and the other only snored. There were no significant differences between infants from either group.

In contrast, Franklin *et al.* (2000) noted in a study of 500 Swedish women that habitual snoring was a sign of pregnancy-induced high blood pressure (preeclampsia), and was associated with lower birth weights and lower Apgar scores. The study also noted that women started to snore before any sign of hypertension appeared, and that snoring was related to sleep apnoea. While it may seem reasonable to suppose that the increased abdominal girth of pregnancy (with or without excessive weight gain) underlies the increase in apnoea, there is little evidence to support this. A more likely explanation is that the frequent nasal congestion experienced by pregnant women predisposes to upper airway collapse due to the large negative pressure in the airway needed to overcome the nasal obstruction.

Perimenopause and Menopause

Many researchers and clinicians have noted an increase in complaints of fragmented sleep secondary to the hot flashes of menopause. Women complain of difficulty in falling asleep and experience disrupted sleep, as hot flashes occur frequently at night. The hot flash typically is characterized by peripheral vasodilatation, profuse sweating, and subsequent chilling, and is thought to be a disorder of thermoregulation. Alterations in central catecholamines occur; specifically, levels of plasma 3-methoxy-4-hydroxyphenylgylcol (MHPG) are higher in women who experience hot flashes (Woodward and Freedman, 1994). In a sense, the hot flash is a general alerting mechanism which interrupts sleep and requires time to settle before sleep can comfortably recur, resulting in sleep loss and daytime consequences such as loss of concentration and memory. The addition of oestrogen and oestrogen HRT reduce the hot flash and have been seen to increase SWS in post-menopausal women (Leproult *et al.*, 1998). Furthermore, oestrogen HRT has been shown to reduce the respiratory disturbances more common in post-menopausal women (Pickett *et al.*, 1989).

Menopause is preceded by many years of hormonal changes. This period, called the perimenopause, can stretch for 5–10 years before the onset of the menopause. Perimenopausal women frequently note mood changes and sleep disruption during this time. Baker *et al.* (1997) confirmed these complaints in a study of 15 perimenopausal and 13 premenopausal women. Perimenopausal women had higher anxiety levels and lower vigour than premenopausal women, as measured by the State-Trait Anxiety Inventory (STAI) and the POMS. There was a significant correlation between the STAI scores and sleep arousals, and it was clear that sleep disruption had a mediating role in mood changes.

In another interesting paper, Shaver and Paulsen (1993) reported on subjective and objective studies of 135 healthy women aged 37–59. Women were grouped as premenopausal and menopausal, each with and without 'poor' sleep. The authors noted that women with objectively documented poor sleep had higher psychological distress rather than active menopausal symptoms. This suggests that the sleep disruption in the menopausal years may not be totally due to hormonal changes. This is also an age of life-altering changes that can produce stress. Children are leaving, parents are requiring more care, marriages are being renegotiated and women may be redefining their roles. These stresses add to a hormonally volatile time in women's lives.

DREAMING

Gender differences in dream content begin to emerge during adolescence. Males show more aggression than females, who dream about relationships and pleasant emotions. This difference continues into adulthood, depending upon the socialization developed (Hall *et al.*, 1982). Working women's dreams, especially those of women in traditionally male professions, become more male-like than do those of the homemaker. This suggests that dreams have a role in reflecting experiences of the waking state (Lortie-Lussier *et al.*, 1985).

PREVALENT SLEEP DISORDERS

Insomnia

Far more women than men complain of insomnia; that is, difficulty in falling or staying asleep (Table XXIV-10.2). This increase may be related to the increase of depression in women or at least the reporting of somatic symptoms related to sleep difficulties, which is increased among depressed women both acutely (Angst and Dobler-Mikola, 1984) and chronically (Kornstein *et al.*, 2000). This association has been noted in epidemiological studies (Bliwise *et al.*, 1992). The causation of symptoms is still unclear, that is, whether sleep difficulties precede mood symptoms or not (Browman *et al.*, 1996). Furthermore, women may be subject to the entrainment of poor sleep habits first developed during years of parenting.

The increase of reports of insomnia among women is especially marked during the perimenopausal years when hormone levels are rapidly shifting, and this disorder continues to be prominent as women age. Maggi *et al.* (1998) evaluated by questionnaire 2398 (867 males/1531 females) community-living older (>65 years) subjects. The prevalence of insomnia was 54% in women compared to 36% in men. There was an increased odds ratio for insomnia (1.69) and depression (1.93) in women, even when results were controlled for potential risk factors such as health status and smoking and alcohol habits. Night waking was the most common complaint.

The causes of insomnia are usually multi-factorial and include the major categories of physical changes such as poor health; hormonal status; physiological changes such as jet lag; and psychological, psychiatric, and pharmacological influences. Because sleep loss has a profound effect on quality of life and daytime functioning, recognition and treatment of insomnia are important.

Treatments should be designed to alleviate the cause when possible. In cases of depression, adequate treatment of the depression usually heralds improvement in sleep, as long as poor sleep habits have not begun. In this event, short-term use of hypnotics may be appropriate while better sleep habits and behavioural changes are being reinforced. Ultimately, long-term improvement is best achieved with behavioural techniques (Morin *et al.*, 1999).

Fibromyalgia

Frequently, pain syndromes, more common in women, can negatively influence sleep. In a study of 11 women with fibromyalgia

Table XXIV-10.2 Sleep disorders prevalent in women compared to men Diagnostic Classification Committee, 1990)

Females	ICSD code	ICSD code	Males
Psychobiological insomnia		780.53	Obstructive sleep apnoea
Sleep state misperception	307.49	780.54	Hypersomnia
Restless legs syndrome	780.56	780.51	Central alveolar hypoventilation
Adjustment sleep disorder	307.41	780.55	Delayed sleep phase
Hypnotic dependent syndrome	780.52	307.46	Sleep terrors
Nightmares	307.49	307.3	Rhythmic movement disorders
Familial sleep paralysis	780.56	307.47	Somniloquy
Headaches	346	780.59	REM behaviour disorder
Fibromyalgia	729	788.36	Sleep enuresis
Nocturnal sleep-related eating disorders	780.52	780.59	Sudden unexplained nocturnal death syndrome
		786.09	Primary snoring
		798	SIDS

and 11 matched controls, Shaver *et al.* (1997) studied subjective reports as well as physiological indicators of stress. The study showed that sleep in the early part of the night is more fragmented, with increased arousal but no prominent EEG change in subjects with fibromyalgia. The 11 women with fibromyalgia reported worse sleep and higher psychological stress, as measured with SCL-90, on the somatization, obsessive-compulsive and anxiety subscales, although the scores were still within the normal range, despite showing no changes on measures of sympathetic activity, such as morning levels of cortisol and catecholamines from urine spills. The authors speculate that a disturbance of nocturnal growth hormone secretion may be related to these complaints.

Restless Legs Syndrome

Restless legs syndrome (RLS) is a common sleep disorder affecting more women than men, and it may affect the ability to fall asleep (Lavigne and Montplassir, 1994). RLS is characterized by the irresistible need to move one's limbs (particularly the legs). Feelings can be described as 'creepy crawling' or 'bubbling in the veins'. The constant need to move disrupts sleep. Unfortunately, the circadian rhythm of RLS worsens the symptoms in the evening. Many sufferers also demonstrate periodic leg movements (PLM) during sleep, further disrupting the continuity of sleep. Symptoms generally increase with age but occur frequently during pregnancy as well.

Recent research suggests the association of RLS with low brain ferritin levels (Early and Connors, 1999). Increasing serum levels of iron may be therapeutic. Furthermore, dopaminergic drugs and antispasmotic medications have also proven useful in treating this disorder.

Sleep Apnoea

Another common sleep disorder, the prevalence of which differs between men and women, is obstructive sleep apnoea. Apnoea, or hypopnoea, refers to the cessation of airflow during sleep, usually as a result of complete (apnoea) or incomplete (hypopnoea) closure of the airway. The closure is brief, lasting $\geq$10 s, but may be repeated every minute across the night. Sleep in this condition is disrupted by brief arousals at the end of each respiratory event. Furthermore, depending on the extent of apnoea and the cardiopulmonary health of the subject, significant oxygen desaturations may occur.

The estimated prevalence of sleep-disordered breathing, which is defined as an apnoea-hypopnoea score over 5/h sleep, is 24% in men and 9% in adult women. Four percent of males and 2% of females have the apnoea-hypopnoea syndrome, which includes daytime sleepiness (Young *et al.*, 1993).

The symptoms of obstructive apnoea in both men and women include dramatic snoring (although many women do not know whether they snore), gasping during sleep, restlessness and daytime sleepiness. Unfortunately, despite giving the classic symptoms of apnoea to their health-care provider, many women go undiagnosed. It is not clear whether this results from the bias of the health-care worker or the concurrent reporting of psychologically oriented symptoms, such as insomnia, depression and anxiety, which attract more attention in women (Young *et al.*, 1996). In fact women with sleep apnoea report far more symptoms of depression and anxiety, as measured with the SCL-90, than men regardless of the severity of their apnoea. Furthermore, complaints of depression and anxiety were higher in women with severe apnoea than women with mild apnoea (Pillar and Lavie, 1998).

Much speculation has occurred as to why there is a sexual dimorphism in this disorder. Popovic and White (1998) studied 12 pre- and 12 post-menopausal women. They found an increase in pharyngeal dilator muscle activity, probably related to levels of progesterone in awake females, such that the genioglossis tone is increased in the luteal menstrual phase, as well as in those post-menopausal women taking oestrogen HRT. However, during sleep, Thurnheer *et al.* (2000) noted no such difference. This group studied two age groups (18–35 years and 40–70 years) of both men and women with nocturnal polysomnography, measuring airway resistance during sleep, and saw no differences in airway tone between genders and across age. They did note an increase in total respiratory resistance at sleep onset in men compared to women. The authors suggested that the waking increase in upper airway resistance previously seen in women reflected the narrower size of their airway.

Obesity tends to be a major factor in the development of obstructive apnoea. However, for equal degrees of obesity, a man would probably have more sleep apnoea than a woman, perhaps because of the placement of male fat in the mid-torso area. However, women who are severely overweight are at risk at any age. They may not have apnoea from airway obstruction, but they may suffer from hypoventilation, a decreased effort to breathe, particularly in REM, allowing significant hypoxia to develop (O'Connor *et al.*, 2000). As previously mentioned, women can also develop a temporary form of sleep apnoea during pregnancy.

Treatment of apnoea is essential to good health. Recent data suggest that apnoea is an independent risk factor for hypertension and cardiovascular morbidity in the general public (Peppard *et al.*, 2000). Treatments range from weight loss and positional therapy to mechanical devices such as CPAP, a pressure of air presented to the airway which acts as a pneumatic splint to keep the airway open, and dental devices which increase muscle tone and space in the pharyngeal airway.

CONCLUSION

Subtle differences in sleep architecture exist between males and females, particularly as they age. Most of these differences appear to be influenced by the gonadal hormones oestrogen and progesterone in females, and testosterone around the perinatal period in males. Oestrogen seems to increase REM sleep in humans and improve sleep continuity in menopausal women. Progesterone is known to be sedating and similar to the benzodiazepines in that it decreases REM sleep and increases spindling and stage 2 sleep in humans. Testosterone in males appears to influence REM sleep, and the ratio of testosterone to oestrogen in females appears to influence irritability and sleep fragmentation. Females' cyclic hormonal nature significantly influences sleep architecture across their reproductive lifetime.

Furthermore, certain sleep disorders appear to 'favour' one sex over the other. Women have a risk of depression twice that of men. Anxiety and depression increase the risk of insomnia in this group. Other sleep disorders such as apnoea appear to be twice as common in men. Significant respiratory disturbance during sleep lessens REM sleep and fragments NREM sleep, resulting in excessive daytime sleepiness.

It is sensible to take this information into consideration when attempting to evaluate or improve sleep in both men and women.

REFERENCES

Angst, J. and Dobler-Mikola, A., 1984. Do the diagnostic criteria determine the sex ratio in depression? *Journal of Affective Disorders*, **7**, 189–198.

Antonijevic, I.A., Murck, H., Frieboes, R.-M., Holsboer, F. and Steiger, A., 1999. On the gender differences in sleep-endocrine regulation in young normal humans. *Clinical Neuroendocrinology*, **70**, 280–287.

Armitage, R., 1995. The distribution of EEG frequencies in REM and NREM sleep stages in healthy young adults. *Sleep*, **18**, 334–341.

Arpels, J.C., 1996. The female brain hypoestrogenic continuum from the premenstrual syndrome to menopause. *Journal of Reproduction Medicine*, **41**, 633–639.

Bach, V., Telliez, F., Leke, A. and Libert, J.-P., 2000. Gender-related sleep differences in neonates in thermoneutral and cool environments. *Journal of Sleep Research*, **9**, 249–254.

Baker, A., Simpson, S. and Dawson, D., 1997. Sleep disruption and mood changes associated with menopause. *Journal of Psychosomatic Research*, **43**, 359–369.

Baker, F.C., Waner, J.I., Vieira, E.F., Taylor, S.R., Driver, H.S. and Mitchell, D., 2001. Sleep and 24 hour body temperatures: a comparison in young men, naturally cycling women and women taking hormonal contraceptives. *Journal of Physiology*, **530**, 565–574.

Bliwise, D.L., King, A.C., Harris, R.B. and Haskell, W.L., 1992. Prevalence of self-reported sleep in a healthy population aged 50–65. *Social Science and Medicine*, **34**, 49–55.

Browman, J.-E., Lundh, L.-G. and Hetta, J., 1996. Insufficient sleep in the general population. *Neurophysiologie Clinique*, **26**, 30–39.

Brunner, D.P., Munch, M., Biedermann, K., Huch, R., Huch, A. and Borbely, A.A., 1994. Changes in sleep and sleep electroencephalogram during pregnancy. *Sleep*, **17**, 576–582.

Buysee, D.J., Monk, T.H., Reynolds, C.F. III, Mesiano, D., Houck, P.R. and Kupfer, D.J., 1993. Patterns of sleep episodes in young and elderly adults during a 36-hour constant routine. *Sleep*, **16**, 632–637.

Campbell, S.S. and Murphy, P.J., 1998. Relationships between sleep and body temperature in middle-aged and older subjects. *Journal of the American Geriatric Society*, **46**, 458–462.

Cornwell, A.C., 1992. A maturational delay in the sleep/wake pattern of male high risk for SIDS infants. IEEE Proceeding of the 14th Annual International Conference of the IEEE Engineering in Medicine and Biology Society.

Diagnostic Classification Steering Committee, Thorpy, M.J. (ed.), 1990. *International Classification of Sleep Disorders Diagnostic and Coding Manual*. American Sleep Disorders Association, Rochester, MN.

Dijk, D.-J., Beersma, D.G.M. and Bloem, G.M., 1989. Sex differences in sleep EEG of young adults: visual scoring and spectral analysis. *Sleep*, **12**, 500–507.

Driver, H.S., Dijk, D.J., Werth, E., Biedermann, K. and Borbely, A.A., 1996. Sleep and the sleep electroencephalogram across the menstrual cycle in young healthy women. *Journal of Clinical Endocrinology and Metabolism*, **81**, 728–735.

Early, C.J. and Connors, J.R., 1999. RLS patients have abnormally reduced CSF ferritin compared to both normals and patient controls. *Sleep*, **22**, S156.

Ehlers, C.L. and Kupfer, D.J., 1997. Slow wave sleep: do young adult men and women age differently? *Journal of Sleep Research*, **6**, 211–215.

Franklin, K.A., Holmgren, P.A., Jonsson, F., Poromaa, N., Stenlund, H. and Svanborg, E., 2000. Snoring, pregnancy-induced hypertension and growth retardation of the fetus. *Chest*, **117**, 137–141.

Fukuda, N., Nonma, H., Kohsaka, M., Kobayashi, R., Sakakibara, S., Kohsaha, S. and Koyama, T., 1999. Gender differences of slow wave sleep in middle-aged and elderly subjects. *Psychiatry and Clinical Neuroscience*, **539**, 151–153.

Hall, C.S., Domhoff, G.W., Blick, K.A. and Weesmer, K.E., 1982. The dream of college men and women in 1950 and 1980: a comparison of dream content and sex differences. *Sleep*, **5**, 188–194.

Hoppenbrowers, T., Hodgman, J., Arakawa, K. and Sterman, M.B., 1989. Polysomnographic sleep and waking states are similar in subsequent siblings of SIDS and control infants during the first six months of life. *Sleep*, **12**, 265–276.

Ito, M., Kohsaka, M., Honma, K., Fukuda, N., Honma, S., Katsuno, Y., Ykawai, I., Honma, H., Morita, N. and Miyamoto, T., 1995. Changes in biological rhythm and sleep structure during the menstrual cycle in healthy women. *Seishin Shinkeigaka Zasshi*, **97**, 155–164.

Kobayashi, R., Kohsaka, M., Fukuda, N., Honma, H., Sakakibara, S. and Koyama, T., 1998. Gender differences in sleep of middle-aged individuals. *Psychiatry and Clinical Neuroscience*, **52**, 861–867.

Kornstein, S.G., Schatzberg, A.F., Thase, M.E., Yonkers, K.A., McCullough, J.P., Keitner, G.I., Gelenberg, A.J., Ryan, C.E., Hess, A.L., Harrison, W., Davis, S.M. and Keller, M.B., 2000. Gender differences in chronic major and double depression. *Journal of Affective Disorders*, **60**, 1–11.

Lancel, M., Faulhaber, J., Schiffelholz, T., Romeo, E., Di Michele, F., Holsboer, F. and Rupprecht, R., 1997. Allopregnanolone affects sleep in a benzodiazepine-like fashion. *Journal of Pharmacological and Experimental Therapeutics*, **282**, 1213–1218.

Lavigne, G.J. and Montplassir, J.Y., 1994. Restless legs syndrome and sleep bruxism, prevalence and association among Canadians. *Sleep*, **17**, 739–743.

Lee, K.A. and Zaffke, M.E., 1999. Longitudinal changes in fatigue and energy during pregnancy and the postpartum period. *Journal of Obstetric, Gynecologic, and Neonatal Nursing*, **28**, 183–191.

Leproult, R., Hofmann, E. and Van Cauter, E., 1998. Slow wave activity: effects of gender and oestrogen replacement therapy. *Sleep*, **21**(Suppl), 590H.

Lortie-Lussier, M., Schwab, C. and DeKoninck, J., 1985. Working mothers versus homemakers: do dreams reflect the changing roles of women? *Sex Roles*, **12**, 1009–1921.

Loube, D.I., Poceta, J.S., Morales, M.C., Peacock, M.D. and Mitler, M.M., 1996. Self-reported snoring in pregnancy. Association with fetal outcome. *Chest*, **109**, 885–889.

Maggi, S., Langlois, J.A., Minicuci, N., Grigoletto, F., Pavan, M., Foley, D.J. and Enzi, G., 1998. Sleep complaints in community dwelling older persons: prevalence, associated factors and reported causes. *Journal of the American Geriatric Society*, **46**, 161–168.

Manber, R. and Armitage, R., 1999. Sex, steroids and sleep: a review. *Sleep*, **22**, 540–555.

Mellon, S.H., 1994. Neurosteriods: biochemistry, modes of action and clinical relevance. *Journal of Clinical Endocrinology and Metabolism*, **78**, 1003–1008.

Moldofsky, H., Lue, F.A., Shahal, B., Jiang, C.-G. and Gorczynski, R.M., 1995. Diurnal sleep/wake-related immune functions during the menstrual cycle of healthy young women. *Journal of Sleep Research*, **4**, 150–159.

Morin, C.M., Colecchi, C., Stone, J., Sood, R. and Brink, D., 1999. Behavioral and pharmacological therapies for late-life insomnia. *Journal of the American Medical Association*, **281**, 991–999.

Moore, T. and Ucko, L.E., 1957. Night waking in early infancy. I. *Archives of Disease in Childhood*, **32**, 333–342.

National Sleep Foundation, 1998. *Poll on Women and Sleep*. Washington, DC.

O'Connor, C., Thornley, K.S. and Hanly, P.J., 2000. Gender differences in the polysomnographic features of obstructive sleep apnoea. *American Journal of Respiratory and Critical Care Medicine*, **161**, 1465–1472.

Parmalee, A.H., Schulz, H.R. and Disbrow, M.A., 1961. Sleep patterns of the newborn. *Journal of Pediatrics*, **58**, 241–250.

Parry, B.L., Berga, S.L., Mostofi, N., Klauber, M.R. and Resnick, A., 1997. Plasma melatonin circadian rhythms during the menstrual cycle and after light therapy in premenstrual dysphoric disorder and normal control subjects. *Journal of Biological Rhythms*, **12**, 47–64.

Peppard, P.E., Young, T., Palta, M. and Skatrud, J., 2000. Prospective study of the association between sleep-disordered breathing and hypertension. *New England Journal of Medicine*, **342**, 1378–1384.

Pfefferbaum, A. and Rosenbloom, M., 1987. Skull thickness influences P3 amplitude. *Psychopharmacology Bulletin*, **23**, 493–496.

Pickett, C.K., Regensteiner, J.G., Woodard, W.D., Hagerman, D.D., Weil, J.V. and Moore, L.G., 1989. Progestin and oestrogen reduce sleep disordered breathing in post-menopausal women. *Journal of Applied Physiology*, **66**, 1656–1661.

Pillar, G. and Lavie, P., 1998. Psychiatric symptoms in sleep apnoea syndrome: effects of gender and respiratory disturbance index. *Chest*, **114**, 697–703.

Popovic, R.M. and White, D.P., 1998. Upper airway muscle activity in normal women: influence of hormonal status. *Journal of Applied Physiology*, **84**, 1055–1062.

Rechtschaffen, A. and Kales, A. (eds), 1968. *A Manual of Standardized Terminology, Techniques and Scoring System for Sleep Stages of Human Subjects*. UCLA Brain Information Service/Brain Research Institute, Los Angeles.

Reyner, L.A. and Horne, J.A., 1995. Gender and age-related differences in sleep determined by home-recorded sleep logs and actimetry from 400 adults. *Sleep*, **18**(5), 391; **18**(2), 127–134.

Schoor, S.J., Chawla, A., Devidas, M., Sullivan, C.A., Naef, R.W. III and Morrison, J.C., 1998. Sleep patterns in pregnancy: a longitudinal study of polysomnography recordings during pregnancy. *Journal of Perinatology*, **18**(6) Part 1, 427–430.

Shaver, J.L. and Paulsen, V.M., 1993. Sleep, psychological distress and somatic symptoms in perimenopausal women. *Family Practice Research*, **13**, 373–384.

Shaver, J.L., Lentz, M., Landis, C.A., Heitkemper, M.M., Buchwald, D.S. and Woods, N.F., 1997. Sleep, psychological distress and stress arousal in women with fibromyalgia. *Research in Nursing and Health*, **20**, 247–257.

Stone, A.B. and Pearlstein, T.B., 1994. Evaluation and treatment of changes in mood, sleep and sexual functioning associated with menopause. *Obstetrics and Gynecology Clinics of North America*, **21**, 391–403.

Thurnheer, R., Wraith, P.K. and Douglas, N.J., 2001. Influence of age and gender in upper airway resistance in NREM and REM sleep. *Journal of Applied Physiology*, **90**, 981–988.

Wiedemann, K.M., Lauer, C.J., Hirschmann, M., Knaudt, K. and Holsboer, F., 1998. Sleep-endocrine effects of mifepristone and megestrol acetate in healthy men. *American Journal of Physiology*, **274**, E139–E145.

Williams, R.L., Karacan, J. and Hursch, C.J., 1974. *Electroencephalography of Human Sleep: Clinical Applications*. Wiley, New York.

Woodward, S. and Freedman, R.R., 1994. The thermoregulatory effects of menopausal hot flashes on sleep. *Sleep*, **17**, 497–501.

Young, T., Palta, M., Dempsey, J., Skatrud, J., Weber, S. and Badr, S., 1993. The occurrence of sleep-disordered breathing among middle-aged adults. *New England Journal of Medicine*, **328**, 1230–1235.

Young, T., Hutton, R., Finn, L., Badr, S. and Palta, M., 1996. The gender bias in sleep apnoea diagnosis. Are women missed because they have different symptoms? *Archives of Internal Medicine*, **156**, 2445–2451.

XXIV-11

Sleep Disorders — Therapeutic Armamentarium

Malcolm Lader

INTRODUCTION

We spend a third of our lives asleep and yet sleep remains an enigma. The numerous and complex disorders of sleep have been dealt with in several previous chapters. The most common complaint is that of insufficient and unsatisfying sleep. Problems with excessive sleep are much less common. Abnormal sleep is also noted on occasion, usually manifested as aberrant behaviour such as night terrors or sleepwalking.

A range of medications is available to treat insomnia, ranging from folk remedies such as valerian to the most recently introduced compound, zaleplon. Many medications possess sedative and sleep-inducing properties as a side effect, such as many tricyclic antidepressants and the first-generation antihistamines. Fewer remedies exist to treat excessive or qualitatively abnormal sleep, but progress is being made.

The purpose of this chapter is to review the available remedies, concentrating on the newest introductions that are of both theoretical interest and practical utility. The emphasis will be on the remedies for insufficient sleep — the hypnotic drugs — as these are among the most-widely prescribed medications, particularly by primary care practitioners (Simon and VonKorff, 1997).

SLEEP HYGIENE

Before dealing with hypnotic medication, it is useful to outline the stratagems that people use to induce and maintain sleep (Table XXIV-11.1). A regular bedtime routine is conducive to sleep, and many people follow a time-hallowed sequence of events, almost a ritual, before they retire at night. Regular hours for going to bed and for rising in the morning help consolidate sleep, and this routine should be maintained at the weekends and during vacations as well. Many people read before going to sleep, but arousing or disturbing material should be avoided. Rehearsing the next day's agenda or worrying about finances, family, etc. is unhelpful.

Exercise late at night is used by many people to hasten the onset of sleep although it is probably the routine that is most important. However, the optimum is moderate exercise in the afternoon or early evening, as anyone taking a vigorous sport-oriented vacation can testify. By contrast, heavy, exhausting exercise may be unhelpful (Horne, 1981).

The bedroom should be quiet, so that sound-attenuation may be needed if it abuts on a noisy street or lies under the flight path to an all-night airport. The room should not be too hot nor too cold. Many people take a milky drink at bedtime and there are many on the market. Tea and coffee may induce insomnia (Stradling, 1993). Coffee was once dubbed an 'antihypnotic' (Miller, 1722). Tolerance to the effects of the active principles, caffeine and, to a lesser extent, theobromine, tends to get lost as the individual ages.

Table XXIV-11.1 Elements of sleep hygiene

A. Regular bedtime routine
B. Standard hours of retiring and getting up
C. Avoid worry
D. Exercise in late afternoon/early, but not late, evening
E. Quiet, warm, comfortable bedroom
F. Avoid caffeine-containing drinks and too much alcohol

Table XXIV-11.2 Behavioural techniques

A. Stimulus control
B. Sleep restriction
C. Sleep hygiene education
D. Paradoxical intention
E. Attention-focusing procedures: thought-stopping, imagery training, meditation, yoga
F. Relaxation: progressive muscular relaxation, autogenic training, biofeedback

Alcohol is also used by many people, the traditional 'nightcap'. However, too much may disturb sleep due to its diuretic effect and to rebound insomnia later on.

RELAXATION AND NON-PHARMACOLOGICAL TECHNIQUES

Some people find formal relaxation techniques very helpful, especially if meditation techniques have been learnt for daytime use (Table XXIV-11.2). Nevertheless, meditation and the induction of sleep are distinct physiological and psychological processes, and it is the muscular relaxation that is most relevant. Simple relaxation exercises in which the person relaxes muscle groups progressively from toes to legs, trunk, arms, neck and head are appropriate.

More elaborate behavioural techniques have been advocated (Bootzin and Perlis, 1992; Sloan and Shapiro, 1993). Although not widely available, a variety of techniques have been developed. Morin and his colleagues evaluated 59 treatment studies involving over 2000 patients. These were predominantly women, and the mean age was 44. Most suffered from chronic primary insomnia, on average, of 11 years' duration. Most subjects received sleep-focused interventions with an average treatment time of 5 h. Follow-up lasted a mean of 6 months.

Of four outcome variables assessed, two in the meta-analysis — sleep-onset latency and time awake after sleep onset — were significantly improved following behavioural interventions. The absolute number of awakenings and total sleep time

Biological Psychiatry: Edited by H. D'haenen, J.A. den Boer and P. Willner. ISBN 0-471-49198-5

were not significantly improved. The average effect size for sleep-onset latency was 0.88, signifying that patients with insomnia were better off after treatment than 81% of untreated control subjects. The average effect size for time awake after sleep onset was lower at 0.65, indicating that patients with insomnia were sleeping better than 74% of the untreated sample. Stimulus control and sleep restriction were the most effective therapy procedures given alone, whereas education about sleep hygiene was not effective when used alone. These improvements were well maintained at follow-up assessments.

What are these apparently useful therapies? *Stimulus control* comprises a set of instructions designed to help the insomniac avoid sleep-incompatible behaviours and to regulate sleep-wake schedules (Bootzin *et al.*, 1991). Such manipulations include instructions to go to bed only when sleepy; that the bedroom is to be used only for sleep and sex, and not to work or watch television; that whenever unable to sleep for 15–20 min, patients are to get up and go into another room, and return only when feeling sleepy again; that patients are to rise every morning at the same preset time regardless of quality and quantity of sleep the previous night; that there is to be no daytime napping.

Sleep restriction consists of curtailing the amount of time the insomniac is allowed in bed to the actual duration of sleep (Spielman *et al.*, 1987). Thus, the insomniac who reports sleeping only 5/8 h in bed is allowed to stay in bed for only 5 h. Once 90% sleep efficiency is achieved, the allotted time is increased by 15–20 min for the next week. If sleep efficiency is below 80%, the time window is decreased by 15–20 min. Between 80% and 90% efficiency, the time in bed is kept constant. Constant monitoring is carried out by means of a sleep diary, and appropriate adjustments are made.

Sleep hygiene education is essentially informing insomniacs about the factors that influence sleep, as set out above. It also involves exploring individual sleep expectations and setting realistic targets. A regular routine, avoidance of napping, and advice concerning substance use and medication are the components of sleep hygiene that are easiest to modify.

Paradoxical intention is somewhat akin to the implosion therapies used in phobias. It consists of persuading the insomniac to confront the feared behaviour, i.e., failing to fall or stay asleep. Often patients become 'insomnophobic', worrying about staying awake and thereby instituting a vicious circle of anxiety, insomnia and further insomnia. The theory is that if the patient stops trying to fall asleep but tries to stay awake instead, sleep will supervene more easily. However, rather like implosion treatment, paradoxical intention treatment has been disappointing.

Attention-focusing procedures use techniques such as thought-stopping, imagery training and meditation to focus the mind away from concerns about staying awake. *Relaxation* therapies focus on the body rather than cognition and comprise techniques such as progressive muscular relaxation, autogenic training and biofeedback.

Most studies evaluating non-pharmacological therapies rely on sleep diary records. This is not necessarily a limitation, as insomnia is a subjective complaint and coordinations with polysomnographic data are disappointing. Where objective techniques have been used as outcome criteria, some efficacy is still seen but less than that relating to subjective reports.

In conclusion, although psychological treatments are time-consuming and should be provided by trained personnel, benefits do accrue with some of the therapies and tend to persist. The long-term drawbacks of drug therapies do not apply. Behavioural and cognitive methods, rather than analytically based psychotherapies, are preferred. Sleep hygiene education is not enough without more specific techniques.

Table XXIV-11.3 Some benzodiazepines and similar hypnotics

Benzodiazepine	Elimination half-life (h)
Long-acting	
Nitrazepam	25–35
Flunitrazepam	10–20
Flurazepam	40–100
Quazepam	40–100
Intermediate-acting	
Temazepam	10–15
Lormetazepam	8–15
Short-acting	
Triazolam	3–5
Non-benzodiazepine	
Zopiclone	4–6
Zolpidem	2–4
Zaleplon	0.8–1.5

HYPNOTIC DRUGS

A wide range of drugs is used to treat insomnia (Table XXIV-11.3). They can be divided into two groups: a) those whose primary purpose is to induce, consolidate or prolong sleep; b) those where side effects of sedation are exploited. In the former group, the benzodiazepines still dominate the market despite misgivings concerning adverse effects, tolerance and dependence (Lader, 1994). Long experience of usage and cheapness still commend them to many practitioners. The properties of the ideal hypnotic include rapid onset of action, dependable onset or prolongation of sleep, minimal residual daytime sedation, safety in overdosage, lack of rebound dependence and abuse potential, and flexible dosage formulation. Safety in the elderly is particularly desirable, as they are heavy users of hypnotics.

Several effects of benzodiazepine hypnotics are clearly dose-related. Efficacy is increased at higher doses, as are side effects on psychomotor and cognitive function. Severe adverse reactions such as aggressive outbursts and episodes of amnesia also increase in frequency as the dosage increases: this is apparent with triazolam and flunitrazepam. Discontinuation effects, such as rebound and dependence, are also dose-dependent. Finally, abuse generally involves very high doses of hypnotic benzodiazepines.

BENZODIAZEPINE HYPNOTICS

Many of these compounds are available throughout the world, the range varying from country to country. The commonest ones encountered are temazepam, flurazepam, triazolam, nitrazepam and flunitrazepam. The last two are not available in the USA. These drugs can be divided for convenience into long-, intermediate- and short-acting, depending on their duration of action in normal dose. This in turn, mostly reflects the mean elimination half-life.

LONG-ACTING COMPOUNDS

As sleep is a night-time phenomenon, averaging 8 out of the 24 h, a long-acting hypnotic raises questions of desirability and logicality. Inevitably drug effects will persist the next day and accumulation is very likely. The development of tolerance will lessen such residual effects, but it is impossible to predict whether any particular individual will remain affected. Furthermore, objective effects may occur with subjective effects so the patient may be impaired unwittingly. The advantage of a long-acting hypnotic benzodiazepine is that an anxiolytic effect will be present during the day. Thus, if the insomnia is a component symptom of an anxiety disorder, the latter will also receive symptomatic treatment. However, there are less contentious drug treatments for anxiety disorders (see Chapter XIX-13).

Nitrazepam was the first benzodiazepine marketed as a hypnotic. Its half-life ranges between 25 and 35 h (Breimer *et al.*, 1977). Residual effects are quite marked the next day, even after doses of 5 mg. Accumulation is likely, but, generally speaking, it is well tolerated and has been widely used in Europe.

Flunitrazepam is a similar compound with a duration of action of at least 24 h, reflecting an elimination half-life of 10–20 h (Boxenbaum *et al.*, 1978). The recommended dosage is 0.5–1 mg, but adverse events such as amnesia have attended the use of higher doses. Flunitrazepam is associated with two types of notoriety. It has a very rapid onset of action and powerful effects. It has been used as a 'date-rape drug', administered clandestinely in alcoholic drinks to unsuspecting women (and men). Usually, the victim is amnesic after the period during which the sexual assaults took place. The formulation has been changed in many countries to obviate surreptitious administration. The second problem is illicit abuse 'on the street'. In this respect, it has given rise to the greatest problem worldwide of all the benzodiazepines, even in the USA, where it is not licensed. It is taken orally, intranasally and by injection. Its scheduling has been strengthened because of its particular menace.

Flurazepam (and the closely related *quazepam*) (Ankier and Goa, 1988) are long-acting drugs with a half-life of 40–100 h. This reflects its metabolism to the long-acting *N*-dealkylflurazepam (Greenblatt, 1991). Residual daytime sedation is marked, particularly at the upper, marketed dose of 30 mg. Accumulation is also marked (Mamelak *et al.*, 1989).

Loprazolam is best regarded as a long-acting compound, as its absorption can be erratic and slow (Clark *et al.*, 1986).

INTERMEDIATE-ACTING COMPOUNDS

Temazepam is the most-widely used of these compounds. It has a half-life of about 10–15 h and is devoid of active metabolites (Greenblatt, 1991). It is generally well tolerated, and residual effects are not usually a problem even in the elderly. A wide dose range is available (7.5–30 mg). Temazepam was originally marketed in the UK in liquid-filled capsules which were extensively abused by addicts. Reformulation as a gel was unsuccessful; therefore, the drug is available in the UK only as a tablet. Its scheduling has also been strengthened.

Lormetazepam is somewhat shorter-acting but is otherwise similar to temazepam (Pierce *et al.*, 1984).

Lorazepam is also licensed as a hypnotic in many countries at higher doses than those recommended for anxiolytic effects.

SHORT-ACTING COMPOUNDS

The major member of this group is *triazolam*. This hypnotic has been the focus of much controversy since the late 1970s. It is rapidly absorbed and has a half-life of 3–5 h (Greenblatt, 1991). Residual day-time sedation is not usually a problem unless the recommended dose of 0.25 mg is exceeded. The other problem at higher dosages is an increased incidence of anterograde amnesia, and aggressive and suicidal behaviour. This resulted in much concern in the early 1990s. The UK Licensing Authority took the hardest line, withdrawing the drug from the market. It was never reinstated. In other countries, notably the USA, triazolam has remained available but with cautions regarding monitoring and recommendations that the appropriate dose be 0.25 mg in adults and 0.125 mg in the elderly.

Midazolam is generally available as an intravenous anaesthetic induction agent. In a few countries it is formulated for use orally as an hypnotic.

UNWANTED EFFECTS

These have been catalogued many times (e.g., Lader, 1994). As emphasized earlier, many adverse effects with hypnotic medication are strongly dose-related (Roth and Roehrs, 1992). The main problems are as follows:

1. There is residual sedation, which may be associated with psychomotor and cognitive impairment. Practical activities, such as driving, may be quite markedly affected so that the accident rate of benzodiazepine hypnotic users is substantially elevated (Ray *et al.*, 1992).
2. Sedation is easily detectable following administration of most hypnotics and is often associated with muscle relaxation. In its most severe form, the sedation is manifested as confusion and the muscle relaxation as ataxia. Both can present major difficulties in the elderly, who often wake at night to urinate. For this reason, some geriatricians eschew the use of benzodiazepines in the very elderly.
3. Memory, particularly for current events, can be impaired by benzodiazepines such as lorazepam. Another problem is amnesic episodes, often accompanied by nocturnal wanderings.
4. Discontinuation syndromes have been well-documented although their clinical significance is difficult to establish. Rebound insomnia and dependence syndromes can occur, the former more commonly with short-acting compounds such as triazolam, and the latter with long-acting drugs.
5. Abuse is often overlooked but can be iatrogenic with escalation of dose or as a feature of illicit use. Benzodiazepines are generally among the most important drugs of abuse, but usually in the context of polydrug abuse or alcohol problems. The combination with alcohol is particularly dangerous, with major psychological impairments, amnesia and aggressive behaviour.

OVERVIEW

The benzodiazepines continue to be the most-widely prescribed of hypnotics, having supplanted the barbiturates because of their relative safety in overdosage. They are effective drugs, at least in the short term before tolerance sets in. Residual sedation is a problem with many of these compounds but is often overlooked although the insomniac patient feels exhausted the next day. Adverse behavioural events, such as amnesia and aggression, have led to much concern. The major problems of rebound, dependence and abuse have curtailed the recommended duration of usage of these drugs. Nevertheless, long-term administration is the rule rather than the exception. Dosage is an important consideration but minimal dosage is not usually adhered to. The advent of more selective compounds has opened up the debate about the risk/benefit ratio of the various benzodiazepine hypnotics.

BENZODIAZEPINE-LIKE HYPNOTICS

Three compounds currently available as hypnotics are chemically non-benzodiazepine although pharmacologically similar; however, they are more selective. They will be reviewed in some detail.

Zopiclone

Zopiclone has been available in most countries for over a decade. The major exception is the USA, where, apparently, the company that developed the drug had no facilities for registration and marketing at the crucial time. Zopiclone can be regarded as the first of the more selective benzodiazepine-type hypnotics

Chemically, zopiclone is a cyclopyrrolone compound that potentiates the inhibitory effects of GABA at $GABA_A$ receptors. However, it differs in some ways from a typical benzodiazepine in the nature of its binding. For example, tolerance is not seen in the $GABA_A$ receptors of mice, in contrast to benzodiazepine effects (Serra *et al.*, 1996).

The other point of interest is its relatively short elimination half-life. Zopiclone is rapidly and extensively absorbed after oral administration, with a bioavailability of about 75% after the standard dose of 7.5 mg. Protein binding is low, but concentrations in the saliva can be quite high, resulting in an unpleasant, bitter taste. It is metabolized in the liver by cytochrome P450 enzymes to essentially inactive metabolites. The elimination half-life is generally accepted to be about 5 h, but it is prolonged in the elderly, particularly those aged over 75 (Gaillot *et al.*, 1987). Half-strength formulations are usually available for the elderly and for patients with impaired liver function. The main drug interaction of clinical relevance is that carbamazepine increases the plasma concentrations of zopiclone.

The hypnotic efficacy of zopiclone has been evaluated in numerous studies comparing it with placebo and with standard hypnotics, mostly benzodiazepines (for detailed reviews, see Goa and Heel, 1986; Noble *et al.*, 1998). Zopiclone shows effects on sleep induction superior to placebo and at least equivalent to short- and intermediate-acting benzodiazepines. It does not generally prolong total sleep time; therefore, some trials have shown long-acting benzodiazepines to be superior to zopiclone in this respect (e.g., Ponciano *et al.*, 1990). In general, zopiclone 7.5 mg is equivalent to 30 mg flurazepam or 5 mg nitrazepam with respect to sleep onset (e.g., Anderson, 1987). A large-scale study in primary care involving 1507 patients showed zopiclone, but not flunitrazepam 1 mg, to be significantly superior to placebo with respect to various measures of sleep quality (Hajak *et al.*, 1994). This study also included a triazolam arm: zopiclone, but not triazolam, separated from placebo. However, in general, zopiclone 7.5 mg is equivalent to or better than triazolam in the high dose of 0.5 mg (e.g., Autret *et al.*, 1987).

Zopiclone has variable effects on sleep architecture, but, in general, changes are minor (Parrino and Terzano, 1996). Tolerance to polysomnographic effects of zopiclone is usually minor, although few long-term studies have been carried out (Fleming *et al.*, 1988). An early review of short-term clinical studies lasting up to 8 weeks concluded that the hypnotic effects of zopiclone were maintained over this period for both younger and older insomniacs (Brun, 1988).

Hypnotics are generally licensed for short-term use, and a substantial proportion of users are middle-aged and elderly. Studies in elderly subjects have shown zopiclone 5 mg to be superior to placebo (Elie *et al.*, 1990), as was 7.5 mg (Klimm *et al.*, 1987). However, nitrazepam 5 mg was superior to zopiclone 7.5 mg with respect to onset latency on day 12 (Klimm *et al.*, 1987), and flunitrazepam 1 mg was superior to zopiclone 5 mg for difficulty in falling asleep (Dehlin *et al.*, 1995). Zopiclone has also shown useful efficacy in facilitating withdrawal from benzodiazepine hypnotics (Shapiro *et al.*, 1995).

Zopiclone, like the other newer hypnotics, is less likely to produce psychomotor and cognitive impairment than benzodiazepines such as nitrazepam or temazepam (Agnoli *et al.*, 1989; Ngen and Hassan, 1990). In particular, although immediate impairments can be detected following zopiclone, effects the next day are generally minor or undetectable. Subjective effects such as difficulty in waking, impaired well-being and reduced morning concentration are minimal providing a period of 5–8 h has elapsed since ingestion (Broadhurst and Cushnaghan, 1987).

Zopiclone is generally well tolerated, the commonest complaint being a bitter aftertaste (Allain *et al.*, 1991). Elderly patients tolerate the drug well, particularly in the lower doses of 3.75 and 5 mg.

Rebound following abrupt withdrawal of zopiclone is much less of a problem than with benzodiazepines such as triazolam (Bianchi and Musch, 1990). Dependence and withdrawal also seem to be far less common (Lader, 1998). However, some cases of dependence have been reported, often a transfer from a pre-existing benzodiazepine dependence. Occasional instances of street abuse have also been documented.

The usual dosage for short-term usage in patients with primary insomnia is 7.5 mg, with lower doses in the elderly. Zopiclone is now established (outside the USA) as a commonly used, well-tolerated drug with particular effects on shortening delay to sleep onset. Residual effects are generally not troublesome.

Zolpidem

The second of these new selective benzodiazepine-like hypnotic drugs is zolpidem (Holm and Goa, 2000). It has been marketed successfully for several years in many countries of the world including the USA (Langtry and Benfield, 1990). It is chemically an imidazopyridine agent and acts as a selective agonist on subtypes of benzodiazepine receptors (Sanger and Depoortere, 1998). This is believed to confer some advantage with respect to adverse effects, as compared with non-selective agonists such as the benzodiazepines.

Zolpidem has a very short half-life (Fraisse *et al.*, 1996), averaging about 2.5 h. The drug is rapidly absorbed; it has a bioavailability of around 70% and is highly protein-bound. It is largely metabolized by P450 isoenzymes, predominantly, CYP3A4, to inactive metabolites. Elimination is somewhat reduced in the elderly so that lower doses, such as 5 mg, are recommended. The pharmacokinetics are linear over the dose range 5–20 mg. The area under the curve is increased in individuals with liver or renal impairment.

The numerous clinical trials comparing zolpidem with placebo and with active comparators, mainly benzodiazepines, have been reviewed in detail by Holm and Goa (2000). The usual dosage was 10 mg in younger adults and 5 mg in the elderly. Most were primary insomniacs with sleep-onset latency beyond 30 min, and/or a total sleep time less than 6 h and/or more than three nocturnal awakenings. As is now standard, the primary outcome variables were derived from questionnaires, visual analogue scales and sleep diaries. Some polysomnographic data are also available.

Several placebo-controlled inpatient trials with acute and chronic insomnia have established the efficacy of zolpidem, mainly with respect to shortening of sleep-onset latency (Scharf *et al.*, 1991; Dockhorn *et al.*, 1996; Lahmeyer *et al.*, 1997). It was also efficacious in patients receiving concomitant selective serotonin reuptake inhibitors (SSRI) therapy (Asnis *et al.*, 1999). Zolpidem generally has equivalent efficacy to benzodiazepines. For example, the effects of 10-mg doses were similar to nitrazepam 5 mg with respect to sleep latency, number of awakenings and total sleep time (Kazamatsuri *et al.*, 1993), but it was preferred in another trial (Kudo *et al.*, 1993). Conversely, patients receiving flurazepam 30 mg reported better sleep than patients given zolpidem 10 or 20 mg (Fleming *et al.*, 1995). Comparisons with intermediate- and short-acting benzodiazepines have generally shown equivalence (e.g., Rosenberg and Ahlstrom, 1994). Studies with triazolam have used both 0.25 and 0.5 mg. In one study, zolpidem 10 mg was more effective than triazolam 0.5 mg in prolonging sleep duration (Monti *et al.*, 1994).

Zolpidem 10 mg had equivalent efficacy to zopiclone 7.5 mg in one large-scale study (see Holm and Goa, 2000: Table IV, p. 877).

In view of increasing concern about the efficacy and safety of hypnotics in the elderly, comparative efficacy data are available from some well-controlled studies in elderly insomniacs. In one placebo-controlled study, zolpidem 5 mg was equivalent to triazolam 0.125 mg and temazepam 15 mg (Leppik *et al.*, 1997). Zolpidem 5 mg is the preferred dose in the elderly (Roger *et al.*, 1993).

Zolpidem does not significantly affect sleep architecture in younger or older subjects (e.g., Blois *et al.*, 1993; Scharf *et al.*, 1991). Indeed, zolpidem tends to increase slow-wave sleep rather than diminish it. Tolerance to the effects of zolpidem was not detected in early studies (Langtry and Benfield, 1990). Later studies have tended to confirm this.

Because of concerns about long-term nightly administration of hypnotics, attempts have been made to prescribe zolpidem on an intermittent or 'as-needed basis'. Studies have shown efficacy for zolpidem in both regimens (Cluydts *et al.*, 1995).

Numerous studies have been conducted on the psychomotor and cognitive effects of zolpidem, both immediate and present the next day. Some impairments are usually detectable immediately following 10-mg doses, and they are definitely present, particularly with respect to memory at higher-than-recommended doses. As predictable from the short elimination half-life, deficits the next day tend to be minimal (Unden and Schechter, 1996). Clinical tolerability is good, as found in clinical trials and postmarketing studies (Allain and Monti, 1997). As with most of these agents interacting with the $GABA_A$ systems, the commonest adverse effects are nausea and dizziness, malaise, headache and nightmares. Reports of amnesic episodes, which have so bedevilled the use of triazolam, are rare with zolpidem.

Rebound discontinuation is uncommonly reported with zolpidem treatment (Soldatos *et al.*, 1999). Dependence and abuse are also quite rare (Lader, 1994), and probably less common than with benzodiazepines. Nonetheless, careful monitoring continues to be a wise procedure.

The recommended dosage in adults is 10 mg–5 mg in the elderly. At these doses, zolpidem is an effective inducer of sleep with little effect on sleep patterns. It is well tolerated with few residual effects. Rebound and withdrawal are not a problem. Intermittent and/or 'as-needed' administration seems feasible and widens the prescriber's choice of stratagems.

Zaleplon

Zaleplon has been recently licensed in several countries as a short-acting hypnotic. It has easily the shortest half-life of licensed hypnotics — only 1 h. This opens up new avenues for therapy, which are explored later in this chapter.

Chemically, zaleplon is quite complex; it is a pyrazolopyrimidine derivative. It has agonist activity at a subtype of the benzodiazepine receptor in the $GABA_A$–chloride-ionophore complex. This selectivity, as with zopiclone and zolpidem, may confer some clinical advantages (Hurst and Noble, 1999). It is rapidly absorbed after oral administration of the usual doses of 10 mg, with 5 mg in the elderly. Its bioavailability is about 30%. Peak plasma levels are achieved within 1 h (Greenblatt *et al.*, 1998), and the elimination half-life is about the same. Kinetics are linear within the usual dosage range (Beer *et al.*, 1994). The major metabolites, 5-oxo-zaleplon and 5-oxo-desethyl zaleplon, appear to be inactive. Pharmacokinetic parameters are only minimally altered in the elderly, but lower dosages are still recommended.

The efficacy of zaleplon was established by standardized questionnaire responses, backed up by polysomnographic data. Subjective sleep latency with 5, 10 and 20 mg of zaleplon was significantly lower than with placebo 1 week into a 4-week trial in 574 patients with insomnia (Elie *et al.*, 1998). This effect continued throughout the trial for the two high doses, but not for zolpidem 10 mg used as the active control. Similar data were obtained in another comparison of zaleplon, zolpidem, and placebo, with 20 mg of zaleplon being superior to 10 mg of zolpidem (Fry *et al.*, 1998). However, in general, zaleplon and zolpidem are equipotent with respect to effects on subjective sleep latency.

A polysomnographic comparison of zaleplon 5 or 10 mg, triazolam 0.25 mg, or placebo for 14 nights found the 10-mg, but not the 5-mg, dose to shorten sleep-onset latency (Walsh *et al.*, 1998). The effects of triazolam were significant for the first two nights only. Zaleplon leaves the sleep architecture unaffected.

A study in 422 elderly insomniac patients compared zaleplon 5 and 10 mg with placebo (Hedner *et al.*, 1998). Both doses significantly reduced subjective sleep latency during both the first and second weeks of treatment. Sleep quality was also improved.

Zaleplon 10 mg was associated with a small but significant reduction in time to return to sleep after a middle-of-the-night wakening (cited in Hurst and Noble, 1999). Flurazepam 30 mg did not show this effect but did prolong residual sleep duration.

In a phase 1 study in normal volunteers, zaleplon 10 mg and 20 mg was compared with 2 mg of lorazepam with respect to psychomotor and memory function (Allen *et al.*, 1993). The effects of zaleplon were ephemeral and also not very marked, compared with those of lorazepam.

A series of studies has examined next-day psychomotor, memory and driving ability in both normal volunteers and insomniac patients. In contrast to various benzodiazepines used as active controls, zaleplon caused no impairments in comparison to placebo (e.g., Walsh *et al.*, 1998; Ware *et al.*, 1998). Lack of residual effects occurs even when zaleplon is given 4 h prior to testing (Vermeeren *et al.*, 1998). This was in contrast to zopiclone 7.5 mg.

Zaleplon is well tolerated in general, adverse effects usually being no greater than following placebo. Headache is the commonest adverse effect, but this is a notoriously difficult complaint to assess. Subjective residual effects the next day are minimal or undetectable, even at 20-mg doses. Daytime anxiety is not increased (Elie *et al.*, 1998).

Discontinuation of zaleplon is not associated with any notable rebound or withdrawal effects. A study in subjects with histories of social drug use suggested that higher doses (25, 50 and 75 mg) significantly increased drug-liking ratings above those for placebo (Rush *et al.*, 1999). Triazolam 0.5 and 0.75 mg had similar effects.

In summary, the available published data shows that zaleplon shortens subjective sleep latency at doses of 10 mg (5 mg in the elderly). It does not alter sleep architecture. It is not associated with rebound or dependence, but abuse liability at high doses cannot be ruled out.

Because of its very brief duration of action, alternative therapeutic strategies can be adopted and are reviewed later.

IMPLICATIONS OF SUBTYPE-SELECTIVE BENZODIAZEPINE RECEPTOR LIGAND HYPNOTICS

Recent work on subtypes of benzodiazepine receptors has resulted in the discovery of numerous subtypes of receptor depending on a rather complex subunit composition (Griebel *et al.*, 2000). The commonest are designated $GABA_{A1a}$, $GABA_{A2a}$, $GABA_{A3a}$ and $GABA_{A5a}$. Benzodiazepines in general are non-selective agonists at all these receptors. Zopiclone has not yet been evaluated in detail for its selectivity but may bind somewhat atypically to a variety of subtypes.

Zolpidem and zaleplon, among the hypnotics, are selective for the $GABA_{A1a}$ subtype. A second consideration is the degree of agonism ('intrinsic efficacy') at the receptor. Zolpidem has high activity at the 1a subtype. When it does bind to the other subtypes, it does so with low efficacy. Zaleplon is also a full agonist at the 1a subtype but also has high intrinsic activity at the high concentrations needed for binding to the other subtypes.

What benefits might the selective binding confer? The cognitive effects of zolpidem and zaleplon appear to be less than for equivalent hypnotic doses of benzodiazepines. Some animal evidence supports this notion, with the acquisition of conditional fear being disrupted at high doses only (Sanger *et al.*, 1986).

Discriminative stimulus studies also suggest that selectivity on subtypes of receptors plays a part. Zolpidem and zaleplon only partly substitute for chlordiazepoxide as a discriminative cue, and only at high sedative doses (Sanger *et al.*, 1999). Tolerance to depressant effects in animals, such as impaired locomotion, is also minimal with the selective compounds as compared with non-selective benzodiazepines (Sanger and Zivkovic, 1992). Similarly, discontinuation effects are not detectable following withdrawal of zolpidem or zaleplon (e.g., Von Voigtlander and Lewis, 1991).

The animal data outlined above are consistent with clinical findings that zolpidem and zaleplon are associated with less psychomotor and cognitive impairment, less tolerance and fewer discontinuation effects than doses of benzodiazepines equipotent for hypnotic effects. The position of zopiclone is unclear. The implication is that compounds selected for development as an hypnotic (and as an anxiolytic) should display some selectivity at the 1a subtype. The consequences of selectivity at other benzodiazepine receptor subtypes remain unexplored.

COMPOUNDS USED AS HYPNOTICS EXPLOITING SECONDARY PROPERTIES

Lorazepam is licensed both as an anxiolytic and as an hypnotic. It is quite useful as a general tranquillizer and sedative, and is even advocated for use in psychotic agitation.

Diazepam is long-acting in view of its own duration of action and that of its very long-acting metabolite, *N*-desmethyldiazepam. However, it also has a marked redistribution phase, with sedative effects lasting a few hours. These can be exploited for use as an hypnotic where daytime anxiolysis is also required.

Barbiturates are still available in some countries but are restricted to use in insomniac patients long habituated to them. They should never be used ab initio.

Clomethiazole is a powerful sedative, which is sometimes used as an hypnotic, particularly in the elderly. However, it has most of the drawbacks of the barbiturates — paradoxical excitement, confusion, dependence, and marked interaction with alcohol.

Chloral and its derivatives are cheap, obsolescent hypnotics, with a dependence liability and a high incidence of gastrointestinal upset.

Antihistamines, such as diphenhydramine and promethazine, are on sale to the public for occasional insomnia. Their prolonged duration of action may cause residual effects the next day. Tolerance is often quite marked. Although dependence does not supervene, polydrug addicts use these drugs as adjuncts to opioids.

Other drugs can be dosed in such a way that their side effects of sedation and torpor can be used to induce sleep. The classic examples are the *tricyclic antidepressants*, trimipramine, amitriptyline and dothiepin (dosulepin) in particular being given at night to help patients sleep. This is quite appropriate when insomnia is secondary to depression.

Antipsychotic drugs are sometimes used in the same way but carry the risk of extrapyramidal syndromes such as tardive dyskinesia.

Melatonin has its advocates as a 'natural hypnotic'. It is the major hormone produced by the pineal gland and is mainly secreted during the hours of darkness (Brown, 1995). Its production falls off with age, so that the elderly often secrete very little. Some preliminary trials have shown encouraging results in the elderly, mainly with respect to quality of sleep. Various formulations of melatonin are being developed, as are synthetic analogues. Melatonin has also been used, often effectively, as a phase-shift agent in sleep disorders associated with jet lag, shift work, periodic sleep disorder in the blind and brain-damaged children. Further trials are required in all these indications, but, meanwhile, melatonin preparations of variable pharmaceutical purity are available in health-food shops and pharmacies in some countries.

HYPERSOMNIA

The commonest disorder under this rubric is narcolepsy. The treatment of narcolepsy can be divided into the management of the daytime sleepiness and that of the cataplexy. Stimulant drugs such as amphetamine and methylphenidate lessen the incidence of daytime drowsiness but are attended by the usual problem of tolerance, dependence, and rebound hypersomnia and depression on withdrawal. The minimal effective dosage must be sought assiduously; for example, methylphenidate 5–20 mg, three times a day. Part of the problem is the difficulty patients have in assessing their own difficulties, and a careful observer is invaluable in establishing the extent of any therapeutic effect. As tolerance develops, the stimulant can be withdrawn to allow a 'drug holiday' before reinstitution of the drug at a lower dose.

The treatment of cataplexy is more satisfactory. Antidepressants, both tricyclics and monoamine-oxidase inhibitors (MAOIs), suppress episodes of rapid-eye-movement sleep and are effective in lessening cataplectic attacks. Clomipramine seems to be currently favoured in the usual antidepressant dosage of 25–50 mg three times a day. The usual unwanted effects are sometimes troublesome. MAOIs have also been used but are less acceptable because of their dietary and drug interactions. They must *never* be combined with clomipramine. *Modafinil* has been recently licensed for the treatment of narcolepsy. The dose is 200–400 mg^{-1} per day, but lower in the elderly. It should be used cautiously in patients with liver impairment or hypertension. The main side effects are those of central nervous system stimulation, such as insomnia, euphoria, and anxiety.

PARASOMNIAS

These comprise a wide variety of behavioural disturbances occurring at various stages of sleep. Diazepam can be used to reduce slow-wave sleep in somnambulists and children with night terrors, and to control excessive nightmares. Otherwise, drug treatments are relatively ineffective.

CONCLUSIONS

A whole range of compounds is available for the treatment of sleep disorders, particularly insomnia of various types. However, the treatment of insomnia largely revolves around drugs that act on benzodiazepine receptors. Recent developments have produced hypnotics which are more selective than the older compounds such as the barbiturates and the widely used benzodiazepines. Whether this selectivity in biochemical terms is translated into clinical advantages, such as reduced impairment of cognitive and psychomotor function and lowered dependence potential, remains to be proved in practice.

The advent of very short-acting compounds, such as zolpidem and zaleplon, has allowed different strategies for the usage of these drugs. Thus, they can be given after the patient has gone to bed and found sleep elusive. In this way, patients recover control of their drug taking and can revert to 'as-required' medication instead of taking the medication 'prophylactically' every night on the presumption that insomnia will occur. The next step will be the use of these very short-acting compounds for middle-of-the-night wakening, when, say, a period of 4 h remains before the sufferer has to rise. Whether or not this changes prescribing practice noticeably will depend on such factors as the conservatism of the medical profession and the concern that patients have that they will have a full night's sleep.

Meanwhile, the use of hypnotics remains a controversial subject, and the development of new compounds and of new strategies to improve the benefit/risk ratio of these compounds remains an important issue.

REFERENCES

Agnoli, A., Manna, V. and Martucci, N., 1989. Double-blind study on the hypnotic and antianxiety effects of zopiclone compared with nitrazepam in the treatment of insomnia. *International Journal of Clinical Pharmacological Research*, **9**, 277–281.

Allain, H., Delahaye, C., Le Coz, F. *et al.*, 1991. Postmarketing surveillance of zopiclone in insomnia: analysis of 20,513 cases. *Sleep*, **14**, 408–413.

Allain, H. and Monti, J., 1997. General safety profile of zolpidem: safety in elderly, overdose and rebound effects. *European Psychiatry*, **12**(Suppl 1), 21s–29.

Allen, D., Curran, H.V. and Lader, M., 1993. The effects of single doses of CL284, 846, lorazepam, and placebo on psychomotor and memory function in normal male volunteers. *European Journal of Clinical Psychiatry*, **45**, 313–320.

Anderson, A.A., 1987. Zopiclone and nitrazepam: a multicentre placebo controlled comparative study of efficacy and tolerance in insomniac patients in general practice. *Sleep*, **10**(Suppl 1), 54–62.

Ankier, S.I. and Goa, K.L., 1988. Quazepam. A preliminary review of its pharmacodynamic and pharmacokinetic properties, and therapeutic efficacy in insomnia. *Drugs*, **35**, 42–62.

Asnis, G.M., Chakraburty, A., DuBoff, E.A. *et al.*, 1999. Zolpidem for persistent insomnia in SSRI-treated depressed patients. *Journal of Clinical Psychiatry*, **60**, 668–676.

Autret, E., Maillard, F. and Autret, A., 1987. Comparison of the clinical hypnotic effects of zopiclone and triazolam. *European Journal of Clinical Pharmacology*, **31**, 621–623.

Beer, B., Ieni, J.R., Wu, W.-H. *et al.*, 1994. A placebo-controlled evaluation of single, escalating doses of CL284, 846, a non-benzodiazepine hypnotic. *Journal of Clinical Pharmacology*, **34**, 335–344.

Bianchi, M. and Musch, B., 1990. Zopiclone discontinuation: a review of 25 studies assessing withdrawal and rebound phenomena. *International Clinical Psychopharmacology*, **5**(Suppl 2), 139–145.

Blois, R., Gaillard, J.-M., Attali, P. *et al.*, 1993. Effect of zolpidem on sleep in healthy subjects; a placebo-controlled trial with polysomnographic recordings. *Clinical Therapeutics*, **15**, 797–809.

Bootzin, R.R., Epstein, D. and Wood, J.M., 1991. Stimulus control instructions in case studies in insomnia. In: Hauri, P. (ed.), *Sleep*. Plenum, New York.

Bootzin, R.R. and Perlis, M.L., 1992. Nonpharmacologic treatments of insomnia. *Journal of Clinical Psychiatry*, **53**(Suppl 6), 37–41.

Boxenbaum, H.G., Postmanter, H.N. Macasieb, T. *et al.*, 1978. Pharmacokinetics of flunitrazepam following single- and multiple-dose administration to healthy human subjects. *Journal of Pharmacokinetics and Biopharmaceutics*, **6**, 283–293.

Breimer, D.D., Bracht, H. and de Boer, A.G., 1977. Plasma level profile of nitrazepam ('Mogadon') following oral administration. *British Journal of Clinical Pharmacology*, **4**, 709–711.

Broadhurst, A. and Cushnaghan, R.C., 1987. Residual effects of zopiclone (Imovane). *Sleep*, **10**(Suppl 1), 48–53.

Brown, G.M., 1995. Melatonin in psychiatric and sleep disorders. Therapeutic implications. *CNS Drugs*, **3**, 209–226.

Brun, J.P., 1988. Zopiclone, a cyclopyrrolone hypnotic: review of properties. *Pharmacology, Biochemistry and Behaviour*, **29**, 831–832.

Clark, B.G., Jue, S.G., Dawson, G.W. and Ward, A., 1986. Loprazolam: a preliminary review of its pharmacodynamic and pharmacokinetic properties and therapeutic efficacy in insomnia. *Drugs*, **31**, 500–516.

Cluydts, R., De Roeck, J., Cosyns, P. *et al.*, 1995. Antagonizing the effects of experimentally induced sleep disturbance in healthy volunteers by lormetazepam and zolpidem. *Journal of Clinical Psychopharmacology*, **15**, 132–137.

Dehlin, O., Rubin, B. and Rundgren, A., 1995. Double-blind comparisons of zopiclone and flunitrazepam in elderly insomniacs with special focus on residual effects. *Current Medical Research Opinion*, **13**, 317–324.

Dockhorn, R.J. and Dockhorn, D.W., 1996. Zolpidem in the treatment of short-term insomnia: a randomized, double-blind, placebo-controlled clinical trial. *Clinical Neuropharmacology*, **19**, 330–340.

Elie, R., Davignon, M. and Emilien, G., 1998. Zaleplon decreases sleep latency in outpatients without producing rebound insomnia after 4 weeks of treatment [Abstract No. 15]. *Journal of Sleep Research*, **7**(Suppl 2), 76.

Elie, R., Frenay, M., Le Morvan, P. *et al.*, 1990. Efficacy and safety of zopiclone and triazolam in the treatment of geriatric insomniacs. *International Clinical Psychopharmacology*, **5**(Suppl 2), 39–46.

Fleming, J.A., Bourgouin, J. and Hamilton, P., 1988. A sleep laboratory evaluation of the long-term efficacy of zopiclone. *Canadian Journal of Psychiatry*, **33**, 103–107.

Fleming, J. Moldofsky, H., Walsh, J.K. *et al.*, 1995. Comparison of the residual effects and efficacy of short term zolpidem, flurazepam and placebo in patients with chronic insomnia. *Clinical Drug Investigation*, **9**, 303–313.

Fraisse, J., Garrigou-Gadenne, D. and Thenot, J.P., 1996. Pharmacokinetic and metabolic profiles of zolpidem. In: Freeman, H., Puech, A.J. and Roth, T. (eds), *Zolpidem: An Update of its Pharmacological Properties*, pp. 45–57, Elsevier, Paris.

Fry, J., Scharf, M.B., Berkowitz, D.V. *et al.*, 1998. A phase III, 28 day, multicentre, randomized, double-blind comparator- and placebo-controlled, parallel-group safety, tolerability, and efficacy study of 5, 10, and 20 mg of zaleplon, compared with 10 mg of zolpidem or placebo, in adult outpatients with insomnia [Abstract No. 312.C], *Sleep*, **21**(Suppl), 262.

Gaillot, J., Le Roux, Y., Houghton, G.W. *et al.*, 1987. Critical factors for pharmacokinetics of zopiclone in the elderly and in patients with liver and renal insufficiency. *Sleep*, **10**(Suppl 1), 7–21.

Goa, K.L. and Heel, R.C., 1986. Zopiclone: a review of its pharmacodynamic and pharmacokinetic properties and therapeutic efficacy as an hypnotic. *Drugs*, **32**, 48–65.

Greenblatt, D.J., 1991. Benzodiazepine hypnotics: sorting the pharmacological facts. *Journal of Clinical Psychiatry*, **52**(Suppl 10), 4–10.

Greenblatt, D.J., Harmatz, J.S., von Moltke, L.L. *et al.*, 1998. Comparative kinetics and dynamics of zaleplon, zolpidem and placebo. *Clinical Pharmacological Therapeutics*, **64**, 553–561.

Griebel, G., Perrault, G. and Sanger, D.J., 2000. Subtype-selective benzodiazepine receptor ligands. In: Briley, M. and Nutt, D. (eds), *Anxiolytics*, pp. 77–94, Birkhauser Verlag, Basel.

Hajak, G., Clarenbach, P., Fischer, W. *et al.*, 1994. Zopiclone improves sleep quality and daytime well-being in insomniac patients: comparison with triazolam, flunitrazepam and placebo. *International Clinical Psychopharmacology*, **9**, 251–261.

Hedner, J., Emilien, G. and Salinas, E., 1998. Improvement in sleep latency and sleep quality with zaleplon in elderly patients with primary insomnia [Abstract No. 229]. *Journal of Sleep Research*, **7**(Suppl 2), 115.

Holm, K.J. and Goa, K.L., 2000. Zolpidem. An update of its pharmacology, therapeutic efficacy and tolerability in the treatment of insomnia. *Drugs*, **59**, 865–889.

Horne, J.A., 1981. The effects of exercise upon sleep: a critical review. *Biological Psychology*, **12**, 241–290.

Hurst, M. and Noble, S., 1999. Zaleplon. *CNS Drugs*, **11**, 387–392.

Kazamatsuri, H., Yamashsita, I., Sato, M. *et al.*, 1993. Clinical evaluation of zolpidem on insomnia of patients with schizophrenia and manic-depressive psychosis: double-blind trial in comparison with nitrazepam [in Japanese]. *Rinsho Lyaku*, **9**, 107–136.

Klimm, H.D., Dreyfus, J.F. and Delmotte, M., 1987. Zopiclone versus nitrazepam: a double-blind comparative study of efficacy and tolerance in elderly patients with chronic insomnia. *Sleep*, **10**(Suppl 1), 73–78.

Kudo, Y., Kawakita, Y., Saito, M. *et al.*, 1993. Clinical efficacy and safety of zolpidem on insomnia — a double-blind comparative study with zolpidem and nitrazepam [in Japanese]. *Rinsho Lyaku*, **9**, 79–105.

Lader, M., 1994. Benzodiazepines. A risk-benefit profile. *CNS Drugs*, **1**, 377–387.

Lader, M., 1998. Withdrawal reactions after stopping hypnotics in patients with insomnia. *CNS Drugs*, **10**, 425–440.

Lahmeyer, H., Wilcox, C.S., Kann, J. *et al.*, 1997. Subjective efficacy of zolpidem in outpatients with chronic insomnia: a double-blind comparison with placebo. *Clinical Drug Investigation*, **13**, 134–144.

Langtry, H.D. and Benfield, P., 1990. Zolpidem: a review of its pharmacodynamic and pharmacokinetic properties and therapeutic potential. *Drugs*, **40**, 291–313.

Leppik, I.E., Roth-Schechter, G.B., Gray, G.W. *et al.*, 1997. Double-blind, placebo-controlled comparison of zolpidem, triazolam, and temazepam in elderly patients with insomnia. *Drug Development Research*, **40**, 230–238.

Mamelak, M., Csima, A., Buck, L. and Price, V., 1989. A comparative study on the effects of brotizolam and flurazepam on sleep and performance in the elderly. *Journal of Clinical Psychopharmacology*, **9**, 260–267.

Miller, J., 1722. *Botanicum Officinale, or a Compendious Herbal*. Bell, Senex, Taylor & Osborne, London, p. 144.

Monti, J.M., Attali, P., Monti D. *et al.*, 1994. Zolpidem and rebound insomnia — a double-blind, controlled polysomnographic study in chronic insomniac patients. *Pharmacopsychiatry*, **27**, 166–175.

Morin, C.M., Culbert, J.P. and Schwartz, S.M., 1994. Nonpharmacological interventions for insomnia: a meta-analysis of treatment efficacy. *American Journal of Psychiatry*, **151**, 1172–1180.

Ngen, C.C. and Hassan, R., 1990. A double-blind placebo-controlled trial of zopiclone 7.5 mg and temazepam 20 mg in insomnia. *International Clinical Psychopharmacology*, **5**, 165–171.

Noble, S., Langtry, H.D. and Lamb, H.M., 1998. Zopiclone. An update of its pharmacology, clinical efficacy and tolerability in the treatment of insomnia. *Drugs*, **55**, 277–302.

Ohayon, M.M., Caulet, M., Priest, R.G. and Guilleminault, C., 1998. Psychotropic medication consumption patterns in the UK general population. *Journal of Clinical Epidemiology*, **51**, 273–283.

Parrino, L. and Terzano, M.G., 1996. Polysomnographic effects of hypnotic drugs: a review. *Psychopharmacology*, **126**, 1–16.

Pierce, D.M., Franklin, R.A., Harry, T.V.A. and Nicholson, A.N., 1984. Pharmacodynamic correlates of modified absorption: studies with lormetazepam. *British Journal of Clinical Pharmacology*, **18**, 31–35.

Ponciano, E., Freitas, F., Camara, J. *et al.*, 1990. A comparison of the efficacy, tolerance and residual effects of zopiclone, flurazepam and placebo in insomniac outpatients. *International Clinical Psychopharmacology*, **5**(Suppl 2), 69–77.

Ray, W.R., Fought, R.L. and Decker, M.D., 1992. Psychoactive drugs and the risk of injurious motor vehicle crashes in elderly drivers. *American Journal of Epidemiology*, **136**, 873–883.

Roger, M., Attali, P. and Coqueline, J.-P., 1993. Multicenter, double-blind, controlled comparison of zolpidem and triazolam in elderly patients with insomnia. *Clinical Therapeutics*, **15**, 127–136.

Rosenberg, J. and Ahlstrom, F., 1994. Randomized double blind trial of zolpidem 10 mg versus triazolam 0.25 mg for treatment of insomnia in general practice. *Scandinavian Journal of Primary Health Care*, **12**, 88–92.

Roth, T. and Roehrs, T.A., 1992. Issues in the use of benzodiazepine therapy. *Journal of Clinical Psychiatry*, **53**(Suppl), 14–18.

Rush, C.R., Frey, J.M. and Griffiths, R.R., 1999. Zaleplon and triazolam in humans: acute behavioral effects and abuse potential. *Psychopharmacology*, **145**, 39–51.

Sanger, D.J. and Depoortere, H., 1998. The pharmacology and mechanism of action of zolpidem. *CNS Drug Review,* **4**, 323–340.

Sanger, D.J., Griebel, G., Perrault, G., Claustre, Y. and Schoemaker, H., 1999. Discriminative stimulus effects of drugs acting at $GABA_A$ receptors: differential profiles and receptor selectivity. *Pharmacology, Biochemistry and Behaviour*, **64**, 269–273.

Sanger, D.J., Joly, D. and Zivkovic, B., 1986. Effects of zolpidem, a new imidazopyridine hypnotic, on the acquisition of conditioned fear in mice: Comparison with triazolam and CL218, 872. *Psychopharmacology*, **90**, 207–210.

Sanger, D.J. and Zivkovic, B., 1992. Differential development of tolerance to the depressant effects of benzodiazepine and non-benzodiazepine agonists at the ω (BZ) modulatory sites of $GABA_A$ receptors. *Neuropharmacology*, **31**, 693–700.

Scharf, M.B., Mayleben, D.W., Kaffeman, M. *et al.*, 1991. Dose response effects of zolpidem in normal geriatric subjects. *Journal of Clinical Psychiatry*, **52**, 77–83.

Scharf, M., Vogel, G. and Kaffeman, M. *et al.*, 1991. Dose-response of zolpidem in elderly patients with chronic insomnia [Abstract]. *Sleep Research*, **20**, 84.

Serra, M., Concas, A. and Biggio, G., 1996. Failure of long-term administration of zopiclone and zolpidem to induce tolerance in mice. *Neuroscience Research Communication*, **19**, 1678.

Shapiro, C.M., Sherman, D. and Peck, D.F., 1995. Withdrawal from benzodiazepines by initially switching to zopiclone. *European Psychiatry*, **10**(Suppl 3), 145–151.

Simon, G.E. and VonKorff, M., 1997. Prevalence, burden, and treatment of insomnia in primary care. *American Journal of Psychiatry*, **154**, 1417–1423.

Sloan, E.P. and Shapiro, C.M. (ed.), 1993. Impact and epidemiology of sleep disorders. *British Medical Journal*, **306**, 1604–1607.

Soldatos, C.R., Dikeos, D.J. and Whitehead, A., 1999. Tolerance and rebound insomnia with rapidly eliminated hypnotics: a meta-analysis of sleep laboratory studies. *International Clinical Psychopharmacology*, **14**, 287–303.

Spielman, A.J., Saskin, P. and Thorpy, M.J., 1987. Treatment of chronic insomnia by restriction of time in bed. *Sleep*, **10**, 45–56.

Stradling, J.R., 1993. Recreational drugs and sleep. *British Medical Journal*, **306**, 573–575.

Unden, M. and Schechter, B.R., 1996. Next day effects after night time treatment with zolpidem: a review. *European Psychiatry*, **11**(Suppl 1), 21–30.

Vermeeren, A., Danjou, P.E. and O'Hanlon, J.F., 1998. Residual effects of evening and middle-of-the-night administration of zaleplon 10 and 20 mg on memory and actual driving performance. *Human Psychopharmacology*, **13**(Suppl 2), 98–107.

Von Voigtlander, P.F. and Lewis, R.A., 1991. A rapid screening method for the assessment of benzodiazepine receptor-related physical dependence in mice. Evaluation of benzodiazepine-related agonists and partial agonists. *Journal of Pharmacology and Methodology*, **26**, 1–5.

Walsh, J.K., Fry, J., Erwin, C.W. *et al.*, 1998. Efficacy and tolerability of 14-day administration of zaleplon 5 mg and 10 mg for the treatment of primary insomnia. *Clinical Drug Investigation*, **16**, 347–354.

Walsh, J.K., Vogel, G.W., Scharf, M., Erman, M., Erwin, C.W., Schweitzer, P.K., Mangano, R.M. and Roth, T., 2000. A five week, polysomnographic assessment of zaleplon 10 mg for the treatment of primary insomnia. *Sleep Medicine*, **1**, 41–49.

Ware, J.C., Allen, R., Scharf, M.B. *et al.*, 1998. An evaluation of residual sedation following night time administration of 10 or 20 mg of zaleplon, 30 mg of flurazepam, or placebo in healthy subjects [Abstract No. 313]. *Sleep*, **21**, 263.

XXV

Psychobiology of Impulse-Control Disorders Not Otherwise Specified (NOS)

Stefano Pallanti, Nicoló Baldini Rossi, Jennifer Friedberg and Eric Hollander

Impulsivity can be defined as the failure to resist an impulse, drive or temptation that is harmful to oneself or others (Hollander *et al.*, in press). Impulsivity is a measurable aspect of behaviour, manifesting as impatience (including the inability to delay rewards), carelessness, risk-taking, sensation- and pleasure-seeking, an underestimated sense of harm, and extraversion. The subjective experience of an impulse involves also an increasing sense of arousal or tension before committing/engaging in the act and an experience of pleasure, gratification or release of tension at the time of committing the act. Aggressive behaviour is a conduct that inflicts harm upon oneself or others. Behaviour can be impulsive without being aggressive (for example, a person who engages in pathological gambling is behaving in an impulsive manner, but not in an aggressive manner). Likewise, aggressive behaviour can lack impulsivity (as in a premeditated murder). Impulsive disorders cause large costs to society, and are associated with substantial morbidity, mortality, social/family/job dysfunction, accidents, suicide, violence, aggression, criminality, and excessive utilization of health-care, government and financial resources (Hollander *et al.*, in press).

Largely on the basis of the varying theoretical and clinical approaches of the myriad scientific and professional disciplines studying impulsivity and aggressive behaviours in animal models or in humans, impulsivity and aggressiveness are conceptualized and diagnosed in an unusually broad and disparate fashion. Just as anxiety and depression may be conceptualized either as symptoms or as specific disorders, impulsivity may be distinguished as a symptom or as a distinct disorder.

In psychiatric classification, impulsivity is a core symptom of a broad spectrum of disorders, including the impulse-control disorders (impulse-control disorders not elsewhere classified, comprising pathological gambling [PG], intermittent explosive disorder, pyromania, kleptomania, and trichotillomania, and impulse-control disorder not otherwise specified [NOS]), the impulsive-aggressive personality disorders (borderline, antisocial), the neurological disorders that can be associated with disinhibition of behaviour (such as epilepsy), and substance abuse (Hollander and Rosen, 2000). Of interest, addictive behaviour could also be described as conduct resulting from failure to inhibit impulses that urge and seek tension relief or pleasure. Furthermore, other psychiatric conditions also contribute to the expression of impulsivity, notably attention deficit/hyperactivity disorder (ADHD), mania, and eating disorders (Hollander and Rosen, 2000). The impulse-control disorders may belong to a family of compulsive-impulsive spectrum disorders lying at opposite ends of the dimension of risk avoidance, with impulsive disorders driven by pleasure or arousal, and compulsive disorders driven by reduction of anxiety (Hollander, 1998). Both impulsive and compulsive disorders involve a failure to resist a drive to act in a way that is potentially self-damaging, escalation of anxiety before engaging in the act, and relief of anxiety following the act. In fact, one of the few differences between the two types of disorders is that most compulsive behaviour disorders are perceived by the patient as ego-dystonic, whereas impulsive behaviours are usually viewed as ego-syntonic, at least in the impulsive setting. Rather than being the dimensional opposite of obsessive-compulsive disorders, impulse-control disorders may represent a different phenomenological manifestation of a group of disorders sharing the feature of decreased ability to inhibit motor responses to affective states.

We are at a very early stage in our understanding of the neurobiology of impulsivity and aggression (Kavoussi *et al.*, 1997). Thus, it is noteworthy that meanings and definitions of impulsivity and aggressiveness differ greatly in psychiatry and in neurobiology. Moreover, no simple extrapolation of animal subtypes to humans is possible, mainly because of the influence of complex cultural variables on behaviour. On the whole, research into the subtypes of human impulsivity has been rather limited. Much of this has been conducted in children. Clinical observation, experimental paradigms in the laboratory, and cluster/factor analytical statistics have all been used in an attempt to subdivide impulsivity and aggression. A consistent dichotomy can be identified for aggression between an impulsive-reactive-hostile-affective subtype and a controlled-proactive-instrumental-predatory subtype. Although good internal consistency and partial descriptive validity have been shown, these constructs still need full external validation, especially regarding their predictive power for comorbidity, treatment response, and long-term prognosis (Vitiello and Stoff, 1997).

In attempting to find parallels between aggression in humans and aggression in animals, Gregg and Siegel (2001) observed that whereas both humans and animals exhibit aggressive behaviour, animals do not engage in the premeditated aggressive acts that humans often display. Vitiello *et al.*, (1990), in distinguishing between affective aggression and predatory aggression, emphasize that the first is impulsive, occurring as a result of autonomic arousal, while the second is cold-blooded and premeditated, and is not a result of arousal. Due to the presence of the frontal cortex, humans have the capacity to engage in both affective and predatory aggression, while animals engage only in affective aggression, which is aggression related to survival and increased arousal. Impulsivity has been classified in to three different types: motor impulsivity, impulsivity without programming, and attentive impulsivity; the last may be represented by an exaggerated alert reaction (Barratt and Stanford, 1995).

Biological Psychiatry: Edited by H. D'haenen, J.A. den Boer and P. Willner. ISBN 0-471-49198-5

NEUROLOGICAL STRUCTURES INVOLVED IN IMPULSIVITY

The neurobiological basis of impulsivity is not fully understood. Frontal lobe abnormalities are associated with an inability to delay or inhibit acting on impulse, and an inability to calculate the odds of negative risk or outcome. Aspects of impulsivity are core symptoms of a number of frontal lobe syndromes, and frontal lobe hypofunction has been observed in impulsive individuals. Studies in subjects with borderline personality disorder have confirmed a fundamental, biologically based, affective hyperresponsiveness in borderline personality disorder (BPD), whereas autonomic underarousal may seriously interfere with a flexible adaptation to environmental stimuli (Herpertz *et al.*, 1999). Damasio (1996) hypothesized that 'somatic states', or emotional changes that occur in response to a stimulus, influence the cognitive process that occurs when an individual decides how to respond to the stimulus. Damasio found that patients with ventromedial frontal damage do not respond to emotionally charged stimuli, thus indicating that the frontal cortex is involved in the decision.

Bechara *et al.* (2000b), investigating gambling, have suggested that gamblers with ventromedial prefrontal cortex lesions are insensitive to future consequences, positive or negative, and are primarily guided by immediate prospects. This 'myopia for the future' in ventromedial prefrontal cortex-lesioned patients persists in the face of severe adverse consequences, as in risking future punishment or declining future reward.

Patients with lesions of the ventromedial prefrontal cortex display decision-making impairment similar to that observed in abusers of cocaine, opiates, and alcohol (Rogers *et al.*, 1999). They also evidence a disregard for or insensitivity to future consequences that is related to, but not entirely explained by, the construct of impulsivity (Bechara *et al.*, 2000a). Metabolic abnormalities have been observed in the orbital frontal, adjacent ventral medial, and cingulate cortex of impulsive-aggressive individuals (Siever *et al.*, 1999). Previous research has implicated the anterior cingulate cortex (ACC) and medial prefrontal cortex (mPFC) in impulsivity and in processes regulating choice between alternative reinforcers, and their abnormal function has been observed in some individuals with ADHD (Ernst *et al.*, 1998). Decreased regional cerebral blood flow to the ACC and frontal cortex has been observed in pathological gambling (Goyer *et al.*, 1999). Lesions of the amygdala reveal a complex modulation of aggressive and impulsive behaviours.

Recent lesion studies in animals and humans have begun to elucidate the neurocircuitry of impulsivity. Cardinal *et al.* (2001) reported induction of persistent impulsive choice in rats following lesions of the nucleus accumbens core (AcbC), a key brain region of reward and reinforcement. These lesioned rats consistently chose small or poor rewards that were immediately available in preference to larger delayed rewards. The group also exhibited locomotor hyperactivity, another sign of the hyperactive-impulsive subtype of ADHD, and so this may represent an animal model of the disorder. In contrast to earlier studies, lesions of two of the AcbC's cortical afferents, the ACC and the mPFC, did not induce impulsive choice, suggesting that ventromedial or orbitofrontal afferents may play a role. This finding complements recent work in humans with bilateral ventromedial prefrontal cortical lesions who, in a gambling test, opt for choices that yield high immediate gains in spite of high future losses (Bechara *et al.*, 2000b). Lesions in the amygdala have also been associated with impaired decision-making (Bechara *et al.*, 1999). Thus, the orbitofrontal, nucleus accumbens and amygdala regions appear to play an important role in mediating at least one aspect of impulsivity. Lesion studies to improve the localization of the neurocircuitry of specific impulsive behaviours may be helpful, and Cardinal *et al.*'s tentative localization of the neuroanatomical basis for delayed reinforcement may eventually lead to new diagnostic imaging or therapeutic procedures. Pharmacological manipulation of neurotransmitter peptide systems specifically targeted at the AcbC and/or relevant afferent pathways may moderate impulsive behaviours more specifically than do current therapies. However, while previous lesion and imaging studies suggest a role for the ACC and mPFC in impulsivity (Ernst *et al.*, 1998; Goyer *et al.*, 1999), Cardinal *et al.*'s study suggests that neither the ACC nor the mPFC contribute to the AcbC's ability to promote the choice of delayed reinforcers. Therefore, the obvious next step is to elucidate the afferent paths by which information concerning the value of delayed reinforcers is supplied to the AcbC. It has been suggested that the basolateral amygdala and/or the orbitofrontal cortex may play such a role. Orbital lesions of the prefrontal cortex have elsewhere been associated with increases in reflexive emotional responses to environmental stimuli (Luria, 1980).

NEUROLOGICAL STRUCTURES INVOLVED IN AGGRESSION

There are many literature data linking specific brain structures to aggressive behaviour in mammals and non-human primates (Hess, 1957). It is commonly observed that patients with neurological lesions may present with symptoms of aggression (Weiger and Bear, 1988). Several investigators hypothesize that, for a subgroup of chronically aggressive persons, the root of the aggressive behaviour is brain damage. Lewis *et al.* (1982) reported that every death-row inmate studied by her team had a history of head injury, often inflicted by abusive parents. Her study concluded that death-row inmates constitute an especially neuropsychiatrically impaired prison population. Although the connection between physical abuse, head injury, and aggression is uncertain, many studies do show an association between physical abuse and later aggressive behaviour. Clinical reports of aggressive patients with specific neurological lesions may help delineate the structures that mediate these symptoms. In patients presenting with aggressive symptoms, researchers have demonstrated neurological 'soft signs', a marker of subtle neurological dysfunction (Shaffer *et al.*, 1985).

It has been shown that antisocial personality disorder patients that engage in aggressive behaviour without exhibiting autonomic arousal have a reduction in prefrontal grey matter and less autonomic activity than healthy controls, psychiatric controls, and patients with substance dependence when presented with a social stressor (Raine *et al.*, 2000). Larson and Summers have recently observed that social stress from aggressive interaction is expressed differently in specific brain regions of dominant and subordinate male lizards (Anolis carolinensis). Prior to aggressive behaviour, the outcome is predictable via the celerity of postorbital colouration: dominant males exhibit more rapid eyespot darkening. Serotoninergic activation is manifested rapidly (1 h) in the hippocampus, nucleus accumbens and brainstem of subordinate males, and is expressed more rapidly in dominant males. Amygdalar serotoninergic activation responds rapidly (1 h) in dominant males, but is expressed slowly (1 week) in chronically subordinate males (Larson and Summers, 2001); these data seem to suggest that aggressive behaviour may play a role in ranking the dominance status.

We should also consider that impulsive and aggressive behaviour corresponds to a wide range of adaptative patterns, such as the self-mutilation of trapped wolves or the cannibalism of the praying mantis, and the aggressive component of reproductive behaviour in certain mammals.

Hypothalamus

The hypothalamus monitors internal status and regulates neuroendocrine responses via sympathetic arousal. It is involved in the regulation of the sleep-wake cycle, appetite, body temperature, and sexual activity. In association with the pituitary, it is the major regulator of the autonomic nervous system. The mesolimbic dopamine (DA) pathway and the ascending serotonergic, noradrenergic, and cholinergic pathways from the brainstem have terminations in the hypothalamus.

The hypothalamus plays a major role in the expression of aggression in animals (Eichelman, 1971; Wasman and Flynn, 1962). Stimulation of the anterior hypothalamus causes predatory attacks in cats, whereas activation of the dorsomedial aspect produces aggression in which the animal ignores the presence of a rat and attacks the experimenter. Destruction of aggression-inhibitory areas, such as the ventromedial nucleus of the hypothalamus, produces permanently aggressive cats and rats (Bard, 1928; Reeves and Plum, 1969). Following cortical ablation, stimulation of the posterior lateral hypothalamus of the cat elicits sham-rage, a posture of preparation for attack. Stimulation of the posterior lateral portion of the hypothalamus shortens the latency of the attack, whereas stimulation of the medial ventral area prolongs it (Eichelman, 1971; Wasman and Flynn, 1962). Hamsters tested for offensive aggression after microinjections of arginine vasopressin (AVP) directly within the anterior hypothalamus in combination with a 5-HT_{1B} agonist have increased aggression, while those injected with AVP and a 5-hydroxytryptamine $(HT)_{1A}$ agonist have a dose-dependent inhibition of AVP-affiliated offensive aggression (Ferris *et al.*, 1999). In humans, structural lesions of the hypothalamus may be associated with unplanned and undirected aggressive behaviours that often appear to be unprovoked but may be in response to physical discomfort (Reeves and Plum, 1969; Killeffer and Stern, 1970; Haugh and Markesbery, 1983; Ovsiew and Yudofsky, 1983).

Recently, Gregg and Siegel (2001), using techniques of electrical brain stimulation, anatomical-immunohistochemical techniques and behavioural pharmacology, have investigated the neural systems and circuits underlying aggressive behaviour in the cat. The authors demonstrate that the medial hypothalamus and midbrain periaqueductal grey (PAG) are the most important structures mediating defensive rage behaviour, and that the fornical lateral hypothalamus clearly mediates predatory attack behaviour. The hippocampus, amygdala, bed nucleus of the stria terminalis, septal area, cingulate gyrus, and prefrontal cortex project to these structures directly or indirectly, and thus can modulate the intensity of attack and rage. Evidence suggests that several neurotransmitters facilitate defensive rage within the PAG and medial hypothalamus, including glutamate, substance P (SP), and cholecystokinin, and that opioid peptides suppress it; these effects usually depend on the subtype of receptor that is activated. A key recent discovery was a GABAergic projection that may underlie the often-observed reciprocally inhibitory relationship between these two forms of aggression. Recently, SP has come under scrutiny as a possible key neurotransmitter involved in defensive rage, and the mechanism by which it plays a role in aggression and rage is still under investigation (Gregg and Siegel, 2001). The possible hypothalamic role of SP in the intraspecific aggressive behaviour of isolated male mice was previously investigated by Bigi *et al.*, who evaluated the effects of a single intravenous administration of this neuropeptide on isolation-induced aggressive behaviour: SP treatment (0.25, 1.0, or 2.5 $mg\,kg^{-1}$ dose injected 15 min before testing) induced a decrease in offensive scores, a longer latency to the first attack episode and enhanced defensive displays. In no case did SP treatment affect locomotor activity levels or freezing behaviour (Bigi *et al.*, 1993).

The possible role of the hypothalamus in aggressiveness is also confirmed by Kim *et al.*, who examined the effects of intracerebroventricular injection of pertussis toxin, a specific inhibitor of G(i)/G(o) proteins, on plasma corticosterone levels, aggressiveness, and hypothalamic and hippocampal monoamines and their metabolite levels in mice. Plasma corticosterone levels were markedly increased after injection of pertussis toxin, which induced a progressive increase in aggressiveness, that is, a decrease in attack latency and an increase in number of attacks, on days 1 and 6 after injection. Brain monoamines and their metabolite levels changed on days 1 and 6 after toxin injection: in the hypothalamus, the levels of dopamine and 3,4-dyhydroxyphenylacetic acid were increased, the norepinephrine level was decreased, and the 5-hydroxyindole acetic acid (5-HIAA) level was markedly increased, with no changes in 5-HT level, whereas, in the hippocampus, the 5-HT level was significantly decreased, with no changes in 5-HIAA and catecholamines (Kim *et al.*, 2000).

According to Kim *et al.*, Van Goozen *et al.* have underlined the possible relationship between adrenal androgens and aggressive behaviour occurring in children with oppositional defiant disorder (ODD), showing that children with ODD had higher dehydroepiandrosterone sulphate (DHEAS) levels than either psychiatric control or normal control groups, and hypothesizing that the mechanism should be a shift in balance of ACTH-beta-endorphin functioning in the hypothalamic-pituitary-adrenal axis due to early stress or genetic factors (Van Goozen *et al.*, 2000).

Finally, it has been documented that maternal and mating-induced aggression is associated with elevated citrulline immunoreactivity in the hypothalamic paraventricular nucleus (PVN) in prairie voles. In the monogamous prairie vole, *Microtus ochrogaster*, the males are parental and exhibit a dramatic increase in aggression, termed mating-induced aggression, in association with reproduction. In mice, the gas, nitric oxide (NO), inhibits the males' aggression, but may have an excitatory role in the production of maternal aggression. Gammie and Nelson have combined aggressive behavioural testing of female and male prairie voles with immunohistochemistry for citrulline, a marker of NO synthesis, to examine NO synthesis indirectly during maternal and mating-induced aggression. A significant increase in the number of citrulline-positive cells was identified in the PVN of the hypothalamus in aggressive lactating females compared with unstimulated lactating females. A significant increase in the number of citrulline-positive cells was also observed in the PVN of aggressive mated males compared with nonaggressive unmated males and unstimulated mated males. In other regions of the brain, no changes in the number of citrulline-positive cells were observed. These data suggest that NO is released specifically in the PVN during both maternal and mating-induced aggression in prairie voles (Gammie and Nelson, 2000). Moreover, the intraperitoneal injections of the neuronal NO synthase (nNOS) inhibitor, 3-bromo-7-nitroindazole, significantly impaired the expression of maternal aggression in terms of the average time in aggressive encounters, the average number of attacks and the average latency to the attack first. These data suggest that the central release of NO may play an important role in the production of maternal aggression in prairie voles (Gammie *et al.*, 2000).

Amygdala

The amygdala consists of an anatomically defined region located within the temporal lobe of the brain in mammals. Along with other limbic system structures, the amygdala responds to changing environmental conditions by inducing emotive behaviours that are linked to past experiences. The amygdala is an important component of the limbic system and, as such, is considered a pivotal region for mediating the perception and the expression of fear and anxiety. The limbic system encompasses the amygdala and the temporal cortex. The amygdala activates and/or suppresses the hypothalamus and modulates input from the neocortex. It also has efferents to the extrapyramidal system. The amygdala may have a role in associating sensory experience with (hypothalamically directed) affects and behaviours, including anger (Bear, 1991). In a study using positron-emission tomography, the amygdala was shown to be more activated during the processing of visually presented linguistic threats than during the processing of neutral words (Isenberg *et al.*, 1999).

Bilateral lesions of the amygdala tame a variety of hostile and vicious animals (Kluver and Bucy, 1939), whereas irritative lesions or electrical stimulation can lead to rage outbursts. Removal of the amygdala from monkeys results in decreased aggression (Downer, 1961). However, amygdalectomy in submissive monkeys may result in increased aggression (Dicks *et al.*, 1969). Aggressive behaviour following stimulation of the amygdala in cats varies accordingly to their pre-existing temperament (Adamac 1990). These findings suggest that the amygdala may not simply function to increase regulatory affects and behaviours, but that it may mediate and balance their control. Moreover, it seems that there is an association between intermale social aggression and cellular density within the central amygdaloid nucleus in rats with lithium/pilocarpine-induced seizures, suggesting that seizure-induced damage within proximal amygdaloid nuclei disinhibits the central nucleus and encourages aggression (Desjardin and Persinger, 1995).

Recently, it has been shown that the monoaminergic activities of limbic regions are elevated during aggression in the lizard *Anolis carolinensis* (Korzan *et al.*, 2000). In monkeys, bilateral temporal lobectomy leads to hyperorality, hypersexuality, absence of fear response, increased touching, and visual agnosia (Kluver-Bucy syndrome). Bilateral temporal lobe damage in humans leads to similar symptoms, including hypersexuality and visual and auditory agnosia. In addition, humans exhibit placidity, apathy, bulimia, and aphasia (Terzian and Ore, 1955; Marlowe *et al.*, 1975; Isern, 1987). This syndrome appears to be a disconnection between sensory information about the environment and the regulation of affects and behaviours (e.g., aggression, sex, food) that usually help the person or animal negotiate that environment.

It has been known since the classical work of Kluver and Bucy (1939) that amygdaloid lesions markedly reduce emotional responsiveness. More localized amygdaloid lesion studies indicate that a specific part of the amygdala, the central nucleus, is important for mediation of autonomic changes associated with stress. Bilateral ablation of the central amygdaloid nucleus attenuates learned heart-rate responses in the rabbit (Kapp *et al.*, 1985). Cryogenic treatment of the central amygdaloid nucleus blocked learned blood pressure and respiratory response in the cat (Zhang *et al.*, 1986). In rats, lesions of the central amygdala impede the increases in heart rate and blood pressure that occur to a tone associated with shock (Iwata *et al.*, 1986). The increases in heart rate and blood pressure to the shock alone were unaffected by amygdaloid lesions. Destruction of the central amygdala in rats also reduced stimulus-induced exaggerated increases in cardiovascular responses (Folkow *et al.*, 1982).

Seizure studies of the limbic area in humans may explain the possible neuroanatomical underpinnings of aggression. Whereas bilateral temporal lobe damage in humans may lead to Kluver-Bucy syndrome, with a decrease in regulatory affects and behaviours, disorders of temporal lobe excitation may result in increased affect and aggression (Serafetinides, 1965; Nachson, 1988). Associations between aggression and temporal lobe epilepsy has been reported: 30% of 286 patients with intermittent violent outbursts had temporal lobe epilepsy (TLE) (Elliot, 1992); 18 of 97 incarcerated delinquent boys with a history of violence presented psychomotor epilepsy (Lewis *et al.*, 1982). TLE patients may demonstrate hyperemotionality and increased aggression. Interictal aggression is much more common than ictal or postictal aggression in TLE. Interictal aggression is often characterized by intense affect in response to environmental stimuli, whereas ictal and postictal aggression is spontaneous and unfocused. In humans, reports of surgical intervention for the relief of mental or structural brain disease or epilepsy have shown that both the amygdala and other temporal lobe and limbic system structures contribute to modulation of aggression. Two patients who underwent bilateral amygdalotomy for intractable aggression showed a reduction in autonomic arousal in response to stressful stimuli and a decrease in aggressive outbursts (Lee and Coccaro, 2001). Limbic system tumours, infections, and blood vessel abnormalities have also been associated with violence and impulsivity. Although it is clear that various limbic system structures have an inhibitory or excitatory effect on aggression, the precise mechanism of the aggression pathway is still far from established.

It has been hypothesized that the amygdala probably does not function in normal homeostatic functions, as it is not active during sleep or anaesthetic states. In addition, the amygdala is not necessary for mediation of cardiovascular response to physical stressors. Rather, the amygdala probably functions to alter autonomic activity during responses to threatening or anxiety-provoking stimuli. Finally, a high density of benzodiazepine receptors has been localized within the amygdala, suggesting that it is an important site for anxiolytic drug actions (Niehoff and Kuhar, 1983). The benzodiazepine receptors are localized within the basolateral amygdaloid nucleus, an important intra-amygdaloid input to the central amygdaloid nucleus.

Prefrontal Cortex

The prefrontal cortex modulates limbic and hypothalamic activity, and is associated with the social and judgement aspects of aggression. The frontal cortex coordinates the timing of social cues, often before the expression of associated emotions. Lesions in this area give rise after minimal provocation to disinhibited anger characterized by an individual's showing little regard for the consequences of affect and behaviour. Weiger and Bear (1988) hypothesize that, whereas TLE patients may express deep remorse over an aggressive act, patients with prefrontal lesions often indicate indifference. Patients with violent behaviour have been found to have a high frequency of frontal lobe lesions (Kandel and Freed, 1989; Lishman, 1968). In a study of Vietnam veterans with a history of penetrating head injuries, patients with ventromedial lesions had higher verbal aggression scores than controls and those with lesions in other brain areas (Grafman *et al.*, 1996). Frontal lesions may result in the sudden discharge of limbic- and/or amygdala-generated affects no longer modulated, processed, or inhibited by the frontal lobe. Patients consequently respond with rage or aggression upon feelings that would have ordinarily been modulated by the individual. Prefrontal damage may cause aggression by a secondary process involving lack of inhibition of the limbic area. Dorsal lesions of the prefrontal cortex are associated with impairment in long-term planning and increased apathy. Orbital lesions of the prefrontal cortex are associated with increases in reflexive emotional responses to environmental stimuli (Luria, 1980).

Recently, neuroimaging studies suggest a role for the prefrontal cortex, along with other regions of the brain, in the expression of aggression, as shown by Lee and Coccaro (2001). Using positron-emission tomography, studies have documented reduced serotonergic function in specific brain regions in subjects with increased aggression and impulsivity. One imaging study showed that in contrast to controls, patients with borderline personality disorder have diminished response to serotonergic stimulation (*d*,1-fenfluramine) in areas of the prefrontal cortex associated with impulsive behaviour regulation, specifically the medial and orbital regions of the right prefrontal cortex, left middle and superior temporal gyri, left parietal lobe and left caudate body (Soloff *et al.*, 2000). Siever *et al.* (1999) found that impulsive-aggressive patients had significantly blunted metabolic responses in the orbital frontal, adjacent ventral medial and cingulate cortex compared to controls. Finally, impulsive murderers have been shown to have lower left and right prefrontal functioning and higher right subcortical functioning in comparison to predatory murderers (Raine *et al.*, 1998). Van Erp and Miczek (2000) investigated the dynamic changes in DA and serotonin during aggressive confrontations in the corticolimbic areas of rats: DA and serotonin levels in the prefrontal cortex changed in opposite directions, with a sustained decrease of serotonin to 80% of baseline levels during and after the confrontation and an increase of DA by up to 120% after the confrontation. The temporal pattern of monoamine changes, which followed rather than preceded the confrontation, points to a significant role of accumbal and cortical DA and 5-HT in the consequences as opposed to the triggering of aggressive acts. The increase in accumbal DA in aggressive animals supports the hypothesis that this neural system is linked to the execution of biologically salient and demanding behaviour.

Other areas implicated in impulsivity and aggression include the midline thalamus, lateral preoptic region, mammillary bodies, hippocampus and basal ganglia.

PSYCHOBIOLOGY

Transmitter Systems

Several recent studies in genetics, neuropsychopharmacology and neuroimaging have helped to clarify the biological contributions to impulsivity and aggression in humans and animals. Various neurotransmitter systems modulate impulsive disorders. Evidence of serotonergic dysregulation and a presynaptic deficit of available 5-HT has been observed in humans with a variety of impulsive disorders, as well as animal models of impulsivity and aggression. Knockout mice lacking 5-HT_{1B} receptors display increased impulsive aggression, cocaine self-administration and alcohol consumption (Brunner and Hen, 1997), and polymorphisms of tryptophan hydroxylase (the rate-limiting enzyme for 5-HT synthesis) have been associated with impulsive-aggressive behaviours (New *et al.*, 1998). Specific impulse-control disorders, such as pathological gambling, probably involve abnormalities of DA receptors and reward pathways, as well as noradrenergic and serotonergic dysfunction (Hollander *et al.*, 2000). DA function, particularly within the mesocorticolimbic pathways, is critical in the mediation of reward and reinforcement behaviours (reviewed in Hollander *et al.*, 2000). Association studies of genes related to DA receptors have supported a genetic influence in impulsive behaviours (reviewed in Hollander *et al.*, 2000), and μ-opioid receptors are involved in the regulation of these pathways. Peptides such as vasopressin have also been implicated in aggressive behaviours. A better understanding of the role of neurotransmitters in modulating relevant neurocircuitry (i.e., the ventromedial cortex and nucleus accumbens) is needed to develop specific treatments for pathological impulsivity across various conditions.

Various approaches involving pharmacological manipulation of neurotransmitters have been undertaken in an attempt to ameliorate pathological impulsivity in several psychiatric disorders. Much research to date has focused on modulation of 5-HT transmission. Selective serotonin reuptake inhibitors (SSRIs) and other enhancers of serotonergic transmission have reduced impulsive behaviours in a wide range of different disorders, including pathological gambling, borderline personality disorder (BPD), sexual addictions and obsessive-compulsive spectrum disorders (Hollander *et al.*, 1998, Hollander and Rosen, 2000). While serotonin dysregulation and hypofunction appear to play a central role in these disorders, it is likely that impulsivity is influenced to differing degrees by the highly interconnected 5-HT, noradrenergic, dopaminergic, opiate and GABAergic systems. Nevertheless, the neuronal mechanisms producing behaviour are complex and irreconcilable with simplistic constructs, and it is impossible to manipulate one neurotransmitter system to the exclusion of surrounding neurons.

Serotonin Function

Animal and human research suggests that the central serotonin system is involved in the inhibition of impulsive behaviour, and reduced levels of cerebrospinal fluid (CSF) 5-HIAA seem to be associated with impulsive aggression.

A decrease in brain 5-HT has been found in the brainstems of muricidal rats (aggressive rats that spontaneously kill mice introduced into their cages) and other animals made aggressive by isolation. The administration of tryptophan, a 5-HT precursor, reduces or abolishes the violence (Depue and Spoont, 1987).

In primate studies, researchers have noted higher blood 5-HT and 5-HIAA CSF concentration in monkeys who tend to be dominant and high-ranking in their colonies (Higley *et al.*, 1992), and lower 5-HIAA CSF concentration as an antecedent to greater alcohol consumption (Higley *et al.*, 1996). Social stress from aggressive interaction is expressed differently in specific brain regions of dominant and subordinate male *A. carolinensis* lizards. Prior to aggressive behaviour, the outcome is predictable via the celerity of postorbital colouration: dominant males exhibit more rapid eyespot darkening. Serotoninergic activation is manifest rapidly (1 h) in the hippocampus, nucleus accumbens and brainstem of subordinate males, and is expressed more rapidly in dominant males. Amygdalar serotoninergic activation responds rapidly (1 h) in dominant males, but is expressed slowly (1 week) in chronically in subordinate males (Larson and Summers, 2001).

Mice deficient in monoamine oxidase A (MAO-A) have increased brain levels of serotonin and norepinephrine, and they show enhanced aggression (Shih *et al.*, 2000). Pruus *et al.* (2000) demonstrated that the 5-HT_{1A} receptors may be involved in the mediation of the apomorphine-induced aggressive behaviour in adult male Wistar rats; nevertheless, the prominent antiaggressive effect of the 5-HT_{1A} receptor agonist buspirone seems to be mediated by some other mechanisms, evidently via the DA D_2 receptors.

Fairbanks *et al.* (2001) provided evidence for serotonergic influences on social impulsivity in vervet monkeys. Svensson *et al.* (2000) have demonstrated that gonadectomy reduced disinhibitory behaviour in 5-HT-depleted rats, and that gamma-amino-butyric acid (A)/benzodiazepine receptor complexes ($GABA_A$/BDZ-RC) may be involved in this effect.

Studies of genetically engineered mice with targeted disruption of the neuronal nitric oxide synthase (nNOS) gene have established the inhibitory role of nitric oxide (NO) in male impulsive-aggressive behaviour. The molecular mechanism accounting for the aggressive behaviour caused by the lack of neuronally derived NO is not known; the excessive aggressiveness and impulsiveness of nNOS knockout mice is caused by selective decrements in serotonin turnover and deficient receptor function in the brain regions regulating emotion, indicating — as already mentioned — an important role for NO in normal brain 5-HT function (Chiavegatto *et al.*, 2001).

For dogs with dominance aggression, the addition of tryptophan to high-protein diets or change to a low-protein diet may reduce aggression; for dogs with territorial aggression, triptophan supplementation of a low-protein diet may be helpful in reducing aggression (De Napoli *et al.*, 2000).

Thus, there is significant evidence for the role of serotonergic (5-HT) dysregulation or dysfunction in impulsive aggression in both animals and humans (Asberg *et al.*, 1976; Brown *et al.*, 1979, 1982; Sabrie, 1986). In an attempt to dissect the contribution of individual 5-HT receptor subtypes to behaviour, Ramboz *et al.* (1996) have generated mutant mice lacking the 5-HT_{1B} receptor. These mice did not exhibit any obvious developmental or behavioural defect; however, the hyperlocomotor effect of the $5\text{-HT}_{1A/1B}$ agonist, RU24969, was completely absent in mutant mice, indicating that this effect is mediated by 5-HT_{1B} receptors; moreover, when confronted with an intruder, isolated mutant mice attacked the intruder faster and more intensely than wild-type mice, suggesting an involvement of 5-HT_{1B} receptors in the modulation of aggressive behaviour. These data might be related to the fact that a class of 5-HT_1 agonists, termed serenics, have antiaggressive properties, and to the findings that certain impulsive-aggressive behaviours are associated with deficits in central serotonin (Saudou *et al.*, 1994; Ramboz *et al.*, 1996). Furthermore, Brunner and Hen (1997), using a knockout mouse that lacks 5-HT_{1B} receptors, observed that this animal shows more impulsive aggression, acquires cocaine self-administration faster, and drinks more alcohol than the corresponding wild-type control; for Brunner and Hen, these impulsive characteristics are not due to a change in cognitive functions, since in a cognitive task involving a choice between a small immediate reward and a larger, more delayed reward, knockout mice showed intact choice and timing capabilities and good discrimination of reward amounts.

Scearce-Levie *et al.* (1999) have evaluated the behavioural effects of 3,4-methylenedioxymethamphetamine (MDMA), a psychoactive drug of abuse, which in rats stimulates locomotion while decreasing exploratory behaviour, on knockout mice lacking the 5-HT_{1B} receptor: these animals show a reduced locomotor response to MDMA, although delayed locomotor effects of MDMA are present in these animals. These findings indicate that the locomotor effects of MDMA are dependent upon the 5-HT_{1B} receptor, at least in part. In contrast, MDMA eliminates exploratory behaviour in both normal and knockout mice, suggesting that the exploratory suppression induced by MDMA occurs through mechanisms other than activation of the 5-HT_{1B} receptor.

Moreover, according to Ramboz, the 5-HT_{1A} receptors should be involved in the modulation of exploratory and fear-related behaviours, suggesting that reductions in 5-HT_{1A} receptor density due to a genetic defect or environmental stressors might result in heightened anxiety (Ramboz *et al.*, 1998). These results seem to be confirmed by other authors who observed that 5-HT_{1B} knockout mice are more aggressive, more reactive and less anxious than the wild types, whereas the 5-HT_{1A} knockouts are less reactive, more anxious, and possibly less aggressive than the wild types (Zhuang *et al.*, 1999).

Animal studies suggest that 5-HT_1-receptor stimulation results in a decrease in aggressive behaviour, whereas, in humans, aggressive, personality-disordered patients show a blunted prolactin response to the 5-HT_{1A} agonist buspirone. Antagonism of the 5-HT_2 receptors appears to decrease aggression, and this effect may explain the ability of newer antipsychotics agents (which, unlike older antipsychotic medications, block 5-HT_2 receptors) to produce a dramatic reduction in aggression and agitation independent of the effects on psychotic symptoms (Kavoussi *et al.*, 1997).

In humans, Asberg *et al.* (1976) initially noted an inverse relationship between violent/lethal suicidal behaviour and the 5-HT metabolite 5-HIAA CSF concentration in depressed patients. Subsequent studies on populations in eight different countries confirmed that suicidal depressed patients have lower 5-HIAA CSF than non-suicidal depressed patients. For example, Lidberg *et al.* (2000) found that homicide offenders with a history of suicide attempts had a lower concentration of spinal fluid 5-HIAA than the remaining murderers. This correlation is particularly strong in those with violent suicide attempts. Low concentration of CSF 5-HIAA has also been shown to be related to aggressive behaviour independent of suicidal behaviour in patients with Axis I disorders (Stanley *et al.*, 2000). In addition, Brown *et al.* (1982) demonstrated a decrease in 5-HIAA CSF in patients with personality disorders and found that this decrease correlated with scores on a lifetime aggression scale. Many studies have confirmed an inverse relationship between 5-HIAA CSF level and impulsive and violent behaviours (Bioulac, 1980; Brown *et al.*, 1982; Linnoila *et al.*, 1983; Lidberg *et al.*, 1984). The individual cases and small study populations studied include psychopathic military personnel, arsonists, murderers, violent suicidal patients, and behaviourally disruptive children and adolescents. Linnoila *et al.* (1983) have reported reduced CSF 5-HIAA concentration in both impulsive violent offenders and impulsive arsonists compared with premeditated violent offenders, suggesting that it is specifically nonpremeditated ('impulsive') aggression that correlates with reduced central 5-HT function in these individuals.

Investigators have also correlated abnormal 5-HT platelet studies with impulsivity and aggression (Biegon *et al.*, 1990; Marazziti and Conti, 1991). Decreased numbers of platelet 5-HT transporter sites are found in aggressive conduct-disordered subjects and in 'aggressive' institutionalized psychiatric subjects (Stoff *et al.*, 1991). In addition, an inverse correlation between platelet 5-HT uptake and the Barratt 'impulsivity' score has been reported in aggressive adult males (Brown *et al.*, 1989). In children and adolescents with conduct disorder, there is a negative correlation between platelet imipramine binding and impulsive aggression (Stoff *et al.*, 1987). In individuals with personality disorders, platelet titrated paroxetine binding has been shown to be inversely correlated with the Life History of Aggression total score and aggression score, and with the Buss-Durkee Hostility Inventory Assault score (Coccaro *et al.*, 1996).

Researchers have noted consistently reduced imipramine binding (Brown *et al.*, 1989) and increased platelet 5-HT_2 binding in suicide victims (Biegon *et al.*, 1990). The reduced imipramine binding may reflect decreased 5-HT release. Increased 5-HT_2 binding may reflect the brain's compensatory response to a decrease in functional serotonergic neurons, with consequent upregulation of postsynaptic 5-HT_2 binding sites. Additional findings that suggest the role of 5-HT in impulsivity and aggression include reports of low serum ratios of tryptophan to other neutral amino acids in alcoholics arrested for assaultive behaviour compared with other alcoholics or nonalcoholic control subjects (Lewis, 1991). Type 2 alcoholism is associated with both violent behaviour and serotonergic deficit (LeMarquand *et al.*, 1994, Virkkunen and Linnoila, 1990). Individuals with a family history of alcoholism may be more sensitive to impulsivity in response to low serotonin levels, as tryptophan-depleted individuals with a family history of alcoholism made more errors in a modified Taylor task than did those with no family history of alcoholism (LeMarquand *et al.*, 1999).

Biver has studied gender differences in the living human brain 5-HT_2 receptor, using positron-emission tomography and a selective radiotracer: he found significantly higher 5-HT_2 receptor-binding capacity in men than in women, especially in the frontal and cingulate cortices; this finding suggests that distinct liability for men and women to suffer from some psychiatric disorders responding to serotonergic agents may be related to differences in brain serotonin receptors (Biver *et al.*, 1996).

Other Neurotransmitter Systems

Neurotransmitters other than serotonin probably influence aggressive and impulsive behaviour; for example, GABA, norepinephrine and DA (Oquendo and Mann, 2000). An alpha-amino-3-hydoxy-5-methylisoxadole-4-propionate (AMPA) receptor antagonist, NBQX, was found to increase impulsivity in rats which was restored by injection of a positive allosteric modulator of AMPA receptors, indicating that the AMPA receptor, a type of glutamate receptor, is involved in the regulation of impulsivity (Nakamura *et al.*, 2000). Some studies demonstrate that increasing norepinephrine levels correlate with impulsive aggression, whereas other studies demonstrate an opposite relationship; thus, the role of norepinephrine in impulsive-aggressive behaviour is still unclear (Oquendo and Mann, 2000).

It has been shown that brain GABA levels are involved in intermale aggression in mice, and that mice selected for differences in sensitivity to a benzodiazepine receptor inverse agonist vary in intermale aggression (Guillot *et al.*, 1999). Moreover, the acute $GABA_A$ receptor agonist THIP and the $GABA_B$ receptor agonist baclofen attenuate the apomorphine-induced aggressive behaviour, indicating the involvement of both $GABA_A$ and $GABA_B$ receptor subtypes in the neurobiology of apomorphine-induced aggressiveness, as this phenomenon is evidently subject to the general inhibitory effect of GABAergic neurotransmission (Rudissar *et al.*, 2000). The involvement of GABA as a possible neurotransmitter of aggressive behaviour is indirectly confirmed by the effect of alcohol: in fact, the aggressive behaviour of certain individual animals can be greatly increased when they are under the influence of low doses of alcohol. One of alcohol's neurochemical actions that may be relevant to alcohol-heightened aggression is its positive modulation of the $GABA_A$ receptor complex. Alcohol prolongs 'bursts' of aggressive acts, and displays and disrupts communication between the aggressive animal and the opponent who defends itself, submits or flees. Pharmacological modulation of the $GABA_A$ receptor with benzodiazepines and neuroactive steroids (allopregnanolone) results in dose-dependent biphasic changes in aggressive behaviour that mimic the dose-effect function of alcohol; benzodiazepines potentiate the aggression-heightening effects of alcohol as well as the behaviourally suppressive effects, and antagonists of benzodiazepine receptors prevent the aggression-heightening effects of alcohol (Miczek *et al.*, 1997). Although alcohol induces aggressive behaviour in mice, it has a suppressive effect upon predatory attack behaviour in the cat. Han's studies support the hypothesis that ethanol's suppressive effects in the cat are mediated, at least in part, by $GABA_A$ receptors in the lateral hypothalamus (Han *et al.*, 1997). Moreover, activation of the mesolimbic DA pathway appears to promote drug- and alcohol-seeking behaviour in laboratory animals (Hill *et al.*, 1999).

The possible role of DA in aggressiveness is suggested by the fact that the blockade of the D_1/D_2 DA receptor produces an antiaggressive action commonly associated with an impairment of other motor behaviours, and the D_3 receptor seems to present opposite actions to D_1 and D_2, since the blockade of this receptor produces a stimulation of motor activity, which has been associated with an increase in DA neurotransmission (Rodriguez-Arias *et al.*, 1999).

Several reports suggest that when there is a dysfunction in a person's brain reward cascade — a dysfunction which could be caused by certain genetic variants, especially in the DA system — leading to a hypodopaminergic trait, that person requires a DA fix to feel good. This trait leads to multiple drug-seeking behaviour. This is so because alcohol, cocaine, heroin, marijuana, nicotine and glucose all cause an activation and neuronal release of brain DA, which may satisfy the abnormal cravings. It seems certain that carriers of the DAD_2 receptor A1 allele have compromised D_2 receptors. Therefore, the lack of D_2 receptors causes individuals to have a high risk of multiple addictive, impulsive and compulsive behavioural propensities, such as severe alcoholism; cocaine, heroin, marijuana, and nicotine addiction; glucose bingeing; pathological gambling; sex addiction; ADHD; Tourette's syndrome; autism; chronic violence; conduct disorder; and antisocial behaviour (Blum *et al.*, 2000).

Shih *et al.* (2000) have observed that mice deficient in MAO-A have increased brain levels of serotonin and norepinephrine and show enhanced aggression, and that the administration of Gingko biloba extract to MAO-A knockout mice reduces their aggressive behaviour in resident-intruder confrontations; this effect on aggression is not due to sedation and may be mediated by $5\text{-}HT_{2A}$ receptors. All these contradictory results suggest the complexity of neuronal mechanisms in producing behaviour. One point to consider is that MAO is relatively nonspecific, as it is involved in the breakdown of a number of monoamines, and the activity of MAO in platelets may not reflect MAO activity in the central nervous system.

The observation that naloxone and naltrexone ameliorate self-injurious behaviour (SIB) has suggested that impairment of opioid secretion may be involved in the physiopathology of this aggressive behaviour (Richardson and Zaleski, 1983). In patients with SIB, Met-enkephalin plasma levels are increased and return to normal after improvement of the disease. Beta-endorphin plasma levels, however, are lower than normal in children with SIB and higher than normal in adults (Sandman *et al.*, 1987). There have been studies of the functional effect of enkephalins isolated from the avian brain on preoptic and hypothalamic neurons in male Japanese quails. Behavioural changes have been observed following injection of naloxone, a non-selective opioid receptor antagonist, and D-Ala2-Met5-enkephalinamide (DALA), a selective delta opioid receptor agonist, into the preopti and anterior hypothalamic regions. Naloxone treatment showed a significant increase in the frequency of several aggressive actions and the effect was dose dependent, whereas DALA treatment significantly decreased the frequency of aggressive actions in a dose-dependent manner (Kotegawa *et al.*, 1997).

Finally, it has been reported that the μ-opioid receptor upregulation in limbic areas is consistent with increased emotional and aggressive behaviours observed in enkephalin knockout mice (Brady *et al.*, 1999). Taken together, all these data seem to suggest that the opioid system may play a role in the neurobiology of aggressiveness.

NEUROENDOCRINOLOGY

Endocrine Studies

Animal studies show that the testosterone levels of male rhesus monkeys correlate positively with behavioural dominance and aggression. If a single male monkey is placed with other aggressive males, he becomes submissive and shows a decrease in plasma testosterone, revealing that endogenous hormone production can be affected by behavioural variables. King's recent data seem to support the hypothesis that early androgen treatment may support the neurobiology of animals with genetic predisposition to hyperactivity, impulsivity and inattention in a manner consistent with the enhanced expression of ADHD-like behaviours (King *et al.*, 2000).

The connection between the endocrine system and aggression and impulsivity is not clear. Some researchers have hypothesized that androgens may play a role in aggression. They suggest that the androgen insensitivity syndrome and the androgenital syndrome are examples of androgen excesses and deficiencies associated with aggressive and inhibited behaviour, respectively. In one study, plasma testosterone levels were elevated in juvenile prisoners who had committed violent crimes. CSF free testosterone has been shown to be correlated with overall aggressiveness, but not with measures of impulsivity (Higley *et al.*, 1996). Oestrogens and antioandrogens have been used to reduce aggressiveness effectively in some violent sex offenders, although these cases clearly need to be better studied. Low salivary cortisol levels have been associated with persistence and early onset of aggression in school-aged boys, suggesting that low hypothalamic-pituitary-adrenal axis activity correlates with aggressive activity (McBurnett *et al.*, 2000).

Van Goozen has recently examined the relationship between adrenal androgens and aggression in children with oppositional and antisocial behaviour, and compared their levels with those of psychiatric and normal controls. Children with oppositional defiant disorder (ODD) had higher dehydroepiandrosterone sulphate (DHEAS) levels than either psychiatric control or normal control groups; DHEAS levels between the last two groups did not differ; in Van Goozen *et al.*'s opinion, it is possible to classify children as having either ODD or ADHD on the basis of their DHEAS levels, whereas this was not the case on the basis of the Child Behaviour Checklist (CBCL) data. These data indicate that adrenal androgen functioning is specifically elevated in children with ODD, and it is speculated that the mechanism could be a shift in balance of ACTH-beta-endorphin functioning in the hypothalamic-pituitary-adrenal axis due to early stress or genetic factors (Van Goozen *et al.*, 2000).

A positive relationship has been reported in boys between testosterone blood level and acting/receiving aggression in 'social interactions' (serious aggression), but not in playing contests (playful aggression). This indicates that radioimmunoassay testosterone samples in saliva can be a useful biological marker for the risk of serious aggression in preschool boys, reflecting that various levels of sociability are linked to different behavioural patterns (Sanchez-Martin *et al.*, 2000).

Moreover, it has been noted that the ability of estradiol to facilitate transcription from six genes whose products are important for lordosis behaviour in female mice (a typical mating behaviour) proved that hormones can turn on genes in specific neurons at specific times, with sensible behavioural consequences. The use of a gene knockout for oestrogen receptor alpha (ERalpha) revealed that homozygous mutant females simply would not do lordosis and instead were extremely aggressive, thus identifying a specific gene as essential for a mammalian social behaviour. In dramatic contrast, (ERbeta) knockout female mice can exhibit normal lordosis behaviour (Pfaff *et al.*, 2000).

A randomized, double-blinded, placebo-controlled, crossover clinical trial has been used to determine the role of sex steroids on the development of aggressive behaviours in 35 boys and 14 girls. Depot testosterone (to boys) or conjugated oestrogens (to girls) was administered in 3-month blocks, alternating with placebo at three dose levels approximating to early, middle and late pubertal amounts. The Olweus Multifaceted Aggression Inventory was administered after each placebo and treatment period to ascertain the effect of steroids on self-reported aggressive behaviours. The data demonstrated significant hormone effects on physical aggressive behaviours and aggressive impulses, but not on verbal aggressive behaviours nor on aggressive inhibitions in both boys and girls (Finkelstein *et al.*, 1997).

Finally, the impairment of the purinergic system, characterized by reduced adenosinergic activity, has been implicated in the neurobiology of aggressive behaviour. Since there are no direct adenosine agonists available for human use, inhibition of purine degradation by allopurinol was conceived as a possible strategy: Lara *et al.* (2000) reports two cases of adults with refractory aggressive behaviour due to a neurological condition with dramatic response to therapy with allopurinol, 300 mg per day p.o., suggesting the involvement of the purinergic system in the neurobiology of aggression.

Pharmacological Challenge Studies

Animal models have been used to define more clearly the role of specific 5-HT receptors in impulsivity and aggression. To define the contribution of 5-HT receptor subtypes to behaviour, mutant mice lacking the 5-HT_{1B} receptor were generated by homologous recombination. As reported above, these mice did not exhibit any obvious developmental or cognitive defects. They were, however, noted to be extremely aggressive — they attacked intruders faster and more intensely than did wild-type mice (Hen, 1994) — to have increased impulsive aggression, to acquire cocaine self-administration faster, and to exhibit increased alcohol consumption (Brunner and Hen, 1997), suggesting a role for the 5-HT_{1B} receptors in modulating aggressive, impulsive and addictive behaviour (Hen, 1994).

Another research approach involves the use of challenge agents, such as m-chlorophenylpiperazine (m-CPP), that simulate or block serotonin receptors. M-CPP, a non-selective serotonin (5-HT) receptor agonist, has a complex effect on the brain with potent binding to the 5-HT_{2C} receptors and weaker affinity for the 5-HT_{1A} receptors (Kahn and Wetzler, 1991). Neuroendocrine changes following m-CPP stimulation have been represented by increased prolactin, adrenocorticotrophic hormone (ACTH), and corticosterone/cortisol responses in rodents, monkeys and humans (Fuller, 1981; Aloi *et al.*, 1984; Yatham and Steiner, 1993; Meltzer and Maes, 1995). Postsynaptic 5-HT_{1A} and 5-$HT_{2A/2C}$ receptors are thought to mediate these effects (Meltzer and Maes, 1995).

Studies have found that aggressive antisocial subjects had significantly lower excretions of baseline urinary free cortisol and lower CSF ACTH concentration than controls. These findings suggest an inverse relationship between the activity of the hypothalamic-pituitary-adrenal (HPA) axis at baseline and aggressive behaviour (Virkkunen, 1985; Virkkunen *et al.*, 1994). Our group (De Caria *et al.*, submitted) studied 5-HT metabolism alteration, examining behavioural ('high') and neuroendocrine (prolactin and cortisol) responses to single dose ($0.5\,mg\,kg^{-1}$) oral m-CPP and placebo in pathological gamblers and matched controls, and the relationship with clinical severity. Pathological gamblers had significantly increased prolactin response compared to controls at 180 and 210 min post m-CPP. Greater gambling severity correlated with increased neuroendocrine responsiveness to m-CCP, suggesting greater 5-HT dysregulation. Pathological gamblers had significantly increased 'high' response to m-CPP compared to placebo. M-CPP challenge, via the HPA axis, provided a dynamic index of central serotonergic function. An enhanced response to direct postsynaptic serotonergic receptor stimulation is consistent with hypersensitive postsynaptic serotonergic function in male pathological gamblers compared to healthy controls. This would be consistent with a net deficiency of presynaptic 5-HT availability at baseline, and a compensatory increase in postsynaptic 5-HT receptor sensitivity.

Similar results were reported in trichotillomanic (Stein *et al.*, 1995a), alcoholic (Benkelfat *et al.*, 1991), and impulsive and antisocial patients (Moss *et al.*, 1990; Maes *et al.*, 2001). These results are also consistent with reported increased prolactin response and a prolonged peak following m-CPP administration in paedophilics, compared to placebo, relative to healthy controls (Maes *et al.*, 2001).

Pathological gamblers reported that the 'high' that they experienced in response to m-CPP was similar to the 'high' they experience while gambling. An increased 'high' response in other impulsive disorders, such as borderline personality disorder (Hollander *et al.*, 1994) and trichotillomania (Stein *et al.*, 1995a), following m-CPP stimulation has been found. These findings suggest that m-CPP elicits an increased euphoric effect in patients with various types of impulsive behaviours/disorders relative to healthy controls and placebo. In disorders of substance abuse, male alcoholics, some of whom had comorbid antisocial personality disorder (Benklefat *et al.*, 1991), cocaine addicts (Buydens-Branchey *et al.*, 1993), and alcoholics (Krystal *et al.*, 1994) also experienced increased 'high' feelings in response to m-CPP stimulation.

Hollander *et al.* (1992) observed that also a subgroup of patients with obsessive-compulsive disorder (OCD) experienced exacerbation of obsessive symptoms following m-CPP challenge studies. M-CPP has affinity for the 5-HT_{1A}, 5-HT_{2C}, and 5-HT_{1D} receptor subtypes. Patients who underwent challenge studies with MK212, a 5-HT agonist with affinity for the 5-HT_{1A} and 5-HT_{2C} receptor subtypes, but not the 5-HT_{1D} subtype, did not manifest exacerbation of obsessions and compulsions. Because there are behavioural changes in a subgroup of OCD patients following m-CPP, but not following MK212, and because the activity of these two agonists differ with regard to only one receptor subtype, the 5-HT_{1D} receptor, it has been suggested that this receptor may modulate obsessions, of which sexual and aggressive symptoms may be prominent.

Dynamic changes of DA and serotonin have also been assessed: rats were implanted with a microdialysis probes aimed at the nucleus accumbens or medial prefrontal cortex, and, as already mentioned, DA and serotonin levels in the prefrontal cortex changed in opposite directions. Serotonin decreased to 80% from baseline levels during and after the confrontation, whereas DA increased by up to 120% after the confrontation. The temporal pattern of monoamine changes points to a significant role of accumbal and cortical DA and 5-HT in the consequences, as opposed to the triggering, of aggressive acts. The increase in accumbal DA in aggressive animals supports the hypothesis that this neural system is linked to the execution of biologically salient and demanding behaviour (Van Erp and Miczek, 2000).

NEUROGENETICS

Genetic studies in humans and animals have not yet supported a definitive association among impulsivity, aggression, and reduced 5-HT activity. The Maudsley rat study, however, was an example of genetic breeding for aggressive behaviour. Two groups of rats were bred. The first group (MNR) included rats that had low measures of impulsivity and high measures of inhibition. The second group (MR) had the opposite features. The MR strains bred from the second group were significantly more impulsive and demonstrated increased aggressive behaviour compared with the MNR rats (Eichelman, 1971). Neurochemically, the MNR strain showed lower limbic brain 5-HT levels than the MR strain (Sudack and Maas, 1964).

At the synaptic level, reuptake of serotonin is accomplished by a plasma membrane carrier called the serotonin transporter (5-HTT). The gene for 5-HTT has been mapped to chromosome 17 (Collier *et al.*, 1996). Preliminary evidence for a genetic disturbance in serotonergic function that might predispose individuals to impulsive-aggressive behaviour includes a study of the gene for the rate-limiting enzyme for serotonin synthesis, tryptophan hydroxylase (TPH). The gene for TPH has been mapped to the short arm of chromosome 11 and is one of the major candidate genes for psychiatric and behavioural disorders. Part of the gene for TPH has been discovered to exist as two alleles: U or L, with certain genotypes (UL and LL) being associated with impulsive-aggressive behaviour and suicidal behaviour, and with low levels of CSF 5-HIAA in violent offenders (Nielsen *et al.*, 1994). Persons having the TPH U allele scored significantly higher on measures of aggression than individuals homozygous for the L allele, and peak prolactin response was attenuated among male subjects, but not female subjects, having any U allele relative to LL homozygotes (Manuck *et al.*, 1999). In another study, the TPH genotype was found to be associated with impulsive-aggressive behaviours in male, but not female, patients who had personality disorders (New *et al.*, 1998). There have been reported polymorphisms in the regulatory region of the serotonin transporter, in intron 7 of the TPH gene, and in the MAO-A gene, associated with mood and anxiety disorders, impulsivity and aggression (New *et al.*, 1997; 1998). Nolan *et al.* (2000) examined these polymorphisms in schizophrenic and schizoaffective patients, suggesting the association between the TPH L allele and impulsive aggression in males with personality disorder. Turecki *et al.* (2001), instead, investigated the correlation between TPH and suicidal behaviour: haplotype analysis revealed that one haplotype (−6526G −5806T 218C) was significantly more frequent among suicide subjects than in normal controls, and this haplotype was particularly more frequent among subjects who committed suicide by violent methods. Further studies are needed to clarify the role of TPH alleles in aggression and the differences between the sexes.

Genetic studies involving the 5-HT_{1B} receptor gene in human subjects have been equivocal. In one study, a polymorphism of the 5-HT_{1B} receptor gene was linked to aggressive and impulsive behaviour in alcoholics (Lappalainen *et al.*, 1998). However, Huang *et al.* (1999) found no relationship between suicide, alcoholism or pathological aggression with 5-HT_{1B} receptor-binding indices or a genotype using two common polymorphisms. In summary, serotonin synthesis and regulation are at least partially regulated by genetic controls that probably contribute to an individual's propensity for impulsive and aggressive behaviours.

Homozygosity of a low-enzyme-activity variant of the catechol-*O*-methyltransferase (COMT) gene has been reported to be associated with aggressive behaviour in a group of schizophrenic patients. A similar tendency has been observed by Kotler *et al.* (1999) in a group of 30 schizophrenic subjects who were confined to a maximum-security psychiatric facility for homicide; significant excess (46.7% versus 21.0%) homozygosity of the low activity COMT Met/Met genotype was observed in 30, mostly male (28 of 30), homicidal schizophrenic patients compared with 415 control subjects, and no difference in COMT genotype has been found between nonviolent schizophrenic patients and control subjects. Moreover, the COMT genotype has been determined in 62 impulsive violent recidivist offenders with early-onset (type 2) alcoholism, 123 late-onset nonviolent alcoholics (type 1) and 267 race- and gender-matched controls. The allele and genotype frequencies of these groups were compared with each other and also with previously published data from 3130 Finnish blood donors. The type 2 alcoholics did not differ from either the blood donors or the controls. The low activity (L) allele frequency was higher among type 1 alcoholics than type 2. The odds ratio for type 1 alcoholism as compared with type 2 alcoholism for those subjects with the LL genotype versus the HH was 3.0 (95% confidence interval 1.1–1.84). These results suggest that the COMT genotype has no major role in the development of early-onset alcoholism with severe antisocial behaviour (Hallikainen *et al.*, 2000).

Currently, there are no controlled family history studies of individuals with impulse-control disorders (i.e., intermittent explosive disorder, kleptomania, pyromania, pathological gambling, and trichotillomania). There are studies supporting associations between major mood disorder and alcohol and substance abuse in first-degree relatives of individuals with kleptomania and in first-degree relatives of pathological gamblers (Linden *et al.*, 1986; Ramirez *et al.*, 1983; Saiz *et al.*, 1992).

The relationship between mood swing and impulse control represents a field of great relevance to the understanding and therapy of impulse-control disorders. Other findings include associations between anxiety disorders in the families of individuals with kleptomania and violent behaviour and ADHD in the families of individuals with intermittent explosive disorder (McElroy *et al.*, 1991).

Research involving monozygotic twins reveals a hereditary aspect of aggressive behaviour, with concordance rates for monozygotic twins greater than those for dizygotic twins. Twin studies suggest that antisocial behaviour in adult life is related more to genetic factors than to environmental factors (Cadoret *et al.*, 1995). Twin studies have established that there are substantial genetic influences on alcoholism in both men and women, and it seems that the heritability of alcoholism is substance-specific; the relationship between this and behaviours predisposing to alcoholism, including impulsivity, is still challenging. Refinement of clinical phenotypes and use of intermediate phenotypes will improve the changes of gene identification (Enoch and Goldman, 2001).

Chromosomal studies have looked at the influence of chromosomal abnormalities in aggression, particularly the XYY syndrome (Bioulac *et al.*, 1980). However, the link between XYY and violence has not been confirmed. Inborn metabolic disorders that affect the nervous system can be associated with aggressive personalities. These disorders, which diffusely affect the central nervous system and are inherited, include phenylketonuria, Lesch-Nyhan syndrome, Prader-Willi syndrome, Vogt syndrome (a neuronal storage disorder), and Sanfilippo's syndrome (increased mucopolysaccharide storage).

THERAPEUTIC INTERVENTIONS

Impulsivity and aggression are behavioural characteristics that encompass a broad range of clinical problems. Studies on impulsivity and aggression have focused on a heterogeneous group of disorders with varied responses to pharmacotherapeutic interventions. In this chapter, we do not focus on the treatment of patients with epilepsy and patients with drug-induced aggression. These areas are reviewed elsewhere.

Controlled studies suggest that a number of medications may be useful in the treatment of impulsivity and aggression. Given the evidence for decreased 5-HT function in impulsive and aggressive behaviours, many, but not all, of these medications involve direct 5-HT mechanisms.

SSRIs have been shown to reduce impulsive, aggressive behaviours in various psychiatric disorders. For example, fluvoxamine resulted in improvement in gambling severity in patients with pathological gambling compared to placebo in one double-blind study (Hollander *et al.*, 2000b). However, in some disorders characterized by impulsivity, SSRIs have a quick onset, but these effects maybe transient, and some patients may require augmentation with compounds such as lithium, buspirone, and anticonvulsants (Hollander and Wong, 1995). Preliminary data from an open-label study conducted by our group reported that nefazodone (100–500 mg per day) is also an effective treatment in a sample of 12 pathological gamblers.

BPD is a common clinical problem in which researchers have used pharmacological interventions to target the characteristic symptoms of impulsivity, aggression, lability, and hostility. Fluoxetine is the best-studied SSRI for the treatment of impulsivity and aggression. A number of open trials of fluoxetine in BPD suggest its efficacy in the treatment of impulsivity and aggression in BPD. Markowitz (1990) reported that BPD patients showed significant decreases in self-injurious behaviour after treatment with fluoxetine 80 mg per day for 12 weeks. Three subsequent double-blind, placebo-controlled trials of fluoxetine confirmed the findings of the open trials (Markowitz, 1992). Overall, controlled studies of fluoxetine, sertraline, and fluvoxamine suggest that these medications are of benefit to patients with impulsivity and aggression in the context of BPD. More studies are needed to assess further which behaviours are associated with responsivity to an SSRI, and to determine the appropriate dosage, and longitudinal efficacy of those agents. The tricyclic antidepressants (TCAs) have been extensively studied in BPD for their effects on depression in BPD patients. Although clearly effective for depressive symptoms, TCAs have not been shown to be particularly helpful in decreasing aggression and impulsivity in BPD (Soloff *et al.*, 1986). Some BPD patients actually experienced increased anger, hostility, and aggression while taking imipramine (Klein, 1968) and amitriptyline (Soloff *et al.*, 1986). There are case reports of using desipramine and clomipramine effectively to treat violent outbursts in some patients, and of using amitriptyline, trazodone, and fluoxetine for aggression associated with brain injury and anoxic encephalopathy. The potential for worsening impulsive, aggressive symptoms and the danger of overdose in patients who have impaired self-control may limit the use of TCAs. The same limits apply to MAOIs, which also have not been shown to decrease the behavioural dyscontrol or impulsivity seen in BPD.

Medications that are not serotonergically mediated, such as carbamazepine and other anticonvulsant mood stabilizers, have also proven to be useful (Haller *et al.*, 1994). Although evidence suggests that impulsivity and aggression are serotonergically mediated, a 5-HT hypothesis of impulsivity is not a definitive model. The complete role of 5-HT activity and its complex interactions with other neurotransmitters and receptors in impulsivity and aggression have not yet been fully delineated. The antagonism of 5-HT2 receptors appears to decrease aggression and may explain the efficacy of newer antipsychotic agents in the reduction of aggression and agitation independently of effects on psychotic symptoms.

The neurotransmitter effects of lithium are complex and include an effect on second-messenger systems related to the 5-HT system. A recent single-blind, randomized study (Pallanti *et al.*, in press) suggests the efficacy of both lithium carbonate and valproate in the treatment of PG. Further studies on psychopharmacological treatments of pathological gambling should be performed, as preliminary studies involving medication in the treatment of this disorder have shown promising results. Researchers and clinicians have used lithium, carbamazepine, valproic acid, and, more recently, gabapentin, lamotrigine, and topiramate to treat the impulsivity, aggression, and mood instability seen in bipolar patients, and they subsequently reasoned that it might stabilize these same symptoms in BPD. In a double-blind placebo-controlled trial (Cowdry and Gardner, 1988), carbamazepine decreased impulsivity in a group of BPD patients.

Our group (Stein *et al.*, 1995b) found that valproate led to significant overall improvement in 50% of a small sample of BPD patients who completed an 8-week, open-label trial, and that valproate may be more effective than placebo was shown in a 10-week, double-blind study (Hollander *et al.*, 2001). The medication was helpful for impulsivity, anger, and irritability, as well as for mood instability and anxiety. The potential efficacy of valproate in the treatment of BPD raises the question of the neurobiological underpinnings of the core features of BPD, namely, impulsivity and aggression. A number of points are relevant. First, a link between impulsive aggression and limbic abnormality has long been postulated. Although only a small percentage of BPD patients have seizure activity, more subtle neuropsychiatric abnormalities have been found in this population, including increased neurological soft signs. The hypothesis that valproate alters limbic dysfunction by interrupting neuronal kindling is therefore of interest. Second, there is increasing evidence that 5-HT hypofunction may play a role in the mediation of BPD symptoms. Although valproate has multiple effects on neurotransmission, it is notable that it increases 5-HIAA levels. Further studies and larger sample sizes for the use of valproate in the treatment of BPD are warranted.

Neuroleptics are among the most studied medications for the treatment of BPD, and they have been effective in treating violence associated with psychosis. Although they are the most commonly used medications for violence and aggression related to psychosis, neuroleptics are often misused as chronic sedatives. In BPD patients, moreover, neuroleptics were not well tolerated and were statistically no better than placebo in the reduction of hostility, anger, and aggression (Goldberg *et al.*, 1986; Soloff *et al.*, 1986). In one 8-week, open-label, pilot study, BPD patients treated with olanzapine had lower Barratt Impulsivity Scale and Buss-Durkee Hostility Inventory scores then those treated with placebo (Schulz *et al.*, 1999). Neuroleptics may result in a number of adverse side effects. They may cause tolerance to sedation and lead to increased doses and thereby increased side effects such as akathisia, extrapyramidal side effects, and anticholinergic toxicity. These specific side effects can worsen aggression in predisposed patients, particularly those with organic brain injury.

Kim has employed the opioid antagonists in the treatment of impulse-control disorders, prescribing naltrexone for up to 9 months to 15 patients who had impulse-control disorder: naltrexone was generally well tolerated, and there were no hepatic side effects. Naltrexone appears to reduce urge-related symptoms and decrease the problematic behaviours such as PG; the effects appear to be sustained. In general, 50 mg per day of naltrexone was not effective, and most patients required higher doses. These data suggest that naltrexone may be of use in selected impulse-control disorder patients (Kim, 1998).

Moreover, it seems that the disinhibitory behaviour of 5-HT-lesioned rats can be reversed by the commonly used opiate receptor-antagonist naloxone at doses that do not significantly affect behaviour in sham-lesioned controls. Moreover, this effect of naloxone is reversed by a low inert dose of amobarbital. Thus, naloxone may represent a new pharmacological principle for the treatment of impulse-control disorders (Soderpalm and Svensson, 1999).

SUMMARY

Impulsivity is a core symptom of a broad spectrum of psychiatric disorders including impulse-control disorders (pathological gambling, intermittent explosive disorder, pyromania, kleptomania, trichotillomania, and impulse-control disorder NOS), impulsive aggressive personality disorders (borderline, antisocial), neurological disorders that can be associated with disinhibition of behaviour (such as epilepsy), and substance abuse. Moreover, impulsive disorders entail large costs to society, and are associated with substantial morbidity, mortality, social/family/job dysfunction, accidents, suicide, violence, aggression, criminality, and excessive utilization of health-care, government and financial resources.

While the concept of impulsivity has been widely studied and reviewed in clinical psychiatry, our understanding of the neurobiology of impulsivity is still at a very early stage. No simple extrapolation of animal subtypes to humans is possible, mainly because of the influence of complex cultural variables on behaviour. On the whole, research into subtypes of human impulsivity has been rather limited. Much of this has been conducted in children, by clinical observation, experimental paradigms in the laboratory, and cluster/factor analytical statistics.

Animal models have recently helped to clarify both the neuroanatomical and biological basis of specific impulse behaviours. Brain regions such as the nucleus accumbens core, the basolateral amygdala, the hypothalamus, and the prefontal cortex may play an important role in impulsivity, as well as genetic and environmental factors. Serotonin dysregulation and hypofunction seem also to play a central role in impulse-control disorders, with the influence of the highly interconnected noradrenergic, dopaminergic, opioid, and GABAergic systems. Pharmacological therapeutic approaches have focused for this reason on serotonin transmission (serotonin reuptake inhibitors), but various classes of medication acting on different neurotransmitter systems, mood stabilizers, and opioid antagonists have also had encouraging results.

Further and more sophisticated research is needed to elucidate the localization of impulsive choice in animal and human models, and to understand this core behavioural symptom domain that cuts across various disorders and plays an important role not only in clinical psychiatry but also in everyday life.

REFERENCES

Adamac, R., 1990. Does the kindling model reveal anything clinically significant? *Biol Psychiatry*, **27**, 249–279.

Aloi, J.A., Insel, T.R., Mueller, E.A. and Murphy, D.L., 1984. Neuroendocrine and behavioural effects of m-chlorophenylpiperazine administration in rhesus monkeys. *Life Sci*, **34**, 1325–1331.

Asberg, M., Traskman, L. and Thoren, P., 1976. 5-HIAA in the cerebrospinal fluid. A biochemical suicide predictor? *Arch Gen Psychiatry*, **33**, 1193–1197.

Bard, P., 1928. A diencephalic mechanism for the expression of rage with special reference to the sympathetic nervous system. *Am J Psychol*, **84**, 490–515.

Barratt, E.S. and Stanford, M.S., 1995. Impulsiveness. In: Costello, C.G. (ed.), *Personality Characteristics of the Personality Disordered Client*, pp. 76–89. Wiley, New York.

Bear, D., 1991. Neurological perspectives on aggressive behaviour. *J Neuropsychiatry Clin Neurosci*, **3**, S3–S8.

Bechara, A., Damasio, H., Damasio, A.R. and Lee, G.P., 1999. Different contributions of the human amygdala and ventromedial prefrontal cortex to decision-making. *J Neurosci*, **19**, 5473–5481.

Bechara, A., Damasio, H. and Damasio, A.R., 2000a. Emotion, decision making and the orbitofrontal cortex. *Cereb Cortex*, **10**, 295–307.

Bechara, A., Tranel, D. and Damasio, H., 2000b. Characterization of the decision-making deficit of patients with ventromedial prefrontal cortex lesions. *Brain*, **123**, 2189–2202.

Benkelfat, C., Murphy, D.L., Hill, J.L., George, D.T., Nutt, D. and Linnoila, M., 1991. Ethanol-like properties of the serotonergic partial agonist m-chlorophenylpiperazine in chronic alcoholic patients. *Arch Gen Psychiatry*, **48**, 383.

Biegon, A., Grinspoon, A., Blumenfeld, B., Bleich, A., Apter, A. and Mester, R., 1990. Increased serotonin $5\text{-}HT_2$ receptor binding on blood platelets of suicidal men. *Psychopharmacology (Berl)*, **100**, 165–167.

Bigi, S.S., De Acetis, L.L., Chiarotti, F.F. and Alleva, E.E., 1993. Substance P effects on intraspecific aggressive behaviour of isolated male mice: an ethopharmacological analysis. *Behav Pharmacol*, **4**, 495–500.

Bioulac, B., Benezech, M., Renaud, B., Noel, B. and Roche, D., 1980. Serotoninergic dysfunction in the 47, XYY syndrome. *Biol Psychiatry*, **15**, 917–923.

Biver, F., Lotstra, F., Monclus, M., Wikler, D., Damhaut, P., Mendlewicz, J. and Goldman, S., 1996. Sex differences in $5\text{-}HT_2$ receptor in the living human brain. *Neurosci Lett*, **204**, 25–28.

Blum, K., Braverman, E.R., Holder, J.M., Lubar, J.F., Monastra, V.J., Miller, D., Lubar, J.O., Chen, T.J. and Comings, D.E., 2000. Reward deficiency syndrome: a biogenetic model for the diagnosis and treatment of impulsive, addictive and compulsive behaviours. *J Psychoactive Drugs*, **32**, 1–112.

Brady, L.S., Herkenham, M., Rothman, R.B., Partilla, J.S., Konig, M., Zimmer, A.M. and Zimmer, A., 1999. Region specific up-regulation of opioid receptor binding in enkephalin knockout mice. *Brain Res Mol Brain Res*, **68**, 193–197.

Brown, C.S., Kent, T.A., Bryant, S.G., Gevedon, R.M., Campbell, J.L., Felthous, A.R., Barratt, E.S. and Rose, R.M., 1989. Blood platelet uptake of serotonin in episodic aggression. *Psychiatry Res*, **27**, 5–12.

Brown, G.L., Goodwin, F.K., Ballenger, J.C., Goyer, P.F. and Major, L.F., 1979. Aggression in humans correlates with cerebrospinal fluid amine metabolites. *Psychiatry Res*, **1**, 131–139.

Brown, G.L., Ebert, M.H., Goyer, P.F., Jimerson, D.C., Klein, W.J., Bunney, W.E. and Goodwin, F.K., 1982. Aggression, suicide, and serotonin: relationships to CSF amine metabolites. *Am J Psychiatry*, **139**, 741–746.

Brunner, D. and Hen, R., 1997. Insights into the neurobiology of impulsive behaviour from serotonin receptor knockout mice. *Ann N Y Acad Sci*, **836**, 81–105.

Buydens-Branchey, L., Branchey, M., Fergeson, P., Hudson, J. and McKernin, C., 1993. Euphorogenic properties of the serotonergic partial agonist m-chlorophenylpiperazine in cocaine addicts. *Arch Gen Psychiatry*, **50**, 1001–1002

Cadoret, R.J., Yates, W.R., Troughton, E., Woodworth, G. and Stewart, M.A., 1995. Genetic-environmental interaction in the genesis of aggressivity and conduct disorders. *Arch Gen Psychiatry*, **52**, 916–924.

Cardinal, R., Pennicott, D., Sugathapala, C., Robbins, T. and Everitt, B., 2001. Impulsive choice induced in rats by lesions of the nucleus accumbens core. *Science*, **292**, 2499–2501.

Chiavegatto, S., Dawson, V.L., Mamounas, L.A., Koliatsos, V.E., Dawson, T.M. and Nelson, R.J., 2001. Brain serotonin dysfunction accounts for aggression in male mice lacking neuronal nitric oxide synthase. *Proc Natl Acad Sci USA*, **98**, 1277–1281.

Coccaro, E.F., Kavoussi, R.J., Sheline, Y.I., Lish, J.D. and Csernansky, J.G., 1996. Impulsive aggression in personality disorder correlates with tritiated paroxetine binding in the platelet. *Arch Gen Psychiatry*, **53**, 531–536.

Collier, D.A., Stober, G., Li, T., Heils, A., Catalano, M., Di Bella, D., Arranz, M.J., Murray, R.M., Vallada, H.P., Bengel, D., Muller, C.R., Roberts, G.W., Smeraldi, E., Kirov, G., Sham, P. and Lesch, K.P., 1996. A novel functional polymorphism within the promoter of the serotonin transporter gene: possible role in susceptibility to affective disorders. *Mol Psychiatry*, **1**, 453–460.

Cowdry, R.W. and Gardner, D.L., 1988. Pharmacotherapy of borderline personality disorder. Alprazolam, carbamazepine, trifluoperazine, and tranylcypromine. *Arch Gen Psychiatry*, **45**, 111–119.

Damasio, A.R., 1996. The somatic marker hypothesis and the possible functions of the prefrontal cortex. *Philos Trans R Soc Lond B Biol Sci*, **351**(1346), 1413–1420.

De Caria, C.M., Pallanti, S., Baldini Rossi, N., Nora, R., Birnbaum, M. and Hollander, E. (Submitted). Increased m-CPP-induced 'high' and prolactin response in pathological gamblers.

De Napoli, J.S., Dodman, N.H., Shuster, L., Rand, W.M. and Gross, K.L., 2000. Effect of dietary protein content and tryptophan supplementation on dominance, aggression, territorial aggression, and hyperactivity in dogs. *J Am Vet Med Assoc*, **217**, 504–508.

Depue, R.A. and Spoont, M.R., 1987. Conceptualizing a serotonin trait: a behavioural dimension of constraint. In: Mann, J.J. and Stanley, M. (eds), *Psychobiology of Suicidal Behaviour*, pp. 71–73. New York Academy of Sciences, New York.

Desjardin, D. and Persinger, M.A., 1995. Association between intermale social aggression and cellular density within the central amygdaloid nucleus in rats with lithium/pilocarpine-induced seizures. *Percept Mot Skills*, **81**, 635–641.

Dicks, P., Meyers, R.E. and Kling, A., 1969. Uncus and amygdala lesions: effects on social behaviour in free-ranging monkey. *Science*, **165**, 69–71.

Downer, J.L., 1961. Changes in visual gnostic functions and emotional behaviour following unilateral temporal pole damage in the 'split brain' monkey. *Nature*, **191**, 50–51.

Eichelman, B.S. Jr, 1971. Effect of subcortical lesions on shock-induced aggression in the rat. *J Comp Physiol Psychol*, **74**, 331–339.

Elliot, F.A., 1992. Violence: the neurological contribution: an overview. *Arch Neurol*, **49**, 595–603.

Enoch, M.A. and Goldman, D., 2001. The genetics of alcoholism and alcohol abuse. *Curr Psychiatry Rep*, **3**, 144–151.

Ernst, M., Zametkin, A., Matochik, J., Jons, P. and Cohen, R., 1998. DOPA decarboxylase activity in attention deficit hyperactivity disorder adults. A [fluorine-18]fluorodopa positron-emission tomographic study. *J Neurosci*, **18**, 5901–5907.

Fairbanks, L.A., Melega, W.P., Jorgensen, M.J., Kaplan, J.R. and McGuire, M.T., 2001. Social impulsivity inversely associated with CSF 5-HIAA and fluoxetine exposure in vervet monkeys. *Neuropsychopharmacology*, **24**, 370–378.

Ferris, C.F., Stolberg, T. and Delville, Y., 1999. Serotonin regulation of aggressive behaviour in male golden hamsters (*Mesocricetus auratus*). *Behav Neurosci*, **113**, 804–815.

Finkelstein, J.W., Susman, E.J., Chinchilli, V.M., Kunselman, S.J., D'Arcangelo, M.R., Schwab, J., Demers, L.M., Liben, L.S., Lookingbill, G. and Kulin, H.E., 1997. Estrogen or testosterone increases self-reported aggressive behaviours in hypogonadal adolescents. *J Clin Endocrinol Metab*, **82**, 2433–2438.

Folkow, B., Hallback-Nordlander, M., Martner, J. and Nordborg, C., 1982. Influence of amygdala lesions on cardiovascular responses to alerting stimuli, on behaviour and on blood pressure development in spontaneously hypertensive rats. *Acta Physiol Scand*, **116**, 133–139.

Fuller, R.W., 1981. Serotonergic stimulation of pituitary-adrenocortical function in rats. *Neuroendocrinology*, **32**, 118–127.

Gammie, S.C. and Nelson, R.J., 2000. Maternal and mating-induced aggression is associated with elevated citrulline immunoreactivity in the hypothalamic paraventricular in prairie voles. *J Comp Neurol*, **418**, 182–192.

Gammie, S.C., Olaghere-da Silva, U.B. and Nelson, R.J., 2000. 3-Bromo-7-7-nitroindazole, a neuronal nitric oxide synthase inhibitor, impairs maternal aggression and citrulline immunoreactivity in prairie voles. *Brain Res*, **870**, 80–86.

Goldberg, S.C., Schulz, S.C., Schulz, P.M., Resnick, R.J., Hamer, R.M. and Friedel, R.O., 1986. Borderline and schizotypal personality disorders treated with low-dose thiothixene vs placebo. *Arch Gen Psychiatry*, **43**, 680–686.

Goyer, P.F., Semple, W.E., Rugle, L., McCormick, R., Lewis, C., Kowaliw, S. and Berridge, M.S., 1999. Brain blood flow and dopamine receptor PET imaging in pathological gamblers. In: *National Conference on Problem Gambling*, Detroit, MI.

Grafman, J., Schwab, K., Warden, D., Pridgen, A., Brown, H.R. and Salazar, A.M., 1996. Frontal lobe injuries, violence, and aggression: a report of the Vietnam Head Injury Study. *Neurology*, **46**, 1231–1238.

Gregg, T.R. and Siegel, A., 2001. Brain structures and neurotransmitters regulating aggression in cats: implications for human aggression. *Prog Neuropsychopharmacol Biol Psychiatry*, **1**, 91–140.

Guillot, P.V., Sluyter, F., Crusio, W.E. and Chapothier, G., 1999. Mice selected for differences in sensitivity to a benzodiazepine receptor inverse agonist vary in intermale aggression. *Neurogenetics*, **2**, 171–175.

Hallikainen, T., Lachman, H., Saito, T., Volavka, J., Kauhanen, J., Salonen, J.T., Ryynanen, O.P., Koulu, M., Karvonen, M.K., Pohjalainen, T., Syvalahti, E., Hietala, J. and Tiihonen, J., 2000. Lack of association between the functional variant of the catechol-*O*-methyltransferase (COMT) gene and early onset alcoholism associated with severe antisocial behaviour. *Am J Med Genet*, **96**, 348–352.

Han, Y., Shaik, M.B. and Siegel, A., 1997. Ethanol enhances medial amygdaloid induced inhibition of predatory attack behaviour in the cat: role of the $GABA_A$ receptors in the lateral hypothalamus. *Alcohol Alcohol*, **32**, 657–670.

Haugh, R.M. and Markesbery, W.R., 1983. Hypothalamic astrocytoma. Syndrome of hyperphagia, obesity, and disturbances of behaviour and endocrine and autonomic function. *Arch Neurol*, **40**, 560–563.

Hen, R., 1994. Enhanced aggressive behaviour in mice lacking HT1B receptor. *Science*, **265**, 119–123.

Herpertz, S.C., Kunert, H.J., Schwenger, U.B. and Ass, H., 1999. Affective responsiveness in borderline personality disorder: a psychophysiological approach. *Am J Psychiatry*, **16**, 1550–1556.

Hess, W.R., 1957. *The Functional Organization of Diencephalon*, p. 180. Grune & Stratton, New York.

Higley, J.D., Mehlman, P.T., Taub, D.M., Higley, S.B., Suomi, S.J., Vickers, J.H. and Linnoila, M., 1992. Cerebrospinal fluid monoamine and adrenal correlates of aggression in free-ranging rhesus monkeys. *Arch Gen Psychiatry*, **49**, 436–441.

Higley, J.D., Mehlman, P.T., Poland, R.E., Taub, D.M., Vickers, J., Suomi, S.J. and Linnoila, M., 1996. CSF testosterone and 5-HIAA correlate with different types of aggressive behaviours. *Biol Psychiatry*, **40**, 1067–1082.

Hill, S.Y., Zezza, N., Wipprecht, G., Locke, J. and Neiswanger, K., 1999. Personality traits and dopamine receptors (D_2 and D_4): linkage studies in families of alcoholics. *Am J Med Genet*, **88**, 634–641.

Hollander, E., 1998. Treatment of obsessive-compulsive spectrum disorders with SSRIs. *Br J Psychiatry*, **173**(Suppl 35), 7–12.

Hollander, E. and Evers, M., 2001. New developments in impulsivity. *Lancet*, **358**, 949–950.

Hollander, E. and Rosen, J., 2000. Impulsivity. *J Psychopharmacol*, **14**(Suppl 1), S39–S44.

Hollander, E. and Wong, C.M., 1995. Obsessive-compulsive spectrum disorders. *J Clin Psychiatry*, **56**(Suppl 4), 3–6; discussion 53–55.

Hollander, E. and Wong, C.M., 1995. Body dysmorphic disorder, pathological gambling, and sexual compulsions. *J Clin Psychiatry*, **56**(Suppl 4), 7–12; discussion, 13.

Hollander, E., DeCaria, C.M., Nitescu, A., Gully, R., Suckow, R.F., Cooper, T.B., Gorman, J.M., Klein, D.F. and Liebowitz, M.R., 1992. Serotonergic function in obsessive-compulsive disorder. Behavioural and neuroendocrine responses to oral m-chlorophenylpiperazine and fenfluramine in patients and healthy volunteers. *Arch Gen Psychiatry*, **49**, 21–28.

Hollander, E., Stein, D.J., DeCaria, C.M., Cohen, L., Saoud, J.B., Skodol, A.E., Kellman, D., Rosnick, L. and Oldham, J.M., 1994. Serotonergic sensitivity in borderline personality disorder: preliminary findings. *Am J Psychiatry*, **151**, 277–280.

Hollander, E., DeCaria, C.M., Mari, E., Wong, C.M., Mosovich, S., Grossman, R. and Begaz, T., 1998. Short-term single-blind fluvoxamine treatment of pathological gambling. *Am J Psychiatry*, **155**, 1781–1783.

Hollander, E., Buchalter, A. and DeCaria, C., 2000. Pathological gambling. *Psychiatr Clin North Am*, **23**, 629–642.

Hollander, E., DeCaria, C.M., Finkell, J.N., Begaz, T., Wong, C.M. and Cartwright, C., 2000b. A randomized double-blind fluvoxamine/placebo crossover trial in pathologic gambling. *Biol Psychiatry*, **47**, 813–817.

Hollander, E., Allen, A., Lopez, R., Bienstock, C., Grossman, R., Siever, L., Merkatz, L. and Stein, D.J., 2001. A preliminary double-blind, placebo-controlled trial of divalproex sodium in borderline personality disorder. *J Clin Psychiatry*, **62**, 199–203.

Hollander, E., Posner, N. and Cherkasky, S. (2002 in press). The neuropsychiatry of aggression and impulse-control disorders. In: Yudofsky, S.C. and Hales, R.E. (eds), *American Psychiatric Press Textbook of Neuropsychiatry*. American Psychiatric Press, Washington, DC.

Huang, Y.Y., Grailhe, R., Arango, V., Hen, R. and Mann, J.J., 1999. Relationship of psychopathology to the human serotonin1B genotype and receptor binding kinetics in postmortem brain tissue. *Neuropsychopharmacology*, **21**, 238–246.

Isenberg, N., Silbersweig, D., Engelien, A., Emmerich, S., Malavade, K., Beattie, B., Leon, A.C. and Stern, E., 1999. Linguistic threat activates the human amygdala. *Proc Natl Acad Sci USA*, **96**, 10456–10459.

Isern, R.D. Jr, 1987. Family violence and the Kluver-Bucy syndrome. *South Med J*, **80**, 373–377.

Iwata, J., LeDoux, J.E., Meeley, M.P., Arneric, S. and Reis, D.J., 1986. Intrinsic neurons in the amygdaloid field projected to by the medial geniculate body mediate emotional responses conditioned to acoustic stimuli. *Brain Res*, **383**(1–2), 195–214.

Kahn, R.S. and Wetzler, S., 1991. m-Chlorophenylpiperazine as a probe of serotonin function. *Biol Psychiatry*, **30**, 1139–1166.

Kandel, E. and Freed, D., 1989. Frontal-lobe dysfunction and antisocial behaviour: a review. *J Clin Psychol*, **45**, 404–413.

Kapp, B.S., Schwaber, J.S. and Driscoll, P.A., 1985. Frontal cortex projections to the amygdaloid central nucleus in the rabbit. *Neuroscience*, **15** 327–346.

Kavoussi, R., Armstead, P. and Coccaro, E., 1997. The neurobiology of impulsive aggression. *Psychiatr Clin North Am*, **20**, 395–403.

Killeffer, F.A. and Stern, W.E., 1970. Chronic effects of hypothalamic injury. Report of a case of near total hypothalamic destruction resulting from removal of a craniopharyngioma. *Arch Neurol*, **22**, 419–429.

Kim, D.H., Jung, J.S., Yan, J.J., Suh, H.W., Son, B.K., Kim, Y.H. and Song, D.K., 2000. Increased plasma corticosterone, aggressiveness and brain monoamine changes induced by central injection of pertussis toxin. *Eur J Pharmacol*, **409**, 67–72.

Kim, S.W., 1998. Opioid antagonists in the treatment of impulse control disorders. *J Clin Psychiatry*, **59**, 159–164.

King, J.A., Barkley, R.A., Delville, Y. and Ferris, C.F., 2000. Early androgen treatment decreases cognitive function and catecholamine innervation in an animal model of ADHD. *Behav Brain Res*, **107**, 35–43.

Klein, D.F., 1968. Psychiatric diagnosis and a typology of clinical drug effects. *Psychopharmacologia*, **13**, 359–386.

Kluver, H. and Bucy, P.C., 1939. Preliminary analysis of functions of the temporal lobes in monkeys. *Arch Neurol Psychiatry*, **42**, 979–1000.

Korzan, W.J., Summers, T.R., Ronan, P.J. and Summers, C.H., 2000. Visible sympathetic activity as a social signal in *Anolis carolinensis*: changes in aggression and plasma catecholamines. *Horm Behav*, **38**, 193–199.

Kotegawa, T., Abe, T. and Tsutsui, K., 1997. Inhibitory role of opioid peptides in the regulation of aggressive and sexual behaviour in male Japanese quails. *J Exp Zool*, **277**, 146–154.

Kotler, M., Barak, P., Cohen, H., Averbuch, I.E., Grinshpoon, A., Gritsenko, I., Nemanov, L. and Ebstein, R.P., 1999. Homicidal behaviour in schizophrenia associated with a genetic polymorphism determining low catechol *O*-methyltransferase (COMT) activity. *Am J Med Genet*, **88**, 628–633.

Krystal, J.H., Webb, E., Cooney, N., Kranzler, H.R. and Charney, D.S., 1994. Specificity of ethanol-like effects elicited by serotonergic and noradrenergic mechanisms. *Arch Gen Psychiatry*, **51**, 898–911.

Lappalainen, J., Long, J.C., Eggert, M., Ozaki, N., Robin, R.W., Brown, G.L., Naukkarinen, H., Virkkunen, M., Linnoila, M. and Goldman, D., 1998. Linkage of antisocial alcoholism to the serotonin 5-HT_{1B} receptor gene in 2 populations. *Arch Gen Psychiatry*, **55**, 989–894.

Lara, D.R., Belmonte-de Abreu, P. and Souza, D.O., 2000. Allopurinol for refractory aggression and self-inflicted behaviour. *J Psychopharmacol*, **14**, 81–83.

Larson, E.T. and Summers, C.H., 2001. Serotonin reverses dominant social status. *Behav Brain Res*, **121**, 95–102.

Lee, R. and Coccaro, E., 2001. The neuropsychopharmacology of criminality and aggression. *Can J Psychiatry*, **46**, 35–44.

LeMarquand, D., Pihl, R.O. and Benkelfat, C., 1994. Serotonin and alcohol intake, abuse, and dependence: clinical evidence. *Biol Psychiatry*, **36**, 326–337.

LeMarquand, D.G., Benkelfat, C., Pihl, R.O., Palmour, R.M. and Young, S.N., 1999. Behavioural disinhibition induced by tryptophan depletion in nonalcoholic young men with multigenerational family histories of paternal alcoholism. *Am J Psychiatry*, **156**, 1771–1779.

Lewis, C.E., 1991. Neurochemical mechanisms of chronic antisocial behaviour (psychopathy). A literature review. *J Nerv Ment Dis*, **179**, 720–727.

Lewis, D.O., Pincus, J.H., Shanok, S.S. and Glaser, G.H., 1982. Psychomotor epilepsy and violence in a group of incarcerated adolescent boys. *Am J Psychiatry*, **139**, 882–887.

Lidberg, L., Asberg, M. and Sundqvist-Stensman, U.B., 1984. 5-Hydroxyindoleacetic acid levels in attempted suicides who have killed their children. *Lancet*, **2**(8408), 928.

Lidberg, L., Belfrage, H., Bertilsson, L., Evenden, M.M. and Asberg, M., 2000. Suicide attempts and impulse control disorder are related to low cerebrospinal fluid 5-HIAA in mentally disordered violent offenders. *Acta Psychiatr Scand*, **101**, 395–402.

Linden, R.D., Pope, H.G., Jr and Jonas, J.M., 1986. Pathological gambling and major affective disorder: preliminary findings. *J Clin Psychiatry*, **47**, 201–203.

Linnoila, M., Virkkunen, M., Scheinin, M., Nuutila, A., Rimon, R. and Goodwin, F.K., 1983. Low cerebrospinal fluid 5-hydroxyindoleacetic acid concentration differentiates impulsive from nonimpulsive violent behaviour. *Life Sci*, **33**, 2609–2614.

Lishman, W.A., 1968. Brain damage in relation to psychiatric disability after head injury. *Br J Psychiatry*, **114**, 373–410.

Luria, A.R., 1980. *Higher Cortical Functions in Man*. Basic Books, New York.

Maes, M., van West, D., De Vos, N., Westenberg, H., Van Hunsel, F., Hendriks, D., Cosyns, P. and Scharpe, S., 2001. Lower baseline plasma cortisol and prolactin together with increased body temperature and higher mCPP-induced cortisol responses in men with pedophilia. *Neuropsychopharmacology*, **24**, 37–46.

Manuck, S.B., Flory, J.D., Ferrell, R.E., Dent, K.M., Mann, J.J. and Muldoon, M.F., 1999. Aggression and anger-related traits associated with a polymorphism of the tryptophan hydroxylase gene. *Biol Psychiatry*, **45**, 603–614.

Marazziti, D. and Conti, L., 1991. Aggression, hyperactivity and platelet imipramine binding. *Acta Psychiatr Scand*, **84**, 209–211.

Markowitz, P.I., 1990. Fluoxetine treatment of self-injurious behaviour in mentally retarded patients [letter]. *J Clin Psychopharmacol*, **10**, 299–300.

Markowitz, P.I., 1992. Effect of fluoxetine on self-injurious behaviour in the developmentally disabled: a preliminary study. *J Clin Psychopharmacol*, **12**, 27–31.

Marlowe, W.B., Mancall, E.L. and Thomas, J.J., 1975. Complete Kluver-Bucy syndrome in man. *Cortex*, **11**, 53–59.

McBurnett, K., Lahey, B.B., Rathouz, P.J. and Loeber, R., 2000. Low salivary cortisol and persistent aggression in boys referred for disruptive behaviour. *Arch Gen Psychiatry*, **57**, 38–43.

McElroy, S.L., Hudson, J.I., Pope, H.G. and Keck, P.E., 1991. Kleptomania: clinical characteristics and associated psychopathology. *Psychol Med*, **21**, 93–108.

Meltzer, H.Y. and Maes, M., 1995. Pindolol pretreatment blocks stimulation by meta-chlorophenylpiperazine of prolactin but not cortisol secretion in normal men. *Psychiatry Res*, **58**, 89–98.

Miczek, K.A., De Bold, J.F., Van Erp, A.M. and Tornatzky, W., 1997. Alcohol, $GABA_A$-benzodiazepine receptor complex and aggression. *Recent Dev Alcohol*, **13**, 139–171.

Moss, H.B., Yao, J.K. and Panzak, G.L., 1990. Serotonergic responsivity and behavioural dimensions in antisocial personality disorder with substance abuse. *Biol Psychiatry*, **28**, 325–338.

Nachson, I., 1988. Hemisphere function in violent offenders. In: Moffitt, T.E. and Mednick, S.A. (eds), *Biological Contributions to Crime Causation*, pp. 55–67. Martinus Nijhoff, Dordrecht, Germany.

Nakamura, K., Kurasawa, M. and Shirane, M., 2000. Impulsivity and AMPA receptors: aniracetam ameliorates impulsive behaviour induced by a blockade of AMPA receptors in rats. *Brain Res*, **17**(1–2), 266–269.

New, A.S., Trestman, R.L., Mitropoulou, V., Benishay, D.S., Coccaro, E., Silverman, J. and Siever, L.J., 1997. Serotonergic function and self-injurious behaviour in personality disorder patients. *Psychiatry Res*, **69**, 17–26.

New, A.S., Gelernter, J., Yovell, Y., Trestman, R.L., Nielsen, D.A., Silverman, J., Mitropoulou, V. and Siever, L.J., 1998. Tryptophan hydroxylase genotype is associated with impulsive-aggression measures: a preliminary study. *Am J Med Genet*, **81**, 13–17.

Niehoff, D.L. and Kuhar, M.J., 1983. Benzodiazepine receptors: localization in rat amygdala. *J Neurosci*, **3**, 2091–2097.

Nielsen, D.A., Goldman, D., Virkkunen, M., Tokola, R., Rawlings, R. and Linnoila, M., 1994. Suicidality and 5-hydroxyindoleacetic acid concentration associated with a tryptophan hydroxylase polymorphism. *Arch Gen Psychiatry*, **51**, 34–38.

Nolan, K.A., Volavka, J., Lachman, H.M. and Saito, T., 2000. An association between a polymorphism of the tryptophan hydroxylase gene and aggression in schizophrenia and schizoaffective disorder. *Psychiatr Genet*, **10**, 109–115.

Oquendo, M.A. and Mann, J.J., 2000. The biology of impulsivity and suicidality. *Psychiatr Clin North Am*, **23**, 11–25.

Ovsiew, F. and Yudofsky, S., 1983. *Aggression: A Neuropsychiatric Perspective*. In: Glick, R.A. and Roose, S.P. (eds), *Rage, Power, and Aggression: The Role of Affect in Motivation, Development and Adaptation*, pp. 213–230. Yale University Press, New Haven CT.

Pallanti, S., Quercioli, L., Sood, E. and Hollander, E. (2002 in press). Lithium and valproate treatment of pathological gambling: a randomized single-blind study. *J Clin Psychiatry*.

Pfaff, D.W., Vasudevan, N., Kia, H.K., Zhu, Y.S., Chan, J., Garey, J., Morgan, M. and Ogawa, S., 2000. Estrogens, brain and behaviour: studies in fundamental neurobiology and observations related to women's health. *J Steroid Biochem Mol Biol*, **74**, 365–373.

Pruus, K., Skrebuhhova-Malmros, T., Rudissaar, R., Matto, V. and Allikmets, L., 2000. 5-HT_{1A} receptor agonists buspirone and gepirone attenuate apomorphine-induced aggressive behaviour in adult male Wistar rats. *J Physiol Pharmacol*, **51**(4 Pt 2), 833–846.

Raine, A., Meloy, J.R., Bihrle, S., Stoddard, J., LaCasse, L. and Buchsbaum, M.S., 1998. Reduced prefrontal and increased subcortical brain functioning assessed using positron emission tomography in predatory and affective murderers. *Behav Sci Law*, **16**, 319–332.

Raine, A., Lencz, T., Bihrle, S., LaCasse, L. and Colletti, P., 2000. Reduced prefrontal gray matter volume and reduced autonomic activity in antisocial personality disorder. *Arch Gen Psychiatry*, **57**, 119–127; discussion 128–289.

Ramboz, S., Saudou, F., Amara, D.A., Belzung, C., Segu, L., Misslin, R., Buhot, M.C. and Hen, R., 1996 5-HT_{1B} receptor knock-out behavioural consequences. *Behav Brain Res*, **73**, 305–312.

Ramboz, S., Oosting, R., Amara, D.A., Kung, H.F., Blier, P., Mendelsohn, M., Mann, J.J., Brunner, D. and Hen, R., 1998. Serotonin receptor 1A knockout: an animal model of anxiety related disorder. *Proc Natl Acad Sci USA*, **95**, 14476–14481.

Ramirez, L.F., McCormick, R.A., Russo, A.M. and Taber, J.I., 1983. Patterns of substance abuse in pathological gamblers undergoing treatment. *Addict Behav*, **8**, 425–428.

Reeves, A.G. and Plum, F., 1969. Hyperphagia, rage, and dementia accompanying a ventromedial hypothalamic neoplasm. *Arch Neurol*, **20**, 616–624.

Richardson, J.S. and Zaleski, W.A., 1983. Naloxone and self-mutilation. *Biol Psychiatry*, **18**, 99–101.

Rodriguez-Arias, M., Felip, C.M., Broseta, I. and Minarro, J., 1999. The dopamine D_3 antagonists U-99194A maleate increases social behaviours of isolation-induced aggressive male mice. *Psychopharmacology*, **144**, 90–94.

Rogers, R.D., Everitt, B.J., Baldacchino, A., Blackshaw, A.J., Swainson, R., Wynne, K., Baker, N.B., Hunter, J., Carthy, T., Booker, E. and London, M., 1999. Dissociable deficits in the decision-making cognition of chronic amphetamine abusers, opiate abusers, patients with focal damage to prefrontal cortex, and tryptophan-depleted normal volunteers: evidence for monoaminergic mechanisms. *Neuropsychopharmacology*, **20**, 322–339.

Rudissaar, R., Pruus, K., Skrebuhkova-Malmros, T., Allikmets, L. and Matto, V., 2000. Involvement of GABAergic neurotransmission in the neurobiology of the apomorphine-induced aggressive behaviour paradigm, a model of psychotic behaviour in rats. *Methods Find Exp Clin Pharmacol*, **22**, 637–640.

Sabrie, P., 1986. Reconciling the role of central serotonin neurons in human and animal behaviour. *Behav Brain Sci*, **9**, 319–364.

Saiz, J., Moreno, I. and Lopez-Ibor, J.J., 1992. Ludopatia: estudio clinico y terapeutico-evolutivo de un grupo de jugadores patologicos. *Acta Luso Esp Neurologia Psiquiatrica*, **46**, 1429–1435.

Sanchez-Martin, J.R., Fano, E., Ahedo, L., Cardas, J., Brain, P.F. and Azpiroz, A., 2000. Relating testosterone levels and free play social behaviour in male and female preschool children. *Psychoneuroendocrinology*, **25**, 773–783.

Sandman, C.A., Barron, J.L., Crinella, F.M. and Donelly, J.F., 1987. Influence of naloxone on brain and behaviour of a self-mutilating woman. *Biol Psychiatry*, **22**, 899–906.

Saudou, F., Amara, D.A., Dierih, A., LeMeur, M., Ramboz, S., Segu, L., Buhot, M.C. and Hen, R., 1994. Enhanced aggressive behaviour in mice lacking 5-HT_{1B} receptor. *Science*, **265**, 1875–1878.

Scearce-Levie, K., Viswanathan, S.S. and Hen, R., 1999. Locomotor response to MDMA is attenuated in knockout mice lacking the 5-HT_{1B} receptor. *Psychopharmacology*, **141**, 154–161.

Schulz, S.C., Camlin, K.L., Berry, S.A. and Jesberger, J.A., 1999. Olanzapine safety and efficacy in patients with borderline personality disorder and comorbid dysthymia. *Biol Psychiatry*, **46**, 1429–1435.

Serafetinides, E.A., 1965. The EEG effects of LSD-25 in epileptic patients before and after temporal lobectomy. *Psychopharmacologia*, **7**, 453–460.

Shaffer, D., Schonfeld, I., O'Connor, P.A., Stokman, C., Trautman, P., Shafer, S. and Ng, S., 1985. Neurological soft signs. Their relationship to psychiatric disorder and intelligence in childhood and adolescence. *Arch Gen Psychiatry*, **42**, 342–351.

Shih, J.C., Chen, K., Ridd, M.J. and Seif, I., 2000. *Ginkgo biloba* abolishes aggression in mice lacking MAO A. *Antioxid Redox Signal*, **2**, 467–471.

Siever, L.J., Buchsbaum, M.S., New, A.S., Spiegel-Cohen, J., Wei, T., Hazlett, E.A., Sevin, E., Nunn, M. and Mitropoulou, V., 1999. d,l-Fenfluramine response in impulsive personality disorder assessed with [18F]fluorodeoxyglucose positron emission tomography. *Neuropsychopharmacology*, **20**, 413–423.

Soderpalm, B. and Svensson, A.I., 1999. Naloxone reverses disinhibitory/aggressive behavior in 5,7-DHT-lesioned rats; involvement of GABAA receptor blockade? *Neuropharmacology*, **38**, 1851–1859.

Soloff, P.H., George, A., Nathan, R.S., Schulz, P.M., Ulrich, R.F. and Perel, J.M., 1986. Progress in pharmacotherapy of borderline disorders. A double-blind study of amitriptyline, haloperidol, and placebo. *Arch Gen Psychiatry*, **43**, 691–697.

Soloff, P.H., Meltzer, C.C., Greer, P.J., Constantine, D. and Kelly, T.M., 2000. A fenfluramine-activated FDG-PET study of borderline personality disorder. *Biol Psychiatry*, **47**, 540–547.

Stanley, B., Molcho, A., Stanley, M., Winchel, R., Gameroff, M.J., Parsons, B. and Mann, J.J., 2000. Association of aggressive behavior with altered serotonergic function in patients who are not suicidal. *Am J Psychiatry*, **157**, 609–614.

Stein, D.J., Hollander, E., Cohen, L., Simeon, D. and Aronowitz, B., 1995a. Serotonergic responsivity in trichotillomania: neuroendrocrine effects of m-chlorophenylpiperazine. *Biol Psychiatry*, **37**, 414–416.

Stein, D.J., Simeon, D., Frenkel, M., Islam, M.N. and Hollander, E., 1995b An open trial of valproate in borderline personality disorder. *J Clin Psychiatry*, **56**, 506–510.

Stoff, D.M., Pollock, L., Vitiello, B., Behar, D. and Bridger, W.H., 1987. Reduction of (3H)-imipramine binding sites on platelets of conduct-disordered children. *Neuropsychopharmacology*, **1**, 55–62.

Stoff, D.M., Ieni, J., Friedman, E., Bridger, W.H., Pollock, L. and Vitiello, B., 1991. Platelet 3H-imipramine binding, serotonin uptake, and plasma alpha 1 acid glycoprotein in disruptive behaviour disorders. *Biol Psychiatry*, **29**, 494–498.

Sudak, H.W. and Maas, J.W., 1964. Behavioural neurochemical correlation in reactive and nonreactive strains of rats. *Science*, **146**, 418–420.

Svensson, A.I., Berntsson, A., Engel, J.A. and Soderpalm, B., 2000. Disinhibitory behaviour and GABAA receptor function in serotonin-depleted adult male rats are reduced by gonadectomy. *Pharmacol Biochem Behav*, **67**, 613–620.

Terzian, H. and Ore, J.D., 1955. Syndrome of Kluver and Bucy reproduced in man by bilateral removal of the temporal lobes. *Neurology*, **5**, 373–380.

Turecki, G., Zhu, Z., Tzenova, J., Lesage, A., Seguin, M., Tousignant, M., Chawky, N., Vanier, C., Lipp, O., Alda, M., Joober, R., Benkelfat, C. and Rouleau, G.A., 2001. TPH and suicidal behaviour: a study in suicide completers. *Mol Psychiatry*, **6**, 98–102.

Van Erp, A.M. and Miczek, K.A., 2000. Aggressive behavior, increased accumbal dopamine, and decreased cortical serotonin in rats. *J Neurosci*, **20**, 9320–9325.

Van Goozen, S.H., Van den Ban, E., Matthys, W., Cohen-Kettenis, P.T., Thijssen, J.H. and van Engeland, H., 2000. Increased adrenal androgen functioning in children with oppositional defiant disorder. A comparison with psychiatric and normal controls. *J Am Acad Child Adolesc Psychiatry*, **39**, 1446–1451.

Virkkunen, M., 1985. Urinary free cortisol secretion in habitually violent offenders. *Acta Psychiatr Scand*, **72**, 40–44.

Virkkunen, M. and Linnoila, M., 1990. Serotonin in early onset, male alcoholics with violent behaviour. *Ann Med*, **22**, 327–331.

Virkkunen, M., Rawlings, R., Tokola, R., Poland, R.E., Guidotti, A., Nemeroff, C., Bissette, G., Kalogeras, K., Karonen, S.L. and

Linnoila, M., 1994. CSF biochemistries, glucose metabolism, and diurnal activity rhythms in alcoholic, violent offenders, fire setters, and healthy volunteers. *Arch Gen Psychiatry*, **51**, 20–27.

Vitiello, B., Behar, D., Hunt, J., Stoff, D. and Ricciuti, A., 1990. Subtyping aggression in children and adolescents. *J Neuropsychiatry Clin Neurosci*, **2**, 189–192.

Vitiello, B. and Stoff, D.M., 1997. Subtypes of aggression and their relevance to child psychiatry. *J Am Acad Child Adolesc Psychiatry*, **36**, 307–315.

Wasman, M. and Flynn, J.P., 1962. Directed attack elicited from the hypothalamus. *Arch Neurol*, **6**, 220–227.

Weiger, W.A. and Bear, D.M., 1988. An approach to the neurology of aggression. *J Psychiatr Res*, **22**, 85–98.

Yatham, L.N. and Steiner, M., 1993. Neuroendocrine probes of serotonergic function: a critical review. *Life Sci*, **53**, 447–463.

Zhang, J.X., Harper, R.M. and Ni, H.F., 1986. Cryogenic blockade of the central nucleus of the amygdala attenuates aversively conditioned blood pressure and respiratory responses. *Brain Res*, **386**(1–2), 136–145.

Zhuang, X., Gross, C., Santarelli, L., Compan, V., Trillat, A.C. and Hen, R., 1999. Altered emotional states in knockout mice lacking 5-HT_{1A} or 5-HT_{1B} receptors. *Neurpsychopharmacology*, **21**(Suppl. 2), 52S–60S.

XXVI

Personality Disorders

XXVI-1

Animal Models of Personality

A.R. Cools and B.A. Ellenbroek

PERSONALITY AND ITS DISORDERS

In practice, we need to be able to assess personality in order to predict how patients will respond to illness and to treatment. We also need to be able to manage people with personalities that cause serious problems to themselves or other people. As elaborated in the next paragraph on 'basic dimensions of personality', the term 'personality' refers to the balance between various traits. If one or more dominant traits are strong enough to cause difficulties to the person or to other people, the person is said to have a personality disorder. However, the borderline between normal personality and personality disorders is hard to define. In fact, there is no reliable and valid measure that allows a cut-off for distinguishing between normality and disorder. In clinical practice, therefore, a personality is said to be disordered when it causes suffering to the person or to other people. It is evident that such a criterion is impossible to model in animals. Indeed, animal models of personality disorders are not available, unless one adheres to the traditional classification system for personality disorders: in that case, we are dealing with animal models for anxiety disorders, mood disorders, etc., as discussed in several other chapters of this textbook.

Recently, however, Cloninger *et al.* (1994) have introduced a new classification system that allows differential diagnosis of personality disorders with the help of temperament and character descriptors. As outlined below, it is possible to model a number of these temperament descriptors in animals. In this chapter, we will focus on these and related studies.

BASIC DIMENSIONS OF PERSONALITY

In the first place we should clarify what we want to model. Thus, we should delineate the basic units of personality. As elaborated by Zuckerman (1991), the basic unit in personality psychology is the trait, defined as a group of related habits that, in turn, are defined as consistent behaviours in specific situations. Using this definition, Zuckerman suggests that the term 'basic dimensions of personality' should refer to

> supertraits that have internal reliability and can be identified in terms of their constituent traits across methods, genders, and cultures; these supertraits should be identifiable in childhood but not necessarily in infancy; the basic personality traits should show consistency over time (but because the phenotype and environment interact throughout life, one would not expect perfect or even near perfect consistency over long periods of time); they should be identifiable in species other than the human on the assumption that they have been shaped by natural selection; they should show at least moderate heritability and be related to significant biological markers; and, eventually, their biological basis in the structure and physiology of the nervous system should be identifiable, though classification is a necessary first step in biological bases of traits (pp. 40–41).

Unfortunately, there is no general agreement about the kind of classification system to be used for classifying fundamental traits. In psychiatry, there are at least two types of classification systems: the traditional system that distinguishes 5–7 dimensions resulting from factor analyses of the phenotypic structure of personality, and a more recently introduced functional classification system that is based on largely hypothetical characteristics of central nervous system functioning. The traditional classification system has resulted, among others, in the three-factor model of Eysenck (1947), encompassing the factors introversion-extraversion (E), neuroticism (N) (or emotional instability), and psychoticism (P); the five-factor model of Fiske (1949) and, later, Norman (1963), encompassing the factors extraversion, agreeableness, consciousness, emotional stability, and culture; and the seven personality dimensions of Zuckerman, which are activity, sociability, impulsivity, socialization, sensation seeking, emotionality (subdivided into general, anxiety, and hostility), and social desirability (Zuckerman *et al.*, 1988). As elaborated elsewhere, this traditional classification system suffers from several shortcomings (Cloninger *et al.*, 1994; van Praag, 1986; Tuinier and Verhoeven, 1995), the most important one being the fact that the entities classified are still complex behaviours that are not yet sufficiently broken down into specific and elementary items that are mutually exclusive and, in addition, theoretically tractable in the brain. Anyhow, animal models for some of these dimensions, especially anxiety in particular and emotionality in general, are discussed elsewhere in this book.

More recently, Cloninger has developed a neurobiologically based model to guide the rational development of descriptors for temperament and character (Cloninger, 1994). Temperament refers to those components of personality that are heritable, developmentally stable, emotion-based, or uninfluenced by sociocultural learning (Goldsmith *et al.*, 1987), whereas character refers to those components of personality that are weakly heritable, and are moderately influenced by sociocultural learning (Loehlin, 1982). His model is based on the synthesis of information from twin and family studies, studies on longitudinal development, and neuropharmacological and neurobehavioural studies of learning in human and other animals, as well as psychometric studies of personality in individuals and twin pairs. Though the neurobiological processes are not yet identified, he proposes four temperament dimensions on the basis of individual differences in associative learning that are postulated to be genetically homogeneous and independent of one another: 'novelty seeking', which is associated with the behavioural activation system; 'harm avoidance', which is associated with the behavioural inhibition system; 'reward dependence', which is associated with the behavioural dependence system; and 'persistence', which is associated with the behavioural persistence system. The dimension 'novelty seeking' nicely corresponds with Zuckerman's dimension 'sensation seeking' (McCourt *et al.*, 1983). Cloninger complements his model of personality with three character dimensions, self-directed behaviour, cooperativeness, and self-transcendence.

Biological Psychiatry: Edited by H. D'haenen, J.A. den Boer and P. Willner. ISBN 0-471-49198-5

Because this definition of character refers to self-concepts and individual differences in goals and values, which influence voluntary choices, intentions, and the meaning of what is experienced in life, it is evident that these character dimensions are difficult to model in animals. For that reason, they are not considered in this chapter.

The authors of this chapter regard Cloninger's classification system as a very powerful model that provides four temperament dimensions that fulfil all criteria summarized by Zuckerman (1991): among others, they are moderately heritable, stable from childhood through adulthood, and structurally consistent in different cultures and ethnic groups (Cloninger *et al.*, 1994). Furthermore, it is interesting to note that Cloninger's four temperaments to some extent correspond to the four basic emotions of anger (*novelty seeking*), fear (*harm avoidance*), love (*reward dependence*), and tenacity (*persistence*), as well as with a modern interpretation of the ancient temperaments the choleric (*novelty seeking*), the melancholic (*harm avoidance*), the sanguine (*reward dependence*), and the phlegmatic (*persistence*). The model of Cloninger *et al.* (1994) is especially powerful, because it has given rise to the development of a validated guide that allows a clear-cut definition of personality disorders with the help of the so-called 'temperament and character inventory' (TCI) scales. In other words, each individual personality disorder is defined as a configural function of all seven temperament and character dimensions. The correlations between TCI scales and various symptoms for individual personality disorders according to DSM-IV classification are illustrated in Table XXVI-1.1 (Svrakic *et al.*, 1993). This table also shows that individuals can fall into disorders in multiple clusters because the temperament dimensions are independent, not mutually exclusive. To what extent Cloninger's dimensions of temperament are identifiable in species other than the human is discussed below. We will also discuss whether the biological basis of these dimensions can be identified in the structure and physiology of the nervous system.

CRITERIA FOR ANIMAL MODELS

Modelling aspects of human personality in animals should result in animal models that meet criteria that allow validation of the models. Though such generally accepted criteria for animal models of normal human behaviour are missing, such criteria are formulated for animal models of abnormal human behaviour. In the latter field, it is quite common to subdivide animal models by specifying the presumed validity of the models. This has led to three different sets of models, which are hierarchically related (Willner, 1984):

1. animal models with predictive validity of the lowest class
2. animal models with face validity of the second class
3. animal models with construct validity of the highest class.

By modifying the set of criteria for each of these models, we can try to formulate criteria for animal models of normal human behaviour. By analogy with the predictive validity of the animal models for human disorders (that is, predicated on the prediction they make with respect to pharmacotherapy), the predictive validity of animal models for normal human behaviour should be based on the prediction they make with respect to treatments and/or environmental conditions that are known to alter specifically the behaviour in question. Though early environmental factors, brain injury, delay in brain development, childhood experience, and the use of alcohol or drugs are assumed to contribute to the occurrence of abnormal behaviour in people with personality disorders, there is no convincing evidence that these factors alter a particular behaviour in a specific and selective manner. Indeed, animal models with predictive validity for normal human behaviour are not yet available. By analogy with the face validity of animal models for human disorders (which are predicated on symptom similarity), the face validity of normal human behaviour should be based on convincing similarity of the behavioural phenomenon between the model and the target behaviour. As mentioned below, there are animal models that fit into this category. Finally, by analogy with the construct validity of animal models for human disorders, the construct validity of animal models for normal human behaviour should be based on convincing similarity of causes and (neuro)biology of the behavioural phenomenon between the model and the target behaviour. In our opinion, the animal models of *novelty seeking* that are discussed below, appear to fit into this category.

Table XXVI-1.1 Correlations between Cloninger's Temperament and Character Inventory (TCI) Scales and number of symptoms for individual personality disorders (Modified from Svrakic *et al.*, 1993)

TCI scale scores Personality disorder symptoms	NS	HA	RD	P	SD	C	ST
Antisocial (adult)	H	—	L	—	L	L	—
Histrionic	H	—	—	—	L	L	—
Borderline	H	H	—	—	L	L	—
Passive-aggressive	H	—	—	L	L	L	—
Avoidant	L	H	—	—	L	—	—
Obsessive-compulsive	—	H	—	—	L	L	—
Dependent	—	H	H	—	L	—	—
Schizoid	—	—	L	—	L	L	L
Schizotypal	—	H	L	—	L	L	—
Paranoid	H	—	L	—	L	L	—

H = high scores.
L = low scores.
P = persistence.
NS = novelty seeking.
SD = self-directedness.
HA = harm avoidance.
C = cooperativeness.
RD = reward dependence.
ST = self-transcendence.

INDIRECT APPROACHES IN ANIMAL STUDIES

In the traditional biological approach to personality, the independent variables are behavioural and the dependent variables biological. Because there are also other approaches in this field that can shed light on selected aspects of personality, it is worthwhile to consider these approaches as well.

Gene-Oriented Approach

Following human studies on the association of various gene alleles with a particular trait or temperament dimension, animal models are developed by assessing behavioural or molecular genetic strategies to trace the genes and their involvement in the trait or dimension under study. The following can illustrate this approach. Studies on the association of dopamine-receptor genes and human behaviour including personality traits have provided evidence that the *Taq* I A D2 dopamine-receptor (DRD2) minor (A1) allele and the 7-repeat (7R) allele of the D4 dopamine-receptor (DRD4) gene D2 polymorphisms individually associate with *novelty-seeking* behaviour (Benjamin *et al.*, 1996; Noble *et al.*, 1998; Noble, 2000; cf. Herbst *et al.*, 2000). Predicated on these findings, two types of animal models are of interest. By the quantitative trait loci (QLT) technique in recombinant inbred mouse strains, it has become possible to show that the QTLs for alcohol preference drinking are localized in the region of the DRD2 (Tarantino *et al.*, 1998). The next question, of course, is whether or not this gene is also associated with the animal counterpart of human novelty seeking. Another animal model in this respect involves mice that lack functional dopamine D2 receptors: such mice are marked by a severe reduction of alcohol- and opiate-related behaviours (Maldonado *et al.*, 1997). In this case, it is also important to know whether these mice are marked by a reduced amount of the animal counterpart of human novelty seeking. These models can be very helpful in laying the foundation for new hypotheses about the involvement of particular genes in personality dimensions, but at the same time they are less suitable for elucidating the genetic complexity of personality dimensions, because the independent variables are biological rather than behavioural.

Substrate-Oriented Approach

Following human studies in which biological correlates and/or substrates of a particular behaviour, trait, or temperament dimension have been mapped, animal models are developed by manipulating the biological correlate or substrate in question, in the hope that the resulting models can help to elucidate the biological mechanisms of the phenomenon under study, and even to discover new treatments for abnormal behaviours that are inherent in a disorder of that trait or temperament dimension. For example, human studies have shown that there is relationship between sensation seeking (*novelty seeking*), violent suicide, homicide, arson, psychopathology or substance abuse with decreased cerebrospinal fluid levels of the main serotonin metabolite 5-hydroxyindoleacetic acid (Lewis, 1991; Virkkunen *et al.*, 1994). Given these findings, together with the notion that serotonin (5-HT) deficiency may be associated with impulsive, disinhibited, and aggressive behaviours (cf. Soubrie, 1986), two kinds of animal models have been developed. One model involves extensive depletion of brain 5-HT by means of 5-HT synthesis inhibition or selective neurotoxic lesioning of 5-HT neurons (Söderpalm and Svensson, 1999). Given the therapeutic efficacy of the opiate receptor antagonist naloxone in this model, it is suggested that this drug may represent a new pharmacological principle for the treatment of impulse-control disorders (Söderpalm and Svensson, 1999). Another animal model involves the selective breeding of rat lines that show a differential physiological response to stimulation of the 5-HT1A receptors, namely, the high and low sensitivity responding lines (HDL and LDS, respectively), since these receptors have been implicated in a variety of disorders, including anxiety and alcoholism. This approach has generated data suggesting that the HDL line is a useful model for a type of high trait anxiety linked to susceptibility to depression (Knapp *et al.*, 1998). Though such models can certainly provide new insights into the relevance of certain biological mechanisms involved in the traits or temperament dimensions under discussion, they are primarily of heuristic value because the independent variables are biological, but not behavioural. Nevertheless, these models can be very helpful in laying the foundation for new hypotheses about the biological mechanisms that underlie the particular personality dimension under discussion.

Physiology-Oriented Approach

Following the finding in human studies (Zuckerman *et al.*, 1974) that high sensation seekers (*high novelty seekers*) show increasing amplitudes of visual evoked potentials (VEP) as a function of flash intensity (VEP augmenters), in contrast to low sensation seekers (*low novelty seekers*), who show decreasing VEP amplitudes as a function of flash intensity (VEP reducers), Siegel and co-workers have looked at animals with a bimodal distribution of certain behavioural features. Initially, VEP responses were compared in cats that vary in terms of their behavioural response to novel and threatening stimuli: active and explorative cats showing approach behaviour even to threatening stimuli turned out to be VEP augmenters, whereas less active cats showing withdrawal responses turned out to be VEP reducers (Saxton *et al.*, 1987a). An additional interesting finding was that VEP augmenter cats learn a novel and simple bar press task much faster than VEP reducer cats (Saxton *et al.*, 1987b). In this context, it is interesting to note that high responders to novelty, considered as the rodent counterpart of novelty seekers (see below), also learn a simple radial-maze task much faster than low responders to novelty (Cools *et al.*, 1993c). Siegel later reported that the Swiss line of the Roman high avoidance (RHA) rats are VEP augmenters, in contrast to the Swiss line of the Roman low avoidance (RLA) rats, who are VEP reducers (Siegel *et al.*, 1993). Again, these animal models are primarily of heuristic value, because in these models the independent variables are biological rather than behavioural. Still, these models can help us to formulate new hypotheses about the biological mechanisms that underlie the particular personality dimension under discussion.

Behaviour-Oriented Approach

Given the enormous individual variation in human behaviour, traits, or temperaments, animal research has focused attention on individual differences in behaviour in its broadest sense. In practice, three research strategies are assessed:

1. comparing features of individuals belonging to different inbred strains of animals, usually rodents (e.g., RHA vs. RLA rats [Driscoll *et al.*, 1998], Lewis vs. Fischer rats [Sternberg *et al.*, 1989] or C57BL/6 vs. DBA/2 mice [Cabib and Puglisi-Allegra, 1988]);
2. comparing features of intrastrain individuals that are selected on the basis of a particular behaviour or trait (e.g., winner vs. loser rats [Masur *et al.*, 1995]);
3. comparing features of intrastrain individuals that differ in terms of behaviour because of known individual-specific features of the physiological state of the brain (Cools *et al.*, 1990).

The first approach has the disadvantage that one is dealing with different inbred strains, each of them marked by a genotypic uniformity that is not only greater than it is in the initial outbred population, but also accompanied by a loss of the originally present variation that is necessary for survival in changing environments. This does not match the human situation. The second approach is far better in this respect, but has the disadvantage that it remains unknown whether the variable used for the selection is a primary feature or just an intervening variable. The final approach lacks these shortcomings, since in this strategy the behavioural variable that is used for the selection is not an intervening variable but, instead, a basic feature, the consequence of a well-delineated and known physiological state of the brain. As discussed in the next paragraph, the latter approach has resulted in an animal that seems to be a highly interesting animal counterpart of the human novelty seeker. In general, the behaviour-oriented approach has provided a large amount of data that are primarily descriptive and correlative by nature. In principle, individual animals, related lines, or related strains are selected on the basis of a particular behavioural variant. The extent to which the behavioural variant is associated with other behavioural features that are considered to be features of a particular trait or temperament dimension is then investigated. Apart from this, one commonly investigates to what extent the behavioural variant is associated with physiological, neurochemical, and neuroendocrine and pharmacological variables. Using this approach, Gentsch *et al.* (1988) have shown that three distinct kind of pairings of rats resulted in a remarkably similar dichotomy across these pairings: RHA, spontaneously hypertensive (SHR) rats and individually housed Wistar rats are marked by lower emotionality (shown in factors such as decreased defecation and corticosterone secretion) than their respective counterparts, RLA,

Wistar-Kyoto rats and group-housed rats. Of course, the question arises why rats selected for extremes in the shuttle box performance (RHA/RLA), blood pressure (SHR/Wistar Kyoto rat), or variation in housing conditions show similar intrapair differences. Though these findings may lead to the hypothesis that these rats are all characterized by a similar idiosyncrasy in relation to emotionality, the similarities in the differences between the various pairings have to be considered as merely coincidences if there is no evidence that the distinct variables used for the selection are part of a cross-situational consistency in brain and behavioural physiology. Thus, the animal models that belong to this category can provide very useful information, although these models should not be considered as animal models for aspects of personality.

Construct-Oriented Approach

Though this approach does not deal with animal models as such, it assesses animal studies to provide insight into neurobiological processes that underlie various aspects of personality. In general, basic constructs about the functioning of the brain and body that are based on theoretical and empirical knowledge are used to relate temperament dimensions to processes and circuitries in the body and brain. Once such a relationship is hypothesized, animal experiments can be performed to (in)validate such hypotheses. An example that clearly illustrates this approach is provided by studies recently reviewed by Davidson (1999). In short, on the basis of a large number of human studies, Davidson developed a model that features individual differences in prefrontal asymmetry as a reflection of a diathesis that modulates reactivity to emotionally significant events. It was then hypothesized that if individual differences in prefrontal asymmetry are associated with a dispositional affective type, such differences should be related to cortisol levels, since individual differences in baseline cortisol levels have been related to various aspects of trait-related stressful behaviour (Davidson, 1999). They indeed found that individual differences in cortisol levels in nonhuman primates predict biological measures that are related to affective style (Kalin *et al.*, 1998). Though our present-day knowledge about the functioning of the brain is limited and, consequently, the available hypotheses in this respect are by definition speculative, this approach is very promising, because it helps us to develop new constructs about the functional anatomy of fundamental dimensions of personality.

DIRECT APPROACH IN ANIMAL STUDIES

As already mentioned above, in the traditional approach to personality the independent variables are behavioural and the dependent variables biological: we label this strategy the 'trait-oriented approach'. A description of the behavioural features of a particular trait or temperament is used to model these features in animals. The demonstration of a convincing similarity in the behavioural phenomenon between the model and the target behaviour provides an animal model with face validity and perhaps even with construct validity.

As clarified above, the authors of this chapter regard the classification system of Cloninger as the most powerful system for two reasons. First, the resulting four temperaments meet all criteria that are set for basic dimensions of personality. Second, the classification system provides the basis for differential diagnosis of personality disorders. Below we consider animal models for the four temperament dimensions delineated by Cloninger (1994).

Persistence

This dimension is hypothesized to be a heritable tendency to maintain behaviour in response to a) signals of anticipated reward, b) intermittent punishment, and c) intermittent frustrative non-reward. Today, animal models of *persistence* are not yet available. According to Cloninger, this dimension is mediated and modulated by the behavioural persistence system that encompasses the hippocampal subiculum, the anterior cingulate cortex and the orbitomedial cortex. Assessment of the above-mentioned construct-approach might help us to develop new constructs about the functional anatomy of this fundamental dimension of personality.

Reward Dependence

This dimension is hypothesized to be a heritable tendency to respond intensely to signals of reward and to maintain or resist extinction of behaviour that has previously been related to rewards or relief from punishment. It can be suggested that individuals of the monogamous vole species serve as animal model, because they show a greater social affiliation with their partner, a larger distress in response to isolation, and a larger sensitivity to social cues than individuals of the polygamous vole species (cf. Insel *et al.*, 1993). According to Cloninger (1994), this dimension is mediated and modulated by the behavioural dependence system that encompasses the lateral amygdala, the bed nucleus of the stria terminalis, the nucleus accumbens, the midline thalamus, and the prelimbic cortex in which oxytocin plays a key role. Thus, a theoretical and empirical analysis of the function of these structures might help us to develop new constructs about the functional anatomy of this fundamental dimension of personality.

Harm Avoidance

This dimension is hypothesized to be a heritable tendency to respond intensely to signals of aversive stimuli, thereby learning to inhibit behaviour in order to avoid punishment, novelty, and frustrated non-reward. If one regards high frequency of defecation under bright lights in a novel environment and/or immobility with bradycardia in response to foot shock as indicators of *harm avoidance* in animals, one can suggest that individuals of the Maudsley reactive rat line (MR) (cf. Broadhurst, 1975) serve as animal models for a high degree of harm avoidance, because they are higher defecators in a novel environments (MR) than their counterparts, individuals of the Maudsley nonreactive rat line (MNR). In this context, it is interesting to note that the MR share this feature with individuals of the Syracuse low avoidance rat line (SLA) (cf. Brush *et al.*, 1988), the Roman low avoidance rat line (RLA) (cf. Driscoll and Bättig, 1982), the Tsukuba high emotional rat line (THE) (Fujita and Nakamura, 1976), and the Flinders sensitive rat line (FLS) (Russell *et al.*, 1982), although the latter rat lines were selected for a different biological variable, namely, performance in a two-way active avoidance task (SLA and RLA), entering a bright runway (THE) and sensitivity to the anticholinesterase dipropyl fluorophosphates (FLS). Although there is hardly any information about the neurochemical, neuroendocrine, physiological, behavioural, and pharmacological features of the MR, Driscoll and his colleagues have invested an enormous amount of research in analysing these features in the RLA (Driscoll *et al.*, 1998). Ongoing research with the RLA and their counterparts, the RHA, investigates to what extent the biological features in question should be conceptualized as substrates of the various traits of these animals rather than just biological correlates. The finding that neonatal handling produces changes in certain behavioural and endocrine responses of the RLA that are line-specific (Escorihuela *et al.*, 1995) strongly suggests that at least these responses reflect basic aspects of the underlying psychobiology of the feature in question. Still, it is important to note that none of these rat lines are selected for *harm avoidance*: they are selected for a feature of which breeding has resulted in a correlated difference in behaviour that is related to *harm avoidance*. Thus, it remains to be proven that the feature used for the selective breeding is consistently and causally coupled to *harm avoidance* or to related aspects of this dimension. If so, the available knowledge about the neurochemical, neuroendocrine, physiological, behavioural, and pharmacological differences between the RLA and their counterparts, the RHA, provide unique information for constructing a functional anatomy of the temperament dimension, *harm avoidance*.

Novelty Seeking

This dimension is hypothesized to be a heritable tendency to intense excitement in response to novel stimuli or cues for potential reward, and it is quite likely to correspond with Zuckerman's *sensation seeking* (McCourt *et al.*, 1983). At least two important animal models are available: a) mice that are selectively bred on the basis of their behavioural response to novelty (Gerschenfeld and Paul, 1998; Hall, 1938; Simmel and Bagwell, 1983; Walsh and Cummins, 1976), and b) Wistar rats that are selected on the basis of their behavioural response to novelty (Cools *et al.*, 1990; Dellu *et al.*, 1996; Piazza *et al.*, 1990). Whereas the mouse model can help us to trace the contribution of the heritable component, the rat model can help us to study the biological processes that underlie this trait. Because the latter model is a very basic one that has provided a wealth of biological data, it will be discussed below under a separate heading. Here we discuss the mouse model, a relatively simple behavioural assay, in which the mouse is placed in a brightly lit, novel environment, and its behaviour serves as indicator. The mouse model is generally seen as an animal model for temperament or emotionality. Zuckerman has rejected the possibility that the mouse behaviour actually models *sensation seeking*, because of the negative correlation usually found between activity and defecation at both the phenotypic and genotypic levels. The reader is referred to Zuckerman for a detailed discussion about the pros and cons of open-field activity in mice as a model for *sensation seeking* (Zuckerman, 1984; cf. Gershenfeld and Paul, 1998). Irrespective of the precise nature of the temperament dimension that is modelled by open-field activity in mice, there is little doubt that it does reflect a particular aspect of personality. Although the interpretation of mouse behaviour under these conditions is difficult and ambiguous, it has been found to represent a well-defined, innate behavioural response, and to have broad generalization across species from chickens to infants. In addition, it has been found to differ between individuals and strains, due to heritable components. With this mouse model, it has become possible to partition the behavioural variance into genetic, environmental, and interaction components, and the heritable component has been further demonstrated by selectively breeding mice that differ in their open-field behaviour. By the above-mentioned QTL technique, it has even become possible to map the QTLs for initial ambulation in the open field: these are localized on chromosomes 1 and 15 (Flint *et al.*, 1995; Gershenfeld and Paul, 1998). This approach should help us to narrow down the human chromosomal regions in order to define human candidate genes and to define polymorphisms.

ANIMAL MODEL OF NOVELTY SEEKING

The best animal model for the temperament dimension *novelty seeking* is the so-called high responder to novelty (HR) (Cools, 2000; Dellu *et al.*, 1996), namely, rats that are selected for their intense behavioural response to novelty in an open-field test. According to Cloninger, the following traditional personality dimensions are marked, among others, by a high degree of novelty seeking: antisocial, histrionic, passive-aggressive, and explosive (Cloninger *et al.*, 1994). When in childhood such a high degree of *novelty seeking* is associated with low *reward dependence*, low *harm avoidance* and high *persistence*, these persons are likely to display antisocial behaviour, to become addicted to alcohol and other drugs of abuse, and to develop criminal behaviour as adults (Cloninger *et al.*, 1994). Because the HR are also marked by low *reward dependence*, low *harm avoidance*, and high *persistence*, we regard these animals as a very important source of information for understanding the psychobiology of humans with a predisposition to the latter behaviours. For that reason, particular attention is paid to this animal model.

The animal studies in question are performed with the HR and their counterparts, the low responders to novelty (LR). These two types of rat occur in any population of Wistar rats, and are characterized by individual-specific differences in the structure, function, and reactivity of the limbic-mesolimbic-striatal axis and the hypothalamic-pituitary-adrenal (HPA) axis. These differences underlie the fully distinct behavioural, physiological, and endocrine responses to stress shown by the HR and the LR, respectively. Genetic factors direct the way to cope with stressors during the early postnatal and, probably, prenatal period: the nature and intensity of the stressor to which the individual is exposed, during the perinatal period, appears to direct the structure and function of the brain and the body of these individuals. The available animal studies reveal that three factors direct the behaviour of this personality variant: a) genetic predisposition, b) the early postnatal and, probably, prenatal factors that direct the phenotypic expression of the genotype in question, and c) the degree of stress to which the individual is exposed immediately before, and during the onset of, the performance of the behaviour (Cools and Gingras, 1998). Knowledge about the structure, function, and reactivity of the brain and the body of the HR and the LR might help us to understand which factors can underlie the behavioural lapses that occur in certain individuals under particular conditions. Below we will provide a short summary of the outcome of animal studies on the HR and the LR.

Selection Procedure

The Nijmegen outbred population of Wistar rats has been found to contain at least two distinct types of individual, each of them marked by their own structure, function, and reactivity of the brain and body. There are three validated methods to select these types of rat.

First, we have the assessment of the open-field test (Cools *et al.*, 1990; Cools *et al.*, 1993c; Cools and Gingras, 1998; cf. Piazza *et al.*, 1989), which allows the separation of the HR and the LR. Both the dimensions of our open field — 160 × 160 cm — and the absence of external cues are important features of this open-field test. The HR and the LR behave differently in this novel environment: the HR are bound to the only available external stimulus, the edge of the open field, and they continue their exploratory behaviour for a very long period of time (>840 s). As in the intruder test (see below), the HR interrupt their ongoing behaviour only when a change in their environment occurs: this is considered to reflect a high degree of context-dependency. In contrast, the LR start to explore their novel environment and, after about 480 s, stop their exploratory activity in an otherwise undisturbed environment. Thus, as in the intruder test, the LR can interrupt their ongoing behaviour by themselves: this is considered to reflect a high degree of self-control.

Second, we have the assessment of the so-called intruder test in which 'freezing', defined as 'sitting motionless for over 45 s' and 'fleeing', defined as 'number of fleeing spells seen during the whole observation period of 6 min', serve as dependent variables (Cools, 1988; Cools *et al.*, 1990; Schuurman, 1981). This test allows the separation of rats that primarily flee (FLEE rats) and rats that primarily freeze (NON-FLEE rats). Since FLEE rats — being the intruders — primarily flee during the direct confrontation with the resident (coping situation), but freeze as long as the intruders can only see and smell the resident without being able to attack him (non-coping situation), and because NON-FLEE rats freeze during the coping situation, but actively explore during the non-coping situation, the nature of the selected coping strategy (active or passive) varies according to the context and therefore is not a trait of the individual.

Third, we have the apomorphine test (Cools *et al.*, 1990), which allows the separation of apomorphine-susceptible rats (APO-SUS) and apomorphine-unsusceptible rats (APO-UNSUS): APO-SUS display more than 500 gnawing spells/45 min following an injection of 1.5 mg kg^{-1} apomorphine (s.c.), and APO-UNSUS display less than 10 gnawing spells/45 min following such an injection. Since 1985, the latter rats have also been bred, using a particular breeding schedule to prevent inbreeding and to maintain the original genotypic heterogeneity, apart from the alleles at the loci (or locus) involved in the determination of the chosen traits. Nevertheless, inbreeding, which reduces the genotypic heterogeneity and, ultimately, creates new substrains and strains, cannot be prevented in the long run; given our interest in the individual variability that occurs within a single strain in order to maintain a situation that approaches the human situation as closely as possible, it became necessary to restart the breeding of these lines, once every 5–8 years.

We have been able to show that the bimodal variation in apomorphine-susceptibility, the original selection criterion for the breeding, is consistently coupled to a bimodal variation in various neuroanatomical, neurochemical, endocrinological, immunological, and behavioural features. Evidence has been provided that rats marked by a high apomorphine-susceptibility (APO-SUS) are high responders to novelty in terms of both their behavioural response and their endocrinological responses, and that rats marked by a low apomorphine-susceptibility (APO-UNSUS) are low responders to novelty in terms of their behavioural and endocrinological responses (Cools *et al.*, 1990, 1993a–c; Rots, 1995; Rots *et al.*, 1996a–c). This individual consistency in behaviour and physiology has revealed that any of the biological or behavioural variables known to differ between these rats can be used as a criterion for selecting these two types of rat. For example, APO-SUS and APO-UNSUS rats can be selected from outbred strains of Wistar rats by establishing their response to novelty and selecting the HR and LR rats, respectively (Cools *et al.*, 1990; 1993). In sum, the male HR, FLEE rats and APO-SUS are marked by idiosyncratic features of one and the same type of individual; the same holds true for male LR, NON-FLEE rats and APO-UNSUS. In other words, there are two distinct types of individuals whose genetic make-up is reflected in the above three responses (Cools *et al.*, 1990).

The HR and LR are not tails of the population, but each group (HR and LR) represents a major part (40–45%) of our outbred strain of Nijmegen Wistar rats; the remaining 10–20% of rats form a heterogeneous group of rats, showing a mixture of HR and LR features, of which no details about the behavioural, neurochemical, and endocrinological features are known. As mentioned below, the ultimate neurochemical and behavioural phenotype of these two types of animal is determined, among others, by early postnatal factors. Owing to this factor and owing to distinct selection procedures, one has to be aware of the fact that the HR and LR that are studied in different research centres are not necessarily fully identical. Nevertheless, it is important to note that the HR/LR studied in other laboratories (Exner and Clark, 1993; Piazza *et al.*, 1989, 1991; Rouge-Pont *et al.*, 1993; Hooks *et al.*, 1991, 1991) share the following features with the Nijmegen HR/LR (Cools *et al.*, 1997; Saigusa *et al.*, 1999; Rots, 1995; Ranaldi *et al.*, 2001):

1. There is a positive correlation between the locomotor response to novelty and the acute behavioural response to dexamphetamine.
2. Environmental or pharmacological stressors produce a greater increase in the extracellular concentration of accumbal dopamine in the HR than in the LR.
3. The HR show a greater release of corticosteroids in response to stressors than the LR.
4. The HR acquire self-administration of psychostimulants such as cocaine and dexamphetamine much faster than LR.

In this chapter, we use the labels HR and LR for the Nijmegen HR (APO-SUS) and the Nijmegen LR (APO-UNSUS), respectively, whereas we refer to 'high responders to novelty' and 'low responders to novelty', respectively, when we refer to the studies of other groups.

CHARACTERISTIC FEATURES OF THE ANIMAL COUNTERPART OF THE *NOVELTY-SEEKING* PERSONALITY DIMENSION: GLOBAL SURVEY

Adult HR and LR animals are male rats that normally occur in every outbred strain of Wistar rats: these rats are neither mutants nor members of different substrains or strains. As mentioned above, these rats are marked by the genotypic heterogeneity that is originally present in every outbred strain of Wistar rats. However, characteristic features differ remarkably between these rats. The most characteristic ones are mentioned below.

1. *Novelty seeking*. The HR explore unfamiliar novel objects and novel environments: they enter the open arms of an elevated plus-maze to an extent that is only displayed by the LR when treated with benzodiazepines (Cools *et al.*, unpublished data). They readily self-administer cocaine (Ranaldi *et al.*, 2001). In sum, there are many features that are characteristic of the high novelty seekers.
2. *Reward dependence*. In studies on the intake of a variety of rewarding solutions, we found that HR consume far less sucrose than LR, possibly indicating that HR respond far less intensely to signals of reward than LR do. In other words, HR may have a low degree of *reward dependence* (Gingras, 1997).
3. *Persistence*. If one regards the repetition of aimless behaviour in response to novelty or psychostimulants as an indicator of *persistence* in animals, it is evident that HR have a high degree of *persistence*, because they show a far more stereotyped response to novelty and dexamphetamine than LR do (Gingras and Cools, 1997a).
4. *Harm avoidance*. If one regards a high frequency of defecation under bright lights in a novel environment and/or immobility with bradycardia in response to foot shock as indicators of *harm avoidance* in animals, HR have a relatively small degree of harm avoidance, because HR produce far fewer droppings in a novel open field than LR (Sluyter *et al.*, unpublished data). In addition, HR show also far less immobility in this open field than LR do (Cools *et al.*, 1990).
5. *Stress-sensitivity*. HR are more stress-sensitive in terms of behavioural (locomotor activity) and endocrine (release of ACTH and corticosteroids) responses than LR. In this context, stress refers to novelty-induced stress as well as to stress measured in the so-called conditioned emotional test (Rots, 1995; Rots *et al.*, 1995, 1996): the locomotor response to novelty, as well as the release of plasma release of ACTH and corticosteroids in response to stress, is far greater and longer-lasting in HR than LR.
6. *Rate of acquiring a new task*. HR that are not habituated to a four-arm radial-maze start to learn a simple cued four-arm radial-maze task during the three initial test days, whereas LR only later start to acquire that task: the overall rate of acquisition, however, does not differ between HR and LR (Cools *et al.*, 1993c, 1994). In fact, it seems that HR need stress

in order to acquire a new task, in contrast to LR, which need to be habituated to stress before learning. This holds especially for tasks known to involve the basolateral part of the amygdala (Tuinstra, 2000).

7. *Retrieval of recently stored information.* Once HR have learned to find a platform that is invisible and submersed in a so-called Morris water maze, with the help of cues around the swimming pool, they have severe difficulty in retrieving the stored information when returning to the pool 24 h after the last trial on the first test day; however, after 2 min, they perform very well. In contrast, LR have no problem in retrieving the stored information under these conditions: in fact, their performance is even better than that shown on the first day. In sum, it seems that stress inhibits HR in retrieving recently stored information, in contrast to LR, in which stress facilitates the retrieval of recently stored information. This holds especially for tasks known to involve the ventral subiculum of the hippocampus (Tuinstra *et al.*, 2000c).
8. *Context-dependency.* HR are very dependent on spatial and contextual stimuli, whereas LR are relatively independent of these stimuli (see sections on Selection procedure and on Early life events).
9. *Self-control.* HR have less self-control than LR do (see sections on Selection procedure and on Early life events).
10. *Predisposition to mental illness.* HR, but not LR, show patterns of behaviour in animal models with construct validity for certain cognitive deficits of schizophrenic patients (Ellenbroek *et al.*, 1995). HR show a reduced latent inhibition as well as a reduced pre-pulse inhibition, whereas LR show normal latent inhibition and pre-pulse inhibition. However, HR display less parkinsonian symptoms in animal models of Parkinson's disease than LR (van Oosten and Cools, unpublished data).
11. *Predisposition to somatoform diseases.* HR respond negatively in animal models for autoimmune diseases such as experimental allergic encephalomyelitis (EAE model), whereas LR respond positively in such models (Cools *et al.*, 1993b; Kavelaars *et al.*, 1997). However, HR show a vigorous, Th2-dependent IgE response after infection with the nematode *Trichinella spiralis*, whereas LR do not (Kavelaars *et al.*, 1997). In other words, HR are relatively insensitive to autoimmune diseases, but very sensitive to infections, whereas LR reveal the opposite pattern.
12. *Predisposition to 'therapeutic' and unwanted effects of drugs.* HR are more sensitive to anti-parkinsonian agents than LR, whereas LR are more sensitive to antipsychotics than HR (Cools *et al.*, 1990; 1993c): systemic administration of dopaminergic agonists such as apomorphine produce a greater and longer-lasting behavioural response in HR than in LR, whereas intra-accumbens administration of neuroleptics, such as sulpiride, produces a behavioural response in HR that is smaller than that seen in LR.
13. *Sensitivity to psychostimulant and/or reinforcing effects of orally or otherwise administered agents.* During absence of stress, HR are far less sensitive to psychostimulant and/or reinforcing effects of ethanol, dexamphetamine, sucrose, and quinine than LR (Cools and Gingras, 1998; Ellenbroek and Cools, 1993; Gingras and Cools, 1995, 1997). Under stress, however, the situation is fully reversed: HR are behaviourally far more sensitive to ethanol, dexamphetamine, and cocaine, and under stress, HR self-administer far more cocaine than LR (cf. Cools and Gingras, 1998).
14. *Structure of the brain.* There are numerous differences in number of receptors (e.g., mineralocorticoid and dopamine receptors: [Rots, 1995; Rots *et al.*, 1995, 1996a–c; Sutanto *et al.*, 1989]), concentrations of neurotransmitters (e.g., noradrenaline and dynorphin: [Cools *et al.*, 1993c; Rots, 1995]), number of synapses (nucleus paraventricularis hypothalami: [Mulders *et al.*, 1995a–b]), etc.
15. *Reactivity of the brain.* The reactivity of both the limbic-mesolimbic-striatal axis and the HPA axis is far greater in HR than in LR. These differences underlie, among others, the fact that during stress HR have a relatively active basolateral part of the amygdala and a relatively inactive ventral subiculum of the hippocampus, with the consequence that HR can easily acquire new information, but have difficulty with retrieving recently stored information. In contrast, LR have a relatively inactive basolateral part of the amygdala and a relatively active subiculum of the hippocampus, with the result that LR show the behavioural mirror image under these conditions (Roozendaal and Cools, 1994; Tuinstra, 2001; Tuinstra *et al.*, 2000b).
16. *Early postnatal development.* A rat of the LR genotype that is deprived of its mother for 24 h on the ninth postnatal day develops into an adult animal with characteristic features of the HR, whereas a rat of the HR genotype raised with an LR foster mother develops into an adult animal with characteristic features of the LR phenotype (Ellenbroek and Cools, 1996). These findings show that the biological variables in question have to be considered as biological substrates rather than biological correlates. These findings also indicate that each distinct genotype is sensitive to a type-specific set of stressors: what is fully harmless for one type appears to have large consequences for the other type. In sum, the nature of the stressors that are present during the early postnatal period have a far-reaching influence upon the phenotypic expression of the genotype.

CHARACTERISTIC FEATURES OF THE ANIMAL COUNTERPART OF THE *NOVELTY-SEEKING* PERSONALITY DIMENSION: BRAIN, BODY, AND BEHAVIOUR

Given the role of telencephalic dopamine and that of corticosteroids in the neurochemical and behavioural responses to novelty (stress) and drugs of abuse (Cools, 1988; Di Chiara and Imperato, 1988; Fahlke *et al.*, 1994, 1995; Goeders and Guerin, 1996; Marinelli *et al.*, 1994; Roberts and Koob, 1982; Shoaib *et al.*, 1995; Wise and Rompré, 1989; Yoshimoto *et al.*, 1991), the most salient type-specific differences in this respect are summarized.

As mentioned, HR are far more sensitive to the dopaminergic agonist apomorphine than LR (Cools *et al.*, 1990). Furthermore, unchallenged HR are more sensitive to noradrenergic agonists. In fact, unchallenged HR behave as if they were sensitized by dexamphetamine; Piazza *et al.* (1990) have also found that their 'high responders to novelty' show this phenomenon. Surprisingly, HR are less sensitive to dopaminergic antagonists such as sulpiride than LR (Cools *et al.*, 1993c). In fact, there are neurochemical features that can explain these differences in susceptibility to aminergic agents (Cools *et al.*, 1990, 1993a; Rots, 1995; Rots *et al.*, 1995, 1996a and c); for example, unchallenged HR have a smaller amount of mesolimbic noradrenaline in the nucleus accumbens than unchallenged LR (Cools *et al.*, 1990; Rots *et al.*, 1996c). As discussed elsewhere in detail (Cools *et al.*, 1987), this explains why unchallenged HR are more sensitive to the accumbal administration of the alpha-adrenergic agonist phenylephrine (Ellenbroek and Cools, 1993). Furthermore, unchallenged HR have more striatal dopamine D1 receptor mRNA and more tyrosine hydroxylase mRNA in the A9 (substantia nigra, pars compacta) and A12 (nucleus arcuatus) cell groups than unchallenged LR, implying that the capacity to enhance the formation of dopamine in response to stress is greater in HR than in LR. Indeed, when the rats are challenged by novelty or tested in the conditioned emotional response test, behavioural and physiological responses mediated by dopamine are greater in HR than LR (Cools *et al.*, 1990; Rots, 1995; Rots *et al.*, 1995, 1996a). The following example nicely illustrates this dopamine hyperreactivity in HR: the dopaminergic, tuberoinfundibular system that arises in A12 normally inhibits prolactin, and this response is far more strongly inhibited in HR than in LR, when the rats are exposed to stress (Rots, 1995; Rots *et al.*, 1996a).

Given the difference in the behavioural response to stress, it could be predicted that this difference extends to the HPA axis. This is indeed the case. First, the amount of corticotrophin-releasing hormone (CRH) mRNA in the nucleus paraventricularis hypothalami (PVN) of HR is greater than that in the PVN of LR (Rots *et al.*, 1995), implying that these cells in HR have also a greater capacity to generate CRH. Because CRH, which is under the stimulatory control of dopamine (Plotsky *et al.*, 1989), stimulates the release of plasma ACTH, especially during exposure to stress, it is logical to expect a HR-LR difference in the ACTH plasma release in response to stressors such as novelty. This is indeed the case: the stress-induced release of ACTH as well as that of plasma corticosteroids, of which the release is stimulated by ACTH, are greater and longer-lasting in HR than in LR (Rots *et al.*, 1995), a finding that fits in with those reported by Piazza *et al.* (1991). Apart from these data, we found that plasma levels of ACTH in HR are greater than those in LR under baseline conditions, but that the plasma release of free corticosteroids in HR is lower than those in LR under these conditions (Rots *et al.*, 1995; 1996a).

NOVELTY AND THE NEUROCHEMICAL STATE OF THE NUCLEUS ACCUMBENS IN THE ANIMAL COUNTERPART OF THE *NOVELTY-SEEKING* PERSONALITY DIMENSION

As elaborated elsewhere in detail (Cools *et al.*, 1991, 1993a, 1994; Cools and Gingras, 1998; Roozendaal and Cools, 1994), there is anatomical, electrophysiological, pharmacobehavioural, and neurochemical evidence that the neurochemical state of the nucleus accumbens of an unchallenged HR is marked by the following features when compared with LR:

1. The functional activity at the level of beta-adrenergic receptors that can stimulate the release of dopamine at the level of dopamine D2 receptors is relatively low.
2. The functional activity at the level of these dopamine D2 receptors, presynaptically localized on glutamatergic hippocampus-accumbens neurons, is relatively low.
3. The functional activity at the level of alpha-adrenergic receptors that can inhibit the release of dopamine at the level of so-called inhibitory dopamine receptors (DAi) — a subtype of dopamine receptors not yet linked to the two more recently discovered families of dopamine D1 and D2 receptors (Cools and van Rossum, 1980) — is relatively low.
4. The functional activity at the level of these DAi receptors — localized on glutamatergic amygdala-accumbens neurons — is relatively high.
5. The neurochemical state of the nucleus accumbens of an unchallenged HR greatly differs from that of an unchallenged LR: for all neurotransmitters, functional activity that is relatively low in HR is relatively high in LR, and vice versa.

Very recently biochemical evidence gained by the microdialysis technique has shown that the noradrenaline-dopamine interaction in the nucleus accumbens differs completely between HR and LR (Saigusa *et al.*, 1999; Tuinstra and Cools, 2000a and b). Finally, under challenge by a mild physiological, pharmacological, or environmental stressor, the neurochemical state of the nucleus accumbens and, probably, of other parts of the brain and body as well, is temporarily reversed (Roozendaal and Cools, 1994; Tuinstra and Cools, 2000a and b). Thus, the state of a challenged HR goes in the direction of that of an unchallenged LR, whereas that of a challenged LR goes in the direction of that of an unchallenged HR.

EARLY LIFE EVENTS AND THE DEVELOPMENT OF THE ADULT PHENOTYPE OF THE ANIMAL COUNTERPART OF THE *NOVELTY-SEEKING* PERSONALITY DIMENSION

Before discussing the consequences of early postnatal life events, it is important to consider characteristic changes that occur during the normal development of HR and LR (Rots *et al.*, 1996b). In 10-day-old rats, type-specific differences in dopaminergic variables (e.g., D1 receptor mRNA and TH mRNA) and in variables of the HPA axis (e.g., ACTH and corticosteroids) are not yet present. However, in 18-day-old rats, variables of the HPA axis already show some type-specific differences known to occur in 60-day-old, adult rats. For instance, the ACTH plasma level under baseline conditions is greater in HR than in LR, and a trend towards lower free corticosterone plasma levels is present in HR; in contrast, there are still no type-specific differences in the dopaminergic variables in 18-day-old rats (Rots, 1995; Rots *et al.*, 1996b). Thus, the divergence in the dopamine phenotype of HR and LR develops subsequent to distinct differences in the HPA axis.

To investigate to what extent early experiences direct the development of the adult phenotype, two paradigms were used (Ellenbroek *et al.*, 2000): cross-fostering on day 1 and maternal deprivation on day 9. These manipulations are chosen because they are known to function as mild stressors at that time. Remarkably, cross-fostering influences only the adult phenotype of HR, and not of LR (Ellenbroek and Cools, 1996), whereas maternal deprivation influences only the adult phenotype of LR (Ellenbroek *et al.*, 2000). In fact, cross-fostering reverses HR into LR, whereas maternal deprivation reverses LR into HR, as far as their apomorphine-susceptibility is concerned. In addition, we found that maternal deprivation affects various characteristics of the biochemical phenotype: adult rats that were deprived show a higher ACTH plasma level under baseline conditions and a greater amount of TH mRNA in A9 cells than their controls (Rots, 1995; Rots *et al.*, 1996b). Very recently, we found that this reversal also holds for the individual-specific sensitivity to diseases such as periodontitis (Sluyter *et al.*, unpublished). These data together suggest that this early life experience reverses the biochemical, immunological, and behavioural phenotype of LR into that of HR.

EPILOGUE

This review reveals that there are many animal studies that deal with animal analogues of various aspects of personality dimensions of the recently introduced functional classification system of personality. However, most of the approaches are indirect in the sense that the independent variables are biological, but not behavioural. Nevertheless, these animal models can be very helpful in laying foundations for new hypotheses about the biological mechanisms and substrates that underlie particular personality dimensions. However, there is only one mouse model and one rat model that use behavioural measures as independent variables, and biological ones as dependent variables. These two models deal with *novelty seeking*. The available mouse model has made it possible to partition the behavioural variance into genetic, environmental, and interaction components. However, the available rat model has made it possible to provide basic insights into various biological processes and substrates that underlie the personality dimension in question. As summarized below, the rat model also helps us to understand to what extent genetic background, perinatal conditions, and the currently present environment determine the individual-specific set of personality dimensions of an individual.

The rat studies on *novelty seeking* show that the animal counterpart of a high novelty seeker, namely, the high responder to novelty (HR), and the animal counterpart of a low novelty seeker, namely, the low responder to novelty (LR), are characterized by individual-specific differences in structure, function, and reactivity of both the limbic-mesolimbic-striatal axis and the HPA axis. These differences underlie the individual-specific manner of coping with stress. The features of these individuals at adult age are determined by a) genetic predisposition, b) early postnatal and, probably, prenatal factors that direct the phenotypic expression of the genotype, and c) the degree of stress to which the individual is exposed immediately before, and during the onset of, the performance of the behaviour.

Available data show that the structure, function, and reactivity of the brain, the endocrine system, and the immune system differ completely between both types of individual. Analysis of behaviour as in the open-field test, the intruder test, the swimming task, the radial-maze task, etc., has clearly revealed that these two types of individuals organize their ongoing behaviour in a fully distinct manner: HR predominantly display extrinsically directed behaviour: they have a very well-developed capacity to use external cues for organizing their behaviour and are, in practice, dependent on these cues. In contrast, LR predominantly display intrinsically organized behaviour: they have a very well-developed capacity to control their own behaviour and are relatively independent of external cues. It is due to these features that HR perform optimally in tasks in which contextual stimuli have to be used for solving problems, but have severe problems with tasks in which internal cues have to be used for solving the problem. This also explains why LR display the mirror behaviour in these tasks. In other words, each of these types has its own optimal niche in which it can flourish, but also its own niche in which it will perish. This explains why this disruptive selection, in which more than just one phenotypic expression of a particular trait has surplus value, is present in such a stable balance within non-selected strains of Wistar rats. This makes it possible that dimorphisms, such as HR and LR, in rat populations and polymorphisms in humans exist.

One of the most remarkable findings is that both these types of individuals deteriorate as soon as they end up in each other's niche. This illustrates that certain stressors are harmful for one type, but not for the other. Nevertheless, one should not forget that a challenged HR behaves as an unchallenged LR, and vice versa. In short, the statement 'once a HR, always a HR' is incorrect. The key message of these findings is that genetic predisposition and early life events are decisive for the psychobiology of the personality dimensions, but that it is ultimately the current situation that gives rise to behavioural lapses.

Finally, HR are marked not only by a high degree of *novelty seeking*, but also by low degree of *harm avoidance*, a low degree of *reward dependence*, and a high degree of *persistence*. The coexistence of this particular configuration of scores on these dimensions is rather unexpected, because the human counterparts of these dimensions are genetically independent. To what extent these findings imply that one is dealing with a species-specific difference in this respect remains to be investigated. Anyhow, persons with a high degree of novelty seeking are marked, among others, by traditional personality dimensions such as the antisocial, histrionic, passive-aggressive, and explosive. When in childhood such a high degree of novelty seeking is associated with low *reward dependence*, low *harm avoidance*, and high *persistence*, these persons are likely to display antisocial behaviour, to become addicted to alcohol and other drugs of abuse, and to develop criminal behaviour at adult age. In view of these considerations, we believe that HR might help us to understand the biological processes and substrates that underlie the behaviour of persons marked by this particular (dys)balance of personality dimensions.

REFERENCES

Benjamin, J., Li, L., Patterson, C., Greenberg, B.D., Murphy, D.L. and Hamer, D.H., 1996. Population and familial association between the D4 dopamine receptor gene and measures of novelty seeking. *Nature Genetics*, **12**, 81–84.

Broadhurst, P.L., 1975. The Maudsley reactive and nonreactive strains of rats: a survey. *Behavior Genetics*, **5**, 299–319.

Brush, F.R., Del Paine, S.H., Pellegrino, L.J., Rykaszewski, I.M., Dess, N.K. and Collins, P.Y., 1988. CER suppression, passive-avoidance learning, and stress-induced suppression of drinking in the Syracuse high- and low-avoidance strains of rats (*Rattus norvegicus*). *Journal of Comparative Psychology*, **102**, 337–349.

Cabib, S. and Puglisi-Allegra, S., 1988. A classical genetic analysis of two apomorphine-induced behaviors in the mouse. *Pharmacology, Biochemistry and Behavior*, **30**, 143–147.

Cloninger, C.R., 1994. Temperament and personality. *Current Opinion in Neurobiology*, **4**, 266–273.

Cloninger, C.R., Przybeck, T.R., Svrakic, D.M. and Wetzel, R.D., 1994. *The Temperament and Character Inventory (TCI): A Guide to Its Development and Use Center for Psychobiology of Personality*, pp. 1–184. Washington University, St. Louis, Missouri.

Cools, A.R., 1988. Transformation of emotion into motion: role of mesolimbic noradrenaline and neostriatal dopamine. In: Hellhamer, D., Florin, I. and Weiner, H. (eds), *Neurobiological Approaches to Human Disease*, pp. 15–28. Hans Huber, Toronto.

Cools, A.R., 1991. Differential role of mineralocorticoid and glucocorticoid receptors in the genesis of dexamphetamine-induced sensitization of mesolimbic, $\alpha 1$ adrenergic receptors in the ventral striatum. *Neuroscience*, **43**, 419–428.

Cools, A.R., 2000. Psychobiologie van persoonlijkheidsvarianten. In: Tuinier, S., Verhoeven, W.M.A. and Van Panhuis, P.J.A. (eds), *Behandelingsstrategieën Bij Agressieve Gedragsstoornissen*, pp. 1–106. Bohn Stafleu van Loghum, Houten.

Cools, A.R. and Gingras, M.A., 1998. Nijmegen high and low responders to novelty: a new tool in the search after the neurobiology of drug abuse liability. *Pharmacology, Biochemistry and Behavior*, **60**, 151–159.

Cools, A.R. and van Rossum, J.M., 1980. Multiple receptors for brain dopamine in behavioral regulation: concept of dopamine-e and dopamine-i receptors. *Life Science*, **27**, 1237–1253.

Cools, A.R., Rots, N. and De Kloet, E.R., 1994. Apomorphine-susceptible and apomorphine-unsusceptible Wistar rats: a new tool in the search for the function of the striatum in switching behavioral strategies. In: Percheron, G. (ed.), *The Basal Ganglia IV*, pp. 507–515. Plenum Press, New York.

Cools, A.R., Ellenbroek, B.A., van den Bos, R. and Gelissen, M., 1987. Mesolimbic noradrenaline/specificity, stability and dose dependency of individual specific responses to mesolimbic injections of α-noradrenergic agonists. *Behavioral Brain Research*, **25**, 49–61.

Cools, A.R., van den Bos, R., Ploeger, G. and Ellenbroek, B., 1991. Gating function of noradrenaline in the ventral striatum: its role in behavioral responses to environmental and pharmacological challenges. In: Willner, P. and Scheel-Kruger, J. (eds), *The Mesolimbic Dopamine System: from Motivation to Action*, pp. 141–173. Wiley, New York.

Cools, A.R., Rots, N., Ellenbroek, B. and De Kloet, E.R., 1993b. Bimodal shape of individual variation in behavior of Wistar rats. *Neuropsychobiology*, **28**, 100–105.

Cools, A.R., Ellenbroek, B., Heeren, D. and Lubbers, L., 1993c. Use of high and low responders to novelty in rat studies on the role of the ventral striatum in radial maze performance. *Canadian Journal of Physiology and Pharmacology*, **71**, 335–342.

Cools, A.R., Brachten, R., Heeren, D., Willemen, A. and Ellenbroek, B., 1990. Search after the neurobiological profile of individual-specific features of Wistar rats. *Brain Research Bulletin*, **24**, 49–69.

Cools, A.R., Ellenbroek, B.A., Gingras, M.A., Engbersen, A. and Heeren, D., 1997a. Difference in vulnerability to dexamphetamine in Nijmegen high and low responders to novelty: a dose-effect analysis of spatio-temporal programming of behavior. *Psychopharmacology*, **132**, 181–188.

Cools, A.R., Gingras, M.A., Tuinstra, T., Ellenbroek, B.A. and Saigusa, T., 1997b. High and low responders to novelty: differences in development of drug dependence. *Alcohol Alcohol*, **32**, 309.

Cools, A.R., Dierx, J., Coenders, C., Heeren, D., Ried, S., Jenks, B. and Ellenbroek, B., 1993a. Apomorphine-susceptible and apomorphine-unsusceptible Wistar rats differ in novelty-induced changes in hippocampal dynorphin B expression and two-way active avoidance: a new key in the search for the role of the hippocampal-accumbens axis. *Behavioral Brain Research*, **55**, 213–221.

Davidson, R.J., 1999. The neurobiology of personality and personality disorders. In: Charney, D.S., Nestler, E.J. and Bunney, B.S. (eds), *Neurobiology of Mental Illness*, pp. 841–854. Oxford University Press, New York.

Dellu, R., Piazza, P.V., Mayo, W., Le Moal, M. and Simon, H., 1996. Novelty seeking in rats' biobehavioral characteristics and possible relationship with the sensation seeking trait in man. *Neuropsychobiology*, **34**, 136–145.

Di Chiara, G. and Imperato, A., 1988. Drugs abused by humans preferentially increase synaptic dopamine concentrations in the mesolimbic system of freely moving rats. *Proceedings of the National Academy of Sciences of the United States of America*, **85**, 274–5278.

Driscoll, P. and Bättig, K., 1982. Behavioral, emotional and neurochemical profiles of rats selected for extreme differences in active, two-way avoidance performance. In: Lieblich, D. (ed.), *Genetics of the Brain*, pp. 95–123. Elsevier, Amsterdam.

Driscoll, P., Escorihuela, R.M., Fernandez-Teruel, A., Giorgi, O., Schwegler, H., Steimer, T., Wiersma, A., Corda, M.G., Flint, J., Koolhaas, J.M., Langhans, W., Schulz, P.E., Siegel, J. and Tobena, A., 1998. Genetic selection and differential stress responses. The Roman lines/strains of rats. *Annals of the New York Academy of Sciences*, **851**, 501–510.

Ellenbroek, B.A. and Cools, A.R., 1993. Apomorphine-susceptible and apomorphine-unsusceptible rats differ in the amphetamine induced sensitization of α-receptors in the nucleus accumbens. *Society of Neurosciences Abstracts*, **19**, 823.

Ellenbroek, B.A. and Cools, A.R., 1996. Dopamine susceptibility and information processing. In: Beninger, R.J., Palomo, T. and Archer, T. (eds), *Dopamine Disease States*, pp. 447–462. Editorial CYM, Madrid.

Ellenbroek, B.A., Geyer, M.A. and Cools, A.R., 1995. The behavior of APO-SUS rats in animal models with construct validity for schizophrenia. *Neuroscience*, **15**, 7604–7611.

Ellenbroek, A., Sluyter, F. and Cools, A.R., 2000. The role of genetic and early environmental factors in determining apomorphine susceptibility. *Psychopharmacology*, **148**, 124–131.

Escorihuela, R.M., Tobena, A., Driscoll, P. and Fernadez-Teruel, A., 1995. Effects of training, early handling, and perinatal flumazenil on shuttle box acquisition in Roman low-avoidance rats: toward overcoming a genetic deficit. *Neuroscience of Behavioral Reviews*, **19**, 353–367.

Exner, E. and Clark, D., 1993. Behavior in the novel environment predicts responsiveness to *d*-amphetamine in the rat: a multivariate approach. *Behavioral Pharmacology*, **4**, 47–56.

Eysenck, H.J., 1947. *Dimensions of Personality*. Praeger, New York.

Fahlke, C., Hard, E., Eriksson, P., Engel, J.A. and Hansen, S., 1994. Consequence of long-term exposure to corticosterone or dexamethasone on ethanol consumption in the adrenalectomized rat, and the effect of type 1 and type II corticosteroid receptor antagonists. *Psychopharmacology*, **48**, 977–981.

Fahlke, C., Jorgen, A., Engel, J.A., Eriksson, P., Hard, E. and Söderpalm, B., 1995. Involvement of corticosterone in the modulation of ethanol consumption in the rat. *Alcohol*, **2**, 195–202.

Fiske, D.W., 1949. Consistency of factorial structures for personality ratings from different sources. *Journal of Abnormal and Social Psychology*, **44**, 329–344.

Flint, J., Corley, R., De Fries, J.C., Fulker, D.W., Gray, J.A., Mille, S. and Collins, A.C., 1995. A simple genetic basis for a complex psychological trait in laboratory mice. *Science*, **269**, 1432–1435.

Fujita, O. and Nakamura, N., 1976. Selection for high and low emotionality based on the runway test in the rat: the first seven generations of selection. *Hiroshima Forum on Psychology*, **3**, 57–62.

Gentsch, C., Lichtsteiner, M. and Feer, H., 1988. Genetic and environmental influences on behavioral and neurochemical aspects of emotionality in rats. *Experientia*, **44**, 482–490.

Gershenfeld, H.K. and Paul, S.M., 1998. Towards a genetics of anxious temperament: from mice to men. *Acta Psychiatrica Scandinavica*, **98**, 56–65.

Gingras, M.A., 1997. Individual Differences in Behavioural Responses to Drugs of Abuse. Thesis Katholieke Universiteit Nijmegen, Nijmegen, pp. 1–152.

Gingras, M.A and Cools, A.R., 1995. Differential ethanol intake in high and low responders to novelty. *Behavioral Pharmacology*, **6**, 718–723.

Gingras, M.A. and Cools, A.R., 1997a. Different behavioral effects of daily or intermittent dexamphetamine administration in Nijmegen high and low responders. *Psychopharmacology*, **132**, 188–194.

Gingras, M.A. and Cools, A.R., 1997b. Nijmegen high and low responders to novelty and differences in intake of sucrose, quinine and ethanol. *Alcohol Alcohol*, **32**, 394.

Goeders, N.E. and Guerin, G.F., 1996. Effects of surgical and pharmacological adrenalectomy on the initiation and maintenance of intravenous cocaine self-administration. *Brain Research*, **22**, 145–152.

Goldsmith, H.H., Buss, A.H., Plomin, R., Rothbart, M.K., Thomas, A., Chess, S., Hinde, R.A. and McCall, R.B., 1987. What is temperament? *Child Development*, **58**, 505–529.

Hall, C.S., 1938. The inheritance of emotionality. *Sigma Xi Quarterly*, **26**, 17–27.

Herbst, J.H., Zonderman, A.B., McCrae, R.R. and Costa, P.T., 2000. Do the dimensions of the temperament and character inventory map a simple genetic architecture? evidence from molecular genetics and factor analysis. *American Journal of Psychiatry*, **157**, 1285–1290.

Hooks, M.S, Jones, G.H., Neill, D.B. and Justice, J.B. Jr., 1991. Individual differences in amphetamine sensitization: dose-dependent effects. *Pharmacology, Biochemistry and Behavior*, **41**, 203–210.

Hooks, M.S., Jones, G.H., Liem, B.J. and Justice, J.B. Jr, 1992. Sensitization and individual differences to i.p. amphetamine, cocaine, or caffeine following repeated intracranial amphetamine infusions. *Pharmacology, Biochemistry and Behavior*, **43**, 815–823.

Insel, T.R., Winslow, J.T., Williams, J.R., Hastings, N., Shapiro, L.E. and Carter, C.S., 1993. The role of neurophypopyseal peptides in the central mediation of complex social processes — evidence from comparative studies. *Regulatory Peptides*, **45**, 127–131.

Kalin, N.H., Larson, C., Shelton, S.E. and Davidson, R.J., 1998. Asymmetric frontal brain activity, cortisol, and behavior associated with fearful temperament in Rhesus monkeys. *Behavioral Neuroscience*, **112**, 286–292.

Kavelaars, A., Heijnen, C.J., Ellenbroek, B., Van Loveren, H. and Cools, A.R., 1997. Apomorphine-susceptible and apomorphine-unsusceptible Wistar rats differ in their susceptibility to inflammatory and infectious diseases: a study on rats with group-specific differences in structure and reactivity of the hypothalamic-pituitary-adrenal axis. *Journal of Neurosciences*, **17**, 2580–2584.

Knapp, D.J., Overstreet, D.H. and Crews, F.T., 1998. Brain 5-HT_{1A} receptor autoradiography and hypothermic responses in rats bred for differences in 8-OH-DPAT sensitivity. *Brain Research*, **782**, 1–10.

Lewis, C.E., 1991. Neurochemical mechanisms of chronic antisocial behavior (psychopathy). A literature review. *Journal of Nervous and Mental Disorders*, **179**, 720–727.

Loehlin, J.C., 1982. Are personality traits differentially heritable? *Behavioral Genetics*, **12**, 417–428.

Maldonado, R., Salardi, A., Valverd, O., Samad, T.A., Roques, B.P. and Borrelli, E., 1997. Absence of opiate rewarding effects in mice lacking dopamine D2 receptors. *Nature*, **388**, 586–589.

Marinelli, M., Piazza, P.V., Deroche, V., Maccari, S., LeMoal, M. and Simon, H., 1994. Corticosterone circadian secretion differentially facilitates dopamine mediated psychomotor effect of cocaine and morphine. *Journal of Neuroscience*, **14**, 2724–2734.

Masur, J., Maroni, J.B. and Benedito, M.A.C., 1975. Genetically selected winner and loser rats in the tunnel competition: influence of apomorphine and DOPA. *Behavioral Biology*, **14**, 21–30.

McCourt, W.F., Gurrera, R.J. and Cutter, H.S., 1983. Sensation seeking and novelty seeking. Are they the same?. *Journal of Nervous and Mental Disease*, **181**, 309–312.

Mulders, W., Meek, J., Hafmans, T. and Cools, A.R., 1995a. The hypothalamic paraventricularis nucleus in two types of Wistar rats with different stress responses. I. Morphometric comparison. *Brain Research*, **689**, 47–60.

Mulders, W., Meek, J., Schmidt, E., Hafmans, T. and Cools, A.R., 1995b. The hypothalamic paraventricular nucleus in two types of Wistar rats with different stress responses. II. Differential fos-expression. *Brain Research*, **689**, 61–70.

Noble, E.P., 2000. Addiction and its reward process through polymorphisms of the D2 dopamine receptor gene: a review. *European Psychiatry*, **15**, 79–89.

Noble, E.P., Ozkaragoz, T.Z., Ritchie, T., Zhang, X., Belin, T.R. and Sparkes, R.S., 1998. D2 and D4 dopamine receptor polymorphisms and personality. *American Journal of Medicinal Genetics*, **81**, 257–267.

Norman, W.T., 1963. Toward an adequate taxonomy of personality attributes: replicated factor structure. *Journal of Abnormal and Social Psychology*, **66**, 574–583.

Piazza, P.V., Deminière, J.M., Le Moal, M. and Simon, H., 1989. Factors that predict individual vulnerability to amphetamine self-administration. *Science*, **245**, 1511–1513.

Piazza, P.V., Deminière, J.M., Maccari, S., Mormède, P., Le Moal, M. and Simon, H., 1990. Individual reactivity to novelty predicts probability of amphetamine self-administration. *Behavioral Pharmacology*, **1**, 339–345.

Piazza, P.V., Maccari, S., Deminière, J., Le Moal, M., Mormède, P. and Simon, H., 1991. Corticosterone levels determine individual vulnerability to amphetamine self-administration. *Proceedings of National Academy of Sciences of the United States of America*, **88**, 2088–2092.

Plotsky, P.M., Cunningham, E.T. Jr and Widmaier, E.P., 1989. Catecholaminergic modulation of corticotropin-releasing factor and adrenocorticotropin secretion. *Endocrinology Reviews*, **10**, 437–458.

Ranaldi, R., Bauco, P., McCormick, S., Cools, A.R. and Wise, R.A., 2001. Equal sensitivity to cocaine reward in addiction-prone and addiction-resistant rat genotypes. *Behavioral Pharmacology*, **12**, 527–534.

Roberts, D.C.S. and Koob, G.F., 1982. Disruption of cocaine self-administration following 6-hydroxydopamine lesions of the ventral tegmental area in rats. *Pharmacology, Biochemistry and Behavior*, **17**, 901–904.

Robinson, T.E. and Becker, J.B., 1986. Enduring changes in the brain and behavior produced by chronic amphetamine administration: a review and evaluation of animal models of amphetamine psychosis. *Brain Research Reviews*, **11**, 157.

Roozendaal, B. and Cools, A.R., 1994. Influence of the noradrenergic state of the nucleus accumbens in basolateral amygdala mediated changes in neophobia of rats. *Behavioral Neurosciences*, **108**, 1107–1118.

Rots, N.Y., 1995. *Dopamine and Stress: Studies with Genetically Selected Rat Lines*. Thesis, State University of Leiden, The Netherlands, pp. 1–128.

Rots, N.Y., Cools, A.R., De Jong, J. and De Kloet, E.R., 1995. Corticosteroid feedback resistance in rats genetically selected for increased dopamine responsiveness. *Journal of Endocrinology*, **7**, 153–161.

Rots, N.Y., Cools, A.R., Oizl, M.S., De Jong, J., Sutanto, W. and De Kloet, E.R., 1996a. Divergent prolactin and pituitary-adrenal activity in rats selectively bred for different dopamine responsiveness. *Endocrinology*. **137**, 1678–1687.

Rots, N.Y., Cools, A.R., Berod, A., Voorn, P., Rostene, W. and De Kloet, E.R., 1996c. Rats bred for enhanced apomorphine susceptibility have elevated tyrosine hydroxylase mRNA and dopamine D2-receptor binding sites in nigrostriatal and tuberoinfundibular systems. *Brain Research*, **70**, 189–196.

Rots, N.Y., Workel, J., Oizl, M.S., Berod, A., Rostene, W., Cools, A.R. and De Kloet, E.R., 1996b. Development in divergence in dopamine responsiveness in genetically selected rats lines is preceded by changes in pituitary-adrenal activity. *Developmental Brain Research*, **92**, 164–172.

Rouge-Pont, F., Piazza, P.V., Kharouby, M., Le Moal, M. and Simon, H., 1993. Higher and longer stress-induced increase in dopamine concentrations in the nucleus accumbens of animals predisposed to amphetamine self-administration. A microdialysis study. *Brain Research*, **602**, 169–174.

Russell, R.W., Overstreet, D.H., Messenger, M. and Helps, S.C., 1982. Selective breeding for sensibility to DFP. Generalization of effects beyond criterion variables. *Pharmacology, Biochemistry and Behavior*, **17**, 885–891.

Saigusa, T., Tuinstra, T., Koshikawa, N. and Cools, A.R., 1999. High and low responders to novelty: effects of a catecholamine synthesis inhibitor on novelty-induced changes in behaviour and release of accumbal dopamine. *Neuroscience*, **4**, 1153–1163.

Saxton, P., Siegel, J. and Lukas, J., 1987a. Visual evoked potential augmenting/reducing slopes in cats. I. Reliability as a function of flash intensity range. *Personal Individual Differences*, **8**, 499–509.

Saxton, P., Siegel, J. and Lukas, J., 1987b. Visual evoked potential augmenting/reducing slopes in cats. II. Correlations with behavior. *Personal Individual Differences*, **8**, 511–519.

Schuurman, T., 1981. Endocrine Processes Underlying Victory and Defeat in the Male Rat. Thesis, State University of Groningen, The Netherlands.

Shoaib, M., Spanagel, R., Stohr, T. and Shippenberg, T.S., 1995. Strain differences in the rewarding and dopamine-releasing effects of morphine in rats. *Psychopharmacology*, **117**, 240–247.

Siegel, J., 1997. Augmenting and reducing of visual evoked potentials in high- and low-sensation seeking humans, cats, and rats. *Behavior Genetics*, **27**, 557–563.

Siegel, J., Sisson, D.F. and Driscoll, P., 1993. Augmenting and reducing of visual evoked potentials in Roman high- and low-avoidance rats. *Physiology and Behavior*, **54**, 707–711.

Simmel, E.C. and Bagwell, M., 1983. Genetics of exploratory behavior and activity. In: Fuller, J.L. and Simmel, E.C. (eds), *Behavior Genetics: Principles and Applications*, pp. 89–115. Hillsdale, NJ, Lawrence Erlbaum Associates.

Söderpalm, B. and Svensson, A.I., 1999. Naloxone reverses disinhibitory/aggressive behavior in 5,7-DHT-lesioned rats; involvement of $GABA_A$ receptor blockade? *Neuropharmacology*, **38**, 1851–1859.

Soubrié, P., 1986. Reconciling the role of central serotonin neurons in human and animal behaviour. *Behavioral Brain Sciences*, **9**, 319–364.

Sternberg, E.M., Hill, J.M., Chrousos, G.P., Kamilaris, T., Listwak, S.J., Gold, P.W. and Wilder, R.L., 1989. Inflammatory mediator-induced hypothalamic-pituitary-adrenal axis activation is defective in streptococcal cell wall arthritis-susceptible Lewis rats. *Proceedings of the National Academy of Sciences of the United States of America*, **86**, 2374–2378.

Sutanto, W., De Kloet, E.R., De Bree, F. and Cools, A.R., 1989. Differential corticosteroid binding characteristics to the mineralocorticoid and glucocorticoid receptors in the brain of pharmacogenetically-selected apomorphine-susceptible and apomorphine-unsusceptible Wistar rats. *Neuroscience Research Communications*, **5**, 19–26.

Svrakic, D.M., Whitehead, C., Przybeck, T.R. and Cloninger, C.R., 1993. Differential diagnosis of personality disorders by the seven factor model of temperament and character. *Archives of General Psychiatry*, **50**, 991–999.

Tarantino, L.M., McClearn, G.E., Rodiguez, L.A. and Plomin, R., 1998. Confirmation of quantitative trait loci for alcohol preference in mice. *Alcohol Clinical Experimental Research*, **22**, 1099–1105.

Tuinier, S. and Verhoeven, W.M.A., 1995. Dimensional classification and behavioral pharmacology of personality disorders; a review and hypothesis. *European Neuropsychopharmacology*, **5**, 135–146.

Tuinstra, T., 2001. *The Role of Noradrenaline and Dopamine in the Nucleus Accumbens, Individual Differences*, pp. 1–148. PrintPartners Ipskamp, Enschede.

Tuinstra, T. and Cools, A.R., 2000a. High and low responders to novelty: effects of adrenergic agents on the regulation of accumbal dopamine under challenged and non-challenged conditions. *Neuroscience*, **1**, 55–64.

Tuinstra, T. and Cools, A.R., 2000b. Newly synthesized dopamine in the nucleus accumbens is regulated by α-adrenergic, but not β-adrenergic, receptors. *Neuroscience*, **4**, 743–747.

Tuinstra, T., Verheij, M., Willemen, A., Iking, J., Heeren, D.J. and Cools, A.R., 2000c. Retrieval of spatial information in Nijmegen high and low responders: involvement of α-adrenergic mechanisms in the nucleus accumbens. *Behavioural Neuroscience*, **114**, 1088–1095.

Tuinstra, T., Cobelens, P., Lubbers, L., Verheij, M. and Cools, A.R., 2001. High and low responders to novelty. Effects of noradrenergic agents on the acquisition of radial-maze performance. In: *The Role of Noradrenaline and Dopamine in the Nucleus Accumbens. Individual Differences*, pp. 41–59. PrintPartners Ipskamp, Enschede.

van Praag, H.M., 1986. Psychiatrists, beware of dichotomies! *Biological Psychiatry*, **21**, 247–248.

Virkkunen, M., Rawlings, R., Tokola, R., Poland, R.E., Guidotti, A., Nemeroff, C., Bissette, G., Kalogeras, K., Karonen, S.L. and Linnoila, M., 1994. CSF biochemistries, glucose metabolism, and diurnal activity rhythms in alcoholic, violent offenders, fire setters, and healthy volunteers. *Archives of General Psychiatry*, **51**, 20–27.

Walsh, R.N. and Cummins, R.A., 1976. The open-field test: a critical review. *Psychology Bulletin*, **83**, 482–504.
Willner, P., 1984. The validity of animal models of depression. *Psychopharmacology*, **83**, 1–16.
Willner, P., 1984. Animal models of depression. *Psychopharmacology (Berl.)*, **83**, 1–16.
Wise, R.A. and Rompré, P.P., 1989. Brain dopamine and reward. *Annual Reviews of Psychology*, **40**, 191–225.
Yoshimoto, K., McBride, W.J., Lumeng, L. and Li, T.K., 1991. Alcohol stimulated the release of dopamine and serotonin in the nucleus accumbens. *Alcohol*, **9**, 17–22.
Zuckerman, M., 1991. *Problems in the Behavioural Sciences*. Cambridge University Press, Cambridge.
Zuckerman, M., Murtaugh, T. and Siegel, J., 1974. Sensation seeking and cortical augmenting-reducing. *Psychophysiology*, **11**, 535–542.
Zuckermann, M., 1984. Sensation seeking: a comparative approach to a human trait. *Behavioral Brain Sciences*, **7**, 413–417.
Zuckerman, M., Simons, R.F. and Como, P.G., 1988. Sensation seeking and stimulus intensity as modulators of cortical, cardiovascular, and electrodermal response: a cross-modality study. *Personality and Individual Differences*, **9**, 361–372.

XXVI-2

Neurotransmitter Systems in the Personality Disorders

Matt Eks, Harold W. Koenigsberg and Larry J. Siever

INTRODUCTION

According to DSM-IV (American Psychiatric Association, 1994), a personality disorder is 'an enduring pattern of inner experience and behaviour that deviates markedly from the expectations of the individual's culture'. This enduring pattern is 'inflexible and pervasive over a broad range of personal and social situations'. It 'leads to clinically significant distress or impairment in important areas of functioning'. The pattern is 'stable', 'of long duration' and 'its onset can be traced back to adolescence or early adulthood'.

Personality disorders represent a relatively new field of research within psychiatry, particularly with a neurobiological approach. People intuitively react and adapt differently to their surroundings. Hippocrates explained these differences in terms of the 'four humors', different combinations and balances of which led to different personality traits. Bumps on the head, shape of the skull, hair colour, and body stature are among other traits that have been studied in the search for biological correlates of personality. Biological factors, such as the ones mentioned above, and environmental factors, such as family environment, social class, or early life experiences, have been considered to be factors which contribute to 'create' our personalities. Psychoanalysts point to 'drives' and defence mechanisms to explain individual differences. Psychologists have defined psychometric dimensional factors in normal personality and proposed that their measures correlate with biological differences. Investigators are now focusing on finding these biological correlates in relation to different temperamental and character traits. This does not necessary imply that personality disorders are explainable by biology alone. A more likely perspective is that we inherit basic traits or endophenotypes that predispose to psychiatric disorders in interaction with the environment.

Clearly defined diagnostic criteria are an important prerequisite for studying the role of biology and environment in the personality disorders. To clearly demarcate them from the more symptom-oriented psychiatric disorders, personality disorders were placed on Axis II in the DSM axial system. Personality disorders are categorized into three clusters: A, B, and C. Cluster A represents a group of personality disorders that are marked by isolation and eccentricity. Disorders in Cluster B are characterized by behaviours of acting out in a dramatic, emotional, and erratic way. Diagnoses in Cluster C include individuals who are anxious and fearful. It is important to emphasize that the DSM criteria are clinically derived schema for categorizing personality disorders. While we seek external validators for the diagnostic system, our knowledge of the biological correlates, pathophysiology, genetics, or aetiological factors has not yet progressed to the point that we can obtain biological validation of the personality disorder diagnoses. The DSM has, however, made it possible to diagnose personality disorders in a more uniform way and in that way identify more homogeneous patient populations for research studies. The advances in neuroscience and its adaptation to study the pathophysiology of the Axis I disorders also have benefited these research efforts. With the help of neuroimaging and neuroendocrine measurements, the mapping of the brain and the activity of its neurotransmitters is possible.

What makes this area interesting and difficult is the fact that what we are trying to study is the essence of what makes all of us who we are. What are the underlying reasons for the extreme problems some people have in relation to themselves and/or their surroundings? These are fundamental questions regarding personality and particularly personality disorders. As our knowledge about the central nervous system is increasing rapidly, evidence of correlations between personality traits and brain function is also increasing. We can see resemblances between Axis I disorders and personality disorders on Axis II, both in personality traits and in brain function (or dysfunction). We can see the therapeutic effects of medication on dysfunctional personality traits, but we still do not have a comprehensive knowledge of the exact mechanisms underlying personality and personality disorders.

DIMENSIONAL APPROACHES TO PERSONALITY

Personality dysfunction may be conceptualized from either a categorical or a dimensional perspective. The categorical model defines a set of specific personality disorder diagnostic categories to which an individual belongs or does not belong. DSM-IV uses this approach with a polythetic system in which individuals may fit into a diagnostic category if they possess a subset of criteria characteristics from a larger set. Thus, individuals with differing clusters of symptoms may share the same diagnosis. In contrast to a categorical system, a dimensional approach identifies a set of features which vary in magnitude among individuals. Individual personality disorders are characterized by high levels of one or more of these dimensions. The temperamental traits that are critical in the different personality disorders show strong evidence of heritability (Torgersen, 1994). Patients rarely represent 'clear-cut' cases; they often demonstrate a mix of traits that do not fit under one single diagnosis. This makes it more fruitful to evaluate personality traits rather then specific disorders to identify such associations. However, the nature of the key traits or dimensions in personality and personality disorders and the specific neurotransmitters and brain systems that can be associated with these key dimensions have not been definitively established. While researchers do not fully agree on what dimensions are critical to the study of personality, there is a fair correspondence between different dimensional systems. Our knowledge of abnormalities in neurotransmitter function in psychiatric disorders such as depression, bipolar disorder, and anxiety has suggested avenues of approach in understanding the biology of the personality disorders (Ressler and Nemeroff, 2000).

Biological Psychiatry: Edited by H. D'haenen, J.A. den Boer and P. Willner. ISBN 0-471-49198-5

There are a number of dimensional approaches to personality disorder. Some of these are derived from studies of normal personality such as the systems of Eysenck (Eysenck, 1991) or the five factor model of personality (Costa and Widiger, 1994). Other approaches have identified key dimensions from analyses of personality disorders. Finally, other schema, such as the temperament and character (TCI) model of Cloninger (Cloninger *et al.*, 1993), are based on a theoretical construct of the psychobiology of personality disorder as well as a framework for describing the relationship of character to temperament. For the purposes of this review, we employ a broad, face-valid model of key domains of personality disorders that may be dimensional and that cut across the boundaries of specific disorders. For example, cognitive disorganization is the hallmark of Cluster A, the schizophrenia spectrum personality disorders, including schizotypal, schizoid, and paranoid personality disorder, and is manifest in traits of suspiciousness, social isolation, and paranoid thinking, and, in some cases, psychotic-like phenomena. More extreme forms of cognitive disorganization are found in schizophrenia, where reality testing is severely distorted. Cluster B is characterized by impulsivity, defined as a relative disinhibition of action-oriented, particularly aggressive responses to the environment, and affective instability, defined as intense affective shifts in response to environmental precipitants. Anxiety, defined as apprehension and anticipation of negative consequences of behaviour often associated with autonomic arousal, is most characteristic of the anxious cluster, Cluster C. These dimensions have been related to specific neurotransmitters in brain systems on the basis of research of Axis I disorders (Siever and Davis, 1991; Kirrane and Siever, 2000). These clinical domains are consistent with those derived from factor models of personality disorders. They may also be related to other models of personality disorders, such as the temperament and character model of Cloninger, in that low harm avoidance could be considered to be coincident with impulsive aggression, while high novelty seeking may map into impulsivity and high reward dependence into affective instability (see Chapter XXVI-6).

THE ECCENTRIC CLUSTER

The eccentric cluster (Cluster A) consists of paranoid, schizoid, and schizotypal personality disorders. Patients that are diagnosed with these disorders share odd and eccentric behaviour as well as unusual thinking. The temperament and character model characterizes this group as having a temperament of low reward dependence (Cloninger *et al.*, 1993; Svrakic *et al.*, 1993). Cognitive disorganization in these patients is a central problem because it interferes with effective interaction with others in social and occupational arenas. Research suggests that the dopaminergic system, an important neurotransmitter system, is involved in cognition. Cognitive function in schizotypal personality disorder has been studied because these patients have a well-demonstrated association with schizophrenia, in both their cognitive symptoms (Siever and Davis, 1991) and their genetic basis (Kendler *et al.*, 1981), yet they are free from the potential confounding effects of chronic neuroleptic treatment and downward social drift. The major metabolite of dopamine, homovanillic acid (HVA), measured in plasma and cerebrospinal fluid (CSF), has been shown to correlate with psychotic-like symptoms in both schizotypal and non-schizotypal personality disorder subjects (Siever *et al.*, 1991a; 1993). Studies using SPECT imaging of IBZM displacement by amphetamine-stimulated dopamine release and studies of plasma HVA responses to 2-deoxyglucose (2-DG) indicate that subcortical dopamine activity in schizotypal patients is comparable to or lower than that seen in normal subjects, and is markedly lower than that seen in schizophrenic patients (Siever *et al.*, 2002). Thus, schizotypal personality disorder patients may be spared from psychosis because of reduced subcortical dopaminergic activity. Among schizotypal patients, those with higher dopaminergic activity tend to have more psychotic-like symptoms.

THE DRAMATIC CLUSTER

The dramatic cluster (Cluster B) consists of antisocial, borderline, histrionic, and narcissistic personality disorders. Common to these disorders are dramatic, emotional, and erratic behaviours. Individuals with these disorders are impulsive and aggressive, as well as affectively unstable. The TCI describes their temperament as one of high novelty seeking and low harm avoidance (Cloninger *et al.*, 1993; Svrakic *et al.*, 1993). Associations have been found between the traits of impulsivity, aggression, and affective liability and the monoaminergic systems, but other systems, such as the cholinergic system, also seem to play a role (Gurvits *et al.*, 2000).

IMPULSIVITY AND AGGRESSION

Aggressive behaviour is common in the personality disorders (Berman *et al.*, 1998), in part because of the interaction between irritability and the interpersonal environment. Borderline personality disorder (BPD) is characterized by prominent impulsive/aggression.

Early evidence suggested that borderline personality disorder (BPD) runs in families (Loranger *et al.*, 1982). Later it was shown that it is not BPD, but the personality trait of impulsive aggression, common in BPD, that is heritable (Torgersen, 1994). Impulsive aggression has been shown to be heritable in the general population through identical twin studies (Coccaro *et al.*, 1993; 1994), adoptive studies of criminal offenders and antisocial personality-disordered subjects (Cloninger *et al.*, 1975; Crowe, 1974), and family studies. The risk of having affective and impulsive personality disorder traits is greater in relatives of BPD than in relatives of people with other personality disorders (Silverman *et al.*, 1991). In order to understand the underlying biology of impulsivity and aggression, a number of neurotransmitter systems have been studied.

Serotonin

Serotonin is involved in self-directed, restitutive behaviours, such as grooming, feeding, and sleeping. Animal studies show that these behaviours are associated with increases in the firing of serotonergic neurons, neurons that normally fire at a consistent, continuous rate (Jacobs and Fornal, 1995). Low levels of the serotonin metabolite 5-HIAA in the CSF have been associated with impulsive, violent crimes and suicide attempts, examples of externally and internally directed aggressive behaviour.

Violent offenders who committed impulsive crimes had a lower concentration of 5-HIAA in the CSF than violent offenders who committed premeditated crimes (Linnoila *et al.*, 1983). It is interesting that the lowest levels were found in the subjects who had attempted suicide. Later several other studies confirmed the hypothesis that a low level of serotonergic activity correlates with an increased risk of suicide or parasuicide. Asberg *et al.* (1987) showed that low serotonin metabolite levels increased the risk of later suicide attempts. This association was confirmed in a short-term prospective study (Nordstrom *et al.*, 1994) and appears to occur regardless of psychiatric diagnosis (Siever *et al.*, 1991b). Reduced 5-HT levels were also found in parasuicidal patients (Coccaro and Astill, 1990). A meta-analyses of 27 research reports (Lester, 1995) and later a review of 20 studies (Asberg, 1997) concluded that low levels of 5-HIAA in the CSF are strongly correlated to suicidal behaviour. Mann *et al.* (1996d) found that low 5-HIAA correlated with a history of planned suicide and with suicide attempts that resulted in greater medical damage, suggesting a more violent method.

Externally directed aggression also correlates to reduced serotonergic metabolites, although not as consistently. Subjects with antisocial personality disorder responded with more aggression when using alcohol than subjects without antisocial personality disorder (Virkkunen and Linnoila, 1993; Moeller *et al.*, 1998b). Finnish alcoholic, impulsive, habitually violent offenders have been found to have low brain serotonin concentrations (Virkkunen *et al.*, 1996). Decreased serotonin metabolism correlates with externally directed aggressive behaviour in criminal offenders and in clinical and normal populations (Coccaro *et al.*, 1990b). Lower concentrations of 5-HIAA in the CSF are found in people with a history of problematic aggressive behaviour (Brown *et al.*, 1979; 1982). Other studies have, however, shown the opposite, that is, that aggression scores correlate with high levels of 5-HIAA in the CSF (Moller *et al.*, 1996). The same study found that low levels of 5-HIAA in the CSF correlate with internally directed aggression scores (Moller *et al.*, 1996). Another study found that homicide offenders did not differ from control subjects in the concentrations of 5-HIAA in the CSF (Lidberg, 2000). However, the group of homicide offenders that had made one or more suicide attempts had a significantly lower concentration of 5-HIAA in the CSF than the rest of the group, with the exception of subjects with impulse-control disorder, suggesting that serotonin regulates suicidal tendencies and impulse control. Thus, the most consistent finding is that serotonergic activity has a strong inverse relationship with internally directed aggression.

It is relatively difficult to obtain CSF samples in order to study serotonergic activity, and these measures reflect only the presynaptic component of serotonergic activity. Since prolactin secretion is regulated by serotonergic neurotransmission (Coccaro *et al.*, 1998a), measurement of prolactin in response to a serotonergic agent could provide an indirect measure of serotonergic activity. It has been suggested that this method might be a more sensitive measurement of serotonergic activity than the measurement of 5-HIAA levels in the CSF in that it also reflects the postsynaptic responsiveness of the serotonergic system (Coccaro *et al.*, 1997a). Studies using the neuroendocrine paradigm report a consistent correlation between blunted prolactin response to serotonergic agents and impulsivity or aggression in the personality disorders.

A blunted prolactin response to *d*-fenfluramine, a serotonin releaser and reuptake inhibitor, was found in personality disorder subjects compared to controls and was associated with a history of suicide attempts and impulsive aggression in the personality disorder subjects (Coccaro *et al.*, 1989; Coccaro, 1989; Siever and Trestman, 1993). A blunted response to fenfluramine was also found in subjects with antisocial personality disorder convicted of murder (O'Keane *et al.*, 1992), and it correlated to both self-reported and behavioural measures of aggression (Coccaro *et al.*, 1996a). In a study employing m-CPP (*m*-chlorophenylpiperazine), a 5-HT_{1a} and 5-HT_{2c} agonist, the prolactin response varied inversely with assaultiveness (Coccaro *et al.*, 1997c) and was blunted in antisocial personality disorder (Moss *et al.*, 1990). Buspirone and ipsapirone, two 5-HT_{1a} agonists, also produced blunted prolactin responses that varied inversely with aggressiveness (Coccaro *et al.*, 1990a; Moeller *et al.*, 1998a). Thus, a blunted prolactin response to a serotonergic challenge seems to be a consistent correlate of impulsive aggression in personality disorder patients.

The 5-HT_{2a} and -$_{2c}$ receptors appear to mediate the prolactin response to *d*-fenfluramine (Coccaro *et al.*, 1996c), while 5-HT_3 receptors seem to play little if any role in the prolactin response (Coccaro *et al.*, 1996b; Mann *et al.*, 1996a). An increase of 5-HT_2-receptor density has been reported in depressed patients and in suicidal patients (Pandey *et al.*, 1990). The increase was localized to the prefrontal cortex in a group of suicide victims (Arango *et al.*, 1990). This could reflect a compensatory increase due to reduced 5-HT release (Mann *et al.*, 1990). The density of 5-HT postsynaptic receptors correlates with the tendency to assaultive behaviour in non-criminally aggressive, personality-disordered subjects (Coccaro *et al.*, 1997c). The density of 5-HT_{2a} receptors positively correlates to assaultiveness in personality-disordered subjects. However, the affinity seems to be decreased (Coccaro *et al.*, 1997b). The number of 5-HT transporter (SERT) sites has been shown to vary inversely with self-mutilation in patients with personality disorder (Simeon *et al.*, 1992). The SERT sites in the brain are coded for by the same single-copy gene as the platelet 5-HT uptake site (Lesch *et al.*, 1993), a fact which makes it possible to study SERT in psychiatric disorders by studying platelets. Coccaro and colleagues have found a correlation between life history of aggressive behaviour and a reduced number of platelet 5-HT transporter sites in personality disorder patients (Coccaro *et al.*, 1996d).

These studies of serotonergic activity pointed the way to candidate gene studies of serotonin-related genes. One candidate gene (Burmeister, 1999) codes for the rate-limiting enzyme, TPH, in the synthesis of serotonin. A particular polymorphism of the TPH gene has been found to be associated with suicide, but not with CSF 5-HIAA concentration, in criminal offenders (Nielsen *et al.*, 1994; 1998). However, this association with suicide was not duplicated in a more general suicidal population (Abbar *et al.*, 1995). There are two alleles of the TPH gene, the 'L' and 'U' alleles. One study has shown that the 'L' allele of the TPH gene appears to be associated with impulsive aggression (New *et al.*, 1998). However, another study contradicted this by showing an association between the presence of at least one 'U' allele of the TPH gene and overt aggression in men (Manuck *et al.*, 1999). Thus, it remains unclear to what extent the TPH gene is involved in aggression. Other studies have shown association between the 'G' allele of the 5-HT_{1b} receptor gene and a history of suicide attempts in Caucasian patients with personality disorders (New *et al.*, 2001), and an association between alleles of the 5-HT_{2a} receptor gene and self-directed aggression (New *et al.*, 1999).

Positron emission tomography (PET) studies can demonstrate activity in regions of interest in the brain through measuring glucose metabolism. Patients with impulsive-aggressive behaviours show decreased activity in orbital frontal cortex at baseline and after fenfluramine compared to controls (Goyer *et al.*, 1994; Siever *et al.*, 1999). By giving subjects fenfluramine, a serotonin releaser and reuptake inhibitor, and measuring the metabolic activity of regions of interest with a PET scan, one can obtain an index of that region's serotonergic responsiveness. Fenfluramine caused an increase in metabolic activity in an area centred on the anterior cingulate and an area in the lateral prefrontal cortex involving the inferior, middle, and superior frontal gyri in the left prefrontal cortex and in the left temporoparietal cortex in normal subjects (Mann *et al.*, 1996c), but no increase in activity was found in depressed inpatients by the same method (Mann *et al.*, 1996b). Raine *et al.* (1994) showed that seriously violent offenders pleading not guilty by reason of insanity or incompetent to stand trial had a reduced metabolic activity in both the lateral and medial prefrontal cortex. Patients with impulsive-aggressive personality disorders have reduced metabolic activity compared to healthy volunteers in the orbital frontal, ventral medial frontal, and cingulate cortex after administration of *d*,l-fenfluramine (Siever *et al.*, 1999).

Pharmacotherapeutic studies have shown that fluoxetine hydrochloride, a selective serotonin-uptake inhibitor, reduced the aggressiveness in impulsive-aggressive personality disorder subjects (Coccaro and Kavoussi, 1997; Salzman *et al.*, 1995), again supporting a relationship between serotonin and aggression.

Dopamine

Animal studies have suggested a connection between dopaminergic activity and aggression (Coccaro, 1996). Human studies show either a negative correlation or no correlation between the dopamine metabolite HVA in the CSF and aggression. CSF HVA levels have been observed to be closely linked to 5-HIAA levels in the CSF, which are known to be reduced in impulsive aggression (Coccaro, 1998), and CSF HVA may thus be reduced as well (Linnoila, 1983). A positive correlation between plasma HVA and novelty seeking among subjects with an anxious cluster personality disorder has been found in our laboratory (Siever *et al.*, unpublished data). The dopamine receptor D4DR gene has been shown to relate to novelty seeking in volunteers in some studies (Benjamin *et al.*, 1996; Ebstein *et al.*, 1996), but not in others (Malhotra *et al.*, 1996). In schizotypal and non-schizotypal personality disorder subjects, HVA concentrations in the CSF and plasma correlate with psychotic-like symptoms rather than aggressive behaviours (Siever *et al.*, 1993; Siever *et al.*, 1991a).

Vasopressin

Animal studies report a correlation between CSF vasopressin levels in the central nervous system (CNS) and aggression (Ferris and Delville, 1994). Vasopressin is associated with aggressive behaviour in humans in that a positive correlation has been reported with a life history of aggression even when controlling for the decreased serotonergic activity (Coccaro *et al.*, 1998b).

Other Peptides

While opiate withdrawal often elicits aggressive behaviour, there has been little study of the relationship of opiates to aggression although some inconsistent correlations have been found (Coccaro and Siever, 2002). Testosterone appears to play a facilitative role for aggressive behaviours in non-psychiatric subjects (Archer, 1991; Rubinow and Schmidt, 1996).

Norepinephrine

While lower concentrations of the serotonin metabolite (5-HIAA) have been found in the CSF of people with a history of problematic aggressive behaviour, a higher level of the norepinephrine metabolite [methoxy-4-hydroxy-phenylglycol (MHPG)] has been found in aggressive subjects than controls, and is correlated with a life history of aggression (Brown *et al.*, 1979; 1982). Plasma norepinephrine has also been correlated with self-reported impulsivity in personality disorder patients (Siever and Trestman, 1993), but reductions in CSF MHPG have also been reported in one study (Virkkunen *et al.*, 1987), although this was not replicated in another later study by the same group (Virkkunen *et al.*, 1994). Increased responses to clonidine were reported to be associated with self-reported 'irritability', but not with assaultiveness (Coccaro *et al.*, 1991).

AFFECTIVE INSTABILITY

In bipolar and depressed patients, PET studies have shown decreased activity in the prefrontal cortex, ventral to the genu of the corpus callosum, a finding partly explained by a corresponding reduction in the grey matter, raising the possibility of reduced cortical activity in relationship to affective symptoms (Drevets *et al.*, 1997). Pleasant and unpleasant emotions both increased cerebral blood flow (CBF) in the vicinity of the medial prefrontal cortex (Brodmann's area 9), thalamus, hypothalamus, midbrain, and head of the left caudate nucleus in healthy women (Lane *et al.*, 1997a; 1997b). Unpleasant affects also activated the bilateral occipitotemporal cortex and cerebellum, and left parahippocampal gyrus, hippocampus, and amygdala (Lane *et al.*, 1997a). Thus, intense affects have been associated with limbic and subcortical activity. Both in healthy sadness and in depressive illness, there is a decrease of CBF in the neocortical (right dorsolateral prefrontal, inferior parietal) and the limbic-paralimbic (subgenual cingulate, anterior insula) regions (Mayberg, 1997; 1999). In remission of depression, a decrease of paralimbic blood flow and an increase of neocortical blood flow was observed (Mayberg, 1997; 1999). These considerations suggest that the cortex may play an inhibitory modulatory role in relation to limbic activation associated with intense affects. Thus, affective instability in patients with BPD may reflect increased paralimbic activity, possibly in response to poor modulation by higher cortical structures.

Acetylcholine

Cholinergic neurons are found in limbic structures, paralimbic structures, the cortex, and the nucleus basalis (Ketter *et al.*, 1996). Acetylcholine is ubiquitous in the CNS and is involved in modulating REM sleep and autonomic nervous system activity. Animal studies suggest a role for central nicotinic receptors in depression (Tizabi *et al.*, 1999).

Procaine activates limbic structures, in part, by means of cholinergic activation (Kellner *et al.*, 1987; Kling *et al.*, 1987). When procaine was administered to healthy volunteer subjects, it induced fear in one-third and euphoria in one-third of the subjects. These effects correlated with the degree of activation of the left amygdala in PET studies (Ketter *et al.*, 1996). When physostigmine, a cholinesterase inhibitor, was given to healthy male volunteers, it induced a dysphoric and cardiovascular response that correlated with high emotional lability, high irritability, feelings of stress, and low life contentment (Fritze *et al.*, 1990). Physostigmine also induced a stronger depressive response in BPD patients than in normal controls and non-BPD patients (Steinberg *et al.*, 1997). The depressive symptoms in response to physostigmine correlated to BPD traits related to affective instability (affective instability, identity disturbances, chronic feelings of emptiness and boredom, and turbulent relationships), but they did not correlate to traits related to impulsivity. Exaggerated affective responses to cholinergic agonists have been shown in affective disorder patients compared to normal controls (Janowsky *et al.*, 1994). BPD patients without current depression showed a decrease in REM latency, similar to depressed patients, as compared to non-BPD and non-psychiatric controls (Akiskal *et al.*, 1985; Bell *et al.*, 1983; McNamara *et al.*, 1984). This is consistent with the possibility of altered cholinergic activity in BPD.

Norepinephrine (NE)

Animal models show an increase of noradrenergic activity in the locus coeruleus when the rodent is confronted with threatening stimuli (Levine *et al.*, 1990). Noradrenergic neuronal function is increased in anxiety and fear states in human subjects (Charney *et al.*, 1992). Administration of dextroamphetamine, a norepinephrine and dopamine releaser/reuptake inhibitor, to healthy subjects induces a dysphoric response (Kavoussi and Coccaro, 1993). This response correlated proportionally to measures of affective lability. By using the neuroendocrine measure of growth hormone response to a clonidine challenge, Coccaro *et al.* (1991) showed that central alpha$_2$-adrenergic receptors play a role in irritability, but not in assaultiveness. Gerra *et al.* (1999) found a positive correlation between sensation seeking, and NE and NE-dependent hormones.

GABA (Gamma-Aminobutyric Acid)

GABA-receptors are found in the amygdala and seem to be involved in the intense affects induced by procaine (Ketter *et al.*, 1996). Medications that successfully treat patients with affective instability, such as lithium, valproate, and carbamazepine, increase GABAminergic neurotransmission (Shatzberg and Nemeroff, 1989), suggesting that GABA plays a role in affective instability.

CLUSTER C

The anxious cluster consists of avoidant, dependent, and obsessive-compulsive personality disorders. Anxious and fearful personality features are common to these disorders. Individuals with these disorders try to avoid situations that can lead to embarrassment, but at the same time they want to be part of their social group and long for close relationships. According to the TCI, they have a temperament of high harm avoidance (Cloninger *et al.*, 1993; Svrakic *et al.*, 1993). Harm avoidance has been hypothesized to be associated with the neurotransmitters serotonin and dopamine.

Serotonin

Blunted prolactin responses to fenfluramine were found in males with compulsive personality disorder compared with males with non-compulsive personality disorders, but these responses correlated with impulsivity in these patients (Stein *et al.*, 1996). A blunted prolactin response to fenfluramine has been shown in obsessive-compulsive disorder (OCD) patients and in patients with major depression compared to normal controls (Lucey *et al.*, 1992). An inverse correlation between harm avoidance and 5-HT_2 receptor sensitivity has also been demonstrated (Pierson *et al.*, 1999). The s/s genotype, but not the s/l or l/l genotypes, of the serotonin transporter is associated with higher scores of neuroticism on the NEO personality inventory, a measurement that includes anxiety (Greenberg *et al.*, 2000; Murakami *et al.*, 1999).

CONCLUSIONS

In general, surprisingly strong correlations have been shown between neurotransmitter activity and the personality disorders, particularly dimensions of personality such as impulsive/aggression, cognitive disorganization, and affective instability. New imaging techniques may permit more specific delineation of the circuits that may be altered in relation to these disturbances in neurotransmitters. As the genome is mapped in more detail, we may have better means of identifying specific candidate genes. Linkage techniques may also help to develop specific identification of altered genes. Not only will such studies inform our clinical interventions with these difficult-to-treat individuals, but they may also help us to understand better the relationship between individual differences in behaviour and personality and neurotransmitter activity.

REFERENCES

American Psychiatric Association APA, 1994. *Diagnostic and Statistical Manual of Mental Disorders (DSM-IV)*, 4th edn. Washington, DC.

Abbar, M., Courtet, P., Amadeo, S., Caer, Y., Mallet, J., Baldy-Moulinier, M., Castelnau, D. and Malafosse, A., 1995. Suicidal behaviors and the tryptophan hydroxylase gene. *Arch Gen Psychiatry*, **52**, 846–849.

Akiskal, H.S., Yerevanian, B.I., Davis, G.C., King, D. and Lemmi, H., 1985. The nosologic status of borderline personality: clinical and polysomnographic study. *Am J Psychiatry*, **142**, 192–198.

Arango, V., Ernsberger, P., Marzuk, P.M., Chen, J.S., Tierney, H., Stanley, M., Reis, D.J. and Mann, J.J., 1990. Autoradiographic demonstration of increased serotonin 5-HT2 and beta-adrenergic receptor binding sites in the brain of suicide victims. *Arch Gen Psychiatry*, **47**, 1038–1047.

Archer, J., 1991. The influence of testosterone on human aggression. *Br J Psychiatry*, **82**(pt 1), 1–28.

Asberg, M., Schalling, D., Traskman-Bendz, L. and Wagner, A., 1987. Psychobiology of suicide, impulsivity and related phenomena. In: Meltzer, H.Y. (ed.), *Psychopharmacology: Third Generation of Progress*, pp. 655–668. Raven Press, New York.

Asberg, M., 1997. Neurotransmitters and suicidal behavior. The evidence from cerebrospinal fluid studies. *Ann NY Acad Sci*, **836**, 158–181.

Bell, J., Lycaki, H., Jones, D., Kelwala, S. and Sitaram, N., 1983. Effect of preexisting borderline personality disorder on clinical and EEG sleep correlates of depression. *Psychiatry Res*, **9**, 115–123.

Benjamin, J., Li, L., Patterson, C., Greenberg, B.D., Murphy, D.L. and Hamer, D.H., 1996. Population and familial association between the D4 dopamine receptor gene and measures of novelty seeking. *Nat Genet*, **12**, 81–84.

Berman, M.E., Fallon, A.E. and Coccaro, E.F., 1998. The relationship between personality psychopathology and aggressive behavior in research volunteers. *J Abnorm Psychol*, **107**, 651–658.

Brown, G.L., Goodwin, F.K., Ballenger, J.C., Goyer, P.F. and Major, L.F., 1979. Aggression in humans correlates with cerebrospinal fluid amine metabolites. *Psychiatry Res*, **1**, 131–139.

Brown, G.L., Ebert, M.H., Goyer, P.F., Jimerson, D.C., Klein, W.J., Bunney, W.E. and Goodwin, F.K., 1982. Aggression, suicide, and serotonin: relationships to CSF amine metabolites. *Am J Psychiatry*, **139**, 741–746.

Burmeister, M., 1999. Basic concepts in the study of diseases with complex genetics. *Biol Psychiatry*, **45**, 522–532.

Charney, D.S., Woods, S.W., Krystal, J.H., Nagy, L.M. and Heninger, G.R., 1992. Noradrenergic neuronal dysregulation in panic disorder: the effects of intravenous yohimbine and clonidine in panic disorder patients. *Acta Psychiatr Scand*, **86**, 273–282.

Cloninger, R.C., Reich, T. and Guze, S.B., 1975. The multifactorial model of disease transmission. II. Sex differences in the familial transmission of sociopathy (antisocial personality). *Br J Psychiatry*, **127**, 11–22.

Cloninger, C.R., Svrakic, D.M. and Przybeck, T.R., 1993. A psychobiological model of temperament and character. *Arch Gen Psychiatry*, **50**, 975–990.

Coccaro, E.F., 1989. Central serotonin and impulsive aggression. *Br J Psychiatry Suppl*, **8**, 52–62.

Coccaro, E.F., 1996. Neurotransmitter correlates of impulsive aggression in humans. *Ann NY Acad Sci*, **794**, 82–89.

Coccaro, E.F., 1998. Impulsive aggression: a behavior in search of clinical definition. *Harv Rev Psychiatry*, **5**, 336–339.

Coccaro, E.F. and Astill, J.L., 1990. Central serotonergic function in parasuicide. *Prog Neuropsychopharmacol Biol Psychiatry*, **14**, 663–674.

Coccaro, E.F. and Kavoussi, R.J., 1997. Fluoxetine and impulsive aggressive behavior in personality-disordered subjects. *Arch Gen Psychiatry*, **54**, 1081–1088.

Coccaro, E.F. and Siever, L.J., 2002. Pathophysiology and treatment of aggression. In: *ACNP's Fifth Generation of Progress*. Lippincott Williams & Wilkins, Philadelphia, PA.

Coccaro, E.F., Siever, L.J., Klar, H.M., Maurer, G., Cochrane, K., Cooper, T.B., Mohs, R.C. and Davis, K.L., 1989. Serotonergic studies in patients with affective and personality disorders. Correlates with suicidal and impulsive-aggressive behavior. *Arch Gen Psychiatry*, **46**, 587–599.

Coccaro, E.F., Gabriel, S. and Siever, L.J., 1990a. Buspirone challenge: preliminary evidence for a role for central 5-HT1a receptor function in impulsive aggressive behavior in humans. *Psychopharmacol Bull*, **26**, 393–405.

Coccaro, E.F., Siever, L.J., Owen, K.R. and Davis, K.L., 1990b. Serotonin in mood and personality disorder. In: Coccaro, E.F., Murphy, D.L. (eds), *Serotonin in Major Psychiatric Disorder*, pp. 71–97. American Psychiatric Press, Washington, DC.

Coccaro, E.F., Lawrence, T., Trestman, R., Gabriel, S., Klar, H.M. and Siever, L.J., 1991. Growth hormone responses to intravenous clonidine challenge correlate with behavioral irritability in psychiatric patients and healthy volunteers. *Psychiatry Res*, **39**, 129–139.

Coccaro, E.F., Bergeman, C.S. and McClearn, G.E., 1993. Heritability of irritable impulsiveness: a study of twins reared together and apart. *Psychiatry Res*, **48**, 229–242.

Coccaro, E.F., Silverman, J.M., Klar, H.M., Horvath, T.B. and Siever, L.J., 1994. Familial correlates of reduced central serotonergic system function in patients with personality disorders. *Arch Gen Psychiatry*, **51**, 318–324.

Coccaro, E.F., Berman, M.E., Kavoussi, R.J. and Hauger, R.L., 1996a. Relationship of prolactin response to *d*-fenfluramine to behavioral and questionnaire assessments of aggression in personality-disordered men. *Biol Psychiatry*, **40**, 157–164.

Coccaro, E.F., Kavoussi, R.J., Cooper, T.B. and Hauger, R., 1996b. 5-HT3 receptor antagonism by ondansetron does not attenuate prolactin response to *d*-fenfluramine challenge in healthy human subjects. *Psychopharmacology (Berl)*, **127**, 108–112.

Coccaro, E.F., Kavoussi, R.J., Oakes, M., Cooper, T.B. and Hauger, R., 1996c. 5-HT2a/2c receptor blockade by amesergide fully attenuates prolactin response to *d*-fenfluramine challenge in physically healthy human subjects. *Psychopharmacology (Berl)*, **126**, 24–30.

Coccaro, E.F., Kavoussi, R.J., Sheline, Y.I., Lish, J.D. and Csernansky, J.G., 1996d. Impulsive aggression in personality disorder correlates with tritiated paroxetine binding in the platelet. *Arch Gen Psychiatry*, **53**, 531–536.

Coccaro, E.F., Kavoussi, R.J., Cooper, T.B. and Hauger, R.L., 1997a. Central serotonin activity and aggression: inverse relationship with prolactin response to *d*-fenfluramine, but not CSF 5-HIAA concentration, in human subjects. *Am J Psychiatry*, **154**, 1430–1435.

Coccaro, E.F., Kavoussi, R.J., Sheline, Y.I., Berman, M.E. and Csernansky, J.G., 1997b. Impulsive aggression in personality disorder correlates with platelet 5-HT2A receptor binding. *Neuropsychopharmacology*, **16**, 211–216.

Coccaro, E.F., Kavoussi, R.J., Trestman, R.L., Gabriel, S.M., Cooper, T.B. and Siever, L.J., 1997c. Serotonin function in human subjects: intercorrelations among central 5-HT indices and aggressiveness. *Psychiatry Res*, **73**, 1–14.

Coccaro, E.F., Kavoussi, R.J., Cooper, T.B. and Hauger, R., 1998a. Acute tryptophan depletion attenuates the prolactin response to *d*-fenfluramine challenge in healthy human subjects. *Psychopharmacology (Berl)*, **138**, 9–15.

Coccaro, E.F., Kavoussi, R.J., Hauger, R.L., Cooper, T.B. and Ferris, C.F., 1998b. Cerebrospinal fluid vasopressin levels: correlates with aggression and serotonin function in personality-disordered subjects. *Arch Gen Psychiatry*, **55**, 708–714.

Costa, P.T. and Widiger, T.A. (eds), 1994. *Personality Disorders and the Five Factor Model of Personality*. American Psychological Association, Washington, DC.

Crowe, R.R., 1974. An adoption study of antisocial personality. *Arch Gen Psychiatry*, **31**, 785–791.

Drevets, W.C., Price, J.L., Simpson, J.R. Jr, Todd, R.D., Reich, T., Vannier, M. and Raichle, M.E., 1997. Subgenual prefrontal cortex abnormalities in mood disorders. *Nature*, **386**(6627), 824–827.

Ebstein, R.P., Novick, O., Umansky, R., Priel, B., Osher, Y., Blaine, D., Bennett, E.R., Nemanov, L., Katz, M. and Belmaker, R.H., 1996. Dopamine D4 receptor (D4DR) exon III polymorphism associated with the human personality trait of novelty seeking. *Nat Genet*, **12**, 78–80.

Eysenck, H.J., 1991. Genetic and environmental contributions to individual differences: the three major dimensions of personality. *J Pers*, **58**, 245–261.

Ferris, C.F. and Delville, Y., 1994. Vasopressin and serotonin interactions in the control of agonistic behavior. *Psychoneuroendocrinology*, **19**(5–7), 593–601.

Fritze, J., Sofic, E., Muller, T., Pfuller, H., Lanczik, M. and Riederer, P., 1990. Cholinergic-adrenergic balance: Part 2. Relationship between drug sensitivity and personality. *Psychiatry Res*, **34**, 271–279.

Gerra, G., Avanzini, P., Zaimovic, A., Sartori, R., Bocchi, C., Timpano, M., Zambelli, U., Delsignore, R., Gardini, F., Talarico, E. and Brambilla, F., 1999. Neurotransmitters, neuroendocrine correlates of sensation-seeking temperament in normal humans. *Neuropsychobiology*, **39**, 207–213.

Greenberg, B.D., Li, Q., Lucas, F.R., Hu, S., Sirota, L.A., Benjamin, J., Lesch, K.P., Hamer, D. and Murphy, D.L., 2000. Association between the serotonin transporter promoter polymorphism and personality traits in a primarily female population sample. *Am J Med Genet*, **96**, 202–216.

Goyer, P.F., Andreason, P.J., Semple, W.E., 1994. Positron-emission tomography and personality disorders. *Neuropsychopharmacology*, **10**, 21–28.

Gurvits, I.G., Koenigsberg, H.W. and Siever, L.J., 2000. Neurotransmitter dysfunction in patients with borderline personality disorder. *Psychiatr Clin North Am*, **23**, 27–40, vi.

Jacobs, B.L. and Fornal, C.A., 1995. Serotonin and behavior: a general hypothesis. In: Bloom, F.E., Kupfer, D.J. (eds), *Psychopharmacology: The Fourth Generation of Progress*, pp. 461–469. Raven Press, New York.

Janowsky, D.S., Overstreet, D.H. and Nurnberger, J.I., Jr., 1994. Is cholinergic sensitivity a genetic marker for the affective disorders? *Am J Med Genet*, **54**, 335–344.

Kavoussi, R.J. and Coccaro, E.F., 1993. The amphetamine challenge test correlates with affective lability in healthy volunteers. *Psychiatry Res*, **48**, 219–228.

Kellner, C.H., Post, R.M., Putnam, F., Cowdry, R., Gardner, D., Kling, M.A., Minichiello, M.D., Trettau, J.R. and Coppola, R., 1987. Intravenous procaine as a probe of limbic system activity in psychiatric patients and normal controls. *Biol Psychiatry*, **22**, 1107–1126.

Kendler, K.S., Gruenberg, A.M. and Strauss, A.J., 1981. An independent analysis of the Copenhagen sample of the Danish Adoption Study of Schizophrenia. II. The relationship between schizotypal personality disorder and schizophrenia. *Arch Gen Psychiatry*, **38**, 982–984.

Ketter, T.A., Andreason, P.J., George, M.S., Lee, C., Gill, D.S., Parekh, P.I., Willis, M.W., Herscovitch, P. and Post, R.M., 1996. Anterior paralimbic mediation of procaine-induced emotional and psychosensory experiences. *Arch Gen Psychiatry*, **53**, 59–69.

Kirrane, R.M. and Siever, L.J., 2000. New perspectives on schizotypal personality disorder. *Curr Psychiatry Rep*, **2**, 62–66.

Kling, M.A., Kellner, C.H., Post, R.M., Cowdry, R.W., Gardner, D.L., Coppola, R., Putnam, F.W. and Gold, P.W., 1987. Neuroendocrine effects of limbic activation by electrical, spontaneous, and pharmacological modes: relevance to the pathophysiology of affective dysregulation in psychiatric disorders. *Prog Neuropsychopharmacol Biol Psychiatry*, **11**, 459–481.

Lane, R.D., Reiman, E.M., Bradley, M.M., Lang, P.J., Ahern, G.L., Davidson, R.J. and Schwartz, G.E., 1997a. Neuroanatomical correlates of pleasant and unpleasant emotion. *Neuropsychologia*, **35**, 1437–1444.

Lane, R.D., Reiman, E.M., Ahern, G.L., Schwartz, G.E. and Davidson, R.J., 1997b. Neuroanatomical correlates of happiness, sadness, and disgust. *Am J Psychiatry*, **154**, 926–933.

Lesch, K.P., Wolozin, B.L., Murphy, D.L. and Reiderer, P., 1993. Primary structure of the human platelet serotonin uptake site: identity with the brain serotonin transporter. *J Neurochem*, **60**, 2319–2322.

Lester, D., 1995. The concentration of neurotransmitter metabolites in the cerebrospinal fluid of suicidal individuals: a meta-analysis. *Pharmacopsychiatry*, **28**, 45–50.

Levine, E.S., Litto, W.J. and Jacobs, B.L., 1990. Activity of cat locus coeruleus noradrenergic neurons during the defense reaction. *Brain Res*, **531**(1–2), 189–195.

Lidberg, L., Belfrage, H., Bertilsson, L., Evenden, M.M. and Asberg, M., 2000. Suicide attempts and impulse control disorder are related to low cerebrospinal fluid 5-HIAA in mentally disordered violent offenders. *Acta Psychiatr Scand*, **101**, 395–402.

Linnoila, M., Virkkunen, M., Scheinin, M., Nuutila, A., Rimon, R. and Goodwin, F.K., 1983. Low cerebrospinal fluid 5-hydroxyindoleacetic acid concentration differentiates impulsive from nonimpulsive violent behavior. *Life Sci*, **33**, 2609–2614.

Loranger, A.W., Oldham, J.M. and Tulis, E.H., 1982. Familial transmission of DSM-III borderline personality disorder. *Arch Gen Psychiatry*, **39**, 795–799.

Lucey, J.V., O'Keane, V., Butcher, G., Clare, A.W. and Dinan, T.G., 1992. Cortisol and prolactin responses to *d*-fenfluramine in non-depressed patients with obsessive-compulsive disorder: a comparison with depressed and healthy controls. *Br J Psychiatry*, **161**, 517–521.

Malhotra, A.K., Virkkunen, M., Rooney, W., Eggert, M., Linnoila, M. and Goldman, D., 1996. The association between the dopamine D4 receptor (D4DR) 16 amino acid repeat polymorphism and novelty seeking. *Mol Psychiatry*, **1**, 388–391.

Mann, J.J., Arango, V. and Underwood, M.D., 1990. Serotonin and suicidal behavior. *Ann NY Acad Sci*, **600**, 476–484; discussion 484–485.

Mann, J.J., Arango, V., Henteleff, R.A., Lagattuta, T.F. and Wong, D.T., 1996a. Serotonin 5-HT3 receptor binding kinetics in the cortex of suicide victims are normal. *J Neural Transm*, **103**(1–2), 165–171.

Mann, J.J., Malone, K.M., Diehl, D.J., Perel, J., Cooper, T.B. and Mintun, M.A., 1996b. Demonstration *in vivo* of reduced serotonin responsivity in the brain of untreated depressed patients. *Am J Psychiatry*, **153**, 174–182.

Mann, J.J., Malone, K.M., Diehl, D.J., Perel, J., Nichols, T.E. and Mintun, M.A., 1996c. Positron emission tomographic imaging of serotonin activation effects on prefrontal cortex in healthy volunteers. *J Cereb Blood Flow Metab*, **16**, 418–426.

Mann, J.J., Malone, K.M., Psych, M.R., Sweeney, J.A., Brown, R.P., Linnoila, M., Stanley, B. and Stanley, M., 1996d. Attempted suicide characteristics and cerebrospinal fluid amine metabolites in depressed inpatients. *Neuropsychopharmacology*, **15**, 576–586.

Manuck, S.B., Flory, J.D., Ferrell, R.E., Dent, K.M., Mann, J.J. and Muldoon, M.F., 1999. Aggression and anger-related traits associated with a polymorphism of the tryptophan hydroxylase gene. *Biol Psychiatry*, **45**, 603–614.

Mayberg, H.S. and 1997. Limbic-cortical dysregulation: a proposed model of depression. *J Neuropsychiatry Clin Neurosci*, **9**, 471–481.

Mayberg, H.S., Liotti, M., Brannan, S.K., McGinnis, S., Mahurin, R.K., Jerabek, P.A., Silva, J.A., Tekell, J.L., Martin, C.C., Lancaster, J.L. and Fox, P.T., 1999. Reciprocal limbic-cortical function and negative mood: converging PET findings in depression and normal sadness. *Am J Psychiatry*, **156**, 675–682.

McNamara, E., Reynolds, C.F. 3rd, Soloff, P.H., Mathias, R., Rossi, A., Spiker, D., Coble, P.A. and Kupfer, D.J., 1984. EEG sleep evaluation of depression in borderline patients. *Am J Psychiatry*, **141**, 182–186.

Moeller, F.G., Allen, T., Cherek, D.R., Dougherty, D.M., Lane, S. and Swann, A.C., 1998a. Ipsapirone neuroendocrine challenge: relationship to aggression as measured in the human laboratory. *Psychiatry Res*, **81**, 31–38.

Moeller, F.G., Dougherty, D.M., Lane, S.D., Steinberg, J.L. and Cherek, D.R., 1998b. Antisocial personality disorder and alcohol-induced aggression. *Alcohol Clin Exp Res*, **22**, 1898–1902.

Moller, S.E., Mortensen, E.L., Breum, L., Alling, C., Larsen, O.G., Boge-Rasmussen, T., Jensen, C. and Bennicke, K., 1996. Aggression and personality: association with amino acids and monoamine metabolites. *Psychol Med*, **26**, 323–331.

Moss, H.B., Yao, J.K. and Panzak, G.L., 1990. Serotonergic responsivity and behavioral dimensions in antisocial personality disorder with substance abuse. *Biol Psychiatry*, **28**, 325–338.

Murakami, F., Shimomura, T., Kotani, K., Ikawa, S., Nanba, E. and Adachi, K., 1999. Anxiety traits associated with a polymorphism in the serotonin transporter gene regulatory region in the Japanese. *J Hum Genet*, **44**, 15–17.

New, A.S., Gelernter, J., Yovell, Y., Trestman, R.L., Nielsen, D.A., Silverman, J., Mitropoulou, V. and Siever, L.J., 1998. Tryptophan hydroxylase genotype is associated with impulsive-aggression measures: a preliminary study. *Am J Med Genet*, **81**, 13–17.

New, A.S., Gelernter, J., Mitropoulou, V. and Siever, L.J., 1999. Serotonin related genotype and impulsive aggression. Presented at the 54th Annual Meeting of the Society of Biological Psychiatry. Washington, DC, May.

New, A.S., Gelernter, J., Goodman, M., Mitropoulou, V., Koenigsberg, H., Silverman, J. and Siever, L.J., 2001. Suicide, impulsive aggression and the HTR1B genotype. *Biol Psychiatry*, **50**, 62–65.

Nielsen, D.A., Goldman, D., Virkkunen, M., Tokola, R., Rawlings, R. and Linnoila, M., 1994. Suicidality and 5-hydroxyindoleacetic acid concentration associated with a tryptophan hydroxylase polymorphism. *Arch Gen Psychiatry*, **51**, 34–38.

Nielsen, D.A., Virkkunen, M., Lappalainen, J., Eggert, M., Brown, G.L., Long, J.C., Goldman, D. and Linnoila, M., 1998. A tryptophan hydroxylase gene marker for suicidality and alcoholism. *Arch Gen Psychiatry*, **55**, 593–602.

Nordstrom, P., Samuelsson, M., Asberg, M., Traskman-Bendz, L., Aberg-Wistedt, A., Nordin, C. and Bertilsson, L., 1994. CSF 5-HIAA predicts suicide risk after attempted suicide. *Suicide Life Threat Behav*, **24**, 1–9.

O'Keane, V., Moloney, E., O'Neill, H., O'Connor, A., Smith, C. and Dinan, T.G., 1992. Blunted prolactin responses to *d*-fenfluramine in sociopathy. Evidence for subsensitivity of central serotonergic function. *Br J Psychiatry*, **160**, 643–646.

Pandey, G.N., Pandey, S.C., Janicak, P.G., Marks, R.C. and Davis, J.M., 1990. Platelet serotonin-2 receptor binding sites in depression and suicide. *Biol Psychiatry*, **28**, 215–222.

Peirson, A.R., Heuchert, J.W., Thomala, L., Berk, M., Plein, H. and Cloninger, C.R., 1999. Relationship between serotonin and the temperament and character inventory. *Psychiatry Res*, **89**, 29–37.

Raine, A., Buchsbaum, M.S., Stanley, J., Lottenberg, S., Abel, L. and Stoddard, J., 1994. Selective reductions in prefrontal glucose metabolism in murderers. *Biol Psychiatry*, **36**, 365–373.

Ressler, K.J. and Nemeroff, C.B., 2000. Role of serotonergic and noradrenergic systems in the pathophysiology of depression and anxiety disorders. *Depress Anxiety*, **12**(Suppl 1), 2–19.

Rubinow, D.R. and Schmidt, P.J., 1996. Androgens, brain and behavior. *Am J Psychiatry*, **153**, 974–984.

Salzman, C., Wolfson, A.N., Schatzberg, A., Looper, J., Henke, R., Albanese, M., Schwartz, J. and Miyawaki, E., 1995. Effect of fluoxetine on anger in symptomatic volunteers with borderline personality disorder. *J Clin Psychopharmacol*, **15**, 23–29.

Shatzberg, A.F. and Nemeroff, C.B., 1989. *The American Psychiatric Press Textbook of Psychopharmacology*. pp. 301–306. American Psychiatric Press, Washington, DC.

Siever, L.J. and Davis, K.L., 1991. A psychobiological perspective on the personality disorders. *Am J Psychiatry*, **148**, 1647–1658.

Siever, L.J. and Trestman, R.L., 1993. The serotonin system and aggressive personality disorder. *Int Clin Psychopharmacol*, **8**(Suppl 2), 33–39.

Siever, L.J., Amin, F., Coccaro, E.F., Bernstein, D., Kavoussi, R.J., Kalus, O., Horvath, T.B., Warne, P., Davidson, M. and Davis, K.L., 1991a. Plasma homovanillic acid in schizotypal personality disorder. *Am J Psychiatry*, **148**, 1246–1248.

Siever, L.J., Kahn, R.S., Lawlor, B.A., Trestman, R.L., Lawrence, T.L. and Coccaro, E.F., 1991b. Critical issues in defining the role of serotonin in psychiatric disorders. *Pharmacol Rev*, **43**, 509–525.

Siever, L.J., Amin, F., Coccaro, E.F., Trestman, R.L., Silverman, J., Horvath, T.B., Mahon, T.R., Knott, P., Altstiel, L., Davidson, M. and Davis, K.L., 1993. CSF homovanillic acid in schizotypal personality disorder. *Am J Psychiatry*, **150**(1), 149–151.

Siever, L.J., Buchsbaum, M.S., New, A.S., Spiegel-Cohen, J., Wei, T., Hazlett, E.A., Sevin, E., Nunn, M. and Mitropoulou, V., 1999. *d*,l-fenfluramine response in impulsive personality disorder assessed with [18F]fluorodeoxyglucose positron emission tomography. *Neuropsychopharmacology*, **20**, 413–423.

Siever, L.J., Koenigsberg, H.W., Harvey, P., Mitropoulou, V., Laruelle, M., Abi-Dargham, A., Goodman, M. and Buchsbaum, M., 2002. Cognitive and brain function in schizotypal personality disorder. *Schizophr Res*, **54**(1–8), 157–167.

Silverman, J.M., Pinkham, L., Horvath, T.B., Coccaro, E.F., Klar, H., Schear, S., Apter, S., Davidson, M., Mohs, R.C. and Siever, L.J., 1991. Affective and impulsive personality disorder traits in the relatives of patients with borderline personality disorder. *Am J Psychiatry*, **148**, 1378–1385.

Simeon, D., Stanley, B., Frances, A., Mann, J.J., Winchel, R. and Stanley, M., 1992. Self-mutilation in personality disorders: psychological and biological correlates. *Am J Psychiatry*, **149**, 221–226.

Stein, D.J., Trestman, R.L., Mitropoulou, V., Coccaro, E.F., Hollander, E. and Siever, L.J., 1996. Impulsivity and serotonergic function in compulsive personality disorder. *J Neuropsychiatry Clin Neurosci*, **8**, 393–398.

Steinberg, B.J., Trestman, R., Mitropoulou, V., Serby, M., Silverman, J., Coccaro, E., Weston, S., de Vegvar, M. and Siever, L.J., 1997. Depressive response to physostigmine challenge in borderline personality disorder patients. *Neuropsychopharmacology*, **17**, 264–273.

Svrakic, D.M., Whitehead, C., Przybeck, T.R. and Cloninger, C.R., 1993. Differential diagnosis of personality disorders by the seven-factor model of temperament and character. *Arch Gen Psychiatry*, **50**, 991–999.

Tizabi, Y., Overstreet, D.H., Rezvani, A.H., Louis, V.A., Clark, E. Jr, Janowsky, D.S. and Kling, M.A., 1999. Antidepressant effects of nicotine in an animal model of depression. *Psychopharmacology (Berl)*, **142**, 193–199.

Torgersen, S., 1994. Genetics in borderline conditions. *Acta Psychiatr Scand Suppl*, **379**, 19–25.

Virkkunen, M. and Linnoila, M., 1993. Brain serotonin, type II alcoholism and impulsive violence. *J Stud Alcohol Suppl*, **11**, 163–169.

Virkkunen, M., Goldman, D. and Linnoila, M., 1996. Serotonin in alcoholic violent offenders. *Ciba Found Symp*, **194**, 168–177; discussion 177–182.

Virkkunen, M., Nuutila, A., Goodwin, F.K. and Linnoila, M., 1987. Cerebrospinal fluid monoamine metabolite levels in male arsonists. *Arch Gen Psychiatry*, **44**, 241–247.

Virkkunen, M., Nuutila, A., Goodwin, F.K. and Linnoila, M., 1987. Cerebrospinal fluid monoamine metabolite levels in male arsonists. *Arch Gen Psychiatry*, **44**, 241–247.

XXVI-3

Neuroendocrinology of Personality Disorders

Roger T. Mulder and Peter R. Joyce

INTRODUCTION

Disorders of personality are currently defined as categories of deeply ingrained and enduring behaviour patterns that are persistently maladaptive and encompass multiple domains of behaviour and psychological functioning. Personality types were described in ancient Greece, yet, despite this lengthy history, it may be argued that we are still far from adequate in describing the phenomena that constitute the clinical core of personality disturbance (Tyrer, 1995). Personality pathology has been conceptualized in a number of ways, including categories, dimensions and clusters, but none of the classification systems have been validated from an aetiological or a biological perspective. We begin by discussing ways of classifying personality pathology and measurement of central nervous system monoamines since the patterns of association are critically influenced by these factors.

CLASSIFICATION OF PERSONALITY PATHOLOGY

Personality Categories

The separation of personality disorders (PDs) as a discrete axis of classification by the American Psychiatric Association (APA) in DSM-III (American Psychiatric Association, 1980) has focused attention on this neglected group of disorders and stimulated research in this area. However, the large increase in literature (Gorton and Akhtar, 1990) has not been accompanied by a corresponding increase in systematic models to aid in understanding the underlying behavioural abnormalities. The 10 current DSM-IV categories — paranoid, schizoid, schizotypal, antisocial, borderline, narcissistic, histrionic, avoidant, dependent and obsessive compulsive — are derived from a mixture of theory, opinion and historical precedent. The *10th Revision of The International Classification of Diseases* (World Health Organization [WHO], 1992) has replicated most features of DSM-IV. Diagnoses in both systems involve a list of operational criteria, of which a specific number must be present for an individual to receive a diagnosis of personality disorder.

Although it is implied that the categories group patients into mutually exclusive diagnostic entities, most studies have reported high rates of co-occurrence (e.g., Pfohl *et al.*, 1986; Joffe and Regan, 1988; Mulder *et al.*, 1994), and the measured behaviours appear to be distributed dimensionally with no evidence of the discontinuity a categorical model would imply (Zimmerman and Coryell, 1990). The overlap and clinical heterogeneity which result hamper attempts to link personality disorder diagnoses with specific neurobiological processes.

Personality Dimensions

Unfortunately, the dimensional models have fared little better. Many have emerged from academic psychology, the most important being the work of Eysenck and the five-factor model currently being refined by Costa and McCrae (1992). Eysenck's model initially consisted of two dimensions labelled introversion/extraversion (E) (sociability, stability, activity) and neuroticism (N) (temperamental sensitivity to negative stimuli). His model included a biological explanatory schema based on autonomic nervous system reactivity and ease of conditionability. He suggested that arousal stems from the ascending reticular activating system and is linked with E, while N reflects activation from the limbic system (Eysenck, 1967). Later critics have noted that these two systems of brain circuitry are interconnected and are thus unlikely to explain two supposedly independent dimensions (e.g., Claridge, 1986; Gray, 1982), but it remains an initial attempt to link behavioural dimensions to underlying biological processes. In 1976, Eysenck added a third dimension, psychoticism (P), defined as tender-minded versus tough-minded (high P is similar to psychopathy) (Eysenck *et al.*, 1976).

Costa and McCrae's (1992) five-factor model consists of five dimensions — neuroticism, extraversion (both similar to Eysenck's dimensions), agreeableness (trust, altruism), conscientiousness (self-discipline, competence, order) and openness to experience (aesthetics, fantasy, values). Although this model is being increasingly related to the DSM PD classification (Nestadt *et al.*, 1994; Widiger and Costa, 1994), it has only recently been linked with biological processes, and then mainly genetics.

More recently, a model of temperament with specific theoretical relationships to neurobiology was proposed by Cloninger (1986; 1987). This model began by postulating brain systems based on animal and genetic studies and then worked out their behavioural manifestations (Carey and DiLalla, 1994). There are three temperament dimensions, namely, novelty seeking (NS), harm avoidance (HA) and reward dependence (RD). Initially, NS was hypothesized to reflect heritable differences in the behavioural activation system and to be associated with central nervous system (CNS) dopaminergic activity, HA was said to reflect individual differences in behavioural inhibition and to be associated with serotonergic neural firing, and RD was held to reflect differences in behavioural maintenance and was associated with noradrenergic activity. More recently, Cloninger's theory has been modified, so that HA is related to gamma-aminobutyric acid (GABA), as well as serotonin; RD is related to serotonin (median raphe) as well as noradrenaline; and persistence (a new temperament dimension based on a reward-dependence subscale) is related to serotonin (dorsal raphe). The tridimensional model of

Biological Psychiatry: Edited by H. D'haenen, J.A. den Boer and P. Willner. ISBN 0-471-49198-5

temperament has been related to DSM PD categories (Cloninger, 1987; Svrakic *et al.*, 1993; Mulder *et al.*, 1999) and has been useful in describing personality pathology (Svrakic *et al.*, 1993; Mulder and Joyce, 1997) and comorbidity (Mulder *et al.*, 1994; Battaglia *et al.*, 1996).

Clusters and Factors

A third approach to classification has been to group PD diagnoses into broad clusters with the aim of decreasing redundancy and creating more valid categories. At one extreme, Rutter (1987) suggested that, since all PDs have a pervasive and persistent abnormality in maintaining social relationships, there should be one overall category defined in terms of relationship abnormalities. More commonly, researchers, using a variety of factor and cluster-analytical methods, have identified three or four major groups with reasonable consistency (Walton and Presly, 1973; Tyrer and Alexander, 1979; Kass *et al.*, 1985; Hyler and Lyons, 1988; Tyrer and Seivewright, 1988; Dowson and Berrios, 1991; Schroeder and Livesley, 1991; Livesley and Jackson, 1992). DSM has also suggested three clusters named A, B and C. In a recent study, we identified four factors we named the 'Four As' — antisocial, asocial, asthenic and anankastic — from an item level factor analysis of DSM-III-R Axis II symptoms (Mulder and Joyce, 1997).

The possible relationships of these four factors to other empirically derived groups and the DSM-IV clusters are shown in Table XXVI-3.1, while the relationship of the 'Four As' to dimensional models of personality is shown in Table XXVI-3.2.

In this chapter, we will present the neuroendocrinology of PDs using the four groups — antisocial, asocial, asthenic and anankastic. This retains the accumulated clinical experience and meaning to clinicians of PD symptoms and signs, as well as a relationship to dimension models. The prototype PDs of the Four As are borderline PD (antisocial), schizoid PD (asocial), avoidant PD (asthenic) and obsessive-compulsive PD (anankastic).

NEUROENDOCRINE MEASUREMENT

Accessing brain function in human subjects presents significant methodological problems. Despite this, a variety of approaches have been used, including measuring monoamines and their metabolites in cerebrospinal fluid (CSF), plasma and urine; neuroendocrine probes of monoamine function; and the use of platelets and other cells as models for CNS monoamine function. Each technique has limitations, and they are all indirect estimates of what it is occurring in the CNS.

Many studies do not consider potentially important interactions between neurotransmitters or physiologically significant relationships with other compounds (Linnoila *et al.*, 1988). For example, CSF 5-hydroxyindoleacetic acid (5-HIAA), a serotonin metabolite, and CSF homovanillic acid (HVA), a dopamine metabolite, are usually significantly correlated. This suggests that when studies report serotonergic abnormalities related to PDs, there are probably dopaminergic abnormalities as well.

If monoamine measures are to be used as an index of personality, they should represent stable biological traits. It is not always clear whether such measures reflect temporary reactions to stressful or pleasant events, that is, state rather than trait.

Finally, there is evidence that neuroendocrine measures are influenced by seasonality, clinical variation, diet and weight,

Table XXVI-3.1 Relationship of Four As to DSM clusters and other factor analyses

Four As 1997	DSM-III R PDs (Mulder and Joyce, 1997)	DSM-III R Clusters	Walton and Presly (1973)	Tyrer and Alexander (1979)	Schroeder and Livesley (1991)
Antisocial	Antisocial Borderline Narcissistic Histrionic Paranoid	B Antisocial Borderline Narcissistic Histrionic	Hysterical	Sociopathy	Psychopathic entitlement
Asocial	Schizoid	A Paranoid Schizoid Schizotypal	Social avoidance	Schizoid	Social avoidance
Asthenic	Avoidant, Dependent	C Avoidant Dependent Obsessive-compulsive	Submissiveness	Passive Dependent	Dependent emotionality
Anankastic	Obsessive-compulsive		Obsessional/schizoid	Anankastic	Compulsiveness

Table XXVI-3.2 Relationship of Four As to personality dimensions

Four As	Descriptors	Eysenck (Mulder and Joyce, 1997)	Cloninger (Mulder and Joyce, 1997)	Costa and McCrae, 1992 (theoretical)
Antisocial	Impulsive, unstable, easily bored	↑Psychoticism	↑Novelty seeking	↓Agreeableness ↓Conscientiousness
Asocial	Socially indifferent, lacks empathy	↑Psychoticism	↓Reward dependence	↓Extraversion
Asthenic	Fearful, anxious, insecure	↑Neuroticism ↓Extraversion	↑Harm avoidance	↑Neuroticism ↓Extraversion
Anankastic	Rigid, conscientious, perfectionistic		↑Persistence ↓Reward dependence	↑Conscientiousness

gender, and menstrual cycle, as well as other variables (Mulder, 1992). Given all these factors, results need to be viewed sceptically, and these considerations may, in part, also explain some of the inconsistencies and contradictory results found in this review.

ANTISOCIAL FACTOR

Most neuroendocrine research into PDs is focused on subjects who would fall within the antisocial personality factor. The behaviours studied have been impulsivity, aggression and affective lability. The principal finding, indeed the major finding, in the neuroendocrinology of PDs, is in the relationship of impulsivity and aggression to CNS serotonin. Much of the initial evidence of a link came from animal studies that had repeatedly demonstrated that serotonin-depleted animals are more aggressive, impulsive and disinhibited (e.g., Brody, 1969; Miczek *et al.*, 1975). The first published study in humans was in 1976, when Asberg *et al.* (1976) reported lower levels of CSF 5-HIAA in those who had made violent suicide attempts than in a control group. Since then, there have been a number of studies linking reduced levels of CSF 5-HIAA in personality-disordered men with a history of aggressive behaviours (Brown *et al.*, 1979), violent prison offenders (Linnoila *et al.*, 1983), impulsive arsonists (Virkkunen *et al.*, 1987) and impulsive suicide attempters (Roy, 1996). Pharmacochallenge studies have reported similar results. Coccaro and others reported a blunted prolactin response to fenfluramine in depressed patients with a history of suicide attempts and/or aggression (Coccaro *et al.*, 1989), and in aggressive and personality-disordered men (Coccaro *et al.*, 1996). There have been reports of reduced prolactin response to fenfluramine in patients with PDs (New *et al.*, 1997) and criminal offenders (O'Keane *et al.*, 1992).

There are some conflicting results. Wetzler *et al.* (1991) failed to find a relationship between self-reported aggression and the prolactin response to fenfluramine in depressed and panic disorder subjects, while Fishbein (1989) reported a positive relationship between prolactin response to fenfluramine and aggression in substance abusers. We have recently found no relationship between repeated self-harm, antisocial or borderline PD, and the prolactin response to fenfluramine in depressed subjects (Mulder and Joyce, 2002, in press).

Another neurotransmitter increasingly studied in relation to antisocial and impulsive behaviour is CNS dopamine. Overall, the evidence is weaker, with some studies showing a relationship between CSF HVA and antisocial and recidivist violent offending (Linnoila *et al.*, 1983; Virkkunen *et al.*, 1989), while others have demonstrated no relationship between this measure and aggression (Brown *et al.*, 1979; Virkkunen *et al.*, 1987). As discussed earlier, this evidence is complicated by the fact that CSF 5-HIAA and CSF HVA are usually correlated. There is some debate over which metabolite is more relevant. Agren (1983), for example, has suggested that suicidal behaviours correlated more closely with low CSF HVA than with low CSF 5-HIAA levels. Animal studies clearly suggest a direct relationship between dopamine function and aggression (Coccaro *et al.*, 1996).

Cloninger's dimension of NS, which is correlated with the antisocial factor, should also theoretically be related to dopaminergic activity. One study (Wiesbeck *et al.*, 1995) reported an association between growth hormone response to apomorphine (an indirect measure of CNS dopamine) and NS scores, but a later study by Hansenne and Ansseau (1998) failed to replicate this finding. Patients at risk of Parkinson's disease have low premorbid NS scores (Menza *et al.*, 1995), a finding which can be seen as support for the importance of dopamine in incentive activation of pleasurable activity. Other behaviours associated with the antisocial cluster, such as hyperactivity, sexual hedonism, drinking and smoking, have also been associated with high NS scores (Bardo *et al.*, 1996; Fergusson and Lynskey, 1996; Downey *et al.*, 1996). However, there is very little study of the relationship of these behaviours to indices of dopaminergic functioning. A study in depressed patients found a correlation between CSF dopamine and extraversion (King *et al.*, 1986).

There have also been some reports linking decreased dopamine β-hydroxylase (DBH) (an enzyme that catalyses the conversion of dopamine to noradrenaline in the brain) with unsocialized conduct disorder in boys (Rogeness *et al.*, 1982; Rogeness *et al.*, 1987; Bowden *et al.*, 1988).

Hyperactivity of noradrenergic functioning has been found to correlate with aggressive behaviour in human beings as well. Increased beta-adrenergic receptor binding has been found in the brains of violent suicide victims compared with accident victims (Stanley and Mann, 1983). Brown *et al.* (1979) reported a positive correlation between CSF 3-methyl-4-hydroxyphenolglycol (MHPG) concentrations and a history of aggression in male subjects with PDs. CSF MHPG levels have also been reported to be elevated in violent suicide attempters compared with non-violent suicide attempters (Traskman-Bendz *et al.*, 1992).

Androgens may also play a role in aggressive behaviour. Violent criminals appear to have higher testosterone levels than criminals who commit non-violent crimes, and are also more aggressive in prison settings (Dabbs *et al.*, 1995). Among violent alcohol offenders, those with antisocial personality disorder (ASPD) and increased aggressiveness appear to have higher CSF testosterone concentration (Virkkunen *et al.*, 1987).

In summary, all three major neurotransmitters and male androgens have been implicated in the impulsive and aggressive behaviour found within the antisocial cluster. The most convincing evidence is for serotonin abnormalities. These biological abnormalities may be confined to individuals with extreme and persistent impulsive/aggressive behaviours.

ASOCIAL FACTOR

The most interesting findings related to asocial behaviour come from animal studies, particularly those on prairie voles (Insel, 1997). The neurohypophysial neuropeptides, oxytocin and vasopressin, appear to be important for the formation of long-term social attachments and some aspects of infant attachment behaviour. For example, blocking oxytocin neurotransmission results in a significant inhibition of maternal behaviour, while a vasopressin antagonist administered to male prairie voles blocks the development of particular mate preference and selective aggression. The pathways appear to be species-specific, but these data suggest that the study of these neuropeptides in highly asocial individuals might be rewarding. There are some inconsistent findings that oxytocin levels may be abnormal in subjects with autism (Gilberg and Coleman, 1992).

There are also suggestions that opioid pathways may be involved in social attachment. There is some literature on an opioid model of autism, although therapeutic trials with opiate agonists have been disappointing (Insel *et al.*, 1996).

The asocial factor may be associated with low reward dependence (Mulder and Joyce, 1997). One study has reported that the noradrenaline metabolite MHPG was significantly correlated with TPQ reward-dependence scores (Garvey *et al.*, 1996). Another has related higher reward dependence scores with increased excretion of harman (a by-product of monoamines) in alcoholics (Wodarz *et al.*, 1996). Neither of these studies utilized measures of asocial behaviour.

Overall, despite the evidence that asocial behaviour or social indifference is consistently reported as a stable and persistent human personality trait, there is remarkably little research on its underlying neurobiology.

ASTHENIC FACTOR

The pathophysiology of this cluster of PDs has also seldom been investigated and is poorly understood (Kirrane and Siever, 1998). There are a few studies in social phobia, which, it could be argued, overlaps with and may not be distinct from avoidant PD. Patients with social phobia may have a greater fenfluramine-induced rise in cortisol than controls (Uhde, 1994), suggesting serotonin receptor supersensitivity. The hypothalamic-pituitary-adrenal (HPA) axis appears to be normal (Tancer *et al.*, 1990), but reduced dopamine metabolism has been suggested in one study (Potts and Davidson, 1992). The fact that the monoamine oxidase inhibitors (MAOIs) and selective serotonin reuptake inhibitors (SSRIs) sometimes reduce symptoms of avoidant personality disorder has led some to suggest that the monoamines, particularly serotonin, are implicated, although the evidence beyond this is vague.

The asthenic cluster is consistently associated with higher Eysenck's neuroticism (N) scores and Cloninger's harm-avoidance (HA) scores. Despite the importance of these dimensions, particularly in predicting the severity and course of mood and anxiety disorders, their neuroendocrinological underpinning has barely been researched. Two studies (Nelson *et al.*, 1996; Pfohl *et al.*, 1990) reported no significant correlation between platelet imipramine binding (an indicator of serotonergic function) and TPQ scores. However, in the Nelson *et al.* study, an alternative measure of serotonin functioning, L-lysergic acid diethylamide (^{125}L-LSD), was strongly related to HA scores. In patients with eating disorders, there was no relationship between blood serotonin and HA (Waller *et al.*, 1993).

Studies of the relationship between biochemical measures and N scores are few. Ballenger *et al.* (1983) reported that serum cortisol correlated negatively with N, as did plasma MHPG and CSF calcium. Recently, McCleery and Goodwin (2001) reported that individuals with high N scores had a smaller cortisol response to the combined dexamethasone–corticotrophin-releasing hormone (CRH) test. This suggests that individuals with a high N may have downregulation of the HPA axis.

ANANKASTIC FACTOR

Specific neurobiological research into the anankastic, or obsessive-compulsive, personality is essentially non-existent. There is some research into the obsessive-compulsive spectrum disorders, which include anankastic personality as well as obsessive-compulsive disorder, Tourette's syndrome, and other stereotypic movement disorders. Whether this characterization of such a varied range of psychopathology is valid remains contentious (e.g., Rasmussen, 1994), but it does hint at possible directions for further research into anankastic personality.

The possible importance of the serotonin system is supported by the response of this obsessive-compulsive spectrum, including anankastic personality, to clomipramine and SSRIs. However, the few studies using CSF 5-HIAA measures or pharmacological challenge techniques do not show evidence of a consistent serotonergic abnormality (Stein, 2000). Although dopamine metabolism may play a part in tics and abnormal movements associated with the obsessive-compulsive spectrum, it seems less likely to have a role in anankastic personality (Stein, 2000).

One interesting hypothesis is that, while impulsivity is associated with decreased serotonergic function, compulsiveness is associated with hyperresponsivity of the serotonergic receptors. This contrast may be overly simplistic in that both impulsive and compulsive disorders have been reported to show neuroendocrine blunting on serotonergic challenge and both respond to serotonergic antidepressants (Stein, 1996).

Millon and Davis (1996) have speculated that the neural connections in the limbic system that control fear and anger may contribute to the indecisiveness and excessive conflict that characterizes decision-making in this personality style. This is an interesting but untested speculative hypothesis.

DISCUSSION

We have noted limitations to formal classifications of personality pathology. These limitations have restricted identification and quantification of behaviours that may be associated with neuroendocrinology. PDs, as currently defined, are non-specific diagnostic categories with no theoretical relationship to neuroendocrinology. Trying to find patterns of associations between such categories and specific neurochemical processes is unlikely to be successful.

Grouping PDs into clusters such as the 'Four As', creates more valid categories from a psychometric point of view, but there is limited evidence that these clusters are related to neuroendocrine abnormalities. The monoamine abnormalities reported in violent, impulsive individuals seem to relate to a broad cluster of personality pathology, including antisocial, borderline, narcissistic, histrionic and paranoid symptoms, rather than to individual personality disorder categories, so that the 'antisocial' cluster has superior face validity. However, the lack of biological research into the other personality groups (i.e., asocial, asthenic and anankastic) means that we do not know whether each has a distinct neuroendocrinology, and whether such groups are likely to be helpful for biological research.

Dimensional classifications appear to offer the most promising model for biological processes. However, most current models are derived through the statistical modelling of answers to questionnaires with little thought given to underlying biological principles. The exception is Cloninger's tridimensional model, which was specifically designed to encompass knowledge about the biology of behaviour. However, there is only limited evidence that CNS neuroendocrinology is related systematically to Cloninger's dimensions, as we have already reported. More convincing evidence is in the neuroanatomical and genetic studies related to TPQ measures (Cloninger, 1998).

It may be time to question whether biological research is building on an adequate base. There are increasingly accurate and sophisticated means for measuring brain processes, but what seems to be lacking is an adequate system for personality description. The current DSM categories may be useful for certain tasks, but they reflect simplistic static notions that seem to relate distantly, if at all, to the core processes involved in psychopathology. The self-report questionnaires used in dimensional models are more self-representations than accurate personality descriptions (Kagan, 1994; Hogan, 1996) and lack any behavioural observation.

The move toward objectification in psychiatric diagnosing was a necessary first step but appears to have come to a premature closure (van Praag, 1992). To advance research into the biology of PDs, detailed scrutiny outside our current symptom representation may be necessary. There are some hints of this already. For example, the serotonin abnormalities correlated with impulsive aggression are largely found in individuals whose aggressive behaviour is not premeditated (Linnoila *et al.*, 1983; Virkkunen *et al.*, 1987). This suggests that the key component may be lack of behavioural inhibition rather than aggression or impulsivity.

It may be better to have skilled clinicians closely observing behaviour and assessing detailed personality pathology rather than using structured interviews and questionnaires. Hypotheses derived from clinical models, genetic studies and brain imaging could provide more specific testable models for linking behaviour and neuroendocrinology. For example, selecting a group of very socially indifferent individuals for study, regardless of their clinical psychopathology (some may have adapted very well to their temperament), might be useful. This could involve using a screening tool such as low RD scores on Cloninger's TPQ questionnaire and then validating these scores by behavioural observation. Animal and genetic studies suggest that neurochemicals such as vasopressin, oxytocin, serotonin and the opioids would be of interest.

The potential significance of finding consistent links between neurochemistry and personality lies in three main areas. First, if maladaptive personality traits can be shown to be shaped by neurotransmitter functions which relate to an individual's ability to regulate impulse, anxiety, mood, sociability and so on, then a sound theoretical basis for pharmacotherapy becomes possible (Soloff, 1990). Rather than targetting PDs, medications could target specific biological trait vulnerabilities and help to modify and regulate the particular behavioural symptoms that make up the psychopathology of PDs.

Second, there is the possibility that much of the relationship between neuroendocrinology and Axis I disorders is mediated by personality traits. There is considerable evidence that certain Axis I disorders are associated with specific personality pathology. For example, individuals with antisocial personality traits are more likely to have alcohol and substance-abuse disorders but less likely to suffer from generalized anxiety disorder, while those with anankastic personality traits are more likely to have obsessive-compulsive disorder, and anxiety and mood disorders but less likely to have alcohol or substance-abuse disorders (Nestadt *et al.*, 1989). These associations may reflect neuroendocrine abnormalities. For example, the serotonergic abnormalities sometimes reported in depressed patients may be largely confined to those with impulsive suicidal behaviours (De Meo *et al.*, 1989). Samples with a high proportion of such individuals report differences in serotonin functioning compared with a control group; those with a low proportion do not. In other words, serotonin disturbances may be non-specific from a functional/categorical perspective but specific from a functional/dimensional perspective, correlating with particular personality traits such as aggression, impulsivity or obsessionality across diagnoses (van Praag, 1986).

Third, linking personality with neuroendocrinology may be a way to integrate biology and psychosocial experience. There is a small but increasing literature reporting associations between negative early life experiences and abnormalities in adult neuroendocrinology. Measuring urinary catecholamine excretion showed that sexually abused girls secreted greater amounts of HVA (De Bellis *et al.*, 1994), and that abused children had higher concentrations of noradrenaline and dopamine than healthy controls (De Bellis *et al.*, 1999). Hospitalized boys who had experienced neglect in the first 3 years of life have been found to have reduced DBH (Galvin *et al.*, 1991), a finding also associated with antisocial cluster behaviour (Galvin *et al.*, 1995; Rogeness *et al.*, 1987), and, in particular, a low valuation of authority and peer-derived rules of conscience (Galvin *et al.*, 1995). Here is a link between an experience (neglect), through a particular behaviour (lack of conscience), to a personality abnormality (conduct disorder).

HPA axis regulation also appears to be related to the quality of early maternal care (Caldji *et al.*, 1998). De Bellis *et al.* (1994) found a reduced adrenocorticotrophic hormone (ACTH) response to CRH stimulation in their sexually abused girls, and Stein *et al.* (1997) reported enhanced dexamethasone suppression in women with a history of childhood sexual abuse. High neuroticism (and its associated reduced cortisol response to dexamethasone-CRH), while partly heritable, may be a measurable vulnerability factor linking such experiences with later post-traumatic stress disorder (PTSD) and depression (McCleery and Goodwin, 2001).

SUMMARY AND CONCLUSION

Over the past 20 years, there has been increasing interest in the neuroendocrinology of PDs. Early results related CSF monoamine metabolites to specific behaviours. There has been a gradual expansion in the types of neuroendocrine measures and behavioural subtypes studied. Despite this, most research has focused on the broad area of antisocial behaviour, particularly impulsivity and lack of inhibition. These behaviours have been linked with abnormalities in all three major CNS biogenic amines and changes in male androgens. Other consistently identified human behavioural traits — asociality or social indifference, asthenic or neurotic behaviours, and anankastic or obsessive-compulsive behaviour — have been much less studied.

Plausible, testable, aetiological models of personality pathology are a necessary step for the science of neuroendocrinology to contribute to an integrated understanding of personality. Attempts to find patterns of association between current DSM PD categories and specific neurochemicals have had limited success. Broader empirical groupings with less overlap such as the 'Four As' may be more useful, but until increased research on the non-antisocial factors is undertaken, it is difficult to be sure. Cloninger's biosocial model is the most sophisticated attempt so far to construct a theoretical, testable model relating biology to behaviour. Results have been somewhat inconsistent, but it offers a base for future research. New developments in measuring the temperament dimensions while incorporating behavioural factors may lead to more valid parameters. Results from animal and imaging studies have already helped refine the initial model of the three monoamines as 'emblematic' neurotransmitters into more complex theoretical relationships between neurochemistry, neuroanatomy and behaviour.

The neuroendocrine abnormalities associated with some adverse early life experiences offer another potentially important model for research. Personality pathology might form the link between such experiences and later psychopathology. Enduring changes in CNS neurochemistry and HPA axis function associated with abuse may be correlated with personality characteristics such as high N or conduct disorder, which in turn make an individual vulnerable to PTSD, depression and ASPD as an adult. Screening a large population for high and low behavioural measures, such as N, NS or RD, and studying these individuals' neurochemistry, early life experiences and current psychopathology might lead to useful results.

The neuroendocrinology of PDs remains an important area of psychiatric research. It could lead to more rational treatment for both Axis I and Axis II disorders, help construct a more valid classification for psychopathology, and provide a link between early life experience and adult development.

REFERENCES

Agren, H., 1983. Life at risk: markers of suicidality in depression. *Psychiatric Developments*, **1**, 87–103.

American Psychiatric Association, 1980. *Diagnostic and Statistical Manual of Mental Disorders — DSM-III*. American Psychiatric Association, Washington, DC.

Asberg, M., Traskman, L. and Thoren, P., 1976. 5-HIAA in the cerebrospinal fluid. A biochemical suicide predictor? *Archives of General Psychiatry*, **33**, 1193–1197.

Ballenger, J., Post, R., Jimerson, D., Lake, C., Murphy, D., Zuckerman, M. and Cronin, C., 1983. Biochemical correlates of personality traits in normals: an exploratory study. *Personality and Individual Differences*, **4**, 615–625.

Bardo, M.T., Donohew, R.L. and Harrington, N.G., 1996. Psychobiology of novelty seeking and drug seeking behaviour. *Behavioural Brain Research*, **77**, 23–43.

Battaglia, M., Przybeck, T.R., Bellodi, L. and Cloninger, C.R., 1996. Temperament dimensions explain the comorbidity of psychiatric disorders. *Comprehensive Psychiatry*, **37**, 292–298.

Bowden, C., Deutsch, C. and Swanson, J., 1988. Plasma dopamine-beta-hydroxylase and platelet monoamine oxidase in attention deficit disorder and conduct disorder. *Journal of the American Academy of Child and Adolescent Psychiatry*, **27**, 171–174.

Brody, J.F., Jr., 1969. Behavioral effects of serotonin depletion and of *p*-chlorophenylalanine (a serotonin depletor) in rats. *Psychopharmacology*, **7**, 14–33.

Brown, G.L., Goodwin, F.K., Ballenger, J.C., Goyer, P.F. and Major, L.F., 1979. Aggression in humans correlates with cerebrospinal fluid amine metabolites. *Psychiatry Research*, **1**, 131–139.

Caldji, C., Tannenbaum, B., Sharma, S., Francis, D., Plotsky, P.M. and Meaney, M.J., 1998. Maternal care during infancy regulates the development of neural systems mediating the expression of fearfulness in the rat. *Proceedings of the National Academy of Sciences of the United States of America*, **95**, 5335–5340.

Carey, G. and DiLalla, D.L., 1994. Personality and psychopathology: genetic perspectives. *Journal of Abnormal Psychology*, **103**, 32–43.

Claridge, G., 1986. In: Modgil, S.H. and Modgil, C. (eds), *Hans Eysenck. Consensus and Controversy*, pp. 73–85. Falmer Press, Philadelphia.

Cloninger, C., 1986. A unified biosocial theory of personality and its role in the development of anxiety states. *Psychiatric Developments*, **4**, 167–226.

Cloninger, C., 1987. A systematic method for clinical description and classification of personality variants. A proposal. *Archives of General Psychiatry*, **44**, 573–588.

Cloninger, C.R., 1998. In: Silk, K.R. (ed.), *Biology of Personality Disorders*, pp. 63–92. American Psychiatric Press, Washington, DC.

Coccaro, E., Siever, L., Klar, H., Maurer, G., Cochrane, K., Cooper, T., Mohs, R. and Davis, K., 1989. Serotonergic studies in patients with affective and personality disorders. Correlates with suicidal and impulsive aggressive behavior. *Archives of General Psychiatry*, **46**, 587–599.

Coccaro, E.F., Berman, M.E., Kavoussi, R.J. and Hauger, R.L., 1996. Relationship of prolactin response to *d*-fenfluramine to behavioral and questionnaire assessments of aggression in personality-disordered men. *Biological Psychiatry*, **40**, 157–164.

Costa, P. and McCrae, R., 1992. The five-factor model of personality and its relevance to personality disorders. *Journal of Personality Disorders*, **6**, 343–359.

Dabbs, J.M., Carr, T.S., Frady, R.L. and Riad, J.K., 1995. Testosterone, crime, and misbehavior among 692 male prison inmates. *Personality and Individual Differences*, **18**, 627–633.

De Bellis, M.D., Chrousos, G.P., Dorn, L.D., Burke, L., Helmers, K., Kling, M.A., Trickett, P.K. and Putnam, F.W., 1994. Hypothalamic-pituitary-adrenal axis dysregulation in sexually abused girls. *Journal of Clinical Endocrinology and Metabolism*, **78**, 249–255.

De Bellis, M.D., Keshavan, M.S., Clark, D.B., Casey, B.J., Giedd, J.N., Boring, A.M., Frustaci, K. and Ryan, N.D., 1999. A.E. Bennett Research Award. Developmental traumatology. II. Brain development. *Biological Psychiatry*, **45**, 1271–1284.

De Meo, M.D., McBridge, P.A. and Chen, J.-S., 1989. Relative contribution of MDD and borderline personality disorder to 5-HT responsivity. *Biological Psychiatry*, **25**, 84A–89A.

Downey, K.K., Pomerleau, C.S. and Pomerleau, O.F., 1996. Personality differences related to smoking and adult attention deficit hyperactivity disorder. *Journal of Substance Abuse*, **8**, 129–135.

Dowson, J.H. and Berrios, G.E., 1991. Factor structure of DSM-III-R personality disorders shown by self-report questionnaire: implications for classifying and assessing personality disorders. *Acta Psychiatrica Scandinavica*, **84**, 555–560.

Eysenck, H.J., 1967. *The Biological Basis of Personality*. Springfield, Chasler and Thomas, London.

Eysenck, S.B., White, O. and Eysenck, H.J., 1976. Personality and mental illness. *Psychological Reports*, **39**, 1011–1022.

Fergusson, D.M. and Lynskey, M.T., 1996. Alcohol misuse and adolescent sexual behaviors and risk taking. *Pediatrics*, **98**, 91–96.

Fishbein, D.H., Lozovsky, D. and Jaffe, J.H., 1989. Impulsivity, aggression, and neuroendocrine responses to serotonergic stimulation in substance abusers. *Biological Psychiatry*, **25**, 1049–1066.

Galvin, M., Shekhar, A., Simon, J., Stilwell, B., Ten Eyck, R., Laite, G., Karwisch, G. and Blix, S., 1991. Low dopamine-beta-hydroxylase: a biological sequela of abuse and neglect? *Psychiatry Research*, **39**, 1–11.

Galvin, M., Ten Eyck, R., Shekhar, A., Stilwell, B., Fineberg, N., Laite, G. and Karwisch, G., 1995. Serum dopamine beta hydroxylase and maltreatment in psychiatrically hospitalized boys. *Child Abuse and Neglect*, **19**, 821–832.

Garvey, M.J., Noyes, R., Jr., Cook, B. and Blum, N., 1996. Preliminary confirmation of the proposed link between reward-dependence traits and norepinephrine. *Psychiatry Research*, **65**, 61–64.

Gilberg, C. and Coleman, M., 1992. *The Biology of the Autistic Syndromes*. MacKeith Press, London.

Gorton, G. and Akhtar, S., 1990. The literature on personality disorders, 1985–88: trends, issues, and controversies. *Hospital and Community Psychiatry*, **41**, 39–51.

Gray, J.A., 1982. *The Neuropsychology of Anxiety*. Oxford University Press, New York.

Hansenne, M. and Ansseau, M., 1998. Catecholaminergic function and temperament in major depressive disorder: a negative report. *Psychoneuroendocrinology*, **23**, 477–483.

Hogan, R., 1996. A socioanalytical perspective on the five-factor model. In: Wiggins, M. (ed.), *The 5-Factor Model of Personality: Theoretical Perspectives*, pp. 163–179. Guilford Press, New York.

Hyler, S. and Lyons, M., 1988. Factor analysis of the DSM-III personality disorder clusters: a replication. *Comprehensive Psychiatry*, **29**, 304–308.

Insel, T.R., 1997. A neurobiological basis of social attachment. *American Journal of Psychiatry*, **154**, 726–735.

Insel, T.R., Winslow, J.T., Wang, Z.X., Young, L. and Hulihan, T.J., 1996. Oxytocin and the molecular basis of monogamy. *Advances in Experimental Medicine and Biology*, **395**, 227–234.

Joffe, R. and Regan, J., 1988. Personality and depression. *Journal of Psychiatric Research*, **22**, 279–286.

Kagan, J., 1994. *Galen's Prophecy: Temperament in Human Nature*. Basic Books, New York.

Kass, F., Skodol, A., Charles, E., Spitzer, R. and Williams, J., 1985. Scaled ratings of DSM-III personality disorders. *American Journal of Psychiatry*, **142**, 627–630.

King, R., Mefford, I., Wang, C., Murchison, A., Caligari, E. and Berger, P., 1986. CSF dopamine levels correlate with extraversion in depressed patients. *Psychiatry Research*, **19**, 305–310.

Kirrane, R. and Siever, L.J., 1998. Biology of personality disorders. In: Schatzberg, A. and Nemeroff, C.B. (eds), *The American Psychiatric Press Textbook of Psychopharmacology*, pp. 691–702. American Psychiatric Press, Washington, DC.

Linnoila, M., Oliver, J., Adinoff, B. and Potter, W.Z., 1988. High correlations of norepinephrine, dopamine, and epinephrine and their major metabolite excretion rates. *Archives of General Psychiatry*, **45**, 701–704.

Linnoila, M., Virkkunen, M., Scheinin, M., Nuutila, A., Rimon, R. and Goodwin, F., 1983. Low cerebrospinal fluid 5-hydroxyindoleacetic acid concentration differentiates impulsive from nonimpulsive violent behaviour. *Life Sciences*, **33**, 2609–2614.

Livesley, W.J. and Jackson, D.N., 1992. Guidelines for developing, evaluating, and revising the classification of personality disorders. *Journal of Nervous and Mental Disease*, **180**, 609–618.

McCleery, J.M. and Goodwin, G.M., 2001. High and low neuroticism predict different cortisol responses to the combined dexamethasone-CRH test. *Biological Psychiatry*, **49**, 410–415.

Menza, M.A., Mark, M.H., Burn, D.J. and Brooks, D.J., 1995. Personality correlates of [18F]dopa striatal uptake: results of positron-emission tomography in Parkinson's disease. *Journal of Neuropsychiatry and Clinical Neurosciences*, **7**, 176–179.

Miczek, K.A., Altman, J.L., Appel, J.B. and Boggan, W.O., 1975. Parachlorophenylalanine, serotonin and behaviour. *Journal of Pharmacology, Biochemistry and Behaviour*, **3**, 961–968.

Millon, T. and Davis, R.D., 1996. *Disorders of Personality: DSM-IV and Beyond*. John Wiley & Sons, New York.

Mulder, R.T., 1992. The biology of personality. *Australian and New Zealand Journal of Psychiatry*, **26**, 364–376.

Mulder, R.T. and Joyce, P.R., 1997. Temperament and the structure of personality disorder symptoms. *Psychological Medicine*, **27**, 99–106.

Mulder, R.T. and Joyce, P.R., 2002. The relationship of temperament and behavior measures to the prolactin response to fenfluramine in depressed men. *Psychiatry Research* (in press).

Mulder, R.T., Joyce, P.R. and Cloninger, C.R., 1994. Temperament and early environment influence comorbidity and personality disorders in major depression. *Comprehensive Psychiatry*, **35**, 225–233.

Mulder, R.T., Joyce, P.R., Sullivan, P.F., Bulik, C.M. and Carter, F.A., 1999. The relationship among three models of personality psychopathology: DSM-III-R personality disorder, TCI scores and DSQ defences. *Psychological Medicine*, **29**, 943–951.

Nelson, E.C., Cloninger, C.R., Przybeck, T.R. and Csernansky, J.G., 1996. Platelet serotonergic markers and Tridimensional Personality Questionnaire measures in a clinical sample. *Biological Psychiatry*, **40**, 271–278.

Nestadt, G., Eaton, W.W., Romanoski, A.J., Garrison, R., Folstein, M.F. and McHugh, P.R., 1994. Assessment of DSM-III personality structure in a general-population survey. *Comprehensive Psychiatry*, **35**, 54–63.

Nestadt, G., Romanski, A.J. and Brown, C.H., 1989. The relationship of personality disorders and axis I disorders in the general population. *Biological Psychiatry*, **25**, 84A–85A.

New, A.S., Trestman, R.L., Mitropoulou, V., Benishay, D.S., Coccaro, E., Silverman, J. and Siever, L.J., 1997. Serotonergic function and self-injurious behavior in personality disorder patients. *Psychiatry Research*, **69**, 17–26.

O'Keane, V., Moloney, E., O'Neill, H., O'Connor, A., Smith, C. and Dinan, T.G., 1992. Blunted prolactin responses to *d*-fenfluramine in sociopathy. Evidence for subsensitivity of central serotonergic function. *British Journal of Psychiatry*, **160**, 643–646.

Pfohl, B., Black, D., Noyes, R., Kelley, M. and Blum, N., 1990. A test of the tridimensional personality theory: associated with diagnosis and platelet imipramine binding in obsessive-compulsive disorder. *Biological Psychiatry*, **28**, 41–46.

Pfohl, B., Coryell, W., Zimmerman, M. and Stangl, D., 1986. DSM-III personality disorders: diagnostic overlap and internal consistency of individual DSM-III criteria. *Comprehensive Psychiatry*, **27**, 21–34.

Potts, N.L. and Davidson, J.R., 1992. Social phobia: biological aspects and pharmacotherapy. *Progress in Neuro-Psychopharmacology and Biological Psychiatry*, **16**, 635–646.

Rasmussen, S.A., 1994. Obsessive compulsive spectrum disorders. *Journal of Clinical Psychiatry*, **55**, 89–91.

Rogeness, G., Javors, M., Maas, J., Macedo, C. and Fischer, C., 1987. Plasma dopamine-beta-hydroxylase, HVA, MHPG, and conduct disorder in emotionally disturbed boys. *Biological Psychiatry*, **22**, 1158–1162.

Rogeness, G.A., Hernandez, J.M., Macedo, C.A. and Mitchell, E.L., 1982. Biochemical differences in children with conduct disorder socialized and undersocialized. *American Journal of Psychiatry*, **139**, 307–311.

Roy, A., 1996. HPA axis function and temperament in depression: a negative report. *Biological Psychiatry*, **39**, 364–366.

Rutter, M., 1987. Temperament, personality and personality disorder. *British Journal of Psychiatry*, **150**, 443–458.

Schroeder, M.L. and Livesley, W.J., 1991. An evaluation of DSM-III-R personality disorders. *Acta Psychiatrica Scandinavica*, **84**, 512–519.

Soloff, P., 1990. What's new in personality disorders?: an update on pharmacologic treatment. *Journal of Personality Disorders*, **4**, 233–243.

Stanley, M. and Mann, J.J., 1983. Increased serotonin-2 binding sites in frontal cortex of suicide victims. *Lancet*, **1**, 214–216.

Stein, D.J., 1996. The philosophy of psychopathy. *Perspectives in Biology and Medicine*, **39**, 569–580.

Stein, D.J., 2000. Neurobiology of the obsessive-compulsive spectrum disorders. *Biological Psychiatry*, **47**, 296–304.

Stein, M.B., Yehuda, R., Koverola, C. and Hanna, C., 1997. Enhanced dexamethasone suppression of plasma cortisol in adult women traumatized by childhood sexual abuse. *Biological Psychiatry*, **42**, 680–686.

Svrakic, D.M., Whitehead, C., Przybeck, T.R. and Cloninger, C.R., 1993. Differential diagnosis of personality disorders by the seven-factor model of temperament and character. *Archives of General Psychiatry*, **50**, 991–999.

Tancer, M.E., Stein, M.B., Gelernter, C.S. and Uhde, T.W., 1990. The hypothalamic-pituitary-thyroid axis in social phobia. *American Journal of Psychiatry*, **147**, 929–933.

Traskman-Bendz, L., Alling, C., Oreland, L., Regnell, G., Vinge, E. and Ohman, R., 1992. Prediction of suicidal behavior from biologic tests. *Journal of Clinical Psychopharmacology*, **12**, 21S–26S.

Tyrer, P., 1995. Are personality disorders well classified in DSM-IV? In: Livesley, W.J. (ed.), *The DSM-IV Personality Disorders*, pp. 29–42. Guilford Press, New York.

Tyrer, P. and Alexander, J., 1979. Classification of personality disorder. *British Journal of Psychiatry*, **135**, 163–167.

Tyrer, P. and Seivewright, N., 1988. Pharmacological treatment of personality disorders. *Clinical Neuropharmacology*, **11**, 493–499.

Uhde, T.W., 1994. Anxiety and growth disturbance: is there a connection? A review of biological studies in social phobia. *Journal of Clinical Psychiatry*, **55**(Suppl), 17–27.

van Praag, H., 1986. Biological suicide research: outcome and limitations. *Biological Psychiatry*, **21**, 1305–1323.

van Praag, H.M., 1992. Reconquest of the subjective. Against the waning of psychiatric diagnosing. *British Journal of Psychiatry*, **160**, 266–271.

Virkkunen, M., De Jong, J., Bartko, J., Goodwin, F.K. and Linnoila, M., 1989. Relationship of psychobiological variables to recidivism in violent offenders and impulsive fire setters. A follow-up study. *Archives of General Psychiatry*, **46**, 600–603 [erratum **46**, 913].

Virkkunen, M., Nuutila, A., Goodwin, F.K. and Linnoila, M., 1987. Cerebrospinal fluid monoamine metabolite levels in male arsonists. *Archives of General Psychiatry*, **44**, 241–247 [erratum 1989; **46**, 960].

Waller, D., Gullion, C., Petty, F., Hardy, B., Murdock, M. and Rush, A., 1993. Tridimensional Personality Questionnaire and serotonin in bulimia nervosa. *Psychiatry Research*, **48**, 9–15.

Walton, H. and Presly, A., 1973. Use of a category system in the diagnosis of abnormal personality. *British Journal of Psychiatry*, **122**, 259–268.

Wetzler, S., Kahn, R.S., Asnis, G.M., Korn, M. and van Praag, H.M., 1991. Serotonin receptor sensitivity and aggression. *Psychiatry Research*, **37**, 271–279.

Widiger, T.A. and Costa, P.T., Jr., 1994. Personality and personality disorders. *Journal of Abnormal Psychology*, **103**, 78–91.

Wiesbeck, G.A., Mauerer, C., Thome, J., Jakob, F. and Boening, J., 1995. Neuroendocrine support for a relationship between 'novelty seeking' and dopaminergic function in alcohol-dependent men. *Psychoneuroendocrinology*, **20**, 755–761.

Wodarz, N., Wiesbeck, G.A., Rommelspacher, H., Riederer, P. and Boning, J., 1996. Excretion of beta-carbolines harman and norharman in 24-hour urine of chronic alcoholics during withdrawal and controlled abstinence. *Alcoholism: Clinical and Experimental Research*, **20**, 706–710.

World Health Organization (WHO), 1992. *ICD-10 Classification of Mental and Behavioural Disorder: Diagnostic Criteria for Research*. WHO, Geneva.

Zimmerman, M. and Coryell, W.H., 1990. DSM-III personality disorder dimensions. *Journal of Nervous and Mental Disease*, **178**, 686–692.

XXVI-4

The Psychophysiology of Personality Disorders

Angela Scarpa and Adrian Raine

The Diagnostic and Statistical Manual of Mental Disorders (DSM-IV) (American Psychiatric Association, 1994), defines a personality disorder (PD) as 'an enduring pattern of inner experience and behavior that deviates markedly from the expectations of the individual's culture, is pervasive and inflexible, has an onset in adolescence or early adulthood, is stable over time, and leads to distress or impairment (p. 629)'. In general, PDs involve personality traits that have become severe and rigid enough to be dysfunctional or maladaptive, and are typically manifested in at least two of the following areas: cognition, affectivity, interpersonal functioning, or impulse control.

The DSM-IV distinguishes 10 specific PDs that are grouped into three broad clusters, based upon similarities in descriptive features. Cluster A includes the paranoid, schizoid, and schizotypal PDs, which describe individuals who often appear odd, eccentric, or suspicious. Cluster A PDs are also thought to be part of the schizophrenia-spectrum disorders due to their similarity in symptoms with schizophrenia, though milder in form. Cluster B includes the antisocial, borderline, histrionic, and narcissistic PDs, which describe individuals who appear dramatic, emotional, impulsive, or erratic. Finally, Cluster C includes the avoidant, dependent, and obsessive-compulsive PDs, which describe individuals who often appear anxious or fearful. Clusters B and C have been described as reflecting externalizing (i.e., dramatic, reactive, and aggressive) or internalizing (i.e., anxious, avoidant, and withdrawn) dimensions of personality, respectively, based upon their primary symptomatology (Scarpa *et al.*, 1999).

Psychophysiology involves the study of cognitions, emotions, and behaviour as related to physiological principles and events (Cacioppo and Tassinary, 1990; see also Chapter IX in this volume). As such, psychophysiology can provide unique information on the cognitive, affective, interpersonal, and impulsive features of PDs that is relatively objective in nature. This chapter will describe psychophysiological studies of PDs, as grouped by cluster. Although such studies provide rich information on psychological processes related to PDs, relatively few PDs have been examined by psychophysiological techniques. Specifically, the schizotypal and antisocial PDs have been most abundantly studied in relation to psychophysiology; thus, this chapter must necessarily focus on these two. Whenever possible, this information will be supplemented with psychophysiological studies of the other PDs. Findings related to characteristics associated with the Cluster C PDs are also discussed.

CLUSTER A PERSONALITY DISORDERS

As described above, Cluster A includes the paranoid, schizoid, and schizotypal PDs, which are thought to reflect psychosis-proneness or schizophrenia-spectrum disorder. In the DSM-IV, paranoid PD is defined as a pattern of suspiciousness whereby others' motives are interpreted as hostile or malevolent; schizoid PD is defined as a pattern of social detachment or indifference with a restricted range of affect; and schizotypal PD is defined as a pattern of cognitive and perceptual distortions, interpersonal deficits, and odd behaviour (American Psychiatric Association, 1994). Indeed, schizotypal and paranoid PDs are found with greater frequency in the relatives of probands with schizophrenia, although not all studies have been consistent (see Webb and Levinson, 1993 for a review).

Schizotypal PD, in particular, has been a focus of attention due to its symptoms seeming to reflect a milder form of those seen in schizophrenia. These include negative (or deficit) symptoms, such as social withdrawal or blunted affect, and positive (or excess) symptoms, such as perceptual aberrations or magical ideation. Social anhedonia (i.e., social indifference) and magical ideation seem most predictive of later psychosis (Chapman *et al.*, 1995). As such, researchers have focused on comparing schizotypal PD to findings in schizophrenia, with the hope of discovering either a common genetic marker for vulnerability or a factor protective against the progression to full-blown schizophrenia. In this vein, the primary psychophysiological variables that have been studied in schizotypal PD are the skin conductance orienting response (SCOR), smooth pursuit eye movement (SPEM), and event-related potential (ERP), all of which have been found to be deviant in individuals with schizophrenia. Each of these variables and research on their relationship to schizotypal PD will be summarized in turn below.

The Skin Conductance Orienting Response (SCOR) and Schizotypal PD

Changes in the electrical activity of the skin generally occur in response to the presentation of novel stimuli in one's environment. For example, the presentation of a new tone generally causes an orienting response that is accompanied by increased electrical activity in the skin, and thus, a change in skin conductance levels called the SCOR. One useful model for understanding the SCOR has been that of template-matching (Ohman, 1979; 1985). In this model, novel stimuli are stored in short-term memory where they create neural 'templates'. Subsequent stimuli are matched against the template currently stored in short-term memory. If the two stimuli differ, preattentive mechanisms will fail to recognize the newly presented stimulus, thus requiring controlled processing of the new stimulus. However, if the stimuli match, habituation occurs. In addition to cases in which there is a mismatch between the 'stored' stimulus and the novel stimulus, controlled processing also occurs when the novel stimulus is recognized as significant, necessitating further processing. In either case, augmented controlled processing of information would produce a SCOR. Thus, the SCOR is a useful index of how one attends to and processes novel environmental stimuli (Dawson and Nuechterlein, 1984; Dawson *et al.*, 1989).

Biological Psychiatry: Edited by H. D'haenen, J.A. den Boer and P. Willner. ISBN 0-471-49198-5

A review of previous studies that have assessed the relationship between SCOR and schizotypy reveals diverse and sometimes inconsistent findings (see Raine *et al.*, 1995 and Yaralian and Raine, in press, for reviews). As in findings with schizophrenia (Dawson and Nuechterlein, 1984), significant effects have shown that negative-symptom schizotypy is marked by hyporesponding while positive-symptom schizotypy is marked by hyperresponding. For example, Simons (1981) and Bernstein and Riedel (1987) both found a greater incidence of SC non-responding in a group of individuals characterized by high scores on physical anhedonia. Whereas neither of these studies found associations with positive symptoms, others have indeed found a significant association between hyperresponsive SCOR amplitudes and positive symptoms of schizotypy, such as cognitive distractibility and distortions (Lipp and Vaitl, 1992; Nielsen and Petersen, 1976). However, significant findings also indicated that positive-symptom schizotypy, as reflected by schizophrenism, perceptual aberrations, and cognitive distortions, is also sometimes associated with non-responding or hyporesponding (Lencz *et al.*, 1991; Raine, 1987; Simons *et al.*, 1983). While the above findings clearly indicate some abnormal orienting in individuals with schizotypal features, it must be noted that none of these studies directly assessed for the syndrome or diagnosis of schizotypal PD. This is particularly noteworthy for studies of negative-symptom schizotypy, where the primary index of physical anhedonia is not even listed as a DSM-IV symptom of schizotypal PD. Thus, the finding of most relevance to DSM-IV symptoms of schizotypy is that either hypo- or hyper-SC responding may characterize cognitive and perceptual deficits.

There is also evidence of a link between erratic responding and schizotypy. One example involved an analysis of SCORs over nine orienting trials for normal subjects characterized by high scores on schizophrenism and physical anhedonia and a group of controls (Wilkins, 1988). The results indicated normal habituation over trials 1–3 for the control and schizophrenism groups, but increased response amplitudes from trials 1–2 in the physical anhedonia group. Similarly, the physical anhedonia group showed an increase in amplitudes, rather than normal habituation, from trials 4–5, which comprised a reorienting set of trials. Thus, negative-symptom schizotypal subjects, characterized in this study by physical anhedonia, failed to display the expected SCOR habituation patterns seen in normal controls. As mentioned above, physical anhedonia is not a DSM-IV symptom of schizotypal PD, and thus it was unclear how these results might generalize to the categorical classification of schizotypy.

To address this issue, this study was replicated, using both a sample of 13 DSM-III-R clinically diagnosed schizotypals (i.e., categorical approach) and a sample of 30 subjects who self-reported on a screening scale for schizotypy (i.e., dimensional approach) (Raine *et al.*, 1997a). The results indicated a similar failure to habituate over orienting trials, regardless of whether schizotypy was defined categorically or dimensionally. Cluster analysis of the 13 diagnosed schizotypals revealed two subclusters, the cognitive-perceptual and the interpersonal deficits subclusters, which respectively reflect positive and negative symptoms of schizotypal PD. The failure to habituate was noted only for the cognitive-perceptual subcluster, as reflected by an initial low orienting response followed by increasingly larger responses for both an orienting trial (i.e., over trials 1–3) and a reorienting trial (over trials 4–6). The interpersonal deficits subcluster, however, showed an expected pattern of habituation, with a large initial SCOR followed by diminished responses. This suggests that erratic SCORs may be associated primarily with positive, rather than negative, symptom features of diagnosed schizotypal PD.

Several interpretations of SC orienting abnormalities have been proposed (see Raine *et al.*, 1995 for a review). One interpretation involves deficits in working memory and frontal brain systems, since reduced SC orienting has been shown to be correlated with both of these indices. In addition, template mismatching has been speculated to underlie abnormal orienting. Template mismatching may result from either the degradation of the accurate representation of the initial stimulus, or from difficulty in initially generating the neuronal template. Inhibitory deficits have also been proposed to explain abnormal orienting. It is possible that the underlying deficit lies in the balance between excitatory and inhibitory processes; too much inhibition would account for the high incidence of SC non-responding in schizotypals, while a failure of inhibitory mechanisms would explain erratic orienting and hyperresponding. It is also thought that the balance between these two contrasting processes affects the particular syndrome. Positive syndrome schizotypy may result from disinhibition, while negative syndrome schizotypy may occur because of an excess of inhibition.

Smooth Pursuit Eye Movement (SPEM) and Schizotypal PD

SPEM measures an individual's visual tracking of a smoothly moving target, such as a pendulum. It can be assessed either qualitatively (by visually inspecting the number of saccadic intrusions and visual lags) or quantitatively (by computerized assessments of tracking accuracy, such as the log of the signal-to-noise ratio). SPEM has been thought to reflect cognitive difficulties with nonvoluntary attention and inhibition (Holzman *et al.*, 1976; 1978) and with working memory and prefrontal disorder (Park *et al.*, 1991), all of which are often seen in schizophrenia.

Indeed, impaired SPEM is one of the most consistent findings in schizophrenia, having been observed in 50–85% of patients with chronic schizophrenia compared with 8% of a control population (Holzman *et al.*, 1974; 1984). Impaired SPEM is also greater in relatives of probands with schizophrenia (Holzman *et al.*, 1974) and in patients whose schizophrenia has remitted (Iacono *et al.*, 1981), and is thus speculated to be a genetic marker or diathesis for schizophrenia-spectrum disorders. As such, an interest arose in its relationship to schizotypal PD.

A relationship between SPEM impairment and schizotypal PD first came from studies of individuals selected from the general population on the basis of either poor tracking ability (Siever *et al.*, 1984) or physical/social anhedonia and perceptual aberration scores (Simons and Katkin, 1985). In the former study, volunteers who were selected on the basis of qualitatively poor eye-tracking accuracy had a greater prevalence of diagnosed schizotypal PD than a control group with high eye-tracking accuracy (11% versus 29%). The difference was even more pronounced for individuals whose eye tracking was reassessed quantitatively, with a prevalence rate of 54% with schizotypal PD. No differences were observed between the two groups on other non-schizophrenia psychopathology, including other PDs. This finding suggested that impaired SPEM was specific to the schizophrenia-spectrum disorder of schizotypal PD.

In the study by Simons and Katkin (1985), subjects were selected by dimensional scores on anhedonia and perceptual aberration. Those with high scores on anhedonia demonstrated heightened prevalence of poor SPEM compared to those with low anhedonia, a finding which suggests a relationship of SPEM to negative symptoms of schizotypy. However, impaired eye tracking has also been noted in relationship to positive psychotic symptoms (Siever *et al.*, 1989). Since this study was not conducted on individuals with clinically diagnosed schizotypal PD, it was still unclear how findings would generalize to the classification of the disorder.

To address the issue of eye-tracking abnormalities in clinically identified schizotypal PD, a study was conducted that compared patients who met DSM criteria for the disorder with three other comparison groups — a group with other non-schizophrenia-related PDs, a group with no psychopathology, and a group with schizophrenia (Siever *et al.*, 1990). The results indicated that the groups with schizotypal PD and schizophrenia displayed greater impairment of SPEM than the other PD group and the normal control group. This finding of poor SPEM in diagnosed schizotypal PD was replicated by Lencz *et al.* (1993), who showed impaired eye tracking in a group of undergraduates who met DSM criteria for the disorder.

In the study by Siever *et al.* (1990), an analysis of specific symptoms showed that impaired SPEM was predicted only by the criterion of social isolation, with low accuracy trackers also reporting reduced desire for social contact. This would seem to support the notion of impaired SPEM in relation to negative-symptom schizotypy. Other studies, however, show a relationship between eye-tracking abnormalities and positive-symptom schizotypy. Raine *et al.* (1995), for example, reported a reanalysis of the data by Lencz *et al.* (1993), finding that those diagnosed with schizotypal PD who displayed cognitive/perceptual symptoms showed significantly poorer eye tracking than those with interpersonal deficit symptoms. These same individuals exhibited a loss of normal SC habituation (described in the above section on SCOR), and Raine *et al.* speculated that this reflected a loss of inhibitory functions related to both saccadic intrusions in eye tracking and SC attentional deficits.

On the basis of these studies, it is still unclear whether impaired SPEM is specific to certain types of symptoms (i.e., negative versus positive) or instead reflects the entire schizotypal syndrome more generally. It is clear, however, that poor eye tracking is consistently found in individuals with clinically diagnosed schizotypal PD. Together with the literature on SPEM in schizophrenia, this finding supports the notion of impaired SPEM as a marker for schizophrenia-spectrum disorders that may reflect a common genetic vulnerability.

Event-Related Potentials and Startle-Blink

Despite the emphasis on SCOR and SPEM presented above, there has more recently been research on event-related potential (ERPs) and eye-blink correlates of Cluster A PDs. Perhaps the best-replicated electrophysiological correlate of schizotypal personality is reduced amplitude of the P300 ERP. At least five studies find evidence of P300 amplitude reduction in DSM diagnosed schizophrenia-spectrum disorders (Salisbury *et al.*, 1996; Trestman *et al.*, 1996; Black *et al.*, 1992) and individuals high on schizotypal personality (Kimble *et al.*, 2000; Klein *et al.*, 1999). However, Blackwood *et al.* (1992) did not find reduced P300 in individuals who had been diagnosed as schizoid in childhood, suggesting that schizoid PD, unlike schizotypal and paranoid PDs, may not be part of the schizophrenia-spectrum of disorders. P300 deficits have been repeatedly found in schizophrenics and relatives of schizophrenics, and reflect a broad attentional deficit.

Three other ERP findings are of note. First, high scorers on the schizotypal personality questionnaire have failed to show the right-sided predominance in the post-imperative negative variation (PINV) observed in normals (Klein *et al.*, 1998). Second, individuals with schizotypal PD show less gating (suppression) of the P50 ERP to the second of a pair of click stimuli than controls (Cadenhead *et al.*, 2000), indicating a failure of sensory gating at a relatively early stage of information processing, and consequently reduced central nervous system (CNS) inhibition. The same deficits have been observed in both schizophrenics and their relatives. Third, there is growing evidence in schizotypal individuals of a deficit in N400, an ERP component that reflects the degree of search for a semantic match to a word. Two recent studies have shown reduced N400 amplitudes in both individuals high on schizotypy and those with schizotypal PD (Kimble *et al.*, 2000; Niznikiewicz *et al.*, 1999). These two studies suggest a language-processing deficit in schizotypals that is similar to that observed in schizophrenics.

Research has also been conducted on startle eye-blink modification (SEM) and psychosis-proneness (Cadenhead *et al.*, 1993; Dawson *et al.*, 1995; Simons and Giardina, 1992). These findings again show some consistency with findings in schizophrenia, whereby SEM is impaired in subjects with schizotypal features. Findings are inconsistent, however, regarding whether the deficits occur in the controlled or automatic attentional components of SEM. Nevertheless, deficits in sensorimotor gating are consistent with the P50 ERP deficit outlined above, indicating a failure to gate stimuli.

Summary

Overall, two primary findings emerge on the relationship between psychophysiological measures and schizotypal PD. First, they are generally consistent with those found in schizophrenia. That is, SCOR hyporesponding and hyperresponding; failure to habituate; and deficits in SPEM, P300, P400, P50, and SEM have paralleled the literature on schizophrenia. These findings imply an underlying psychophysiological commonality between schizophrenia and schizotypal PD, and suggest that the latter does indeed reflect part of the schizophrenia-spectrum of disorders. Second, all of these psychophysiological measures tap some cognitive capacity, primarily related to attentional, inhibitory, and working-memory processes. They converge in suggesting specific deficits in such cognitive processes in individuals with schizotypal PD. The findings are not consistent, however, in regard to whether the impairments are related to positive or negative symptoms, and this issue needs to be further examined. It is possible, for example, that three-factor models of symptomatology in schizophrenia and schizotypal personality may provide clearer findings than the two-factor positive-negative model (Raine *et al.*, 1994). Moreover, the relationship to the other Cluster A PDs is still understudied.

CLUSTER B PERSONALITY DISORDERS

Cluster B includes the antisocial, borderline, histrionic, and narcissistic PDs. Antisocial PD is defined as a pattern of disregarding and violating the rights of others; borderline PD is defined as a pattern of unstable relationships, self-image, affect, and behaviour in the form of impulsivity; histrionic PD is defined as a pattern of excessive emotionality and seeking of attention; and narcissistic PD is defined as a pattern of grandiosity, need for admiration by others, and lack of empathy with others (American Psychiatric Association, 1994). These PDs seem to share symptoms that reflect dramatic, erratic, and highly emotional behaviours, although antisocial PD may also be associated with a lack of emotionality.

Of this cluster, antisocial PD has been most extensively studied in relation to psychophysiology, especially in regard to heart rate (HR), skin conductance (SC), and electroencephalogram (EEG) as a reflection of underarousal (see Chapter 7 in Raine, 1993 for a comprehensive review). As such, this will be the focus of the following review. It should be noted, however, that the majority of these studies do not use DSM criteria for measurement of PD, but instead use measures of psychopathy or repetitive antisocial behaviour. Thus, though obviously related, the exact nature of the findings in regard to clinically diagnosed antisocial PD is blurred. There has also been some limited psychophysiological research on borderline PD and one known psychophysiological study of narcissism, and this information will be included as well.

HR Studies and Antisocial Behaviour

HR reflects both sympathetic and parasympathetic nervous system activity and can be measured both tonically (i.e., beats per minute at rest) or phasically (i.e., change in response to a stimulus). Accelerations in HR to a stimulus are thought to reflect sensory rejection or 'tuning out' of noxious environmental events, while decelerations are thought to reflect sensory intake or an environmental openness (Lacey and Lacey, 1974). Emotionally, HR has been associated with the experience of anxiety. As such, high tonic HR is thought to reflect fear, while low tonic HR may reflect fearlessness.

Regarding studies on tonic HR, one of the best-replicated findings to date is that of reduced resting HR in antisocial individuals. In his review of this topic, Raine (1993) noted that of 14 relevant studies, there were no failures to replicate the finding of reduced resting HR in the antisocial groups. Low HR is a robust marker independent of cultural context, with the relationship having been established in the UK (e.g., Farrington, 1987), Germany (Schmeck and Poustka, 1993), New Zealand (Moffitt and Caspi, 2001), the USA (e.g., Rogeness *et al.*, 1990), Mauritius (Raine *et al.*, 1997b), and Canada (Mezzacappa *et al.*, 1997). It is also diagnostically specific (i.e., it is not found in other disorders), and multiple confounds have been ruled out (Raine *et al.*, 1997b).

All of these studies used child or adolescent samples, but consistent with this finding, low HR recently has also been associated with self-reported aggression in uninstitutionalized young adults (Scarpa *et al.*, 2000). In addition, 21 adult individuals from the community with a diagnosis of antisocial PD were found to have low HR during a social stressor (Raine *et al.*, 2000). However, this effect seems specific to antisocial behaviour and personality in general rather than psychopathic personality in particular. Reviews by Hare (1970; 1975; 1978) revealed no successes and at least 15 failures to obtain low resting HR in institutionalized, psychopathic criminals.

Low resting HR has recently been found to characterize life-course persistent offenders (Moffitt and Caspi, 2001), as well as those with diagnoses in institutionalized psychopathy, indicating that low HR is related to a pervasive pattern of severe rule violations. It also characterizes milder forms of antisocial and aggressive behaviour in children and adolescents that preface more serious criminal violations later in life. For example, in one of the few prospective studies examining this issue, psychophysiological measures were obtained at age 15 years in an unselected sample of male students, and government records were obtained 9 years later to measure any criminal violations. Only relatively serious offences were registered, ranging from theft to wounding, with the most common offence being burglary. By this criterion, 17 of the 101 subjects were found to have a criminal record. These 17 criminals were found to have significantly lower resting HR than the non-criminal controls, indicating reduced cardiovascular arousal as measured 9 years earlier. Low HR at age 3 years is also predictive of aggressive behaviour at age 11 years in both males and females (Raine *et al.*, 1997b). Reduced HR may reflect autonomic underarousal, as suggested by Raine *et al.* (1990a), or, alternatively, fearlessness in novel situations (Kagan, 1989; Venables, 1987), which theoretically could predispose a child to early social transgressions that cycle into later serious antisocial behaviour.

Regarding studies on phasic HR changes, the literature is less extensive, but suggests that psychopathic criminals exhibit anticipatory HR acceleration prior to an aversive event. In general, the findings of early studies indicated that psychopaths gave significantly larger acceleratory HR responses in anticipation of a signalled aversive stimulus such as a loud noise or electric shock, followed by reduced SC responses to the aversive stimulus itself (Hare, 1982; Hare and Craigen, 1974; Hare *et al.*, 1978). Hare (1978) interpreted these findings to suggest that psychopathic individuals have a very proficient active coping mechanism that allows them to 'tune out' aversive events. Although interesting, there has been very little further research on this phenomenon. Again, the relationship has not been studied specifically in relationship to antisocial PD, but it would be predicted that these individuals may engage in similar sensory rejection of aversive events. In terms of theories of socialization, this pattern may lead to poor conditioning in response to cues of punishment and thus decreased learning of appropriate social behaviour (Eysenck, 1977).

SC Studies and Antisocial Behaviour

Besides measuring SC phasically, as discussed above in the description of the SCOR, SC can also be measured tonically or in a resting state. In this regard, SC is measured in terms of resting level (SCL) or number of nonspecific SC fluctuations (NSF). NSFs are changes in SC that look like orienting responses, but do not occur in response to a known stimulus. Both SCL and NSF are thought to reflect some baseline level of physiological sympathetic arousal, and thus have often been associated with fear emotions in the fight/flight response.

Recent reviews of SC studies (Raine, 1993; Scarpa and Raine, 1997) indicate that

1. There is some evidence for SC underarousal in antisocial individuals, particularly with respect to nonviolent and non-impulsive forms of crime.
2. SCOR deficits seem specific to antisocial individuals with concomitant schizotypal personality features.
3. Prior findings up to 1978 of reduced SC responsivity to aversive stimuli in psychopaths generally have not been observed in more recent studies, either in psychopathic or non-psychopathic antisocial populations.
4. The strongest findings lie with respect to reduced SC classical conditioning in antisocial populations.

These findings are summarized below.

With regard to SC underarousal, both SCL and NSFs have been found to be reduced in antisocial groups in a number of studies, though this has not been entirely consistent. As with HR, the findings are primarily in uninstitutionalized subjects with mild forms of aggressive or other antisocial behaviour. Again, however, in the prospective study by Raine *et al.* (1990a), it was found that a reduced number of NSFs at age 15 years predicted criminal behaviour 9 years later. Raine and colleagues suggested that this pattern, along with low resting HR, reflected autonomic underarousal in criminals-to-be. In an early review of the literature on psychopathy, Hare (1978) concluded that these individuals are characterized by reduced SCL, but not NSFs. Thus, it is possible that reduced SC arousal is also related to antisocial PD in adulthood. This has recently been confirmed in a study showing that individuals with antisocial PD show reduced SC activity during a social stressor (Raine *et al.*, 2000).

Regarding SCORs, Hare (1978) had concluded that the research to that date showed reduced SC responses to aversive, but not neutral tones (i.e., a reduced defensive response, but no difference in orienting response). This pattern of findings, however, has not been consistently replicated in research conducted after that review. Nevertheless, deficits in SCOR have been consistently observed in individuals who display both antisocial behaviour and features of schizotypal PD. For example, antisocial adolescents with schizotypal features had significantly lower SCORs than those with only schizotypal features (Raine and Venables, 1984). In his review, Raine (1993) also noted that, with the exception of one study, reduced frequency of SCORs was found only in studies where antisocial behaviour was combined with schizotypal or schizoid characteristics. Thus, it seems that SCOR deficits may be specific to schizotypal criminals. Since the number of SCOR responses may be related to frontal lobe functioning (Raine *et al.*, 1991), Raine interpreted these results as possibly reflecting frontal dysfunction in this particular subgroup of antisocial individuals. Further support for interpreting reduced SC activity in terms of prefrontal deficits comes from a recent study showing that individuals with antisocial PD have both reduced prefrontal grey matter and reduced SC activity (Raine *et al.*, 2000). Furthermore, when antisocials were divided into those with and those without reduced prefrontal grey, it was the subgroup with prefrontal grey deficits who showed SC deficits compared to those without prefrontal deficits.

Perhaps the strongest findings for SC activity lie with respect to reduced classical conditioning in antisocial populations. Classical conditioning involves learning that an initially neutral event (i.e., a conditioned stimulus [CS]), when closely followed in time by an aversive event (i.e., an unconditioned stimulus [UCS]), will develop the properties of this UCS. Eysenck (1977) argued that the socialization process and development of a 'conscience' stems from a set of classically conditioned negative emotional responses to situations that have previously led to punishment. In this way, socialized individuals develop a feeling of uneasiness at even contemplating antisocial behaviour, presumably because such thoughts elicit representations of punishment earlier in life. Furthermore, according to Eysenck's theory, arousal levels are related to conditionability, such that low levels of arousal predispose to poor conditionability and high levels to good conditionability.

The central idea in Eysenck's theory is that antisocials are characterized by poor classical conditioning. Classical conditioning has frequently been assessed with SC: a neutral tone (CS) is presented to the subject, followed a few seconds later by either a loud tone or an electric shock (UCS). The key measure is the size of the SCR elicited by the CS after a number of CS-UCS pairings. In a review by Hare (1978), 13 out of 14 studies reported significantly poorer SC conditioning in antisocial populations. In a review of studies since 1978 by Raine (1993), all six studies showed some evidence of significantly poorer SC conditioning in antisocials, including psychopathic gamblers, other psychopaths, conduct-disordered children from high social-class backgrounds, and criminals from good homes. These results are also consistent with findings of reduced SC arousal in antisocial populations, as presented above.

EEG, ERPs, and Antisocial Behaviour

The EEG reflects the electrical activity of the brain recorded from electrodes placed at different locations on the scalp according to the standardized international 10–20 system. The EEG can be broken down into different frequency components, most commonly delta (0–4 Hz), theta (4–8 Hz), alpha (8–12 Hz), and beta (13–30 Hz). Alpha and beta are also often subdivided into slow and fast components. The EEG can be either clinically scored by observing the chart record to detect excessive theta or slow-wave activity, or subjected to a more quantitative computerized analysis, which more objectively delineates the EEG into different components.

EEG frequency has been aligned with a continuum of consciousness, with delta associated with sleep, theta associated with drowsiness and low levels of alertness, alpha associated with relaxed wakefulness, and beta associated with alertness and vigilance. As such, individuals with a predominance of theta or slow alpha activity would be viewed as having relatively reduced levels of cortical arousal, while those with relatively more fast alpha and beta activity would be viewed as relatively more aroused.

In a review by Mednick *et al.* (1982), the authors concluded that there is a high prevalence (25–50%) of EEG abnormalities in violent criminals, especially recidivistic offenders, compared with the 10–15% normally found in the general population. Volavka (1987) and Milstein (1988) drew similar conclusions for crime in general and violent crime in particular. Reviews of the EEG literature on psychopathy are less consistent. Hare (1970) initially concluded that psychopaths are characterized by excessive slow-wave activity. Later reviews, however, concluded that the evidence of EEG abnormalities in psychopaths is inconsistent (Blackburn, 1983; Syndulko, 1978), with one study even showing the opposite pattern that primary psychopaths were *more* aroused than secondary (schizoid) psychopaths.

The ERP refers to averaged changes of electrical activity of the brain in response to specific stimuli. ERP responses typically follow a sequence of early, middle, and late components which are thought to reflect the psychological processes of environmental filtering, cortical augmenting, and attention, respectively. ERP studies of antisocial behaviour have primarily involved psychopathic populations, and a review of this literature (conceptually broken down into early, middle, and late latency studies) was presented by Raine (1989). The main conclusions of this review are findings of

1. long early latency brainstem averaged evoked responses, reflecting excessive environmental filtering and reduced arousal
2. increased middle latency ERP amplitudes to stimuli of increasing intensity, which has been linked to sensation seeking
3. enhanced late latency ERP P300 amplitudes to stimuli of interest, suggesting enhanced attention to stimulating events.

Raine suggested that these processes may be causally linked, such that individuals with chronically low levels of arousal (possibly caused by excessive filtering of stimuli) would seek out stimulating events (including risky situations) in order to increase their levels of arousal to more optimal levels. This stimulation-seeking may partly account for the enhanced attention shown to events of interest.

While the evidence is unclear in terms of antisocial PD, there is again some reason to believe that impaired EEG and ERPs may reflect an early risk of later criminal behaviour. As reflected in the prospective study by Raine *et al.* (1990a; 1990b), criminals had significantly more slow-frequency EEG theta activity and larger N100 ERPs to target stimuli, as measured nine years earlier, than non-criminals. These findings are consistent with notions of underarousal and enhanced early stimulus attention in criminals and psychopaths.

Psychophysiological Study of Borderline PD

There are only two known studies examining the psychophysiological correlates of borderline PD. In the first study, a group of female patients with borderline PD were compared to female controls with no psychopathology on emotional reactions to pleasant, neutral, and unpleasant slides as measured by self-report, HR, SC, and eye-blink startle response (Herpertz *et al.*, 1999). In the second study, a comparison group of patients with avoidant PD was added to the borderline PD and normal control groups (Herpertz *et al.*, 2000). It is unclear whether the same individuals were used in both studies to form the borderline PD and normal control groups. The eye-blink startle response measures the automatic blink response that occurs to a startling probe, and is typically magnified when viewing unpleasant stimuli, but diminished when viewing pleasant stimuli. On the basis of previous theories of borderline PD, the authors predicted heightened affective responsivity in the subjects with this diagnosis.

Contrary to predictions, the borderline PD and control groups did not differ in startle response or HR responsivity in both studies, and the borderline PD group exhibited significantly reduced SC responses to all three stimulus categories. Moreover, the borderline PD group reported less pleasant affect to pleasant and neutral stimuli and less arousal to neutral stimuli. Self-report ratings on impulsivity, sensation seeking, and aggressiveness also did not account for the findings of SC hyporesponsivity. The authors speculated that this finding of decreased electrodermal responsiveness instead reflected problems in attentional processing.

Psychophysiological Study of Narcissism

There is one known study relating psychophysiological variables to narcissism (Kelsey *et al.*, 2001). As with many of the other studies reviewed here, narcissism was measured by a dimensional scale in this study, and the diagnostic syndrome of narcissistic PD was not assessed. Nonetheless, this study provides an initial peek at the psychophysiology of the major features of this disorder, including egocentricity, grandiosity, arrogance, a need for admiration, and a lack of empathy.

In this study, 40 undergraduate men who scored high or low on the Narcissistic Personality Inventory were compared on measures of pre-ejection period (PEP), frequency of SC responses, and HR reactivity in anticipation of an aversive stimulus. PEP was included as a measure of beta-adrenergic cardiac reactivity, primarily reflecting sympathetic cardiac activity; SC was included as a measure of sympathetic activity; and HR was included as a measure of both sympathetic and parasympathetic influences. Because narcissism has been posited to be an underlying feature of psychopathy, the authors hypothesized reduced sympathetic activity overall and enhanced parasympathetic control of the heart.

The results indicated greater PEP shortening, HR deceleration, and SC response habituation in the high narcissism group in anticipation of the aversive stimulus. Consistent with one hypothesis, the cardiac deceleration was interpreted as reflecting parasympathetic dominance. Contrary to the other hypotheses, however, the PEP and SC results suggested a fractionation of the sympathetic response. Shortened PEP reflects heightened sympathetic reactivity, while reduced SC activity reflects reduced sympathetic activity. The authors interpreted these findings according to a model of arousal proposed by Pribram and McGuinness (1975), suggesting that low SC activity in narcissism reflects physiological underarousal, HR deceleration reflects internally generated attention and activity, and PEP reactivity reflects heightened effort during the processing of aversive information.

Summary

For antisocial, psychopathic personality, the psychophysiological results suggest several conclusions. First, psychophysiological underarousal may reflect an early predisposition to mild antisocial behaviour that cycles into more serious recidivistic crime later in life. Second, as suggested by poor SC classical conditioning and low tonic SC, psychopathic and antisocial personality may be characterized by poor passive avoidance learning, which would interfere with the ability to learn to avoid misbehaviour in response to the anticipation of punishment. Because SC and HR have been associated with anxiety and fear, it is conceivable that these findings, along with underarousal, may also reflect the callousness and unemotionality that is characteristic of the psychopathic personality. Parallel findings of reduced SC responsivity in borderline PD and in narcissism suggest that they instead may relate to behaviour that is characterized by impulsivity and risk-taking (common to both antisocial and borderline PD) or may reflect an attentional ‘tuning out’ of aversive environmental stimuli in order to manage negative affect or maintain self-esteem (common to both antisocial and narcissistic PD). Third, low resting HR is the best-replicated psychophysiological correlate of antisocial behaviour. Fourth, findings in antisocial personality using ERPs are consistent with the notions of both increased sensation seeking and focus on events of interest, a fact which could explain the increase in impulsivity and risky behaviour seen in this personality style. Lastly, findings suggest that antisocial individuals with schizotypal PD may reflect a special subgroup of criminality characterized by frontal lobe dysfunction which is reflected in SCOR hyporesponsivity. Further study is necessary to see how the above findings generalize to clinically diagnosed antisocial PD, and a clear need is present to study the psychophysiology of the other Cluster B PDs.

CLUSTER C PERSONALITY DISORDERS

Cluster C includes the avoidant, dependent, and obsessive-compulsive PDs. Avoidant PD is defined as a pattern of social inhibition, feelings of inadequacy, and hypersensitivity to negative evaluation; dependent PD is defined as a pattern of submissive and clinging behaviour related to a need be taken care of; and obsessive-compulsive PD is defined as a pattern of preoccupation with orderliness, perfectionism, and control (American Psychiatric Association, 1994). Each of these PDs has some association with underlying feelings of anxiety and internalizing behaviours. To the authors’ knowledge, the only Cluster C PD that has been studied psychophysiologically is avoidant PD, which will begin the following section. Inhibited temperament in children, which includes shy and cautious behaviour, along with fear of novel or unfamiliar people and situations, is also discussed as a possible developmental precursor to avoidant PD. No studies are known that directly assess obsessive-compulsive PD in relation to psychophysiological measures, but the DSM-IV notes that many features of this PD overlap with ‘type A’ personality (e.g., hostility, competitiveness, and time urgency). Type A personality has been studied extensively in relation to cardiovascular disease risk. As such, a brief review of this literature is also provided.

Psychophysiological Studies of Avoidant PD

As described above, avoidant PD involves a pervasive pattern of social inhibition or avoidance of social situations that seems to revolve around feelings of being inadequate and fears of consequent criticism and rejection by others. According to DSM-IV, there appears to be a great deal of overlap between this PD and the Axis I disorder of social phobia, generalized type. As such, several studies have been conducted to assess for differences or similarities between social phobia with and without avoidant PD, and they do indeed suggest a distinction between these two forms of social phobia in terms of severity.

In general, studies which compare these subgroups of social phobia on measures of subjective and behavioural anxiety find greater reports of anxiety and behavioural impairment in those diagnosed with avoidant PD or the generalized subtype of social phobia (Herbert *et al.*, 1992; Holt *et al.*, 1992). If social phobia with avoidant PD indeed reflects a more severe form of social phobia, one would predict greater psychophysiological reactivity to fearful social situations in these individuals. There seems to be a discrepancy, however, between the subjective anxiety reported and the psychophysiological profile exhibited in this population. For example, one study compared groups with discrete social phobias, generalized social phobia with avoidant PD, and generalized social phobia without avoidant PD on HR recorded during an impromptu speech (Turner *et al.*, 1992). The results indicated no HR differences among these three groups. Similarly, two other studies showed no HR differences during a public-speaking task between socially phobic individuals with avoidant PD and normal controls, but those with a specific social phobia did show higher HR with the task (Heimberg *et al.*, 1990; Hofmann *et al.*, 1995). Interestingly, in these studies, the group with avoidant PD reported the greatest subjective anxiety and fear, although their HR responses did not differ from controls and were lower than the group without avoidant PD.

Overall, these findings indicate a discordance between the subjective and HR responses in socially phobic individuals with avoidant PD. Although the reason for this discordance is unknown, Hofmann *et al.* (1995) suggest several possibilities — that social phobias with avoidant PD have a less coherent cognitive fear structure, that other emotions may be blending with fear to attenuate HR responses, or that the tonic presence of fearful cognitions in avoidant PD may inhibit further processing of fearful material because the feared event provides no new emotional information. A possibility that was not considered is that excessive tonic worry in avoidant PD may inhibit the information processing of feared stimuli because it simply serves as an attentional distraction, thus leading to reduced HR reactivity. Either of the latter two interpretations is supported by a study by Herpertz *et al.* (2000) in which eye-blink startle, HR, and SC responses to emotional stimuli were compared in groups with avoidant PD and borderline PD, or normal controls. Relevant to avoidant PD, the results showed increased startle magnitude relative to the borderline PD and control groups, but only at baseline (i.e., before the emotional stimuli were presented). No group differences were found for SC and HR responses. Since the eye-blink startle response is specifically sensitive to anxious/fearful mood, this finding suggests that individuals with avoidant PD may have a tonically high level of anxiety that interferes with ongoing information processing.

Psychophysiological Studies of Inhibited Temperament in Children

Behavioural inhibition in childhood reflects a temperamental style of avoidance in situations that are novel or unfamiliar. According to DSM-IV, avoidant PD is described as often starting in infancy or childhood with characteristics of shyness, isolation, and fear of strangers and new situations. Thus, inhibited temperament in children may reflect a developmental precursor to avoidant PD, although it is clear that not all children with such shyness will go on to develop the PD.

In a series of studies, Kagan and his colleagues examined children who were classified as either behaviourally inhibited or uninhibited at 21 months of age by their tendency consistently to withdraw or interact respectively across various experimental situations. At 21 months, inhibited relative to uninhibited children were found to have higher and more stable HR while looking at unfamiliar pictures and listening to unfamiliar sounds (Garcia-Coll *et al.*, 1984). These children were again examined at ages 31 months, and 4, 5.5, and 7.5 years. At every age, it was observed that the behavioural differences which originally led to the classification as inhibited or uninhibited at age 21 months were still maintained between the two groups, and the inhibited children showed higher and more stable HR to a series of cognitive procedures than the uninhibited children (Kagan *et al.*, 1984; Kagan *et al.*, 1988; Reznick *et al.*, 1986). The results were replicated on a second cohort of children who were tested at ages 2, 3.5, 5.5, and 7.5 years, suggesting a stability of inhibited/uninhibited temperament over time, with those classified as inhibited having higher HR at each age than those classified as uninhibited (Kagan, 1989; Kagan, *et al.*, 1987). Taken together, these results indicate that high HR is associated with increased behavioural inhibition.

Kagan (1989; 1994) has suggested that this heightened sympathetic reactivity in inhibited children stems from a lower threshold of excitability in limbic sites, particularly the amygdala and hypothalamus. If behavioural inhibition is thus reflected in increased sympathetic activity, other sympathetic measures should show similar group differences in inhibited individuals. Indeed, Kagan (1994) reports findings of increased sympathetic activity reflected in other measures such as salivary cortisol, urinary norepinephrine, and facial skin temperature. Furthermore, in a study of 3-year-old children, those who were inhibited exhibited heightened levels of both resting HR and SC relative to those who were uninhibited (Scarpa *et al.*, 1997), again providing support for the relationship between inhibition and physiological arousal through limbic activation.

If behavioural inhibition does developmentally precede avoidant PD in adulthood, similar sympathetic arousal and reactivity would be expected in adults with avoidant PD. As described in the preceding section, however, there is no evidence for increased sympathetic levels or responsivity in adults with avoidant PD. In fact, of the few studies examining psychophysiology of avoidant PD, all indicated similar levels and reactivity of HR and/or SC compared to normal controls (Herpertz *et al.*, 2000; Hofmann *et al.*, 1995; Turner *et al.*, 1992). It is possible, therefore, that inhibited temperament in children is not a childhood precursor of adulthood avoidant PD. Alternative explanations could also be that the physiological responses of inhibited children who grow up to develop avoidant PD differ from those who do not develop the disorder, or that their physiological responsivity changes as they grow into adulthood.

Psychophysiological Studies of Type A Personality

As originally described by Friedman and Rosenman (1959), the type A behaviour pattern is characterized by excessive competitiveness; impatience; hostility; overcommitment to work; and a loud, rapid, and pressured vocal style. This pattern has many behavioural similarities to the symptoms of obsessive-compulsive PD, suggesting a possible overlap. We are aware of no psychophysiological studies of obsessive-compulsive PD; however, psychophysiological reactivity in relation to type A personality has been extensively studied (see Houston, 1983 and Harbin, 1989 for reviews). Although other measures have been included, blood pressure (BP) and HR have been the foci of these investigations due to the link between type A behaviour and coronary heart disease (e.g., Cooper *et al.*, 1981). A brief summary of this literature follows.

Results from reviews have generally concluded that, relative to type B individuals (i.e., people who are easy-going, patient, and soft-spoken), type A individuals show greater BP and HR responses to stressors (Houston, 1983; Harbin, 1989). In a re-examination of the same data presented by Houston (1983), Holmes (1983) emphasized that the most consistent findings were with respect to systolic BP and that this effect was of small magnitude. That is, 13 out of 20 experiments revealed reliable differences in systolic BP, while only 4 of 18 experiments revealed reliable diastolic BP effects and only 6 of 24 experiments revealed reliable HR effects. Moreover, the median group difference in systolic BP was 6 mmHg, a difference that is not typically considered to be physiologically meaningful.

Despite some inconsistency in findings and the suggestion that this relationship is weak to moderate at best, the quantitative review by Harbin (1989) still showed an overall effect for increased cardiovascular activity in those with the type A behaviour pattern. It appears that more consistent findings are obtained when the individual is faced with a stressor task that is challenging, where there is an intermediate chance of failure, where there is moderate external incentive to do well, or where there is an interpersonal encounter that is annoying or harassing to the subject (Houston, 1992). Moreover, the most reliable BP responses have been found when type A behaviour is measured according to a structured interview that assesses behavioural qualities, rather than by self-report measures. Finally, it may be that not all aspects of type A personality are equally related to physiological reactivity. Hostility, for example, has been identified as the most powerful type A characteristic to predict coronary heart disease (Dembroski and Costa, 1987), and it has been associated with increased cardiovascular reactivity in response to stress (see Smith and Leon [1992] for a summary).

As summarized by Smith and Leon (1992), several psychological explanations have been posited for the increased cardiovascular reactivity found in type A personality. In general, these explanations imply that the stressor tasks activate a relevant type A characteristic that leads these individuals to increase their efforts, and this is associated with increased sympathetic nervous system activity. Such a behavioural response on the part of the person with type A personality may be due to excessively high standards for success, perceptions of threat of loss of control over the environment or other people, or a high level of self-involvement. It is also possible that these individuals simply create more frequent stressful situations in their lives, the net result of which is more frequent physiological reactivity and consequent increased risk of coronary heart disease.

Summary

None of the Cluster C PDs have been studied extensively enough to form substantive conclusions in relation to psychophysiological variables. Nonetheless, studies on associated features, such as inhibited temperament and the type A behaviour pattern, as well as the few studies of avoidant PD, suggest some directions. Sympathetic reactivity is implicated in both inhibited temperament and type A personality. However, it is more pervasive in relation to behavioural inhibition, and seems to be primarily associated with systolic BP in relation to type A behaviour. Moreover, no studies found HR differences between avoidant PD, in particular, and normal control groups. Thus, it appears that inhibited temperamental style, avoidant PD, and type A personality (which is the closest personality analogue to obsessive-compulsive PD) are distinct constructs with distinct psychophysiological profiles. As such, one suggested direction for further research in this area includes the study of whether behavioural inhibition does indeed serve as a developmental precursor to adult avoidant PD, and, if so, why is there a change in psychophysiological response over time? Another suggested direction is to examine whether the cardiovascular findings in type A personality generalize to obsessive-compulsive PD. Lastly, more work overall needs to be done on the psychophysiology of all of the Cluster C PDs.

CONCLUSIONS

As can be seen from the above review, the psychophysiological findings with respect to PD are quite diverse. While this might be expected given the diverse characteristics of each of the 10 PDs described in the DSM-IV, it is also notable given the high degree of overlap in PD symptomatology and the resulting high PD comorbidity. As such, this psychophysiological research provides some insight into the differences that may underlie the various PDs. Caution, however, is warranted due to the fact that there has been little work on the diagnostic syndromes of *any* of the PDs. That is, what work has been done typically has focused on dimensional characteristics, specific symptoms, or associated features of the disorders rather than the clinical diagnosis as a syndrome. Further research is definitely needed in this area, but despite this major limitation, the following conclusions are suggested.

First, the psychophysiological findings generally indicate cognitive abnormalities in Cluster A disorders, especially schizotypal PD, that mirror findings in schizophrenia and thus suggest a common underlying biological marker. Second, the findings generally indicate arousal and cognitive learning deficits as well as emotional deficits in Cluster B disorders, which particularly reflect impulsive, antisocial behavioural styles. Third, primarily emotional contributions are suggested in relation to Cluster C PDs, particularly to fear in avoidant PD and to hostility/anger in obsessive-compulsive PD. These findings suggest that the behavioural similarities within PD clusters and differences across clusters may indeed be reflected in corresponding psychophysiological profiles.

It is also noted, however, that certain paradigms for measuring psychophysiology do not cut across the study of PDs. SC conditioning, for example, has in the past been extensively studied in relation to antisocial behaviour, but not in the other PDs. Similarly, SPEM has been studied in relation to schizotypal PD, but not specifically in the other PDs. As such, psychophysiology still has much to offer in terms of elucidating the cognitive and emotional psychology of PDs. This review establishes a clear need for further work on the psychophysiology of PDs.

Finally, probably the most striking and consistent finding in the field of the psychophysiology of PDs is the low autonomic arousal of antisocial behaviour and personality. Furthermore, low autonomic arousal is diagnostically specific to antisocial personality within the diagnostic subfield of PDs in that no other PD is characterized by low autonomic arousal. In particular, low resting HR is the best-replicated biological correlate of antisocial behaviour in community samples. A challenge for future research lies in placing this finding, linked to impairments of the prefrontal cortex, within a wider, neurophysiological, neuropsychological, and psychosocial context. A similar challenge exists with respect to the larger literature on the psychophysiology of PDs overall.

ACKNOWLEDGEMENT

This chapter was written with the support of an Independent Scientist Award to the second author from the National Institute of Mental Health (K02 MH01114-01).

REFERENCES

American Psychiatric Association, 1994. *Diagnostic and Statistical Manual of Mental Disorders* (4th edn, revised). American Psychiatric Association, Washington, DC.

Bernstein, A.S. and Riedel, J.A., 1987. Psychophysiological response patterns in college students with physical anhedonia: scores appear to reflect schizotypy rather than depression. *Biological Psychiatry*, **22**, 829–847.

Black, J.L., Mowry, B.J., Barton, D.A. and De Roach, J.N., 1992. Auditory P300 studies in schizophrenic subjects and their first degree relatives. *Australasian Physical and Engineering Sciences in Medicine*, **15**, 65–73.

Blackburn, R., 1983. Psychopathy, delinquency, and crime. In: Gale, A. and Edwards, J.A. (eds), *Physiological Correlates of Human Behavior*, vol. 3, pp. 187–205. Academic Press, London.

Blackwood, D.H., Muir, W.J., Roxborough, H.M., Walker, M.R., Townshend, R., Glabus, M.F. and Wolff, S., 1994. 'Schizoid' personality in childhood: auditory P300 and eye tracking responses at follow-up in adult life. *Journal of Autism and Developmental Disorders*, **24**, 487–500.

Cacioppo, J.T. and Tassinary, L.G., 1990. Psychophysiology and psychophysiological inference. In: Cacioppo, J.T. and Tassinary, L.G. (eds), *Principles of Psychophysiology: Physical, Social, and Inferential Elements*, pp. 3–33. Cambridge University Press, New York.

Cadenhead, K.S., Geyer, M.A. and Braff, D.L., 1993. Impaired startle prepulse inhibition in schizotypal patients. *American Journal of Psychiatry*, **150**, 1862–1867.

Cadenhead, K.S., Light, G.A., Geyer, M.A. and Braff, D.L., 2000. Sensory gating deficits assessed by the P50 event-related potential in subjects with schizotypal personality disorder. *American Journal of Psychiatry*, **157**, 55–59.

Chapman, J.P., Chapman, L.J. and Kwapil, T.R., 1995. Scales for the measurement of schizotypy. In: Raine, A., Lencz, T. and Mednick, S.A. (eds), *Schizotypal Personality*, pp. 79–106. Cambridge University Press, New York.

Cooper, T., Detre, T. and Weiss, S.M., 1981. Coronary-prone behavior and coronary heart disease: a critical review. *Circulation*, **63**, 1199–1215.

Dawson, M.E., Filion, D.L. and Schell, A.M., 1989. Is elicitation of the autonomic orienting response associated with the allocation of processing resources? *Psychophysiology*, **26**, 560–572.

Dawson, M.E. and Nuechterlein, K.H., 1984. Psychophysiological dysfunction in the developmental course of schizophrenic disorders. *Schizophrenia Bulletin*, **10**, 204–232.

Dawson, M.E., Schell, A.M., Hazlett, E.A., Filion, D.L. and Nuechterlein, K.H., 1995. Attention, startle eye-blink modification, and psychosis proneness. In: Raine, A., Lencz, T. and Mednick, S.A. (eds), *Schizotypal Personality*, pp. 250–271. Cambridge University Press, New York.

Dembroski, T.M. and Costa, P.T., 1987. Coronary prone behavior: components of the type A pattern and hostility. *Journal of Personality*, **55**, 211–235.

Eysenck, H.J., 1977. *Crime and Personality* (3rd edn). Paladin, St Albans.

Farrington, D.P., 1997. The relationship between low resting heart rate and violence. In: Raine, A., Brennan, P.A., Farrington, D.P. and Mednick, S.A. (eds), *Biosocial Bases of Violence*, pp. 89–106. Plenum Press, New York.

Friedman, M. and Rosenman, R.H., 1959. Association of a specific overt behavior pattern with blood and cardiovascular findings. *Journal of the American Medical Association*, **169**, 1286–1296.

Garcia-Coll, C., Kagan, J. and Reznick, J.S., 1984. Behavioral inhibition in young children. *Child Development*, **55**, 1005–1019.

Harbin, T.J., 1989. The relationship between type A behavior pattern and physiological responsivity: a quantitative review. *Psychophysiology*, **26**, 110–119.

Hare, R.D., 1970. *Psychopathy: Theory and Practice*. Wiley, New York.

Hare, R.D., 1975. Psychophysiological studies of psychopathy. In: Fowles, D.C. (ed.), *Clinical Applications of Psychophysiology*, pp. 77–105. Cambridge University Press, New York.

Hare, R.D., 1978. Electrodermal and cardiovascular correlates of psychopathy. In: Hare, R.D. and Schalling, D. (eds), *Psychopathic Behavior: Approaches to Research*, pp. 107–144. Wiley, New York.

Hare, R.D., 1982. Psychopathy and physiological activity during anticipation of an aversive stimulus in a distraction paradigm. *Psychophysiology*, **19**, 266–271.

Hare, R.D. and Craigen, D., 1974. Psychopathy and physiological activity in a mixed motive game situation. *Psychophysiology*, **11**, 197–206.

Hare, R.D., Frazelle, J. and Cox, D., 1978. Psychopathy and physiological responses to threat of an aversive stimulus. *Psychophysiology*, **15**, 165–172.

Heimberg, R.G., Hope, D.A., Dodge, C.S. and Becker, R.E., 1990. DSM-III-R subtypes of social phobia. Comparison of generalized social phobics and public-speaking phobics. *Journal of Nervous and Mental Diseases*, **178**, 172–179.

Herbert, J.D., Hope, D.A. and Bellack, A.S., 1992. Validity of the distinction between generalized social phobia and avoidant personality disorder. *Journal of Abnormal Psychology*, **101**, 332–339.

Herpertz, S.C., Kunert, H.J., Schwenger, U.B. and Sass, H., 1999. Affective responsiveness in borderline personality disorder: a psychophysiological approach. *American Journal of Psychiatry*, **156**, 1550–1556.

Herpertz, S.C., Schwenger, U.B., Kunert, H.J., Lukas, G., Gretzer, U., Nutzmann, J., Schuerkens, A. and Sass, H., 2000. Emotional responses in patients with borderline as compared with avoidant personality disorder. *Journal of Personality Disorders*, **14**, 339–351.

Hofmann, S.G., Newman, M.G., Ehlers, A. and Roth, W.T., 1995. Psychophysiological differences between subgroups of social phobia. *Journal of Abnormal Psychology*, **104**, 224–231.

Holmes, D.S., 1983. An alternative perspective concerning the differential psychophysiological responsivity of persons with the type A and type B behavior patterns. *Journal of Research in Personality*, **17**, 40–47.

Holt, C.S., Heimberg, R.G. and Hope, D.A., 1992. Avoidant personality disorder and the generalized subtype of social phobia. *Journal of Abnormal Psychology*, **101**, 318–325.

Holzman, P.S., Levy, D.L. and Proctor, L.R., 1976. Smooth-pursuit eye movements, attention, and schizophrenia. *Archives of General Psychiatry*, **33**, 1415–1420.

Holzman, P.S., Levy, D.L. and Proctor, L.R., 1978. The several qualities of attention in schizophrenia. *Journal of Psychiatric Research*, **14**, 99–110.

Holzman, P.S., Proctor, L.R., Levy, D.L., Yasillo, N.J., Melzer, H.Y. and Hurt, S.W., 1974. Eye tracking dysfunction in schizophrenic patients and their relatives. *Archives of General Psychiatry*, **31**, 143–151.

Holzman, P.S., Solomon, C.M., Levin, S. and Waternaux, C.S., 1984. Pursuit eye movement dysfunctions in schizophrenia. *Archives of General Psychiatry*, **41**, 136–139.

Houston, B.K., 1983. Psychophysiological responsivity and the type A behavior pattern. *Journal of Research in Personality*, **17**, 22–39.

Houston, B.K., 1992. Personality characteristics, reactivity, and cardiovascular disease. In: Turner, J.R., Sherwood, A. and Light, K.C. (eds), *Individual Differences in Cardiovascular Response to Stress*, pp. 103–124. Plenum Press, New York.

Iacono, W.G., Tuason, V.B. and Johnson, R.A., 1981. Dissociation of smooth pursuit and saccadic eye tracking in remitted schizophrenics. *Archives of General Psychiatry*, **38**, 991–996.

Kagan, J., 1989. Temperamental contributions to social behavior. *American Psychologist*, **44**, 668–674.

Kagan, J., 1994. *Galen's Prophecy: Temperament in Human Nature*. Basic Books, New York.

Kagan, J., Reznick, J.S., Clarke, C., Snidman, N. and Garcia-Coll, C., 1984. Behavioral inhibition to the unfamiliar. *Child Development*, **55**, 2212–2225.

Kagan, J., Reznick, J.S. and Snidman, N., 1987. The physiology and psychology of behavioral inhibition. *Child Development*, **58**, 1459–1473.

Kagan, J., Reznick, J.S. and Snidman, N., 1988. Biological bases of childhood shyness. *Science*, **240**, 167–171.

Kelsey, R.M., Ornduff, S.R., McCann, C.M. and Reiff, S., 2001. Psychophysiological characteristics of narcissism during active and passive coping. *Psychophysiology*, **38**, 292–303.

Kimble, M., Lyons, M., O'Donnell, B., Nestor, P., Niznikiewicz, M. and Toomey, R., 2000. The effect of family status and schizotypy on electrophysiologic measures of attention and semantic processing. *Biological Psychiatry*, **47**, 402–412.

Klein, C., Andresen, B., Berg, P., Krueger, H. and Rockstroh, B., 1998. Topography of CNV and PINV in schizotypal personality. *Psychophysiology*, **35**, 272–282.

Klein, C., Berg, P., Rockstroh, B. and Andresen, B., 1999. Topography of the auditory P300 in schizotypal personality. *Biological Psychiatry*, **45**, 1612–1621.

Lacey, B.C. and Lacey, J.I., 1974. Studies of heart rate and other bodily processes in sensorimotor behavior. In: Obrist, P.A., Black, A.H., Brener, J. and DiCara, L.V. (eds), *Cardiovascular Psychophysiology: Current Issues in Response Mechanisms, Biofeedback, and Methodology*, pp. 538–564. Aldine, Chicago.

Lencz, T., Raine, A., Scerbo, A.S., Redmon, M. and Brodish, S., 1993. Impaired eye tracking in undergraduates with schizotypal personality disorder. *American Journal of Psychiatry*, **150**, 152–154.

Lencz, T., Raine, A., Sheard, C. and Reynolds, G., 1991. Two neural bases of electrodermal hypo-responding in schizophrenia. *Psychophysiology*, **28**, 37.

Lipp, O.V. and Vaitl, D., 1992. Latent inhibition in human Pavlovian conditioning: effects of additional stimulation after preexposure and relation to schizotypal traits. *Personality and Individual Differences*, **13**, 1003–1012.

Mednick, S.A., Volavka, J. and Gabrielli, W.F., 1982. EEG as a predictor of antisocial behavior. *Criminology*, **19**, 219–231.

Mezzacappa, E., Tremblay, R.E., Kindlon, D., Saul, J.P., Arseneault, L., Seguin, J., Pihl, R.O. and Earls, F., 1997. Anxiety, antisocial behavior, and heart rate regulation in adolescent males. *Journal of Child Psychology and Psychiatry*, **38**, 457–469.

Milstein, V., 1988. EEG topography in patients with aggressive violent behavior. In: Moffitt, T.E. and Mednick, S.A. (eds), *Biological Contributions to Crime Causation*, pp. 40–54. Martinus Nijhoff, Dordrecht.

Moffitt, T.E. and Caspi, A., 2001. Childhood predictors differentiate life-course persistent and adolescent limited pathways among males and females. *Development and Psychopathology*, **13**, 355–375.

Nielsen, T.C. and Petersen, K.E., 1976. Electrodermal correlates of extraversion, trait anxiety, and schizophrenism. *Scandinavian Journal of Psychology*, **17**, 73–80.

Niznikiewicz, M.A., Voglmaier, M., Shenton, M.E., Seidman, L.J., Dickey, C.C., Rhoads, R., Teh, E. and McCarley, R.W., 1999. Electrophysiological correlates of language processing in schizotypal personality disorder. *American Journal of Psychiatry*, **156**, 1052–1058.

Ohman, A., 1979. The orienting response, attention, and learning: an information processing perspective. In: Kimmel, H.D., van Olst, E.H. and Orlebeke, J.F. (eds), *The Orienting Reflex in Humans*, pp. 443–471. Lawrence Erlbaum, Hillsdale, NJ.

Ohman, A., 1985. Face the beasts and fear the face: animal and social fears as prototypes for evolutionary analyses of emotions. *Psychophysiology*, **23**, 123–145.

Park, S., Holzman, P.S. and Levy, D.L., 1991. Spatial working memory deficit in the relatives of schizophrenic patients is associated with their smooth pursuit eye tracking performance. *Schizophrenia Research*, **9**, 185.

Pribram, K. and McGuinness, D., 1975. Arousal, activation, and effort in the control of attention. *Psychological Review*, **82**, 116–149.

Raine, A., 1987. Effect of early environment on electrodermal and cognitive correlates of schizotypy and psychopathy in criminals. *International Journal of Psychophysiology*, **4**, 277–287.

Raine, A., 1989. Evoked potentials and psychopathy. *International Journal of Psychophysiology*, **8**, 1–16.

Raine, A., 1993. *The Psychopathology of Crime: Criminal Behavior as a Clinical Disorder*. Academic Press, San Diego, CA.

Raine, A., Benishay, D.S., Lencz, T. and Scarpa, A., 1997a. Abnormal orienting in schizotypal personality disorder. *Schizophrenia Bulletin*, **23**, 75–82.

Raine, A., Lencz, T. and Benishay, D.S., 1995. Schizotypal personality and skin conductance orienting. In: Raine, A., Lencz, T. and Mednick, S.A. (eds), *Schizotypal Personality*, pp. 219–249. Cambridge University Press, New York.

Raine, A., Lencz, T., Bihrle, S., Lacasse, L. and Colletti, P., 2000. Reduced prefrontal gray matter volume and reduced autonomic activity in antisocial personality disorder. *Archives of General Psychiatry*, **57**, 119–127.

Raine, A., Reynolds, C., Lencz, T., Scerbo, A., Triphon, N. and Kim, D., 1994. Cognitive-perceptual, interpersonal and disorganized features of schizotypal personality. *Schizophrenia Bulletin*, **20**, 191–201.

Raine, A., Reynolds, G.P. and Sheard, C., 1991. Neuroanatomical mediators of electrodermal activity in normal human subjects: a magnetic resonance imaging study. *Psychophysiology*, **28**, 548–558.

Raine, A., Venables, P.H. and Mednick, S.A., 1997b. Low resting heart rate at age 3 years predisposes to aggression at age 11 years: findings from the Mauritius Joint Child Health Project. *Journal of the American Academy of Child and Adolescent Psychiatry*, **36**, 1457–1464.

Raine, A., Venables, P.H. and Williams, M., 1990a. Relationships between CNS and ANS measures of arousal at age 15 and criminality at age 24. *Archives of General Psychiatry*, **47**, 1003–1007.

Raine, A., Venables, P.H. and Williams, M., 1990b. Relationships between N1, P300, and CNV recorded at age 15 and criminal behavior at age 24. *Psychophysiology*, **27**, 567–575.

Reznick, J.S., Kagan, J., Snidman, N., Gersten, M., Baak, K. and Rosenberg, A., 1986. Inhibited and uninhibited children: a follow-up study. *Child Development*, **57**, 660–680.

Rogeness, G.A., Cepada, C., Macedo, C.A., Fischer, C. and Harris, W.R., 1990. Differences in heart rate and blood pressure in children with conduct disorder, major depression, and separation anxiety. *Psychiatry Research*, **33**, 199–206.

Salisbury, D.F., Voglmaier, M.M., Seidman, L.J. and McCarley, R.W., 1996. Topographic abnormalities of P3 in schizotypal personality disorder. *Biological Psychiatry*, **40**, 165–172.

Scarpa, A., Fikretoglu, D. and Luscher, K.A., 2000. Community violence exposure in a young adult sample. II. Psychophysiology and aggressive behavior. *Journal of Community Psychology*, **28**, 417–425.

Scarpa, A., Luscher, K.A., Smalley, K.J., Pilkonis, P.A., Kim, Y. and Williams, W.C., 1999. Screening for personality disorders in a nonclinical population. *Journal of Personality Disorders*, **13**, 345–360.

Scarpa, A. and Raine, A., 1997. Psychophysiology of anger and violent behavior. *Psychiatric Clinics of North America*, (Special Issue on Anger, Aggression, and Violence), **20**, 375–394.

Scarpa, A., Raine, A., Venables, P.H. and Mednick, S.A., 1997. Heart rate and skin conductance in behaviorally inhibited Mauritian children. *Journal of Abnormal Psychology*, **106**, 182–190.

Schmeck, K. and Poustra, F., 1993. Psychophysiologische Reacktionsmuster und psychische auffälligkeiten im kindesalter. In: Baumann, P. (ed.), *Bioloogische Psychiatrie der gegenwart.* Springer-Verlag, Vienna.

Siever, L.J., Coursey, R.D., Alterman, I.S., Buchsbaum, M.S. and Murphy, D.L., 1984. Impaired smooth pursuit eye movement: vulnerability marker for schizotypal personality disorder in a normal volunteer population. *American Journal of Psychiatry*, **141**, 1560–1566.

Siever, L.J., Coursey, L.D., Alterman, I.S. and Zahn, T., 1989. Clinical, psychophysiological, and neurological characteristics of volunteers with impaired smooth pursuit eye movements. *Biological Psychiatry*, **26**, 35–51.

Siever, L.J., Keefe, R., Bernstein, D.P., Coccaro, E.F., Klar, H.M., Zemishlany, Z., Peterson, A.E., Davidson, M., Mahon, T., Horvath, T. and Mohs, R., 1990. Eye tracking impairment in clinically identified patients with schizotypal personality disorder. *American Journal of Psychiatry*, **147**, 740–745.

Simons, R.F., 1981. Electrodermal and cardiac orienting in psychometrically defined high-risk subjects. *Psychiatry Research*, **4**, 347–356.

Simons, R.F. and Giardina, B.D., 1992. Reflex modification in psychosis-prone young adults. *Psychophysiology*, **29**, 8–16.

Simons, R.F. and Katkin, W., 1985. Smooth pursuit eye movements in subjects reporting physical anhedonia and perceptual aberrations. *Psychiatry Research*, **14**, 275–289.

Simons, R.F., Losito, B.D., Rose, S.C. and MacMillan, F.W., 1983. Electrodermal nonresponding among college undergraduates: temporal stability, situational specificity, and relationship to heart rate change. *Psychophysiology*, **20**, 498–506.

Smith, T.W. and Leon, A.S., 1992. Psychosocial risk factors. In: *Coronary Heart Disease: A Behavioral Perspective*, chapter 5, pp. 49–66. Research Press, Champaign, IL.

Syndulko, K., 1978. Electrocortical investigations of sociopathy. In: Hare, R.D. and Schalling, D. (eds), *Psychopathic Behavior: Approaches to Research*, pp. 145–156. Wiley, Chichester.

Trestman, R.L., Horvath, T., Kalus, O., Peterson, A.E., Coccaro, E., Mitropoulou, V., Apter, S., Davidson, M. and Siever, L.J., 1996. Event-related potentials in schizotypal personality disorder. *Journal of Neuropsychiatry and Clinical Neurosciences*, **8**, 33–40.

Turner, S.M., Beidel, D.C. and Townsley, R.M., 1992. Social phobia: a comparison of specific and generalized subtypes of avoidant personality disorder. *Journal of Abnormal Psychology*, **101**, 326–331.

Venables, P.H., 1987. Autonomic and central nervous system factors in criminal behavior. In: Mednick, S.A., Moffitt, T.E., Stack, S.A. (eds), *The Causes of Crime: New Biological Approaches*, pp. 110–136. Cambridge University Press, Cambridge.

Volavka, J., 1987. Electroencephalogram among criminals. In: Mednick, S.A., Mofitt, T.E. and Stack, S. (eds), *The Causes of Crime: New Biological Approaches*, pp. 137–145. Cambridge University Press, Cambridge.

Webb, C.T. and Levinson, D.F., 1993. Schizotypal and paranoid personality disorder in the relatives of patients with schizophrenia and affective disorders: a review. *Schizophrenia Research*, **11**, 81–92.

Wilkins, S., 1988. Behavioral and Psychophysiological Aspects of Information Processing in Schizotypics. PhD dissertation, University of York, UK.

Yaralian, P. and Raine, A. (2002, in press). Schizotypal personality and skin conductance orienting. In: Klein, C. (ed.). *Schizotypal Personality*.

Neuropsychology of Personality Disorders

Martina M. Voglmaier

INTRODUCTION

Intuitively, one might expect individuals with personality disorders to have neuropsychological deficits. The hypersensitivity of the paranoid and avoidant personalities, the rigidity of the obsessive-compulsive personality, the perceptual distortions of the schizotypal personality, and the limited social and emotional responsiveness of the schizoid personality suggest areas of deficit fascinating to the researcher interested in brain–behaviour relationships. Yet the study of neuropsychological functioning in personality disorders is in its infancy, primarily because of methodological problems associated with studying these disorders. The focus of this chapter is a general review of studies of clinical neuropsychological test performance in DSM-IV personality disorders as well as a description of the methodological problems associated with their study. Information processing, psychophysiological, and structural anatomical studies are dealt with elsewhere in this text.

GENERAL METHODOLOGICAL CONSIDERATIONS

Before reviewing empirical studies of neuropsychological test performance in personality-disordered individuals, a number of general methodological concerns must be addressed. Typically, in such studies, personality disorders are diagnosed by structured clinical interview, and subjects are administered a battery of neuropsychological tests measuring one or more cognitive domains, such as attention, memory, language, visuospatial perception, executive functions, and motor skills. Test performance of a group of individuals with a personality disorder of interest is then compared to that of one or more groups of subjects with either a different personality disorder, a mixed group of 'other' personality disorders, another psychiatric disorder, or no psychiatric disorder.

Research in this area is fraught with methodological difficulties. Samples differing in selection criteria, inpatient status, medications, and gender may result in inconsistent findings. Moreover, diagnosing personality disorders is a decidedly unclear science (Strack and Lorr, 1997). The clinical definition of character traits, severity, and impact on functional ability can be subjective, and whether a personality disorder can be diagnosed by self-report to an examiner in a preset period of time has been questioned (Oldham and Skodol, 1992). The DSM-IV requires a specific number of character traits to meet clinical diagnostic criteria for a personality disorder, and some studies include individuals who have fewer than the cut-off number of traits, such as those defined as having a 'probable' disorder.

Another concern is determining the specificity of any cognitive deficits given the co-occurrence of the 10 personality disorders with each other (Stuart *et al.*, 1998), the co-morbidity of personality disorders with Axis I disorders (Oldham and Skodol, 1992), and the possibility of misdiagnosis of behavioural traits associated with neurological disorders, such as head trauma, substance abuse, and temporolimbic epilepsy (Devinsky and Najjar, 1999). For example, increased rates of depression have been associated with a number of personality disorders (Table XXVI-5.1). Even with detailed historical and diagnostic information, it could be difficult to determine whether cognitive deficits evinced by a group of subjects are related to the personality disorder under examination, to concurrent symptoms of depression, to cognitive vulnerabilities related to the predisposition to depression, or to treatments for depression. A related concern is that individuals with personality disorders may be vulnerable to neuropsychological dysfunction from secondary sources such as precursors or lifestyle behaviours associated with maladaptive personality traits. For example, risk-taking behaviours, substance use, impulsivity, and aggression in antisocial personality disorder (ASPD) may increase the risk of head trauma in this population, and childhood trauma (physical, emotional, or sexual) may predispose an individual to head injury, borderline personality traits, symptoms of post-traumatic stress, and dissociative disorders (Paris, 1997).

The battery of neuropsychological tests employed in research studies is also of importance. Often, only a few tests or cognitive domains are examined, resulting in a limited view of cognitive functioning. For example, if only executive-function tasks are employed, it cannot be determined whether any weaknesses in this domain are due to a generalized deficit associated with having a psychiatric illness, or to a domain-specific deficit associated with the personality disorder being examined. Finally, there is some evidence for sex differences in cognitive functioning in some personality disorders (Voglmaier *et al.*, submitted). Grouping males and females together in such studies may result in inconsistent findings.

DSM-IV CLUSTER A: THE ODD/ECCENTRIC PERSONALITY DISORDERS

General Findings

Schizotypal, paranoid, and schizoid personality disorders make up this cluster of odd and eccentric personalities. By far, the most research on cognitive functioning in this cluster has been on schizotypal personality disorder (SPD). SPD is characterized by oddities in appearance, perception, and behaviour, as well as marked discomfort in close relationships. On the hypothesis that this disorder is biologically related to schizophrenia, studies have focused on cognitive domains known to be impaired in schizophrenic subjects, that is, abstraction, attention, language, and verbal learning and memory (e.g., Gur *et al.*, 1991; Saykin *et al.*, 1991).

Biological Psychiatry: Edited by H. D'haenen, J.A. den Boer and P. Willner. ISBN 0-471-49198-5

Table XXVI-5.1 Methodological considerations in the study of personality disorders

	Axis I	Axis II	Precursors	Lifestyle
Cluster A				
Schizotypal (SPD)	Depression, dysthymia, social phobia, agoraphobia	Cluster A BPD, OCP	—	—
Schizoid (SZD)	Depression, substance abuse	Cluster A APD	—	—
Paranoid (PPD)	Depression, delusional disorder, agoraphobia, bulimia	Cluster A	—	—
Cluster B				
Borderline (BPD)	Depression, bipolar, PTSD, substance abuse, dissociative disorders	Cluster B SPD, OCP, DPD	Physical/sexual abuse, emotional trauma, head trauma	Reduced impulse control, substance abuse
Antisocial (ASPD)	Substance abuse, depression, anxiety	Cluster B ADHD, OCP	Conduct disorder	Reduced impulse control, increased risk taking, violence, substance abuse
Histrionic (HPD)	Depression	Cluster B	—	—
Narcissistic (NPD)	Depression	Cluster B	—	—
Cluster C				
Avoidant (APD)	Depression, anxiety disorders, social phobia, GAD, panic disorder	Cluster C SZD	—	—
Dependent (DPD)	Depression, anxiety disorders	Cluster C	—	—
Obsessive-compulsive (OCP)	Anxiety disorders, bulimia	Cluster C SPD, BPD, ASPD	—	—

PTSD [post-traumatic stress disorder], GAD [generalized anxiety disorder], and ADHD [attention deficit hyperactivity disorder].

There have been relatively few comprehensive studies of neuropsychological function in individuals who meet full DSM diagnostic criteria for SPD. Generally, the extant studies have shown deficits in sustained attention (Roitman *et al.*, 1997), working memory (Farmer *et al.*, 2000; Roitman *et al.*, 2000), abstract reasoning (Voglmaier *et al.*, 1997), and verbal learning (Voglmaier *et al.*, 1997; Bergman *et al.*, 1998) that are similar to but less severe than those evident in schizophrenic subjects (Table XXVI-5.2). These findings have been hypothesized to reflect involvement of similar frontal, left hemisphere, and temporal-limbic brain areas.

My colleagues and I examined the neuropsychological profile of SPD (Voglmaier *et al.*, 1997). We studied a wide array of cognitive functions in 10 right-handed men with DSM-IIIR-defined SPD and 10 matched non-psychiatric comparison subjects (Voglmaier *et al.*, 1997). All subjects were unmedicated and were carefully screened for Axis I disorders, neurological disorders, and substance abuse. Cognitive domains included abstraction, verbal and spatial intelligence, language, learning, memory, attention, and motor skills. Analyses covaried the effects of general ability (IQ) and symptoms of depression, variables that were found to differ between subject groups. The resultant profile revealed a mild, general decrement in most cognitive domains, as well as more severe dysfunction in verbal learning and abstract reasoning. Specifically, SPD subjects showed significant decrements in performance on the California Verbal Learning Test (CVLT) (Delis *et al.*, 1987), a word-list learning measure which requires semantic organization for efficient performance, and on the Wisconsin Card Sort Test (WCST) (Heaton, 1981), a measure requiring concept formation, abstraction, and mental flexibility. The CVLT involves five presentations of a list of 16 'shopping items', which can be grouped into four semantic clusters (fruits, spices, clothing, and tools) to enhance learning. The SPD subjects learned significantly fewer words over the five trials, and used the clustering strategy less frequently than comparison subjects. There was no evidence of increased rate of forgetting. On the WCST, subjects were asked to sort cards by category (number of items, shape, or colour) and shift the categorical set based on limited feedback from the examiner. SPD subjects formed significantly fewer categories and made more perseverative responses than control subjects. Overall performance by male SPD subjects was similar to but less severe than in schizophrenic subjects. Females with SPD were found to have less severe cognitive deficits than males (Voglmaier *et al.*, submitted).

Questions were raised about the source of the apparent deficit in verbal learning in SPD. Because the CVLT requires intact language, verbal learning, and memory, and semantic organization skills for efficient performance, it was unclear to us whether the SPD group's reduced performance on this task reflected a primary deficit in language processes, learning, or concept formation and organization. For further examination of the verbal learning deficit in SPD, we evaluated selected components of verbal and non-verbal attention; learning and memory, including short-term retention (trigram versus pattern recall); supraspan learning (serial digit learning versus spatial block span); persistence (verbal versus design fluency); learning (CVLT versus Continuous Visual Memory Test [Trahan and Larrabee, 1988]); and memory retention (WMS-R Logical Memory versus Visual Reproductions [Wechsler, 1987]). In addition to a mild generalized deficit, 16 carefully screened and matched male SPD subjects revealed deficits on verbal measures of persistence, short-term retention, and learning (Voglmaier *et al.*, 2000). Non-verbal analogues of these tests, supraspan learning, and long-term retention of newly learned information were relatively preserved. The results suggested that the verbal learning deficit apparent on the CVLT is at least in part the result of a deficit in the early processing (encoding) stages of verbal learning, and not solely due to a primary deficit in organization or conceptualization.

Language functioning in SPD remains unclear. Standard neuropsychological tests of language ability have not revealed specific deficits in this domain, such as naming, repetition, comprehension, reading, and spelling (Voglmaier *et al.*, 1997). Reduced WAIS-R (Wechsler, 1981a) Vocabulary subtest performance was found in our group of 16 male SPD subjects, and we speculated that a primary deficit in verbal learning could account for such performance (Voglmaier *et al.*, 2000). Based on language samples, we have documented an increased amount of thought disorder in male SPD subjects that is qualitatively similar to that of schizophrenics

Table XXVI-5.2 Neuropsychological test performance in personality disorders

	General ability/IQ	Attention/working memory	Learning	Memory	Language	Visuoperception/ construction	Abstraction/executive functions	Sensory and motor skills
CLUSTER A Schizotypal (SPD)	(+)Mild General Decrement, WAIS-R VIQ < PIQ	(+)CPT-IP (+)COWAT (CFL) (+)Trigram Recall (+/−)Visuospatial Working Memory (−)Design Fluency (−)Digit Span (−)Pattern Recall (−)HRB Trail-Making Test	(+)CVLT, total words learned; semantic clusters (−)CVMT (−)Serial Digit Learning (−)Corsi Block Tapping	(−)WMS-Logical Memory, % retained (−)WMS-Visual Reproductions, %retained	(+/−)WAIS-R Vocabulary (−)BNT (−)BDAE-Complex Ideation (−)Sentence Repetition (−)WRAT-R Spelling (−)WRAT-R Reading	(−)WAIS-R Block Design (−)WAIS-R Picture Arrangement (−)Judgment of Line Orientation	(+)WCST, fewer categories (+)WCST, perseverative responses	(−)Finger Tapping Test
CLUSTER B[a]		(+)Serial 7's (−)Digit Span Forward		(+)Delayed Memory for 3 items at 10 min (−)Orientation	(+)Naming Common Objects (−)Word Repetition		(+)Similarity/ Dependence Comparisons (+)Proverb Interpretation	
Borderline (BPD)	(+/−)WAIS-R	(+/−)Stroop Color-Word Test (−)Trail-Making Test, Part B (−)Digit Span (−)Digit Symbol Test		(−)WMS-R Logical Memory (−)WMS-R Figural Memory (−)Story Recall (−)Verbal Recall with Interference	(−)WAIS-R Vocabulary	(+/−)Rey-Osterreith Copy/Recall (+)Matching Familiar Figures Test (−)WAIS-R Block Design (−)Embedded Figures Test	(−)Porteus Mazes	(+)Left side soft signs
Antisocial (ASPD)		(+)Object Alternation (+)Stroop Color Naming (+)Divergent Thinking (+/−)COWAT (+/−)Visual GoNoGo (−)Mental Rotation (−)Trail-Making Test		(+)Sequential Matching Memory	(+)Visual Naming (+)Token Test (−)Aural Comprehension of Words	(+)Necker cube	(+/−)WCST (+)perseverative errors (+)Porteus Mazes Q-scores (e.g., rule-breaking errors)	(+)Odour identification

(+) Deficits evident in at least one study; (−) no deficits evident in at least one study; BDAE indicates Boston Diagnostic Aphasia Examination (Goodglass and Kaplan, 1983); BNT, Boston Naming Test (Kaplan *et al.*, 1983); COWAT, Controlled Oral Word Association Test; CPT-IP, Continuous Performance Test, Independent Pairs; CVLT, California Verbal Learning Test (Delis *et al.*, 1987); CVMT, Continuous Visual Memory Test (Trahan and Larrabee, 1988); HRB, Halstead Reitan Battery (Reitan and Wolfson, 1985); MAE, Multilingual Aphasia Examination (Benton and Hamsher, 1976); WCST, Wisconsin Card Sorting Test (Heaton, 1981); WAIS-R, Wechsler Adult Intelligence Scale-Revised (Wechsler, 1981b), WRAT-R, Wide Range Achievement Test-Revised (Jastak and Wilkinson, 1984); WMS-R, Wechsler Memory Scale-Revised (Wechsler, 1987); [a]Burgess (1992), mixed Cluster B 'dramatic' personality disorder.

(Voglmaier *et al.*, 1996). Overall, neuropsychological test results from our laboratory imply involvement of frontal and left temporal brain structures and suggest a specific deficit in the early processing stages of verbal learning in SPD. The results support hypotheses of a dysfunctional semantic language network in schizophrenia (Spitzer *et al.*, 1993). Dysfunction, inefficiency, or reduced inhibition of such a system could result in verbal learning deficits, deficient facilitation by semantic context, magical thinking, and thought disorder.

The paranoid and schizoid personality disorders are also thought to have some biological connection to schizophrenia, but neuropsychological test performance has not been studied independently in these groups. It is noteworthy that schizoid personality traits (e.g., limited social and emotional responses) are similar to those seen in social-emotional or 'right-hemisphere' learning disabilities (Weintraub and Mesulam, 1983), making this disorder worth a detailed study of neuropsychological test performance.

Methodological Concerns

There are several additional methodological concerns that are specific to the study of SPD. First, there is considerable overlap between SPD and major depression and borderline personality disorder (Siever, 1992) (Table XXVI-5.1), disorders that may be associated with cognitive deficits. Second, many studies have assessed neuropsychological function in populations thought to be at higher risk of developing schizophrenia, in an attempt to elucidate markers of vulnerability to the disease. Studying these groups is considered preferable because they do not include the confounding factors of chronic institutionalization and medications. These high-risk samples include the non-psychotic first-degree relatives of schizophrenic probands, and the so-called 'psychosis-prone' populations, non-clinical groups who have abnormally high scores on one or more measures thought to assess schizotypal symptoms (such as the Chapman scales [Chapman and Chapman, 1985]). These samples are often described as 'schizotypal' or their results as indicative of 'schizotypy'. However, it is not clear how such groups are related to clinically defined SPD or how many (if any) of the DSM-IV diagnostic criteria are actually met by each subject. Although the results of these studies also suggest similar deficits in information processing (Chen *et al.*, 1998), abstraction (e.g., Tallent and Gooding, 1999), and left-hemisphere function (Overby, 1992), it is possible that relatives of schizophrenics and 'psychosis-prone' samples differ from SPD in phenomenology as well as severity.

A related concern is the possibility of heterogeneous subgroups among individuals who meet diagnostic criteria for SPD. Those with a family history of schizophrenia have been found to have more 'negative' symptoms (e.g., constricted affect, anhedonia, and no close friends) than those without such a family history. Moreover, some SPD samples may share a genetic link with mood disorders. These 'familial' and 'clinical' samples may represent different SPD subtypes (Bergman *et al.*, 2000) with differing neuropsychological test profiles. Finally, it is unclear how subject groups should be matched in terms of general ability. As in schizophenic subjects, because education, IQ and verbal skills may be reduced in SPD groups as a result of the disorder, matching patient and control groups on these indices may artificially dilute the extent of any deficits (e.g., the 'matching fallacy' [Meehl, 1970], matching high-functioning patients with low-functioning controls). In our laboratory, we have found that matching groups on age, sex, handedness, parental socio-economic status, and non-verbal general ability (e.g., the WAIS-R Block Design subtest) yields the most consistent results without affecting the cognitive domains of particular interest.

DSM-IV CLUSTER B: THE DRAMATIC PERSONALITY DISORDERS

General Findings

This cluster includes the borderline, histrionic, narcissistic, and antisocial personality disorders. Burgess (1992) studied neuropsychological test performance in a mixed group of 37 subjects who met diagnostic criteria for at least one of the 'dramatic' personality disorders and 40 non-psychiatric control subjects. Of the 37 patients, 30 patients had borderline personality disorder and seven had another Cluster B disorder. On a 16-item neuropsychiatric scale, the dramatic patient group showed relative deficits on tasks requiring multistep or multielement associative procedures (Table XXVI-5.2).

Within Cluster B, only the borderline and antisocial personalities have been studied independently with regard to neuropsychological function. In patients with borderline personality disorder (BPD), the results of cognitive studies have been inconsistent, perhaps due to heterogeneous samples. Some studies have found deficits on memory and executive tasks, suggesting that the behaviours and interpersonal problems associated with BPD result from deficits in attention, impulsivity, memory, and processing complex information (e.g., O'Leary *et al.*, 1991), and have hypothesized frontotemporal brain involvement in at least a subgroup of patients (Swirsky-Sacchetti *et al.*, 1993). Performance deficits may be exacerbated by stress or increased emotional arousal (Farrell and Shaw, 1994). Stein *et al.* (1993) found increased left-sided neurological soft signs in a group of 28 patients with 'impulsive' personality disorders: all 28 subjects met criteria for BPD, and 10 subjects also met criteria for antisocial personality disorder (ASPD). Increased soft signs correlated with reduced performance on the Trail-Making Test and Matching Familiar Figures Test, and the authors suggested the possibility of right-hemisphere and/or frontal network dysfunction. However, these results are difficult to interpret given the heterogeneity of the patient group, which included males, females, inpatients, and outpatients. Eight subjects met current diagnostic criteria for major depression and 25 subjects had histories of substance abuse.

van Reekum *et al.* (1996) found evidence of a high proportion of cerebral insults among borderline patients (including developmentally based and acquired insults) and a neuropsychological profile reminiscent of traumatic brain injured patients. It is unclear whether borderline samples in earlier studies had been carefully screened for such insults. A recent study of females that carefully controlled for history of neurological insult and symptoms of depression found essentially no deficits on neuropsychological tests of frontal executive and memory tests. Sprock *et al.* (2000) studied a group of 18 women with BPD, and compared them to female depressed patients and a non-psychiatric control group. They employed a battery of tests thought to tap frontal-executive (e.g., the Trail-Making Test, Part B; Stroop Color-Word Test; Porteus Mazes; and Rey-Osterreith Complex Figure) and memory functions (e.g., Rey-Osterreith Figure immediate and delayed memory, Wechsler Memory Scale-Revised Logical Memory, Figural Memory, Digit Span subtests, Story Recall Task, and Verbal Recall with Interference). There were essentially no differences in test performance between the BPD and control groups, and only the depressed patients showed evidence of cognitive dysfunction. Similarly, in a study that revealed abnormal hippocampal volumes in females with BPD and history of trauma, neuropsychological performance was related to symptoms of depression, but not to hippocampal volume (Driessen *et al.*, 2000). The results suggest there may be considerable heterogeneity in the cognitive functioning of BPD patients. Moreover, evidence of abnormal neuropsychological test performance may be confounded by affective state and/or history of cerebral insult.

The neuropsychology of antisocial personality disorder (ASPD) is also unclear. The results of studies have been conflicting (Table XXVI-5.2), and this may also be related to sampling differences and comorbid disorders. Executive dysfunction has been associated with antisocial behaviour in adolescent females with conduct disorder (Giancola *et al.*, 1998). In another study, deficient language skills, but not executive functions, were associated with conduct disorder in a mixed group of male and female adolescents (Dery *et al.*, 1999). Some studies have indicated that ASPD may be characterized by deficits in self-modulation of executive functions and verbal skills, suggesting that frontal and left-hemisphere abnormalities may be related to impulsive aggression (Miller, 1987). A recent meta-analytical review of 39 studies supported the hypothesis that executive-function deficits (e.g., planning, organization, goal-formulation and follow-through, self-monitoring, and problem-solving) are associated with antisocial personality (Morgan and Lilienfeld, 2000), implying involvement of frontal networks and dorsolateral/prefrontal brain structures. In a community sample of adults with ASPD that were screened for neurological disorders, deficits were evident on measures sensitive to orbitofrontal function (e.g., object alternation and spatial working memory), but not on standard measures of frontal-executive function (Dinn and Harris, 2000).

Methodological Concerns

The study of neuropsychological function in BPD is complicated by the high incidence of developmental and/or acquired brain insults (van Reekum *et al.*, 1996), and comorbid disorders such as depression, bipolar illness (Atre-Vaidya and Hussain, 1999), post-traumatic stress, and substance use (McGlashan *et al.*, 2000). Many studies mix male and female subjects, and often include medicated and/or hospitalized patients or those with current mood disorders and substance abuse. Similarly, the study of ASPD is confounded by overlap with substance abuse, attention deficits, depression, and anxiety (see Widiger *et al.*, 1993). Moreover, the aggressive, violent, and impulsive lifestyle of these patients may also increase their risk of head trauma.

DSM-IV CLUSTER C: THE ANXIOUS PERSONALITY DISORDERS

This cluster comprises the avoidant, dependent, and obsessive-compulsive personality types. There has been little research on these disorders, which are often comorbid with anxiety disorders (Alpert *et al.*, 1997; Paris, 1998). Neuropsychological function has not been studied directly in this cluster, although these subjects have made up 'other' or 'mixed' personality groups for comparison. The relationship of obsessive-compulsive personality (OCP) and obsessive-compulsive disorder (OCD) is unclear, although one study found that 36% of its sample of OCD patients also had OCP (Bejerot *et al.*, 1998). Neuropsychological deficits have been found in OCD (e.g., Bolton *et al.*, 2000) and sub-clinical compulsive samples (Matai-Cols *et al.*, 1997; Roth and Baribeau, 1996). It is unclear whether similar deficits could be expected in OCP, but this represents another untapped area for neuropsychological research.

CONCLUSION: FUTURE NEEDS AND NEW RESEARCH

The DSM-IV personality disorders represent a fascinating area of study for the neuropsychologist, yet their comprehensive study is in its infancy. The available data imply involvement of frontal, temporal, and left-hemisphere structures in schizotypal personality disorder, and orbitofrontal, dorsolateral/prefrontal, and possibly left-hemisphere structures in ASPD. Findings in patients with BPD have been inconsistent, with some studies showing involvement of frontal networks. In particular, the schizoid and OCP disorders represent interesting untapped areas worthy of comprehensive neuropsychological evaluation.

Methodological concerns such as sampling criteria, gender differences, comorbid disorders, and neurological risk factors limit the interpretation of the neuropsychological performance of individuals with personality disorders, and there is evidence that some personality disorders may include heterogeneous subtypes. In future studies, detailed assessment of Axis I and Axis II disorders and careful screening for head trauma, substance abuse, and current mood disorders will help to clarify the specificity of any neuropsychological deficits. It is recommended that subject groups include unmedicated individuals who meet full diagnostic criteria for the personality disorder under study, and that multiple cognitive domains be evaluated, with attention to the possibility of gender effects in cognitive functioning. Matching study groups for age, handedness, and parental socio-economic status, rather than education or IQ, may reveal the most accurate picture of cognitive functioning. Careful evaluation of verbal ability, education, and IQ as possible areas of secondary deficit will also be informative. Use of statistical procedures such as analysis of covariance (ANCOVA) will help in evaluating the effect of these factors, as well as the variance associated with comorbid disorders. Whenever possible, use of psychiatric control groups is advised. It may be most informative to employ a comparison group of individuals who meet full diagnostic criteria for a specific personality disorder from a different diagnostic cluster than the one under study.

REFERENCES

Alpert, J.E., Uebelacker, L.A., McLean, N.E., Nierenberg, A.A., Pava, J.A., Worthington, J.J., Tedlow, J.R., Rosenbaum, J.F. and Fava, M., 1997. Social phobia, avoidant personality disorder and atypical depression: co-occurrence and clinical implications. *Psychological Medicine*, **27**, 627–633.

Atre-Vaidya, N. and Hussain, S., 1999. Borderline personality disorder and bipolar mood disorder: two distinct disorders or a continuum? *Journal of Nervous and Mental Disease*, **187**, 313–315.

Bejerot, S., Ekselius, L. and von Knorring, L., 1998. Comorbidity between obsessive-compulsive disorder (OCD) and personality disorders. *Acta Psychiatrica Scandinavica*, **97**, 398–402.

Benton, A.L. and Hamsher, K., 1976. *Multilingual Aphasia Examination*. University of Iowa, Iowa City, IA.

Bergman, A.J., Harvey, P.D., Roitman, S.L., Mohs, R.C., Marder, D., Silverman, J.M. and Siever, L.J., 1998. Verbal learning and memory in schizotypal personality disorder. *Schizophrenia Bulletin*, **24**, 635–641.

Bergman, A.J., Silverman, J.M., Harvey, P.D., Smith, C.J. and Siever, L.J., 2000. Schizotypal symptoms in the relatives of schizophrenia patients: an empirical analysis of the factor structure. *Schizophrenia Bulletin*, **26**, 577–586.

Bolton, D., Raven, P., Madronal-Luque, R. and Marks, I.M., 2000. Neurological and neuropsychological signs in obsessive-compulsive disorder: interaction with behavioral treatment. *Behaviour Research and Therapy*, **38**, 695–708.

Burgess, J.W., 1992. Neurocognitive impairment in dramatic personalities: histrionic, narcissistic, borderline, and antisocial disorders. *Psychiatry Research*, **42**, 283–290.

Chapman, L.J. and Chapman, J.P., 1985. Psychosis proneness. In: Alpert, M. (ed.), *Controversies in Schizophrenia*, pp. 157–174. Guilford Press, New York.

Chen, W.J., Liu, S.K., Chang, C.J., Lien, Y.J., Chang, Y.H. and Hwu, H.G., 1998. Sustained attention deficit and schizotypal personality features in nonpsychotic relatives of schizophrenic patients. *American Journal of Psychiatry*, **155**, 1214–1220.

Delis, D., Kramer, J.H., Kaplan, E. and Ober, B.A., 1987. *California Verbal Learning Test Manual—Research Edition*. The Psychological Corporation. San Diego, CA.

Dery, M., Toupin, J., Pauze, R., Mercier, H. and Fortin, L., 1999. Neuropsychological characteristics of adolescents with conduct disorder: association with attention-deficit-hyperactivity and aggression. *Journal of Abnormal Child Psychology*, **27**, 225–236.

Devinsky, O. and Najjar, S., 1999. Evidence against the existence of a temporal lobe epilepsy personality syndrome. *Neurology*, **53**(Suppl), S13–S25.

Dinn, W.M. and Harris, C.L., 2000. Neurocognitive function in antisocial personality disorder. *Psychiatry Research*, **97**, 173–190.

Driessen, M., Herrmann, J., Stahl, K., Zwaan, M., Meier, S., Hill, A., Osterheider, M. and Petersen, D., 2000. Magnetic resonance imaging volumes of the hippocampus and the amygdala in women with borderline personality disorder and early traumatization. *Archives of General Psychiatry*, **57**, 1115–1122.

Farmer, C.M., O'Donnell, B.F., Niznikiewicz, M.A., Voglmaier, M.M., Mccarley, R.W., Shenton, M.E., 2000. Visual perception and working memory in schizotypal personality disorder. *American Journal of Psychiatry*, **157**, 781–786.

Farrell, J.M. and Shaw, I.A., 1994. Emotional awareness training: a prerequisite to effective cognitive-behavioral treatment of borderline personality disorder. *Cognitive and Behavioral Practice*, **1**, 71–91.

Giancola, P.R., Mezzich, A.C. and Tarter, R.E., 1998. Executive cognitive functioning, temperament, and antisocial behavior in conduct-disordered adolescent females. *Journal of Abnormal Psychology*, **107**, 629–641.

Goodglass, H. and Kaplan, E., 1983. *The Assessment of Aphasia and Related Disorders* (2nd edn). Lea & Febiger, Philadelphia.

Gur, R.C., Saykin, A.J. and Gur, R.E., 1991. Neuropsychological study of schizophrenia. In: Tamminga, C.A. and Schulz, S.C. (eds), *Advances in Neuropsychiatry and Psychopharmacology, Vol 1: Schizophrenia Research*, pp. 153–162. Raven Press, New York.

Heaton, R.K., 1981. *Wisconsin Card Sorting Test, Manual*. Psychological Assessment Resources, Odessa, FL.

Jastak, S. and Wilkinson, G.S., 1984. *Wide Range Achievement Test-Revised, Manual*. Jastak Associates, Wilmington, DE.

Kaplan, E.F., Goodglass, H. and Weintraub, S., 1983. *The Boston Naming Test* (2nd edn). Lea & Febiger, Philadelphia.

Matai-Cols, D., Junque, C., Vallejo, J., Sanchez-Turet, M., Verger, K. and Barrios, M., 1997. Hemispheric functional imbalance in a sub-clinical obsessive-compulsive sample assessed by the Continuous Performance Test, Identical Pairs Version. *Psychiatry Research*, **72**, 115–126.

McGlashan, T.H., Grilo, C.M., Skodol, A.E., Gunderson, J.G., Shea, M.T., Morey, L., Zanarini, M.C. and Stout, R.L., 2000. The Collaborative Longitudinal Personality Disorders Study: baseline Axis I/II and II/II diagnostic co-occurrence. *Acta Psychiatrica Scandinavica*, **102**, 256–264.

McKay, D., Kulchycky, S. and Danyko, S., 2000. Borderline personality and obsessive compulsive symptoms. *Journal of Personality Disorders*, **14**, 57–63.

Meehl, P., 1970. Nuisance variables and the ex post facto design. In: Radner, M. and Winoker, S. (eds), *Minnesota Studies of the Philosophy of Science*, pp. 373–402. University of Minnesota Press, Minneapolis, MN.

Miller, L., 1987. Neuropsychology of the aggressive psychopath: an integrative review. *Aggressive Behavior*, **13**, 119–140.

Morgan, A.B., Lilienfield, S.O., 2000. A meta-analytic review of the relation between antisocial behavior and neuropsychological measures of executive function. *Clinical Psychological Review*, **20**, 113–136.

O'Leary, K.M., Brouwers, P., Gardner, D.L., Cowdry, R.W., 1991. Neuropsychological testing of patients with borderline personality disorder. *American Journal of Psychiatry*, **148**, 106–111.

Oldham, J.M. and Skodol, A.E., 1992. Personality disorders and mood disorders. In: Tasman, A. and Riba, M.B. (eds), *Review of Psychiatry*, Vol. 11, pp. 418–435. American Psychiatric Press, Washington, DC.

Overby, L.A., 1992. Perceptual asymmetry in psychosis-prone college students: evidence for left hemisphere overactivation. *Journal of Abnormal Psychology*, **101**, 96–103.

Paris, J., 1997. Childhood trauma as an etiological factor in the personality disorders. *Journal of Personality Disorders*, **11**, 34–49.

Paris, J., 1998. Anxious traits, anxious attachment, and anxious-cluster personality traits. *Harvard Review of Psychiatry*, **6**, 42–48.

Reitan, R.M. and Wolfson, D., 1985. *The Halstead-Reitan Neuropsychological Test Battery: Theory and Clinical Interpretation*. Neuropsychology Press, Tucson, AZ.

Roitman, S.E., Cornblatt, B.A., Bergman, A., Obuchowski, M., Mitropoulou, V., Keefe, R.S., Silverman, J.M. and Siever, L.J., 1997. Attentional functioning in schizotypal personality disorder. *American Journal of Psychiatry*, **154**, 655–660.

Roitman, S.E., Mitropoulou, V., Keefe, R.S., Silverman, J.M., Serby, M., Harvey, P.D., Reynolds, D.A., Mohs, R.C. and Siever, L.J., 2000. Visuospatial working memory in schizotypal personality disorder patients. *Schizophrenia Research*, **41**, 447–455.

Roth, R.M. and Baribeau, J., 1996. Performance of subclinical compulsive checkers on putative tests of frontal and temporal lobe memory functions. *Journal of Nervous and Mental Disease*, **184**, 411–416.

Saykin, A.J., Gur, R.C., Gur, R.E., Mozley, D., Mozley, L.H., Resnick, S.M., Kester, B. and Stefiniak, P., 1991. Neuropsychological function in schizophrenia: selective impairment in memory and learning. *Archives of General Psychiatry*, **48**, 618–624.

Siever, L., 1992. Schizophrenia spectrum personality disorders. In: Tasman, A. and Riba, M.B. (eds), *Review of Psychiatry*, Vol. 11, pp. 25–42. American Psychiatric Press, Washington, DC.

Spitzer, M., Braun, U., Hermle, L. and Maier, S., 1993. Associative semantic network dysfunction in thought disordered schizophrenic patients: direct evidence from indirect semantic priming. *Biological Psychiatry*, **34**, 864–877.

Sprock, J., Rader, T.J., Kendall, J.P. and Yoder, C.Y., 2000. Neuropsychological functioning in patients with borderline personality disorder. *Journal of Clinical Psychology*, **56**, 1587–1600.

Stein, D.J., Hollander, E., Cohen, L., Frenkel, M., Saoud, J.B., Decaria, C., Aronowitz, B., Levin, A., Liebowitz, M.R., Cohen, L., 1993. Neuropsychiatric impairment in impulsive personality disorders. *Psychiatry Research*, **48**, 257–266.

Strack, S. and Lorr, M., 1997. Invited essay: the challenge of differentiating normal and disordered personality. *Journal of Personality Disorders*, **11**, 105–122.

Stuart, S., Pfohl, B., Battaglia, M., Bellodi, L., Grove, W. and Cadoret, R., 1998. The co-occurrence of DSM-III-R personality disorders. *Journal of Personality Disorders*, **12**, 302–315.

Swirsky-Sacchetti, T., Gorton, G., Samuel, S., Sobel, R., Genetta-Wadley, A. and Burleigh, B., 1993. Neuropsychological function in borderline personality disorder. *Journal of Clinical Psychology*, **49**, 385–396.

Tallent, K. and Gooding, D.C., 1999. Working memory and Wisconsin Card Sorting Test performance in schizotypic individuals: a replication and extension. *Psychiatry Research*, **89**, 161–170.

Trahan, D.E. and Larrabee, G.J., 1988. *Continuous Visual Memory Test, Professional Manual*. Psychological Assessment Resources, Odessa, FL.

van Reekum, R., Links, P.S., Finlayson, M.A., Boyle, M., Boiago, I., Ostrander, L.A. and Moustacalis, E., 1996. Repeat neurobehavioral study of borderline personality disorder. *Journal of Psychiatry and Neuroscience*, **21**, 13–20.

Voglmaier, M.M., Shenton, M.E., Seidman, L.J., Salisbury, D., Sollinger, J. and McCarley, R.W., 1996. Thought Disorder Index (TDI) in schizotypal personality disorder. Presented at the annual meeting of the American Psychiatric Association, New York City.

Voglmaier, M.M., Seidman, L.J., Salisbury, D. and McCarley, R.W., 1997. Neuropsychological dysfunction in schizotypal personality disorder: a profile analysis. *Biological Psychiatry*, **41**, 530–540.

Voglmaier, M.M., Seidman, L.J., Niznikiewicz, M.A., Dickey, C.C., Shenton, M.E. and McCarley, R.W., 1998. Sex differences in cognitive function in schizotypal personality disorder. Paper presented at the annual meeting of the Society of Biological Psychiatry, Toronto.

Voglmaier, M.M., Seidman, L.J., Niznikiewicz, M.A., Dickey, C.C., Shenton, M.E. and McCarley, R.W., 2000. Verbal and nonverbal neuropsychological test performance in schizotypal personality disorder. *American Journal of Psychiatry*, **157**, 787–793.

Voglmaier, M.M., Seidman, L.J., Niznikiewicz, M.A., Dickey, C.C., Shenton, M.E. and McCarley, R.W., 2002. A comparative profile analysis of neuropsychological function in men and women with schizotypal personality disorder. Submitted.

Wechsler, D., 1981a. *WAIS-R Manual*. The Psychological Corporation, New York.

Wechsler, D., 1981b. *Wechsler Adult Intelligence Scale-Revised, Manual*. The Psychological Corporation, Cleveland, OH.

Wechsler, D., 1987. *Wechsler Memory Scale-Revised, Manual*. The Psychological Corporation, Cleveland, OH.

Weintraub, S. and Mesulam, M.M., 1983. Developmental learning disabilities of the right hemisphere: emotional, interpersonal, and cognitive components. *Archives of Neurology*, **40**, 463–468.

Widiger, T.A., Corbitt, E.M. and Millon, T., 1992. Antisocial personality disorder. In: Tasman, A. and Riba, M.B. (eds), *Review of Psychiatry*, Vol. 11, pp. 63–79. American Psychiatric Press, Washington, DC.

XXVI-6

Functional Neuroanatomy and Brain Imaging of Personality and its Disorders

C. Robert Cloninger

People differ markedly in their personality traits, but there is a stable organizational structure of the brain circuits regulating personality traits. In this chapter, a clinical model of personality will be described that corresponds well with DSM-IV categories of personality disorder and also with available data about the functional neuroanatomy of temperament and character. Temperament refers to the emotional aspects of personality that are regulated by subdivisions of the limbic system and centrally integrated in the hypothalamus. Character refers to the higher cognitive aspects of personality that are regulated by subdivisions of the thalamo-neocortical system and centrally integrated in the frontal cortex. In this chapter, quantifiable personality traits will be related to a model of their functional neuroanatomy derived from classical and comparative neuroanatomy, along with supporting clinical data and experimental findings from brain imaging.

Temperament will be considered in terms of four dimensions of personality that are related to specific subdivisions of the limbic system. These traits are called 'harm avoidance' (anxiety-proneness versus libido, which is outgoing vigour and daring), 'novelty seeking' (exploratory impulsivity and irritable aggression versus frugality and stoicism), 'reward dependence' (social sensitivity attachment versus insensitivity and aloofness), and 'persistence' (industrious determination versus underachievement). A quantitative dimensional approach is used because this corresponds well with the functional neuroanatomy and because there is no evidence of discrete boundaries between traditional syndromes of personality disorder, as in DSM-IV. Instead, traditional syndromes emerge from the interaction of multiple dimensions, which give rise to specific configurations of temperament that distinguish developmentally stable subtypes (Cloninger, 1987; Cloninger and Svrakic, 2000).

Character will be considered in terms of higher cognitive functions that regulate an individual's goals and values. In other words, character refers to mental self-government, which includes executive, legislative, and judicial functions. These traits are called 'self-directedness' (purposeful and resourceful versus aimless and helpless in executive functions), 'cooperativeness' (helpful and principled versus hostile and opportunistic in legislative functions), and 'self-transcendence' (inventive and insightful versus unimaginative and undiscerning judgement) (Cloninger *et al.*, 1993).

Each of the seven dimensions of personality considered here has been shown to have genetic variability that is unique from all the others, indicating that a model with seven dimensions is needed to describe the organization of human personality (Gillespie *et al.*, in press). The correlations among the temperament dimensions are weak, as are the correlations among the character dimensions, but there are moderate non-linear relations between temperament and character. This is expected because character (i.e., higher cognitive functions) modulates temperament (i.e., emotionality). A well-integrated character allows coherence of personality by modulation of emotional conflicts. In contrast, to the degree that character is not well integrated, emotional conflicts arise from the interplay of competing urges from various temperament dimensions. Likewise, the dynamics of complex adaptive systems oscillates between multiple states as a result of small contextual influences on dissociable circuits whenever such circuits are coordinated by a self-organized interplay, as has been suggested as a model of brain systems (Bressler and Kelso, 2001). Consequently, different dimensions of temperament are correlated with differences in the activity of specific brain circuitry that is partially overlapping but functionally dissociated when character is not coherent in its guidance.

All individuals with personality disorders have immature character development, particularly low self-directedness and low cooperativeness (Svrakic *et al.*, 1993; Cloninger and Svrakic, 2000). Individuals with different DSM-IV categories of personality disorder are distinguished primarily by their temperament profiles. Descriptive labels for the personality subtypes defined by the temperament dimensions of novelty seeking, harm avoidance, and reward dependence are shown in Figure XXVI-6.1. For example, borderline personality disorder is associated with a temperament configuration comprising high novelty seeking, high harm avoidance, and low reward dependence. Individuals with antisocial personality disorder are also high in novelty seeking and low in reward dependence, but they are low in harm avoidance. Consequently, the brain images of individuals with antisocial and borderline personality disorder are similar in many, but not all, ways. Specifically, individuals with either borderline or antisocial personality disorder have brain images expected from low self-directedness (i.e., low activity in the medial prefrontal network) and low cooperativeness (i.e., low activity in the orbital prefrontal network) (Kuruoglu *et al.*, 1996; Raine *et al.*, 1998; London *et al.*, 2000; Soloff *et al.*, 2000). Likewise, both groups of individuals have brain images expected from high novelty seeking (e.g., high activity in the right insula) and low reward dependence (e.g., high activity in the right superior temporal gyrus) (Sugiura *et al.*, 2000; Soloff *et al.*, 2000). However, they differ in activity associated with harm avoidance, which is negatively correlated with activity in paralimbic regions such as the left parahippocampal gyrus, left orbitoinsular junction, and some neocortical regions such as the fusiform gyrus (Sugiura *et al.*, 2000). Borderline subjects have the brain correlates of high harm avoidance (Herpertz *et al.*, 2001), whereas antisocial subjects have the brain correlates of low harm avoidance (Raine *et al.*, 1998; Schneider *et al.*, 2000). Each of the dimensions of personality distinguished here has unique genetic variability and brain circuitry, so it is more informative to describe personality dimensionally than categorically. Studies of categorically defined groups of patients

Biological Psychiatry: Edited by H. D'haenen, J.A. den Boer and P. Willner. ISBN 0-471-49198-5

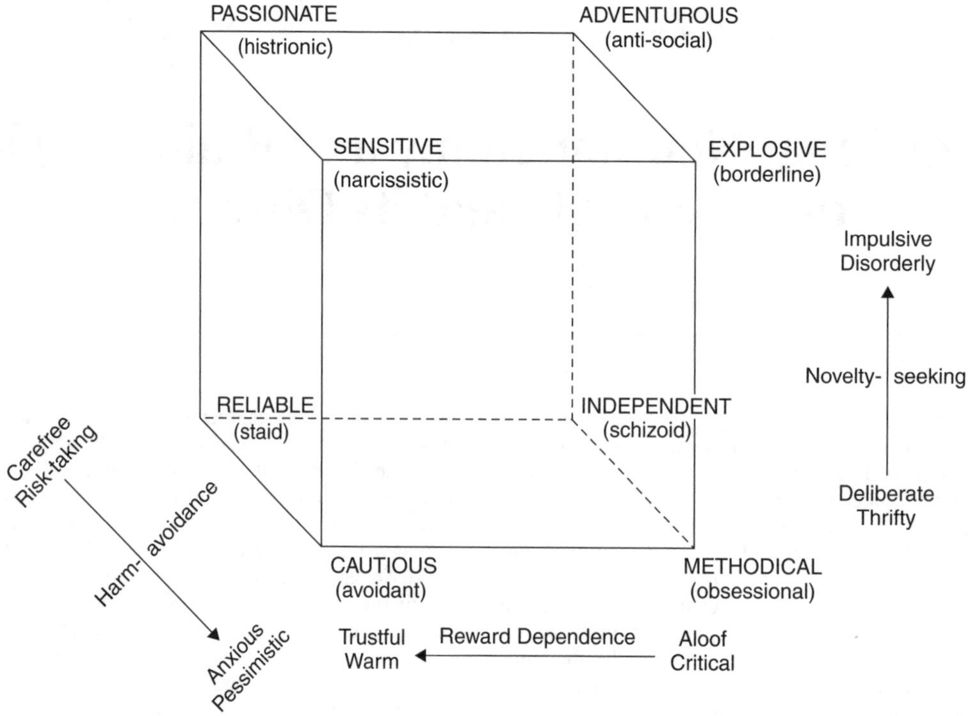

Figure XXVI-6.1 Subtypes of personality disorder defined by various combinations of novelty seeking, harm avoidance, and reward dependence (Reproduced by permission of Centre for Psychobiology of Personality, directed by C.R. Cloninger)

with personality disorder can be informative, nevertheless, and they support the findings based on dimensional studies of both clinical and general population samples.

TEMPERAMENT AND SUBDIVISIONS OF THE LIMBIC SYSTEM

Temperament is often defined as those aspects of personality that are emotion-based, heritable, and developmentally stable regardless of social and cultural influences. Four such dimensions of personality have been distinguished, and each has been shown to be moderately heritable and stable over time (Cloninger *et al.*, 1994). This same structure for temperament has been observed regardless of culture by studies throughout the world (Cloninger and Svrakic, 2000). Descriptors of individuals who score high versus low on each dimension are summarized in Table XXVI-6.1.

Activity of any or all of the brain networks involved in information processing, from sensory input to motor output, could vary with temperament. Sensory input into the primary sensory cortex is processed hierarchically, then is integrated within the multimodal association cortex, and finally reaches the limbic system via the paralimbic cortex. The limbic system is regarded as the anatomical basis for the regulation of emotion, motivation, and autonomic-endocrine functions. The paralimbic cortex plays a critical role in organizing motivated behaviour toward relevant intrapsychic and extrapersonal targets (Mesulam, 1998). Two partially dissociated networks have been distinguished in the paralimbic cortex by their connections with each another and other brain regions (Ongur and Price, 2000). The orbital network receives sensory inputs from several modalities, including olfaction, taste, visceral afferents, somatic sensation and vision. In contrast, the medial network provides the major cortical output to the visceromotor structures in the hypothalamus and the brainstem.

Table XXVI-6.1 Descriptors of individuals who score high and low on the four temperament dimensions

Temperament dimension	Descriptors of extreme variants	
	High	Low
Harm avoidance	Pessimistic Fearful Shy Fatigable	Optimistic Daring Outgoing Vigorous
Novelty seeking	Exploratory Impulsive Extravagant Irritable	Reserved Rigid Frugal Stoical
Reward dependence	Sentimental Open Warm Sympathetic	Critical Aloof Detached Independent
Persistence	Industrious Determined Ambitious Perfectionist	Apathetic Spoiled Underachiever Pragmatist

The limbic system itself has multiple subdivisions that are partly overlapping but functionally dissociable based on anatomical connections and physiology (MacLean, 1990). According to modern understanding, the limbic system is a distributed network of structures with synaptic proximity to the hypothalamus, which serves as the central integrator of the system (Nauta and Feirtag, 1986). MacLean distinguished three subdivisions of the limbic system with regulatory nodes in the septum, amygdala, and thalamus. More recent work has also distinguished a fourth subdivision involving the ventral striatum. Here I propose the hypothesis that individual differences in harm avoidance, novelty seeking, reward dependence, and persistence are regulated by individual differences within the septal, amygdaloid, thalamo-cingulate, and striato-thalamic subdivisions, respectively.

The hypothalamus centrally integrates input from the limbic subdivisions and regulates the tonic opposition of the sympathetic and parasympathetic branches of the autonomic nervous system. The autonomic nervous system maintains homeostasis by the opposition of its parasympathetic functions (such as sexual arousal, feeding, digestion and storage of nutrients, elimination, and sleep) and its sympathetic functions (such as sexual orgasm, preparation for fighting or flight, and wakefulness). Accordingly, it is not surprising that each of the limbic subdivisions also regulates the tonic opposition of pairs of such psychodynamic drives, each of which has advantages and disadvantages depending on the context. Specifically, there are opposing drives for sexuality versus preservation of safety in the septal subdivision, feeding and aggression versus satiety and satisfaction in the amygdaloid subdivision, social attachment versus aloofness in the thalamo-cingulate subdivision, and industriousness versus impersistence in the striato-thalamic subdivision.

For clarity, I will describe each limbic subdivision individually, but it should be understood that they are partially overlapping and may be dissociated or integrated in function depending on the degree of coherence from higher cortical function. Then I will relate the functional neuroanatomy to available clinical and neurophysiological information.

THE SEPTAL SUBDIVISION AND HARM AVOIDANCE

The septal subdivision of the limbic system is hypothesized to regulate sexuality and the preservation of safety (MacLean, 1990). In humans and other mammals, stimulation of the septum, medial preoptic area, and anterior hypothalamus is pleasurable, with sexual arousal (Heath, 1963; Margules and Olds, 1962; MacLean, 1958, 1962, 1990; Mink *et al.*, 1983). Conversely, lesions in the anterior hypothalamus abolish sexual interest.

In addition, the septum projects to the entire hippocampal formation, but is strongly reciprocally connected with the giant pyramids of the CA3 and CA4 fields. The septal division also includes parts of the paralimbic cortex near the segments of the hippocampus to which it most heavily projects, namely, the caudal part of the entorhinal cortex (Brodmann's area 28) (BA 28), the postrhinal hippocampal gyrus, the presubicular part of the lingual gyrus (BA 27), and the retrosplenial cortex (BA 29) (MacLean, 1990). The septal subdivision also includes the pericallosal hippocampal rudiment and a narrow strip of preseptal cortex continuous with it. These areas are all closely interconnected with one another and the hippocampal formation in the medial aspects of the limbic system (Sanides, 1969; Reep, 1984). In turn, fibres from the hippocampal formation (primarily from the rostral subiculum) terminate in the medial prefrontal cortical network, including BA 24, 25, 32, and parts of 11 through 14 (Ongur and Price, 2000). This medial prefrontal network is the major source of cortical output to the visceromotor structures in the hypothalamus and brainstem. The hypothalamus also receives input directly from lateral septum and hippocampal formation.

Individual differences in harm avoidance have been observed to be significantly negatively correlated with individual differences in activity in the medial prefrontal network at rest (Sugiura *et al.*, 2000). This includes significant negative correlations between regional blood flow and the score for harm avoidance in paralimbic regions such as the left parahippocampal gyrus and the left orbitoinsular junction, and various neocortical regions in the frontal, parietal, and temporal cortex. Likewise, patients with familial pure depressive disorder, which is specifically associated with high harm avoidance, have a decrease in blood flow in the subgenual part of BA 24 (Drevets *et al.*, 1997). This decrease in blood flow is associated with a reduced volume of this area ventral to the genu of the corpus callosum in the medial prefrontal network. This decrease in volume is associated with a reduction in the number and density of glial cells in this area (Ongur and Price, 2000).

Gray (1982) has shown in detailed neurobehavioural studies that the septo-hippocampal-hypothalamic connections of the septal subdivision are essential in the inhibition of behaviour to preserve safety. According to Gray (1982), this circuit is essential in passive-avoidance learning, which is manifest as anticipatory anxiety in response to conditioned signals of punishment or frustrative non-reward. In particular, input to the lateral septum from the hippocampal CA3 field results in habituation and inhibition of unrewarded behaviour. Other aspects of Gray's model of anxiety involve interactions between the septal and thalamo-cingulate subdivisions, which are described later.

Key elements in the neuroanatomy of the septal subdivision include sensory input via the entorhinal cortex and internal sensory input from the midbrain limbic area, such as the dopaminergic ventral tegmental area and the serotonergic raphe nuclei. The septal connections with the dentate gyrus and hippocampal CA3 fields are involved in habituation of unpleasant or unrewarded behaviour. The connections of the subiculum and the lateral septum with the medial prefrontal network and the hypothalamus influence visceromotor output.

The significance of these neuroanatomical connections can be understood in behavioural and psychodynamic terms, which help to reveal their evolutionary and developmental significance. Individuals who are low in harm avoidance are described as outgoing, vigorous, and daring optimists, as shown in Table XXVI-6.1. Harm avoidance is hypothesized to be a behavioural manifestation of individual differences in the septal subdivision of the limbic system regulating the tonic opposition of sexual drive necessary for reproduction versus the preservation of personal safety (MacLean, 1958, 1962, 1990). Likewise, in his theory of libido, Freud (1938) described such vigorous and outgoing optimists as having a strong libido, which leads to anxiety when unsatisfied. Libido does not refer to sexual appetite or conscious sexual desires, although it does energize such desires. Rather, libido refers more broadly to quantitative differences between individuals in their vigour or energy derived from their procreative drive. Consequently, low harm avoidance is a valid measure of libido as originally conceived by Freud.

Freud noted that libido is essential for the preservation of the species by sexual reproduction. However, high harm avoidance is associated with anxiety-proneness, sensitivity to contextual stress, and concern about the preservation of personal safety. At the most basic reflex level, harm avoidance modulates the human startle reflex, which abruptly interrupts behaviour that is potentially harmful and causes withdrawal by widespread contraction of the flexor muscles (Graham, 1979; Corr *et al.*, 1995, 1997; Cloninger, 1998). When compared to the magnitude of the eye-blink startle to a loud noise while the subject is viewing a neutral foreground stimulus, high harm avoidance potentiates startle while viewing an unpleasant stimulus whereas low harm avoidance reduces startle while viewing a pleasant stimulus (Corr *et al.*, 1995, 1997). Other temperament dimensions are uncorrelated with the modulation of startle when subjects are viewing pleasant and unpleasant pictures (Corr *et al.*, 1995, 1997). Anxiety can also be induced in animals by prolonged exposure to bright light or intraventricular administration of the stress peptide corticotrophin-releasing hormone. These anxiety-producing effects depend on a brain area called the bed nucleus of the stria terminalis, rather than the central nucleus of the amygdala, which is involved in the fight or flight response (Davis *et al.*, 1999).

AMYGDALOID SUBDIVISION AND NOVELTY SEEKING

The amygdaloid subdivision of the limbic system regulates the tonic opposition of feeding and aggression versus satiety and satisfaction. Stimulation of the lateral hypothalamus is satisfying, but only if the human or other mammal is hungry (Heath, 1963; Margules and Olds, 1962; Hoebel and Teitelbaum, 1962). In contrast, stimulation of the septum is sexually arousing regardless of feeding status (Heath, 1963; Margules and Olds, 1962; Hoebel and Teitelbaum, 1962). Stimulation of the lateral hypothalamus leads to overeating, whereas stimulation of the ventromedial hypothalamus produces satiety. Conversely, lesions in these same areas have opposite results: lesions of the ventromedial hypothalamus produce hyperphagia whereas those in the lateral hypothalamus lead to aphagia and adipsia. The ventromedial hypothalamus seems to inhibit the activity of the lateral hypothalamus because destruction of both produces anorexia.

In cats and monkeys, activation of the lateral hypothalamus by stimulation of the basal amygdaloid nucleus also produces a defence reflex or rage reaction. This is characterized by pupillary dilation, snarling and aggressive gestures, piloerection, elevation of blood pressure with cardiac deceleration, generally lower amplitude and increased rate of breathing, and changes in gastric motility and acidity (Brodal, 1981; FitzGerald, 1985). This reflex prepares an individual for fight or flight by muscle vasodilation, increased muscle blood flow, and decreasing sensitivity to aversive stimulation (Kelly *et al.*, 1973; Graham, 1979; Deakin and Graeff, 1991). The defence reflex or its autonomic components are elicited from a neural circuit that extends from the basal amygdaloid nucleus, through the central nucleus and the lateral hypothalamus, and into the pontomedullary brainstem, ending approximately at the level of the dorsal vagal complex (Price and Amaral, 1981; Price *et al.*, 1987). Hypothalamic stimulation is ineffective if the amygdalas have been removed (FitzGerald, 1985). In humans, the defence response is usually more modulated, so stimulation of the amygdala most often produces a sensation of fear, occasionally anger, and rarely a full rage reaction (Brodal, 1981). However, in humans with frequent temper tantrums or severely violent rage reactions, surgical lesions in the amygdaloid or hypothalamic components of the defence reflex circuit produce clinical improvement with decreases in aggression, anxiety, restlessness, and sympathetic overactivity (Kelly *et al.*, 1973; Sano and Mayanagi, 1988).

The defence reflex circuit is also involved in fear-potentiated startle in which the startle reflex is potentiated by a conditioned aversive stimulus, as when a human subject is anticipating a painful shock. Fear-potentiated startle depends on the integrity of the central nucleus of the amygdala, and not on the bed nucleus of the stria terminalis (Davis *et al.*, 1999). Increasing the intensity of the threat of harm leads to a switch to active responses (which depend on the integrity of the dorsolateral periaqueductal grey) from more passive responses (which depend on the integrity of the ventral periaqueductal grey) (Davis *et al.*, 1999).

The amygdaloid subdivision of the limbic system receives highly processed sensory input through the orbital prefrontal network. The orbital prefrontal network in humans includes most of the areas on the posterior, central, and lateral orbital surface, including the agranular insular areas Ial, Iam, Iapl, and Iapm, and the orbital areas 11l, 12m, 12l, 13b, 13l, and 13m (Ongur and Price, 2000). Significant positive correlations are observed between scores on novelty seeking and cerebral blood flow in the orbital prefrontal network, particularly the right anterior and right posterior insula (Sugiuri *et al.*, 2000). Other temperament dimensions do not show such positive correlations.

Stimulation of the basal amygdaloid nucleus produces feeding, like the lateral hypothalamus, whereas stimulation of the central amygdaloid nucleus produces satiety, like the ventromedial hypothalamus. When hunger or hunting urges are unsatisfied, there is irritability and impulsive aggressive behaviour, so the amygdaloid subdivision is involved in both feeding and attack behaviour (Chi and Flynn, 1971; Siegel and Brutus, 1990). In cats, synaptic transmission within the amygdaloid subdivision has been experimentally manipulated to cause stable changes in fight or flight behaviour (Adamec and Stark-Adamec, 1983a; b).

The neuroanatomy of the amygdaloid subdivision of the limbic system can be considered functionally in relation to clinical and psychodynamic descriptions of novelty seeking. Individuals who are high in novelty seeking are supposed to have a strong psychodynamic drive for exploratory hunting and feeding, which leads to aggression rather than anxiety if unsatisfied (Freud, 1938). The novelty-seeking dimension is hypothesized to be regulated by the amygdaloid subdivision of the limbic system, which regulates the tonic opposition of drives for feeding and aggression versus satiety and satisfaction (MacLean, 1958, 1990; Kelly *et al.*, 1973; Kelly, 1980). Novelty seeking involves a tonic opposition of craving and desire for novel stimuli and avoidance of fear-inducing stimuli. Experimentally, the amygdaloid subdivision can be activated in humans by negative stimuli, such as exposure to faces expressing fear, or positive stimuli, such as pictures of erotic nudes (Davidson and Irwin, 1999; LaBar *et al.*, 1998). Likewise, individuals high in novelty seeking are particularly prone to thrill-seeking behaviour, overeating, and substance dependence, as well as to irritability and impulsive aggression when they are unsatisfied (Cloninger *et al.*, 1994). Individuals who are high in novelty seeking are quick-tempered, that is, they have a low threshold for the defence reflex.

THE THALAMO-CINGULATE SUBDIVISION AND REWARD DEPENDENCE

The thalamo-cingulate subdivision of the limbic system is also called the circuit of Papez in recognition of James W. Papez, who described it as the 'mechanism of emotion' (Papez, 1937). More specifically, the thalamo-cingulate subdivision is hypothesized here to regulate the tonic opposition of social attachment and aloofness by its role in selective attention to salient emotional events.

The thalamo-cingulate subdivision involves connections between the posterior hypothalamus, anterior thalamus, cingulate gyrus, and hippocampal subiculum. This subicular loop (subiculum to mammillary body to anterior thalamus to anterior cingulate and back to the subiculum) has been studied physiologically in detail (Parmeggiani *et al.*, 1971). For example in the curarized cat, conduction around the entire loop occurs within 50–60 ms and involves no other relay sites until there is transfer of information beyond this simple circuit (Parmeggiani *et al.*, 1974). The subiculum receives information from the outside world, as it is already processed when it reaches the entorhinal cortex or hippocampal CA3-CA1 fields. The subiculum compares the information it receives with what was expected, and then projects to the cingulate cortex and to the septal subdivision via the entorhinal cortex so as to select responses that should habituate and be inhibited (Gray, 1982) as well as what is useful to enter into long-term memory (Eccles, 1989). Information reaching the subicular circuit has already been extensively processed, and its potential importance or salience has already been tagged by processing in the septal or amygdaloid subdivisions (Gray, 1982). By acting as a comparator of observed and expected stimuli, the subicular circuit can modulate orienting responses.

Sensory input about the external context and internal milieu also enters this subdivision through the sensory association cortex and midbrain limbic area, respectively. Papez (1937) showed that connections among the posterior hypothalamus, anterior thalamus, cingulate gyrus, and hippocampus formed a two-way circuit by which emotions could be elicited either by ideational association in the neocortex or by visceral activation of the hypothalamus, which in turn provides central control of the autonomic nervous system.

MacLean (1990) showed that differentiation of the thalamo-cingulate subdivision in mammals is associated with the emergence of a behavioural triad of social interactions, including parental nursing, play, and audiovocal communication, to maintain communication between mother and offspring. This was a major advance in capacity for social attachment in mammals over reptiles and more primitive vertebrates.

Individuals who are high in reward dependence are sentimental and emotionally warm, whereas those who are low in reward dependence are aloof and emotionally cold. In psychodynamic terms, individuals who are high in reward dependence are sympathetic to emotional distress in others and attribute their own positive emotions onto others. However, individuals low in reward dependence do not form social attachments readily because they project or attribute their own negative emotions onto others and remain unresponsive to the positive emotions of others.

Accordingly, reward dependence is hypothesized to be regulated by the thalamo-cingulate subdivision of the limbic system (MacLean, 1990). More specifically, the subicular circuit is hypothesized to modulate the magnitude of the orienting reflex, which alerts and orients a person to information to which they need to pay selective attention (Graham, 1979; Gray, 1982). More specifically, it is hypothesized that the orienting reflex is potentiated in individuals who are high in reward dependence when they are stressed and responding to high-intensity stimuli, particularly stimuli of social interest, such as frowns and signs of distress in others. However, individuals low in reward dependence are expected to have greater orienting responses in the absence of stress when responding to low-intensity stimuli. Empirically, this expected interaction between intensity of stimulus and reward dependence is empirically supported by the results of personality measures with reward dependence as their major common correlate, such as high extraversion and low psychoticism, but not neuroticism (Fowles *et al.*, 1977; Wigglesworth and Smith, 1976; O'Gorman, 1983).

It should be noted that the initial magnitude and the rate of habituation of orienting responses are only weakly correlated (O'Gorman, 1983). Habituation of the orienting response may be more closely modulated by the septal subdivision, as proposed by Gray (1982), so harm avoidance would interact with reward dependence. Specifically, individuals with high reward dependence and low harm avoidance are expected to habituate slowly to unpleasant social cues, such as a frown, whereas individuals with low reward dependence and high harm avoidance are expected to habituate rapidly to pleasant social cues, such as a smile. Consequently, studies of the orienting reflex with extraversion as a measure may have had inconsistent results because extraversion confounds high reward dependence and low harm avoidance. More empirical research is therefore needed to test the tentative hypotheses about the orienting reflex suggested here.

Nevertheless, the hypothesis that reward dependence modulates the magnitude of the orienting reflex is suggested by the sentimentality and preference for social closeness of individuals who are high in reward dependence, in contrast to the preference for social distance in individuals who are low in reward dependence. It is supported empirically by the particular sensitivity of the thalamo-cingulate subdivision to facial cues and visceral (autonomic) variability through exteroceptive and interoceptive sensory inputs to the mesocortical ring. This concentric ring of mesocortex links the anterior cingulate (area 24) with the infralimbic (area 25), medial and ventrolateral orbital, insula, perirhinal (area 35), and retrosplenial (area 29) mesocortex (Reep, 1984). Individual differences in reward dependence are negatively correlated with cerebral blood flow in this mesocortical ring (Sugiura *et al.*, 2000).

THE STRIATO-THALAMIC SUBDIVISION AND PERSISTENCE

Persistence despite partial reinforcement has been poorly explained by the functional neuroanatomy of the preceding three subdivisions of the limbic system (Gray, 1982). Persistence can be measured by the partial reinforcement extinction effect (PREE), which means that behaviour is more persistent despite non-reward after an initial period of intermittent reinforcement than after an initial period of continuous reinforcement. This persistence effect is abolished after lesions of the nucleus accumbens, which interrupts an excitatory projection from the hippocampal subiculum to the ventral striatum (Tai *et al.*, 1991).

Phenomena that are closely related to PREE are the greater resistance to extinction after continuous small rewards than after continuous large rewards and the greater approach speeds during acquisition with intermittent rewards than with continuous rewards. The latter is called the partial reinforcement acquisition effect (PRAE) or eagerness reflex. Therefore, the temperament dimension of persistence is not simply a form of perseverative behaviour. Instead, it involves persistence in behaviour to achieve long-term goals with eagerness, enthusiasm, and industry, which may require flexible adaptation of routines. In fact, neurons in the ventral striatum selectively respond to motivationally significant stimuli that are rewarding or punishing (Rolls and Williams, 1987; Schneider and Lidsky, 1981; Schultz *et al.*, 1998). This reward-guided behaviour in animals involves activation in a circuit connecting the ventral striatum and the prefrontal cortex. In humans, this striatal-prefrontal circuit is known to include intermediate connections between the ventromedial striatum, pallidum, certain medial thalamic nuclei, and the prefrontal cortex (Knight, 1964; Kelly *et al.*, 1973; Modell *et al.*, 1989; Hay *et al.*, 1993; Joseph, 1999).

Individual differences in persistence in humans are strongly correlated with responses measured by fMRI in a circuit involving the ventral striatum, orbitofrontal cortex/rostral insula, and prefrontal/cingulate cortex (BA 32) (Gusnard *et al.*, 2001). Subjects low in persistence exhibited relative decreases in activity within this circuit whereas those high in persistence exhibited relative increases. Persistence scores also correlated with an apparent selection bias such that subjects with high persistence scores made relatively more pleasant judgements at the expense of neutral judgements when viewing pictures from the International Affective Picture System.

The neuroanatomy of this ventral striatal-prefrontal circuitry can be appreciated functionally in terms of its clinical and developmental significance for the temperament dimension of persistence. Individuals who are high in persistence are industrious overachievers. In contrast, those who are low in persistence are described as apathetic underachievers who are easily discouraged when their expectations are not quickly and consistently satisfied. More specifically, when individuals are intermittently reinforced, those who are high in persistence remain eager and industrious despite discouragement by others, whereas those low in persistence quit quickly despite encouragement by others. In terms of functional neuroanatomy, the ventral striato-thalamic-prefrontal circuit is likely to be involved in reward-guided choice behaviour (Schultz *et al.*, 1998). Striatal neurons are almost silent at rest, whereas nigro-striatal and pallido-thalamic projections are tonically active and inhibitory. The motivation to initiate behaviour is associated with increases in both striatal and pallidal activity, which selectively disinhibits thalamo-frontal activity (Penney and Young, 1983). In turn, the increased thalamo-frontal activity completes the fronto-striato-pallido-thalamo-frontal circuit, so that a positive fronto-striatal feedback loop can maintain activity in a persistent goal-directed manner. However, decreased nigro-striatal activity may lead to tonic inhibition of the pallidum, which produces akinesia, rigidity, and tremor in the dorsolateral striatum. It is hypothesized that the analogous effect of tonic inhibition of the ventral pallidum on motivation mediated by the ventromedial striatum is low persistence, characterized by amotivation (apathy, underachievement, and discouragement), inflexibility (spoiled behaviour — wanting your way regardless of consequences and subjectively complaining without adapting efforts), and lability (mood swings).

Patients with bipolar mood swings are often low in persistence, even when euthymic (Osher *et al.*, 1996; 1999). Moreover, subcaudate tractotomy is frequently beneficial in such patients when they are chronically or recurrently depressed (Mindus and Jenike, 1992). The target of this surgery is the substantia innominata below the head of the caudate, which is the location of the ventral pallidum. The treatment produces a relief of amotivation, that is, an increase in industry with improved mood and work capacity (Strom-Olsen and Carlisle, 1971; Goktepe *et al.*, 1975; Lovett and Shaw, 1987).

HIGHER COGNITIVE FUNCTIONS OF FRONTAL CORTEX

Character has long been regarded as what human beings make of themselves intentionally (Cloninger, 1994). In contrast to temperament, which involves basic emotional responses, character involves our concepts of self and our relations with other people and the world as a whole. In other words, character involves our conceptual or propositional learning about goals and values that allow us to organize and integrate the behavioural drives motivated by temperament. The subdivisions of the limbic system produce a variety of responses, often producing conflict. For example, individuals may be high in both harm avoidance and novelty seeking, so when they encounter unfamiliar situations or strangers, they will have conflicting impulses to experience something new (thereby producing a thrill or relieving boredom) and to avoid the unfamiliar (thereby playing it safe). The way such emotional conflicts are organized and resolved defines a person's character or style of higher cognitive processing.

Empirically, individual differences in temperament do not tell us whether or not a person is integrated in character (that is, mature as opposed to having a character disorder). However, individual differences in maturity can be well described by three dimensions of character called self-directedness, cooperativeness, and self-transcendence (Cloninger *et al.*, 1993; Svrakic *et al.*, 1993). Descriptors of individuals who are high or low on each of these character dimensions are summarized in Table XXVI-6.2.

Table XXVI-6.2 Descriptors of individuals who score high and low on the three character dimensions

Character dimension	Descriptors of extreme variants	
	High	Low
Self-directed	Responsible	Blaming
	Purposeful	Aimless
	Resourceful	Inept
	Self-accepting	Vain
	Generative	Unproductive
Cooperative	Reasonable	Prejudiced
	Empathic	Insensitive
	Helpful	Hostile
	Compassionate	Revengeful
	Principled	Opportunistic
Self-transcendent	Judicious	Undiscerning
	Insightful	Superficial
	Intuitive	Dualistic
	Inventive	Unimaginative
	Spiritual	Materialistic

These dimensions allow quantitative ratings of the degree of maturity as well as the severity of personality disorder. The presence of personality disorder can be defined by those individuals who are in about the lowest 10% of the distribution of the sum of self-directedness and cooperativeness (Svrakic *et al.*, 1993). Even those in the bottom third of this distribution are noticeably immature and disorganized. However, there is more clinical information in considering the full distribution of scores. Likewise, consideration of quantitative variation in these dimensions is more helpful as a way of understanding the functional neuroanatomy of personality.

Empirical findings showed temperament and character to be interactive aspects of personality in which each influences the other. Specifically, the relations are non-linear, as expected in a self-organizing adaptive system in which temperament influences the emotional salience of events, and character influences the higher cognitive processing of the meaning of events (Cloninger *et al.*, 1997). Furthermore, character, but not temperament, was observed to be correlated with individual differences in event-related potentials of healthy adults that are characteristic of higher cognitive processes subserved by the prefrontal cortex and sensory association cortex (Fuster, 1984, 1997). Specifically, P300 is positively correlated with self-directedness and no other temperament or character dimension; in parietal leads, the correlations are +0.3 to +0.4 in healthy adults (Cloninger, 1998; Vedeniapin *et al.*, 2001). The P300 is a positive potential recorded at the scalp surface and elicited by an unexpected event that has been awaited while a subject deals with another repetitive, highly structured task. Likewise, contingent negative variation (CNV) is negatively correlated with cooperativeness and self-transcendence, and not with temperament dimensions (Cloninger, 1998; Vedeniapin *et al.*, 2001). CNV is a scalp-recorded, slow negative potential recorded at the scalp in the interval between two events that lead to a motor act. In recordings from single neurons in the prefrontal cortex, Fuster (1984, 1997) has shown that CNV originates in the prefrontal cortex. In delayed response tasks, large numbers of prefrontal neurons increase in their discharge rate, and this discharge is measured as the CNV surface potential.

It has long been recognized that higher cognitive functions depend on the integrity of the thalamo-neocortical system, and are centrally integrated in the prefrontal cortex (Freeman and Watts, 1942; Nauta, 1971; Fuster, 1984, 1997; Cloninger, 1994; Joseph, 1999). The prefrontal cortex is seen as the peak in a hierarchy of structures modulating goal-directed behaviour. These higher cognitive functions have a delayed experience-dependent maturation, just as the prefrontal cortex and sensory association areas have a delayed onset of myelination, not maturing until puberty (Sanides, 1969; Stuss, 1992). Likewise, social deprivation and psychological trauma during early childhood can disrupt normal neocortical development and higher cognitive processing (Meares *et al.*, 1999). These observations suggest the hypothesis that the maturation of higher cognitive functions, which I will call character development, involves the integration of the interactions among the areas of neocortex that supervise the individual limbic subdivisions.

A useful metaphor for the integrative activity of the thalamo-neocortical system is the government of a large and complex country. To manage a country effectively, it is useful to have executive, legislative, and judicial branches of government (Sternberg, 1990). Likewise, as previously described on empirical clinical grounds, higher cognitive functions can be measured as three dimensions of character that have been shown to distinguish individuals with personality disorder from those who are mature (Cloninger *et al.*, 1993; Svrakic *et al.*, 1993; Cloninger and Svrakic, 2000). These dimensions involve executive functions (self-directedness), legislative functions (cooperativeness), and judicial functions (self-transcendence).

Alterations in personality and cognitive processing caused by frontal lobe lesions have been described in detail (Freeman and Watts, 1942; Damasio, 1985; Milner and Petrides, 1984; Stuss and Benson, 1986; Joseph, 1999). Three syndromes of frontal lobe dysfunction have been described that can be systematically related to the three character dimensions of self-directedness, cooperativeness, and self-transcendence, as shown in what follows.

The prefrontal cortex is not homogeneous in its connectivity, cytoarchitecture, ontogeny, and phylogeny, or its function (Sanides, 1969; Nauta, 1971; Reep, 1984; Joseph, 1999; Ongur and Price, 2000). Most recent research on the prefrontal cortex distinguishes regions including the medial, orbital, dorsolateral, and polar areas (Ongur and Price, 2000; Joseph, 1999; Bechara *et al.*, 1998; Roland, 1984). The medial prefrontal network includes all the areas on the medial wall of the cerebrum (areas 25, 32, 14r, 14c, 24a, and 24b) and related areas on the orbital surface (areas 11m, 13a, Iai, and 12o). The orbital prefrontal network includes most of the areas on the posterior, central, and lateral orbital surface (agranular insular areas Ial, Iam, Iapl, and Iapm, and orbital areas 13b, 13l, 13m, 11l, 12r, 12m, and 12l) (Ongur and Price, 2000). The frontal poles and dorsolateral prefrontal cortex are designated as areas 10 and 11, respectively.

Furthermore, there are prominent functional differences related to hemispheric specialization or laterality. Whereas the left side is usually dominant for verbal analysis and speech, some observations suggest that the right side is usually dominant for the integrative and modulatory functions described here as character (Joseph, 1999). It is suggested that the right frontal lobe has a greater attentional capacity than the left and exerts bilateral inhibitory influences on arousal (Joseph, 1999; Pardo *et al.*, 1991). In contrast, the left frontal lobe appears to exert unilateral excitatory influences on arousal and attention (Davidson and Irwin, 1999). Finally, it is useful to distinguish the frontal pole (area 10) from other prefrontal regions since it has distinct patterns of development, connectivity, and coactivation (Roland, 1984), such as receiving projections from the mediodorsal thalamus, but not the amygdala (Reep, 1984).

Patients with left-sided or bilateral lesions in the medial prefrontal network show deficits suggestive of the executive functions associated with self-directedness, as indicated by apathy, abulia, or lack of initiative, and inability to organize or prioritize activities in their life (Damasio, 1985; Joseph, 1999). In recent brain-imaging research, individual differences in Self-directedness, as measured by the Temperament and Character Inventory, were strongly correlated with fMRI response magnitudes in BA 9/10 when subjects were carrying out simple executive tasks (Gusnard *et al.*, 2001). Self-directedness was also negatively correlated with reaction times in the same tasks.

Likewise, Bechara *et al.* (1994, 1996, 1997, 1998) have found that patients with bilateral medial prefrontal lesions cannot anticipate future positive or negative consequences of their actions, although their behaviour is influenced appropriately by immediately available contingencies. The same patients fail to show anticipatory electrodermal responses when confronted by a risky choice, whereas normal controls generate such anticipatory autonomic responses even before they are able to declare this explicitly. Patients with medial prefrontal lesions who were unable to anticipate future positive or negative consequences had normal working memories, whereas other patients with dorsolateral prefrontal lesions had impaired working memories but were able to anticipate future positive or negative consequences on a gambling task (Bechara *et al.*, 1998).

Right-sided or bilateral medial prefrontal lesions usually produce a deficit in a subjects' concept of temporal self-continuity in which they have difficulty thinking about themselves as having a continuity from the past to the future (Freeman and Watts, 1942). This leads to severe impairment of self-directedness and sometimes to bizarre ideation. This has led some to suggest that the right prefrontal cortex is dominant over the left in character functions (Joseph, 1999). The right-sided dominance in self-directedness is also shown by the release of inhibitory control over limbic impulses, as manifest by the emergence of impulsivity, distractibility, hypertalkativeness, and overactivity. The mood is usually hyperthymic and labile, with an increased risk of hypomania and manic episodes (Joseph, 1999). However, self-directedness, as measured by the Temperament and Character Inventory, has been correlated with medial prefrontal activity in both hemispheres (Gusnard *et al.*, 2001).

In contrast, lesions in the orbital network cause deficits in legislative function indicative of low cooperativeness. Low cooperativeness is indicated by reduced empathy and social sensitivity, ethical unreliability, and poor social judgement in which patients seem to lack principles and compassion regarding the effects of their behaviour on others (Damasio, 1985; Stuss and Benson, 1986; Joseph, 1999). This can lead to criminality, promiscuity, profane speech, and a crude, immature social manner that is inconsiderate of the feelings of others. In addition, as in right medial lesions, there is often excessive eating, drinking, and hypersexuality (Joseph, 1999).

Although right-sided lesions of either the medial or orbitofrontal cortex produce behavioural disinhibition, there is still a difference in their impact on the capacity for self-directedness (which is impaired by medial lesions) and cooperativeness (which is impaired by orbital lesions), a finding which illustrates the distinction between executive and legislative functions. Patients with low cooperativeness as a result of orbital lesions do not make rules to moderate their social interactions; they are unprincipled and opportunistic, and show pervasive impairment in social judgement according to the standards of others because they make no standards for themselves (a legislative function). In contrast, patients with only right medial lesions do have standards and principles of which they are consciously aware, but are undisciplined, have difficulty in conforming to rules (an executive function), and tend to be hyperthymic and impulsive (Joseph, 1999). Thus, there are interactions between mood and character effects.

The frontal poles are uniquely increased in human beings compared to other primates, and are the latest to myelinate of all parts of neocortex (Sanides, 1969; Eccles, 1989). Lesions to the frontal pole (BA 10 or the part of the mediodorsal thalamus that projects to area 10) may possibly impair Self-transcendence, but relevant observations are old, limited, and no studies have used the Temperament and Character Inventory (Cloninger *et al.*, 1993) to test this. Nevertheless, low self-transcendence may be indicated by early reports of impairment in creativity, spirituality, and the capacity for abstract fantasy after surgery to the frontal poles (Freeman and Watts, 1942). These are characteristics that distinguish human beings from all other primates (Eccles, 1989; Mithen, 1996). Consequently various artists, theatrical performers, writers, musicians or scientists lost their capacity for creative insight and judgement after bilateral lesions of the frontal pole, even though they remained self-directed and cooperative (Freeman and Watts, 1942). This impairment can be understood as the loss of judicial function, that is, the ability to know when a particular rule should be applied. Such judgement is intuitive in the sense that it cannot be taught algorithmically.

CONCLUSIONS

Substantial progress has been made toward the development of a functional neuroanatomy of personality and its disorders based on classical neuroanatomy, neurophysiology, and recent brain-imaging studies using reliable quantitative measures of personality or related cognitive and emotional functions. Reliable clinical measures of temperament are available to quantify personality traits that correspond well to functional subdivisions of the limbic system. Likewise, dimensions of character may distinguish the executive, legislative, and judicial functions of different regions of the frontal cortex.

The temperament and character dimensions are now being investigated by brain imaging, but much more work is needed. Modern methods of brain imaging and psychophysiology offer excellent opportunities to relate individual differences in personality to regional brain activity. These methods can provide rigorous tests of the hypotheses and findings described here, which are often based on limited data or the synthesis of diverse observations from animals and humans. Nevertheless, the multidimensional model of temperament and character is well tested clinically and psychometrically. Accordingly, the remarkable correspondences described here between personality and available data on functional neuroanatomy are much too extensive and systematic to be coincidental.

The functional neuroanatomy of personality described here offers hope that psychiatry can progress beyond a purely descriptive approach to diagnosis and treatment. Psychiatry can become a science of functional psychobiology only when it approaches individual patients in terms of assessments based on the psychodynamics and neurodynamics of specific brain systems as described here for personality and its disorders.

REFERENCES

Adamec, R.E. and Stark-Adamec, C., 1983a. Partial kindling and emotional bias in the cat: lasting aftereffects of partial kindling of the ventral hippocampus. *Behavioral and Neural Biology*, **38**, 205–239.

Adamec, R.E. and Stark-Adamec, C., 1983b. Limbic kindling and animal behavior — implications for human psychopathology associated with complex partial seizures. *Biological Psychiatry*, **18**, 269–293.

Bechara, A., Damasio, A.R., Damasio, H. and Anderson, S.W., 1994. Insensitivity to future consequences following damage to human prefrontal cortex. *Cognition*, **50**, 7–15.

Bechara, A., Damasio, H., Tranel, D., Damasio, A.R., 1997. Deciding advantageously before knowing the advantageous strategy. *Science*, **275**, 1293–1295.

Bechara, A., Tranel, D., Damasio, H., Damasio, A.R., 1996. Failure to respond autonomically to anticipated future outcomes following damage to prefrontal cortex. *Cerebral Cortex*, **6**, 215–225.

Bechara, A., Damasio, H., Tranel, D. and Anderson, S.W., 1998. Dissociation of working memory from decision making within the human prefrontal cortex. *Journal of Neuroscience*, **18**, 428–437.

Bressler, S.L. and Kelso, J.A.S., 2001. Cortical coordination dynamics and cognition. *Trends in Cognitive Sciences*, **5**, 26–36.

Brodal, A., 1981. *Neurological Anatomy in Relation to Clinical Medicine* (3rd edn). Oxford University Press, New York.

Chi, C.C., Flynn, J.P., 1971. Neural pathways associated with hypothalamically elicited attack behaviour in cats. *Science*, **171**, 703–706.

Cloninger, C.R., 1987. A systematic method for clinical description and classification of personality variants: a proposal. *Archives of General Psychiatry*, **44**, 573–587.

Cloninger, C.R., 1994. Temperament and personality. *Current Opinion in Neurobiology*, **4**, 266–273.

Cloninger, C.R., 1998. The genetics and psychobiology of the seven-factor model of personality. In: Silk, K.R. (ed.), *Biology of Personality Disorders*, pp. 63–92. American Psychiatric Press, Washington, DC.

Cloninger, C.R., Svrakic, D.M. and Przybeck, T.R., 1993. A psychobiological model of temperament and character. *Archives of General Psychiatry*, **50**, 975–990.

Cloninger, C.R., Przybeck, T.R., Svrakic, D.M. and Wetzel, R.D., 1994. *The Temperament and Character Inventory (TCI): A Guide to Its Development and Use*. Washington University Centre for Psychobiology of Personality, St Louis, MO.

Cloninger, C.R. and Svrakic, D.M., 2000. Personality disorders. In: Sadock, B.J. and Sadock, V.A. (eds), *Comprehensive Textbook of Psychiatry* (7th edn), pp. 1723–1764. Lippincott Williams & Wilkins, New York.

Cloninger, C.R., Svrakic, N.M. and Svrakic, D.M., 1997. Role of personality self-organization in development of mental order and disorder. *Development and Psychopathology*, **9**, 681–906.

Corr, P.J., Kumari, V., Wilson, G.D., Checkley, S. and Gray, J.A., 1997. Harm avoidance and affective modulation of the startle reflex: a replication. *Personality and Individual Differences*, **22**, 591–593.

Corr, P.J., Wilson, G.D., Fotiadou, M., Kumari, V., Gray, N.S., Checkley, S. and Gray, J.A., 1995. Personality and affective modulation of the startle reflex. *Personality and Individual Differences*, **19**, 543–553.

Damasio, A.R., 1985. The frontal lobes. In: Heilman, K.M. and Valenstein, E. (eds), *Clinical Neuropsychology*, pp. 339–375. Oxford University Press, New York.

Davidson, R.J. and Irwin, W., 1999. The functional neuroanatomy of emotion and affective style. *Trends in Cognitive Sciences*, **3**, 11–21.

Davis, M., Walker, D.L. and Lee, Y., 1999. Neurophysiology and neuropharmacology of startle and its affective modulation. In: Dawson, M.E., Schnell, A.M. and Bohmelt, A.H. (eds), *Startle Modification: Implications for Neuroscience, Cognitive Science, and Clinical Science*, pp. 95–113. Cambridge University Press, New York.

Deakin, J.F.W. and Graeff, F.G., 1991. 5-HT and mechanisms of defense. *Journal of Psychopharmacology*, **5**, 305–315.

Drevets, W.C., Price, J.L., Simpson, J.R., Todd, R.D., Vannier, M. and Raichle, M.E., 1997. Subgenual prefrontal cortex abnormalities in mood disorders. *Nature*, **386**, 824–827.

Eccles, J.C., 1989. *Evolution of the Brain: Creation of the Self*. Routledge, New York.

FitzGerald, M.J.T., 1985. *Neuroanatomy: Basic and Applied*. Bailliére Tindall, London.

Fowles, D.C., Roberts, R. and Nagel, K.E., 1977. The influence of introversion/extraversion on the skin conductance response to stress and stimulus intensity. *Journal of Research in Personality*, **11**, 129–146.

Freeman, W. and Watts, J.W., 1942. *Psychosurgery: Intelligence, Emotion, and Social Behavior Following Prefrontal Lobotomy for Mental Disorders*. C.C. Thomas, Springfield, IL.

Freud, S., 1938. *A General Introduction to Psychoanalysis*. Riviere, J. (trans.). Garden City Publishing, Garden City, NY.

Fuster, J.M., 1984. Behavioral electrophysiology of the prefrontal cortex. *Trends in Neurosciences*, **7**, 408–414.

Fuster, J.M., 1997. *The Prefrontal Cortex: Anatomy, Physiology, and Neuropsychology of the Frontal Lobes*. Lippincott-Raven, New York.

Gillespie, N., Cloninger, C.R., Heath, A.C. and Martin, N.G. (2002, in press). The genetic and environmental relationship between Cloninger's dimensions of temperament and character. *Personality and Individual Differences*.

Goktepe, E.O., Young, L.B., Bridges, P.K., 1975. A further review of the results of stereotactic subcaudate tractotomy. *British Journal of Psychiatry*, **126**, 270–280.

Graham, F.K., 1979. Distinguishing among orienting, defense, and startle reflexes. In: Kimmel, H.D., Van Olst, E.H. and Orlebeke, J.F. (eds), *The Orienting Reflex in Humans*, pp. 137–167. Lawrence Erlbaum Associates, Hillsdale, NJ.

Gray, J.A., 1982. *The Neuropsychology of Anxiety*. Oxford University Press, Oxford.

Gusnard, D.A., Ollinger, J.M., Shulman, G.L., Cloninger, C.R., Raichle, M.E., 2001. Personality differences in functional brain imaging. *Society of Neuroscience Abstracts*, **27**, no. 80.11.

Hay, P., Sachdev, P., Cummings, S., Cummins, S., Smith, J.S., Lee, T., Kitchener, P. and Matheson, J., 1993. Treatment of obsessive-compulsive disorder by psychosurgery. *Acta Psychiatrica Scandinavica*, **87**, 197–207.

Heath, R.G., 1963. Electrical self-stimulation of the brain in man. *American Journal of Psychiatry*, **120**, 571–577.

Herpertz, S.C., Dietrich, T.M., Wenning, B., Krings, T., Erberich, S.G., Willmes, K., Thron, A. and Sass, H., 2001. Evidence of abnormal amygdala functioning in borderline personality disorder: a functional MRI study. *Biological Psychiatry*, **50**, 292–298.

Hoebel, B.G. and Teitelbaum, P., 1962. Hypothalamic control of feeding and self-stimulation. *Science*, **135**, 375–377.

Joseph, R., 1999. Frontal lobe psychopathology: mania, depression, confabulation, perseveration, obsessive compulsions, and schizophrenia. *Psychiatry*, **62**, 138–172.

Kelly, D., 1980. *Anxiety and Emotions: Physiological Basis and Treatment*. Charles C. Thomas, Springfield, IL.

Kelly, D., Richardson, A. and Mitchell-Heggs, N., 1973. Stereotactic limbic leucotomy: neurophysiological aspects and operative techniques. *British Journal of Psychiatry*, **123**, 133–140.

Knight, G., 1964. The orbital cortex as an objective in the surgical treatment of mental illness. *British Journal of Surgery*, **51**, 114–124.

Kuruoglu, A.C., Arikan, Z., Vural, G., Karatas, M., Arac, M. and Isik, E., 1996. Single photon emission computerised tomography in chronic alcoholism. Antisocial personality disorder may be associated with decreased frontal perfusion. *British Journal of Psychiatry*, **169**, 348–354.

LaBar, K.S., Gatenby, J.C., Gore, J.C., LeDoux, J. and Phelp, E.A., 1998. Role of the amygdala in emotional picture evaluation as revealed by fMRI. *Journal of Cognitive Neuroscience*, **10**(Suppl 5), 108–121.

London, E.D., Ernst, M., Grant, S., Bonson, K. and Weinstein, A., 2000. Orbitofrontal cortex and human drug abuse: functional imaging. *Cerebral Cortex*, **10**, 334–342.

Lovett, L.M. and Shaw, D.M., 1987. Outcome in bipolar affective disorder after stereotactic tractomy. *British Journal of Psychiatry*, **151**, 113–116.

MacLean, P.D., 1949. Psychosomatic disease and the visceral brain: recent developments bearing on the Papez theory of emotion. *Psychosomatic Medicine*, **11**, 338–353.

MacLean, P.D., 1958. The limbic system with respect to self-preservation and the preservation of the species. *Journal of Nervous and Mental Disease*, **127**, 1–11.

MacLean, P.D., 1962. New findings relevant to the evolution of psychosexual functions of the brain. *Journal of Nervous and Mental Disease*, **135**, 289–301.

MacLean, P.D., 1990. *The Triune Brain in Evolution: Role in Paleocerebral Functions*. Plenum Press, New York.

Margules, D.L. and Olds, J., 1962. Identical feeding and rewarding systems in the lateral hypothalamus of rats. *Science*, **135**, 374–375.

Meares, R., Stevenson, J. and Gordon, E., 1999. A Jacksonian and biopsychosocial hypothesis concerning borderline related phenomena. *Australian and New Zealand Journal of Psychiatry*, **33**, 831–840.

Mesulam, M.M., 1998. From sensation to cognition. *Brain*, **121**, 1013–1052.

Milner, B. and Petrides, M., 1984. Behavioral effects of frontal lobe lesions in man. *Trends in Neurosciences*, **7**, 403–407.

Mindus, P. and Jenike, M.A., 1992. Neurosurgical treatment of malignant obsessive compulsive disorder. *Psychiatric Clinics of North America*, **15**, 921–938.

Mink, J.W., Sinnamon, H.M. and Adams, D.B., 1983. Activity of basal forebrain neurons in the rat during motivated behaviors. *Behavioral Brain Research*, **8**, 85–108.

Mithen, S., 1996. *The Prehistory of the Mind: The Cognitive Origins of Art, Religion and Science*. Thomas and Hudson, London.

Modell, J.G., Mountz, J.M., Curtis, G.C. and Greden, J.F., 1989. Neurophysiological dysfunction in basal ganglia/limbic striatal and thalamocortical circuits as a pathogenetic mechanism of obsessive–compulsive disorder. *Journal of Neuropsychiatry*, **1**, 28–36.

Nauta, W.J.H., 1971. The problem of the frontal lobe: a reinterpretation. *Journal of Psychiatric Research*, **8**, 167–187.

Nauta, W.J.H. and Feirtag, M., 1986. *Fundamental Neuroanatomy*. W.H. Freeman, New York.

O'Gorman, J.G., 1983. Individual differences in the orienting response. In: Siddle, D. (ed.), *Orienting and Habituation: Perspectives in Human Research*, pp. 431–448. Wiley, New York.

Ongur, D. and Price, J.L., 2000. The organization of networks within the orbital and medial prefrontal cortex of rats, monkeys and humans. *Cerebral Cortex*, **10**, 206–219.

Osher, Y., Cloninger, C.R. and Belmaker, R.H., 1996. TPQ in euthymic manic depressive patients. *Journal of Psychiatric Research*, **30**, 353–357.

Osher, Y., Lefkifer, E. and Kotler, M., 1999. Low persistence in euthymic manic-depressive patients: a replication. *Journal of Affective Disorders*, **53**, 87–90.

Papez, J.W., 1937. A proposed mechanism of emotion. *Archives of Neurology and Psychiatry*, **38**, 725–743.

Pardo, J.V., Fox, P.T. and Raichle, M.E., 1991. Localization of a human system for sustained attention by positron emission tomography. *Nature*, **349**, 61–63.

Parmeggiani, P.L., Lenzi, P. and Azzaroni, A., 1974. Transfer of the hippocampal output by the anterior thalamic nuclei. *Brain Research*, **67**, 267–278.

Penney, J.B. and Young, A.B., 1983. Speculations on the functional anatomy of basal ganglia disorders. *Annual Review of Neuroscience*, **6**, 73–94.

Price, J.L. and Amaral, D.G., 1981. An autoradiographic study of the projections of the central nucleus of the monkey amygdala. *Journal of Neuroscience*, **1**, 1242–1259.

Price, J.L., Russchen, F.T. and Amaral, D.G., 1987. The limbic region. II. The amygdaloid complex. In: Borklund, A., Hokfelt, T. and Swanson, L.W. (eds), *Handbook of Chemical Neuroanatomy, Vol. 5: Integrated Systems of the CNS*. Part I, pp. 270–388. Elsevier Science Publishers, Amsterdam.

Raine, A., Phil, D., Stoddard, J., Bihrle, S. and Buchsbaum, M., 1998. Prefrontal glucose deficits in murderers lacking psychosocial deprivation. *Neuropsychiatry, Neuropsychology, and Behavioral Neurology*, **11**, 1–7.

Reep, R., 1984. *Relationship Between Prefrontal and Limbic Cortex. A Comparative Anatomical Review*, pp. 1–80. Karger, Basel, Switzerland.

Roland, P.E., 1984. Metabolic measurements of the working frontal cortex in man. *Trends in Neurosciences*, **7**, 430–435.

Rolls, E.T. and Williams, G.V., 1987. Neuronal activity in the ventral striatum of the primate. In: Carpenter, M.B. and Jayaraman, A. (eds), *The Basal Ganglia*, pp. 137–148. Plenum, New York.

Sanides, F., 1969. Comparative architectonics of the neocortex of mammals and their evolutionary interpretation. *Annals of the New York Academy of Sciences*, **167**, 404–423.

Sano, K. and Mayanagi, Y., 1988. Posteromedial hypothalamotomy in the treatment of violent, aggressive behavior. *Acta Neurochirurgica*, **44**(Suppl), 145–151.

Schneider, F., Habel, U., Kessler, C., Posse, S., Grodd, W. and Muller-Gartner, H.W., 2000. Functional imaging of conditioned aversive emotional responses in antisocial personality disorder. *Neuropsychobiology*, **42**, 192–201.

Schneider, J.S. and Lidsky, T.I., 1981. Processing of somatosensory information in striatum of behaving cats. *Journal of Neurophysiology*, **45**, 841–851.

Schultz, W., Tremblay, L. and Hollerman, J.R., 1998. Reward prediction in primate basal ganglia and frontal cortex. *Neuropharmacology*, **37**, 421–429.

Siegel, A. and Brutus, M., 1990. Neural substrates of aggression and rage in the cat. *Progress in Psychobiology and Physiological Psychology*, **14**, 135–233.

Soloff, P.H., Meltzer, C.C., Greer, P.J. Constantine, D. and Kelly, T.M., 2000. A fenfluramine-activated FDG-PET study of borderline personality disorder. *Biological Psychiatry*, **47**, 540–547.

Sternberg, R.J., 1990. *Wisdom: Its Origin, Nature, and Development*. Cambridge University Press, New York.

Strom-Olsen, K. and Carlisle, S., 1971. Bifrontal stereotactic tractotomy: a follow-up study of its effects on 210 patients. *British Journal of Psychiatry*, **118**, 141–154.

Stuss, D.T. and Benson, D.F., 1986. *The Frontal Lobes*. Raven Press, New York.

Stuss, D.T., 1992. Biological and psychological development of executive functions. *Brain and Cognition*, **20**, 8–23.

Sugiura, M., Kawashima, R., Nakagawa, M., Okada, K., Sato, T., Goto, R., Sato, K., Ono, S., Schormann, T., Zilles, K. and Fukuda, H., 2000. Correlation between human personality and neural activity in cerebral cortex. *Neuroimage*, **11**, 541–546.

Svrakic, D.M., Whitehead, C., Przybeck, T.R. and Cloninger, C.R., 1993. Differential diagnosis of personality disorders by the seven factor model of temperament and character. *Archives of General Psychiatry*, **50**, 991–999.

Tai, C.T., Clark, A.J.M., Feldon, J. and Rawlins, J.N., 1991. Electrolytic lesions of the nucleus accumbens in rats which abolish the PREE enhance the locomotor response to amphetamine. *Experimental Brain Research*, **86**, 333–340.

Vedeniapin, A.B., Anokhin, A.A., Sirevaag, E., Rohrbaugh, J.W. and Cloninger, C.R., 2001. Visual P300 and the self-directedness scale of the temperament-character inventory. *Psychiatry Research*, **101**, 145–156.

Wigglesworth, M.J. and Smith, B.D., 1976. Habituation and dishabituation of the electrodermal orienting reflex in relation to extraversion and neuroticism. *Journal of Experimental Research in Personality*, **10**, 437–445.

XXVI-7

Neurogenetics of Personality Disorders

Andreas Reif and Klaus-Peter Lesch

INTRODUCTION

The behavioural predisposition of an individual is commonly referred to as temperament or personality. In genetics, personality is generally defined as the characteristic manner and style of an individual's behaviour and encompasses the emotional expression, such as fearfulness, exuberance, aggressiveness, and self-restraint, as well as the vigour, temper, and persistence of the resulting behaviour (Benjamin *et al.*, 1998; Ebstein *et al.*, 2000). Personality disorder (PD) is an umbrella term covering a plethora of conditions characterized by a persistent pattern of abnormal behaviour, dysfunctioning in social contexts, and suffering of either the individual or the environment. Despite problems of classification, epidemiological research involving family, twin, and adoptee studies has gathered persuasive evidence that several categories of PD including antisocial, anxious/avoidant, and schizoid-schizotypal personalities are influenced by genetic factors, and that the genetic component is highly complex, polygenic, and epistatic (Coolidge *et al.*, 2001; Eley *et al.*, 1999; Jang *et al.*, 1996; Kendler *et al.*, 1991; McGuffin and Thapar, 1992; O'Connor *et al.*, 1998; Vernon *et al.*, 1999).

The analysis of genetic contributions to normal personality and behaviour as well as to PDs is both conceptually and methodologically difficult, so that consistent findings remain sparse. The documented heterogeneity of both genetic and environmental determinants suggests the ineffectiveness of searching for unitary causes. This vista has therefore increasingly encouraged the pursuit of dimensional and quantitative approaches to personality and behavioural genetics, in addition to the traditional strategy of studying individuals with categorically defined psychiatric entities (Plomin *et al.*, 1994). While quantitative genetics has focused on complex, quantitatively distributed traits and their origins in naturally occurring variation caused by multiple genetic and environmental factors, molecular genetics has begun to identify specific genes for quantitative traits, called quantitative trait loci (QTLs) (Eley and Plomin, 1997). In this polygenic model, behavioural disorders are extremes of continua in which various genes interact additively or nonadditively. The QTL concept thus implies that there may not be genes for psychiatric disorders, just genes for behavioural dimensions. In line with this notion, Livesley *et al.* (1998) have recently suggested that personality disorders are best classified by dimensional scales and are not qualitatively distinct from normal personality traits. Underlying genes of extremes of normal personality traits may therefore contribute to a range of psychopathology including psychoses (Tien *et al.*, 1992).

Any attempt to provide a comprehensive overview would be futile; however, an appraisal of the genetics of PDs requires the consideration of several critical caveats. This chapter therefore describes fundamental aspects of the genetics of personality and focuses on topics undergoing particularly rapid progress. Conceptual and methodological issues in the search for candidate genes of personality traits and PDs as well as for the development of mouse models of human PDs will also be reviewed.

PERSONALITY DISORDERS — A DIAGNOSTIC DILEMMA

The diagnosis of PD is evidently not as clear-cut as is desirable. In a continuum ranging from reasonably well-characterized brain disorders with a defined genetic cause, such as Huntington's disease or fragile-X syndrome, to wider and more unspecific diagnoses such as bipolar affective or schizophrenic disorders, extreme variants of personality represent disorder entities which are the least well defined and accessible to psychobiological research. DSM-IV (American Psychiatric Association, 1994) lists the following criteria of PD: a persistent pattern of abnormal behaviour, dysfunctioning in social contexts, suffering of either the patient or the environment, and early onset in childhood or adolescence. When the first three DSM-IV criteria are inverted, (pattern of normal behaviour, functioning, and no suffering), and the last is kept, one might see this as a definition of 'normal' personality, or behaviour, as human personality is mainly what is constructed from an individual's actions. It is conceivable that the DSM-IV definition of PD covers a wide range of disorders; may be subdivided in almost infinite different ways, just as human personality; and depends not only on the patient, but also the environment. The social context is of substantial importance when the diagnosis of PD is applied; individuals functioning perfectly in some societies may fail to do so in others. Thus, we have the media stereotype of a workaholic German manager, who could be indexed as neurotic and anankastic in other socio-economic models; the temperamental stereotype of a young lady from Sicily, readily regarded as highly histrionic in Norway; and that revered eccentric English gentlemen, in DSM-IV euphemisms the archetype of a schizotype personality. Accordingly, PD, in part, lies in the eye of the beholder.

What leads to the term 'disorder', is the suffering of the individual or — as is sometimes more common in PDs — the environment. Otherwise, this 'disorder' could easily be described as 'personality variation', the outer limits of a Gaussian distribution of personality traits. Thus, the presence of PDs could be viewed as an evolutionary strategy to adapt to different environmental conditions. Dysfunctioning and abnormal behaviour might be appropriate attributes for a certain kind of personality structure in a given culture; but cultures and societies vary and, even more meaningfully, constantly change, and what was abnormal or dysfunctional yesterday might be successful and perfectly normal today. PDs therefore may be the price a given society has to pay for the flexibility to adapt to different environments and for the variation of behaviour which helps it to maintain reproductive success and to ensure survival. Furthermore, the genes underlying behavioural traits have been shaped

Biological Psychiatry: Edited by H. D'haenen, J.A. den Boer and P. Willner. ISBN 0-471-49198-5

throughout evolution for success in primordial societies, and not in contemporary civilization. Humans still bear the constraints of this genetic background, and it has to be kept in mind that some of the features now regarded as 'disordered', such as exaggerated anxiety, novelty seeking and risk-taking hyperactivity, or straightforward aggression, might represent behavioural strategies that were, in the evolutionarily perspective, highly successful in ancient times. For further reading, several monographs are recommended to the interested reader (Allman, 1994; Hamer and Copeland, 1998; Nesse and Williams, 1995; Weiner, 1999; Wilson, 1998).

The current classification systems of DSM-IV (American Psychiatric Association 1994) and ICD-10 (World Health Organization 1992) distinguish three distinct subgroups of PD: paranoid, histrionic, and avoidant. While an operationalized diagnostic procedure is laborious to obtain, these subgroups are familiar and intuitively comprehensible in the clinical setting. However, rating scales often fail to identify a specific PD, or the results are contrary to the experienced clinician's view. This is likely to be due to the fact that PDs arise in social contexts hardly to be reflected in standardized interviews.

Furthermore, a distinct PD, according to DSM-IV or ICD-10, does not represent a categorical unit of human behaviour but rather a blend of temperamental traits, cognitive plans, mental 'master' attitudes, patterns of behaviour, and so on. Some of these features have a substantial genetic component, while others do not. Biological background mingles with environmental factors and education — both nature and nurture shape personality and PDs alike. Due to the heterogeneity of PD diagnoses, it appears to be naive and futile to search for a single genetic cause resulting in exactly one specific PD. In DSM-IV, PDs have been grouped in three clusters (withdrawn, flamboyant, and fearful), which might be a reasonable starting point in the search for genetic influences. Several authors assign PDs of the so-called Cluster A (paranoid, schizoid, and schizotype) to the schizophrenia spectrum disorders, with an overlapping genetic background; Cluster B, the flamboyant group, appears to be influenced more by environmental than genetic factors (Kendler and Eaves, 1986). Cluster C, comprising obsessive-compulsive, avoidant, and dependent traits, seems to share genetic and environmental causes in equal parts.

In order to avoid the inherent problems of multidimensional diagnosis of PDs, it is sensible to identify the temperamental and behavioural traits, such as anxiety, novelty seeking, impulsivity, aggressiveness, and antisocial behaviour, that underlie PDs. These traits can be assessed by rating scales for humans (e.g., the Revised NEO Personality Inventory NEO-PI-R [Costa and McCrae, 1992], the Tridimensional Personality Questionnaire/Tridimensional Character Inventory TPQ/TCI [Cloninger *et al.*, 1993], and the Karolinska Scales of Personality [KSP] [Schalling *et al.*, 1987] questionnaires), as well as by specific behavioural paradigms in animal models, making it possible to investigate specific genetic influences. A specific PD could then be dissected into behavioural features, with known genetic components and non-genetic contributions, by cognitive schemes and strategies. The search for the genetics of PD thus closely resembles the search of the genetics of behaviour.

TOWARDS GENETIC DISSECTION OF PDs

It is now widely accepted that human temperament and personality is a multigene product. There is no single gene or major gene effect, respectively, for a specific behavioural trait, and, consequently, there is no single gene for a PD subtype. Rather these characteristics are polygenic, a fact which results in the failure of classical genome-wide linkage studies to detect the genes accounting for personality traits or PDs. Many genes, with only modest phenotypic effects, add up to account for the full variance of a particular personality dimension. This implies also that single variation in a given gene might lead to only a minimal change in the phenotype, but another variation in the same gene might have deleterious effects, resulting in an apparent 'one gene, one disorder (OGOD)' type of disease. This notion becomes even more complicated when gene–environment interactions and epistatic phenomena are taken into account.

A gene variant which is associated with a PD in one population may not be so associated in another ethnic group — a problem which is increasingly being encountered in behavioural genetics. Since a given gene influences distinct personality traits only to a small extent — for instance, allelic variation in 5HTT function, which is described in more detail below, accounts for approximately 8% of the genetic variance of traits related to anxiety and aggression — and since the genetic component of PD is polygenic, classical linkage analysis has failed to identify relevant genomic variation. Because the power of linkage analysis to detect small gene effects is quite limited, at least with realistic samples, QTL research relies on association analysis using DNA variants in or near candidate genes that are presumably functional. The first QTL analysis was conducted 1988 by Paterson *et al.*, who searched for the genes responsible for the phenotypes of tomato fruits (Paterson *et al.*, 1988). While this study demonstrated that a set of six genes controls fruit mass, it highly likely that personality traits are defined by sets of at least 10–20 different genes, and that both pleiotropy and epistasis play an critical role in the molecular basis of personality.

The pace of integration of quantitative and molecular genetics has been accelerated remarkably as a result of the *Drosophila*, mouse, and human genome projects, which have brought neuroscience to the threshold of the postgenomic era in which the human genome and those of other species are known. While several million DNA variations (polymorphisms) have been identified in the genomic sequence, most importantly for the analysis of complex traits, roughly 30 000–60 000 common polymorphisms are located in coding and regulatory regions of genes that are the ultimate causes of the heritability of complex traits (McPherson *et al.*, 2001; Sachidanandam *et al.*, 2001). These advances have generated new technologies, such as DNA microarrays, that make it possible to investigate the role of thousands of DNA variants in complex traits. The rate of discovery of genes associated with complex traits, such as personality and behaviour, will also increase, as systematic QTL scans can be conducted using functional DNA variants in the brain that affect coding regions or gene regulation. Of the nearly 40 000 genes, approximately 50% are expressed in the brain, but a substantial proportion of these are housekeeping genes. Thus, fewer than 15 000 tissue-specific genes may be expressed in the brain. Identifying the estimated 8000–16 000 functional DNA variants in coding regions of these genes and the DNA variants that regulate the expression of these genes is now a high priority for behavioural genetic research. Several classes of genomic variations in coding and regulatory regions of genes, commonly referred to as candidate genes, are of particular interest. The variety of these functionally relevant variations ranges from single nucleotide polymorphisms (SNPs) to microdeletions (or insertions), and polymorphic simple sequence repeats (SSRs) of 2–50+ nucleotides in length.

Quantitative genetic research on animal models consists primarily of inbred strain and selection studies. While comparisons between different inbred strains of mice expose remarkable differences in measures of anxiety-related behaviour, such as performance in the Open Field or Elevated Plus Maze paradigm, differences within strains can be attributed to environmental influences. Inbred and recombinant inbred strain studies are highly efficient in dissecting genetic influences, for investigating interactions between genotype and environment, and for testing the disposition-stress model. Selective breeding of mice for many generations produces differences between high and low anxiety lines that steadily increase from generation to generation. Selection studies of behavioural traits strongly suggest a genetic influence and that many genes contribute to variation in behaviour. Mice strains that have been selectively bred to display a phenotype of interest are currently being used to identify genetic loci that contribute to behavioural traits. The QTL approach has been applied with some success to a trait in mice called 'emotionality' (Flint *et al.*, 1995). Crosses between the high- and low-activity selected mouse lines yielded three QTL regions that appear to be related to various measures of fearfulness. A modified QTL strategy that uses recombinant inbred mouse strains produced candidate QTLs for Open Field fearfulness (Phillips *et al.*, 1995).

Regrettably, such linkage analyses provide only a rough chromosomal localization, whereas the next step, identifying the relevant genes by positional cloning, remains a challenging task (Tecott and Barondes, 1996). Since mice and humans share many orthologous genes mapped to synthenic chromosomal regions, it is conceivable that individual genes identified for behaviour may be developed as animal models. After chromosomal mapping of polymorphic genes and evaluation of gene function with knockout mutants, behavioural parameters are investigated. Thus, the combination of elaborate genetic and behavioural analyses results in the identification of many genes with effects on the variation and development of murine behaviour; ultimately, mouse QTL research is likely to generate candidate genes for human behavioural disorders.

CANDIDATE GENES

A complementary approach to quantitative genetic studies is investigation of whether certain candidate genes are involved in the manifestation of a specific phenotype, and whether such genes are involved in the pathogenesis of disease states. While this approach was restricted until recently to a relatively small number of genes, identification of new candidates will be facilitated by the new tools of the postgenomic era. Because it is hypothesis-driven, the investigation of candidate genes is a powerful means to examine the biological basis of personality and behaviour. In this context, psychobiology accumulated a thorough knowledge of neurotransmitter networks; consequently, the first candidate genes investigated were components of the monoamine neurotransmitter pathways. Interest has primarily been focused on the serotonergic, dopaminergic, and — to a lesser extent — noradrenergic systems. Almost no information is available on the role of genetic variations of the constituents of second and third messenger pathways, transcription factors, or other morphoregulators.

Nevertheless, several caveats have to be kept in mind with respect to candidate gene studies. First of all, negative studies might be underrepresented due to publication bias, an error with declining impact, since this problem is increasingly acknowledged by scientists, reviewers, and editors. Also of importance seems to be the problem that initial false-negative association studies impede further research, as they are unlikely to be replicated (Cardon, 2001a; b). This emphasizes the importance of further research on known or hypothesized candidate genes. Further issues are the artefacts due to population stratification as well as to gene–gene and gene–environment interactions. However, as QTL loci mostly require very large sets of sib-pairs to gain enough statistical power in linkage analyses (Speer, 1998), candidate gene studies are currently more feasible despite these limitations.

Serotonergic Gene Pathway

In view of the converging lines of evidence that 5-HT and serotonergic gene expression is involved in a myriad of processes during brain development as well as synaptic plasticity in adulthood, temperamental predisposition and complex behaviour are likely to be influenced by genetically driven variability of 5-HT function. Originating from the raphe nuclei in the brainstem, the serotonergic system innervates multiple regions throughout the brain. For instance, serotonergic neurons are found in the basal ganglia, amygdala, hippocampus, nucleus accumbens, cingulum, thalamus, cortex, and many other areas. The central 5-HT system is thought to function as a behavioural inhibition system, and to be involved in the regulation of motor activity, food intake, sleep and other circadian rhythms, cognition, mood, anxiety, aggression, and impulsivity. It exerts its actions by the modulation of various other transmitter systems, such as the noradrenergic, dopaminergic, glutamatergic, GABAergic, and cholinergic systems. The 5-HT system integrates and connects these spatially separated systems and thus forms a global meta-network of distinct local networks, thereby coordinating and balancing common brain functions. Moreover, 5-HT not only acts as a neurotransmitter but is also involved in the regulation of neurogenesis and synaptic plasticity in the pre- and post-natal period, as well as in the adult brain.

Serotonergic system dysfunction has been implicated in various psychiatric disorders, including depression, bipolar disorder, panic and generalized anxiety disorder (GAD), seasonal affective disorder (SAD), obsessive-compulsive disorder (OCD), eating disorders, and possibly also schizophrenic and neurodegenerative disorders (Lucki, 1998). Regarding PDs, a pivotal role of the serotonergic system has been hypothesized in the pathogenesis of emotional instability syndrome, commonly referred to as borderline personality disorder (BPD) (Goodman and New, 2000; Gurvits *et al.*, 2000). Consequently, psychoactive drugs targetting the serotonergic neurocircuitries, such as selective 5-HT reuptake inhibitors (SSRIs) and 5-HT (ant)agonists, including atypical neuroleptics, have been proven to be beneficial in most of these diseases. Low 5-HT concentrations or turnover — as measured by the metabolite 5-hydroxyindole acetic acid (5-HIAA) in cerebrospinal fluid (CSF) — are correlated with suicide, impulsivity, aggression (Asberg *et al.*, 1986; Higley *et al.*, 1996; Higley *et al.*, 1992a), and — in neonates — a family history of antisocial PD (Constantino *et al.*, 1997). In line with these findings, patients suffering from severe PDs of the high aggression/low impulse-control type (e.g., antisocial PD) exhibit decreased 5-HIAA levels (Brown *et al.*, 1982; Brown *et al.*, 1979; Coccaro *et al.*, 1992). A landmark study by Raleigh *et al.* (1991) elegantly demonstrated that male vervet monkeys with low social status also have low CSF 5-HIAA concentrations. Correspondingly, high 5-HIAA levels are associated with high social status. Intriguingly, pharmacological alterations of serotonergic function influence social rank, a fact which further underscores the critical role 5-HT plays in controlling temperament and behavioural traits. Hence, 5-HT appears to be a stabilizer of neural circuits as well as of social networks.

In a two-step reaction, 5-HT is synthesized from the essential amino acid, tryptophan. The first and rate-limiting step, the hydroxylation at the 5-position, is catalysed by the enzyme tryptophan hydroxylase (TPH) and is restricted to raphe neurons. Decarboxylation of 5-hydroxytryptophan represents the second step, which is catalysed by an amino acid decarboxylase. This non-specific enzyme is expressed not only in serotonergic neurons but also in catecholamine-synthesizing cells. Once formed, 5-HT is transported into synaptic vesicles by a nonselective monoamine transporter (VMAT). When intracellular free calcium levels reach a certain threshold, 5-HT is released into the synaptic cleft by fusion of the vesicle with the cell membrane. It may act thereafter as a paracrine hormone with effects also on non-excitable cells, as well as a classical neurotransmitter; up to now, 14 receptor subtypes are known. The reuptake of extracellular 5-HT is performed by the selective 5-HT transporter (5-HTT). 5-HT is thereafter recycled for repetitive release or degraded to 5-HIAA by the enzyme monoamine oxidase A (MAO-A), which is localized at the outer membrane of mitochondria. For several of the genes involved in the regulation and function of the serotonergic pathway, various polymorphisms have been identified that may influence personality traits and related disorders.

Tryptophan Hydroxylase

Tryptophan hydroxylase (TPH), the rate-limiting enzyme in the synthesis of 5-HT, is a tetrahydrobiopterin (H_4Bip)-dependent mono-oxygenase which, in the CNS, is localized exclusively in raphe neurons. It is a member of the superfamily of aromatic amino acid hydroxylases, which also comprises the tyrosine and phenylalanine hydroxylases (Ledley *et al.*, 1987). The TPH gene has been assigned to human chromosome 11p15.3-p14, comprises 11 exons, and is subject to alternative splicing (Boularand *et al.*, 1995; Craig *et al.*, 1991). Besides polymorphisms in the upstream regulatory region, intron 7 is the site of two variations, although their functional relevance remains elusive (Nielsen *et al.*, 1997). Both are A to C transversions at the base pairs 218 and 779, respectively. 779A is termed allele U, and 779 C allele L (Nielsen *et al.*, 1992). Since low 5-HT system function is known to correlate with (violent) suicide, aggression, and impulsivity, a link between TPH gene variants and these traits had been predicted.

In a pioneering study by Nielsen *et al.* (1994), it was shown in a Finnish sample that the L variant of intron 7 of the TPH gene is associated with decreased CSF 5-HIAA concentrations, and that this polymorphism may predispose to suicidal behaviour. However, no association between this genetic variation and impulsivity was found. In a replication study by the same group, the TPH L allele was again linked to suicidality, history of suicide attempts, and alcohol dependence (Nielsen *et al.*, 1998). Siever and associates (New *et al.*, 1998) reported an association of the TPH gene L allele with measures of impulsivity and aggression with the Buss-Durkee Hostility Inventory (BDHI). However, it was demonstrated that in a non-patient sample 'outward bound' aggression is correlated with the U allele of TPH (Manuck *et al.*, 1999) and low CSF 5-HIAA levels (Jonsson *et al.*, 1997a). In depressed patients, the U allele was shown to be linked to a history of suicide attempt (Mann *et al.*, 1997); in schizophrenic patients, the L allele was more frequent in male subjects with a history of violent behaviour (Nolan *et al.*, 2000b). Regarding the A218 C polymorphism, the results are similarly equivocal, with both positive (Tsai *et al.*, 1999) and negative (Geijer *et al.*, 2000) findings. Recently, a negative report on the relation between both TPH polymorphisms and suicidality was published (Bennett *et al.*, 2000) in line with the findings by Abbar *et al.* (1995) and Bellivier *et al.* (1998), who argued that TPH polymorphisms are not causally linked to suicide, but that the reported associations are due to ethnic stratification. As both investigated polymorphisms are non-coding, it seems likely that they are linked with functional polymorphisms in some, but not all, populations. This possibility may explain the observed inconsistencies and thus warrants further research. In conclusion, it seems that at least in some populations, or in connection with psychiatric disease states, TPH polymorphism may play a role in the predisposition to suicidality, aggression, and possibly alcoholism. To resolve these apparent discrepancies, studies with large and ethnically matched samples need to be conducted to clarify the role of the TPH gene in personality traits and related disorders.

5-HT Receptors

Fourteen 5-HT receptor subtypes are known and are distinguished pharmacologically, structurally, functionally, and/or by molecular biologic means (for reviews, see Hoyer and Martin, 1996; Saxena, 1995). They probably derive from a common primordial 5-HT receptor, which developed in the course of evolution more than a billion years ago. The 5-HT receptors are subdivided in seven families, the largest being the 5-HT_1 family with five 5-HT receptor subtypes termed 5-HT_{1A-F} (5-HT_{1C} has been reassigned as 5-HT_{2C}). The 5-HT_2 family has three members, the 5-HT_5 family two subtypes; with respect to 5-$HT_{4,6,7}$, only a single member is known. 5-HT_3 comprises two subunits, A and B. The diversity of 5-HT receptors is probably due to the ontogenetically old role of 5-HT in neuromodulation; the apparent complexity of serotonergic subsystems allows fine tuning. Regarding personality and behaviour, a large body of evidence suggests that 5-HT receptors are involved in anxiety, impulsivity, and aggression (Goldman *et al.*, 1996; Roth, 1994). While 5-HT_{1A} and 5-$HT_{1B/D}$ (which share a high degree of similarity), 5-HT_{2A}, and 5-HT_{2C} have been extensively investigated, little is known about subtypes 5-HT_{4-7}.

5-HT_{1A} receptors are expressed on neurons as well as on astrocytes. They act presynaptically as somatodendritic autoreceptors in the raphe complex and postsynaptically in the hippocampus, septum, and the amygdala, where they initiate neuronal inhibition by hyperpolarization. The 5-HT_{1A} receptor gene is located on human chromosome 5q11.2-q13. Studies employing pharmacological techniques suggested that 5-HT_{1A} activation decreases aggressive behaviour in humans as well as rodents (Coccaro *et al.*, 1990; De Vry, 1995; Kavoussi *et al.*, 1997). In line with these findings, mice with a targetted inactivation of the 5-HT_{1A} receptor gene display increased anxiety-related behaviours in three independent studies (Heisler *et al.*, 1998; Parks *et al.*, 1998; Ramboz *et al.*, 1998). While other mechanisms for the observed behavioural changes could be excluded, a link between serotonergic and GABAergic transmission was recently reported. Mice with a targetted inactivation of the 5-HT_{1A} receptor consistently display a spontaneous phenotype that is associated with a gender-modulated and gene/dose-dependent increase of anxiety-related behaviours. With the exception of an enhanced sensitivity of terminal 5-HT_{1B} receptors and downregulation of GABA-A receptors (Sibille *et al.*, 2000), no major neuroadaptational changes were detected. Activation of presynaptic 5-HT_{1A} receptors provide the brain with an autoinhibitory feedback system controlling 5-HT neurotransmission. Thus, enhanced anxiety-related behaviour probably represents a consequence of increased terminal 5-HT availability resulting from the lack or reduction in presynaptic somatodendritic 5-HT_{1A} autoreceptor negative feedback function. Indirect evidence for increased presynaptic serotonergic activity is provided by the compensatory upregulation of terminal 5-HT_{1B} receptors. This mechanism is also consistent with recent theoretical models of fear and anxiety that are primarily based upon pharmacologically derived data. The cumulative reduction in serotonergic impulse flow to septohippocampal and other limbic and cortical areas involved in the control of anxiety is believed to explain the anxiolytic effects of ligands with selective affinity for the 5-HT_{1A} receptor in some animal models of anxiety-related behaviour. This notion is based, in part, on evidence that 5-HT_{1A} agonists (e.g., 8-OH-DPAT) and antagonists (e.g., WAY 100635) have anxiolytic or anxiogenic effects, respectively. However, to complicate matters further, 8-OH-DPAT has anxiolytic effects when injected in the raphe nucleus, whereas it is anxiogenic when applied to the hippocampus. Thus, stimulation of postsynaptic 5-HT_{1A} receptors has been proposed to elicit anxiogenic effects, while activation of 5-HT_{1A} autoreceptors is thought to induce anxiolytic effects via suppression of serotonergic neuronal firing, resulting in attenuated 5-HT release in limbic terminal fields.

Taken together, these findings lead to the conclusion that the 5-HT_{1A} receptor is a key player in the modulation of anxiety-related behaviour and thus behavioural inhibition. Anxiety-related behaviour in 5-HT_{1A}-deficient mice seems to be caused by an increased serotonergic tone due to the absent negative feedback of the 5-HT_{1A} autoreceptor. Interestingly, when wild house mice were divided into those with high and those with low-aggression scores, the aggressive mice showed high levels of 5-HT_{1A} receptor expression in the dorsal hippocampus compared with low-aggression mice (Korte *et al.*, 1996). This finding supports the notion of a contraposition of aggression and anxiety and the critical role of the serotonergic system in balancing both.

The 5-HT_{1B} receptor (like the structurally similar 5-HT_{1D} receptor) serves as an inhibitory autoreceptor on serotonergic terminals but also as a postsynaptic heteroceptor on non-5-HT neurons. It is expressed in the basal ganglia, striatum, hippocampus, amygdala, and frontal cortex. 5-HT_{1B} has been assigned to human chromosome 6q13 (Demchyshyn *et al.*, 1992). Based on rather indirect pharmacological evidence, it is thought to play a role in aggressive as well as reproductive behaviour. Accordingly, 5-HT_{1B} knockout mice show increased exploratory behaviour and are more aggressive in the resident-intruder paradigm (Brunner *et al.*, 1999; Malleret *et al.*, 1999; Ramboz *et al.*, 1996; Saudou *et al.*, 1994). As for 5-HT_{1A} knockout mice, this was not due to changes in locomotor activity. Mice lacking the 5-HT_{1B} receptor were also more prone to develop cocaine (Rocha *et al.*, 1998) and alcohol dependence (Brunner and Hen, 1997), a finding which suggests a role of this receptor in the pathophysiology of substance abuse. Two polymorphisms in the human 5-HT_{1B} gene, C129T and G861C, were not associated with depression, suicidality, or alcoholism (Huang *et al.*, 1999). However, in Finnish antisocial alcoholics, as well as a Southwest Native American tribe with a high rate of alcoholism, a significant association with G861C was demonstrated (Lappalainen *et al.*, 1998).

The human 5-HT_{2A} receptor gene is located on chromosome 13q14-q21 near the genes for retinoblastoma-1 and esterase D (Hsieh *et al.*, 1990) and consists of three exons and two introns (Chen *et al.*, 1992). There is reason to assume that 5-HT_{2A} is subject to genomic imprinting; only the maternal allele is expressed (Kato *et al.*, 1996). The hallucinogenic effects of LSD have been attributed to its 5-HT_{2A} agonism (Aghajanian and Marek, 1999); consequently, an association between the T102C polymorphism of the 5-HT_{2A} receptor and schizophrenia has been suggested by several, but not all, studies (He *et al.*, 1999; Spurlock *et al.*, 1998; Williams *et al.*, 1996; 1997). However, Holmes *et al.* (1998) reported that the 102 C allele is linked to the presence of hallucinations in late-onset Alzheimer's disease. No association between suicide attempts and 5-HT_{2A} polymorphism was detected (Geijer *et al.*, 2000) when suicide attempters were split into different categories including Cluster B, but not Cluster C, PD. In a study with patients suffering from bipolar affective disorder and healthy controls, no major effect of the T102C polymorphism on the TPQ personality dimension 'harm avoidance' was found (Blairy *et al.*, 2000). All in all, there is, as yet, no clear-cut evidence for a role of this polymorphism in PDs.

The physiological function of the 5-HT_{2C} receptor, which is located in the cortex, hippocampus and striatum, remains elusive. It has been mapped to Xq24 (Milatovich *et al.*, 1992). A functional knockout mouse model, in which the carboxy-terminal half of the receptor is removed, has been generated by Tecott *et al.* (1995). In addition to increased vulnerability of these mice to die from seizures, they were also overweight, hinting at a role for 5-HT_{2C} in the regulation of food intake (Tecott *et al.*, 1995). In humans, the Cys23Ser polymorphism in the N-terminal end of the 5-HT_{2C} receptor protein has attracted considerable attention (Lappalainen *et al.*, 1995). The 23Ser allele was associated with hallucinations and, interestingly, hyperphagia in Alzheimer's disease (Holmes *et al.*, 1998). Furthermore, an association between the Cys23Ser polymorphism and violent alcoholism was reported (Virkkunen *et al.*, 1996), although failure of replication casts some doubt on the initial finding (Himei *et al.*, 2000; Lappalainen *et al.*, 1999; Schuckit *et al.*, 1999).

Based on a personality assessment with the TPQ questionnaire, an interesting gene–gene interaction between a polymorphism of the dopamine receptor DRD4 (also see below) and the 5-HT_{2C} Cys23Ser polymorphism was demonstrated. When both polymorphisms were present, they accounted for 13% of the variance of TPQ 'reward dependence' and 30% of the variance for 'persistence' — a subscore of 'reward dependence' (Ebstein *et al.*, 2000; Ebstein *et al.*, 1997c; Kuhn *et al.*, 1999). No influence of the Cys23Ser polymorphism alone was found (Kuhn *et al.*, 1999); no replication studies have been performed to date.

With respect to 5-HT_{3-7} receptors, little evidence for involvement of these molecules in behaviour has been presented to date. Clearly, more research on these, in part, poorly understood and characterized receptors is needed. An interesting finding has been presented by Grailhe *et al.* (1999), who demonstrated that 5-HT_{5A} knockout mice, just like 5-HT_{1B}-deficient mice, display increased explorative behaviour, as well as altered response to hallucinogens, such as LSD. In a Finnish group of antisocial alcoholics, an association with a polymorphism of the 5-HT_7 receptor gene has been suggested, but this finding still awaits confirmation (Pesonen *et al.*, 1998).

5-HT Transporter

In contrast to the remarkable diversity of 5-HT receptors, only a single protein, the 5-HT transporter (5-HTT), mediates the reuptake of 5-HT from the synaptic cleft and thus the termination of its action. The 5-HTT is structurally and functionally similar to the dopamine (DAT) and norepinephrine (NET) transporter proteins (Blakely *et al.*, 1994; Borowsky and Hoffman, 1995). The exchange of intracellular sodium against extracellular potassium generates the energy necessary for transport of 5-HT against the extra-intracellular gradient. When intracellular 5-HT levels are very high — for instance, as a consequence of VMAT2 inhibition following MDMA ('ecstasy') intake — the 5-HTT reverses its action by releasing 5-HT into the synaptic cleft. 5-HTT is an initial target for antidepressant drugs, either with relatively low specificity, such as the TCAs (e.g., imipramine and clomipramine) or high selectivity, such as the SRIs (e.g., fluoxetine, sertraline, and citalopram), as well as for psychostimulants, including amphetamines and cocaine (Schloss and Williams, 1998). The efficacy and versatility of 5-HTT-inhibiting drugs underscores the outstanding role of the 5-HTT in the fine regulation of the serotonergic system.

The human 5-HTT is encoded by a single gene on chromosome 17q11 adjacent to the CPD and NF1 genes (Shen *et al.*, 2000). It is composed of 14–15 exons spanning approximately 35 kb (Lesch *et al.*, 1994). In humans, the transcriptional activity of the 5-HTT gene, 5-HTT availability, and ultimately 5-HT reuptake are modulated by a polymorphic repetitive element, the 5-HTT gene-linked polymorphic region (5-HTTLPR), located upstream of the transcription start site (for review, see Lesch, 1997). Additional variations have been described in the 5′ untranslated region (5′UTR) due to alternative splicing of exon 1B (Bradley and Blakely, 1997), and in intron 2 (variable number of a 16/17-base-pair tandem repeat, VNTR-17) (Lesch *et al.*, 1994), and 3′UTR (Battersby *et al.*, 1999). Comparison of different mammalian species confirmed the presence of the 5-HTTLPR in Platyrrhini and Catarrhini (hominoids, cercopithecoids), but not in prosimian primates and other mammals (Lesch *et al.*, 1997). The 5-HTTLPR is unique to humans and simian primates. The majority of alleles are composed of either 14-or 16-repeat elements in humans (short and long allele, respectively), while alleles with 15, 18, 19, 20, or 22 repeat elements, and variants with single-base insertions/deletions or substitutions within individual repeat elements are rare. A predominantly Caucasian population displayed allele frequencies of 57% for the long (*l*) allele and 43% for the short (*s*) allele with a 5-HTTLPR genotype distribution of 32% *l*/*l*, 49% *l*/*s*, and 19% *s*/*s* (Lesch *et al.*, 1996); different allele and genotype distributions are found in other populations (Gelernter *et al.*, 1998). Consequently, the contribution of the 5-HTTLPR to individual phenotypic differences in personality traits was explored in independent population- and family-based genetic studies (for review, see Lesch, 2001a). Anxiety-related and other personality traits were assessed by the NEO Personality Inventory — Revised (NEO-PI-R), a self-report inventory based on the five-factor model of personality ('Big Five') (Costa and McCrae, 1992), and by the 16PF Personality Inventory (Cattell, 1989). The five factors assessed by the NEO are 'neuroticism' (emotional instability), 'extraversion', 'agreeableness' (cooperation and reciprocal alliance formation), 'openess' (intellect and problem-solving), and 'conscientiousness' (will to achieve).

In an initial study, population and within-family associations were discovered between the low-expressing s allele and 'neuroticism', a trait related to anxiety, hostility, and depression, on the NEO-PI-R in a primarily male population ($n = 505$) (Lesch *et al.*, 1996). Individuals with either one or two copies of the short 5-HTTLPR variant (group S) had significantly greater levels of neuroticism, defined as proneness to negative emotionality, including anxiety, hostility, and depression, than those homozygous for the long genotype (group L) in the sample as a whole and also within sibships. Individuals with 5-HTTLPR S genotypes also had significantly decreased NEO 'agreeableness'. In addition, the group S individuals had increased scores on 'anxiety' on the separate 16PF personality inventory, a trait related to NEO 'neuroticism'. In a more recent investigation, this association was tested in an independent sample ($n = 397$, 84% female, primarily sib-pairs) (Greenberg *et al.*, 2000). The findings replicated the association between the 5-HTTLPR and NEO 'neuroticism'. Combined data from the two studies ($n = 902$), which were corrected for ethnicity and age, gave a highly significant association between the *s* allele and anxiety-related traits both across individuals and within families, reflecting a genuine genetic influence rather than an artefact of ethnic admixture.

Another association encountered in the original study between the *s* allele and lower scores of NEO 'agreeableness' was also replicated and was even more robust in the primarily female replication sample. Gender-related differences in 5-HTTLPR-personality trait associations are possible, since several lines of evidence demonstrate gender-related differences in central 5-HT system function in humans and in animals. These findings include the effects of gonadal steroids on 5-HTT expression in rodent brain and differences in anxiety-related behaviours in male and female 5-HTT knockout mice (Li *et al.*, 2000).

Analysis of NEO subscales further defined the specific aspects of personality that were reproducibly associated with the 5-HTTLPR genotype. For the NEO 'neuroticism' subscales, the combined samples from Lesch *et al.* (1996) and Greenberg *et al.* (2000) demonstrated significant associations between 5-HTTLPR S group genotypes and the facets of 'depression' and 'angry hostility', two of the three facets that showed the most significant associations in the initial sample (Lesch *et al.*, 1996). In contrast, the NEO 'neuroticism anxiety' facet, which was associated with genotype in the first study at a weaker significance level, was not significantly associated with the 5-HTTLPR genotype in the new cohort. With regard to the NEO 'agreeableness' subscales, the previously observed associations of 5-HTTLPR S group genotypes with decreased 'straightforwardness' and 'compliance' were consistently replicated. It therefore appears more accurate to state that the 5-HTTLPR is associated with traits of negative emotionality related to interpersonal hostility and depression. The relationship between these two aspects of negative emotionality is not unexpected in view of the previously observed negative correlation between 'angry hostility', a facet of 'neuroticism', and 'agreeableness' (Costa and McCrae, 1992), indicating that both measures assess a behavioural predisposition to uncooperative interpersonal behaviour (Greenberg *et al.*, 2000).

The effect sizes for the 5-HTTLPR-personality associations, which were comparable in the two samples, indicate that this gene variation has only a modest influence on the behavioural predisposition of approximately 0.30 standard deviation units. This corresponds to 3–4% of the total variance and 7–9% of the genetic variance, based on estimates from twin studies using these and related measures that have consistently demonstrated that genetic factors contribute 40–60% of the variance in neuroticism and other related personality traits. Although the genetic effect suggests that the 5-HTTLPR represents an above-average size QTL, the associations represent only a small portion of the genetic contribution to anxiety-related personality traits. If additional genes were hypothesized to contribute similar gene-dose effects to anxiety, at least 10–15 genes are predicted to be involved. Additive contributions of comparable size based on epistatic epigenetic interactions have, in fact, been found in studies of other quantitative traits. Thus, the results are consistent with the view that the influence of a single, common polymorphism on continuously distributed traits is likely to be small in humans, and possibly to influence different quantitative characteristics in other species (Plomin *et al.*, 1994).

At first glance, association between the high-activity 5-HTTLPR *l* allele and lower 'neuroticism' and related traits seems to be counter-intuitive with regard to the known antidepressant and anxiolytic effects of 5-HTT inhibitors (SRIs). Likewise, Knutson *et al.* (1998) reported that long-term inhibition of the 5-HTT by the SRI paroxetine reduced indices of hostility through a more general decrease in negative affect, a personality dimension related to neuroticism. The same individuals also demonstrated an increase in directly measured social cooperation after paroxetine treatment, an interesting finding in view of the replicated association between 5-HTTLPR genotype and agreeableness. That a drug which inhibits 5-HTT lessened negative emotionality and increased social cooperation appears to conflict with findings that the 5-HTTLPR long allele, which confers higher 5-HTT expression, is associated with lower NEO 'neuroticism' and higher NEO 'agreeableness'. However, this apparent contradiction may be due to the fact that both 5-HT and 5-HTT play critical roles in brain development that differ from their functions in regulating neurotransmission in the adult.

The conclusion that the 5-HTT may affect personality traits via an influence on brain development and synaptic plasticity is strongly supported by recent findings in rodents and nonhuman primates. Studies in rats confirmed that the 5-HTT gene is expressed in brain regions central to emotional behaviour during foetal development, but not later in life (Hansson *et al.*, 1998), hence enduring individual differences in personality could result from 5-HTTLPR-driven differential 5-HTT expression during pre- and perinatal life. In support of this notion, mice with a targetted disruption of 5-HTT display enhanced anxiety-related behaviours (also see section on mouse models of anxiety-related traits) in models of avoidance and anxiety (Wichems *et al.*, 2000).

Together with DRD4, the 5-HTTLPR is the best-investigated candidate gene polymorphism with regard to personality dimensions, with 22 studies directly or indirectly targetting this subject. The results are controversial, for manifold reasons. The limiting factor in QTL analysis often is sample size, because studies including small samples lack the statistical power to detect QTL gene effects, which account typically for 2–10% of the genetic variance. In subsequent investigations, only two attempts have been reported to replicate the original finding using large

Table XXVI-7.1 Overview of published data on the association between the 5-HT transporter gene-linked polymorphic region (5HTTLPR) and anxiety-related traits in general populations and patient samples

	n	Population and study design	Trait assessment/inventory	Association of *s* allele, *P*	Family-based studies, *P*
Lesch *et al.*, 1996	505	General, USA, males, two subsamples	NEO-PI-R, 16PF	0.02–0.002	0.03–0.004
Ebstein *et al.*, 1997	120	General, Israeli	TPQ	0.75, n.s.	—
Ball *et al.*, 1997	106	General, German, 5% of highest vs. lowest N scores	NEO-FFI	0.89, n.s.	—
Nakamura *et al.*, 1997	203	General, Japanese, females	NEO-PI, TCI	*s* increased, *l* rare	—
Mazzanti *et al.*, 1998	655	Controls, alcoholic violent offenders, Finnish	TPQ	n.s.	0.45, but 0.003 for HA1 + HA2
Ebstein *et al.*, 1998	81	General, Israeli, neonates (2 weeks old)	NBAS	interaction with DRD4#	—
Ricketts *et al.*, 1998	84	Controls, Parkinson's disease, USA	TPQ	0.04–0.003	—
Gelernter *et al.*, 1998	185/322	Controls, substance dependence, personality disorder, USA	NEO-PI TPQ	0.47, n.s. 0.87, n.s.	—
Jorm *et al.*, 1998	759	General, European Australian	EPQ-R	n.s.	—
Seretti *et al.*, 1999	132	Depression, bipolar disorder	HAMD, anxiety	0.01	—
Murakami *et al.*, 1999	189	General, Japanese	SRQ-AD	0.05	—
Flory *et al.*, 1999	225	General, USA	NEO-PI-R	0.97	—
Kamakiri *et al.*, 1999	144	General, Japanese	NEO-PI-R, TPQ	n.s.	—
Katsuragi *et al.*, 1999	101	General, Japanese	TPQ	0.007	—
Auerbach *et al.*, 1999	76	General, Israeli, infants (2 months old), follow-up of Ebstein *et al.*, 1998	IBQ	0.05–0.005, interaction with DRD4#	—
Menza *et al.*, 1999	32	Parkinson's disease	HAMD	0.05	—
Dreary *et al.*, 1999	204	General, Scottish, 20% of highest vs. lowest N scores	NEO-FFI	n.s.	—
Gustavsson *et al.*, 1999	305	General, Swedish	KSP	n.s.	—
Osher *et al.*, 2000	148	General, Israeli	NEO-PI-R TPQ	—	0.06 0.07
Greenberg *et al.*, 2000	397	General, USA, females	NEO-PI-R, 16PF	0.03–0.01	0.01
Melke *et al.*, 2001	251	General, Swedish, females, same age	KSP	0.002–0.04	—
Du *et al.*, 2000	186	General, Canadian, males	NEO-PI-R	0.018	—

NEO-PI-R and NEO-FFI: Costa and McCrae's NEO Personality Inventory; TPQ/TCI: Cloninger's Tridimensional Personality Questionnaire/Temperament and Character Inventory; 16PF: Catell's 16 Personality Factor Inventory; EPQ-R: Eysenck Personality Questionnaire; KSP: Karolinska Scales of Personality; SRQ-AD: Self-Rating Questionnaire for anxiety and depression; HAMD: Hamilton Depression Rating Scale; IBQ: Rothbart's Infant Behaviour Questionnaire; NBAS: Brazelton's Neonatal Assessment Scale.
#Dopamine receptor D4.
n.s.: not significant; —: not determined.

populations with samples sizes of >400 individuals (Jorm *et al.*, 1998; Mazzanti *et al.*, 1998) (Table XXVI-7.1). Two of the three available large studies found evidence congruent with an influence of the 5-HTTLPR on 'neuroticism' and related traits (Lesch *et al.*, 1996; Mazzanti *et al.*, 1998), whereas a large population study not employing a within-family design (Jorm *et al.*, 1998) did not. Smaller population-based studies have had variable, but generally negative results (Table XXVI-7.1). Interpretation of these studies is complicated by their use of relatively small or unusual samples, and the lack of within-family designs that minimize population stratification artefacts. Other efforts to detect associations between the 5-HTTLPR and personality traits have been complicated by the use of small sample sizes, heterogeneous subject populations, and differing methods of personality assessment, that is, the use of other questionnaires as the original report, rendering between-study comparison difficult or even impossible. This may explain the conflicting results of Jorm *et al.* (1998), since this group utilized the EPQ-R questionnaire, which was not used in any of the other studies (Table XXVI-7.1). Furthermore, the subject selection in two studies (Ball *et al.*, 1997; Deary *et al.*, 1999) was unusual in that subjects at the high or low ends of the distribution for 'neuroticism' were selected on the assumption that the 5-HTTLPR affects the trait uniformly across its distribution. However, reanalysis of the data from the initial study revealed that the contribution of the 5-HTTLPR to NEO 'neuroticism' is greatest in the central range of the distribution and actually decreases at the extremes (Sirota *et al.*, 1999). This illustrates the need to obtain genotypes from individuals across the distribution of a trait, and suggests caution in the use of extreme populations in attempting to establish genetic influences on traits that are continuously distributed in the population.

Finally, difficulties in interpretation of population-based association studies due to ethnic differences in 5-HTTLPR allele frequencies have also been raised by recent studies. One found no association between the 5-HTTLPR and NEO 'neuroticism' in a sample of 191 Japanese, or between 5-HTTLPR genotype and TCI 'harm avoidance' in a subsample (Kumakiri *et al.*, 1999). In addition to its relatively small sample size, a major difficulty with this study is that the frequency of the *l*/*l* genotype (corresponding to group L) was only 6% of the total population, giving very low statistical power to detect a genotype-related difference. Another study of association between the 5-HTTLPR and TPQ 'harm avoidance' in a Japanese population is also difficult to interpret due to differences in genotypes related to ethnicity (Katsuragi *et al.*, 1999b). In that case, the small sample ($n = 101$) had a frequency of l/l genotypes of only 4%. From an evolutionary psychological perspective, anxiety is a pervasive and innately driven form of distress that arises in response to actual or threatened exclusion from social groups (Baumeister and Tice, 1990; Buss, 1995). Notably, Nakamura *et al.* (1997) have discussed the higher prevalence of the anxiety and depression-related l/s and s/s genotypes in the context of the extraordinary emotional restraint and interpersonal sensitivity in the Japanese as a possible population-typical adaptation to prevent social exclusion (Ono *et al.*, 1996).

Nevertheless, spurious results due to population stratification cannot be ruled out entirely. It is, however, important to note that, while population stratification may lead to false-positive results, false-negative findings occur due to background factors masking QTL effects (Cardon, 2001a; Pericak-Vance, 1998). Studies which incorporate large samples of different population groups, the assessment of genetic background markers, and within-family study designs, such as the Transmission Disequilibrium Test (TDT), might help to minimize the bidirectional effects of stratification (Cardon, 2001b). In addition to regional or ethnic variations of allele frequency, epistatic and gene–environment interactions may well influence the possible phenotypic effect of a given genotype, especially in behavioural genetics, where roughly equal proportions of genetic effects and non-genetic effects contribute to trait variance. With respect to the 5-HTTLPR, further studies aiming at these questions are clearly needed to resolve these issues, which should include large, community-based cohorts of different populations. Of course, the same is true for other target genes such as DRD4.

The 5-HTTLPR has also been extensively studied in other psychiatric conditions, with both positive and negative findings (for review, see Lesch, 2001b). Especially the link between depression, suicidality, violent suicide attempts, and the 5-HTTLPR remains controversial. Seasonality and seasonal affective disorder (SAD) also seem to be associated with the 5-HTTLPR s allele (Rosenthal *et al.*, 1998; Sher *et al.*, 1999). This effect was shown to be independent of the gene effect on neuroticism, thus arguing for genetic pleiotropy of the 5-HTTLPR gene (Sher *et al.*, 2000). Furthermore, the 5-HTTLPR is thought to be associated with an increased vulnerability to develop nicotine (Hu *et al.*, 2000; Lerman *et al.*, 2000) and alcohol (Sander *et al.*, 1997b) dependence, the latter being comorbid with antisocial PD (Hallikainen *et al.*, 1999; Sander *et al.*, 1998).

As in the 5-HT_{1A} knockout mouse, exaggerated serotonergic neurotransmission has been implicated in the increased anxiety-related behaviours recently reported in 5-HT transporter-deficient mice (Wichems *et al.*, 2000). These findings are consistent with other evidence suggesting that increased 5-HT availability may contribute to increased anxiety in rodents, and the studies reporting that anxiety-related traits in humans are associated with allelic variation of 5-HTT function (Lesch *et al.*, 1996). Mice with a disrupted 5-HTT gene have been suggested as an alternative model to pharmacological studies of SSRI-evoked antidepressant and anxiolytic mechanisms to assess the hypothesized association between 5-HT uptake function and 5-HT_{1A} receptor desensitization (Bengel *et al.*, 1998). Excess serotonergic neurotransmission in mice lacking 5-HT transport results in desensitized and — unlike observations following SSRI administration — downregulated 5-HT_{1A} receptors in the midbrain raphe complex, but not in the hippocampus (Li *et al.*, 2000), and is suspected to play a role in the increased anxiety-related and antidepressant-like behaviours in these mice shown by the Light-Dark and Elevated Zero Maze paradigms, and the Tail Suspension paradigms. In contrast to that of 5-HT_{1A}-deficient mice, the anxiety-related behaviour, which can be reversed by anxiolytics of the benzodiazepine type, is more pronounced in female 5-HTT null mutants.

Dopaminergic Gene Pathway

While the 5-HT system exerts global, brain-wide modulatory functions, the action of the dopamine (DA) system is mediated via four distinct tracts, namely, the nigro-striatal, tubero-infundibular, meso-limbic, and fronto-cortical tract. The nigro-striatal tract, which originates in the substantia nigra and projects to the nucleus caudatus, is involved in motor control and has been implicated in the pathophysiology of Parkinson's disease; the tubero-infundibular system regulates prolactin secretion. While both systems participate in the common side effects of DA receptor antagonists, such as the classic neuroleptic drugs (e.g., dyskinesia, akathisia, and hyperprolactinaemia), they do not appear to be particularly relevant to the psychobiological aspects of dopaminergic neurotransmission. More outstanding in this regard are both the meso-limbic and fronto-cortical tracts, formerly termed the meso-cortico-limbic system. The two systems are thought to play important roles in a variety of psychiatric disease states. According to the DA hypothesis of schizophrenic disorders, functional alterations in the meso-limbic and fronto-cortical tracts underlie specific symptoms observed in schizophrenic psychoses. The meso-limbic system appears to be involved in 'positive' or 'productive' symptoms, such as hallucinations, paranoia, and delusions, whereas the fronto-cortical tract may cause 'negative' symptoms such as disorganization and lack of initiative. Furthermore, the DA system is involved in the brain's reward system and consequently in the pathogenesis of addictive behaviour. Pharmacological disinhibition of dopaminergic neurons in the ventral tegmental area, which project to the nucleus accumbens, results in the activation of the reward mechanism, while blockade of the reward system provokes symptoms similar to drug withdrawal.

Based on its functional neuroanatomy, the DA system seems to be involved in Cluster A PDs, associated in some cases with 'soft signs' of schizophrenic disorders and hence they are labelled by some authors as 'schizophrenia spectrum disorders' (Kety *et al.*, 1971), 'schizoid disease' (Heston, 1970), or 'schizotaxia'. A dysfunctional reward system in conjunction with dopaminergic abnormalities, as reflected by high novelty-seeking behaviour seems to play a role in PDs.

DA is synthesized from tyrosine in two steps. The first step is catalysed by the rate-limiting enzyme tyrosine hydroxylase, and the resulting L-DOPA is then decarboxylated by an aromatic amino acid decarboxylase (DOPA decarboxylase). Dopamine acts on at least five subtypes of receptors termed D1 to D5; the reuptake is performed by a specific DA transporter. Metabolic pathways involve two non-specific enzymes, monoamine oxidase (MAO) and catechol-*O*-methyltransferase (COMT). A critical appraisal of the key components of dopaminergic transmission implicated in PDs follows.

Tyrosine Hydroxylase

Tyrosine hydroxylase (TH) is central to the function of the dopaminergic as well as noradrenergic neurotransmission. In a series of elegant experiments, Zhou *et al.* (1995) showed that targetted inactivation of both TH genes results in an embryonic lethality that was prevented by prenatal administration of L-DOPA. It was also demonstrated that TH-deficient mice pups may be rescued with restored with wild-type noradrenergic cells, although marked behavioural abnormalities persist (Zhou and Palmiter, 1995): TH knockout mice remained hypoactive and refused to eat and drink. Upon acute L-DOPA injection, the behavioural deficits were reversed, and by continuous L-DOPA administration normal growth was restored.

The human TH gene has been assigned to chromosome 11p15 (Craig *et al.*, 1986) near the insulin and IGF1 gene. Several polymorphisms have been identified in the TH gene which cause different forms of Segawa syndrome, an inborn, autosomal, recessive, parkinsonism-like disorder starting in early childhood. Linkage of TH polymorphisms to several psychiatric Axis 1 disorders, including bipolar illness or schizophrenia, has been hypothesized, but the results to date are equivocal. Recently, a seemingly functional tetranucleotide repeat polymorphism ($TCAT_n$) in intron X of the TH gene (M) has been investigated for association with personality traits as assessed by the NEO-PI-R questionnaire in a Swedish population (Persson *et al.*, 2000b). Carriers of the T8 allele of $TCAT_n$ displayed significantly elevated 'neuroticism' scores, which were most prominent in the 'neuroticism' subitems 'angry hostility' and 'vulnerability'. Furthermore, a correlation of the T8 allele with both suicide attempts among subjects suffering from adjustment disorders (Persson *et al.*, 1997) and late-onset alcoholism among other patients was reported (Geijer *et al.*, 1997). It was concluded that the $TCAT_n$ polymorphism is linked to anxiety-related traits, and that the search for gene–gene interactions between $TCAT_n$ and 5-HTTLPR could be promising.

Dopamine (DA) Receptors

Although genomic variations have been identified in all five DA receptor genes, only the role of the D_2, D_3, and D_4 receptor genes (DRD2, DRD3, and DRD4, respectively) has been studied in normal personality and PDs. However, each receptor subtype has been investigated for a possible pathogenetic role in several psychiatric disease states, especially schizophrenic disorders, with inconclusive results (Wong *et al.*, 2000).

The human DRD2 gene, which has been located on chromosome 11q22–23, is subject to alternative splicing, and comprises eight exons. Interestingly, it is able to form a heterodimer with the somatostatin receptor upon binding of the respective ligand (Rocheville *et al.*, 2000). Several polymorphisms of the DRD2 have been studied in personality genetics, especially a *Taq*I restriction fragment length polymorphism (*Taq*I A) in the 3′-untranslated region of the gene (Grandy *et al.*, 1989). Several lines of evidence indicate that the A1 allele is associated with decreased dopaminergic tone in the CNS. A second *Taq*I site, identified between the first intron and the second exon has been termed *Taq*I B (Hauge *et al.*, 1991). Furthermore, a single nucleotide polymorphism (SNP) was found in intron 6 (*Hph* I site) (Sarkar *et al.*, 1991) and a functionally relevant Ser311Cys polymorphism in exon 7, which impairs D2 signal transduction, has been described (Cravchik *et al.*, 1996).

DRD2, the target for neuroleptic agents such as haloperidol or risperidone, has been suggested to be involved in a 'spectrum of DA-related disorders', including substance abuse, pathological gambling, obesity, and Tourette's syndrome (Comings *et al.*, 1996a, b; Noble *et al.*, 1994). Although this hypothesis is controversial, especially severe alcoholism seems to be associated with the *Taq*I A1 allele (Blum *et al.*, 1990). In line with a possible association of DRD2 with addictive behaviour, DRD2 knockout mice do not respond with reward behaviour following administration of morphine (Maldonado *et al.*, 1997), in addition to locomotor disturbances (Baik *et al.*, 1995).

The DRD2 gene locus has also been studied for a possible association with personality traits as well as PDs. Corresponding with the hypothesis of a schizophrenia spectrum disorder as a result of a DA neurotransmission impairment, Blum *et al.* (1997) found an association of the DRD2 *Taq*1 A1 allele with schizoid and avoidant behaviour, suggesting an involvement of DRD2 in PDs of Cluster A. By means of the TPQ questionnaire, it was shown that *Taq*1 A1, *Taq*2 B1, intron 6 alleles alone, and, even more robustly, the corresponding haplotype resulted in higher TPQ 'novelty-seeking' (NS) scores than other allele combinations. When the 7-repeat allele of DRD4 (see below) was present, a further increase of the difference was observed. This DRD2 haplotype also resulted in higher 'persistence' scores, while no influence of DRD4 7-repeat allele was detected; neither polymorphism was associated with 'harm avoidance' (Noble *et al.*, 1998). If replicated, these findings further support the notion of a link between dopaminergic function and NS (Cloninger, 1987). However, de Brettes *et al.* (1998) failed to find any association between *Taq*1 A1 and TPQ NS scores, suggesting that reports on associations between this polymorphism and personality traits should be considered preliminary. The only study investigating the Ser311Cys polymorphism in healthy individuals also yielded negative results regarding a relationship between DRD2 and scores of the TCI, a modified version of the TPQ (Cloninger *et al.*, 1993).

An interesting gene–environment interaction was reported by Ozkaragoz and Noble (2000). Children with the A1 DRD2 allele had higher extraversion scores when living in an alcoholic home; DRD2 A2 allele subjects tended to have lower extraversion levels. This result may link the DRD2 effect on alcohol dependence to environmental factors and personality. Another preliminary finding is the report on an association between DRD2 alleles and the age at first sexual intercourse, explaining the variance by 23% alone and by 55% in combination with DRD1 alleles (Miller *et al.*, 1999). These interesting, but hitherto incompletely understood data on the impact of DRD2 on personality warrant further investigation of gene–gene as well as gene–environment interactions.

Only a few data are available concerning personality traits and DRD3, which is expressed almost exclusively in limbic structures (Sokoloff *et al.*, 1990). Preliminary findings suggest a role for a functional DRD3 polymorphism (*Bal*I) influencing the TPQ NS scores of bipolar patients (Staner *et al.*, 1998); opiate-dependent subjects with high NS scores were found to carry *Bal*I significantly more often (Duaux *et al.*, 1998). As noted above, gene–gene interactions of the Glyc/Ser substitution of DRD3 with both the DRD4-7 repeat allele and the $5HT_{2C}$ Cys23Ser substitution were demonstrated by Ebstein *et al.* (1997c) regarding TPQ 'persistence' and 'reward dependence' scores. In a large population study ($n = 2752$), the *Bal*I polymorphism was investigated for a possible association with personality traits, psychiatric symptoms, and life events (Henderson *et al.*, 2000). Since the EPQ-R (Eysenck's Revised Personality Questionnaire) (Eysenck *et al.*, 1985) and the BIS/BAS (Behavioural Inhibition System/Behavioural Activation System scales) (Carver and White, 1994) were used to assess personality scores, comparison with similar studies investigating DRD3 is difficult. In an initial subsample (including 30% of the final sample), the authors found subjects with at least one serine allele to have higher scores for neuroticism, behavioural inhibition, depression, and anxiety, when experiencing more than one life event recently. However, the gene–environment interaction became non-significant when the full sample was evaluated. A study on the association between the DRD3 polymorphism and alcoholism yielded negative results (Gorwood *et al.*, 1995). All in all, the relevance of the DRD3 in personality traits remains inconclusive, but the search for a possible association and the assessment of environmental factor such as psychosocial stress seem promising.

The potential role of the D4 receptor in the personality traits related to NS behaviour has attracted considerable attention. DRD4 has been mapped to the human chromosome 11p15.5 (Gelernter *et al.*, 1992). Several atypical neuroleptics, including clozapine and olanzapine, preferentially bind to DRD4, making this receptor an attractive therapeutic target. In exon 3 of the DRD4 gene, which codes for the third cytoplasmatic loop, a polymorphic 48-bp repeat was found (Lichter *et al.*, 1993; Van Tol *et al.*, 1992). It varies between 2 and 10 repeat units, resulting in a corresponding length variation of the receptor protein and differential receptor function (Asghari *et al.*, 1994; 1995). The polymorphism has been termed DRD4-*n*R, with *n* being the number of repeats. The 2-, 4-, and 7-repeat alleles are most common; however, allele frequencies show substantial ethnic variability. In addition, several SNPs have been described in the upstream promoter region of DRD4 and examined with respect to their relevance for personality traits and behaviour.

Cloninger and associates have suggested that the personality trait of NS, as defined by the TPQ, is exclusively based on dopaminergic function (Cloninger, 1987). While likely to be rather simplistic, this notion provided a starting point to assess the role of DRD4 in the trait of NS. The initial study and several follow-up studies were conducted by Ebstein and co-workers (reviewed in Ebstein *et al.*,1997b; 2000). In a cohort of 124 Israeli volunteers, higher TPQ NS scores were associated with the DRD-7R allele independently of age or sex (Ebstein *et al.*, 1996) with a case-control design. No association between DRD4 alleles and TPQ 'harm avoidance', 'reward dependence', or 'persistence' was found. Simultaneously, the DRD4 polymorphism and a NS equivalent of the NEO-PI-R were studied in a North American sample that included sib-pairs to allow a complementary within-family design. The concurring results further substantiated the association between DRD4-7R and NS (Benjamin *et al.*, 1996).

These findings prompted a considerable number of groups to follow-up on these studies, with both positive and negative results (Table XXVI-7.2). Several groups succeeded in replicating the effect of the DRD4 polymorphism on NS. An association between DRD4-7R and NS could be found in populations from Finland ($n = 190$, with the TCI, a modified TPQ questionnaire [Ekelund *et al.*, 1999]), Germany ($n = 136$; TPQ) (Strobel *et al.*, 1999), and Japan ($n = 153$; TCI and $n = 69$, females, respectively) (Ono *et al.*, 1997; Tomitaka *et al.*, 1999). Noble *et al.* (1998) found an influence of DRD4-*n*R on NS alone, and an even more pronounced effect in concert with DRD2 polymorphisms.

In contrast, Gelernter *et al.* (1997) studied the DRD4-*n*R polymorphism in a North American sample of mixed ethnicity subdivided into substance-abusing, personality-disordered, and healthy individuals. As reported earlier, addicted subjects had higher NS scores; however, in neither subgroup was a relationship between DRD4 alleles and NS detected. Likewise, in a German sample, the DRD4-*n*R status did not differ between patients with alcohol dependence and controls, even when they were selected for high and low TPQ NS scores (Sander *et al.*, 1997a). Similarly, in two samples from New Zealand — one being rather small ($n = 86$) from a depression treatment trial, and the other from 14 pedigrees with alcoholism ($n = 181$) — no significant correlation between DRD4 genotype and NS was found (Sullivan *et al.*, 1998).

Moreover, in studies of populations from Finland ($n = 193$; TPQ) (Malhotra *et al.*, 1996), Sweden ($n = 126$ and 167, respectively; Karolinska Scale of Personality [KSP] [Jonsson *et al.*, 1997b; Jonsson *et al.*, 1998]), the USA ($n = 200$, NEO-PI-R [Vandenbergh *et al.*, 1997]; $n = 256$, NEO-PI-R [Persson *et al.*, 2000a]; and $n = 58$, TCI [Herbst *et al.*, 2000], respectively), Brazil ($n = 110$ patients with alcohol dependence, TPQ [Bau *et al.*, 1999]), Austria ($n = 109$, TCI [Gebhardt *et al.*, 2000]), and Germany ($n = 190$, TPQ [Kuhn *et al.*, 1999]), no association between DRD4-*n*R and the trait of NS was uncovered. The latter group, however, reported a significant interaction between DRD4 and $5HT_{2C}$ polymorphisms on reward dependence. Finally, a thorough twin study (92 monozygotic and 61 dizygotic twin pairs; TPQ and NEO-PI-R) conducted by Pogue-Geile *et al.* (1998) also did not reveal an influence of DRD4 repeat length on NS as well as positive emotional experience. Of note, several studies had been conducted in similar populations as the positive studies.

The DRD4 polymorphisms were also investigated for association with several psychiatric disorders, with substance abuse and attention deficit hyperactive disorder (ADHD) being the most extensively studied. In ADHD, several, but not all, investigators using case-control and family-based study designs found an increased disease risk associated with DRD4-7R (Castellanos *et al.*, 1998; LaHoste *et al.*, 1996; Rowe *et al.*, 1998; Smalley *et al.*, 1998; Swanson *et al.*, 1998). The findings were also inconsistent in alcoholism. While some researchers reported an association with the DRD4 exon 3 repeat polymorphism (George *et al.*, 1993; Vandenbergh *et al.*, 2000), others failed to do so (Adamson *et al.*, 1995; Geijer *et al.*, 1997; Parsian and Zhang, 1999).

Based on these inconsistent findings, it was concluded that DRD4-*n*R itself is not a susceptibility gene for NS, but rather another gene variant in linkage disequilibrium with DRD4-*n*R (Ekelund *et al.*, 1999). Indeed, a polymorphism in the DRD4 promoter region, which is located at the nucleotide position −521 of the DRD4 gene, and which comprises a C to G transition, was shown to be associated with NS scores (Okuyama *et al.*, 2000). Several follow-up studies either replicated (Ronai *et al.*, 2001) this finding or failed to do so (Mitsuyasu *et al.*, 2001; Strobel *et al.*, in press).

Evidently, efforts to detect associations between the DRD4-*n*R or promoter polymorphism and personality traits have been complicated by the use of small sample sizes (with only two of 33 studies incorporating more than 400 subjects, one being positive and one negative), heterogeneous subject populations, unusual subject selection, and differing methods of personality assessment (Table XXVI-7.2). As mentioned above, gene–gene or gene–environment interactions may also play a role, both within and among different populations. Another major concern is the lack of a within-family design in that study, raising the possibility of artefacts due to ethnic admixture. Thus, it remains controversial whether variation in DRD4 expression and function contributes to the phenotype of NS. Interestingly, DRD4 knockout mice are less active than the wild-type animals, and display supersensitivity to ethanol, cocaine, and methamphetamine (Rubinstein *et al.*, 1997). Furthermore, it was shown that DRD4-deficient mice exhibit a decreased response to novel stimuli, as tested in three paradigms including the open field, emergence, and novel objects test (Dulawa *et al.*, 1999). These results argue for a role of this receptor in explorative and addictive behaviour which appears to represent facets of NS. Whether the investigated polymorphisms are relevant to differences in NS, or whether they are in linkage disequilibrium with alternative, as yet unknown, genetic variations remains to be elucidated.

Dopamine Transporter

Similar to the 5-HT system, only a single transporter protein mediates reuptake of dopamine. The dopamine transporter (DAT, SLC6A3) is structurally similar to other monoamine transporters, and several polymorphisms, including a polymorphic 40-base-pair VNTR in the 3′ untranslated region of the DAT gene, have been identified (Byerley *et al.*, 1993; Sano *et al.*, 1993). While this VNTR-based gene variation seems to play a role in ADHD and addiction, especially cigarette smoking and alcoholism (Barr *et al.*, 2001; Daly *et al.*, 1999; Parsian and Zhang, 1997; Sabol *et al.*, 1999; Ueno *et al.*, 1999), few data are available with respect to personality traits. A weak association between the VNTR 10/10 genotype and schizoid/avoidant behaviour was found in a pilot study by Blum *et al.* (1997). In the context of research on the genetic basis of cigarette smoking, Sabol *et al.* (1999) found the SLC6A3-9 polymorphism of DAT to be associated with lower NS scores, although this was not replicated in a follow-up study (Jorm *et al.*, 2000). Thus, the role of DAT polymorphisms in personality traits is still unclear and warrants further research.

Table XXVI-7.2 Overview of published data on the association between the dopamine DRD4 polymorphisms and temperament or personality traits in general populations and patient samples

Study	n	Population and study design	Tested polymorphism, if different from DRD4-nR	Trait assessment/ inventory	Association of the polymorphism with trait, P	Remarks
Ebstein *et al.*, 1996	124	General, Israeli		TPQ	NS with 7R: $P = 0.013$	
Benjamin *et al.*, 1996	315	General, US, of mixed ethnicity: mostly male		NEO-PI-R	Extraversion with 7R: $P = 0.001$; consciousness, $P = 0.03$	NS (calculated) with 7R, $P = 0.002$; within-sibship analysis positive
Malhotra *et al.*, 1996	193/138	General and alcoholic offenders, Finnish		TPQ	n.s. for controls, for alcoholics *lower* NS with 7R, $P = 0.02$	
Ebstein *et al.*, 1997	120	General, Israeli	Interaction with DRD3 and 5-HT_{2C}	TPQ	5HT2C effect on RD and 'persistence' higher with long DRD4-nR alleles	
Jonsson *et al.*, 1997	126	General, Swedish	DRD4n-R, exon I 12-bp repeat, exon I 13-bp del	KSP	n.s. for all polymorphisms and all traits	
Sander *et al.*, 1997	197/252	General and alcoholics, subgrouped; German		TPQ	n.s. for any trait	
Ono *et al.*, 1997	153	General, Japanese; females		TCI	0.045: L with 'exploratory excitability'	
Gelernter *et al.*, 1997	72/162/107	Controls, substance abuse, PD; US, of mixed ethnicity	DRD4n-R, exon I 13-bp del, 12-bp ins/del, exon III gly194 SNP	TPQ	NS: n.s. for all polymorphisms, except for subgroups (lower NS)	
Vandenbergh *et al.*, 1997	200	General, US; subjects stratified for high and low NS scores from $n = 1143$ sample		NEO-PI-R	n.s. for NS	
Ebstein *et al.*, 1997	94	General, Israeli		TPQ	No significant difference, but NS range differed ($P = 0.01$)	In combination with expanded cohort sign. diff. ($P = 0.01$)
Sullivan *et al.*, 1998	86/181	Depressive patients, alcoholics; New Zealand		TCI	n.s. for NS	
Pogue-Geile *et al.*, 1998	306	General, US, twins (monozygotic 92, dizygotic 61 pairs)	DRD4n-R, exon I 12-bp repeat	TPQ, NEO-PI, EES, SSST	n.s. for NS	Within-sibship analysis also n.s.
Noble *et al.*, 1998	119	General, Caucasian, mean age of 12 years	Interaction with DRD2	TPQ	0.049 for NS	Interaction with minor alleles of DRD2 on NS
Ebstein *et al.*, 1998	81	2 week-old neonates, Israeli	Interaction with 5HTT	NBAS	$P = 0.00026$–0.07, depending on cluster	Significant interaction with 5HTTLPR on orientation
Jonsson *et al.*, 1998	167	General, Swedish	DRD4n-R, exon I 12-bp-R, exon I 13-bp del	KSP	n.s.	
Poston *et al.*, 1998	115	Obese patients, US		KSP	n.s.	n.s. with respect to BMI; L significantly assoc. with high-risk patients

(*continued overleaf*)

Table XXVI-7.2 (*continued*)

Study	n	Population and study design	Tested polymorphism, if different from DRD4-nR	Trait assessment/ inventory	Association of the polymorphism with trait, P	Remarks
Kuhn *et al.*, 1999	190	General, middle European; males	Interaction with 5-HT_{2C}	TPQ	n.s.	Significant interaction of DRD4 with 5HT2c on RD
Auerbach *et al.*, 1999	76	2 month-old infants, Israeli; follow-up of Ebstein *et al.*, 1998	Interaction with 5HTT	IBQ	'Negative emotionality', 0.005; 'distress to limitations', 0.03	Significant interaction with 5HTTLPR
Strobel *et al.*, 1999	136	General, German		TPQ, NEO-FFI, EPQ-R, I7, SSS V	$P = 0.001$ for NS, explaining 8% of the variance	$P = 0.022$ for 'persistence', 0.013 for HA1
Ekelund *et al.*, 1999	190	Finnish with extreme NS scores from cohort of 4773 persons		TCI	2-repeat: 0.01 5-repeat: 0.03	
Tomitaka *et al.*, 1999	69	General, Japanese; females		TCI	0.014 for NS	Significant differences in NS1 and NS3
Bau *et al.*, 1999	110	Alcoholics, Brazilian; males		TPQ	n.s. for NS, RD; $P = 0.001$ for 7R with lower HA	No genotype differences in antisocial PD
Hill *et al.*, 1999	204	Alcoholics with families, US	Interaction with DRD2 and DAT	TPQ, MPQ	No linkage of either polymorphism with NS	Linkage of D2 and D4 polymorphisms with HA and corresponding MPQ scales
Okuyama *et al.*, 1999	86	General, Japanese	Six promoter polymorphisms	TCI	-521C/T polymorphism associated with NS ($P = 0.0001$)	DRD4-nR n.d.
Benjamin *et al.*, 2000	455	General, Israeli	Interactions with 5HTT and COMT	TPQ	5-HTTLPR × D4DR, $P = 0.03$ COMT × 5-HTTLPR, $P = 0.03$ on NS	
Herbst *et al.*, 2000	587	General, US, of mixed ethnicity	5HTT (interaction n.d.)	TCI	n.s.	
Persson *et al.*, 2000	256	General, Caucasian		NEO-PI-R	n.s. for extraversion	
Gebhardt *et al.*, 2000	109	General, Austrian	DRD2 Cys311Ser	TCI	n.s. for any polymorphism and any trait	
Comings *et al.*, 2000	81/119	General, addictives; US, males		TCI	$P < 0.001$ for seven TCI summary scores	Largest effect on self-transcendence
Ronai *et al.*, 2001	109	General, Hungarian	−521 C/T SNP	TCI	NS and CC genotype: n.s. for males; $P < 0.01$ for females	DRD4-nR n.d.
Mitsuyasu *et al.*, 2001	173	General, Japanese	DRD4n-R, five promoter polymorphisms	TCI	NS and any polymorphism: n.s.	−768G > A polymorphism associated with RD ($P = 0.044$)
De Luca *et al.*, 2001	122	Neonates at 1 and 5 months, Italian		EITQ/RITQ	Correlation with adaptability ($P < 0.02$) at $t = 1$ month	Differences not detected at $t = 5$ months
Strobel *et al.*, 2001, submitted	276	General, German	−521 C/T SNP	TPQ	n.s.	

NEO-PI-R and NEO-FFI: Costa and McCrae's NEO Personality Inventory; TPQ/TCI: Cloninger's Tridimensional Personality Questionnaire/Temperament and Character Inventory; KSP: Karolinska Scales of Personality; IBQ: Rothbart's Infant Behaviour Questionnaire; NBAS: Brazelton's Neonatal Assessment Scale; EITQ/RITQ: Early and Revised Infancy Temperament Questionnaires; MPQ: Multidimensional Personality Questionnaire; EES: Eysenck's Extraversion Scale; SSST: Zuckerman's Sensation Seeking Scale; SSS V: Sensation Seeking Scale form V; EPQ: Eysenck's Personality Questionnaire; I7: Eysenck's Impulsivity Questionnaire. NS: 'novelty seeking'; RD: 'reward dependence'; HA: 'harm avoidance'; 7R: 7-repeat allele of DRD4-nR; n.s.: not significant; n.d.: not determined.

Monoamine Metabolic Gene Pathway

Monoamines involved in neurotransmission (5-HT, dopamine, and norepinephrine) share common metabolic pathways: deamination, accomplished by MAO-A and, in the case of the catecholamines, methylation of the 3-hydroxy group, catalysed by the enzyme COMT. An increasing body of evidence indicates that both enzymes are relevant to genetic variation of behaviour.

Monoamine Oxidase (MAO) A

MAO, the enzyme which degrades 5-HT, dopamine, and norepinephrine by oxidative removal of the amino group, occurs in two isoforms, MAO-A and MAO-B, which are encoded by distinct genes. They are located close together on chromosome Xp11.23 (Lan *et al.*, 1989). In the brain, MAO-A is the prevailing isoform and is thought to be crucial for the catabolic metabolism of monoamine neurotransmitters. MAO-A thus links three important transmitter systems. Norrie's disease, the result of an X-chromosomal deletion which includes the MAO-A gene, causes mental retardation, autistic behaviour, motor hyperactivity, and sleep disturbances. These symptoms may, at least in part, be attributed to the lack of MAO activity in the affected individuals (Sims *et al.*, 1989).

A MAO-A-deficient mouse was found to display — as predicted by the function of this enzyme — increased brain concentrations of 5-HT (ninefold), dopamine, and norepinephrine (twofold) (Cases *et al.*, 1995). In addition, cytoarchitectural alterations of the cerebral cortex were demonstrated in these animals: like 5-HTT knockout mice, they show malformation of barrels in the somatosensory cortex (Cases *et al.*, 1996), thus highlighting the morphogenetic role of 5-HT in CNS development. MAO-A knockout mice are also characterized by markedly altered behaviour. Adult mice were more aggressive (Cases *et al.*, 1995; Shih *et al.*, 1999), as tested by the resident-intruder paradigm, and this offensive-aggressive behaviour resulted in an increased number of woundings under standard housing conditions (Popova *et al.*, 2000). Furthermore, male mice had modified sexual behaviour with enhanced "offensive" sexuality. As the behavioural changes, at least in part, could be antagonized by an inhibitor of 5-HT synthesis, parachlorophenylalanine, but not by inhibitors of catecholamine synthesis, the aggressive-offensive behavioural phenotype in MAO-A knockout mice is probably due to altered 5-HT degradation, further underscoring the role of this transmitter system in the balance of fearfulness and aggression and other outward directed behaviours.

In accordance with the observations made in the rodent model, a rare mutation in the human MAO-A gene results in noticeably changed temperament and behaviour. The disorder, termed 'Brunner syndrome' after its first describer, represents an example of transmissible genetic influence on human behaviour. In a large Dutch kindred, all affected males could be shown to suffer from mild, non-dysmorphic mental retardation along with prominent abnormal behavioural changes. This included impulsive-aggressive behaviour, sometimes shown as hypersexuality and attempted rape and exhibitionism, as well as arson and attempted suicide. The disorder is X-linked and was demonstrated to result from a point mutation in the MAO-A gene, changing a glutamine-coding triplet into a stop codon (Brunner *et al.*, 1993a; b). This leads to measurable changes in monoamine metabolism with increased 5-HT levels, as assessed by urinary examinations, as well as the absence of MAO-A activity (Brunner *et al.*, 1993b). These features largely resemble the data obtained from MAO-A knockout mice. Thus, this MAO-A mutation is the only disorder in behavioural genetics nearly to fulfil the criteria of an OGOD type of disorder, albeit there has been a considerable controversy as to the derivation of this notion (Hebebrand and Klug, 1995). Brunner (1996) later made it clear that 'the concept of a gene that directly encodes behaviour is unrealistic', and that MAO-A deficiency results in complex effects on neurotransmitter function as well as behavioural phenotypes.

At first sight, these findings contrast with the antidepressant and aggression-related effects of MAO-A inhibitors such as tranylcypromine. This apparent discrepancy is resolved when brain cytoarchitectural changes are assumed in MAO-A-deficient individuals as reported for MAO-A-deficient mice (Cases *et al.*, 1996). Moreover, drug-induced MAO-A inhibition occurs rapidly, whereas antidepressant effects require approximately 2 weeks and are probably due to neuroadaptional changes which compensate MAO-A inhibition. Nevertheless, Brunner's disease and MAO-A deficiency states are rare, as shown by a thorough screening of a large cohort (Schuback *et al.*, 1999).

The MAO-A gene consists of 15 exons and spans approximately 60 kb. Several polymorphisms have been described in the human MAO-A gene (Black *et al.*, 1991; Hinds *et al.*, 1992). Two single base-pair mutations in the last base of a triplet codon have been described that do not alter the amino acid sequence of the primary transcript but result in the absence or presence of a restriction enzyme site, thus influencing the expression of MAO-A and resulting in 30-fold increase in total enzyme activity (Hotamisligil and Breakefield, 1991). A dinucleotide repeat length polymorphism (MAOCA-1) was not associated with increased aggressivity scores (Vanyukov *et al.*, 1995). Several studies have been conducted on the association of MAO-A polymorphisms and affective disorders, but despite initially promising findings (Lim *et al.*, 1995) only controversial (Lin *et al.*, 2000) or negative results could be found (Furlong *et al.*, 1999; Muramatsu *et al.*, 1997; Parsian and Todd, 1997; Rubinsztein *et al.*, 1996).

In addition, a 30-bp VNTR polymorphism of the MAO-A promotor region has been shown to alter the expression of the enzyme (Deckert *et al.*, 1999; Sabol *et al.*, 1998) and to influence CSF 5-HIAA levels in women, but not men (Jonsson *et al.*, 2000). The longer allele (four repeats) could be shown to be associated with panic disorder in a combined German and Italian sample (Deckert *et al.*, 1999) and unipolar depression (Schulze *et al.*, 2000), both in females only. Regarding bipolar affective disorder, no association was found (Furlong *et al.*, 1999; Syagailo *et al.*, 2001). To date, only two studies have dealt with the MAO-A promotor VNTR polymorphism (MAOALPR) in PDs and provided evidence that this polymorphism is associated with antisocial behaviour in alcohol-dependent patients (Samochowiec *et al.*, 1999) and enhanced impulsivity and aggression in healthy, male subjects (Manuck *et al.*, 2000). More research is needed to clarify the apparently gender-specific effects of MAOALPR on behaviour. Nonetheless, these data again point to a role of the 5-HT system in the regulation of aggression, impulsivity, and negative emotionality.

Catechol-O-Methyltransferase

COMT is an enzyme which, alternatively or subsequentially to MAO, degrades catecholamines by methylation of the 3-hydroxy group of the catecholamine ring scaffold. *S*-Adenosylmethionine is utilized as a methyl group donor in this reaction. The human COMT gene has been mapped to 22q11.1-q11.2 (Grossman *et al.*, 1992), and three different COMT phenotypes have been described with respect to activity and stability differences resulting in low, intermediate, and high levels of enzymatic activity (Weinshilboum and Raymond, 1977). The mode of inheritance suggests the presence of autosomal dominant or codominant alleles. Accordingly, two alleles were identified (G158A). Carrying two 158A alleles results in an up to fourfold decrease of enzymatic activity when compared to homozygosity for 158G, while both alleles appear to be distributed equally (Lachman *et al.*, 1996; Syvanen *et al.*, 1997). Tiihonen and co-workers suggested an association between this polymorphism and alcohol consumption among social drinkers (Kauhanen *et al.*, 2000) as well as the risk of developing 'late-onsets' alcoholism (type 1) (Tiihonen *et al.*, 1999), but not type-2 alcoholism, a form with severe antisocial behaviour (Hallikainen *et al.*, 2000).

Altered COMT activity in affective and schizophrenic disorders has long been suspected, but the results of studies have been equivocal (Dunner *et al.*, 1977; Fahndrich *et al.*, 1980; Gershon and Jonas, 1975; Shulman *et al.*, 1978), so that the enzyme went out of focus for a while. However, in the last 4 years, evidence has accumulated of a role for COMT polymorphisms in self- and outward directed aggression. Male schizophrenic patients were shown to have a higher risk of aggressive and dangerous behaviour when they were homozygous for the low-activity 158A allele (Kotler *et al.*, 1999; Lachman *et al.*, 1998; Strous *et al.*, 1997). Any interaction with both DRD4 and 5-HTTLPR polymorphisms could be excluded (Kotler *et al.*, 1999). Additionally, the suicidal behaviour of male schizophrenic patients again was associated with the 158A allele (Nolan *et al.*, 2000a). In females, the low-activity L allele seems to be associated with OCD (Karayiorgou *et al.*, 1997). In line with these findings, female COMT knockout mice displayed impairment in emotional reactivity; in contrast, male heterozygous mice showed increased aggressive behaviours (Gogos *et al.*, 1998), thus suggesting gender-specific effects of COMT on behaviour similar to MAOALPR variants. Because meticulous investigations of subjects who do not suffer from a psychiatric Axis 1 disorder are lacking, there is obviously a demand for further studies investigating the role of COMT polymorphisms in personality.

The influence of the COMT polymorphism on personality was investigated by Benjamin *et al.* (2000a; b) with the TPQ. An interesting gene–gene interaction was demonstrated. When the individual was homozygous for either 158A or 158G, the presence of the short allele of the 5-HTTLPR raised 'persistence' scores; COMT polymorphism alone had a significant effect as well. When the short 5-HTTLPR allele was absent in combination with both alleles of the high-activity allele of COMT, NS scores could be significantly increased by the presence of the DRD4 7-repeat allele. However, a population study from Australia failed to find any association between the COMT polymorphism (both alleles occurred in the same frequency) and personality traits or psychiatric symptoms (Henderson *et al.*, 2000). As noted above, EPQ-R and BIS/BAS were utilized, a fact which renders comparison with results derived by the TPQ or NEO-PI-R questionnaires difficult. All in all, COMT polymorphisms appear to play a role in aggressive behaviour in male schizophrenic patients and in the behavioural trait of NS, in concert with other genetic variations that have yet to be investigated in greater detail.

Miscellaneous Genes

In contrast to the remarkable amount of genetic research on the 5-HT and dopamine systems, and although there are both functional data and animal models for almost all neurotransmitter and modulator systems (e.g., noradrenergic, GABAergic, adenosinergic, and peptidergic transmission), signalling cascades as well as regulatory and structural proteins, with respect to their influence on behaviour, behavioural genetic studies of other neurotransmitter systems are largely lacking.

Noradrenergic Genes

The noradrenergic system of the brain, which originates primarily in the locus coeruleus, acts as a central arousal system and is thought to play a modulatory role in the 'fight or flight' response and, according to Cloninger, in reward dependence, albeit the latter claim requires further validation. Norepinephrine is synthesized from dopamine by the enzyme dopamine β-hydroxylase (DBH), of which the human gene is located on chromosome 9q34 (Perry *et al.*, 1991). DBH activity has been investigated as a biological marker for various psychiatric disease states, and appears to be correlated with the MMPI (Minnesota Multiphasic Personality Inventory) score (Major *et al.*, 1980). Enzyme activity varies widely among individuals, with a part of the population having very low DBH activity, a variation which has been ascribed to a functional polymorphism in the 5′-flanking region of the gene, resulting in a C to G transition and explaining up to 50% of the activity variation (Zabetian *et al.*, 2001). No linkage of DBH polymorphisms to Axis 1 disorders was found, although DBH seems to play a role in nicotine dependence (McKinney *et al.*, 2000). While DBH activity measures in serum and CSF appear to link DBH to personality traits, as well as to life events, education, and even response to psychotherapy, no data on DBH polymorphisms and personality (disorders) have been reported to date. DBH thus remains an attractive candidate gene.

Although several polymorphisms in adrenergic receptor genes have been identified, and both ADRA2A and ADRA2C gene polymorphisms have been shown to be involved in ADHD and learning disorders (Comings *et al.*, 1999), only a single study deals with the influence of adrenoceptors on personality traits. Comings *et al.* (2000c) reported that a single base-pair *Msp*I polymorphism in the promoter region of the ADRA2A is associated with irritability (as assessed by the Brown Adult Attention Deficit Disorder [BADD] scale), indirect hostility, negativity, irritability, and verbal hostility (as measured by the Buss-Durkee Hostility Inventory [BDHI]) in two populations ($n = 123$ and 204, respectively), but not with aggressiveness subscales. These results argue for a role of ADRA2A in irritability, as proposed by Coccaro *et al.* (1991). In this study, which awaits replication, the polymorphism accounted for 2–8% of the variance; however, no significant association with TCI subscales was found, underscoring the importance of using appropriate questionnaires. No studies investigating the role of norepinephrine transporter (NET1) polymorphisms in personality or behaviour have been published to date, even though NET1 is an outstanding candidate gene.

GABAergic Genes

Following ground-breaking studies by Mohler and co-workers (Crestani *et al.*, 1999), who generated mice lacking the γ_2 subunit of the GABA-A (gamma-aminobutyric acid type A) receptor, a notable body of evidence has been accumulated that GABA-A function is compromised in anxiety disorders. Preliminary data suggest that GABA receptor polymorphisms might be involved in the pathogenesis of alcoholism (Parsian and Zhang, 1999; Sander *et al.*, 1999a, b), as well as the glutamate transporter gene EAAT2 (Sander *et al.*, 2000). However, studies on PDs are largely lacking, although one group found a polymorphism in the γ_2 subunit of the GABA-A receptor to be associated with antisocial PD (Loh *et al.*, 2000).

Nitric Oxide

Nitric oxide (NO) was the first to be discovered substance in a class of novel gaseous messenger molecules, acting as paracrine and highly diffusible neurotransmitters. NO or a precursor molecule is synthesized by a family of three H_4Bip-dependent enzymes termed NO synthases (NOS-I, II, and III). NO appears to play a role in learning, memory, and long-term potentiation in the hippocampus (for a review, see Snyder and Ferris, 2000). By the modulation of oxytocin release, NO inhibits maternal behaviour in female rats (Okere *et al.*, 1996); however, male mice in which the neuronal NOS isoform has been knocked out (nNOS$^{-/-}$ rats), like mice treated with an NO inhibitor (Demas *et al.*, 1997), show a clear increase in aggressive and sexual behaviour (Nelson *et al.*, 1995). Moreover, it was recently demonstrated that the aggressive behaviour of $NOS^{-/-}$ mice is apparently due to deficient $5\text{-}HT_{1A}$ and $5\text{-}HT_{1B}$ receptor functioning and a selective decrease in 5-HT turnover, especially in the cortex, hippocampus, amygdala, and midbrain (Chiavegatto *et al.*, 2001). NO thus seems to have a modulatory effect on the serotonergic system, a finding which functionally couples two ontogenetically old and major signalling pathways. Unfortunately, no data on NOS functioning and/or NOS polymorphisms with respect to human behaviour are available yet.

Finally, Comings *et al.* (2000a) reported that a dinucleotide polymorphism in the 5′ region of the neutral endopeptidase gene (coding for membrane metalloendopeptidase [MME]) is significantly associated with SCL-90 scores for (phobic) anxiety and obsessive compulsivity. MME is one of the major enzymes for enkephalin degradation; the report thus argues for a role of enkephalin pathway polymorphisms in the genetic variation of anxiety. Clearly, further studies are needed to strengthen this hypothesis. A tetranucleotide polymorphism of the human transcription factor AP-2β gene was shown to be gender-specifically associated with guilt, anxiety, psychasthenia, and indirect aggression, as measured by the Karolinska Scales of Personality (KSP; $n = 137$) (Damberg *et al.*, 2000). Mothers with a son suffering from fragile-X syndrome, and who themselves had a full mutation or a premutation of the FMR-1 gene, which is responsible for the fragile-X syndrome, were found to have social phobia as well as avoidant and schizotypal PD more often than controls (Franke *et al.*, 1998; Levitas, 1996; Sobesky *et al.*, 1994), although this was not evident in MMPI testing (Steyaert *et al.*, 1994).

GENE–GENE INTERACTION

Since a considerable number of genes appear to contribute to the phenotypic expression of anxiety-related behaviour, dissection of gene–gene interaction (i.e., epistasis) in the development of personality and behavioural traits is a pertinent and exciting avenue of research. Moreover, in the evaluation of complex genetic effects, it seems to be essential to control for environmental factors. Recent studies have therefore focused on the neonatal period, a time in early development when environmental influences may be minimal, and least likely to confound associations between temperament and genes. In this context, the term ‘temperament’ is used to refer to the psychological qualities of infants that display considerable variation and have a relatively, but not indefinitely, stable biological basis in the individual's genotype, even though different phenotypes may emerge as the child grows (Kagan, 1989).

Ebstein *et al.* (1998) investigated the behavioural effects of the VNTR polymorphism in exon 3 of the dopamine D4 receptor (DRD4), which had previously been linked to the TPQ personality trait of NS, as discussed in detail above (Benjamin *et al.*, 1996; Ebstein *et al.*, 1996), and of 5-HTTLPR, which seems to influence NEO ‘neuroticism’ and TPQ ‘harm avoidance’, in 2-week-old neonates ($n = 81$). Neonate temperament and behaviour were assessed by the Brazelton neonatal assessment scale (NBAS). In addition to a significant association of the DRD4 polymorphism across four behavioural clusters relevant to temperament (orientation, motor organization, range of state, and regulation of state), an interaction was observed between the DRD4 polymorphism and 5-HTTLPR. The presence of the 5-HTTLPR *s/s* genotype decreased the orientation score for the group of neonates lacking the long variant of DRD4. The D4DR polymorphism–5-HTTLPR interaction was also assessed in a sample of adult subjects. Interestingly, there was no significant effect of the L-DRD4 genotype in those subjects homozygous for 5-HTTLPR s, whereas in the group without the homozygous genotype, the effect of L-DRD4 was significant and represented 13% of the variance in NS scores between groups. Furthermore, the $5\text{-}HT_{2C}$ polymorphism in conjunction with DRD-*n*R accounted for 30% of the variance for persistence and 13% of ‘reward dependence’ assessed by the TPQ (Ebstein *et al.*, 1997c), and DRD2 and DRD4 polymorphisms seem to exert synergistic effects on NS (Noble *et al.*, 1998).

In this series of landmark studies by Ebstein and his group, temperament and behaviour of the infants were re-examined at 2 months with Rothbart's Infant Behaviour Questionnaire (IBQ) as well as at 1 year with a structured play situation and an information-processing task (Auerbach *et al.*, 1999; 2001). There were significant negative correlations between neonatal orientation and motor organization as measured by the NBAS at 2 weeks and negative emotionality, especially distress in daily situations, at 2 months of age. Furthermore, grouping of the infants by DRD4 polymorphism and 5-HTTLPR revealed significant main effects for negative emotionality and distress. Infants with long DRD4 alleles had lower scores on ‘negative emotionality’ and ‘distress to limitations’ than infants with short DRD4 alleles. In contrast, infants homozygous for the 5-HTTLPR s allele had higher scores on ‘negative emotionality’ and ‘distress’ than infants with the *l/s* or *l/l* genotypes. Infants with the *s/s* genotype who also were lacking the NS-associated long DRD4 alleles showed most ‘negative emotionality’ and ‘distress’, temperament traits that possibly contribute to the predisposition to adult neuroticism.

In addition, an interaction between the 5-HTT gene and the COMT gene has been shown to influence the trait of ‘persistence’ (RD2), a subscale of TPQ major personality factor ‘reward dependence’. ‘Persistence’ is considered to be highly adaptive in the presence of stable intermittent reward patterns. Persistent individuals are eager, ambitious, and determined overachievers (Cloninger *et al.*, 1993). In the presence of COMT Val/Val or Met/Met homozygosity, the low 5-HTT function 5-HTTLPR *s* allele significantly raised TPQ RD2 scores, including ‘perfectionism’, in a sample of 577 healthy subjects (Benjamin *et al.*, 2000b). Benjamin *et al.* (2000a) also investigated the interaction of three different gene variants, DRD4, 5-HTT, and COMT, and TPQ personality factors in 455 individuals. In the absence of the 5-HTTLPR *s* allele and in the presence of the high enzyme activity COMT Val/Val genotype, NS scores were higher in the presence of the DRD4 7-repeat allele. In a within-family design, siblings who shared identical genotype groups for all three polymorphisms had significantly correlated TPQ NS scores, whereas sibs with dissimilar genotypes in at least one polymorphism showed no correlation.

Since a large number of epistatic interactions are anticipated to bear a considerable potential of false-positive findings that may lead to meaningless conclusions, gene–gene interaction analyses should at this stage be limited to polymorphisms known to be functional, preferentially within a single neural circuit, such as the 5-HT system, or demonstrated to be associated with behavioural phenotypes of interest.

GENE–ENVIRONMENT INTERACTION

It is no longer controversial whether nature or nurture shapes personality development, but it remains elusive how complex genetic and environmental factors interact in the formation of a behavioural phenotype. While genetic research has typically focused either on normal personality characteristics or on PDs, with few investigations evaluating the genetic and environmental relationship between the two, it is of critical importance to answer the questions of whether a certain quantitative trait aetiopathogenetically influences the disorder, or whether the trait is a syndromal dimension of the disorder.

Under the influence of the sociobiological concept of Edward O. Wilson (Wilson, 1978), there has also been an increasing interest in human personality, particularly the ‘big five’ personality dimensions, from the evolutionary perspective (Buss, 1995). These five dimensions may define the framework for adapting to other people, a crucial task in long-term reproductive success. Extraversion and agreeableness are important to the formation of social structures ranging from pair-bonds to coalitions or groups; emotional stability and conscientiousness are critical to the endurance of these structures; openness may reflect the capacity for innovation. Since the genetic basis of present-day personality dimensions may reflect selective forces among our remote ancestors, we have recently focused our research efforts on rhesus monkeys. In this non-human primate model, environmental influences are probably less complex, can be more easily controlled, and are thus less likely to confound associations between temperament and genes.

Human and non-human primate behaviour is similarly affected by deficits in 5-HT function. In rhesus monkeys, 5-HT turnover, as measured by cerebrospinal (CSF) 5-HIAA concentrations, has a strong heritable component and is traitlike, with demonstrated stability over an individual's lifespan (Higley *et al.*, 1991; 1992b). Moreover, CSF 5HIAA concentrations are subject to the long-lasting influence of deleterious events early in life as well as of situational stressors. Monkeys separated from their mothers and reared in the absence of conspecific adults (peer-reared) have altered serotonergic function and exhibit behavioural deficits throughout their lifetimes when compared to their mother-reared counterparts.

Comparison of different mammalian species indicates that the 5-HTTLPR is unique to humans and simian primates. In hominoids, all alleles originate from variation at a single locus (polymorphic locus 1, PL1), whereas an alternative locus for a 21-bp length variation (PL2) was found in the 5-HTTLPR of rhesus monkeys (rh5-HTTLPR) (Lesch *et al.*, 1997). The fact that the 5-HTTLPR is encountered in hominoids and the cercopithecoids, represented by the macaques, indicates remarkable conservation of this part of the 5-HTT gene promoter throughout the different lineages of these two superfamilies, and suggests that a progenitor 5-HTTLPR sequence, possibly representing viral DNA, was introduced into the genome some 40 million years ago. The appearance of the 5-HTTLPR is therefore an example of a one-time event in the evolutionary history of a species. The 5-HTTLPR sequence may be informative in the comparison of closely related species, and it reflects the phylogeny of the old world monkeys, great apes, and humans. The presence of an analogous rh5-HTTTLPR and the resulting allelic variation of 5-HTT activity in rhesus monkeys provides a unique model to dissect the relative contribution of genes and environmental sources to central serotonergic function and related behavioural outcomes.

In order to study this genotype–environment interaction, the association between central 5-HT turnover and the rh5-HTTLPR genotype was tested in rhesus monkeys with well-characterized environmental histories. This sample of rhesus monkeys ($n = 177$) showed allele frequencies of 83% for the 24-repeat allele (long, [l]) and 16% for the 23-repeat (short, [s]) rh5-HTTLPR variant with a genotype distribution of 68% l/l, 31% l/s, and 1% s/s; one individual was heterozygous for a rare allele with an additional repeat unit ($\times l$) similar to longer alleles found occasionally in humans (Lesch *et al.*, 1997). The monkeys' rearing fell into one of the following categories: mother-reared, either reared with the biological mother or cross-fostered; or peer-reared, either with a peer group of 3–4 monkeys or with an inanimate surrogate and daily contact with a playgroup of peers. Peer-reared monkeys were separated from their mothers, placed in the nursery at birth, and given access to peers at 30 days of age, either continuously or during daily play sessions. Mother-reared and cross-fostered monkeys remained with the mother, typically within a social group. At roughly 7 months of age, mother-reared monkeys were weaned and placed together with their peer-reared cohort in large, mixed-gender social groups. The frequency of the l/l genotype was 70% for mother-reared ($n = 79$) and 68% for peer-reared monkeys ($n = 95$), respectively; subjects with the rare genotypes s/s and $l/\times l$ were excluded from subsequent analyses.

Since the monkey population comprised two groups that received dramatically different social and rearing experience early in life, the interactive effects of environmental experience and the rh5-HTTLPR on cisternal CSF 5-HIAA levels and 5-HT-related behaviour was assessed. CSF 5-HIAA concentrations were significantly influenced by genotype for peer-reared, but not for mother-reared, subjects (Bennett *et al.*, 2001). Peer-reared rhesus monkeys with the low-activity rh5-HTTLPR s allele had significantly lower concentrations of CSF 5-HIAA than their homozygous l/l counterparts. Low 5-HT turnover in monkeys with the s allele is congruent with *in vitro* studies that show reduced binding and transcriptional efficiency of the 5-HTT gene to be associated with the 5-HTTLPR s allele (Lesch *et al.*, 1996). This suggests that the rh5-HTTLPR genotype is predictive of CSF 5-HIAA concentrations, but that early experiences make unique contributions to variation in later 5-HT functioning. This finding is the first to provide evidence of an environment-dependent association between a polymorphism in the 5′-regulatory region of the 5-HTT gene and a direct measure of 5-HT functioning, cisternal CSF 5HIAA concentration, thus revealing an interaction between rearing environment and rhHTTLPR genotype. Similar to the 5-HTTLPR's influence on NEO 'neuroticism' in humans, however, the effect size is small, with 4.7% of variance in CSF 5-HIAA accounted for by the rh5-HTTLPR–rearing environment interaction.

Previous work has shown that monkeys' early experiences have long-term consequences for the functioning of the central 5-HT system, as indicated by robustly altered CSF 5-HIAA levels, as well as anxiety and depression-related behaviour, in monkeys deprived of their parents at birth and raised only with peers (Higley *et al.*, 1991; 1992b). Intriguingly, the biobehavioural results of deleterious early experiences of social separation are consistent with the notion that the 5-HTTLPR may influence the risk of affective spectrum disorders. Evolutionary preservation of two prevalent 5-HTTLPR variants and the resulting allelic variation in 5-HTT expression may be part of the genetic mechanism resulting in the emergence of temperamental traits that facilitate adaptive functioning in the complex social worlds most primates inhabit. The uniqueness of the 5-HTTLPR among humans and simian non-human primates, but not among prosimians or other mammals, along with the role 5-HT plays in complex primate sociality, forms the basis for the hypothesized relationship between the 5-HTT function and the personality traits that mediate individual differences in social behaviour. Accumulating evidence demonstrates the complex interplay between individual differences in the central 5-HT system and social success. In monkeys, lowered 5-HT functioning, as indicated by decreased CSF 5-HIAA levels, is associated with lower rank within a social group, less competent social behaviour, and greater impulsive aggression (Higley *et al.*, 1992b; Mehlman *et al.*, 1995). It is well established that, while subjects with low CSF 5-HIAA concentrations are no more likely to engage in competitive aggression than other monkeys, when they do engage in aggression it frequently escalates to violent and hazardous levels.

Association between the rh5-HTTLPR genotype and aggressive behaviour was studied by analysing the joint effects of genotype and early rearing environment on competition-elicited aggression. Socially dominant mother-reared monkeys were more likely than their peer-reared counterparts to engage in competitive aggression. Moreover, under both rearing conditions, monkeys with the low-activity s allele exhibited more aggressive behaviours than their l/l counterparts. The lack of a genotype for competitive aggression in rearing interaction indicates that subjects with the s allele, while unlikely to win in a competitive encounter, are more inclined to persist in aggression once it begins. A role of s

allele-dependent low-5HTT function in non-human primate aggressive behaviour is in remarkable agreement with the association in humans between the NEO subscales 'neuroticism' (increased 'angry hostility') and 'agreeableness' (decreased 'compliance' = increased aggressiveness and hostility) and 5-HTTLPR *s* genotypes.

As the scope of human studies has been extended to the neonatal period, a time in early development when environmental influences are modest and least likely to confound gene–temperament associations, complementary approaches have recently been applied to non-human primates. Rhesus monkey infants heterozygous for the *s* and *l* variant of the rhHTTLPR (*l/s*) displayed higher behavioural stress-reactivity than infants homozygous for the long variant of the allele (*l/l*) (Champoux *et al.*, 1999). Mother-reared and peer-reared monkeys ($n = 36$ and $n = 83$, respectively) were assessed on days 7, 14, 21, and 30 of life, on a standardized primate neurobehavioural test designed to measure orienting, motor maturity, reflex functioning, and temperament. The main effects of genotype, and, in some cases, interactions between rearing condition and genotype, were demonstrated for items indicative of orienting, attention, and temperament. In general, heterozygote animals demonstrated diminished orientation, lower attentional capabilities, and increased affective responding relative to *l/l* homozygotes. However, the genotype effects were more pronounced for animals raised in the neonatal nursery than for animals reared by their mothers. These results demonstrate the contributions of rearing environment and genetic background, and their interaction, in a non-human primate model of behavioural development.

As in humans, the neonatal period in rhesus monkeys represents a time when environmental influences are only starting to gain influence on the genetic make-up, thus rendering relationships between temperament, behaviour and genetic variants less complex. When tested early in life at post-natal days 7–30, rhesus monkey infants with the low-expression rh5-HTTLPR *s* allele displayed higher behavioural stress-reactivity than infants homozygous for the *l* allele (Champoux *et al.*, 1999). Thus, non-human primate models are consistent with the finding in humans that it is the low-activity *s* allele that is associated with increased negative emotionality. The findings are intriguing in light of speculations that the recent appearance of the 5-HTTLPR-associated genetic variation may have helped permit more sophisticated modulation of social behaviours during the evolution of higher-order primates (Lesch *et al.*, 1997). The 5-HTT-personality association data also emphasize the advantage of the five-factor NEO-PI-R and the lexical tradition of personality theory on which it is based. This view of personality is consistent with evolutionary perspectives on personality, and the trait terms in natural language may best reflect individual behavioural differences important to group survival and reproductive success (Buss, 1995).

Another well-defined behavioural pattern among non-human primates that seems to be directly related to CSF 5-HIAA concentrations is dispersal from the natal group (Mehlman *et al.*, 1995). Most male rhesus monkeys leave their natal group and either visit or join other social groups or form small, transient all-male groups before returning to their birth group. While natal dispersal occurs at a highly variable age and is almost always associated with loss of social status and an increase in stress, injury, and mortality, its cause and intention remain controversial. Interestingly, a recent study by Trefilov *et al.* (2000) showed a gene-dose effect of the rh5-HTTLPR *s* variant on the age of dispersal, with s/s homozygotes leaving earlier than carriers of the *l* allele. This finding further supports the notion that impaired 5-HTT function resulting in low 5-HT turnover is associated with impulsive behaviour together with a high tendency to risk-taking activity that leads to early dispersal.

Taken together, these findings provide evidence of an environment-dependent association between allelic variation of 5-HTT expression and central 5-HT function, and suggest that specific genetic factors play a role in 5-HT-mediated social competence in primates. The objective of further studies will be the elucidation of the relationship between the rh5-HTTLPR genotype and sociability in monkeys, as this behaviour is expressed with characteristic individual differences both in daily life and in response to challenge. Because rhesus monkeys exhibit temperamental and behavioural traits that parallel anxiety, depression, and aggression-related personality dimensions associated in humans with the low-activity 5-HTTLPR variant, it may be possible to search for evolutionary continuity in this genetic mechanism for individual differences. Nonhuman primate studies may also be useful to help identify environmental factors that either compound the vulnerability conferred by a particular genetic make-up or, conversely, act to improve the behavioural outcome associated with that genotype.

CONCLUSIONS

The integration of emerging tools and technologies for genetic analysis will further prepare the ground for an advanced stage of gene identification and functional studies in personality and behavioural genetics. Several refined concepts should therefore be adopted.

First, future studies will require extended, homogeneous, and ethnically matched population and patient samples in conjunction with family-based designs. In order to control for non-independence within cohorts and thus to minimize the risk of population stratification bias, rigorous methods of 'genomic control' have been designed. These statistical strategies are based on the assessment of 60 SNPs or genotypes of 100 unlinked microsatellite markers spread throughout the genome to adjust the significance level of a candidate gene polymorphism (Bacanu *et al.*, 2000; Pritchard *et al.*, 2000). With recent advances in molecular genetics, the rate-limiting step in identifying candidate genes has nevertheless become the definition of phenotype.

Second, more functionally relevant polymorphisms in genes within a single neurotransmitter system, or in genes that comprise a developmental and functional unit in their concerted actions, need to be identified and investigated in large association studies both to avoid stratification artefacts and to elucidate complex epistatic and epigenetic interactions of multiple loci with the environment. Not only will DNA variants in coding and regulatory regions of genes be useful in systematic genome scans to identify genes associated with personality and behaviour, but they will also make it possible to study integrated systems of gene pathways as an important step on the route to behavioural genomics. Although great strides have been made in understanding the diversity of the human genome, including the frequency, distribution, and type of genetic variation that exists, the feasibility of applying this information to uncover useful genomic markers of behavioural traits remains uncertain. The implications of using SNPs to uncover markers for behavioural traits and disorders, as well as treatment response, such as population and patient sample size, SNP density and genome coverage, SNP functionality, and data interpretation that will be important for determining the suitability of genomic information are, however, rarely addressed. Success will eventually depend on the availability of SNPs in the coding or regulatory regions (cSNPs or rSNPs, respectively) of a large number of candidate genes as well as knowledge of the average extent of linkage disequilibrium between SNPs, the development of high-throughput technologies for genotyping SNPs, identification of protein-altering SNPs by DNA and protein microarray-assisted expression analysis, and collection of DNA from well-assessed cohorts. As more appreciation of the potential for polymorphisms in gene regulatory regions to affect gene expression is gained, knowledge of novel functional variants is likely to emerge.

Third, genetic influences are not the only pathways that lead to individual differences in personality dimensions, behaviour, psychopathology, and drug response. Complex traits are most likely to be generated by a complex interaction of environmental and experiential factors with a number of genes and their products. Even pivotal regulatory proteins of cellular pathways and neurocircuits are likely to have only a very modest, if not minimal, impact, while noise from non-genetic mechanisms obstructs identification of relevant gene variants. Although current methods for the detection of gene–gene and gene–environment interaction in behavioural genetics are largely indirect, the most relevant consequence of gene identification for behavioural traits and psychotropic drug effects may be that it will provide the tools required to clarify systematically the effects of gene–environment interaction on brain development and plasticity.

Finally, future benefits will stem from novel techniques in molecular cell biology, transgenics, and gene-transfer technologies. However, in the postgenomic world, behavioural genetic research will require integration of the entire spectrum of genomics, DNA variants, gene expression, proteomics, brain development, structure, and function, as well as behaviour, in a wide range of species. Although bioinformatics resources are evolving in most of these areas, the incorporation of these resources from the perspective of the functional genomics of personality and behaviour will greatly facilitate research.

REFERENCES

Abbar, M., Courtet, P., Amadeo, S., Caer, Y., Mallet, J., Baldy-Moulinier, M., Castelnau, D. and Malafosse, A., 1995. Suicidal behaviors and the tryptophan hydroxylase gene. *Arch Gen Psychiatry*, **52**, 846–849.

Adamson, M.D., Kennedy, J., Petronis, A., Dean, M., Virkkunen, M., Linnoila, M. and Goldman, D., 1995. DRD4 dopamine receptor genotype and CSF monoamine metabolites in Finnish alcoholics and controls. *Am J Med Genet*, **60**, 199–205.

Aghajanian, G.K. and Marek, G.J., 1999. Serotonin and hallucinogens. *Neuropsychopharmacology*, **21**, 16S–23S.

Allman, W.F., 1994. *The Stone Age Present*. Simon & Schuster, New York.

American Psychiatric Association, 1994. *Diagnostic and Statistical Manual of Mental Disorders*, 4th edn. American Psychiatric Association, Washington, DC.

Asberg, M., Eriksson, B., Martensson, B., Traskman-Bendz, L. and Wagner, A., 1986. Therapeutic effects of serotonin uptake inhibitors in depression. *J Clin Psychiatry*, **47**(Suppl), 23–35.

Asghari, V., Sanyal, S., Buchwaldt, S., Paterson, A., Jovanovic, V. and Van Tol, H.H., 1995. Modulation of intracellular cyclic AMP levels by different human dopamine D4 receptor variants. *J Neurochem*, **65**, 1157–1165.

Asghari, V., Schoots, O., van Kats, S., Ohara, K., Jovanovic, V., Guan, H.C., Bunzow, J.R., Petronis, A. and Van Tol, H.H., 1994. Dopamine D4 receptor repeat: analysis of different native and mutant forms of the human and rat genes. *Mol Pharmacol*, **46**, 364–373.

Auerbach, J., Geller, V., Lezer, S., Shinwell, E., Belmaker, R.H., Levine, J. and Ebstein, R., 1999. Dopamine D4 receptor (D4DR) and serotonin transporter promoter (5-HTTLPR) polymorphisms in the determination of temperament in 2-month-old infants. *Mol Psychiatry*, **4**, 369–373.

Auerbach, J.G., Benjamin, J., Faroy, M., Geller, V. and Ebstein, R., 2001. DRD4 related to infant attention and information processing: a developmental link to ADHD? *Psychiatr Genet*, **11**, 31–35.

Bacanu, S.A., Devlin, B. and Roeder, K., 2000. The power of genomic control. *Am J Hum Genet*, **66**, 1933–1944.

Baik, J.H., Picetti, R., Saiardi, A., Thiriet, G., Dierich, A., Depaulis, A., Le Meur, M. and Borrelli, E., 1995. Parkinsonian-like locomotor impairment in mice lacking dopamine D2 receptors. *Nature*, **377**, 424–428.

Ball, D., Hill, L., Freeman, B., Eley, T.C., Strelau, J., Riemann, R., Spinath, F.M., Angleitner, A. and Plomin, R., 1997. The serotonin transporter gene and peer-rated neuroticism. *Neuroreport*, **8**, 1301–1304.

Barr, C.L., Xu, C., Kroft, J., Feng, Y., Wigg, K., Zai, G., Tannock, R., Schachar, R., Malone, M., Roberts, W., Nothen, M.M., Grunhage, F., Vandenbergh, D.J., Uhl, G., Sunohara, G., King, N. and Kennedy, J.L., 2001. Haplotype study of three polymorphisms at the dopamine transporter locus confirm linkage to attention-deficit/hyperactivity disorder. *Biol Psychiatry*, **49**, 333–339.

Battersby, S., Ogilvie, A.D., Blackwood, D.H., Shen, S., Muqit, M.M., Muir, W.J., Teague, P., Goodwin, G.M. and Harmar, A.J., 1999. Presence of multiple functional polyadenylation signals and a single nucleotide polymorphism in the 3′ untranslated region of the human serotonin transporter gene. *J Neurochem*, **72**, 1384–1388.

Bau, C.H., Roman, T., Almeida, S. and Hutz, M.H., 1999. Dopamine D4 receptor gene and personality dimensions in Brazilian male alcoholics. *Psychiatr Genet*, **9**, 139–143.

Baumeister, R.F. and Tice, D.M., 1990. Anxiety and social exclusion. *J Soc Clin Psychol*, **9**, 165–195.

Bellivier, F., Leboyer, M., Courtet, P., Buresi, C., Beaufils, B., Samolyk, D., Allilaire, J.F., Feingold, J., Mallet, J. and Malafosse, A., 1998. Association between the tryptophan hydroxylase gene and manic-depressive illness. *Arch Gen Psychiatry*, **55**, 33–37.

Bengel, D., Murphy, D.L., Andrews, A.M., Wichems, C.H., Feltner, D., Heils, A., Mossner, R., Westphal, H. and Lesch, K.P., 1998. Altered brain serotonin homeostasis and locomotor insensitivity to 3,4-methylenedioxymethamphetamine ('Ecstasy') in serotonin transporter-deficient mice. *Mol Pharmacol*, **53**, 649–655.

Benjamin, J., Ebstein, R.P. and Lesch, K.P., 1998. Genes for personality traits: implications for psychopathology. *Int J Neuropsychopharmacol*, **1**, 153–168.

Benjamin, J., Li, L., Patterson, C., Greenberg, B.D., Murphy, D.L. and Hamer, D.H., 1996. Population and familial association between the D4 dopamine receptor gene and measures of novelty seeking. *Nat Genet*, **12**, 81–84.

Benjamin, J., Osher, Y., Kotler, M., Gritsenko, I., Nemanov, L., Belmaker, R.H. and Ebstein, R.P., 2000a. Association between Tridimensional Personality Questionnaire (TPQ) traits and three functional polymorphisms: dopamine receptor D4 (DRD4), serotonin transporter promoter region (5-HTTLPR) and catechol *O*-methyltransferase (COMT). *Mol Psychiatry*, **5**, 96–100.

Benjamin, J., Osher, Y., Lichtenberg, P., Bachner-Melman, R., Gritsenko, I., Kotler, M., Belmaker, R.H., Valsky, V., Drendel, M. and Ebstein, R.P., 2000b. An interaction between the catechol *O*-methyltransferase and serotonin transporter promoter region polymorphisms contributes to Tridimensional Personality Questionnaire persistence scores in normal subjects. *Neuropsychobiology*, **41**, 48–53.

Bennett, A.J., Lesch, K.P., Heils, A., Long, J., Lorenz, J., Shoaf, S.E., Champoux, M., Suomi, S.J., Linnoila, M. and Higley, J.D., 2002. Early experience and serotonin transporter gene variation interact to influence primate CNS function. *Mol Psychiatry*, **7**, 118–122.

Bennett, P.J., McMahon, W.M., Watabe, J., Achilles, J., Bacon, M., Coon, H., Grey, T., Keller, T., Tate, D., Tcaciuc, I., Workman, J. and Gray, D., 2000. Tryptophan hydroxylase polymorphisms in suicide victims. *Psychiatr Genet*, **10**, 13–17.

Black, G.C., Chen, Z.Y., Craig, I.W. and Powell, J.F., 1991. Dinucleotide repeat polymorphism at the MAOA locus. *Nucleic Acids Res*, **19**, 689.

Blairy, S., Massat, I., Staner, L., Le Bon, O., Van Gestel, S., Van Broeckhoven, C., Hilger, C., Hentges, F., Souery, D. and Mendlewicz, J., 2000. 5-HT2a receptor polymorphism gene in bipolar disorder and harm avoidance personality trait. *Am J Med Genet*, **96**, 360–364.

Blakely, R.D., De Felice, L.J. and Hartzell, H.C., 1994. Molecular physiology of norepinephrine and serotonin transporters. *J Exp Biol*, **196**, 263–281.

Blum, K., Braverman, E.R., Wu, S., Cull, J.G., Chen, T.J., Gill, J., Wood, R., Eisenberg, A., Sherman, M., Davis, K.R., Matthews, D., Fischer, L., Schnautz, N., Walsh, W., Pontius, A.A., Zedar, M., Kaats, G. and Comings, D.E., 1997. Association of polymorphisms of dopamine D2 receptor (DRD2), and dopamine transporter (DAT1) genes with schizoid/avoidant behaviors (SAB). *Mol Psychiatry*, **2**, 239–246.

Blum, K., Noble, E.P., Sheridan, P.J., Montgomery, A., Ritchie, T., Jagadeeswaran, P., Nogami, H., Briggs, A.H. and Cohn, J.B., 1990. Allelic association of human dopamine D2 receptor gene in alcoholism. *JAMA*, **263**, 2055–2060.

Borowsky, B. and Hoffman, B.J., 1995. Neurotransmitter transporters: molecular biology, function, and regulation. *Int Rev Neurobiol*, **38**, 139–199.

Boularand, S., Darmon, M.C. and Mallet, J., 1995. The human tryptophan hydroxylase gene. An unusual splicing complexity in the 5′-untranslated region. *J Biol Chem*, **270**, 3748–3756.

Bradley, C.C. and Blakely, R.D., 1997. Alternative splicing of the human serotonin transporter gene. *J Neurochem*, **69**, 1356–1367.

Brown, G.L., Ebert, M.H., Goyer, P.F., Jimerson, D.C., Klein, W.J., Bunney, W.E. and Goodwin, F.K., 1982. Aggression, suicide, and serotonin: relationships to CSF amine metabolites. *Am J Psychiatry*, **139**, 741–746.

Brown, G.L., Goodwin, F.K., Ballenger, J.C., Goyer, P.F. and Major, L.F., 1979. Aggression in humans correlates with cerebrospinal fluid amine metabolites. *Psychiatry Res*, **1**, 131–139.

Brunner, D., Buhot, M.C., Hen, R. and Hofer, M., 1999. Anxiety, motor activation, and maternal-infant interactions in 5HT1B knockout mice. *Behav Neurosci*, **113**, 587–601.

Brunner, D. and Hen, R., 1997. Insights into the neurobiology of impulsive behavior from serotonin receptor knockout mice. *Ann NY Acad Sci*, **836**, 81–105.

Brunner, H.G., 1996. MAOA deficiency and abnormal behaviour: perspectives on an association. *Ciba Found Symp*, **194**, 155–164.

Brunner, H.G., Nelen, M., Breakefield, X.O., Ropers, H.H. and van Oost, B.A., 1993a. Abnormal behavior associated with a point mutation in the structural gene for monoamine oxidase A. *Science*, **262**, 578–580.

Brunner, H.G., Nelen, M.R., van Zandvoort, P., Abeling, N.G., van Gennip, A.H., Wolters, E.C., Kuiper, M.A., Ropers, H.H. and van Oost, B.A., 1993b. X-linked borderline mental retardation with prominent behavioral disturbance: phenotype, genetic localization, and evidence for disturbed monoamine metabolism. *Am J Hum Genet*, **52**, 1032–1039.

Buss, D., 1995. Evolutionary psychology: a new paradigm for psychological science. *Psychol Inquiry*, **6**, 1–30.

Byerley, W., Khan, A.S., Holik, J., Hoff, M. and Sikela, J.M., 1993. Dinucleotide repeat polymorphism in the 3′ untranslated region of an anonymous brain cDNA mapping to chromosome 2 (D2S230). *Hum Mol Genet*, **2**, 1329.

Cardon, L.R., 2001a. Association study designs for complex traits. *Nat Rev Genet*, **2**, 91–99.

Cardon, L.R., 2001b Practical barriers to identify complex trait loci. In: Plomin, R.D.J, Craig, I., McGuffin, P. (eds), *Behavioural Genetics in a Postgenomic World*, American Psychiatric Association, Washington, DC, in press.

Carver, C.S. and White, T.L., 1994. Behavioural inhibition, behavioral activation, and affective responses to impending reward and punishment: the BIS/BAS scales. *J Personal Soc Psychol*, **67**, 319–333.

Cases, O., Seif, I., Grimsby, J., Gaspar, P., Chen, K., Pournin, S., Muller, U., Aguet, M., Babinet, C., Shih, J.C. and De Maeyer, E., 1995. Aggressive behavior and altered amounts of brain serotonin and norepinephrine in mice lacking MAOA. *Science*, **268**, 1763–1766.

Cases, O., Vitalis, T., Seif, I., De Maeyer, E., Sotelo, C. and Gaspar, P., 1996. Lack of barrels in the somatosensory cortex of monoamine oxidase A-deficient mice: role of a serotonin excess during the critical period. *Neuron*, **16**, 297–307.

Castellanos, F.X., Lau, E., Tayebi, N., Lee, P., Long, R.E., Giedd, J.N., Sharp, W., Marsh, W.L., Walter, J.M., Hamburger, S.D., Ginns, E.I., Rapoport, J.L. and Sidransky, E., 1998. Lack of an association between a dopamine-4 receptor polymorphism and attention-deficit/hyperactivity disorder: genetic and brain morphometric analyses. *Mol Psychiatry*, **3**, 431–434.

Cattell, H.B., 1989. *The 16PF: Personality in Depth*. IPAT, Champaign, IL.

Champoux, M., Bennett, A., Lesch, K.P., Heils, A., Nielsen, D.A., Higley, J.D. and Suomi, S.J., 1999. Serotonin transporter gene polymorphism and neurobehavioral development in rhesus monkey neonates. *Soc Neurosci Abstr*, **25**, 69.

Chen, K., Yang, W., Grimsby, J. and Shih, J.C., 1992. The human 5-HT2 receptor is encoded by a multiple intron-exon gene. *Brain Res Mol Brain Res*, **14**, 20–26.

Chiavegatto, S., Dawson, V.L., Mamounas, L.A., Koliatsos, V.E., Dawson, T.M. and Nelson, R.J., 2001. Brain serotonin dysfunction accounts for aggression in male mice lacking neuronal nitric oxide synthase. *Proc Natl Acad Sci USA*, **98**, 1277–1281.

Cloninger, C.R., 1987. A systematic method for clinical description and classification of personality variants. A proposal. *Arch Gen Psychiatry*, **44**, 573–588.

Cloninger, C.R., Svrakic, D.M. and Przybeck, T.R., 1993. A psychobiological model of temperament and character. *Arch Gen Psychiatry*, **50**, 975–990.

Coccaro, E.F., Gabriel, S. and Siever, L.J., 1990. Buspirone challenge: preliminary evidence for a role for central 5-HT1a receptor function in impulsive aggressive behavior in humans. *Psychopharmacol Bull*, **26**, 393–405.

Coccaro, E.F., Kavoussi, R.J. and Lesser, J.C., 1992. Self- and other-directed human aggression: the role of the central serotonergic system. *Int Clin Psychopharmacol*, **6**(Suppl 6), 70–83.

Coccaro, E.F., Lawrence, T., Trestman, R., Gabriel, S., Klar, H.M. and Siever, L.J., 1991. Growth hormone responses to intravenous clonidine challenge correlate with behavioral irritability in psychiatric patients and healthy volunteers. *Psychiatry Res*, **39**, 129–139.

Comings, D.E., Dietz, G., Gade-Andavolu, R., Blake, H., Muhleman, D., Huss, M., Saucier, G. and MacMurray, J.P., 2000a. Association of the neutral endopeptidase (MME) gene with anxiety. *Psychiatr Genet*, **10**, 91–94.

Comings, D.E., Gade-Andavolu, R., Gonzalez, N., Blake, H., Wu, S. and MacMurray, J.P., 1999. Additive effect of three noradrenergic genes (ADRA2a, ADRA2C, DBH) on attention-deficit hyperactivity disorder and learning disabilities in Tourette syndrome subjects. *Clin Genet*, **55**, 160–172.

Comings, D.E., Gonzales, N., Saucier, G., Johnson, J.P. and MacMurray, J.P., 2000b. The DRD4 gene and the spiritual transcendence scale of the character temperament index. *Psychiatr Genet*, **10**, 185–189.

Comings, D.E., Johnson, J.P., Gonzalez, N.S., Huss, M., Saucier, G., McGue, M. and MacMurray, J., 2000c. Association between the adrenergic alpha 2A receptor gene (ADRA2A) and measures of irritability, hostility, impulsivity and memory in normal subjects. *Psychiatr Genet*, **10**, 39–42.

Comings, D.E., Rosenthal, R.J., Lesieur, H.R., Rugle, L.J., Muhleman, D., Chiu, C., Dietz, G. and Gade, R., 1996a. A study of the dopamine D2 receptor gene in pathological gambling. *Pharmacogenetics*, **6**, 223–234.

Comings, D.E., Wu, S., Chiu, C., Ring, R.H., Gade, R., Ahn, C., MacMurray, J.P., Dietz, G. and Muhleman, D., 1996b. Polygenic inheritance of Tourette syndrome, stuttering, attention deficit hyperactivity, conduct, and oppositional defiant disorder: the additive and subtractive effect of the three dopaminergic genes — DRD2, D beta H, and DAT1. *Am J Med Genet*, **67**, 264–288.

Constantino, J.N., Morris, J.A. and Murphy, D.L., 1997. CSF 5-HIAA and family history of antisocial personality disorder in newborns. *Am J Psychiatry*, **154**, 1771–1773.

Coolidge, F.L., Thede, L.L. and Jang, K.L., 2001. Heritability of personality disorders in childhood: a preliminary investigation. *J Personal Disord*, **15**, 33–40.

Costa, P.T. and McCrae, R.R., 1992. *Revised NEO Personality Inventory (NEO PI-R) and NEO Five Factor Inventory (NEO-FFI) Manual*. Psychological Assessment Resources, Odessa, FL.

Craig, S.P., Boularand, S., Darmon, M.C., Mallet, J. and Craig, I.W., 1991. Localization of human tryptophan hydroxylase (TPH) to chromosome 11p15.3-p14 by *in situ* hybridization. *Cytogenet Cell Genet*, **56**, 157–159.

Craig, S.P., Buckle, V.J., Lamouroux, A., Mallet, J. and Craig, I., 1986. Localization of the human tyrosine hydroxylase gene to 11p15: gene duplication and evolution of metabolic pathways. *Cytogenet Cell Genet*, **42**, 29–32.

Cravchik, A., Sibley, D.R. and Gejman, P.V., 1996. Functional analysis of the human D2 dopamine receptor missense variants. *J Biol Chem*, **271**, 26013–26017.

Crestani, F., Lorez, M., Baer, K., Essrich, C., Benke, D., Laurent, J.P., Belzung, C., Fritschy, J.M., Luscher, B. and Mohler, H., 1999. Decreased GABAA-receptor clustering results in enhanced anxiety and a bias for threat cues. *Nat Neurosci*, **2**, 833–839.

Daly, G., Hawi, Z., Fitzgerald, M. and Gill, M., 1999. Mapping susceptibility loci in attention deficit hyperactivity disorder: preferential transmission of parental alleles at DAT1, DBH and DRD5 to affected children. *Mol Psychiatry*, **4**, 192–196.

Damberg, M., Garpenstrand, H., Alfredsson, J., Ekblom, J., Forslund, K., Rylander, G. and Oreland, L., 2000. A polymorphic region in the human transcription factor AP-2beta gene is associated with specific personality traits. *Mol Psychiatry*, **5**, 220–224.

Deary, I., Battersby, S., Whiteman, M., Connor, J., Fowkes, F. and Harmar, A., 1999. Neuroticism and polymorphisms in the serotonin transporter gene. *Psychol Med*, **29**, 735–739.

de Brettes, B., Berlin, I., Laurent, C., Lépine, J.P., Mallet, P. and Puech, A.P., 1998. The dopamine D2 receptor gene *TaqI* A polymorphism is not associated with novelty seeking, harm avoidance and reward dependence in healthy subjects. *Eur Psychiatry*, **13**, 427–430.

Deckert, J., Catalano, M., Syagailo, Y.V., Bosi, M., Okladnova, O., Di Bella, D., Nothen, M.M., Maffei, P., Franke, P., Fritze, J., Maier, W.,

Propping, P., Beckmann, H., Bellodi, L. and Lesch, K.P., 1999. Excess of high activity monoamine oxidase A gene promoter alleles in female patients with panic disorder. *Hum Mol Genet*, **8**, 621–624.

Demas, G.E., Eliasson, M.J., Dawson, T.M., Dawson, V.L., Kriegsfeld, L.J., Nelson, R.J. and Snyder, S.H., 1997. Inhibition of neuronal nitric oxide synthase increases aggressive behavior in mice. *Mol Med*, **3**, 610–616.

Demchyshyn, L., Sunahara, R.K., Miller, K., Teitler, M., Hoffman, B.J., Kennedy, J.L., Seeman, P., Van Tol, H.H. and Niznik, H.B., 1992. A human serotonin 1D receptor variant (5HT1D beta) encoded by an intronless gene on chromosome 6. *Proc Natl Acad Sci USA*, **89**, 5522–5526.

De Luca, A., Rizzardi, M., Torrente, I., Alessandroni, R., Salvioli, G.P., Filograsso, N., Dallapiccola, B. and Novelli, G., 2001. Dopamine D4 receptor (DRD4) polymorphism and adaptability trait during infancy: a longitudinal study in 1- to 5-month-old neonates. *Neurogenetics*, **3**, 79–82.

De Vry, J., 1995. 5-HT1A receptor agonists: recent developments and controversial issues. *Psychopharmacology (Berl)*, **121**, 1–26.

Du, L., Bakish, D. and Hrdina, P.D., 2000. Gender differences in association between serotonin transporter gene polymorphism and personality traits. *Psychiatr Genet*, **10**, 159–164.

Duaux, E., Gorwood, P., Griffon, N., Bourdel, M.C., Sautel, F., Sokoloff, P., Schwartz, J.C., Ades, J., Loo, H. and Poirier, M.F., 1998. Homozygosity at the dopamine D3 receptor gene is associated with opiate dependence. *Mol Psychiatry*, **3**, 333–336.

Dulawa, S.C., Grandy, D.K., Low, M.J., Paulus, M.P. and Geyer, M.A., 1999. Dopamine D4 receptor-knock-out mice exhibit reduced exploration of novel stimuli. *J Neurosci*, **19**, 9550–9556.

Dunner, D.L., Levitt, M., Kumbaraci, T. and Fieve, R.R., 1977. Erythrocyte catechol-O-methyltransferase activity in primary affective disorder. *Biol Psychiatry*, **12**, 237–244.

Ebstein, R.P., Benjamin, J. and Belmaker, R.H., 2000. Personality and polymorphisms of genes involved in aminergic neurotransmission. *Eur J Pharmacol*, **410**, 205–214.

Ebstein, R.P., Gritsenko, I., Nemanov, L., Frisch, A., Osher, Y. and Belmaker, R.H., 1997a. No association between the serotonin transporter gene regulatory region polymorphism and the Tridimensional Personality Questionnaire (TPQ) temperament of harm avoidance. *Mol Psychiatry*, **2**, 224–226.

Ebstein, R.P., Levine, J., Geller, V., Auerbach, J., Gritsenko, I. and Belmaker, R.H., 1998. Dopamine D4 receptor and serotonin transporter promoter in the determination of neonatal temperament. *Mol Psychiatry*, **3**, 238–246.

Ebstein, R.P., Nemanov, L., Klotz, I., Gritsenko, I. and Belmaker, R.H., 1997b. Additional evidence for an association between the dopamine D4 receptor (D4DR) exon III repeat polymorphism and the human personality trait of novelty seeking. *Mol Psychiatry*, **2**, 472–477.

Ebstein, R.P., Novick, O., Umansky, R., Priel, B., Osher, Y., Blaine, D., Bennett, E.R., Nemanov, L., Katz, M. and Belmaker, R.H., 1996. Dopamine D4 receptor (D4DR) exon III polymorphism associated with the human personality trait of novelty seeking. *Nat Genet*, **12**, 78–80.

Ebstein, R.P., Segman, R., Benjamin, J., Osher, Y., Nemanov, L. and Belmaker, R.H., 1997c. 5-HT2C (HTR2C) serotonin receptor gene polymorphism associated with the human personality trait of reward dependence: interaction with dopamine D4 receptor (D4DR) and dopamine D3 receptor (D3DR) polymorphisms. *Am J Med Genet*, **74**, 65–72.

Ekelund, J., Lichtermann, D., Jarvelin, M.R. and Peltonen, L., 1999. Association between novelty seeking and the type 4 dopamine receptor gene in a large Finnish cohort sample. *Am J Psychiatry*, **156**, 1453–1455.

Eley, T.C., Lichtenstein, P. and Stevenson, J., 1999. Sex differences in the etiology of aggressive and nonaggressive antisocial behavior: results from two twin studies. *Child Dev*, **70**, 155–168.

Eley, T.C. and Plomin, R., 1997. Genetic analyses of emotionality. *Curr Opin Neurobiol*, **7**, 279–284.

Eysenck, S.B.G., Eysenck, H.J. and Barrett, P., 1985. A revised version of the psychoticism scale. *Pers Indiv Differ*, **6**, 21–29.

Fahndrich, E., Coper, H., Christ, W., Helmchen, H., Muller-Oerlinghausen, B. and Pietzcker, A., 1980. Erythrocyte COMT-activity in patients with affective disorders. *Acta Psychiatr Scand*, **61**, 427–437.

Flint, J., Corley, R., DeFries, J.C., Fulker, D.W., Gray, J.A., Miller, S. and Collins, A.C., 1995. A simple genetic basis for a complex psychological trait in laboratory mice. *Science*, **269**, 1432–1435.

Flory, J.D., Manuck, S.B., Ferrell, R.E., Dent, K.M., Peters, D.G. and Muldoon, M.F., 1999. Neuroticism is not associated with the serotonin transporter (5-HTTLPR) polymorphism. *Mol Psychiatry*, **4**, 93–96.

Franke, P., Leboyer, M., Gansicke, M., Weiffenbach, O., Biancalana, V., Cornillet-Lefebre, P., Croquette, M.F., Froster, U., Schwab, S.G., Poustka, F., Hautzinger, M. and Maier, W., 1998. Genotype-phenotype relationship in female carriers of the premutation and full mutation of FMR-1. *Psychiatry Res*, **80**, 113–127.

Furlong, R.A., Ho, L., Rubinsztein, J.S., Walsh, C., Paykel, E.S. and Rubinsztein, D.C., 1999. Analysis of the monoamine oxidase A (MAOA) gene in bipolar affective disorder by association studies, meta-analyses, and sequencing of the promoter. *Am J Med Genet*, **88**, 398–406.

Gebhardt, C., Leisch, F., Schussler, P., Fuchs, K., Stompe, T., Sieghart, W., Hornik, K., Kasper, S. and Aschauer, H.N., 2000. Non-association of dopamine D4 and D2 receptor genes with personality in healthy individuals. *Psychiatr Genet*, **10**, 131–137.

Geijer, T., Frisch, A., Persson, M.L., Wasserman, D., Rockah, R., Michaelovsky, E., Apter, A., Jonsson, E.G., Nothen, M.M. and Weizman, A., 2000. Search for association between suicide attempt and serotonergic polymorphisms. *Psychiatr Genet*, **10**, 19–26.

Geijer, T., Jonsson, E., Neiman, J., Persson, M.L., Brene, S., Gyllander, A., Sedvall, G., Rydberg, U., Wasserman, D. and Terenius, L., 1997. Tyrosine hydroxylase and dopamine D4 receptor allelic distribution in Scandinavian chronic alcoholics. *Alcohol Clin Exp Res*, **21**, 35–39.

Gelernter, J., Kennedy, J.L., van Tol, H.H., Civelli, O. and Kidd, K.K., 1992. The D4 dopamine receptor (DRD4) maps to distal 11p close to HRAS. *Genomics*, **13**, 208–210.

Gelernter, J., Kranzler, H., Coccaro, E., Siever, L., New, A. and Mulgrew, C.L., 1997. D4 dopamine-receptor (DRD4) alleles and novelty seeking in substance-dependent, personality-disorder, and control subjects. *Am J Hum Genet*, **61**, 1144–1152.

Gelernter, J., Kranzler, H., Coccaro, E.F., Siever, L.J. and New, A.S., 1998. Serotonin transporter protein gene polymorphism and personality measures in African American and European American subjects. *Am J Psychiatry*, **155**, 1332–1338.

George, S.R., Cheng, R., Nguyen, T., Israel, Y. and O'Dowd, B.F., 1993. Polymorphisms of the D4 dopamine receptor alleles in chronic alcoholism. *Biochem Biophys Res Commun*, **196**, 107–114.

Gershon, E.S. and Jonas, W.Z., 1975. Erythrocyte soluble catechol-*O*-methyl transferase activity in primary affective disorder. A clinical and genetic study. *Arch Gen Psychiatry*, **32**, 1351–1356.

Gogos, J.A., Morgan, M., Luine, V., Santha, M., Ogawa, S., Pfaff, D. and Karayiorgou, M., 1998. Catechol-*O*-methyltransferase-deficient mice exhibit sexually dimorphic changes in catecholamine levels and behavior. *Proc Natl Acad Sci USA*, **95**, 9991–9996.

Goldman, D., Lappalainen, J. and Ozaki, N., 1996. Direct analysis of candidate genes in impulsive behaviours. *Ciba Found Symp*, **194**, 139–152.

Goodman, M. and New, A., 2000. Impulsive aggression in borderline personality disorder. *Curr Psychiatry Rep*, **2**, 56–61.

Gorwood, P., Martres, M.P., Ades, J., Sokoloff, P., Noble, E.P., Geijer, T., Blum, K., Neiman, J., Jonsson, E., Feingold, J. and Schwartz, Y.C., 1995. Lack of association between alcohol-dependence and D3 dopamine receptor gene in three independent samples. *Am J Med Genet*, **60**, 529–531.

Grailhe, R., Waeber, C., Dulawa, S.C., Hornung, J.P., Zhuang, X., Brunner, D., Geyer, M.A. and Hen, R., 1999. Increased exploratory activity and altered response to LSD in mice lacking the 5-HT(5A) receptor. *Neuron*, **22**, 581–591.

Grandy, D.K., Litt, M., Allen, L., Bunzow, J.R., Marchionni, M., Makam, H., Reed, L., Magenis, R.E. and Civelli, O., 1989. The human dopamine D2 receptor gene is located on chromosome 11 at q22-q23 and identifies a *TaqI* RFLP. *Am J Hum Genet*, **45**, 778–785.

Greenberg, B.D., Li, Q., Lucas, F.R., Hu, S., Sirota, L.A., Benjamin, J., Lesch, K.P., Hamer, D. and Murphy, D.L., 2000. Association between the serotonin transporter promoter polymorphism and personality traits in a primarily female population sample. *Am J Med Genet*, **96**, 202–216.

Grossman, M.H., Emanuel, B.S. and Budarf, M.L., 1992. Chromosomal mapping of the human catechol-*O*-methyltransferase gene to 22q11.1 — q11.2. *Genomics*, **12**, 822–825.

Gurvits, I.G., Koenigsberg, H.W. and Siever, L.J., 2000. Neurotransmitter dysfunction in patients with borderline personality disorder. *Psychiatr Clin North Am*, **23**, 27–40, vi.

Gustavsson, J.P., Nothen, M.M., Jonsson, E.G., Neidt, H., Forslund, K., Rylander, G., Mattila-Evenden, M., Sedvall, G.C., Propping, P. and

Asberg, M., 1999. No association between serotonin transporter gene polymorphisms and personality traits. *Am J Med Genet*, **88**, 430–436.

Hallikainen, T., Lachman, H., Saito, T., Volavka, J., Kauhanen, J., Salonen, J.T., Ryynanen, O.P., Koulu, M., Karvonen, M.K., Pohjalainen, T., Syvalahti, E., Hietala, J. and Tiihonen, J., 2000. Lack of association between the functional variant of the catechol-*O*-methyltransferase (COMT) gene and early-onset alcoholism associated with severe antisocial behavior. *Am J Med Genet*, **96**, 348–352.

Hallikainen, T., Saito, T., Lachman, H.M., Volavka, J., Pohjalainen, T., Ryynanen, O.P., Kauhanen, J., Syvalahti, E., Hietala, J. and Tiihonen, J., 1999. Association between low activity serotonin transporter promoter genotype and early onset alcoholism with habitual impulsive violent behavior. *Mol Psychiatry*, **4**, 385–388.

Hamer, D. and Copeland, P., 1998. *Living with our Genes*. Doubleday, New York.

Hansson, S.R., Mezey, E. and Hoffman, B.J., 1998. Serotonin transporter messenger RNA in the developing rat brain: early expression in serotonergic neurons and transient expression in non-serotonergic neurons. *Neuroscience*, **83**, 1185–1201.

Hauge, X.Y., Grandy, D.K., Eubanks, J.H., Evans, G.A., Civelli, O. and Litt, M., 1991. Detection and characterization of additional DNA polymorphisms in the dopamine D2 receptor gene. *Genomics*, **10**, 527–530.

He, L., Li, T., Melville, C., Liu, S., Feng, G.Y., Gu, N.F., Fox, H., Shaw, D., Breen, G., Liu, X., Sham, P., Brown, J., Collier, D. and St Clair, D., 1999. 102T/C polymorphism of serotonin receptor type 2A gene is not associated with schizophrenia in either Chinese or British populations. *Am J Med Genet*, **88**, 95–98.

Hebebrand, J. and Klug, B., 1995. Specification of the phenotype required for men with monoamine oxidase type A deficiency. *Hum Genet*, **96**, 372–376.

Heisler, L.K., Chu, H.M., Brennan, T.J., Danao, J.A., Bajwa, P., Parsons, L.H. and Tecott, L.H., 1998. Elevated anxiety and antidepressant-like responses in serotonin 5-HT1A receptor mutant mice. *Proc Natl Acad Sci USA*, **95**, 15049–15054.

Henderson, A.S., Korten, A.E., Jorm, A.F., Jacomb, P.A., Christensen, H., Rodgers, B., Tan, X. and Easteal, S., 2000. COMT and DRD3 polymorphisms, environmental exposures, and personality traits related to common mental disorders. *Am J Med Genet*, **96**, 102–107.

Herbst, J.H., Zonderman, A.B., McCrae, R.R. and Costa, P.T., Jr., 2000. Do the dimensions of the temperament and character inventory map a simple genetic architecture? Evidence from molecular genetics and factor analysis. *Am J Psychiatry*, **157**, 1285–1290.

Heston, L.L., 1970. The genetics of schizophrenic and schizoid disease. *Science*, **167**, 249–256.

Higley, J.D., Mehlman, P.T., Higley, S.B., Fernald, B., Vickers, J., Lindell, S.G., Taub, D.M., Suomi, S.J. and Linnoila, M., 1996. Excessive mortality in young free-ranging male nonhuman primates with low cerebrospinal fluid 5-hydroxyindoleacetic acid concentrations. *Arch Gen Psychiatry*, **53**, 537–543.

Higley, J.D., Mehlman, P.T., Taub, D.M., Higley, S.B., Suomi, S.J., Vickers, J.H. and Linnoila, M., 1992a. Cerebrospinal fluid monoamine and adrenal correlates of aggression in free-ranging rhesus monkeys. *Arch Gen Psychiatry*, **49**, 436–441.

Higley, J.D., Suomi, S.J. and Linnoila, M., 1991. CSF monoamine metabolite concentrations vary according to age, rearing, and sex, and are influenced by the stressor of social separation in rhesus monkeys. *Psychopharmacology*, **103**, 551–556.

Higley, J.D., Suomi, S.J. and Linnoila, M., 1992b. A longitudinal assessment of CSF monoamine metabolite and plasma cortisol concentrations in young rhesus monkeys. *Biol Psychiatry*, **32**, 127–145.

Hill, S.Y., Zezza, N., Wipprecht, G., Locke, J. and Neiswanger, K., 1999. Personality traits and dopamine receptors (D2 and D4): linkage studies in families of alcoholics. *Am J Med Genet*, **88**, 634–641.

Himei, A., Kono, Y., Yoneda, H., Sakai, T., Koh, J., Sakai, J., Inada, Y. and Imamichi, H., 2000. An association study between alcoholism and the serotonergic receptor genes. *Alcohol Clin Exp Res*, **24**, 341–342.

Hinds, H.L., Hendriks, R.W., Craig, I.W. and Chen, Z.Y., 1992. Characterization of a highly polymorphic region near the first exon of the human MAOA gene containing a GT dinucleotide and a novel VNTR motif. *Genomics*, **13**, 896–897.

Holmes, C., Arranz, M.J., Powell, J.F., Collier, D.A. and Lovestone, S., 1998. 5-HT2A and 5-HT2C receptor polymorphisms and psychopathology in late onset Alzheimer's disease. *Hum Mol Genet*, **7**, 1507–1509.

Hotamisligil, G.S. and Breakefield, X.O., 1991. Human monoamine oxidase A gene determines levels of enzyme activity. *Am J Hum Genet*, **49**, 383–392.

Hoyer, D. and Martin, G.R., 1996. Classification and nomenclature of 5-HT receptors: a comment on current issues. *Behav Brain Res*, **73**, 263–268.

Hsieh, C.L., Bowcock, A.M., Farrer, L.A., Hebert, J.M., Huang, K.N., Cavalli-Sforza, L.L., Julius, D. and Francke, U., 1990. The serotonin receptor subtype 2 locus HTR2 is on human chromosome 13 near genes for esterase D and retinoblastoma-1 and on mouse chromosome 14. *Somat Cell Mol Genet*, **16**, 567–574.

Hu, S., Brody, C.L., Fisher, C., Gunzerath, L., Nelson, M.L., Sabol, S.Z., Sirota, L.A., Marcus, S.E., Greenberg, B.D., Murphy, D.L. and Hamer, D.H., 2000. Interaction between the serotonin transporter gene and neuroticism in cigarette smoking behavior. *Mol Psychiatry*, **5**, 181–188.

Huang, Y.Y., Grailhe, R., Arango, V., Hen, R. and Mann, J.J., 1999. Relationship of psychopathology to the human serotonin1B genotype and receptor binding kinetics in postmortem brain tissue. *Neuropsychopharmacology*, **21**, 238–246.

Jang, K.L., Livesley, W.J., Vernon, P.A. and Jackson, D.N., 1996. Heritability of personality disorder traits: a twin study. *Acta Psychiatr Scand*, **94**, 438–444.

Jonsson, E.G., Goldman, D., Spurlock, G., Gustavsson, J.P., Nielsen, D.A., Linnoila, M., Owen, M.J. and Sedvall, G.C., 1997a. Tryptophan hydroxylase and catechol-*O*-methyltransferase gene polymorphisms: relationships to monoamine metabolite concentrations in CSF of healthy volunteers. *Eur Arch Psychiatry Clin Neurosci*, **247**, 297–302.

Jonsson, E.G., Norton, N., Gustavsson, J.P., Oreland, L., Owen, M.J. and Sedvall, G.C., 2000. A promoter polymorphism in the monoamine oxidase A gene and its relationships to monoamine metabolite concentrations in CSF of healthy volunteers. *J Psychiatr Res*, **34**, 239–244.

Jonsson, E.G., Nothen, M.M., Gustavsson, J.P., Neidt, H., Brene, S., Tylec, A., Propping, P. and Sedvall, G.C., 1997b. Lack of evidence for allelic association between personality traits and the dopamine D4 receptor gene polymorphisms. *Am J Psychiatry*, **154**, 697–699.

Jonsson, E.G., Nothen, M.M., Gustavsson, J.P., Neidt, H., Forslund, K., Mattila-Evenden, M., Rylander, G., Propping, P. and Asberg, M., 1998. Lack of association between dopamine D4 receptor gene and personality traits. *Psychol Med*, **28**, 985–989.

Jorm, A.F., Henderson, A.S., Jacomb, P.A., Christensen, H., Korten, A.E., Rodgers, B., Tan, X. and Easteal, S., 1998. An association study of a functional polymorphism of the serotonin transporter gene with personality and psychiatric symptoms. *Mol Psychiatry*, **3**, 449–451.

Jorm, A.F., Henderson, A.S., Jacomb, P.A., Christensen, H., Korten, A.E., Rodgers, B., Tan, X. and Easteal, S., 2000. Association of smoking and personality with a polymorphism of the dopamine transporter gene: results from a community survey. *Am J Med Genet*, **96**, 331–334.

Kagan, J., 1989. Temperamental contributions to social behavior. *Am Psychol*, **44**, 664–668.

Karayiorgou, M., Altemus, M., Galke, B.L., Goldman, D., Murphy, D.L., Ott, J. and Gogos, J.A., 1997. Genotype determining low catechol-*O*-methyltransferase activity as a risk factor for obsessive-compulsive disorder. *Proc Natl Acad Sci USA*, **94**, 4572–4575.

Kato, M.V., Shimizu, T., Nagayoshi, M., Kaneko, A., Sasaki, M.S. and Ikawa, Y., 1996. Genomic imprinting of the human serotonin-receptor (HTR2) gene involved in development of retinoblastoma. *Am J Hum Genet*, **59**, 1084–1090.

Katsuragi, S., Kunugi, H., Sano, A., Tsutsumi, T., Isogawa, K., Nanko, S. and Akiyoshi, J., 1999b. Association between serotonin transporter gene polymorphism and anxiety-related traits. *Biol Psychiatry*, **45**, 368–370.

Kauhanen, J., Hallikainen, T., Tuomainen, T.P., Koulu, M., Karvonen, M.K., Salonen, J.T. and Tiihonen, J., 2000. Association between the functional polymorphism of catechol-*O*-methyltransferase gene and alcohol consumption among social drinkers. *Alcohol Clin Exp Res*, **24**, 135–139.

Kavoussi, R., Armstead, P. and Coccaro, E., 1997. The neurobiology of impulsive aggression. *Psychiatr Clin North Am*, **20**, 395–403.

Kendler, K.S. and Eaves, L.J., 1986. Models for the joint effect of genotype and environment on liability to psychiatric illness. *Am J Psychiatry*, **143**, 279–289.

Kendler, K.S., Ochs, A.L., Gorman, A.M., Hewitt, J.K., Ross, D.E. and Mirsky, A.F., 1991. The structure of schizotypy: a pilot multitrait twin study. *Psychiatry Res*, **36**, 19–36.

Kety, S.S., Rosenthal, D., Wender, P.H. and Schulsinger, F., 1971. Mental illness in the biological and adoptive families of adopted schizophrenics. *Am J Psychiatry*, **128**, 302–306.

Knutson, B., Wolkowitz, O.M., Cole, S.W., Chan, T., Moore, E.A., Johnson, R.C. and Terpstra, J., 1998. Selective alteration of personality and social behavior by serotonergic intervention. *Am J Psychiatry*, **155**, 373–379.

Korte, S.M., Meijer, O.C., de Kloet, E.R., Buwalda, B., Keijser, J., Sluyter, F., van Oortmerssen, G. and Bohus, B., 1996. Enhanced 5-HT1A receptor expression in forebrain regions of aggressive house mice. *Brain Res*, **736**, 338–343.

Kotler, M., Barak, P., Cohen, H., Averbuch, I.E., Grinshpoon, A., Gritsenko, I., Nemanov, L. and Ebstein, R.P., 1999. Homicidal behavior in schizophrenia associated with a genetic polymorphism determining low catechol *O*-methyltransferase (COMT) activity. *Am J Med Genet*, **88**, 628–633.

Kuhn, K.U., Meyer, K., Nothen, M.M., Gansicke, M., Papassotiropoulos, A. and Maier, W., 1999. Allelic variants of dopamine receptor D4 (DRD4) and serotonin receptor 5HT2 c (HTR2c) and temperament factors: replication tests. *Am J Med Genet*, **88**, 168–172.

Kumakiri, C., Kodama, K., Shimizu, E., Yamanouchi, N., Okada, S., Noda, S., Okamoto, H., Sato, T. and Shirasawa, H., 1999. Study of the association between the serotonin transporter gene regulatory region polymorphism and personality traits in a Japanese population. *Neurosci Lett*, **263**, 205–207.

Lachman, H.M., Nolan, K.A., Mohr, P., Saito, T. and Volavka, J., 1998. Association between catechol *O*-methyltransferase genotype and violence in schizophrenia and schizoaffective disorder. *Am J Psychiatry*, **155**, 835–837.

Lachman, H.M., Papolos, D.F., Saito, T., Yu, Y.M., Szumlanski, C.L. and Weinshilboum, R.M., 1996. Human catechol-*O*-methyltransferase pharmacogenetics: description of a functional polymorphism and its potential application to neuropsychiatric disorders. *Pharmacogenetics*, **6**, 243–250.

LaHoste, G.J., Swanson, J.M., Wigal, S.B., Glabe, C., Wigal, T., King, N. and Kennedy, J.L., 1996. Dopamine D4 receptor gene polymorphism is associated with attention deficit hyperactivity disorder. *Mol Psychiatry*, **1**, 121–124.

Lan, N.C., Heinzmann, C., Gal, A., Klisak, I., Orth, U., Lai, E., Grimsby, J., Sparkes, R.S., Mohandas, T. and Shih, J.C., 1989. Human monoamine oxidase A and B genes map to Xp 11.23 and are deleted in a patient with Norrie disease. *Genomics*, **4**, 552–559.

Lappalainen, J., Long, J.C., Eggert, M., Ozaki, N., Robin, R.W., Brown, G.L., Naukkarinen, H., Virkkunen, M., Linnoila, M. and Goldman, D., 1998. Linkage of antisocial alcoholism to the serotonin 5-HT1B receptor gene in 2 populations. *Arch Gen Psychiatry*, **55**, 989–994.

Lappalainen, J., Long, J.C., Virkkunen, M., Ozaki, N., Goldman, D. and Linnoila, M., 1999. HTR2 C Cys23Ser polymorphism in relation to CSF monoamine metabolite concentrations and DSM-III-R psychiatric diagnoses. *Biol Psychiatry*, **46**, 821–826.

Lappalainen, J., Zhang, L., Dean, M., Oz, M., Ozaki, N., Yu, D.H., Virkkunen, M., Weight, F., Linnoila, M. and Goldman, D., 1995. Identification, expression, and pharmacology of a Cys23-Ser23 substitution in the human 5-HT2c receptor gene (HTR2C). *Genomics*, **27**, 274–279.

Ledley, F.D., Grenett, H.E., Bartos, D.P., van Tuinen, P., Ledbetter, D.H. and Woo, S.L., 1987. Assignment of human tryptophan hydroxylase locus to chromosome 11: gene duplication and translocation in evolution of aromatic amino acid hydroxylases. *Somat Cell Mol Genet*, **13**, 575–580.

Lerman, C., Caporaso, N.E., Audrain, J., Main, D., Boyd, N.R. and Shields, P.G., 2000. Interacting effects of the serotonin transporter gene and neuroticism in smoking practices and nicotine dependence. *Mol Psychiatry*, **5**, 189–192.

Lesch, K.P., 1997. Molecular biology, pharmacology, and genetics of the serotonin transporter: psychobiological and clinical implications. In: Baumgarten, H.G., Göthert, M. (eds), *Serotonergic Neurons and 5-HT Receptors in the CNS*, pp. 671–705. Springer, Berlin.

Lesch, K.P., 2001a. Molecular foundation of anxiety disorders. *J Neural Transm*, **108**, 717–746.

Lesch, K.P., 2001b. Serotonin transporter: from genomics and knockouts to behavioral traits and psychiatric disorders. In: Briley, M., Sulser, F. (eds), *Molecular Genetics of Mental Disorders*, pp. 221–267. Martin Dunitz, London.

Lesch, K.P., Balling, U., Gross, J., Strauss, K., Wolozin, B.L., Murphy, D.L. and Riederer, P., 1994. Organization of the human serotonin transporter gene. *J Neural Transm Gen Sect*, **95**, 157–162.

Lesch, K.P., Bengel, D., Heils, A., Sabol, S.Z., Greenberg, B.D., Petri, S., Benjamin, J., Muller, C.R., Hamer, D.H. and Murphy, D.L., 1996. Association of anxiety-related traits with a polymorphism in the serotonin transporter gene regulatory region. *Science*, **274**, 1527–1531.

Lesch, K.P., Meyer, J., Glatz, K., Flugge, G., Hinney, A., Hebebrand, J., Klauck, S.M., Poustka, A., Poustka, F., Bengel, D., Mossner, R., Riederer, P. and Heils, A., 1997. The 5-HT transporter gene-linked polymorphic region (5-HTTLPR) in evolutionary perspective: alternative biallelic variation in rhesus monkeys. *J Neural Transm*, **104**, 1259–1266.

Levitas, A., 1996. Neuropsychiatric aspects of fragile X syndrome. *Semin Clin Neuropsychiatry*, **1**, 154–167.

Li, Q., Wichems, C., Heils, A., Lesch, K.P. and Murphy, D.L., 2000. Reduction in the density and expression, but not G-protein coupling, of serotonin receptors (5-HT1A) in 5-HT transporter knock-out mice: gender and brain region differences. *J Neurosci*, **20**, 7888–7895.

Lichter, J.B., Barr, C.L., Kennedy, J.L., Van Tol, H.H., Kidd, K.K. and Livak, K.J., 1993. A hypervariable segment in the human dopamine receptor D4 (DRD4) gene. *Hum Mol Genet*, **2**, 767–773.

Lim, L.C., Powell, J., Sham, P., Castle, D., Hunt, N., Murray, R. and Gill, M., 1995. Evidence for a genetic association between alleles of monoamine oxidase A gene and bipolar affective disorder. *Am J Med Genet*, **60**, 325–331.

Lin, S., Jiang, S., Wu, X., Qian, Y., Wang, D., Tang, G. and Gu, N., 2000. Association analysis between mood disorder and monoamine oxidase gene. *Am J Med Genet*, **96**, 12–14.

Livesley, W.J., Jang, K.L. and Vernon, P.A., 1998. Phenotypic and genetic structure of traits delineating personality disorder. *Arch Gen Psychiatry*, **55**, 941–948.

Loh, E.W., Higuchi, S., Matsushita, S., Murray, R., Chen, C.K. and Ball, D., 2000. Association analysis of the GABA(A) receptor subunit genes cluster on 5q33-34 and alcohol dependence in a Japanese population. *Mol Psychiatry*, **5**, 301–307.

Lucki, I., 1998. The spectrum of behaviors influenced by serotonin. *Biol Psychiatry*, **44**, 151–162.

Major, L.F., Lerner, P., Goodwin, fnmF.K., Ballenger, J.C., Brown, G.L. and Lovenberg, W., 1980. Dopamine beta-hydroxylase in CSF. Relationship to personality measures. *Arch Gen Psychiatry*, **37**, 308–310.

Maldonado, R., Saiardi, A., Valverde, O., Samad, T.A., Roques, B.P. and Borrelli, E., 1997. Absence of opiate rewarding effects in mice lacking dopamine D2 receptors. *Nature*, **388**, 586–589.

Malhotra, A.K., Virkkunen, M., Rooney, W., Eggert, M., Linnoila, M. and Goldman, D., 1996. The association between the dopamine D4 receptor (D4DR) 16 amino acid repeat polymorphism and novelty seeking. *Mol Psychiatry*, **1**, 388–391.

Malleret, G., Hen, R., Guillou, J.L., Segu, L. and Buhot, M.C., 1999. 5-HT1B receptor knock-out mice exhibit increased exploratory activity and enhanced spatial memory performance in the Morris water maze. *J Neurosci*, **19**, 6157–6168.

Mann, J.J., Malone, K.M., Nielsen, D.A., Goldman, D., Erdos, J. and Gelernter, J., 1997. Possible association of a polymorphism of the tryptophan hydroxylase gene with suicidal behavior in depressed patients. *Am J Psychiatry*, **154**, 1451–1453.

Manuck, S.B., Flory, J.D., Ferrell, R.E., Dent, K.M., Mann, J.J. and Muldoon, M.F., 1999. Aggression and anger-related traits associated with a polymorphism of the tryptophan hydroxylase gene. *Biol Psychiatry*, **45**, 603–614.

Manuck, S.B., Flory, J.D., Ferrell, R.E., Mann, J.J. and Muldoon, M.F., 2000. A regulatory polymorphism of the monoamine oxidase-A gene may be associated with variability in aggression, impulsivity, and central nervous system serotonergic responsivity. *Psychiatry Res*, **95**, 9–23.

Mazzanti, C.M., Lappalainen, J., Long, J.C., Bengel, D., Naukkarinen, H., Eggert, M., Virkkunen, M., Linnoila, M. and Goldman, D., 1998. Role of the serotonin transporter promoter polymorphism in anxiety-related traits. *Arch Gen Psychiatry*, **55**, 936–940.

McGuffin, P. and Thapar, A., 1992. The genetics of personality disorder. *Br J Psychiatry*, **160**, 12–23.

McKinney, E.F., Walton, R.T., Yudkin, P., Fuller, A., Haldar, N.A., Mant, D., Murphy, M., Welsh, K.I. and Marshall, S.E., 2000. Association between polymorphisms in dopamine metabolic enzymes and tobacco consumption in smokers. *Pharmacogenetics*, **10**, 483–491.

McPherson, J.D., Marra, M., Hillier, L., Waterston, R.H., Chinwalla, A., Wallis, J., Sekhon, M., Wylie, K., Mardis, E.R., Wilson, R.K., Fulton, R., Kucaba, T.A., Wagner-McPherson, C., Barbazuk, W.B., Gregory, S.G., Humphray, S.J., French, L., Evans, R.S., Bethel, G., Whittaker, A., Holden, J.L., McCann, O.T., Dunham, A., Soderlund, C.,

Scott, C.E., Bentley, D.R., Schuler, G., Chen, H.C., Jang, W., Green, E.D., Idol, J.R., Maduro, V.V., Montgomery, K.T., Lee, E., Miller, A., Emerling, S., Kucherlapati, R., Gibbs, R., Scherer, S., Gorrell, J.H., Sodergren, E., Clerc-Blankenburg, K., Tabor, P., Naylor, S., Garcia, D., de Jong, P.J., Catanese, J.J., Nowak, N., Osoegawa, K., Qin, S., Rowen, L., Madan, A., Dors, M., Hood, L., Trask, B., Friedman, C., Massa, H., Cheung, V.G., Kirsch, I.R., Reid, T., Yonescu, R., Weissenbach, J., Bruls, T., Heilig, R., Branscomb, E., Olsen, A., Doggett, N., Cheng, J.F., Hawkins, T., Myers, R.M., Shang, J., Ramirez, L., Schmutz, J., Velasquez, O., Dixon, K., Stone, N.E., Cox, D.R., Haussler, D., Kent, W.J., Furey, T., Rogic, S., Kennedy, S., Jones, S., Rosenthal, A., Wen, G., Schilhabel, M., Gloeckner, G., Nyakatura, G., Siebert, R., Schlegelberger, B., Korenberg, J., Chen, X.N., Fujiyama, A., Hattori, M., Toyoda, A., Yada, T., Park, H.S., Sakaki, Y., Shimizu, N., Asakawa, S. *et al.*, 2001. A physical map of the human genome. *Nature*, **409**, 934–941.

Mehlman, P.T., Higley, J.D., Faucher, I., Lilly, A.A., Taub, D.M., Vickers, J., Suomi, S.J. and Linnoila, M., 1995. Correlation of CSF 5-HIAA concentration with sociality and the timing of emigration in free-ranging primates. *Am J Psychiatry*, **152**, 907–913.

Melke, J., Landen, M., Baghei, F., Rosmond, R., Holm, G., Bjorntorp, P., Westberg, L., Hellstrand, M. and Eriksson, E., 2001. Serotonin transporter gene polymorphisms are associated with anxiety-related personality traits in women. *Am J Med Genet*, **105**, 458–463.

Menza, M.A., Palermo, B., DiPaola, R., Sage, J.I. and Ricketts, M.H., 1999. Depression and anxiety in Parkinson's disease: possible effect of genetic variation in the serotonin transporter. *J Geriatr Psychiatry Neurol*, **12**, 49–52.

Milatovich, A., Hsieh, C.L., Bonaminio, G., Tecott, L., Julius, D. and Francke, U., 1992. Serotonin receptor 1c gene assigned to X chromosome in human (band q24) and mouse (bands D-F4). *Hum Mol Genet*, **1**, 681–684.

Miller, W.B., Pasta, D.J., MacMurray, J., Chiu, C., Wu, H. and Comings, D.E., 1999. Dopamine receptor genes are associated with age at first sexual intercourse. *J Biosoc Sci*, **31**, 43–54.

Mitsuyasu, H., Hirata, N., Sakai, Y., Shibata, H., Takeda, Y., Ninomiya, H., Kawasaki, H., Tashiro, N. and Fukumaki, Y., 2001. Association analysis of polymorphisms in the upstream region of the human dopamine D4 receptor gene (DRD4) with schizophrenia and personality traits. *J Hum Genet*, **46**, 26–31.

Murakami, F., Shimomura, T., Kotani, K., Ikawa, S., Nanba, E. and Adachi, K., 1999. Anxiety traits associated with a polymorphism in the serotonin transporter gene regulatory region in the Japanese. *J Hum Genet*, **44**, 15–17.

Muramatsu, T., Matsushita, S., Kanba, S., Higuchi, S., Manki, H., Suzuki, E. and Asai, M., 1997. Monoamine oxidase gene polymorphisms and mood disorder. *Am J Med Genet*, **74**, 494–496.

Nakamura, T., Muramatsu, T., Ono, Y., Matsushita, S., Higuchi, S., Mizushima, H., Yoshimura, K., Kanba, S. and Asai, M., 1997. Serotonin transporter gene regulatory region polymorphism and anxiety-related traits in the Japanese. *Am J Med Genet*, **74**, 544–545.

Nelson, R.J., Demas, G.E., Huang, P.L., Fishman, M.C., Dawson, V.L., Dawson, T.M. and Snyder, S.H., 1995. Behavioural abnormalities in male mice lacking neuronal nitric oxide synthase. *Nature*, **378**, 383–386.

Nesse, R.M. and Williams, G.C., 1995. *Why We Get Sick. The New Science of Darwinian Medicine*. Times Books (Random House), New York.

New, A.S., Gelernter, J., Yovell, Y., Trestman, R.L., Nielsen, D.A., Silverman, J., Mitropoulou, V. and Siever, L.J., 1998. Tryptophan hydroxylase genotype is associated with impulsive-aggression measures: a preliminary study. *Am J Med Genet*, **81**, 13–17.

Nielsen, D.A., Dean, M. and Goldman, D., 1992. Genetic mapping of the human tryptophan hydroxylase gene on chromosome 11, using an intronic conformational polymorphism. *Am J Hum Genet*, **51**, 1366–1371.

Nielsen, D.A., Goldman, D., Virkkunen, M., Tokola, R., Rawlings, R. and Linnoila, M., 1994. Suicidality and 5-hydroxyindoleacetic acid concentration associated with a tryptophan hydroxylase polymorphism. *Arch Gen Psychiatry*, **51**, 34–38.

Nielsen, D.A., Jenkins, G.L., Stefanisko, K.M., Jefferson, K.K. and Goldman, D., 1997. Sequence, splice site and population frequency distribution analyses of the polymorphic human tryptophan hydroxylase intron 7. *Brain Res Mol Brain Res*, **45**, 145–148.

Nielsen, D.A., Virkkunen, M., Lappalainen, J., Eggert, M., Brown, G.L., Long, J.C., Goldman, D. and Linnoila, M., 1998. A tryptophan hydroxylase gene marker for suicidality and alcoholism. *Arch Gen Psychiatry*, **55**, 593–602.

Noble, E.P., Noble, R.E., Ritchie, T., Syndulko, K., Bohlman, M.C., Noble, L.A., Zhang, Y., Sparkes, R.S. and Grandy, D.K., 1994. D2 dopamine receptor gene and obesity. *Int J Eat Disord*, **15**, 205–217.

Noble, E.P., Ozkaragoz, T.Z., Ritchie, T.L., Zhang, X., Belin, T.R. and Sparkes, R.S., 1998. D2 and D4 dopamine receptor polymorphisms and personality. *Am J Med Genet*, **81**, 257–267.

Nolan, K.A., Volavka, J., Czobor, P., Cseh, A., Lachman, H., Saito, T., Tiihonen, J., Putkonen, A., Hallikainen, T., Kotilainen, I., Rasanen, P., Isohanni, M., Jarvelin, M.R. and Karvonen, M.K., 2000a. Suicidal behavior in patients with schizophrenia is related to COMT polymorphism. *Psychiatr Genet*, **10**, 117–124.

Nolan, K.A., Volavka, J., Lachman, H.M. and Saito, T., 2000b. An association between a polymorphism of the tryptophan hydroxylase gene and aggression in schizophrenia and schizoaffective disorder. *Psychiatr Genet*, **10**, 109–115.

O'Connor, T.G., McGuire, S., Reiss, D., Hetherington, E.M. and Plomin, R., 1998. Co-occurrence of depressive symptoms and antisocial behavior in adolescence: a common genetic liability. *J Abnorm Psychol*, **107**, 27–37.

Okere, C.O., Wang, Y.F., Higuchi, T., Negoro, H., Okutani, F., Takahashi, S. and Murata, T., 1996. The effect of systemic and central nitric oxide administration on milk availability in lactating rats. *Neuroreport*, **8**, 243–247.

Okuyama, Y., Ishiguro, H., Nankai, M., Shibuya, H., Watanabe, A. and Arinami, T., 2000. Identification of a polymorphism in the promoter region of DRD4 associated with the human novelty seeking personality trait. *Mol Psychiatry*, **5**, 64–69.

Ono, Y., Manki, H., Yoshimura, K., Muramatsu, T., Mizushima, H., Higuchi, S., Yagi, G., Kanba, S. and Asai, M., 1997. Association between dopamine D4 receptor (D4DR) exon III polymorphism and novelty seeking in Japanese subjects. *Am J Med Genet*, **74**, 501–503.

Ono, Y., Yoshimura, K., Sueoka, R., Yamauchi, K., Mizushima, H., Momose, T., Nakamura, K., Okonogi, K. and Asai, M., 1996. Avoidant personality disorder and taijin kyoufu: Sociocultural implications of the WHO/ADAMHA international study of personality disorders in Japan. *Acta Psychiatr Scand*, **93**, 172–176.

Osher, Y., Hamer, D. and Benjamin, J., 2000. Association and linkage of anxiety-related traits with a functional polymorphism of the serotonin transporter gene regulatory region in Israeli sibling pairs. *Mol Psychiatry*, **5**, 216–219.

Ozkaragoz, T. and Noble, E.P., 2000. Extraversion. Interaction between D2 dopamine receptor polymorphisms and parental alcoholism. *Alcohol*, **22**, 139–146.

Parks, C.L., Robinson, P.S., Sibille, E., Shenk, T. and Toth, M., 1998. Increased anxiety of mice lacking the serotonin1A receptor. *Proc Natl Acad Sci USA*, **95**, 10734–10739.

Parsian, A. and Todd, R.D., 1997. Genetic association between monoamine oxidase and manic-depressive illness: comparison of relative risk and haplotype relative risk data. *Am J Med Genet*, **74**, 475–479.

Parsian, A. and Zhang, Z.H., 1997. Human dopamine transporter gene polymorphism (VNTR) and alcoholism. *Am J Med Genet*, **74**, 480–482.

Parsian, A. and Zhang, Z.H., 1999. Human chromosomes 11p15 and 4p12 and alcohol dependence: possible association with the GABRB1 gene. *Am J Med Genet*, **88**, 533–538.

Paterson, A.H., Lander, E.S., Hewitt, J.D., Peterson, S., Lincoln, S.E. and Tanksley, S.D., 1988. Resolution of quantitative traits into Mendelian factors by using a complete linkage map of restriction fragment length polymorphisms. *Nature*, **335**, 721–726.

Pericak-Vance, M.A., 1998. Linkage disequilibrium and allelic association. In: Haines, J.L., Pericak-Vance, M.A. (eds), *Approaches to Gene Mapping in Complex Human Diseases*, pp. 321–334. Wiley-Liss, New York.

Perry, S.E., Summar, M.L., Phillips, J.A., 3rd and Robertson, D., 1991. Linkage analysis of the human dopamine beta-hydroxylase gene. *Genomics*, **10**, 493–495.

Persson, M.L., Wasserman, D., Geijer, T., Frisch, A., Rockah, R., Michaelovsky, E., Apter, A., Weizman, A., Jonsson, E.G. and Bergman, H., 2000a. Dopamine D4 receptor gene polymorphism and personality traits in healthy volunteers. *Eur Arch Psychiatry Clin Neurosci*, **250**, 203–206.

Persson, M.L., Wasserman, D., Geijer, T., Jonsson, E.G. and Terenius, L., 1997. Tyrosine hydroxylase allelic distribution in suicide attempters. *Psychiatry Res*, **72**, 73–80.

Persson, M.L., Wasserman, D., Jonsson, E.G., Bergman, H., Terenius, L., Gyllander, A., Neiman, J. and Geijer, T., 2000b. Search for the influence of the tyrosine hydroxylase (TCAT)(n) repeat polymorphism on personality traits. *Psychiatry Res*, **95**, 1–8.

Pesonen, U., Koulu, M., Bergen, A., Eggert, M., Naukkarinen, H., Virkkunen, M., Linnoila, M. and Goldman, D., 1998. Mutation screening of the 5-hydroxytryptamine7 receptor gene among Finnish alcoholics and controls. *Psychiatry Res*, **77**, 139–145.

Phillips, T.J., Huson, M., Gwiazdon, C., Burkhart-Kasch, S. and Shen, E.H., 1995. Effects of acute and repeated ethanol exposures on the locomotor activity of BXD recombinant inbred mice. *Alcohol Clin Exp Res*, **19**, 269–278.

Plomin, R., Owen, M.J. and McGuffin, P., 1994. The genetic basis of complex human behaviors. *Science*, **264**, 1733–1739.

Pogue-Geile, M., Ferrell, R., Deka, R., Debski, T. and Manuck, S., 1998. Human novelty-seeking personality traits and dopamine D4 receptor polymorphisms: a twin and genetic association study. *Am J Med Genet*, **81**, 44–48.

Popova, N.K., Vishnivetskaya, G.B., Ivanova, E.A., Skrinskaya, J.A. and Seif, I., 2000. Altered behavior and alcohol tolerance in transgenic mice lacking MAO A: a comparison with effects of MAO A inhibitor clorgyline. *Pharmacol Biochem Behav*, **67**, 719–727.

Poston, W.S., 2nd, Ericsson, M., Linder, J., Haddock, C.K., Hanis, C.L., Nilsson, T., Astrom, M. and Foreyt, J.P., 1998. D4 dopamine receptor gene exon III polymorphism and obesity risk. *Eat Weight Disord*, **3**, 71–77.

Pritchard, J.K., Stephens, M., Rosenberg, N.A. and Donnelly, P., 2000. Association mapping in structured populations. *Am J Hum Genet*, **67**, 170–181.

Raleigh, M.J., McGuire, M.T., Brammer, G.L., Pollack, D.B. and Yuwiler, A., 1991. Serotonergic mechanisms promote dominance acquisition in adult male vervet monkeys. *Brain Res*, **559**, 181–190.

Ramboz, S., Oosting, R., Amara, D.A., Kung, H.F., Blier, P., Mendelsohn, M., Mann, J.J., Brunner, D. and Hen, R., 1998. Serotonin receptor 1A knockout: an animal model of anxiety-related disorder. *Proc Natl Acad Sci USA*, **95**, 14476–14481.

Ramboz, S., Saudou, F., Amara, D.A., Belzung, C., Segu, L., Misslin, R., Buhot, M.C. and Hen, R., 1996. 5-HT1B receptor knock out — behavioral consequences. *Behav Brain Res*, **73**, 305–312.

Ricketts, M.H., Hamer, R.M., Sage, J.I., Manowitz, P., Feng, F. and Menza, M.A., 1998. Association of a serotonin transporter gene promoter polymorphism with harm avoidance behaviour in an elderly population. *Psychiatr Genet*, **8**, 41–44.

Rocha, B.A., Scearce-Levie, K., Lucas, J.J., Hiroi, N., Castanon, N., Crabbe, J.C., Nestler, E.J. and Hen, R., 1998. Increased vulnerability to cocaine in mice lacking the serotonin-1B receptor. *Nature*, **393**, 175–178.

Rocheville, M., Lange, D.C., Kumar, U., Patel, S.C., Patel, R.C. and Patel, Y.C., 2000. Receptors for dopamine and somatostatin: formation of hetero-oligomers with enhanced functional activity. *Science*, **288**, 154–157.

Ronai, Z., Szekely, A., Nemoda, Z., Lakatos, K., Gervai, J., Staub, M. and Sasvari-Szekely, M., 2001. Association between Novelty Seeking and the −521 C/T polymorphism in the promoter region of the DRD4 gene. *Mol Psychiatry*, **6**, 35–38.

Rosenthal, N.E., Mazzanti, C.M., Barnett, R.L., Hardin, T.A., Turner, E.H., Lam, G.K., Ozaki, N. and Goldman, D., 1998. Role of serotonin transporter promoter repeat length polymorphism (5-HTTLPR) in seasonality and seasonal affective disorder. *Mol Psychiatry*, **3**, 175–177.

Roth, B.L., 1994. Multiple serotonin receptors: clinical and experimental aspects. *Ann Clin Psychiatry*, **6**, 67–78.

Rowe, D.C., Stever, C., Giedinghagen, L.N., Gard, J.M., Cleveland, H.H., Terris, S.T., Mohr, J.H., Sherman, S., Abramowitz, A. and Waldman, I.D., 1998. Dopamine DRD4 receptor polymorphism and attention deficit hyperactivity disorder. *Mol Psychiatry*, **3**, 419–426.

Rubinstein, M., Phillips, T.J., Bunzow, J.R., Falzone, T.L., Dziewczapolski, G., Zhang, G., Fang, Y., Larson, J.L., McDougall, J.A., Chester, J.A., Saez, C., Pugsley, T.A., Gershanik, O., Low, M.J. and Grandy, D.K., 1997. Mice lacking dopamine D4 receptors are supersensitive to ethanol, cocaine, and methamphetamine. *Cell*, **90**, 991–1001.

Rubinsztein, D.C., Leggo, J., Goodburn, S., Walsh, C., Jain, S. and Paykel, E.S., 1996. Genetic association between monoamine oxidase A microsatellite and RFLP alleles and bipolar affective disorder: analysis and meta-analysis. *Hum Mol Genet*, **5**, 779–782.

Sabol, S.Z., Hu, S. and Hamer, D., 1998. A functional polymorphism in the monoamine oxidase A gene promoter. *Hum Genet*, **103**, 273–279.

Sabol, S.Z., Nelson, M.L., Fisher, C., Gunzerath, L., Brody, C.L., Hu, S., Sirota, L.A., Marcus, S.E., Greenberg, B.D., Lucas, F.Rt., Benjamin, J., Murphy, D.L. and Hamer, D.H., 1999. A genetic association for cigarette smoking behavior. *Health Psychol*, **18**, 7–13.

Sachidanandam, R., Weissman, D., Schmidt, S.C., Kakol, J.M., Stein, L.D., Marth, G., Sherry, S., Mullikin, J.C., Mortimore, B.J., Willey, D.L., Hunt, S.E., Cole, C.G., Coggill, P.C., Rice, C.M., Ning, Z., Rogers, J., Bentley, D.R., Kwok, P.Y., Mardis, E.R., Yeh, R.T., Schultz, B., Cook, L., Davenport, R., Dante, M., Fulton, L., Hillier, L., Waterston, R.H., McPherson, J.D., Gilman, B., Schaffner, S., Van Etten, W.J., Reich, D., Higgins, J., Daly, M.J., Blumenstiel, B., Baldwin, J., Stange-Thomann, N., Zody, M.C., Linton, L., Lander, E.S. and Attshuler, D., 2001. A map of human genome sequence variation containing 1.42 million single nucleotide polymorphisms. *Nature*, **409**, 928–933.

Samochowiec, J., Lesch, K.P., Rottmann, M., Smolka, M., Syagailo, Y.V., Okladnova, O., Rommelspacher, H., Winterer, G., Schmidt, L.G. and Sander, T., 1999. Association of a regulatory polymorphism in the promoter region of the monoamine oxidase A gene with antisocial alcoholism. *Psychiatry Res*, **86**, 67–72.

Sander, T., Ball, D., Murray, R., Patel, J., Samochowiec, J., Winterer, G., Rommelspacher, H., Schmidt, L.G. and Loh, E.W., 1999a. Association analysis of sequence variants of GABA(A) alpha6, beta2, and gamma2 gene cluster and alcohol dependence. *Alcohol Clin Exp Res*, **23**, 427–431.

Sander, T., Harms, H., Dufeu, P., Kuhn, S., Hoehe, M., Lesch, K.P., Rommelspacher, H. and Schmidt, L.G., 1998. Serotonin transporter gene variants in alcohol-dependent subjects with dissocial personality disorder. *Biol Psychiatry*, **43**, 908–912.

Sander, T., Harms, H., Dufeu, P., Kuhn, S., Rommelspacher, H. and Schmidt, L.G., 1997a. Dopamine D4 receptor exon III alleles and variation of novelty seeking in alcoholics. *Am J Med Genet*, **74**, 483–487.

Sander, T., Harms, H., Lesch, K.P., Dufeu, P., Kuhn, S., Hoehe, M., Rommelspacher, H. and Schmidt, L.G., 1997b. Association analysis of a regulatory variation of the serotonin transporter gene with severe alcohol dependence. *Alcohol Clin Exp Res*, **21**, 1356–1359.

Sander, T., Ostapowicz, A., Samochowiec, J., Smolka, M., Winterer, G. and Schmidt, L.G., 2000. Genetic variation of the glutamate transporter EAAT2 gene and vulnerability to alcohol dependence. *Psychiatr Genet*, **10**, 103–107.

Sander, T., Samochowiec, J., Ladehoff, M., Smolka, M., Peters, C., Riess, O., Rommelspacher, H. and Schmidt, L.G., 1999b. Association analysis of exonic variants of the gene encoding the GABAB receptor and alcohol dependence. *Psychiatr Genet*, **9**, 69–73.

Sano, A., Kondoh, K., Kakimoto, Y. and Kondo, I., 1993. A 40-nucleotide repeat polymorphism in the human dopamine transporter gene. *Hum Genet*, **91**, 405–406.

Sarkar, G., Kapelner, S., Grandy, D.K., Marchionni, M., Civelli, O., Sobell, J., Heston, L. and Sommer, S.S., 1991. Direct sequencing of the dopamine D2 receptor (DRD2) in schizophrenics reveals three polymorphisms but no structural change in the receptor. *Genomics*, **11**, 8–14.

Saudou, F., Amara, D.A., Dierich, A., LeMeur, M., Ramboz, S., Segu, L., Buhot, M.C. and Hen, R., 1994. Enhanced aggressive behavior in mice lacking 5-HT1B receptor. *Science*, **265**, 1875–1878.

Saxena, P.R., 1995. Serotonin receptors: subtypes, functional responses and therapeutic relevance. *Pharmacol Ther*, **66**, 339–368.

Schalling, D., Asberg, M., Edman, G. and Oreland, L., 1987. Markers for vulnerability to psychopathology: temperament traits associated with platelet MAO activity. *Acta Psychiatr Scand*, **76**, 172–182.

Schloss, P. and Williams, D.C., 1998. The serotonin transporter: a primary target for antidepressant drugs. *J Psychopharmacol*, **12**, 115–121.

Schuback, D.E., Mulligan, E.L., Sims, K.B., Tivol, E.A., Greenberg, B.D., Chang, S.F., Yang, S.L., Mau, Y.C., Shen, C.Y., Ho, M.S., Yang, N.H., Butler, M.G., Fink, S., Schwartz, C.E., Berlin, F., Breakefield, X.O., Murphy, D.L. and Hsu, Y.P., 1999. Screen for MAOA mutations in target human groups. *Am J Med Genet*, **88**, 25–28.

Schuckit, M.A., Mazzanti, C., Smith, T.L., Ahmed, U., Radel, M., Iwata, N. and Goldman, D., 1999. Selective genotyping for the role of 5-HT2A, 5-HT2C, and GABA alpha 6 receptors and the serotonin transporter in the level of response to alcohol: a pilot study. *Biol Psychiatry*, **45**, 647–651.

Schulze, T.G., Muller, D.J., Krauss, H., Scherk, H., Ohlraun, S., Syagailo, Y.V., Windemuth, C., Neidt, H., Grassle, M., Papassotiropoulos, A., Heun, R., Nothen, M.M., Maier, W., Lesch, K.P. and Rietschel, M., 2000. Association between a functional polymorphism in the monoamine oxidase A gene promoter and major depressive disorder. *Am J Med Genet*, **96**, 801–803.

Serretti, A., Cusin, C., Lattuada, E., Di Bella, D., Catalano, M. and Smeraldi, E., 1999. Serotonin transporter gene (5-HTTLPR) is not associated with depressive symptomatology in mood disorders. *Mol Psychiatry*, **4**, 280–283.

Shen, S., Battersby, S., Weaver, M., Clark, E., Stephens, K. and Harmar, A.J., 2000. Refined mapping of the human serotonin transporter (SLC6A4) gene within 17q11 adjacent to the CPD and NF1 genes. *Eur J Hum Genet*, **8**, 75–78.
Sher, L., Greenberg, B.D., Murphy, D.L., Rosenthal, N.E., Sirota, L.A. and Hamer, D.H., 2000. Pleiotropy of the serotonin transporter gene for seasonality and neuroticism. *Psychiatr Genet*, **10**, 125–130.
Sher, L., Hardin, T.A., Greenberg, B.D., Murphy, D.L., Li, Q. and Rosenthal, N.E., 1999. Seasonality associated with the serotonin transporter promoter repeat length polymorphism. *Am J Psychiatry*, **156**, 1837.
Shih, J.C., Chen, K. and Ridd, M.J., 1999. Monoamine oxidase: from genes to behavior. *Annu Rev Neurosci*, **22**, 197–217.
Shulman, R., Griffiths, J. and Diewold, P., 1978. Catechol-*O*-methyl transferase activity in patients with depressive illness and anxiety states. *Br J Psychiatry*, **132**, 133–138.
Sibille, E., Pavlides, C., Benke, D. and Toth, M., 2000. Genetic inactivation of the serotonin(1A) receptor in mice results in downregulation of major GABA(A) receptor alpha subunits, reduction of GABA(A) receptor binding, and benzodiazepine-resistant anxiety. *J Neurosci*, **20**, 2758–2765.
Sims, K.B., de la Chapelle, A., Norio, R., Sankila, E.M., Hsu, Y.P., Rinehart, W.B., Corey, T.J., Ozelius, L., Powell, J.F. and Bruns, G., 1989. Monoamine oxidase deficiency in males with an X chromosome deletion. *Neuron*, **2**, 1069–1076.
Sirota, L.A., Greenberg, B.D., Murphy, D.L. and Hamer, D.H., 1999. Non-linear association between the serotonin transporter promoter polymorphism and neuroticism: a caution against using extreme samples to identify quantitative trait loci. *Psychiatr Genet*, **9**, 35–38.
Smalley, S.L., Bailey, J.N., Palmer, C.G., Cantwell, D.P., McGough, J.J., Del'Homme, M.A., Asarnow, J.R., Woodward, J.A., Ramsey, C. and Nelson, S.F., 1998. Evidence that the dopamine D4 receptor is a susceptibility gene in attention deficit hyperactivity disorder. *Mol Psychiatry*, **3**, 427–430.
Snyder, S.H. and Ferris, C.D., 2000. Novel neurotransmitters and their neuropsychiatric relevance. *Am J Psychiatry*, **157**, 1738–1751.
Sobesky, W.E., Hull, C.E. and Hagerman, R.J., 1994. Symptoms of schizotypal personality disorder in fragile X women. *J Am Acad Child Adolesc Psychiatry*, **33**, 247–255.
Sokoloff, P., Giros, B., Martres, M.P., Bouthenet, M.L. and Schwartz, J.C., 1990. Molecular cloning and characterization of a novel dopamine receptor (D3) as a target for neuroleptics. *Nature*, **347**, 146–151.
Speer, M.C., 1998. Sample size and power. In: Haines, J.L., Pericak-Vance, M.A. (eds), *Approaches to Gene Mapping in Complex Human Diseases*, pp. 161–200. Wiley-Liss, New York.
Spurlock, G., Heils, A., Holmans, P., Williams, J., D'Souza, U.M., Cardno, A., Murphy, K.C., Jones, L., Buckland, P.R., McGuffin, P., Lesch, K.P. and Owen, M.J., 1998. A family based association study of T102 C polymorphism in 5HT2A and schizophrenia plus identification of new polymorphisms in the promoter. *Mol Psychiatry*, **3**, 42–49.
Staner, L., Hilger, C., Hentges, F., Monreal, J., Hoffmann, A., Couturier, M., Le Bon, O., Stefos, G., Souery, D. and Mendlewicz, J., 1998. Association between novelty-seeking and the dopamine D3 receptor gene in bipolar patients: a preliminary report. *Am J Med Genet*, **81**, 192–194.
Steyaert, J., Decruyenaere, M., Borghgraef, M. and Fryns, J.P., 1994. Personality profile in adult female fragile X carriers: assessed with the Minnesota Multiphasic Personality Profile (MMPI). *Am J Med Genet*, **51**, 370–373.
Strobel, A., Lesch, K.P., Hohenberger, K., Jatzke, S., Gutzeit, H.O., Anacker, K. and Brocke, B., 2002. No association between polymorphism of the dopamine D4 receptor gene and novelty seeking. *Mol Psychiatry* (in press).
Strobel, A., Wehr, A., Michel, A. and Brocke, B., 1999. Association between the dopamine D4 receptor (DRD4) exon III polymorphism and measures of novelty seeking in a German population. *Mol Psychiatry*, **4**, 378–384.
Strous, R.D., Bark, N., Parsia, S.S., Volavka, J. and Lachman, H.M., 1997. Analysis of a functional catechol-*O*-methyltransferase gene polymorphism in schizophrenia: evidence for association with aggressive and antisocial behavior. *Psychiatry Res*, **69**, 71–77.
Sullivan, P.F., Fifield, W.J., Kennedy, M.A., Mulder, R.T., Sellman, J.D. and Joyce, P.R., 1998. No association between novelty seeking and the type 4 dopamine receptor gene (DRD4) in two New Zealand samples. *Am J Psychiatry*, **155**, 98–101.
Swanson, J.M., Sunohara, G.A., Kennedy, J.L., Regino, R., Fineberg, E., Wigal, T., Lerner, M., Williams, L., LaHoste, G.J. and Wigal, S., 1998. Association of the dopamine receptor D4 (DRD4) gene with a refined phenotype of attention deficit hyperactivity disorder (ADHD): a family-based approach. *Mol Psychiatry*, **3**, 38–41.
Syagailo, Y.V., Stöber, G., Grässle, M., Reimer, E., Jungkunz, G., Okladnova, O., Meyer, J. and Lesch, K.P., 2001. Association analysis of the functional monoamine oxidase A gene promoter polymorphism in psychiatric disorders. *Am J Med Genet*, **105**, 168–171.
Syvanen, A.C., Tilgmann, C., Rinne, J. and Ulmanen, I., 1997. Genetic polymorphism of catechol-*O*-methyltransferase (COMT): correlation of genotype with individual variation of S-COMT activity and comparison of the allele frequencies in the normal population and parkinsonian patients in Finland. *Pharmacogenetics*, **7**, 65–71.
Tecott, L.H. and Barondes, S.H., 1996. Genes and aggressiveness. Behavioural genetics. *Curr Biol*, **6**, 238–240.
Tecott, L.H., Sun, L.M., Akana, S.F., Strack, A.M., Lowenstein, D.H., Dallman, M.F. and Julius, D., 1995. Eating disorder and epilepsy in mice lacking 5-HT2c serotonin receptors. *Nature*, **374**, 542–546.
Tien, A.Y., Costa, P.T. and Eaton, W.W., 1992. Covariance of personality, neurocognition, and schizophrenia spectrum traits in the community. *Schizophr Res*, **7**, 149–158.
Tiihonen, J., Hallikainen, T., Lachman, H., Saito, T., Volavka, J., Kauhanen, J., Salonen, J.T., Ryynanen, O.P., Koulu, M., Karvonen, M.K., Pohjalainen, T., Syvalahti, E. and Hietala, J., 1999. Association between the functional variant of the catechol-*O*-methyltransferase (COMT) gene and type 1 alcoholism. *Mol Psychiatry*, **4**, 286–289.
Tomitaka, M., Tomitaka, S., Otuka, Y., Kim, K., Matuki, H., Sakamoto, K. and Tanaka, A., 1999. Association between novelty seeking and dopamine receptor D4 (DRD4) exon III polymorphism in Japanese subjects. *Am J Med Genet*, **88**, 469–471.
Trefilov, A., Berard, J., Krawczak, M. and Schmidtke, J., 2000. Natal dispersal in rhesus macaques is related to serotonin transporter gene promoter variation. *Behav Genet*, **30**, 295–301.
Tsai, S.J., Hong, C.J. and Wang, Y.C., 1999. Tryptophan hydroxylase gene polymorphism (A218C) and suicidal behaviors. *Neuroreport*, **10**, 3773–3775.
Ueno, S., Nakamura, M., Mikami, M., Kondoh, K., Ishiguro, H., Arinami, T., Komiyama, T., Mitsushio, H., Sano, A. and Tanabe, H., 1999. Identification of a novel polymorphism of the human dopamine transporter (DAT1) gene and the significant association with alcoholism. *Mol Psychiatry*, **4**, 552–557.
Vandenbergh, D.J., Rodriguez, L.A., Hivert, E., Schiller, J.H., Villareal, G., Pugh, E.W., Lachman, H. and Uhl, G.R., 2000. Long forms of the dopamine receptor (DRD4) gene VNTR are more prevalent in substance abusers: no interaction with functional alleles of the catechol-*O*-methyltransferase (COMT) gene. *Am J Med Genet*, **96**, 678–683.
Vandenbergh, D.J., Zonderman, A.B., Wang, J., Uhl, G.R. and Costa, P.T., Jr., 1997. No association between novelty seeking and dopamine D4 receptor (D4DR) exon III seven repeat alleles in Baltimore Longitudinal Study of Aging participants. *Mol Psychiatry*, **2**, 417–419.
Van Tol, H.H., Wu, C.M., Guan, H.C., Ohara, K., Bunzow, J.R., Civelli, O., Kennedy, J., Seeman, P., Niznik, H.B. and Jovanovic, V., 1992. Multiple dopamine D4 receptor variants in the human population. *Nature*, **358**, 149–152.
Vanyukov, M.M., Moss, H.B., Yu, L.M. and Deka, R., 1995. A dinucleotide repeat polymorphism at the gene for monoamine oxidase A and measures of aggressiveness. *Psychiatry Res*, **59**, 35–41.
Vernon, P.A., McCarthy, J.M., Johnson, A.M., Jang, K.L. and Harris, J.A., 1999. Individual differences in multiple dimensions of aggression: a univariate and multivariate genetic analysis. *Twin Res*, **2**, 16–21.
Virkkunen, M., Goldman, D. and Linnoila, M., 1996. Serotonin in alcoholic violent offenders. *Ciba Found Symp*, **194**, 168–177.
Weiner, J., 1999. *Time, Love, Memory*. A.A. Knopf, New York.
Weinshilboum, R.M. and Raymond, F.A., 1977. Inheritance of low erythrocyte catechol-*O*-methyltransferase activity in man. *Am J Hum Genet*, **29**, 125–135.
Wichems, C.H., Li, Q., Holmes, A., Crawley, J.N., Tjurmina, O., Goldstein, D., Andrews, A.M., Lesch, K.P. and Murphy, D.L., 2000. Mechanisms mediating the increased anxiety-like behavior and excessive responses to stress in mice lacking the serotonin transporter. *Soc Neurosci Abst*, **26**, 400.

Williams, J., McGuffin, P., Nothen, M. and Owen, M.J., 1997. Meta-analysis of association between the 5-HT2a receptor T102C polymorphism and schizophrenia. EMASS Collaborative Group. European Multicentre Association Study of Schizophrenia. *Lancet*, **349**, 1221.

Williams, J., Spurlock, G., McGuffin, P., Mallet, J., Nothen, M.M., Gill, M., Aschauer, H., Nylander, P.O., Macciardi, F. and Owen, M.J., 1996. Association between schizophrenia and T102C polymorphism of the 5-hydroxytryptamine type 2a-receptor gene. European Multicentre Association Study of Schizophrenia (EMASS) Group. *Lancet*, **347**, 1294–1296.

Wilson, E.O., 1978. *On Human Nature*. Harvard University Press, Cambridge, MA.

Wilson, E.O., 1998. *Consilience. The Unity of Knowledge*. A.A. Knopf, New York.

Wong, A.H., Buckle, C.E. and Van Tol, H.H., 2000. Polymorphisms in dopamine receptors: what do they tell us? *Eur J Pharmacol*, **410**, 183–203.

World Health Organization, 1992. *International statistical classification of diseases and related health problems, 10th Revision*. World Health Organisation, Geneva.

Zabetian, C.P., Anderson, G.M., Buxbaum, S.G., Elston, R.C., Ichinose, H., Nagatsu, T., Kim, K.S., Kim, C.H., Malison, R.T., Gelernter, J. and Cubells, J.F., 2001. A quantitative-trait analysis of human plasma-dopamine beta-hydroxylase activity: evidence for a major functional polymorphism at the DBH locus. *Am J Hum Genet*, **68**, 515–522.

Zhou, Q.Y. and Palmiter, R.D., 1995. Dopamine-deficient mice are severely hypoactive, adipsic, and aphagic. *Cell*, **83**, 1197–1209.

Zhou, Q.Y., Quaife, C.J. and Palmiter, R.D., 1995. Targeted disruption of the tyrosine hydroxylase gene reveals that catecholamines are required for mouse foetal development. *Nature*, **374**, 640–643.

XXVI-8

Gene–Environment Interactions in Personality Disorders

Joel Paris

PERSONALITY DISORDERS AND THE STRESS-DIATHESIS MODEL

Personality disorders are clinical syndromes in which personality traits cause psychopathology. Disorders are diagnosed when traits interfere with occupational and personal adjustment, leading to distress and/or dysfunction. Patients meeting these criteria develop abnormalities of behaviour, affect, and cognition that begin early in life, are pervasive in many contexts, and remain consistent over time.

The roots of personality disorders lie both in genetic vulnerability and environmental adversity. Research in every category of mental disorder demonstrates genetic predispositions associated with psychopathology (Paris, 1999). These vulnerabilities are then uncovered and unleashed by environmental stressors. Predisposition and stress have an interactive relationship: genetic variability influences the way individuals respond to their environment, while environmental factors determine whether genes are expressed.

These principles describe a general theory of the aetiology of mental disorders, the stress-diathesis model (Monroe and Simons, 1991; Paris, 1999). This model provides a frame for understanding the role of gene–environment interactions in personality disorders.

One of the main problems in identifying genetic and biological factors in personality disorders concerns how to define the phenotype (Jang *et al.*, 2001). Diagnoses, as defined in the current psychiatric classification, are not very useful in this regard. Each of the present categories of personality disorders has some relationship to biological variables, but only to the extent that these disorders reflect traits. When we apply a wide range of research strategies (genetic associations, imaging, biological markers, or neuropsychological testing), relationships with measures of biological function are consistently stronger with traits, and weaker with disorders.

The relationship between traits and disorders is crucial to understanding the nature of personality pathology. Trait vulnerabilities, by themselves, do not explain why patients develop clinical symptoms. Instead, interactions between genetic and environmental factors, leading to pathological feedback loops, are responsible for the amplification of traits to dysfunctional levels.

TEMPERAMENT, PERSONALITY TRAITS AND PERSONALITY DISORDERS

Personality disorders, personality traits, and temperament have a hierarchical relationship (Rutter, 1987). Temperament refers to behavioural dispositions present at birth. Personality traits are individual differences in behaviour that remain stable over time and context. These characteristics represent an amalgam of inborn characteristics and the effects of life experiences. Personality disorders describe dysfunctional outcomes arising from traits.

In trait psychology, personality is measured as 'dimensions' with a normal distribution. Therefore, each personality profile should be common in the general population, and be compatible with normality. Disorders occur when these traits are amplified, and used in rigid and maladaptive ways.

Using current criteria, some studies (Weissman, 1993) have estimated that approximately 10% of the general population have a diagnosable personality disorder. Clearly, the precise figure depends on the cut-off point one uses. If personality is dimensional, one would expect to find no sharp break between traits and disorders. Research in clinical and community populations (Livesley and Jang, 2000) consistently supports this principle.

Personality disorders are even more common in treatment settings (Loranger *et al.*, 1994). But they are not always recognized as such, since patients present clinically when they also have Axis I symptoms. Moreover, there are serious problems in the classification of personality disorders.

CATEGORICAL AND DIMENSIONAL MODELS OF PERSONALITY DISORDERS

DSM-IV (American Psychiatric Association, 1994) divides personality disorders into 10 categories. ICD-10 (World Health Organization, 1992) uses a similar system of classification, describing most of the same types. DSM groups these diagnoses into three clusters (A, B, and C) that share common characteristics. A patient who meets the overall criteria for a disorder, but who does not fall into any specific category, is classified as 'personality disorder, not otherwise specified' (NOS). Many patients fail to fit prototypically into any single category, and about a third of all cases fall into the 'NOS' group (Loranger *et al.*, 1994).

Cluster A, described as 'odd', includes schizoid, paranoid, and schizotypal disorders, all of which lie in the 'schizophrenic spectrum' (Siever and Davis, 1991). Cluster B, which can be called either 'dramatic' or impulsive, includes antisocial, borderline, narcissistic, and histrionic disorders. Cluster C, described as 'anxious', includes avoidant, dependent, and compulsive disorders.

Many of these categories exist largely on the basis of clinical tradition, and their validity is suspect. The constructs describing schizotypal, antisocial, and borderline personality are the most useful, since each of these diagnoses communicates crucial clinical information in a compact fashion. Thus, typical patients in each of these categories have a characteristic outcome and a characteristic treatment response.

One of the most serious difficulties with the existing categories is that they overlap, with most patients earning more than one diagnosis (Pfohl *et al.*, 1986). Many (but not all) of these overlaps occur within clusters. The clusters therefore reflect underlying dimensions, which may be more valid than individual categories. In

Biological Psychiatry: Edited by H. D'haenen, J.A. den Boer and P. Willner. ISBN 0-471-49198-5

support of this hypothesis, family history methods demonstrate that personality traits within clusters are often shared with first-degree relatives (Siever and Davis, 1991).

In the European tradition, personality disturbances have been thought to be milder versions, or 'formes frustes', of major mental disorders. Some evidence supports this view. For example, schizotypal personality shares biological markers with schizophrenia, suggesting that it represents a less severe form of the illness (Siever and Davis, 1991). Similarly, antisocial and borderline personality disorders share markers with substance abuse and other Axis I impulsive disorders (Zanarini, 1993). Avoidant and compulsive personality have common family histories with Axis I anxiety disorders (Paris, 1998).

The largest body of empirical research has focused on the antisocial and borderline categories. The only category to have been examined systematically in epidemiological surveys is antisocial personality. (The forthcoming International Comorbidity Survey will also measure the prevalence of borderline personality.) About 2–3% of the population (mostly males) meet criteria for antisocial personality (Robins and Regier, 1991). By indirect evidence, 2% of the population (mostly females) can probably be diagnosed with borderline personality (Swartz *et al.*, 1990).

Traits provide an alternate way to measure personality disorders. Trait dimensions are generally derived from the factor analysis of self-report data. The most influential system has been the 'five factor model' (FFM)(McCrae and Costa, 1999), which describes personality profiles with scores measuring 'neuroticism', 'extraversion', 'openness to experience', 'conscientiousness', and 'agreeableness'. In a related schema, Livesley *et al.* (1993) described personality through 18 narrow dimensions that can also be grouped into superfactors that closely resemble four of the five factors in the FFM. Cloninger *et al.*'s (1993) model attempts to unite factor analysis and biological theory. His schema describes seven factors in personality, of which four are posited to be 'temperamental' (novelty seeking, reward dependence, harm avoidance, and persistence), and three are posited to be 'characterological'.

Biological researchers tend to favour dimensional measures of personality. This preference arises from the relationship between biological variability and traits. Moreover, dimensional systems describe pathology as rooted in unusually high levels of traits, concordant with the concept that disorders are amplified versions of these characteristics. However, it is not certain which schema provides the best description of personality. To answer this question, we require more research into the mechanisms that shape traits. Although factor analytical data can be useful in searching for genetic factors, dimensions should ultimately be rooted in biology (Paris, 2000a).

GENETIC FACTORS IN PERSONALITY

To the extent that personality dimensions represent normally distributed individual differences, they should be heritable. However, single genes will not often be associated with single traits. The heritable component of personality emerges from complex and interactive polygenetic mechanisms associated with variations in multiple alleles (Livesley and Jang, 2000).

It is nonetheless striking that virtually every personality dimension that has been studied has been found to have a heritable component, with genetic factors accounting for nearly half the variance on every trait (Plomin *et al.*, 1997). This conclusion has emerged consistently from behavioural genetic studies comparing concordance in traits between monozygotic (MZ) and dizygotic (DZ) twins. Twin methodology is based on the equal-environments assumption, that is, that there is no consistent difference in the environment of MZ and DZ twins, a conclusion in accord with a large body of evidence (Kendler *et al.*, 1993). However, the percentage of the variance accounted for by genetic variability is not that precise, since twin methodology tends to exaggerate the heritable component, and is subject to error variance. Another limitation of twin studies is that they do not readily identify gene–environment correlations.

Adoption studies (Plomin *et al.*, 1997), as well as studies of twins separated at birth (Tellegen *et al.*, 1988), confirm the heritability of traits. Moreover, the degree of heritability is about the same irrespective of which schema is used to define personality dimensions. It therefore seems safe to conclude that individual differences in personality have a strong basis in heredity and temperament.

Associations between personality traits and genetic variations derive from many different genes, and are therefore measurable as quantitative trait loci. But, thus far, this line of investigation has been disappointing. Promising earlier reports (e.g., Lesch *et al.*, 1996) have not been consistently replicated (Gelertner *et al.*, 1998). The main reason is that single alleles account for only a small percentage of the variance on any trait. These studies also suffer from the lack of a precise phenotype for personality traits.

The presence of a genetic component in personality also implies that traits should be linked to biological markers. Research in this area is at an early stage. Thus far, the strongest finding has been a strong relationship, established in clinical populations, between low levels of central serotonin activity and impulsivity (Mann, 1998).

ENVIRONMENTAL FACTORS IN PERSONALITY

The other half of the variance in personality derives from the environment. Again, behaviour genetic studies shed light on the nature of this influence. The variance affecting traits is almost all 'unshared', meaning that it does not depend on being raised in the same family (Plomin *et al.*, 2001). In fact, siblings demonstrate little similarity in personality.

This finding points to the importance of gene–environment interactions. Moreover, the environment is also complex and interactive. In contrast to classical ideas in developmental and clinical psychology, parenting is not the only factor shaping personality development. Since temperament affects the response of others in the environment, parents respond differently to different children. In a recent large-scale study of adolescents (Reiss *et al.*, 2000), using a combination of twin and family methods, multivariate analyses showed that the temperament of the child was the underlying factor driving differential parenting. This interaction is one of several reasons why family environment is unshared.

The other explanation for unshared environment concerns the unique nature of each person's experience. Thus, the environmental factors affecting personality are often extrafamilial. Every child has shaping experiences with peers, with teachers, or with community leaders (Rutter and Maughan, 1997). Harris (1998), who emphasizes these importance of these factors, has criticized the traditional view of parenting in psychology, which minimizes the role of social factors in personality development.

It is also important to note that developmental psychology has often failed to take into account the influence of genetic factors on measures of environmental influence. As Harris (1998) points out, almost all the literature claiming to establish links between life experiences and personality has to be questioned in this light. Personality traits can be latent variables affecting how the environment is perceived and how it affects development. For example, Plomin and Bergeman (1991) showed that standard measures of life stress, past and present, contain a heritable component that can best be accounted for by the influence of genetically influenced traits.

GENETIC FACTORS IN PERSONALITY DISORDERS

Whereas the heritability of personality traits is firmly established, evidence for the presence of genetic factors in personality disorders has been more equivocal. Research has been limited by a lack of diagnostic precision, and by the rarity of large-scale behavioural genetic studies.

Yet if disorders are amplified traits, one would expect them to demonstrate similar levels of heritability. Some writers (Nigg and Goldsmith, 1995) have argued that disorders represent extremes on a continuum, extremes less open to genetic influence and reflecting a larger environmental component. But this supposition seems illogical, since extremes on any normally distributed dimension should be more, not less, heritable.

In any case, the concept that environmental factors are more predominant in personality disorders has been overturned by recent data. Torgersen *et al.* (2000) located a large sample of twins in which one proband met criteria for at least one categorical diagnosis in the DSM classification. All personality disorders had heritabilities resembling those observed for traits (i.e., close to half the variance). Although these numbers lack precision (due to sample size), the heritability coefficient for disorders as a whole was 0.60 (0.37 for Cluster A, 0.60 for Cluster B, and 0.62 for Cluster C). There were no antisocials in the cohort, but in the borderline category, heritable factors accounted for over 69% of the variance, while in the narcissistic category, heritability was 77%.

These observations are highly consistent with the findings of family history studies (Siever and Davis, 1991). The heritability of mental disorders is generally greater when spectra including both Axis I and Axis II diagnoses are considered. Thus, first-degree relatives of patients with personality disorders tend to suffer from disorders lying within a closely related spectrum of pathology. For example, relatives of patients with disorders in Cluster A have pathology in the schizophrenic spectrum.

Similarly, patients in Cluster B tend to have relatives with other impulsive disorders. These observations led Zanarini (1993) to describe an 'impulsive spectrum', (including antisocial and borderline personality, as well as addictive disorders such as substance abuse or bulimia nervosa). Biological markers support these relationships, with the most robust findings linking decreased serotonin levels with aggression, impulsivity, and suicide attempts (Mann, 1999), all of which are characteristic features of the antisocial and borderline categories.

Parallel findings apply to Cluster C, where first-degree relatives tend to suffer from anxiety disorders. These relationships could be described as forming an 'anxious spectrum' (Paris, 1998). Temperamental anxiety has consistent physiological correlates, and it is heritable. An ongoing prospective study by Kagan (1994), following children with 'behavioural inhibition' (unusual levels of anxiety beginning in infancy) into adulthood, will shed further light on these links.

In summary, personality disorders have biological correlates related to underlying traits. Neurophysiological and neuropsychological correlates of personality disorders confirm these relationships. For example, functional abnormalities in the prefrontal cortex are associated with traits of impulsive aggression. Raine *et al.* (2000) has reported decreases in the mass of frontal grey matter in subjects with antisocial personality. On standard measures such as the Wisconsin Card Sorting Test, patients with antisocial and borderline personality demonstrate deficits in executive function (O'Leary *et al.*, 2000).

ENVIRONMENTAL FACTORS IN PERSONALITY DISORDERS

Psychotherapists have traditionally considered personality pathology to be the outcome of defective parenting. This belief was based on the assumption that disorders that begin early in life must be the result of adversities occurring even earlier in development.

Patients with personality disorders frequently report serious adversities during childhood. In borderline personality disorder, histories of sexual abuse, physical abuse, and gross neglect are particularly common (Zanarini, 2000). The common factor behind all these experiences is usually severe family dysfunction.

However neither trauma nor family pathology, by themselves, necessarily cause personality disorders. For example, community surveys of the impact of childhood sexual abuse (Browne and Finkelhor, 1986; Rind *et al.*, 1999) and physical abuse (Malinovsky-Rummell and Hansen, 1993) show that only a minority of those exposed suffer measurable sequelae. Single traumatic events are not strongly associated with pathology, while continuously adverse circumstances lead to cumulative effects that are much more consistent (Rutter, 1987). In general, patients experiencing multiple adversities, which also tend to be associated with more severe trauma, are at the greatest risk.

The retrospective methodologies used in most studies of childhood risks of personality disorders have also made firm conclusions about causality problematic. Almost all findings reported in the literature are based on reports of life experiences occurring many years in the past. Memories are coloured by recall bias, that is, the tendency for individuals with symptoms in the present to remember more adversities in the past.

Prospective studies are clearly needed to confirm these relationships. The best available longitudinal data concern the development of antisocial personality. Robins' (1966) study showed that the strongest predictor of adult antisocial outcome among conduct-disordered children (usually boys) is parental psychopathy, usually in a father. This association was later supported by Farrington's (1998) British follow-up studies.

These findings parallel data showing that close family members of patients with borderline personality disorder have increased levels of psychopathology, usually within the impulsive spectrum (Links *et al.*, 1988; Zanarini, 1993). The presence of impulsivity in parents reflects genetic risk factors, but impulsive parents (and their partners) are also more likely to be inconsistent, neglectful, or even abusive in their parenting behaviours.

A recent prospective longitudinal study has confirmed the relationship between childhood adversity and personality disorders. The Albany-Saratoga study has been following a large community cohort of children into young adulthood. In one report, Johnson *et al.* (1999) observed that early adversities, including neglect, physical abuse, and sexual abuse, were significant predictors of the number of personality disorder symptoms. (The researchers used this continuous variable to measure outcome, since few subjects in this study had a diagnosable personality disorder.) However, this relationship accounted for only part of the variance. The study design should have obtained more data on temperamental factors, which could have helped to account more precisely for outcome.

INTERACTIONS BETWEEN RISK FACTORS FOR PERSONALITY DISORDERS

Personality disorders can best be understood by using multifactorial models. The complexity and multitude of aetiological factors in these categories requires a biopsychosocial theory and a diathesis-stress model (Paris, 1996; 1999). The diatheses for personality disorders consist of abnormal temperament, while the stressors for these disorders consist of adverse life events.

The role of temperament as a risk factor is supported by observations that children with early behavioural disturbances are more likely to develop parallel forms of pathology later in life. Strikingly, children at the age of 3 years with high levels of aggression and irritability have been shown to be at risk of antisocial personality disorder in early adulthood (Caspi *et al.*, 1996). Moreover, when conduct symptoms during childhood begin earlier and are more pervasive, they are more likely to continue as antisocial personality (Zoccolillo *et al.*, 1992).

In the same way, infants with unusual shyness and reactivity ('behavioural inhibition') are at risk of either anxiety disorders (Kagan, 1994) or anxious cluster personality disorders (Paris, 1998). Although many in Kagan's cohort of behaviourally inhibited children eventually overcame their temperamental difficulties, none became extroverted or impulsive. When the group was followed into early adolescence, a minority still had significant social anxiety. It will be interesting to see whether this population is at risk of avoidant personality disorder in adulthood.

Some authors (e.g., Kernberg *et al.*, 2000) have suggested that personality disorders can be diagnosed in adolescence, or even in childhood. Although specific categories of disorder are unstable over time, overall personality disturbance has significant continuities. One longitudinal follow-up study (Lofgren *et al.*, 1991) showed that children with a wide range of behavioural disturbances (often termed 'borderline children') develop personality disorders in early adulthood.

The course of personality pathology over time provides a clue to its causes. Disorders beginning early in life are more likely to have a heritable biological component (Childs and Scriver, 1986). Moreover, most patients with personality disorders have a chronic course, with the exception of antisocial and borderline personality, which tend to 'burn out' by middle age (Paris, 1994).

Genetic-temperamental factors in personality disorders shed light on the relationship between childhood adversities and adult psychopathology. In community surveys of adults who report trauma and neglect during their development, associations between childhood trauma and sequelae are consistently much stronger in clinical than in community populations (Paris, 1997). While adverse events in development lead to psychopathology only in a minority of those exposed, some are more vulnerable than others (Rutter, 1989; Paris, 2000).

The explanation depends on interactions between genes and environment. The effects of adversity are greatest in individuals who are predisposed to psychopathology. In this respect, associations between reported adversities in childhood and personality disorders in adulthood are a classic example of the principle that correlation does not prove causation. Childhood adversity increases the risk of psychopathology in adulthood, but these effects are largely accounted for by vulnerable subpopulations.

Abnormal temperament is associated with a greater sensitivity to environmental risk factors. At the same time, individuals with problematic temperaments also experience more trauma and conflict during development (Rutter and Maughan, 1999). Children with difficult temperaments elicit responses from others that tend to amplify their most problematic characteristics. Specifically, those with high levels of aggression and irritability are in chronic conflict with their parents, as well as with their peers and teachers. These children respond to these conflicts with even greater aggression, creating a positive feedback loop. In a parallel fashion, children with behavioural inhibition elicit overprotective responses from their parents, which only amplify the problem (Kagan, 1994).

Thus, childhood adversities reflect positive feedback loops which are strongly influenced by personality traits. The more affected children are by these experiences, the more their traits become amplified. The more traits are amplified, the more likely children are to experience adversity.

In adult life, no specific relationship exists between stressors and symptoms (Paris, 1999). Instead, predispositions and vulnerabilities unique to each individual determine what type of disorder will develop. Personality traits lie at the core of these differences in susceptibility.

Finally, personality disorders are a social phenomenon. The prevalence of antisocial personality varies widely across cultures, suggesting that social forces play an important aetiological role in this condition. Similar considerations apply to other disorders characterized by impulsivity, such as borderline personality. The mechanisms could involve direct effects of social stressors, or indirect effects, due to the failure of the social community to buffer biological risks and/or psychological adversities (Paris, 1996).

Personality disorders are not the only possible outcome of temperamental vulnerability or psychosocial adversities. A spectra of disorders, including Axis I diagnoses, is associated with each of the Axis II clusters (schizophrenic, impulsive, and anxious). In cases where the dysfunction arising from the Axis I condition is extensive, one will not be able to diagnose a personality disorder. In other cases, Axis I and Axis II pathology will be 'comorbid'. But in either of these scenarios, common biological factors are mediated by personality trait profiles.

In summary, none of the risk factors associated with personality disorders are sufficient conditions for their development. Biological factors increase risk, but do not determine outcome. Psychosocial factors have little specificity, with similar forms of adversity being associated with many categories of disorder, or with no disorder at all.

Only a combination of risks, that is, a 'two-hit' or 'multiple hit' mechanism, can account for the data. While the cumulative effects of multiple risk factors determine whether psychopathology develops, the specific disorder that ultimately emerges depends on temperament (Kagan, 1994; Paris, 1996). Thus, only those with impulsive temperamental characteristics will develop Cluster B disorders, such as antisocial or borderline personality. Similarly, only those with introverted temperament will develop Cluster C disorders, such as avoidant personality.

SUMMARY

We can summarize the application of a stress-diathesis model to the personality disorders as follows:

1. Biological vulnerability and environmental adversity are necessary conditions, but neither is sufficient for the development of personality disorders.
2. The genetic factors in personality disorders are associated with temperamental predispositions.
3. Personality traits, which reflect both temperament and experience, are the underlying factors behind personality disorders.
4. Personality disorders are most likely to develop when environmental stressors, particularly multiple adversities with cumulative and interactive effects, amplify traits.
5. Environmental adversities have greater effects on those who are temperamentally vulnerable.
6. Once established, personality disorders are supported by positive feedback loops that lead to chronicity.

REFERENCES

American Psychiatric Association, 1994. *Diagnostic and Statistical Manual of Mental Disorders*, 4th edn. American Psychiatric Press, Washington, DC.

Benjamin, J., Patterson, C., Greenberg, B.D., Murphy, D.L. and Hamer, D.L., 1996. Population and familial association between the D4 receptor gene and measures of novelty seeking. *Nat Genet*, **12**, 81–84.

Browne, A. and Finkelhor, D., 1986. Impact of child sexual abuse: a review of the literature. *Psychol Bull*, **99**, 66–77.

Caspi, A., Moffitt, T.E., Newman, D.L. and Silva, P.A., 1996. Behavioral observations at age three predict adult psychiatric disorders: longitudinal evidence from a birth cohort. *Arch Gen Psychiatry*, **53**, 1033–1039.

Childs, B. and Scriver, C.R., 1986. Age at onset and causes of disease. Perspect *Biol Med*, **29**, 437–460.

Cloninger, C.R., Svrakic, D.M. and Pryzbeck, T.R., 1993. A psychobiological model of temperament and character. *Arch Gen Psychiatry*, **50**, 975–990.

Farrington, D.P., 1998. Youth crime and antisocial behavior. In Campbell, A., Muncer, S., (eds), *The Social Child*, pp. 353–392. Hove, Psychology Press.

Gelertner, J., Kranzler, H. and Lacobelle, J., 1998. Population studies of polymorphisms at loci of neuropsychiatric interest (tryptophan hydroxylase (TPH), dopamine transporter protein (SLC6A3), D3 dopamine receptor (DRD3), apolipoprotein E (APOE), mu opioid receptor (OPRM1), and ciliary neurotrophic factor (CNTF)). *Genomics*, **52**, 289–297.

Harris, J.R., 1998. *The Nurture Assumption*. Free Press, New York.

Jang, K., Vernon, P.A. and Livesley, W.J., 2001. Behavioural genetic perspectives on personality function. *Canad J Psychiatry*, **46**, 234–244.

Johnson, J.J., Cohen, P., Brown, J., Smailes, E.M. and Bernstein, D.P., 1999. Childhood maltreatment increases risk for personality disorders during early adulthood. *Arch Gen Psychiatry*, **56**, 600–606.

Kagan, J., 1994. *Galen's Prophecy*. Basic Books, New York.

Kendler, K.S., Neale, M.C., Kessler, R.C., Heath, A.C. and Eaves, L.J., 1993. A test of the equal-environment assumption in twin studies of psychiatric illness. *Behav Genet*, **23**, 21–27.

Kernberg, P.F., Weiner, A.S. and Bardenstein, K.K., 2000. *Personality Disorders in Children and Adolescents*. Basic Books, New York.

Lesch, K.P., Bengel, D., Heils, A., Sabol, S.Z., Greenberg, B.D., Petri, S., Benjamin, J., Muller, C.R., Hamer, D.H. and Murphy, D.L., 1996. Association of anxiety-related traits with a polymorphism in the serotonin transporter gene regulatory region. *Science*, **274**, 1527–1531.

Links, P.S., Steiner, B. and Huxley, G., 1988. The occurrence of borderline personality disorder in the families of borderline patients. *J Pers Disord*, **2**, 14–20.

Livesley, W.J., Jang, K.L., Jackson, D.N. and Vernon, P.A., 1993. Genetic and environmental contributions to dimensions of personality disorders. *Am J Psychiatry*, **150**, 1826–1831.

Livesley, W.J. and Jang, K.L., 2000. Toward an empirically based classification of personality disorder. *J Pers Disord*, **14**, 137–151.

Lofgren, D.P., Bemporad, J., King, J., Lindem, K. and O'Driscoll, G., 1991. A prospective follow-up study of so-called borderline children. *Am J Psychiatry*, **148**, 1541–1545.

Loranger, A.W., Sartori, N., Andreoli, A. and Berger, P., 1994. The International Personality Disorder Examination. *Arch Gen Psychiatry*, **51**, 215–224.

Malinovsky-Rummell, R. and Hansen, D.J., 1993. Long-term consequences of physical abuse. *Psychol Bull*, **114**, 68–79.

Mann, J.J., 1998. The neurobiology of suicide. *Nat Med*, **4**, 425–430.

McCrae, R.R. and Costa, P.T., 1999. A five-factor theory of personality. In: Pervin, L.A. and John, O.P., (eds), *Handbook of Personality: Theory and Research*, 2nd edn, pp. 139–153. Guilford, New York.

Monroe, S.M. and Simons, A.D., 1991. Diathesis-stress theories in the context of life stress research. *Psychol Bull*, **110**, 406–425.

Nigg, J.T. and Goldsmith, H.H., 1994. Genetics of personality disorders: perspectives from personality and psychopathology research. *Psychol Bull*, **115**, 346–380.

O'Leary, K.M., 2000. Neuropsychological testing results. *Psychiatr Clin North Am*, **423**, 1–60.

Paris, J., 1994. *Borderline Personality Disorder: A Multidimensional Approach*. American Psychiatric Press, Washington, DC.

Paris, J., 1996. *Social Factors in the Personality Disorders*. Cambridge University Press, Cambridge.

Paris, J., 1997. Childhood trauma as an etiological factor in the personality disorders. *J Pers Disord*, **11**, 34–49.

Paris, J., 1998. Anxious traits, anxious attachment, and anxious cluster personality disorders. *Harvard Rev Psychiatry*, **6**, 142–148.

Paris, J., 1999. *Nature and Nurture in Psychiatry*. American Psychiatric Press, Washington, DC.

Paris, J., 2000a. The classification of personality disorders should be rooted in biology. *J Pers Disord*, **14**, 127–136.

Paris, J., 2000b. *Myths of Childhood*. Brunner/Mazel, Philadelphia.

Pfohl, B., Coryell, W., Zimmerman, M. and Stangl, D., 1986. DSM-III personality disorders: diagnostic overlap and internal consistency of individual DSM-III criteria. *Compr Psychiatry*, **27**, 21–34.

Plomin, R. and Bergeman, C.S., 1991. The nature of nurture: genetic influence on 'environmental' measures. *Behav Brain Sci*, **14**, 373–427.

Plomin, R., DeFries, J.C., McClearn, G.E. and Rutter, M., 1997. *Behavioral Genetics*, 3rd edn. Freeman, New York.

Plomin, R., Asbury, K. and Dunn, J., 2001. Why are children in the same family so different? Nonshared environment a decade later. *Can J Psychiatry*, **46**, 225–233.

Raine, A., Lencz, T. and Bilhul, S., 2000. Reduced prefrontal gray matter and reduced autonomic activity in antisocial personality disorder. *Arch Gen Psychiatry*, **37**, 119–127.

Reiss, D., Hetherington, E.M. and Plomin, R., 2000. *The Relationship Code*. Harvard University Press, Cambridge, MA.

Rind, B. and Tromofovitch, P., 1997. A meta-analytic review of findings from national samples on psychological correlates of child sexual abuse. *J Sex Res*, **34**, 237–255.

Robins, L.N., 1966. *Deviant Children Grown Up*. Williams and Wilkins, Baltimore.

Robins, L.N. and Regier, D.A. (eds), 1991. *Psychiatric Disorders in America*. Free Press, New York.

Rutter, M., 1987. Temperament, personality, and personality development. *Br J Psychiatry*, **150**, 443–448.

Rutter, M., 1989. Pathways from childhood to adult life. *J Child Psychol Psychiatry*, **30**, 23–51.

Rutter, M. and Maughan, B., 1997. Psychosocial adversities in psychopathology. *J Pers Disord*, **11**, 19–33.

Siever, L.J. and Davis, K.L., 1991. A psychobiological perspective on the personality disorders. *Am J Psychiatry*, **148**, 1647–1658.

Swartz, M., Blazer, D., George, L. and Winfield, I., 1990. Estimating the prevalence of borderline personality disorder in the community. *J Pers Disord*, **4**, 257–272.

Tellegen, A., Lykken, D.T., Bouchard, T.J., Wilcox, K.J., Segal, N.L. and Rich, S., 1988. Personality similarity in twins reared apart and together. *J Pers Soc Psychol*, **54**, 1031–1039.

Torgersen, S., Lygren, S., Oien, P.A., Skre, I., Onstad, S., Edvardsen, J., Tambs, K. and Kringlen, E., 2000. A twin study of personality disorders. *Compr Psychiatry*, **41**, 416–425.

Weissman, M.M., 1993. The epidemiology of personality disorders: a 1990 update. *J Pers Disord*, **7**, (Suppl) 44–62.

World Health Organization, 1992. *International Classification of Diseases*, 10th edn. World Health Organization, Geneva.

Zanarini, M.C., 1993. Borderline personality as an impulse spectrum disorder. In: Paris, J. (ed.), *Borderline Personality Disorder: Etiology and Treatment*, pp. 67–86. American Psychiatric Press, Washington, DC.

Zanarini, M.C., 2000. Childhood experiences associated with the development of borderline personality disorder. *Psychiatr Clin North Am*, **23**, 89–101.

Zoccolillo, M., Pickles, A., Quinton, D. and Rutter, M., 1992. The outcome of childhood conduct disorder: implications for defining adult personality disorder and conduct disorder. *Psychol Med*, **22**, 971–986.

XXVI-9

The Psychopharmacological Treatment of Personality Disorders

Royce Lee and Emil Coccaro

INTRODUCTION

This chapter will present available evidence on the psychopharmacological treatment of personality disorders. Clinical and theoretical implications of axis I/II and Axis II/II comorbidity in the treatment of patients with personality disorders will be discussed. Biological correlates of some of the major symptoms of personality disorders will provide the rationale for a review of the evidence for psychopharmacological treatment of personality disorders. These will be presented by medication class to facilitate an understanding of the evidence for the efficacy of these treatments.

PERSONALITY DISORDERS IN THE CLINICAL SETTING

The estimated prevalence of personality disorders in the community is approximately 6–11% (Samuels *et al.*, 1994; Reich *et al.*, 1989), with Cluster B personality disorders being the most common (4–5.4%), followed by cluster C (1.7–3.4%) and Cluster A (<0.1%). Evidence suggests that many personality-disordered people in the community who could benefit from treatment do not receive it. This holds true in clinical settings, where personality disorders, in general, are underdiagnosed (Zimmerman and Mattia, 1999).

Paradoxically, personality disorders may be disproportionately represented in outpatient and inpatient treatment settings (Zimmerman and Coryell, 1989). This may be due to the significant morbidity associated with them. Personality-disordered patients tend to function at lower levels than those without such disorders (Mehlum *et al.*, 1991), report more frequent adverse events in their lives (Maier *et al.*, 1992), and have elevated rates of divorce, substance abuse, and suicide (Zimmerman and Coryell, 1989). This is the case despite relatively heavy use of clinical services by some, but not all, persons with Axis II diagnoses. A recent study of treatment utilization by patients with personality disorder found that those with borderline personality disorder, compared to depressives, were more likely to have received every class of psychopharmacological medication, from twice as many trials of antidepressants to 10 times as many trials of antipsychotic medications. They had also received more psychosocial treatments than the depressive comparison group with the exception of family/couples therapy and self-help groups (Bender *et al.*, 2001). These results were consistent with earlier reports in persons diagnosed with borderline personality disorder (BPD) of more frequent hospitalization, a 20% lifetime incidence of suicide attempt (McGlashan *et al.*, 1986), and extensive use of outpatient mental health services (Perry and Cooper, 1985; Skodol *et al.*, 1983). Patients with personality disorders may also be more difficult to treat than most patients, with less treatment compliance (Bender *et al.*, 2001), less favourable Axis I treatment outcomes (Reich *et al.*, 1991), and more frequently aborted treatments. In research settings, it is not uncommon for up to two-thirds or more of personality-disordered subjects to drop out of treatment studies (Skodol *et al.*, 1983), a finding which mirrors clinical reports of their intensive but intermittent contact with outpatient services (McGlashan *et al.*, 1986).

COMORBIDITY IN PERSONALITY DISORDERS

Comorbidity in personality disorders may represent the random co-occurrence of independent disorders, co-occurrence of different disorders sharing a common aetiology or pathophysiology, or different disorders that have a causal relation between them (McGlashan *et al.*, 2000). The frequency of Axis II/Axis II comorbidity may be in part due to the fact that psychiatric nosology since DSM-III has favoured a trend towards more frequent comorbidity through the use of operationalized criteria, structured diagnostic interviews, and less stringent exclusionary rules. In some cases as well, Axis I/II and Axis II/II comorbidity could reflect the limitations of categorical diagnoses in characterizing the behavioural dimensions, that may underlie them.

Clinically, the possibility of the existence of comorbid conditions in the personality-disordered patient must be carefully evaluated for the following reasons:

1. to identify other conditions with relatively well-defined treatments — for example, the presence of a medical disorder, mood disorder, or anxiety disorder
2. to identify other conditions whose symptoms may be aggravated by proposed treatments — for example, the presence of bipolar I disorder in a patient considering the trial of an antidepressant
3. to identify disorders whose symptoms may account for the set of behaviours in questions, including such disorders as post-traumatic stress disorder (PTSD) or social anxiety disorder
4. to identify conditions whose course may be complicated by the presence of a personality disorder, such as refractory depression
5. because comorbidity may be markedly more frequent in clinical settings than community settings, as shown by comparisons between the two (Samuels *et al.*, 1994), possibly due to the selection for treatment of patients with more than one disorder and more functional impairment.

CLUSTER A

Schizotypal personality disorder is the most commonly encountered Cluster A personality disorder in clinical settings. It frequently

Biological Psychiatry: Edited by H. D'haenen, J.A. den Boer and P. Willner. ISBN 0-471-49198-5

occurs in the context of other personality disorders, with most affected patients meeting the criteria for at least two other personality disorders. The most frequently comorbid personality disorder may be paranoid personality disorder, with 36.1% of patients with schizotypal personality disorder meeting the criteria for paranoid personality disorder (McGlashan *et al.*, 1986). Fulton found that 4/17 (23.5%) of subjects diagnosed by chart review with paranoid personality disorder met the criteria for schizotypal personality disorder (Fulton *et al.*, 1993). Although schizoid personality disorder is not frequently diagnosed even in clinical settings, it has been found in 10.5% of patients diagnosed with schizotypal personality disorder (McGlashan *et al.*, 1986). In contrast, Fulton found that only one out of 33 (3%) patients with schizoid personality disorder met the criteria for schizotypal personality disorder (Fulton *et al.*, 1993). Evidence suggests that despite some degree of comorbidity, schizotypal, schizoid, and paranoid personality disorders categorize distinct groups of patients. The nature and extend of the comorbidity relationships between schizoid and avoidant personality disorder (West *et al.*, 1995) and between schizotypal and borderline personality disorder are unclear.

CLUSTER B

Borderline personality disorder (BPD) is the most common of the Cluster B disorders. Like schizotypal personality disorder, BPD represents a heterogeneous group of individuals with frequent Axis I and Axis II comorbidities. The most frequent Axis I comorbidity with personality disorders is substance-abuse disorder, which is found in approximately 53% of BPD patients (McGlashan *et al.*, 2000). Affective disorders are also frequently comorbid. Approximately 41% of patients with BPD may meet research diagnostic criteria for cyclothymia (Levitt *et al.*, 1990). BPD is frequently comorbid with major depression, but major depression is frequently comorbid in nearly all personality disorders (Alnaes *et al.*, 1988), with some evidence suggesting that approximately 70–80% of patients with any Axis II disorder have at least one episode of major depression during their life (McGlashan *et al.*, 1986). However, depressive disorders associated with BPD may be more chronic and severe, and have an earlier onset (Skodol *et al.*, 2000). Curiously, some BPD patients with major depression may cope better than those without it, perhaps due to more robust medication responses (Pope, 1983).

BPD and PTSD share phenomenological and developmental risk factors, but may be separable by their longitudinal course (Gunderson *et al.*, 1993). Comorbidity is frequent. About 30–47% of patients with BPD meet the criteria for PTSD (Swartz *et al.*, 1990, McGlashan, 2000), compared to 25% of patients with schizotypal, obsessive-compulsive, and avoidant personality disorder (McGlashan, 2000).

CLUSTER C

Although measurements of personality traits are affected by state factors (Reich *et al.*, 1986), evidence to date suggests that as many as 40–90% of patients with social phobia also meet the criteria for avoidant personality disorder (McGlashan, 2000; Widiger, 1992). It remains unclear whether social phobia and avoidant personality disorder represent two frequently co-occurring conditions or different aspects of a single underlying psychopathology (Perugi *et al.*, 1999).

The extent of comorbidity between obsessive-compulsive personality disorder (OCPD) and obsessive-compulsive disorder (OCD) is unknown, with rates from 2–6% to 30–60% reported in the literature (Diaferia *et al.*, 1997). The relationship between OCD and OCPD may not be specific to OCPD but may simply reflect an overall increase in the risk of personality disorders, as approximately half of patients with OCD meet the criteria for various personality disorders (Baer *et al.*, 1990). Additionally, the majority of patients with comorbid OCD and OCPD meet criteria for at least one other personality disorder (Bejerot *et al.*, 1998).

THE ROLE OF PSYCHOPHARMACOLOGICAL TREATMENT IN PERSONALITY DISORDERS

The treatment of some personality disorders, such as BPD, with psychopharmacological agents is not uncommon in clinical practice, and in fact may be in excess of treatment in comparable populations (Bender *et al.*, 2001). Some patients, especially high-risk patients, undergo polypharmacy (Zanarini, personal communication), despite the lack of controlled evidence to validate the practice in this population. However, the severity of psychosocial dysfunction and dramatic nature of some of these patients' symptoms often warrant therapeutic intervention and may make discontinuing possibly ineffective treatment difficult.

On the whole, psychopharmacological treatments for personality disorders are considered to be adjunctive to psychotherapy, but the relative contributions of psychopharmacological treatment versus psychosocial interventions such as psychotherapy, and the interactions between the two, remain important topics for future study.

PSYCHOPHARMACOLOGICAL TREATMENT STUDIES

Three main patterns in treatment studies of personality disorders emerge. One is a relative lack of evidence for syndromal improvement, or remission, in response to pharmacological treatment. The second pattern is that pharmacotherapy may show effects on a specific range of symptoms. Modern studies emphasize treating specific symptom dimensions with agents that possess selective psychopharmacological properties. Some of these studies look within specific diagnostic categories, while others look across diagnostic categories. The third pattern that emerges is the non-specific effects that many psychopharmacological compounds have. For example, some neuroleptics seem to have a global, sedating effect on patients with personality disorders, leading to changes in a wide range of outcome measures. Even selective agents, such as the serotonin selective reuptake inhibitors (SSRIs), have effects on a range of symptoms such as mood, anxiety, obsessionality, and impulsive aggression. Sometimes these non-specific effects may also be detrimental, especially when they are unpredictable or paradoxical.

NEUROLEPTICS

The predominantly antidopaminergic effects of neuroleptics and their proven ability to treat symptoms of psychosis in schizophrenia and affective illnesses have led to studies in personality disorders with psychotic-like symptoms. These include the schizophrenia-related personality disorders of DSM-IV: schizotypal, paranoid, and schizoid personality disorders, in addition to DSM-IV BPD. The rationale for the use of dopaminergic antagonists in these patients is provided by findings of increased cerebrospinal fluid (CSF) and plasma levels of dopamine metabolites in selected schizotypal subjects (Siever *et al.*, 1991; 1993b), more frequent dyskinetic-like movements following amphetamine challenge compared to normal controls (Fenton *et al.*, 1994), genetic relationships to schizophrenia (Kendler *et al.*, 1982), and psychotic-like symptoms in BPD patients exposed to amphetamine challenge (Schulz *et al.*, 1985).

The relative rarity of paranoid and schizoid personality disorders, the frequent comorbidity of schizotypal personality disorder and BPD, the importance of psychotic symptoms in BPD and schizotypal personality disorder, and the initial conceptualization of schizotypal personality disorder and BPD as being related to each other and to schizophrenia have led to the overwhelming majority of neuroleptic trials being dedicated to these two personality-disorder populations.

Three early studies failed to find evidence for syndromal improvement with neuroleptic treatment in comparison to other medications in patients with what today would be considered Cluster B personality disorders. In a double-blind trial by Vilkin (1964) of trifluoperazine, diazepam, and meprobamate/benactyzine in BPD patients, diazepam was more effective than trifluoperazine in relieving overall symptoms, and trifluoperazine was marginally better than mebrobamate/benactyzine. Fink *et al.* (1964) reported improvement in patients with emotionally unstable character disorder (EUCD), who today might be diagnosed as having histrionic personality disorder, using relatively high doses of chlorpromazine (up to 1200 mg) when compared to placebo and imipramine. While imipramine was found to reduce affective instability and agitation, chlorpromazine's global effects were not different from those of placebo. Hedberg *et al.* (1971) noted some improvement in 22% of pseudoneurotic schizophrenics treated with moderately high doses of trifluoperazine (up to 32 mg) and in 28% of patients with trifluoperazine and tranylcypromine (up to 30 mg), but the largest number of patients in this study, as in the study of Fink *et al.* (1964), did better on the antidepressant.

The first placebo-controlled, double-blind study of a neuroleptic in DSM-III-diagnosed BPD showed some improvement with treatment on specific dimensions. In a subgroup of DSM-III-diagnosed BPD patients with at least one psychotic symptom, Goldberg *et al.* (1986) studied low-dose thiothixene (average dose 8.7 mg) compared to placebo, noting significant improvement in cognitive disturbances, ideas of reference, obsessive-compulsive symptoms, and panic-anxiety symptoms. No improvement in depressive symptoms was found, and no improvement was found in global functioning as measured by global assessment of function (GAF). The marked reductions of psychosis in this study may be partially explained by the higher levels of psychosis in the study population.

Some studies have found evidence of global improvement in BPD and schizotypal patients with neuroleptic treatment. Two controlled comparison trials in schizotypal/BPD subjects comparing low-dose chlorpromazine (105–120 mg d^{-1}) versus loxapine (13.5–14.5 mg d^{-1}) (Leone, 1982) and low-dose thiothixene (mean 9.4 mg d^{-1}) versus haloperidol (mean 3 mg d^{-1}) (Serban and Siegel, 1984) reported improvement in suspiciousness, hostility, depressed mood, and anxiety. An open-label study of pimozide in DSM-II personality-disordered subjects showed that pimozide was associated with good to excellent global improvement in 69% of subjects. Paranoid or schizoid personality disorder predicted response to the neuroleptic (Reyntjens, 1972).

In a randomized, placebo-controlled trial of haloperidol versus amitriptyline, Soloff *et al.* (1986) found that haloperidol at 4–16 mg per day (mean 7.24 mg d^{-1}) had significant effects on depression, anxiety, hostility, paranoid ideation, impulsive behaviour, and global function in hospitalized patients with DSM-III-diagnosed BPD or comorbid BPD and schizotypal personality disorder. Responding patients ended the study reporting clear improvement but remained moderately symptomatic by observer-rated measures. Patients' subjective reports on the Beck Depression Inventory distinguished between groups, while the observer-rated Hamilton Depression Rating Scale differences between groups were not significantly different. The patients most likely to respond to low-dose haloperidol had both affective and schizotypal symptoms. Diagnostic category did not predict outcome with haloperidol. However, a dimension of schizotypy, which included psychoticism, did predict a more favourable result with haloperidol. Haloperidol seemed to be useful for a subset of patients, but drug response could not identify a subgroup of BPD patients with an underlying 'schizotypal' illness.

Two large, placebo-controlled studies found less favourable results. Cowdry and Gardner (1988) studied alprazolam, carbamazepine (mean 820 mg d^{-1}), trifluoperazine (mean 7.8 mg d^{-1}), and tranylcypromine sulphate (mean 40 mg d^{-1}) in a double-blind, placebo-controlled trial. Patients were female; met five of eight DSM-III criteria for BPD; had histories of overdoses, self-mutilation, or physical violence; and had no current Axis I comorbidity. Physicians rated significant improvement in patient's depression and anxiety with trifluoperazine treatment, but subjective ratings were variable. Although physicians did not rate subjects on trifluoperazine as being less impulsive, they did rate suicidality as decreased. Non-significant trends were seen for less behavioural dyscontrol. On the whole, trifluoperazine seemed to be slightly less efficacious than tranylcypromine and carbamazepine on the behavioural and affective measures used in the study, and only 50% of the trifluoperazine trials could be completed due to clinical worsening or medical complications.

Soloff *et al.* (1993) compared phenelzine and haloperidol versus placebo in hospitalized, DSM-III-R-diagnosed BPD, with or without comorbid schizotypal personality disorder. Pre-treatment depression scores were high (Ham D-24 $= 25.3 \pm 5.9$). Although improvement with haloperidol therapy was seen, there were considerable residual depressive symptoms at the end of the study. Significant improvement was found with phenelzine. Surprisingly, mood reactivity increased in all three groups, although both phenelzine and haloperidol resulted in modest improvements in hostility. Only phenelzine produced a statistically significant but clinically modest improvement in impulsivity. Soloff *et al.* concluded that neuroleptic medications functions as a non-specific tranquillizer in BPD, with significant effects only in the most severely impaired borderlines (Soloff *et al.*, 1993).

A 16-week continuation follow-up study on the same group of patients also failed to find evidence for haloperidol's efficacy on syndromal measures. In fact, treatment with haloperidol was associated with a significant increase in the 'hopelessness' item of the Hamilton Depression Scale. Of the subjects treated with haloperidol, 64.3% dropped out of the continuation study, compared to 45.5% of phenlzine-treated subjects. The drop-out rate for the entire 22 weeks of study was 87.5 for the haloperidol-treated subjects. The study failed to find demonstrable value of continuation therapy with haloperidol in this population.

Although prolonged treatment with neuroleptics probably does not improve syndromal or affective measures, Montgomery and Montgomery (1982) found that over a 6-month period depot flupenthixol in comparison to placebo decreased suicidal and parasuicidal behaviour in patients with past histories of suicide attempts and self-destructive behaviour. This finding may be due to the tranquillizing effects of neuroleptics in this study population.

ATYPICAL ANTIPSYCHOTICS

The adverse side effects, high rates of drop out and non-compliance, and lack of consistent efficacy data associated with neuroleptics make the newer, atypical antipsychotics promising candidates for evaluation in the treatment of personality-disorder symptoms. Atypical antipsychotics may address affective symptoms in bipolar disorder and deficit symptoms in schizophrenia, which have similarities to the affective dysregulation in Cluster B disorders and the deficit symptoms of Cluster A disorders.

Deficit symptoms in Cluster A personality disorders are associated with impairments in working memory (Roitman *et al.*, 2000) and sustained attention (Siever *et al.*, 1991; Meritt *et al.*, 1989). Neuropsychological evidence that the cortical deficits in Cluster A personality disorders may be selective (Raine *et al.*, 1992; Siever *et al.*, 1991) has been corroborated by neurobiological findings of altered CSF homovanillic acid (HVA) levels (Siever *et al.*, 1991) and volumetric neuroimaging findings of increased ventricular size (Raine *et al.*, 1992; Cazzullo *et al.*, 1991; Siever *et al.*, 1991), abnormally shaped corpus callosum (Downhill *et al.*, 2000), and decreased pulvinar size (Byne *et al.*, 2001). These abnormalities may be intermediate in severity between schizophrenics and normal controls (Byne *et al.*, 2001; Downhill *et al.*, 2000), indicating that these disorders may exist on a continuum with schizophrenia, and thus may be amenable to treatment with atypical antipsychotics.

The efficacy of atypical antipsychotics in the treatment of bipolar affective disorder for affective symptoms suggests they may have similar efficacy for affective symptoms in 'dramatic cluster' disorders such as BPD.

Three open trials of clozapine in BPD suggest that it may have efficacy on a range of symptom dimensions. An open trial of clozapine in 15 DSM-III-R-diagnosed BPD patients with symptoms of psychosis, seven of whom also met the criteria for schizotypal personality disorder, found significant improvement of psychosis and global function (Frankenburg and Zanarini, 1993). Benedetti *et al.* (1998) gave 12 inpatients with BPD and severe 'psychotic-like' symptoms low doses of clozapine (25–100 mg d^{-1}) and found improvement in psychosis, depression, impulsive behaviours, and global functioning. Most patients suffered from some side effects of clozapine treatment, and on follow-up, one patient at week 24 developed reversible granulocytopaenia. Chengappa *et al.* (1999) treated seven subjects with BPD, psychosis, and a history of severe self-mutilation and/or violence serious enough to warrant hospitalization. All subjects had previous trials with conventional neuroleptics in combination with other psychotropic agents with equivocal benefits. Clozapine (mean dose 421 mg d^{-1}) led to significant improvements in self-mutilation, behavioural dyscontrol leading to seclusion, global function, and need for p.r.n. medications. However, one patient experienced leukopaenia, two patients gained 9 kg, and one patient gained 17.7 kg during the trial with clozapine. Although the study was limited by that absence of a control group, it is significant because of the severity of the subjects' borderline pathology. The risk-to-benefit ratio of the use of clozapine in personality-disordered patients remains unclear without the availability of placebo-controlled data.

No conclusive data on the newer atypical antipsychotics olanzapine, risperdal, seroquel, and ziprasidone are available yet. Their relatively low side-effect profiles and efficacy in treating psychotic as well as affective symptoms make them appealing alternatives to 'typical' neuroleptics. Preliminary data with olanzapine indicate that it shows promise as an agent that may be able to address several different symptom dimensions in patients with BPD. Case reports with olanzapine 5 mg d^{-1} suggest it may have efficacy in reducing the frequency and intensity of self-injurious behaviour (SIB) in BPD (Hough, 2001). One open trial in BPD with dysthymia suggests that it may lead to syndromal improvement. In an 8-week open trial in BPD conducted, by Schulz *et al.* (1999), olanzapine led to decreases in psychosis, impulsivity, anger and interpersonal sensitivity, and depression, and improvements in global function. Patients in this study had comorbid dysthymia and were in continuing psychotherapy. Also notable was a low drop-out rate, and a lack of the extrapyramidal symptoms and the statistically significant weight gain of patients taking olanzapine (mean 2.7 kg). Preliminary results from a not yet published placebo-controlled trial of olanzapine in BPD outpatients show that, in comparison to placebo, olanzapine (5 mg d^{-1}) demonstrates efficacy on a variety of symptom dimensions as well as global function, as assessed by GAF score (Zanarini *et al.*, 2002).

Controlled data in children and adolescents with borderline intellectual functioning suggest that risperidone is effective in comparison with placebo in the treatment of behavioural disturbances and aggression (Van Bellinghen *et al.*, 2001; Buitelaar *et al.*, 2001). Data regarding the usefulness of risperdone in the treatment of adult, personality-disordered patients are limited. A case report suggests that risperidone 4 mg d^{-1} may be helpful in the treatment of self-mutilation in BPD (Khouzam *et al.*, 1997). Szigethy and Schulz (1997) found that risperdone 2 mg d^{-1}, in conjunction with fluovoxamine 200 mg d^{-1}, was helpful in treating psychosis and depression in a BPD patient with comorbid dysthymia. A single case report has described the successful treatment of a patient with antisocial personality disorder and impulsive aggression with risperidone 3 mg d^{-1} in conjunction with 9 mg biperiden, 60 mg propranolol, and 30 mg diazepam per day to treat akathisia. In an unpublished pilot study, Schulz and associates treated BPD in a double-blind, placebo-controlled trial of risperidone versus placebo. Treatment with risperidone led to improvements in psychoticism and global function. However, the 8-week study was unable to show a statistically significant superiority of risperidone over placebo. This may have been due to the small number of subjects, robust placebo response, and coadministered weekly psychotherapy in both the placebo and treatment groups.

Atypical antipsychotics show promise and controlled data are forthcoming. In general, evidence for the use of 'typical' neuroleptics indicates that some improvement may be seen in impulsivity, aggression, and psychoticism. Improvement may depend on the severity of symptoms before treatment, with psychoticism standing out as a dimensional symptom that predicts better neuroleptic response. The value of maintenance treatment with typical neuroleptics remains unclear, but evidence suggests that the risk of worsened depression must be balanced against a non-specific sedative effect that may decrease impulsive aggressive behaviours.

MOOD STABILIZERS AND ANTICONVULSANTS

The use of lithium and the anticonvulsants carbamazepine and valproate in the treatment of acute mania has prompted interest in examining their efficacy in treating the prominent affective symptoms of the Cluster B disorders. In addition, the EEG-normalizing effect of the anticonvulsants and early studies showing the therapeutic behavioural effects of the anticonvulsant diphenylhydantoin (Klein and Greenberg, 1967; Stephens and Schaffer 1970) have made them candidates for the treatment of impulsivity in disorders with 'soft' neurological signs and personality disorders.

The rationale for the treatment of affective symptoms in Cluster B personality disorders with mood stabilizers as well as with antidepressants is based on a limited set of data. Biological studies of the affective component of personality disorders have found conflicting evidence on whether or not findings of thyroid and HPA axis abnormalities persist (Korezekwa *et al.*, 1991; Kavoussi *et al.*, 1993) or disappear (Loosen and Prange, 1982) if the presence of comorbid depression is taken into account. Similar discrepancies have been found in heritability studies (Torgersen *et al.*, 1984; Schulz *et al.*, 1986; Riso *et al.*, 2000). Affective instability, a hallmark of BPD, has been associated with cholinergic receptor responsiveness in volunteers (Fritze *et al.*, 1990) and BPD patients (Steinberg *et al.*, 1997). Evidence from a family history study suggests that trait affective lability, in conjunction with trait impulsivity, may have a greater familial relation to BPD than to affective disorders in general (Silverman *et al.*, 1991).

Lithium

Two controlled trials in two markedly different populations have found lithium to be effective at reducing anger and/or impulsive aggression. Links compared lithium (mean dose $985\,\mathrm{mg\,d^{-1}}$) to placebo and desipramine (mean $162.5\,\mathrm{mg\,d^{-1}}$) for 6-week intervals with a 2-week washout period between each arm (Links, 1998). Patients in the study were moderately impaired BPD outpatients who remained in psychotherapy with their referring clinicians. Lithium was superior to desipramine and placebo on observer ratings of anger and suicidality, but the patients did not notice any change in how they felt, and no improvement was seen on objective measures of depression.

In a double-blind, placebo-controlled study of the effect of lithium on aggressive behaviour in 66 chronically aggressive prisoners in a medium-security institution, Sheard (1976) found that lithium compared to placebo was associated with a reduction in the frequency of serious aggressive incidents. Many of these patients today would be considered to have, among other DSM-IV diagnoses, antisocial personality disorder, making this one of the few controlled trials of any psychopharmacological intervention in this kind of patient population. In this study, 80–90% of the subjects had been incarcerated for longer than 1 year between the ages of 12 and 18 years; had committed crimes such as manslaughter, rape, murder, and assault; and had a history of chronic assaulting behaviour and/or impulsive antisocial behaviour. The group was described as being an 'extremely manipulative, hostile group of young men who were extroverted, highly impulsive, and action oriented' (p 1411). Lithium serum levels were maintained between $0.6–1.0\,\mu\mathrm{g\,m^{-1}}$. One weakness of this study was that subjects could reliably guess which treatment they were receiving.

Two studies have found that lithium may have therapeutic effects on affective symptoms in Axis II disorders. LaWall and Cassie (1982), reported a case series of five DSM-III-diagnosed BPD patients who demonstrated relief from labile affect, decreased aggression, and decreased depression with lithium therapy. A double-blind, randomized, crossover study comparing lithium to placebo in the treatment of patients with what would today be considered BPD or histrionic personality disorder (Rifkin, 1972) found that lithium therapy significantly reduced the range of daily or hourly mood swings.

Carbamazepine

Studies to date with carbamazepine have focused on the treatment of impulsive aggression. Mattes (1990) found that carbamazepine, in comparison with propranolol, in subjects who met the first two criteria of intermittent explosive disorder but who could also have shown episodes of aggressiveness between severe outbursts, was effective at reducing the severity of outbursts by non-blind ratings by the psychiatrist, patient, and family member. Serum levels were $8–12\,\mu\mathrm{g\,kg^{-1}}$. In general, a history of attention-deficit disorder predicted better response to propranolol, while a history of intermittent explosive disorder and/or epilepsy predicted response to carbamazepine. In a study more generalizable to the treatment of personality-disorder patients seen in the typical clinical setting, Cowdry and Gardner (1988), in the crossover study of tranylcypromine, carbamazepine, alprazolam, and trifluoperazine already mentioned, found carbamazepine (mean dose $820\,\mathrm{mg\,d^{-1}}$), in a group of BPD patients with histories of self-destructive behaviour, to be beneficial in suppressing episodes of impulsive aggression, compared to alprazolam, trifluoperazine, tranylcypromine, and placebo. The authors suggested that treatment with carbamazepine produced a 'reflective delay', allowing patients to pause before reacting to an emotional stimulus. Although objective raters noted a significant improvement in mood, patients themselves did not, a finding that was attributed to a halo effect on the part of clinicians, who may have seen an improvement in impulsive aggression as improved mood. This is consistent with the additional finding that 3 of the 17 (18%) patients taking carbamazepine actually noticed worsening of their mood. Their depressive symptoms resolved after cessation of carbamazepine. Thus, carbamazepine's usefulness in treating affective symptoms of personality disorder, such as affective instability or depressive symptoms remains uncertain. However, preliminary evidence suggests that it attenuates impulsive aggression in personality-disordered patients.

Valproate

Valproate has been found to be efficacious in the treatment of bipolar disorder. There is also evidence that it might be effective in reducing impulsive aggression. A double-blind, placebo-controlled trial in 20 children and adolescents with either oppositional defiant disorder or conduct disorder found that divalproex, with a mean blood level of $82.2\,\mu\mathrm{g\,ml^{-1}}$, compared to placebo, was efficacious in reducing mood lability and explosive temper (Donovan *et al.*, 2000).

Two open trials of valproate have found benefit in personality-disordered subjects. Stein *et al.* (1995) found that valproate, in 11 DSM-III-R-diagnosed BPD patients, was moderately effective at reducing anger, impulsivity, anxiety, and rejection sensitivity. The mean serum valproate level in this study was $78.8\,\mu\mathrm{g\,ml^{-1}}$. Although dramatic improvements were not seen, patients at baseline were only mildly impaired with respect to depressive symptoms and aggression. Both patients and raters noted improvement in mood and irritability, with 50% of subjects taking valproate showing change scores for mood and 38% showing change scores for anxiety, anger, impulsivity, and rejection sensitivity. Kavoussi *et al.* (1998) studied valproate in 10 patients meeting DSM-IV criteria for at least one personality disorder who had failed an SSRI trial for impulsive aggressive behaviour. Patients in this trial had higher baseline OAS-M scores (mean = 27.2, SD = 17.9); met criteria for a range of Cluster A, B, and C personality disorders; had frequent Axis II comorbidity; and were treated with a maximum of 2000 mg per day of valproic acid. Systematic assessments of mood were not made in this trial. Improvements were seen on mean OAS-M scores at weeks 2, 4, 6, and 9. At week 4, OAS-M irritability scores were significantly lower. Of the eight completers in the study, six had a 50% or more reduction on the OAS-M.

A single placebo-controlled trial of valproate in BPD has been published (Hollander *et al.*, 2001). In a 10-week, parallel-group, double-blind, placebo-controlled, comparison trial, 16 outpatients with DSM-IV-diagnosed BPD received valproate, with a mean serum level of $64.57\,\mu\mathrm{g\,ml^{-1}}$. Patients in this study showed global improvement as measured by global assessment of symptoms (GAS) and clinical global inventory (CGI). Significant changes in aggression were not detected in this study, perhaps because subjects did not begin the study with high aggression. Unfortunately, none of the patients randomized to placebo completed the trial. In the intent-to-treat analysis (ITT), measures made in the study failed to reach statistical significance, with the principal finding being a non-significant trend of the GAS from serious to moderate impairment.

Evidence supporting the use of valproate in personality-disordered patients for impulsivity, aggression, and mood instability is promising but incomplete. Pilot data suggests that it may have efficacy for these dimensions and may even lead to global, syndromal improvement, although this finding needs replication in a larger, controlled trial with sufficient power. A multicentre, placebo-controlled trial of valproate in a heterogeneous group of subjects with impulsive aggression is currently under way.

NEURONTIN (GABAPENTIN)

Although gabapentin's efficacy as a mood stabilizer is equivocal, a randomized, placebo-controlled study (Pande *et al.*, 1999) indicates that it may be an effective treatment for generalized social phobia. Because of the frequent comorbidity of social phobia with avoidant personality disorder, it may be an agent to consider in patients with generalized social anxiety and avoidant personality disorder. No data is available on gabapentin's efficacy in treating impulsive aggression or affective instability. Topiramate and lamotrigene, two anticonvulsants tested in the treatment of affective disorders, have not yet been tested in personality-disordered patients.

ANTIDEPRESSANTS

Antidepressants have been studied in personality disorders because of the similarity of the mood complaints of the Cluster B disorders to affective syndromes such as cyclothymia and atypical depression, substantial comorbidity with affective disorders, the efficacy of antidepressants in treating anxiety and obsessive symptoms, and the serotonergic abnormalities linked to impulsive aggression and suicide.

The rationale for the use of antidepressants for affective symptoms in personality disorders was touched on in the section on mood stabilizers. The rationale for the use of antidepressants in the treatment of impulsive aggression is based on data relating diminished serotonergic function to impulsive aggression in personality-disordered patients. Deficits in serotonergic function have been associated with suicide in depressives (Åsperg *et al.*, 1976); aggression towards oneself and others (Brown, 1979); impulsive, rather than premeditated aggression (Linnoila *et al.*, 1983); and self-injurious behaviour (SIB) in depressives (Lopez-Ibor *et al.*, 1985) and SIB in personality-disordered subjects (New *et al.*, 1997). Neuropsychopharmacological challenge studies with the serotonergic agent fenfluramine (both *d*,l- and *d*-stereoisomer forms) have found blunted prolactin responses in association with impulsive aggression, implicating reduced serotonergic function in BPD (Coccaro, 1989a) and antisocial personality-disordered subjects (O'Keane *et al.*, 1992). Neuroimaging studies have discovered reduced metabolic activity in the areas of the prefrontal cortex in aggressive prisoners (Raine *et al.*, 1997). Using the positron emission tomography (PET) scan in personality-disordered subjects with histories of impulsive aggression, Siever *et al.* (1999) found blunted metabolic responses to *d*,l-fenfluramine in the orbital frontal, adjacent medial, and cingulate cortex when compared to matched controls, findings that were partially replicated by Soloff *et al.* (2000). These brain regions rely heavily on serotonergic neurotransmission.

In addition to abnormalities in the serotonergic system, reduced CSF levels of norepinephrine metabolites (Brown *et al.*, 1979) and dopamine metabolites (Linnoila, 1983), and increased levels of CSF vasopressin (Coccaro *et al.*, 1996) have been correlated with measures of aggression.

TRICYCLIC ANTIDEPRESSANTS

Early studies of the tricyclic antidepressants (Klein, 1968) found some efficacy in the treatment of 'pseudoneurotic schizophrenics'. Soloff *et al.* 1987 found modest benefits in depressed mood with amitriptyline (mean dose 147 $mg\,d^{-1}$) compared to placebo in a 5-week study of hospitalized BPD and schizotypal personality patients. Although some patients seemed to benefit primarily on affective measures, a subgroup of patients on amitriptyline showed increases in ratings of impulsive and aggressive behaviour. These patients were characterized as having higher levels of aggression, psychoticism, negativism, impulsivity, and schizotypal symptoms.

Three other studies (Klein 1968; Rampling, 1978; Links *et al.*, 1990) have also found that a subgroup of patients with BPD or schizotypal personality disorder seemed to worsen after treatment with tricyclic antidepressants with respect to suicidality and physical assaultiveness. This may be due to the noradrenergic actions of these agents, which could increase the likelihood of acting on aggressive impulses or increase their intensity.

MONOAMINE-OXIDASE INHIBITORS (MAOIs)

MAOIs, which are useful in the treatment of atypical depression, have been studied in personality-disorder patients in the hope that they would improve atypical mood symptoms such as the mood reactivity of histrionic personality disorder, rejection sensitivity in dependent and avoidant personality disorder, and depressive symptoms in BPD. The serotonergic effects of the MAOIs inhibitors also make them candidates for the treatment of impulsive aggressive behaviour.

The studies to date have produced conflicting results. Hedberg *et al.* (1971) found phenelzine to be effective in treating a subset of patients with pseudoneurotic schizophrenia, patients who, under DSM-IV, might be considered to have Cluster B or C personality disorders. In a retrospective study of patients with atypical depression (Parsons *et al.*, 1989), patients with comorbid BPD were three times as likely to benefit from therapy with phenelzine than imipramine in the treatment of mood symptoms. However, patients with atypical depression without comorbid BPD were no more likely to respond to phenelzine than imipramine. Cowdry and Gardner's (1989) double-blind, placebo-controlled, crossover comparison of tranylcypromine (40 $mg\,d^{-1}$), alprazolam, and carbamazepine found efficacy in mood symptoms in a group of treatment-resistant subjects with BPD without a comorbid affective disorder. Although improvement was seen in rated suicidality and impulsivity, there was no change in the severity of aggressive behaviours during the study, and the authors concluded that the improvement seen was multidimensional and mood-related, with little or no effect on impulsivity.

In a double-blind, placebo-controlled comparison of phenelzine and haloperidol in DSM-III-R borderlines, Soloff *et al.* (1993) found phenelzine (60 $mg\,d^{-1}$) to be modestly effective for symptoms of depression, anxiety, anger, and hostility compared to placebo and haloperidol. However, they did not replicate Parson *et al.* (1989) findings of efficacy against atypical depressive symptoms. The magnitude of change for all arms of the study were relatively low, leaving the patients still substantially impaired at the end. One possible explanation for their failure to replicate earlier more positive results with MAOIs was that the dose range in the study was slightly lower than previous studies due to treatment side effects. In their 16-week continuation study, Cornelius *et al.* (1993) found that continued phenelzine demonstrated only minor efficacy for treatment of the mood symptoms of irritability and depression. In these subjects, phenelzine had an activating effect, showing increased, rather than decreased, mood reactivity, although the authors note that activation was an improvement in the overall well-being of the patients suffering from anergia.

In summary, treatment of BPD patients with MAOIs may lead to improvements in mood if atypical mood symptoms are prominent, and may lead to improvements in impulsivity. Therapeutic effects may be modest, and their magnitude may be determined by the presence of comorbid atypical depression. There is no clear evidence that treatment with an MAOI leads to global or syndromal improvement.

Although not studied in the treatment of avoidant personality disorder specifically, MAOIs have been shown to be effective in the treatment of generalized social phobia. In an 8-week study comparing phenelzine to cognitive-behavioural group therapy and placebo, phenelzine treatment was more effective than either (Heimberg *et al.*, 1998). However, evidence to date suggests that the more specific monoamine-oxidase-B inhibitor, selegiline, is not efficacious in generalized social phobia (Simpson *et al.*, 1998).

SELECTIVE SEROTONIN REUPTAKE INHIBITORS (SSRIs)

SSRIs have been shown to be effective in treating depressive disorders and anxiety disorders. Preliminary evidence that SSRIs are effective in reducing impulsive aggression and affective symptoms in personality-disorder patients comes from several open trials of fluoxetine (Cornelius, 1991; Norden, 1989; Markovitz *et al.*, 1991; Coccaro *et al.*, 1990) and one of sertraline (Kavoussi, 1994).

In a double-blind, placebo-controlled trial of fluoxetine (20–60 mg), Coccaro *et al.* (1997) treated 40 non-depressed DSM-III-R-diognosed personality-disorder individuals with impulsive aggressive behaviour with fluoxetine or placebo, and found significant decreases in observed aggression scale — modified (OAS-M) irritability at week 6, and OAS-M verbal aggression and aggression against objects subscale decreases at week 10 of treatment. The effect of fluoxetine was mainly on verbal aggression, with most subjects responding at in the 20–40 mg d^{-1} dose range. No patients worsened while on fluoxetine. Notably, this study demonstrated that the treatment of a dimensional symptom (impulsive aggression) could occur across a categorical Axis II diagnosis. Patients in the study had an average of 1.8 ± 1.1 Axis II personality disorders, with the three most common diagnoses being BPD (33%), paranoid personality disorder (25%), and OCPD (23%). If SSRIs in these treatment responders were ameliorating a 'serotonin deficit', it might be hypothesized that patients with abnormalities in peripheral measures of serotonergic function would be the most likely to respond to fluoxetine. However, in a companion study, 15 of the patients underwent *d*-fenfluramine challenge prior to the start of the treatment trial. Among all of the subjects, there were positive correlations between pre-treatment prolactin response to *d*-fenfluramine challenge (PRL [*d*-FEN]) and percent improvement in the Overt Aggression Scale — Modified (OAS-M) scores in fluoxetine-treated versus placebo-treated subjects. Subjects with smaller responses to serotonergic challenge showed less improvement with SSRI treatment. Since PRL [*d*-FEN] response is thought to be an indirect measure of central nervous system serotonergic functioning, these results might indicate that impulsive aggressive subjects with the most severe serotonergic abnormalities are the ones least likely to benefit from SSRIs, possibly due to a blunted 5-HT-2 response to them (Coccaro and Kavoussi, 1997).

There is preliminary evidence that SSRIs may be able to improve depressive symptoms in BPD. Salzman *et al.* (1995) compared fluoxetine (mean dose 40 mg d^{-1}) to placebo in a 13-week, double-blind study of subjects with BPD diagnosed by DSM-III-R criteria. Patients in this study were mild to moderately symptomatic volunteers with no history of psychiatric hospitalization, recent suicidal behaviour, or self-mutilation. Significant improvement was found in anger and depression on the Profile of Mood States (POMS). There were trends for improvement in OAS and Hamilton Depression Inventory (HAM-D) scores. Although results from this trial were positive, it is unclear whether these results may be generalizable to more impaired BPD patients.

No controlled studies are available yet on the new, 'atypical' antidepressants such as mirtazepine, nefazadone, venlafaxine, and buproprion. In an open trial of venlafaxine in patients with BPD, Markovitz and Wagner (1995) found that venlafaxine seemed to be effective in treating depressive symptoms. Further work is needed with the newer antidepressants. It is unknown whether these agents, which also have effects on norepinephrine, will have tricyclic-like effects in patients with impulsive aggression.

SSRIs have been shown to be effective in the treatment of social phobia, and may be of benefit in patients with comorbid avoidant personality disorder. Controlled trials of paroxetine (Stein *et al.*, 1998), fluvoxamine (Stein *et al.*, 1999; van Vliet *et al.*, 1994), and sertraline (Katzelnick *et al.*, 1995) have all shown efficacy compared to placebo. Open trials of citalopram (Bouwer *et al.*, 1998), fluoxetine (van Ameringen *et al.*, 1993), venlafaxine (Altamura *et al.*, 1999), and nefazadone (van Ameringen *et al.*, 1999) show promising results.

BENZODIAZEPINES

Although an early comparison study of diazepam and trifluoperazine found that diazepam was more effective than the neuroleptic in relieving symptoms of BPD (Vilkin, 1964), Cowdry and Gardner found an increase in the frequency of episodes of serious dyscontrol in patients with BPD and histories of behavioural dyscontrol randomized to receive alprazolam (average dose 4.7 mg d^{-1}) in comparison to trifluoperazine, tranylcypromine, alprazolam, carbamazepine, or placebo. This troubling 'disinhibiting' effect occurred in the context of reduced anxiety and overall benefit to some patients. Although commonly used and generally considered to be safe and efficacious in the treatment of acute agitation and anxiety, the benzodiazepines remain relatively untested in the treatment of personality-disordered patients.

BUSPIRONE

There are no controlled trials to date in the use of buspirone, a 5-HT-1a selective partial agonist, in the treatment of impulsive aggression in personality-disordered patients. While it is an effective agent in the treatment of generalized anxiety disorder, its efficacy in generalized social phobia remains unclear. Although an open trial found buspirone to be effective at higher doses (average dose of responders was approximately 60 mg per day) (Schneier *et al.*, 1993), a controlled trial of buspirone at 30 mg per day in the treatment of generalized social phobia failed to find efficacy compared to placebo (van Vliet *et al.*, 1997). Further work should be done with higher doses of buspirone in patients with comorbid social phobia/avoidant personality disorder.

OPIATE ANTAGONISTS

There are no controlled data in the use of opiate antagonists to treat self-injurious behaviour (SIB) in personality-disordered patients. A few controlled data regarding the use of naltrexone in the treatment of SIB in patients with developmental disorders and mental retardation suggest that naltrexone in moderate doses ($<$1.5 mg per kg d^{-1}) may be effective (Pies and Popli, 1995), but not all trials to date have found positive results (Willemsen-Swinkels *et al.*, 1995).

In an open trial of naltrexone (50 mg d^{-1}), six of seven patients with histories of SIB experienced remissions of self-injury (Roth *et al.*, 1996). Patients in this trial exhibited striking self-destructive behaviours but had a heterogeneous set of diagnoses. A second open trial of naltrexone (50 mg d^{-1}) in five patients with BPD showed that treatment reduced the number of self-injurious thoughts and actions (Sonne *et al.*, 1996).

A single open trial of naltrexone for the treatment of dissociation and flashbacks in BPD patients by Bohus *et al.* (1999) found that treatment was associated with a decrease in intensity of, and total amount of time in, dissociative states in all patients. In the group of nine patients evaluated for flashbacks, six reported a reduction in the number of flashbacks in a dose-dependent fashion, while three reported no change. Doses in this study ranged from 25 to 100 mg per day, and approximately one-third of the patients were receiving concomitant antidepressant therapy.

Open trials in the use naltrexone for the treatment of SIB and dissociation show promising results that need to be verified with placebo-controlled data.

ECT (ELECTROCONVULSIVE THERAPY)

Data on the ECT of personality-disordered patients are limited to comparisons of subjects with major depressive disorder (MDD) with a comorbid personality disorder and subjects with MDD only. These echo pharmacological treatment trials of MDD with comorbid personality disorders, which have found, in general, that comorbid personality disorders are associated with a less robust treatment response (DeBattista *et al.*, 2001).

Two prospective correlational studies have provided somewhat conflicting evidence. Pfohl (1984) found that patients with MDD + PD, as diagnosed by the Structured Interview for DSM-III Personality Disorders (SCID-P), did not differ significantly in treatment response to ECT, with 79% of MDD + PD subjects versus 75% of MDD-only subjects responding to ECT.

Zimmerman *et al.* (1986) found that at completion of ECT, 20% of MDD + PD versus 53% of MDD-only subjects had recovered at the completion of treatment. At 6 months, 33% of MDD + PD subjects versus 61% of MDD-only patients had recovered. Although most patients in both groups at the end of treatment experienced some symptomatic recovery, within 6 months, 62% of MD + PD subjects, versus only 8% of MD only subjects, were rehospitalized.

Evidence to date suggests that patients with comorbid major depressive disorder and personality disorders may respond to ECT but less robustly, may be left with considerable residual psychopathology, and may relapse at a higher rate. However, evidence also suggests that ECT may still have therapeutic effects in this population of patients, and is not contraindicated.

CONCLUSION

Evidence to date does not support the efficacy of psychopharmacological treatments in personality disorder, but does support their efficacy in treating specific symptom dimensions. There is not yet enough information available to make evidence-based treatment recommendations for every Axis II disorder. This is less true regarding BPD, which has been comparatively well studied.

For the neuroleptics, selection of appropriate patients with psychotic or psychotic-like symptoms for acute treatment produces tangible results, although these must be weighed against the lack of evidence for continuation or maintenance therapy, the risk of extrapyramidal side effects, high drop-out rates due to side effects, and possibly deleterious effects on mood with prolonged usage. The newer atypical antipsychotic agents may have better efficacy across a broader range of symptoms with fewer side effects. Mood stabilizers show promise in the treatment of impulsive aggression and possibly affective instability. These effects may occur even if subjective effects are less prominent. Benzodiazepines may help with some symptoms commonly encountered in Axis II disorders such as acute anxiety; however, they may also lead to behavioural dyscontrol in certain patients with histories of impulsive aggressive behaviour. Antidepressants may be effective in treating commonly encountered comorbid Axis I anxiety disorders in patients with Cluster C personality disorders. Tricyclics in patients with histories of behavioural dyscontrol may lead to worsening. Evidence for the efficacy of MAOIs in treating impulsive aggression, anxiety, and affective symptoms must be weighed against the risk of hypertensive crisis. For patients with histories of impulsive aggression, and without comorbid bipolar disorder, SSRIs are among the most promising agents. SSRIs may also be beneficial if mood symptoms are present. Their relatively benign side-effect profile and positive effects on mood may lead to improved compliance.

At this point, it is unclear how the effects of psychopharmacological treatment and psychotherapeutic treatment may interact. Some recent studies have kept subjects in pre-existing psychotherapy; other have not. It is also unclear whether the specific targets and efficacy measurements of the two treatment modalities are comparable. These are relevant questions, given that some patient groups with Axis II disorders are heavy utilizers of both psychotherapy and psychopharmacological treatment. It is also unclear what effect different combinations of medications may have on one another. For example, it is unclear whether the use of an SSRI or mood stabilizer lessens the risk of behavioural dyscontrol associated with benzodiazepines. Newer agents, such as the atypical antipsychotics, highly selective agents such as buspirone, and dual serotonergic/noradrenergic antidepressants, show promise for their improved side-effect profiles and atypical actions, but are untested in personality-disordered populations.

REFERENCES

Alnaes, R. and Torgerson, S., 1988. The relationship between DSM III symptoms disorders (Axis I) and personality disorders (Axis II) in an outpatients populations. *Acta Psychiatr Scand*, **78**, 485–492.

Altamura, A.C., Pioli, R., Vitto, M. and Mannu, P., 1999. Venlafaxine in social phobia: a study in selective serotonin reuptake inhibitor non-responders. *Int Clin Psychopharmacol*, **14**, 239–245.

Asperg, M., Traskman, L. and Thoren, P., 1976. 5-HIAA in the cerebrospinal fluid. A biochemical suicide predictor? *Arch Gen Psychiatry*, **33**, 1193–1197.

Baer, L., Jenike, M.A., Ricciardi, J.N., Holand, A.D., Seymour, R.S. and Minichiello, W.E., 1990. Standardized assessment of personality disorders in OCD. *Arch Gen Psychiatry*, **47**, 826–830.

Baldwin, D., Bobes, J., Stein, D.J., *et al.*, 1999. Fluvoxamine treatment of social phobia (social anxiety disorder); a double-blind, placebo controlled study. *Am J Psychiatry*, **175**, 120–126.

Bejerot, S., Eskelius, L. and von Knorring, L., 1998. Comorbidity between obsessive-compulsive disorder and personality disorders. *Acta Psychiatr Scand*, **97**, 398–402.

Bender, D.S., Dolan, R.T., Skodol, A.E., Sanislow, C.A., Dyck, I.R., McGlashan, T.H., Shea, M.T., Zanarini, M.C. and Oldham, J.M., 2001. Gunderson JG: Treatment utilization by patients with personality disorders. *Am J Psychiatry*, **158**, 295–302.

Benedetti, F., Sforzini, L., Colombo, C., Maffei, C. and Smeraldi, E., 1998. Low-dose clozapine in acute and continuation treatment of severe borderline personality disorder. *J Clin Psychiatry*, **59**, 103–7.

Bohus, M.J., Landwehrmeyer, G.B., Stiglmayr, C.E., Limberger, M.F., Bohme, R. and Schmahl, C.G., 1999. Naltrexone in the treatment of dissociative symptoms in patients with borderline personality disorder: an open-label trial. *J Clin Psychiatry*, **60**, 598–603.

Bouwer, C. and Stein, D.J., 1998. Use of the selective serotonin reuptake inhibitor citalopram in the treatment of generalized social phobia. *J Affect Disorder*, **49**, 79–82.

Brinkley, J.R., Beitman, B.D. and Friedel, R.O., 1979. Low dose neuroleptic regimes in the treatment of borderline patients. *Arch Gen Psychiatry*, **36**, 319–326.

Brown, G.L., Goodwin, F.K., Ballenger, J.C., Goyer, P.F. and Major, L.F., 1979. Aggession in humans correlates with cerebrospinal fluid amine metabolites. *Psychiatry Res*, **1**, 131–139.

Buitelaar, J.K., van der Gaag, R.J., Cohen-Kettenis, P. and Melman, C.T., 2001. A randomized controlled trial of risperidone in the treatment of aggression in hospitalizedadolescents with suibaverage cognitive abilities. *J Clin Psychiatry*, **62**, 239–48.

Byne, W., Bucsbaum, M.S., Kemether, E., Hazlett, E.A., Shinwari, A., Mitropoulou, V. and Siever, L.J., 2001. Magnetic Resonance imaging of the thalamic mediodorsal nucleus and pulvinar in schizophrenia and schizotypal personality disorder. *Arch Gen Psychiatry*, **58**, 133–40.

Cassady, S.L., Adami, H., Moran, M., Kunkel, R. and Thaker, G.K., 1998. Spontaneous dyskinesia in subjects with schizophrenia spectrum personality. *Am J Psychiatry*, **155**, 70–75.

Cazzullo, C.L., Vita, A., Giobbio, G.M., Diecie, M. and Sacchetti, E., 1998. Cerebral structural abnormalities in schizophreniform disorder in schizophrenia spectrum personality disorders. In: Tamminga, C.A., Schultz, S.C. (eds), *Schizophrenia Research: Advances in Neuropsychiatry and Psychopharmacology*, Vol. 1, pp. 209–217. Raven Press, New York.

Chengappa, K.N., Ebeling, T., Kang, J.S., Levine, J. and Parepally, H., 1999. Clozapine reduces severe self-mutilation and aggression in psychotic patients with borderline personality disorder. *J Clin Psychiatry Jul*, **60**, 477–84.

Coccaro, E.F., Siever, L.J., Klar, H., Maurer, G., Cochrane, K., Cooper, T.B., Mohs, R.C. and Davis, K.L., 1989a. Serotonergic studies in patients with affective and personality disorders: correlates with suicidal and impulsive aggressive behaviour. *Arch Gen Psychiatry*, **46**, 587–599.

Coccaro, E.F., Astill, J.L., Herbert, J.L. and Schut, A.G., 1989b. Fluoxetine treatment of impulsive aggression in DSM-III-R personality disorder patients. *J Clin Psychopharmacol*, **10**, 373–5.

Coccaro, E.F., Astill, J.L., Herbert, J.L. and Schut, A.G., 1990. Fluoxetine treatment of impulsive aggression in DSM-III-R personality disorder patients. *J Clin Psychopharmacol*, **10**, 373–5.

Coccaro, E.F., Kavoussi, R.I.J., Hauger, R., Cooper, T.B. and Ferris, C.F., 1996. CSF vasopressin: correlates with indices of aggression and serotonin function in personality disordered subjects. In: Abstracts of the 35th Annual Meeting of the American Meeting of the American College of Neuropsychopharmacology, San Juan 243.

Coccaro, E.F., Kavoussi, R.J. and Hauger, R.L., 1997. Serotonin function and antiaggressive response to fluoxetine: a pilot study. *Biol Psychiatry*, Oct, **42**, 546–52.

Coccaro, E.F. and Kavoussi, R.J., 1997. Fluoxetine and impulsive aggressive behaviour in personality-disordered subjects. *Arch Gen Psychiatry*, **54**, 1081–8.

Cornelius, J.R., Soloff, P.H.M. Perel, J.M. and Ulrich, R.F., 1993. Continuation pharmacotherapy of borderline personality disorder with haloperidol and phenlzine. *Am J Psychiatry*, **150**, 1843–1848.

Cornelius, J.R., 1991. A Preliminary trial of fluoxetine in refractory borderline personality disorder. *J Clin Psychopharmacolog*, **11**, 116–120.

Cowdry, R.W. and Gardner, D.L., 1988. Pharmacotherapy of borderline personality disorder. Alprazolam, carbamazepine, trifluoperazine, and tranylcypromine. *Arch Gen Psychiatry*, **45**, 111–29.

DeBattista, C. and Mueller, K., 2001. Is electroconvulsive therapy effective for the depressed patient with comorbid borderline personality disorder? *J ECT*, **17**, 91–8.

Diaferia, G., Bianchi, I., Bianchi, M.L., Cavedini, P., Erzegovesi, S. and Bellodi, L., 1997. Relationship between obsessive-compusive personality disorder and obsessive-compulsive disorder. *Comprehensive Psychiatry*, **38**, 31–42.

Donovan, S.J., Stuart, J.W., Nenes, E.V., Quitkin, F.M., Michael, P., William, D., Susser, E. and Klein, D.F., 2000. Divalproex Treatment for youth with explosive temper and mood lability: a double-blind, placebo-controlled crossover design. *Am J Psychiatry*, **157**, 818–820.

Downhill, J.E., Buchsbaum, M.S., Wei, T., Speigel-Cohen, J., Hazlett, E.A., Haznedar, M.M., Silverman, J. and Siever, L.J., 2000. Shape and size of the corpus callosum in schizophrenia and schizotypal personality disorder. *Schizophr Res*, **42**, 193–208.

Fenton, W.S., Wyatt, R.J. and McGlashan, T.H., 1994. Risk factors for spontaneous dyskinesia in schizophrenia. *Arch Gen Psych*, **51**, 643–650.

Fink, M., Pollack, M., Klein, D.F., Blumburg, A.G., Belmont, I., Karp, E., Kramer, J.C. and Willner, A., 1964. Comparative studies of chlorpromazine and imipramine. I. Drug discriminating patterns. *Neuropsychopharmacology*, **3**, 370–372.

Frankenburg, F.R. and Zanarini, M.C., 1993. Clozapine treatment of borderline patients: a preliminary study. *Compr Psychiatry*, **34**, 402–5.

Fritze, J., Sofic, E., Muller, T., Pfuller, H., Lanczik, M. and Riederer, P., 1990. Cholinergic-adrenergic balance, Part 2: Relationship between drug sensitivity and personality. *Psychiatry Res*, **34**, 271–279.

Fulton, M. and Winokur, G., 1993. A comparative study of paranoid and schizoid personality disorders. *Am J Psychiatry*, **50**, 1363–7.

Gardner, D.L. and Cowdry, R.W., 1985. Suicidal and parasuicidal behavior in borderline personality disorder. *Psychiatr Clin North America*, **8**, 389–403.

Gardner, D.L. and Cowdry, R.W., 1986. Development of melancholia during carbamazepine treatment in borderline personality disorder. *J Clin Psychopharmacol*, **6**, 236–239.

Gardner, D.L. and Cowdry, R.W., 1989. Pharmacotherapy of borderline personality disorder: A review. *Psychopharmacology Bulletin*, **25**, 515–523.

Goldberg, S.C., Schulz, S.C., Shculz, P.J.M., Resnick, R.J., Hamer, R.M. and Friedel, R.O., 1986. Borderline and schizotypal personality disorders treated with low-dose thiothixene vs. placebo. *Arch Gen Psychiatry*, **43**, 680–686.

Gunderson, J.G. and Sabo, A.N., 1993. The phenomenological and conceptual interface between borderline personality disorder and PTSD. *Am J Psychiatry*, **150**, 19–27.

Hedberg, D.L., Houck, J.H. and Glueck, B.C., 1971. Tranylcypromine-trifluoperazine combination in the treatment of schizophrenia. *Am J Psychiatry*, **127**, 1141–1146.

Heimberg, R.G., Liebowitz, M.R., Hope, D.A., Schneier, F.R., Holt, C.S., Welkowitz, L.A., Juster, H.R., Campeas, R., Bruch, M.A., Cloitre, M., Fallon, B. and Klein, D.F., 1998. Cognitive-behavioral group therapy vs. phenelzine therapy for social phobia: 12-week outcome. *Arch Gen Psychiatry*, **195**, 113–114.

Hirose, S., 2001. Effective treatment of aggression and impulsivity in antisocial personality disorder with risperidone. *Psychiatry and Clinical Neurosciences*, **55**, 161–162.

Hollander, E., Allen, A., Lopez, R.P., Bienstock, C.A., Grossman, R., Siever, L.J., Merkatz, L. and Stein, D.J., 2001. A preliminary double-blind, placebo-controlled trial of divalproex sodium in borderline personality disorder. *J Clin Psychiatry*, **62**, 199–203.

Hough, D.W., 2001. Low-dose olanzapine for self-mutilation behavior in patients with borderline personality disorder. *J Clin Psychiatry*, **62**, 296–297.

Katzelnick, D.J., Kobak, K.A., Greist, J.H., Jefferson, J.W., Mantle, J.M. and Serlin, R.C., 1995. Sertraline for social phobia: a double-blind, placebo-controlled crossover study. *Am J Psychiatry*, **152**, 1368–1371.

Kavoussi, R.J. and Coccaro, E.F., 1993. The amphetamine challenge test correlates with affective lability in healthy volunteers. *Psychiatry Res*, **48**, 219–228.

Kavoussi, R.J., Coccaro, E.F., Klar, H.M., Lesser, J. and Siever, L.J., 1993. The TRH stimulation test in DSM-III personality disorder. *Biol Psychiatry*, **34**, 234–23.

Kavoussi, R.J., 1994. Open trail of sertraline in personality disorders with impulsive aggression. *J Clin Psychiatry*, **55**, 137–141.

Kavoussi, R.J. and Coccaro, E.F., 1998. Divalproex sodium for impulsive aggressive behavior in patients with personality disorder. *J Clin Psychiatry*, **59**, 676–680.

Kelsey, J.E., 1995. Venlafaxine in social phobia. *Psychopharmacol Bull*, **31**, 767–771.

Kendler, K.S. and Gruenberg, A.M., 1982. Genetic relationship between paranoid personality disorder and the 'schizophrenic spectrum' disorders. *Am J Psychiatry*, **139**, 1185–1186.

Khouzam, H.R. and Donnelly, N.J., 1997. Remission of self-mutilation in a patient with borderline personality disorder during risperidone therapy. *J Nerv Ment Dis*, **185**, 348–9.

Klein, D.F. and Greenberg, I.M., 1967. Behavioral effects of diphenylhydantoin in severe psychiatric disorders. *Am J Psychiatry*, **124**, 847–849.

Klein, D.F., 1968. Psychiatric diagnosis and a typology of clinical drug effects. *Psychopharmacology*, **13**, 359–386.

Korzekwa, M., Steiner, M., Links, P. and Eppel, A., 1991. The dexamethasone suppression test in borderlines: is it useful? *Can J Psychiatry*, **36**, 26–28.

Kringlen, E., 1965. Obsessional neurotics: a long-term follow-up. *Br J Psychiatry*, **111**, 709–722.

LaWall, J.S. and Cassie, L.W., 1982. The use of lithium carbonate in borderline patients. *Journal of Psychiatric Teatment and Evaluations*, **4**, 265–267.

Leone, N.F., 1982. Response of borderline patients to loxapine and chlorpromazine. *J Clin Psychiatry*, **43**, 148–150.

Levitt, A.J., Russel, T.J., Ennis, J., MacDonald, C. and Kutcher, S.P., 1990. The prevalence of cyclothymia in borderline personality disorder. *J Clin Psychiatry*, **51**, 335–339.

Links, P.S., Steiner, M., Boiago, I. and Irwin, D., 1990. Lithium therapy for borderline patients: preliminary findings. *Journal of Personality Disorders*, **4**, 173–181.

Links, P.S., 1998. Developing effective services for patients with personality disorders. *Can J Psychiatry*, **43**, 251–259.

Linnoila, M., Virkkunen, M., Scheinin, M., Nuutila, A., Rimon, R. and Goodwin, F.K., 1983. Low cerebrospinal fluid 5-hydroxyindolacetic acid concentration differentiates impulsive from nonimpulsive violent behavior. *Life Sci*, **33**, 2609–14.

Loosen, P.T. and Prange, A.J., 1982. Serum thyrotropin response to thyrotropine-releasing hormone in psychiatric patients. *Am J Psychiatry*, **139**, 405–950.

Lopez-Ibor, J.J., Saiz-Ruiz, J. and Perez de los Cobos, J.C., 1985. Biological correlates of suicide and agessivity in major depressions (with melancholia) *Neuropsychobiology*, **14**, 67–74.

Maier, W., Lichtermann, D., Linger, T., Heun, R. and Hallmayer, J., 1992. Prevalence of personality disorders (DSM-III-R) in the community. *J Personality Disorders*, **6**, 187–196.

Markovitz, P.J., Calabrese, J.R., Schulz, S.C. and Meltzer, H.Y., 1991. Fluoxetine in the treatment of borderline and schizotypal personality disorders. *Am J Psychiatry*, **148**, 1064–1067.

Markovitz, P.J. and Wagner, S.C., 1995. Venlafaxine in the treatment of borderline personality disorder. *Psychopharmacol Bull*, **31**, 773–7.

Mattes, J.A., 1990. Comparative effectiveness of carbamazepine and propranolol for rage outbursts. *Journal of Neuropsychiatry and Clinical Neurosciences*, **2**, 159–164.

McGlashan, T., 1986. The Chestnut Lodge follow-up study III. Long-term outcome of borderline personalities *Arch Gen Psychiatry*, **43**, 20–30.

McGlashan, T.H., Grilo, C.M., Skodol, A.E., Gunderson, J.G., Shea, M.T., Morey, L.C., Zanarini, M.C. and Stout, R.L., 2000. The Collaborative Longitudinal Personality Disorders Study: baseline Axis I/II and II/II diagnostic co-occurrence. *Acta Psychiatr Scand*, **102**, 256–64.

Mehlum, L., Friis, S., Irion, T., Johns, S., Karerud, S. and Vaglum, S., 1991. Personality disorders 2–5 years after treatment: a prospective follow-up study. *Acta Psychiatr Scand*, **84**, 72–77.

Meritt, R.D. and Balogh, D.W., 1989. Backward masking spatial frequency defects among hypothetically schizotypal individuals. *Schizophr Bull*, **15**, 573–583.

Montgomery, S.A. and Montgomery, D., 1982. Pharmacological prevention of suicidal behavior. *J Affective Disorder*, **4**, 291–298.

Norden, M.J., 1989. Fluoxetine in borderline personality disorder. *Progress in Neuropsychopharmacol Biol Psychiatry*, **13**, 885–893.

O'Keane, V., Moloney, E., O'Neill, H., O'Connor, A., Smith, C. and Dinan, T.G., 1992. Blunted prolactin responses to d-fenfluramine in sociopathy: evidence for subsensitivity of central serotonergic function. *Br J Psychiatry*, **160**, 643–646.

New, A.S., Trestman, R.L., Mitropoulou, V., Benishay, D.S., Coccaro, E.F., Silverman, J. and Siever, L.J., 1997. Serotonergic function and self-injurious behavior in personality disorder patients. *Psychiatry Research*, **69**, 17–26.

Pande, A.C., Davidson, J.R., Jefferson, J.W., Janney, C.A., Katzelnick, D.J., Weisler, R.H., Greist, J.H. and Sutherland, S.M., 1999. Treatment of social phobia with gabapentin: a placebo-controlled study. *J Clin Psychopharmacol*, **19**, 341–8.

Parsons, B., Quitkin, F.M. and McGrath, P.J., 1989. Phenelzine, imipramine, and placebo in borderline patients meeting criteria for atypical depression. *Psychopharmacol Bull*, **25**, 524–534.

Perry, J.C. and Cooper, S.H., 1985. Psychodynamics, symptoms, and outcome in borderline personality disorders and bipolar type II affective disorder. In: McGlashan, T.H. (ed.), *The Borderline: Current Empirical Research*, pp. 19–41. American Psychiatric Press, Washington, DC.

Perugi, C., Nassini, S., Socci, C., Lenzi, M., Toni, C., Simonini, E. and Akiskal, H.S., 1985, 1999. Avoidant personality in social phobia and panic-agoraphobic disorder: a comparison. *Journal of Affective Disorders*, **54**, 277–282.

Pfohl, B., Stangl, D. and Zimmerman, M., 1984. The implications of DSM-III personality disorders for patients with major depression. *J Affect Disord*, **7**, 309–18.

Pies, R.W. and Popli, A.P., 1995. Self-injurious behavior: Pathophysiology and implications for treatment. *J Clin Psychiatry*, **56**, 580–588.

Pope, H.G. Jr., Jonas, J.M., Hudson, J.I., Cohen, B.M. and Gunderson, J.G., 1983. The validity of DSM-III borderline person disorder. *Arch Gen Psych*, **40**, 23–30.

Potter, W.Z., 1990. Cerebrospinal fluid and plasma monoamine metabolites and their relation to psychosis. *Arch Gen Psychiatry*, **47**, 641–648.

Raine, A., Sheard, C., Reynolds, G.P. and Lencz, T., 1992. Prefrontal structural and functional deficits associated with individual differences in schizotypal personality. *Schiz Res*, **7**, 237–247.

Raine, A., Buichsbaum, M.S. and La Casse, L., 1997. Brain abnormalities in murderers indicated by positron emission tomography. *Biol Psychiatry*, **42**, 495–508.

Rampling, D., 1978. Aggression: a paradoxical response to tricyclic antidepressants. *Am J Psychiatry*, **135**, 117–118.

Rassmussen, S.A. and Tsuang, M.T., 1986. Clinical characteristics and family history in DSM-III obsessive-compulsive disorder. *Am J Psychiatry*, **143**, 317–320.

Reich, J., Noyes, R., Jr, Coryell, W. and O'Gorman, T.W., 1986. The effect of state anxiety on personality measurement. *Am J Psychiatry*, **143**, 760–3.

Reich, J., Yates, W. and Nudaguba, M., 1989. Prevalence of DSM-III personality disorders in the community. *Soc Psychiatry Psychiatr Epidemiolog*, **24**, 12–16.

Reich, J.H., 1991. Avoidant and dependent personality traits in relatives of patients with panic disorder, patients with dependent personality disorder, and normal controls. *Psychiatry Res*, **39**, 89–98.

Reyntjens, A.M., 1972. A series of multicentric pilot trials with pimozide in psychiatric practice, I: pimozide in the treatment of personality disorders. *Acta Psychiatr Belg*, **72**, 653–661.

Rifkin, A., Quitkin, F., Carrillo, C., Blumberg, A.G. and Klein, D.F., 1972. Lithium carbonate in emotionally unstable character disorder. *Arch Gen Psychiatry*, **27**, 519–23.

Riso, L.P., Klein, D.N., Anderdson, R.L. and Ouimette, P.C.L., 2000. A family study of outpatients with borderline personality disorder and no history of mood disorder. *J Personal Disord*, **14**, 2008–17.

Roitman, S.E., Mitropoulou, V., Keefe, R.S., Silverman, J.M., Serby, M., Harvey, P.D., Reynolds, D.A., Mohs, R.C. and Siever, L.J., 2000. Visuospatial working memory in schizotypal personality disorder patients *Schizophr Res*, **41**, 447–55.

Roth, A.S., Ostroff, R.B. and Hoffman, R.E., 1996. Naltrexone as a treatment for repetitive self-injurious behavior: an open-label trial. *J Clin Psychiatry*, **5**, 6.

Salzman, C., Wolfson, A.N., Schatzberg, A., Looper, J., Henke, R., Albanese, M., Schwartz, J. and Miyawaki, E., 1995. Effect of fluoxetine on anger in symptomatic volunteers with borderline personality disorder. *J Clin Psychopharmacol*, **15**, 23–9..

Samuels, J., Nestad, G., Folstein, M.F. and McHugh, P.R., 1994. DSM III Personality disorders in the community: *Am J Psychiatry*, **151**, 1055–1062.

Schneier, F.R., Saoud, J.B., Campeas, R., Fallon, B.A., Hollander, E., Coplan, J. and Liebowitz, M.R., 1993. Buspirone in social phobia. *J Clin Psychopharmacol*, **13**, 251–256.

Schulz, S.C., Cornelius, J., Schulz, P.M. and Soloff, P.H., 1988. The amphetamine challenge test in patients with bpd. *Am J Psychiatry*, **145**, 809–814.

Schulz, P.M., Schulz, S.C., Goldberg, S.C., Prakesh, E., Resnick, R.J. and Friedel, R.O., 1986. Diagnoses of the relatives of schizotypal outpatients. *J Nerv Ment Dis*, **174**, 457–463.

Schulz, S.C., Schulz, P.M., Dommisse, C., Hamer, R.M., Blackard, W.G., Narasimhachari, N. and Friedel, R.O., 1985. Amphetamine response in borderline patients. *Psychiatry Research*, **15**, 97–108.

Schulz, P.M., Soloff, P.H., Kelly, T., Morgenstern, M., DiFranco, R. and Schulz, S.C., 1989. A family history of borderline subtypes. *J Personality Disorders*, **3**, 217–229.

Schulz, S.C., Camlin, K.L., Berry, S.A. and Jesberger, J.A., 1999. Olanzapine safety and efficacy in patients with borderline personality disorder and comorbid dysthymia. *Biol Psychiatry*, **15**, 1429–35.

Seiver, L.J. and Davis, K.L., 1991. A psychobiological perspective on the personality disorders. *Am J Psychiatry*, **148**, 1647–1658.

Serban, G. and Siegel, S., 1984. Responses of borderline and schizotypal patients to small doses of thiothixene and haloperidol. *Am J Psychiatry*, **141**, 1455–1458.

Sheard, M.H., Marini, J.L., Bridges, C.I. and Wagner, E., 1976. The effect of lithium on impulsive aggressive behavior in men: *Am J psychiatry*, **33**, 1409–1413.

Siever, L.J., Amin, F. and Coccaro, E.F., 1991. Plasma homovanillic acid in schizotypal personality disorder. *Am J Psychiatry*, **148**, 1246–1248.

Siever, L.J. and Davis, K.L., 1991. A psychobiolgoical perspective on the personality disorders *Am J Psychiatry*, **148**, 1647–1658.

Siever, L.J. and Kalus, O.F. and Keefe, R.S., 1993a. The boundaries of schizophrenia. *Psychiatr Clin North Am*, **16**, 217–244.

Siever, L.J., Amin, F., Coccaro, E.F., Trestman, R., Silverman, J., Hovath, T.B., Mahon, T.R., Knott, P., Altstiel, L., Davidson, M. and

Davis, K.L., 1993b. CSF homovanillic acid in schizotypal personality disorder. *Am J Psychiatry*, **150**, 149–151.

Siever, L.J., Buchsbaum, M.S., New, A.S., Spiegel-Cohen, J., Wei, T., Hazlett, E.A., Sevin, E., Nunn, M. and Mitropoulou, V., 1999. d,l-fenfluramine response in impulsive personality disorder assessed with [18F]flourodeoxyglucose positron emission tomography. *Neuropsychopharmacology*, **20**, 413–23.

Silverman, J.M., Pinkham, L., Horvath, T.B., Coccaro, E.F., Klar, H., Schear, S., Apter, S., Davidson, M., Mohs, R.C. and Siever, L.J., 1991. Affective and impulsive personality disorder traits in the relatives of borderline personality disorder. *Am J Psychiatry*, **148**, 1378–1385.

Simpson, H.B., Schneier, F.R., Marshall, R.D., Campeas, R.B., Vermes, D., Silvestre, J., Davies, S. and Liebowitz, M.R., 1998. Low dose selegiline (L-deprenyl) in social phobia. *Depress Anxiety*, **7**, 126–129.

Skodol, A.E., Bucley, P. and Charles, E., 1983. Is there a characterstic pattern to the treatment history of clinical outpatients with borderline personality? *J Nerv Ment Dis*, **171**, 405–410.

Skodol, A.E., Stout, R.L., McGlashan, T.H., Grilo, C.M., Gunderson, J.G., Shea, M.T., Morey, L.C., Zanarini, M.C., Dyck, I.R. and Oldham, J.M., 2000. Co-occurrence of mood and personality disorders: a report from the Collaborative Longitudinal Personality Disorders Study (CLPS). *Depress Anxiety*, **10**, 175–82.

Soloff, P.H., 1981. Pharmacotherapy of borderline disorders. *Compr Psychiatry*, **22**, 535–543.

Soloff, P.H., George, A., Nathan, R.S., Schulz, P.M., Ulrich, R.F. and Perel, J.M., 1986. Progress in pharmacotherapy of borderline disorders. *Arch Gen Psychiatry*, **43**, 691–697.

Soloff, P.H., George, A., Swami Nathan, R., Schulz, P.M. and Perel, J.M., 1987. Behavioral dyscontrol in borderline patients treated with amitriptyline. *Psychology Bulletin*, **23**, 177–181.

Soloff, P.H., George, A., Nathan, R.S., Schulz, P.M. and Cornelius, J., 1988. Patterns of response to amitriptyline and haloperidol among borderline patients. *Psychopharmacol Bull*, **28**, 264–268.

Soloff, P.H., Meltzer, C.C., Greer, F.J., Constantine, D. and Kelly, T.M., 2000. A fenfluramine activated FDG-PET study of borderline personality disorder. *Biol Psychiatry*, **47**, 540–7.

Soloff, P.H., George, A., Nathan, R.S., Schulz, P.M., Cornelius, J.R., Herring, J. and Perel, J.M., 1989. Amitryiptyline versus hloperidol in borderlines: final outcomes and predictors of response. *J Clin Psychopharmacol*, **9**, 238–246.

Soloff, P.H., Cornelius, J., Anselm, G., Nathan, S., Perel, J.M. and Ulrich, R.F., 1993. Efficacy of phenelzine and haloperidol in borderline personality disorder. *Arch Gen Psychiatry*, **50**, 377–385.

Sonne, S., Rubey, R., Brady, K., Malcolm, R. and Morris, T., 1996. Naltrexone treatment of self-injurious thoughts and behaviors. *J Nerv Ment Dis*, **184**, 192–5..

Stein, D.J., Simeon, D., Frenkel, M., Islam, M.N. and Hollander, E., 1995. An open trial of valproate in borderline personality disorder. *J Clin Psychiatry*, **56**, 506–510.

Stein, M.B., Liebowitz, M.R., Lydiard, B., *et al.*, 1998. Paroxetine treatment of generalized social phobia (social anxiety disorder) a randomized controlled trial. *JAMA*, **280**, 708–713.

Stein, M.B., Fyer, A.J. and Davidson, J.R.T., 1999. Fluvoxamine treatment of social phobia (social anxiety disorder) a double-blind placebo-controlled study. *Br J Psychiatry*, **175**, 756–760.

Steinberg, B.J., Trestman, R., Mitropoulou, V., Serby, M., Silverman, J., Coccaro, E., Weston, S., de Vegvar, M. and Siever, L.J., 1997. Depressive response to physostigmine challenge in borderline personality disorder patients. *Neuropsychopharmacology*, **17**, 264–73.

Stephens, J.H. and Schaffer, J.W., 1970. A controlled study of the effects of diphenylhydantoin on anxiety, irritability, and anger in neurotic outpatients. *Psychopharmacology*, **17**, 169–181.

Sternbach, H.A., 1990. Fluoxetine treatment of social phobia. *J Clin Psychopharmacol*, **10**, 230–1.

Swartz, M., Blazer, D., George, L. and Windfield, I., 1990. Estimating the prevalence of bpd in the community. *J Personality Disorders*, **4**, 257–272.

Szigethy, E.M. and Schulz, S.C., 1997. Risperidone in comorbid borderline personality disorder and dysthymia. *J Clin Psychopharmacol*, **17**, 326–7.

Tancer, M.E., Stein, M.B., Gelernter, C.S. and Uhde, T.W., 1990. The hypothalmic-pituitary-thyroid axis in social phobia. *Am J Psychiatry*, **147**, 929–933.

Torgerson, S., 1984. Genetic and nosological aspects of schizotypal and borderline personality disorders. *Arch Gen Psychiatry*, **41**, 546–554.

Turner, S.M., Beidel, D.C. and Townsley, R.M., 1992. Social phobia a comparison of specific and generalized subtypes and avoidant personality disorder. *J Abnorm Psychol*, **101**, 326–331.

van Ameringen, M., Mancini, C. and Streiner, D.L., 1993. Fluoxetine efficacy in social phobia. *J Clin Psychiatry*, **54**, 27–32.

van Ameringen, M., Mancini, C. and Oakman, J.M., 1999. Nefazadone in social phobia. *J Clin Psychiatry*, **14**, 239–245.

Van Bellinghen, M. and De Troch, C., 2001. Risperidone in the treatment of behavioural disturbances in children and adolescents with borderline intellectual functioning: a double-blind, placebo-controlled pilot trial. *J Child Adolesc Psychopharmacol*, **11**, 5–13.

van Vliet, I.M., den Boer, J.A. and Westenberg, H.G., 1994. Psychopharmacological treatment of social phobia: a double blind placebo controlled study with fluvoxamine. *Psychopharmacolgy (Berl)*, **115**, 128–134.

van Vliet, I.M., den Boer, J.A., Westenberg, H.G.M., *et al.*, 1997. Clinical effects of buspirone in social phobia: a double-blind placebo-controlled study. *J Clin Psychiatry*, **58**, 164–168.

Vilkin, M.I., 1964. Comparative chemotherapeutic trial in treatment of chronic borderline patients. *Am J Psychiatry*, **120**, 1004–1015.

West, M., Rose, M.S. and Sheldon-Keller, A., 1995. Interpersonal disorder in schizoid and avoidant personality disorders: an attachment perspective. *Can J Psychiatry*, Sep **40**, 411–4.

Widiger, T.A., 1992. Generalized social phobia versus avoidant personality disorder: a commentary on three studies. *J Abnorm Psychol*, **101**, 340–343.

Willemsen-Swinkels, S.H., Buitelaar, J.K., Nijhof, G.J. and van England, H., 1995. Failure of naltrexone hydrochloride to reduce self-injurious and autistic behaviour in mentally retarded adults. *Arch Gen Psychiatry*, **52**, 766–773.

Zanarini, M.C., Frankenburg, F.R., Khera, G.S. and Bleichmar, J., 2001. Treatment histories of borderline inpatients. *Comprehensive Psychiatry*, **42**, 144–150.

Zanarini, M.C. and Frankenburg, F.R., 2001. Olanzapine treatment of female borderline personality disorder patients: a double-blind, placebo-controlled pilot study. *J Clin Psychiatry*, **62**, 849–54.

Zimmerman, M., Coryell, W. and Pfohl, B., 1986. ECT response in depressed patients with and without a DSM-III personality disorder. *American Journal of Psychiatry*, **143**, 1030–2.

Zimmerman, M. and Coryell, W., 1989. DSM-III personality disorder diagnoses in a nonpatient sample. Demographic correlates and comorbidity. *Arch Gen Psychiatry*, **46**, 682–9.

Zimmerman, M. and Mattia, J.I., 1999. Differences between clinical and research practices in diagnosing borderline personality disorder. *Am J Psychiatry*, **156**, 1570–4.

Index